eighth edition

Introductory
Medical-Surgical
Nursing

eighth edition

Introductory Medical-Surgical Nursing

Barbara K. Timby, RN, BC, BSN, MA
Nursing Professor
Medical-Surgical Nursing
Glen Oaks Community College
Centreville, MI

Nancy E. Smith, MS, RN
Chairperson
Department of Nursing
Southern Maine Technical College
South Portland, ME

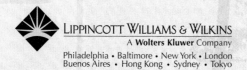

LIPPINCOTT WILLIAMS & WILKINS
A **Wolters Kluwer** Company

Philadelphia • Baltimore • New York • London
Buenos Aires • Hong Kong • Sydney • Tokyo

Acquisitions Editor: Lisa Stead
Developmental Editor: Renee Gagliardi
Production Editor: Debra Schiff
Senior Production Manager: Helen Ewan
Art Director: Carolyn O'Brien
Manufacturing Manager: William Alberti
Indexer: Alexandra Nickerson
Compositor: Circle Graphics
Printer: Quebecor Versailles

8th edition

9 8 7 6 5 4 3 2 1

Library of Congress Cataloging-in-Publication Data

Timby, Barbara Kuhn.
    Introductory medical-surgical nursing / Barbara K. Timby, Nancy E. Smith.—8th ed.
        p. ; cm.
    Includes bibliographical references and index.
    ISBN 0-7817-3553-X (alk. paper)
        1. Nursing. 2. Surgical nursing. I. Smith, Nancy E. (Nancy Ellen), 1949-II. Title.
    [DNLM: 1. Nursing Care. 2. Perioperative Nursing. WY 150 T583i 2003]
    RT41 .S38 2003
    610.73—dc21   2002069435

LWW.com

This edition is dedicated to those who lost their lives or loved ones in the tragedy of September 11th and to the many nurses and nursing students who cared and will care for victims of tragic events.

Contributors

Susan Dudek, RD, CDN, BS
Dietitian in Private Practice
Buffalo, New York

Pamela Gwin, RNC
Director, Vocational Nursing Program
Brazosport College
Lake Jackson, Texas

Mary Jo Kirkpatrick, RN, MSN
Director, Associate of Science in Nursing
Mississippi University for Women
Columbus, Mississippi

Kristine Kirsch, RNC, MPA, NMCC
Chief Executive Officer
Community Mental Health St. Joseph County
Three Rivers, Michigan

Sharon Powell-Laney, BSN, RN, MSN
Director of Practical Nursing
Jefferson County-DuBois AVTS
Reynoldsville, Pennsylvania

Nancy Rayhorn, BSN, RN, BN, CGBN
Nurse Clinician
Pediatric Gastroenterology
Arizona State University
Tempe, Arizona

Sally S. Roach, MSN, RN
Associate Professor
University of Texas at Brownsville & Texas Southmost College
Brownsville, Texas

Patricia L. Schneider, MSN, RN
Formerly of Glen Oaks Community College
Three Rivers, Michigan

Bonnie Smith, BSN, RN
39 Gould Street
Kewanee, Missouri

Reviewers

Carol Ann Alexander, MSN, RN
Associate Professor, Department of Nursing
Palm Beach Community College
Lake Worth, Florida

Nancy T. Hatfield, RNC, MA
Director, Practical Nursing Program
Albuquerque Public Schools–Career Enrichment Center
Albuquerque, New Mexico

Merilee (Misty) McDuffie, BSN, MPH
Program Director, Practical Nursing
Department of Business and Health
Front Range Community College, Longmont Campus
Longmont, Colorado

Lazette Nowicki, RN, MSN
Department of Nursing
Sacramento City College
Sacramento, California

Beverly Peoples, BS
Department Head, Practical Nursing
Louisiana Technical College, Northeast Campus
Winnsboro, Louisiana

Sharon Powell-Laney, BSN, RN, MSN
Director of Practical Nursing
Jefferson County-DuBois AVTS
Reynoldsville, Pennsylvania

Esther Salinas, RN, MSN, MS, ED
Associate Professor of Nursing
Vocational Nursing and Registered Nursing Departments
Del Mar College
Corpus Christi, Texas

Preface

In today's changing health care environment, nurses face many challenges and opportunities. The 8th edition of *Introductory Medical-Surgical Nursing* was written to help nurses meet these challenges and take advantage of expanding opportunities.

NEW TO THIS EDITION

- **Full, four-color art program.** This edition contains a brilliant design and new illustrations and photographs **in full color.** The addition of color will assist visual learners to understand important concepts.
- **Stop, Think, and Respond boxes.** Found in all chapters, these boxes ask students to consider scenarios related to pertinent topics and to respond quickly based on their understanding. The boxes are numbered for quick reference, with answers provided in Appendix A so students can check their learning.
- **Client and Family Teaching boxes.** These new specially numbered boxes are found throughout clinical chapters and highlight essential education points for nurses to communicate to clients and their families.
- **New content.** The entire text has been reviewed, revised, and updated to reflect current medical and nursing practice. Additionally, several chapters and sections contain brand new content. The following are some highlights:
  - Chapter 6, *Leadership Roles and Management Functions,* is a new chapter addressing these important topics for today's nurses, who are assuming more responsibilities that require delegation, accountability, and prioritization.
  - Chapter 7, *Biopsychosocial Aspects of Caring for Young Adults,* has been recreated to present many problems that adults may face across their adult lifespan, including issues related to sexual concerns and violence.

- Chapter 12, *Interaction of Body and Mind,* targets the importance of the growing field of complementary and alternative medicine with a brand new section covering specific modalities, such as Chinese medicine, biofeedback, imagery, spiritual healing, herbal therapy, aromatherapy, yoga, reiki, and many more. Additionally, important considerations related to the use of complementary and alternative modalities are found throughout the text.
- Chapter 21, *Caring for Clients With Pain,* has been rewritten to adhere to the latest research findings and guidelines of accrediting organizations, such as the JCAHO.
- Unit 7, *Caring for Clients With Cardiovascular Disorders,* discusses many new diagnostic and treatment modalities. Examples include coronary arteriography, enhanced external counterpulsation, percutaneous transluminal coronary angioplasty, coronary stent, atherectomy, automatic implanted cardiac defibrillator, transcutaneous and transvenous pacemakers, radiofrequency catheter ablation, cardiac resynchronization therapy, ventricular assist device, cardiomyoplasty, artificial heart, off-pump coronary artery bypass, minimally invasive direct coronary artery bypass, and port access coronary artery bypass.
- Chapter 58, *Caring for Clients With Diabetes Mellitus,* is fully updated, with the latest dietary management and newest oral agents used to treat this increasingly prevalent condition.
- Chapter 70, *Caring for Clients With Burns,* is a new chapter with a full discussion of the needs and management of such clients.
- The 8th edition contains **more than 30 Nursing Care Plans**—triple the number in the 7th edition! The additional plans address the care of clients with such diverse issues and problems as rape, Alzheimer's disease, cancer, myocardial infarction, cerebrovascular accident, diabetes mellitus, modified radical mastectomy, and chronic renal failure. Furthermore, Chapter 3, *The Nurs-*

ing Process, contains a Sample Nursing Care Plan that introduces students to the structure and components of these important tools.

- **Rationales for Interventions.** In this new edition, both Nursing Care Plans and Nursing Process sections include easily identifiable rationales with interventions. The rationales assist students to know not only what to do but also why doing so is important.

REVISED AND REFOCUSED CONTENT

- **Expanded emphasis on pathophysiology.** The authors have expanded discussions of pathophysiology and etiology in several chapters to connect each disorder with its assessment findings, medical and surgical management, and nursing management.
- **Added Drug Therapy tables.** This edition contains more Drug Therapy tables. As an extra bonus, they are clearly labeled and numbered for easy reference. They address the major categories of medications prescribed for the treatment of common disorders discussed. The tables include categories of drugs, an example of generic and trade names, their mechanism of action, common side effects, and nursing considerations. This feature reinforces the beginning student's knowledge of drug therapy and coordinates pharmacology for students whose nursing curricula integrate this content rather than teach it as a separate course.
- **Reorganized Nursing Process format.** As in the 7th edition, the 8th edition emphasizes the nursing process extensively throughout the text. In this edition, each step is clearly separated from the others and easy to read. Each diagnosis and expected outcome are clearly matched with the interventions (and rationales!) most likely to help the client achieve the intended goal. The text has incorporated diagnoses from the most recently approved NANDA list, a copy of which is found in the back end page of the text. It also includes collaborative problems.
- **Additional Resource Appendix.** Appendix B contains many addresses, phone and fax numbers, and Web links for numerous healthcare-related resources and organizations.

STRUCTURE OF THE TEXT

The 8th edition addresses the common adult disorders that are treated medically and surgically in the following format:

- Unit 1, *Nursing Roles and Responsibilities,* includes chapters on *Concepts and Trends in Healthcare, Nursing in Various Settings, The Nursing Process, Interviewing and Physical Assessment, Legal and Ethical Issues,* and *Leadership and Management.*
- Unit 2, *Development Across the Lifespan,* contains chapters on *Biopsychosocial Aspects of Caring for Young Adults, Biopsychosocial Aspects of Caring for Middle-Aged Adults,* and *Biopsychosocial Aspects of Caring for Older Adults.*
- Unit 3, *Psychosocial Aspects of Nursing,* contains chapters on *Nurse–Client Relationships* and *Caring for Culturally Diverse Clients.*
- Unit 4, *Psychobiologic Disorders* contains chapters on *Interaction of Body and Mind, Caring for Clients With Somatoform Disorders, Caring for Clients With Anxiety Disorders, Caring for Clients With Mood Disorders, Caring for Clients With Eating Disorders, Caring for Chemically Dependent Clients,* and *Caring for Clients With Dementia and Thought Disorders.*
- Unit 5, *Common Medical-Surgical Problems,* includes chapters on *Caring for Clients With Infectious Disorders; Caring for Clients With Cancer; Caring for Clients With Pain; Caring for Clients With Fluid, Electrolyte, and Acid-Base Imbalances; Caring for Clients in Shock; Caring for Clients Requiring Intravenous Therapy; Caring for Perioperative Clients;* and *Caring for Dying Clients.*
- Units 6 through 17 present information on disorders according to body systems. Each unit begins with an introductory chapter that includes a general review of anatomy and physiology, a discussion of client assessment, and common diagnostic and laboratory tests that pertain to particular disorders.

FEATURES AND LEARNING TOOLS

Many of the features that long-time users of Timby and Smith love are found in the 8th edition as well:

- **Words to Know.** These words are listed at the beginning of each chapter and are set in bold type within the text where they appear with or near their definition. Additional technical terms are italicized throughout the text.
- **Learning Objectives.** These student-oriented objectives appear at the beginning of each chapter to serve as guidelines for acquiring specific information within each chapter.
- **General Nutritional, Pharmacologic, and Gerontologic Considerations.** Included at the end of most chapters, the content has been developed by experts in their fields. These are identified by the following icons:

- **Nursing Guidelines.** These boxed displays present essential nursing information related to caring for a client with a specific disorder.
- **Critical Thinking Exercises.** These questions, which follow each chapter summary, aim to facilitate application of the material contained within the chapter, using clinical situations or rhetorical questions.
- **Summary of Key Concepts.** Located in the study guide, the summary condenses the chapter's content and integrates information that corresponds with the learning objectives as well. The summation can be used as a preview of the chapter and a later resource for quick review.
- **Selected Readings.** These are intended to provide a guide to current literature that has been cited as references within the chapter or to encourage further independent learning about disorders discussed in the text.
- **Appendices.** These include the answers to the Stop, Think, and Respond boxes, a list of important Nursing Resources, a guide to Commonly Used Medical Abbreviations, and a list of laboratory tests and their normal values.
- **Glossary.** Found at the back of the book, this is a quick reference of definitions for Words to Know that are used throughout the text.
- **Detailed Table of Contents.** Located at the beginning of the textbook, this provides an outline of each unit's and chapter's subject matter.
- **Quick Table of Contents.** Printed on the front end page, this feature facilitates prompt location of specific chapters.
- **Quick Reference to NANDA-Approved Nursing Diagnoses.** This list is printed on the back end page to help students become familiar with the ex-

panding taxonomy of problems that falls within nursing's domain.

INSTRUCTOR'S ANCILLARY PACKAGE

The ancillary package includes the *Instructors' Resource Manual and Testbank to Accompany Introductory Medical-Surgical Nursing,* 8th edition. Included in the Instructors' Manual are chapter overviews, words to know, chapter resources, and case study exercises. Also included are multiple-choice testbank questions on CD-ROM. All material for testbank questions are derived from the textbook.

STUDENT STUDY GUIDE

The *Study Guide to Accompany Introductory Medical-Surgical Nursing,* 8th edition, is designed for use with this text. The study guide now includes practice exercises of all question types, an answer key, and a student self-study CD-ROM. All questions in the study guide are also based on information in the textbook.

PRONUNCIATIONS CD-ROM

In the back of this text is included a free CD-ROM that contains all the terms found in the "Words to Know" and Glossary, sorted by chapter. Students can click on each term to hear its correct pronunciation. This tool will be helpful for learning how to say unfamiliar medical terminology. It also will be especially helpful for ESL and foreign students.

Acknowledgments

The authors wish to thank all those who helped in the preparation of this edition. To those at Lippincott Williams & Wilkins, especially Renee Gagliardi, Development Editor, and Lisa Stead, Acquisitions Editor, we say thank you for all your support, encouragement, and willingness to help. To Debra Schiff, Production Editor, we appreciate the work on the final editing process.

We are also grateful to Susan G. Dudek, RD, CDN, BS, for her contribution of the Nutritional Considerations and review of the nutritional content within chapters. We thank Mary Jo Kirkpatrick, RN, MSN, for her contribution of the Pharmacologic Considerations and review of the pharmacologic content within chapters. We thank Sally Roach, RN, MSN, for her contribution of the Gerontologic Considerations and review of gerontologic content within chapters. Sally also prepared many of the drug tables throughout the book.

We would like to extend thanks to Sheila Timby for assisting with the literature searches and Michael Porter for work on the Appendices and Glossary.

There are several contributors to whom we are grateful: Pamela Gwin, RNC; Kristine Kirsch, RNC, MPA, NMCC; Sharon Powell-Laney, BSN, RN, MSN; Nancy Rayhorn, BSN, RN, BN, CGBN; Patricia L. Schneider, MSN, RN; and Bonnie Smith, BSN, RN.

We hope that *Introductory Medical-Surgical Nursing,* 8th edition, provides the readers with the practical knowledge and skills to manage the nursing care of clients in today's changing health care environments. We also hope that our contributions provide students with similar joys and rewards that we experience in our nursing careers.

Barbara K. Timby, RN, BC, BSN, MA
Nancy E. Smith, MS, RN

Contents

chapter 1

Concepts and Trends in Healthcare

Words to Know

capitation
client
critical pathways
diagnosis-related group
disease
health
healthcare delivery
   system
healthcare team
health maintenance
health maintenance
   organization
health promotion
holism

illness
integrated delivery
   system
managed care
   organization
preferred provider
   organization
primary care
prospective payment
   systems
secondary care
tertiary care
wellness

Learning Objectives

On completion of this chapter, the reader will:

- Define holism.
- Explain the concepts of health, wellness, illness, disease, and the health–illness continuum.
- Identify how those with chronic illness may still be considered healthy.
- Differentiate between health maintenance and health promotion.
- Discuss members of the healthcare team.
- Describe the three levels of care that the healthcare delivery system provides.
- Describe problems related to access to healthcare.
- Describe Medicare, Medicaid, and Medigap insurance.
- Explain how health maintenance organizations and preferred provider organizations work.
- Discuss the difference between capitation and fee-for-service insurance.
- Identify trends that will influence future healthcare policy.
- Discuss methods for monitoring quality of care.
- Describe healthcare goals that were identified in *Healthy People 2000*.
- Identify the five sets of overall health indicators created by *Healthy People 2010*.
- List six priorities for global health.

The roles of nurses in the healthcare delivery system are multiple and complex. Nurses collect data, diagnose human responses to health problems, and plan, provide, and evaluate outcomes of care. They work in various settings, adhering to facility policies and state nurse practice acts. Nurses educate clients, families, and staff; manage resources; and act as advocates for clients. In addition, they participate in disease prevention and health promotion activities for clients, families, and communities. Nurses practice from the perspective of holism. **Holism** means viewing a person's health as a balance of body, mind, and spirit. Treating only the body will not necessarily restore optimal health. In addition to physical needs, nurses must also consider the client's psychological, sociocultural, developmental, and spiritual needs.

HEALTH AND WELLNESS

The constitution of the World Health Organization (WHO) defines **health** as "a state of complete physical, mental, and social well-being and not merely the absence of disease and infirmity" (WHO, 1997). Although this definition of health is useful, it presents health and illness in absolute terms: if a person is not functioning optimally in every way, he or she is not healthy. It also implies that an infirmity negates the possibility of health. A holistic definition of health considers all aspects of the person: physical, emotional, mental, social, and spiritual.

Wellness involves a state of being. Good physical self-care, prevention of illness and injury, use of one's full intellectual potential, expression of emotions, appropriate management of stress, comfortable and congenial interpersonal relationships, and concern about one's environment and conditions throughout the world are components of wellness (Rosdahl, 1999).

A state of wellness is highly individual, as are personal definitions of health and illness.

Illness and Disease

Theoretically, **illness** refers to a state of being sick. Illness may be viewed as catastrophic (sudden, traumatic), acute, chronic, or terminal. **Disease** refers to a pathologic condition of the body that presents with clinical signs and symptoms and changes in laboratory values. The term *disease* has related terminology and concepts. Table 1-1 provides a list of these terms with brief definitions.

The major difference between illness and disease is that illness is highly individual and personal, whereas disease is something more definitive and measurable. For example, a client with arthritis presents with distinct pathologic changes associated with the disease. A person, however, may or may not be ill with arthritis. The degree of pain, suffering, and immobility varies with each person.

TABLE 1-1	DISEASE-RELATED TERMINOLOGY
TERM	**DEFINITION**
Etiology	The cause of a disease
Incidence	The frequency of a particular disease in a specific population during a specific period
Morbidity	The number of sick persons with a particular disease in a specific population
Mortality	The death rate or the ratio of the number of deaths for a specific population
Pathophysiology	Study of how disease alters normal physiologic processes
Prevalence	The number of cases of a disease in a specific population during a specific period
Primary prevention	Prevention of the development of disease in a susceptible or potentially susceptible population; includes health promotion and immunization
Secondary prevention	Early diagnosis and treatment to shorten duration and severity of an illness, reduce contagion, and limit complications
Sign	Objective manifestation of a disease; can be seen, heard, measured, or felt
Symptom	Subjective manifestation of a disease or illness; what the client relates is happening
Tertiary prevention	Healthcare to limit the degree of disability or promote rehabilitation in chronic, irreversible diseases

The Health–Illness Continuum

In contrast to definitions of health and illness, the health–illness continuum considers levels of health, which vary for each person. This continuum provides a broad range for determining a client's health status. Dunn (1961) described health as a dynamic state that ranges from high-level wellness to very poor health and death (Fig. 1-1). This concept allows for many levels of health and illness. Other theorists expanded this idea to describe health as the ability to adapt physically, emotionally, and socially, enabling maintenance of comfort, stability, and self-expression. Embedded in this definition of health is the idea that a client with chronic illness can achieve a high level of wellness if he or she can experience a high quality of life within the limits of that illness. For example, physically disabled people are considered healthy if they are physiologically stable and engaged in personal and social activities that they find meaningful.

Health Maintenance and Promotion

Many people now believe they have control over their well-being and are taking more responsibility for their health status. **Health maintenance** refers to protecting one's current level of health by preventing illness or deterioration, such as by complying with medication regimens, being screened for such diseases as breast and colon cancer, or practicing safe sex. **Health promotion** refers to engaging in strategies to enhance health. Such strategies include eating a diet high in grains and complex carbohydrates, exercising regularly, balancing work with leisure activities, and practicing stress reduction techniques. The use of the term *client* in this textbook reflects the attitude of personal responsibility for health. A **client** is an

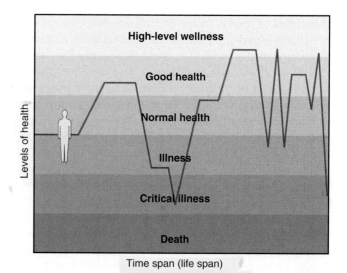

FIGURE 1-1 The health–illness continuum.

active partner in nursing care. Thus, the person receiving healthcare services no longer plays a passive, ill role but is an active purchaser of healthcare services. Clients may or may not be ill, but they take great responsibility for meeting their health maintenance and promotion needs and actively participate in treatment decisions regarding health restoration.

HEALTHCARE

Just as the concept of health has changed in recent decades, so too has the healthcare industry. Rapid advances in science and technology have contributed to the development of highly sophisticated methods for diagnosing and treating disease. At the same time, escalating healthcare costs have created difficult economic conditions, disparity in access to care, and brief lengths of stays in hospitals. The healthcare system has grown to include multiple outpatient, short-term, and long-term care facilities with care given by various providers.

Healthcare Providers

The **healthcare team** consists of specially trained personnel who work together to help clients meet their healthcare needs. The team includes physicians, nurses, psychologists, pharmacists, dietitians, social workers, respiratory and physical therapists, occupational therapists, nursing assistants, technicians, and insurance company staff. All members of this team collaborate on client issues (medical, social, and financial) to achieve the best possible outcomes. Figure 1-2 shows personnel who are part of the healthcare team.

The Healthcare Delivery System

The **healthcare delivery system** refers to the full range of services available to people seeking prevention, identification, treatment, or rehabilitation of health problems. The first resource person or agency that clients contact about a health need provides **primary care.** This initial contact is often with a family practitioner, internist, or nurse practitioner. **Secondary care** includes referrals to facilities for additional testing such as cardiac catheterization, consultation, and diagnosis. **Tertiary care** is provided in hospitals where specialists and complex technology are available. Skilled nursing care occurs in facilities or units that offer prolonged health maintenance or rehabilitative services, such as long-term care or extended care facilities. Examples include nursing homes, skilled nursing facilities, rehabilitation centers, and subacute care units. Home care is an important adjunct to inpatient care;

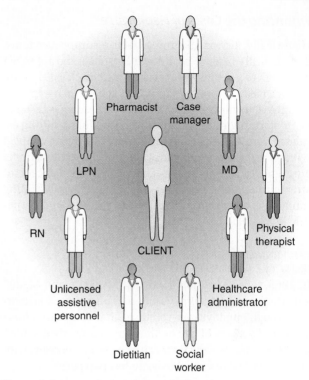

FIGURE 1-2 Members of the healthcare team.

visiting nurses and home health aides are the personnel who make earlier discharge to home possible by providing services formerly done in hospitals or long-term care facilities. Hospices and home hospice care are resources for terminally ill clients and their families.

Stop, Think, and Respond ● BOX 1-1

A client in an acute tertiary care setting is ready for discharge. Where will this client go?

Access to Care

As the types of health services expand, the healthcare delivery system becomes more complex, costly, and, in many cases, inaccessible. An estimated 43.4 million citizens in the United States do not have access to healthcare because of the economic burden it poses. Another 25 million citizens have inadequate healthcare coverage (U.S. Census Bureau, 1998). For many, health maintenance and health promotion are unaffordable luxuries. Groups such as children, the elderly, ethnic minorities, and the poor are most likely to be underserved. Many of these people delay seeking early treatment for their health problems because they cannot afford to pay for services. When an illness becomes so severe that the only choice is to seek medical attention, many turn to their local hospital emergency departments for primary care. This expensive alternative usually involves long waits and no follow-up care.

Financing the Costs of Healthcare

Historically, private insurance, self-insurance systems, and Medicare paid for healthcare. Hospitals and approved providers received payment for what they charged; more charges meant more revenues. Thus, these plans had no incentives to control costs. Not only did charges escalate at an alarming rate, but abuse and fraudulent billing escalated as well. Disparities in access to healthcare coupled with its high costs prompted evaluation of spending in the entire healthcare industry. The 1990s were a decade of streamlining government payment systems and finding innovative approaches from private insurers and corporate health plans.

GOVERNMENT-FUNDED HEALTHCARE: MEDICARE AND MEDICAID

In 1965, federal legislation created Medicare and Medicaid. Medicare is a federally run program financed primarily through employee payroll taxes. It covers individuals who are 65 years of age or older, permanently disabled workers of any age and their dependents, and persons with end-stage renal disease. Medicare has two parts:

- Part A—Mostly free; covers acute hospital care, rehabilitative care, hospice, and home care services
- Part B—Purchased for a fee; covers physician services, outpatient hospital care, laboratory tests, durable medical equipment, and other selected services

Although Medicare is for older Americans, it does not cover long-term care and limits coverage for health promotion and illness prevention. It also does not cover outpatient medications, a significant expense for seniors. For these reasons, individuals with adequate resources purchase private Medigap insurance to cover these expenditures.

Medicaid is a state-administered entitlement program designed to serve the poor. Funds come from federal, state, and local sources; each state determines how funds will be spent. In general, Medicaid programs cover hospitalization, diagnostic tests, physician visits, rehabilitation, and outpatient care. They also may cover long-term care when a person no longer has private funds.

PROSPECTIVE PAYMENT SYSTEMS

In 1983, Medicare implemented a **prospective payment system (PPS).** PPS uses financial incentives to decrease total charges by reimbursing on a fixed-rate basis. Medicare reimburses predetermined amounts to hospitals based on the **diagnosis-related group (DRG)** in which the client's condition falls. The DRG system is a method of grouping clients with similar diagnoses. For example, all clients receiving a hip, knee, or shoulder replacement fall into DRG 209, Total Joint Replacement, and their

surgeries are reimbursed at basically the same rate. If actual costs are less than the reimbursed amount, the hospital makes money; if costs exceed the reimbursed amount, the hospital loses money.

This reimbursement system was largely responsible for the marked decreases in hospital lengths of stay since the early 1980s. The possible premature discharge of clients and increased responsibility for family members who may be unable to provide adequate care created much criticism of the PPS/DRG system. Another criticism has been the shift in costs from clients with Medicare to those who have private insurance. Providers charge privately insured clients inflated amounts to make up for the losses in Medicare revenues. In response to this cost shifting and other economic forces, insurance companies began to challenge hospital charges aggressively, refuse payment when hospital level of care was not provided, and shift their clients into cost-containment reimbursement systems now known as *managed care.*

MANAGED CARE

Managed care organizations (MCOs) are insurers who carefully plan and closely supervise the distribution of healthcare services. Although it is a business venture that emphasizes cost of services and economic use of resources, managed care focuses on prevention as the best way to manage healthcare costs (Box 1-1). The two most common types of managed care systems are health maintenance organizations (HMOs) and preferred provider organizations (PPOs). Capitation is a third emerging MCO financing structure.

Health Maintenance Organizations. Health maintenance organizations are group insurance plans in which each participant pays a preset, fixed fee in exchange for healthcare services. This fee does not fluctuate with the type or frequency of care. The financial stability of HMOs is based on their ability to keep their members healthy and out of the hospital through periodic screening, health education, and preventive services.

Health maintenance organizations provide ambulatory, hospitalization, and home care services. Some HMOs have their own facilities; others use community agencies

---

BOX 1-1 ● **Goals of Managed Care**

- Use healthcare resources efficiently.
- Deliver high-quality care at a reasonable cost.
- Measure, monitor, and manage fiscal and client outcomes.
- Prevent illness through screening and health promotion activities.
- Provide client education to decrease risk of disease.
- Case manage clients with chronic illness to minimize number of hospitalizations.

for services. A member of an HMO must receive authorization (referral) for secondary care, such as second opinions from specialists or diagnostic testing. If members obtain unauthorized care, they are responsible for the entire bill. In this way, HMOs serve as gatekeepers for healthcare services.

Preferred Provider Organizations. Preferred provider organizations operate on the principle that competition can control costs. Acting as agents for health insurance companies, PPOs create a community network of providers who are willing to discount their fees for service in exchange for a steady supply of referred customers. Consumers can lower their healthcare costs if they receive care from the preferred providers. If they select providers outside the network, they pay a higher percentage of the costs.

Capitation. Capitation is a fundamentally different concept in healthcare financing. Instead of paying a fee for services provided, as in traditional insurance plans (including HMOs and PPOs), **capitation** plans pay a preset fee per member per month to the healthcare provider, usually a hospital or hospital system. This fee covers all medical costs incurred and is paid regardless of whether the member requires healthcare services. If members do not require much high-cost care, the provider makes money; if members use many high-cost resources, the provider loses money. This method of financing provides the strongest incentives for limiting use of expensive services and focusing healthcare on health maintenance and health promotion.

Evolution of Healthcare

The changes in reimbursement structures and practices have created a shift in economic and decision-making power from hospitals, nurses, and physicians to insurance companies. Much criticism and concern accompany this shift, as physicians, nurses, other providers, and consumers find themselves unable to obtain or provide care free from the insurer's economic pressure. As a result of managed care's influence, hospitals downsized, restructured, or sometimes closed. Consequently, many regions are left with fewer hospitals, higher nurse/client ratios, and higher client acuity levels on general medical–surgical units, skilled nursing facilities, long-term care facilities, and home health settings. Thus, many claim that the profits posted by large insurance companies come at the expense of quality care and jobs of healthcare providers.

Changes in the healthcare industry have also affected employment for healthcare workers. Hospitals are using unlicensed assistive personnel (UAPs) to perform some duties practical and registered nurses once provided. Many are concerned that the use of UAPs will jeopardize the quality of care. In addition, physicians' income decreased in recent years. This trend will most likely continue, partly because of the growth of nurse practitioners and physician assistants. The predicted decreased income may lead to fewer men and women entering the medical profession. In many rural areas of the United States, medical care already is inadequate—an unfortunate situation that is unlikely to improve.

These changes also may affect the client's experience and satisfaction with healthcare. A single episode of illness can involve negotiating for a referral, receiving testing at a site other than the hospital, staying a short time in the hospital, transferring to a rehabilitation or skilled nursing facility (or both), and obtaining outpatient rehabilitation and home health services. Although much effort is made to coordinate care, particularly by nurse case managers (see Chap. 2), this fragmentation forces clients repeatedly to build therapeutic relationships and may leave them unsure of who is in charge.

The cost-driven changes have had positive effects as well. In an attempt to reduce redundancy of healthcare services and increase economic leverage, hospitals and other healthcare facilities are forming networks, known as **integrated delivery systems (ICDs)** (Box 1-2). ICDs provide a full range of healthcare services that should result in highly coordinated, cost-effective care. Shorter hospital stays may result in fewer nosocomial (acquired in the hospital) complications and quicker return to self-care. In some ways, nurses have greater ability to take an active role in advocating for high-quality, nurse-provided care. Nurses work in new and expanded positions in the healthcare industry (see Chap. 2).

BOX 1-2 ● Integrated Delivery Systems

Fully integrated healthcare delivery systems will provide:
- Wellness programs
- Preventive care
- Ambulatory care
- Outpatient diagnostic and laboratory services
- Emergency care
- General and tertiary hospital services
- Rehabilitation
- Long-term care
- Assisted living facilities
- Psychiatric care
- Home healthcare services
- Hospice care
- Outpatient pharmacies

Adapted from Buerhas, P. (1996). Creating a new place in a competitive market: The value of nursing care. In E. Hein (Ed.), *Contemporary nursing leadership: Selected readings.* Philadelphia: Lippincott Williams & Wilkins.

EMERGENCY DEPARTMENT CRITICAL PATH: PNEUMONIA Exclusion Criteria: Clients with HIV, neutropenia, severe hypotension, steroid dependency > 20mg/day, those requiring mechanical ventilation, or clients on immunosuppressive or chemotherapy.

	2ND HOUR	3RD HOUR	4TH HOUR
ASSESSMENTS	REASSESSMENT/ASSESSMENT RESPONSE TO TREATMENT	REASSESSMENT/ASSESSMENT RESPONSE TO TREATMENT	REASSESSMENT/ASSESSMENT RESPONSE TO TREATMENT
CONSULTS	IF INDICATED NOTIFY ADMITTING RESIDENT		
LABS, DIAGNOSTICS PROCEDURES	1. AP/LAT CXR RESULTED 2. CBC, SMA7 3. BLOOD CULTURES X2 4. SPUTUM C + S/gmst. Y__N__ 5. ABG IF PULSE OX <92% RA 6. EKG FEMALE >55 MALE >45 OR CLINICALLY INDICATED		
INTERVENTIONS	SAFETY MEASURES AS PER STANDARD		
IV/MEDICATION	1. SALINE LOCK 2. O2 THERAPY AS PER ORDER 3. ANTIBIOTIC AS PER ALGORITHM AFTER BLOOD CULTURE AND ATTEMPT AT SPUTUM CULTURE		

Community Acquired Is the client allergic to PCN?		Institutional Is the client allergic to PCN?	
No	Yes	No	Yes
Ceftriaxone 1gm q24 •	TMP/SMX 2amps (320mg/1600mg) IV q12 •	Ticarcillin/Clavulanate 3.1gm q6 •	Ciprofloxacine 400mg IV q12 • and Clindamycin 600mg IV q8 •
CIRCLE MEDICATION: TIME OF ADMINISTRATION _____		**CIRCLE MEDICATION: TIME OF ADMINISTRATION _____**	

	2ND HOUR	3RD HOUR	4TH HOUR
TEACHING	1. REASSURE AND INFORM PT/SO RE: TX PLAN AND INTERVENTIONS 2. PROVIDE CLIENT WITH PSYCHOLOGICAL SUPPORT 3. PT/FAMILY CAN VERBALIZE DISCHARGE INSTRUCTIONS? Y__N__ 4. PT/FAMILY RECEIVED WRITTEN DISCHARGE INSTRUCTIONS? Y__N__	1. REASSURE AND INFORM PT/SO RE: TX PLAN AND INTERVENTIONS 2. PROVIDE CLIENT WITH PSYCHOLOGICAL SUPPORT 3. PT/FAMILY CAN VERBALIZE DISCHARGE INSTRUCTIONS? Y__N__ 4. PT/FAMILY RECEIVED WRITTEN DISCHARGE INSTRUCTIONS? Y__N__	1. REASSURE AND INFORM PT/SO RE: TX PLAN AND INTERVENTIONS 2. PROVIDE CLIENT WITH PSYCHOLOGICAL SUPPORT 3. PT/FAMILY CAN VERBALIZE DISCHARGE INSTRUCTIONS? Y__N__ 4. PT/FAMILY RECEIVED WRITTEN DISCHARGE INSTRUCTIONS? Y__N__
D/C PLANNING AND FOLLOW-UP	DISPOSITION: 1. ADMITTED RM#____ 2. TREATED AND REFERRED 3. TX TO OTHER INSTITUTION 4. NOT EXAMINED OR TREATED 5. LEFT AMA 6. DOA/DIED IN ED TIME OF DISCHARGE_____	DISPOSITION: 1. ADMITTED RM#____ 2. TREATED AND REFERRED 3. TX TO OTHER INSTITUTION 4. NOT EXAMINED OR TREATED 5. LEFT AMA 6. DOA/DIED IN ED TIME OF DISCHARGE_____	DISPOSITION: 1. ADMITTED RM#____ 2. TREATED AND REFERRED 3. TX TO OTHER INSTITUTION 4. NOT EXAMINED OR TREATED 5. LEFT AMA 6. DOA/DIED IN ED TIME OF DISCHARGE_____
OUTCOMES	1. CLINICALLY STABLE 2. PULSE OX > 92% (W OR W/O O2) Y__N__ 3. HR 60–135 Y__N__ 4. RR 12–35 Y__N__ 5. SBP >90 Y__N__ 6. RECEIVED FIRST DOSE OF ANTIBIOTICS Y__N__	1. CLINICALLY STABLE 2. PULSE OX > 92% (W OR W/O O2) Y__N__ 3. HR 60–135 Y__N__ 4. RR 12–35 Y__N__ 5. SBP >90 Y__N__ 6. RECEIVED FIRST DOSE OF ANTIBIOTICS Y__N__	1. CLINICALLY STABLE 2. PULSE OX > 92% (W OR W/O O2) Y__N__ 3. HR 60–135 Y__N__ 4. RR 12–35 Y__N__ 5. SBP >90 Y__N__ 6. RECEIVED FIRST DOSE OF ANTIBIOTICS Y__N__

SIGNATURE	TIME	INITIAL	SIGNATURE	TIME	INITIAL

**Shaded Area Represents MD Decision Point

FIGURE 1-3 An emergency department (ED) critical pathway for pneumonia. This generic critical pathway covers the first hour of care, which includes the general interventions and baseline diagnostics that lead to a working diagnosis and a specific critical pathway. ABG = arterial blood gas; AMA = against medical advice; AP/LAT CXR = anterior, posterior, and lateral chest x-rays; CBC = complete blood count; DOA = dead on arrival; EKG = electrocardiogram; HR = heart rate; pulse ox = pulse oximetry; PT/SO = patient/significant other; RR = respiratory rate; SBP = systolic blood pressure; SMA7 = electrolytes, glucose; Sputum C & S/gmst = sputum culture, sensitivity, and Gram stain; Tx = treatment or transfer; W or W/O = with or without.

In addition, the economic burden imposed on society by out-of-control healthcare costs had to be addressed. Another indirect positive result of the cost-containment initiatives is increased attention given to what constitutes quality in healthcare and how hospitals, practitioners, and insurance companies measure, monitor, and manage quality.

Quality of Care

Demand for evidence that hospitals and practitioners provide high-quality, cost-effective care comes from insurers, regulatory bodies such as the Joint Commission for Accreditation of Healthcare Organizations (JCAHO), and consumers. To meet this demand, hospitals have formed performance improvement committees. These groups or hospital departments also may be called *quality improvement* or *outcomes management committees.* They assess such factors as readmission to the hospital within 30 days of discharge, average cost per case, wound infection rates, incidence of hospital-acquired pressure ulcers, and various other measures. Because insurers have so much say about the type and quantity of care provided, they too have quality improvement departments that monitor similar outcomes.

As concern for cost meets concern for quality, practitioners search for ways to ensure that they accomplish all care, teaching, and preparation before the discharge date without overusing expensive resources. Stemming from such concerns, protocols (also known as *guidelines* or *standards*) for managing care have been developed. One method gaining widespread use is the critical or clinical pathway. Multidisciplinary teams develop **critical pathways** for specific diagnoses or procedures, which standardize important aspects of care such as diagnostic work-ups, nursing care, education, physical therapy, and discharge planning across the estimated length of stay. By analyzing variances from the pathway (unexpected events such as delayed discharge or transfer to a more intensive level of care), clinicians can identify trends that are beneficial or detrimental. The team who develops the pathway can then redesign care to address the identified trend. Critical pathways often are considered a tool of case management (see Chap. 2). Figure 1-3 is an example of a critical pathway for a client with pneumonia.

Many other methods exist for determining quality of care. Patient satisfaction surveys, quality-of-life questionnaires, functional assessment tools, number of hospital admissions per year for clients with chronic illnesses, and morbidity (complications) and mortality (deaths) rates are a few important measures assessed when examining quality.

Future Trends and Goals for Healthcare

The United States Department of Health and Human Services (2000) identifies national health goals. *Healthy*

BOX 1-3 ● Leading Health Indicators

1. Physical activity
2. Overweight and obesity
3. Tobacco use
4. Substance abuse
5. Responsible sexual behavior
6. Mental health
7. Injury and violence
8. Environmental quality
9. Immunization
10. Access to healthcare

U.S. Department of Health and Human Services. (2000). *Healthy people 2010: Understanding and improving health.* (2nd ed.). (On-line.) Available: http://www.health.gov/healthypeople.

People 2010 is the initiative that provides an overall action plan to improve the health and quality of life for people living in the United States. There are two overall goals identified by *Healthy People 2010*:

- Help individuals of all ages increase life expectancy and improve their quality of life
- Eliminate health disparities among segments of the population, including differences that occur by gender, race or ethnicity, education or income, disability, geographic location, or sexual orientation (U.S. Department of Health and Human Services, 2000).

The Healthy People initiative targets the improvement of health for all. It promotes a systematic approach to health improvement by setting goals, objectives, determinants of health, and general health status. Focus areas include specific concerns, such as diseases (diabetes, arthritis), environmental issues (environmental health, food safety), and social issues (substance abuse, family planning).

In addition, the *Healthy People 2010* initiative developed leading health indicators for measuring the overall health of the U.S. population (Box 1-3). These include outcomes for health and disease, preventive health behaviors, indicators of mental health, access to healthcare, and ecologic factors such as injuries and deaths related to firearms.

As the 21st century begins, economics, consumer satisfaction, effectiveness of traditional medical care, alternative medicine, disease prevalence, global emergence of drug-resistant organisms, and cultural diversity are all forces that will influence the direction of healthcare around the world. The WHO foresees the continued effects of infectious diseases on global health, particularly in developing nations. Epidemics of cancer and other chronic diseases are likely as life expectancies continue to increase because people are at increased risk for chronic illnesses as they age (WHO, 1997). Box 1-4 outlines the WHO's priorities for international health, which can be applied to any individual nation or community. In the midst of these

BOX 1-4 ● Priorities for International Health

- Integrated, comprehensive disease control that incorporates prevention, diagnosis, treatment, and rehabilitation
- Improved training of healthcare professionals
- Wider use of cost-effective methods for disease prevention and management, including screening
- Intense and sustained global efforts to encourage healthy lifestyles to modify risk factors such as poor diet, lack of exercise, and smoking, especially among children and young adults
- Development of health-enhancing public policy, including policy on financing, pricing, and taxation, that will support disease prevention programs
- Alleviation of pain, reduction of suffering, and provision of palliative (comfort) care to those who cannot be cured

World Health Organization (1997). *World health report 1997–executive summary: Conquering suffering, enriching humanity.* [On-line.] Available: http://www.who.ch/whr/1997/exsum97e.htm.

dramatic changes and challenges, nurses must continue to provide safe, high-quality, cost-effective care to individuals, families, and communities. It also is imperative that nurses distinguish and communicate to clients the various choices that they may make about their healthcare.

Critical Thinking Exercises

1. *Interview a person who has had experience with traditional healthcare insurance and with managed care. Explore the advantages and disadvantages of both systems.*

2. *Select a healthcare facility where you have had student clinical experiences. Have any cost reduction measures occurred? What effect have these actions had?*
3. *Discuss how economic conditions affect working conditions for nurses.*

References and Suggested Readings

Dunn, H. L. (1961). *High-level wellness.* Arlington, VA: Beatty.

Ellis, J. R. & Hartley, C. L. (2001). *Nursing in today's world: Challenges, issues, and trends* (7th ed.). Philadelphia: Lippincott Williams & Wilkins.

Medicare learning network for outpatient PPS. [On-line.] Available: http://www.hcfa.gov/medlearn/faqs.htm.

Rosdahl, C. B. (1999). *Textbook of basic nursing* (7th ed.). Philadelphia: Lippincott Williams & Wilkins.

Schaffner, J. W. (1999). Developing a patient care model for an integrated delivery system. *Journal of Nursing Administration, 29*(9), 43–50.

U.S. Census Bureau. (1998). In S. M. Wolfe (Ed.), *Third World traveler: Going bare* (1999). [On-line.] Available: http://www.thirdworldtraveler.com/Health/GoingBare.html.

U.S. Department of Health and Human Services. (1999). *18-Month outcomes.* [On-line.] Available: www.dhhd.gov/progorg/oei.

U.S. Department of Health and Human Services. (2000). *Healthy people 2010: Understanding and improving health.* (2nd ed.). (On-line.) Available: http://www.health.gov/healthypeople.

World Health Organization. (1997). World health report 1997— Executive summary: Conquering suffering, enriching humanity. [On-line.] Available: http://www.who.ch/whr/1997/exsum97e.htm.

Zerwekh, J. & Claborn, J. C. (2000). *Nursing today: Transitions and trends.* Philadelphia: W.B. Saunders.

Nursing in Various Settings

Words to Know

assisted living
boarding homes
case management
case method
congregate housing

functional nursing
home healthcare
patient-focused care
primary nursing
team nursing

Learning Objectives

On completion of this chapter, the reader will:
- Define nursing.
- Compare six nursing care delivery models.
- Describe the types of clients served in various settings in which nurses practice.
- Differentiate congregate housing, boarding homes, and assisted living.
- Identify the functions of the home health nurse.
- List six services provided by home health agencies.
- Define case management.
- Explain the nurse case manager's role.

Today's dynamic healthcare environment challenges the traditional territory, roles, and responsibilities of healthcare providers. Registered nurses (RNs) used to provide care in hospital intensive care units for conditions that clients and their significant others now may manage at home with the support of visiting nurses. Clients undergoing procedures that formerly required a 2-week hospital stay now are discharged in fewer than 5 days. In many instances, insurance companies and case managers dictate choice of services, treatment options, and hospital lengths of stay, all traditional decisions of the attending physician. Such changes have called on nursing to provide high-quality nursing care wherever it is needed and to function in both traditional and evolving roles.

NURSING CARE

Nursing is concerned with caring for the individual, family, or community and requires nurses to play a significant role in health education, prevention, and promotion. Nurses attend to client needs related to hygiene, activity, diet, the environment, medical treatment, and physical, emotional, and spiritual comfort. People with different

educational levels provide care in diverse settings, which includes various activities. The licensed practical or vocational nurse (LP/LVN) provides care to clients under the direction of an RN or physician in a structured healthcare setting. LP/LVNs care for clients with well-defined, common problems that often require a high level of technical competency and expertise. They frequently work in settings in which RN supervision is available but must be sought after the LP/LVN determines the need to do so. The RN's role is more complex, involving the management and coordination of all the care provided to a group of clients. As healthcare delivery models continue to change, the roles of the LP/LVN and RN are likely to change as well.

Definitions of Nursing

Arriving at a clear and comprehensive definition of nursing is difficult. Florence Nightingale (1859) described the role of the nurse as putting "the patient in the best condition for nature to act upon him." Virginia Henderson (1966), one of the first nursing theorists, envisioned the nurse's role as helping people (sick or well) to carry out those activities contributing to health, recovery, or a peaceful death that they would do for themselves if they had the necessary strength, will, or knowledge. Her definition also focused on regaining independence.

The American Nurses Association (ANA) traditionally defined nursing as "the diagnosis and treatment of human responses to actual or potential health problems" (ANA, 1995, p. 9). In response to an increased emphasis on the science of care, the ANA now acknowledges four essential features of contemporary nursing practice:

- Attention to the full range of human experiences and responses to health and illness without resorting to a problem-focused orientation
- Integration of objective data with knowledge gained from an understanding of the client's or group's subjective experience
- Application of scientific knowledge to the processes of diagnosis and treatment
- Promotion of a caring relationship that facilitates health and healing (ANA, 1995, p. 6).

Other definitions of nursing by selected theorists are given in Table 2-1.

Stop, Think, and Respond ● BOX 2-1

Imogene King stated that clients are open systems in constant interaction with their environment. Compare King's definition with Virginia Henderson's. What is different? What is the same?

Settings and Models for Nursing Care

Nursing care is provided in various settings. Although hospitals employ all levels of nurses in outpatient care areas (e.g., dialysis units, clinics, same-day surgery units, related diagnostic departments), inpatient units have been the traditional site for much of the nursing work force. Although trends in financing suggest decreased reliance on hospitals as the future location for nursing care delivery, there is a great deal of interest in determining the best, most cost-effective method for providing that care. Many models for care delivery exist and can coexist within hospitals based on need.

Hospital-Based Nursing

CASE METHOD

Nursing care was historically provided on a **case method** basis, by which one nurse provided all the services that a particular client required. Although the nurse would accompany the client to the hospital if necessary, the nurse provided care in the home and performed many household duties as well. As times changed and care became more complex, this method become impractical, and different models for the hospital-based delivery of nursing care evolved. A modern version of the case method is private duty nursing.

FUNCTIONAL NURSING

Functional nursing, a task-oriented method, evolved during the 1930s. In **functional nursing,** distinct duties are assigned to specific personnel. For example, one nurse takes all the vital signs, someone else makes all the beds, a third nurse does all the dressing changes, and so on. Tasks are divided, and the client sees several people during the shift. Although efficient, functional nursing fragments care and is confusing for the client.

TEAM NURSING

Team nursing emerged in the 1950s, partially in response to the fragmented care of functional nursing and to accommodate staff with varying levels of education and skill. In **team nursing,** teams are made up of an RN team

TABLE 2-1	DEFINITIONS OF NURSING BY SELECTED THEORISTS
THEORIST	**DEFINITION**
Florence Nightingale (1859)	Nurses alter the environment to put the client in the best condition for nature to act.
Virginia Henderson (1966)	Nurses assist clients to carry out those activities that they would perform unaided if they possessed the necessary strength, will, or knowledge.
Ernestine Weidenbach (1964)	Nursing is a helping, nurturing, and caring service delivered sensitively with compassion, skill, and understanding.
Dorothea Orem (1980)	Nursing care is directed at restoring self-care abilities, which are activities that clients initiate on their own behalf in maintaining health, life, and well-being.
Imogene M. King (1981)	Nursing is the care of human beings; individuals and groups are viewed as open systems in continual interaction with the environment.

leader, other RNs, LP/LVNs, and nursing assistants who provide care to a group of clients. The RN team leader directs the care provided by the RNs, LP/LVNs, and aides, and works with them in various capacities. The team conference for discussion and care planning is a feature of team nursing.

TOTAL CARE

Total care refers to assignments in which a nurse assumes all the care for a small group of clients. This method focuses more on the client as a whole rather than the collection of nursing tasks that need to be accomplished. Total care often is practiced in intensive care units where nurses are assigned one or two clients.

PRIMARY NURSING

In **primary nursing,** an RN assumes 24-hour accountability for the client's care and has total responsibility for the nursing care of assigned clients during his or her shift. Secondary nurses carry out the plan of care in the primary nurse's absence. This approach, which was initiated in the 1970s, is expensive because it relies entirely on RNs. An advantage, however, is that the client is assured of having a caregiver who sees to all of his or her needs and who provides holistic and comprehensive care. Some settings still use this model effectively, such as home care.

PATIENT-FOCUSED CARE

An updated version of primary care and team nursing called **patient-focused care** uses an RN partnered with one or more assistive personnel to care for a group of clients. The RN may work with an LP/LVN and an assistant, a respiratory therapist and an assistant, or a similar combination of staff. The licensed and unlicensed assistants are cross-trained to do many functions formerly done by separate departments, such as drawing blood or obtaining electrocardiograms. The RN may have a role in resource management and may be held accountable for outcomes of nursing care such as skin breakdown (negative outcome) or early ambulation (positive outcome).

COMMUNITY-BASED NURSING

Many facilities and settings besides acute care hospitals provide all levels of nursing care. Nursing homes, skilled nursing facilities, rehabilitation centers, schools, single- and multiple-physician practices, surgicenters, industries, adult day-care centers, homes, insurance companies, and hospices are some locations in which nurses practice.

Skilled nursing facilities provide skilled nursing and rehabilitative care to people who have the potential to regain function but need skilled observation and nursing care during an acute illness. Clients using these facilities also require invasive procedures and therapies (e.g., tube feedings, intravenous fluids, and sterile dressing changes).

Intermediate care facilities (ICFs) are nursing homes that provide custodial care for people who cannot care for themselves because of mental or physical disabilities. ICFs do not receive reimbursement from Medicare because they are not considered medical facilities.

Rehabilitation centers provide physical and occupational therapy to clients and families to help individuals regain as much independence with activities of daily living (ADLs) as possible.

Hospices provide care for clients diagnosed with a terminal illness whose life expectancy is less than 6 months. Hospice allows terminally ill clients to live as fully as possible while pain, discomfort, and other symptoms are controlled. Hospice staffs are specially trained to help families with the grief process. Medicare covers many of the services provided by hospice.

Community health centers and local health departments provide a range of services to the districts, counties, or communities they serve. These agencies receive partial or complete funding from federal, state, and local governments. Community mental health centers also are part of this network. Neighborhood health clinics make healthcare more accessible, and when health facilities are more accessible, people are more likely to seek prompt treatment and reduce the need for acute care.

In addition to the community-based settings described previously, other facilities and services are available for seniors and adults with physical or mental disabilities. These individuals are relatively healthy and not in need of extended care, but may need some assistance with ADLs. The goal of alternative care facilities is to provide the least restrictive living arrangements, while maintaining safety and quality. These facilities include congregate housing, boarding homes, and assisted living facilities.

CONGREGATE HOUSING

Congregate housing provides independent to minimal assistance for seniors or disabled adults. There are free-standing apartments, private rooms, or both. Often residents must meet certain qualifications and may have subsidized rent based on income. Some congregate housing centers may provide other services such as one or more meals per day in a common dining room and recreational activities. In general, congregate housing is affordable, but residents may not have any other resources to purchase extra services or goods. They are assured of appropriate housing, but may lack the resources, ability, or opportunity to participate in outside activities.

BOARDING HOMES

Boarding homes usually are small homes with individual rooms where residents pay for room and board and minimal nursing services. Residents often share rooms. Boarding homes usually have a common dining area for all meals. Often, boarding homes also oversee employment for disabled adults and provide a stable environment for those who cannot live independently. In this type of setting, residents have needed supervision but may relinquish independence and privacy.

ASSISTED LIVING

Assisted living facilities provide care to residents who require assistance with up to three ADLs. Residents maximize their independence in a setting that maintains their privacy and dignity. These facilities are not regulated like long-term care facilities, and there is some concern that the quality of care is not at an appropriate level. The Joint Commission on Accreditation of Healthcare Organizations is developing a voluntary accrediting process for assisted living facilities to ensure consistency and quality of care. In many instances, this type of living arrangement is very expensive. Residents must provide a large up-front investment and then a high monthly fee. The facility may or may not provide such services as housekeeping, laundry, transportation, and meals. Residents can, however, maintain a lifestyle more similar to that which they previously enjoyed. They also are more able to participate in the decisions that affect their future care needs.

Home Health Nursing

Cost containment measures in the last 20 years have resulted in the expansion of home healthcare services. **Home healthcare** can cover both long-term and short-term health needs and can provide comprehensive services. Home health nurses provide specialized care such as intravenous infusion of fluids, medications, and chemotherapy; hospice care; postcardiac surgery care; and care to ventilator-dependent clients (Fig. 2-1). The RN manages and coordinates the care the client receives and has a high level of competency in assessment, skills, communi-

cation, teaching, management, and documentation abilities. The RN encourages the client and the family to develop self-care skills, with support from community resources. Box 2-1 lists other functions of the home health nurse. Besides nursing, home health agencies provide many other services (Table 2-2).

Case Management

A new role and responsibility for nurses is case management. **Case management** maximizes fiscal outcomes without sacrificing quality through careful oversight of a client's healthcare. The person responsible for overseeing the client's care, usually an RN with a bachelor's or mas-

---

BOX 2-1 ● Functions of the Home Healthcare Nurse

- Plan, coordinate, and provide care in consultation with hospital and physician.
- Teach client and family to perform procedures, monitor symptoms, administer medications, and report to physician.
- Assess client and consult with physician as needed.
- Evaluate the home environment for safety hazards, cleanliness, ability to safely store medication, family support, and adequacy of food supplies.
- Connect client and family with community resources.
- Advocate for the client when additional services are needed.
- Document care and teaching provided.
- Complete forms required for reimbursement.

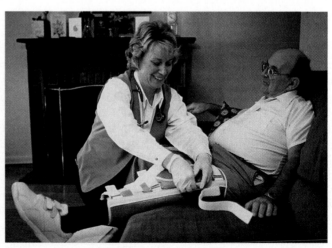

FIGURE 2-1 Home health nurses. (From Taylor, C., Lillis, C., & LeMone, P. [2001]. *Fundamentals of nursing: The art and science of nursing care* [4th ed., p. 204]. Philadelphia: Lippincott Williams & Wilkins.)

TABLE 2-2	SERVICES PROVIDED BY HOME HEALTH AGENCIES
TYPE OF SERVICE	**DESCRIPTION**
Physical therapy	Therapist assesses the client's mobility after orthopedic surgery, injury, or stroke. He or she assesses the need for assistive devices. Client must meet Medicare requirements to receive physical therapy.
Speech therapy	Therapist provides rehabilitation to clients with speech or swallowing disorders. Client must meet Medicare requirements.
Occupational therapy	Therapist assesses need for assistive devices to aid in activities of daily living and identify issues related to fine motor movements and muscle retraining.
Social services	Social worker meets with client and family to identify difficulties with managing illness at home and provides information about financial assistance and community services.
Home health aides	Aides provide personal care such as bathing and dressing and basic skills such as taking vital signs.
Homemakers	Homemakers clean, do laundry, and shop for groceries.

ter's degree, is called the *case manager* (Fig. 2-2). Insurance companies and hospitals employ case managers. A hospital-based case manager may have a caseload of 15 to 25 clients, depending on the acuity (degree of illness) of the clients. Not every client is aggressively case managed; those who are sickest, experience complications, or have chronic illnesses require more intensive case management. The case manager follows clients when they are scheduled for admission until the day of discharge. An insurance-based case manager often maintains contact with the client, especially one with a chronic illness, in the home. Regardless of the employer, case managers plan and coordinate the client's progress through the various phases of care to avoid delays, unnecessary diagnostic testing, and overuse of expensive resources. An important function of the case manager is early, thorough discharge planning. Case

managers often use tools such as critical pathways (see Chap. 1), practice guidelines, and standards of care to help them plan and coordinate care. Hospitals and insurance companies may develop their own or rely on published protocols for guidance. (A cautionary note: Experts using published research should develop all protocols.)

Along with the increase in responsibility, autonomy, and power, nurse case managers have increased accountability for the financial and health outcomes of care. Many employers, particularly insurance companies, measure the costs of services provided to the case manager's clients as a means of assessing his or her effectiveness. One of the complaints about case management, and its parent, managed care, is that the "bottom line" will become more important than quality. For this reason, and because they are in the best position to collect outcome data, case

FIGURE 2-2 Functions of the nurse case manager.

managers often are integral members of hospital-based and insurance-based quality improvement programs.

Critical Thinking Exercises

1. *How do you think nurses will practice in 2010?*
2. *What is your definition of nursing?*
3. *Discuss the pros and cons of case management for both the client and the nurse case manager.*

References and Suggested Readings

American Nurses Association. (1995). *Nursing's social policy statement.* Washington, DC: Author.

Ellis, J. R. & Hartley, C. L. (1999). *Managing and coordinating nursing care* (3rd ed.). Philadelphia: Lippincott Williams & Wilkins.

Ellis, J. R. & Hartley, C. L. (2001). *Nursing in today's world: Challenges, issues, and trends* (7th ed.). Philadelphia: Lippincott Williams & Wilkins.

Henderson, V. (1966). *The nature and science of nursing.* New York: Macmillan.

Hunt, R. & Zurek, E. L. (2001). *Introduction to community-based nursing* (2nd ed.). Philadelphia: Lippincott Williams & Wilkins.

Nightingale, F. (1859). *Notes on nursing: What it is and what it is not.* London: Harrison. [Commemorative edition. (1992). Philadelphia: J.B. Lippincott].

The Nursing Process

Words to Know

actual diagnosis	interventions
assessment	nursing diagnosis
client database	nursing orders
collaborative problems	nursing process
critical thinking	planning
documentation	possible diagnosis
evaluation	risk diagnosis
expected outcomes	syndrome diagnosis
implementation	wellness diagnosis

Learning Objectives

On completion of this chapter, the reader will:

- State the purpose of the nursing process.
- Describe the five steps of the nursing process.
- Define assessment.
- Discuss the parts of a nursing diagnostic statement.
- Differentiate the types of nursing diagnoses.
- Explain the five levels of human needs as identified by Maslow.
- Explain how nurses use the hierarchy of needs to establish nursing priorities.
- Define expected outcomes.
- Analyze how the nurse evaluates a client's plan of care.
- Explain the implementation phase of the nursing process and its relationship with documentation.
- Explain the role of evaluation.
- Give reasons why expected outcomes may not be accomplished.
- Define critical thinking.
- Explain how critical thinking is similar to the nursing process.
- List characteristics of critical thinkers.

The provision of healthcare is a process of problem-solving. Clients present with multiple healthcare needs that the caregiver must approach in an organized, systematic manner to provide efficient and effective care. The purpose of the **nursing process** is to provide a systematic method for nurses to plan and implement client care to achieve desired outcomes. The nursing process for making clinical decisions grew from problem-solving techniques and the scientific process. It includes collecting information, identifying problems, developing an outcome-based plan, carrying out the plan, and evaluating the results. The nursing process provides the framework for nursing care in all healthcare settings. Most states' nurse practice acts include the nursing process as part of the definition of nursing. Nursing educators use the nursing process in the organizational structure of nursing curricula.

STEPS OF THE NURSING PROCESS

The nursing process begins when a client enters the healthcare system. It consists of five steps:

- Assessment
- Diagnosis (nursing)
- Planning
- Implementation
- Evaluation

ADPIE

The nurse collects data (assessment), defines problems or needs (diagnosis), establishes outcomes and actions that will help achieve the overall goals (planning), puts the plan into action (implementation), and determines the client's responses to the care provided (evaluation). Figure 3-1 depicts these five steps in a dynamic, circular model, showing that each component not only is

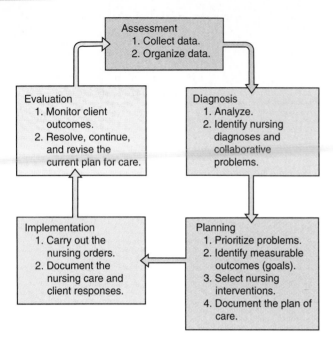

FIGURE 3-1 Steps in the nursing process.

separate and distinct, but interrelated and continuous with the others.

Assessment

Assessment is the careful observation and evaluation of a client's health status. During assessment, the nurse collects information to determine abnormal function and risk factors that contribute to health problems, as well as client strengths (Alfaro-LeFevre, 1998). Not only is assessment the first step in the nursing process, it is an important, recurring nursing activity that continues as long as a need for healthcare exists. During assessment, the nurse methodically obtains data about the client's health and illness. The nurse documents the data in the medical record, which contributes to the client database. The **client database** includes all the information obtained from the medical and nursing history, physical examination (see Chap. 4), and diagnostic studies. Baseline data serve as a comparison for future signs and symptoms and provide a reference for determining if a client's health is improving. Initial and ongoing assessment is essential to the provision of nursing care.

Nursing Diagnosis

During the second phase of the nursing process, **nursing diagnosis,** the nurse reports or analyzes data, according to his or her level of practice, to identify and define problems. Licensed practical nurses (LPNs) report information that suggests actual or potential health problems. Regis-

tered nurses (RNs) examine and analyze the client database to formulate nursing diagnoses. Table 3-1 compares the roles of the LPN and RN in the nursing process and nursing diagnosis.

A nursing diagnosis identifies and defines a health problem that independent or physician-prescribed nursing actions can prevent or solve. Table 3-2 presents the different types of diagnoses. The North American Nursing Diagnosis Association (NANDA) developed the classification system for client problems and nursing diagnoses. NANDA meets every 2 years to review and update the list, the most recent version of which is on the inside cover of this text. Nurses should use NANDA-approved nursing diagnoses whenever possible. If a client's problem does not fit into any of the NANDA-approved diagnoses, the nurse can use her or his own terminology. The NANDA-approved diagnoses are very comprehensive, however, and provide student nurses with the appropriate terminology to formulate nursing diagnoses.

Nursing Diagnostic Statement

A diagnostic statement includes one to three parts: (1) the name, or label, of the problem; (2) the cause of the problem; and (3) the signs and symptoms, or data, that indicate the problem. The name or label portion of the statement is linked to the cause with the phrase *related to,* and the data are linked to the name/label and cause by the phrase *as manifested by* or *as evidenced by.* The following is an example of a nursing diagnostic statement:

> *Constipation* (name of the problem) *related to decreased fluid intake, lack of dietary fiber, and lack of exercise* (causes) *as manifested by no bowel movement for the past 3 days, abdominal cramping, and straining to pass stools* (signs and symptoms).

Sometimes the cause is explained in more depth using the term *secondary to,* as in *decreased fluid intake secondary to nausea.* Different types of diagnoses also have different prefixes or stems. Table 3-3 lists examples related to the type of nursing diagnosis.

Actual diagnoses identify existing problems, such as Constipation or Anxiety. **Risk diagnoses** identify potential problems and use the stem *risk for,* as in Risk for Impaired Skin Integrity related to inactivity. **Possible diagnoses** use the stem *possible* to indicate uncertainty, as in Possible Sexual Dysfunction. Potential and possible diagnoses do not include the third part of the statement, the data, because the data are undeveloped or incomplete. Sometimes the cause of a possible diagnosis may be unknown; in such cases, the nurse can omit the second part of the statement as well. **Collaborative problems** denote complications with a physiologic origin. Nurses monitor the client to detect physiologic changes or the onset of physiologic problems. "Nurses manage collaborative problems using physician-prescribed interventions and

TABLE 3-1	COMPARISON OF THE ROLE OF LICENSED PRACTICAL/VOCATIONAL NURSE (LPN/LVN) AND REGISTERED NURSE (RN) IN THE NURSING PROCESS	
NURSING PROCESS PHASE	**ROLE OF LPN/LVN**	**ROLE OF RN**
Assessment	Gathers data, performs assessment, identifies client's strengths	Gathers more extensive biopsychosocial data, groups and analyzes data, researches additional data needed, identifies client resources
Nursing diagnosis	Not applicable	Draws conclusions, uses judgment, makes diagnosis
Planning	Contributes to development of care plans	Establishes priorities, sets short- and long-term client outcomes, collaborates and refers
Implementation	Provides basic therapeutic and preventive nursing measures, provides client education, records information	Manages client care (performs and delegates), provides client and family teaching, provides referrals, records and exchanges information with health-care team
Evaluation	Evaluates effects of care given	Evaluates effectiveness of overall plan, analyzes new data, modifies and redesigns plan, collaborates with health team members

Adapted from Harrington, N., Smith, N. E., & Spratt, W. E. (1996). *LPN to RN transitions.* Philadelphia: Lippincott-Raven.

nursing-prescribed interventions to minimize the complications of the events" (Carpenito, 1999, p.7). Collaborative problems begin with the stem *potential complication* (abbreviated PC), as in PC: Pulmonary Embolism. Nurses do not include related factors and supporting data when writing collaborative problems. **Wellness diagnoses** begin with the stem *potential for enhanced* and do not include related factors or supporting data. An example of a wellness diagnosis is Potential for Enhanced Family Coping. **Syndrome diagnoses** identify a diagnosis associated with a cluster of other diagnoses. NANDA identifies five syndrome diagnoses: Disuse Syndrome, Impaired Environmental Interpretation Syndrome, Post-trauma Syndrome, Rape Trauma Syndrome, and Relocation Stress Syndrome. (Refer to Table 3-2 for an example of Disuse Syndrome.)

TABLE 3-2	TYPES AND EXAMPLES OF NURSING DIAGNOSES
TYPE	**EXPLANATION AND EXAMPLE**
Actual diagnosis	A problem that already exists *Feeding Self-Care Deficit related to right hemiparesis as manifested by inability to grasp utensils*
Risk diagnosis	A problem that the client is at high risk for developing *Risk for Disturbed Sleep Pattern related to changed environment (intensive care unit)*
Possible diagnosis	A problem that is suspected but more data are needed before making a decision *Possible Parental Role Conflict related to impending divorce*
Collaborative problem	A problem that is monitored and managed by the nurse using physician-prescribed and nursing-prescribed interventions *Potential Complication (PC): Phlebitis*
Wellness diagnosis	No problem exists; the client desires a higher level of wellness *Potential for Enhanced Physical Fitness**
Syndrome diagnosis	Used when the diagnosis is associated with a cluster of other diagnoses *Disuse Syndrome: Impaired Physical Mobility, Risk for Constipation, Risk for Ineffective Breathing Pattern, Risk for Infection, Risk for Activity Intolerance, Risk for Injury, Risk for Disturbed Thought Processes, Risk for Disturbed Body Image, Risk for Powerlessness, Risk for Impaired Tissue Integrity*

*Not an approved NANDA diagnosis.

TABLE 3-3	NURSING DIAGNOSTIC STATEMENTS
TYPE OF DIAGNOSIS	**DIAGNOSTIC STATEMENT**
Actual	Impaired Verbal Communication related to hearing deficit as evidenced by inability to hear or read lips
Risk	Risk for Impaired Skin Integrity related to prescribed bed rest and decreased sensation and mobility of the lower extremities
Possible	Possible Ineffective Airway Clearance related to excessive mucus
Collaborative problem	PC: Pneumothorax
Wellness	Readiness for Enhanced Spiritual Well-Being
Syndrome	Disuse Syndrome

Planning

The third step of the nursing process is planning. **Planning** involves several steps: setting priorities, defining expected (desired) outcomes (goals), determining specific nursing interventions, and recording the plan of care. Respecting the client's right to participate in her or his healthcare is an important ethical principle. An actively involved client is more committed to carrying out the plan and achieving the outcomes. Thus, the nurse ensures that the client and family participate in care planning as much as possible. The nurse consults with the client about specific activities that are equally effective in achieving the outcomes.

For example, a woman client has a nursing diagnosis of Imbalanced Nutrition: Less than Body Requirements related to poor appetite and medication side effects as manifested by an intake of less than 1000 calories per day and weight loss of 3 kg in 10 days. When planning care for this client, the nurse must talk with her about the importance of increased caloric intake and ways to accomplish it, including types of foods, frequency of meals, and timing of medications. If the nurse simply decides to add certain high-calorie foods to the client's food tray, it is highly possible that the client will reject the foods because she may not like them.

Establishing Priorities

The nurse prioritizes the client's multiple problems by ranking first the diagnoses that are related to the client's most important, serious, or immediate needs, followed by the remainder in descending order of importance. A framework that nurses frequently use when prioritizing client problems is the hierarchy of human needs developed by Abraham Maslow (1968). Maslow proposed five levels of needs that motivate human behavior and grouped them as follows, according to their significance:

- Physiologic needs (first level)
- Safety and security needs (second level)
- Love and belonging needs (third level)
- Esteem and self-esteem needs (fourth level)
- Self-actualization needs (fifth level)

The first-level needs, sometimes called *baseline survival needs,* have the highest priority. These activities, such as eating, breathing, and drinking, sustain life. Maslow believed humans could not or would not seek to fulfill higher-level needs until physiologic needs were satisfied. Thus, nurses must rank any problem that poses a threat to physiologic functioning first. For example, nursing diagnoses such as Ineffective Breathing Pattern and Deficient Fluid Volume demand the nurse's attention more than other diagnoses because these conditions may be life-threatening.

Nursing diagnoses such as Anxiety or Risk for Injury address second-level needs of safety and security. Parental Role Conflict and Social Isolation are examples of nursing diagnoses that apply to the third level of love and belonging needs. Examples of nursing diagnoses that affect the fourth level of esteem and self-esteem needs are Powerlessness and Ineffective Coping. Delayed Growth and Development and Spiritual Distress are examples of nursing diagnoses that interfere with an individual's ability to achieve fifth-level, self-actualization needs.

Defining Expected Outcomes

Defining **expected outcomes** is an important part of the care planning process. The nurse includes the client and family in establishing outcomes. Outcomes are specific and realistic, so the client can attain them and not become frustrated, and measurable so the nurse can reliably determine to what extent the client is meeting the goals.

The nurse determines client-centered outcomes from the nursing diagnoses, so that the focus is on the treatments and results, as opposed to what the nurse hopes to achieve. For example, a nurse may desire the outcome that the client understands everything the nurse teaches. Instead, the outcome needs to focus on the essential care techniques for the client to master before leaving the healthcare facility. Thus, an appropriate outcome in this scenario would be "Before discharge, the client will demonstrate clean technique when changing the dressing on his left calf wound."

Specifically, outcomes are as follows:

- Derived from nursing diagnoses
- Documented as measurable goals
- Developed with the client and family and other healthcare providers when possible
- Realistic in relation to the client's present and potential capabilities
- Achievable in relation to the client's available resources
- Written to include:
  - Time estimate for achievement
  - Direction for continuity of care (Alfaro-LeFevre, 1998)

When writing expected outcomes, the nurse should relate them directly to the nursing diagnoses and make them clear and specific. For example, if the nursing diagnosis is "Acute Pain related to left knee replacement surgery, movement, and physical therapy," an expected outcome is that "the client will experience minimal pain throughout hospitalization." Table 3-4 provides examples of client-centered outcomes for each type of nursing diagnosis.

In some settings, it may be necessary to identify short-term outcomes and long-term outcomes. For example, in a rehabilitation center, clients may be involved in therapy for weeks or months. The expected outcomes need to reflect this length of treatment. In this situation, a short-term outcome is "the client will ambulate 20 feet on the first postoperative day," whereas a long-term outcome is "the client will ambulate with a walker by the end of 3 weeks."

Determining Specific Interventions

The plan of care identifies **interventions** or actions for achieving the outcomes. Relieving the cause of the prob-lem directs the interventions. If the cause cannot be fixed, such as in permanent injury, reducing the consequences of the problem itself becomes the focus for the interventions.

For example, if a client has the nursing diagnosis of Impaired Skin Integrity related to the effects of pressure secondary to decreased mobility as manifested by a 2-cm ulcer on the right heel, the nurse needs to identify measures directed at relieving pressure and its effects (decreased circulation). Such interventions would include elevating the heel off the bed to relieve pressure and having the client do ankle-pumping exercises to increase blood flow to the area. If the diagnosis is Feeding Self-Care Deficit related to right hemiparesis (paralysis affecting one side of the body) secondary to stroke as manifested by inability to grasp utensils, the nurse may provide utensils with large rubber grips as a means to decrease the effects of the problem.

Recording the Plan of Care

Once the RN determines the interventions, he or she writes the interventions in the written plan as nursing orders. **Nursing orders** are specific nursing directions so that all healthcare team members understand exactly what to do for the client (Box 3-1). Different people are likely to interpret a vague nursing order such as "Encourage fluids" differently, resulting in inconsistent care. In such cases, if outcomes are not met, determining whether the nursing measures themselves were ineffective or whether they were carried out ineffectively becomes difficult. A more appropriate nursing order would be "Give the client 100 mL of juice, water, tea, or milk every hour while awake." The interventions in the nursing care plan also must be compatible with the medical orders. For instance, if the physician has prescribed complete bed rest, a nursing order for ambulation conflicts with it.

TABLE 3-4	EXAMPLES OF EXPECTED OUTCOMES DERIVED FROM NURSING DIAGNOSES
NURSING DIAGNOSIS	**EXPECTED OUTCOME**
Ineffective Airway Clearance related to excessive secretions secondary to inflammation	The client will demonstrate optimal positioning to facilitate drainage of secretions on day of admission.
Risk for Deficient Fluid Volume related to nausea and vomiting and increased loss of fluids and electrolytes from gastrointestinal tract	The client will maintain fluid balance as evidenced by total intake greater than or equal to 2500 mL with output equal to intake or differing from intake by no more than 500 mL.
Possible Constipation	The client will have soft bowel movements as evidenced by client report.
PC: Congestive Heart Failure	The nurse will monitor the client for shortness of breath, dyspnea on exertion, and orthopnea.
Disuse Syndrome: Impaired Physical Mobility related to mechanical immobilization	The client will demonstrate ability to turn with assistance, maintaining restrictions, by second postoperative day.

> ### BOX 3-1 ● Characteristics of Nursing Interventions and Orders
>
> Nursing interventions and orders are:
> - Directed at preventing or minimizing the underlying causes of a problem
> - Directed at minimizing problems when the cause cannot be changed
> - Compatible with medical orders and other therapies
> - Compatible with professional and facility standards of care
> - Specific and outline what, how, when, how often, and how much
> - Safe
> - Individualized
> - Supported by scientific rationales

Many agencies have preprinted or computer-generated care plans that help identify nursing interventions for specific nursing or medical diagnoses. They save time by providing general suggestions for common conditions. The nurse selects appropriate interventions from the list, makes the orders specific for the individual client, and eliminates whatever is unnecessary.

A complete plan of care provides a means to communicate to all shifts of nursing personnel. This communication establishes a basis for continuity of care.

Implementation

As the fourth step of the nursing process, **implementation** means carrying out the written plan of care, performing the interventions, monitoring the client's status, and assessing and reassessing the client before, during, and after treatments. Carrying out the plan involves the client and one or more members of the healthcare team. It also may include the client's family and the community. It requires that the nurse not only acts but also thinks before acting. For example, the nurse looks for any changes in the client's condition, reviews the client's responses to changes or care, and determines if changes need to be made in the plan of care.

An important element of implementation is documentation. Accurate and thorough **documentation** in the medical record serves five functions:

1. Communicates care
2. Shows trends and patterns in client status
3. Creates a legal document
4. Supplies validation for reimbursement
5. Provides a foundation for evaluation, research, and quality improvement (Alfaro-LeFevre, 1998)

By law, nurses must document all nursing actions, observations, and client responses in a permanent record. This record of nursing actions should be a mirror image of the written plan. Appropriate documentation is essential in maintaining communication among members of the healthcare team and ensuring that nurses monitor the client's progress.

Evaluation

Evaluation, the fifth step of the nursing process, is assessment and review of the quality and suitability of care given and the client's responses to that care (Box 3-2). During evaluation, nurses compare the actual outcomes to the expected outcomes. This process enables the nurse to revise the expected outcomes or select alternative plans of action when expected outcomes are not met. The nurse may reach one of several conclusions during evaluation:

1. The outcome is achieved, the problem is solved, and the nursing orders are discontinued.
2. The outcome is not met, but progress is being made and the plan of care is continued or revised with minor changes.
3. The outcome is not achieved, and the plan requires critical re-evaluation and major revision.

A client's lack of progress may result from unrealistic expectations, incorrect diagnosis of the original problem, development of additional problems, ineffective nursing measures, or a premature target date. Once nurses identify the deficiency in the plan, they may implement a revision.

THE NURSING PROCESS AND CRITICAL THINKING

Critical thinking is intentional, contemplative, and outcome-directed thinking. In nursing, critical thinking:

- Involves purposeful, outcome-directed thinking
- Considers client, family, and community needs
- Is based on principles of nursing process and scientific method
- Requires knowledge, skills, and experience
- Is guided by professional standards and codes of ethics
- Makes judgments based on evidence rather than conjecture
- Involves constant re-evaluation, revision, and striving for improvement
- Requires strategies that maximize human potential (using individual strengths) and compensate for problems (Alfaro-LeFevre, 1998, 1999)

When caring for clients, nurses continually assess their clients' needs and frequently confront situations that

> ### BOX 3-2 ● Evaluating Care
>
> Evaluation includes the following components:
> - Determining if expected outcomes have been met
> - Identifying factors that interfered with achieving expected outcomes
> - Deciding whether to continue, modify, or discontinue the plan

require multiple interventions. Developing good critical thinking skills will make nurses more efficient and effective at resolving these situations. This careful, deliberate, outcome-directed thinking has predictable features that nurses can practice and learn. One key feature is the ability to maintain a questioning attitude. "Why is this occurring?," "Do I have all the information I need?," and "What does this mean?" are examples of questions that critical thinkers ask themselves (Alfaro-LeFevre, 1998). Box 3-3 outlines other characteristics of critical thinkers.

The use of the nursing process in nursing combines critical thinking with problem-solving methods. Nurses identify client problems and develop and implement plans of care with a logical, purposeful, and outcome-based method. The nursing process assists nurses to acquire critical thinking and problem-solving skills, because it entails scientific problem-solving in a systematic, client-centered, outcome-based way. It also is a dynamic continuous process.

Nurses must use specific cognitive and mental activities when thinking critically:

- Ask questions to determine why a situation occurred and if more information is needed.
- Gather relevant information to consider all factors.
- Validate information for accuracy, ensuring that it is not just supposition or opinion—it needs to be factual and based on evidence.
- Analyze information to determine what it means—does it form patterns that lead to specific conclusions?
- Use past clinical experience and knowledge to explain what is happening and to anticipate what may occur.
- Acknowledge personal bias and cultural influences.
- Maintain a flexible attitude so that facts guide thinking.
- Consider all possibilities.
- Determine all possible options, considering the advantages and disadvantages of each.
- Make decisions that are creative and show independent decision-making (Smeltzer & Bare, 2000).

BOX 3-3 ● **Characteristics of Critical Thinkers**

Critical thinkers are:

- Aware of their strengths and capabilities (show confidence)
- Aware of their own limitations (know when to ask for help)
- Open minded (listen to new ideas and other viewpoints)
- Humble (do not have to know everything all the time)
- Creative (look for ways to improve performance)
- Proactive (anticipate problems and prevent them)
- Flexible (can modify priorities and adapt to change)
- Aware that mistakes lead to new knowledge (learn from errors)
- Willing to persevere (accept that answers may not come easily)
- Aware that the world is not ideal (realize that the best solution may not be perfect)
- Logical thinkers (establish facts, determine what is relevant, search for cause and effect, avoid jumping to conclusions)
- Able to weigh advantages and disadvantages before making decisions (foresee probable outcomes)

Nurses use critical thinking skills in all practice settings. Each client presents with unique and dynamic issues. The nurse considers all factors and interprets the information to focus on the most needed elements and make decisions relevant to the individual client's care. Developing critical thinking skills requires knowledge, practice, and experience. This text presents critical thinking exercises at the end of each chapter, as well as "Stop, Think, and Respond" situations in many chapters. These exercises encourage the reader to begin the process of critical analysis and interpretation, as well providing a foundation for critical decision-making.

Stop, Think, and Respond ● **BOX 3-1**

A do not resuscitate (DNR) order was just added to a terminally ill client's plan of care. Using critical thinking skills, what must the nurse consider when adapting the nursing care plan? What types of nursing diagnoses should the nurse consider adding to the care plan?

---

*Sample Nursing Care Plan 3-1**

POSTOPERATIVE ABDOMINAL SURGERY CARE

Assessment

- Check the client's abdominal dressing.
- Assess the Hemovac drain.
- Check the nasogastric tube.
- Assess the Foley catheter.
- Review the intravenous (IV) infusion rate.

(continued)

Sample Nursing Care Plan 3-1 (Continued)*

POSTOPERATIVE ABDOMINAL SURGERY CARE

■ Assess the patient-controlled analgesia (PCA).

■ Evaluate the IV insertion site.

■ Take the client's vital signs.

■ Determine the client's ability to ambulate.

■ Assess the client's level of consciousness.

■ Assess the client's pain.

Nursing Diagnosis: **Risk for Ineffective Airway Clearance** related to depressed respiratory function, pain, and bed rest

Expected Outcomes: Client maintains a patent airway at all times.

Client's breath sounds remain clear.

Interventions	*Rationales*
Monitor breath sounds at least every 4 hours for 48 hours.	Breath sounds with crackles and wheezes indicate retained secretions.
Instruct client to deep breathe and cough every 2 hours.	Lung expansion prevents atelectasis and keeps secretions cleared.
Turn client at least every 2 hours.	Movement promotes lung expansion and movement of secretions.

Evaluation of Expected Outcomes:

■ Client's respirations are unlabored and regular.

■ Client's bilateral breath sounds are clear.

■ Client performs deep breathing and coughing exercises with coaching.

■ Client turns every 2 hours with maximum assistance.

Collaborative Problem: **PC: Wound Infection**

Expected Outcome: The nurse will minimize the client's potential for a wound infection.

Interventions	*Rationales*
Observe incision for signs and symptoms of infection.	Redness, warmth, fever, or swelling indicates a wound infection.
Monitor wound drainage, dressing, and Hemovac drain.	Changes in wound drainage from serosanguinous to purulent indicate a wound infection.
Maintain sterile technique for dressing changes.	Sterile technique reduces potential for development of infection.

Evaluation of Expected Outcomes

■ Incision remains free of redness, warmth, and swelling.

■ Drainage is decreased and serosanguinous.

■ The nurse changes the dressing every 8 hours, with scant serosanguinous drainage on old dressings.

---

*Sample care plan only. See more complete care plan for postoperative clients in Chapter 25.

Critical Thinking Exercises

1. *List several reasons why including clients in care planning is important.*
2. *Explain the importance of the five steps of the nursing process. Give examples of what problems might arise if the nurse skips steps.*
3. *Think of a client problem and a personal problem you encountered recently, and refer to the characteristics of critical thinkers to determine which characteristics you demonstrated. Apply the other characteristics to the problems, and discuss how the outcomes might have been different.*

References and Suggested Readings

Alfaro-LeFevre, R. (1998). *Applying nursing diagnosis and nursing process: A step-by-step guide* (4th ed.). Philadelphia: Lippincott Williams & Wilkins.

Alfaro-LeFevre, R. (1999). *Critical thinking in nursing: A practical approach* (2nd ed.). Philadelphia: W. B. Saunders Company.

Carpenito, L. J. (1999). *Nursing care plans and documentation: Nursing diagnoses and collaborative problems* (3rd ed.). Philadelphia: Lippincott Williams & Wilkins.

Lunney, M. (2000). *Critical thinking and nursing diagnoses: Case studies and analyses.* Philadelphia: North American Nursing Diagnosis Association.

Maslow, A. (1968). *Toward a psychology of being* (2nd ed.). New York: Von Nostrand.

North American Nursing Diagnosis Association. (2001). *Nursing diagnoses: Definitions and classifications 2001–2002.* Philadelphia: Author

Powers, P. H., Goldstein, C., Plank, G., et al. (2000). The value of patient- and family-centered care. *American Journal of Nursing, 100*(5), 84–86, 88.

Rosdahl, C. B. (1999). *Textbook of basic nursing* (7th ed.). Philadelphia: Lippincott Williams & Wilkins.

Rubenfield, M. G. & Scheffer, B. K. (1999). *Critical thinking in nursing: An interactive approach* (2nd ed.). Philadelphia: Lippincott Williams & Wilkins.

Smeltzer, S. C. & Bare, B. G. (2000). *Brunner & Suddarth's textbook of medical–surgical nursing* (9th ed.). Philadelphia: Lippincott Williams & Wilkins.

Interviewing and Physical Assessment

Words to Know

auscultation
chief complaint
closed questions
cultural history
focus assessment
functional assessment
head-to-toe method
inspection
objective data
open-ended questions

palpation
past health history
percussion
physical assessment
psychosocial history
signs
subjective data
symptoms
systems method

Learning Objectives

On completion of this chapter, the reader will:

- Explain the purpose of the interview and the physical assessment.
- Define subjective data, objective data, symptoms, and signs.
- Summarize the three phases of the interview process.
- Explain the components of an interview.
- Differentiate a systems method of assessment from a head-to-toe method of assessment.
- Identify four assessment techniques.
- Describe general assessment measures that all nurses can perform.

Assessment is the process of gathering information about a client's health (see Chap. 3). Through systematic assessment, the nurse identifies the client's:

- Current and past health status
- Current and past functional status
- Coping patterns
- Health beliefs and relevant cultural practices
- Risks for potential health problems
- Responses to care
- Nursing care needs
- Referral needs

Assessment includes obtaining a health history and doing a physical examination. The nurse first assesses the client when he or she is admitted to the healthcare system. Findings from this comprehensive initial assessment establish a database that gives all team members relevant client information and becomes a yardstick for measuring effectiveness of care. The initial assessment consists of two parts: the interview and the physical examination.

Nurses gather subjective data during the interview and objective data during the physical assessment. **Subjective data** are statements the client makes about what he or she feels. When the client tells the nurse about nau-

sea, pain, fear, bloating, or other feelings of discomfort, he or she is providing subjective data. These feelings of discomfort are called **symptoms.**

Objective data are facts obtained through observation, physical examination, and diagnostic testing. When the nurse assesses blood pressure or heart rate or examines results from urinalysis, he or she obtains objective data. When objective data are abnormal, they are called **signs.** Objective data often support the subjective data.

THE INTERVIEW PROCESS

The length of the interview depends on variables such as the severity of the client's condition, level of discomfort, ability to cooperate, age, and mental state. The interview process is divided into three parts: the preinterview period, the interview, and the postinterview period (Box 4-1).

Preinterview Period

The preinterview period determines the direction of the interview process. The nurse should start by establishing rapport with the client and family members and ensuring that the client is comfortable. Putting the client physically and emotionally at ease facilitates the exchange of information and helps to establish a bond between the client and the nurse. When making introductions, the nurse should address the client by his or her surname. A private setting for the interview is essential to eliminate interruptions and maintain the client's confidentiality (Fig. 4-1). The nurse should explain that the information obtained during the interview helps with planning care. He or she should tell the client that all information is kept confidential, although all members of the healthcare team share the data.

Stop, Think, and Respond ● BOX 4-1

Describe approaches you would use in the pre-interview period for a client who is hearing or vision impaired.

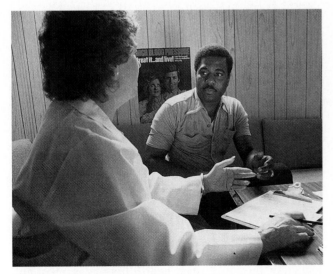

FIGURE 4-1 The nurse should provide a relaxed and private atmosphere when conducting an interview. (From Smeltzer, S. C. & Bare, B. G. [2000]. *Brunner & Suddarth's textbook of medical–surgical nursing* [9th ed.]. Philadelphia: Lippincott Williams & Wilkins.)

The Interview

The components of the interview include the following (Box 4-2):

1. The psychosocial and cultural history
2. The **chief complaint** or the reasons that the client is seeking care at this time
3. Functional status—self-care ability
4. A history of the present illness
5. The past health history
6. The family history
7. A review of body systems

Following a specific pattern when conducting an interview is unnecessary. The examiner can rearrange the order in which topics are discussed, digress from an established format if additional information seems pertinent, or omit areas that are not applicable. Many institutions have assessment forms that help ensure that the database is complete.

The nurse should avoid using medical terms. He or she should ask **open-ended questions** that require discussion rather than **closed questions** that require only "yes" or "no" answers. Giving the client ample time to answer each question and maintaining frequent eye contact are important measures. Reading and writing by the client should be minimized as much as possible. If the nurse asks the client to complete the assessment form, he or she should clarify information that the client gives during the interview.

Psychosocial and Cultural History

The **psychosocial history** and **cultural history** include the client's age, occupation, religious affiliation, cultural background and health beliefs (see Chap. 11), marital status, and home and working environments. Although some of this material is found on the face sheet of the client's chart, specific aspects may need further exploration. If, for example, the client is a factory worker, the examiner would ask if the client works around hazardous chemicals or has had job-related injuries.

Chief Complaint

The primary purpose of the interview is to discover what the client perceives as the health problem that needs treatment. Recording the information in the client's own words is best. For example, "I had a terrible pain in the right side of my stomach after I ate. I never had it so bad. The doctor said maybe it's my gallbladder."

Functional Assessment

A **functional assessment** is a determination of how well the client can manage activities of daily living (ADLs). ADLs include self-care activities such as walking moderate distances, bathing, and toileting, and instrumental

BOX 4-2 ● Interview Guide

The interviewer establishes a database by asking the client questions about his or her health.

PSYCHOSOCIAL AND CULTURAL HISTORY

Age; gender; marital status; number of children; occupation; highest level of education; religious affiliation; place of residence; country of origin; primary language; military service; date, location, and length of foreign travel or residence

CHIEF COMPLAINT

Reason for seeking care; type, location, and severity of symptoms

FUNCTIONAL ASSESSMENT

Ability to walk, get in and out of bed, bathe, dress, eat, and get to and from the bathroom; ability to drive, take public transportation, get groceries, or prepare meals

HISTORY OF PRESENT ILLNESS

Chronologic description of the onset, frequency, and duration of current symptoms; attempts and outcomes of self-treatment; what the client thinks caused the problem; how the illness affects the client's life at home, at work, and socially

PAST HEALTH HISTORY

Childhood diseases, physical injuries, major illnesses, previous medical or psychiatric hospitalizations, surgical procedures, drug history, use of alcohol and tobacco, allergy history

FAMILY HISTORY

Health problems among relatives living and deceased, longevity and cause of death among deceased blood relatives

REVIEW OF SYSTEMS

General. Usual weight, recent weight change, weakness, fatigue, fever
Skin. Rashes, lumps, sores, itching, dryness, color change, changes in hair or nails
Head. Headache, head injury
Eyes. Vision, glasses or contact lenses, last eye examination, pain, redness, excessive tearing, double vision, blurred vision, spots, specks, flashing lights, glaucoma, cataracts
Ears. Hearing, tinnitus, vertigo, earaches, infection, discharge, use of hearing aids
Nose and sinuses. Frequent colds; nasal stuffiness, discharge, or itching; hay fever; nosebleeds; sinus trouble
Mouth and throat. Condition of teeth and gums; bleeding gums; dentures, if any, and how they fit; last dental examination; sore tongue; dry mouth; frequent sore throats; hoarseness
Neck. Lumps; "swollen glands," goiter, pain or stiffness in the neck

Breasts. Lumps, pain or discomfort, nipple discharge, self-examination
Respiratory. Cough; sputum (color, quantity); hemoptysis, wheezing, asthma, bronchitis, emphysema, pneumonia, tuberculosis, pleurisy, last chest x-ray film
Cardiac. Heart trouble, high blood pressure, rheumatic fever, heart murmurs, chest pain or discomfort, palpitations, dyspnea, orthopnea, paroxysmal nocturnal dyspnea, edema, past electrocardiogram or other heart test results
Gastrointestinal. Trouble swallowing, heartburn, appetite, nausea, vomiting, regurgitation, vomiting of blood, indigestion, frequency of bowel movements, color and size of stools, change in bowel habits, rectal bleeding or black tarry stools, hemorrhoids, constipation, diarrhea, abdominal pain, food intolerance, excessive belching or passing of gas, jaundice, liver or gallbladder trouble, hepatitis
Urinary. Frequency of urination, polyuria, nocturia, burning or pain on urination, hematuria, urgency, reduced caliber or force of the urinary stream, hesitancy, dribbling, incontinence, urinary infections, stones
Genital. Male: Hernias, discharge from or sores on the penis, testicular pain or masses, history of sexually transmitted diseases and their treatments, sexual preference, interest, function, satisfaction, and problems. *Female:* Age at menarche; regularity, frequency, and duration of periods; amount of bleeding; bleeding between periods or after intercourse; last menstrual period; dysmenorrhea; premenstrual tension; age at menopause; menopausal symptoms; postmenopausal bleeding. If the client was born before 1971, exposure to diethylstilbestrol from maternal use during pregnancy. Discharge, itching, sores, lumps, sexually transmitted diseases and their treatments. Number of pregnancies, deliveries, or abortions (spontaneous and induced); complications of pregnancy; birth control methods. Sexual preference, interest, function, satisfaction; any problems, including dyspareunia (painful intercourse)
Peripheral vascular. Intermittent claudication, leg cramps, varicose veins, past history of blood clots in the veins
Musculoskeletal. Muscle or joint pains, stiffness, arthritis, gout, backache. If present, describe location and symptoms (e.g., swelling, redness, pain, tenderness, stiffness, weakness, limitation of motion or activity)
Neurologic. Fainting, blackouts, seizures, weakness, paralysis, numbness or loss of sensation, tingling or "pins and needles," tremors or other involuntary movements
Hematologic/immunologic. Anemia, easy bruising or bleeding, past transfusions and any reactions to them, status for human immunodeficiency virus infection autoimmune disorders
Endocrine. Thyroid trouble, heat or cold intolerance, excessive sweating, diabetes, excessive thirst or hunger, polyuria
Psychobiologic. Nervousness, tension, mood, memory

Adapted from Bickley, L. S., & Hoekelman, R. A. (2003). *Bates' guide to physical examination and history taking* (8th ed.). Philadelphia: Lippincott Williams & Wilkins.

---

activities such as preparing meals, obtaining transportation, and dialing the telephone. This assessment component is particularly important when assessing older adults or physically challenged clients of any age.

History of Present Illness

The nurse should ask the client to describe all present problems, including the onset, frequency, and duration of symptoms. Asking for more detailed information about one body system or problem is called a **focus assessment** because it adds depth to the original data. For example, a

client may reveal that he or she has experienced abdominal pain for the past several weeks. The questioning then addresses what causes the pain, how long the pain lasts, what the quality of the pain is, and what makes it better or worse.

Past Health History

Obtaining the client's **past health history** is important. This component includes identifying childhood diseases, previous injuries, major illnesses, prior hospitalizations, surgical procedures, and drug history. When discussing the client's past medical problems, the nurse should ask the age at which the problem was diagnosed, the treatment prescribed, and whether the problem still exists. Information about past surgeries includes the types, when each was done, and whether recoveries were uneventful or accompanied by complications.

The nurse identifies any current and past use of prescription and nonprescription drugs. He or she asks about the client's use of alcohol and tobacco because these drugs can create or contribute to other health problems.

The nurse compiles a list of the client's allergies, including sensitivities to drugs, foods, and environmental substances. If the client has a drug allergy, the drug and the client's reaction are described; some clients confuse a drug's side effects with an allergic response. If the client or family cannot remember the name of the drug, the nurse should try to identify it from another source, such as the prescribing physician or past hospital records.

Family History

The family history is important because many disorders are hereditary. The nurse asks if parents, siblings, and grandparents are living or dead. If any blood relatives in the immediate family have died, the nurse documents the causes of their deaths and the ages at which they died. He or she identifies health problems that affect other living relatives.

Review of Body Systems

The nurse asks general questions about each body system to trigger the client's memory of inadvertently overlooked health problems. For example, when reviewing the gastrointestinal system, the nurse should ask if the client has a history of nausea, vomiting, food intolerance, bowel irregularity, stomach ulcer, changes in the color of stool, and similar questions that suggest a current or past health problem. Asking an exhaustive number of questions for each system may be unnecessary, but the review should include a few questions about each system. If the client affirms that a problem exists, the nurse asks more focused questions until he or she has obtained all data about the problem.

Postinterview Period

An effective way of ending the interview is to summarize what occurred and thank the client for cooperating. Asking the client if he or she needs more information provides an opportunity for the client to express concerns and ask questions.

THE PHYSICAL EXAMINATION

The second part of the assessment process is the collection of objective data through a physical examination. During the **physical assessment,** the nurse examines body structures and observes the client's physical appearance, mood, mental status, behaviors, and ability to interact. The examination is conducted using one of two methods: the systems method of assessment or the head-to-toe method of assessment. The **systems method** approaches the examination by assessing each body system separately. See Box 4-3 for an overview of the systems approach to a complete physical examination. The **head-to-toe method** approaches the examination beginning at the top of the body and progressing downward. Sometimes, healthcare providers use parts of both methods.

Assessment Techniques

The nurse performs a physical assessment using four assessment techniques: inspection, palpation, percussion, and auscultation.

Inspection

Inspection is the systematic and thorough observation of the client and specific areas of the body (Fig. 4-2A). The nurse uses the senses of vision, smell, and hearing to inspect a client. Inspection includes examining the client for changes in skin color, temperature, or both; observing a wound for signs of healing or infection; or generally noting color, size, location, texture, symmetry, odors, and sounds. The technique of inspection includes the following measures:

- Expose the area being inspected while draping the rest of the client.
- Look before touching.
- Use adequate lighting.
- Provide a warm room for examination (Weber, 2001).

Palpation

Palpation is assessing the characteristics of an organ or body part by touching and feeling it with the hands or fingertips (see Fig. 4-2B). The process of palpation provides nurses with knowledge about texture, temperature, moisture, motion, and consistency or firmness of structures (solid vs. fluid). Palpation detects abnormal conditions, such as enlarged organs, tumors, or fluid in a cavity. When palpating, the nurse uses the fingertips to detect pulsations or to differentiate surfaces, the surface of the palm to sense vibrations, and the back of the hand to determine temperature. Techniques for palpation include using first light then deep palpation and palpating tender areas last (Weber, 2001).

Percussion

Percussion is tapping a portion of the body to determine if there is tenderness or to elicit sounds that vary accord-

BOX 4-3 ● Components of the Physical Examination

Using inspection, palpation, percussion, and auscultation, the examiner assesses and records findings about the following attributes, body functions, and systems:

GENERAL APPRAISAL

Physical appearance, age, overall physical development, hygiene, grooming, posture, mobility, use of ambulatory devices, weight, height, and vital signs

SKIN AND RELATED STRUCTURES

Color, moisture, temperature, texture, turgor, skin integrity, rash, edema (swelling caused by the collection of fluid in the tissues), warts, moles, petechiae (hemorrhagic spots on the skin), distribution of body hair, condition and shape of fingernails and toenails

HEAD

Shape and size of head; texture, color, and distribution of hair

EYES

External structures of the eyes (upper and lower lids, eyelashes, cornea, conjunctiva, sclera, iris, and pupil), pupil size and reaction to light, eye movement, anterior chambers of the eye, visual acuity

LIPS AND MOUTH

Condition of the teeth and gums, oral cavity and mucous membranes, oral pharynx, tonsils, uvula

EARS

External ear (the earlobe, auricle, and surrounding tissues), tympanic membrane, hearing

NECK

Lymph nodes, thyroid, position of trachea, carotid arteries, neck veins

THORAX AND LUNGS

Shape of the chest, expansion, axilla (armpits), breathing patterns, respiratory rate and depth, use of accessory muscles, breath sounds

BREASTS

Appearance, skin characteristics, nipples, presence of lumps or masses

CARDIOVASCULAR SYSTEM

Radial pulse rate; apical pulse rate; heart sounds; blood pressure measurement in both arms while standing, sitting, and lying down; pedal pulses

ABDOMEN

Bowel sounds, tenderness, pain, muscle resistance or rigidity, masses, scars, hernia, liver size, spleen, kidneys, abdominal aorta

RECTUM

Hemorrhoids, fissures, prostate gland in male clients, stool

GENITALIA

Male: penis, scrotum, inguinal lymph nodes. *Female:* external genitalia (labia, clitoris, urethral orifice, and vaginal opening), internal structures (vaginal wall and the cervix), inguinal lymph nodes

MUSCULOSKELETAL SYSTEM

Contour and size of joints, range of motion, muscle size and strength

NEUROLOGIC SYSTEM

Level of consciousness; orientation; intellectual functioning; emotional state; speech patterns; short-term and long-term memory, perception of pain, heat, cold, light touch, and vibration; gait; reflexes; cranial nerves; muscle strength; movement; coordination; tendon reflexes; proprioception (or position awareness)

---

ing to the density of underlying structures (see Fig. 4-2C). Table 4-1 provides a description of sounds that may be heard with percussion. The procedure for percussion is as follows:

1. Place the index or middle finger of the nondominant hand firmly on the surface to be percussed. Only the finger should have contact with the skin surface. Raise the other fingers and the heel of the hand off the surface.
2. Use quick, light, firm strikes with the tip of the middle finger of the dominant hand against the distal end of the nondominant finger. Use wrist motion to make the tapping movements—keep the forearm stable.
3. Deliver one to three taps, then move the nondominant finger to another area.

Auscultation

Auscultation means listening with a stethoscope for normal and abnormal sounds generated by organs and structures such as the heart, lungs, intestines, and major arteries (see Fig. 4-2D). When performing auscultation, nurses describe normal and abnormal sounds using descriptive terms such as *high-pitched, low-pitched, harsh,* *blowing, crackling, loud, distant,* and *soft.* They auscultate the lungs, heart, and abdomen.

Performing the Examination

In-depth physical examination requires practice and skill. Nurse practitioners or physicians perform some components of the physical examination. The extent of the examination performed by the licensed practical nurse or registered nurse depends on the nurse's skill, the client's condition, and facility practices. In any case, the nurse should give the client an examination gown or drape and maintain the client's privacy. He or she should ensure that there is adequate lighting in the examination area and gather all equipment, such as a penlight, stethoscope, and sphygmomanometer. Another important nursing measure is to maintain Standard Precautions (see Chap. 19).

Clients often feel anxiety, embarrassment, and fear when undergoing a physical examination. They are concerned about the findings and the implication of those findings for their future well-being. Explaining what will happen helps the client prepare for the examination and assists in obtaining the most valid information. The nurse should avoid showing surprise or concern at any findings to prevent increasing the client's anxiety level. At the

FIGURE 4-2 Assessment techniques. (**A**) Inspection, (**B**) palpation, (**C**) percussion, and (**D**) auscultation. (A from Taylor, C., Lillis, C., & LeMone, P. [2001]. *Fundamentals of nursing: The art and science of nursing care* [4th ed.]. Philadelphia: Lippincott Williams & Wilkins. B, C, and D from Smeltzer, S. C. & Bare, B. G. [2000]. *Brunner & Suddarth's textbook of medical–surgical nursing* [9th ed.]. Philadelphia: Lippincott Williams & Wilkins.)

TABLE 4-1	PERCUSSION SOUNDS		
PERCUSSION SOUNDS	**ORIGIN**	**SOUND**	**EXAMPLES**
Tympany	Enclosed air	Drumlike	Puffed-out cheek, air in bowel
Resonance	Part air and part solid tissue	Hollow	Normal lung
Hyperresonance	Mostly air	Booming	Lung with emphysema
Dullness	Mostly solid tissue	"Thud" sound	Liver, spleen, heart
Flatness	Very dense tissue	Flat	Muscle, bone

From Weber, J. R. (2001). *Nurses' handbook of health assessment* (4th ed, p. 41). Philadelphia: Lippincott Williams & Wilkins.

conclusion of the examination, the nurse should help the client dress and get in a comfortable position and ask if he or she has any questions. Finally, the nurse should inform the client and family that data will be shared with the physician.

 GENERAL GERONTOLOGIC CONSIDERATIONS

Avoid tiring the client—allow rest periods during the physical examination.
Keep the room warm and free from drafts.
Make sure the client has easy access to the rest room.
Allow time for the client to respond to directions and change position.
Use silence to allow more time for the client to respond to questions.
If possible, observe the client performing ADLs.
Provide sufficient space to accommodate wheelchairs and other devices (Weber, 2001).
Be certain that assistive sensory devices (e.g., glasses, hearing aids) are in place and functioning.
Data obtained from the interview may need to be validated with family or significant others involved in the client's care.

Critical Thinking Exercises

1. *How might you handle a situation in which a client's spouse answers questions asked of the client? Role-play a possible nurse–client scenario.*
2. *How might room temperature, lighting, lack of privacy, or limited time affect the assessment of a client?*

References and Suggested Readings

Bickley, L. S. & Hoekelman, R. A. (2003). *Bates' guide to physical examination and history taking* (8th ed.). Philadelphia: Lippincott Williams & Wilkins.

Burgener, S. C. (1999). Assessing patients in the early stages of irreversible dementia: The relevance of patient perspectives. *Journal of Gerontological Nursing, 25*(2), 33–41.

Hayes, K. S. (2000). Challenges in emergency care: The geriatric patient: Geriatric assessment in the emergency department. *Journal of Emergency Nursing, 26*(5), 430–435.

Weber, J. R. (2001). *Nurses' handbook of health assessment* (4th ed.). Philadelphia: Lippincott Williams & Wilkins.

Legal and Ethical Issues

Words to Know

administrative law
advance directives
advocacy
anecdotal record
board of nursing
civil law
common law
constitutional law
criminal law
deontology
duty
ethics
Good Samaritan laws
incident report
informed consent
intentional tort
laws

liability
living will
malpractice
medical durable power
   of attorney
negligence
nurse practice acts
rights
risk management
statute of limitations
statutory law
tort
tort law
unintentional torts
utilitarianism
values

Learning Objectives

On completion of this chapter, the reader will:

- Explain the differences between laws and ethics.
- Differentiate sources of U.S. law.
- Differentiate intentional and unintentional torts.
- Summarize negligence, malpractice, and liability.
- Explain the elements of risk management and other methods to avoid malpractice suits.
- Discuss informed consent, advance directives, and do not resuscitate orders.
- Interpret utilitarianism, deontology, duties, and rights.
- Summarize the characteristics of ethical values.
- Define six professional values.
- Describe factors that affect healthcare ethics.
- Explain an ethical decision-making model.

A system of laws and ethical beliefs help to establish and maintain order and harmony within a society. **Laws** are written rules for conduct and actions. They are binding for all citizens and ensure the protection of rights. **Ethics** are moral principles and values that guide the behavior of honorable people. Ethical standards dictate the rightness or wrongness of human behavior. Box 5-1 highlights the differences between laws and ethics.

The healthcare delivery system affects and is affected by societal beliefs, values, and laws. It is accountable to society for maintaining established legal and ethical standards. In turn, legal and ethical situations that healthcare personnel face also may become issues for society. Nurses today require a basic understanding of laws and ethics that may affect their practice. Issues related to competence, safety, optimal care, protecting clients' rights, and practicing according to professional standards of care are of most concern to nurses. This chapter provides an introduction to the legal and ethical dimensions of nursing practice.

LEGAL ISSUES IN NURSING PRACTICE

Federal and state legislation directly affects the healthcare industry. Laws and regulations that affect nursing practice and the safety of clients are essential for nurses to know.

Sources of Law

Laws stem from several sources. Types of law discussed in this section include constitutional, statutory, common, administrative, criminal, and civil law.

Constitutional Law

The constitution guarantees fundamental freedoms to all people in the United States. **Constitutional law** affects

BOX 5-1 ● Laws Versus Ethics

LAWS
Serve as rules of conduct
Guide actions and interactions within a society
Are regulated by authorized organizations and law officers

ETHICS
Deal with right and wrong
Consider beliefs about morals and values
Do not have a formal enforcement system

Adapted from Harrington, N., Smith, N. E., & Spratt, W. E. (1996). *LPN to RN transitions.* Philadelphia: Lippincott-Raven.

nurses in that it protects their basic rights, just as it protects the rights of clients. For example, freedom of speech and right to privacy are rights that nurses and clients have as citizens of the United States.

Statutory Law

Statutory law is law that any local, state, or federal legislative body enacts. These laws can significantly affect healthcare providers. For example, the "DRG law" described in Chapter 1 greatly influenced healthcare reimbursement and length of hospital stays. Another example of statutory law is the nurse practice act in each state.

NURSE PRACTICE ACT
Nurse practice acts define nursing practice and set standards for nurses in each state. These legal statutes regulate the practice of nursing to protect the health and safety of citizens. Although each state has its own nurse practice act, they all share common components:

- Define the scope of practice
- Establish requirements for licensure and entry into practice
- Create a board of nursing to oversee nursing practice
- Identify legal titles for nurses, such as *registered nurse* and *licensed practical nurse*
- Determine what constitutes grounds for disciplinary action

STATE BOARD OF NURSING
The primary responsibility of a state **board of nursing** is to protect the public. Other responsibilities include reviewing and approving nursing education programs in the state, forming criteria for granting licensure, overseeing procedures for licensure examinations, issuing or transferring licenses, and implementing disciplinary procedures.

Common Law

Common law, also known as *judicial law,* is based on earlier court decisions, judgments, and decrees. These earlier decisions set precedents for interpretation of laws.

Common law evolved when courts began to present written decisions based on prior court cases. Stated another way, if one court has previously decided on a particular case and another court reviews a similar case, the second court will make the same decision, citing the precedent of the previous case. The court will make new rules if the precedent is outdated.

Administrative Law

Statutory law empowers regulatory agencies to create and carry out the laws. These federal and regulatory agencies practice **administrative law,** which means they enforce the rules and regulations that concern the health, welfare, and safety of federal and state citizens. For example, the Occupational Safety and Health Administration (OSHA) is the federal agency that develops the rules and regulations that govern workplace safety. State statutory law forms nurse practice acts, but the authority to regulate that act is given to an administrative agency, usually called the State Board of Nursing.

Criminal Law

Criminal law concerns offenses that violate the public's welfare. A crime is a violation of criminal law. There are two categories of offenses: (1) misdemeanors, which are minor offenses; and (2) felonies, which are serious offenses. Misdemeanors involving healthcare workers are similar to those for all citizens (e.g., driving violations). Examples of felonies involving healthcare workers include falsification of medical records, insurance fraud, and theft of narcotics. If an individual misrepresents himself or herself as a licensed nurse, this person commits the crime of practicing without a license.

Civil Law

Civil law applies to disputes that arise between individual citizens. Civil laws protect each individual's personal freedoms and property rights. Some civil laws include the right to be left alone, freedom from threats of injury, freedom from offensive contact, and freedom from character attacks. The plaintiff is the individual who brings a dispute to the court; the complaint is the formal written dispute and the restitution that the plaintiff seeks. The individual or party against whom the complaint is filed is the defendant. **Liability** means legal responsibility. If a client receives the wrong medication and is harmed as a result, the nurse is liable, or held responsible, for that harm.

Although there are various branches of civil law, tort law is most likely to affect nurses. **Tort law** is the body of law that governs breaches of duty owed by one person to another. A **duty** is an expected action based on moral or legal obligations. A **tort** is an injury that occurred because of another person's intentional or unintentional actions, or failure to act. This injury can be physical, emotional, or financial. If the defendant is found to have breached his or her duty and that breach causes harm, he or she must pay restitution for damages. The types of torts that involve nurses are intentional and unintentional.

INTENTIONAL TORTS

An **intentional tort** is a deliberate and willful act that infringes on another person's rights or property. Examples of intentional torts include assault, battery, false imprisonment, invasion of privacy, and defamation.

Assault. Assault is an act that involves a threat or attempt to do bodily harm. Types of assault include physical intimidation, verbal remarks, or gestures that lead the client to believe that force or injury may be forthcoming. For example, a nurse is frustrated because a client constantly turns on the call light. The nurse threatens to restrain the client's hands if he or she continues this action. This verbal threat constitutes assault.

Battery. Battery is actual physical contact with another person without that person's consent. The contact can include touching a person's body, clothing, chair, or bed. A charge of battery can be made even if the contact did not cause physical harm to the individual. To protect healthcare workers from being charged with battery, clients sign a general permission for care and treatment at the time of admission (Fig. 5-1). They also sign a written consent before undergoing special tests, procedures, or surgery. A parent or guardian must provide consent if the client is a minor, mentally retarded, or mentally incompetent. In an emergency, healthcare providers can infer consent, meaning the law assumes that in life-threatening circumstances clients would provide consent.

Nonconsensual physical contact sometimes is justified. When mentally ill or intoxicated clients are endangering their own safety or the safety of others, health professionals may use physical force to subdue them. The nurse must clearly document that the situation required the degree of restraint used. Excessive force never is appropriate when less force would have been just as effective. When recording these incidents, the nurse must document the behavior that resulted in the use of force and the client's response when the nurse tried lesser forms of restraint first.

False Imprisonment. False imprisonment occurs when healthcare workers physically or chemically restrain an individual from leaving a healthcare institution. Mentally impaired, confused, or disoriented clients may be restrained if their safety or the safety of others is at risk. This confinement requires restraining orders, court-ordered commitments, or medical orders. A nurse, however, cannot detain a competent client who wishes to leave a hospital or long-term care facility before being discharged by the physician. If a client wishes to leave the facility against medical advice, he or she signs a form (Fig. 5-2) that releases the healthcare facility from responsibility.

The unnecessary or unprescribed application of physical or chemical restraints also creates potential liability for battery and false imprisonment. If the nurse must apply restraints and no current medical order exists, the best legal defense is to show just cause through accurate documentation. Because confined and restrained clients cannot protect themselves or meet their own needs, charting must show that the nurse assessed the client frequently, offered fluids and nourishment, and provided an opportunity for bowel and bladder elimination. It is expected that the restraints will be discontinued when the client no longer poses a threat to self or others.

Invasion of Privacy. The right to privacy means that persons have the right to expect that they and their property will be left alone. Failure to do so is an invasion of privacy. Nonmedical torts of this nature generally include trespassing, illegal search and seizure, or wiretapping. Invasion of privacy also applies to releasing private information about a person, regardless of whether the information is true.

Medical examples of invasion of privacy include photographing an individual without consent, revealing a client's name in a public report or research paper, and allowing unauthorized persons to observe a client during treatment or care. Health professionals protect a client's privacy by:

- Obtaining a signed release for recognizable photographs for publications or presentations
- Using initials or code numbers instead of names in written reports or research papers
- Closing bedside curtains when giving personal care
- Obtaining a client's permission for a nursing student or other healthcare person to be present as an observer during treatment

Defamation. Defamation is an act that harms a person's reputation and good name. If a person orally utters a character attack in the presence of others, the action is called *slander.* If the damaging statement is written and read by others, it is called *libel.* Nurses must avoid offering unfounded or exaggerated negative opinions about clients, the expertise of physicians, or other coworkers. Injury occurs because the derogatory remarks may mar a person's public image or keep potential clients from seeking the services of the defamed person. If a client accuses a nurse of defamation of character, the client must prove that there was malice, misuse of privileged information, and spoken or written untruths. Nurses are at risk for defamation of character suits if they make negative comments in public areas (elevators, cafeterias) or assert opinions regarding a client's character in the medical record.

UNINTENTIONAL TORTS

Unintentional torts involve situations that result in injuries, although the person responsible did not mean to cause any harm. Negligence is the principal form of

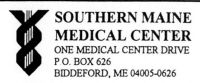

SOUTHERN MAINE
MEDICAL CENTER
ONE MEDICAL CENTER DRIVE
P.O. BOX 626
BIDDEFORD, ME 04005-0626

NOTICE
You are being admitted to SMMC as an inpatient.

CONSENT TO TREAT AND/OR ADMIT
When I sign this form, I agree to let SMMC treat me in the emergency department, or as an outpatient, or to admit and treat me as an inpatient at this hospital.

1. SMMC may examine me and perform tests and treatments to help learn about, and care for, my injury or illness.
2. This could mean emergency care or outpatient services with more visits.
3. It could also mean hospital care with a need for inpatient hospital services.

I know that inpatient hospital treatment may mean medications, tests, and nursing care. I agree to this.

I know I can stop all or part of my treatment at any time.

I know my consent is needed to have me take part in any experiments or research.

I know that medicine and surgery have risks. Some tests and treatments could cause harm even death. In some cases I may be asked to sign a separate consent form. SMMC has not told me that any test or treatment will guarantee a certain result.

I know that many staff doctors are not employed by SMMC, but may use the hospital as a place to care for their patients. Other doctors at SMMC may be in post-graduate training programs. Some other health care workers at SMMC may also not be employees of SMMC.

MEDICAL RECORDS RELEASE
I know that, under Maine law, SMMC may give parts of my medical record to those who pay for health care services, check for insurance claims or do medical reviews. SMMC may also release my medical record to other people who may be responsible for my further care. Only parts of my record that relate to these purposes may be released. Maine law also allows SMMC to share health care information about me with my family and household members, unless I instruct SMMC not to do so.

I know that Maine Worker's Compensation law gives my employer(s) and their agents the right to review my record if I may have an injury or illness covered by that law. I know also, that state and federal laws may provide additional protection against giving out information regarding HIV status, mental health services, or services received from an alcohol or drug abuse treatment program.

I know that Maine law gives me the right to decide whether certain health care information may be disclosed to others. I may tell SMMC if I wish to exercise this right. If I do, one of my choices is to have my name left out of the directory that lists people being cared for at SMMC. Leaving my name out of this directory may prevent SMMC from directing visitors and telephone calls to me.

ASSIGNMENT OF INTEREST AND FINANCIAL AGREEMENT
I know I must pay any charges not covered by insurance. I agree to have the payments of insurance and plan benefits (including Medicare) go directly to SMMC. If the payment is in keeping with the provisions of the insurance policy or plan, this will end the claim on the payor to the extent of the payment. If charges are denied, or are not covered by my insurance or plan, I must pay SMMC for these charges. If my account is referred for collection, I may be responsible for all fees required to collect it (including attorney's fees).

ADVANCE APPROVAL FOR MEDICAL SERVICES
If my insurance or health plan says I need an OK for a test or treatment before it is provided, SMMC will try to help me. SMMC cannot, however, promise to get this OK for me. If some services are denied later by my payor, I must pay the balance of my bill.

MEDICARE
_____ I have received a copy of the *Important Message from Medicare*.
(Initial)

_____   _____
Patient   Date

_____   _____   _____
Legal Representative   Relationship to Patient   Date

INPATIENT

_____
Witness

FIGURE 5-1 Consent for treatment.

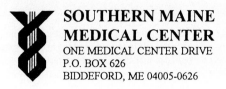

SOUTHERN MAINE MEDICAL CENTER
ONE MEDICAL CENTER DRIVE
P.O. BOX 626
BIDDEFORD, ME 04005-0626

LEAVING HOSPITAL AGAINST MEDICAL ADVICE

I certify that I am leaving the hospital voluntarily, against the advice and recommendation of the attending physician and the hospital. I acknowledge that I have been informed of the following risks and possible medical consequences involved:

_____

_____

_____

I release the attending physician, his associates or assistants, the hospital, and its personnel from any and all responsibility for any ill effects which may result from this action.

_____   _____
Witness   Patient Signature

_____   _____ A.M. / P.M.
Date   Time

* Because the above patient is an unemancipated minor, _____ years of age, or is unable to sign for the following reasons:

_____

_____

the above consent is given on the patient's behalf by:

_____   _____
Witness   Closest Relative or Legal Guardian

_____   _____ A.M. / P.M.   _____
Date   Time   Relationship

FIGURE 5-2 Release form for leaving against medical advice.

unintentional tort. Negligence involving licensed health-care workers is referred to as *malpractice.*

Negligence. Negligence describes the failure to act as a reasonable person would have acted in a similar situation. If harm results from the action (or failure to act),

a person may sue that individual for negligence. For example, a homeowner fails to repair a broken step or warn a visitor to be careful. The visitor falls and suffers an injury. The jury decides if another reasonable, prudent person would have repaired the step or warned the visitor to be careful.

Malpractice. The law defines **malpractice** as professional negligence. It refers to harm that results from a licensed person's actions or lack of action. A jury must determine if the responsible person's conduct deviated from the standard expected of others with similar education and experience. This type of tort holds healthcare workers to a higher standard than that used in negligence cases. Rather than being held accountable for acting as an ordinary, reasonable lay person, the court will determine if a nurse acted in a manner comparable with that of his or her peers. For example, if a client sustains a burn from warm soaks, the nurse who failed to check the water temperature could be found liable because he or she violated professional standards by not checking the temperature of the water before applying the soak to the skin. Published standards (Box 5-2), the testimony of expert witnesses, written agency policies and procedures, A Patient's Bill of Rights (Box 5-3), and standardized care plans are examples of documents that establish professional standards of care (Fig. 5-3). These help familiarize the jury with the scope of a nurse's practice.

Stop, Think, and Respond ● BOX 5-1

An elderly client refuses to take his medication for hypertension. The nurse informs him that if he does not take it, his blood pressure will skyrocket and he will have a stroke that may kill him or leave him severely disabled. The nurse also states that she may need to restrain the client so that he will take his medication as ordered.

Consider this nurse's actions. Is the nurse threatening the client or merely providing important information?

BOX 5-2 ● Standards of Care

STANDARD I. ASSESSMENT
The nurse collects client health data.

STANDARD II. DIAGNOSIS
The nurse analyzes the assessment data in determining diagnoses.

STANDARD III. OUTCOME IDENTIFICATION
The nurse identifies expected outcomes individualized to the client.

STANDARD IV. PLANNING
The nurse develops a plan of care that prescribes interventions to attain expected outcomes.

STANDARD V. IMPLEMENTATION
The nurse implements the interventions identified in the plan of care.

STANDARD VI. EVALUATION
The nurse evaluates the client's progress toward attainment of outcomes.

Reprinted with permission from Standards of Clinical Nursing Practice, 2nd ed. 1998. Washington, D.C.: American Nurses Association.

BOX 5-3 ● A Patient's Bill of Rights

1. The patient has the right to considerate and respectful care.
2. The patient has the right to and is encouraged to obtain from physicians and other direct caregivers relevant, current, and understandable information concerning diagnosis, treatment, and prognosis.
3. The patient has the right to make decisions about the plan of care prior to and during the course of treatment and to refuse a recommended treatment or plan of care to the extent permitted by law and hospital policy and to be informed of the medical consequences of this action.
4. The patient has the right to have an advance directive (such as a living will, health care proxy, or durable power of attorney for health care) concerning treatment or designating a surrogate decision maker with the expectation that the hospital will honor the intent of that directive to the extent permitted by law and hospital policy.
5. The patient has the right to every consideration of privacy. Case discussion, consultation, examination, and treatment should be conducted so as to protect each patient's privacy.
6. The patient has the right to expect that all communications and records pertaining to his/her care will be treated as confidential by the hospital, except in cases such as suspected abuse and public health hazards when reporting is permitted or required by law.
7. The patient has the right to review the records pertaining to his or her medical care and to have the information explained or interpreted as necessary, except when restricted by law.
8. The patient has the right to expect that, within its capacity and policies, a hospital will make reasonable response to the request of a patient for appropriate and medically indicated care and services. The hospital must provide evaluation, service, and/or referral as indicated by the urgency of the case.
9. The patient has the right to ask and be informed of the existence of business relationships among the hospital, educational institutions, other health care providers, or payers that may influence the patient's treatment and care.
10. The patient has the right to consent to or decline to participate in proposed research studies or human experimentation affecting care and treatment or requiring direct patient involvement, and to have those studies fully explained prior to consent.
11. The patient has the right to expect reasonable continuity of care when appropriate and to be informed by physicians and other caregivers of available and realistic patient care options when hospital care is no longer appropriate.
12. The patient has the right to be informed of hospital policies and practices that relate to patient care, treatment, and responsibilities.

American Hospital Association. (1992). [On-line.] Available: http://www.aha.org/resource/pbillofrights.asp.

Limiting Liability

Some measures protect nurses and other healthcare workers from litigation (lawsuits) or provide a foundation for legal defense. Good Samaritan laws, statutes of limitations, principles regarding assumption of risk, documentation, risk management, anecdotal records, and liability insurance can limit or reduce a nurse's liability.

Good Samaritan Laws

Many states have enacted **Good Samaritan laws,** which provide legal immunity for rescuers who provide first aid

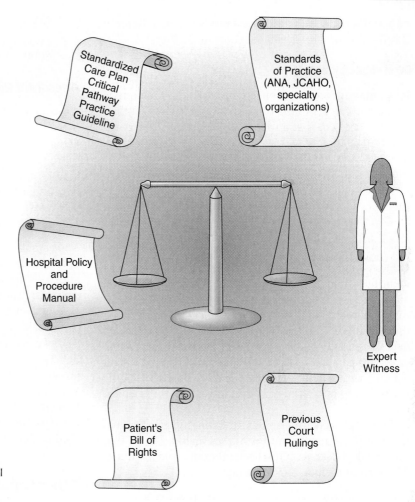

FIGURE 5-3 How the court establishes professional standards of care.

in an emergency to accident victims. The law defines an emergency as one occurring outside a hospital, not in an emergency department.

None of the Good Samaritan laws provides absolute exemption from prosecution in the event of an injury. The law still holds paramedics, emergency medical technicians, physicians, nurses, and other healthcare providers who stop to provide assistance to a higher standard of care because they have training above and beyond that of lay persons. In cases where there has been gross negligence (total disregard for another's safety), individuals may be charged with a criminal offense.

Statute of Limitations

Each state establishes statutes of limitations related to civil laws. A **statute of limitations** is the designated time in which a person can file a lawsuit. The time usually is calculated from when the incident occurred. When the injured party is a minor, however, the statute of limitations sometimes does not commence until the victim reaches adulthood. Once the period expires, an injured party can no longer sue.

Assumption of Risk

If a client is forewarned of a potential hazard to his or her safety and chooses to ignore the warning, the court may hold the client responsible. For example, if the client objects to having the side rails up or lowers the rails independently, the nurse or healthcare facility may not be held fully accountable if an injury occurs. It is essential that the nurse document that he or she warned the client and that the client disregarded the warning. The same recommendation applies when nurses caution clients about ambulating only with assistance.

Documentation

A major component in limiting liability is accurate, thorough documentation. Nurses are held responsible or liable for information that they either include or exclude in reports and documentation. Each healthcare setting requires accurate and complete documentation. The medical record is a legal document and is used as evidence in court. Records must be timely, objective, accurate, complete, and legible. The quality of the documentation, including neatness and spelling, can influence a jury's decision. Refer to Box 5-4 for rules for legally safe documentation.

Risk Management

Risk management, a concept developed by insurance companies, refers to the process of identifying and then reducing the costs of anticipated losses. Healthcare institutions that employ risk managers now use this term. The risk manager has responsibility for reviewing all the problems that occur at the workplace, identifying common elements, and then developing methods to reduce the risk of their occurrence.

One of the primary tools of risk management is the **incident report**. Healthcare workers complete incident reports when they make or discover errors, or when an event occurs that results in harm. The incident report identifies the nature of the incident (who, what, where, and when), witnesses, what actions were taken at the time, and the client's condition. The incident report is not intended to be a punitive tool but rather a means to collect data. It is factual and complete and does not include excuses for behaviors or actions. The nurse records the incident in the client's record, but does not refer to the incident report, because it is not part of the medical record.

Risk management also is a function of the individual nurse. Risk management for nurses includes steps that nurses take to reduce harm to clients and avoid litigation. These steps include the following:

- Complying with the state's nurse practice act
- Following institutional procedures and policies
- Acknowledging personal strengths and weaknesses
- Seeking means of growth, education, and supervised experiences
- Discussing issues or problems with colleagues
- Evaluating proposed assignments and refusing to accept responsibilities for which one is not prepared
- Keeping knowledge and skills up to date
- Respecting client rights and developing rapport with clients
- Documenting client care accurately and thoroughly

BOX 5-4 ● Rules for Legally Safe Documentation

- Chart promptly.
- Write legibly.
- Chart objectively, accurately, and concisely.
- Use only standard abbreviations.
- Do not leave vacant lines.
- Sign every entry.
- Keep charting free of criticism or complaints.
- Make no mention of an incident report.
- Do not destroy or attempt to obliterate documentation.
- Record the date of a return visit, cancellation, or missed appointments.
- Document all telephone conversations and follow-up instructions.

- Working within the institution to develop and support management policies (Taylor, Lillis, & LeMone, 2000)

Anecdotal Records

An **anecdotal record** is a handwritten, personal account of an incident made at the time of occurrence and updated as needed. Such records are not official but are useful in refreshing the nurse's memory. Anecdotal records may be used as evidence in court, particularly if testimony about the events that transpired is conflicting.

Liability Insurance

Today, all healthcare professionals need liability or malpractice insurance. Liability insurance provides funds for attorneys' fees and damages awarded in malpractice lawsuits. All healthcare institutions carry liability insurance, and some may insure their employees. Nurses also should carry their own personal malpractice insurance, however, so they have a separate attorney working on their sole behalf. Because the damages sought in malpractice lawsuits are so high, the attorneys hired by healthcare institutions sometimes are more committed to defending the institution rather than the nurse against liability. There also have been instances in which healthcare facilities have countersued negligent nurses for reimbursement of damages.

Other Legal Issues

Some legal issues and regulations affect client care. Two prominent issues are informed consent and advance directives. Another issue involves do not resuscitate orders.

Informed Consent

Informed consent is the voluntary permission granted by a client, or the client's assigned *medical proxy* (a person who legally may make medical decisions for a client), for medical staff to perform an invasive procedure or surgery on the client. The physician obtains the informed consent and must inform the client of the following:

- Description of treatment, procedure, or surgery proposed
- Potential benefits
- Material risk involved
- Acceptable alternatives available
- Expected outcome
- Consequences if treatment, procedure, or surgery is not done

Only competent adults may sign the informed consent form. If a person is not competent, a guardian or medical proxy may sign for the client. In an emergency, physicians may invoke implied consent if the client cannot sign but is at great risk if a procedure is not done. The physician

TO MY FAMILY, MY PHYSICIAN, MY LAWYER, MY CLERGYMAN
TO ANY MEDICAL FACILITY IN WHOSE CARE I HAPPEN TO BE
TO ANY INDIVIDUAL WHO MAY BECOME RESPONSIBLE FOR MY
HEALTH, WELFARE OR AFFAIRS

Death is as much a reality as birth, growth, maturity and old age—it is the
one certainty of life. If the time comes when I, _____
can no longer take part in decisions for my own future, let this statement
stand as an expression of my wishes, while I am still of sound mind.

If the situation should arise in which there is no reasonable expectation of
my recovery from physical or mental disability, I request that I be allowed to
die and not kept alive by artificial means or "heroic measures." I do not fear
death itself as much as the indignities of deterioration, dependence and
hopeless pain. I therefore, ask that medication be mercifully administered to
me to alleviate suffering even though this may hasten the moment of death.

This request is made after careful consideration. I hope you who care for me
will feel morally bound to follow its mandate. I recognize that this appears to
place a heavy responsibility upon you, but it is with the intention of relieving
you of such responsibility and of placing it upon myself in accordance with
my strong convictions, that this statement is made.

Signed _____

Date _____

Witness _____

Witness _____

Copies of this request have been given to _____
_____
_____
_____

FIGURE 5-4 A living will. (From Ellis, J. R., &
Hartley, C. L. [2001]. *Nursing in today's world:
Challenges, issues and trends* (7th ed.). Phila-
delphia: Lippincott Williams & Wilkins.)

documents these facts in the medical record, and in most
facilities another physician must verify the need for the
emergency procedure (Marquis & Huston, 1998).

Nurses may witness the client's signature on the consent form. The nurse must be certain that the client has
the necessary information before signing. If it appears
that the client is uncertain or lacks the appropriate information, the nurse must notify the physician. Sometimes the nurse just needs to clarify the information and
teach the client more about the procedure.

Advance Directives

The federal Patient Self-Determination Act of 1990 mandates that all federally funded healthcare facilities inform
clients of their right to have and prepare advance directives. The **advance directives** provide an opportunity for
clients to determine in advance their wishes regarding life-
sustaining treatment and other medical care, so that their
significant others will know what decisions clients desire.

The two types of advance directives are the living will and
medical durable power of attorney.

LIVING WILL

A **living will** is a document that states a client's wishes
regarding healthcare if he or she is terminally ill. It is specific about what the client will accept and not accept for
medical treatment if he or she is no longer competent or
able to make medical decisions. Figure 5-4 provides an example of a living will. The living will does not necessarily
mean legal consent, but it does indicate the client's wishes
(Ellis & Hartley, 2001).

MEDICAL DURABLE POWER OF ATTORNEY

A client may designate another person to be the **medical
durable power of attorney** or healthcare proxy. This
person has the authority to make healthcare decisions for
the client if he or she is no longer competent or able to
make these decisions. Although durable power of attorney

forms are available in office supply stores, it is desirable to consult a lawyer when making these arrangements. The document may simply name the appointed person, or it may also include the client's preferences for end-of-life care.

Do Not Resuscitate Orders

Legally, nurses cannot act on a patient's advance directive without a physician's order. Do not resuscitate (DNR) orders involve a written medical order for end-of-life instructions. If a DNR order is written, the client wishes to have no resuscitative action taken if he or she experiences a cardiac arrest. Often DNR instructions may be part of an advance directive, but when a client is in the hospital or other healthcare facility there must be a written medical order for a "no code." Each facility should have a policy regarding DNR orders.

Stop, Think, and Respond ● BOX 5-2

A physician tells the nurse that he informed the client about his lung biopsy scheduled for the following day and that the client just needs to sign the form for the procedure to move forward. The doctor asks the nurse to take the form to the client for his signature. When the nurse asks the client if he understands what the lung biopsy will involve, the client states that after the biopsy the spot on his lung will be gone.

Should the nurse allow the client to sign the form at this time or take other action?

ETHICAL ISSUES IN NURSING PRACTICE

Nurses frequently encounter complex situations that require decisions based on determining not what is legally right or wrong, but what is morally good or bad. Ethical issues do not have absolute answers. Conflicts may arise related to the desire to maintain the client's rights, and yet uphold professional values and institutional policies.

For example, a mildly confused, elderly client has liver cancer but is expected to live at least several more months. The client eats and drinks some, but overall her intake is poor. Efforts to help the client drink and eat more have failed. The physician obtains consent from the client's medical durable power of attorney to place a feeding tube in the client. The physician asks the nurse to assist while the tube is placed. The client resists placement and the nurse must restrain the client's hands to place the feeding tube. Because the client makes frequent attempts to remove the feeding tube, the restraints remain in place, with frequent checks by the nursing staff. In such a situation, knowing the ethically right course of action is difficult. The client receives better nutrition this way but must endure the discomfort of the tube and wrist restraints. What are the benefits and harms of the feeding tube and the wrist restraints? Should the client be forced to accept a treatment that necessitates the use of physical restraints? In the following material, theories of ethical practice and an ethical decision-making model provide essential information to consider situations such as the one just described. Refer to Box 5-5 for definitions of terms related to ethics.

Theories of Ethics

Ethical theories provide a means to determine if a particular action is good or bad. In nursing ethics, two systems or theories predominate: utilitarianism and deontology.

Utilitarianism

Utilitarianism, also referred to as *teleologic theory,* is an outcome-oriented approach for decision-making. There are two important principles: "the greatest good for the greatest number" and "the end justifies the means." When individuals or groups use utilitarianism to make ethical decisions, they consider the consequences of their actions and make decisions that benefit the greatest number and outweigh the harm for a few. Furthermore, an action is not good or bad in and of itself. Instead, the consequences of the action determine if the action was good or bad. Utilitarianism compels the individual or group to evaluate consequences. Theorists suggest that:

BOX 5-5 ● Definitions Related to Ethics

ETHICS
Decisions regarding what is right and wrong; often a system that is used to protect the rights of individuals or groups

CODE OF ETHICS
Standards of conduct and values as defined by a profession; forms the basis for ethical decision-making by a profession.

VALUES
The ideals and beliefs held by an individual or group; usually influenced by family, society, and religion; greatly influence behavior

MORALS
An individual's standards of right and wrong; formed in childhood; also influenced by family, society, and religion

BIOETHICS
Ethical questions surrounding life and death questions and concerns regarding quality of life as it relates to advanced technology

ETHICAL DILEMMA
A situation in which an individual must choose between two undesirable alternatives; often involves examining rights and obligations of particular individuals; choice frequently defended

---

Adapted from Harrington, N., Smith, N. E., & Spratt, W. E. (1996). *LPN to RN transitions.* Philadelphia: Lippincott-Raven.

- Consequences are good if they bring pleasure.
- The primary consideration is the outcome desired by those who are most affected.

Allocation of healthcare dollars provides an example of the use of utilitarianism. If a group is considering funding vaccines for many children or organ transplants for a few, the group will decide to give the money to the vaccines because a greater number will benefit.

Deontology

Another theory of ethics, **deontology,** argues that consequences are not the only important consideration in ethical dilemmas. Deontology states that duty is equally important. Duties are part of our understanding of the situations and relationships in which we find ourselves. We know intuitively that we must keep promises, return borrowed items, or help an injured person (Quinn & Smith, 1987). We have an obligation to perform or avoid some actions, regardless of the consequences, because of our duties to others. For example, the deontologist would say that lying is never acceptable because it disregards one's duty to tell the truth. He or she would believe abortion is unethical because it violates the duty to respect and preserve life (Zerwekh & Claborn, 2000).

Implied in the concept of duties is the idea of rights. **Rights** are freedoms or actions to which individuals have a just moral or legal claim. Another individual is entitled to what we have a duty to provide. For example, a person has a right to have his or her belongings returned or to have promises kept. This concept is particularly important in nursing practice. Nurses have a professional duty to their clients, and those clients have a right to expect that the nurse will perform his or her duties (see Box 5-3).

The deontologic approach considers the rights of each person—a distinct advantage. A second advantage is that the obligation to duty and moral thinking is foremost, and thus the decisions for similar situations are the same. Applying the deontologic method may be difficult, however, when the consequence of the decision can be harmful to an individual. For example, the decision to maintain life for all infants regardless of the outcome may be difficult when the infant is severely deformed and will require many invasive and expensive procedures to survive in a vegetative state.

Factors That Influence Ethical Decision-Making

Selecting a system for ethical decision-making should simplify the process; however, most nurses do not necessarily use one system or another. Other factors influence their decisions, not just knowledge of ethical theory.

Professional Values

Values are the beliefs that individuals find most meaningful. People value many different ideas, and not all ideas are ethical. Ethical values are rules or principles a person uses to make decisions about right and wrong. They share four characteristics. Ethical values:

- Are consistent
- Take priority over other values
- Concern the treatment of others
- Are well thought out (Quinn & Smith, 1987)

Professional values are principles intended to support the ethical conduct of the profession. Some of those values do not differ from personal values, whereas some may come from a person's professional education. Several professional values guide the decisions that nurses make.

BENEFICENCE

Beneficence is the duty to do good for the clients assigned to the nurse's care. This "good" includes technical competence and a humanistic, holistic approach. Stated another way, a nurse ought to prevent or remove harm, and promote or do good. The nurse has a duty to remove wrist restraints whenever possible (removing a harm) and to help the client regain independence (promoting and doing good). The principle of beneficence directly supports the nurse's role of client advocacy. **Advocacy** is safeguarding clients' rights and supporting their interests. For example, if a client is being discharged before mastering a complicated dressing change, the nurse advocates for an additional day in the hospital or home health visits.

NONMALEFICENCE

Nonmaleficence is the duty to do no harm to the client. If a nurse fails to check an order for an unusually high dose of insulin and administers it, he or she has violated the principle of nonmaleficence. Sometimes it is difficult to reconcile nonmaleficence with medical care because the choice of treatment may initially cause harm, even though the outcome is potentially good. For example, a client with colon cancer has a resection with a colostomy and endures the pain of surgery. In addition, the client undergoes unpleasant chemotherapy and radiation treatments. Although the client is harmed in many ways, the ultimate goal is for the client to be free of cancer. In these cases, the treatment still is ethically right because the intended effect is good and outweighs the bad effect. If the outcome is likely to be poor despite the treatment, what is ethically right may be difficult to determine.

AUTONOMY

Autonomy refers to a client's right to self-determination or the freedom to make choices without opposition. Nurses respect the client's right of autonomy even if the client's decision conflicts with the nurse's values. Through their advocacy role, nurses support clients' autonomy.

JUSTICE

Justice is the duty to be fair to all people regardless of age, sex, race, sexual orientation, or other factors. The American Nurses Association Code of Ethics (Box 5-6) has the

BOX 5-6 ● American Nurses Association Code of Ethics for Nurses

1. The nurse, in all professional relationships, practices with compassion and respect for the inherent dignity, worth, and uniqueness of every individual, unrestricted by considerations of social or economic status, personal attributes, or the nature of health problems.
2. The nurse's primary commitment is to the patient, whether an individual, family, group, or community.
3. The nurse promotes, advocates for, and strives to protect the health, safety, and rights of the patient.
4. The nurse is responsible and accountable for individual nursing practice and determines the appropriate delegation of tasks consistent with the nurse's obligation to provide optimum patient care.
5. The nurse owes the same duties to self as to others, including the responsibility to preserve integrity and safety, to maintain competence, and to continue personal and professional growth.
6. The nurse participates in establishing, maintaining, and improving health care environments and conditions of employment conducive to the provision of quality health care and consistent with the values of the profession through individual and collective action.
7. The nurse participates in the advancement of the profession through contributions to practice, education, administration, and knowledge development.
8. The nurse collaborates with other health professionals and the public in promoting community, national, and international efforts to meet health needs.
9. The profession of nursing, as represented by associations and their members, is responsible for articulating nursing values, for maintaining the integrity of the profession and its practice, and for shaping social policy.

From American Nurses Association. (2001). *Code for nurses with interpretive statements*. Washington, DC: Author.

principle of justice as its first statement. A conflict can occur if healthcare resources are limited or when fairness to one means discrimination to another.

FIDELITY

Fidelity is the duty to maintain commitments of professional obligations and responsibilities. Such obligations and responsibilities usually are defined by nurse practice acts.

VERACITY

Veracity is the duty to tell the truth. The nurse must provide factual information to the client so that he or she may exercise autonomy. There are potential conflicts if the family or physician withholds information from the client. The issues of beneficence and nonmaleficence can enter into this ethical conflict.

Legislative and Judicial Influences

Society's struggles with ethical issues result in legislative and judicial decisions that affect ethical decisions. For example, the issue of declaring death and removing life support has become more difficult with advances in technology. Formerly, the loss of cardiac and respiratory

function was the deciding factor in determining death. With greater abilities to maintain cardiac and respiratory function, however, society has had to redefine death. Definitions of death now include brain criteria, including lack of movements or breathing, absence of reflexes, a flat reading on an electroencephalogram, and unresponsiveness. Most states accept such criteria. The ethical issues for many nurses are related to their own beliefs about the dignity of life, harvesting of donor organs from an individual who is brain dead, and supporting the family members who may be asked to make decisions. The legality of brain death has removed some of the uncertainties for nurses regarding ethical issues.

Another topic that creates debate is physician-assisted suicide and euthanasia. Many people fear a prolonged and painful death. This has given rise to a movement for a legally sanctioned, medically assisted, peaceful death as an option for clients of sound mind with terminal illnesses. Nurses are committed to preserving life and also to maintaining quality of life. Nurse practice acts prohibit nurses from assisting clients to die; however, nurses have a unique understanding of their clients' wishes and suffering. Some nurses may face dilemmas in advocating for their clients.

Influence of Technology

Developments in science and technology produce ethical issues that were unheard of even 10 years ago. Some examples include the following:

- Successful impregnation of a woman past menopause—some governments are considering age limitations for such procedures.
- Genetic engineering—such procedures may potentially harm humans, create a "perfect" being, or lead to discrimination.
- Cloning animals, humans, or both—this raises difficult questions about the creation of life and individuality.

These advances, once in the realm of science fiction, now pose serious ethical dilemmas. Nurses definitely will play a key role in the decisions involved with these issues. They also will have particular problems if the need to promote science and progress obscures the nurse's duty to clients.

Healthcare Reform

Cost control, decreased hospital stays, increased client acuity, and interest in alternative healthcare are factors that affect ethical decision-making. The discharge of clients to their homes when they are sicker and more vulnerable is of great concern. Issues related to the allocation of healthcare dollars to those who need it the most or who have the greatest potential to have a positive outcome also are ethically challenging. Nurses will face questions that make them examine their own values as they relate to providing quality care to clients and their families.

Ethical Decision-Making

Nurses use a problem-solving method (the nursing process) to provide care to clients. Healthcare providers use a similar problem-solving approach for ethical dilemmas. Nurses can use the following steps when making ethical decisions:

1. Obtain as much information as possible to understand the situation. Identify the problem and describe it. Determine what values are involved and whom the decision will affect. A statement of the dilemma (after considering all the data) helps to define the issue as clearly as possible.
2. List all the possible options for solving the dilemma; this process is referred to as *brainstorming*. Do not determine the consequences at this point.
3. Examine the pros and cons of each option, foreseeing possible consequences from both a utilitarian and a deontologic approach. Consider the effects on the individual.
4. Make the decision and follow through on it.
5. Evaluate the decision in terms of effects and results.

Stop, Think, and Respond ● BOX 5-3

A kidney becomes available for transplantation. The tissue matches that of an adolescent and a middle-aged client, both of whom need the organ. If you were responsible for deciding which client receives the kidney transplant, how would you decide?

Ethics Committees

Hospitals and other healthcare institutions often have ethics committees to help resolve ethical dilemmas and make decisions on a per case basis. Ethics committees are composed of individuals with diverse backgrounds. They often include physicians, nurses, clergy, social workers, and community members. Ethics committees establish guidelines and policies before an ethical dilemma develops. They also may be called on to act as an advocate for clients who no longer are mentally capable of making their own decisions. Having a resource for reviewing difficult cases by a committee of individuals with different perspectives helps to ensure a careful and unbiased decision.

GENERAL GERONTOLOGIC CONSIDERATIONS

The ability to give informed consent is an issue every time an older adult is asked to agree to treatment or to execute an advanced directive or living will.

Cognitive impairment does not automatically constitute incapacity. Older people with fluctuating cognitive status may retain sufficient ability to make some, if not all, their healthcare decisions. For example, an older adult may be unable to decide to have a feeding tube but can appoint a daughter or son to make such decisions.

Older adults depend more than younger people on the healthcare provider to deliver care that optimizes health. The unique needs of older adults present meaningful legal and ethical questions.

Because of the vulnerability of older adults, federal and state governments carefully regulate the treatment given in licensed healthcare facilities. These regulations address almost every aspect of life in a nursing facility and include sanctions to force compliance.

Critical Thinking Exercises

1. *A confused client has attempted to get out of bed by climbing over the side rails. What actions would you take to protect yourself from being sued?*
2. *Consider the case of the client who needed to be restrained to have tube feedings (presented earlier in this chapter). Discuss the ethical issues involved from the standpoint of values. Assess the situation from a utilitarian and a deontologic viewpoint using the ethical decision-making model. Do you think inserting the feeding tube and using wrist restraints were ethically good decisions?*

References and Suggested Readings

Andrews, P. (1999). Side rails: The ups and downs. *Nursing, 30*(6), 8.

Brown, S. M. (1999). Legally speaking: Good Samaritan laws: Protection and limits. *RN, 62*(11), 65–67,68.

Ellis, J. R. & Hartley, C. L. (2001). *Nursing in today's world: Challenges, issues, and trends* (7th ed.). Philadelphia: Lippincott Williams & Wilkins.

Haddad, A. (2000). Acute care decisions: Ethics in action. *RN, 63*(3), 21–22, 24, 82–83.

Haddad, A. (2001). Acute care decisions: Ethics in action. *RN, 64*(3), 21–24.

Kennedy-Schwartz, J. (2000). The "ethics" of instinct. *American Journal of Nursing, 100*(4), 71–73.

Lenehan, G. P. (1999). Patients' Bill of Rights offers welcomed protection of patients, nurses, and emergency department. *Journal of Emergency Nursing, 25*(1), 3–4.

Marquis, B. L. & Huston, C. J. (1998). *Management decision making for nurses* (3rd ed.). Philadelphia: Lippincott Williams & Wilkins.

Quinn, C. A. & Smith, M. D. (1987). *The professional commitment: Issues and ethics in nursing.* Philadelphia: Saunders.

Sullivan, G. H. (2000). Keep your charting on course. *RN, 63*(5), 75–79.

Taylor, C., Lillis, C., & LeMone, P. (2000). *Fundamentals of nursing: The art and science of nursing care* (4th ed.). Philadelphia: Lippincott Williams & Wilkins.

Wolfe, S. (2000). Clinical trials: How informed should consent be? *RN, 63*(6), 77–82.

Zerwekh, J. & Claborn, J. C. (2000). *Nursing today: Transitions and trends* (3rd ed.). Philadelphia: Saunders.

Leadership Roles and Management Functions

Learning Objectives

On completion of this chapter, the reader will:

- Differentiate leadership and management.
- Define three styles of leadership.
- Outline the purpose of power in the leadership role.
- Describe the role of the LPN/LVN in managing client care.
- Distinguish delegation and supervision.
- Compare responsibility and accountability.
- Discuss problems that may occur with delegation and supervision.
- Describe the role of the LPN/LVN in collaboration and advocacy.
- Explain the role of the LPN/LVN in resource management.
- Discuss methods to manage time effectively.

Licensed practical/vocational nurses (LPN/LVNs), in their role of providing care to clients, must have skills in organizing client care, supervising care provided by unlicensed personnel, collaborating with other healthcare personnel, managing time and resources, and being accountable for assigned client care. Although they are primarily educated to provide direct client care, LPN/LVNs need a basic understanding of management and supervisory principles to function in leadership roles in various healthcare settings. This chapter provides an overview of theory related to leadership and management, with a focus on the role of the LPN/LVN in delegation and supervision.

LEADERSHIP AND MANAGEMENT

In many ways, leadership and management are interrelated concepts; discussing one is impossible without reference to the other. These terms, however, are not synonymous, as the following paragraphs explain.

Leadership

Leadership involves qualities related to a person's character and behaviors, as well as roles within a group or organization. It requires that a person has the ability to guide and influence another person, group, or both to think in a certain way, achieve common goals, or provide inspiration for change. Marquis and Huston (1998) state that leaders:

1. May or may not have delegated authority, but are capable of obtaining their power through means other than delegated authority
2. Have a wider variety of roles than do managers
3. Frequently are not part of a formal organization
4. Focus on the group process, information gathering, feedback, and empowering others (p. 37)

Any healthcare provider has the potential to be a leader in terms of influencing a group or exercising power in a particular situation. Accordingly, LPN/LVNs also may be leaders, informally or formally. For example, an LPN working on a medical–surgical unit may assume responsibility for organizing social events for fellow employees.

A more formal leadership role would be acting as co-chairperson of the unit's staffing policy committee.

Management

Management entails assigned functions such as planning, organizing, directing, and controlling to meet specific objectives within an organization (Ellis & Hartley, 2000). The manager's overall goal is to coordinate and direct resources, which include work space, supplies, equipment, budgetary concerns, and services (Harrington et al., 1996). In addition, managers direct and coordinate the work of assigned employees. Managers (1) are assigned a position in an organization, (2) have a legitimate source of power owing to the delegated authority that accompanies their position, (3) are expected to carry out specific functions, and (4) emphasize control, decision-making, decision analysis, and results (Marquis and Huston, 1998). A key feature is the individual manager's responsibility and accountability for the accomplishment of tasks (Ellis & Hartley, 2000).

The Relationship of Leadership and Management

To be effective, leaders and managers must possess certain qualities:

- An ability to gain the respect of others through competence and shared goals
- Expertise in communication skills, both oral and written
- A capacity to motivate others to achieve a particular purpose or accomplish goals

Ideally, a good manager is also a good leader, and a good leader is a good manager. In reality, some managers do not possess good leadership skills, and some leaders are ineffective managers. People can learn leadership and management skills. Improving and developing skills through education and experience enhances a person's ability to lead and manage.

Integrated leaders/managers (Marquis & Huston, 2000) have traits that distinguish them from just leaders or managers:

- Thinking in the long term
- Seeing the big picture
- Influencing others outside their own group
- Emphasizing vision, values, and motivation
- Being politically astute
- Embracing change and modification (Gardner, 1990)

In addition, integrated leaders/managers set reasonable goals, think positively, and are willing to take risks.

Leadership Styles

Lewin (1951) identified three prevalent leadership styles that managers use, either consciously or unconsciously, to accomplish certain goals and tasks. These styles vary in the amount of control that the manager exerts and the degree of input that subordinates have in the decision-making process.

The first leadership style is the authoritarian or **autocratic leadership** style. Strong control by the manager over the work group characterizes this style. The manager gives and asks for little input from staff for decisions. Communication flows from top to bottom. The focus is on accomplishing tasks.

The second leadership style, **democratic leadership,** involves more participation in decision-making by the work group. Leaders with this style often see themselves as coworkers or colleagues, as opposed to superiors. They emphasize communication, consensus, and teamwork (Ellis & Hartley, 2000).

The third leadership style is **laissez-faire leadership,** or permissive management. This style involves the least structure and control. The manager leaves the work group to set goals, make decisions, and take responsibility for their own management (Ellis & Hartley, 2000).

Table 6-1 provides information about the advantages and disadvantages of the three styles of leadership. Each leadership style may be effective, depending on the particular situation. A good leader can determine which approach is best for a particular circumstance. Ellis and Hartley (2000) refer to this ability as **multicratic leadership.** This so-called multicratic style combines the best of all styles, mediated by the requirements of the situation at hand. The multicratic leader provides maximum structure when appropriate to the situation, asks for maximum group participation when needed, and gives support and encouragement to subordinates in all instances.

Stop, Think, and Respond ● BOX 6-1

A new LPN/LVN works on a long-term care unit where the nurse manager typically uses an autocratic style of leadership. What are the advantages and disadvantages of this style for the new LPN/LVN?

Power and Leadership

The leader/manager has the potential to provide guidance, direction, and support to coworkers. The leader/manager also exerts a certain power. **Power** is the ability to control, influence, or hold authority over an individual or group. People in leadership/management posi-

TABLE 6-1	ADVANTAGES AND DISADVANTAGES OF LEADERSHIP STYLES	
LEADERSHIP STYLE	**ADVANTAGES**	**DISADVANTAGES**
Autocratic	Tasks are accomplished without questions. Communication is directive and flows downward. Lines of authority and policies are clear. Decisions are made quickly. Autocratic leadership works best in bureaucracies and with employees who have limited education or training.	Subordinates have little input into decision- or policy-making and receive little feedback or recognition. Staff members are not invested in management's goals. Leaders may create hostility and dependency. Work is highly controlled and dictated.
Democratic	Subordinates contribute to decision- and policy-making. Staff members are invested in planning and accomplishing goals. Communication is mutual—back and forth. Employees receive regular feedback. Democratic leadership works well with competent and motivated employees.	Decisions may not occur in a timely way. Staff members may fail to acknowledge the manager's role. Employees do not recognize the need for urgent decisions that are made without staff input.
Laissez-faire	Coworkers can develop their own goals, make their own decisions, and take full responsibility for their actions. Managers provide support and freedom for employees. Subordinates perform at high levels because of their independence. Staff members share the process of making decisions for the group. Laissez-faire leadership works well with professional employees.	Employees receive little direction or guidance. Generally, decisions are not made because managers are unable or unwilling to make them Staff members do not receive feedback regarding their performance. Communication is limited to memos. Change is rare.

tions are in a position to exert power in an organization. If leadership is to be effective, a degree of power must support it.

Each type of power has a particular source or base (Table 6-2). The first type of power is *reward power,* which a person attains through the ability to grant favors or rewards. For example, organizational leaders have the ability to grant financial rewards or special favors.

Coercive or *punishment power* is the ability to threaten or punish someone who fails to meet expectations. In using such power, a manager may threaten undesirable schedules, denial of vacation time, or layoff if an employee is not compliant.

A manager exercises *legitimate power* through a designated position, which also may be referred to as *authority.* A manager has legitimate power by virtue of the management position.

Expert power results from knowledge, expertise, or experience in a particular area. Managers typically possess expert power through education and work experience.

TABLE 6-2	SOURCES OF POWER	
TYPE OF POWER	**SOURCE OF POWER**	**EXAMPLE**
Reward power	Ability to grant favors	Team leader making assignments
Coercive power	Fear	Head nurse scheduling vacations
Legitimate power	Position	Director of nursing
Expert power	Knowledge and skill	An LPN/LVN with 20 years' experience working on a medical unit
Referent power	Association with others	Shift supervisor
Informational power	Need for information to accomplish a goal	Merit raise information related to annual evaluations

(Adapted from Marquis, B. L. & Huston, C. J. [2000]. *Leadership roles and management functions in nursing: Theory and application.* [3rd ed.]. Philadelphia: Lippincott Williams & Wilkins.)

Referent power concerns the power a person has because of his or her association with others who are powerful. For example, society perceives that physicians are powerful. A new physician may use this referent power to his or her advantage. Referent power also may be called *charismatic* or *connection power,* referring to personal characteristics, such as charisma, the way a person talks or acts, the people he or she associates with, or the organizations to which he or she belongs.

Another type of power is *informational power,* which exists when a person has information that others need to accomplish certain goals. Examples may relate to budget preparation, planning for educational events, or making changes in an organization.

Leaders and managers may exercise power to accomplish assigned tasks. They also must have the authority or legitimate right to direct and guide work. A nurse in an authorized position (e.g., team leader, charge nurse) can exert power in a positive way.

THE LPN/LVN AS LEADER/MANAGER

Usually, managers are appointed to or hired for a specific management position. In healthcare, however, the term *manager* may be used more broadly, in that nurses manage the care of clients. This role involves overseeing the care that a client receives. Other healthcare providers may actually care for the clients. In acute care settings, registered nurses (RNs) are assigned to a group of clients. An LPN/LVN and certified nurse's aide (CNA) may work with the RN and be responsible for certain aspects of client care. The RN, as the manager of care, ensures that the LPN/LVN and CNA complete all assigned tasks, assess the clients, and evaluate the effects of all nursing interventions.

In other healthcare settings, the role of the LPN/LVN may be extended. For example, in long-term care settings LPN/LVNs may be team leaders and thus assigned to oversee the work of unlicensed assistive personnel (UAPs). In medical offices, an LPN/LVN may be the office manager, coordinating certain aspects of the office work, such as scheduling and coordinating work assignments. These roles require the LPN/LVN to delegate responsibility for certain tasks and then supervise the accomplishment of the work. The next sections delineate the terms *delegation, supervision, responsibility,* and *accountability.*

Delegation

The National Council of State Boards of Nursing (NCSBN) (1995) states that **delegation** is "transferring to a competent individual the authority to perform a selected nursing

task in a selected situation. The nurse retains the accountability for the delegation" (p. 3). Delegation also is a means of accomplishing work through others (Marquis & Huston, 1998). The ability to guide, teach, and direct others is integral to the ability to delegate.

Nurses need to learn delegation skills. The NCSBN (1995) identified the Five Rights of Delegation:

1. Right task
2. Right circumstances
3. Right person
4. Right direction/communication
5. Right supervision/evaluation

Ellis and Hartley (2000) suggest that carrying out the five rights of delegation requires following certain steps similar to those of the nursing process:

- *Assess the situation*—know the client's needs, the skills of the UAPs, and the priorities. Match the UAPs' skills with the tasks to be completed.
- *Plan actions*—identify the UAPs who will best handle the delegated tasks.
- *Implement the plan*—communicate expectations clearly to UAPs, including what they need to do, what to watch for, and potential problems.
- *Evaluate the results*—ensure that tasks are completed according to standards.

Box 6-1 provides tips for delegating successfully. Part of succeeding at delegating involves the process of supervision.

Supervision

Supervision is the process of guiding, directing, evaluating, and following-up on tasks delegated to others (NCSBN, 1995). Delegation and supervision are tightly connected, because once a nurse has delegated a task, he or she is obligated to supervise the person to whom he or

---

BOX 6-1 ● Tips for Delegating Successfully

Know the abilities of unlicensed assistive personnel (UAPs).
Plan ahead to prevent problems.
Match tasks to be accomplished to the skills of UAPs.
Communicate expectations and directions clearly.
Trust the UAP to complete the task.
Supervise the UAP to determine progress in completing the task.
Assess results.
Provide positive feedback to the UAP as appropriate.

(Adapted from Ellis, J. R. & Hartley, C. L. [2000]. *Managing and coordinating nursing care* [3rd ed.]. Philadelphia: Lippincott Williams & Wilkins.)

she has assigned that task. In reviewing the steps of delegation described in the previous section, supervision begins when the LPN/LVN implements the plan. The implementation step includes giving instructions about what needs to be done, and when. The nurse must include any specific issues, such as telling the UAP that a client must complete morning care before going for physical therapy at 10:00 AM. In addition, the nurse needs to tell the UAP about any potential problems, such as a client who may experience dizziness when getting up secondary to antihypertensive medications.

Supervision also is necessary throughout the implementation step. The LPN/LVN must check with UAPs during the shift to assess if tasks are complete, the results, if something has changed that may interfere with the work, or if the UAP is having problems accomplishing the task safely.

The evaluation step of delegation also includes supervision of the UAP, in that the LPN/LVN ensures that the client received the appropriate care, all the client's needs were met, and that problems were addressed. Providing feedback to UAPs also is important, in terms of letting them know that they did a good job or asking questions about the client's response to the care provided.

Delegation and supervision imply that the people carrying out these functions assume responsibility and accountability for their actions as well as the actions of those to whom they delegate. The next section defines these concepts.

Responsibility and Accountability

Responsibility is a duty or assignment related to a specific job. It means being obligated to perform certain activities and duties. When a person is responsible for something, he or she is obligated to ensure that the task or job is completed (Ellis & Hartley, 2000).

Accountability means being answerable for the consequences of one's actions or inactions. The term *liability* (see Chap. 5) is closely associated with accountability, because of the legal implications. "Although the tasks may be delegated, the nurse who delegates that task to others remains accountable—or legally liable—for the outcome" (Ellis & Hartley, 2000, p. 32).

An LPN/LVN who delegates to a UAP is responsible for ensuring that the task is appropriate for the UAP and that the UAP has the skills to complete the task. The LPN/LVN is accountable for determining if the task is accomplished, and if there are any issues associated with completing or not completing the task. In addition, the LPN/LVN also is accountable for evaluating the results of the tasks. The UAP is responsible for performing the actual task. The following exercise clarifies these concepts.

Stop, Think, and Respond ● BOX 6-2

An LPN is the team leader for 20 clients on a long-term care unit. She delegates to a UAP the task of feeding supper to an older client. When the UAP feeds this client, the client begins to cough and choke, aspirating some food. The client eventually develops pneumonia and must be hospitalized for 1 week. Who is responsible for this incident?

Confronting Problems

LPN/LVNs may experience some problems with delegation and supervision of tasks. In part this is because LPN/LVNs may not be well prepared for the role of team leader. Schools of practical/vocational nursing traditionally have focused primarily on the direct caregiver role. In turn, employers may not plan for LPN/LVNs to be team leaders or other managers of care, but out of necessity place LPN/LVNs in these roles. Other factors that may interfere with effective delegation and supervision are as follows:

- Reluctance to delegate from fear of overloading a coworker or desire to do everything
- Inability to move out of the role of direct caregiver— "It is easier to do it myself"
- Miscommunication regarding specific directions and desired outcomes
- Desire to be liked by coworkers, which interferes with ability to delegate, supervise, or both

In addition, LPN/LVNs are not strictly supervisors, in that they do not have the authority to hire or fire. They may have responsibility for overseeing and directing the care that UAPs provide, but they do not have responsibility for disciplining them.

Solutions for improving one's ability to delegate and direct UAPs include obtaining education for this role. In addition, LPN/LVNs must focus on client care needs first. In this way, the LPN/LVN ensures that the clients receive appropriate care and that tasks are carried out efficiently and in a caring manner. If an LPN/LVN remains responsible and accountable for his or her actions, it assists him or her to delegate and direct responsibly.

Other Functions

Although LPN/LVNs as team leaders have primary responsibility for delegating tasks to UAPs, other functions are important for the LPN/LVN leader/manager. These functions include collaboration, advocacy, resource management, and time management.

Collaboration

Collaboration involves a team effort to achieve client care outcomes. Although RNs often direct collaborative efforts, LPN/LVNs are responsible to direct the care of UAPs. As a team member and leader, LPN/LVNs maintain open and effective communication with all team members. They also assist in solving problems related to client care. LPN/LVNs may contribute to decisions about client care and unit activities by participating in client care conferences and unit meetings. Last, collaborative behavior for the LPN/LVN involves participating in the management of the unit by following the appropriate channels of communication and supporting the group in collaborative efforts.

Advocacy

Advocacy means promoting the cause of another person or organization. In healthcare, advocates support the needs of a client or organization. Nurses in general act on behalf of their clients. Ethically, nurses support a client's right to be autonomous and to make informed decisions (American Nurses Association, 1998). LPN/LVNs function as client advocates by:

- Understanding the rights of all clients
- Remaining informed about diagnoses, treatments, prognoses, and choices
- Contributing to the provision of information and education
- Supporting the client's decisions
- Communicating with other professionals (Ellis & Hartley, 2000)

Resource Management

Resource management, the responsibility of all who work in healthcare, means using resources, which include not only actual money but supplies, equipment, buildings, and personnel, optimally. Nurses who provide direct care may not have a direct role in formulating budgets, but they are responsible for controlling the use of resources and recognizing when resources are inadequate. In addition, they must know the costs of resources and the importance of using cost-effective measures when caring for clients.

Many factors are related to the rising costs of healthcare (Box 6-2). In general, new technologies increase costs, which leads to the need for better facilities and, it is hoped, better outcomes for client care. Related costs are salaries for healthcare personnel, newer and more expensive medications, and equipment. As a result of increased costs, healthcare providers are expected to be more cost-conscious. Cost-conscious measures, or resource management, include prudent use of expensive supplies, knowledgeable operation of medical equip-

---

BOX 6-2 ● Factors Involved in Rising Healthcare Costs

Higher prices for new technology
New construction of facilities
Increased survival rate of clients (leads to more costly care)
Growing elderly population who require healthcare
Rising salaries of healthcare personnel
Higher prices for medications
Increased costs for medical equipment

(Adapted from Ellis, J. R. & Hartley, C. L. [2000]. *Nursing in today's world: Challenges, issues, and trends* [7th ed.]. Philadelphia: Lippincott Williams & Wilkins.)

---

ment, careful monitoring of clients to reduce potential complications and lengths of stay, heightened awareness of practicing measures that reduce costs, essential knowledge of all costs of caring for clients, and deliberate reduction of waste of limited resources.

LPN/LVNs also may be involved in controlling costs by participation in a client acuity system. Acute care and long-term care facilities may use an acuity system to determine staffing needs. Acuity measures the degree of a client's illness and what care is required to meet the client's needs. Often systems use categories to designate the level of care needed. For example, one category may reflect the need for complex dressing changes, another the need for special monitoring, such as neurologic checks. Each category has assigned points—at the end, the points are totaled to ascertain the acuity level of the client. This information may then be used to determine what nursing staff is needed to provide adequately for the needs of the unit (Ellis & Hartley, 2001).

Time Management

Time is an essential resource, particularly in today's fast-paced healthcare environment. **Time management** involves organizing time, as well as delegating tasks to other personnel and essentially "making optimal use of what time you have" (Marquis & Huston, 1998, p. 257). Figure 6-1 provides three basic steps for managing time. In the first step the nurse makes time to plan and establish priorities. The second step involves completing the highest-priority task and moving from completing one task to beginning another. The final step requires that the nurse reassess and reprioritize tasks based on any changes.

The onset of managed care increased the focus on efficiency and productivity. Making the most of one's time is an important skill that takes effort to achieve. Although on chaotic days it may seem that nothing works, those who are most effective at managing time will have the most success in accomplishing the work that needs to be done. New nurses usually need to learn to organize their

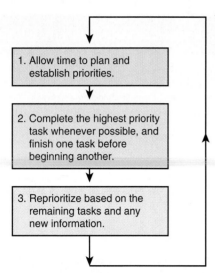

FIGURE 6-1 The three basic steps in time management. (Adapted from Marquis, B. L. & Huston, C. J. [1998]. *Management decision making for nurses* [3rd ed.]. Philadelphia: Lippincott Williams & Wilkins.)

BOX 6-3 ● Criteria for Setting Priorities

1. Items critical to maintaining life: Think in terms of your cardiopulmonary resuscitation basics.
  - Essential assessment
  - Airway management
  - Breathing support
  - Circulation needs
  - Neurologic stability

2. Critical symptom management: What is important to the client?
  - Pain management
  - Relief of nausea
  - Relief of diarrhea
  - Relief of severe anxiety

3. Items needed to progress in health restoration: What orders has the physician written? What nursing plans have been developed?
  - Medication and intravenous fluid administration
  - Completing treatments
  - Preventing complications
  - Meeting nutritional needs

4. Items needed to move toward self-care
  - Teaching
  - Contacting referral needs
  - Meeting psychosocial needs
  - Creating comfort and feelings of well-being
  - Bathing
  - Changing linens

(Adapted from Ellis, J. R. & Hartley, C. L. [2000]. *Managing and coordinating nursing care* [3rd ed.]. Philadelphia: Lippincott Williams & Wilkins.)

---

time. The following techniques are useful in learning to manage time:

- Assess expectations for the shift. Do so in a chart that identifies specific periods (e.g., 30-minute increments). This also can be done after a shift to determine how one spent time that particular day and how it might help to organize another shift.
- Use a worksheet to identify specific tasks and important assessments that need to be done for that particular shift. This works very well with multiple client assignments. Organize the worksheet according to each client. Many nurses refer to this as a "to do" list or "brain sheet." They use the worksheet to identify tasks, but also to write quick notes to jog their memories for further tasks or assessments.
- Prioritize tasks that need to be accomplished (Box 6-3). Reprioritize as needed.
- Write things down to remember later for charting and reporting. Many nurses use their worksheet as a report sheet for the oncoming shift.
- Develop efficiency and the ability to multitask, which means engaging in more than one task at a time. For example, if a client requests pain medication and you need to assess his roommate's vital signs, bring needed equipment as well as pain medication.
- Delegate appropriate tasks to appropriate personnel.

Most people readily admit that they do not always make good use of their time and then have to scramble to complete tasks. Box 6-4 identifies some "time wasters." These essentially include an inability to plan, procrastination, chatting, allowing low-priority tasks to take precedence, inability to delegate appropriately, and difficulty

---

BOX 6-4 ● Time Wasters

Poor planning
Inability to delegate
Procrastination
Socializing
Unwillingness to say no
Poor communication
Inefficient use of time
Failure to write things down
Haste
Repetitive paperwork
Unclear direction
Management by crisis

---

saying no. Assessing what wastes one's time is an important step in using time more effectively.

Critical Thinking Exercises

1. *An LPN is a team leader on a skilled care unit. When she returns from her dinner break, the UAP reports the following:*
   - *One client vomited after receiving her 6 PM medications.*
   - *A family member is upset that his mother pulled out her feeding tube and that it is not replaced.*
   - *A client's catheter seems to be leaking.*

- *A physician wants to order medications for the new client who had hip replacement surgery 2 weeks ago.*

Prioritize these tasks—indicate what the LPN should attend to and what she can delegate.

2. *An LVN is planning to change jobs from an acute care setting to a long-term care facility. He is concerned about his role in the new job as a team leader. He knows that he will be working with UAPs. What should he know about his role in delegating tasks to UAPs if he takes this new job?*

References and Suggested Readings

American Nurses Association. (1998). *Standards of clinical nursing practice* (2nd ed.). Washington, DC: Author.

Crowell, D. M. (1998). Organizations are relationships: A new view of management. *Nursing Management, 29*(5), 28–29.

Elder, K. N., O'Hara, N., Crutcher, T., Wells, N., Graham, C., & Hefline, W. (1998). Managed care: The value you bring. *American Journal of Nursing, 98*(6), 34–40.

Ellis, J. R. & Hartley, C. L. (2000). *Managing and coordinating nursing care* (3rd ed.). Philadelphia: Lippincott Williams & Wilkins.

Gardner, J. W. (1990). *On leadership.* New York: The Free Press.

Harrington, N., Smith, N. E., & Spratt, W. (1996). *LPN to RN transitions.* Philadelphia: Lippincott-Raven.

Lewin, K. (1951). *Field theory in social sciences.* New York: Harper & Row.

Marquis, B. L. & Huston, C. J. (1998). *Management decision making for nurses* (3rd ed.). Philadelphia: Lippincott Williams & Wilkins.

Marquis, B. L. & Huston, C. J. (2000). *Leadership roles and management functions in nursing: Theory and application* (3rd ed.). Philadelphia: Lippincott Williams & Wilkins.

National Council of State Boards of Nursing. (1995). *Delegation: Concepts and decision making process.* Chicago: Author.

chapter 7

Biopsychosocial Aspects of Caring for Young Adults

Words to Know

adolescent moratorium
androgeny
autonomy
blended family
development
developmental stage
developmental tasks
domestic violence
doubt
ego identity
extended family
gender role
Generation X
Generation Y
growth
guilt
industry

inferiority
initiative
intimacy
isolation
mistrust
nuclear family
personal protection
 order
psychosocial stages
rape
role confusion
shame
single-parent family
temporary restraining
 order
traditional family
trust

Learning Objectives

On completion of this chapter, the reader will:

- Differentiate growth from development.
- Explain the terms *developmental stage* and *developmental task*.
- Name Erikson's eight psychosocial stages of development.
- Describe the attributes associated with each stage of psychosocial development from infancy to young adulthood.
- Give three components that are used to determine if a person meets or exceeds a safe weight.
- Describe the national goal for adult exercise by 2010.
- Give examples of drugs used to facilitate smoking cessation.
- Name two growing practices among young adults that affect the integrity and safety of the integument.
- List examples of life events that mark the transition from adolescence to young adulthood.
- Cite at least one benefit of androgeny.
- Describe the current status of sexuality among young adults.
- Name four types of family structures in which young adults may be members.
- Name two consequences young adults experience in relation to unemployment and downsizing.
- Name three types of rape.
- List three drugs that potentiate the commission of rape.
- Identify two principles that are followed when caring for rape victims.
- List six aspects of nursing care when treating a rape victim.
- Identify the most dangerous period for victims of domestic violence.
- Discuss at least three areas for health teaching when caring for young adults.

Nurses provide care to all individuals from birth to old age. An important nursing intervention is to prepare clients for the physical changes and common life experiences that occur at various life stages. To do this, nurses must be knowledgeable about how aging affects health and familiar with social changes that are characteristic of each period in the life cycle.

The first part of this chapter discusses growth and development and reviews the tasks and crises commonly encountered in the developmental stages from birth to young adulthood (roughly between ages 18 to 35 years). The second part of the chapter focuses on the physical and psychosocial development of the young adult, with an exploration of common societal problems that have their first appearance or are especially prevalent in young adulthood.

GROWTH AND DEVELOPMENT

Growth refers to an increase in body size and is measured by changes in height and weight. **Development** refers to the ability to perform physical, intellectual, social, and psychological tasks. Development is measured by evaluating a person's physical coordination, language skills, problem-solving abilities, relationships, and methods of coping during crises. Although development depends heavily on physical growth and maturation, social relationships and life experiences also affect development.

At one time, it was commonly believed that growth and development ceased after adolescence. Now development is considered a lifelong process of transitions during which people change according to their unique age-related experiences.

Developmental Stages and Tasks

A **developmental stage** is a period of life during which unique physical and behavioral changes occur. The human life span is a continuous series of developmental stages. Each stage is separate and distinct from the previous stage and from the stage that follows. All individuals develop in the same cycle and pattern of progression.

During each stage, individuals are challenged to complete specific **developmental tasks,** activities unique to a particular stage. Accomplishing the tasks in each stage is critical to future development. Handling a task out of sequence, either prematurely or belatedly, can cause frustration and emotional crisis. For example, consider the impact of trying to toilet train a child too soon, having a first child close to menopause, or being forced to retire early because of health problems. These situations create psychic stress because the tasks occur during atypical periods of life. Finally, a person's degree of success in accomplishing the tasks of a particular developmental stage

influences the outcome of each successive stage. Failure to complete the developmental tasks in a timely manner makes eventual achievement difficult. Conversely, mastery of the tasks empowers one to succeed in future challenges.

Erikson's Psychosocial Stages

Erik Erikson divided developmental stages into eight periods that span the life cycle. He suggested that social relationships influence each stage and coined the term **psychosocial stages.** Erikson proposed that a person acquires one of two opposing attributes at each psychosocial stage (Fig. 7-1). The outcome is either positive or negative, depending on the person's success or failure in accomplishing the developmental tasks.

The following discussion presents a brief overview of Erikson's psychosocial stages up to and including young adulthood. Chapters 8 and 9 discuss the stages of middle and older adulthood.

Infancy and Trust vs. Mistrust

During infancy (birth to approximately age 18 months), a baby's developmental tasks are to communicate and satisfy basic needs. Infants indicate they are hungry, cold, hot, wet, or tired primarily through crying, pointing, and using other body language. When parents or caretakers consistently respond to their needs, infants develop a sense of **trust** or reliance on others. When adults ignore a baby's physical and emotional needs, the infant acquires a general **mistrust** of others that stems from uncertainty that caretakers will meet his or her needs. If an infant does not acquire trust, he or she will have difficulty progressing through future developmental stages.

Early Childhood and Autonomy vs. Shame and Doubt

Erikson observed that a major developmental task during the toddler years, 18 months to 3 years of age, is eliminating urine and feces in a socially acceptable manner. The

Infancy birth-18 months	Early childhood 18 months to 3 years	Pre-school age 3-6 years	School age 6-12 years	Adolescence 12-18 years	Young adult 18-35 years	Middle-aged adult 35-65 years	Older adult 65+ years
Trust vs. Mistrust	Autonomy vs. Shame, Doubt	Initiative vs. Guilt	Industry vs. Inferiority	Identity vs. Role Confusion	Intimacy vs. Isolation	Generativity vs. Stagnation	Ego Integrity vs. Despair

FIGURE 7-1 Erikson's psychosocial stages of development.

emotional consequences, as Erikson saw them, depended on the approval or disapproval of significant persons, usually the parents. Erikson proposed that when toddlers learn to suppress immediate gratification, such as delaying urinating or defecating until an appropriate time, they are praised and accepted. The approval results in **autonomy,** a sense of pride in self, which lays a positive foundation for the next developmental stage. When toddlers are met with impatience or criticism for toileting accidents, **shame** or **doubt** develops. Shame may result from having disappointed parents, whereas doubt may surround the child's inability to live up to parental expectations.

The Preschooler and Initiative vs. Guilt

During ages 3 to 6 years, the child seeks to perform tasks modeled by parents and identifies with the same-sex parent. Little girls imitate their mothers; little boys behave like their fathers. **Initiative,** the positive result of this stage, develops when children feel that others appreciate and encourage their efforts. Constant, unwarranted, or harsh discipline without praise can create overwhelming feelings of **guilt** and low self-esteem.

Parents or caregivers can enhance a child's development during this stage by supervising the child in appropriate activities and praising accomplishments. Giving the preschool child opportunities to complete tasks within his or her ability helps to prepare the child to acquire industry, a characteristic of the next developmental stage.

The School-Age Child and Industry vs. Inferiority

The tasks during early school age, 6 to 12 years, include paying attention, following directions, cooperating with others, and completing work in a timely and acceptable manner. If the child developed the negative attributes of mistrust, shame or doubt, and guilt in the previous stages, his or her self-confidence is diminished. This child appears withdrawn, feels inadequate, and experiences failure, all of which contribute to a sense of **inferiority** at this stage. Contrast this experience with the child who has acquired the positive attributes of trust, autonomy, and initiative during previous stages. This child enjoys new challenges and is eager to engage in efforts to produce work of high quality—examples of **industry.**

Adolescence and Ego Identity vs. Role Confusion

In adolescence, 12 to 18 years of age, the child strives to establish self-identity, or **ego identity.** Before adolescence, children identify themselves primarily in terms of their position in the family, such as son or daughter, brother or sister. During adolescence, the healthy child explores alternative value systems, develops a sense of self beyond the family, and eventually adopts values that are compatible with his or her personal beliefs. Adolescents must perceive that they are valuable parts of society and find satisfactory roles in it.

In contrast, some adolescents are reluctant to oppose or question parental or adult views. This leads to **role confusion** because these adolescents never develop true self-identity, and they attempt to fulfill the dreams and expectations of others. Confusion over role identity, substance abuse, and family stress are factors that contribute to suicidal behaviors. Some adolescents consider suicide, the third leading cause of death in this age group, as an escape from hopelessness and depression.

Young Adulthood and Intimacy vs. Isolation

Erikson observed that the developmental tasks during young adulthood, 18 to 35 years of age, involve leaving the home, forming lasting relationships with nonrelatives, and committing to a career (Fig. 7-2). If the young adult forms friendships with others and has a significant, intimate relationship with one individual, a basis for closeness with others results. The young adult then acquires the positive attribute of **intimacy,** the ability to enter into personal relationships that reaffirm one's own identity. Acquiring intimacy during this period enhances the young adult's ability to become a productive and happy member of society. The inability to form a close relationship with others results in loneliness and **isolation.**

YOUNG ADULTHOOD

Young adults who graduated from college in 1998 are commonly described as belonging to **Generation Y.** They may also be called Echo Boomers to differentiate them from older young adults, who are labeled as **Generation X.** Age, alphabetical designations of X and Y, and euphemistic labels, however, fail fully to explain today's young adults.

Physical Characteristics

Most people are healthiest and attain peak physical performance as young adults. Physical condition begins to decline, however, after 20 years of age (Vander Zanden, 2000). Chronic diseases are very rare among young adults. This age group is more likely to experience acute infectious illnesses and trauma from injuries. The success in treating victims of major trauma has increased the numbers of survivors with varying degrees of disability. The following is a brief overview of the typical physical characteristics of the young adult.

Weight

Weight fluctuates in relation to activity. Young adults consume more calories in relation to the energy expenditures they once had as adolescents. Consequently, overweight and obesity become new problems for many young adults. The National Institutes of Health (NIH) (1998) reports

FIGURE 7-2 Developmental tasks of the young adult involve establishing intimate relationships and beginning an occupation. (From Taylor, C., Lillis, C., & LeMone, P. [2001]. *Fundamentals of nursing: The art and science of nursing care* [4th ed., p. 151]. Philadelphia: Lippincott Williams & Wilkins.)

that approximately 55% of the adult population in the United States is overweight. In response, the NIH released the first federal obesity clinical guidelines that now recommend three components for determining if a person meets or exceeds a safe weight. They include (1) body mass index (BMI), (2) waist circumference, and (3) risk factors for diseases and conditions associated with obesity. One method for calculating BMI is to multiply 703 times weight in pounds and then divide by height in inches, squared. According to the NIH guidelines, a BMI of 25 to 29.9 is considered overweight; a person is considered obese if the BMI is 30 or greater. A waist circumference that measures more than 40 inches in men and more than 35 inches in women increases health risks. When the first two mea-

surements exceed desirable limits (Table 7-1) and the person has a personal or family history of hypertension, diabetes, high cholesterol, heart disease, and respiratory disorders, the probability for a premature death increases.

DIETS

An obvious technique used to control weight or promote weight loss is dieting. Approximately 40% of young adult women and 24% of young adult men diet (Vander Zanden, 2000). Young adults are prone to follow fad diets rather than make low-calorie selections from among the categories of foods within the Food Guide Pyramid (see Chap. 16). Characteristics of fad diets include the following:

TABLE 7-1	HEALTH RISK ACCORDING TO BODY MASS INDEX (BMI) AND WAIST SIZE		
		HEALTH RISK	
RANGE IN BMI	**WEIGHT INDICATOR**	Waist Size <40 in. (Men) or <35 in. (Women)	Waist Size >40 in. (Men) or >35 in. (Women)
<18.5	Underweight	—	—
18.5–24.9	Normal	—	—
25.0–29.9	Overweight	Increased	High
30.0–34.9	Obese	High	Very high
35.0–39.9	Obese	Very high	Very high
≥40	Extremely obese	Extremely high	Extremely high

From Office of Consumer Information. (2000). Partnership for healthy weight management: Body mass index. [On-line.] Available: http://www.consumer.gov/weightloss/bmi.htm.

- Prolonged periods of fasting
- Severe restrictions of amounts of food
- Restrictions of particular food groups
- Claims for fast and easy weight loss

Strict dieting can cause nutritional deficits and a "yo-yo" effect of weight loss followed by weight gain. Some young adults develop eating disorders (see Chap. 16). The healthiest way to lose weight is to exercise, limit calories, and consume a variety of foods. These measures help to supress the appetite, enhance loss of body fat, increase lean body mass, improve self-image, reduce anxiety and depression, and facilitate stress management.

EXERCISE

Many people begin to exercise because of the benefits of aerobic exercise in preventing cardiovascular diseases. Young adults use indoor fitness centers and outside settings for walking, jogging, cycling, swimming, and rollerblading. The number of adults who exercise, however, is still below the national goals set in *Healthy People 2010* (see Chap. 1). By 2010, the goal is to increase from the current 15% to 30% the proportion of adults who engage in regular, preferably daily, moderate physical activity for at least 30 minutes (U.S. Department of Health and Human Services, 2000). Moderate activity includes walking at approximately 3 to 4 miles per hour, easy cycling, leisurely swimming, golfing without a cart, playing table tennis, canoeing at 2 to 4 miles per hour, and mowing the yard with a power mower (Vander Zanden, 2000).

Respiratory System

With the exceptions of upper or lower respiratory tract infections, the lungs remain highly functional throughout young adulthood among nonsmokers and persons who are not chronically exposed to significant levels of air pollution. Young adults with scoliosis, a lateral curvature of the spine, may have diminished respiratory volumes.

Smokers and those who inhale smoke passively (i.e., those who inhale the air emitted from exhaled smoke or smoke from a burning cigarette, pipe, or cigar) are exposed to harmful chemicals such as nicotine, tar, carbon monoxide, and hydrogen cyanide. Chronic exposure increases the rate of respiratory infections, pulmonary and cardiovascular diseases, and lung cancer. The number and severity of attacks of asthma, a chronic lung disorder, is much higher among smokers and those who inhale smoke passively. Maternal smoking lowers infant birth weight. A link exists between low birth weight and the incidence of sudden infant death syndrome. Although many smokers continue to perpetuate their habit into later years of adulthood, various drugs can assist with smoking cessation (Drug Therapy Table 7-1).

Cardiovascular System

Minor changes occur in the heart and vascular system. One percent of myocardial strength is lost with each year of adulthood. Blood pressure gradually increases after 20 years of age. Early narrowing of the coronary arteries and other vascular changes begin as well. A diet high in saturated fat contributes to the building of plaque on the walls of the coronary arteries, beginning the pathologic process of atherosclerosis (see Chap. 33). Effects of this process, however, are not evident for many years.

Cognition and Sensory Perception

The young adult's brain is totally developed although it continues to change in structure and complexity. For example, additional life experiences refine the person's ability to problem-solve. According to Vander Zanden (2000, p. 633), young adults become more adaptive and knowledgeable about themselves, form values, and develop increased depth in thinking, logical reasoning, and using imagination. As a result, they acquire characteristics of adult maturity (Box 7-1).

DRUG THERAPY TABLE 7-1	DRUGS FOR SMOKING CESSATION	
DRUG CLASS AND EXAMPLES	**SIDE EFFECTS**	**NURSING CONSIDERATIONS**
Antidepressants buproprion (Zyban)	Weight loss, insomnia, restlessness, agitation, dry mouth, headache, tremors, excessive sweating, seizures, hypertension	Dose is different when used to treat depression. Begin drug therapy 1 week before cessation of smoking. Drug is contraindicated for pregnant or breast-feeding women. Use with alcohol increases seizure potential. Blood pressure increases when used with smoking or nicotine products for smoking cessation. This drug can induce psychotic behavior when combined with marijuana.
Nicotine Products Nicotine patch *(Nicoderm, Nicotrol, Habitrol)*	Itching, burning, or tingling at site of patch when first applied; tachycardia; increased blood pressure, redness at site when patch is removed Nicotine overdose: headaches, dizziness, upset stomach, vomiting, diarrhea, mental confusion, weakness, or fainting	Consult the physician if application site becomes swollen or very red. Caution client against wearing the patch and smoking or using tobacco products. Avoid if client is allergic to adhesive tape. Monitor blood pressure and heart rate. Keep away from children.
Nicotine gum *(Nicorette)*	Tachycardia, elevated blood pressure	Advise client to chew the gum slowly until a slight tingling occurs or a peppery taste is noted, then place it between the cheek and gum until the taste or tingling is almost gone. Explain that 9 to 12 pieces of gum per day usually control the urge to smoke, but up to 20 to 30 pieces of gum are safe depending on the strength of the gum. Use an alternate product if there is evidence of temporomandibular joint disease or the person has dentures or vulnerable dental work. Monitor blood pressure and heart rate. Keep away from children.
Nicotine inhaler	Cough and throat irritation, cardiac and central nervous system stimulation	Nicotine is delivered to the mouth and throat, where it is absorbed through the mucous membranes; the inhaler does not deliver nicotine to the lungs. Caution is necessary for people who have bronchospastic disease; drugs for asthma may need to be adjusted. Monitor blood pressure and heart rate. Keep away from children.
Nicotine nasal spray *(Nicotrol)*	Nasal and sinus irritation, cardiac and central nervous system stimulation	Instruct client to inhale when compressing the nasal pump to distribute nicotine to nasal mucosa. This is not to be used longer than 6 months. Monitor blood pressure and heart rate. Drug-seeking people may abuse this system. Keep away from children.

Sensory organs undergo slight changes. Hearing, which is most acute at approximately 14 years of age, gradually declines. Significant hearing loss, if identified at this time, is more likely associated with a history of childhood middle ear infections or exposure to loud music during adolescence.

Pregnancy-Related Changes

Pregnancy causes unique physical changes. The breasts and uterus enlarge. Circulatory volume increases. Skin pigmentation changes occur, the most obvious of which are darkening of the nipples and a brown line, called

BOX 7-1 ● Characteristics of Adult Maturity

- Developing personal self-reliance
- Learning from past experiences
- Communicating feelings
- Respecting others
- Coping with stressors
- Restraining impulses
- Being accountable
- Accepting consequences of decisions

the *linea nigra,* in the midline of the pregnant abdomen. In some women, a dark area across the cheeks and forehead develops, called *chloasma* or *mask of pregnancy.* The thyroid gland may increase in size because of metabolic changes. Posture and gait compensate for the shift in the center of gravity caused by the enlarging fetus. The lumbar curve is accentuated to resemble lordosis to accommodate the increasing abdominal girth.

Musculoskeletal System

Young adults in general are physically strong and resilient. They enjoy remarkable agility and stamina because the musculoskeletal system is functioning optimally. *Proprioception,* the ability to sense and coordinate body movements, and speed of reaction time reach their peak between 20 and 30 years of age. By approximately 20 years of age, changes in general appearance no longer take place as rapidly as during adolescence. Growth for nonpregnant women and most men is complete. Some men grow a few more inches between 18 and 20 years of age.

Upper body strength is greater among men than women because of their higher percentage of muscle fibers. Men also have athletic and fitness advantages because the greater size of their heart, lungs, and blood volume facilitates greater aerobic capacity. Because women have more subcutaneous fat than men, they have an advantage in using fat stores when necessary for additional energy (Murray & Zentner, 2001).

Integumentary System

Skin blemishes, a problem during puberty and adolescence, tend to resolve. Facial hair for young men is more widely distributed and requires daily shaving. Wisdom teeth or third molars, if present, erupt during early young adulthood. Men who inherit male pattern baldness may note early thinning or loss of hair at the hairline.

TATTOOS

Micropigmentation, the application of pigment to the skin, is used medically as an adjunct to procedures such as breast reconstruction surgery (see Chap. 60). It also has been used to recreate the appearance of eyebrows on persons who have lost their facial hair (see Chap. 69). A growing trend among young adults is to have a tattoo, a graphic design using permanently colored pigments, applied to their skin. Because the pigments in tattoo inks are not subject to regulation by the U.S. Food and Drug Administration (FDA) (2000), the nonmedical use poses several health risks. Allergies to the pigments can occur; once applied, the pigments are difficult or impossible to remove. The pigments also can interfere with the quality of magnetic resonance imaging (MRI) when the metallic components of the pigment interact during the procedure. Some have experienced swelling or burning in the area of the tattoo when undergoing an MRI.

Infection is another potential complication. Unless the equipment, including components that hold the needles, is sterilized, the potential exists for transmitting bloodborne infectious diseases, such as hepatitis (see Chap. 55) and acquired immunodeficiency syndrome (AIDS; see Chap. 43). For this reason, the American Association of Blood Banks rejects potential blood donors who have received a tattoo in the past year.

Other consequences of tattooing are physiologic consequences of traumatized integument. A granuloma, an inflammatory nodular lesion, may form as the result of a cellular attack waged against the particles in the tattoo pigment, which the body senses as foreign (see Chap. 41). Some persons, especially those with darkly pigmented skin, have a tendency to form keloids, an overgrowth of scar tissue (Fig. 7-3).

A common problem is that the person regrets ever having had a tattoo or is dissatisfied with its appearance. Although tattoos can be removed, the skin rarely returns to its pretattoo appearance. Some techniques for changing the skin's appearance include the following:

- Laser treatments, which tend only to lighten tattoos
- Dermabrasion, which mechanically rubs away the skin layers, sometimes leaving scar tissue in its place
- Salabrasion, which uses a salt solution rather than a sanding disc or wire brush to abrade the skin
- Scarification of the skin with an acid solution
- Plastic surgery, in which fluid-filled balloons are inserted under the skin to stretch it so that once the tattooed skin is removed, the wound edges can be approximated
- Retattooing to camouflage the existing tattoo

BODY PIERCING

Body piercing, the act of inserting a metal ring, barbell, or other device through the lips, cheeks, nose, tongue, eyebrow, or other areas, is a growing trend among young adults. Infection, allergic reactions, and bleeding are potential complications. The airway may become obstructed from swelling when the tongue is pierced. Oral devices can damage the teeth, interfere with speaking and swallowing, and cause respiratory complications if the objects are inhaled.

FIGURE 7-3 Ear keloid. (From Weber, J. & Kelley, J. [1998]. *Health assessment in nursing* (p. 145). Philadelphia: Lippincott Williams & Wilkins.)

Social Characteristics

The young adult's social network undergoes major changes: relationships with high school classmates dwindle after graduation; peer conformity loses its importance; and new acquaintances at college, work, or in the community replace former close friendships. Eventually, young persons establish their independence; develop their own lifestyles; form new relationships with friends, coworkers, and a significant other; and take on increasing responsibilities, such as working full-time and raising children. Education after high school and employment offer the means for achieving greater independence.

Marking the Transition

In the United States, identifying the end of adolescence and the beginning of young adulthood is difficult. The transition is less clear than it is in other, less industrialized cultures, where rituals provide formal rites of passage. For example, when boys are 16 years of age in aboriginal Australia, tradition dictates that they leave the village of their youth for a *walkabout*. A walkabout is a test of survival in which the solitary person must rely on his own skills and cunning to stay alive in the outback areas of the country for approximately 6 months. On return, the societal group accepts the adolescent as a mature adult.

Traditionally, the ultimate mark of adulthood in the United States was a person's ability to live independently of parental support. Before World War II, most adolescents were forced into assuming the role of adults very quickly. That trend has changed. Sociologists have observed that an immediate compulsion for adolescents to become independent members of society no longer exists. Instead, a

period called an **adolescent moratorium** seems to pass, during which persons aged 18 to 27 years may continue to live at home and be supported by their parents while working or going to school.

Society encourages individuals to prove they are ready for adulthood by participating in activities outside the home and school. Some become youth ministers in their churches; others do community service such as assisting older adults with minor repairs and yard work. Others experience a sense of indoctrination from life events that help demonstrate passage into maturity (Box 7-2).

Stop, Think, and Respond ● BOX 7-1
How is initiation into a gang or fraternity similar to a rite of passage like a walkabout?

Gender Roles

Developing the qualities that transform adolescents into mature adults is a gradual process. The development of gender roles is an example of an area that may become modified over time. **Gender role,** the set of behaviors ascribed by society as either feminine or masculine, continues to be refined during young adulthood. During this period, young adults may cling to or reject society's stereotypical notions about gender differences, such as men must make more money than women and women are the primary nurturers. Those who rigidly conform to established stereotypes may experience extreme conflict when circumstances, such as a traumatic injury or chronic disease, interfere with their perception of gender role. The best outcome occurs when young adults develop a perspective of androgeny. **Androgeny** is the belief that it is acceptable to perform roles that have been traditionally ascribed to men or women regardless of gender.

The feminist movement raised the consciousness of America to social and gender inequities. It liberated women from being homemakers to working full-time or part-time outside the home. Both sexes now feel more comfortable seeking employment in what were previously

---

BOX 7-2 ● Transitional Events From Adolescence to Adulthood

- Staying at home while parents are out of town
- Graduating from high school
- Enrolling in college
- Enlisting in the military
- Moving away from home
- Registering to vote
- Purchasing alcohol legally
- Applying for a personal loan
- Obtaining a credit card
- Getting married
- Parenting a child

gender-specific occupations and professions. For example, men are accepted in nursing, and women are accepted as physicians. Financial inequities still exist among women in male-dominated positions, however, and not nearly the same number of women are heads of businesses and corporations as are men.

Sexuality

Young adults are very sexually active and abortion is more common. By age 22 years, 90% of young adults have had a sexual relationship with one or more partners (Vander Zanden, 2000). Although AIDS is the leading cause of death among 25- to 44-year-old African-American men and the fifth leading cause of death among all races and both sexes in this age group (see Chap. 43), AIDS has had little effect on whether couples have unprotected sex. Many unmarried and nonmonogamous young adults use condoms only to prevent pregnancy. Consequently, if a woman is using a reliable contraceptive (e.g, taking an oral contraceptive), neither she nor her male partner is likely to use a condom during intercourse. The result is that many young adults are acquiring and spreading sexually transmitted diseases (STDs).

On a positive note, sexual promiscuity has decreased, meaning that when sexual intercourse occurs, it usually is between individuals who are involved in an ongoing social relationship. And, although young adults have multiple sex partners before marriage, the number of sexual contacts they have is fewer than those of previous generations. A small number of young adults are vowing to remain sexually abstinent until married.

Although heterosexuality is the norm, homosexuality does not carry the stigma it once did. Many gay men and lesbians have committed monogamous relationships.

Family Structures

Although some cohabiting adults choose to remain childless, most young adults marry and have children. More young adults, however, are marrying later in life than age mates of previous generations. The average age for marriage is now 25 to 26 years (Vander Zanden, 2000). Later age at marriage contributes to smaller family sizes. Many women wait until their 30s and even 40s to have their first child. State-of-the-art reproductive technology is facilitating pregnancies for women who previously would have been childless, such as perimenopausal women, single women, and lesbians. Some couples with infertility may feel unfulfilled. Nurses can refer childless couples to local and international agencies that provide adoptive services.

A **nuclear family,** or **traditional family,** consists of a married man and woman with biologic offspring. Other family variations are common. A **single-parent family** is one in which one biologic parent provides for the well-being of one or more children. A **blended family** refers to a married couple who are caretakers of children from each spouse's previous marriage(s). An **extended family** is multigenerational.

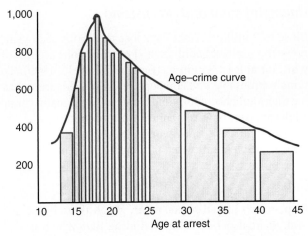

FIGURE 7-4 Age–crime curve. (Source: http://www.urban.org/crime/module/butts/youth_violence.html)

Prevalent Psychosocial Problems

Young adults face many crises, including job insecurity, unemployment, and sexual harassment. Crime and violence are national problems that involve young adults to a high degree (Fig. 7-4). The highest rates of violent crime (i.e., murder, forcible rape, aggravated assault, robbery) occur among those aged 15 to 25 years (Butts, 1999). The fact that the leading cause of death among 18- to 35-year-olds is homicide supports the validity of crime statistics (Fig. 7-5). In 1995, 77% of murder victims were male, and 88% were 18 years of age or older (U.S. Department of Justice, 1996). Crime also includes such problems as rape and domestic violence.

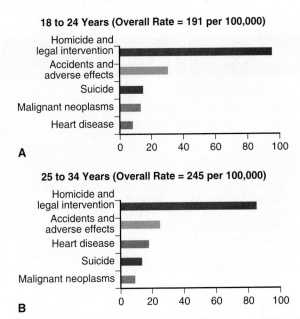

FIGURE 7-5 Top five causes of death among young adults (**A**) age 18 to 24, and (**B**) age 25 to 34. Note that homicide greatly surpasses other causes of death. (Source: http://iihe.org/information/Datebook1996/T17_DeathCausesLeadingAge.htm)

Unemployment and Downsizing

Close to 2 million Americans lose their jobs each year; more than 20% of adults who lose their jobs are out of work for at least 6 months (Carson & Arnold, 1999). To remain profitable and competitive, employers are reducing their numbers of full-time workers. Thus, many young adults are part-time, temporary, and subcontracted workers. Consequently, many working young adults do not receive health insurance and other full-time benefits.

Rape

Rape is any forced sexual act in which there is vaginal, oral, or anal penetration, including that which is performed with an inserted object. Rape occurs even if the victim consents out of fear of violence or death. Rape is a crime. It is not motivated by a desire for sex. Rather, it is a manifestation of a need for dominance and control and uses sex as a weapon.

Although women are the usual victims and men are the usual perpetrators, rape can occur regardless of gender. Rape even occurs among gays and lesbians. Rape statistics are unreliable because an estimated 84% of cases are unreported. Researchers believe that one of every three women will be raped in her lifetime (District of Columbia Rape Crisis Center, 1998).

TYPES OF RAPE

There are three general types of rape: (1) *stranger rape,* in which the victim does not know the perpetrator; (2) *marital rape,* which involves spouses; and (3) *date rape,* also called *acquaintance rape,* in which the victim knows the assailant. Date rapes account for more than 60% of all rapes (University of Nebraska Extension Center, 2001).

BOX 7-3 ● Advice for Rape Prevention

- Install deadbolt locks on doors.
- Keep ground floor windows and patio doors secured.
- Use a door viewer to identify visitors.
- Do not let a stranger into your home or apartment.
- Avoid going alone to a basement laundry room in an apartment building.
- Use your first initial and last name on your mailbox and phone listing.
- Ask a friend to accompany you on walks; some colleges and universities have volunteers that will escort students to and from their dormitory to other places on campus such as the library.
- Carry a whistle and keys in your hand while walking alone.
- Yell, "Call 911. I'm being attacked" rather than "Help," to which few people respond.
- Avoid listening to tapes, compact discs, or radios with earphones while walking; it may distract your attention.
- Park in well-lit areas.
- Stay in your locked car when there is a mechanical problem and put on flashing hazard lights.
- Ask someone to call the police rather than leave your car.
- Keep your distance if someone asks for information from a car.

Gang rape, which is less common, involves several perpetrators (Fontaine & Fletcher, 1997). Box 7-3 gives information on methods of preventing rape.

Stop, Think, and Respond ● BOX 7-2

A female college student returns to her apartment after spending the evening at the library. Her boyfriend, who has been waiting there, accuses her of being out with another man. He pulls her into the bedroom and insists on having sex. The woman resists, but her boyfriend says, "If you love me, prove it." They have sex. Has a rape occurred?

DATE-RAPE DRUGS

Of all the drugs that potentiate date rape, alcohol is the most common substance involved. From one half to two thirds of all rapes occur when one or both people are drinking alcohol, which causes disinhibition and impaired judgment.

Since 1993, the combination of alcohol and flunitrazepam (Rohypnol), known as the *date-rape drug,* has increased the ease with which rape can occur. Rohypnol, sometimes called "Rophie" for short, potentiates alcohol and interferes with memory. Rapists often give Rohypnol, which is illegal in the United States, to unknowing victims. The drug is tasteless, colorless, odorless, and dissolves quickly in drinks. Sedation occurs within 15 to 20 minutes after ingestion and lasts for approximately 6 hours (U.S. Department of Justice, Drug Enforcement Agency, 2001). There is temporary paralysis of the limbs, an inability to speak, and finally unconsciousness. Some awaken briefly during an assault but cannot defend themselves. For 1 to 2 days after the drug-induced stupor, victims experience the equivalent of a very bad hangover.

Without the ability to recall the event—or just a dreamlike quality to the memory—these types of rapes go unreported. If a victim reports that he or she suspects having been raped, proving that flunitrazepam was used is difficult because the drug becomes undetectable in the blood 4 hours after its ingestion. Its metabolites can be identified in urine for up to 72 hours, but blood is tested more often than urine in rape cases. If the victim waits too long to act on his or her suspicion of rape, the delay may extend beyond the window of opportunity to detect the drug's metabolites.

A third drug that has been used to incapacitate a victim for the commission of sexual assault is gamma-hydroxybutyrate (GHB). GHB is an abused central nervous system depressant that produces drowsiness, dizziness, unconsciousness, seizures, severe respiratory depression, and coma. GHB has a salty taste when consumed in a drink. As of March 2000, the FDA has classified GHB as a Schedule I controlled substance, making GHB illegal to possess, buy, or sell. See Client and Family Teachings 7-1.

7-1 *Client and Family Teaching*
Avoiding Rape Drugs

To avoid being drugged and subsequently raped, the nurse can teach clients the following:

- Do not accept alcoholic beverages from strangers.
- Report seeing someone dropping any substance into a drink.
- Open all cans or bottles of beverages yourself.
- Avoid mixed drinks served in glasses.
- Never leave a drink unattended while dancing or using the rest room.
- Watch as any mixed drink is being prepared.
- Seek medical attention if you think you have been drugged.

RAPE AVOIDANCE TECHNIQUES

Predicting rape is difficult. Rapists, however, often are controlling men who lose their tempers easily, are jealous, become physically or verbally abusive, and do not tolerate differences of opinion very well. What may seem to be minimal faults early in a relationship can escalate into something more serious later.

Trusting one's instincts always is best. If a person has the slightest premonition that a situation may become dangerous, it is important to leave. The longer a possible victim remains in the immediate environment, the greater is the potential for rape. If there is no avenue for escape, the person should say "No!" with conviction. Potential victims of rape should avoid smiling when saying "No" because it may send a mixed message. They should say the word "rape" to emphasize the seriousness of what may happen. Emotionally charged words often cause a potential rapist to reconsider the consequences of persisting. If aborting an attack is impossible, the victim should resist if it is safe to do so. Resisting is foolhardy, however, if the rapist may have a weapon.

CARING FOR RAPE VICTIMS

Rape victims need treatment as soon as possible after the assault. Feelings of shame, fear, and disbelief often interfere with obtaining appropriate care. Those who do seek medical attention often display one of two emotional responses: expressive or controlled. The *expressive style* of response is one in which the victim cries or sobs and is restless, hyperalert, and tense. The *controlled style* of response is one in which the victim is calm, composed, and subdued (Carson & Arnold, 1999). Because a controlled response contradicts the stereotypical expectation, victims with controlled responses are sometimes less likely to be believed than those who are intensely emotional. Nurses should not assume that a person who remains controlled has been any less traumatized by the rape than one who is expressive. Above all, healthcare workers and law enforcement officers must believe all victims who say

they have been raped and convey that the rape was not the victim's fault.

The rape victim must not bathe or shower, douche, or destroy clothing. Initial treatment involves attending to injuries, providing prophylaxis against pregnancy and STDs, giving emotional support, and collecting legal evidence. Nursing Care Plan 7-1 provides extensive information on nursing care and management of rape.

Rape victims sometimes experience long-term consequences of their attack, especially those who refuse counseling or are not referred for counseling. Clients who have been raped are at risk for the development of post-traumatic stress disorder (see Chap. 14).

Domestic Violence

The notion that all couples and families "live happily ever after" is false. Unfortunately, some loving relationships turn violent. **Domestic violence** is a pattern of physical, sexual, and psychological attacks that adults use to control their intimate relationships (Gerard, 2000). Domestic violence involves:

- Couples who are or were formerly married, living together, or dating
- People related by blood, marriage, or adoption
- Couples who have one or more minor children in common

The statistics on domestic violence are staggering. Although men are battered, in approximately 95% of cases, men are the batterers. One woman in four is physically abused by her partner (Gerard, 2000), resulting in 2 to 3 million severe assaults every year. A woman is beaten every 15 seconds, and 2000 to 4000 women are murdered every year by their husbands or live-in boyfriends (Fontaine & Fletcher, 1997). Abusive partners often have lived with and observed their own parents' violent relationships, which conditions them to believe that violence in a relationship is normal. Other reasons that cause a person to become violent include feelings of inadequacy, depression, and substance abuse.

Physical abuse is obvious by the resulting injuries. If physical abuse is occurring, other types of abuse usually are too. Psychological abuse includes verbal insults, threats that create fear for one's life (especially if the victim reveals the abuse to others), isolation, and control over daily activities. Batterers of spouses or partners commonly abuse children as well.

PATTERN OF DOMESTIC VIOLENCE

Most cases of domestic violence follow a three-stage pattern: tension-building, acute battering, and a honeymoon period. During the *tension-building phase,* which may last several years, there is verbal abuse and minor forms of physical abuse such as slapping and shoving. The *acute battering phase* is manifested by overt violence like choking, breaking bones, or using a weapon. This phase usu-

Nursing Care Plan 7-1

THE CLIENT WHO HAS BEEN RAPED

Assessment

- Ask the client:
  - Time, location, and circumstances of the attack
  - Identity of perpetrator, if known
  - Description of perpetrator, if unknown
  - Type of sexual assault: oral, vaginal, anal
  - For female client, date of last menstrual period
  - Current use of condom or other contraceptive by victim or perpetrator
  - Date of last consensual intercourse
  - Current or recent treatment for sexually transmitted disease (STD)
  - Who to call for emotional support and safety after treatment
  - If a rape crisis advocate can be contacted
  - If the client needs temporary shelter on discharge
- Examine the client for physical injuries.

Nursing Diagnosis: Rape Trauma Syndrome

Expected Outcome: Client will work through feelings associated with rape and recover from the experience.

Interventions	Rationales
Ensure privacy but remain with client at all times.	Privacy ensures client's dignity. Staying with client reduces fear and anxiety.
Convey that the rape was not the client's fault.	Many rape victims blame themselves; dispel this false belief.
Remain nonjudgmental.	Clients often feel unjustifiably ashamed and guilty.
Ask permission to photograph client and areas of injury.	Giving the opportunity to decide restores a sense of control for client; photographs demonstrate the magnitude of rape and physical assault to a jury.
Identify each person involved in client's care and treatment and the purpose for his or her involvement.	Client may feel revictimized when approached by strangers. Information reduces anxiety.
Explain the process of collecting evidence.	Evidence is necessary for future legal prosecution. Even if the client does not want to prosecute the perpetrator, he or she may change that decision in the future.
Obtain a rape evidence kit.	Successful prosecution of the perpetrator depends on collecting physical evidence.
Assist client with removing outer garments and underwear, and place them in evidence bag.	Semen, blood, and hairs can be used to match the DNA of the rapist.
Assist physician to collect hair from client's head and pubic area.	Samples of client hair can be differentiated from that of the rapist and matched for DNA evidence.
Help obtain swabs and smears from vagina, penis, mouth, and anus.	Body fluids such as semen can be used to identify the DNA of the rapist. Specimens also are needed to diagnose and treat STDs.
Collect saliva and blood samples. Scrape or clip fingernails and deposit specimens in the evidence kit.	Saliva and blood are used for comparing the client's DNA with DNA of the rape suspect.

(continued)

Nursing Care Plan 7-1 (Continued)

THE CLIENT WHO HAS BEEN RAPED

Interventions	*Rationales*
Seal and mark all specimens placed in the evidence kit.	A rapist may go free if the identification or its chain of custody are questionable.
Perform tests for STDs.	A potential outcome of rape is infection.
Offer and explain the purpose of postcoital contraception.	Postcoital contraception prevents implantation of a fertilized ovum and avoids pregnancy.
Notify a support person, rape crisis counselor, or both.	The support of a significant other and encouragement to process the rape verbally help reduce the potential for post-traumatic stress disorder.
Offer client an opportunity to shower after physical evidence has been obtained.	Meeting hygiene needs helps to eliminate the physical and emotional trauma of being sexually violated.
Provide disposable underwear and a scrub suit until client has access to personal clothing.	Clean clothing restores dignity.
Arrange for temporary shelter in a safe house if client fears returning home.	Client may have flashbacks of the rape if he or she returns to the place of the assault before feeling a measure of safety.
Arrange a referral for long-term counseling.	Individual and group therapy helps clients recover from psychological trauma.
Schedule a date for medical follow-up.	Postdischarge assessment will verify prevention of pregnancy and prevention or appropriate management of STDs.

Evaluation of Expected Outcome: Client returns to a level of functioning similar to that before the rape.

---

ally lasts for 24 hours or less. During the *honeymoon phase,* which shortly follows the acute battering phase, the batterer appears remorseful and behaves in ways to convince the victim that he or she will be nonviolent. For example, the batterer may send flowers or give some other token of affection. Most victims want to believe that the relationship will improve, and they may even blame themselves for triggering the violent episode. As tension returns, however, the cycle of violence is repeated.

CARING FOR VICTIMS OF DOMESTIC VIOLENCE

Nurses are likely to see female victims of domestic violence in emergency departments. These women often come alone and present with repeated injuries (particularly to the head, upper body, and breasts) or stress-related disorders. Previous hospital records may be linked to repeated abuse; in fact, acts of violence and subsequent injuries tend to escalate in severity over time. During the history, the client's explanation for the injury may be incompatible with the extent of the trauma.

Unlike cases of child abuse, nurses are not obligated to report their suspicions of abuse between partners to legal authorities. But nurses can intervene in other ways, as discussed in Nursing Guidelines 7-1.

NURSING IMPLICATIONS

When caring for young adults, nurses must be aware of common patterns of behavior that affect the health and well-being of individuals in this age group. Because they are seeking healthcare for the first time as adults, clients in this age group have minimal knowledge of community healthcare resources. In addition, nurses are likely to find that young adults tend to seek healthcare only when they experience an emergency. In many cases, young adults delay seeking medical care because they cannot pay for treatment.

Health Promotion

Nurses should understand that young adults perceive themselves as perpetually healthy and invincible. Consequently, many disregard early warning signs of diseases. They often do not consider preventive health measures a priority and disregard healthy behaviors such as obtaining early prenatal care, performing breast or testicular self-examinations, or scheduling regular health and dental examinations. Nurses can distribute educational materials about important health promotion measures at local

NURSING GUIDELINES 7-1

Interventions in Cases of Domestic Violence

- Ask the client directly if the injuries are the result of physical abuse.

- Assess if the client wants help in leaving the batterer. A woman may choose to remain in an abusive relationship for several reasons (Table 7-2), and nurses must respect her choice. Danger is actually greatest when a woman attempts to terminate the relationship with the batterer. According to Gerard (2000, p. 56), "About 70% of intimate partner violence victims who are murdered die either as they're trying to leave or after they've moved."

- Discuss safe places to which the person can retreat when there is a potential for future violence. If escape is impossible, rooms to avoid include the bathroom (where no exit is possible) and rooms where weapons may be kept (kitchen or bedroom).

- Tell the victim to memorize the phone numbers of people who can help during an altercation to eliminate the time it takes to look them up. The victim should develop a "code word" with phone contacts to alert them to the need for assistance.

- Provide the address and phone number of one or more domestic assault shelters; shelters house victims and their children for 4 to 6 weeks while providing food, counseling, and help with finding employment, alternative housing, and financial assistance.

- Explain the process of obtaining an emergency **personal protection order,** a document that forbids contact between the batterer and victim for a specified period, or a **temporary**

restraining order, a legal directive issued by a court that requires that the batterer avoid all contact with the victim.

- Advise the client to call the local police if her physical safety has been threatened. Police are more likely to arrest a person who violates a court-ordered directive.

- Recommend that the client insist that the responding police officers complete an official report and write down the number of the report before leaving so it can be accessed in the future.

- Encourage the client to press charges against the batterer; however, the prosecuting attorney makes the final decision about whether to prosecute a batterer based on whether the evidence is sufficient to win the case.

- Tell the victim to contact the Legal Aid Office or Friend of the Court for legal assistance. A batterer may be tried in a civil court more successfully than in a criminal court (as was the case involving O. J. Simpson).

- Suggest that the police or a friend photograph any evidence of physical injury that may be used in court if the victim brings criminal charges against the batterer.

- Offer the phone number of the community mental health association where therapists are available for crisis intervention and group and family therapy.

- Recommend discussing personal safety with an employer and the employer's security officer; provide a photograph of the abuser.

community health fairs. They may also speak to members of service organizations like the Rotary Club, Big Brothers and Big Sisters, and 4-H leaders.

Illness and Hospitalization

Young adults continue to adjust to their physical characteristics and to work through feelings about sexuality.

They are apt to develop great anxiety when faced with a medical examination or need for surgery. Carefully explaining necessary procedures is essential, as is providing privacy. Such measures convey to young adults that the nurse is concerned about their welfare, understands their feelings, and respects their need for dignity. During database interviews, the nurse often finds that young adult clients have no knowledge about their family's health history or their personal history of childhood diseases. For

TABLE 7-2	REASONS PEOPLE REMAIN IN ABUSIVE RELATIONSHIPS	
EMOTIONAL	**FINANCIAL**	**SOCIAL**
Fear for life	Lack of employment	Lack of support from friends and family
Hope that the batterer will change	No access to cash or bank assets	Acceptance of responsibility for saving the relationship
Belief that batterer is basically a good person		Blame of batterer's behavior on substance abuse, finances, or job-related stressors
Belief that batterer has more good qualities than bad		Correlation of ending the relationship with failure
		Protection of public image of family
		Belief that it is better for children to be raised by two people rather than one
		Lack of knowledge about a means to end the relationship
		Desire to protect children from greater harm

this reason, nurses need to collaborate with a family member or rely on past medical records to obtain a comprehensive health history.

During hospitalization, young adults are as frightened as younger clients but show their fear in less obvious ways. The nurse must realize that young adults also require reassurance, even though they tend to conceal their need for it. The nurse is especially supportive of young adults by allowing them to express ideas and ask questions about matters that interest or concern them, and by conveying respect for them as individuals. The nurse also helps young adults cope with their illness, whether temporary or permanent, and teaches them preventive healthcare measures.

Human Immunodeficiency Virus

Nurses who work in public health agencies, acute care settings, and long-term healthcare facilities are likely to see an increase in young adults diagnosed with human immunodeficiency virus (HIV) infection. Individuals infected with HIV can remain asymptomatic for 10 years or more, yet they are capable of transmitting the virus to others. This information indicates a need for nurses to educate teenagers and adults about the advantages of sexual abstinence, maintaining monogamous relationships with uninfected partners, or using other safer sex practices. Unfortunately, when HIV becomes active, infected adults succumb to and need treatment for opportunistic infections and eventually require terminal care (see Chap. 43).

 GENERAL NUTRITIONAL CONSIDERATIONS

Lean body mass and basal metabolic rate peak in early adulthood and then gradually decline each successive decade. If a person does not decrease calorie intake or physical activity decreases, he or she will experience gradual weight gain.

Because peak bone mass is not attained until 30 to 35 years of age, young adults must consume adequate calcium to maximize bone density. The Recommended Daily Allowance (RDA) for calcium and other bone-building nutrients was replaced in the fall of 1997 with new Dietary Reference Intakes (DRIs). For young adults, the recommendation for calcium intake increased to 1000 mg daily or at least three servings from the Milk Group.

Young adults may outgrow irregular eating habits, reliance on fast food, and frequent fad dieting as they mature and adopt a more stable lifestyle.

Despite counseling for wellness promotion, young adults may not recognize the long-term value of a healthful diet.

Vitamin supplements are widely used, though only a few groups actually need them: people on very low-calorie diets, strict vegetarians, pregnant and lactating women, people with malabsorption disorders and certain other chronic diseases, and people who use specific medications that interfere with vitamin absorption or metabolism.

 GENERAL PHARMACOLOGIC CONSIDERATIONS

Caution all clients who take medication after discharge from the hospital about combining the use of prescription drugs with nonprescription drugs unless approved by the physician. Interactions of various drugs can cause serious adverse effects.

Although the incidence of acne declines in young adults, some cases persist. Warn young women prescribed isotretinoin (Accutane) for severe acne that this drug has been associated with birth defects. Under no circumstances should pregnancy occur while a woman is taking this drug. Effective contraception is essential during administration of and for 1 month after discontinuing the drug. If pregnancy is suspected, the client must stop the medication and notify the healthcare provider immediately.

Caution all young adults about mixing medications (both over-the-counter and prescription) with alcohol. Alcohol potentiates the action of many drugs.

If pregnant, women must not take any drug, legal or illegal, prescription or nonprescription, unless a healthcare provider prescribes or recommends the use of the drug.

Critical Thinking Exercises

1. *What data would suggest that a person has positively adjusted to young adulthood?*
2. *When planning a health promotion program for a group of young adults, what topics are most important to include?*

References and Suggested Readings

Brown, J. K., Whittemore, K. T., Knapp, T. R., et al. (2000). Is arm span an accurate measure of height in young and middle-age adults? *Clinical Nursing Research, 9*(1), 84–94.

Butts, J. (1999). Youth violence: Perception versus reality. [On-line.] Available: http://www.urban.org/crime/module/butts/youth_violence.html.

Carson, V. B., & Arnold, E. N. (1999). *Mental health nursing.* Philadelphia: W.B. Saunders.

District of Columbia Rape Crisis Center. (1998). [On-line.] Available: http://dcrcc.org/. Accessed February 5, 2001.

Fontaine, K. L., & Fletcher, J. S. (1997). *Essentials of mental health nursing* (3rd ed.). Redwood City, CA: Addison-Wesley.

Gerard, M. (2000). Domestic violence, how to screen and intervene. *RN, 63*(12), 52–56.

LePage, J. P., et al. (2000). The impact of the number of young adults on an inpatient psychiatric unit. *Journal of Psychosocial Nursing and Mental Health Services, 38*(1), 33–36, 38–39.

Murray, R. B., & Zentner, J. P. (2001). *Health promotion strategies through the life span* (7th ed.). Upper Saddle River, NJ: Prentice Hall.

National Institutes of Health. (1998). First federal obesity clinical guidelines released. [On-line.] Available: http://www.nih.gov/news/pr/jun98/nhlbi-17.htm.

Patterson, D. L., et al. (1999). Adolescent health transitions: focus group study of teens and young adults with special health needs. *Family and Community Health, 22*(2), 43–58.

University of Nebraska Cooperation Extension (2001). [On-line.] Available: http://www.ianr.unl.edu/pubs/family/nf244.htm.

U.S. Department of Health and Human Services, Office of Disease Prevention and Health Promotion. (2000). *Healthy people 2010.* [On-line.] Available: http:www.health.gov. healthypeople/.

U.S. Department of Justice, Federal Bureau of Investigation. (1996). Uniform crime reporting program press release. [On-line.] Available: http://www.fbi.gov/ucr/ucr95prs.htm.

U.S. Department of Justice, Drug Enforcement Agency. (2001). Gamma hydroxybutyrate (GHB). [On-line.] Available: http:// usdoj.gov/dea/concern/ghb.htm

U.S. Food and Drug Administration. (2000). Tattoos and permanent makeup. [On-line.] Available: http://vm.cfsan.fda. gov/~dms/cos-204.html.

Vander Zanden, J. W. (2000). *Human development* (7th ed.). Boston: McGraw-Hill.

Biopsychosocial Aspects of Caring for Middle-Aged Adults

Words to Know

basal metabolic rate (BMR)
climacteric
generativity
keratotic lesion
menopause
midlife crisis
osteoporosis
presbycusis
presbyopia
sandwich generation
stagnation

Learning Objectives

On completion of this chapter, the reader will:

- List the developmental tasks associated with middle age.
- Discuss the two characteristics associated with the tasks of middle-age development.
- Describe the physical, social, and emotional characteristics of middle-aged adults.
- Discuss at least three unique problems that nurses deal with when caring for middle-aged adults.

Middle age, generally from ages 35 to 65 years, is characterized as the "established years." During this period, the person has a chance to actualize the earlier struggles of youth, adolescence, and young adulthood to establish a home and career. Middle-aged adults have the opportunity to analyze their assets and channel their energies into accomplishing life goals that remain unfulfilled. The middle years are characterized by the pursuit of activities that provide self-satisfaction and community responsibility.

GROWTH AND DEVELOPMENT

Demographics

Currently, middle-aged Americans comprise about one fifth of the U.S. population. Many of these Americans entered the job market and made their way in the labor force during the late 1960s and 1970s. Now, one American turns 50 years old every 7.6 seconds. Each middle-aged adult is experiencing life stresses and major changes. Many are feeling the psychological pressures associated with the shift from the industrial age to the information age.

Developmental Stages and Tasks

The task of terminating early adulthood involves reviewing the past, considering how one's life is going, and deciding the future. Many people begin to experience the gap between earlier life aspirations and current achievements. They may wonder if they should continue with earlier life choices. During this period, a person may choose a different career path or redefine his or her current roles. This is a time when people take "stock" of current life situations, analyze, and make necessary adjustments.

Triggered by the realization that life is rapidly advancing, the middle years are a time when adults take inventory of their lives. As young adults, these people focused on setting goals. As middle adults, they evaluate if, and how well, they are achieving their goals.

Middle-aged adults are more likely to philosophically ponder the purpose for and value of their existence. With the knowledge that their remaining years are limited, they want to survey their achievements and pursue opportunities for self-fulfillment, a characteristic referred to as **generativity.** Middle-aged adults become more caring, giving, and productive. Many spend time comforting, advising, and listening to younger family members or close friends and volunteering in civic activities to contribute to the community.

On self-examination, however, some middle-aged adults are disappointed to find that they have not invested their energies wisely. The feeling that they have accomplished nothing of true significance, along with a lack of commitment to future endeavors, is referred to as **stagnation.** Box 8-1 summarizes the major developmental tasks of the middle-aged adult.

MIDDLE ADULTHOOD

Physical Characteristics

The middle years are productive years, yet the pace of living changes subtly. Evidence of declining physical abilities becomes apparent. The incidence of various health problems increases with age. About 35 million Americans (1 in 7) have disabilities ranging from arthritis, diabetes, and emphysema to mental disorders. People can maximize their chances for a healthy, long life by altering their lifestyles to include various health-conscious practices such as exercising regularly and eating a healthy diet.

The human body, which has been functioning optimally for several decades, tends to work less efficiently. Early signs of aging appear, which can be traumatic, especially in the U.S. culture, which emphasizes youth and glamour.

Weight

As a person moves into middle adulthood, weight becomes a concern. About 50% of the adult population weighs above the upper limit of normal. About 40% become overweight as a result of genetics. Others become overweight from changes in the **basal metabolic rate (BMR),** the minimum energy a person uses in a resting state. Sex and age affect BMR, which decreases quickly during adolescence and then more slowly during adulthood. Decreased BMR is caused by a change in the ratio of lean body mass to fat. Thus, if a person continues to eat the same foods, he or she will gain weight.

BOX 8-1 ● Major Developmental Tasks of the Middle-Aged Adult

- Reassessing life accomplishments and goals
- Adjusting to role changes
- Accepting physical, emotional, and social changes associated with middle age
- Planning for retirement
- Strengthening relationships with spouse, family, friends, or companions
- Adjusting to responsibilities for aging parents
- Developing skills, hobbies, or activities that provide satisfaction

---

Adults tend not to exercise routinely, which compounds weight gain. Added weight is responsible for many health problems. Adults with weight problems need to work closely with their physicians and a nutritionist who can assist with meal planning. Adults should avoid fad diets and crash diets because they do more harm than good. Eating properly and following a routine exercise program can ward off unwanted pounds.

Respiratory System

The lungs begin to change. The extent of such changes depends on lifestyle, predisposition to illnesses such as asthma, and environmental hazards. Staying active and either walking or engaging in some form of aerobic exercise will maintain lung function.

Smoking is a serious problem in the United States and leads to many health deficits such as emphysema, lung cancer, and chronic lung changes and conditions. Smoking is the number one controllable cause of cancer, responsible for at least 30% of cancer deaths. Various smoke reduction programs are available to those who wish to make this lifestyle change.

Cardiovascular System

Cardiovascular disease is the leading killer of adults today. Genetics and lifestyle play important roles. Men are at higher risk compared with premenopausal women; however, the risks equalize for men and women after menopause. African-American men are at a higher risk of heart disease than are white men.

Arteries continue to fill with deposits of fat, while calcium infiltrates the fatty plaque, making the arteries hard and inelastic. Mild hypertension (high blood pressure) is a common sign of early heart disease and also can affect the kidneys and brain. Diet, exercise, and medications can help reduce high blood pressure. Regular blood pressure screenings several times a year are recommended during the middle years.

Cholesterol, a white, waxy fat that occurs naturally in the body, has become the "buzzword" in health since the 1990s. The National Cholesterol Education Program suggests regular testing of cholesterol levels starting at 20 years of age. Dietary changes to reduce consumption of saturated fats and increasing the activity level through regular exercise can raise the beneficial high-density lipoprotein cholesterol and lower the damaging low-density lipoprotein cholesterol. Educating adults about maintaining a healthy lifestyle by watching their weight, decreasing salt intake, decreasing cholesterol and fats, decreasing alcohol intake, decreasing or stopping smoking, learning stress management techniques, and increasing exercise can reduce the risk of hypertension and cardiac problems.

Neurologic System

Intellectual and stimulating hobbies, such as reading, working with computer programs, and solving crossword puzzles, can slow the process of brain cell loss. Other factors can affect brain activity, such as alcohol intake or a physical disease such as cerebrovascular accident (stroke), Parkinson's disease, or Alzheimer's disease. A cerebrovascular accident occurs when blood circulation to the brain fails. Brain cells can die from decreased blood flow and the resulting lack of oxygen. Both blockage and bleeding can be involved. Stroke is the third leading killer of Americans and the most common cause of disability. Each year more that 500,000 Americans have a stroke, with about 145,000 dying. Strokes occur in all age groups, both sexes, and all races.

Cognition and Sensory Perception

Visual accommodation, the ability to focus an image on the retina, gradually declines. Between 40 and 50 years of age, many people notice difficulty in reading small print or performing other tasks that require close vision. This condition, called **presbyopia,** results from a loss of elasticity in the lens of the eye. Because the lens tends to be more rigid, middle-aged adults need more time to adjust to rapid changes in light and darkness. Changes in the lens, such as thickening, decreased flexibility, and increased opacity, cause glare sensitivity. Other eye conditions, such as glaucoma, dry eye, or floaters, can appear. Another condition called *macular degeneration* can fade, distort, or blur vision. Annual eye examinations may prevent many of these eye conditions.

Presbycusis is hearing loss associated with aging. High-pitched sounds diminish first. Some people, particularly those in their later middle years, find that the decrease interferes with hearing and communicating with others.

Teeth strength may begin to decline, which can cause tooth loss. Dental examinations every 6 months are recommended.

Taste buds are replaced at a slower rate, which may account for changes in food-related tastes. Smell receptors begin to deteriorate, also affecting the sense of taste.

Reproductive System

Couples have a variety of contraceptive measures available to limit family size during their reproductive years. The use of oral contraceptives, however, especially among middle-aged women who smoke, increases the risk for blood clot formation.

Climacteric refers to abrupt changes in the body caused by alterations in the secretion and balance of reproductive hormones. Women between 40 and 55 years of age experience a dramatic physiologic change in the reproductive system known as **menopause** (see Chap. 59). Ovulation becomes irregular toward late middle life and eventually ceases. Reduced estrogen also causes changes in female secondary sex characteristics (Box 8-2).

As men age, the ability to achieve and sustain an erection slightly diminishes, and the prostate gland enlarges. Male fertility extends long past that of women.

BOX 8-2 ● **Secondary Sex Changes With Decreased Estrogen**

- Breasts begin to droop and sag.
- Vaginal mucous membranes become dry and easily irritated.
- Pubic hair becomes sparse and gray.
- Vaginal lubrication decreases.
- Mood swings are common.
- Hot flashes and headaches occur.
- Bones become more brittle as a result of loss of calcium.
- Vascular changes are accelerated.

Midlife men and women remain at risk for human immunodeficiency virus (HIV) infection and acquired immunodeficiency syndrome (AIDS). The number of cases among middle-aged and older women has been steadily increasing, mainly among postmenopausal women who no longer use barrier forms of birth control. Because of their age or monogamous marital status, these women do not see themselves as being at risk for HIV/AIDS or other sexually transmitted diseases (STDs). Health providers also do not regularly ask for sexual histories or test for HIV/AIDS/STDs in this population. Anyone who is sexually active with multiple partners, however, is at risk for HIV/AIDS (see Chap. 43).

Urinary System

Men older than 50 years of age begin to notice slight changes in urinary patterns, such as hesitancy, reduced force of urinary stream, or fullness in the bladder. These signs are indicators of prostatic hypertrophy (see Chap. 61). Women who have had several children often experience stress incontinence from a relaxation of the pelvic floor muscles. Coughing, sneezing, or laughing may cause leakage of urine.

Musculoskeletal System

Height remains constant until the late stages of middle adulthood, when there is a slight decline. Adipose and connective tissues gradually replace muscle mass, which compromises strength. Muscles can begin to atrophy, although this development is less noticeable in men. Regular exercise that combines both cardiovascular techniques with strength training can prevent most muscle aging.

Range of joint motion diminishes from a sedentary lifestyle or damage to joints from hard work. Bone mass becomes increasingly porous, particularly in women after menopause, leading to osteoporosis. Women should begin a regimen of calcium supplements or drugs that prevent bone resorption as recommended by their physician. For some, these debilitating processes can go unnoticed until a simple injury has serious consequences, such as a fracture or delayed healing.

Another disorder that surfaces in middle age is rheumatoid arthritis (RA), an inflammatory disease that causes pain, swelling, and loss of joint function (see Chap. 67). Some people have mild forms of RA; others live with serious disability. Physicians classify RA as an autoimmune disease, which means that the person's own immune system is attacking his or her own body tissue (see Chap. 42). Although no single test for RA is available, especially in its early stages, laboratory and radiographic tests can determine the extent of bone damage and monitor the progression of this disease. See Chapter 67 for more detail about treatment and nursing management of RA.

Integumentary System

Subcutaneous fat disappears toward the end of the middle-age period, giving the face a bony appearance. Age lines or wrinkles are evident at the forehead, corners of the eyes, and mouth. The skin appears wrinkled and dry from chronic exposure to the sun.

Keratotic lesions, elevated, darkly pigmented skin plaques, appear as moles on the scalp, face, neck, or trunk (Fig. 8-1). The hair loses texture and color. Baldness becomes more evident among men. Change in the balance of estrogen and testosterone causes facial hair or hair growth about the nipples and chest area in postmenopausal women.

Stop, Think, and Respond ● BOX 8-1

What advice would you give to "sun worshippers?"

Social Characteristics

During middle age, most adults remain socially involved with many relatives and friends. As their children marry, the social network of middle-aged adults expands to include sons- and daughters-in-law. When children leave home, middle-aged couples have more time to spend with

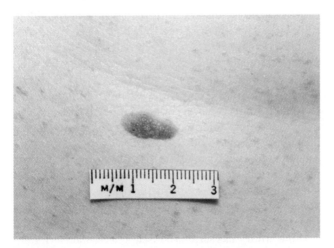

FIGURE 8-1 Keratotic lesion. (Courtesy of Ken Timby)

each other. For many couples, this strengthens the relationship. Others, however, find that the relationship has changed since the years of childrearing, causing them to feel distant and estranged from each other. Irreconcilable differences may lead to separation or divorce.

Couples who remain together tend to be more financially secure than they were during early adulthood. Many start to focus on ensuring that their savings will be adequate during their retirement years.

Adults in this age group often are described as the **sandwich generation,** because many of them are raising their children while assuming increasing responsibility for their aging parents. As a result, they are "sandwiched" between two generations. Some middle-aged adults also must care for their grandchildren. These added responsibilities can thwart the middle-aged adult's independence and create a crisis. Well-adjusted middle adults, however, view the added responsibilities of aging parents and children as part of life.

Stop, Think, and Respond ● BOX 8-2

In addition to being called the "established years" and the "sandwich generation," middle adulthood also has been labeled as the "empty nest years," symbolizing the departure of children from the parental home. What are some potential problems that may result from the "empty nest?"

Prevalent Psychosocial Issues and Problems

Personality is viewed as the combination of particular dynamic traits that continue to develop and change throughout adulthood. For many middle-aged adults, new events and challenges influence their personality.

Aging tends to be emotionally difficult in the U.S. culture. Many Americans value youth and energy more than the experience and wisdom that accompany passing years. As a result, many people tend to associate midlife with change and loss. Depression in midlife is common but often unrecognized and untreated. Suicide risk increases with age, especially for adult men.

As a consequence of feeling unfulfilled and unappreciated, some middle-aged clients develop a **midlife crisis,** in which they view themselves as less likely to accomplish the goals of their youth. Even those who have accomplished their goals and seem successful have feelings of dissatisfaction. To relieve their feelings of insecurity and unhappiness over the loss of their youth, some have cosmetic surgery, wear clothing styles more characteristic of younger adults, have extramarital affairs, or abandon their current lifestyle to seek a more meaningful existence.

Financial insecurity also continues to stress middle-aged adults. Unemployment jeopardizes pension plans, retirement packages, and health insurance benefits. Without insurance coverage, serious illness or injury can mean financial ruin. Another financial burden includes caring for elderly parents, formerly the pillars of security and support, now dependent on their middle-aged children. Some middle-aged adults struggle with guilt for being unable to assume the care that aging parents require and worry about finding an adequate caregiver or nursing home.

NURSING IMPLICATIONS

Many middle-aged clients become concerned about their physical condition after the illness or death of a friend. They recognize the negative effects of neglecting their health and seek to reform poor health habits. Nurses must identify health risks and teach clients ways to modify or refrain from behaviors that contribute to preventable diseases. Health teaching includes smoking cessation, refraining from excessive alcohol, eating a low-fat diet, exercising regularly, and obtaining regular screening for colorectal, prostate, breast, and cervical cancer. Monthly breast self-examination is important for women in this age group to aid in early detection of breast cancer. Nurses also stress the importance of routine annual examinations, blood work, and other tests to assist in the early detection of many diseases, which is the key to treatment and recovery.

Nutrition

As discussed earlier, weight tends to increase in middle age, usually from a combination of excessive calories, decreased metabolic rate, and less activity. A person's diet should include all nutrients he or she needs to maintain and repair body tissue; however, decreased caloric intake is necessary to compensate for decreased activity levels and metabolism.

Because calcium in the bone is constantly being broken down and replenished, calcium requirements remain high. A regular exercise program helps to prevent weight gain, maintains bone mass, and compensates for lowered metabolism.

As adults age, poor dentition may affect the ability to chew food. If the diet is deficient in whole grains, fresh fruits, and uncooked vegetables to compensate for the inability to chew, stool volume and moisture are reduced, which contributes to a pattern of bowel irregularity and constipation. Nurses should assess for such problems and help the client address them as necessary.

Sleep

Many middle-aged adults fill every hour of the day with activity; consequently, many also are sleep deprived. Several factors can affect the quality of sleep, including use of caffeine, stimulants, or other medications. Changes in circadian rhythms also can affect sleep patterns. Many middle-aged adults commonly go to sleep, then wake a few hours later and cannot return to sleep. For parents of teenagers, waiting for them to come home is another factor that may disrupt sleep during these years.

Nurses should assess all clients for sleep disturbances. A few simple techniques such as limiting or eliminating caffeine, engaging in stress reduction techniques (see Chap. 12), attending to stressful issues earlier in the day, cooling the room temperature, taking a warm bath or reading before bed, or listening to soft music may help.

Sexuality

Although sexuality exists throughout the life span, the frequency and vigor of intercourse are likely to decrease during middle adulthood. Sexual effectiveness, however, does not automatically disappear as humans age. Healthy men and women often enjoy sexual functioning well into their 80s. Unfortunately, many clients accept social definitions of themselves as sexless. Believing that they will naturally lose their sexual effectiveness becomes a self-fulfilling prophecy, even though their bodies have not lost the capacity for sex.

Nurses should take the time to address issues related to sexuality for all adults. They should answer questions honestly and provide information and referrals that will help clients continue to enjoy this part of life for as long as they desire. For more information on particular issues, treatments, and teaching, see Unit 14.

GENERAL NUTRITIONAL CONSIDERATIONS

By middle adulthood, food preferences and eating habits are well established, making it difficult for some clients to accept special diets or dietary restrictions. Some clients view a "diet" as punishment or not worthwhile.

Promoting a healthful diet during the midlife years, before evidence of chronic disease is apparent, may help reduce the risk of several disorders. From a psychological standpoint, modifying eating habits to prevent disease may be easier than doing so to treat disease. Urge clients to eat more fruits and vegetables, choose foods lower in fat and higher in fiber, and avoid overeating. Maintaining an active lifestyle, with both aerobic activity and weight training, helps promote weight management.

Because aging causes everyone to lose bone mass, new calcium requirements for all adults older than 50 years of age are increased to 1200 mg/day, or about four servings from the milk group.

GENERAL PHARMACOLOGIC CONSIDERATIONS

Clients must thoroughly understand drug use: quantity of the drug (number of capsules or tablets, amount of liquid); the time to take it; and any instruction relating to a specific drug.

Noncompliance is a problem with adults who perceive themselves as healthy. Appropriate and thorough client teaching helps diminish non-compliance.

Menopausal women face a decision concerning hormone replacement therapy (HRT). Provide up-to-date information on the risks and benefits of HRT to assist the client to make an informed choice.

To diminish the possibility of osteoporosis in postmenopausal women who do not elect HRT, a bone resorption inhibitor such as alendronate (Fosamax) often is prescribed. Instruct women taking alendronate to ingest the drug in the morning with 6 to 8 ounces of water and to remain upright for 30 minutes after ingestion.

Caution men with prostate hypertrophy that some medications can exacerbate urinary retention. Instruct these men to check with the primary care provider before taking over-the-counter or prescription medications.

Critical Thinking Exercises

1. *A middle-aged client is admitted for observation after an incidence of chest pain. Based on what you know about the physical, emotional, and social characteristics of a person in this age group, what assessments are important to make? Why?*

2. *One of your clients is a 72-year-old man and his family. The client's health is generally good, but he needs assistance with activities of daily living because he is blind in one eye and has only partial vision in the other. He lives with his 51-year-old son and daughter-in-law, who also are responsible for their 3-year-old granddaughter. Explain how this situation represents the "sandwich generation." What are some potential problems? What would be the 51-year-old son's greatest stressor? What suggestions would you offer?*

References and Suggested Readings

Akram, G. (2000). Over-the-counter medication: An emerging and neglected drug abuse? *Journal of Substance Use, 5,* 136–142.

Arslanian-Engoren, C. (2000). Gender and age bias in triage decisions. *Journal of Emergency Nursing, 26,* 117–124.

Benetos, A., Thomas, F., Safar, M. E., et al. (2001). Should diastolic and systolic blood pressure be considered for cardiovascular risk evaluation: A study in middle-aged men and women. *Journal of the American College of Cardiology, 37,* 163–168.

Childs, H. W., Hayslip, B., Jr., Radika, L. M., et al. (2000). Young and middle-aged adults' perceptions of elder abuse. *Gerontologist, 40*(1), 75–85.

Chisholm, J. F. (1999). The sandwich generation. *Journal of Social Distress and the Homeless, 8,* 177–191.

DeLaune, S. C. & Ladner, P. K. (1998). *Fundamentals of nursing: Standards and practice.* Albany, NY: Delmar.

Dudek, S. (2000). *Nutrition essentials for nursing practice* (4th ed.). Philadelphia: Lippincott Williams & Wilkins.

Edelman, C. L. (2002). *Health promotion throughout the lifespan* (5th ed.). St. Louis: Mosby–Year Book.

Fournier, R. A. (1999). The sandwich generation: A continuing education offering. *DNA Reporter, 23*(4), 16–19.

Kenney, J. W. (2000). Women's "inner-balance": A comparison of stressors, personality traits, and health problems by age groups. *Journal of Advanced Nursing, 31,* 639–650.

Lakka, T. A., Laukkanen, J. A., Rauramaa, R., et al. (2001). Cardiorespiratory fitness and the progression of carotid atherosclerosis in middle-aged men. *Annals of Internal Medicine, 134,* 12–20, 34.

Lauer, J. C. & Lauer, R. H. (1999). *How to survive and thrive in an empty nest.* Oakland: U.S. New Harbinger Publications.

Martin, M., Grünendahl, M., & Martin, P. (2001). Age differences in stress, social resources, and well-being in middle and older age. *Journal of Gerontology. Series B: Psychological Sciences and Social Sciences, 56B,* 214–222.

Peacock, J. M., Folsom, A. R., Knopman, D. S., et al. (2000). Dietary antioxidant intake and cognitive performance in middle-aged adults. *Public Health Nutrition, 3,* 337–343.

Rosdahl, C. B. (2003). *Textbook of basic nursing* (8th ed.). Philadelphia: Lippincott Williams & Wilkins.

Ryan, C. M. & Geckle, M. O. (2000). Circumscribed cognitive dysfunction in middle-aged adults with type 2 diabetes. *Diabetes Care, 23,* 1486–1493.

Schott-Baer, D. & Kotal, B. (2000). Frequency and effectiveness of self-care actions and menopause symptoms of middle-aged working women. *MEDSURG Nursing, 9,* 302–307.

Seward, M. R. (1999). The sandwich generation copes with elder care. *Benefits Quarterly, 15*(2), 41–48.

Biopsychosocial Aspects of Caring for Older Adults

Words to Know

ageism
antioxidants
autophagocytosis
despair
ego integrity
elder abuse
free radicals
gerontology

kyphosis
life review
pet therapy
reality orientation
reminiscence therapy
senescence
validation therapy

Learning Objectives

On completion of this chapter, the reader will:

- List five trends for which society should prepare in view of the growing population of aging adults.
- Identify developmental tasks for older adults.
- Contrast the developmental characteristics of ego integrity and despair.
- Define gerontology.
- Discuss three theories of aging.
- Discuss physical characteristics that are unique to adults older than 65 years of age.
- Identify social characteristics of older adults.
- Discuss factors that affect the emotional health of older adults.
- Define ageism and how it affects older adults.
- Discuss ways that a nurse's attitude concerning the aged can affect their care.
- List approaches the nurse can use when teaching older adults.
- Identify nursing care measures that are especially important when providing physical care for an older adult.
- Describe pet therapy, reality orientation, and reminiscence therapy.

Older adults play a vital role in society, the home, the workplace, and the community. They offer others with less maturity the wisdom of life experiences. Healthcare workers play an important role in helping older adults maintain their independence, health, and productivity.

GROWTH AND DEVELOPMENT

Senescence is the last stage in the life cycle. During senescence, body processes gradually deteriorate. Diet, exercise, stress reduction, and health promotion activities play a role in slowing the rate of senescence. This developmental period is subdivided into three categories: the young-old, ages 65 to 74 years; the middle-old, ages 75 to 84 years; and the old-old, older than age 85 years.

Demographics

According to the United States Bureau of the Census, the number of people older than age 65 is increasing rapidly. Life expectancy has been extended for both sexes. Males can expect to live an average of 73 years, and females can expect to live an average of 79 years (National Institute on Aging, 1996). By 2050, the population of Americans who live to be 85 years of age will represent almost 5% of the U.S. population (Federal Interagency Forum on Aging-Related Statistics, 2000). By 2000, centenarians (those 100 years of age or older) increased 35% above the number in 1990 (Administration on Aging, 2001). The federal government has identified 10 major trends in the aging population, which are presented in Box 9-1.

Developmental Stages and Tasks

During late adulthood, older adults have developmental tasks to complete (Box 9-2). They must discover activities to fill the time previously spent at work and raising families. These activities must sustain a sense of usefulness and self-worth. In addition, older adults must adjust to many losses such as the loss of friends or a spouse, loss of income, loss of health and agility, and loss of independence. Aging adults must face their own death.

As aging adults deal with life's remaining challenges, they acknowledge the permanency of past decisions and actions. They develop either a sense of ego integrity or despair as they reflect on their lives. **Ego integrity** is a feeling of personal satisfaction that life has been happy and fulfilling. **Despair,** on the other hand, results when a person views life as disappointing and unfulfilling and anguishes over what might have been.

Most older adults engage in **life review,** which is a process of looking back at one's life and reviewing decisions, choices, conflicts, and resolutions. For integrity to emerge in the older adult, a life review results in the belief that life has been meaningful and well spent. Despair is the predominant feeling if, after a life review, the older adult feels that life has been ineffective, decisions were poor, and life has been filled with unresolved conflict.

OLDER ADULTHOOD

Gerontology is the study of aging, including physiologic, psychological, and social aspects. Gerontology is considered a young science because most significant advances in this field have been made since 1950. Research findings enhance the understanding of the nature of aging and how older people function. Scientists are conducting much research to determine the actual causes of the aging processes. The goal of this extensive research is to find ways to extend both the quantity and the quality of life.

Theories of Aging

It is an established fact that physical characteristics change throughout the life cycle. As one ages, the hair turns gray, skin wrinkles, bones demineralize, and blood vessels become hard and inelastic. The biologic mechanisms that trigger these changes, however, remain a mystery. Some theories that attempt to explain the aging process include autophagocytosis, the stress response, impairment of the immune response, alterations in DNA replication, and cellular damage by free radicals. No one theory fully explains the aging process; it is likely that aging is a combination of physiologic phenomena. Although the effects of aging often are confounded by the effects of disease, aging is a phenomenon that occurs even in relatively healthy people.

Autophagocytosis

Autophagocytosis literally means "to eat self." This does not mean that cells are totally consumed, but portions of them are consumed to reduce their size. This process is used when the cell senses adverse conditions. A smaller cell results in a temporary decrease in energy needs and increases the potential for survival. During this process, a brown-colored residue called *lipofuscin* forms. Scientists have noted that this cellular pigment accumulates as people age. Cell shrinkage caused by autophagocytosis contributes to the decreased weight and height of older adults and to the atrophy of tissues and organs.

Stress Response

Hans Selye, a gifted physician of the early 20th century, pioneered a theory concerning stress and its effects on the body. He proposed that physical, psychological, and social changes produce biologic stress. Regardless of the stress-producing stimulus, Selye maintained that the physiologic response, which he called the *general adaptation syndrome,* is always the same (see Chap. 12). Gerontologists hypothesize that the defense mechanisms associated with the stress response eventually weaken, leading to death.

Decline of the Immune System

One of the most important mechanisms for preserving health is the immune system. Scientists have discovered that as people age, the immune system becomes impaired and the body's defenses are weakened, leaving it vulnerable to overwhelming infection and cancer, an increased incidence of both being associated with advancing age. Others theorize that as the immune system declines, the body misidentifies normal cells as foreign. The autoimmune theory of aging is that the body's defenses attack the healthy cells, advancing the aging process.

Faulty DNA Replication

The deoxyribonucleic acid (DNA) molecule present in each cell programs cellular reproduction. DNA is susceptible to damaging agents such as free radicals (see later discussion). A damaging agent locked onto the DNA molecule has the potential to scramble the genetic code. The dysfunctional DNA then cannot program the continued, orderly synthesis of proteins. When this happens repeatedly, fewer cells are capable of replication. In the young, cells resist agents that damage DNA or repair the damage efficiently. Because billions of cells are damaged in the aging process, tissue disorganization occurs and leads to organ failure.

Free Radicals

Free radicals are unstable atoms with excessive energy capable of damaging DNA molecules. It is possible that free radicals are responsible for changes associated with aging. Chronic exposure to substances such as radiation and environmental toxins damages DNA, causing cellular changes. Healthy cells resist the damaging effects of free radicals using chemicals called **antioxidants** that block the chemical reactions that cause free radicals. Scientists are investigating the antioxidant properties of vitamins C and E, and provitamin A, known as *beta carotene* and found in the pigments of deep yellow and dark green fruits and vegetables.

Physical Characteristics

In older adults, functional decline occurs without any specific illness. In caring for older clients, nurses must recognize the normal physiologic variations that accompany aging. In addition, older adults often manifest diseases with milder or atypical symptoms. Many of the physical changes seen in the older adult are a progression of the changes that occur during middle age (see Chap. 8). Because aging is not a uniform process, organ systems age at different rates, producing varying alterations in functions. Norms for health and illness have not been established for older adults as they have for younger age groups. Landmarks of normal aging are not thoroughly understood. The nurse can compare the older person's patterns of health and illness with current ability, using the client as the standard. The nurse also considers capabilities, social support, and the environment as to the effects on overall functioning. Knowledge about the client's particular situation provides an approach to care and helps ensure accurate assessment, interpretation of data, interventions, and evaluations.

Respiratory System

The lungs of the older adult have been exposed for many years to smoke, bacteria, and multiple irritants in the environment. The age-related changes that do affect the respiratory system are so gradual that most older adults compensate for their effects. Normal aging includes a reduction of alveolar surface area, loss of elastic recoil, decrease in vital capacity and oxygen saturation, decline in host defense, and reduction in tolerance for exercise.

The rib cage becomes rigid as cartilage calcifies. The thoracic spine shortens and osteoporosis may cause stooped posture, which decreases available lung space and limits the older adult's ability to take deep breaths. The abdominal muscles become weaker, causing a decrease in inspiratory and expiratory effort. The alveoli enlarge and become thin, although their numbers remain constant in the absence of chronic pulmonary disease.

Cardiovascular System

Important cardiovascular changes that accompany aging include decreased cardiac output (volume of blood pumped by the heart). The aorta and arteries stiffen and become less flexible with age, and the circulatory system responds less efficiently to the demands of activity and exercise. Common changes in vital signs include increased blood pressure, irregular pulse, and shortness of breath on exertion. Older adults also experience postural hypotension (rapid drop in blood pressure when rising or standing from a lying or sitting position).

Impaired arterial circulation makes the skin feel cool and causes the feet to appear purplish or bluish when in a sitting or standing position. Varicose veins (bulging, twisted veins in the legs) cause the lower extremities to swell and fatigue easily.

The classic symptoms of cardiovascular diseases are altered or absent in older adults, so that accurate assessment and diagnosis are imperative. Nursing interventions should focus on prevention of further disease by helping the older person to minimize risk factors. Examples of ways to reduce risks are stopping smoking, lowering cholesterol, eating well-balanced meals, limiting salt intake, performing stress reduction techniques, and exercising regularly.

Neurologic System

Sooner or later, all adults worry about whether they are thinking, remembering, and making decisions with the same acuity as when they were younger. As early as 40 years of age, adults begin to notice occasional mental lapses. A decline in cognition may accompany normal aging; however, there is less decline or no decline for people with favorable lifestyles and good health.

The incidence of serious cognitive deficits, like Alzheimer's disease (see Chap. 18), increases with age. Most older adults have better long-term memory than short-term memory. The older adult responds less quickly to questions in an interview. Nurses should not assume, however, that the client is cognitively impaired. Diminished hearing or anxiety slows a client's responses.

Clinical depression, common among older adults, often is mistaken for dementia. Age-related changes in the nervous system are different from disease states. The normal changes that take place have little effect on thinking and cognition. Structural changes that accompany aging include loss of neurons and brain weight, accumulations of lipofuscin in the neuronal cytoplasm, slowed synaptic transmissions, and loss of peripheral nerve function. Functional changes include slowed reaction time, impaired thermoregulation, and changes in sleep wave patterns.

Stop, Think, and Respond ● BOX 9-1

Do you think learning stops or changes as a person ages?

Sensory Perception

Most older adults wear glasses. The *presbyopia* (age-related loss of visual acuity for near vision) that began in the middle years becomes more pronounced. Visual acuity declines at an accelerated rate as structures of the eye degenerate. Most people older than age 70 years have some degree of cataract formation. Many avoid driving at night because of the difficulty in adjusting to the glare of oncoming headlights.

Hearing loss also becomes more pronounced. *Presbycusis* (age-related hearing loss) that began in the middle years progresses. Presbycusis is gradual, with initial loss of ability to hear high-pitched sound, followed by a decreased ability to hear middle- and low-pitched sounds. The nurse must look for signs of hearing loss because older adults do not always report hearing difficulties.

Position sense and reaction time decline gradually until about 70 years of age, when the rate of decline becomes rapid. The deterioration of these two faculties, together with diminished vision, is a common cause of accidents. Consequently, many older adults are injured in falls.

Stop, Think, and Respond ● BOX 9-2

What are the signs of hearing loss that an older adult may display?

Gastrointestinal System

Changes in the gastrointestinal (GI) system usually are not life-threatening; however, they may cause the greatest concern and often are the source of many complaints for older adults. GI problems such as constipation, indigestion, diarrhea, nausea, vomiting, weight gain or loss, or increased flatulence (gas) are bothersome and become more pronounced even without organic disease. The incidence of gallbladder disease and cancer of the GI tract increases with age. Poor nutrition, medications, emotions, inactivity, and various health factors influence the status of the GI system.

Age affects virtually every area of the GI tract. In the oral cavity, taste buds decrease in number and saliva production diminishes. Poor dental hygiene can cause problems with chewing. The older adult is at increased risk for aspiration because food remains in the esophagus for a longer time and the gag reflex is weaker. Decreased gastric acid secretions impair the absorption of iron, vitamin B_{12}, and proteins. The cells of the colon atrophy and peristalsis slows, resulting in constipation and flatulence.

Older adults are aware of their various GI complaints and use a variety of measures to treat them. Self-treatment can delay assessment and diagnosis of GI problems. Good health habits can prevent several GI problems. Dental hygiene and regular visits to the dentist can prevent many disorders that can threaten nutritional intake. The proper quantity and quality of food can enhance general health and minimize the risk of indigestion and constipation. The nurse also should educate older adults on the relationship between medications and GI health.

Reproductive Changes

Changes in sexual response may dramatically alter genitourinary function and contribute to embarrassment and general discomfort for older adults. The breasts of older women lose their suppleness and hang flat against the chest wall. Men appear to have more prominent breasts as a result of slightly decreased testosterone. Clients remain sexually active, but both men and women need more stimulation to become aroused. In men, the penis and testes shrink, whereas the prostate gland enlarges. Erections are briefer. In women, the vagina becomes shorter and narrower, and the walls become thin and less elastic. The vulva may atrophy. Vaginal secretions diminish, which may cause discomfort and bleeding during intercourse.

Urinary System

Both men and women develop urinary problems as they age. The bladder capacity decreases in both sexes. The bladder also loses muscle tone; emptying may be incomplete. Men awaken at night to void because the enlarged prostate gland blocks complete emptying of urine. It becomes necessary to urinate more frequently. For women, ligaments and muscles stretched during pregnancy fail to keep the bladder suspended. As elastic tissue and pelvic floor muscles weaken, stress incontinence, leakage of urine with increased abdominal pressure during coughing, sneezing, laughing, or lifting, occurs. Another type of chronic incontinence is urge incontinence, leakage of urine because of an inability to delay voiding. There also is a decrease in renal blood flow because of decreased cardiac output and reduced glomerular filtration rate.

Musculoskeletal System

The older adult continues to experience a decrease in height that began in middle adulthood as a result of compression of the disks between the vertebrae. This, combined with a weakening of the chest muscles, causes the spine to take on an obvious thoracic curve known as **kyphosis** or *humpback*. With a change in the center of gravity, the older adult assumes a wider stance when standing and walking. The hips and the knees tend to be flexed at all times. There may be stiffness in the weight-bearing joints and limitation in their range of motion. Muscles atrophy, yet they are more clearly defined because of the loss of subcutaneous fat. There is a general, progressive loss of muscle fibers that leads to flabby, thin muscles, particularly of the arms and legs.

The physical limitations seen in older adults are the result of inactivity, not degenerative changes. Remaining as active as possible helps slow the loss of physical ability. Arthritis is the leading chronic condition that affects the musculoskeletal system among people older than 65 years of age. Arthritis results in joint stiffness, limitation of movement, and deformity. Osteoporosis causes a loss of bone mass, particularly in older women, and places the older adult at increased risk for spontaneous fractures (see Chap. 67).

Integumentary System

Gradual changes in the skin and in the body's ability to adjust to heat and cold occur with age. The skin is drier, is prone to wrinkling, and becomes thin, flaky, and susceptible to irritation. Small, brown-pigmented freckles called *lentigines,* or *liver spots,* appear about the hands, arms, and face or other areas exposed to sun and weather (Fig. 9-1). Older adults bruise easily because of fragile capillaries. Di-

FIGURE 9-1 Senile lentigines. (Courtesy of Ken Timby)

abetes and vascular disease predispose older adults to poor healing.

Skin disorders are found in more than 90% of older adults. The major cause of pathologic skin changes is sunlight, which directly affects the skin and causes kerato-acanthomas, premalignant diseases, basal cell and squamous cell epitheliomas, and malignant melanomas. The most common skin disorders in older adults are keratoses and skin cancers. Other lesions frequently seen are liver spots, cherry angiomas, skin tags, and senile purpura. Minor trauma can cause bruising and often tearing of the skin (see Chap. 69).

Facial features change as the result of loss of subcutaneous tissue. Wrinkles appear and the face seems to sag. The most obvious change in aging is hair color. Fifty percent of the population older than age 50 years experiences hair graying, starting at the temples and working its way back. The hair also becomes drier and thinner. Hair changes become more noticeable after 60 years of age. Gray hair is determined by an autosomal dominant gene and results from a loss of melanin production. Hair growth begins to slow and its distribution becomes more restricted. Men also experience a general thinning of hair, except at the eyebrows, ears, and nose. Hairs in these areas become longer and coarser. Often, the hair line recedes in men as well as women. Baldness in men is inherited from the mother.

Nails, particularly toenails, often thicken and become brittle from poor circulation to the extremities (Fig. 9-2). Nail growth rate diminishes by 30% to 50% after age 50 years. Aging nails show increased longitudinal striation, which causes splitting of the nail surface.

Older clients may lose their teeth from neglected oral hygiene. The gums recede and teeth loosen as the bones in the jaw shrink.

The body gradually loses its ability to adjust to extremes of temperature. It is harder for older people to keep warm because their metabolism is lower. In hot weather,

A. Onychauxis

B. Onychorrhexis

FIGURE 9-2 (A) Onychauxis is characterized by nail hypertrophy which may be a consequence of aging. **(B)** Onychorrhexis, associated with aging, results in brittle, fragile, uneven nail edges.

they do not lose heat as well as younger people because the blood vessels in their skin dilate slowly and their sweating mechanism does not function as effectively.

Social Characteristics

Healthy older adults usually maintain fairly active lives. Some become more active than they were when younger, learning new hobbies and socializing with new friends, because they simply have time that they used to spend on work or other activities. For many, old age is a period of continued learning and emotional growth. Working and raising a family previously provided many social contacts for the older adult. Some older adults feel bored and lonely when they retire, with a loss of self-esteem because their former activities and contacts are curtailed. The outcome of this period is directly linked to the person's overall attitude about life in general. There is growing evidence that staying active and maintaining social contacts or acquiring new acquaintances is simply another way to stay healthy, both mentally and physically.

Prominent Psychosocial Issues and Problems

Although personality continues to evolve throughout life, basic temperament is stable into old age. Thus, if a client's temperament was cheerful and optimistic during youth, he or she usually keeps that demeanor in old age. A bitter, complaining young person often carries that attitude into old age.

The ability to cope with the crises of diminished health, dependence, leisure time, fixed income, and alternative housing depends on the coping skills established much earlier in life. Many older adults experience loss, and the ability to cope effectively becomes apparent. Effective cop-

ing skills acquired throughout life assist the older adult to overcome grief and accept his or her losses. This also is a time to plan for life-end decision making, such as burial arrangements, living wills, and advance directives.

Ageism

Ageism describes behaviors and beliefs that depict older adults in negative, inaccurate, or stereotypical ways. Ageism results in the older adult being characterized as a sick, feeble, rigid, disagreeable, opinionated, or demented person who lives in the past. According to most experts in gerontology, older adults are remarkably healthy and productive until the extremes of old age. Some Americans believe that the significant part of life is over after middle age. This view undermines the dignity of older people, who sense that they are not expected to remain physically or mentally healthy. Ageism can prevent older adults from obtaining new jobs or force them into early retirement. In some situations, older adults are avoided, treated disrespectfully, or ignored.

Dependence

Approximately 67% of older persons continued to live alone or in a family setting in 1998 (American Association of Retired Persons, 1999). The others lived with a companion or in supervised living arrangements, such as an extended care facility or a nursing home. Many older adults find dependence on others difficult to accept, even though they recognize the need for it. Some deny that they need assisted living and insist on remaining at home even when it jeopardizes their safety.

Housing

Finding safe and affordable living accommodations is difficult for many older people. Retirement communities combine smaller residences with conveniences such as an infirmary, shopping services, and recreational facilities. The older adult must part with treasured objects to accommodate a smaller dwelling. Familiar objects and mementos are extremely comforting to the older adult because they are reminders of past accomplishments and relationships.

Economic Concerns

For many, retirement is a time of freedom and an opportunity to experience many activities. The timing and quality of retirement depend on how well the person planned financially. Working after retirement should be a choice, but some people experience financial problems, and continued work becomes a necessity. Older adults face economic concerns related to decreased income. Compulsory retirement or serious and chronic illnesses are major factors contributing to financial worries. Although studies show that older workers tend to be conscientious, careful, accurate, and dependable, many employers are reluctant to hire them. There is significant growth in the number of older adults engaged in part-time employment, and employers may be recognizing the value of older adults because trends suggest that more retired people are re-entering the work force.

Medical expenses increase for older adults, adding to economic concerns. The enactment of Medicare, federal legislation providing health benefits to the aged, has been an important advance in helping older adults meet health-care costs.

Older adults also need to use others to carry out tasks they no longer can perform, such as caring for the lawn, painting, and cleaning. Most older adults rely on Social Security, a fixed income that does not increase at the same rate as the cost of living. Consequently, as older adults live longer, their money does not stretch as far. They are less able to buy material goods as costs continue to rise.

Loneliness

All people have emotional needs for love, companionship, and acceptance. Hobbies or other special interests and so-cial contacts help older adults cope. Some become involved in community volunteer work or take advantage of activities and meeting places specifically for older adults.

The problem of loneliness is acute for many older people. Besides facing a lack of contact with former coworkers, the older adult also faces separation from family and friends and the death of a spouse. Community meal sites and senior centers try to meet the older adult's need for companionship by providing opportunities for socialization.

Pets also fill the void (Fig. 9-3). For older adults living alone, pets serve as family substitutes, provide comfort, and decrease feelings of loneliness. Many extended care facilities are using **pet therapy** and have a resident cat or dog. The activity and playfulness of the animal stimulate aged persons who are uncommunicative. Pets can decrease anxiety and depression and provide the older adult with the feeling of being needed and loved.

Depression and Suicide

Many older adults experience depression. Symptoms such as fatigue, irritability, loss of interest in surroundings, de-creased ability to concentrate, or feelings of worthlessness often are viewed as natural consequences of aging, and many older adults with depression receive no treatment. This is unfortunate because older adults respond well to antidepressants such as amitriptyline (Elavil), nortripty-line (Aventyl, Pamelor), trazodone (Desyrel, Trazone), and fluoxetine (Prozac).

Although older adults represent only 13% of the pop-ulation, they account for 20% of all suicide attempts. More suicide attempts occur in individuals 65 years of age

FIGURE 9-3 Pets provide companionship to many older adults.

or older than in any other age group. The risk for suicide is greater among those who live alone, have health prob-lems, or abuse alcohol. Death of a spouse also is associated with an increased risk of suicide. The nurse or health care provider investigates any expressions of hopelessness or helplessness. It is appropriate to ask older adults who seem depressed if they are considering harming them-selves or ending their life.

Fear for Safety

Many older adults who live alone, particularly those liv-ing in urban settings, are vulnerable to crimes against their property and person. Some cope with these fears by becoming isolated prisoners in their own homes. Older adults also are the victims of fraud or confidence games.

Older adults may become victims of **elder abuse** when they depend on others for care and support. Abuse may be physical, in the form of beatings; psychological, in the form of threats; social, in the form of abandonment or un-reasonable confinement; and material, in the form of theft or mismanagement of money. The abuser often is a care-taker or family member. Older adults at risk for abuse are frail, dependent, and cognitively or physically impaired. Adult Protective Services, a division of each state's De-partment of Social Services, investigates and safeguards older adults who are suspected victims of abuse.

NURSING IMPLICATIONS

Nurses will care for greater numbers of older adults in various healthcare settings as this population continues to increase. The plan of care includes accurate assessments, interventions, restorative care to support independence, early discharge planning, and appropriate use of community resources.

Older adults retain the ability to learn new information but require more time during the teaching process. The nurse proceeds slowly to allow time for the client to think about and respond to new ideas. He or she speaks slowly and distinctly if the client has a hearing deficit and ensures that the older client is wearing glasses (if necessary) and that lighting is adequate. The nurse provides ample opportunity for questions to clarify misunderstood information. If he or she uses visual aids such as graphs, pictures, or printed material, the nurse makes sure such materials are clear, uncluttered, and large enough to be seen. If the client uses a hearing aid, the nurse makes certain that the client is wearing it and that it is working properly. If possible, the nurse includes another person who will assist the client after discharge. He or she asks about past experiences and relates the new information to these past experiences. The older client has a vast fund of knowledge, and helping him or her draw on this knowledge facilitates learning new information.

Addressing Psychosocial Issues

It is extremely important for nurses to be aware of the high incidence of depression and the potential for suicide in older adults. This is true both in the home setting and extended care facility. The nurse assesses for signs of increased alcohol consumption, decreased interest in friends and social activities, complaints of fatigue, anger, and feelings of hopelessness. He or she asks depressed clients about suicidal thoughts or intentions. If an older adult confides suicidal thoughts, the nurse reports those intentions immediately to the nursing supervisor and primary care physician. He or she immediately removes any potential articles that the client could use to commit suicide, such as guns, razors, knives, scissors, and medications (both prescription and nonprescription). The nurse has someone stay with the client. The number of suicides in the older population can be decreased significantly by recognizing and treating depression in the elderly in appropriate and effective ways. (See Chap. 15 for more information on depression and suicide.)

Assessing Nutrition and Modifying the Diet

Nutritional deficiencies are serious problems for older adults. Dietary insufficiencies are related to loss of or changes in teeth, boredom at eating alone, fatigue, or lack of money. The diet of older adults tends to be high in carbohydrates, which are more affordable on a fixed income. In addition, because many shop irregularly, they may depend on a stockpile of processed foods that have an extended shelf life. Older adults benefit from a diet lower in calories but high in nutrients because absorption of the nutrients is diminished.

Some older clients require a soft diet and foods that are easy to digest. Chewing is difficult for some because of diminished production of saliva or improperly fitted dentures. Many benefit from supplemental vitamins and minerals or nourishing between-meal snacks. Tracking body weight is a good assessment tool for evaluating the nutritional status of older adults. The nurse reports weight gain or loss of 5% in a 4-week period to the primary care provider for analysis.

Giving Physical Care

The nurse helps older adults maintain their dignity and self-respect by promoting hygiene and grooming. Clients feel better about themselves when their hair is neatly arranged, their skin is clean and healthy, and they are dressed attractively.

Older adults must learn to adjust to their increasing physical limitations, but nurses always encourage self-care. Older adults quickly lose their ability to care for themselves when someone does it for them. If the nurse performs activities of daily living for clients when they are capable of performing these activities without help, clients may think they no longer are considered capable of managing such tasks. Surrendering self-care functions that help maintain their independence and contact with reality leads to unnecessary dependence on others, as well as a loss of self-esteem.

Some older adults are slower in their movements and responses. Attempts to make them hurry result in confusion, anxiety, and accidents. The thoughtful nurse prepares everything clients need for self-care and then lets them proceed at their own pace to complete those aspects of care that they can perform.

Skin and Nail Care

Decreased circulation to the extremities results in prolonged healing time for injuries or infections. If the skin on the legs and feet is very dry, cream or lotion is necessary after bathing. Thickened, brittle toenails are carefully trimmed after soaking the feet in water. If the older adult has very thick nails, diabetes, or a peripheral vascular disease, professional nail care is indicated.

Bathing and Hygiene

A daily partial bath and a biweekly tub bath are adequate because frequent bathing dries the skin. The nurse helps the older client get in and out of a tub. A stall shower is desirable because it avoids the need to step over an elevated edge and lower oneself into the tub. A shower chair is ideal for the weak and unsteady client. The shower offers the most thorough rinsing of soap from the skin, thus helping to minimize skin irritations. Whatever method of bathing is used, care is taken to ensure privacy.

Some older women have a vaginal discharge or urinary incontinence. The vaginal mucous membrane becomes thin and subject to infection. If the nurse or family member detects this problem, he or she should consult the physician regarding use of a cleansing douche or appropriate medication. The nurse keeps the client clean and comfortable with good perineal care and uses disposable pads.

Assisting With Elimination

Bowel and urinary elimination may pose problems for older adults. Urinary frequency is common. The nurse takes care to prevent falls when the client gets up during the night to use the toilet. He or she sees that the call button is nearby so that the client can obtain assistance. For those who cannot wait for assistance, the nurse leaves a commode, bedpan, or urinal in easy reach.

Constipation is more likely in those who are immobile, who fail to drink sufficient fluids, or whose diet lacks sufficient bulk. Helping the client maintain adequate fiber and fluid intake and to have a regular time for evacuation helps restore regularity. The physician can order enemas, mild laxatives, or stool softeners if other methods of relieving constipation are ineffective.

Assisting With Mobility

Confinement in bed causes adverse effects among older people. Because older adults expand their chests less fully, confinement in bed, which accentuates this problem, often leads to the development of hypostatic pneumonia (pneumonia that occurs as a result of shallow breathing).

Pressure ulcers (bed sores) are common among older adults because they have diminished subcutaneous fat. Frequent position changes and pressure-relieving devices are necessary for clients who are inactive. Muscle tone is readily lost during prolonged bed rest; extreme weakness results and is difficult to overcome. To combat these complications, the nurse promotes alternative activity such as active or passive exercises.

Promoting Safety

The nurse ensures that the environment is safe for the older client. Beds that are left in a high position are a potential danger because older adults can misjudge the distance to the floor and fall when getting out of bed. The bed is left in the low position except when direct nursing care

is administered. A dim night light helps the older person become oriented to the surroundings and prevents falling or tripping over objects when the client gets out of bed. The call button is placed within reach.

Nighttime agitation and confusion are common among older adults, particularly when they are moved from familiar surroundings to a hospital or nursing home. Unfortunately, this problem commonly is mismanaged. Physical restraints increase the individual's frustration and distress. As an alternative, the nurse tries to determine the cause of the client's confusion and then attempts to reduce or eliminate it. Causes of agitation include the need to urinate, the discomfort of constipation, being too hot or cold, fatigue, pain, fear, or loneliness. Meeting physical or emotional needs often is all that is needed to quiet a restless client.

Promoting Sleep

Older adults usually require less sleep than younger adults. Keeping older clients awake and active during the day facilitates sleep at night. Sedatives and hypnotics, even when administered in low doses, can result in wakefulness, excitement, and confusion. The nurse can provide a warm, caffeine-free beverage, an extra blanket, or soft music to promote restful sleep.

Orienting the Client

Measures to help older clients maintain contact with reality can prevent episodes of confusion. The older adult benefits from **reality orientation** (Nursing Guidelines 9-1). Reality orientation involves using various techniques that reinforce the client's awareness of the date, time, place, names or roles of individuals involved in their care, and current events.

NURSING GUIDELINES 9-1

Reality Orientation

- Prominently display the date.
- Identify yourself and address the client by name each time you interact with him or her.
- Reinforce the time of day during routine activities (e.g., "Mrs. Green, it's 2 PM and time for your pill.")
- Give the client a few pages of the newspaper to read.
- Discuss current events.
- Compare events from day to day.
- Routinely tune in radio or television news programs.
- Encourage social interaction with other clients.

Communicating With Older Adults

An important aspect of encouraging communication involves stimulating older adults to talk about past experiences and events. This is referred to as **reminiscence therapy** and is a good technique for reinforcing self-esteem. Older adults have a need to talk about past events, achievements, and losses. Asking them to recall their personal history encourages communication between the older adult, health care personnel, and the family.

Validation therapy, developed by Naomi Feil (1992), is a method of communicating with the elderly who are confused, disoriented, and act out in inappropriate ways because of a permanent and progressive loss of cognitive ability. Feil believes these individuals are seeking to communicate feelings through their behavior. In validation therapy, the nurse seeks to reassure the client and gain understanding of the client's behavior or words spoken. For example, the woman who cares for and nurtures a doll may need validation of her role as a mother or the assurance of the love of her children. In this case the nurse says, "I know you love your children" or "You are such a good mother." To say "That is not a baby, but a doll," is presenting reality, but would cause emotional pain or agitation in many older adults. By seeking to validate feelings, the nurse provides comfort and affirming feelings.

GENERAL NUTRITIONAL CONSIDERATIONS

Limited income, inadequate cooking facilities, social isolation, and poor dentition are factors that affect the eating habits of older adults. Older adults, particularly those living alone, are at risk for nutritional deficiencies. Nutritional care of older adults is client centered and based on the person's physical and psychosocial status. Rigid dietary restrictions are bypassed in favor of quality of life and independent functioning.

Physical activity may help improve calcium balance, energy balance, bowel elimination, and sense of well-being. Encourage the client to be as active as possible.

Increasing fiber and fluid intake may help alleviate constipation. Clients with altered dentition who cannot chew fresh fruits and vegetables may find using wheat bran and whole-grain breads and cereals the most practical method of increasing fiber intake. A soft, ground, or pureed diet may be necessary if chewing or swallowing is impaired.

Thirst is not a reliable indicator of need in older adults. Encourage ample fluid intake of six to eight glasses daily to maintain hydration and normal urinary and fecal output.

GENERAL PHARMACOLOGIC CONSIDERATIONS

Because older adults excrete drugs more slowly, lower doses of many pharmacologic agents, particularly narcotics, sedatives, hypnotics, and other central nervous system depressants, are indicated. In some instances, toxicity results when normal doses are administered.

Many medications cause confusion in older adults. When an older adult experiences sudden confusion, an evaluation of the medication regimen is necessary to identify the drug or drugs that cause or contribute to the confusion. All older adults need a periodic review of their medication regimen. In some situations, polypharmacy is practiced (the taking of a large number of prescription and nonprescription drugs). Some of these drugs could be inappropriate and cause needless adverse reactions.

Some medications cause depression in older adults. Antipsychotics, hypnotics, some antihypertensives and cardiovascular drugs, and the narcotic analgesics are drugs associated with the development of depression. Careful monitoring of the older client who takes these drugs is essential. Clients must take antidepressants for up to 8 weeks before a therapeutic effect is observed. Warn family members and caregivers to take precautions against suicide until a therapeutic effect is achieved.

GENERAL GERONTOLOGIC CONSIDERATIONS

Older clients with arthritis or other conditions that cause loss of strength or coordination may request that prescriptions be filled without using childproof caps.

Nurses caring for older adults must dispel stereotypical thinking and view their clients as individuals with unique qualities and characteristics.

Critical Thinking Exercises

1. *An 82-year-old client sits alone all day in the nursing home. He spends his time staring at the television with no obvious interest. When the nursing staff try to involve him in various activities, he becomes irritated or says that he is too tired. What are some possible reasons for the client's behavior? What actions(s) could you take to help him?*
2. *The nursing home asks you to help organize a reality orientation program for the older adults in the facility. Many of the nursing assistants are unaware of the intervention. How would you explain reality orientation to the nurse assistants? What are some suggestions you could make to reinforce reality for the elderly clients in the nursing home?*

References and Suggested Readings

Administration on Aging. (2001). A profile of older Americans. Department of Health and Human Services. [On-line.] Available: http://www.aoa.dhhs.gov/aoa/stats/profile/2002/1.html.

American Association of Retired Persons. (1999). A profile of older Americans. [On-line.] Available: http:www.research.aarp.org/.

Conner, L. T. (2001). Memory in old age: Patterns of decline and preservation. *Seminars in Speech and Language, 22,* 117–125, 157–158.

Courts, N. F., Barba, B. E., & Tesh, A. (2001). Family caregivers' attitudes toward aging, caregiving, and nursing home placement. *Journal of Gerontological Nursing, 27*(8), 44–52.

Derry, A. D. (2000). Substance use in older adults: A review of current assessment, treatment and service provision. *Journal of Substance Use, 5,* 252–262.

Dudek, S. G. (2001). *Nutrition handbook for nursing practice* (5th ed.). Philadelphia: Lippincott Williams & Wilkins.

Eliopoulos, C. (2001). *Gerontological nursing* (5th ed.). Philadelphia: Lippincott Williams & Wilkins.

Federal Interagency Forum on Aging-Related Statistics. (2000). Older Americans 2000: Key indicators of well-being. Administration on Aging, Agency for Healthcare Research and Quality, Bureau of Labor Statistics. [On-line.] Available: http:www.agingstats.gov/chartbook2000/population.html.

Feil, N. (1992). *Validation: The Feil method.* Cleveland, OH: Edward Feil Productions.

Feldt, K. S. & Oh, H. L. (2000). Pain and hip fracture outcomes for older adults. *Orthopaedic Nursing, 19*(6), 35–44.

Gomez, R. G. & Madey, S. F. (2001). Coping with hearing loss model for older adults. *Journal Of Gerontology. Series B: Psychological Sciences and Social Sciences, 56B,* 233–235.

Hirst, S. P. & Raffin, S. (2001). "I hated those darn chickens..." The power in stories for older adults and nurses. *Journal of Gerontological Nursing, 27*(9), 24–29, 55–56.

Kurlowicz, L. & Wallace, M. (2001). Try this: Best practices in nursing care to older adults. The Mini Mental State Examination (MMSE). *Update: Society of Otorhinolaryngology and Head-Neck Nurses, 23*(3), 12–13.

Matteson, M. A., McConnell, E. S., & Linton, A. D. (1997). *Gerontological nursing: Concepts and practice* (2nd ed.). Philadelphia: W. B. Saunders.

McBean, L. D., Groziak, S. M., Miller, G. D., et al. (2001). Healthy eating in later years. *Nutrition Today, 36,* 192–201.

McInnis, G. J. & White, J. H. (2001). A phenomenological exploration of loneliness in the older adult. *Archives of Psychiatric Nursing, 15,* 128–139.

National Institute on Aging. (1996). The secrets of aging. Department of Health and Human Services. [On-line.] Available: http://www.originalghr15.com/secrets.html.

Pinquart, M. & Srensen, S. (2001). How effective are psychotherapeutic and other psychosocial interventions with older adults? *Journal of Mental Health and Aging, 7,* 207–243.

Resnick, B. (2001). Skills workshop: Motivating older adults to engage in self-care. *Patient Care for the Nurse Practitioner, 4*(9), 13–14, 16, 19.

Roy, R. (2001). Old age, pain, and loss. *Topics in Geriatric Rehabilitation, 16*(3), 66–76.

Taaffe, D. R. & Marcus, R. (2000). Musculoskeletal health and the older adult. *Journal of Rehabilitation Research and Development, 37,* 245–254.

U.S. Department of Health and Human Services. (1992). *Healthy people 2000: National health promotion and disease prevention objectives.* Boston: Jones and Bartlett.

Van Wynen, E. A. (2001). Healthy people 2010. A key to successful aging: Learning-style patterns of older adults. *Journal of Gerontological Nursing, 27*(9), 6–15.

Walsh, K. & Bennett, G. (2000). Financial abuse of older people. *Journal of Adult Protection, 2*(1), 21–29.

Zeiss, A. M. & Kasl-Godley, J. (2001). Sexuality in older adults' relationships. *Generations, 25*(2), 18–25.

Nurse–Client Relationships

Words to Know

affective learner
affective touch
caregiver
cognitive learner
collaborator
comfort zone
delegator
educator
empathy
formal teaching
hearing
informal teaching
intimate space
introductory phase
kinesics
learning capacity
learning needs
learning readiness
learning style

listening
motivation
nonverbal
  communication
nurse–client
  relationship
paralanguage
personal space
proxemics
psychomotor learner
public space
social space
task-oriented touch
teaching plan
terminating phase
therapeutic
  communication
verbal communication
working phase

Learning Objectives

On completion of this chapter, the reader will:

- List four roles that nurses perform within the nurse–client relationship.
- Name three phases in a nurse–client relationship.
- Differentiate between verbal, nonverbal, and therapeutic communication.
- Give at least two examples of therapeutic and nontherapeutic communication techniques.
- List and explain five components of nonverbal communication.
- Give the names of four proxemic zones.
- Explain what is meant by a client's "comfort zone."
- Differentiate between task-oriented and affective touch.
- Explain the learning styles of cognitive, affective, and psychomotor learners.
- Name three variables that affect learning.
- Compare informal with formal learning.
- Discuss at least five nursing guidelines for teaching adult clients.

The word *relationship* refers to an association between two or more people. Nurses form relationships with clients, families, and community groups. In this chapter, the term *relationship* is used in its strictest sense—that is, one between nurses and the clients for whom they care.

THE NURSE–CLIENT RELATIONSHIP

The **nurse–client relationship** exists during the period when the nurse interacts with clients, sick or well, to promote or restore their health, help them to cope with their illness, or assist them to die with dignity. Communicating therapeutically, listening empathetically, sharing information, and providing client education are among the most basic processes that occur in the context of the nurse–

client relationship. As in any effective relationship, each party has unique responsibilities to the other (Box 10-1).

Nursing Roles Within the Nurse–Client Relationship

The nurse–client relationship requires the nurse to respond to the client's needs. The National Council of State Boards of Nursing, which develops the national licensing examination for practical nurses (NCLEX-PN), identifies four categories of client needs as the structure for its test plan. These categories include (1) safe, effective care environment, (2) health promotion and maintenance, (3) psychosocial integrity, and (4) physiologic integrity. These content areas within nursing practice are consistently applied regardless of the stage in the client's life span or the setting for healthcare delivery.

BOX 10-1 ● Nurse–Client Responsibilities

NURSING RESPONSIBILITIES
Possess current knowledge.
Be aware of unique age-related differences.
Perform technical skills safely.
Be committed to the client's care.
Be available and courteous.
Allow client to participate in decisions.
Remain nonjudgmental.
Advocate on the client's behalf.
Provide explanations in language that is easily understood.
Promote independence.

CLIENT RESPONSIBILITIES
Identify current problem.
Describe desired outcomes.
Answer questions honestly.
Provide accurate historic and subjective data.
Participate to the fullest extent possible.
Be open and flexible to alternatives.
Comply with the therapeutic regimen.
Keep follow-up appointments.

To meet client needs, nurses perform four basic roles: caregiver, educator, collaborator, and delegator (see Chap. 6). Refer to Table 10-1 for an example of how the NCLEX-PN test categories integrate with these basic nursing roles.

The Nurse as Caregiver

A **caregiver** is one who performs health-related activities that a sick person cannot perform independently. The nurse's caregiving skills help to restore wellness, especially during an acute illness, or maintain as much function and independence as possible among those who have chronic physical or mental health problems.

Traditionally, nurses have been providers of physical care; however, caring also involves a close emotional relationship. Contemporary nurses understand that illness and injuries cause feelings of insecurity that may threaten a person's ability to cope. Consequently, the nurse becomes the client's guide, companion, and interpreter. The supportive relationship that develops establishes trust and reduces fear and worry.

TABLE 10-1	INTEGRATION OF NCLEX-PN TEST CATEGORIES WITH NURSING ROLES	
CATEGORY	**SUBCATEGORIES**	**NURSING ROLE**
Safe, Effective Care Environment	Coordinated Care *Example:* Using assistive personnel in client care	• Collaborator • Delegator
	Safety and Infection Control *Example:* Controlling exposure to sources of radiation and hazardous substances	• Caregiver • Collaborator • Educator
Health Promotion and Maintenance	Growth and Development Through the Life Span *Example:* Facilitating the transition from independent living to living with assistance	• Caregiver • Collaborator • Educator
	Prevention and Early Detection of Disease *Example:* Minimizing risk factors related to the development of acute or chronic illnesses	• Educator • Caregiver • Collaborator
Psychosocial Integrity	Coping and Adaptation *Example:* Using principles of therapeutic communication	• Caregiver • Collaborator
	Psychosocial Adaptation *Example:* Promoting the expression of feelings within established boundaries	• Caregiver • Collaborator
Physiologic Integrity	Basic Care and Comfort *Example:* Encouraging fluid intake	• Caregiver • Educator • Collaborator • Delegator
	Pharmacologic Therapies *Example:* Identifying therapeutic and nontherapeutic reactions to medications	• Caregiver • Educator
	Reduction of Risk Potential *Example:* Performing blood glucose finger sticks	• Caregiver • Delegator • Collaborator
	Physiologic Adaptation *Example:* Maintaining a patent airway	• Caregiver • Delegator • Collaborator

Nurses use **empathy,** an intuitive awareness of what the client is experiencing, to perceive the client's emotional state and need for support. Empathy helps the nurse become effective in providing for the client's needs while remaining compassionately detached.

> **Stop, Think, and Respond ● BOX 10-1**
>
> *When you are assigned to one or more clients during clinical experience, what kinds of caregiving skills do you perform?*

The Nurse as Educator

An **educator** is one who provides information. Nurses offer health teaching that is pertinent to each client's needs and knowledge base. Some examples include explanations about diagnostic test procedures, self-administration of medications, techniques for managing wound care, and restorative exercises like those performed after a mastectomy.

When it comes to treatment decisions, the nurse avoids giving advice, reserving the right of each person to make his or her own choices on matters affecting health and illness care. The nurse shares information on potential alternatives, allows the client the freedom to choose, and supports the client's ultimate decision.

Because nursing is considered a practice "without walls" (i.e., extending beyond the original treatment facility), nurses are resources for information about health services available in the community. This type of information empowers clients to become involved with self-help groups or those that offer rehabilitation, financial assistance, or emotional support.

The Nurse as Collaborator

A **collaborator** is one who works with others to achieve a common goal. Usually, many people are involved in a client's care (Fig. 10-1). The most obvious example of collaboration occurs between the nurse who is responsible for managing care and those to whom the care is delegated. Collaboration also takes place when the nurse and physician share information and when they exchange information with other healthcare workers, such as the dietitian, physical therapist, respiratory therapist, and discharge planner.

> **Stop, Think, and Respond ● BOX 10-2**
>
> *What healthcare workers might be involved in managing the care of a client with a stroke?*

The Nurse as Delegator

A **delegator** is one who assigns a task to someone. Before the nurse assumes the role of delegator, he or she must know what tasks are appropriate for particular healthcare

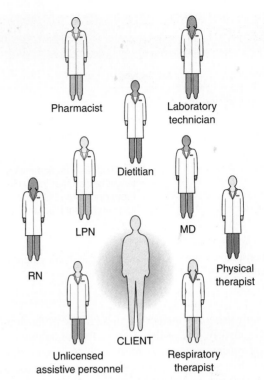

FIGURE 10-1 Collaboration may involve many members of the health-care team.

workers. It is unsafe to delegate a task to someone who does not have the knowledge or expertise to perform it correctly. Once a task has been assigned, it is still the delegator's responsibility to check that the task has been performed and determine the resulting outcome. For example, if a nurse asks a nursing assistant to change a client's position, the nurse must verify that the assistant has completed the job and obtain other pertinent information such as the condition of the client's skin. If the delegated task is not performed or is performed incorrectly, the nurse is held accountable for the inadequate client care.

> **Stop, Think, and Respond ● BOX 10-3**
>
> *What tasks might a staff nurse delegate to a student nurse?*

Phases of the Nurse–Client Relationship

The nurse–client relationship progresses through three phases: the introductory phase, the working phase, and the terminating phase. Table 10-2 shows an example of the activities that occur in each of the three phases.

Introductory Phase

The **introductory phase** starts when the nurse and the client get acquainted and the client identifies one or more health problems for which he or she is seeking care. Both the nurse and client bring preconceived ideas about the other to the initial interaction, and these assumptions

TABLE 10-2	EXAMPLES OF PHASE-RELATED ACTIVITIES
CLIENT	**NURSE**
Introductory Phase	
Seeks help in managing → diabetes	Determines what the client needs to learn ↓
Working Phase	
Practices skills and returns the demonstrations to the nurse ↓	←Develops and implements a teaching plan that includes monitoring blood glucose level and insulin administration
Termination Phase ↓	
Demonstrates desired → competencies	Refers client to diabetic clinic for future follow-up

eventually are confirmed or dismissed. The nurse demonstrates courtesy, active listening, empathy, competence, and appropriate communication skills to convey that he or she values the client. Nurses demonstrate partnership and advocacy in the client's healthcare by:

- Treating each client as a unique person
- Respecting the client's feelings
- Striving to promote the client's physical, emotional, social, and spiritual well-being
- Encouraging the client to participate in problem-solving and decision-making
- Accepting that a client has the potential for change
- Communicating in terms and language that the client understands
- Using the nursing process to individualize the client's care
- Involving those persons to whom the client turns for support, such as family and friends, when providing care
- Implementing healthcare techniques that are compatible with the client's value system and cultural heritage

Working Phase

The **working phase** involves mutually planning the client's care and putting the plan into action. Both the nurse and the client participate. Each shares in performing those tasks that will lead to the desired outcomes identified by the client. During the working phase, the nurse supports the client's independence. Doing too much is as harmful as doing too little.

Terminating Phase

The **terminating phase** occurs when the nurse and client mutually agree that the client's immediate health problems have improved and the nurse's services are no longer necessary. The nurse uses compassion and a caring attitude when facilitating the client's transition to other healthcare services or return to independent living.

COMMUNICATION

Communication is an exchange of information. It involves both sending and receiving messages between two or more individuals. It is followed by feedback indicating that the information is understood or needs further clarification (Fig. 10-2).

Therapeutic Communication

Communication occurs on a social or therapeutic level. **Therapeutic communication** refers to using words and gestures to promote a person's physical and emotional well-being. Techniques that are helpful are identified in Table 10-3.

> ### Stop, Think, and Respond ● BOX 10-4
> *Give an example of a therapeutic response to the following statement made by a client: "My family didn't visit me last evening."*

In situations in which clients are quiet and uncommunicative, the nurse must avoid assuming that the client has no problems or understands everything. On the other hand, it is never appropriate to probe or press an unwilling client to communicate. It is advantageous to wait because it is not unusual for reticent clients to share their feelings and concerns after they feel that the nurse is sincere and trustworthy.

The nurse also must respond delicately to a vocal and emotional client. For instance, when clients are angry or cry, the best nursing approach is to allow them to express their emotions without fear of retaliation or censure.

Although nurses have the best intentions of interacting therapeutically with clients, some fall into traps that block

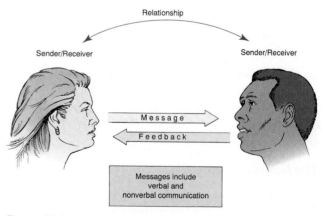

FIGURE 10-2 Communication is a two-way process.

TABLE 10-3	THERAPEUTIC COMMUNICATION TECHNIQUES

TECHNIQUE	USE	EXAMPLE
Broad opening	Relieves tension before getting to the real purpose of the interaction	"Wonderful weather we're having."
Giving information	Provides facts	"Your surgery is scheduled at noon."
Direct questioning	Acquires specific information	"Do you have any allergies?"
Open-ended questioning	Encourages the client to elaborate	"How are you feeling?"
Reflecting	Confirms that the nurse is following the conversation	*Client:* "I haven't been sleeping well." *Nurse:* "You haven't been sleeping well."
Paraphrasing	Restates what the client has said to demonstrate listening	*Client:* "After every meal, I feel like I will throw up." *Nurse:* "Eating makes you nauseous, but you don't actually vomit."
Verbalizing what has been implied	Shares how the nurse has interpreted a statement	*Client:* "All the nurses are so busy." *Nurse:* "You're feeling that you shouldn't ask for help."
Structuring	Defines a purpose and sets limits	"I have 15 minutes. If your pain is relieved, I could go over how your test will be done."
Giving general leads	Encourages the client to continue	"Uh, huh," or "Go on."
Sharing perceptions	Shows empathy for how the client is feeling	"You seem depressed."
Clarifying	Avoids misinterpretation	"I'm afraid I don't quite understand what you're asking."
Confronting	Calls attention to manipulation, inconsistencies, or lack of responsibility	"You're concerned about your weight loss, but you didn't eat any breakfast."
Summarizing	Reviews information that has been discussed	"You've asked me to check on increasing your pain medication and getting your diet changed."
Silence	Allows time for considering how to proceed or arouses the client's anxiety to the point that it stimulates more verbalization	

or hinder therapeutic communication. Table 10-4 lists common examples of nontherapeutic communication.

Verbal Communication

Verbal communication is communication that uses words. It includes speaking, reading, and writing. The following variables affect verbal communication:

- Attention and concentration
- Language compatibility
- Verbal skills
- Hearing and visual acuity
- Motor functions involving the throat, tongue, and teeth
- Noise and distracting activity
- Interpersonal attitudes
- Literacy
- Cultural similarities
- Listening

Listening is as important during communication as speaking. In contrast to **hearing,** which is perceiving sounds, **listening** is an activity that includes attending to and becoming fully involved in what the client says. Empathetic listening implies that the nurse attempts to perceive the client's emotions and meanings. When the nurse conveys empathy to clients, it helps them to feel both understood and valued. How empathetically one listens often is demonstrated through nonverbal means.

When communicating with most American clients, it is best to position oneself at the client's level and make frequent eye contact (see cultural exceptions in Chap. 11). Nodding and encouraging the client to continue with comments, such as "Yes, I see," conveys interest in what the client is saying. The nurse guards against sending messages that indicate boredom, such as looking out a window or interrupting a comment.

Nonverbal Communication

Nonverbal communication is the exchange of information without using words. It is what is not said. Nonverbal communication consists of components such as kinesics, paralanguage, proxemics, touch, and silence.

TABLE 10-4	NONTHERAPEUTIC COMMUNICATION TECHNIQUES	
TECHNIQUE AND CONSEQUENCE	**EXAMPLE**	**IMPROVEMENT**
Giving False Reassurance Trivializes the client's unique feelings and discourages further discussion	"You've got nothing to worry about. Everything will work out just fine."	"Tell me about your specific concerns."
Using Clichés Provides worthless advice and curtails exploring alternatives	"Keep a stiff upper lip."	"It must be difficult for you right now."
Giving Approval or Disapproval Holds the client to a rigid standard; implies that future deviation may lead to subsequent rejection or disfavor	"I'm glad you're exercising so regularly." "You should be testing your blood sugar each morning."	"Are you having any difficulty fitting regular exercise into your schedule?" "Let's explore some ways that will help you test your blood sugar each morning."
Agreeing Does not allow the client flexibility to change his or her mind	"You're right about needing surgery immediately."	"Having surgery immediately is one possibility. What others have you considered?"
Disagreeing Intimidates the client; makes the person feel foolish or inadequate	"That's not true! Where did you get an idea like that?"	"Maybe I can help clarify that for you."
Demanding an Explanation Puts the client on the defensive; the client may be tempted to make up an excuse rather than risk disapproval for an honest answer	"Why didn't you keep your appointment last week?"	"I see you couldn't keep your appointment last week."
Giving Advice Discourages independent problem-solving and decision-making; provides a biased view that may prejudice the client's choice	"If I were you, I'd try drug therapy before having surgery."	"Share with me the advantages and disadvantages of your options as you see them."
Defending Indicates such a strong allegiance that any disagreement to the contrary is not acceptable	"Ms. Johnson is my best nursing assistant. She wouldn't have let your light go unanswered that long."	"I'm sorry you had to wait so long."
Belittling Disregards how the client is responding as an individual	"Lots of people learn to give themselves insulin."	"You're finding it especially difficult to stick yourself with a needle."
Patronizing Treats the client condescendingly, as less than capable of making an independent decision	"Are we ready for our bath yet?"	"Would you like your bath now, or should I check with you later?"
Changing the Subject Alters the direction of the discussion to a topic that is safer or more comfortable	*Client:* "I'm so scared that a mammogram will show I have cancer." *Nurse:* "Tell me more about your family."	"It is a serious disease. What concerns you the most?"

Kinesics

Kinesics refers to body language, or those collective nonverbal techniques such as facial expressions, postures, gestures, and body movements. Even clothing style and accessories (e.g., jewelry) can affect the context of communication.

Stop, Think, and Respond ● BOX 10-5

What nonverbal message is communicated when a person wears a white lab coat, a ring on the third finger of the left hand, or a badge and gun?

Paralanguage

Paralanguage is vocal sounds (not actually words) that communicate a message. Some examples include drawing in a deep breath to indicate surprise, clucking the tongue to show disappointment, and whistling to get someone's attention. Crying, laughing, and moaning are additional forms of paralanguage. Vocal inflections, volume, pitch, and rate of speech add yet another dimension to communication.

Proxemics

Proxemics refers to the use of space when communicating. In general, four proxemic zones are common when Americans communicate. They include **intimate space, personal space, social space,** and **public space** (Table 10-5).

Most Americans tolerate strangers up to an area of 2 to 3 feet. Determining the circumference of a person's **comfort zone,** the area that when intruded does not create anxiety, is important because physical closeness is common during nursing care. Approaches that relieve a client's anxiety about being close include explaining beforehand how a nursing procedure will be performed and ensuring that the client is properly draped.

Touch

Touch is a tactile stimulus produced by personal contact with another person or object. In the context of nursing, touch is either task-oriented, affective, or both. **Task-oriented touch** involves the personal contact that is required when performing nursing procedures (Fig. 10-3). **Affective touch** is used to demonstrate concern or affection (Fig. 10-4). Its intention is to communicate caring and support. Most people respond positively to being touched; however, a nurse should use affective touching cautiously because there is a great deal of variation among individu-

FIGURE 10-3 Task-oriented touch. (Courtesy of Nursing Spectrum.)

als. In general, nurses use affective touch therapeutically when a client is lonesome; uncomfortable; near death; anxious, insecure, or frightened; disoriented; disfigured; semiconscious or comatose; visually impaired; or sensory deprived.

Silence

Silence is the art of remaining quiet. One of its therapeutic uses is to encourage a client's verbal communication. Other therapeutic uses include providing a personal presence and a brief period during which clients can process information or respond to a question.

CLIENT TEACHING

Sharing information and performing client teaching are essential nursing activities that promote a person's ability

TABLE 10-5	PROXEMIC ZONES	
ZONE	**DISTANCE**	**PURPOSE**
Intimate space	Within 6 inches	Lovemaking Confiding secrets Sharing confidential information
Personal space	6 inches to 4 feet	Interviewing Physical assessment Therapeutic interventions involving touch Private conversations Teaching one-on-one
Social space	4 to 12 feet	Group interactions Lecturing Conversations that are not intended to be private
Public space	12 or more feet	Giving speeches Gatherings of strangers

FIGURE 10-4 Affective touch. (Courtesy of Brett Ainsworth.)

FIGURE 10-5 A nurse implements teaching proper lifting technique for a client who is a psychomotor learner. (From Craven, R. F. & Hirnle, C. J. [2000]. *Fundamentals of nursing: Human health and function* [3rd ed., p. 738]. Philadelphia: Lippincott Williams & Wilkins.)

to understand the healthcare environment and independently meet his or her own health needs. Limited hospitalization time demands that nurses begin teaching clients as soon as possible after admission. Teaching continues while nurses care for clients in their homes or present educational programs in community settings. Teaching is either formal or informal, and the most efficient teaching occurs when the nurse presents information compatible with the client's learning style.

Learner Assessment

The nurse performs a learner assessment to determine various components of the client's learning status. Besides determining the style of learning a client prefers, the nurse assesses the client's learning needs, learning capacity, motivation for learning, and learning readiness.

Learning Styles

A **learning style** is the manner in which a person best comprehends new information. Usually people fall into one of three categories: cognitive, affective, or psychomotor learner (Table 10-6). The **cognitive learner** processes information best by listening to or reading facts and descriptions. The **affective learner** is more attuned to learning when presented with information

that appeals to his or her feelings, beliefs, and values. The **psychomotor learner** likes to learn by doing (Fig. 10-5).

One way to determine a client's learning style is to ask, "When you learned to add fractions, what helped you most: listening to the teacher's explanation, recognizing the value of fractions in cooking or carpentry, or actually working on sample problems?" Although most favor one style of learning, presenting information through a combination of the three styles tends to optimize learning.

Learning Needs

Client education begins with an assessment of learning needs. **Learning needs** are those skills and concepts that the client and family must acquire to restore, maintain, or promote health. For example, the client with diabetes needs to learn to self-administer insulin, a skill, and how diabetes affects circulation, a concept. Distinguishing the important skills and concepts a client must learn and then assessing what the client already knows helps in identifying goals, tailoring the teaching plan to the individual, and evaluating outcomes.

TABLE 10-6	ACTIVITIES THAT PROMOTE LEARNING ACCORDING TO STYLES	
COGNITIVE LEARNERS	**AFFECTIVE LEARNERS**	**PSYCHOMOTOR LEARNERS**
Listing	Advocating	Assembling
Identifying	Supporting	Changing
Naming	Accepting	Emptying
Describing	Promoting	Filling
Summarizing	Internalizing	Adding
Selecting	Valuing	Removing

Learning Capacity

Learning capacity refers to a person's intellectual ability to understand, remember, and apply new information. Illiteracy, sensory deficits, and a shortened attention span require special adaptations when implementing client teaching.

Motivation

Motivation is the desire to acquire new information. Learning occurs at an accelerated rate when a person has a purpose or reason for mastering it. Some motivating forces include restoring independence, preventing complications, facilitating discharge, and returning to or remaining in the comfort of home.

Learning Readiness

Learning readiness pertains to the optimal time for learning. Ideally, it occurs when a client is in a state of physical and psychological well-being. For example, a client who is in pain, uncomfortably warm or cold, anxious, or depressed is not in the best condition for learning. In these situations, it is best to restore comfort and then attend to teaching.

Informal and Formal Teaching

Informal teaching is unplanned. It occurs spontaneously, usually at the client's bedside or while caring for the client at home. **Formal teaching** requires a plan to avoid being haphazard. A **teaching plan** is the organized arrangement of content in a specific time frame. It facilitates reaching goals, providing essential information and ensuring the client's comprehension before he or she assumes responsibility for self-care. Developing a plan and implementing it gradually and sequentially avoids overwhelming the client with new information or learning skills that are difficult to perform. The suggestions in Nursing Guidelines 10-1 are useful when teaching adult clients.

GENERAL NUTRITIONAL CONSIDERATIONS

Hunger, thirst, nausea, distention, constipation, or diarrhea interferes with a client's attention and readiness for learning. Restoring physical comfort increases a client's receptiveness for communication and learning.

GENERAL PHARMACOLOGIC CONSIDERATIONS

Some medications dull mental ability and make concentration more difficult. They can affect the client's ability to learn new material and to remember specific details taught during a teaching session.

NURSING GUIDELINES 10-1

Teaching Adult Clients

- Identify the value or purpose for learning new information.
- Determine if the client is comfortable at the moment.
- Make sure the adult is wearing glasses or using a hearing aid, if he or she needs one or the other.
- Reduce noise and distractions in the environment.
- Sit at eye level (unless doing group teaching) and face the client(s).
- Use short sentences of 10 words or fewer.
- Avoid speaking rapidly.
- Minimize technical terms and medical jargon; define words whenever necessary.
- Use words that a seventh- to ninth-grader would understand.
- Present at least one but no more than three new ideas at each teaching session.
- Review frequently.
- Use the active form of the verb rather than passive (e.g., "Wipe straight down the center of the incision," rather than "The incision is wiped down the center.").
- Use examples with which the learner can identify.
- Relate new information to prior learning.
- Build in a learner performance evaluation, such as asking the client to repeat or paraphrase prior information, demonstrate a skill, or apply the information to a hypothetical situation, such as "What would you do if . . . ?"
- Terminate teaching if the client cannot remain attentive.

GENERAL GERONTOLOGIC CONSIDERATIONS

Older adults have a lifetime of past experiences that are useful as a foundation for new learning.

Older adults tend to lose the ability to hear at high-pitched ranges. Therefore, it is best to lower the voice pitch during communication.

Communicate with hearing-impaired adults by inserting a stethoscope into the client's ears and speaking into the bell or using a magic slate, chalkboard, flash cards, or writing tablets.

Before beginning a teaching session, ask the older adult about the need for glasses or a hearing aid. If either is necessary, make sure that glasses are clean or the hearing aid is in good working order.

When teaching older adults, choose printed materials that positively portray persons of similar age.

Avoid using printed materials that are cluttered with extensive information.

Be sure that printed materials are of sufficient size for easy reading. Such materials usually should be in at least 14-point type for older adults.

Booklets, pamphlets, and brochures that are printed in black-on-white matte paper improve visual clarity.

Healthy older adults do not have a significant decrease in cognitive ability and can learn new information. They do, however, learn more efficiently when they are allowed to progress at their own pace.

Learning motor skills may be more difficult for older adults because of physiologic changes. They may need more time to learn new activities.

An appreciation of the older adult as an individual with unique needs and concerns is the foundation of a positive nurse–client relationship with older adults.

When an older adult repeatedly tells the same story or asks the same question, make an effort to see if there is a hidden or unspoken message of fear or concern that the older adult is too apprehensive to discuss.

During the introductory phase of the nurse–client relationship, take time to listen actively to the older adult. Allow ample time for a response to questions. Remember that the health history of an older adult may span more than 80 years.

Clarify any questionable information with a family member or the primary caregiver. Older adults may have short-term memory impairment, even though long-term memory remains intact.

Critical Thinking Exercises

1. *Change the nontherapeutic interaction in the following example to one that is therapeutic:*
   Client: "I'm having second thoughts about having this breast reduction surgery."
   Nurse: "You'll be happy with the results when it's over."
2. *Change the therapeutic interaction in the following example to one that is nontherapeutic:*
   Client: "My pain is worse today than it was right after surgery."
   Nurse: "You're concerned that the increase in pain suggests a complication."

References and Suggested Readings

Barry, C. B. (2000). Teaching the older patient in the home: Assessment and adaptation. *Home Healthcare Nurse, 18*(6), 374–387.

Gannon, B. A. (2000). Caring one day at a time. *Journal of Neonatal Nursing, 19*(5), 25–32.

Giving patients the tools is the first step, ensuring they understand is the next: Focus on teaching materials and techniques that improve comprehension. (2000). *Patient Education Management, 7*(10), 109–112.

Hague, W. (2000). I'm listening. *Nursing Standard, 15*(2), 25.

Hawkins-Walsh, E. (2000). Listening. *American Journal of Nursing (Advanced Practice Extra), 100*(9), 24BBB, 24DDD.

Michelini, C. A. (2000). MIND MAP: A new way to teach patients and staff. *Home Healthcare Nurse, 18,* 318–322.

National Council of State Boards of Nursing, Inc. (1999). *Detailed test plan for the NCLEX-PN Examination.* Chicago: Author.

Rankin, S. H. & Stallings, K. D. (2000). *Patient education: Issues, principles, practices* (4th ed.). Philadelphia: Lippincott Williams & Wilkins.

Tammelleo, A. D. (2000). Failure to "understand"—do your patients "understand" you? Are you sure? *Nursing's Law Regan Report, 41*(1), 3.

Woodring, B. C. (2000). If you have taught—have the child and family learned? *Pediatric Nursing, 26,* 505–509.

Caring for Culturally Diverse Clients

Words to Know

cultural competence
culture
ethnicity
ethnocentrism
generalization
health beliefs

health practices
minority
race
stereotyping
subculture
transcultural nursing

Learning Objectives

On completion of this chapter, the reader will:

- Define terms related to culture.
- List the five population groups delineated in the United States.
- Differentiate race from ethnicity and culture.
- Contrast stereotyping and generalization.
- Describe how cultural background and practices influence actions and behaviors.
- Name three views that societies use to explain illness or disease.
- Discuss biocultural assessment.
- Describe cultural assessment.
- Explain the meaning and characteristics of transcultural nursing.
- List at least five ways to demonstrate culturally sensitive nursing care.
- Describe the culturally competent nurse.

Healthcare providers are becoming increasingly aware that high-quality care involves greater cognizance and appreciation of different linguistic and cultural backgrounds. Healthcare facilities in most large cities and many rural and suburban areas serve diverse populations. Providers and clients bring their respective cultural backgrounds and expectations to any healthcare situation (Diversity Rx, 1997). Thus, nurses must become culturally competent. This chapter provides information about cultural concepts, clinical variations among different ethnic and racial groups, and communication issues for various cultures. Knowledge of cultural differences and the ability to adapt to each client's cultural needs are crucial to provide quality care.

CULTURAL CONCEPTS

To deliver culturally competent care, nurses must understand terms related to culture. They also must view each person as a unique human being who may have a similar or different frame of reference as the nurse.

Culture

Sir Edward Tyler, a British anthropologist, first used the term *culture* in 1871. He stated that culture includes knowledge, beliefs, art, morals, laws, customs, and other capabilities and habits. Andrews and Boyle (1999) state "**Culture** represents a way of perceiving, behaving, and evaluating the world. It provides a blueprint or guide for determining people's values, beliefs, and practices, including those pertaining to health" (p. 3). According to Smeltzer and Bare (2000), four basic concepts characterize culture. Culture is (1) learned from birth through language and socialization; (2) shared by members of the same cultural group; (3) influenced by specific conditions related to environment, technology, and availability of resources; and (4) dynamic and ever-changing.

Subculture

The United States is often referred to as a *melting pot,* implying that culturally diverse groups are assimilated in one society. Subcultures, however, are readily apparent. **Sub-**

culture refers to a particular group that shares characteristics identifying the group as a distinct entity (Smeltzer & Bare, 2000). For example, African Americans, Hispanic Americans, and Native Americans share physical characteristics, language, and ancestry. These groups may have more subcultures related to specific place of origin, such as Latinos or Chicanos within the Hispanic-American group. Other ways to categorize subcultures include region; religion; age; sex; social class; political party; ethnic, racial or cultural identity; and occupation.

Minority

The term **minority** is used to describe a group of people who differ from the majority in a society in terms of cultural characteristics, physical characteristics, or both. Because people from the minority group are "different," the majority group may treat them unfairly. The United States defines five population groups: white, black, Hispanic, Asian/Pacific Islander, and American Indian/Alaskan Native. Whites still are considered the majority; the other groups are referred to as *ethnic minorities.* Other minorities are based on sex or religion. The defining characteristics for a minority group are not based on numbers but rather on powerlessness and lack of control. For example, women in the United States outnumber men, but women remain in lower-paying jobs and less powerful positions, and thus still are considered a minority.

Ethnicity

Ethnicity is the bond or kinship that people feel with their country of birth or place of ancestral origin. It provides a sense of identity. People demonstrate pride in their ethnic heritage by valuing certain physical characteristics, giving children ethnic names, wearing unique items of clothing, appreciating folk music and dance, or eating native food.

Race

The term *race* often is confused with ethnicity and culture. **Race** refers to biologic differences in physical features, such as skin color, bone structure, and eye shape. Many people associate physical differences, particularly skin color, with culture. Although ethnic and racial groups overlap, nurses must not equate skin color and other physical features with culture. Doing so may lead to erroneous assumptions that all people with certain physical attributes share essentially the same culture and ethnicity. This attitude leads to stereotyping.

Stereotyping

Stereotyping means assuming that all people in a particular cultural, racial, or ethnic group share the same values and beliefs, behave similarly, and are basically alike. For example, a nurse who thinks stereotypically may assign a client to a staff member who is of the same culture as the client, simply because the nurse assumes that all people of that culture are alike. This same nurse also may believe that clients with the same skin color have similar social situations. Because stereotypes are preconceived ideas unsupported by facts, they may not be real or accurate. In fact, they can be dangerous because they are dehumanizing and interfere with accepting others as unique individuals.

Generalization

Distinguishing between stereotyping and generalization is important. Stereotyping has an end point; the assumption prevents one from seeing another person as unique. **Generalization,** however, acknowledges common trends in a group while recognizing that more information is needed. As explained by Galanti (2000, p. 1), "If I meet a Mexican woman named Maria and assume that she has a large family, I am stereotyping her. But if I say to myself, 'Mexicans tend to have large families; I wonder if Maria does,' then I am generalizing." Cultural generalizations do not describe each client but provide a broad pattern of beliefs and behaviors for clients from a particular cultural group. This knowledge may assist healthcare providers to provide appropriate care. Nevertheless, generalization can lead to stereotyping, of which nurses must remain cognizant. Increased awareness will assist them to see each client as a unique person.

> ### Stop, Think, and Respond ● BOX 11-1
> *You overhear a nurse talking about a client admitted with diabetes and a leg ulcer. The nurse says, "It figures he doesn't do what the doctors say— he's been in this country for 10 years and still can't speak English well. Those people are just stupid!" How would you respond?*

Ethnocentrism

Ethnocentrism is the belief that one's own ethnic heritage is the "correct" one and superior to others. Nurses are human and certainly enter the nursing profession with their own ethnocentrism. They must be aware that their way is not the only or best way. Clients will sense that a nurse feels superior if he or she approaches with a patronizing or condescending attitude. Clients bring their own values and practices and are not ignorant simply because they have different beliefs. Nurses must appreciate that their values and beliefs are not better than those of clients—they simply are different.

Other Culture-Related Terms

Acculturation is the process by which members of one cultural group adapt to or take on the behaviors of another group. *Cultural blindness* is an inability to recognize the values, beliefs, and practices of others because of strong ethnocentric tendencies. *Cultural imposition* is a tendency to impose one's cultural beliefs, values, and patterns of behavior on persons from a different culture. *Cultural taboos* are activities governed by rules of behavior that a particular cultural group avoids, forbids, or prohibits (Smeltzer & Bare, 2000).

CULTURALLY INFLUENCED CHARACTERISTICS

Cultural upbringing influences a person's actions and behaviors. Socially acceptable conduct for one person may be unacceptable for another. Cultural background affects a person's actions and reactions to his or her environment. When considering cultural background, there is the danger of stereotyping. Issues such as personal space, verbal behaviors, touch, diet, time, and beliefs about the cause of illness are unique for each individual but may be culturally influenced.

Eye Contact

Nurses are taught to maintain eye contact with clients when they are speaking with them, but respecting and understanding behavior and providing a comfortable climate for clients are important considerations. The physical act of making eye contact may be culturally influenced. Anglo-Americans typically value direct eye contact or "looking a person straight in the eye" while speaking. Such eye contact, however, may offend Asian Americans, Native Americans, and other cultural groups who view lingering eye contact as an invasion of privacy. Others, such as Hispanic clients, may avoid eye contact with authority figures as a sign of respect.

Space and Distance

People are not always aware of personal space needs until such needs are threatened. Healthcare situations, such as providing personal care or performing intricate procedures, reduce the accepted personal space, along with causing personal discomfort. Furthermore, nurses often provide comfort and support through close physical proximity, but such closeness may threaten some clients. Nurses must observe how clients position themselves and respect their desire for space as much as possible. Simple explanations of the need for physical proximity during clinical procedures and personal care alleviate the discomfort that some clients may experience.

Verbal Differences

Interpreter may be needed

General communication patterns are found among the major U.S. subcultures. The nurse must carefully observe or tactfully question clients about communication preferences and tailor the interview accordingly.

Anglo-Americans usually are open to providing personal health information and expressing positive and negative feelings. Asian Americans tend to control their emotion and not reveal that they are physically uncomfortable (Giger & Davidhizar, 1995), especially when among people with whom they are unfamiliar. Similarly, Latino men may not show feelings or readily discuss symptoms because they may interpret doing so as less than manly (Andrews & Boyle, 1999). Male Latino behavior can be attributed to *machismo,* the belief that virile men are physically strong and must deal with emotions privately. Thus, many Latino men in general are protective and authoritarian when it comes to women and children. They expect to be consulted in decision-making when a family member is the primary client.

Many Native Americans are rather private and may hesitate to share much personal information with strangers. They also may fear encounters with non-Indian healthcare providers because of the long history of careless treatment of Native Americans. They may interpret questioning as prying or meddling. Nurses should be patient and listen carefully. In Native American cultures, listening is a valued skill, whereas impatience is seen as disrespectful (Lipson et al., 1996). Some Native Americans may be skeptical of Anglo-American nurses who write down what clients say because Native Americans preserve their history through the oral tradition. If possible, writing notes after instead of during the interview may be helpful. Navajos, currently the largest tribe of Native Americans, feel that no person has the right to speak for another; they may refuse to comment on a family member's health problems.

Some clients may distrust healthcare personnel because of poor past experiences. For example, the U.S. healthcare system has a history of victimizing some African Americans as unknowing research subjects or denying them appropriate access to healthcare. Because of such experiences, African Americans may hesitate to give any more information than they are asked. They may not trust healthcare professionals to do the right thing. Nurses can show professionalism by introducing themselves and addressing clients by their last names. Following up thoroughly with requests is essential, as are respecting privacy and asking open-ended rather than direct questions until trust is established. Latinos are characteristically more comfortable sitting close to interviewers and letting interactions slowly unfold. Many Latinos speak English but still may have difficulty with medical terminology. They may be embarrassed to ask the interviewer to speak slowly, so nurses must provide information and ask questions carefully without displaying impatience. If a client requires an interpreter, having a translator of the same sex as the client is best. Asian Americans feel comfortable positioned more than an arm's length from the interviewer. They tend to respond with brief, factual answers and little elaboration. Asian Americans may not openly disagree with authoritarian figures, like physicians and nurses, because of their respect for harmony. Their reticence can conceal a potential for noncompliance when a particular therapeutic regimen is unacceptable from their perspective.

Communication with someone who speaks a different language presents unique challenges. Nurses who speak a client's language are far more likely to connect positively with the client. More than 150 languages are spoken in the United States, so it is unlikely that nurses can converse easily with most non–English-speaking clients. An interpreter is invaluable, but the nurse's actions, cultural respect, and nonverbal communication techniques will promote acceptance and cooperation.

Touch

There are great cultural differences in the use of touch. For example, some Native Americans may interpret the Anglo-American custom of a strong handshake as offensive. They may be more comfortable with just a light passing of the hands. Arab culture prohibits male healthcare providers from physically examining women. Asian Americans consider touching the head impolite because the spirit rests there. Orthodox Jewish women highly value their modesty and must keep their heads and limbs covered (Smeltzer & Bare, 2000). Nurses need to respect and adapt care to honor these and other differences related to touch.

Diet

The relationship between food-related behaviors and culture is complex (Box 11-1). Basically, food is a means of survival—it relieves hunger, promotes health, and prevents disease. Its social meanings encompass love, togetherness, and celebration. Food also has other connotations in terms of its use to reward or punish, relieve stress, and delineate social classes. Culture often dictates the types of food and how frequently a person eats, the types of utensils he or she uses, and the status assigned to particular individuals (e.g., who eats first, who gets the most to eat).

BOX 11-1 ● **Selected Examples of Cultural Meanings of Food**

- Critical life force for survival
- Relief of hunger
- Peaceful coexistence
- Promotion of health and healing
- Prevention of disease or illness
- Expression of caring for another
- Interpersonal closeness or distance
- Promotion of kinship and familial alliances
- Solidification of social ties
- Celebration of life events (e.g., birthday, marriage)
- Expression of gratitude or appreciation
- Recognition of achievement or accomplishment
- Business negotiations
- Information exchange
- Validation of social, cultural, or religious ceremonial functions
- Way to generate income
- Expression of affluence, wealth, or social status

---

dividuals (e.g., who eats first, who gets the most to eat). Religious practices also impose certain rules and restrictions, such as fasting, eliminating some foods, and observing rituals (e.g., Passover dinner; Box 11-2). There are implications for healthcare when a client is diagnosed with diabetes, hypertension, or other disorders that require dietary adjustments. Nurses must consider cultural and religious food preferences/requirements when instructing clients about the dietary restrictions related to a specific condition.

Time

Throughout the world, people view clock time and social time differently (Giger & Davidhizar, 1995). *Clock time* implies the orderly division of time into years, months, weeks, days, hours, minutes, and seconds. Calendars, clocks, sunrises, tides, and moons define clock time. *Social time* is based more on cultural habits, meals, celebrations, and other events and is related to punctuality and waiting. Aspects of social time vary among cultures. For example, some cultures highly value punctuality. A client from such a culture may be on time for an appointment and then have to wait, increasing his or her frustration with the healthcare system. Clients from other cultures may place priority more on activities, such as family needs, and less on punctuality for appointments. Recognizing that clients have different perceptions of time assists the nurse to provide more sensitive care.

Beliefs About Causes of Illness

Societies use three overall views to explain illness or disease (Smeltzer & Bare, 2000):

BOX 11-2 ● Prohibited Foods and Beverages for Selected Religious Groups

HINDUISM
All meats
Animal shortenings

ISLAM
Alcoholic products and beverages (including extracts, such as vanilla and lemon)
Animal shortenings
Gelatin made with pork, marshmallow, and other confections made with gelatin
Pork

JUDAISM (NOTE: NOT NECESSARILY PRACTICED BY ALL JEWISH GROUPS)
Blood by ingestion (e.g., blood sausage, raw meat) (*Note:* Blood by transfusion is acceptable.)
Mixing dairy products and meat dishes at same meal
Pork
Predatory fowl
Shellfish and scavenger fish (e.g., shrimp, crab, lobster, escargot, catfish) (*Note:* Fish with fins and scales are permissible.)
Note: Packaged foods contain labels identifying *kosher* ("properly preserved" or "fitting") and *pareve* (made without meat or milk) items.

MORMONISM (CHURCH OF JESUS CHRIST OF LATTER-DAY SAINTS)
Alcohol
Beverages containing caffeine stimulants (coffee, tea, colas, and selected carbonated soft drinks)
Tobacco

SEVENTH-DAY ADVENTISM
Certain seafood, including shellfish
Fermented beverages
Pork
Note: Optional vegetarianism is encouraged.

(Adapted from Smeltzer, S. C. & Bare, B. G. [2000]. *Brunner & Suddarth's textbook of medical–surgical nursing* [9th ed.]. Philadelphia: Lippincott Williams & Wilkins, p. 106.)

1. *Biomedical or scientific perspective:* This view, shared by many healthcare personnel, embraces a cause-and-effect philosophy of human body functions. An example is the belief that bacterial or viral organisms cause meningitis.
2. *Naturalistic or holistic perspective:* This view espouses that human beings are only one part of nature. Natural balance or harmony is essential for health. Native Americans are one group who share this view. An example is the *Yin/Yang theory,* which promotes the idea that energy forces exist between organisms and objects in the universe. The balance between these forces is health. Many Asian groups embrace Yin/Yang. Another example is the *hot/cold theory,* which says that diseases should be treated by adding or subtracting heat or cold or dryness or moisture to restore balance. Many Hispanic, African-American, and Arab groups embrace beliefs based on hot/cold theory.

3. *Magico-religious perspective:* Supernatural forces dominate. Examples include faith healing in some Christian faiths and voodoo or witchcraft in some Caribbean cultures.

Nurses may disagree with a client's health/illness beliefs; however, they must appreciate these beliefs to assist the client to achieve healthcare goals. These concepts relate to the practice of transcultural nursing.

Stop, Think, and Respond ● BOX 11-2
Hot/cold theory proposes that illnesses caused by heat or cold must be treated with substances having the opposite property. A Puerto Rican client believes she has arthritis because she rinsed her hands in cold water after washing dishes in hot water. She believes that if she eats "hot" foods (e.g., chili peppers), the symptoms will subside. How would you respond?

BIOCULTURAL ASSESSMENT

When assessing any client, the nurse must consider general appearance and obvious physical characteristics, components that make up biocultural assessment. Andrews and Boyle (1999) delineate four areas for consideration:

- Physical appearance: age, sex, level of consciousness, facial features, and skin color, including evenness of tone, pigmentation, intactness, and lesions or other abnormalities
- Body structure: stature, nutrition, symmetry, posture, position, overall body build or contour
- Mobility: gait and range of motion
- Behavior: facial expression, mood and affect, fluency of speech, ability to communicate, appropriateness of word choice, grooming, attire or dress (p. 49)

Table 11-1 provides a brief overview of some biocultural variations; nurses should access more complete sources when caring for clients from culturally diverse backgrounds.

CULTURAL ASSESSMENT

A cultural nursing assessment is a "systematic appraisal or examination of individuals, families, groups, and communities in terms of their cultural beliefs, values, and practices" (Smeltzer & Bare, 2000, p. 107). The nurse should include cultural characteristics along with health practices and beliefs in any initial assessment (Nursing Guidelines 11-1).

TABLE 11-1	BIOCULTURAL VARIATIONS	
	ASSESSMENT	**VARIATIONS**
Skin	Normal colors vary widely; melanin accounts for the shades and tones. Establish baseline tone to note future differences.	*Mongolian spots* are irregular areas of deep-blue pigmentation usually found in the sacral and gluteal areas of children of African, Asian, or Latin descent. They are not to be confused with bruising. *Vitiligo* are unpigmented skin patches. *Cyanosis* is difficult to assess in dark-skinned persons. Assess other factors such as respiratory rate, use of accessory muscles, and nasal flaring. People of Mediterranean descent normally have a dark blue tone around the mouth.
Jaundice	Jaundice is best observed in the sclera; establish normal scleral pigmentation.	African Americans, Filipino Americans, and other groups have heavy deposits of conjunctival fat, which contains carotene and may resemble jaundice.
Pallor	Generalized pallor is best observed in mucous membranes, lips, and nailbeds; nailbeds and conjunctiva are better to assess the pallor of anemia.	Dark-skinned clients may not have underlying red tones and exhibit pallor more as yellowish-brown or ashen-gray skin tones.
Erythema	Localized inflammation is characterized by reddened skin, which may not show in dark-skinned clients. Also assess for increased warmth, tautness, or edema.	Conditions such as carbon monoxide poisoning, in which flushing is present, may be observed in the lips of dark-skinned clients.
Skin changes/normal aging	Light skin tends to show the effects of aging/sun exposure earlier; African Americans, Asian Americans, and Alaskan Natives wrinkle later than whites.	Healthcare providers frequently assess age inaccurately, based on their own cultural assumptions (e.g., African-American nurses often overestimate the age of white clients).
Secretions	Apocrine and eccrine sweat glands are important in fluid balance and thermoregulation. When skin flora contaminates sweat, odor results.	Alaskan Natives sweat less than whites on their trunks and extremities but more on their faces.
Eyes	Biocultural differences are common in eye color and structure. Asians have characteristic epicanthal eye folds.	Dark irises are associated with darker retinas and poorer night vision.
Skeletal system	The long bones of African Americans are longer and more dense; hence, this population has a low incidence of osteoporosis. Bone density of Asians and Alaskan Natives is less than in whites.	Many variations occur among all groups.
Laboratory tests	Biocultural variations occur in some laboratory results, such as hemoglobin/hematocrit, cholesterol, and blood glucose levels.	Be familiar with variations and their clinical significance.
Drug responses	Genetic or environmental factors may influence differences in pharmacokinetics.	Clients may respond differently to the same drug. For example, mydriatic drugs (drugs that cause eye dilation) produce less dilation in dark-colored eyes than in light-colored eyes.

Assessing Cultural Heritage

Cultural ignorance can profoundly affect access to quality healthcare. It can provide the motivation for expanding one's knowledge base about different cultures. Recognizing all the areas in which cultural differences subtly manifest themselves is important. Examples include communication patterns; hygiene practices, including feelings about modesty and accepting help from others; use of special clothing or amulets; food preferences; management of symptoms such as pain, constipation, and depression; rituals surrounding birth and death; spiritual or religious orientation, especially as related to healthcare; family relationships, including expectations of elders and children; and patterns of interacting with healthcare providers (Lipson et al., 1996).

NURSING GUIDELINES 11-1

Performing a Cultural Assessment

Ask about or observe for the following cultural elements:

- Where was the client born? How long has the client lived in this country?

- What is the client's ethnic background? Does the client identify strongly with others from the same cultural background? Does the client live in a neighborhood with others of the same ethnic or cultural background?

- To whom does the client turn for support? Who is the head of the family? Is he or she involved in decision-making about the client?

- What is the client's primary language and literacy level?

- What is the client's religion, and is it important in his or her daily life? Are there religious rituals related to sickness, death, or health that the client observes?

- Has the client sought the advice of traditional healers?

- What are the client's communication styles? Does the client avoid eye contact and maintain physical distance? Is the client open and verbal about symptoms?

- What are the client's food preferences or restrictions?

- Does the client participate in cultural activities such as dressing in traditional clothing and observing traditional holidays and festivals?

(Adapted from Lipson, J. G., Dibble, S. L., & Minarik, P. A. [1996]. *Culture and nursing care: A pocket guide.* San Francisco: UCSF Nursing Press.)

NURSING GUIDELINES 11-2

Assessing Health Beliefs and Practices

Initial assessment of the client should include the following questions:

- What have you done in the past and what do you do now to maintain health?

- How do these activities help you maintain your health?

- What practices could you add to help promote health?

- What is your definition of good health?

- Do you have any difficulties with performing activities that will restore, maintain, or promote health?

- What do you call your health problem?

- What do you think has caused this problem?

- Why do you think it started when it did?

- What does this problem do to you?

- What are the difficulties that this health problem has caused you, personally, in your family, or at work?

- What do you fear most about this health problem?

- What kind of treatment do you think will help? What are the most important results you hope to get from this treatment?

(Adapted from McSweeney, J. C., Allan, J. D., & Mayo, K. [1997]. Exploring the use of explanatory models in nursing research and practice. *Image: Journal of Nursing Scholarship, 29,* 243–248.)

Assessing Health Beliefs and Practices

Health beliefs and **health practices,** ideas about what causes illness, the role of the sick person, how to restore health, and how one stays healthy, are perpetuated and influenced by strong cultural affiliations. To discover a client's health beliefs and practices, the nurse will find it useful to ask specific questions (Nursing Guidelines 11-2). Assessment of these factors helps identify the client's beliefs about his or her health or illness; recognize health-seeking behaviors on which to capitalize to promote health; view the situation from the client's perspective; distinguish behaviors that do not contribute to health restoration, maintenance, or promotion; perceive issues that can compromise the treatment plan; and establish a mutually agreed-on plan of care (McSweeney et al., 1997).

TRANSCULTURAL NURSING

Transcultural nursing, founded by Madeline Leininger (1977), is considered a specialty in nursing. It refers to nursing care that is provided within the context of an-

other's culture. Its characteristics are (1) accepting each client as an individual, (2) possessing knowledge of health problems that affect particular cultural groups, (3) assessing cultural background and health beliefs and practices, and (4) planning care compatible with the client's health belief system.

Leininger (1991) theorizes that *culturally congruent care* (care that fits a person's cultural values) assists a client to achieve better health outcomes. If a nurse respects a client's cultural values and beliefs, he or she can better teach diet modifications or lifestyle changes that promote healthier outcomes, without insulting or patronizing the client. For example, clients of Middle Eastern cultures do not normally drink milk after childhood. They do, however, eat yogurt and also a goat or sheep cheese called *feta.* For such clients who need to increase calcium intake, nurses can inform them that these foods provide needed calcium.

Differences in language can pose significant barriers when providing nursing care. With all the different cultural groups living in the United States, many do not speak English or have learned it as their second language and do not speak it well. In addition, most people prefer to speak in their native tongue, especially when under stress. Nurses should use a translator when the client speaks a different language. They should take care when asking family members to interpret; embarrassment and lack of medical knowledge can result in miscommunication. When a nurse from one culture and a client from another speak the same language, the way they do so may cause miscommunication. An accepted pattern during verbal interactions for one may be unusual, rude, or offensive to the other. Understanding that unique cultural characteristics are related to verbal and nonverbal communication can facilitate the transition to culturally sensitive care. Refer to Nursing Guidelines 11-3 for additional communication techniques.

NURSING GUIDELINES 11-3

Communicating With Non–English-Speaking Clients

When Clients Speak No English

- Learn a second language, especially one spoken by a large ethnic population serviced by the health agency.

- Speak words or phrases in the client's language, even if it is not possible to carry on a conversation.

- Refer to an English/foreign language dictionary for bilingual vocabulary words.

- Construct a loose-leaf folder or file cards with words in one or more languages spoken by clients in the community.

- Develop a list of employees or individuals to contact in the community who speak a second language and are willing to act as translators; in an extreme emergency, international telephone operators may be able to provide assistance.

- Select a translator who is the same sex as the client and approximately the same age, if possible.

- Look at the client, not the translator, when asking questions and listening to the client's response.

When English Is a Second Language

- Determine if the client speaks or reads English, or both.

- Speak slowly, not loudly, using simple words and short sentences.

- Avoid using technical terms, slang, or phrases with a double or colloquial meaning, such as "Do you have to use the john?"

- Ask questions that can be answered by a "yes" or "no."

- Repeat the question without changing the words, if the client appears confused.

- Give the client sufficient time to process the question from English to the native language, and respond back in English.

- Rely heavily on nonverbal communication, and pantomime if necessary.

- Avoid displaying impatience.

- Ask the client to "read this line," to determine the client's ability to follow written instructions, which are provided in English.

Developing Transcultural Sensitivity

Increasing one's awareness that the United States is a multicultural nation is a first step toward transcultural nursing. Examining personal beliefs, communication habits, and healthcare practices is another. The following recommendations will help to develop a growing expertise in culturally sensitive nursing care:

- Learn to speak a second language.
- Use techniques for facilitating interactions: sit within the client's comfort zone and make appropriate eye contact.
- Become familiar with physical differences among ethnic groups.
- Be aware of biocultural aspects of disease (Table 11-2).
- Perform physical assessments, using appropriate techniques that will provide accurate data.
- Perform cultural and health beliefs assessment and plan care accordingly.
- Consult the client about ways to solve health problems.
- Never ridicule a cultural belief or practice, verbally or nonverbally.
- Integrate cultural practices that are helpful or harmless into the plan of care.
- Modify or gradually change unsafe practices.
- Avoid removing religious medals or clothing that hold symbolic meaning for the client; if this must be done, keep them safe and replace them as soon as possible.
- Provide food that is customarily eaten.
- Advocate routine screening for diseases to which clients may be genetically or culturally prone.
- Facilitate rituals by whomever the client identifies as a healer within his or her belief system.
- Apologize if cultural traditions or beliefs are violated.

Being Culturally Competent

Cultural competence means that the nurse understands his or her own worldview as well as the client's. It also may be viewed as a process in which the nurse consistently endeavors to work within the cultural context of the client and his or her family and community (Andrews & Boyle, 1999). In doing so, the nurse must avoid stereotyping clients based on race or culture. The nurse also must listen to clients, acknowledge and respect their beliefs about health and illness, recognize culturally influenced health behaviors, communicate in a culturally sensitive manner, and adapt care to reflect cultural needs.

All individuals grow up with an ethnocentric perspective. The ethnocentrism reflects lack of knowledge and experience. Nurses must personally evolve from an ethnocentric viewpoint and develop a multicultural perspective that includes knowledge of their own as well as other cul-

TABLE 11-2	BIOCULTURAL ASPECTS OF DISEASE
DISEASE	**CONSIDERATIONS**
Alcoholism	Native Americans have twice the rate of whites. Chinese and Japanese Americans have decreased alcohol tolerance.
Anemia	Incidence is high among Vietnamese Americans because of infestations among immigrants and low-iron diets.
Arthritis	Incidence is increased among Native Americans.
Asthma and bronchitis	Incidence is six times greater for Native American infants than the rest of the population.
Cancer	The incidence of nasopharyngeal cancer is high among Chinese and Native Americans. Breast cancer is 1½ times more likely in African-American women than white women. Esophageal cancer is the second leading cause of death for African-American men aged 35 to 54 years. Filipino Hawaiians have the highest rates of liver cancer. The incidence of stomach cancer is twice as high in African-American men than in white men. The incidence of cervical cancer is 120% higher in African-American women than white women, and that of uterine cancer is 53% lower in African-American than in white women. African-American men have the highest incidence of prostate cancer in all groups.
Colitis	Incidence is increased in Japanese Americans.
Diabetes mellitus	Incidence is much higher in Filipino, Hispanic, and Native Americans than whites and African Americans.
Influenza	Death rate is increased among Native Americans 45 years of age and older.
Ischemic heart disease	This condition is responsible for 32% of heart-related deaths in Native Americans. African Americans have the highest related mortality rates.
Lactose intolerance	Incidence is increased in African, Chinese, and Hispanic Americans.
Myocardial infarction	This is the leading cause of heart disease in Native Americans, accounting for 43% of deaths. Incidence is decreased in Japanese Americans.
Otitis media	Incidence in school-aged Navajo children is 7.9%, versus 0.5% in whites. Up to one third of Alaskan Natives younger than 2 years of age have chronic otitis media. Incidence is increased among bottle-fed Native American and Alaskan Native infants.
Pneumonia	Death rate is increased among Native Americans 45 years of age and older.
Renal disease	Incidence is decreased in Japanese Americans.
Sickle cell anemia	Incidence is increased in African Americans.
Trachoma	Incidence is increased in Native American and Alaskan Native children.
Tuberculosis	Incidence is increased in Native Americans.
Ulcers	Incidence is decreased in Japanese Americans.

tures. They also must acknowledge any personal biases to develop a nonjudgmental attitude toward all clients. Developing strategies to avoid *cultural imposition* is absolutely pivotal (Andrews & Boyle, 1999). The culturally competent nurse accepts each client as a unique individual. The first ethical principle in the American Nurses Association (ANA) Code for Nurses states that "The nurse, in all professional relationships, practices with compassion and respect for the inherent dignity, worth, and uniqueness of every individual, unrestricted by considerations of social or economic status, personal attributes, or the nature of health problems" (ANA, 2002). This principle extends to providing culturally competent care to all individuals.

GENERAL NUTRITIONAL CONSIDERATIONS

Culture defines what food is; how it is obtained, stored, prepared, and served; when it is eaten; differences in food habits based on age, sex, and status; and food's meaning. In any cultural or ethnic group, food habits can vary greatly. Generalizations are intended only as a guide.

African Americans are at increased risk for hypertension, stroke, diabetes, and obesity. Limiting fat, sodium, and excess calories may help prevent or treat these disorders. Because lactose intolerance is common, calcium intake may be inadequate. In the South, "soul food" refers to both cooking style (barbecued or fried) and particular foods consumed (e.g., pork, greens).

Throughout Latin America, Indian and Spanish cultures and local food availability influence food practices. Obesity, diabetes, and hypertriglyceridemia are common among Latino Americans. Calcium intake may be inadequate because milk intake often is low.

The traditional Asian diet is plant-based; common foods include rice, noodles, flat bread, potatoes, vegetables, nuts, seeds, beans, and soy foods. It is low in fat, saturated fat, and cholesterol, and rich in fiber and nutrients. Meat serves more as a condiment than as a main entrée. Preparing food usually takes longer than cooking it. Moderation is valued and obesity is rare. Lactose intolerance is common. Because of extensive use of soy sauce, limiting sodium intake is difficult.

Native Americans/Alaskan Natives represent a heterogeneous group of more than 500 tribes and villages. Eating patterns and habits are widely diverse and and influenced by cultural and religious beliefs, geography, and food availability. Although staples vary among tribes, corn, squash, and beans are used extensively. Many plant foods also are used in traditional medicinal practices. Obesity, diabetes, and lactose intolerance are common among Native Americans.

GENERAL PHARMACOLOGIC CONSIDERATIONS

Almost all cultures and ethnic groups have traditional folk remedies. These preparations have pharmacologic actions that can affect physiology and cause drug interactions.

Folk-healing beliefs and practices are important aspects of healing. Nurses should find methods to combine them with medically prescribed treatments. Noncompliance with the pharmaceutical regimen may be a problem with those who use folk remedies unless healthcare providers find ways to incorporate at least some of these remedies into the treatment regimen.

When a drug is prescribed, ask if the client has used or is using any herbal medicines or teas and inform the physician of such use.

Biologic and physiologic variations may influence the absorption and metabolism of drugs. Be alert to any variations in drug action or the appearance of unusual adverse drug reactions, which may or may not be related to the person's inherited characteristics.

GENERAL GERONTOLOGIC CONSIDERATIONS

In many African-American families, a grandmother or an older aunt is considered the matriarch (female head or leader). Include this matriarch in teaching sessions or ask if the client would like this person to be present.

Older adults are more likely to follow the advice of spiritual healers and use folk medicines than are younger generations. For example, some older Hispanics use a traditional folk healer, the curandero, to manage health problems. If they use a folk healer exclusively for healthcare needs, however, problems can arise that need a more conventional medical approach.

Aging Asians tend to be cared for by and live with one of their children. Suggesting the placement of an aging parent in a nursing home is considered rude.

Older Asian women are very modest and often prefer not to be examined or cared for by men. Rather than be touched during physical assessment, they prefer to point to a model to indicate where they are experiencing symptoms (Giger & Davidhizar, 1995). Latino women also are frequently uncomfortable being cared for by male nurses.

Illnesses, especially those that cause obvious physical changes or dependence on a woman for care, may threaten an aging male Latino's self-image and security.

Take time to listen to older adults nonjudgmentally. Failure to be culturally sensitive to an older adult's health beliefs blocks communication and identification of healthcare needs.

Native American older adults may not look directly into a nurse's eyes. Their eyes may move from the floor to the ceiling and around the room. Native Americans believe that the eyes are a window to the soul and consider staring disrespectful because it may harm the spirit.

Older adults who do not speak English well may respond by saying "yes" or nodding even though they do not understand. For example, Asian cultures consider it disrespectful to disagree with a person of authority or one who is more educated. They consider it rude to imply that the person in authority did not teach properly or explain in enough detail.

Critical Thinking Exercises

1. *How could a culturally sensitive nurse prepare for the home care of a non–English-speaking client from Pakistan (or some other foreign country)?*
2. *How could a culturally sensitive nurse respond to a pregnant woman who wears a chicken bone around her neck to protect her unborn child from birth defects?*

References and Suggested Readings

American Nurses Association. (2001). *Code of ethics for nurses.* [On-line.] Available: http://www.ana.org/ethics/chcode.htm.

Andrews, M. M. & Boyle, J. S. (1999). *Transcultural concepts in nursing care* (3rd ed.). Philadelphia: Lippincott Williams & Wilkins.

Diversity Rx. (1997). Why language and culture are important. [On-line.] Available: http://www.diversityrx.org/ (accessed May 22, 2001).

Galanti, G. (2000). An introduction to cultural differences. *Western Journal of Medicine.* [On-line.] Available: http://www.ewjm.com/cgi/content/full/172/5/335(accessed May 22, 2001).

Giger, J. N. & Davidhizar, R. E. (1995). *Transcultural nursing: Assessment and intervention* (2nd ed.). St. Louis: Mosby.

Leininger, M. (1977). Transcultural nursing and a proposed conceptual framework. In M. Leininger (Ed.), *Transcultural nursing care of infants and children: Proceedings from the first transcultural conference.* Salt Lake City: University of Utah.

Leininger, M. (1991). Transcultural nursing: The study and practice field. *Imprint, 38*(2), 55–66.

Leininger, M. (1995). *Transcultural nursing: Concepts, theories, research, and practices.* New York: McGraw-Hill.

Lester, N. (1998). Cultural competence: A nursing dialogue. Part one. *American Journal of Nursing, 98*(8), 26–33.

McSweeney, J. C., Allan, J. D., & Mayo, K. (1997). Exploring the use of explanatory models in nursing research and practice. *IMAGE: Journal of Nursing Scholarship, 29,* 243–248.

Oderkirk, W. (1999). Challenging Spanish: Ways for nurses to become bilingual. *Journal of Continuing Education in Nursing, 30*(2), 88–93.

Rivera-Andino, J. & Lopez, L. (2000). When culture complicates care. *RN, 63*(7), 47–49.

Smeltzer, S. C. & Bare, B. G. (2000). *Brunner & Suddarth's textbook of medical–surgical nursing* (9th ed.). Philadelphia: Lippincott Williams & Wilkins.

Spence, D. G. (2001). Prejudice, paradox, and possibility: Nursing people from cultures other than one's own. *Journal of Transcultural Nursing, 12*(2), 100–106.

chapter **12**

Interaction of Body and Mind

Words to Know

acupuncture	massage therapy
alternative medical	mental status
systems	examination
alternative therapy	mind–body
apitherapy	interventions
aromatherapy	neuropeptides
Ayurvedic medicine	neurotransmitters
biofeedback	placebo
biologic-based therapies	placebo effect
body-based therapies	psyche
brain mapping	psychobiologic disorders
Chinese medicine	psychobiology
chiropractic	psychoneuro-
complementary therapy	endocrinology
coping mechanisms	psychoneuro-
distress	immunology
electromagnetic therapy	psychosomatic diseases
energy therapies	receptors
eustress	reflexology
general adaptation	reiki
syndrome	shiatsu
hardiness	soma
herbal therapy	spiritual healing
humor	stress
hypnosis	stress management
imagery	stress-related disorder
immunopeptides	tai chi
limbic system	yoga

Learning Objectives

On completion of this chapter, the reader will:

- Explain why mental illnesses are now considered psychobiologic disorders.
- Discuss two new areas of neuroscience being studied to learn more about psychobiologic disorders.
- Name two chemical substances transmitted between neurons, giving examples of each.
- Name three psychodynamic factors that affect behavior.
- List four examples of techniques used to assess clients with psychobiologic disorders.
- Distinguish between stress, eustress, and distress.
- Describe the general adaptation syndrome, and name its three stages.
- Explain the purpose of coping mechanisms and the outcomes that may result from their use.
- List the defining features of hardiness.
- Discuss two methods that are sometimes used to predict a person's vulnerability for acquiring stress-related disorders.
- Discuss techniques that the nurse can suggest for helping clients cope with stressors.
- Discuss the rationale for a mind–immune system connection.
- Discuss four explanations for the development of psychosomatic diseases.
- Differentiate between the terms *complementary therapy* and *alternative therapy*.
- List five categories of psychobiologic interventions that the National Center for Complementary and Alternative Medicine investigates.

The mind, the central nervous system (CNS), and the body were once thought of as completely separate structures. Now more than ever, they are viewed as a single communicating entity. Recent research has uncovered anatomic and chemical links between the body and the mind, and new fields of science have emerged that examine these linkages and their effects on health.

Psychobiology is the study of the biochemical basis of thought, behavior, affect, and mood. **Psychobiologic disorders** are those conditions in which evidence sup-

ports a link between biologic abnormalities in the brain and altered cognition, perception, emotion, behavior, and socialization. **Psychoneuroendocrinology** is the study of how fluctuations in pituitary, adrenal, thyroid, and reproductive hormones alter cognition, perception, behavior, and mood. **Psychoneuroimmunology** studies the connections among the emotions, CNS, neuroendocrine system, and immunologic system. Although a new and not completely developed science, psychoneuroimmunology is the focus of much interest. Research in this field studies how stress predisposes to infection (see Chap. 19), autoimmune disorders (see Chap. 42), and cancer (see Chap. 20). All these overlapping fields study the anatomy, physiology, and pathology of the brain.

THE BRAIN AND PSYCHOBIOLOGIC FUNCTION

The brain is a complex organ made up of the cerebrum, brain stem, and cerebellum (Fig. 12-1). The *cerebrum* is the brain's largest component. It is the basis for sensory perception, voluntary movement, personality, intelligence, language, thoughts, judgment, emotions, memory, creativity, and motivation. The outer layer of the cerebrum receives, processes, integrates, and relays information to appropriate functional areas of the brain. The *cerebral cortex* is the major pathway of physiologic intercommunication. The **limbic system** is a network in the brain that contains structures involved in emotions and related physiologic functions. It includes the *thalamus*, which connects many brain centers and modulates movement, sensation, behavior, and emotions. The limbic system also includes the *hypothalamus*, which controls the autonomic nervous system and coordinates the endocrine and immune systems through pituitary–adrenocortical connections (Porth, 2002). Because of its neuroendocrine and neuroimmunologic roles, the limbic system affects and determines many psychobiologic activities.

Stop, Think, and Respond ● **BOX 12-1**

Which two structures in the brain play the greatest role in connecting the mind with physiologic functions?

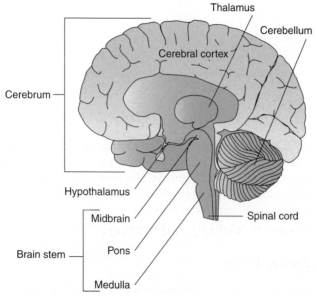

FIGURE 12-1 Brain structures.

Receptors

Receptors are structures found on the surface of cells throughout the body and brain. Each cell has millions of different receptors. These receptors sense and pick up chemical messengers that arrive in the extracellular fluid. A chemical messenger may be thought of as a specific key that fits into and binds with a specific receptor. Only those messengers that have molecules in exactly the right shape can bind with specific receptors. For example, opiate receptors can bind only with chemicals in the opiate group such as heroin, morphine, or endorphins. Once binding occurs, the message is received and the cell begins to respond. Chemical messengers may be natural or synthetic, and the message may cause the cell to perform any number of activities. Neurotransmitters are the messengers that play a significant role in regulating all physical, emotional, and mental processes.

Neurotransmitters

Neurotransmitters (Table 12-1) are chemical messengers. They communicate information that affects thinking, behavior, and bodily functions across the synaptic cleft between neurons (Fig. 12-2). The chemicals, which are synthesized in the neurons and then stored in vesicles in the axons, are released and attach themselves (bind) momentarily to the receptors on postsynaptic neurons. After the chemicals have transmitted their information, they are

- Broken down into inactive substances by enzymes like monoamine oxidase
- Recaptured by the releasing neuron for later use, a process called *reuptake*
- Weakened by becoming diluted in intercellular fluid

Neurons are classified by the type of neurotransmitter they release; for example, cholinergic neurons release acetylcholine, and dopaminergic neurons release dopamine.

Neuropeptides are a separate type of neurotransmitter. They include chemicals such as

- Substance P, which transmits the sensation of pain (see Chap. 21)
- Endorphins and enkephalins, morphine-like neuropeptides that interrupt the transmission of substance P and promote a feeling of well-being
- Neurohormones released by interactions between the hypothalamus, pituitary, and the endocrine glands they stimulate

Different areas of the brain contain different types of neurons with specific neurotransmitters. Each neurotransmitter has either a stimulating or inhibiting effect on neurons. All brain function, including thoughts, emotions, or messages to organs and muscles, depends on these neurotransmitters (Barry, 1996).

TABLE 12-1	SELECTED NEUROTRANSMITTERS	
NEUROTRANSMITTER	**ABBREVIATION**	**EXAMPLES OF FUNCTIONS**
Serotonin (5-hydroxytryptamine)	5-HT	Stabilizes mood Induces sleep Regulates temperature Controls appetite
Dopamine	DA	Integrates thoughts Promotes movement in concert with ACH Stimulates hypothalamic endocrine activity Enhances judgment
Norepinephrine	NE	Affects attention and concentration Raises energy level Heightens arousal
Acetylcholine	ACH	Assists memory storage Promotes movement in concert with DA Prepares for action
Gamma-aminobutyric acid	GABA	Reduces arousal and aggression Inhibits excitatory neurotransmitters like NE and DA Decreases seizure potential

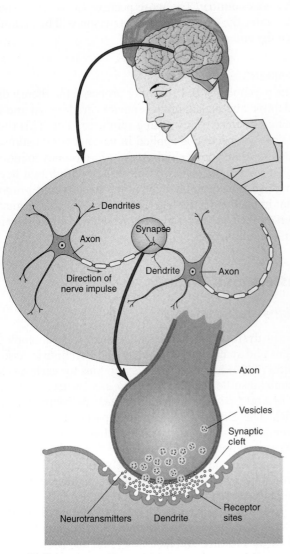

FIGURE 12-2 Neurotransmitter anatomy.

Receptors for neurotransmitters and neuropeptides are located not only throughout the CNS, but also in the endocrine and immune systems. This finding suggests that these systems communicate with each other through chemical messages. This concept has tremendous implications for how the mind and emotions can affect physical well-being and how physical status can affect the mind (Barry, 1996).

PSYCHOBIOLOGIC ILLNESS

Historically, many believed that mental illness resulted from character defects, demonic possession, or punishment by God. These myths persist, which explains why individuals with mental illness sometimes are feared and stigmatized. The study of brain structure, chemistry, and genetics has begun to replace ignorance and misinformation about mental illness with facts. Brain pathology is now seen as the major factor contributing to mental illnesses, now called *psychobiologic disorders.* Three major types of psychobiologic disorders are somatoform and anxiety disorders (see Chaps. 13 and 14), mood disorders (see Chap. 15), and thought disorders (see Chap. 18). Other conditions with a biologic basis include eating disorders (see Chap. 16) and chemical dependency (see Chap. 17).

Pathophysiology and Etiology

Biologic Factors

The neurotransmitters dopamine, norepinephrine, epinephrine, serotonin, and acetylcholine often are implicated in the psychobiology of mental illness. Because the neurotransmitters are concentrated in different areas of the brain, disruption of a neurotransmitter system results in the specific symptoms associated with that area of the brain. For example, dopamine influences movement, memory, thoughts, and judgment. The disorganized thought patterns and bizarre behavior of schizophrenia have been correlated with excess levels of dopamine; the impaired balance and uncontrolled tremors of Parkinson's disease have been linked with low levels of dopamine. Serotonin is found in areas that regulate sleep, appetite, sexual behavior, and mood. Imbalances in serotonin are thought to be responsible for depression, eating disorders, sleep disturbances, and obsessive–compulsive disorder.

Other insights into brain physiology came from observing the effects of medications on behavior and symptoms (psychopharmacology). The theory that depression results from decreased levels of norepinephrine and serotonin was first postulated when the monoamine oxidase inhibitors, which block the inactivation of norepinephrine and serotonin (see Chap. 15), were found to alleviate depression. Similarly, antianxiety medications like the benzodiazepines (see Chap. 14) activate gamma-aminobutyric acid (GABA) receptors that inhibit arousal, excitement, and aggression.

> ### Stop, Think, and Respond ● BOX 12-2
>
> *If norepinephrine binds to its receptor site on cells, what effects would occur?*

Psychological Factors

Psychological factors (forces that shape behavior) also influence psychological equilibrium and may be tied to brain chemistry as well. Some researchers postulate that the neurotransmitter network links emotion, memory, and learned behavior (Pert & Chopra, 1999). Psychological factors have long been components of psychiatric theory and include intrapersonal development, interpersonal interactions, and learning.

INTRAPERSONAL DEVELOPMENT

Sigmund Freud proposed that disordered behavior is the result of intrapersonal (within oneself) conflicts that arise during particular stages of development that occur between infancy and adolescence. For example, Freud correlated compulsive neatness and stinginess with rigid toilet training. Freud greatly emphasized sexual aspects of behaviors between an infant and mother, conflicts surrounding toilet training, awareness of gender differences and genital pleasure, rivalry with the same-sex parent, investment of energy in intellectual pursuits, and efforts

to establish relationships with members of the opposite sex. Although many of Freud's theories have been questioned, negated, rejected, revised, and expanded, he provided the foundation for the current fields of psychiatry and psychology, and thus many of his tenets have withstood the test of time.

> ### Stop, Think, and Respond ● BOX 12-3
>
> *What do you think may be the physiologic and psychological consequences if an infant is not held very much, is not talked to affectionately, or is ignored when hungry?*

INTERPERSONAL INTERACTION

Other theorists, like Erik Erikson (see Chap. 7) and Harry Stack Sullivan, proposed that mental health or illness is a consequence of social relationships and interpersonal interactions. Some theorists go further, suggesting that a person's mental stability is affected not only by significant others, but also by social systems, such as neighborhood, city, and country. The more positive the social system, the better the chances are that a person will be mentally healthy and well adjusted.

LEARNING

The psychologist B. F. Skinner proposed the theory that adaptive and maladaptive behaviors are learned and repeated because of rewarding reinforcement. This theoretical perspective is applied in various circumstances, such as when young children are offered candy to induce toilet training or when privileges are withdrawn to extinguish unacceptable behaviors. Some would propose that hypochondriasis (see Chap. 13) develops because a person received excessive attention and concern during childhood illnesses.

Assessment Findings

Signs and Symptoms

Brain dysfunction can cause a mix of psychobiologic signs and symptoms. The American Psychiatric Association (2000) has established symptoms for each specific mental disorder in the *Diagnostic and Statistical Manual of Mental Disorders* (4th edition, text revision; DSM-IV-TR). The DSM-IV-TR classifies psychiatric disorders. Commonly seen symptoms include anxiety, mood changes, abnormal eating patterns, chemical dependence, or thought disturbances. Ultimately, the client's signs and symptoms affect relationships with others and interfere with age-related role responsibilities.

Besides a comprehensive personal and family medical history, clients undergo a mental status examination, psychological testing, and laboratory and diagnostic testing.

Mental Status Examination

A **mental status examination** is one component of a thorough neurologic examination. It is an array of observations and questions that elicit information about a person's cognitive and mental state. The components of an extensive mental status examination include obtaining data about the client's:

- Physical appearance
- Orientation
- Attention and concentration
- Short-term and long-term memory
- Movement and coordination
- Speech patterns
- Mood
- Intellectual performance
- Perception
- Insight
- Judgment
- Thought content

Nurses regularly conduct Mini-Mental Status Examinations (Box 12-1). Changes in the total score are used to evaluate changes in the client's condition.

Stop, Think, and Respond ● BOX 12-4

How would you evaluate the mental status of a person who achieved a score of 20 on the Mini-Mental Status Examination?

Psychological Tests

Psychological tests are administered to detect personality characteristics, interpersonal conflicts, and self-concept. Table 12-2 gives examples of various psychological tests.

Diagnostic Findings

Measuring levels of neurotransmitters and neuropeptides is difficult, expensive, and sometimes impossible. Un-

BOX 12-1 ● Sample Mini-Mental Status Examination Questions

- What is the year?
- What is today's date?
- In what city (town) are we?
- Spell "globe" backward.
- Repeat the following statement: "A rolling stone gathers no moss."
- Write a sentence of your own choice. (Nurse evaluates whether sentence has a subject, predicate [verb], and object.)

From Folstein, M. E., Folstein, S. E., & McHugh, P. R. (1975). Mini-Mental State: A practical method for grading the cognitive state of patients for the clinician. *Journal of Psychiatric Research, 12*(189). Used with permission.

TABLE 12-2	PSYCHOLOGICAL TESTS
TEST	**DESCRIPTION**
Minnesota Multiphasic Personality Inventory (MMPI)	This true-or-false test of 550 questions is used to analyze which of nine clinical personality traits are manifested by the client's responses.
Beck Depression Inventory	Client rates self according to statements that concern mood.
Draw-a-Person (tree, house, family) Test	Client's drawing is analyzed for symbolism about his or her self-perception or other emotional data.
Word Association Test	Client is asked to quickly provide a response to words, such as "mother . . . work . . .", etc. Responses are analyzed for psychological significance.
Thematic Apperception Test (TAT)	Client is asked to look at pictures and then tell a story about them. Recurring themes in the stories suggest the underlying basis of emotional problems.
Rorschach Test	The client is asked to indicate what he or she sees in each of 10 separate inkblots.

fortunately, a definitive diagnosis for many psychobiologic disorders usually is achieved by ruling out other diseases that manifest similar symptoms. The reader is referred to Chapter 44 for a description of tests such as electroencephalography (EEG), computed tomography scan, magnetic resonance imaging (MRI), and positron emission tomography.

One of the newest diagnostic tools, brain mapping, suggests that the future diagnosis of psychobiologic disorders will be more efficient. **Brain mapping** is a technique that compares a client's brain activity patterns (from an EEG or other electronic image) with a computerized database of electrophysiologic abnormalities. A growing database of distinctive patterns for seizure disorders, schizophrenia, depression, dementia, anxiety disorders, attention deficit/hyperactivity disorder, and others now exists for comparison.

Medical and Nursing Management

Treatment of psychobiologic disorders depends on the specific diagnosis. Modalities include drug therapy, psychotherapy, cognitive therapy, and behavior modification (see Chaps. 13 through 18). Drug therapy aims at correcting the underlying biochemical abnormality and is particularly useful with mood disorders (see Chap. 15), anxiety disorders (see Chaps. 13 and 14), and schizophrenia (see Chap. 18). The goals of psychotherapy, cognitive therapy, and behavior modification are to uncover repressed thoughts and emotions and identify healthier coping mechanisms. Nurses play an active role in all aspects of treatment, including administering and monitoring response to drug therapy, implementing behavior modification plans, and providing individual and group counseling.

THE BRAIN AND PSYCHOSOMATIC FUNCTION

In addition to the study of the biologic basis of mental illness, brain chemistry and its effects on physical health are being widely researched as well. Emotions, which originate in brain structures and chemicals, can powerfully influence an individual's health and sense of well-being.

According to Selye's theory (1956), **stress** is a physiologic response to biologic stressors like surgical trauma or infection, psychological stressors such as worry and fear, or sociologic stressors, including a new job or increased family responsibilities. Stress has been implicated in the development or exacerbation of autoimmune diseases, anorexia nervosa, obsessive–compulsive disorder, panic attacks, thyroid conditions, heart disease, functional and inflammatory disorders of the gastrointestinal tract, chronic pain conditions, and diabetes. Stress is not an entirely negative concept. Just the right amount of stress, called **eustress,** is what maintains a healthy balance in life. Eustress helps individuals to pursue goals, learn to solve problems, or manage life's predictable and unpredictable crises. Excessive, ill-timed, or unrelieved stress is called **distress.** It triggers the **general adaptation syndrome,** a nonspecific physiologic response (Box 12-2). This response, which can cycle many times through the alarm and resistance stages before reaching the exhaustion stage, occurs through the neuroendocrine and autonomic nervous systems.

> ### Stop, Think, and Respond ● BOX 12-5
> *How might failing one test be considered eustress but failing several tests be considered distress?*

Physiologic Stress Response

The autonomic nervous system consists of the sympathetic and the parasympathetic divisions. The most common pathway for the stress response is through the sympathetic division, which uses norepinephrine to stimulate body systems, arousal, and anxiety in response to stress. This response overrides the control of the parasympathetic nervous system, which slows many meta-

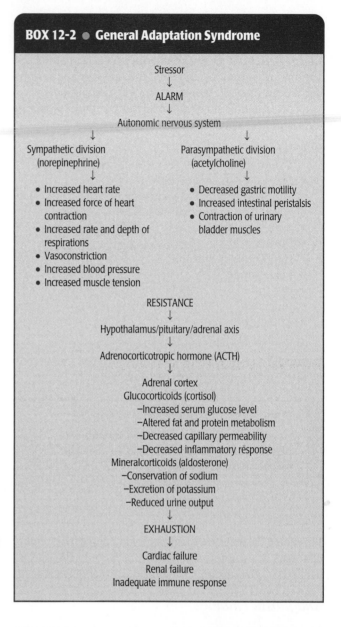

BOX 12-2 ● General Adaptation Syndrome

Stressor
↓
ALARM
↓
Autonomic nervous system
↓   ↓
Sympathetic division   Parasympathetic division
(norepinephrine)   (acetylcholine)
↓   ↓
- Increased heart rate   - Decreased gastric motility
- Increased force of heart   - Increased intestinal peristalsis
  contraction   - Contraction of urinary
- Increased rate and depth of   bladder muscles
  respirations
- Vasoconstriction
- Increased blood pressure
- Increased muscle tension

RESISTANCE
↓
Hypothalamus/pituitary/adrenal axis
↓
Adrenocorticotropic hormone (ACTH)

Adrenal cortex
Glucocorticoids (cortisol)
   –Increased serum glucose level
   –Altered fat and protein metabolism
   –Decreased capillary permeability
   –Decreased inflammatory response
Mineralcorticoids (aldosterone)
   –Conservation of sodium
   –Excretion of potassium
   –Reduced urine output
↓
EXHAUSTION
↓
Cardiac failure
Renal failure
Inadequate immune response

bolic processes. A few individuals respond to stressors through the parasympathetic pathway. Instead of being stimulated to fight or flee, parasympathetic responders become "frozen by fear." Becoming motionless is beneficial among various animals. For example, possums "play dead" when a predator is nearby, which causes the predator to lose interest in its potential prey. Some theorists argue that taking a similarly less aggressive stance could help humans to avoid confrontation.

Psychological Stress Response

Just as the body responds to stressors, the **psyche,** or mind, also reacts to stress. **Coping mechanisms** are unconscious tactics humans use to protect the self from feeling inadequate or threatened. These mechanisms function like "psychological first aid" by helping temporarily to avoid the emotional effects of a stressful situation. When used appropriately and in moderation, coping mechanisms allow maintenance of psychological equilibrium and lead to psychological growth. If a person overuses coping mechanisms, however, he or she becomes dysfunctional. In addition, some individuals develop maladaptive coping mechanisms such as abusing alcohol or other substances.

Some people have developed a particularly effective coping style called **hardiness** (Kobasa, 1979). Characteristics of hardiness are as follows:

- A commitment to something meaningful versus a sense of alienation
- A sense of having control over sources of stress versus a feeling of helplessness
- The perception of life events as a challenge rather than a threat

Refer to Nursing Guidelines 12-1 for interventions that can foster effective coping skills and a sense of hardiness.

PSYCHOSOMATIC ILLNESSES

Psyche refers to the mind, and **soma** refers to the body. The term *psychosomatic* means "pertaining to the mind–

NURSING GUIDELINES 12-1

Fostering Effective Coping Skills

- Explore the coping strategies the client has found helpful in the past and encourage their continued use.

- Encourage clients to re-establish priorities and to strike a healthy balance between work and play.

- Suggest cultivating relationships with family and friends who are supportive.

- Teach the client assertiveness skills by role-playing how to (1) clearly state feelings, and (2) say "no" to unreasonable requests.

- Discuss time management techniques like (1) getting up earlier, (2) avoiding procrastination, (3) performing stressful tasks when the client has maximum energy, and (4) eliminating or delegating unwanted tasks.

- Recommend a daily exercise program to reduce stimulating neurotransmitters and release endorphins and enkephalins such as (1) beginning with a 5- to 10-minute workout, (2) increasing the duration by 5 minutes each day, and (3) building up to a 30- to 45-minute period of exercise.

- Tell the client to avoid using alcohol or other nonprescribed sedative drugs as forms of self-treatment.

- Suggest writing about feelings in a diary if verbalizing traumatic or angry thoughts is difficult.

- Suggest stress management education and joining a support group.

body relationship," and psychosomatic illness refers to illnesses influenced by the mind. The term *psychosomatic illness* often is used interchangeably with **stress-related disorder.** In the past, *psychosomatic* had a negative connotation, suggesting that a client's illness was not legitimate. Psychoneuroimmunologic research since the early 1980s, however, has given the term a much more holistic meaning, reflecting the concept that the mind and the body are not separate. **Psychosomatic diseases** (Box 12-3) are bona fide medical conditions associated with or aggravated by stress. Many healthcare providers now believe that all illnesses, if not psychosomatic in origin, have psychosomatic components.

Pathophysiology and Etiology

Biologic Factors

In addition to the known effects of stress on the autonomic nervous system, studies show that stressful events, such as preparing for examinations or undergoing job strain, also affect the immune system. The purpose of the immune system is to defend the body against cancer and invading microorganisms. Stress can lower the numbers of white blood cells, the immune system's disease fighters. Research also shows that chronic stress or very intense stress, such as the death of a spouse, has a greater effect on health than temporary stressors. This finding seems to be particularly true when a person lacks supportive relationships. A connection seems to exist between poorer immune function and loneliness; when individuals share emotions with others, immune functions improve.

Support for a biologic connection between the mind and the immune system is found in research that demonstrates that the immune system and the brain communicate with each other through the chemical messenger system using neurotransmitters and immunopeptides. **Immunopeptides** (or immunotransmitters) are called *cytokines* (see Chap. 41) and function in the same way as neurotransmitters; they relay messages throughout the immune system and the brain (Pert & Chopra, 1999). Immune cells also can secrete small quantities of neuro-

BOX 12-3 ● Stress-Related Diseases and Disorders

Allergic and hypersensitivity disorders	Hypertension
	Infertility
Anovulation	Irritable bowel syndrome
Bronchial asthma	Low back pain
Bruxism	Multiple sclerosis
Cancer	Psoriasis
Cardiac dysrhythmias	Rheumatoid arthritis
Connective tissue disorders	Temporomandibular joint disorder
Eczema	Tension headaches
Hair loss	Tic disorders
Herpes simplex infection	Ulcerative colitis

chemicals. In addition, nerve cells connecting the organs of the immune system (thymus, spleen, and lymph nodes) to the brain have been identified. This ability to communicate through chemicals implies that the immune system can make the brain aware of processes at distant sites in the body and that the brain can send messages directing the immune system's actions. The powerful actions of neurotransmitters, especially in states of excess or depletion, suggest that the psychological state can significantly affect immune function.

Many psychosomatic or stress-related diseases involve allergic, inflammatory, or altered immune responses (see Chap. 42). They are characterized by physical symptoms that cycle through periods of *remission,* or absence, and *exacerbation,* or recurrence, with the symptomatic episodes often occurring when the client is under stress. The brain–immune system connection suggests that changes in body chemistry during periods of stress trigger an autoimmune (self-attacking) response or result in immunosuppression. Invasion of the body by cancer cells or disease-causing microorganisms, however, is not sufficient cause for disease; disease occurs when defenses are compromised or cannot recognize unnatural cells or pathogens. For this reason, psychological variables that influence immunity have the potential to influence the onset and progression of immune system–mediated diseases.

Psychological Factors

The association of certain psychological characteristics with an increased incidence of illness has been observed for centuries. Research suggests that there may be a generic, disease-prone personality with character traits that include anger and hostility, depression, anxiety, and other features (Pelletier, 1977). The type of disease that develops is related to an individual's health habits, environmental exposure, family history, and other socioeconomic factors.

ANGER

Although anger is a normal emotion, many people fail to express it, perhaps feeling threatened by possible retaliation. They expend vast amounts of energy maintaining a facade of being happy and well adjusted. The effect of chronically suppressing anger and the neurochemical changes that accompany it, however, may be the triggering mechanism for a dysfunctional immune response.

Conversely, evidence suggests that the excess expression of hostility and anger is correlated with an increased incidence of heart attacks and may result from low levels of serotonin. The frequent activation of the sympathetic nervous system in persons prone to anger and hostility is another factor implicated in the development of heart disease.

DEPENDENCE

Some propose that unmet dependency needs and fears of rejection or abandonment provoke feelings of insecurity among some individuals with psychosomatic disorders (Townsend, 1999). Helplessness is related to dependence, and numerous studies have shown that people who feel powerless in their lives have more illnesses than those who have a sense of control.

AMBIVALENCE

Ambivalence means feeling or acting in two opposing ways at the same time. For example, an individual may feel hostility toward the persons from whom they most want love and approval, or he or she may act independently and yet desire dependence. These unresolved conflicts may affect neurotransmitter and immune functioning and be another key to the development of physical disorders.

Assessment Findings

Signs and Symptoms

Many stress-prone individuals seek medical attention when they experience symptoms in one or more organs affected by the autonomic nervous system. Clients may present with heart palpitations, pounding headaches, breathlessness, tightness in the chest, chest pain, chronic pain, irritability, epigastric pain, abdominal discomfort and bloating, or constipation alternating with diarrhea. Many other illnesses, including cancer and cardiovascular disease, are not so obviously related to stress but are thought to have a psychosomatic component. The biopsychosocial effects of stress and mental state should be considered in the evaluation and treatment of all illnesses.

Diagnostic Findings

Diagnostic tests are done to determine the extent of the disease and all physical causes for the client's symptoms. Because other conditions such as excessive intake of caffeine, cocaine use, mitral valve prolapse, hyperthyroidism, hypoglycemia, and lactose intolerance, to name a few, can mimic the signs and symptoms of some stress-related diseases, it is important to conduct tests before assuming that the disorder is stress induced.

Medical and Nursing Management

Treatment involves standard medical care pertinent to the diagnosis, control of the physical symptoms, and implementation of methods effective in managing stress and supporting the immune system. Nurses have an important role in participating in the treatment and education of clients regarding these methods. Stress management and other techniques have gained acceptance based on studies that suggest psychological factors can reduce the effects of stress on the immune system and facilitate healing. **Stress management** programs offer instruction in relaxation techniques and effective coping strategies, including assertiveness training and developing a network of social support.

PSYCHOBIOLOGIC INTERVENTIONS

Psychobiologic interventions are those that use the mind and body to alter disease. The placebo effect often is used as a example of how the mind and body are connected. Consequently, mainstream, traditional medicine is now investigating and, in some cases, integrating broader approaches, known as complementary and alternative therapies, to manage and treat various disorders.

The Placebo Effect

A **placebo** is an inert or inactive substance that by its very nature cannot alter physiology, yet does in a significant number of people. The **placebo effect** refers to the healing or improvement that takes place simply because the individual believes a treatment method will be effective.

The placebo effect was first observed during drug research. In most clinical drug trials, half the research volunteers receive the drug being studied, whereas the other half receive a placebo. None of the volunteers or the researchers know which subjects are receiving the actual drug. When the results of the studies are analyzed, researchers find that 30% or more of the individuals who receive a placebo experience improvement. This is thought to show how a person's belief system positively influences health and that a purely psychological basis for recovery exists. In other words, when clients believe in the treatment regimen or have faith in the prescriber, it potentiates a positive outcome. Harnessing the psychological forces that create a "placebo effect" by communicating caring, optimism about treatment, and the belief that the client has the ability to recover can significantly affect wellness.

Stop, Think, and Respond ● BOX 12-6

What response would you expect if you gave 100 people a red-colored candy that you said would increase their desire for sex?

Complementary and Alternative Therapies

In 1998, the National Center for Complementary and Alternative Medicine (NCCAM) was established as a research unit in the National Institutes of Health. NCCAM defines a **complementary therapy** as one used *in addition to* conventional medical treatment. In contrast, an **alternative therapy** is one used *instead of* conventional medical treatment. The goals of the NCCAM are to (1) study complementary and alternative therapies scientifically, (2) educate scientists and healthcare providers on the nature and principles of complementary and alternative therapies, and (3) distribute the results of research findings to whomever is interested in the information.

The NCCAM subdivides complementary and alternative therapies, which approximately 42% of Americans use, into five general groups:

- Alternative medical systems
- Mind–body interventions
- Biologic-based therapies
- Body-based therapies
- Energy therapies

Alternative Medical Systems

From a conventional American standpoint, **alternative medical systems** are those that evolved from non-Western cultures. Some examples of non-Western medical systems include traditional Chinese medicine, Ayurvedic medicine practiced in India, and Native American medicine in the United States. What most Americans call *alternative,* however, is referred to as *traditional* by those indigenous groups, meaning that their system existed before the beginning of modern medicine. Table 12-3 compares differences between alternative and conventional medical systems.

CHINESE MEDICINE

Although the term **Chinese medicine** is used, this medical system also includes contributions from Japan, Korea, and other Southeast Asian countries. Basically, Chinese medicine proposes that health is the outcome of balancing *yin* and *yang,* opposite forces that must remain equalized to maintain *qi* (or *chi*), life's energy force. Forces that alter *qi,* either by depleting or obstructing it, cause illness. Correcting an imbalance between two attributes like motion and stillness or hot and cold restores harmony and health. Treatment measures such as acupuncture, herbal remedies, diet, exercise, and massage are used to restore *qi.*

AYURVEDIC MEDICINE

Ayurvedic medicine has its roots in India and is the oldest system of medicine in the world. It is based on spiritual practices that developed among Tibetan monks. The object of Ayurvedic medicine is to help individuals become unified with nature to develop a strong body, clear mind, and tranquil spirit. One belief is that the *prana,* or the life force (similar to the *qi* in Chinese medicine), moves through various centers in the body called *chakras* (Fig. 12-3). The Ayurvedic doctor prescribes modalities such as yoga, herbal medicine, fasting and eating cleansing foods, meditation, and massage to maintain or restore the dynamic flow of the *prana.*

TABLE 12-3	DIFFERENCES BETWEEN ALTERNATIVE AND CONVENTIONAL MEDICAL SYSTEMS
ALTERNATIVE MEDICAL SYSTEMS	**CONVENTIONAL MEDICAL SYSTEMS**
Originated approximately 1500 BC or earlier	Originated with Hippocrates in approximately 5 BC
Believe that health results from harmony among the person, his or her environment (nature, universe), and energy force	Believe that health results from normal physiologic function
Focus on maintaining a healthy state	Focus on treating illness or injury
Do not correlate symptoms of disease with any specific organ or anatomic location	Correlate symptoms with the organ or location of the person's disorder
Identify with and are sensitive to cultural traditions	Recognize cultural differences but may not incorporate the client's beliefs into the treatment regimen
Incorporate religious principles	Do not reject spirituality, but do not apply any religious significance to a person's illness or recovery
Rely heavily on medicinal plants	Rely on manufactured pharmaceuticals
Accept the efficacy of treatment approaches based not on specific scientific explanation but rather traditional use	Demand scientific evidence for the mechanisms of treatment and replication of results through unbiased research
Do not have established educational standards for practitioners	Require practitioners to have formal education beyond college
Do not regulate practice	Require formal licensure for practice

NATIVE AMERICAN MEDICINE

Native Americans perceive disease as resulting from disharmony with Mother Earth, possession by an evil spirit, or violation of a taboo. They rely on a *shaman,* a person in the tribal community who is both a medicine man (or woman) and a spiritual figure with the extraordinary ability to heal. The shaman has the power to achieve an altered state of consciousness to journey to the spirit world or assume the persona of another life form, such as an eagle or mountain lion.

Native Americans believe that the shaman obtains knowledge from a higher power during a trance-like state, which is accompanied by chanting, drumming, dancing, and, in some cases, consuming psychoactive botanicals. The knowledge allows the shaman to determine the cause and remedies for sick individuals. Remedies may include herbs, meditation, fasting, and sweating. The shaman may fashion a talisman, a symbolic figure, that the sick individual wears around the neck or another body location to ward off evil spirits or exorcise bad spirits.

Mind–Body Interventions

Mind–body interventions are techniques that rely on the power of the mind to alter body functions or symptoms. Many practices that were once categorized as alternative medicine (e.g., biofeedback, imagery, humor, hypnosis) are now becoming accepted as conventional medical treatments. Spiritual healing is a mind–body technique that the medical community has not yet entirely accepted as legitimately therapeutic.

BIOFEEDBACK

Biofeedback is a technique in which an individual voluntarily controls one or more physiologic functions,

FIGURE 12-3 The chakras and channels of energy.

such as body temperature, heart rate, blood pressure, and brain waves. Initially, clients are attached to a machine that translates a physiologic activity, like heart rate, into a pulsating waveform, digital numbers, or audible sound. While receiving feedback from the machine, clients try to alter a particular function (e.g., decrease heart rate). If the machine's signal changes, it helps them determine if they are successful. Eventually, clients do not need to rely on the response from the device; they can alter their physiology at will. Biofeedback is currently being used in the United States to reduce hypertension and rapid heart rates, manage pain, abort seizures, relieve migraine headaches, and produce dilation of peripheral blood vessels in individuals with vascular disorders.

IMAGERY

Imagery is a psychobiologic technique that uses the mind to visualize a positive physiologic effect. When using imagery, clients conjure up mental images of their body waging and winning a battle with the disease process. For example, clients might visualize their body producing white blood cells in large numbers. They then imagine the white cells destroying cancer cells. Laboratory values of white cell counts taken before and after such imagery sessions often show that the numbers of white blood cells dramatically increase.

HUMOR

Humor can be used therapeutically. Laughter stimulates the immune system by increasing the number of white blood cells and lowering cortisol, which suppresses immune function. Laughter can cause the release of neuropeptides (endorphins and enkephalins). Norman Cousins (1979) shared his own pain-relieving and healing experiences using humor in his book, *Anatomy of an Illness.*

HYPNOSIS

Hypnosis is a therapeutic intervention that facilitates a physiologic change through the power of suggestion. Hypnotism has been used to help individuals overcome habits like smoking, relieve chronic pain, and extinguish irrational fears. Research is needed to find out how hypnotism works and why not everyone can be hypnotized.

SPIRITUAL HEALING

Spiritual healing restores health through a higher power (God or some other metaphysical force). An intermediary person may channel the healing force, acting strictly as a facilitator. Sometimes healing occurs through the sick person's prayers or those said by others on his or her behalf. In "hopeless" cases, some would call the healing a miracle; however, spiritual healing is not limited to miracles. In his book, *Prayer is Good Medicine* (1996), the physician Larry Dossey notes that prayer-like thoughts offered from a distance have increased the healing rate of surgical wounds and sped the recovery of clients who have had surgery.

Biologic-Based Therapies

Biologic-based therapies use natural products such as herbs, aromas, and even bee venom. The specific therapies include herbal therapy, aromatherapy, and apitherapy.

HERBAL THERAPY

For centuries, humans have used ethnobotanicals, plants that grow in a region where specific groups of people live, for food, clothing, shelter, and medicine. The particular plants that are used by the Chinese, Indians, Native Americans, and other groups are different in various world locales, but their general purposes are largely the same. The use of plants as **herbal therapy,** a technique for treating disease and disorders, has been mostly handed down orally from generation to generation. Their use is commonly referred to as *folk medicine* because their benefits are largely anecdotal rather than based on scientific investigation.

Approximately 25% of prescription drugs are derived from plants. Drugs manufactured from plant sources usually contain one or more extracts from the plant or a synthesized, molecularly similar structure. Herbalists argue that using only parts of a plant changes the effects that are achieved from using the whole plant. Consequently, interest in self-treatment using herbs has been renewed (Table 12-4). Clients can use herbs in a variety of forms:

- Liquified juice
- Mashed paste
- Steeped teas
- Compressed powders
- Fermented liquid
- Sweetened syrups
- Tinctures
- Liniments
- Salves

Herbal therapy is not regulated like pharmaceutical drugs are in the United States. The health food industry lobbied federal legislators in the early 1990s to "preserve the consumer's right to choose dietary supplements" (Barrett, 2000). As a result, Congress passed the Dietary Supplement Health and Education Act of 1994. That legislation defines a "dietary supplement" as something that supplies one or more essential nutrients missing from the diet and includes vitamins, minerals, amino acids, herbs, and other botanicals. Consequently, herbs are classified as nutritional supplements and are not held to the same standards of unified dosages, safety, and efficacy as drugs. Manufacturers of herbal preparations, however, cannot claim that the herbal product prevents or treats a disease because that automatically places the substance in the category of a drug, which is highly regulated.

To avoid federal regulation, labels on herbal products can suggest medicinal use as long as they also contain a

TABLE 12-4	POPULAR HERBS USED IN THE UNITED STATES		
HERB	**BOTANICAL NAME**	**CLAIM FOR USE**	**PRECAUTIONS**
Chamomile	*Chamomilla recutita*	Relieves digestive disorders	Avoid if allergic to ragweed, asters, chrysanthemums, or members of the daisy family.
Echinacea	*Echinacea augstifolia*	Boosts immune function and speeds healing	Avoid if allergic to plants in the daisy family; prolonged use may reduce effects.
Ephedra	*Ephedra vulgaris*	Relieves asthma, stimulates the central nervous system, promotes weight loss, increases energy	Action is similar to that of amphetamine; ephedra can cause tachycardia, headache, hypertension, seizures, insomnia, chest pain, decreased intestinal motility, and death from stroke or heart attack.
Garlic	*Allium sativum*	Lowers blood pressure, thins the blood	Possible side effects include intestinal gas; combining garlic with aspirin or other anticoagulants can prolong bleeding.
Ginkgo	*Ginkgo biloba*	Improves memory	Possible side effects include gastrointestinal distress, headaches, and allergic reactions; use with caution if taking aspirin or other blood-thinning drugs.
Ginseng	*Panax gensema*	Increases energy and helps in dealing with stress	Use may raise blood pressure and serum glucose level and can increase the growth of estrogen-dependent cancer.
Kava	*Piper methysticum*	Reduces stress and anxiety	Large doses can produce an intoxicating effect; long-term use can lead to dry, scaly skin.
St. John's Wort	*Hypericum perforatum*	Treats mild depression	Use may cause sensitivity to light; interactions with other drugs can be dangerous.
Saw palmetto	*Serenoa repens*	Relieves enlargement of the prostate gland	Avoid tea versions because the herb dissolves poorly; nausea and gastrointestinal distress are possible.
Valerian	*Valerian officinalis*	Relieves anxiety and insomnia	Possible side effects include blurred vision, excitability, and changes in heartbeat if taken in large doses or for more than 2 weeks.

disclaimer that the Food and Drug Administration has not evaluated the product. As the NCCAM studies herbs more scientifically, it will make more than anecdotal information available. Until then, Dr. Robert Lee, Director of Education at the Beth Israel Center for Health and Healing in New York, advises consumers of herbs to (1) find out what they are using, (2) not use a product if information is unavailable, (3) use the lowest dose initially, (4) increase the dose gradually, and (5) never exceed the maximum dose. Even herbs have possibly lethal side effects. Consulting with a physician before using herbs and disclosing that information before any medication is prescribed are best. Use of herbs also is not recommended for pregnant or lactating women, infants, and children younger than 6 years of age.

AROMATHERAPY

Most people agree that they positively or negatively associate odors of certain substances with various people, places, or feelings. **Aromatherapy** is the use of scents to alter emotions and biologic processes. For therapeutic uses, scents from botanical oils of lavender, peppermint, and the like are released by adding them to bath water, permeating the air where they are inhaled, or rubbing them on the skin. The olfactory nerves carry the scented

molecules and carry them to the limbic system. As discussed earlier in this chapter, the limbic system is the brain area used for learning, memory, and emotions. Once the limbic system is stimulated, it can trigger physiologic and psychological responses through neurotransmitters like serotonin, endorphins (see Chap. 21), or norepinephrine, released by the hypothalamus. The neurotransmitters can, in turn, affect nervous, endocrine, and immune system functions. Some believe that aromatherapy can help control blood pressure and hormone secretions; relieve pain, depression, and anxiety; or promote higher states of alertness. More research is needed to validate the physiologic actions of various scents, evaluate how best to use them, and determine why one type of aroma affects people differently.

Stop, Think, and Respond ● BOX 12-7

Discuss particular scents and the images or feelings they create for you. For example, the smell of the ocean may make you happy because of the pleasant memories that you associate with a holiday or former residence. On the other hand, the antiseptic smell of the dentist's office may create feelings of anxiety or fear because you associate it with discomfort.

APITHERAPY

Apitherapy is the medicinal use of bee venom. To date, apitherapy has been used as an alternative for treating various inflammatory conditions of the joints like rheumatoid arthritis and osteoarthritis. It is also used to treat multiple sclerosis, a neurologic condition. Although reports of the use of bee venom have dated from the mid-1800s, interest in apitherapy gained momentum around 1920. Bee venom does contain various enzymes that may stimulate the adrenal glands and induce the release of cortisol, an anti-inflammatory and immunosuppressant hormone. Physicians currently consider apitherapy an unconventional treatment, however, and do not recommend its use or support a client's request for it. Nevertheless, experiments have demonstrated relief of symptoms among research volunteers (Kuthan, 2000). Under the supervision of the NCCAM, further study may validate (1) if bee venom therapy is efficacious; (2) if so, which types of disorders respond best when apitherapy is used; (3) which yields better results: the actual sting of the bee or chemically prepared apitoxin (bee venom); (4) how many stings or what apitoxin concentrations are necessary to achieve positive results; and (5) besides discomfort and potential allergic reactions, any other side effects to consider.

Body-Based Therapies

Body-based therapies are those healing methods that use manipulation and movement to improve health and restore biologic functions. They include massage therapies (including reflexology and shiatsu), chiropractic, yoga, and tai chi.

MASSAGE THERAPY, REFLEXOLOGY, AND SHIATSU

Massage therapy involves applying pressure and movement to stretch and knead soft body tissues. Massage therapists use the warmth of their hands, elbows, and forearms and lubricating oils to stimulate circulation and relieve physical and psychological tension. The benefits of massage include relief from discomfort and improved mobility or functional use of affected parts of the body.

Reflexology is a complementary health practice in which manual pressure is applied to the feet and hands. The International Academy of Advanced Reflexology (2001) and those who practice reflexology claim that locations in the extremities contain reflex centers composed of more than 7000 nerve endings linked to body organs and tissues. When pressure is applied to a reflex area, the impulse travels from peripheral nerves to the spinal cord and brain. As a result, reflexologists believe that reconditioning or reprogramming the neural reflex improves the body's ability to facilitate natural healing.

Shiatsu is a Japanese word that means "finger pressure." Shiatsu has many similarities to acupressure and acupuncture because practitioners apply pressure to acupoints in various body meridians (energy channels; Fig. 12-4). Each meridian correlates with an organ or its function. Acupoints are locations along the meridians where Asians believe the body's life force, or *qi,* moves. Unblocking and strengthening *qi* rebalances the body's energy and restores health.

CHIROPRACTIC

Chiropractic theory proposes that subluxation (malalignment) of the spinal vertebrae alters nerve activities that regulate body functions in distant organs. To treat various disorders, chiropractors, who are the single largest group of alternative–complementary practitioners in the United States, perform spinal manipulation as a generic method for curing neuromuscular disorders and a host of other diseases. According to William T. Jarvis (2001, p. 2), "chiropractors have not shown that impinging a spinal nerve alters an impulse beyond the zone of impingement, nor have they shown that disrupting a nerve impulse produces disease." Despite the criticisms of Jarvis and many members of the American Medical Association (AMA), millions of people continue to seek chiropractic treatment with obviously some improvement in their symptoms. Chiropractic treatment is further legitimized because (1) many health insurance policies cover it, (2) the federal government provides Medicare and Medicaid reimbursement for it, and (3) the costs are an approved medical income tax deduction (Jarvis, 2001).

FIGURE 12-4 Location of the meridians and acupoints in the body.

Some feel that chiropractic is a form of pseudomedicine that has attracted clients who are disgruntled with the outcomes of conventional medical care. Critics continue to suggest that there is no reason to justify practitioners who use "one cure" for all ailments. In fact, some hold that this type of philosophy can delay appropriate medical treatment. Many agree that spinal manipulation should be limited to medically trained specialists like osteopaths, orthopedists, and physiatrists, physicians who specialize in rehabilitation. But until the NCCAM conducts further scientific research, emotions and conjecture rather than facts will continue to fuel the controversy.

YOGA AND TAI CHI

Yoga developed in India, and **tai chi** has its origins in China. Both incorporate techniques that combine mental and physical exercises for the purpose of integrating body and mind. There are several branches of yoga; hatha yoga is most commonly practiced in the United States. Advocates of hatha yoga attribute the following benefits to its practice:

- Relaxation and centeredness
- Relief of headaches, insomnia, anxiety, and pain
- Increased musculoskeletal flexibility
- Improved breathing
- Overall contentment

The Chinese believe that tai chi exercises restore *qi* or *chi*. The exercises require standing and shifting body weight from one foot to another while performing a series of slow, choreographed arm movements. To obtain full advantage of the physical exercise, it should be accompanied by slow, controlled breathing and visualization of energy circulating throughout the body. Proponents believe that tai chi exercises tone the whole body without the exertion and cardiac risks associated with other aerobic forms of physical exercise, restore health, and prevent disease. In China where a slightly different form of tai chi called *qi gong* is practiced, there are reports that people develop psychokinetic powers, the ability to move objects and people without touching them.

Energy Therapies

Energy therapies are techniques that claim to manipulate electromagnetic fields in the body. Some examples include reiki, acupuncture, and techniques involving magnets and electricity.

REIKI

Reiki (pronounced "ray-key") shares many features with what Westerners may call "therapeutic touch" and spiritual healing. Reiki is a Japanese method of healing that was introduced to the Western world in the 1800s. *Rei* means "spirit" and *ki* is translated like *qi* or *chi*. Basically, those who use reiki believe that *ki* promotes health and healing. They further believe that when *ki* is blocked and

a person is ill, a reiki practitioner can channel energy—not from his or her own body, but from the universe—to the sick person's body. Once *ki* is restored, healing occurs.

The practitioner transfers the energy in the universe by laying-on of hands. Direct contact between the practitioner and client is the usual method of healing; however, healing can also occur from a distance because the Japanese believe that the spirit is not confined by time or space. In other words, the practitioner and ill person can be geographically separate. The practitioner then moves his or her hands on an object that symbolically represents the sick person while visualizing the transmission of energy. The belief is that the recipient draws in the energy, which goes where it is needed.

ACUPUNCTURE

Acupuncture is a healing therapy in which a needle is placed in one or more acupoints to unblock *qi*. Acupuncture is considered a form of energy therapy because its ultimate goal is to restore the balance and free flow of energy in the body. Some acupuncturists take the technique one step further by manipulating the needles with an electric current. When used in this manner, it is referred to as *electroacupuncture*.

ELECTROMAGNETIC THERAPY

Electromagnetic therapy promotes healing using electricity, magnets, or both. Microcurrent therapy, using low-intensity electrical currents to alter cellular physiology, is currently used to treat nonhealing fractures and to relieve pain (see Chap. 21 and the discussion of transcutaneous electrical nerve stimulation). Magnetism is used diagnostically with MRI. Despite the use of electromagnetic therapies, several questions are yet unanswered: (1) how do these two forces produce healing; (2) what is the explanation for the anecdotal reports of symptom relief among people who wear magnets; and (3) if electromagnetic healing is validated, for what disorders is it best used?

The theory concerning electromagnetism is based on the physiologic principle that cellular membranes emit electrical currents. This is verified by the fact that electrical energy can be recorded using electrocardiograms, EEGs, and electromyelograms. Science also has confirmed that nerve stimulation causes the resting membrane potentials of cells to change to action potentials. Furthermore, a magnet can change the direction of an electrical current by separating charged ions. Consequently, speculation is that electromagnetic therapy (1) affects the cell membrane by changing the ion exchange of electrolytes like calcium, sodium, and potassium; (2) stimulates the release of endorphins, naturally produced morphine-like chemicals, or other neurotransmitters through the cell's membrane; or (3) rebalances the electromagnetic field in the body.

Although questions about the what, why, and how of electromagnetic therapy remain largely unanswered, its use has been unscientifically expanded to include static magnet therapy and pulsed magnetic field therapy. Static magnet therapy refers to wearing stationary magnets, which are stronger than everyday refrigerator-type magnets, directly on the body. The static magnets are incorporated in bracelets, necklaces, belts, wraps, and even mattress pads. Pulsed magnetic field therapy uses devices that apply very low frequency electricity (50 Hz) to body areas at intervals of 25 pulses per second for 600 seconds (10 minutes) followed by an interval of rest. Supposedly, the pulsing effect produces rising and falling levels in the body's magnetic field.

Electromagnetic therapeutic devices continue to be used haphazardly for a host of unrelated conditions such as fibromyalgia, postpolio syndrome, peripheral neuropathy, multiple sclerosis, depression, epilepsy, and urinary incontinence. Research as to whether beneficial results can be attributed entirely to the placebo effect or if there is a legitimate scientific basis to its efficacy is long overdue.

GENERAL NUTRITIONAL CONSIDERATIONS

Some people overeat in response to stress, whereas others deny normal hunger. Assess for changes in appetite, eating patterns, and weight. Encourage clients to eat at regular intervals to avoid both overeating and undereating.

Dietary interventions for some psychosomatic diseases may be necessary only during periods of exacerbation, such as avoiding lactose during acute episodes of ulcerative colitis. For other psychosomatic diseases, such as irritable bowel syndrome, dietary interventions are recommended regardless of symptoms.

GENERAL PHARMACOLOGIC CONSIDERATIONS

Obtain a complete current medication history for each client, including nonprescription drugs. Some people who experience stress take over-the-counter drugs, stimulants, and tranquilizers that they may not mention unless asked.

Anti-inflammatory drugs and corticosteroids often are given to treat the symptoms of various psychosomatic diseases. Drug treatment is considered symptomatic rather than curative.

Herbs may interact with over-the-counter and prescribed medications. Most often, such an interaction causes the therapeutic action of the medication to either increase or decrease.

Certain herbs may decrease blood glucose levels, whereas some may potentiate the effects of cardiac glycosides. The client's physician should be aware of all herbs the client uses before any medications are prescribed. The client should read labels on over-the-counter medications for any known contraindications with herbal use, or consult a pharmacist.

GENERAL GERONTOLOGIC CONSIDERATIONS

The function of the immune system diminishes with age, resulting in increased incidences of infection, cancer, and autoimmune disease.

Elderly clients who have developed positive coping skills continue to cope well as they age.

Some older adults feel helpless and cannot cope when released from a healthcare facility without adequate discharge planning.

Emotional distress and impaired self-care abilities have been identified as major contributors to rehospitalization of older adults.

Loss of a network for support increases an older adult's vulnerability and reaction to stressors.

Adults who have chronic psychosomatic diseases are likely to manifest debilitating effects in late adulthood.

Critical Thinking Exercises

1. *What would you say to someone who characterizes mental illness as the manifestation of a poor or weak character?*
2. *What suggestions would you offer to someone who has a stress-related (psychosomatic) disorder?*

References and Suggested Readings

American Psychiatric Association. (2000). *Diagnostic and statistical manual of mental disorders* (4th ed., text revision). Washington, DC: Author.

Barrett, S. (2001). How the dietary supplement health and education act of 1994 weakened the FDA. [On-line.] Available: http://www.quackwatch.com/02Consumer Protection/dshea.html.

Barry, P. (1996). *Psychosocial nursing: Care of physically ill patients and their families* (3rd ed.). Philadelphia: Lippincott-Raven.

Basmajian, J. V. (1999). The third therapeutic revolution: behavioral medicine. *Applied Psychophysiology and Biofeedback, 24*(2), 107–117.

Benson, H. (2000). *The relaxation response.* New York: Avon Books.

Carmagnani, A. (1999). Biofeedback: Present state and future possibilities. *International Journal of Mental Health, 28*(3), 83–86.

Cousins, N. (1979). *Anatomy of an illness.* New York: Norton.

Curtis, M. (1999). The placebo effect. *Survey of Ophthalmology, 44*(1), 31.

Donaldson, V. W. (2000). A clinical study of visualization on depressed white blood cell count in medical patients. *Applied Psychophysiology and Biofeedback, 25*(2), 117–129.

Dossey, L. (1996). *Prayer is good medicine: How to reap the healing benefits of prayer.* San Francisco: Harper.

Dossey, L. (1999). *Reinventing medicine: Beyond mind-body to a new era of healing.* San Francisco: Harper.

Fisher, M. J. (2000). Better living through the placebo effect: Self-delusion as a form of wellness. *The Atlantic, 286*(4), 16–20.

Fox, S., Shephard, T. J., McCain, N. (1999). Neurologic mechanisms in psychoneuroimmunology. *Journal of the American Association of Neuroscience Nurses, 31*(2), 87–97.

Heinonen, T., Lantinen, A., Hakkin, V. (1999). Implementation of three-dimensional EEG brain mapping. *Computers and Biomedical Research, 32*(2), 123–132.

Horwitz, J. (2001). All life is connected: The shaman's journey. [On-line.] Available: http://www.users.dircon.co.uk/~snail/SCSS/Articles/All%20Life.htm.

International Academy of Advanced Reflexology. (2001). Reflexology accurately defined. [On-line.] Available: http://www.reflexology.net/reflexology.htm.

Jarvis, W. T. (2001). Why chiropractic is controversial (1990). [On-line.] Available: http://www.chirobase.org/01General/controversy.html.

Kaye, J., Morton, J., Bowcutt, M., et al. (2000). Stress, depression, and psychoneuroimmunology. *Journal of the American Association of Neuroscience Nurses, 32*(2), 93–101.

Kobasa, S. (1979). Stressful life events, personality and health: an inquiry into hardiness. *Journal of Personality and Social Psychology, 42*(1), 1–11.

Kuthan, F. (2000). Bee venom treatment of rheumatic disorders. [On-line.] Available: http://www.apitherapy.org/aas/kuthan.html and http://www.apitherapy.org/aas/kuthan2.html.

Moerman, C. (2000). Cultural variations in the placebo effect: Ulcers, anxiety, and blood pressure. *Medical Anthropology Quarterly, 14*(1), 51–72.

Pelletier, K. (1977). *Mind as healer, mind as slayer.* New York: Dell.

Pert, C., & Chopra, D. (1999). *Molecules of emotions: Why you feel the way you feel.* New York: Scribner.

Ramey, D. W. (2001). Magnetic and electromagnetic therapy. [On-line.] Available: http://www.hcrc.org/contrib/ramey/magnet.html.

Selye, H. (1956). *The stress of life.* New York: McGraw-Hill.

Townsend, M. C. (1999). *Psychiatric mental health nursing: Concepts of care* (3rd ed.). Philadelphia: F.A. Davis.

Caring for Clients With Somatoform Disorders

Learning Objectives

On completion of this chapter, the reader will:
- Describe the coping mechanism referred to as *somatization.*
- Name five somatoform disorders
- List three characteristics of somatoform disorders.
- Explain why malingering and syndromes classified as factitious disorders are not somatoform disorders.
- Discuss three explanations for the development of somatoform disorders.
- Explain the meaning of insight-oriented therapy.
- Name two nursing diagnoses that are common to clients with somatoform disorders.

The care of clients with somatoform disorders is challenging because the symptoms, which are very real and distressing, do not result from any specific pathology. By understanding the psychological origins of these disorders, nurses can provide better care for clients who suffer physically from underlying emotional factors.

SOMATOFORM DISORDERS

Somatoform disorders are conditions with a basis in the coping mechanism of somatization. **Somatization** is the manifestation of unconscious emotional distress through physical symptoms. Approximately 2% to 15% of the U.S. population has various types of somatoform disorders (Videbeck, 2001); however, because somatoform disorders sometimes are misdiagnosed as medical diseases, the incidence could be higher. Although many people have physical illnesses that are worsened by stress and emotional conflict (see Chap. 12), somatizers (people with somatoform disorders) have no physiologic basis for their

symptoms and often go from doctor to doctor seeking relief. The psychological origin of the somatizer's symptoms is unknown to the client, and the illnesses seem very real. All somatoform disorders share three characteristics:

1. The physical symptoms resemble those of a medical illness, but no medical illness can be objectively identified.
2. Psychological factors promote and maintain the symptoms or cause their periodic recurrence.
3. Unconscious motivators influence the course of the disorder; the client does not consciously control the symptoms (Videbeck, 2001).

Somatoform disorders are not to be confused with **malingering,** which is deliberately faking an illness to acquire financial compensation, obtain drugs, or be relieved of responsibilities from work or school. Nor are they **factitious disorders,** in which people purposefully cause illness-like symptoms. Two examples of factitious disorders are Munchausen's syndrome and Munchausen's syndrome by proxy. In **Munchausen's syndrome,** a person self-induces an illness (e.g., by taking nonlethal amounts of poison) to acquire medical treatment. In **Munchausen's syndrome by proxy,** a person makes another person—usually his or her own child—sick. The motivation for creating a life-threatening situation is to gain attention from medical personnel and sometimes notoriety for being influential in saving the child's life. For example, a mother may inject feces into her child's urinary catheter or intravenous line to cause infection that requires medical attention or revive a child with cardiopulmonary resuscitation after first smothering the child.

Types

Somatization Disorder

A person with **somatization disorder** has combinations of multiple unexplained somatic complaints (Box 13-1) with no medical explanation. The chronic symptoms cause the person repeatedly to seek medical attention, sometimes from more than one physician simultaneously. More women than men develop somatization disorder, which explains why it was formerly referred to as *hysteria* (*hyster* referring to "uterus"). The term *hysteria* has a connotation of high states of emotion, which also is characteristic of affected individuals.

Hypochondriasis

Hypochondriasis is a somatoform disorder in which a person is preoccupied with minor symptoms and develops an exaggerated belief that they signify a life-threatening illness. When medical diagnostic work-ups show normal findings, clients with hypochondriasis may be convinced that their illness is so complex that it eludes diagnosis by their primary physician. As the symptoms continue and their frustration mounts, these individuals become increasingly anxious and invest time, energy, and money to discover a cause for their concerns.

BOX 13-1 ● **Examples of Somatic Complaints**

GASTROINTESTINAL SYMPTOMS
Nausea, bloating, vomiting, diarrhea, food intolerance

PAIN SYMPTOMS
Headache; abdominal discomfort; pain in the back, extremities, chest, or rectum; pain during urination, menstruation, or sexual intercourse

SEXUAL SYMPTOMS
Disinterest in sex, erectile or ejaculatory dysfunction, irregular menses, excessive menstrual bleeding, vomiting throughout pregnancy

PSEUDONEUROLOGIC SYMPTOMS
Impaired coordination or balance, paralysis or localized weakness, difficulty swallowing or lump in the throat, inability to speak, urinary retention, hallucinations, loss of touch or pain sensation, double vision, blindness, deafness, seizures, amnesia, loss of consciousness other than fainting

---

Conversion Disorder

Conversion disorder is characterized by a sudden loss of motor or sensory function, such as paralysis or deafness, after a stressful event or experience. Often the manifestation of the symptom holds some symbolic meaning. For example, blindness developed in several Cambodian women who witnessed the execution of their families in what has become known as the "killing fields" of the Pol Pot regime (1975–1979). Although the anatomic structures in their visual tracts and centers for vision in the brain are normal, they cannot see. Theorists hypothesize that these women used blindness as a defense mechanism to prevent them from ever having to see a similar event. Because the physical malady is a protective mechanism, albeit a strange one, the affected persons appear unconcerned that it exists, a characteristic referred to as *la belle indifference.*

Pain Disorder

Persons with **pain disorder,** formerly known as *somatic pain disorder,* experience pain in one or more anatomic sites that cannot be linked with any identifiable medical condition. As in conversion disorder, the onset, severity, continuation, or recurrence of the pain is related to psychological factors. The person with this disorder generally experiences somewhat perverted beneficial effects because the pain provides an excuse from unwanted responsibilities or garners sympathetic attention from family and social acquaintances. Pain disorder can lead to abuse of analgesic medications and in some cases unnecessary surgery when physicians deal with the condition on a physical rather than a psychological level.

Body Dysmorphic Disorder

People with **body dysmorphic disorder** become obsessed with the idea that some feature of their bodies, such as their nose, ears, lips, arms, abdomen, or breasts, is flawed. Although most people believe that their appearance could be improved in some way, those with body dysmorphic disorder exaggerate the significance of what others would describe as a minor characteristic. According to Carol Watkins (2001), people with body dysmorphic disorder are likely to manifest some of the following behaviors:

- Glancing frequently in reflective surfaces
- Touching or picking at their skin
- Measuring or repeatedly palpating the defect
- Continually requesting reassurance about the defect
- Performing elaborate grooming rituals
- Using various means to disguise the defect, such as with a hat, their hands, or make-up
- Avoiding social situations in which others could observe the defect
- Becoming anxious around other people

Preoccupation with thoughts about what those with body dysmorphic disorder believe is distorted can lead to social isolation, impaired ability to concentrate, cosmetic surgery, depression, and sometimes suicide.

Pathophysiology and Etiology

Several theories exist to explain somatoform disorders. One belief is that the chronic release of neurotransmitters and neuroendocrine hormones in response to stress exhausts or depletes regions in the brain that facilitate adaptation and coping behaviors. Alternatively, the brain may attach exaggerated significance to minor physical symptoms, such as a belief that the symptoms of indigestion are caused by stomach cancer or a heart disorder. Another theory suggests that physical symptoms provide relief from psychological tension when the person cannot deal with it consciously. For example, the disorder may be a consequence of childhood abuse. Yet another explanation is that the conversion of emotional pain into a physical disorder serves as a justifiable way to obtain attention and compassion from others—an outcome referred to as **secondary gain.** Still other theories suggest that either parental failure to respond to an infant's needs or inadvertent reward during routine childhood illnesses lay the groundwork for somatization. Somatization also may be learned behavior modeled after close relatives who manifest similar disorders.

Regardless of the cause, clients with somatoform disorders experience physical distress that interferes with the quality of their lives. In some cases, the disorder impairs social interactions and affects the ability to perform activities of daily living and role responsibilities.

Assessment Findings

Signs and Symptoms

Clients seek diagnosis and treatment for symptoms that usually involve a variety of body systems, pain, or a unique body characteristic. Some may have illnesses that are highly symbolic in nature (e.g., imagined heart ailments after termination of a romance). Some somatizers appear **histrionic,** a term that derives from the word *hysteria,* when describing their symptoms. They are animated, dramatic, and prone to exaggeration. Others, like those with conversion disorder, appear apathetic. They often have multiple symptoms, and many provide a history of extensive medical consultations, diagnostic procedures, and surgical interventions. Despite such measures, the symptoms persist or others replace them. The physical examination usually reveals symptoms that do not fit with known patterns of disease or injury. Often, these symptoms become more distressing during emotional crises, although most somatizers do not acknowledge such a relationship. The symptoms often provide some secondary gain: they distract from dealing with emotional problems, they provide a means for gaining attention, or they relieve the client from performing unwanted responsibilities.

Stop, Think, and Respond ● BOX 13-1

A man who is in a middle management position must make monthly verbal presentations to his company's board of directors. A day or two before the board meetings, he experiences severe diarrhea. On several occasions, he has asked the board to postpone his report or allow him to submit a written report. The manager has visited his physician about the diarrhea on many occasions, and the results of diagnostic tests have been unremarkable. He asked his physician to refer him to a gastroenterologist for a second opinion, but the results were the same. Based on information about somatoform disorders, explain the dynamics that may be involved.

Diagnostic Findings

Despite comprehensive laboratory and diagnostic tests, no etiology or pathology can be identified. In some cases, all current medications are temporarily discontinued to determine if a drug–drug or drug–food interaction or an interaction with some other environmental substance may explain the client's symptoms. When all investigative approaches prove negative, it is presumed that the symptoms are the consequence of a psychobiologic process.

Medical Management

Differentiating the somatizer from a client with a medical illness is important. The physician, of course, attempts to discover the pathologic basis for the disorder while treating the symptoms. Clients with pain disorder are referred to specialty pain clinics to learn nonpharmacologic interventions for the relief of their discomfort (see Chap. 21).

Eventually, repeated diagnostic testing with negative results can reinforce the client's belief that the physician is inept at determining the cause of the disorder. Although many clients with somatoform disorders resist it, they eventually may be referred to psychiatrists or psychologists for insight-oriented psychotherapy.

Insight-oriented psychotherapy helps clients understand the causal relationship between their emotional distress and physical symptoms. Goals of treatment include avoiding further unnecessary procedures and diagnostic testing, minimizing disability, and helping the client find other coping mechanisms that will prevent translating emotional stress into bodily symptoms. Therapy may be brief and can be followed by one or two sessions as needed if extreme stress results in a recurrence. Antianxiety medications such as alprazolam (Xanax) and diazepam (Valium) are avoided or prescribed for only a brief period because of their potential for abuse and addiction among clients with chronic symptoms. Antidepressant drugs are used if the client becomes despondent (see Chap. 15).

NURSING PROCESS

● The Client With a Somatoform Disorder

Assessment

The nurse begins by obtaining a detailed health history. The client often reports a remarkable number of vague health problems and a variety of diagnostic and treatment procedures (including surgery) that outnumber those for most people of a comparable age. Some clients may appear fixated and animated when discussing their physical problems. They may manipulate the focus of any interaction to their physical state. On the other hand, those with a conversion reaction may appear passive and unperturbed by their health status.

During assessment of psychosocial issues, the client may deny that stressors exist now or occurred in the past. He or she may cut short efforts to discuss these areas. It is appropriate to explore the possibility of childhood abuse, although the client may protect revelations of this nature. Most clients are firmly convinced that the nature of their illness is physical and resist suggestions to the contrary.

The nurse should also ask questions related to the client's social history. Clients with somatoform illness may be unemployed, work less than full-time, or have a pattern of frequent absenteeism. Medical expenses may have severely diminished their income or savings. Some may have had to resort to public assistance to meet their basic needs for food and shelter. They may lead a fairly isolated existence, having alienated themselves from relationships with their family and friends. Social interactions are more often limited to those with healthcare providers.

Diagnosis, Planning, and Interventions

Altered Comfort: Somatic complaints related to ineffective coping
Expected Outcome: The client's discomfort will be reduced or eliminated as evidenced by a reduction in the need for medication, fewer medical encounters, and resumption of functional abilities.

- Assess physical complaints matter-of-factly without emphasizing undue concern, yet avoid dismissing them altogether. *Attention to physical symptoms provides secondary gain.*
- Acknowledge that the client's discomfort is real. *Remaining nonjudgmental enhances the nurse–client relationship.*
- Implement pharmacologic and nonpharmacologic measures that may provide symptomatic relief. *Physical needs must be met before the client can deal with the possibility that somatization serves a psychological purpose.*

Ineffective Coping related to unconscious emotional conflict
Expected Outcomes: (1) The client will use coping strategies, other than somatizing, for managing stressors. (2) The client will identify a connection between emotional issues and physical symptoms.

- Express a caring attitude. *Client will be more willing to examine and discuss psychosocial stressors with an empathetic and concerned individual.*
- Accept the client's need to use somatizing as a coping mechanism until he or she has acquired alternative coping strategies. *Eliminating the chief means by which the client protects his or her consciousness of the underlying etiology may worsen symptoms or lead to a more fragile psychological state.*
- Meet the client's needs for symptom relief and attention. *Implementing nursing interventions addresses client's needs for physical care and demonstrates that the client will not be ignored or abandoned.*
- Set gradual limits on the amount of time that the client can discuss physical problems. *Setting limits promotes the realization that physical symptoms cannot remain the main focus of all interactions.*
- Give the client opportunities and encouragement to express feelings, and provide positive feedback when the client discusses emotional issues. *Calling attention to the occasions when the client discusses emotional, rather than physical, issues is rewarding. Clients are likely to repeat rewarded behavior.*
- Offer the suggestion that a link may exist between underlying emotional conflict and the client's physical response. *A new point of view from someone the client trusts may help the client develop some insight.*
- Explore the positive outcomes the client achieves as a result of having physical symptoms. *The client may have thought of his or her physical symptoms only in negative terms, but with supportive encouragement may identify how illness meets emotional needs.*
- Explore alternative strategies for managing needs for dependency, attention, trauma from abuse, insecurity, decreased self-confidence, and low self-esteem. *Identifying alternatives may help the client relinquish the use of somatization, which is maladaptive, and use one or more strategies that promote emotional and psychological maturation.*

Evaluation of Expected Outcomes

Expected outcomes for the client are that physical discomfort significantly decreases and that emotional health improves. The client begins to identify emotional conflicts that he or she subconsciously repressed and admits that physical symptoms protected against dealing with psychological issues. The client develops and uses adaptive coping strategies to manage emotionally traumatic feelings.

GENERAL PHARMACOLOGIC CONSIDERATIONS

Numerous drugs may be prescribed for somatoform disorders. The course of treatment usually is short because of adverse reactions or lack of therapeutic effect.

Psychotropic medications and prescription analgesics usually are avoided in clients with somatoform disorders.

When medications are prescribed for clients with somatoform disorders, careful monitoring is necessary because these clients may overuse or abuse drugs.

GENERAL GERONTOLOGIC CONSIDERATIONS

Loss of a support network increases an older adult's vulnerability and reaction to stressors.

Older adults who are socially isolated may focus on themselves and become preoccupied with bodily illness.

By focusing on somatoform disorders, older adults may obtain more attention and care from family members than they would otherwise.

The incidence of somatoform disorders is increased in older adults. Healthcare providers must carefully evaluate all physical symptoms, however, before treating the older adult for a somatoform disorder.

Critical Thinking Exercises

1. *Discuss the physical, emotional, social, and financial implications that can result from having a somatoform disorder.*
2. *What behaviors might be therapeutic to avoid the development of somatoform disorders?*

References and Suggested Readings

Cunningham, S. J., et al. (2000). Body dysmorphic disorder involving the facial region: A report of 6 cases. *Journal of Oral and Maxillofacial Surgery, 58,* 1180–1183.

Fortinash, K. M. & Holoday-Worret, P. A. (2000). *Psychiatric mental health nursing* (2nd ed.). St. Louis: Mosby.

Mind matters. Fear of being sick can become an illness. (1999). *Health News, 17*(2), 10.

Noyes, R., Jr. (1999). The relationship of hypochondriasis to anxiety disorders. *General Hospital Psychiatry, 21*(1), 8–17.

Peppard, A. & Denegar, C. R. (1999). Depression and somatization as a source of persistent pain. *Athletic Therapy Today, 4*(6), 43–47.

Righter, E. L. & Sansone, R. A. (1999). Managing somatic preoccupation. *American Family Physician, 59,* 3113–3120.

Schatz, D., et al. (2000). The relationship of maternal personality characteristics to birth outcomes and infant development. *Birth: Issues in Perinatal Care and Education, 27*(1), 25–32.

Slaughter, J. R. & Sun, A. M. (1999). In pursuit of perfection: A primary care physician's guide to body dysmorphic disorder. *American Family Physician, 60,* 1738–1742.

Townsend, M. C. (2000). *Psychiatric mental health nursing: Concepts of care* (3rd ed.). Philadelphia: F.A. Davis.

Videbeck, S. L. (2001). *Psychiatric mental health nursing.* Philadelphia: Lippincott Williams & Wilkins.

Watkins, C. E. (2001). Body dysmorphic disorder. [Online.] Available: http://www.baltimorepsych.com/body_dysmorphic_disorder.htm (accessed March 18, 2001).

Caring for Clients With Anxiety Disorders

Words to Know

agoraphobia
anxiety
anxiety disorders
anxiolytics
behavioral therapy
cognitive therapy
compulsion
desensitization
fear
flashbacks
generalized anxiety
   disorder

limbic system
obsession
obsessive–compulsive
   disorder
panic disorder
phobic disorders
post-traumatic stress
   disorder
psychic numbing
psychotherapy
social phobia

Learning Objectives

On completion of this chapter, the reader will:

- Differentiate anxiety from fear.
- Name four levels of anxiety, explaining the differences among each level.
- Give six areas of nursing management that apply to the care of anxious clients.
- Give three examples of anxiety disorders.
- List categories of drugs used to treat anxiety disorders.
- Name and discuss two types of psychotherapy used to treat anxiety disorders.
- List six nursing interventions that are helpful for reducing anxiety.
- Discuss areas of teaching for clients with anxiety disorders.

Although anxiety and fear are normal human responses, anxiety disorders are not. Questions remain whether anxiety disorders are strictly biologic, learned, the result of unconscious emotional conflicts, or a combination of all three. Probably both physical and psychological factors play a role. A person is first genetically predisposed to an anxiety disorder and then manifests a disorder when exposed to situational triggers.

This chapter explores anxiety and fear and discusses how to intervene for an anxious client. It also explores anxiety disorders and nursing care of those who have them.

ANXIETY AND FEAR

Anxiety differs from fear, but these terms often are used interchangeably. **Anxiety** is a vague uneasy feeling, the cause of which is not readily identifiable. It is evoked when a person anticipates nonspecific danger. **Fear** is a feeling of terror in response to someone or something specific that a person perceives as dangerous or threatening. Because it is common for clients to be anxious in

an unfamiliar environment, or to be fearful of pain, suffering, or death, both reactions are common in hospitals and other healthcare agencies.

Because many medical and surgical clients temporarily feel vulnerable, they are prime candidates for experiencing anxiety. Recognizing the signs of escalating anxiety, understanding its consequences, and intervening appropriately are important interventions.

Levels of Anxiety

Anxiety can range from mild, which is constructive, to moderate, severe, and panic (Table 14-1). Mild anxiety prepares an individual to take action in appropriate situations. For example, mild anxiety before a test causes most people to study.

Moderate, severe, and panic levels of anxiety are counterproductive; they provoke responses that interfere with well-being. As a person's level of anxiety escalates:

- Physiologic changes occur, such as elevation of blood pressure and racing heart.

TABLE 14-1	LEVELS OF ANXIETY	
LEVEL	**BEHAVIORAL MANIFESTATIONS**	**PHYSICAL MANIFESTATIONS**
Mild	Attention is heightened. Sensory perception is expanded. Focus is on stimuli. Reality is intact. Information processing is accurate. Person feels in control.	Muscle tone increases. Heart rate, blood pressure, and breathing slightly increase. Perspiration is noticeable.
Moderate	Person is more easily distracted. Concentration is slightly impaired. Person can redirect attention. Learning takes more effort. Perception narrows. Problem-solving becomes difficult. Person is irritable and feels inadequate.	Muscles are tense. Slight leg or hand tremors may occur. Rate, pitch, and volume of speech change. Respiratory depth and vital signs increase. Sleep is disturbed.
Severe	Attention span decreases. Person cannot concentrate or remain focused. Perception is reduced. Ability to learn is impaired. Information processing is inaccurate or incomplete. Person is aware of extreme discomfort. Effort is needed to control emotions. Person feels incompetent.	Symptoms include hyperventilation, dizziness, tachycardia, heart palpitations, and hypertension. Fine motor movement is impaired. Communication is limited.
Panic	Person exaggerates details. Perception is distorted. Learning is disabled. Thoughts are fragmented. Person cannot control emotions and feels helpless.	Speech is incoherent. Movements are haphazard, usually in an effort to escape. Symptoms include dyspnea, fainting, tremors, and diaphoresis.

- Perception of information and events narrows.
- Thinking becomes increasingly disorganized and distorted.
- Physical and emotional fatigue develops from the investment of energy in worrying.

Stop, Think, and Respond ● BOX 14-1

Give examples of situations that provoke mild anxiety and the appropriate outcomes that usually result. Discuss situations that may trigger more extreme levels of anxiety and their potential consequences.

Nursing Management

The nurse can assist the anxious client by implementing interventions that maintain or restore a sense of calm and control.

Building Trust

Building trust is especially critical to developing a therapeutic relationship with an anxious client. Being available and attentive to the client's needs contributes to this trust. The nurse should not leave an anxious client alone, especially during a new or potentially frightening experience.

Restoring Comfort

The nurse's interventions are guided by what will bring relief to a particular person. The nurse should ask the client to suggest methods that may be personally comforting. For example, some clients find it helpful for the nurse to give support in nonverbal ways, like remaining with them without talking, holding a hand, or stroking the skin. Others prefer to talk about how they feel, but are more relaxed if the nurse remains physically distant (Fig. 14-1).

Modifying Communication

The nurse should avoid interrupting anxious clients when they talk. Although verbalizing does not relieve anxiety, it can be beneficial. Talking helps in processing information and exploring methods for dealing with problems. Some clients prefer not to discuss their anxiety and fears with the nurse. In such cases, the nurse respects the client's right to privacy. Offering a referral to a health professional like a psychiatrist or medical social worker with counseling expertise, however, is appropriate.

FIGURE 14-1 A nurse listens to an anxious client.

Adjusting Teaching

Because an anxious client's attention and concentration are limited, directions or explanations must be simple, brief, and repeated frequently. To determine a client's level of comprehension, asking the person to paraphrase what he or she has been taught is helpful. The client also benefits from reductions in sensory stimulation such as dimming the lights and eliminating as much noise as possible. The nurse must avoid expecting the client to show a great deal of self-reliance or independence until the client feels more relaxed and secure.

Helping Problem-Solve

Anxiety impairs problem-solving ability, and clients may look to the nurse for advice in decision-making. Nurses avoid influencing their clients' choices. Instead, they help clients follow a step-by-step problem-solving process to formulate decisions:

1. Identifying problems
2. Determining their causes
3. Exploring possible solutions
4. Examining the pros and cons of each option
5. Selecting the choice that is most compatible with personal values

don't give advice or influence choice

Once the client arrives at a decision, the nurse advocates on the client's behalf for its implementation—even if it is not one the nurse would personally choose. The nurse also respects the client's right to change his or her mind at any time.

Ensuring Safety

Persons experiencing panic-level anxiety can act impulsively and endanger their safety (e.g., jumping out of a window, running into the street). The nurse remains calm to help such individuals reduce anxiety to a more manageable level. Having only one nurse interact with the client usually is best because responding to multiple sources of stimulation adds to a client's agitation. If the client is extremely unstable, it is wise to avoid touching or getting physically close to him or her. Intruding in the client's personal space is likely to increase anxiety.

ANXIETY DISORDERS

Anxiety disorders are a group of psychobiologic illnesses that result from activation of the autonomic nervous system, chiefly the sympathetic division. They tend to be chronic and sometimes appear without any logical explanation.

Types

Some examples of anxiety disorders include generalized anxiety disorder, panic disorder, phobic disorders, post-traumatic stress disorder, and obsessive–compulsive disorder. Anxiety disorders sometimes lead to other psychobiologic conditions such as depression, substance abuse, and eating disorders, which are discussed in subsequent chapters.

Generalized Anxiety Disorder

Generalized anxiety disorder is characterized by chronic worrying on a daily basis for 6 or more months. There usually is more than one focus of worry. For example, a person may be worried about finances, job performance, and personal health. Often, the worrying is out of proportion with reality. In addition to worrying, at least six other signs and symptoms of anxiety accompany the client's distress. When the client seeks medical attention, test results fail to reveal physical disorders that produce signs and symptoms similar to anxiety (Box 14-1).

Panic Disorder

Panic disorder is the most extreme manifestation of anxiety. Those who are affected experience an abrupt onset of

---

BOX 14-1 • **Examples of Conditions That Resemble Generalized Anxiety Disorder**

- Mitral valve prolapse
- Hypoglycemia
- Hyperthyroidism
- Premenstrual syndrome
- Menopause
- Dementia
- Abuse of psychostimulants (cocaine, caffeine, weight loss drugs)
- Sedative (alcohol, opioids, barbiturates) withdrawal

physical symptoms and terror that include intense apprehension; tachycardia, palpitations, chest pain, smothering or choking sensations; hyperventilation; lightheadedness; feeling of impending doom; and fear of fainting, dying, losing control, or going insane.

Episodes of panic may last minutes to less than 1 hour and then spontaneously subside. The episodes are often referred to as *attacks* because they interrupt a period during which the client is asymptomatic. The first instinct during a panic attack is to escape to a safer place. The unexplained flight from work, school, or the like that ensues often strains relationships with others who observe the client's behavior as strange.

The person who experiences a panic attack often is at a loss to identify its cause but associates the location or concurrent activity as the precipitating event. Most affected individuals cope with their disorder by avoiding situations or places where attacks have occurred. As the attacks recur in a variety of circumstances, however, people with panic disorder often develop agoraphobia. **Agoraphobia** is a fear of experiencing a panic attack in a public place where the person may be publicly humiliated by his or her behavior or help may be unavailable. Consequently, many of those with panic disorder permanently confine themselves to their homes.

Phobic Disorders

Phobic disorders are those conditions in which a person manifests an exaggerated fear. Many individuals are irrationally afraid of insects, animals, or various life experiences, some of which are potentially dangerous. When a person with a phobic disorder is exposed to the phobic stimulus, however, he or she experiences symptoms of anxiety that may reach severe or panic levels. He or she usually goes to extremes to avoid the object of the phobia or painfully endures the phobic stimulus despite the fact that it causes severe distress. Most people with phobic disorders are aware of how illogical the phobia is and how unrealistic their disabling response has become.

One common phobic disorder is social phobia. Persons with **social phobia,** also known as *social anxiety,* fear those situations in which they must perform in front of or may capture the attention of others. Examples of situations that may induce social phobia include speaking publicly, entertaining theatrically or musically, eating in a restaurant or at a banquet, attending a party, or being asked to explain a concept in an academic setting. The greatest worry for those with social phobia, which is for the most part imagined, is that they will be embarrassed or criticized for failing to meet acceptable standards.

Post-traumatic Stress Disorder

Post-traumatic stress disorder (PTSD) is a condition that involves a delayed anxiety response 3 or more months after an emotionally traumatic experience (Box 14-2).

BOX 14-2 ● Traumatic Events Associated With Post-traumatic Stress Disorder

- Witnessing a murder or violent crime
- Watching the torture of a person or animal
- Escaping a fiery crash (car, plane, train) or industrial explosion
- Seeing military friends or public servants killed in the line of duty
- Being raped or abused
- Surviving a natural disaster like a flood, earthquake, or tornado
- Being trapped in an automobile, elevator, subway, or underground cave
- Being taken hostage by criminals or terrorists

Although traumatic experiences are somewhat relative, they must be extraordinarily severe to cause PTSD. The circumstances of the traumatic event involve actual or threatened death or injury to self or others and produce fear, helplessness, or horror. Some feel guilty for having survived such an event when others just as deserving of life died.

Initially, the affected person avoids dealing with the tragedy and detaches himself or herself from others using a technique that is referred to as **psychic numbing.** Eventually, however, the person no longer can stifle his or her memories. Months or years later, the memories may resurface in recurrent nightmares or **flashbacks,** in which the person feels as if he or she is reliving the precipitating event. This feeling may also occur when the person is exposed to a situation that resembles the original trauma, like associating the explosive sound of fireworks with military gunfire.

To relieve symptoms of guilt, grief, anger, or sadness, some clients with PTSD abuse substances like alcohol or other mind-altering and mood-altering drugs. When such coping strategies prove ineffective, they may act out aggressively. They may respond violently if startled from sleep. Those who suspect that they may have PTSD should consult a mental health professional for a definitive diagnosis.

Stop, Think, and Respond ● BOX 14-2

Discuss how nurses who care for seriously burned clients may develop PTSD.

Obsessive–Compulsive Disorder

Obsessive–compulsive disorder (OCD) is manifested by the performance of an anxiety-relieving ritual (**compulsion**) to terminate a disturbing, persistent thought (**obsession**). Obsessions may involve concerns about potential danger or being contaminated with germs. They are intrusive, and persons with OCD cannot dismiss them from their consciousness. To relieve their anxiety, clients with OCD repetitively perform a tension-relieving compulsion that usually falls into one or more of the following categories:

- Cleaning, such as repetitiously scrubbing the surface of a dining table
- Washing, such as repeated bathing or handwashing
- Checking, such as verifying that doors have been locked or an iron has been unplugged even though the person has already checked earlier
- Counting, such as a bank teller repeatedly making sure that the money in a cash drawer is accurate
- Touching, such as feeling to make sure that a lucky charm is on one's person or having to touch the door frame before entering a room

Clients with OCD may feel compelled to perform the same act repeatedly for a specific number of times or in a prescribed sequence. The more the person resists performing the compulsive act, the more the anxiety escalates. The same is true if another person interrupts, alters, or forbids the ritual. Because the rituals are often excessive and time-consuming, they may lead to problems in social relationships, failure in school, or loss of employment. Most clients with OCD recognize that their thoughts and behaviors border on the ridiculous, but they are helpless to stop independently.

Pathophysiology and Etiology

Genetic studies suggest that many anxiety disorders have familial patterns. This finding can imply an inherited faulty physiology, maladaptive learning, or acquisition of personality traits modeled after those displayed by significant others.

Symptoms are manifested because the neurotransmitter norepinephrine floods the limbic system; a minority of individuals respond to stress through the parasympathetic route, in which case the neurotransmitter acetylcholine causes symptoms. The **limbic system,** which surrounds the brain stem, is a ring of structures made up of lobes of the cerebrum, thalamus, hypothalamus, and others (Fig. 14-2). This complex neural tissue is a physiologic network for emotions, survival and behavioral responses, motivation, and learning. The biochemical changes brought on by the autonomic nervous system trigger physical arousal in the cortex and the neuroendocrine pathways involving the hypothalamus, pituitary, and adrenal glands.

Other biochemical mechanisms also may contribute to the development of anxiety disorders. A dysregulation of gamma-aminobutyric acid (GABA), a neurotransmitter that should buffer or extinguish the activity of norepinephrine, is one possibility. The second possibility is depletion of serotonin, which would explain why some clients with anxiety disorders develop depression or improve when receiving treatment with antidepressant drugs (see Chap. 15).

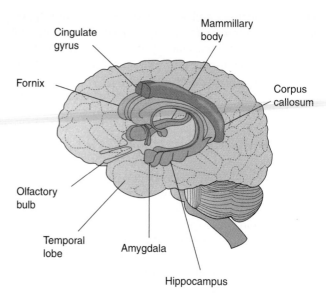

FIGURE 14-2 The limbic system is the center for emotions.

Assessment Findings

Signs and Symptoms

Although anxiety causes behavioral, cognitive, and emotional effects, most clients seek treatment for physical signs and symptoms (cardiovascular, respiratory, neuromuscular, gastrointestinal, integumentary problems; Table 14-2). For example, clients may be concerned about palpitations, breathlessness, chronic fatigue, tension headaches, and sleep disturbances. In many clients, blood pressure is elevated and heart rate is increased. Some clients acknowledge having unrealistic worries or fears or exaggerated startle reactions, experiencing flashbacks of previously traumatic events, avoiding situations that provoke symptoms, or performing ritualistic behaviors.

Diagnostic Findings

Findings from laboratory blood tests and diagnostic tests like electrocardiography are essentially normal. Positron emission tomography and computed tomography scans have shown abnormal brain use of glucose in clients with anxiety disorders. Magnetic resonance imaging has demonstrated atrophy in some brain areas in selected anxiety disorders. Diagnosis of most clients with anxiety disorders, however, is based on symptomatology and history.

Medical Management

The medical management of anxiety disorders includes drug therapy combined with cognitive and behavioral psychotherapy. Drug therapy relieves the symptoms

TABLE 14-2	COMMON SIGNS AND SYMPTOMS OF ANXIETY
RESPONSES	**SIGNS AND SYMPTOMS**
Physical	
Cardiovascular	Hypertension, tachycardia, palpitations, fainting*
Respiratory	Dyspnea, rapid breathing, hyperventilation, choking sensation, tightness in the chest
Neuromuscular	Tremors, restlessness, insomnia, muscle tension, excessive sleep,* generalized weakness, dizziness
Gastrointestinal	Anorexia, nausea, diarrhea,* constipation, feeling of fullness
Urinary	Frequency and urgency of urination*
Integumentary	Diaphoresis, sweaty palms, pallor, blushing,* dry mouth
Behavioral	Crying, rapid speech or mutism, hypervigilance, being easily startled or accident-prone, social isolation, physical escape, avoidance, loss of interest in sexual activity, pacing, fidgeting, nail-biting, picking at skin, seeking comfort in food or alcohol, absenteeism, failure to complete or poor performance of tasks
Cognitive	Forgetfulness, poor judgment, lack of motivation, confusion, nightmares, intrusive thoughts, preoccupation, decreased attention and concentration, inability to recall information
Emotional	Unrealistic fears, mood swings, easily angered, impatient, intolerant, nervous

*Indicates a parasympathetic rather than a sympathetic nervous system response.

associated with anxiety, but it does not eliminate causative factors. Once drug therapy is implemented, however, clients are more capable of dealing with issues affecting their daily lives.

Drug Therapy

Drugs that (1) reduce or block levels of norepinephrine or (2) normalize levels of serotonin are most commonly prescribed for anxiety disorders. They include anxiolytics, beta-adrenergic blockers, central-acting sympatholytics, and occasionally antidepressants (Drug Therapy Table 14-1).

ANXIOLYTICS

Anxiolytics are drugs that relieve the symptoms of anxiety. Sometimes they are referred to as *minor tranquilizers* to differentiate them from major tranquilizers or antipsychotic drugs used to treat thought disorders like schizophrenia. Anxiolytics include benzodiazepines like alprazolam (Xanax), lorazepam (Ativan), and diazepam (Valium) and nonbenzodiazepine drugs like buspirone (BuSpar).

Stop, Think, and Respond ● BOX 14-3

What health teaching is appropriate when a client begins taking an anxiolytic drug?

BETA-ADRENERGIC BLOCKERS

Receptors for norepinephrine are referred to as *alpha-adrenergic* and *beta-adrenergic receptors*. Beta-adrenergic receptors are located primarily in the heart and lungs. When norepinephrine stimulates beta-adrenergic recep-

tors, heart rate, forcefulness of heart contraction, and dilation of bronchi all increase. The ultimate outcome is that the body is prepared for "fight or flight," a function of the sympathetic nervous system. In anxiety disorders, norepinephrine prepares the body for a similar response. Blocking the beta-adrenergic receptors with drugs like propranolol (Inderal), atenolol (Tenormin), or metoprolol (Lopressor) reduces the sympathetic nervous system stimulation that causes some symptoms associated with anxiety.

Beta-adrenergic blocking agents frequently are prescribed for people with social phobia. This category of drugs does not cause sedation, tolerance, or addiction. These drugs do, however, lower blood pressure and subsequently can cause episodes of dizziness or fainting when the client rises quickly from a lying or sitting position. Other major side effects include bradycardia and reduced blood glucose level. Those taking a nonselective beta-adrenergic blocker—one that interferes with bronchodilation—may experience fatigue, dyspnea, and wheezing.

Stop, Think, and Respond ● BOX 14-4

Beta-adrenergic blockers should be cautiously prescribed or avoided for clients with which kinds of concurrent medical conditions?

CENTRAL-ACTING SYMPATHOLYTICS

Central-acting sympatholytics block alpha-2 receptors for norepinephrine in the brain stem. Consequently, they reduce heart rate and blood pressure. Examples of drugs in this category include clonidine (Catapres), methyldopa (Aldomet), and guanabenz (Wytensin). Although these drugs are prescribed more often to control primary hyper-

DRUG THERAPY TABLE 14-1	**DRUGS USED TO TREAT ANXIETY**

DRUG CATEGORY AND EXAMPLES	MECHANISM OF ACTION	SIDE EFFECTS	NURSING CONSIDERATIONS
Benzodiazepines alprazolam (Xanax)	Exact mechanism of action not understood, but is thought to increase the inhibitory effects of GABA, making the cells less responsive to norepinephrine	Transient mild drowsiness, sedation, fatigue, lightheadedness, constipation, diarrhea, nausea, dry mouth, drug dependence	Instruct client to avoid alcohol and other CNS depressants. Warn client that cimetidine, disulfiram, omeprazole, valproic acid, and oral contraceptives increase the effects of these drugs. Tell client to avoid operating machinery, report all side effects, and avoid stopping the drug abruptly.
Nonbenzodiazepine anxiolytics buspirone (BuSpar)	Exact mechanism unknown but does bind with serotonin and dopamine receptors	Dizziness, nervousness, insomnia, headache, lightheadedness, dry mouth, abdominal distress, vomiting, palpitations, chest pain, hyperventilation	Instruct client to avoid alcohol and other CNS depressants and operating machinery, and to report side effects. Inform client that frequent small meals and sucking on ice chips will alleviate gastrointestinal disturbances and dry mouth.
Beta-adrenergic blockers propranolol hydrochloride (Inderal)	Decrease the effects of the sympathetic nervous system by reducing CNS sympathetic outflow and blocking beta-adrenergic receptors	Fatigue, nausea, vomiting, diarrhea, flatulence, constipation, bradycardia, hypotension, congestive heart failure, dysrhythmias, erectile dysfunction, decreased libido, decreased activity tolerance	Monitor heart rate, blood pressure, and postural changes. Instruct client to avoid alcohol, to report all side effects, and not to discontinue the drug abruptly. Review all medications because propranolol can interact with many other drugs. Administer with food. Warn clients with diabetes that propranolol may obscure signs and symptoms of hypoglycemia and thus to manage serum glucose carefully.
Central-acting sympatholytics clonidine hydrochloride (Catapres)	Decrease the sympathetic outflow from the CNS and inhibit sympathetic nervous system effects	Drowsiness, sedation, dizziness, constipation, dry mouth, anorexia, erectile dysfunction, weight gain, weakness, nightmares	Monitor blood pressure and postural changes. Instruct client to avoid alcohol. Inform client to take drug as prescribed and not to miss doses or abruptly discontinue use. Tell client to report any side effects and that side effects will disappear once the drug is discontinued.

CNS = central nervous system; GABA = gamma-aminobutyric acid.

tension, they potentially have beneficial effects among anxious individuals with elevated blood pressure. Clonidine also is used to control hypertension among individuals who experience withdrawal symptoms when abruptly abstaining from alcohol or anxiolytic therapy. Side effects associated with central-acting sympatholytics include sedation, dizziness, dry mouth, constipation, urinary retention, elevated blood glucose level, fatigue, erectile dysfunction, and diminished libido. Some individuals may have a rash or experience depression. Blood pressure should be monitored on a regular basis. The client must learn to rise slowly from a sitting or lying position to avoid postural (orthostatic) hypotension. Clients with diabetes may need to adjust their medication regimen to maintain normal ranges in blood glucose level.

ANTIDEPRESSANTS

Obsessive–compulsive disorder seems to respond to the administration of selective serotonin reuptake inhibitors (SSRIs)—antidepressants such as fluvoxamine (Luvox), sertraline (Zoloft), paroxetine (Paxil), and fluoxetine (Prozac); or tricyclic antidepressants (TCAs) such as clomipramine (Anafranil). Sertraline (Zoloft) also has been approved for the treatment of social phobia. The symptoms of PTSD are somewhat relieved by some SSRIs like citalopram (Celexa) and TCAs such as amitriptyline (Elavil) and imipramine (Tofranil). These antidepressants sustain levels of serotonin, which perhaps is the mechanism by which these medications treat selected anxiety disorders. Antidepressants are discussed in more detail in Chapter 15.

Psychotherapy

Psychotherapy involves talking with a psychiatrist, psychologist, or mental health counselor. Some clients respond better when therapy sessions are conducted one on one; others, such as those with PTSD, respond better to group interactions.

COGNITIVE THERAPY

One type of psychotherapy useful in treating clients with anxiety disorders is cognitive therapy. **Cognitive therapy** is a type of psychotherapy in which the therapist helps clients alter their irrational thinking, correct their faulty belief systems, and replace negative self-statements with positive ones. This therapy is based on the theory that it is not events that provoke anxiety, but the person's interpretation of events. By reshaping a person's viewpoint, the disorder can be minimized or eliminated.

BEHAVIORAL THERAPY

Behavioral therapy attempts to extinguish undesirable responses by learning other adaptive techniques. One example that is sometimes used with clients who have phobic disorders or OCD is desensitization. **Desensitization** involves providing emotional support while gradually exposing a person to whatever it is that provokes anxiety. If anxiety escalates, the therapist coaches the client to perform relaxation or breathing exercises to overcome symptoms. Eventually, the client can tolerate the anxiety-provoking experience independently by learning methods for eliminating physical and emotional discomfort.

N U R S I N G   P R O C E S S

● The Client With an Anxiety Disorder

Assessment

The nurse observes for evidence of various levels of anxiety: pacing, talking excessively, complaining, crying, being withdrawn, or trying to run away. He or she encourages the client to express anxiety by asking open-ended questions such as "How are you feeling now?" Having the client rate his or her anxiety level using a scale from 0 to 10 is helpful. The client should indicate the level at which anxiety is tolerable. The nurse asks the client if he or she has an effective method for controlling anxiety. The nurse observes the client's mood for signs of concurrent depression and assesses the client's use of and knowledge about medications to treat the disorder.

Diagnosis, Planning, and Interventions

Anxiety related to faulty perception of danger
Expected Outcome: The client's anxiety will return to a tolerable level.

- Reduce as many external stimuli, such as noise, bright lights, and activity, as possible. *Numerous stimuli escalate anxiety because they interfere with attention and concentration. Dealing simultaneously with multiple stimuli can tax the client's energy.*
- Maintain a calm manner when interacting with the client. *Anxiety is communicated; an anxious nurse can increase anxiety in a client. Modeling a controlled state promotes a similar response in the client.*
- Take a position at least an arm's length away from the client. *Invading an anxious client's personal space may increase his or her discomfort.*
- Avoid touching the client without first asking permission. *An anxious client may misinterpret unexpected touching as a threatening gesture.*
- Establish trust by being available to the client and keeping promises. *Insecurity can be relieved if the client knows he or she can depend on assistance from the nurse.*
- Advise the client to seek out the nurse or another supportive person when feeling the effects of anxiety. *The earlier that anxiety is de-escalated, the sooner the client will experience relief of symptoms.*
- Stay with the client during periods of severe anxiety. *The nurse's presence can help the client stay in control or restore control to a more comfortable level.*
- Follow a consistent schedule for routine activities. *Unpredictability heightens anxiety; consistency helps a client manage time and cope with personal demands.*
- Encourage the client to identify what he or she perceives to be a threat to emotional equilibrium. *Processing situations verbally may give the client perspective on perceived threats so that they are more realistic and less exaggerated.*
- Use a soft voice, short sentences, and clear messages when exchanging information. *Anxious clients have a short attention span and reduced ability to concentrate; they may be unable to follow lengthy or complicated information.*
- Provide specific, succinct directions for tasks the client should complete or assist the client who becomes agitated. *Anxious clients have difficulty following instructions and performing tasks in correct sequence. Assistance relieves unnecessary distress.*
- Instruct and help the client with moderate or severe anxiety to perform one or more of the following until anxiety is within a tolerable level:
  - Count slowly backward from 100. *Distraction redirects the client's attention from distressing physiologic symptoms to the task at hand.*
  - Breathe slowly and deeply in through the nose and out through the mouth. *Slowing respirations aborts hyperventilation and subsequent potential for fainting, peripheral tingling, and numbness from respiratory alkalosis.*
  - Offer a warm bath or back rub. *Warm running water promotes relaxation; massage relaxes muscles and*

possibly releases endorphins, natural chemicals that promote a sense of well-being.

- Progressively relax groups of muscles from the toes to the head. *Consciously relaxing muscles relieves tension and fatigue.*
- Repeat positive statements such as, "I am in control," "I am safe," "I am relaxed." *Positive self-talk can be transformed into reality.*
- Visualize a pleasant, relaxing place. *Imagery can transform a person's aroused state to one that is more relaxed.*
- Listen to a relaxation tape or soothing music. *Distraction helps to refocus attention to less anxiety-provoking stimuli.*
- Engage in a large-muscle activity such as riding an exercise bicycle or going for a brisk walk. *Activity uses norepinephrine and can reduce it to a more manageable amount.*
- Administer antianxiety medication that has been prescribed on an as-needed (prn) basis if nonpharmacologic approaches are ineffective. *Medication may be necessary to ensure the client's or others' safety if there is a potential for loss of control or violent acting out.*

Risk for Ineffective Therapeutic Regimen Management related to knowledge deficit of drug and dietary modifications

Expected Outcome: The client will safely manage his or her own self-care.

- Explain the routine for self-administering prescribed medications and side effects associated with prescribed drugs. *Identifying the frequency and approximate time during the day when medications should be taken ensures safe self-care. Knowing what to expect as side effects reduces the potential for noncompliance or harm.*
- Emphasize that the client must avoid alcohol and other sedating drugs when taking anxiolytic drugs. *Combining two drugs that cause sedation may have dangerous consequences.*
- Encourage compliance with drug therapy, although it may take several weeks for the client to feel a beneficial effect. *Making the client aware that symptoms will not disappear immediately may create motivation for remaining compliant.*
- Advise the client to first discuss discontinuing drug therapy for whatever reason with the prescribing physician. *Abrupt discontinuation of benzodiazepines can cause withdrawal symptoms that mimic anxiety.*
- Tell the client to avoid caffeine, nicotine, or stimulating drugs such as nonprescription diet pills and cold and allergy medications. *These drugs contain chemicals that stimulate the sympathetic nervous system, which interferes with the desired effect of anxiolytic drug therapy.*
- Inform the client of the process for arranging follow-up appointments with his or her physician. *The client needs periodic contact with the treating physician for*

further assessment, evaluation of treatment outcomes, or adjustment to the therapeutic regimen.

- Provide information on self-help groups for anxiety. *Interacting with others who share similar problems can help clients cope.*

Evaluation of Expected Outcomes

After successful nursing interventions, the client deals with anxiety-provoking stimuli realistically and implements measures to decrease anxiety. He or she has extended periods during which anxiety is at a tolerable level and participates in normal activities without becoming incapacitated by anxiety.

The client accurately repeats information on the dose, frequency, potential side effects, and duration of drug therapy. He or she verbalizes possible consequences if an anxiolytic drug is discontinued abruptly and lists drugs, foods, and beverages that are contraindicated when taking anxiolytic medication. Finally, the client has written instructions for follow-up care and is aware of community-based groups that may help in the management of his or her disorder.

GENERAL NUTRITIONAL CONSIDERATIONS

Clients with anxiety should avoid caffeine.
Although some clients lose their appetite, others may react to stress by overeating. Assess current weight status and recent weight fluctuations.

GENERAL PHARMACOLOGIC CONSIDERATIONS

Obtain a complete current medication history for each client, including nonprescription drugs. Many people who experience anxiety take over-the-counter drugs, herbal remedies, stimulants, and tranquilizers that they may not mention unless asked.
Antianxiety drugs such as alprazolam or diazepam are used in the short-term treatment of anxiety. Long-term treatment is not recommended because prolonged use can result in drug dependence.
Antianxiety drugs may cause drowsiness or blurred vision. Advise the client to use caution while driving or performing tasks requiring mental alertness.
Buspirone, a nonbenzodiazepine, also is recommended for short-term treatment of anxiety. It does not produce muscle relaxation or cause sedation. It takes up to 3 to 4 weeks to produce a desired effect.
The most commonly prescribed antianxiety drugs are the benzodiazepines, but some clients respond better to buspirone than the benzodiazepines.

GENERAL GERONTOLOGIC CONSIDERATIONS

Feelings of vulnerability and limitations associated with age may contribute to anxiety in older adults.

Because the kidneys excrete most antianxiety agents, older adults with impaired kidney function are at increased risk for toxicity when taking these medications.

Anxiety may be manifested in the older adult as confusion, behavior changes, or withdrawal.

Many older adults on fixed incomes experience financial problems related to housing and medical expenses that can produce anxiety.

Antianxiety drugs may cause short periods of memory impairment that can aggravate an already existing cognitive disorder.

Before administering a benzodiazepine to an older adult, assess for sleep problems, especially snoring. These drugs have the potential to exacerbate sleep apnea.

Short-acting benzodiazepines, such as alprazolam, are preferred in older adults because they are less likely than longer-acting benzodiazepines to cause toxicity, leading to excessive sedation and depression.

Buspirone is commonly used to treat anxiety in older adults. The drug does not produce dependence or interact with benzodiazepines or alcohol. A decrease in anxiety may occur in approximately 1 week; however, the drug may take up to 4 weeks before a full therapeutic response occurs.

The drugs used to treat anxiety may cause dizziness or lightheadedness, increasing the risk of falling in older adults.

Critical Thinking Exercises

1. *Discuss nursing interventions that would be appropriate when a client tells you that he or she feels anxious about her upcoming surgery.*
2. *What interventions should a nurse implement if a client suddenly experiences a panic attack?*

References and Suggested Readings

Barstow, D. G. (2000). Post-traumatic stress disorder: A student nurse's personal experience of terror. *Journal of Psychosocial Nursing and Mental Health Services, 38*(4), 29–33.

Deblinger, L. (2000). Antidepressants and cognitive-behavioral therapy effective in panic disorder. *Patient Care, 34*(16), 13, 67.

Fortinash, K. M. & Holoday-Worret, P. A. (2000). *Psychiatric mental health nursing* (2nd ed.). St. Louis: Mosby.

Giger, J. N., Davidhizar, R., Poole, V. L., et al. (2000). Breakthrough in psychiatric care: Pharmacological treatment of obsessive-compulsive disorders with implications for nursing care. *Journal of Practical Nursing, 50*(1), 23, 25–29, 31.

Hollander, E. & Jebuje, M. A. (1999). When OCD takes hold. *Patient Care, 33*(13), 134–140, 145–146, 149–153.

Laidlow, T. M., Falloon, I. R. H., Barnfather, D., et al. (1999). The stress of caring for people with obsessive compulsive disorders. *Community Mental Health Journal, 35*, 443–450.

LoBuono, C. (1999). Social phobia: more prevalent than you think. *Patient Care, 33*(13), 120–124, 127–130.

Maes, M., Lin, A., Verkerk, R., et al. (1999). Serotonergic and noradrenergic markers of post-traumatic stress disorder with and without major depression. *Neuropsychopharmacology, 20*(2), 188.

Raj, A. & Sheehan, D. V. (1999). The use of selective serotonin reuptake inhibitors in panic disorder. *Home Health Care Consultant, 6*(4), 15–19.

Ringel, M. The anxiety spectrum: Which disorder is it? *Patient Care, 33*(13), 73–76, 80, 82.

Spotlight on Zoloft. (1999). *Journal of Psychosocial Nursing and Mental Health Services, 37*(8), 9.

Tan, W. & Tsai, T. W. (2000). Antidepressants and cognitive-behavioral therapy effective in panic disorder. *Patient Care, 34*(16), 13, 67.

Valente, S. M. (1999). Anxiety and panic disorders in older adults. *Home Health Care Management and Practice, 11*(4), 49–59.

VanderZyl, S. K. (1999). Anxious? You're not alone. *Nursingmatters, 10*(11), 4.

Vanin, J. R. & Vanin, S. K. (1999). Blocking the cycle of panic disorder: Ways to gain control of the fear of fear. *Postgraduate Medicine, 105*(5), 141–146, 205–206.

Videbeck, S. L. (2001). *Psychiatric mental health nursing.* Philadelphia: Lippincott Williams & Wilkins.

Zal, H. M. (2000). Social anxiety disorder: How to help. *Consultant, 40*, 1686–1692.

Caring for Clients With Mood Disorders

Words to Know

affect
bipolar disorder
delusions
dexamethasone (cortisol)
  suppression test
dopamine
electroconvulsive
  therapy
euthymic
gamma-aminobutyric
  acid
hallucinations
hypertensive crisis
major (unipolar)
  depression
mania
melatonin

monoamine hypothesis
mood
mood disorders
norepinephrine
photoperiods
phototherapy
psychomotor agitation
psychomotor retardation
psychotherapy
psychotic depression
reactive (secondary)
  depression
reuptake
seasonal affective
  disorder
serotonin
serotonin syndrome

Learning Objectives

On completion of this chapter, the reader will:

- Discuss the signs and symptoms of mood disorders.
- Name three neurotransmitters that, when imbalanced, affect mood.
- Identify the types of drugs that are used to treat mood disorders and nursing considerations related to their administration.
- Give three criteria that indicate a high risk for suicide.
- Discuss nursing measures that are useful in preventing suicide.
- Discuss the nursing management of clients with common mood disorders.

Normal affect - smiles when appropriate

Flat affect - looks w/ gloomy empty expression

Affect - objective
mood - subjective

The term **mood** refers to a person's overall feeling state and may be thought of as a continuum, with extremes of emotion existing at both ends or poles (Fig. 15-1). Mood is displayed in a person's affect, the verbal and nonverbal behavior that communicates feelings (Table 15-1).

People with normal moods are referred to as **euthymic;** they are capable of experiencing a variety of feelings, all of which are situationally appropriate. Individuals with **mood disorders** experience an extreme persistent mood or severe mood swings that interfere with social relationships. The primary mood disturbances include major (unipolar) depression and bipolar disorder, formerly called *manic-depressive syndrome.*

Dysthymia, a feeling of unremitting sadness, is similar to but less severe than major depression. In **psychotic depression,** an extreme form of depressive disorder, some individuals experience **hallucinations,** sensory phenomena like hearing voices or seeing images that do not objectively exist, and **delusions,** fixed false beliefs that

often are persecutory in nature. Cyclothymia, alternating sad and elated moods, resembles bipolar disorder, but the extremes of mood are less pronounced. **Mania** refers to the frenzied state of euphoria exhibited by persons during the manic phase of bipolar disorder. **Seasonal affective disorder** (SAD) is a mood disorder characterized by depressive feelings that develop during darker winter months and then disappear in the spring.

MAJOR DEPRESSION

Everyone experiences depression at some point. In most cases, transient depression is a normal reaction to loss, such as the death of a loved one; disappointment, such as being fired from a job; or overwhelming events, like being heavily in debt. A sad feeling that can be directly attributed to a situation or cause is referred to as **reactive** or **secondary depression.** Usually, reactive depression is

FIGURE 15-1 Mood continuum.

self-limiting; when circumstances change or supportive others provide help, depression is relieved. Nevertheless, many people experience **major** or **unipolar depression,** a sad mood with no obvious relationship to situational events. More than 8 million Americans experience unexplained feelings of depression. Depression is also a comorbid (coexisting) condition among people with anxiety disorders and substance abuse (see Chaps. 14 and 17).

Pathophysiology and Etiology

Brain function, and consequently mood, depends on the dynamic interplay of neurotransmitters (see Chap. 12). Moods are most likely generated by the limbic system, which is the center for emotions (see Chap. 14). Several possible explanations exist for the causes and mechanisms that trigger major depressive symptoms. The most solid evidence at present suggests that mood disorders are related to genetics, dysregulation of neurotransmitters, and neuroendocrine imbalance. Psychological and social theories suggest that infantile rejection or neglect, learned feelings of helplessness, chronic exposure to discrimination, or distorted or false perceptions about oneself contribute to depression. Although these latter factors should not be dismissed, research in brain chemistry gives more support to biologic explanations.

Genetics

Mood disorders tend to be prevalent among close blood relatives, which suggests a genetic link. Even when raised separately, each identical twin has a higher incidence of depressive episodes when the other is affected (Kelsoe, 2000). Researchers are studying the DNA of fairly homogeneous groups (e.g., the Amish) for variations in chromosome patterns among relatives who have mood disorders and those who do not. Preliminary evidence shows that differences exist in at least two chromosomes, but research must continue before a definite conclusion can be reached (Videbeck, 2000).

Stop, Think, and Respond ● **BOX 15-1**
What other reason might explain why people who are related manifest similar disturbances in mood?

Neurotransmitter Dysregulation

The most widely accepted psychobiologic theory for depression is the **monoamine hypothesis,** which proposes that depression results from imbalances in one or more of the monoamine neurotransmitters: serotonin, norepinephrine, and dopamine. The hypothesis is based on the fact that levels of a metabolite of **serotonin,** 5-HIAA, measured in cerebrospinal fluid, are lower in depressed people than in samples taken from euthymic people. Second, **norepinephrine** levels may be low or high among people affected by depression. Low levels of norepinephrine help to explain why some depressed people develop **psychomotor retardation,** which is characterized by a lack of energy, increased sleep, and little interest in daily events or responsibilities. On the other hand, some depressed people may have excessive norepinephrine. They are more likely to experience **psychomotor agitation** with such stimulating manifestations as insomnia, pacing, and distractibility, rather than lethargy. Third, the symptoms of some depressed clients suggest an excess of **dopamine,** which is associated with distortion of thoughts. In moderate to severe depression, this may be evidenced as over-reactive guilt, self-blame, self-pity, and low self-worth.

TABLE 15-1	EXAMPLES OF MOOD AND AFFECT
MOOD	**AFFECT**
Happy	Smiling
	Briskly walking
	Paying attention to appearance
	Showing a positive attitude
	Being cooperative, creative, gregarious
Depressed	Looking gloomy
	Being inactive
	Neglecting appearance
	Feeling empty
	Showing no initiative
	Being insensitive to others' feelings, or isolated

Neuroendocrine Imbalance

Interactions of the pituitary, adrenal cortex, thyroid gland, and ovaries also may play a role in producing depression by altering levels of hormones. These endocrine glands are stimulated and suppressed through the hypothalamus, a structure in the limbic system. Abnormal levels of cortisol, a hormone produced by the adrenal cortex, and variations in thyroid hormones are accompanied by changes in mood and motor activity. The hypothalamus also influences the pituitary gland's stimulation of reproductive hormones. The latter hormonal relationships help to explain the altered mood states associated with premenstrual syndrome (also known as *late luteal phase dysphoric syndrome*), menopause, and postpartum depression.

Assessment Findings

Signs and Symptoms

The predominant feature of major depression is a persistent sad mood accompanied by multiple physiologic and cognitive (thought) changes, represented by the acronym SAD IMAGES (Box 15-1). Because the manifestations of depression may be similar to those of other conditions (Box 15-2), a tentative diagnosis is made while simultaneously investigating and eliminating alternative reasons for the clinical findings.

Diagnostic Findings

Studies that identify 5-HIAA in cerebrospinal fluid and the metabolite of norepinephrine in urine are financially prohibitive except for research purposes. Blood levels of serotonin can be measured more easily, but there is some question whether the level in blood correlates with the level necessary for normal mood in the brain. Furthermore, some managed care groups consider diagnostic laboratory tests of neurotransmitter levels unnecessary. Third-party payers often maintain that a diagnosis of depression can be confirmed or ruled out by the client's clinical presentation and by performing other standard tests for disorders that mimic depression. Findings that would

---

BOX 15-2 ● **Conditions That Mimic Depression**

- Hypothyroidism
- Brain tumor
- Alcohol or sedative abuse
- Stimulant withdrawal
- Chronic hypoxia
- Side effects of drug therapy such as corticosteroids, antihypertensives such as reserpine (Reserfia), methyldopa (Aldomet), propranolol (Inderal)

---

indicate alternative diagnoses to depression include low thyroid function test results, suggesting hypothyroidism (see Chap. 57); abnormal blood glucose levels, suggesting diabetes mellitus (see Chap. 58); low hemoglobin levels, indicative of anemia (see Chap. 39); and detection of drug abuse in a urine drug screen (see Chap. 17).

Occasionally, physicians order a **dexamethasone suppression test** (DST), also called a **cortisol suppression test.** This blood test theoretically indicates major depression if cortisol levels remain elevated despite the administration of an oral dose of dexamethasone, a corticosteroid, the day before. Under normal conditions, increased blood levels of corticosteroid should suppress the pituitary gland's secretion of corticotropin through a negative feedback loop. Statistics show, however, that the level of cortisol remains elevated among depressed clients, suggesting that cortisol is a chemical marker for depression. Many physicians, however, do not believe that the DST is significant; therefore, it is not widely ordered.

Neurologic imaging tests like computed tomography or magnetic resonance imaging may be performed to eliminate diagnoses such as brain tumor or cerebrovascular accident as causes for a client's altered mood. A positron emission tomography scan may show a change in activity in the prefrontal cortex suggestive of a mood disorder (Fig. 15-2). The physician may omit imaging tests if he or she thinks the clinical evidence strongly supports the diagnosis of depression.

Medical Management

The most commonly used treatments for depression are drug therapy (Drug Therapy Table 15-1), psychotherapy, and, in severe cases, electroconvulsive therapy (ECT).

Drug Therapy

The three main categories of drugs that relieve the symptoms of depression are tricyclic antidepressants (TCAs), monoamine oxidase inhibitors (MAOIs), and selective serotonin reuptake inhibitors (SSRIs; see Drug Therapy Table 15-1). A fourth group of medications is called *atypical antidepressants* because they that do not fall in any of the three major chemical families.

BOX 15-1 ● **Signs and Symptoms of Major Depression**

Sad mood
Appetite change (increased or decreased)
Disturbed sleep (insomnia or hypersomnia)
Inability to concentrate
Marked decrease in pleasure
Apathy, including lack of interest in sex
Guilty feelings
Energy changes (restlessness or inactivity)
Suicidal thoughts

FIGURE 15-2 PET scanning is useful in revealing metabolic changes in the cortex on unmedicated and medicated clients. (Courtesy of Monte S. Buchsbaum, MD, The Mount Sinai Medical Center and School of Medicine, New York, New York. From Videbeck, S. [2001]. *Psychiatric mental health nursing* [p. 334]. Philadelphia: Lippincott Williams & Wilkins.)

All antidepressants increase or potentiate levels of serotonin. **Serotonin syndrome** is a potentially life-threatening condition that results from elevated levels of serotonin in the blood. Manifestations include fever, sweating, shivering, feelings of intoxication, confusion, restlessness, anxiety, disorientation, ataxia, tachycardia, hypertension, tremors, and muscular spasms and rigidity. The following factors place a client at risk for serotonin syndrome:

- Antidepressants from different classes such as MAOIs and SSRIs are coprescribed.
- The time between weaning from one antidepressant drug to initiating another is inadequate.
- Other serotonergic agonists, drugs that stimulate serotonin receptors, are combined with antidepressant therapy. Serotonergic agonists include dextromethorphan (Benylin, Pertussin, Delsym), meperidine (Demerol), and lithium (Eskalith, Lithane).

Temporarily withholding the antidepressant is recommended initially. In severe cases, symptoms can be managed with anxiolytic drugs like diazepam (Valium), beta-adrenergic blockers like propranolol (Inderal), or skeletal muscle relaxants like dantrolene (Dantrium), while supporting breathing with mechanical ventilation.

TRICYCLIC ANTIDEPRESSANTS

The TCAs were the first group of drugs used to treat depression; they occasionally are prescribed for clients with chronic pain (see Chap. 21). Tricyclics were so named because they have three chemical attachments in their organic molecular structure. Many variations of drugs in this category have been developed since the first tricyclics. The subsequent modifications are referred to as *bicyclics* and even *heterocyclics* according to the changes in their molecules. Collectively, they may be called *cyclic* antidepressants.

Cyclic antidepressants block the **reuptake** of serotonin and norepinephrine (Fig. 15-3). In other words, they interfere with the reabsorption of these two neurotransmitters by the releasing presynaptic neuron, thereby creating a sustained effect.

One disadvantage of cyclic antidepressants is the lag time between the initiation of drug therapy and relief of the depressive symptoms. It may take from 10 to 28 days or longer, depending on the specific cyclic drug, before a client notes any change in mood. Another disadvantage is that cyclics are highly lethal if taken in an overdose. Because suicide is not uncommon among depressed clients, the physician must consider limiting the number of cyclics that are filled in any one prescription. Regardless of the prescribed class of antidepressant, clients with psychomotor retardation may attempt suicide once their level of energy increases. Nurses should not be lulled into thinking that a depressed client is necessarily nonsuicidal just because he or she is more active. In fact, close observation is even more important at this time.

Side effects of cyclic antidepressants, like postural hypotension, tachycardia, cardiac dysrhythmias, blurred vision, dry mouth, urinary retention, and constipation, make them particularly undesirable for older adults. Some cyclic antidepressants are more sedating than others. Signs of liver toxicity and bone marrow depression require frequent monitoring. The seizure threshold may also be lowered, causing a convulsion in clients who never ex-

DRUG THERAPY TABLE 15-1	ANTIDEPRESSANT DRUG THERAPY

DRUG CATEGORY AND EXAMPLES	MECHANISM OF ACTION	SIDE EFFECTS	NURSING CONSIDERATIONS
Tricyclic antidepressants (TCAs) *amitriptyline (Elavil), nortriptyline (Pamelor), imipramine (Tofranil)*	Block the reuptake of serotonin and norepinephrine	Orthostatic hypotension, sedation, dry mouth, blurred vision, weight gain, constipation, urinary retention, cardiac dysrhythmias	Inform client that symptomatic relief may not occur for 2 to 4 weeks or longer. Caution client to rise slowly from a lying or sitting position. Inform client that blurred vision and dry mouth will decrease over time. Discuss the increased potential for suicide as energy increases before depression resolves. Discontinue the drug gradually.
Monoamine oxidase inhibitors (MAOIs) *phenelzine (Nardil), tranylcypromine (Parnate)*	Block the enzyme that breaks down monoamines	Headache, insomnia, severe hypertension with certain foods and drugs, orthostatic hypotension, transient erectile dysfunction, constipation or diarrhea, dry mouth, blurred vision	Provide information on diet and drug restrictions to avoid hypertensive crisis. Advise client to wear a Medic Alert bracelet. Educate client about potentially lethal interaction with meperidine (Demerol) Explain that there may be a 2- to 6-week delay before symptoms improve. Advise client to take last dose before bedtime to avoid sleep disturbances. Allow at least a 14-day interval between discontinuing a TCA and initiating an MAOI.
Selective serotonin reuptake inhibitors *fluoxetine (Prozac), sertraline (Zoloft), paroxetine (Paxil)*	Block the reuptake of serotonin but not norepinephrine	Weight loss, insomnia, tremor, nervousness, headache, decreased libido, erectile dysfunction, interference with liver enzymes that potentiates the risk for altered metabolism of other drugs	Instruct client to avoid caffeine and other foods or drugs that are cardiac stimulants. Monitor blood pressure and heart rate. Allow at least 14 days before switching to an MAOI. Monitor for serotonin syndrome, which can result from a drug–drug interaction.

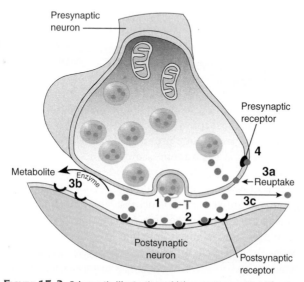

FIGURE 15-3 Schematic illustration of (1) neurotransmitter (T) release, (2) binding of transmitter to postsynaptic receptor; termination of transmitter action by (3a) reuptake of transmitter into the presynaptic terminal, (3b) enzymatic degradation, or (3c) diffusion away from the synapse; and (4) binding of transmitter to presynaptic receptors for feedback regulation of transmitter release. (From Rhoades, R. A. & Tanner, G. A. [1996]. *Medical physiology* [p. 46]. Boston: Little, Brown.)

perienced one before. There must be sufficient time (2 to 4 weeks) between tapering the dosage of a cyclic antidepressant and initiating drug therapy with an MAOI or SSRI.

MONOAMINE OXIDASE INHIBITORS

Monoamine oxidase is an enzyme that breaks down monoamine neurotransmitters. Inhibiting this enzyme allows the neurotransmitters to continue stimulating receptor sites for norepinephrine, serotonin, and, to some extent, dopamine. MAOIs, however, are the least prescribed category of antidepressants because they have a high potential for food–drug and drug–drug interactions (Box 15-3). When an MAOI is combined with foods containing tyramine, another monoamine, clients are likely to develop a potentially fatal **hypertensive crisis** with symptoms such as elevated blood pressure, headache, nausea, vomiting, sweating, palpitations, visual changes, neck stiffness, sensitivity to light, and tachycardia. The nurse, therefore, has a grave responsibility for teaching clients about dietary and drug restrictions, which the client must follow for at least 2 weeks after discontinuing the drug.

Foods aged or fermented

BOX 15-3 ● Food, Beverage, and Drug Restrictions During Monoamine Oxidase Inhibitor Drug Therapy

FOOD AND BEVERAGES TO AVOID

Aged, hard cheese	Pepperoni, sausage
Chocolate	Sour cream
Pickled herring	Broad beans (fava beans)
Overripe bananas	Monosodium glutamate
Chicken liver	Beer
Dried fish	Soy sauce
Fermented meat (salami)	Red wine
Yogurt	Meat tenderizer

DRUGS TO AVOID

Cold and allergy medications	Meperidine (Demerol)
Appetite suppressants	Antidepressants in other categories
Antiasthmatics	Local anesthetics with epinephrine
Antihypertensives	

The physician usually prescribes a low dose at the beginning of MAOI drug therapy and increases the dose according to the client's tolerance of side effects, which include dry mouth, blurred vision, constipation, urinary retention, postural hypotension, insomnia, weight gain, and sexual dysfunction. The lag time is approximately 3 to 6 weeks after beginning MAOI therapy (Fortinash & Holoday-Worret, 2000). Dosages must be tapered when the client no longer needs the drug. At least 2 weeks should elapse after the last dose of a cyclic antidepressant and the initiation of an MAOI drug.

Stop, Think, and Respond ● BOX 15-2

What information would you offer to a person who has just started MAOI therapy and plans to go out for pizza and beer?

SELECTIVE SEROTONIN REUPTAKE INHIBITORS

The SSRIs, as their name implies, interfere primarily with the reabsorption of serotonin. They have lesser effects on other neurotransmitter levels. The accumulated serotonin prolongs the stimulation of neuroreceptor sites. SSRIs are the newest and currently most prescribed group of drugs used to treat depression. They are widely used for several reasons: (1) they have milder side effects; (2) they are unlikely to cause death in cases of overdose; (3) dosages do not need much adjustment after initiation of therapy; and (4) the lag time is short, perhaps 3 to 10 days.

Although SSRIs cause side effects like nausea, weight loss, insomnia, nervousness, tremor, and headache, these problems tend to dissipate within weeks of starting drug therapy. If the side effects do not resolve, they can be managed with additional medications like a mild hypnotic for sleep. Unfortunately, sexual dysfunction (e.g., reduced desire for sex, erectile and ejaculatory dysfunction, in-

ability to reach orgasm) is a frequent and undesirable side effect. Alterations in sexual activity are a leading cause of noncompliance. Lowering the dose of SSRIs can reduce sexual side effects, but many clients, especially men, are reluctant to discuss changes in their sexuality with the prescribing physician.

ATYPICAL ANTIDEPRESSANTS

Several additional drugs relieve depression but do not belong to the major categories of antidepressants. Some examples include nefazodone (Serzone), venlafaxine (Effexor), and maprotiline (Ludiomil). The atypical drugs are used as alternatives for clients who do not respond to trials with other standard classes of antidepressants.

Stop, Think, and Respond ● BOX 15-3

How would you respond to a client who reports feeling just as depressed as when he or she began antidepressant drug therapy 4 days earlier?

Psychotherapy

Psychotherapy, talking with a psychiatrist, psychologist, or mental health counselor, promotes coping with emotional problems, gaining insight into behaviors, and learning techniques that can improve well-being. Various types of psychotherapy are available:

- *Psychodynamic psychotherapy* is patterned after a Freudian model. Clients discuss their early life experiences to raise repressed feelings to a conscious level. Clients often are in psychodynamic psychotherapy for months to years. This form of therapy can be tedious and expensive, but traumatic events buried deep in the unconscious may require extensive therapy.
- *Interpersonal psychotherapy* is facilitated by a bond that develops between the therapist and client. The empathy and trust help clients gain an understanding of their condition and the courage and support to overcome it.
- *Supportive psychotherapy* helps clients learn about their disorder and treatment techniques, improve or develop new social skills, obtain positive reinforcement for progress, and give encouragement to persevere.
- *Cognitive therapy* helps clients replace negative, and often illogical, ways of thinking with more positive outlooks. For example, the therapist might encourage a person who believes a friend purposely avoided speaking to him or her in a store to consider other possibilities (e.g., the friend was preoccupied and did not actually notice the client, the friend did not recognize the client, the friend was in a hurry and could not spend time socializing).

● *Behavioral therapy* endeavors to change unhealthy ways of behaving. Clients are rewarded verbally or in some other way when they alter their behavior positively. For example, when a person who is often taken advantage of at work asserts himself or herself, the therapist praises the client's action. The praise and recognition encourage the client to continually repeat the healthy behavior. Gradually, the resulting changes increase self-esteem and promote further improvement.

Psychotherapy often is more productive after depressed clients respond to antidepressant drug therapy. Clients should be advised that if they feel uncomfortable or dissatisfied with a particular practitioner or style of therapy, they can be referred elsewhere.

Electroconvulsive Therapy

Electroconvulsive therapy uses the application of an electric stimulus to one or both temporal regions of the head to produce a brief, generalized seizure. Although the exact mechanism of action is unknown, the belief is that ECT achieves its effect by either increasing circulating levels of monoamine neurotransmitters or by improving transmission to the receptor site. ECT usually is reserved for depressed clients who:

● Have not responded to drug therapy
● Are intolerant of the side effects of antidepressant medications
● Are so seriously suicidal that waiting for antidepressants to become effective jeopardizes their safety

Except for clients who are extremely suicidal, ECT can be administered on an ambulatory, outpatient basis. Many clients experience aftereffects, including headache, soreness of skeletal muscles, temporary confusion, short-term, patchy memory loss, and brief learning disability. ECT usually is contraindicated for clients with cardiac or neurovascular diseases.

NURSING PROCESS

● The Depressed or Suicidal Client

Assessment

Besides assessing the client physically and monitoring mood and affect, nurses can use various assessment questionnaires as a database for quantifying a person's mood state and tracking changes that occur during treatment. One example is the Beck Depression Inventory, a self-assessment tool, which contains 22 multiple-choice questions that the client reads and answers independently. The second is the Hamilton Rating Scale for Depression (HAMD), which is administered by a mental health worker. Usually the scores on the Beck Depression Inven-

tory correlate closely with the HAMD. The HAMD is used more widely for determining the severity of depression. The National Institute of Mental Health has used the HAMD to evaluate responses to pharmacologic drug treatment; pharmaceutical companies use the HAMD when submitting research results for new antidepressant approval by the U.S. Food and Drug Administration (FDA); and practitioners and researchers alike use the HAMD to compare and validate scores when more than one assessment tool is used.

If a client is depressed, the nurse must assume that he or she also may be suicidal. Suicide is the third leading cause of death among 15- to 24-year-olds. Older adults commit approximately 20% of all suicides, with the greatest incidence among men aged 80 to 84 years (Centers for Disease Control and Prevention, 1996). One of the most reliable suicide assessment techniques is to ask bluntly, "Do you feel like killing yourself?" Unfortunately, some depressed clients conceal their suicidal thoughts, provide only vague verbal or behavior clues (Box 15-4), or assume that others are aware of their despair but have chosen to ignore it.

If a client admits to being suicidal, the nurse must next determine whether the client has a suicide plan, which increases the seriousness of the risk. The nurse must assess if the plan is feasible and whether it is considered of high or low lethality. High-lethality methods are those from which the possibility of rescue is remote. Some examples include shooting or hanging oneself, jumping from a bridge or building, throwing oneself in front of a train or truck, and driving into a tree, wall, or off a cliff. Low-lethality methods are those that allow a window of time for the suicidal person to be found and rescued. They

---

BOX 15-4 ● Clues of Suicidal Intentions

CLEAR VERBAL CLUES
"I'm planning to kill myself."
"I wish I were dead."

VAGUE VERBAL CLUES
"I just can't stand it any longer."
"Nobody needs me anymore."
"Life has lost its meaning for me."
"You won't be seeing me anymore."
"I'm getting out."
"Everybody would be better off without me."

BEHAVIORAL CLUES
Giving away a valued possession
Donating large sums of money to charity
Putting personal affairs in order
Writing poetry with morbid themes
Composing a suicide note
Making funeral arrangements
Buying a gun; stockpiling pills
Lifting of depressed mood (may indicate a plan and energy to carry it out)

include overdosing on medications, cutting the wrists, or inhaling carbon monoxide. In almost all cases, people who are suicidal are ambivalent—they would choose life rather than death if they held some hope for the future. Despite conscientious efforts to prevent suicide, some individuals cannot be stopped.

The nurse must determine the level at which the depressed client can carry out activities of daily living. Depressed clients may not eat, bathe, shave, or shampoo or style their hair. In some cases, they neglect self-care because they lack energy. They also may ignore cleanliness and grooming because of low self-esteem or little concern for social acceptance.

Diagnosis, Planning, and Interventions

Risk for Suicide related to feelings of hopelessness
Expected Outcomes: (1) The client will not harm self. (2) The client will identify a reason for living.

- If hospitalized, move the client close to the nursing station. *Doing so facilitates close and frequent observation.*
- Encourage a client who is not hospitalized to contact a friend or relative rather than remain alone. *The presence of another supportive person can deter a suicide attempt.*
- Talk to a nonhospitalized client on the phone as long as possible while contacting a 911 operator. *Communication with a comforting person can delay a potential suicide attempt or provide time to obtain assistance from emergency personnel who can intervene.*
- Make a verbal or written contract with the client that he or she will not attempt suicide. *Clients often honor such commitments.*
- Confiscate any objects that the client may use for self-harm, such as belts, shoelaces, safety razors, sharp combs, keys, or knives. *Limiting access to items that the client can use for self-destruction reduces the resources he or she has for attempting suicide.*
- Inspect the client's mouth, looking under the tongue and within the buccal cavity, after administering medications. *Suicidal clients may conceal and hoard medications until they stockpile sufficient numbers for an overdose.*
- Observe the client's whereabouts at least every 15 minutes, and spend time interacting with him or her. *These measures reduce the client's potential time for attempting or completing suicide and increase the response time available to resuscitate a person who has attempted suicide.*
- Keep the client busy and involved in activities. *Activity shifts the client's attention away from his or her emotional pain and hopelessness.*

Ineffective Coping related to feelings of helplessness and worthlessness
Expected Outcome: The client will identify one or more alternatives to suicide.

- Acknowledge the client's feeling of despair. *Recognizing a client's mood demonstrates that the nurse has noticed the person and is perceptive.*
- Indicate that you want to help. *Offering assistance is characterized as a therapeutic use of self. Doing so reassures the client that you will not abandon him or her and that he or she is worthy of help.*
- Emphasize hope, previous positive experiences, and outcomes. *Such discussion reinforces that the client has the potential to overcome current difficulties based on past success.*
- Explore other courses of action rather than suicide. *Alternatives help the client consider options for dealing with the current situation.*
- Appeal to the client's ambivalence by indicating that current feelings are likely to change given additional time. *Most suicidal clients will delay or dismiss suicidal activities if they believe that they will feel better eventually.*
- Discuss previous coping strategies and encourage using some that were effective in the past. *Reusing previous methods for managing problems offers the possibility that similar actions can achieve a positive result.*
- Develop a plan for maintaining future safety such as talking with a trusted friend or calling a crisis hotline. *If a plan is developed, there is a possibility that the client will implement it.*

Disturbed Sleep Pattern related to depression
Expected Outcome: The client will sleep a maximum of 8 hours during the night with no napping during the day.

- Keep the client busy during the day, and discourage napping or going to bed early. *Left alone, depressed clients are likely to become more vegetative (i.e., they withdraw by sleeping).*
- Include active exercise during the day, but not before bedtime. *Exercise relieves anxiety, but it may cause stimulation when performed at night.*

Evaluation of Expected Outcomes

Expected outcomes are that the client's suicidal feelings pass. The client implements new or previously successful coping strategies to manage emotional problems. At night, the client falls asleep easily and does not awaken for 6 to 8 hours.

SEASONAL AFFECTIVE DISORDER

Seasonal affective disorder (SAD) is a mood disorder that has its onset during darker winter months and spontaneously disappears in the spring. SAD is more prevalent among people living in states north of 40 to 50 degrees of latitude such as Washington, Oregon, Minnesota, Michigan, New York, and the New England states. Native Alaskans do not manifest the disorder as much as those who move there.

Pathophysiology and Etiology

The best explanation for SAD is that it is a primitive biologic response triggered by **photoperiods,** daytime hours that are short because of fewer hours of sunlight. The condition actually resembles the characteristics of hibernating animals. Theorists believe that light rays follow a visual pathway to the hypothalamus, the center for regulating sleep, hunger, libido, and mood. The hypothalamus relays the light-sensing data to the pineal gland, which regulates the production of a hormone called melatonin. **Melatonin,** which also affects regulation of serotonin, induces sleep during dark hours and is suppressed by daylight (Fig. 15-4). When hours of daylight become fewer, the production of melatonin is extended. In northern latitudes, melatonin secretion is sustained until spring, when days become brighter and longer.

Assessment Findings

Clients with SAD use the terms *sleepy, fatigued,* and *lethargic* to describe themselves in the winter. The lack of energy crosses over into feeling irritable, unable to concentrate, worthless, guilty, depressed—even suicidal. Some also report cravings for carbohydrates, which leads to weight gain, much like an animal preparing to sleep through the winter. As clients with SAD become more depressed and irritable, they are less inclined to interact socially. Many tend to stay indoors and dread leaving home.

The depression is bimodal; it cycles with the seasons. After a prolonged period of winter depression, most report a lifting of spirits in the spring. Some also describe feeling energetic, more motivated, hyperactive, and even euphoric. The cheery mood or absence of depressive symptoms tends to be sustained until late fall, when the depressive pattern repeats itself.

At this time, no diagnostic tests can confirm SAD. Physicians rely on clients' reports of cycling moods that correlate with the ratio of sunlight.

Medical Management

For those who cannot move to a sunnier location, phototherapy is the best alternative for treating SAD. **Phototherapy** is a technique that uses artificial light that simulates the intensity of sunlight. The artificial light is produced by fluorescent bulbs at 2500 to 10,000 lux, the international measurement of illumination. Ten thousand lux is approximately 10 to 20 times as bright as ordinary indoor light.

The frequency and duration for phototherapy can vary, but a common prescription is to sit by the light source from 30 minutes to 2 hours per day, preferably in the early morning hours (Fig. 15-5). The client need not stare at the fluorescent light; in fact, it is best not to look directly at it. Glancing periodically at the light is sufficient to relieve symptoms in 1 to 2 weeks. Other models are available as well. A head-mounted light that shines on the face during daytime activities facilitates mobility. Bedroom phototherapy lights can be set with an automatic timer to come on at a predawn schedule. Even though the sleeper's eyes are closed, it is believed that the light penetrates the eyelids, which triggers a decline in melatonin—much like daybreak naturally activates arousal from sleep.

FIGURE 15-4 Melatonin (and subsequently serotonin) levels depend on exposure to sunlight. Dark months result in seasonal affective disorder for some people.

FIGURE 15-5 Phototherapy products such as a light box relieve the symptoms of seasonal affective disorder. (Courtesy of Light Therapy Products.)

Nursing Management

Because most clients with SAD are outpatients or may soon become so, the nurse provides information on how to implement phototherapy and how to supplement its beneficial effects. One of the most important principles to stress is that natural sunlight is brighter and better than any artificial substitute. The nurse also should teach measures found in Client and Family Teaching Box 15-1.

BIPOLAR DISORDER

Bipolar disorder is characterized by cycling between depression, euthymia, and euphoria. Each dysfunctional mood is likely to last several months, although depressive phases tend to be longer than manic phases. Some individuals experience a mild manic phase, referred to as *hypomania;* others, known as *rapid cyclers,* experience at least four episodes of mania and depression per year.

Pathophysiology and Etiology

Extremes in levels of monoamines—excessive in mania and inadequate during depression—seem to be responsible for the symptoms of bipolar disorder. In severe cases, excess dopamine may cause distorted thinking and hallucinations. Another possibility is that there is insufficient **gamma-aminobutyric acid** (GABA), an inhibitory neurotransmitter, to counteract the effects of the monoamines. Altered blood calcium levels also may contribute to the development of bipolar disorder because calcium is re-

quired for exciting neurons. Genetic predisposition also is implicated in the development of bipolar disorder.

Assessment Findings

Signs and Symptoms

Signs and symptoms of the depressive phase of bipolar disorder are the same as those for major depression. During the manic phase, clients are hyperactive and often display an exaggerated sense of their own importance. They can quickly become angry and aggressive with those who attempt to restrain their burst of energy and wild ideas. Because judgment is impaired—another characteristic of the disorder—reckless and impulsive behavior like sexual promiscuity, criminal activity, spending sprees, gambling, and risky business transactions can occur. The surge of norepinephrine allows clients who are experiencing the manic phase to go without sleep for long periods. It also causes rapid thinking accompanied by racing speech. When extremely ill, some individuals experience psychotic features such as hallucinations. Combined with delusions, which are illogically false beliefs, the client with bipolar disorder can become homicidal or suicidal.

Diagnostic Findings

It eventually may be possible to predict who will develop bipolar disorder with the use of gene mapping. At present, however, no objective tests are available, and the diagnosis is based on the client's history. The key indicator is the client's pattern of emotional "highs" and "lows." A family member with bipolar disorder is a risk factor, as is a history of substance abuse, because undiagnosed individuals naively attempt to self-medicate to relieve the depressive episodes.

Medical Management

Bipolar disorder is managed by the administration of one or more mood-stabilizing medications (Drug Therapy Table 15-2). Lithium (Eskalith, Lithane, Lithobid), a chemical element, usually is the initial drug of choice. It controls both depressive as well as manic symptoms in clients who respond to lithium monotherapy (single-drug treatment). The American Psychiatric Association's Practice Guideline for the Treatment of Bipolar Disorder (1994) now recommends the use of anticonvulsants such as valproic acid derivatives (Depakote, Depakene, Valproate) and others such as carbamazepine (Tegretol), alone or in combination with lithium, for controlling mood swings. Antipsychotics such as haloperidol (Haldol; see Chap. 17) also may be prescribed for a brief period to induce sedation and control hallucinations and delusions. Some have proposed using calcium channel blockers, but little research supports the application of their use for managing bipolar disorder.

15-1 *Client and Family Teaching*
Seasonal Affective Disorder (SAD)

The nurse must teach the client who experiences SAD and his or her family the following:

- Avoid the use of eyeglasses or contact lenses that are coated to shield ultraviolet radiation because the coating interferes with light transmission to the pineal gland.
- Add more lamps and bright fixtures at home and work.
- Install skylights.
- Trim shrubs and trees from around windows.
- Use translucent curtains or shades rather than heavy drapes.
- Sleep and work in an east-facing room.
- Take brief walks outside around noon without sunglasses.
- Jog after sun-up and before sundown.
- Take up an outdoor winter sport.

DRUG THERAPY TABLE 15-2 | MOOD-STABILIZING MEDICATIONS

DRUG EXAMPLES	MECHANISM OF ACTION	SIDE EFFECTS	NURSING CONSIDERATIONS
lithium carbonate (Eskalith, Lithane, Lithobid)	Alters sodium transport in nerve and muscle cells; increases intra-neural stores and inhibits release of norepinephrine and dopamine	Hand tremors, nausea, vomiting, diarrhea, thirst, polyuria, sedation, thyroid dysfunction, wrist and ankle edema at therapeutic level	Administer with meals. Withhold if serum level is >1.5 mEq. Female clients should use contraception and avoid breast-feeding.
valproic acid (Depakote)	May increase levels of GABA	Drowsiness, mild tremor, ataxia, nausea, vomiting, diarrhea, blood dyscrasias, liver toxicity	Administer with meals. Caution client to avoid activities that require alertness and coordination. Monitor blood for therapeutic level.
carbamazepine (Tegretol)	Decreases rate of neuronal impulse transmission	Dizziness, drowsiness, unsteady gait, nausea, vomiting, fluid retention, edema, blood dyscrasias, skin rash, liver toxicity	Administer with meals. Caution client to avoid activities that require alertness and coordination. Risk of central nervous system toxicity increases when given with lithium. Risk of liver toxicity increases when given with a monoamine oxidase inhibitor. Monitor blood for therapeutic levels. Female clients should use contraceptives.
clonazepam (Klonopin)	May increase brain levels of GABA	Drowsiness, dizziness, unsteady gait, nausea, vomiting, constipation, blood dyscrasias, dry mouth, liver toxicity	Collaborate with the physician on baseline blood tests before initiating therapy. Administer drug with food or milk. Drowsiness may be potentiated if combined with alcohol or other sedative drugs. Monitor laboratory findings during therapy and withhold drug if there is bone marrow suppression or serious elevation in liver enzymes. Advise sucking on hard candy or more frequent oral hygiene to relieve dry mouth. Advise women that incidence of birth defects increases if drug is taken during pregnancy, and to use a reliable contraceptive while taking this drug. Never discontinue the drug abruptly.

GABA = gamma-aminobutyric acid.

Lithium

Lithium is a naturally occurring element found in stone and spring water that flows from underground sources. Pharmaceutical preparations are available for those who are lithium-deficient. When ingested, lithium moves easily through cell membranes, but it is less easily removed. Some believe that this feature may stabilize cell membranes, leading to the equalization of moods. Another possibility is that lithium regulates the activity between neurotransmitters like serotonin, norepinephrine, dopamine, and their receptor sites. However, lithium:

- May be ineffective for some
- Has a delay of 5 to 14 days in achieving therapeutic benefits
- Has a narrow range of safety between a therapeutic serum level (0.8 to 1.2 mEq) and toxic levels (1.5 mEq)
- May be nontherapeutic or dangerously elevated when taken in combination with other drugs (Drug Therapy Table 15-3)
- Causes side effects that challenge compliance
- Requires periodic laboratory tests to monitor serum blood levels

Lithium crosses the placental barrier; therefore, its use is contraindicated in pregnant women. Furthermore, lithium is water soluble and present in all body fluids, including breast milk. Lithium administered to infants through breast milk can cause toxicity; thus, breast-feeding mothers should also avoid use. Loss of body fluid from diarrhea, diuretics, and excessive perspiration can lead to concentrated blood levels and lithium toxicity. Because the body always attempts to balance cations with anions, lithium may be retained if sodium levels are low. Providers must stress the importance of maintaining an adequate ingestion of salt to all clients who rely on lithium to control their disorder.

DRUG THERAPY TABLE 15-3	DRUGS AFFECTING SERUM LITHIUM LEVELS	
INCREASE SERUM LITHIUM LEVEL	**DECREASE SERUM LITHIUM LEVEL**	
Tetracycline	Theophylline	
Thiazide diuretics	Aminophylline	
Nonsteroidal anti-inflammatory drugs	Carbamazepine	
Haloperidol	Sodium bicarbonate	
	Osmotic diuretics	

Anticonvulsants

Anticonvulsants may achieve their therapeutic effects by enhancing the action of GABA in much the same way that benzodiazepines reduce anxiety (see Chap. 14). One of the first anticonvulsants used to treat bipolar disorder was carbamazepine (Tegretol). It still is used to manage the symptoms of clients at the onset of acute mania. In addition, it is efficacious for decreasing the incidence and frequency of mood swings among rapid cyclers. Because carbamazepine stimulates drug metabolism by the liver, however, maintaining consistent therapeutic drug levels is difficult. Clients who take carbamazepine also are at risk for infection because the drug impairs white blood cell formation. Consequently, serum drug levels and leukocyte counts must be monitored periodically.

Valproic acid derivatives like Depakote are preferred to carbamazepine most of the time. These derivatives also enhance GABA activity. Clients who take valproic acid tend to experience gastrointestinal symptoms like nausea, vomiting, and diarrhea. Some experience sedation and ataxia, putting them at risk for injury. There must be periodic assessment of liver function and blood cell counts. Although it can be combined with lithium and used for the long-term management of bipolar disorder, valproic acid is unsafe during pregnancy.

Nursing Management

Nursing Care Plan 15-1 provides a detailed discussion of care for the client with bipolar disorder. Before discharge, the nurse educates the client and his or her significant others on these aspects:

- The disease process
- How prescribed drugs help in symptom management
- Drug effects and side effects
- Signs of drug toxicity and actions to take
- Frequency of blood tests
- The advantages of wearing a Medic Alert bracelet

In addition to arranging outpatient therapy, the nurse informs the client and others of support groups that can continue the educational and therapeutic processes. Both the client and those who live in the same environment need to understand the signs of relapse, such as an in-ability to sleep for several days in a row or increasingly impulsive behavior such as making unnecessary purchases. The nurse also reviews the signs of cycling into a depressed mood so that indications for reinitiating medical care are clear.

GENERAL NUTRITIONAL CONSIDERATIONS

Although more than 12 European studies show that St. John's wort relieves some of the symptoms of mild to moderate depression in approximately half the people who take it for at least 3 to 4 weeks, the first large-scale U.S. study failed to show any benefits. Yet millions of Americans take St. John's wort as a "natural" remedy for depression or "the blues." Compared with other antidepressant drugs, St. John's wort produces fewer and less severe side effects, is less expensive, and does not require a prescription. It can, however, interact with certain prescription medications (e.g., SSRIs, antiepilepsy drugs), reducing their effectiveness.

S-adenosylmethionine (SAM-e), a chemical compound formed from the amino acid methionine, is found in protein-rich foods. Low levels of SAM-e have been associated with depression and other disorders. SAM-e has been used in Europe for more than 20 years to treat depression and arthritis pain. Like all other dietary supplements sold in the United States, however, the FDA has not approved it for safety or effectiveness.

Some studies indicate that a high-carbohydrate, low-protein meal or snack alters neurotransmitter levels in the brain and thus affects mood. Insulin secreted by the pancreas in response to eating causes most amino acids to leave the blood and enter muscle cells. Tryptophan is the exception; with the decrease in blood concentration of other competitive amino acids, tryptophan is readily transported across the blood-brain barrier and floods the brain, which converts it to serotonin. Carbohydrate-generated serotonin may promote calmness, fatigue, or sleepiness. In clients with depression, however, a high carbohydrate load may elevate mood. (Starchy meals or snacks that contain significant amounts of protein provide enough competing amino acids to inhibit the brain's uptake of tryptophan and the subsequent production of serotonin.)

GENERAL PHARMACOLOGIC CONSIDERATIONS

Drugs used to treat depression require 2 to 4 weeks before a therapeutic effect is seen. Therefore, monitor the client closely for the first month of therapy, especially if the client has suicidal tendencies.

Nursing Care Plan 15-1

THE CLIENT WITH BIPOLAR DISORDER/ACUTE MANIC PHASE

Assessment

■ It may be necessary to perform the initial assessment and physical examination in brief increments. Bipolar clients have short attention spans and poor concentration; they become easily frustrated if their activity is curtailed. As an alternative, use the family as a more objective resource for necessary information. Their information is valuable because the client's symptoms have usually created multiple crises.

■ Determine what types of prescribed medications the client takes and if he or she has been compliant with the medication regimen. Sometimes antidepressants can trigger manic symptoms because they raise monoamine neurotransmitter levels.

■ Ask about the client's use of alcohol or other controlled substances because many clients with bipolar disorder attempt to self-medicate to control their moods or they use drugs recreationally because of their poor judgment.

■ Obtain information about the client's recent sleep patterns, hydration, and dietary intake.

■ Observe the client's attention to hygiene and manner of dress. Check the female client's last date of menstruation and if she has consistently used contraception.

■ Prepare the client for laboratory and diagnostic tests that are likely to include an electrocardiogram, thyroid function studies, and a profile of blood chemistry tests. Note if the client is voiding in sufficient quantities and inquire as to the client's bowel elimination patterns, including the date of the last bowel movement.

■ Record baseline vital signs.

■ Listen to the client's thought content during verbal interactions. The client is likely to speak loudly and rapidly. At the very least, bipolar clients express expansive and elaborate ideas or schemes. Some may have paranoid ideas or inflate their own importance. They may be experiencing hallucinations.

Nursing Diagnosis: **Disturbed Thought Processes** related to excessive levels of monoamines

Expected Outcome: Client will be oriented and accurately perceive circumstances surrounding admission.

Interventions	Rationales
Orient client to person, place, time, and events.	Racing thoughts often interfere with comprehension.
Provide information in small amounts, using brief sentences.	Brief discussions accommodate for short attention span.
Reduce distracting stimuli such as noise and stimulation.	External stimuli potentiate client's internal activity.
Present reality when client is delusional; do not press the issue if it causes agitation.	Failing to present reality reinforces that client's delusions are real. Persistence may create conflict or cause client to act out violently.
Monitor client's whereabouts to ensure that he or she does not wander from unit or healthcare agency.	Bipolar clients are impulsive and resist being confined. Healthcare personnel are responsible for safety at all times.

Evaluation of Expected Outcome

■ Client becomes oriented.

■ Client interacts appropriately for the situation.

Nursing Diagnoses: **Risk for Other-Directed Violence** and **Risk for Self-Directed Violence**

Expected Outcome: Client will not injure self or others.

(continued)

Nursing Care Plan 15-1 *(Continued)*

THE CLIENT WITH BIPOLAR DISORDER/ACUTE MANIC PHASE

Interventions	*Rationales*
Take client to a room or other secluded area when he or she shows signs of aggression.	Decreased stimulation may restore self-control.
Set firm limits for behavioral expectations using a modulated and controlled tone of voice.	Client remains informed of the kinds of behavior that will not be tolerated. A modulated, controlled voice is less likely to provoke a confrontation.
Offer client a large-muscle activity like playing basketball or riding an exercise bicycle.	Exercise releases energy and reduces the potential for an angry outburst.
Administer a prescribed short-acting sedative if aggressive behavior escalates and endangers others.	A sedate client is more responsive to directions from others and less likely to become physically violent.
Obtain an order to seclude or restrain if client becomes violent.	Legally, restraints must be avoided unless absolutely necessary to protect others because clients have the right to the least restrictive treatment.
Initiate suicide precautions if data suggest vulnerability for self-harm.	The client's safety is a priority of care.

Evaluation of Expected Outcome:

■ Client has no angry outbursts.
■ Client demonstrates self-control.

Nursing Diagnosis: **Imbalanced Nutrition: Less than Body Requirements** related to increased activity and distraction from eating

Expected Outcome: Client will maintain admission weight.

Interventions	*Rationales*
Consult the dietitian about increasing calories at meal times.	Loading calories without loading quantities of food may help maintain weight and nutrition.
Offer liquid nutritional supplements at least three times a day.	Each container of liquid nourishment may provide 350 or more calories. Consuming liquids does not require sitting at a table and interrupting activity.
Provide finger foods that the client may consume throughout the day.	Frequent snacking increases caloric intake and nourishment.

Evaluation of Expected Outcome: Client consumes sufficient food to maintain weight.

Nursing Diagnosis: **Risk for Imbalanced Fluid Volume** related to polyuria secondary to lithium therapy and inattention to thirst

Expected Outcome: Client will be well hydrated as evidenced by moist mucous membranes, light-colored urine, and normal body temperature.

Interventions	*Rationales*
Monitor intake and output if possible.	Urine output of 1500 to 3000 mL indicates an adequate fluid volume.
Offer at least 2500 to 3000 mL of fluid per day.	An adequate volume compensates for polyuria that can occur with lithium therapy. Urination ensures excretion of lithium.
Monitor electrolyte laboratory results.	Electrolytes become elevated when fluid intake is low.

(continued)

Nursing Care Plan 15-1 (Continued)

THE CLIENT WITH BIPOLAR DISORDER/ACUTE MANIC PHASE

Evaluation of Expected Outcome:

■ Client consumes sufficient fluids to maintain hydration.

■ Client has moist mucous membranes, light-colored urine, and normal body temperature.

Nursing Diagnosis: **Bathing/Hygiene Self-Care Deficit** related to decreased attention and concentration

Expected Outcome: Client will be clean and groomed each day.

Interventions	Rationales
Prepare necessities for bathing, grooming, and hygiene for client. Supervise hygiene and provide assistance if needed.	Distractability may interfere with client's ability to organize hygiene items. Client may be less thorough without nurse's supervision.
Spread uncompleted hygiene tasks throughout remainder of the day.	All hygiene needs may not be met at one time.
Help client to dress appropriately and remain dressed.	Bipolar clients may dress flamboyantly or seductively unless supervised. Poor judgment may result in episodes of nudity.

Evaluation of Expected Outcome: Client resumes independent responsibility for self-care and activities of daily living.

Caution the client to avoid alcohol and other central nervous system depressants while taking any psychotropic drug.

Some antidepressants, particularly TCAs, may trigger a manic phase in individuals with bipolar disorder.

Clients must continue dietary and drug restrictions for 2 weeks after stopping use of an MAOI to avoid a hypertensive episode.

Complaints of a headache (especially an occipital headache) may indicate a hypertensive crisis in those receiving MAOIs. Report such episodes to the healthcare provider immediately.

Pregnant women always should consult with their obstetrician before taking any medication. Lithium and the MAOIs are especially hazardous to the fetus.

Monitor for signs and symptoms of lithium toxicity: diarrhea, vomiting, nausea, drowsiness, muscular weakness, twitching, and lack of coordination.

Polyuria can occur with administration of lithium. Unless contraindicated because of a disease condition, the client may require an increase in fluids up to 3000 mL/day to maintain fluid balance.

Monitor the client taking valproic acid (Depakote, Depakene) closely for hepatotoxicity periodically during therapy. Frequent liver function tests and serum ammonia concentrations may be ordered.

Anyone who takes an antidepressant, mood-stabilizing drug, or any other prescribed medication should consult a physician before self-medicating with St. John's wort, ginkgo biloba, kava, tyrosine, or SAM-e. Herbal remedies and dietary supplements can cause adverse reactions when taken alone; when combined with drugs, there may be dangerous interactions.

GENERAL GERONTOLOGIC CONSIDERATIONS

Impaired regulation of neurotransmitters in older adults suggests that they may be biologically predisposed to depression and thought disorders.

Cognitive impairment in the depressed older adult can be easily confused with dementia. It is important to distinguish between the two because depression in the elderly usually can be treated successfully.

In older adults, psychotropic drugs are prescribed at the lowest possible dosage that will produce a therapeutic effect because of the potential for increased adverse reactions and toxicity.

Risk for orthostatic hypotension from psychotropic drugs is increased in older adults because of decreased functioning of the blood pressure–regulating mechanism.

Older adults may require longer administration (up to 8 weeks) than other clients to obtain a therapeutic effect when taking antidepressants.

Antidepressants must be used cautiously in older adults with cardiovascular disease. Older men with prostatic enlargement are more susceptible to urinary retention.

Older adults who seek treatment for subacute physical symptoms, such as loss of appetite, trouble sleeping, lack of energy, and weight loss, may actually be depressed.

The losses that accompany aging and chronic or terminal illness may trigger feelings of hopelessness, which increase the risk for suicide.

The rate of suicide is 50% higher in older adults than in other age groups (Klebanoff & Smith, 1997). Older adults who are depressed often use a lethal means to ensure successful suicide. The highest suicide rate is seen in older adults 75 to 80 years of age.

Suicidal behavior cues such as putting personal affairs in order, giving away possessions, and making funeral plans are a sign of good judgment in the older adult and do not necessarily convey suicidal ideation. Other indicators, such as unsatisfactory relationships, poor or failing health, divorce, losing one's spouse or partner, or addiction may be stronger indicators of suicide in older adults.

As individuals with bipolar disorder age, their depressive episodes may increase in frequency and last longer.

Older adults who are prescribed lithium to treat bipolar disorder require careful monitoring. Because the kidneys eliminate lithium, age-related changes in the elderly may reduce renal clearance, predisposing these clients to lithium toxicity.

Critical Thinking Exercises

1. *Two depressed clients are in a psychiatric hospital. One feels suicidal, but has no plan for carrying it out. The other indicates that he would kill himself with a gun, but has none. Describe the similarities and differences in their nursing care.*
2. *What physical consequences might occur for the client in a manic episode?*
3. *What problems might family members experience as a result of living with a person with a mood disorder?*

References and Suggested Readings

Abrams, A. C. (2000). *Clinical drug therapy* (6th ed.). Philadelphia: Lippincott Williams & Wilkins.

American Psychiatric Association. (1994). Practice guideline for the treatment of patients with bipolar disorder. *American Journal of Psychiatry, 151*(12s), iii–36.

Centers for Disease Control and Prevention. (1996). Suicide among older persons—United States 1980–1992. *Morbidity and Mortality Weekly Report, 4*(01), 3–6.

Challiner, V. & Griffiths, L. (2000). Electroconvulsive therapy: a review of the literature. *Journal of Psychiatric and Mental Health Nursing, 7*(3), 191–198.

Cole, M. R. (1999). Bridging the great divide: Management of the patient with bipolar disorder. *Nursing Spectrum, 11A*(3), 8–9.

Fortinash, K. M. & Holoday-Worret, P. A. (2000). *Psychiatric mental health nursing* (2nd ed.). St. Louis: Mosby.

Gispen-de Wied, C., Christine, C., Lucres, M. C., et al. (2000). Pituitary-adrenal function in adolescent psychiatric patients: impact of depressive symptoms. *Journal of Affective Disorders, 59*(1), 71–77.

Heffern, W. A. (2000). Psychopharmacological and electroconvulsive treatment of anxiety and depression in the elderly. *Journal of Psychiatric and Mental Health Nursing 7*(3), 199–204.

Hotopf, M. (1999). St. John's wort is more effective than placebo for treating depressive disorders. *Evidenced-Based Medicine, 4*(3), 82.

Kaye, J., Morton, J., Bowcutt, M., et al. (2000). Stress, depression, and psychoneuroimmunology. *Journal of Neuroscience Nursing, 32*(2), 93–100.

Kelsoe, J. R. (2000). Mood disorders: Genetics. In B. J. Sadock & V. A. Sadock (Eds.), *Comprehensive textbook of psychiatry* (Vol. 1, 7th ed., pp. 1308–1328). Philadelphia: Lippincott Williams & Wilkins.

Miller, S. M. (2000). One nurse's story of bipolar disease. *Nursing Spectrum, 12A*(15), 21–22.

Oshima, A., Yamashita, S., Owashi, T., et al. (2000). The differential ACTH responses to combined dexamethasone/CRH administration in major depressive and dysthymic disorders. *Journal of Psychiatric Research, 34*, 325–329.

Patient suicide: Court faults nurse's referral of patient to chemical dependency program. (2000). *Legal Eagle Eye Newsletter for the Nursing Profession, 8*(9), 3.

Pollack, L. E. & Cramer, R. D. (2000). Perceptions of problems in people hospitalized for bipolar disorder: Implications for patient education. *Issues in Mental Health Nursing, 21*, 765–778.

Rapp, J. W., Beckwith, M. C., & Reimherr, F. W. (2000). Clinical uses and differences among the selective serotonin reuptake inhibitors. *Journal of Pharmaceutical Care in Pain and Symptom Control, 8*(3), 23–28.

Terman, M. & Terman, J. S. (1999). Bright light therapy: Side effects and benefits across the symptom spectrum. *Journal of Clinical Psychiatry, 60*, 799–808.

Tredgett, J. (2000). Lithium clinic update. *Mental Health Nursing, 20*(5), 13–15.

Videbeck, S. (2000). *Psychiatric mental health nursing*. Philadelphia: Lippincott Williams & Wilkins.

Zauszniewski, J. A. & Rong, J. (1999). Depressive cognitions and psychosocial functioning: A test of Beck's cognitive theory. *Archives of Psychiatric Nursing, 13*, 286–293.

Caring for Clients With Eating Disorders

Words to Know

anorexia nervosa
binge-eating disorder
body mass index
bulimarexia
bulimia nervosa
compulsive overeating
eating disorders
endocannabinoids
food binges
lanugo

leptin
melanin-concentrating
  hormone
normal eating
orexin A
orexin B
purge
satiety
water loading

Learning Objectives

On completion of this chapter, the reader will:

- Differentiate normal eating from eating disorders.
- Name four types of eating disorders.
- Describe two subtypes of anorexia nervosa.
- Name the neurotransmitters, neurohormones, and other chemicals that affect the appetite and satiety center in the brain.
- Discuss two reasons why most clients with anorexia induce self-starvation.
- Give the healthy adult range for body mass index.
- List four components of treatment for clients with anorexia nervosa.
- Name at least two problems that are the focus of nursing management when caring for clients with anorexia nervosa.
- Discuss the nurse's role in managing the nutrition of a client with anorexia nervosa.
- Give two examples of how clients with bulimia compensate for binging.
- Name two problems, besides nutrition, that nurses focus on when caring for clients with bulimia nervosa.
- Differentiate between binge-eating disorder and compulsive overeating.
- Discuss at least three psychosocial problems that may accompany overeating syndromes.
- Name a support group that individuals with overeating syndromes may find particularly helpful.

A rich variety of foods, sufficient for energy needs, growth and repair of cells, and maintenance of a healthy weight, is required to preserve health. Depending on such variables as age, sex, physical condition, activity level, and height, **normal eating** involves consuming approximately 1500 to 2500 calories per day, usually spread over three meals and two to three snacks. Normal eating occurs in response to hunger and ceases when **satiety** (a feeling of comfortable fullness) is attained. This chapter deals with conditions characterized by disordered eating.

Collectively, **eating disorders** are those in which eating

- Is consistently more or less than the client's caloric needs to maintain a healthy weight
- Occurs without hunger or fails to bring about satiety

- Is accompanied by anxiety and guilt
- Results in physiologic imbalances or medical complications

Eating disorders affect 500,000 people in the United States at any given time. They are most prevalent among middle to upper middle class young women 12 to 25 years of age. Often, clients with eating disorders strive to keep their illness secret; family and friends may become aware of the problem only after repeatedly noting emotional and behavioral symptoms (Table 16-1) or when serious health consequences ensue. Box 16-1 is a self-test that can assist individuals in determining if their eating pattern is abnormal.

Anorexia nervosa, bulimia nervosa, binge-eating disorder, and compulsive overeating are eating disorders.

TABLE 16-1	SIGNS AND SYMPTOMS OF EATING DISORDERS		
EATING DISORDER	**PHYSICAL**	**EMOTIONAL**	**BEHAVIORAL**
Anorexia nervosa	Decrease of 25% in body weight; weight is 85% or less of normal; lanugo; alopecia; cold intolerance; amenorrhea; constipation; abdominal pain	Distorted body image; hatred of a particular body part; low self-esteem; depression; isolation; perfectionism	Restriction of food choices and intake; ritualistic handling of food (cutting into tiny pieces, arranging food a certain way, using certain plates and utensils only); weighing oneself frequently; denial of hunger
Bulimia nervosa	Inability to accurately interpret hunger and fullness signals; swelling of parotid glands ("chipmunk cheeks"); frequent weight fluctuations; irregular menses	Feeling unable to control eating; depressive mood and frequent mood swings; black-and-white thinking; exaggerated concern about weight	Excessive exercise, use of diuretics, and laxatives; secret eating of high-calorie, high-carbohydrate foods; alternately binging and fasting
Binge eating and compulsive overeating	Obesity; discomfort after eating	Preoccupation with weight, eating, and dieting; attributes professional and social success and failure to weight; feels disgust or guilt after eating; feels lack of control over eating	Frequent dieting, restricts activities because of embarrassment about weight; eating when not hungry; rapid eating; eating alone

Obesity is a consequence of overeating; therefore, some obese clients also have eating disorders.

ANOREXIA NERVOSA

Anorexia nervosa is an eating disorder characterized by an obsession with thinness that is achieved through self-starvation. It occurs more often in women than in men; anorexia nervosa develops in 1 in 200 girls 12 to 18 years of age. Although eating disorders also develop in men, they are less likely to disclose such problems to a health professional. Even when they do, the information often is dismissed and untreated.

There are two subtypes of clients with anorexia: those who lose weight by exclusively restricting their intake of calories, and those who manifest **bulimarexia,** a pattern of both food restriction and purging discussed later in this chapter, to avoid absorbing the food that is consumed.

Pathophysiology and Etiology

The exact cause of anorexia nervosa is unknown. Many authorities believe that anorexia and other eating disorders result from a combination of cultural, social, physiologic, and psychological factors. Increasing evidence is strengthening the connection between genetics and altered physiology.

Culturally and socially, extremely skinny role models in the media suggest to young women and men that thinness is linked with attractiveness and success. The image portrayed as ideal, however, is unhealthy and unrealistic for most people. Self-starvation, rigorous physical activity, or both is sometimes the only way to achieve a similar appearance. Furthermore, some athletes like gymnasts, figure skaters, and even ballet dancers restrict food intake under the assumption that low body weight improves performance. This belief sometimes induces or contributes to eating disorders in such athletes.

Physiologic influences play a key role in eating disorders. Research suggests that neurotransmitters and neurohormones influence eating by binding with receptors in the appetite center of the hypothalamus. Clients with anorexia may experience a down-regulation or insensitivity to norepinephrine and also may have increased serotonin levels, which fool the brain into believing satiety has occurred despite minimal intake (Kaye & Weltzin, 1991). Evidence supporting this phenomenon is that weight loss is a side effect of drugs that increase the serotonin level, such as the selective serotonin reuptake inhibitors (see Chap. 15). Variations in the gene for serotonin receptors also have been found in clients with anorexia. One of the most recent and exciting discoveries occurred in 1999, when researchers located receptors in the human brain for **melanin-concentrating hormone** (Saito et al., 1999). In animal studies, low levels of this hormone caused weight loss, whereas high levels promoted obesity. Finally, **leptin,** a substance manufactured in human fat cells, acts on receptors in the hypothalamus, where it inhibits food intake. Clients with anorexia may have excessive leptin.

BOX 16-1 ● Eating Behavior Self-Test

_____ Even though people tell me I'm thin, I feel fat.
_____ I get anxious if I can't exercise.
_____ My menstrual periods are irregular or absent (female).
_____ My sex drive is not as strong as it used to be (male).
_____ I worry about what I will eat.
_____ If I gain weight, I get anxious or depressed.
_____ I would rather eat by myself than with family or friends.
_____ Other people talk about the way I eat.
_____ I get anxious when people urge me to eat.
_____ I don't talk much about my fear of being fat because no one understands how I feel.
_____ I enjoy cooking for others, but I don't usually eat what I've cooked.
_____ I have a secret stash of food.
_____ When I eat I'm afraid I won't be able to stop.
_____ I lie about what I eat.
_____ I don't like to be bothered or interrupted when I'm eating.
_____ If I were thinner I would like myself better.
_____ I have missed work or school because of my weight or eating habits.
_____ I tend to be depressed and irritable.
_____ I feel guilty when I eat.
_____ I avoid some people because they bug me about the way I eat.
_____ My eating habits and fear of food interfere with friendships or romantic relationships.
_____ I cut my food into tiny pieces, eat it on special plates, make patterns on my plate with it, or spit it out before swallowing it.
_____ I am hardly ever satisfied with myself.
_____ I have taken laxatives to control my weight.
_____ I have vomited to control my weight.
_____ I want to be thinner than my friends.
_____ I have said or thought, "I would rather die than be fat."
_____ I have fasted to lose weight.
_____ In romantic moments I cannot let myself go because I am worried about my fat and flab.

If you answer yes to any of these questions; discuss your eating habits with your physician.

Adapted from Anorexia Nervosa and Related Eating Disorders, Inc. Are you at risk? Take a self test. (2002). (On-line.) Available: http://www.anred.com/slf_tst.html.

In terms of psychological influences, theorists have noted that persons with anorexia nervosa often are perfectionists, have low self-esteem, and possess an intense desire to please others. Some consider the refusal to eat a form of self-control that clients with anorexia use to cope with stressful life experiences or dysfunctional family relationships.

Assessment Findings

Signs and Symptoms

Despite the use of the term *anorexia,* persons with this disorder do experience hunger, but they control the urge to eat because of a morbid fear of becoming fat. It is not uncommon to find that the client with anorexia consumes an average of 600 to 900 calories per day and often less. Eventually, the weight of clients with anorexia is

85% or less than that of others of similar build, age, and height. Almost universally, they consider themselves obese despite appearing emaciated.

When confronted with the fact that they are in jeopardy of dying, clients deny the seriousness of everyone's concern. They may appear skeleton-like and develop a growth of fine body hair called **lanugo** that, in the absence of subcutaneous fat, helps to maintain body temperature by reducing heat loss. These clients tend to be hypotensive and may have irregular, low pulse rates, making them prone to fainting. Severe malnutrition causes those with anorexia to be constipated, feel cold most of the time, have frequent chronic infections, and cease menstruating. Many conceal their starvation by hiding or disposing of food and dressing in bulky clothing.

Complications

Failure to consume adequate nourishment eventually deprives all body systems of the nutritional elements required for homeostasis, growth, and cellular repair. Low serum estrogen levels lead to osteopenia (low bone mass) and premature osteoporosis (severe demineralization of bones), both of which lead to stress fractures, particularly of the spine and hips (Thrash et al., 2000). Starvation can cause vitamin deficiencies, fluid and electrolyte imbalances, and death from cardiac failure or dysrhythmia.

Diagnostic Findings

Body mass index (BMI), a mathematical computation based on height and weight (Box 16-2), is used to evaluate a person's size in relation to norms in the adult population. Clients with anorexia typically have a BMI of 16 or less. Anemia usually is present, and electrolyte levels,

BOX 16-2 ● Body Mass Index Formula, Calculation, and Interpretation

FORMULA

$$BMI = \frac{weight\ in\ kg}{height\ m^2}$$

CALCULATION

1. Divide pounds by 2.2 = kilograms.
2. Divide height (inches) by 39.4 = meters.
3. Square the answer in step 2 by multiplying the number times itself.
4. Divide weight in kg by m².

INTERPRETATION

Anorectic	BMI = ≤16
Underweight	BMI = 16–18.5
Healthy	BMI = 18.5–24.9
Overweight	BMI = 25–29.9
Obese	BMI = 30–34.9
Severely obese	BMI = 35–39.9
Extremely obese	BMI = ≥40

especially potassium and sometimes sodium, often are dangerously low. Deficiencies in serum proteins are reflected in low albumin, transferrin, and ferritin levels. Cardiac irregularities are identified by electrocardiography. Bone densitometry studies are used to determine if osteopenia has developed, and, if so, its severity.

Stop, Think, and Respond ● BOX 16-1
Besides weighing less than normal for one's height, what other findings suggest that an underweight person has anorexia nervosa?

Medical Management

Treatment involves four aspects: nutritional therapy, psychotherapy, drug therapy, and family counseling. Nutritional therapy includes providing nourishing meals, supplemental vitamins and minerals, intravenous fluids and electrolytes, tube feedings, or total parenteral nutrition. Once the client's weight improves or stabilizes, outpatient treatment begins.

To promote compliance with the weight-gain regimen, behavioral therapy (see Chap. 15) is instituted. By eating, the client earns privileges, such as having visitors and participating in social and physical activities. The privileges are rewards used to reinforce desired behavior. Individual and group psychotherapy (see Chap. 15) is used to help clients gain insight into distorted perceptions of thinness and the motivations for continuing with dangerous weight-loss behaviors. Counseling and involvement in self-help groups for several years often are indicated.

Antidepressant medications such as amitriptyline (Elavil) are administered (see Chap. 15). Bulimarexic clients have responded to drug therapy with the antihistamine cyproheptadine (Periactin), which seems to have antiseritonergic activity. Supplemental vitamins and minerals such as those containing iron, potassium, and calcium may be included in the therapeutic regimen to compensate for natural sources that the client is not consuming as a result of the self-imposed fast. Stool softeners or laxatives may be necessary to counteract constipation resulting from deficient dietary fiber. Family counseling aims at relieving the power struggles between those who try to convince the client to eat and the client who refuses. It also focuses on learning skills for undoing *enmeshment,* a phenomenon in which family members are so involved with one another that personal identities are lost and contacts with others outside the family are excluded.

NURSING PROCESS

● The Client With Anorexia Nervosa

Assessment

The nurse performs a physical assessment, being careful to note signs of malnutrition such as absence of body fat; dry skin, scalp, and hair; fine hair covering the body; edema from hypoproteinemia; and cold hands and feet. The nurse monitors vital signs regularly to detect hypothermia, bradycardia, or hypotension. Cardiac monitoring can detect dysrhythmias caused by hypokalemia. The client is weighed as accurately as possible with minimal clothing, and BMI is calculated.

The nurse obtains a nutritional history and identifies the date of the client's last menstrual period. He or she questions whether the client restricts food intake or combines it with purging. Noting the form of purging is important, and the nurse should keep in mind that excessive exercise is a form of purging. The nurse observes the client's mood and anxiety level and asks about family dynamics or other stressors.

Diagnosis, Planning, and Interventions

Imbalanced Nutrition: Less than Body Requirements related to fear of gaining weight
Expected Outcomes: (1) The client will consume an established amount of calories each day and gain 2 to 5 lbs by a mutually agreed-on target date. (2) The client will attain and maintain a BMI of at least 18.5.

● Consistently assign the same few nurses to the client's care. *Limiting staff relationships promotes a therapeutic alliance, and consistency reduces the potential for manipulation.*
● Establish a contract for expected weight restoration and target date; include the rewards for reaching goals and consequences of failure to achieve goals. *Participating in setting goals promotes self-involvement and a sense of ownership in the plan. Identifying rewards and negative consequences makes the client aware of the management of outcomes in the therapeutic plan.*
● Weigh the client regularly, but randomly. *Random weights usually are more accurate. They prevent the client from falsifying his or her weight by* **water loading,** *a technique in which clients with anorexia attempt to demonstrate weight gain by consuming a large volume of water and avoiding urination before being weighed.*
● Work with the dietitian to provide at least six to eight meals each day with a total caloric value between 1500 to 2000 calories; then gradually increase the total calories to between 2500 to 4000 calories per day. *The client is much more likely to work toward weight gain if food is offered frequently and is not heavily calorie*

loaded. To gain 1 lb of weight, a person must consume 3500 calories that are not used for basic metabolism and activities.

- Set a limit of 30 minutes to consume the meal. *Clients with anorexia practice various rituals such as cutting food into small pieces and rearranging food on the plate without actually eating. Informing clients of the time limit may provide an incentive to consume food.*

- Observe or sit with the client during meals. *Being observed prevents the client from hiding rather than eating food.*

- Remove the dietary tray after 30 minutes without commenting on food that has not been eaten. *Removal of food at the designated time avoids a power struggle. Negative comments reinforce that the client was victorious in resisting the urge to eat. Withholding any comments avoids an adversarial image.*

- Record the type and amount of food consumed. *Documentation provides information by which to evaluate the client's progress and helps the dietitian calculate caloric intake.*

- Restrict the client's use of the bathroom for 2 hours after meals or accompany the client to the bathroom. *A 2-hour restriction allows time for consumed food to enter the small intestine for absorption rather than being vomited.*

- Give the client a liquid nutritional supplement to replace the uneaten calories at meals. *Clients may consume liquids that are calorie-loaded rather than solid food.*

- Implement behavioral rewards or consequences consistently and fairly. *Deviation from or inconsistent application of guidelines reduces the effectiveness of the plan of care.*

- Administer prescribed drug, vitamin, and mineral therapy, and ensure that the client attends group and individual psychotherapy. *Resistance to the therapeutic regimen is common. Anorexia requires management with medical, nutritional, and psychological modalities.*

Disturbed Body Image related to unresolved psychosocial conflicts

Expected Outcome: The client will develop a realistic perception of self and insight into the motivation for thinness.

- Encourage the client to talk about perceptions of body image, but avoid opposing the client's views. *Disagreeing tends further to entrench the client's beliefs.*

- Offer the observation that fixation with weight control diverts attention and energy needed to deal with real issues surrounding psychosocial conflicts. *Offering alternative views can raise awareness.*

- Help the client clarify issues underlying the need to control weight gain and promote weight loss. *Self-examination helps develop insight.*

- Suggest that perfection is impossible and that no body image is worth dying for. *Calling attention to the seri-ousness of the health problem may promote modifications in the client's behavior.*

Evaluation of Expected Outcomes

The client consumes nutritious food, resulting in gradual weight gain and a BMI greater than 18.5. The person no longer perceives himself or herself as fat. Evidence of enhanced insight is based on the client's self-disclosure that withholding consumption of food created a sense of power and provided a way to achieve an unrealistic image of perfection.

Client and Family Teaching Box 16-1 presents education points for families of clients with anorexia nervosa.

BULIMIA NERVOSA

Bulimia nervosa is characterized by two episodes of secret **food binges** (rapid consumption of many calories) per week followed by behaviors intended to prevent weight gain. The abnormal eating pattern persists for at least 6 months. There are two types of clients with bulimia: (1) those who **purge** (eliminate nutrients) after binging, with self-induced vomiting, laxatives, enemas, or diuretics; and (2) those who do not purge but compensate by fasting, using diet pills, or engaging in excessive exercise (see section on binge-eating disorder later in this chapter).

16-1 *Client and Family Teaching*
Anorexia Nervosa

The nurse counsels and educates family members by offering the following suggestions:

- Focus on the person rather than the eating disorder.
- Provide unconditional love.
- Avoid inflicting guilt for the family distress that the disorder causes in daily living.
- Give the client the power to make decisions and facilitate changes in matters other than eating.
- Avoid being manipulated by the person with anorexia nervosa.
- Explain that it is common for clients with anorexia nervosa to discredit the staff of the eating disorder team, the facility, and the treatment approaches.
- Demonstrate united support for one another and the plan for the client's treatment.
- Prepare for rehospitalization if the client becomes medically unstable or experiences a relapse.

Evaluation of Expected Outcomes

The client's caloric intake is in accordance with her or his metabolic needs. Binging and purging are reduced or eliminated. The client successfully implements alternative strategies for managing compulsive behaviors and has positive self-regard.

Stop, Think, and Respond ● BOX 16-2

Where is the appetite center, and what substances stimulate or suppress it?

BINGE-EATING DISORDER AND COMPULSIVE OVEREATING

Binge-eating disorder is characterized as the inability to control overeating, feeling guilty, but not engaging in compensating behaviors to prevent weight gain. **Compulsive overeating** is characterized as eating when not hungry or regardless of feeling full. Some individuals have both problems simultaneously. Either may result in obesity.

Pathophysiology and Etiology

The cause of overeating syndromes is still unknown. Because people with eating disorders suffer from anxiety, depression, and compulsive behavior, evidence is growing that biochemical factors are involved in binge eating and compulsive overeating. Similar to anorexia and bulimia nervosa, there is likely an imbalance of neurotransmitters involving norepinephrine and serotonin, or neurohormones like orexin A and B or leptin, which affect the appetite center in the brain. There also may be additional neuroendocrine disequilibrium involving cortisol, a hormone the adrenal cortex releases in response to stress (see Chap. 12); reduced cholecystokinin, a hormone secreted by the mucosa of the upper small intestine that causes laboratory animals to stop eating when feeling full; and imbalances in neuropeptides Y and YY, psychoactive chemicals that stimulate eating behavior in research animals. In 2001, scientists located brain receptors for **endocannabinoids,** natural chemicals with marijuana-like properties, that activate the appetite center (DiMarzo et al., 2001; Mechoulam & Fride, 2001). The existence of endocannabinoids helps explain why marijuana users experience ravenous hunger, called "the munchies," and why dronabinol (Marinol), synthetic tetrahydrocannabinol—the active ingredient in marijuana—helps those with cancer and acquired immunodeficiency syndrome gain weight. Increased amounts of or increased sensitivity to endocannabinoids may explain some syndromes characterized by overeating. Also, the fact that many overeaters state they use food as a way of coping with stress should not be overlooked.

Assessment Findings

Signs and Symptoms

Overeaters typically are overweight and have a history of unsuccessful attempts at dieting. Clients tend to eat without being hungry. They have preferences for high-sugar and high-fat foods that they may nibble over several hours or gorge on until they feel uncomfortably full. Some report that they overeat or binge when angry, sad, bored, or anxious. They often have a history of other compulsive behaviors such as alcohol or drug abuse. Some reveal that they have considered suicide or have performed self-mutilation, such as cutting and burning themselves, pulling their hair, and interfering with wound healing to cope with their intense feelings, to punish themselves, or to experience physical pain to counteract the consequences of feeling emotionally numb.

Complications

Ultimately, overeating leads to many physical and emotional problems. As a consequence of obesity, many individuals have hyperlipidemia (elevated blood fat levels), hypertension, type 2 diabetes mellitus, degenerative arthritis, and sleep apnea. They are at increased risk for gallbladder disease, heart disease, and some types of cancer. Many feel unhappy, ashamed, and disgusted with themselves. They tend to become socially isolated to avoid being noticed and possibly rejected.

Diagnostic Findings

People with overeating syndromes usually have a BMI of 30 or above. Other laboratory and diagnostic tests reflect secondary complications from obesity such as elevated blood sugar, cholesterol, and serum lipid levels.

Medical Management

A comprehensive approach to treating overeating syndromes involves weight reduction, psychotherapy, and self-help support groups. The first step is a sensible weight-loss regimen prescribed by a dietitian. Strict dieting is discouraged because it tends to worsen binge eating. To help clients lose weight and remain compliant, short-term drug therapy may be used. Prescribed medications include antidepressants such as selective serotonin reuptake inhibitors [e.g., fluoxetine (Prozac)] that promote weight loss (see Chap. 15).

Support groups, like Overeaters Anonymous (see Additional Resources), or group therapy in eating disorder clinics are helpful adjuncts to individual psychotherapy. In some cases, surgery is an option for severely obese clients with medical complications (see Chap. 52).

NURSING   PROCESS

● The Client Who Compulsively Overeats

Assessment

The nurse interviews the client, showing sensitivity to the individual's self-consciousness about weight and emotional problems. He or she performs a comprehensive physical assessment, providing privacy when measuring weight and height. Education points are presented in Client and Family Teaching Box 16-2.

Diagnosis, Planning, and Interventions

Imbalanced Nutrition: More than Body Requirements related to insensitivity to satiety
Expected Outcome: The client will consume only the prescribed number of calories per day.

- Advise the client to follow the meal plan for three meals and three snacks each day that has been developed by a dietitian in conjunction with nutritional counseling. *Compliance with a nutritious food plan promotes gradual weight loss.*
- Emphasize that the client should not deviate from the food plan. *Deviation leads to overeating.*
- Recommend using a scale and measuring utensils to comply with portion sizes. *Estimating amounts increases the potential to consume more calories than the food plan allows.*
- Remind the client to prepare a shopping list and purchase only the size and amount of food that is needed. *Impulse shopping or having leftovers increases the potential for eating more than the planned amount.*
- Suggest planning activities throughout the day that preferably involve others. *Isolation provides an opportunity for secretive binging.*

Risk for Loneliness related to self-consciousness concerning appearance and eating behavior
Expected Outcome: The client will participate in social relationships and activities.

- Accept the client. *Rejection encourages isolation.*
- Seek out the client for verbal interactions. *Attention from others reinforces that the client is a worthwhile person.*
- Encourage the client to contact friends or support persons or join social or self-help groups. *Activities that involve other people reduce feelings of loneliness.*
- Suggest that the client cultivate leisure activities that he or she can share with others. *Mutually shared activities provide opportunities for social relationships.*

Evaluation of Expected Outcomes

The client complies with the food plan and loses weight gradually. The client takes part in group activities and develops a network of friends.

 16-2 *Client and Family Teaching*
Overeating Syndromes

The nurse counsels clients with overeating syndromes as follows:

- Obtain and persist with treatment from professionals who are experienced in treating eating disorders.
- Follow the label directions for taking prescribed medications; report any untoward effects.
- Avoid popular nonprescription diet pills. They usually contain central nervous system stimulants. They can increase heart rate and blood pressure and cause dizziness, irritability, insomnia, and dry mouth.
- Strict dieting or fasting is the leading cause of binging.
- Exercise according to the advice of a physician to reduce appetite and increase weight loss.
- Avoid nutritional and weight loss centers because they usually do not offer the comprehensive services most clients need to keep from gaining weight once reaching the target weight.
- Read food labels and understand that those that say "sugar free" or "contains no cholesterol" do not mean that the ingredients are calorie free or even low calorie.
- Talk to a close friend or support person about feelings.
- Attend an Overeaters Anonymous meeting. This free self-help group is modeled after the 12-step program of Alcoholics Anonymous.
- Remember that recovery is a day-by-day process; it is self-defeating to dwell on the lack of previous success or relapses that may occur.

 ## GENERAL NUTRITIONAL CONSIDERATIONS

The focus of treatment for anorexia nervosa is the resumption of normal eating behaviors, not simply restoring body weight. Initially, as few as 1500 calories may be prescribed because large amounts of food, as well as high-fat foods and gassy vegetables, may cause gastrointestinal discomfort after constipation. No foods are restricted, but the client should avoid "diet" foods (artificially sweetened beverages, fat-free foods). Clients may need ongoing nutritional counseling throughout the maintenance period.

Like clients with anorexia, clients with bulimia nervosa need to resume normal eating behaviors and avoid restrictive practices. They also may need to accept a body weight higher than they would like. Nursing interventions include identifying and correcting fears and misconceptions about food and weight; clients who are persuaded occasionally to eat small amounts of a high-calorie food are less likely to binge later. Advise clients not to skip meals or snacks, to use appropriate utensils, not to pick at food, and not to feel guilty about occasional planned indulgences. Having the client record intake *before* eating adds to a sense of control. Clients with binge-eating disorder need to establish a regular, balanced, healthy eating pattern that includes three daily meals, planned snacks, and decreased avoidance of "trigger" foods. Eating is nonrestrained but self-regulated as clients respond to their internal cues. Discussion of weight management is not appropriate until binge eating is eliminated.

Rather than produce long-term weight management, restrictive low-calorie diets increase preoccupation with food and weight and the risk of binge eating. Estimates are that 95% of people who lose weight regain it within 5 years, and some dieters gain back more than they originally lost. The newer "nondiet" approach to weight management stresses that all foods are acceptable, teaches clients to recognize and differentiate between physiologic and psychological hunger, and emphasizes size acceptance. It is based on the belief that the body will find its natural weight when eating occurs in response to hunger and fullness, not from following a set meal pattern that may not reflect an individual's physiologic state of hunger at any given time.

GENERAL PHARMACOLOGIC CONSIDERATIONS

Adolescent girls with type 1 diabetes mellitus sometimes reduce their dose of insulin to promote weight loss. The practice is unsafe for obvious medical reasons.

Constipation in anorexia nervosa may be treated with a stool softener (e.g., docusate sodium [Colace, Regutol]), but harsh laxatives never should be administered. Administration of such laxatives can lead not only to loss of body fluids and mucosal irritation (which could result in infection), but to imbalanced electrolytes. A possible dangerous consequence is cardiac problems.

Constipation usually is relieved when the client with anorexia begins to eat normally.

No drug therapy is universally given for those with eating disorders; however, some clients with certain types of anorexia nervosa gain weight using cyproheptadine (Periactin). If this drug is given to increase weight, monitor for the following adverse reactions: dry mouth, dry eyes, sedation, photosensitivity, lethargy, and constipation.

If chlorpromazine (Thorazine) is given, the severely emaciated client is at increased risk for hypotension and hypothermia.

GENERAL GERONTOLOGIC CONSIDERATIONS

Older adults may experience severe weight loss as the result of major depression, but it is extremely rare for older adults to have an excessive fear of gaining weight or an excessive desire for weight loss. Assess any adult with significant weight loss for depression.

In addition to depression, weight loss in older adults can be related to bereavement, confusion, ill-fitting dentures, diminished sensations of taste and smell, or inability to self-feed. Consider these factors when assessing any older adult with significant weight loss.

At times, older adults may simply refuse to eat, resulting in self-starvation. Self-starvation over the loss of health, diagnosis of a terminal disease, or inability to cope with life's losses is related to major depression or faulty coping skills and is not classified as an eating disorder.

Critical Thinking Exercises

1. *Based on the food pyramid, explain the components of a healthy daily diet.*
2. *Calculate the BMI of a person who weighs 175 pounds and is 63 inches tall. What conclusion is appropriate based on your calculation?*
3. *What weight loss strategies are appropriate to recommend and discourage for an obese client who is a compulsive overeater?*

References and Suggested Readings

Beals, K., Brey, R., & Gonyou, J. (1999). Understanding the female athlete triad: Eating disorders, amenorrhea, and osteoporosis. *Journal of School Health, 69,* 337–340.

Brewerton, T. D., Dansky, B. S., Kilpatrick, D. G., et al. (2000). Which comes first in the pathogenesis of bulimia nervosa: Dieting or bingeing? *International Journal of Eating Disorders, 28*(3), 259–264.

DiMarzo, V., Goparaju, S., Wang, L., et al. (2001). Leptin-regulated endocannabinoids are involved in maintaining food intake. *Nature, 410,* 822–825.

Drewnowski, A. (1999). Sweetness, appetite, and energy intake: Physiological aspects. *World Review of Nutrition and Dietetics, 85,* 64–76.

Gopel, C., Herrmann, F., & Marcus, A. (2001). Life-threatening tonsil hyperplasia probably induced by severe bulimia nervosa: A case report. *International Journal of Eating Disorders, 29*(1), 100–103.

Jimerson, D. C., Mantzoros, C., Wolfe, B. E., et al. (2000). Decreased serum leptin in bulimia nervosa. *Journal of Clinical Endocrinology and Metabolism, 85,* 4511–4514.

Kaye, W. H. & Weltzin, T. E. (1991). Serotonin activity in anorexia and bulimia nervosa: Relationship to the modulation of feeding and mood. *Journal of Clinical Psychiatry, 52,* 41–48.

Leutwyler, K. (1998). The discovery of two new hormones gives researchers food for thought. *Scientific American.* (Online.) Available: http://www.sciam.com/explorations/1998/030298eating/.

Mechoulam, R. & Fride, E. (2001). Physiology: A hunger for cannabinoids. *Nature, 410,* 763–765.

Montekeibem P., Di Lieto, A., & Tortorella, A. (2000). Circulating leptin in patients with anorexia nervosa, bulimia nervosa, or binge-eating disorder: Relationship to body weight, eating patterns, psychopathology and endocrine changes. *Psychiatry Research, 94,* 121–130.

Orbanic, S. (2001). Understanding bulimia: Signs, symptoms, and the human experience. *American Journal of Nursing, 101*(3), 35–42.

Ricca, V., Mannucci, E., Zucchi, T., et al. (2000). Cognitive-behavioral therapy for bulimia nervosa and binge eating disorder. *Psychotherapy and Psychosomatics, 69,* 287–295.

Saito, Y., Nothacker, H. P., Wang, Z., et al. (1999). Molecular characterization of the melanin-concentrating-hormone receptor. *Nature, 400,* 265–269.

Schmidt, U. (2001). Treating eating disorders: Ethical, legal and personal issues. *Behavior Research and Therapy, 39,* 369.

Striegel-Moore, R. H., Cachelin, R. M., Dohm, F. A., et al. (2001). Comparison of binge eating disorder and bulimia nervosa in a community sample. *International Journal of Eating Disorders, 29*(2), 157–165.

Thrash, L. E. & Anderson, J. (2000). The female athlete triad: Nutrition, menstrual disturbances, and low bone mass. *Nutrition Today, 35*(5), 168–174.

Travis, J. (1999). Feeding hormone finds its partner. *Science News, 156*(9), 139.

Walsh, B., Agras, W., Devlin, M., et al. (2000). Fluoxetine for bulimia nervosa following poor response to psychotherapy. *American Journal of Psychiatry, 157,* 1332–1333.

Caring for Chemically Dependent Clients

Words to Know

alcoholism
aversion therapy
blackouts
chemical dependence
cross-tolerance
detoxification
environmental tobacco
  smoke
methadone maintenance
  therapy

opiate dependence
polydrug abuse
relapse
rule of one hundreds
substance abuse
tolerance
withdrawal

Learning Objectives

On completion of this chapter, the reader will:

- Discuss the health and social consequences of substance abuse.
- Name four commonly abused addictive substances and at least three other categories of abused drugs.
- Discuss the meaning of withdrawal.
- Explain tolerance and give two mechanisms by which it occurs.
- List four steps in the progression toward chemical dependence.
- List two physiologic explanations and two psychosocial factors for the development of chemical dependence.
- Explain two ways abused drugs produce their effects.
- Define alcoholism and list three accompanying symptoms.
- Name four components of treatment for alcoholism.
- Discuss the nursing management of clients with alcoholism.
- List five potential health consequences of tobacco use.
- Discuss the components of a successful smoking cessation program.
- Discuss elements of recovery programs.
- Name drugs commonly abused by persons who use cocaine.
- Give four reasons for methadone maintenance therapy.

Substance abuse and chemical dependence are serious public health and social problems. They contribute significantly to *morbidity* (incidence of disease) and *mortality* (deaths) from liver damage, cardiopulmonary disease, and infectious diseases such as hepatitis and acquired immunodeficiency syndrome (AIDS). Alcohol and drug abuse also are major contributors to domestic violence and child abuse, crime, traffic and boating fatalities, assaults, and murders (see Chap. 7).

SUBSTANCE ABUSE AND CHEMICAL DEPENDENCE

Substance abuse is the use of a drug that is different from its accepted purpose. Usually, it is the consequences of inappropriately taking drugs—primarily mind-altering

and mood-altering substances—that are of major concern. Commonly abused drugs include alcohol, cocaine, heroin, hallucinogens, amphetamines, marijuana, barbiturates, volatile hydrocarbons such as those found in glue, and nicotine. Because of their widespread use, alcohol and nicotine contribute most to morbidity and mortality, and thus are the most harmful substances. Tobacco use is so widely accepted and its psychoactive properties are so subtle that its negative social and occupational effects seem minor. Yet tobacco is an addictive substance that contributes annually to the deaths of 430,000 people—as many as are caused by alcohol, cocaine, heroin, suicide, homicide, motor vehicle accidents, fire, and AIDS combined (National Center for Chronic Disease Prevention and Health Promotion, 2000).

Withdrawal refers to the physical symptoms and craving for a drug that occur when a person abruptly stops using an abused substance (Table 17-1). **Chemical**

TABLE 17-1	COMMONLY ABUSED SUBSTANCES		
DRUG	**EFFECTS**	**SIGNS AND SYMPTOMS OF TOXICITY**	**SIGNS AND SYMPTOMS OF WITHDRAWAL**
Alcohol	Central nervous system depressant • Lethargy • Slurred speech • Slowed motor reaction • Impaired judgment • Decreased social inhibition	Nausea and vomiting, loss of coordination, belligerence, stupor, coma	Anxiety, agitation, elevated vital signs, hyperactive reflexes, tremors, diaphoresis, insomnia, hallucinations, seizures
Cocaine	Central nervous system stimulant • Tachycardia • Hypertension • Increased energy • Feeling of well-being • Insensitivity to pain and fatigue • Weight loss	Restlessness, paranoia, irritability, auditory hallucinations, convulsions, respiratory or cardiac arrest	Depressed mood, lethargy, impaired concentration, craving for drug
Heroin	Central nervous system depressant • Initial brief rush of euphoria • Sedation • Reduced motivation, attention, and concentration • Altered sensitivity to stressors • Pain relief • Lowered vital signs, especially respiratory rate • Slowed peristalsis • Constricted pupils • Decreased interest in sex	Respiratory depression, hypothermia, pinpoint pupils, coma	Yawning, runny nose, perspiration, goose bumps, anorexia, vomiting, diarrhea, dilated pupils, insomnia, elevated vital signs, drug craving

dependence means that a person must take a drug to avoid withdrawal symptoms. *Addiction* sometimes is used interchangeably with *dependence,* but addiction more accurately refers to the drug-seeking behaviors that interfere with work, relationships, and normal activities (Box 17-1). **Tolerance** refers to the reduction in a drug's effect that follows persistent use. Tolerance results because the body develops mechanisms for using the drug more effectively or inactivating the drug more efficiently. Consequently, a person must take increasing amounts of the substance to obtain the desired effect.

Pathophysiology and Etiology

The causes of chemical dependence are complex and involve many psychobiologic factors. Substance abuse often begins with curious experimentation and progresses to habituation, psychological and physical dependence, and finally addiction (Table 17-2). One factor that explains substance abuse is the self-reinforcing pleasurable effects that some substances produce in the limbic system of the brain. Stimulant drugs such as cocaine and amphetamines affect levels of norepinephrine, dopamine, and acetylcholine. Depressant drugs such as alcohol, heroin, and barbiturates cause effects similar to those of gamma-aminobutyric acid (GABA), endorphins, and enkephalins. These drugs either mimic the neurotransmitters by attaching to their receptor sites or block their reuptake (see Chap. 12).

Psychosocial dynamics also are a component in substance use and abuse. Observing family members, peers, and role models who use alcohol, tobacco, and other drugs influences impressionable teenagers and youngsters. The promotion of alcohol in U.S. culture also fosters its use and abuse. Many people abuse drugs in a dysfunctional effort to cope with psychosocial stressors.

Treatment

Initiating treatment is one of the most difficult hurdles in treating chemical dependence. Clients deny their addiction, rationalize substance use, or blame life situations for their drug and drinking habits. Often, dependent individuals must "hit bottom" before they seek help. Once

BOX 17-1 ● Signs of Alcohol or Drug Addiction

Regularly drinking or taking more than was originally planned
Unsuccessfully attempting to reduce or regulate use
Spending excessive time obtaining, consuming, or recovering from the effects of the drug
Continuing use despite negative consequences
Drinking or consuming drugs alone
Failing to fulfill major role obligations at work, school, or home
Exhibiting tolerance to alcohol and sedative drugs
Displaying withdrawal symptoms when drug is not consumed

TABLE 17-2	PATTERNS OF SUBSTANCE ABUSE			
EXPERIMENTATION	**HABITUATION**	**DEPENDENCE**		**ADDICTION**
Initial use	Repeated use	Frequent use		Unremitting use
Low dose	Uniform doses	Doses increase		High doses
Finds experience pleasurable	Seeks to re-experience pleasure	Craves ongoing pleasure from drug		Needs drug to feel "normal"
No discomfort from abstinence	No discomfort from abstinence	Experiences minor physical discomfort if drug is not used		Experiences severe withdrawal symptoms if drug is not used

they seek treatment and withdrawal is managed, recovering individuals must learn new methods of coping with stressors, repair relationships damaged by addiction, and develop new interests and activities to fill the time once devoted to using drugs or alcohol.

Although some individuals quit taking abused substances unassisted, most people benefit from chemical detoxification and a treatment plan that involves abstinence, counseling, and support of peers through a 12-step program. Twelve-step programs are free and provide specific guidelines (steps) for becoming and staying drug or alcohol free. Frequent (daily, if necessary) attendance at meetings is encouraged. During meetings, members share their experiences and discuss the 12 steps and other topics related to recovery.

● ALCOHOL DEPENDENCE

Alcoholism is a chronic, progressive, multisystem disease characterized by an inability to control the consumption of alcohol. Unchecked, alcoholism is fatal. Serious medical consequences of alcoholism are dose related; that is, the more alcohol a person consumes, the sooner he or she will experience health problems. On a drink-by-drink comparison, women are more likely to experience health problems earlier than men because in general they weigh less than men. Consequently, the same amount of alcohol is more concentrated and more toxic to women than to men.

Pathophysiology and Etiology

In alcoholism, accumulating evidence suggests that a genetically determined component alters metabolism of alcohol in those with the disease (Box 17-2) (Li, 2000; Olms, 1983). Instead of acetaldehyde converting to acetic acid, some acetaldehyde combines with dopamine to form an addictive substance called tetrahydroisoquinoline (TIQ). TIQ is formed only in the brains of alcoholics, not in the brains of those who drink socially. Other researchers have identified a variant gene for dopamine among alcoholics that locks onto receptors, triggering sensations of pleasure

and reward (Cowen & Lawrence, 1999; Hill, et al., 1999; Noble, 1996).

Assessment Findings

Signs and Symptoms

Although the client may emphatically deny problem drinking, he or she typically has a history of increasing alcohol consumption. The person may hide containers of alcohol and drink privately at any time during the day. Many clients manifest a great tolerance for alcohol and a **cross-tolerance** (reduced effect) for sedative-hypnotic drugs. **Blackouts,** periods of amnesia involving events and activities during drinking, occur even in the early stages. Family and friends note alcoholic behaviors, and social or legal repercussions occur. A history of marital, financial, and occupational problems reflects the individual's inability to control drinking despite negative consequences. Many clients with alcoholism have been arrested for driving under the influence of liquor.

Acutely intoxicated alcoholics may enter the tertiary care hospital with altered mental status or acute gastric bleeding, or as victims of trauma or violence. When hospitalization occurs, management of alcohol withdrawal is as important as management of the related conditions. Withdrawal from alcohol results in nervous system stimulation manifested by tremors, sweating, hypertension, tachycardia, heart palpitations, craving for alcohol, seizures, and hallucinations.

BOX 17-2 ● Normal and Alcoholic Metabolism of Alcohol

Ethyl alcohol
↓
Acetaldehyde + dopamine → Tetrahydroisoquinoline (TIQ)
↓
Acetic acid (vinegar)
↓
Carbon dioxide + water

Altered alcohol metabolism shown in purple

Stop, Think, and Respond ● BOX 17-1

What assessment findings suggest that a person who consumes alcohol is an alcoholic rather than a social drinker?

Complications

A host of alcohol-related physical symptoms can accompany persistent drinking. Esophagitis, gastritis, enlarged liver, esophageal and rectal bleeding, and pancreatitis are common. Memory is impaired, and clients may experience erectile dysfunction or decreased libido. Studies also implicate alcohol in liver cancer, cerebrovascular accident, metabolic deficiencies, aspiration pneumonia, cardiomyopathy, blood dyscrasias, and neurologic disorders. Infants born to women who drank alcohol during pregnancy sometimes have fetal alcohol syndrome, which causes physical and intellectual deficits.

Diagnostic Findings

A blood alcohol level measures the percentage of alcohol in the blood, indicating the extent of alcohol toxicity (Table 17-3). Elevated levels of gamma-glutamyltransferase, aspartate aminotransferase, and alanine aminotransferase reflect alcohol-induced liver disease. Levels of pancreatic enzymes (amylase and lipase) also may be elevated.

Medical Management and Rehabilitation

To break the progression of alcoholism, clients undergo detoxification, nutritional therapy, psychotherapy, and drug therapy. They are encouraged to continue rehabilitation by joining a support group such as Alcoholics Anonymous (AA).

Detoxification

Alcohol withdrawal without detoxification is a potentially fatal process. **Detoxification** ("detox") involves stabilizing the client with a sedative drug while the alcohol is me-

tabolized from his or her system. Withdrawal symptoms are controlled until they subside. Drugs used in detoxification are lorazepam (Ativan), diazepam (Valium), and chlordiazepoxide (Librium; Drug Therapy Table 17-1). Initially, these medications are administered frequently and in high doses to compensate for the client's cross-tolerance; they are then tapered and discontinued. A beta-adrenergic blocker such as propranolol (Inderal) is given to reduce the dangerously elevated heart rate and blood pressure that can occur. Alcoholism is related to thiamine deficiency, which can lead to dementia. Because thiamine is necessary for the metabolism of glucose, glucose solutions must be avoided until thiamine is administered. Once thiamine is administered, intravenous (IV) hydration with glucose and additional vitamins, such as folic acid, supports the client metabolically until the condition stabilizes.

Nutritional Therapy

Alcoholics often are undernourished and have deficiencies of B vitamins. Injections of thiamine for 3 days followed by oral administration and folic acid supplements often are prescribed. Vitamin therapy prevents neurologic complications known as Wernicke's encephalopathy and Korsakoff's psychosis.

Psychotherapy

Individual or group psychotherapy helps the client to gain greater insight into the emotional problems that have led to or resulted from alcohol dependence. Family therapy with the spouse and children provides an opportunity to share how alcoholism has affected each person so that healing may begin.

Drug Therapy

Disulfiram (Antabuse) is a drug given to recovering alcoholics who cannot control the compulsion to drink. It is a form of **aversion therapy** because it deters drinking by causing unpleasant physical reactions when alcohol is consumed or absorbed through the skin (see Drug Therapy Table 17-1). Health teaching includes a list of products that contain alcohol such as liquid cough suppressants (Box 17-3). The client must be informed that

TABLE 17-3	BLOOD ALCOHOL LEVEL AND ASSOCIATED IMPAIRMENT	
BLOOD ALCOHOL LEVEL	PERCENTAGE OF BLOOD ALCOHOL	PHYSICAL AND BEHAVIORAL EFFECTS
50 mg/dL	0.05%	Mood changes, loosening of inhibition, decreased judgment, slight euphoria
80–100 mg/dL	0.08–0.1%	Reduced muscle coordination, decreased reaction time, impaired vision
200 mg/dL	0.2%	Staggering, poor control of emotions, easily angered
300 mg/dL	0.3%	Mental confusion, stupor
400 mg/dL	0.4%	Coma
500 mg/dL	0.5%	Respiratory depression, death

DRUG THERAPY TABLE 17-1	DRUGS USED IN THE RECOVERY FROM CHEMICAL DEPENDENCE	
DRUG CATEGORY AND EXAMPLES	**SIDE EFFECTS**	**NURSING CONSIDERATIONS**
Benzodiazepine chlordiazepoxide hydrochloride (Librium)—management of acute alcohol withdrawal	Sedation, confusion, restlessness, bradycardia, tachycardia, urinary retention or incontinence, drug dependence	If giving intravenously, use a large vein and monitor vital signs carefully. Intramuscular injection can be quite painful; reconstitute with special diluent only, monitor injection sites, administer slowly. Observe client for excessive sedation, and use cautiously in clients with impaired kidney or liver function.
Antialcoholic Agent disulfiram (Antabuse)—blocks oxidation of alcohol, resulting in the accumulation of acetaldehyde	*If alcohol is used:* flushing, throbbing headaches, dyspnea, vomiting, tachycardia, hypotension, blurred vision; severe reactions can result in convulsions, myocardial infarction, death. *Disulfiram alone:* drowsiness, headache, dermatitis	Do not administer until at least 12 hours have elapsed since last exposure to alcohol. Inform client to avoid all sources of alcohol and to wear a medical identification bracelet. Arrange for follow-up liver and blood studies. Inform client of potential side effects and to report them to a healthcare provider.
Smoking Deterrent nicotine transdermal (Nicotrol)—binds to nicotinic receptors in central and peripheral nervous system	Headache, insomnia, diarrhea, constipation, pharyngitis, burning and itching at site, backache, chest pain, dysmenorrhea	Explain application, site rotation, and disposal of used patches so that pets or children do not come in contact with product. Inform client of side effects and to report any that occur.
Narcotic Antagonist naltrexone hydrochloride (Trexan, ReVia)—blocks the effects of opioids and aids in the abstinence from alcohol	Insomnia, anxiety, nervousness, low energy, abdominal pain, nausea, vomiting, decreased sexual potency, delayed ejaculation, rash, joint and muscle pain, increased thirst	Induces sudden withdrawal so do not use until 7 to 14 days have elapsed since last exposure to opioids. Inform client that small doses of opioids will have no effect. Larger doses may overcome the inhibiting effect, but coma or death may occur. Tell the client to report any side effects.
Narcotic Agonist Analgesic methadone (Dolophine)—binds with opioid receptors in the CNS and produces euphoria, analgesia, and sedation	Light-headedness, dizziness, sedation, nausea, vomiting, respiratory depression, circulatory depression, shock, cardiac arrest	A single liquid oral dose is used for maintenance. Constipation may be severe; ensure that client is taking a stool softener. Use with caution in clients receiving sedatives, hypnotics, tranquilizers, tricyclic antidepressants, and monoamine oxidase inhibitors—respiratory depression, hypotension, and coma can occur.

life-threatening cardiopulmonary complications and even death can occur when disulfiram and alcohol are combined. Naltrexone (Trexan, ReVia), a narcotic antagonist, also is used as an adjunct for recovering alcoholics. It decreases the effects of alcohol should the person **relapse** (return to drinking).

BOX 17-3 ● Obscure Sources of Alcohol

- Liquid cough and cold medications
- Liquid sleep medications
- Flavoring extracts
- Mouthwash
- Rubbing alcohol
- Aftershave lotions
- Fruitcake with alcohol

Support Groups

Alcoholics Anonymous was the first 12-step self-help program. Founded in 1926 by an alcoholic physician, AA is composed of and run by recovering alcoholics to help people who are dependent on alcohol get and stay sober. AA emphasizes personal accountability, spirituality, and powerlessness over alcohol. Family members of clients with alcoholism may benefit from attending meetings of Al Anon, Alateen, or Adult Children of Alcoholics to learn more about how alcoholism has affected them.

Stop, Think, and Respond ● BOX 17-2

Explain why the first of AA's 12 steps leading to recovery from alcoholism is "We admitted we were powerless over alcohol—and that our lives had become unmanageable."

N U R S I N G   P R O C E S S

● The Client With Alcohol Dependence

Assessment

The nurse examines the client from head to toe, noting any signs of fall-related injuries, abdominal enlargement, jaundiced skin or sclera, and blood in any body fluids or stool that may indicate complications from liver damage or portal hypertension (see Chap. 55). The nurse includes questions about the use of alcohol when establishing the client's database. The CAGE Screening Test is helpful in detecting alcoholic behaviors (Box 17-4). If the client admits to consuming alcohol, the nurse determines the type, how much, and when the last drink was consumed. The latter information is important because withdrawal symptoms occur within 3 to 72 hours after a client's last drink. The nurse may administer a breath alcohol concentration test as soon as possible on contact with the client to obtain an approximation of the client's current alcohol level. A history of seizures or other severe symptoms in previous withdrawals merits close observation for a similar reaction.

The nurse monitors the client for signs and symptoms of withdrawal. Nurses often use the **Rule of One Hundreds** as an indicator of escalating withdrawal. It refers to a body temperature of at least 100°F, pulse rate of at least 100 beats per minute, or diastolic blood pressure of at least 100 mm Hg. The rise in any one of these three vital signs suggests the need for sedative medication because the physiologic consequences of withdrawal may be extremely difficult to counteract once they have begun.

Diagnosis, Planning, and Interventions

PC: Alcohol Withdrawal

Expected Outcome: The nurse will manage and minimize alcohol withdrawal.

- Assess the client's vital signs and other data, such as hand tremors, hyperactive tendon reflexes, diaphoresis, anxiety, insomnia, and disorientation, that suggest physiologic stimulation. *As the body metabolizes alcohol, it releases norepinephrine, causing autonomic nervous system stimulation.*

BOX 17-4 ● CAGE Questionnaire for Alcoholism

1. Have you ever felt that you ought to **C**ut down on your drinking?
2. Have people **A**nnoyed you by criticizing your drinking?
3. Have you ever felt **G**uilty about your drinking?
4. Have you ever had a drink first thing in the morning to steady your nerves or get rid of a hangover (**E**ye-opener)?

From Ewing, J. A. (1984). Detecting alcoholism: The CAGE questionnaire. *Journal of the American Medical Association, 252,* 1905–1907.

- Consult with the physician regarding the need for a detoxification drug. *The physician is responsible for prescribing a drug for detoxification and the dose, route, and frequency of administration according to assessment data the nurse obtains.*
- Administer prescribed detoxification medication. *Minor tranquilizers maintain a controlled level of intoxication so withdrawal is not rapid and dangerous.*
- Repeat assessments for withdrawal at least every 2 hours. *Administration of a detoxification drug should control physiologic stimulation; if not, administration of another dose is warranted.*
- Monitor for seizure activity, hallucinations, extreme tremors, and agitation. *If early and minor symptoms of alcohol withdrawal are not managed effectively, the client's withdrawal will progress in severity because of dopamine stimulation.*

Imbalanced Nutrition: Less Than Body Requirements related to inadequate dietary intake

Expected Outcome: The client will consume at least 75% of the food that is served.

- Obtain a baseline weight. *Documenting the client's current weight provides a means of evaluating if the client's subsequent nutritional intake maintains or increases the current weight.*
- Determine the client's food preferences. *A person is more likely to consume food that he or she likes.*
- Collaborate with the dietary department to provide six small meals each day and an ample variety of snacks. *The client is likely to consume more food if the quantity is distributed throughout the day.*
- Monitor dietary intake and record data in the medical record. *Documentation provides an objective means for evaluating the client's progress.*

Anticipatory Grieving related to loss of alcohol use and related social activities and social contacts

Expected Outcomes: (1) The client will verbalize that alcohol abuse is an illness that requires ongoing treatment and support. (2) The client will understand the connection between alcohol and its associated activities and develop non–alcohol-related interests and contacts.

- Let the client express feelings concerning potential losses. *Discussing the effects of abstinence is the first step in working through grief.*
- Explore alternatives that may substitute for potential losses. *Identifying activities and other people with whom to socialize may substitute for the void caused by abstaining from alcohol.*
- Encourage the family or significant others to support one another. *The physical and emotional burden associated with life-altering changes can be lightened if shared among many people who are meaningful to the client.*
- Promote sharing of experiences between the client and others who are further ahead in their recovery. *Role models who are dealing with similar issues can motivate and encourage the client.*

Health-Seeking Behavior: Abstinence From Alcohol related to a desire to manage a chronic, fatal disease
Expected Outcome: The client will formulate a plan for attaining and maintaining sobriety.

- Provide the locations of AA meetings. *Knowing the locations and times of meetings allows the client to make personal choices in pursuing his or her recovery.*
- Explain that a sponsor may be selected from among those who attend AA meetings. *A sponsor provides social and emotional support throughout recovery.*
- Recommend that the client begin reading the "Big Book" of AA. *This book describes the traditional 12 steps that lead to recovery.*
- Prepare the client for possible relapse by role-playing situations that may entice him or her to drink. *Role-playing helps the client prepare for possible barriers to recovery and provides an opportunity to simulate methods for dealing with them.*

Evaluation of Expected Outcomes

Vital signs are stable, and symptoms of withdrawal are controlled. The client eats a well-balanced diet and sleeps an adequate number of hours per night. The client demonstrates a willingness to cope with losses associated with overcoming dependence on alcohol. He or she also moves forward with measures to remain sober, such as participating in AA.

● NICOTINE DEPENDENCE

Nicotine, the stimulant drug in tobacco, is the most heavily used addictive, mood-altering substance in the United States. The drug is absorbed by inhaling the tobacco in cigarettes, cigars, and pipes, or through the mucous membranes of the mouth from loose tobacco. Smoking raises carbon monoxide levels in the blood and causes constriction of peripheral blood vessels. It disrupts the structure of alveoli, causing them to become overstretched and inelastic. It is implicated in the development and recurrence of gastric ulcers. Smokeless tobacco (chewing tobacco) exposes the oral cavity to carcinogens, inhaled tobacco targets the lungs and distant organs, and cigars or pipes repeatedly expose the oral cavity and esophagus to harmful substances.

Although nicotine causes disease and dysfunction throughout the body, U.S. society condones and even endorses tobacco use. Although smoking and tobacco use have decreased in recent decades, approximately 25% of adults use tobacco. Estimates of associated medical costs are $53 billion annually. Passive absorption of smoke also can cause disease in nonsmokers.

Nicotine produces tolerance, resulting in increased use over time and withdrawal symptoms when use is discontinued. Users light up or chew to maintain blood and brain levels; nicotine is then distributed throughout the body, metabolized in the liver, and excreted by the kidneys. Frequency of tobacco use also is governed by conditioned, learned responses, meaning that past patterns of use reinforce the habit of smoking. This factor is important, in that smoking cessation strategies must target both the physical dependence and the conditioned related behaviors.

Consequences

Smoking is responsible for 90% of deaths from lung cancer, 90% of deaths from chronic obstructive lung disease, 35% of all cancer deaths, and 21% of all deaths from coronary artery disease (Munzer, 1997). Tobacco contains more than 40 carcinogenic chemicals. It is the major cause of oropharyngeal cancers and contributes to cerebrovascular disease, peripheral vascular disease, and cancers of the urinary tract, esophagus, and pancreas.

Breathing **environmental tobacco smoke** (also called *secondhand smoke* or *passive smoke*), the smoke given off by the burning end of a cigarette, pipe, or cigar and the exhaled smoke from the lungs of a smoker, is potentially injurious to others. *Epidemiologists,* scientists who study the incidence and causation of illnesses, have identified that breathing secondhand smoke causes headaches and eye, nose, and throat irritation. Nonsmokers exposed to environmental tobacco smoke have increased rates of heart disease, lung and other types of cancer, and lower respiratory infections. Risk of sudden infant death syndrome is increased among infants whose mothers smoked throughout the pregnancy and after delivery. Children with asthma have an increased frequency of and more severe attacks when exposed to an environment with passive smoke.

Medical Management

All smokers and tobacco users are advised to quit and provided with materials that inform them of methods to do so. Various levels of intervention are available and include minimal approaches such as brief counseling and follow-up, or more intense measures such as enrollment in behavior modification programs. These programs help clients manage temptation and extinguish preconditioned cues to smoke. They also provide rewards for goal achievement. Pharmacologic therapy using nicotine substitutes (gum, patch, inhaler; see Drug Therapy Table 17-1 and Chap. 7), which are gradually tapered and stopped, helps clients avoid withdrawal symptoms and is an adjunct to other interventions.

Relapse is common, and only 10% to 15% of smokers who quit remain tobacco free for 1 year. Attempts to quit, however, are a predictor for eventual success; 60% of those who try and fail do ultimately succeed.

Nursing Management

Nurses help clients who smoke by counseling them to quit and providing them with information on various smoking cessation programs. Nurturing the client's belief that he or she can be successful is an important supportive measure. Because many clients fear gaining weight after smoking cessation, the nurse informs them that typical weight gain in the year after cessation is 9 to 10 lbs. The nurse then helps the client plan strategies to offset the tendency for weight gain, such as beginning a walking program, substituting fruits for high-calorie desserts, and reducing dietary fat. Sucking on sugarless hard candy or sugarless chewing gum also may help by keeping the client's mouth busy without adding calories. If the client is unwilling to contemplate quitting, the nurse informs him or her of the dangers of passive smoke to others and encourages abstinence from smoking in the presence of nonsmokers, especially children. The nurse also actively promotes individual and community health by learning smoking cessation techniques and providing seminars to the public.

Based on recommendations from the U.S. Environmental Protection Agency, the nurse can advise nonsmokers on techniques for reducing the inhalation of passive smoke:

- Do not permit others to smoke in one's home or workplace.
- If smoking takes place in the home, increase ventilation by opening windows or using exhaust fans.
- Avoid riding in a car with someone who smokes; the small area contributes to a high concentration of toxic smoke, which increases exposure.

● COCAINE DEPENDENCE

Cocaine is a central nervous system (CNS) stimulant obtained from the leaves of the coca plant. The powder form of cocaine is snorted (inhaled through the nose) or dissolved and injected intravenously. Crack, a purified form of cocaine with a crystalline or rocklike appearance, is smoked either by placing it in a pipe or by sprinkling it onto or mixing it with tobacco or marijuana. Cocaine may be freebased, which reduces the drug to its purest form. The person then smokes freebased cocaine by sprinkling it onto a cigarette or inhaling it through a pipe. Freebased cocaine provides an intense physical experience as the drug is absorbed, more so than when it is taken by other routes. It also increases the risk of toxic effects and overdose reactions. Metabolism of cocaine, which is rapid, usually is followed by an intense craving to use the drug again. Cravings can recur months or years after abstinence.

Assessment Findings

Signs and Symptoms

Signs and symptoms of the drug's effect may be brief (see Table 17-1) because cocaine is fully metabolized in several minutes. Signs correlate with its route of administration and consequences of chronic use. For example, ulceration of the nasal mucosa and perforation of the nasal septum are found in those who snort cocaine. Needle marks are found along the pathways of veins in those who inject cocaine intravenously. Those who smoke or freebase may have burns on their faces, fingertips, or eyebrows from using or leaning over a lighted pipe. Smoking cocaine can cause a chronic cough and pulmonary congestion.

Clients who are addicted to cocaine often have a problem with **polydrug abuse,** abuse of more than one substance. It is common for them also to take sedative drugs such as alcohol, minor tranquilizers, barbiturates, and marijuana to offset their agitation and irritability.

Complications

Long-term abusers of cocaine experience anorexia, weight loss, memory impairment, personality and behavioral changes, paranoia, psychosis, and hallucinations. Medically, stimulant abuse can cause rapid and severe hypertension, cardiac dysrhythmias, seizures, cerebral hemorrhage (stroke), myocardial infarction (heart attack), and respiratory arrest. Some people who use cocaine experience bizarre skin sensations referred to as "cocaine bugs," which lead to scratching and scarring. Newborns also can experience withdrawal symptoms if their mothers have recently used cocaine.

Diagnostic Findings

Drug toxicology tests are done on blood and urine. Metabolites of cocaine can be found in urine up to 36 hours after its use. Other abused substances also are identified.

Medical Management and Rehabilitation

Cocaine toxicity (see Table 17-1) requires immediate treatment because the condition is life-threatening. Referral to Cocaine Anonymous, which is based on the same principles as AA, provides a source of ongoing support for those addicted to cocaine. Participation in individual and group psychotherapy and Cocaine Anonymous is encouraged to help the client eliminate all forms of drug abuse. The recreational use of other drugs can lead to relapse.

To help the person addicted to cocaine with recovery, medications like bromocriptine (Parlodel) and amantadine (Symmetrel) are used temporarily. They increase or mimic the effects of dopamine, the neurotransmitter that is most likely responsible for the rewarding and reinforcing effects of cocaine. Antidepressants are prescribed to relieve the dysphoria (depression) that occurs during withdrawal. Amino acid precursors such as phenylalanine and tyrosine, the substances from which the neurotransmitters norepinephrine and dopamine are made, are included in drug therapy to replace levels depleted by chronic use. Research is underway to develop a drug that can neutralize cocaine in the blood, thus reducing the amount available for brain uptake.

Nursing Management

The nurse assesses the client's history of drug use and his or her current physical condition. The nurse also looks for signs of toxicity and withdrawal. He or she implements medical treatment during a life-threatening emergency. Later, the nurse explains the effects of drug abuse and the risks for continuing drug-taking behaviors. Monitoring the client for suicidal ideation (see Chap. 15) and administering medications that provide support during withdrawal are essential nursing interventions.

● OPIATE DEPENDENCE

Opiate dependence is an addiction to CNS depressant drugs, narcotics, that are either derived from or chemically similar to opium. *Opioid* is a term for synthetic narcotics. Some examples of opiate drugs include heroin (diacetylmorphine), codeine, morphine, meperidine (Demerol), methadone, hydromorphone (Dilaudid), oxycodone, and opium as in tincture of paregoric. Opiates produce sedation after initial euphoria. The rate of tolerance and chemical dependence is related to the drug, dose, and frequency of use.

herion (?)

Assessment Findings

Refer to heroin in Table 17-1 for the effects of opiates. The pupils usually are pinpoint in size. Constipation is associated with slowed peristalsis. Chronic use is evidenced by anorexia, weight loss, constipation, malnutrition, needle marks, and scarring (tracks) along the paths of veins.

Respiratory depression can lead to unconsciousness and death. Sharing needles during the IV administration of any abused substance can lead to AIDS, hepatitis, and septicemia. Abscesses may develop in punctured skin and veins. General debilitation increases susceptibility to tuberculosis and anemia. Neonates in withdrawal are observed to have a high-pitched cry, tremors, insomnia, increased respirations, vomiting, diarrhea, dehydration, and convulsions.

A urine drug screen reveals evidence of opiate use. Rapid recovery (within 2 to 5 minutes) from lethargy, hypotension, and respiratory depression after the IV administration of a narcotic antagonist such as naloxone (Narcan) supports the diagnosis of narcotic overdose.

Medical Management and Rehabilitation

Withdrawal symptoms are treated with the alpha-adrenergic blocker clonidine (Catapres) to inhibit the release of norepinephrine. Methadone (Dolophine), a synthetic narcotic, may be used to eliminate or control withdrawal symptoms.

One method for helping those addicted to heroin avoid IV or street-supplied narcotics is methadone maintenance therapy. **Methadone maintenance** therapy involves substituting one addicting drug for another. The advantage is that because methadone is a synthetic drug prepared by a pharmaceutical company, the drug is untainted and the dose is reliable. The rationale behind methadone maintenance therapy is that it forestalls withdrawal, avoids a toxic overdose, reduces the potential for bloodborne infections, and theoretically reduces crime because the drug is provided legally. Some addicts, however, have been known to combine methadone with their depressant drug of choice, which increases the potential for overdose and death. The practice of testing the urine before providing methadone is one way of screening and eliminating those who are abusing the system.

Naltrexone (Trexan, ReVia) also is used for opiate addiction. If clients return to opiate abuse while taking naltrexone, they do not experience the previous level of opiate effects.

Psychotherapy is an important aspect of rehabilitation. It involves treating the complex web of social problems that accompanies the addiction. Clients also are referred to Narcotics Anonymous, a self-help organization modeled after AA.

Nursing Management

The nurse's role is similar to that discussed for other types of chemical dependence, with a few exceptions that apply to administering drug therapy. If naltrexone is prescribed, the client must be opiate free for at least 7 days before administration begins. The nurse advises the client who takes methadone to tell healthcare providers or wear a Medic Alert tag in case the client needs a narcotic, tranquilizer, or barbiturate. Because methadone is a narcotic, lower doses of other sedative drugs are necessary because the combination can potentiate their depressant action.

● OTHER ABUSED SUBSTANCES

Various other substances are abused and addictive. Some examples include hallucinogens, amphetamines, marijuana, barbiturates, tranquilizers, and volatile hydrocarbons. Signs and symptoms follow the same pattern as with previously discussed substances: experimental use progresses through stages of increased use until dependence and addiction occur; there is failure to meet social, familial, or occupational obligations with increased defensive mechanisms to explain behavior; disturbances in mood and physical function occur as the result of drug abuse. Treatment and recovery include withdrawal, abstinence, and ongoing enrollment in a support group.

GENERAL NUTRITIONAL CONSIDERATIONS

Nutritional interventions for alcoholism include correcting nutrient deficiencies and modifying the diet as needed for complications. Parenteral nutrition may be indicated for clients with acute pancreatitis; a low-fat diet may improve symptoms of chronic pancreatitis. Protein intake is adjusted for clients with acute and chronic liver disease.
Sodium and fluid restrictions are indicated for ascites.
A soft diet is used for esophageal varices.

GENERAL PHARMACOLOGIC CONSIDERATIONS

A reaction to disulfiram can occur up to 2 weeks after discontinuing the drug. Inform the client to avoid all forms of alcohol (e.g., cough syrups, elixirs) for at least 2 weeks after discontinuing the drug.
Used nicotine patches contain enough nicotine to cause serious adverse reactions in children. Advise clients to store nicotine gum out of children's reach.
Obtain a careful drug history from chemically dependent clients because these individuals tend to abuse multiple substances.

GENERAL GERONTOLOGIC CONSIDERATIONS

Alcoholism may be difficult to identify in the older adult because symptoms such as tremors, unsteady gait, or memory loss mimic changes associated with aging.
Older adults who drink alcohol exhibit greater impairment than younger adults and recover more slowly.
Prolonged use of alcohol can result in neurologic deficits such as confusion, ataxia, and loss of cognitive ability.
Older adults may abuse over-the-counter and prescription drugs rather than illicit drugs.
Acute alcohol withdrawal in older adults is serious and may be life-threatening.
Administration of disulfiram to older adults requires caution. This drug interferes with the actions of several drugs (e.g., warfarin, nitroglycerin) that are often a part of the older adult's medication regimen.

Critical Thinking Exercises

1. *What information would you offer to a smoker who claims that "smoke-free environments" violate his or her right to smoke?*
2. *From which type of substance could a person be withdrawing if the following assessments are made? The person has a runny nose and tearing eyes. Frequent yawning is observed.*

The pilomotor muscles around hair follicles produce the appearance of "goose bumps." The person is experiencing nausea, vomiting, abdominal cramps, and diarrhea.

References and Suggested Readings

Bulthius, D. & Dmaz, J. E. (2000). Ultrarapid opiate detoxification. *Annals of Emergency Medicine, 35,* 100–101.
Compton, P. & McCaffery, M. (2001). Controlling pain: Treating acute pain in addicted patients. *Nursing, 31*(1), 17.
Cowen, M. S. & Lawrence, A. J. (1999). The role of opioid-dopamine interactions in the induction and maintenance of ethanol consumption. *Progress in Neuropsychopharmacology and Biological Psychiatry, 23,* 1171–1210.
Henderson-Martin, B. (2000). No more surprises: Screening patients for alcohol abuse. *American Journal of Nursing, 100*(9), 26–33.
Hill, S. Y., Zezza, N., Wipprecht, G., et al. (1999). Linkage studies of D2 and D4 receptor genes and alcoholism. *American Journal of Medical Genetics, 88,* 676–685.
Li, T. (2000). Pharmacogenetics of responses to alcohol and genes that influence alcohol drinking. *Journal of Studies on Alcohol, 61*(1), 5–12.
Mannino, D. M., Moorman, J. E., Kingsley, B., et al. (2001). Health effects related to environmental tobacco smoke exposure in children in the United States. *Archives of Pediatrics and Adolescent Medicine, 155,* 36–41.
McGee, E. M. (2000). Alcoholics Anonymous and nursing: Lessons in holism and spiritual care. *Journal of Holistic Nursing, 18*(1), 6–26.
Munzer, A. (1997). Smoking and smoking cessations. In W. Kelley (Ed.), *Textbook of internal medicine.* Philadelphia: Lippincott-Raven.
National Center for Chronic Disease Prevention and Health Promotion. Office on Smoking and Health. (2000). Reducing tobacco use. A report of the Surgeon General–2000. (On-line.) Available: http://www.cdc.gov/tobacco/.
Noble, E. P. (1996). The gene that rewards alcoholism. *Scientific American Science and Medicine, 3*(2), 52–61.
Olms, D. (1983). *The disease concept of alcoholism.* Belleville, IL: Gary Whiteaker Company.
Powell, A. H. (2000). Alcohol withdrawal in critical care. *Nursing (Critical Care), 30*(8), 32cc1–32cc2, 32cc4, 32cc6–32cc7.
Ryan, L. A. & Ottlinger, A. (1999). Implementation of alcohol withdrawal program in a medical-surgical setting: Improving patient outcomes. *Journal of Addictions Nursing, 11*(3), 102–106.
Sachse, D. S. & Kearney, K. (2000). Emergency. Delirium tremens. *American Journal of Nursing, 100*(5), 41–42.
Schmidt, J. & Williams, E. (1999). When all else fails, try harm reduction. *American Journal of Nursing, 99*(10), 67–70.
Scott, C. M. & Popovich, D. J. (2001). Undiagnosed alcoholism and prescription drug misuse among the elderly: Special considerations for home assessment. *Caring, 20*(1), 20–25.
Stein, R. T., Holberg, C. J., Sherrill, D., et al. (1999). Influence of parental smoking on respiratory symptoms during the first decade of life. *American Journal of Epidemiology, 149,* 1030–1037.
Stewart, K. B. & Richards, A. B. (2000). Recognizing and managing your patient's alcohol abuse. *Nursing, 30*(2), 56–59.

Caring for Clients With Dementia and Thought Disorders

Words to Know

acalculia
acetylcholine
agnosia
agraphia
alexia
Alzheimer's disease
aphasia
apraxia
ataxia
beta amyloid
cognitive functions
conservatorship
delirium
delusions
dementia
depot injections
durable power of
    attorney
extrapyramidal
    symptoms
guardianship
hallucinations
homocysteine
incompetent
mentation
negative symptoms
neuritic plaques
neurofibrillary tangles
positive symptoms
prions
respite care
restraint alternatives
schizophrenia
voice dismissal

Learning Objectives

On completion of this chapter, the reader will:

- Differentiate between delirium and dementia, and give an example of a condition that causes each.
- List five etiologic factors linked to Alzheimer's disease.
- Name four pathologic changes associated with Alzheimer's disease.
- Name the first symptom of Alzheimer's disease.
- Identify two methods for diagnosing Alzheimer's disease.
- Explain the mechanism of drug therapy in Alzheimer's disease.
- Describe the focus of nursing management when caring for clients with Alzheimer's disease.
- List six nursing diagnoses common to clients with Alzheimer's disease.
- Give three characteristics of schizophrenia.
- Describe two psychobiologic explanations for schizophrenia.
- Differentiate between positive and negative symptoms of schizophrenia, and give two examples of each.
- Discuss the medical management of most people with schizophrenia.
- Name three examples of antipsychotic drugs and their mechanisms of action.
- Explain the term *extrapyramidal symptoms,* and list four examples.
- Describe a technique to prevent noncompliance with drug therapy in clients with schizophrenia.
- Summarize the nursing management of clients with schizophrenia.
- List five nursing diagnoses common to clients with schizophrenia.

Changes in **mentation,** mental activity, can occur anytime during the life cycle. **Cognitive functions,** such as short-term memory and learning ability, change gradually as people get older, but many acute, chronic, reversible, and irreversible conditions that impair thinking processes can occur at any age. Although older adults are at greatest risk for cognitive impairment, one should never assume that such impairment is necessarily a normal consequence of aging, nor that it is untreatable. Depression and other medical disorders, such as hypothyroidism, can manifest as mental dysfunction. Consequently, mental changes re-

quire aggressive investigation to determine what, if anything, can reverse the symptoms that clients experience.

DELIRIUM AND DEMENTIA

Delirium is a sudden, transient state of confusion. The period of confusion depends on the cause of the delirium. Clients with delirium may have difficulty processing information. They may be disoriented as to the date, time

175

of day, and location. Their judgment may be impaired, or they may be unable to perform intellectually at the same capacity as in the past. Some clients with delirium may be suspicious or frightened or behave inappropriately.

Delirium can result from high fever, head trauma, brain tumor, drug intoxication or withdrawal, metabolic disorders (e.g., liver or renal failure), or inflammatory disorders of the central nervous system (CNS), such as meningitis or encephalitis. Treating the underlying medical condition usually restores mental functions.

Dementia, which more commonly affects older adults, refers to conditions in which decline in memory and other mental functions is severe enough to affect the daily life of an alert person (Small et al., 1997). Various disorders are characterized by dementia. Alzheimer's disease is the leading example, followed by cerebrovascular disorders (see Chap. 46) and Parkinson's disease (see Chap. 45). In contrast to delirium, dementia is manifested by a gradual, irreversible loss of intellectual abilities. Although clients with dementia display signs and symptoms similar to those of delirium, several differences exist (Table 18-1).

Stop, Think, and Respond ● BOX 18-1

In the descriptions that follow, which client is manifesting delirium, and which is manifesting dementia?

Client A is 60 years of age. He developed a headache and high fever 24 hours ago. When he is aroused, he thinks he is in the city in which he spent his boyhood. He calls for his mother who has been dead for more than 10 years.

Client B is 60 years old. He got lost driving home from work last week. Lately he has had difficulty remembering where he put his keys and wallet. His wife feels he is more argumentative than usual.

TABLE 18-1	COMPARISON OF DEMENTIA AND DELIRIUM
DEMENTIA	**DELIRIUM**
Onset	
Gradual	Sudden
Presentation	
Alert	Blunted
Attentive	Inattentive
Course	
Stable	Unstable
Progressive deterioration	Fluctuations in function
Extended	Brief
Duration	
Permanent	Temporary
Treatment	
Symptomatic or supportive	Specific
Outcome	
Incurable	Curable

ALZHEIMER'S DISEASE

Alzheimer's disease is a progressive, deteriorating brain disorder. Two types exist: early onset (before age 60 years) and late onset (after age 60 years), with late onset being more common. As many as 30% of all adults older than 85 years of age manifest Alzheimer's disease (Small et al., 1997).

Pathophysiology and Etiology

Having a first-degree relative with Alzheimer's disease nearly doubles the risk for acquiring this form of dementia. Inherited genetic abnormalities on chromosomes 14, 19, and 21 have been associated with early-onset Alzheimer's disease. One theory suggests a defective gene (ApoE4) causes weakness in the neuronal cell membranes. This weakness stimulates an immune system response that results in excess **beta amyloid,** a starchy component that accumulates in the brains of clients with Alzheimer's. Beta amyloid injures neurons in the area of the brain responsible for producing **acetylcholine,** the neurotransmitter that is critical for memory and cognition (Lombard & Germano, 1997). Elevated levels of **homocysteine,** an amino acid created during the metabolism of protein, also have been shown to impair memory. Other theories of causation include aluminum toxicity leached from cooking utensils and metal food containers; mercury absorption from the metal amalgam used in dental fillings (Kranhold, 2001); and infection by **prions,** small proteins that cause neurologic diseases like bovine spongiform encephalopathy (mad cow disease) in animals and Creutzfeldt-Jakob disease, a form of dementia, in humans (Prusiner, 1998) (see Chap. 19).

In dementia of the Alzheimer's type, four pathologic changes occur in the brain:

1. The size of the cortex decreases.
2. The neurotransmitter acetylcholine is deficient, especially in the cortex and hippocampus.
3. **Neuritic plaques,** deposits of beta amyloid and degenerating nerve cells, are found.
4. **Neurofibrillary tangles,** twisted bundles of nerve fibers (Fig. 18-1), appear.

The decreased size of the cerebral cortex along with acetylcholine deficiency explain the cognitive deficits and alterations in emotions that accompany the disease. The degree to which plaque and tangles are present is directly related to the severity of disease manifestations.

Assessment Findings

Signs and Symptoms

Alzheimer's disease progresses through seven distinct stages that correspond with those identified in the Global

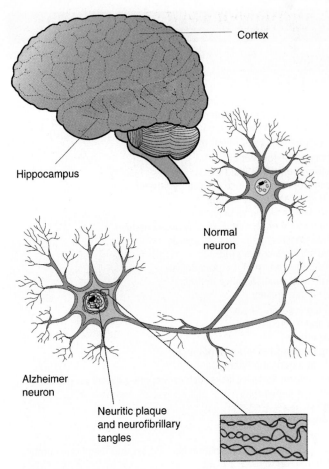

FIGURE 18-1 Neurofibrillary tangling and neuritic plaques in Alzheimer's disease.

Deterioration Scale (Table 18-2). Progression from one stage to another can occur at different rates among affected individuals. The early stages may last 2 to 4 years or longer; it may take as long as 5 to 10 years before a person needs constant care.

Onset usually is insidious, and symptoms may develop slowly over years. Memory loss, the classic symptom, is confined at first to recent information. Eventually, long-term memory and the ability to make appropriate judgments and problem-solve become impaired as well. Disturbances in behavior, personality changes, and depression also occur. As the disease advances, memory, cognition, awareness, and the ability to care for self deteriorate markedly. Clients may wander and become lost. Periodic incidences of violent behavior are possible. Problems with speaking (**aphasia**), reading (**alexia**), writing (**agraphia**), and calculating (**acalculia**) develop. Inability to recognize objects and sounds (visual, tactile, and auditory **agnosia**), difficulty walking (**ataxia**), and tremors occur. In the final stage of the disease, an inability to accomplish activities of daily living (ADLs; **apraxia**), such as grooming, toileting, and eating, despite intact motor function, makes the client totally dependent on others.

Diagnostic Findings

Ruling out Alzheimer's disease in clients who are experiencing similar signs and symptoms can spare them emotional agony, as well as saving time and money spent on nonspecific tests. The diagnosis of Alzheimer's usually is made by excluding other causes for the client's symptoms. A computed tomography (CT) scan shows shrinking of the cerebral cortex, but this is not apparent in the early stages of the disease. Positron emission tomography (PET) and magnetic resonance imaging (MRI) provide structural and metabolic information about the brain. Electroencephalography detects slower-than-normal brain waves. None of these diagnostic tests is specific for Alzheimer's disease, which until recently could be confirmed only during a postmortem examination of the brain. A new diagnostic test called Nymox AD7C detects evidence of beta amyloid protein in cerebrospinal fluid.

Medical Management

No cure exists for Alzheimer's disease; treatment is mainly supportive using one of various drugs currently available. Although maintaining the client's independence in the familiar environment of his or her home for as long as possible is best, the physician continues to assess the client's safety and burden on caregivers. Eventually, clients may be referred to an extended care facility, many of which have a unit dedicated to the care of clients with Alzheimer's or other forms of dementia.

Current drugs approved for the treatment of dementia of the Alzheimer's type include cholinesterase inhibitors like tacrine (Cognex), donepezil (Aricept), and galantamine hydrobromide (Reminyl; Drug Therapy Table 18-1). These drugs increase acetylcholine by inhibiting cholinesterase, the enzyme that degrades it. When administered in the early to middle stages of Alzheimer's disease, some clients improve, some stay the same, some progress more slowly, and some fail to respond. All clients eventually get worse over time.

One new drug, memantine, is in clinical trials. Memantine's mechanism of action is different from the cholinesterase inhibitors. Memantine is a neuroprotective drug classified as an *N*-methyl-D-aspartate (NMDA) antagonist. By blocking NMDA receptors, the drug protects neurons from excessive stimulation by glutamate, an excitatory neurotransmitter responsible for neuronal death. Clients in advanced stages of Alzheimer's disease experienced less deterioration when taking memantine than others who were given a placebo (Merz Pharmaceuticals, 2002).

Working from the premise that high homocysteine levels interfere with memory, some physicians also are prescribing folic acid (folate) supplements. Folate low-

TABLE 18-2	GLOBAL DETERIORATION SCALE	
STAGE	**CHARACTERISTIC**	**MANIFESTATIONS**
1	Normal mentation	None
2	Forgetfulness	Concern for self-identified memory changes such as forgetting location of items, forgetting familiar names No objective demonstration of memory deficit No social consequences for minor memory loss

3	Early confusion	One or more of the following:
		    getting lost in an unfamiliar location
		    decline in work performance noticed by others
		    deficit in word and name finding
		    little retention of what has been read
		    difficulty remembering names of new acquaintances
		    loss or misplacement of valuable objects
		    impaired ability to concentrate
		Objective demonstration of memory deficit
		Denial of memory and cognitive deficits
		Mild to moderate anxiety

4	Late confusion	Deficits in the following areas:
		    current and recent events
		    personal history
		    counting backward in series of numbers
		    traveling and handling finances
		Inability to perform complex tasks such as preparing dinner for guests
		Strong denial of impairment
		Blunted affect
		Retreat from challenges

5	Early dementia	Assistance of others needed Memory loss for important information like address and telephone number Some disorientation to time or place Difficulty counting backward by 4s or 2s May have difficulty choosing proper clothing

6	Middle dementia	May forget name of spouse or significant others
		Unaware of recent events and experiences
		Memory of past sketchy
		Unaware of date and surroundings
		Difficulty counting backward and sometimes forward in 10s
		Requires assistance with activities of daily living
		May be incontinent
		Needs assistance to travel
		Confuses day and night
		Personality and emotional changes such as:
		    delusional thinking
		    repetition of cleaning
		    anxiety, agitation, violence
		    cannot keep a thought long enough to carry it out

7	Late dementia	Loss of verbal ability Grunting may be evident Incontinent; requires help with toileting and feeding Loss of motor skills for walking, sitting, head control, and smiling

Adapted from Reisberg, B., Ferris, S. H., Leon, J. J., & Crook, T. (1982). The global deterioration scale (GDS): An instrument for the assessment of primary degenerative dementia. *American Journal of Psychiatry, 139*, 1136–1139.

ers homocysteine levels; in one study, clients who received folate supplements were better able to recall recent information (Landry, 1998). Because high levels of homocysteine have been correlated with cardiovascular and cerebrovascular disease, some claim that the positive results observed in clients with Alzheimer's are merely the consequence of treating the coexisting cerebrovascular pathology.

Antidepressants or tranquilizers may help agitated or depressed clients.

DRUG THERAPY TABLE 18-1	ALZHEIMER'S DISEASE		
DRUG CATEGORY AND EXAMPLES	MECHANISM OF ACTION	SIDE EFFECTS	NURSING CONSIDERATIONS
Cholinesterase Inhibitor *tacrine (Cognex)*	Provides for increased levels of acetylcholine in the cortex by inhibiting cholinesterase, the enzyme that breaks down acetylcholine	Headache, fatigue, confusion, seizures, dizziness, nausea, vomiting, diarrhea, gastrointestinal upset, abdominal pain, loss of appetite, skin rashes, hepatotoxicity	Administer on an empty stomach on an around-the-clock schedule. Do not abruptly discontinue. Arrange for regular blood tests to determine aminotransferase levels. Inform client and family of side effects and to report any that occur. Tell client to exercise caution if performing tasks that require alertness.
donepezil (Aricept)	Inhibits the breakdown of acetylcholine	Nausea, vomiting, diarrhea, bradycardia, possible exacerbations of asthma and chronic obstructive pulmonary disease, muscle cramps, loss of appetite	Tell client that frequent small meals may minimize gastrointestinal upset. Monitor heart rate, and report bradycardia (heart rate <60 beats per minute).
galantamine hydrobromide (Reminyl)	Increases concentration of acetylcholine by blocking action of acetylcholinesterase	Nausea, vomiting, anorexia, diarrhea, weight loss	Tell client to take drug at morning and evening meals.
N-Methyl-D-Aspartate (NMDA) Antagonist *memantine*	Blocks NMDA receptors		

Nursing Management

The major focus of nursing management is to help the client and caregiver maintain the highest possible quality of life by supporting mental and physical functions and ensuring safety. Most clients initially receive care in their homes, and home health nurses can instruct the family about physical care, the disease process, and treatment. They also provide emotional support and intervene if family caregivers become overburdened. When transfer of the client from the home to an extended care facility becomes necessary, the nurse meets the client's physical needs on a full-time basis and helps the family cope during the client's deterioration (see Client and Family Teaching Box 18-1 and Nursing Care Plan 18-1).

SCHIZOPHRENIA

Schizophrenia is a thought disorder characterized by deterioration in mental functioning, disturbances in sensory perception, and changes in affect (emotion). Clients with schizophrenia improve with drug therapy but, unfortunately, never fully recover. Because the condition is lifelong and appears in young adulthood, it causes considerable anguish for families who must deal with both the burden of healthcare costs and the responsibility for caring for a loved one with this illness.

Pathophysiology and Etiology

Schizophrenia, historically attributed to emotional dysfunction, is now categorized as a psychobiologic disease because of recent findings in brain and neurotransmitter chemistry. Many neurotransmitter imbalances are involved in schizophrenia. Dopamine excess is believed to be

(text continued on page 184)

18-1 *Client and Family Teaching* Cognitive Disorders

The nurse helps the family cope by teaching about the client's illness, the treatment plan, and prognosis:

- Encourage the family to be supportive and involved, while allowing the client to remain as independent as possible.
- Give the family a referral to a social worker and crisis telephone numbers.
- Direct the family to local community mental health associations and support groups.

Nursing Care Plan 18-1

THE CLIENT WITH ALZHEIMER'S DISEASE

Assessment

■ Interview both client and family because the client may be unable to give a complete or objective history regarding memory, sleep patterns, moods, and self-care activities. Assess the caregiver's strengths, limitations, and ability to manage caretaking activities.

■ Perform a complete head-to-toe physical examination. Be especially attentive to muscular strength, balance, and gait.

■ Determine the client's mental status. Identify level of orientation, short-term and long-term memory, social behavior, emotional status, cognitive and motor skills, and ability to perform ADLs.

Nursing Diagnosis: **Caregiver Role Strain** related to being overwhelmed by responsibilities, fatigue, and depression

Expected Outcome: Caregiver will experience less anxiety as knowledge about implementing plans that will provide needed relief increases.

Interventions	Rationales
Assess caregiver's strengths, limitations, and ability to manage caretaking activities.	The spouse (who is the usual caretaker) may experience sleep deprivation, physical injury, and social isolation if no one else is available to assist with client care.
Suggest scheduling **respite care,** brief relief from caretaking responsibilities, with family and friends on a regular rotating basis.	Dividing caretaking responsibilities promotes physical endurance and emotional stability.
Provide a list of agencies that offer social services such as the county's commission on aging and Social Security and Medicare agencies.	Clients may be unaware of services available for assistance or how to contact them.
Develop a list of people to contact in an emergency, including a 24-hour hotline for the home health nursing agency.	Having a plan helps clients obtain assistance in a crisis.
Recommend that caregiver and client take care of legal matters such as wills, transferring titles, and preparing an advanced directive (see Chap. 26).	Attending to legal matters before severe cognitive changes occur is best.
Suggest establishing **durable power of attorney,** designating who may make decisions regarding finances or healthcare when the client becomes **incompetent,** the legal term for the inability to understand the risks or benefits of decisions.	Such measures ensure that the client's spouse or caretaker has access to unencumbered funds and follows the client's wishes regarding healthcare decisions.
Advise caregiver to obtain **guardianship** or **conservatorship,** court-appointed responsibility, for managing the client's care and assets if the client already is incompetent.	The client's financial assets may be frozen unless the court stipulates that another person can have access to private accounts.
Encourage the caregiver to temporarily place the client in a long-term nursing facility to take a well-deserved vacation.	Giving the caregiver a temporary option for a vacation may help to sustain his or her ability to continue caring for the client.

Evaluation of Expected Outcomes:

■ Caregiver seeks relief from responsibilities at least 1 or 2 days a week.

■ Caregiver and client take care of legal issues.

(continued)

Nursing Care Plan 18-1 *(Continued)*

THE CLIENT WITH ALZHEIMER'S DISEASE

Nursing Diagnosis: **Risk for Interrupted Family Processes** related to guilt over placing the client in a care facility

Expected Outcome: Family will remain united and supportive over the decision to transfer the client's care to others.

Interventions	Rationales
Acknowledge and empathize with the family's ambivalent feelings.	Family is more likely to accept transfer of the client's care if the nurse demonstrates empathy.
Emphasize skills and services that the facility provides.	Knowledge that the facility offers many services to promote and maintain the client's well-being enhances acceptance of the decision.
Let the family participate in developing and revising the plan of care.	Family participation promotes a team approach to managing the client's care.
Keep the family informed of the client's progress or lack thereof.	Communication often is the key to good interpersonal relationships.
Encourage the family to visit and participate in the client's care as much as they want.	Promoting continued interactions conveys a sense that family is included rather than excluded from the client's life.
Allow the family privacy during interactions with the client, and make an area available to them for special occasions like birthdays.	Making special accommodations for family activities individualizes care.
Keep a current list of family phone numbers, listing the relationships of members to the client and indications for which they prefer to be called.	Accurate information is important when communication is necessary.
Prepare the family for the client's likely deterioration.	Realistic preparation for the progression of the disease promotes anticipatory grieving and acceptance of the client's potentially terminal condition.

Evaluation of Expected Outcomes:

■ Family members reconcile themselves to the difficult decision to transfer the care of the client to a nursing care facility.

■ They remain involved in the client's care and understand the changes that accompany the disease process.

Nursing Diagnosis: **Impaired Memory** related to global cognitive deficits

Expected Outcome: Client will be reoriented and participate in life experiences to his or her potential.

Interventions	Rationales
Orient client frequently to person, place, and time.	Frequent reminders accommodate for impairment in memory.
Place a large-faced clock and calendars at multiple places in the client's environment.	External clues help the client maintain orientation or become oriented with minimal effort.
Assign consistent caregivers, and maintain a structured daily routine.	Repetition and consistency reduce episodes of confusion.
Attach something the client can recognize to the door of his or her room.	The client is more likely to find his or her room by looking for a familiar clue like his or her name printed in large letters or a brightly colored bow.

(continued)

Nursing Care Plan 18-1 *(Continued)*

THE CLIENT WITH ALZHEIMER'S DISEASE

Interventions	Rationales
Make sure the client wears an identification bracelet with an address and telephone number.	Clients with Alzheimer's disease are known to wander and not recall their current residence.
Maintain a current photograph in the medical record.	Having the means to identify the client aids in search-and-rescue efforts.

Evaluation of Expected Outcome: Client becomes reoriented with techniques such as verbal reminders and environmental clues like a large-faced clock and calendar and can participate in activities that occur at consistent times throughout the day.

Nursing Diagnosis: **Risk for Trauma** related to ataxia and propensity for wandering

Expected Outcome: Client will move about freely and safely in the healthcare facility but will not leave the facility unsupervised.

Interventions	Rationales
Help the client don supportive walking shoes when out of bed.	Supportive shoes promote a stable gait and posture.
Provide assistance with ambulation. Remove hazards, such as foot stools, small tables, or liquid spills, from the ambulatory area.	Assistance reduces the potential for falls. Removing obstacles and slippery surfaces promotes safer ambulation.
Keep the environment well lighted.	The ability to see helps the client avoid environmental hazards.
Maintain the bed in low position.	Should a fall occur, the bed's low position reduces the potential for serious injury.
Use **restraint alternatives,** protective or adaptive devices for fall protection and postural support.	Physical restraints increase the potential for injury; clients have the right to the least restrictive intervention.
Place a bed monitor under the client's mattress.	Bed monitors alert caregivers when a client gets out of bed without signaling for assistance.
Install alarms on exit doors, and respond immediately when one sounds.	An alarm alerts caregivers when someone leaves who is unauthorized to do so.

Evaluation of Expected Outcomes:

■ No injuries occur.

■ The client's whereabouts are known at all times.

Nursing Diagnosis: **Disturbed Sleep Pattern** related to confusion between day and night

Expected Outcome: Client will sleep uninterrupted for at least 6 hours or return to sleep after awakening during the night.

Interventions	Rationales
Keep client active during daytime hours, but avoid excessive fatigue.	Remaining awake during daytime hours helps enhance normal circadian rhythm.
Restrict consumption of coffee, tea, and cola.	Caffeine, a CNS stimulant, interferes with sleep.
Make sure that the room is comfortably warm or cool and that the client has urinated and satisfied his or her thirst just before bedtime.	Meeting basic comfort needs promotes sleep once the client retires for the night.

(continued)

Nursing Care Plan 18-1 (Continued)

THE CLIENT WITH ALZHEIMER'S DISEASE

Interventions	*Rationales*
Dim the lights and reduce unnecessary noise.	A darkened environment increases production of melatonin, which promotes sleep; a quiet environment reduces stimulation of the cerebral cortex.
Provide a lighted clock at the bedside.	A clock provides an environmental clue as to whether it is time to sleep or awaken.
Redirect the client gently, but firmly, to return to bed if nighttime wandering occurs.	Caregivers help reinforce appropriate behavior.

Evaluation of Expected Outcome: Client returns to bed after awakening and wandering and sleeps until an appropriate time for the day's activities.

Nursing Diagnosis: **Impaired Verbal Communication** related to expressive or receptive aphasia

Expected Outcome: Client will communicate with healthcare professional at whatever level is possible.

Interventions	*Rationales*
Approach from the front, make eye contact, and look for a response to your voice.	Obtaining the client's attention promotes verbal interaction.
Get the client's attention by using the name to which he or she is most likely to respond.	Using a client's name increases cognitive awareness and potential for social interaction.
Keep explanations or directions short and simple.	Being succinct makes it easier for the client to process information and respond appropriately.
Give gentle reminders or model the desired response.	Reminding and modeling compensate for failing memory or loss of language skills.
Involve client in one idea or task at a time.	Keeping ideas and tasks to a minimum promotes attention and concentration.
Reduce environmental stimuli like noise and activity.	Excess stimulation interferes with attention and concentration and may agitate the client.
Promote interactions that tap into the client's long-term memory such as reminiscing; offer client verbal cues such as, "I understand you were . . . (a school teacher)."	Long-term memory is retained more than short-term memory; recalling information promotes social interaction and elevates self-esteem.
Give client plenty of time to respond to questions. Try to understand what client wants to convey.	Impaired language skills make communication more difficult.
Repeat information that you believe the client is trying to communicate.	Rephrasing or paraphrasing helps ensure accurate interpretation of the client's thoughts.
Include client in small group activities, even if there is little or no socialization.	Despite the appearance of being uninvolved, participation may stimulate the client's awareness.
Change activities or distract the client if he or she becomes angry, hostile, or uncooperative.	The nurse is responsible for ensuring the safety of the client, other clients, and staff.

Evaluation of Expected Outcome: Client understands spoken works and responds verbally.

the major cause of the symptoms, with imbalances of nor-epinephrine, serotonin (5-HT), and gamma-aminobutyric acid (GABA; see Chap. 12) also playing a role. The disease is known to have a familial or genetic component. Other theories suggest that the anatomic and physiologic changes associated with schizophrenia result from a viral infection experienced by the affected individual's mother during pregnancy. The neurochemical imbalance produces a variety of manifestations characterized by disturbed thinking, with themes that may include suspiciousness; persecution; being controlled; grandiosity (belief in one's importance); religious fixation; or preoccupation with sex, a love interest, illness, or a body part.

Assessment Findings

Symptoms usually begin during late adolescence to early adulthood. Clients manifest a range of symptoms categorized as positive or negative. **Positive symptoms** include delusions, hallucinations, and fluent but disorganized speech. **Negative symptoms,** sometimes called *defect symptoms,* are marked by impoverished speech and an inability to enjoy relationships or express emotions (Box 18-1). Positive symptoms are more easily managed than negative symptoms. Classic symptoms are inexplicable sensory experiences such as hearing voices or seeing apparitions of people who are not there. These occur in combination with peculiar patterns of speaking and odd motor behaviors. The client also tends to abandon rela-tionships and interactions with others and loses motivation for working, going to school, or engaging in other goal-driven behaviors. Hygiene and appearance tend to lose their previous importance.

The diagnosis is made primarily on the symptomatology and by ruling out other possible causes. CT and PET scans, MRIs, and brain mapping (see Chap. 12) may show decreased brain size and activity, especially in the frontal and temporal lobes.

Medical Management

Clients with schizophrenia are referred to the care of psychiatrists. Once the client is in the mental health system, every effort is made to avoid institutionalization. The exception is when the client is dangerous to self or others. In general, community mental health services are selected that meet the client's needs for psychotherapy, drug administration, and social needs, such as housing, job assistance, and money management, in an outpatient setting.

Antipsychotic drugs are the mainstay of treatment. These drugs, also called *major tranquilizers* or *neuroleptics,* belong to several different chemical families, but all block receptors for dopamine. Some examples of antipsychotic drugs are haloperidol (Haldol), fluphenazine (Prolixin), risperidone (Risperdal), clozapine (Clozaril), and olanzapine (Zyprexa; Drug Therapy Table 18-2).

Risperidone, clozapine, and olanzapine, newer drugs called *atypical antipsychotics,* produce their effects with reduced incidence of **extrapyramidal symptoms** (EPS), movement disorders associated with traditional drugs (Box 18-2). Clozapine, however, has the potential adverse effect of dangerously depressing bone marrow function, and clients who take clozapine must undergo a weekly blood count. If the client's white blood cell count drops too low, the drug is discontinued. Anticholinergic drugs such as trihexyphenidyl (Artane) and benztropine (Cogentin) are given to prevent or relieve EPS. Antipsychotics sometimes are combined with anticonvulsant drugs such as clonazepam (Klonopin) and carbamazepine (Tegretol).

Noncompliance with drug therapy is the leading cause for the return of disease symptoms and the need for short-term hospitalization. For this reason, some nonhospitalized clients are given depot injections, intramuscular injections of antipsychotic drugs in an oil suspension that are gradually absorbed over 2 to 4 weeks.

BOX 18-1 ● **Positive and Negative Symptoms of Schizophrenia**

POSITIVE

Delusions, false beliefs that cannot be changed by logical reasoning

Hallucinations, sensory experiences that others do not perceive; can be auditory, visual, tactile, olfactory, or gustatory (involving taste)

Loose associations, a sequence of ideas that are slightly connected

Inappropriate affect, a display of emotional feeling inconsistent with the situation

Peculiarities in speech like *echolalia,* repeating what others say; *rhyming; word salad,* using unrelated words in a sentence; or *neologisms,* inventing new words

Bizarre behavior such as *stereotopy* (repetitive movement) and *echopraxia* (mimicking the movements of others)

NEGATIVE

Concrete thinking, an inability to explain abstract ideas

Thought blocking, an inability to recall information for a time

Symbolism, attaching significance to an insignificant object or idea

Blunted or *flat affect,* little or no display of feeling

Anhedonia, inability to experience pleasure

Catatonia, immobility

Posturing, assuming statuesque positions

Autism, social withdrawal

Self-neglect of hygiene, eating, work, finances, and the like

Poverty of thought, lacking any opinions or ideas

NURSING PROCESS

● The Client With Schizophrenia

Assessment

When caring for clients in acute care or community mental health settings, the nurse performs a Mini Mental Status Examination (see Chap. 12) during the initial contact

DRUG THERAPY TABLE 18-2	TREATMENT OF SCHIZOPHRENIA

DRUG CATEGORY AND EXAMPLES/ MECHANISM OF ACTION	SIDE EFFECTS	NURSING CONSIDERATIONS
Antipsychotics *haloperidol (Haldol)* Blocks postsynaptic dopamine receptors	Drowsiness, pseudoparkinsonism, dystonia, akathisia, neuroleptic malignant syndrome, dysrhythmias, suppression of cough reflex, anaphylactoid reactions, anemia, dry mouth, constipation, urinary retention	Monitor older clients for dehydration and aspiration potential. Withdraw drug gradually. Tell client to avoid driving. Instruct client to drink fluids and report any side effects.
fluphenazine (Prolixin) Blocks postsynaptic dopamine receptors	Drowsiness, extrapyramidal syndromes, dysrhythmias, suppression of cough reflex, dry mouth, constipation, urinary retention	Tell client to avoid alcohol. Do not mix oral concentrate with caffeine-containing beverages, teas, or apple juice. Monitor older clients for signs of dehydration. Tell client to drink plenty of fluids and to report any side effects.
risperidone (Risperdal) Blocks dopamine and serotonin receptors in the brain	Insomnia, agitation, headache, anxiety, drowsiness, nausea, vomiting, constipation, tardive dyskinesias, neuroleptic malignant syndrome, seizures	Monitor client for seizures when initiating therapy or increasing dose. Increase dose gradually until therapeutic effect is achieved. Tell client not to stop taking drug abruptly or to make up missed doses, but to contact the healthcare provider. Instruct client not to take this drug during pregnancy and to report any side effects.
olazapine (Zyprexa) Blocks dopamine and serotonin receptors	Dizziness, drowsiness, headache, weight gain, orthostatic hypotension, extrapyramidal symptoms	Instruct clients in measures to offset orthostatic hypotension, such as rising slowly and doing ankle pumps before standing. Monitor for extrapyramidal symptoms. Initiate anticholinergic drugs. Decrease, discontinue, or switch medications as directed.

and periodically thereafter to monitor for changes. He or she assesses the client for positive and negative symptoms of schizophrenia, including delusions, bizarre speech patterns, hallucinations, agitation, stupor, and social withdrawal. The nurse also assesses the client's physical status, including hygiene and nutritional condition.

BOX 18-2 ● Extrapyramidal Side Effects (EPS)

Movement Disorder	Explanation
Akinesia (pseudoparkinsonism)	The client appears to have symptoms of Parkinson's disease (see Chap. 45) such as hand tremors, stooped posture, stiff shuffling gait.
Akathisia	The client cannot sit or stand still.
Dystonia	Sudden severe muscle spasm occurs, usually in the neck, tongue, or eyes.
Tardive dyskinesia	Client makes involuntary muscle movements, usually in the face, such as tongue thrusting, continuous chewing, grimacing, lip smacking, blinking; irreversible once manifested.

Diagnosis, Planning, and Interventions

Disturbed Thought Processes related to brain changes as manifested by illogical beliefs

Expected Outcome: The client's thoughts will be reality-based as evidenced by a decrease in or absence of delusions.

- Administer antipsychotic drugs as prescribed. *Antipsychotics block dopamine receptors and usually reduce or relieve positive symptoms like delusions.*
- Do not argue about the validity of the client's delusions or try to convince him or her otherwise, but indicate that you do not share the client's delusional belief. *Clients may become more fixated on their delusions, defensive, or hostile if others challenge their delusions. Stating that you do not share the client's belief prevents the client from assuming that the delusion is plausible.*
- Shift the client's focus to what is real in the "here and now" when he or she dwells on the delusion. *Redirecting the client's thoughts to present reality interrupts delusional thinking.*
- Direct the client to a quiet place when he or she becomes agitated. *Reduced stimuli help restore calm and prevent loss of control.*

Disturbed Sensory Perception (Specify: auditory, visual, olfactory, tactile, gustatory) related to brain changes as manifested by hallucinations

Expected Outcome: The client will acknowledge that hallucinations are not real or will minimize their importance.

- Intervene when it appears that the client is experiencing a hallucination such as assuming a listening pose or laughing or talking when others are absent or uninvolved in interaction. *Hallucinations tend to frighten the client. Another person helps the client cope.*
- State that you do not hear or see anyone, but acknowledge that the experience must seem real and frightening to the client. *Stating that you do not share the content of the hallucination helps the client understand that it is not real.*
- Stay with the client throughout the hallucination. *The presence of another trusted person relieves anxiety, facilitates coping, and protects the client from acting dangerously.*
- Avoid touching the client without warning. *Unexpected touching may cause the client to respond violently to what he or she perceives as a threat.*
- Call auditory hallucinations "the voices" rather than using a personal pronoun like "they" or "them." *Personifying the voices suggests the words are coming from real people.*
- Ask the client to share the content of the hallucination. *Obtaining specific information about the hallucination helps to determine if the safety of the client or others is in jeopardy.*
- Distract the client from attending to the hallucination. *Distraction interrupts the perception of the hallucination, thereby reducing the accompanying emotional distress.*
- Teach the client the technique of **voice dismissal,** which refers to saying "stop" or "be gone." *Voice dismissal is a method the client can use to halt the hallucination.*

Self-Care Deficit (Specify type: Bathing/Hygiene, Dressing/Grooming, Feeding, Toileting) related to lack of motivation, illogical fears, emotional withdrawal

Expected Outcome: The client will independently perform ADLs.

- Explain where hygiene is done and how to obtain soap, shampoo, and toothpaste. *Informing the client of the location and resources for bathing and hygiene promotes self-care.*
- Direct the client to care for himself or herself at an appropriate time. *Gentle direction facilitates cooperation.*
- Assist if the client cannot initiate or complete self-care. *The nurse implements a therapeutic use of self when a client is incapable of total self-care.*
- Praise any worthy accomplishments. *Praise is a form of positive reinforcement, which increases the possibility that the client will repeat the activity.*
- Monitor food and fluid intake and toileting patterns. *Data collection facilitates problem identification.*

- Provide nutritious snacks if the client eats insufficiently. *Eating nutritious foods promotes a stable weight and well-being.*

Impaired Social Interaction related to autism as evidenced by absence from group meetings and reluctance to participate in group activities

Expected Outcome: The client will interact independently with one person initially and more than one person as his or her comfort level improves.

- Accompany the client to group meetings and activities. *Support from a trusted other may help the client participate in situations that he or she perceives as threatening or causing social discomfort.*
- Sit by the client, but do not manipulate the client into participating. *The nurse's physical presence reduces anxiety. Pressure to participate may increase the client's anxiety.*
- Share time with the client after the group interaction, and use open-ended questions to explore his or her perception of the experience. *Private discussions promote the client's ability to process the group event and his or her comfort level.*
- Verbally compliment the client when possible for speaking voluntarily with others or acting appropriately in a social situation. *Approval from someone the client respects empowers the client to make further efforts to interact with others.*
- Suggest ways the client can improve interactions with others. *The nurse acts as a mentor to help the client modify social skills.*

Evaluation of Expected Outcomes

Expected outcomes are that the client thinks rationally and realistically and reports fewer delusions and hallucinations. Communication is coherent and understandable. The client manages self-care, takes responsibility for other ADLs, socializes, and interacts in group activities.

Stop, Think, and Respond ● BOX 18-2

Discuss appropriate nursing interventions when a client with schizophrenia expresses a delusional belief or experiences a hallucination.

 GENERAL NUTRITIONAL CONSIDERATIONS

Alzheimer's disease can devastate nutritional status. Forgetfulness, alterations in smell and taste, and decreasing ability to self-feed impair intake. Weight loss is common. Choking may occur if the client forgets to chew food thoroughly or hoards food in his or her mouth.

Increased agitation significantly increases calorie requirements. Nutritionally dense foods that are easy to consume, such as finger foods and liquid supplements, help maximize intake. Minimize distractions at meals and offer one food at a time to avoid overwhelming the client.

Clients in the later stages of Alzheimer's disease may be unable to swallow or may not know what to do when food is placed in their mouths. When such a situation occurs, a decision regarding nutritional support (e.g., percutaneous endoscopic gastrostomy tube feedings) must be made.

GENERAL PHARMACOLOGIC CONSIDERATIONS

Tacrine therapy in clients with Alzheimer's is not curative and becomes ineffective with time.

Achieving maximum benefits with tacrine takes up to 2 months of continuous treatment.

Antipsychotic drugs do not cure mental illness. Rather, they calm unmanageable clients and make some clients more responsive to other forms of therapy.

Monitor the client taking an antipsychotic drug for symptoms of neuroleptic malignant syndrome, and notify the primary healthcare provider immediately if fever, dyspnea, tachycardia, hypertension, severe muscle stiffness, or loss of bladder control occurs.

Advise clients to take all antipsychotic drugs as directed and to avoid double dosing if they miss a dose.

Advise clients not to stop antipsychotic drugs abruptly; nausea, vomiting, sweating, tachycardia, headache, and insomnia can occur.

GENERAL GERONTOLOGIC CONSIDERATIONS

Alzheimer's disease affects approximately 30% of individuals older than 85 years of age.

Tacrine can be dissolved in orange juice or other liquid if the older adult has difficulty swallowing.

Older adult clients require lower dosages of antipsychotic drugs.

The older adult taking haloperidol (Haldol) is at risk for dehydration. Report lethargy, decreased thirst, weakness, and dry mucous membranes.

Older adults are particularly susceptible to tardive dyskinesia while taking antipsychotic drugs. Report symptoms immediately because the drug must be discontinued.

Critical Thinking Exercises

1. *Discuss the similarities and differences between Alzheimer's disease and schizophrenia.*
2. *In what ways are the interventions for altered mentation different for a client with Alzheimer's disease and schizophrenia?*

References and Suggested Readings

Armstrong, M. (2001). The pressures felt by informal carers of people with dementia. *Nursing Standard, 15*(17), 47–55.

Brooker, D. & Duce, L. (2000). Well-being and activity in dementia: A comparison of group reminiscence therapy, structured goal-directed group activity and unstructured time. *Aging and Mental Health, 4,* 354–358.

Fago, J. P. (2001). Care of the elderly. Dementia: Causes, evaluation, and management. *Hospital Practice, 36*(1), 59–66, 69.

Gray, R. & Gournay, K. (2000). What can we do about acute extrapyramidal symptoms? *Journal of Psychiatric and Mental Health Nursing, 7,* 205–211.

Kranhold, K. (2001; May 10). Dentists battle "gag" on warning about mercury. *Wall Street Journal,* Eastern edition 327(92), Section B:1.

Landry, S. (1998). Study reveals folic acid, Alzheimer's disease link. [On-line.] Available: http://www.sptimes.com/Worldandnation/101998/study_reveals_folic_a.html.

Lo, R. & Brown, R. (2000). Caring for family carers and people with dementia. *International Journal of Psychiatric Nursing Research, 6,* 684–694.

Lombard, J. & Germano, C. (1997). *The brain wellness plan: Breakthrough medical, nutritional, and immune-boosting therapies.* New York: Kensington.

Lynch, M. & Wagstaff, C. (1999). Managing care of the patient with schizophrenia—before and after surgery. *Journal of Practical Nursing, 49*(4), 12–15.

Marland, G. R. & Sharkey, V. (1999). Depot neuroleptics, schizophrenia and the role of the nurse: Is practice evidence based? *Journal of Advanced Nursing, 30,* 1255–1262.

Merz Pharmaceuticals. (2002). Memantine. (On-line.) Available at: http://www.memantine.com.

Millar, E., Garland, C., Ross, F., et al. (1999). Practice nurses and the care of patients receiving depot neuroleptic treatment: Views on training, confidence and use of structured assessment. *Journal of Advanced Nursing, 29,* 1454–1461.

NIMH funds study of drugs for schizophrenia and Alzheimer's. (1999). *Journal of Psychosocial Nursing and Mental Health Services, 37*(12), 7.

Petersen, R. C. (2000). Aging, mild cognitive impairment, and Alzheimer's disease. *Neurologic Clinics, 18,* 789–805.

Powell, J. A. (2000). Communication interventions in dementia. *Reviews in Clinical Gerontology, 10*(2), 161–168.

Prusiner, S. B. (1998). The prion diseases. *Brain Pathology, 8,* 499–513.

Rempusheski, V. F. & Hurley, A. C. (2000). Advance directives and dementia. *Journal of Gerontological Nursing, 26*(10), 27–34.

Schafer, C., Sodoma, C., Gonzalez, S., et al. (2000). Your turn. How do you structure the day for individuals with dementia? *Journal of Gerontological Nursing, 26*(10), 52–53.

Small, G. W., Rabins, P. V., Barry, P. B., et al. (1997). Consensus statement of the American Association for Geriatric Psychiatry, the Alzheimer's Association, and the American Geriatrics Society. *Journal of the American Medical Association, 278,* 1363–1371.

Teschinsky, U. (2000). Living with schizophrenia: The family illness experience. *Issues in Mental Health Nursing, 21,* 387–396.

Tredget, J. (1999). Family intervention in the treatment of schizophrenia. *Mental Health Nursing, 19*(4), 25–27.

Valcour, V. G., Masaki, K. H., Curb, J. D., et al. (2000). The detection of dementia in the primary care setting. *Archives of Internal Medicine, 160,* 2964–2968.

Webster, J. (2001). Unraveling Alzheimer's disease and other dementias. *Home Health Care Consultant, 8*(1), 10–18.

Weitzel, C. (2000). Could you spot this psych emergency? *RN, 63*(9), 35–38.

Wuerker, A. K. (1999). The family and schizophrenia. *Issues in Mental Health Nursing, 21*(1), 127–141.

Yeaworth, R. (2000). Coalition to change assisted living regulations governing special units for dementia patients. *Nursing Outlook, 48,* 314–315.

chapter **19**

Caring for Clients With Infectious Disorders

Words to Know

bacteremia
carrier
community-acquired
   infections
culture
fomites
host
infectious process cycle
leukocytosis
means of transmission
microorganisms
multidrug resistance
nonpathogens
nosocomial infections
opportunistic infections

pathogens
phagocytosis
portal of entry
portal of exit
prion
reservoir
sensitivity
sepsis
septicemia
superinfections
susceptibility
transmission-based
   precautions
virulence

Learning Objectives

On completion of this chapter, the reader will:

- List three factors that influence whether an infection develops.
- Describe infectious agents, and list at least three examples.
- Differentiate between nonpathogens and pathogens.
- List at least five factors that increase susceptibility to infection.
- Name the six components of the infectious process cycle.
- Explain the difference between mechanical and chemical defense mechanisms.
- Differentiate localized from generalized infections.
- Describe events during the inflammatory process.
- Name at least three diagnostic tests ordered for clients suspected of having an infectious disorder.
- Discuss the medical management of clients with infectious disorders.
- Name three nursing interventions to prevent or control infectious disorders.
- List three reasons why clients in healthcare agencies are at increased risk for infection.
- Explain the role of an infection control committee.
- List at least four measures that have reduced community-acquired infections.
- Discuss measures to take if a needlestick injury occurs.

Infections have always plagued humankind. This chapter discusses the causes of infections, their transmission, methods to prevent or control them, and techniques for managing the care of clients with infections.

MICROORGANISMS AND INFECTIOUS DISORDERS

Infectious disorders are conditions caused by infectious agents called **microorganisms** (with the exception of prions, discussed later). Microorganisms, commonly called *germs,* are so small they can be seen only with a microscope. Once microorganisms invade, one of three events

occurs: (1) the body's immune defense mechanisms eliminate them (see Chap. 41), (2) they reside in the body without causing disease, or (3) they cause an infection or infectious disease. Factors that influence whether an infection develops are the type of microorganism and its characteristics, and the presence of the components of the infectious process cycle.

Types of Infectious Agents

Infectious microorganisms include bacteria, viruses, fungi, rickettsiae, protozoans, mycoplasmas, and helminths. Prions are a new category of infectious agent. Some infectious agents cause *communicable* or *contagious diseases,* infections that can be transmitted from one person to another. Examples include measles, streptococcal sore throat, sexually transmitted diseases, and tuberculosis (TB).

Bacteria

Bacteria are single-celled microorganisms. They appear in various shapes: round (cocci), rod shaped (bacilli), and spiral (spirochetes) (Fig. 19-1). *Aerobic bacteria* require oxygen to grow and multiply, whereas *anaerobic bacteria* grow and multiply in an atmosphere that lacks oxygen. Some bacteria, such as *Staphylococcus aureus, Streptococcus pneumoniae,* and *Escherichia coli,* are developing **multidrug resistance,** the ability to remain unaffected by antimicrobial drugs such as antibiotics (Box 19-1). Infections with multidrug-resistant microorganisms are very difficult to destroy with pharmacologic agents. Thus, the potential for death from such infections is increased.

Viruses

Viruses are so small they can be seen only with high-powered electron microscopes. They also are filterable, meaning they pass through very small barriers. Viruses are divided into two types: (1) those whose nucleic acid is composed of deoxyribonucleic acid (DNA), and (2) those whose nucleic acid is composed of ribonucleic acid (RNA). Viruses use the metabolic and reproductive materials of living cells or tissues to multiply. Some viral infections, such as the common cold, are minor and *self-limiting;* that is, they terminate with or without medical treatment. Others, such as rabies, poliomyelitis, and viral hepatitis, are more serious and may be fatal. Occasionally, viruses are dormant in a living host, reactivate periodically, and cause the infection to recur. An example is the herpes simplex virus, which causes periodic outbreaks of cold sores (fever blisters) long after the initial infection (see Chap. 69).

Fungi

Fungi are divided into two basic groups: yeasts and molds. Only a small number of fungi appear to produce disease in humans. There are three types of fungal (mycotic) in-

---

BOX 19-1 ● Causes of Antibiotic Resistance

- Bacterial mutations that interfere with the mechanism of antibiotic action
- Inappropriate prescription of antibiotics for viral infections
- Less than full compliance with antibiotic drug regimens
- Prophylactic (preventive) administration of antibiotics without infection
- Environmental dispersal of antibiotic solutions that intermingle with microorganisms, such as when partially empty IV bags are deposited in waste containers or droplets are released when purging IV tubing or removing air from syringes used to inject antibiotics
- Administration of antibiotics to livestock, leaving traces of drug residue after slaughter

---

fections: superficial (dermatophytoses), which affect the skin, hair, and nails; intermediate, which chiefly affect subcutaneous tissues; and deep (systemic), which affect deep tissues and organs.

Rickettsiae

Rickettsiae resemble but are different from bacteria. Like viruses, they invade living cells and cannot survive outside a living organism or host. Arthropods (invertebrate animals with a segmented body, an external skeleton, and jointed, paired appendages) transmit rickettsial diseases. Examples of arthropods include fleas, ticks, lice, and mites.

Protozoans

Protozoans are single-celled animals classified according to their motility (ability to move). Some possess *amoeboid motion,* meaning that they extend their cell walls and their intracellular contents flow forward. Others move by means of *cilia,* hairlike projections, or *flagella,* whiplike appendages. Still others have little or no movement.

Mycoplasmas

Mycoplasmas are single-celled microorganisms that lack a cell wall and, therefore, are pleomorphic (assume many shapes). They are similar to but not related to bacteria. They primarily infect the surface linings of the respiratory, genitourinary, and gastrointestinal (GI) tracts.

Helminths

Helminths are infectious worms, some of which are microscopic. They are divided into three major groups: nematodes or roundworms, cestodes or tapeworms, and trematodes or flukes. Some helminths enter the body in the egg stage, whereas others spend the larval stage in an intermediate host and then enter the human host. The organisms mate and reproduce in the definitive host and are then excreted, after which the cycle begins again.

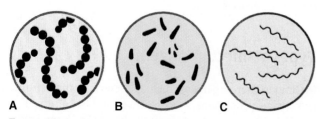

FIGURE 19-1 Classification of bacteria according to shape: (**A**) cocci, (**B**) bacilli, and (**C**) spirochetes.

Prions

Until recently, the scientific community believed all infectious agents contained nucleic acid (DNA or RNA), enabling their replication. The idea of an atypical infectious agent was proposed in 1967. Dr. Stanley Prusiner (1998) won a Nobel Prize in physiology and medicine in 1997 for his discovery of such proteins, called *prions.*

A **prion** is a protein that does not contain nucleic acid. Research suggests that normal prions, present in brain cells, protect against dementia (see Chap. 18). When a prion mutates, however, it is capable of becoming an infectious agent and altering other normal prion proteins into similar mutant copies. The mutant prions, which can either be formed by genetic predisposition or acquired by transmission between the same or similar infected animal species, cause transmissible spongiform encephalopathies (TSEs). TSEs are so named because the brain becomes spongy (full of holes), the brain tissue withers, and uncoordinated movements develop in the affected person or animal. Examples of TSEs include bovine spongiform encephalopathy (mad cow disease), scrapie in sheep, and Creutzfeldt-Jakob disease (CJD). Research is ongoing to determine if prions contribute to Alzheimer's disease (see Chap. 18), Parkinson's disease, and Huntington's disease (see Chap. 45), or if clients with these disorders lack sufficient or have ineffective prions.

Mutant prions clearly have been transmitted from sheep to cattle when cattle are fed waste parts of slaughtered infected sheep. Although one form of CJD is definitely familial, a new-variant form has developed in humans who have consumed beef infected with mad cow disease in Europe. To prevent the transmission of new-variant CJD, infected animals are destroyed, and potentially infected animal tissues are banned from human consumption. The Centers for Disease Control and Prevention (2001) advises Americans traveling to Europe to (1) avoid eating beef or beef products, or (2) eat solid pieces of muscle meat from beef rather than ground meat products, which may contain tissues with infectious prions.

In May 2001, the American Red Cross adopted a new policy concerning blood donations to prevent the potential for collecting prion-contaminated blood (Meckler & Ricks, 2001). The policy bans blood collection from anyone who has lived in the United Kingdom for a total of 3 months or longer since 1980, lived anywhere in Europe for a total of 6 months since 1980, or received a blood transfusion in the United Kingdom.

Characteristics of Microorganisms

Not all microorganisms are dangerous. Some are **nonpathogens** because they generally are harmless to healthy humans. For example, nonpathogens in the intestine help synthesize vitamin B_{12}, biotin, vitamin K, and folic acid. **Pathogens,** on the other hand, have a high potential to cause infectious diseases.

The ability of a microorganism to become pathogenic depends on several factors: ability to move or be moved from one place to another; **virulence** (power to produce disease); how many there are; ability to invade a **host,** the person on or in whom the microorganism will reside; the host's duration of exposure to the infectious agent; and the host's **susceptibility** (ability to be compromised by or infected with disease). Unless and until a supporting host becomes weakened, microorganisms remain in check. Usually, available immunizations and natural body defenses (discussed later) protect most humans from infection. Given the right circumstances, however, both pathogens and nonpathogens can cause infections.

Certain individuals are at increased risk for infection because their defenses are compromised in one or more ways. For example, older adults, premature infants, malnourished and debilitated clients, clients receiving immunosuppressive agents, and clients with impaired skin, bone marrow suppression, or disorders of the immune system are especially susceptible to virulent and nonvirulent strains of microorganisms.

Even benign microorganisms can produce **superinfections,** also called **opportunistic infections,** in which nonpathogenic or remotely pathogenic microorganisms take advantage of favorable situations and overwhelm the host. For example, a prescribed antibiotic sometimes can upset biologic checks and balances. Although the antibiotic destroys one pathogen, other pathogens that the antibiotic does not affect grow and proliferate. Usually, however, common pathogens cause infections.

Infection Transmission

Like the links in a chain, all components in the **infectious process cycle** must be present to transmit an infectious disease from one human or animal to a susceptible host (Fig. 19-2). In addition to the infectious agent and host, an appropriate reservoir, exit route, means of transmission, and portal of entry are necessary.

Reservoir

A **reservoir** is the environment in which the infectious agent can survive and reproduce. It may be human, animal, or nonliving, such as contaminated food and water. A human or animal that harbors (or is the reservoir of) an infectious microorganism but does not show active evidence of infectious disease is a **carrier.** Nonliving reservoirs are **fomites.**

Portal of Exit

The **portal of exit** is the route by which the infectious agent escapes from the reservoir. Examples include the

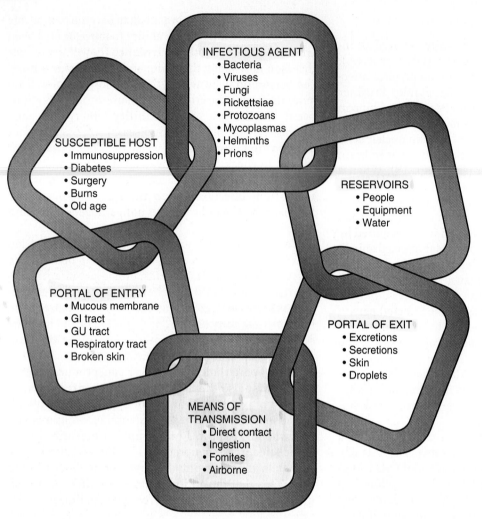

FIGURE 19-2 The infectious process cycle. GI, gastrointestinal; GU, genitourinary.

respiratory, GI, or genitourinary tract; the skin and mucous membranes; and blood and other body fluids.

Means of Transmission

A microorganism's **means of transmission** refers to how it is transferred or moved from its reservoir to the susceptible host. The five potential means of transmis-

sion are contact, droplet, airborne, vehicle, and vector (Table 19-1).

Portal of Entry

An infectious agent gains entrance into a susceptible host through a **portal of entry.** Some infectious agents may have only one portal of entry; others may use sev-

TABLE 19-1	COMMON MEANS OF TRANSMISSION	
ROUTE OF TRANSMISSION	**DESCRIPTION**	**EXAMPLE**
Contact		
Direct	Infected person to susceptible person	Sexual intercourse
Indirect	Contaminated substance to susceptible person	Handling a contaminated paper tissue
Droplet	Spray of moist particles within a 3-foot radius of infected person	Sneezing, coughing, talking
Airborne	Suspension and transport on air currents beyond 3 feet	Inhalation of microorganisms attached to dust particles
Vehicle	On or in contaminated food, water, objects, *or* equipment	Eating or drinking tainted products
Vector	Infected animal or insect to susceptible person	Transfer from bites of mosquitoes, bats, or ticks

cellular response results in leakage of fluid, colloids, and ions from the capillaries into the tissues between the cells, producing swelling. An ensuing vascular response produces redness and heat, whereas a chemical response causes pain. WBCs—neutrophils, macrophages, monocytes, and lymphocytes—move to the injury site to destroy the toxins produced by the pathogens and to remove debris from the area (Fig. 19-4). More WBCs are manufactured as needed.

To prevent the spread of pathogens to adjacent tissues, a fibrin barrier forms around the injured area. Inside the barrier, a thick, white exudate (pus) accumulates. This collection of pus is called an *abscess*, which may break through the skin and drain or continue to enlarge internally.

If the lymph nodes in the area become involved, they become enlarged and tender, an inflammatory condition referred to as *lymphadenitis*. If this defense mechanism cannot contain the infection, the microorganisms begin to travel from node to node (see Chap. 40). Because the lymphatic system drains into the venous system, the microorganisms may eventually reach the bloodstream, causing a condition called **bacteremia** or **septicemia,** which may lead to **sepsis,** a systemic inflammatory response syndrome resulting from infection.

Sepsis

The pathophysiology of sepsis varies, depending on the virulence of the pathogen and condition of the host. Two or more of the following characterize sepsis:

- Temperature greater than 100.4°F (38°C) or less than 96.8°F (36°C)
- Heart rate greater than 90 beats per minute
- Respiratory rate greater than 20 breaths per minute or PaCO₂ less than 32 mm Hg

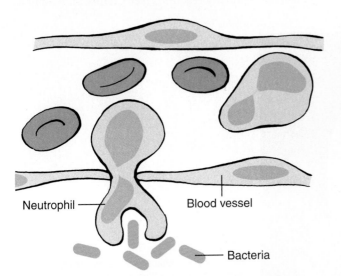

FIGURE 19-4 A neutrophil leaves a blood vessel to engulf infectious bacteria.

Neutrophil

Blood vessel

Bacteria

- WBC count greater than 12,000 cells/mm³ or 10% immature (band) forms (American College of Chest Physicians, 1992)

Fever, which is the body's attempt to destroy the pathogen with heat, occurs in most people as an infection worsens. Exceptions may include older adults and clients who are immunocompromised, debilitated, or addicted to alcohol; have kidney or liver failure; or are receiving corticosteroids or immunotherapy. These clients may have normal or low body temperature. The person with an elevated temperature feels chilled despite the fever because surface blood vessels constrict to prevent loss of body heat. Muscles may contract to produce additional heat, causing uncontrollable shivering. Sweating stops as circulation is diverted to blood vessels deep within the body. The pulse and respiratory rates rise in proportion to the fever. More WBCs are manufactured as needed, a process referred to as **leukocytosis.**

The body uses an inflammatory response to suppress the infectious process. Once the proinflammatory mechanisms achieve a beneficial effect, the body releases anti-inflammatory mediators to restore homeostasis.

Severe Sepsis

Estimates are that 300,000 to 500,000 people per year in the United States develop severe sepsis, a disorder associated with organ dysfunction, hypotension, and hypoperfusion manifested by lactic acidosis, oliguria, and acute alteration in mental status (Porth, 2002). Basically, the system of proinflammatory mechanisms remains unchecked in severe sepsis. The proinflammatory response promotes coagulation of blood (microvascular clots) and suppression of fibrinolysis, the process by which clots are dissolved. Systemic microvascular clotting becomes responsible for multiple organ failure because it interferes with delivery of oxygen to cells.

Some believe that severe sepsis results from deficiency of a substance called *protein C,* an inhibitor of coagulation. Protein C may also be responsible for interrupting the inflammatory cycle. Although sepsis and severe sepsis are treated with one or more antimicrobial drugs, severe sepsis remains quite lethal. Many with severe sepsis develop septic shock (see Chap. 23) and die. A new drug called *drotrecogin alfa* (proposed name, Zovant), however, is being tested in clinical trials (Bernard, et al., 2001). Zovant is a recombinant form of human protein C. Eli Lilly and Company, which developed Zovant, states that "one in five people who would have died from severe sepsis survived due to Zovant" (The Associated Press, 2001).

Diagnostic Tests

A thorough history and physical examination are essential for the diagnosis of an infectious disease. Diagnosis of some infectious diseases, however, requires additional tests and laboratory examinations to identify the microorganism.

White Blood Cell Count and Differential

An elevation in the number and type of WBCs (leukocytes), whose main function is phagocytosis, indicates an inflammatory and possibly infectious process. Although a total WBC count provides important information, a differential—one that indicates the percentage of WBC subtypes—is even more valuable. Elevated neutrophils, the largest subtype of leukocytes, indicate that the body is in the early stages of responding to an invading pathogen. As the number of neutrophils becomes depleted, bone marrow produces additional cells called *band cells* (bands) that eventually mature and replace them. Elevated monocytes, the largest-sized subtype of WBCs, are the body's second line of defense.

Culture and Sensitivity Test

A **culture** is used to identify bacteria in a specimen taken from a person with symptoms of an infection. The source of the specimen may be body fluids or wastes, such as blood, sputum, urine, or feces, or the *purulent exudate,* collection of pus, from an open wound. The specimen is cultured, which involves placing a small amount of it in or on a special growth medium (Fig. 19-5). The specimen is incubated for a specific period (usually 48 to 72 hours), then examined microscopically. To facilitate examination, it is stained or dyed (colored). One stain is the Gram stain. Those bacteria that absorb the color of the stain are classified as *gram positive;* those that do not are classified as *gram negative.* A coagulase test also may be used to test the microorganisms for pathogenicity or virulence. When a culture is reported as *coagulase positive,* it is more virulent than a culture of the same microorganism that produces a negative (*coagulase-negative*) response.

Sensitivity studies are done to determine which antibiotic inhibits the growth of a nonviral microorganism and will be most effective in treating the infection.

Examination for Ova and Parasites

Most ova (eggs) and parasites (those that live at the expense of the host) are intestinal worms. Therefore, the stool is examined for evidence of any forms in the infecting microorganism's life cycle. Usually, three random stools are collected from a bedpan, not the toilet. Urine and toilet paper may alter the specimen and therefore must be disposed of separately. Clients suspected of having intestinal ova and parasites are advised to perform scrupulous handwashing to avoid reinfecting themselves and others.

Skin Tests

Skin testing determines the presence of a specific active or inactive infection. Diseases for which skin testing may be done include histoplasmosis, mumps, TB, diphtheria, and coccidioidomycosis. The material for skin testing is injected intradermally (Fig. 19-6). The reaction is read after a specified period (usually 48 to 72 hours). The size of the *induration* (hard, elevated tissue), not including the surrounding area of *erythema* (redness), is measured in millimeters (mm). The measurement determines whether the reaction is significant. For example, a tuberculin skin test is considered positive if the induration is 15 mm or greater in persons with no known risk factors for TB; smaller measurements are significant in certain risk groups, such as immunocompromised clients.

Immunologic Tests

Immunologic tests may be used to determine the presence of *antigen* (substances that stimulate an immune response) and antibody reactions (see Chap. 41). Examples

FIGURE 19-5 Variability of the macroscopic appearance of bacteria cultured on solid, agar-containing medium. (From Porth, C. M. [2002]. *Pathophysiology: Concepts of altered health states* [6th ed.]. Philadelphia: Lippincott Williams & Wilkins.)

FIGURE 19-6 The Mantoux test for tuberculosis. (**A**) Correct technique for inserting the needle. (**B**) To determine the extent of the reaction, the wheal is measured using a commercially prepared gauge. A wheal measuring 5 mm or more is considered significant.

include *agglutination* tests, such as the cold agglutinins test, which may reveal the presence of high antibody titers confirming immunity to rubella (measles); *precipitation tests,* such as the C-reactive protein test and erythrocyte sedimentation rate, the results of which are elevated in some inflammatory diseases; *complement fixation* tests, which, when results are elevated, indicate an inflammatory process; and *immunofluorescence* tests, which identify immunoglobulins, antibodies formed by the immune system.

Other Tests

Depending on the disease, other diagnostic tests may be used. Radiography (plain films or contrast studies), computed tomography scanning, and magnetic resonance imaging may be used to locate abscesses, identify displacement of organs or structures that may indicate abscess formation, and detect changes in tissues in areas such as the bones or lungs.

Medical Management

In some cases, supportive therapy such as rest, fluids, adequate nutrition, and antipyretics (e.g., aspirin or acetaminophen [Tylenol]) for a significantly elevated fever may be advised while the infectious disease runs its course (Table 19-3). If the etiology is responsive to drug therapy, antimicrobials (e.g., antibiotics, sulfonamides, antiviral drugs) are prescribed.

Infected wounds may be *debrided,* a process of removing dead and damaged tissue. Wound irrigations, hydrotherapy (whirlpool), and application of wet-to-dry dressings may accomplish the same objective.

Treatment of a primary condition may relieve the infectious process. Bone marrow transplantation or administration of drugs that boost WBC production, such as filgrastim (Neupogen), may help immunosuppressed clients.

N U R S I N G   P R O C E S S

● The Client With a Potential or Actual Infection

Assessment

The nurse obtains the client's history, paying particular attention to information that might suggest exposure to someone with an infectious illness or other reservoirs of infection, immunization status, recent travel to a

TABLE 19-3	THE COURSE OF INFECTIOUS DISEASES
STAGE	**CHARACTERISTIC**
Incubation period	The infectious agent reproduces. The host displays no recognizable symptoms; however, the infectious agent may exit the host at this time and infect others.
Prodromal stage	Initial symptoms appear; they may be vague and nonspecific. Possible symptoms include mild fever, headache, and loss of usual energy.
Acute stage	Symptoms become severe and specific to the affected tissue or organ. For example, tuberculosis is manifested by respiratory symptoms.
Convalescent stage	Symptoms subside as the host overcomes the infectious agent.
Resolution	The pathogen is destroyed. Health improves or is restored.

foreign country, treatment with antimicrobial or immuno-suppressive drugs, and current medical disorders. He or she weighs the client to gain information about nutritional status and measures vital signs to detect temperature, heart and respiratory rate, and blood pressure. A head-to-toe physical assessment helps detect manifestations of an inflammatory response, impaired skin, and evidence of unusual drainage. Questioning about feelings of lassitude (tiredness) and anorexia is important. After preparing the client for diagnostic tests and collecting specimens, the nurse monitors the results of the laboratory findings and observes the response to skin tests.

Diagnosis, Planning, and Interventions

The nurse implements measures to prevent or interrupt components of the infectious process cycle. Examples include supporting nutrition and hydration, maintaining intact skin and mucous membranes, and following aseptic principles. The nurse administers drug therapy and observes for evidence of improvement. He or she also implements measures that promote comfort (e.g., reducing fever).

To help prevent and control nosocomial infections, nurses apply principles of medical and surgical asepsis whenever they care for clients. Recommendations from the healthcare agency's infection control committee provide further guidance. Such committees usually consist of representatives from various areas and departments, such as medical staff, nursing service, clinical laboratories, pathology, operating room, housekeeping, and dietary service. Their responsibilities include conducting *surveillance,* the process of detecting, reporting, and recording nosocomial infections; educating personnel about methods to reduce nosocomial infections; providing guidelines for prevention of infectious diseases; and investigating outbreaks of nosocomial infections. Infection control guidelines usually establish policies for pre-employment and postemployment health examinations, sterilization procedures and methods, disposal of garbage and biologic wastes, and housekeeping techniques; designate precautions to follow for specific infections; and define procedures for managing contaminated materials such as linen, equipment, and supplies used in the care of infectious clients.

Many community-acquired (communicable, contagious) infections have been contained or eliminated because of advances in the prevention and treatment of infectious diseases. These advances include the discovery and use of antibiotics, the development of immunizing agents, guidelines for the proper disposal of human wastes, legislation controlling the preparation and sale of foods, immunization programs, and public education. Local, state, and federal public health agencies and the World Health Organization (WHO) cooperate in the detection and control of communicable diseases. Their combined efforts have reduced the incidence of many infectious diseases and virtually eliminated others (e.g., smallpox). To help prevent and control community-acquired infections, nurses encourage childhood immunizations (Table 19-4), vaccines that stimulate the body to produce antibodies against a specific disease organism. Parental apathy, religious beliefs, fear that immunizations will cause illness, or inability to afford healthcare, however, can pose potential barriers to children obtaining immunizations. The immunization of children protects all people—children as well as adults who may not have developed sufficient immunity (Client and Family Teaching Box 19-1).

Diagnoses, expected outcomes, and interventions for clients with infections include the following:

Risk for Infection related to compromised defense mechanisms

Expected Outcome: Client will remain free of infection.

- Follow handwashing guidelines (Box 19-2) using lathered soap and friction for 30 to 60 seconds or at least 2 minutes if hands are grossly contaminated. *Handwashing remains the single most important measure to prevent the spread of infection. It reduces the number of transient and resident microorganisms.*
- Rinse soap from the wrists toward the fingers using running water. *Directing the flow of rinse water toward the fingers avoids transferring microorganisms to cleaner skin areas.*
- Use a paper towel to turn off a hand-operated faucet. *The towel protects against recontamination of the hands.*
- Advise the client to avoid touching any areas of impaired skin. *Hands contain microorganisms that clients can transfer to tissue and blood vessels beneath impaired skin.*
- Monitor food intake; offer nutritious supplements if appetite is suppressed. *Sufficient intake helps restore biologic defense mechanisms (e.g., adequate WBCs, wound healing).*
- Keep dressings clean, dry, and intact. *They act as barriers to environmental microorganisms.*
- Use surgical asepsis when changing dressings or inserting or changing invasive equipment (e.g., urinary catheters, IV access devices). *Pathogens can enter from several different routes.*
- Use a prescribed topical antimicrobial or one approved by the agency during wound care. *Antimicrobials reduce microorganisms at the site of impaired skin.*
- Administer prescribed systemic antimicrobial medications. *Antibiotics may be ordered prophylactically (i.e., to reduce the potential for infection).*
- Monitor for signs of superinfection: diarrhea, vaginal discharge, and inflammation of oral mucous membranes. *Antibiotic therapy may cause microorganisms to overgrow elsewhere in the body.*

PC: Sepsis

Expected Outcome: The nurse will manage and minimize sepsis.

- Follow **transmission-based precautions** (Table 19-5). *They interfere with the ways a particular pathogen is spread.*
- Monitor vital signs every 4 hours or as ordered medically. *Changes may be the earliest indication of sepsis.*

TABLE 19-4	RECOMMENDED CHILDHOOD IMMUNIZATION SCHEDULE	

VACCINE	DOSES	ACCEPTABLE AGE RANGE FOR IMMUNIZATION
Hepatitis B (Hep B)	1st dose	Birth to 2 months
	2nd dose	1–4 months
	3rd dose	6–18 months or 11–12 years if not immunized earlier
Diphtheria, tetanus, pertussis (DTaP or DTP)	1st dose	2 months
	2nd dose	4 months
	3rd dose	6 months
	Booster	15–18 months
	Booster	4–6 years
	Td booster	11–16 years; repeat T every 10 years
Haemophilus influenzae B (HiB)	1st dose	2 months
	2nd dose	4 months
	3rd dose	6 months
	Booster	12–15 months
Inactivated poliomyelitis (IPV)	1st dose	2 months
	2nd dose	4 months
	3rd dose	6–18 months
	Booster	4–6 years
Pneumococcal conjugate (PCV)	1st dose	2 months
	2nd dose	4 months
	3rd dose	6 months
	Booster	12–15 months
Measles, mumps, rubella (MMR)	1st dose	12–15 months
	2nd dose	4–6 years or 11–12 years
Varicella (Var) (chickenpox)	One dose	12–18 months; 11–12 years if not immunized earlier or never acquired the disease
Hepatitis A (Hep A)	2 doses	2–18 years in selected areas

IPV, inactivated (injected) polio vaccine; Td, full dose of tetanus, reduced dose of diphtheria.
Recommendations are based on those approved by the Advisory Committee on Immunization Practices, the American Academy of Pediatrics, and the American Academy of Family Physicians (January–December 2001).

- Observe the client's mental status. *Changes in mentation accompany sepsis.*
- Check skin color and observe for signs of impaired circulation or bleeding. *Microvascular clots accompany sepsis; disseminated intravascular coagulation may develop from alterations in the clotting mechanisms.*
- Administer antimicrobials as prescribed. *Systemic antimicrobial therapy may be necessary to prevent, control, and eliminate an infection.*
- Report hypotension and signs of organ dysfunction to the physician. *Severe sepsis may lead to septic shock and death.*

Evaluation of Expected Outcomes

Expected outcomes include a WBC count below 10,000 cells/mm^3, body temperature less than 99°F, no purulent drainage from impaired skin, wound culture free of virulent pathogens, and no signs of superinfection. The nurse performs early and accurate detection of changes in vital signs, mental status, and leukocyte count. The infection resolves and does not progress to septic shock.

NEEDLESTICK INJURIES

One of the greatest threats to healthcare workers is the potential for acquiring blood-borne infectious diseases such as hepatitis B virus (HBV) infection and acquired immunodeficiency syndrome (AIDS). Following Standard Precautions, techniques used to prevent the potential for transmitting pathogens in blood or other body fluids when a person's infectious status is unknown, reduce this risk (Box 19-3). Gloves, however, are not impervious to

BOX 19-2 • Handwashing Guidelines

Handwashing is performed:
- When arriving at and leaving work
- Before and after contact with each client
- Before and after handling equipment
- Before and after gloving
- Before and after collecting specimens
- Before preparing medications
- After administering medications
- Before serving trays or feeding clients
- Before eating
- After toileting, hair combing, or performing other hygiene
- After cleaning a work area

TABLE 19-5	TRANSMISSION-BASED PRECAUTIONS		
TYPE OF PRECAUTION	**LOCATION**	**PROTECTION**	**EXAMPLES OF DISEASES**
Airborne	Private room Negative air pressure* Room air is discharged to environment or filtered before being circulated	Follow Standard Precautions. Wear a mask for airborne pathogens or particulate air filter respirator in the case of TB. Place a mask on the client if transport is required.	TB Measles Chickenpox
Droplet	Private room, or in a room with similarly infected client(s) or one with at least 3 feet between the client and other client(s) or visitors	Follow Standard Precautions. Wear a mask when entering the room, but especially when within 3 feet of the infected client. Place a mask on the client if transport is required.	Influenza Rubella Streptococcal pneumonia Meningococcal meningitis
Contact	Private room, or in a room with similarly infected client(s), or consult with an infection control professional if the above options are not available	Follow Standard Precautions. Don gloves before entering the room. Remove gloves before leaving the room. Change gloves after contact with infective material. Perform handwashing with an antimicrobial agent immediately after removing gloves. Wear a gown when entering the room if your clothing could touch the client or items in the room, or if the client is incontinent, has diarrhea, an ileostomy, or a colostomy, or wound drainage not contained by a dressing. Avoid transporting the client, but, if required, use precautions that minimize transmission. Clean bedside equipment and client care items daily. Use items such as a stethoscope, sphygmomanometer, and other assessment tools exclusively for the infected client, and terminally disinfect them when precautions are no longer necessary.	Drug-resistant gastrointestinal, respiratory, skin, or wound infections Acute diarrhea Draining abscess

TB, tuberculosis.
*Negative air pressure pulls air from the hall into the room when the door is opened, as opposed to positive air pressure, which pulls room air into the hall.
From Centers for Disease Control and Prevention. (1996). *Guideline for isolation precautions in hospitals.* CDC Publication 96138102. Atlanta, GA: National Center for Infectious Diseases.

penetration by sharp objects (e.g., needles) that may contain blood. Despite following policies and precautions for avoiding blood-borne pathogens and using new needleless access devices on IV lines, needlestick injuries continue to occur. Should an injury occur, healthcare workers are advised to follow postexposure recommendations:

- Report the injury to one's supervisor immediately.
- Document the injury in writing.
- Identify the person or source of blood, if possible.
- Obtain the HIV and HBV statuses of the source of blood, if it is legal to do so. Unless the client gives permission, testing and revealing HIV status are prohibited.
- Obtain counseling on the potential for infection.

- Receive the most appropriate postexposure prophylaxis.
- Be tested for disease antibodies at appropriate intervals.
- Receive instructions on monitoring potential symptoms and medical follow-up.

 ## GENERAL NUTRITIONAL CONSIDERATIONS

Infection changes body metabolism, including increases in metabolic rate and breakdown of glycogen, fat, and protein tissue.
Fever is a major determinant of caloric needs during infection. Basal metabolic rate (BMR) increases 7% for each degree Fahrenheit that tempera-

19-1 *Client and Family Teaching*
Reducing Infections

To reduce potential infections, the nurse teaches the following measures:

- Perform frequent handwashing, especially before eating, after using the toilet, and after contact with nasal secretions.
- Bathe and perform other personal hygiene (e.g., oral care) daily.
- Keep the home environment clean; household bleach diluted 1:10 or 1:100 is an excellent disinfectant.
- Keep immunizations current. Tetanus vaccine is recommended every 10 years, influenza vaccine is repeated yearly, and one dose of pneumococcal pneumonia vaccine lasts a lifetime.
- Investigate the need for vaccinations, water purification techniques, and foods to avoid when traveling outside the United States.
- Eat the recommended servings from the food pyramid (see Chap. 16) and use safe food handling practices.
- Use and immediately discard disposable paper tissues rather than reuse cloth handkerchiefs.
- Avoid sharing washcloths, drinking cups, and other personal care items.
- Follow safe sex practices.
- Stay home from work or school when ill rather than expose others to infectious pathogens.
- Avoid crowds and public places during local outbreaks of influenza.
- Follow posted infection control instructions when visiting hospitalized family members and friends.
- Understand that antibiotic therapy is not appropriate for every infectious disease, but when it is, take the full dose for the prescribed period.

BOX 19-3 ● Standard Precautions

Wear clean gloves when touching:
- Blood, body fluids, secretions, excretions, and items containing these body substances
- Mucous membranes
- Nonintact skin

Perform handwashing immediately:
- When there is direct contact with blood, body fluids, secretions, excretions, and contaminated items
- After removing gloves
- Between client contacts

Wear a mask, eye protection, and face shield during procedures and client care activities that are likely to generate splashes or sprays of blood, body fluids, secretions, and excretions.

Wear a cover gown during procedures and client care activities that are likely to generate splashes or sprays of blood, body fluids, secretions, or excretions or cause soiling of clothing.

Remove soiled protective items promptly when the potential for contact with reservoirs of pathogens is no longer present.

Clean and reprocess all equipment before reuse by another client.

Discard all single-use items promptly in appropriate containers that prevent contact with blood, body fluids, secretions, and excretions; contamination of clothing; and transfer of microorganisms to other clients, healthcare workers, and the environment.

Handle, transport, and process linen soiled with blood, body fluids, secretions, and excretions in such a way as to prevent skin and mucous membrane exposures, contamination of clothing, or transfer to other clients, healthcare workers, and the environment.

Prevent injuries with used needles, scalpels, and other sharp devices by:
- Never removing, recapping, bending, or breaking used needles
- Never pointing the needle toward a body part
- Using a one-handed "scoop" method, special syringes with a retractable protective guard or shield for enclosing a needle, or blunt-point needles
- Depositing disposable and reusable syringes and needles in puncture-resistant containers

Use a private room or consult with an infection control professional for the care of clients who contaminate the environment, or who cannot or do not assist with appropriate hygiene or environmental cleanliness measures.

GENERAL PHARMACOLOGIC CONSIDERATIONS

Antibiotics can cause an overgrowth of microorganisms not affected by these drugs. This overgrowth can cause a superinfection, leading to a serious and potentially life-threatening diarrhea called *pseudomembranous colitis*. Report fever, abdominal cramps, and severe diarrhea immediately.

Antipyretic drugs (e.g., aspirin, acetaminophen) usually are ordered for elevated temperature.

With rectal administration of an antipyretic drug, the suppository is inserted high in the rectum. The client must be checked in 30 minutes to ensure that the suppository has not been expelled.

After administering injections of penicillin, make the client wait at least 30 minutes before allowing him or her to leave the healthcare facility. Reactions are frequent and can be severe enough to be fatal.

Antibiotics are administered on time and regularly around-the-clock to maintain therapeutic blood levels.

When antibiotics are administered, observe the client for adverse drug effects. Nausea, vomiting, anorexia, diarrhea, and rash are adverse

ture is above normal. For instance, the BMR for a person with a temperature of 103.6°F is increased by 35% (5°F above normal × 7% = 35% increase). This translates into an extra 350 to 700 calories needed per day, based on an average BMR of 1000 to 2000 calories per day.

Protein needs can increase to 1.5 to 2.5 g/kg of body weight for severe infections (normal protein requirement is 0.8 g/kg). Milk, milk drinks, and commercial supplements may be used to add significant proteins and calories.

Fluid needs depend on the severity of fever and any complicating factors (e.g., diarrhea, vomiting, excessive sweating). Encourage the intake of ice water, broth, fruit juices, milk, popsicles, and gelatin. Clients should avoid tea, coffee, and carbonated beverages containing caffeine, which promotes diuresis.

Acutely ill clients may accept and tolerate a full liquid diet with in-between-meal supplements better than solid food. Advance the diet as tolerated to maximize intake.

For clients who require transmission-based precautions, meals are served on disposable dinnerware. The tray is made as attractive as possible to encourage eating. Uneaten food is disposed in the toilet, and plastic containers are deposited in sealed bags before removal.

effects of some antibiotics but also are symptoms associated with some infectious diseases. An accurate history and physical examination at the time of admission and ongoing documentation of the client's symptoms help distinguish between symptoms related to the infectious disease and those possibly caused by antibiotic therapy.

GENERAL GERONTOLOGIC CONSIDERATIONS

Chronic diseases and inadequate nutrition predispose older adults to infections.

Infections in older adults are more serious because their defense mechanisms are less efficient. Symptoms of infectious disease are subtle, atypical, or blunted. For example, temperature is less elevated with pneumonia or urinary tract infection. Confusion and changes in behavior often are signs of infection among older adults.

Residents in nursing homes tend to acquire infections involving the urinary tract, skin, and respiratory tracts.

Combined, pneumonia and influenza are the fifth leading cause of death in people older than 65 years of age. Immunizing for pneumococcal pneumonia and influenza can reduce morbidity and mortality.

Tactfully advise those with respiratory infections to avoid visiting older adults until their symptoms are relieved, or provide them with a mask.

When transmission-based precautions are necessary, older adults may become confused because of decreased social contact and lack of environmental stimulation from such sources as television, radio, windows, and reading materials.

Some older adults who had TB as children can experience a reactivation of the disease if they become seriously ill.

Critical Thinking Exercises

1. *Use the infectious process cycle illustrated in Figure 19-2 to trace the viral transmission of a common cold from one person to another.*
2. *Give a specific example of how pathogens are spread among clients and healthcare workers, then identify techniques for preventing their transmission.*
3. *Select any community-acquired infection and identify the type of microorganism that causes it and its usual reservoir, exit route, mode of transmission, and port of entry.*

References and Suggested Readings

American College of Chest Physicians. (1992). Definitions for sepsis and organ failure and guidelines for the use of innovative therapies in sepsis. *Chest 101*(6), 1644–1655.

Baird, V. L. & Hoawley, R. (2000). Methicillin-resistant *Staphylococcus aureus* (MRSA): Is there a need to change clinical practice? *Intensive and Critical Care Nursing, 16*, 357–366.

Bernard, G. R., Vincent, J., & Laterre, P. (2001). Efficacy and safety of recombinant human activated protein C for severe sepsis. *New England Journal of Medicine, 344*, 699–709.

Bielan, B. (1999). What's your assessment? . . . streptococcal sepsis. *Dermatology Nursing, 11*(1), 48.

Bures, S., Fishbain, J. T., Uyehara, C. F. T., et al. (2000). Computer keyboards and faucet handles as reservoirs of nosocomial pathogens in the intensive care unit. *American Journal of Infection Control, 28*, 465–471.

Cardin, P., Taylor, L., & Vorster, K. (2001). Sepsis. *Journal of PeriAnesthesia Nursing, 16*(1), 58–60.

Centers for Disease Control and Prevention. (2001, January 29). Bovine spongiform encephalopathy ("mad cow disease") and new variant Creutzfeldt-Jakob disease (nvCJD). [On-line.] Available: http://www.cdc.gov/travel/other/fmd-europe-mar2001.htm.

Coignard, B., Siegel, J. D., Weinstein, R. A., et al. (2000). Reality check: How should we control antimicrobial use? *Infection Control and Hospital Epidemiology, 21*, 792–795.

Earl, M. L., Jackson, M. M., & Rickman, L. S. (2001). Improved rates of compliance with hand antisepsis guidelines: A three-phase observational study. *American Journal of Nursing, 101*(3), 26–33.

Fletcher, C. E. (2000). Accurate data: An essential component in reducing needlestick injuries. *Policy, Politics, and Nursing Practice, 1*, 316–324.

Gardner, S. E., Frantz, R. A., Troia, C., et al. (2001). A tool to assess clinical signs and symptoms of localized infection in chronic wounds: Development and reliability. *Ostomy/Wound Management, 47*(1), 40–47.

Gordon, L. (1999). The sepsis continuum from systemic inflammatory response syndrome to multiple organ dysfunction syndrome. *Nursing in Critical Care, 4*, 238–244.

Gunn, K. (2001). Infection control in nursing and residential homes. *Nursing Times, 97*(7), IX.

Kennedy, V. S., Steinfeld, S. R., & Sims, G. L. (2001). Improving care practices for patients with multidrug-resistant organisms: One facility's evolution. *Rehabilitation Nursing, 26*(2), 58–60, 63–65, 78.

Lejeune, J. R. & Berkowitz, D. M. (2000). Bad bugs: What you should know about VRE/MRSA. *Journal of Emergency Medical Services, 25*(12), 57–63.

Mason, D. J., Winslow, E. H., & Jacobson, A. (2001). Hand stand: When it comes to patient safety, nurses have the whole world in their hands. *American Journal of Nursing, 101*(3), 7.

McCoy, K. D., Beekman, S. E., Ferguson, K. J., et al. (2001). Monitoring adherence to Standard Precautions. *American Journal of Infection Control, 29*, 24–31.

Meckler, L. & Ricks, C. (2001, May 22). Mad cow scare prompts Red Cross to tighten blood-donation rules. *Kalamazoo Gazette* Section A:2.

Porth, C. M. (1998). *Pathophysiology: Concepts of Altered States* (5th ed.). Philadelphia: Lippincott Williams & Wilkins.

Prusiner, S. B. (1998). The prion diseases. *Brain Pathology, 8*, 499–513.

Shelton, B. K. (1999). Sepsis. *Seminars in Oncology Nursing, 15*, 209–221.

Souweine, B., Traore, O., Aublet-Cuvelier, B., et al. (2000). Role of infection control measures in limiting morbidity associated with multi-resistant organisms in critically ill patients. *Journal of Hospital Infection, 45*, 107–116.

The Associated Press. (2001). Long-sought drug said to fight sepsis. [On-line.] Available: http://usatoday.com/news/health/2001-02-09-sepsis-drug.htm.

Thompson, S. (1999). Nursing care of a patient with fever due to sepsis/SIRS. *Nursing in Critical Care, 4*(2), 63–66.

Wagenlehner, F. M. E. & Naber, K. G. (2000). Hospital-acquired urinary tract infections. *Journal of Hospital Infection, 46*, 171–181.

Ward, D. (2000). Delivering effective infection control in the community setting: Facing the challenge. *Journal of Community Nursing, 14*(10), 22, 24, 26–27.

Caring for Clients With Cancer

Learning Objectives

On completion of this chapter, the reader will:

- Discuss the pathophysiology and etiology of cancer.
- Compare benign and malignant tumors.
- Name factors that contribute to the development of cancer.
- Identify the warning signs of cancer.
- Describe ways to reduce the risks of cancer.
- Explain methods for diagnosing cancer.
- Describe systems for staging and grading malignant tumors.
- Differentiate various treatments and methods for managing cancer.
- Discuss various adverse effects that occur with cancer treatments and methods used to treat those effects.
- Describe emotions associated with the diagnosis of cancer.
- Use the nursing process as a framework for caring for clients with cancer.

Cancer is characterized by abnormal, unrelated cell proliferation. Cancerous tumors invade healthy tissues and compete with normal cells for oxygen, nutrients, and space. Nurses in all settings care for clients of all ages with cancer, a complex and challenging endeavor. The nursing specialty related to care of clients with cancer is **oncology nursing.** A diagnosis of cancer is frightening to most people, although reactions depend on the particular diagnosis, location, stage, treatment, effects on bodily functions, and prognosis.

CANCER

Pathophysiology

The cell is the basic structural unit in plants and animals. Differentiated cells work together to perform specific functions. Cell regeneration occurs through cell division and reproduction. Abnormal changes in cells develop for many reasons. These abnormal cells reproduce in the same way as normal cells, but they do not have the regulatory mechanisms to control growth. Thus, abnormal cell growth proliferates in an uncontrolled and unrestricted way.

New growths of abnormal tissue are called **neoplasms** or *tumors.* Table 20-1 classifies tumor cells. The first part of the tumor's name indicates the particular cell or tissue. The suffix *-oma* indicates it is a tumor. Four main tumor classifications according to tissue type are *carcinomas* (cancers originating from epithelial cells), *lymphomas* (cancers originating from organs that fight infection), *leukemias* (cancers originating from organs that form blood), and *sarcomas* (cancers originating from connective tissue, such as bone or muscle). Tumors also are classified according to their cell of origin and whether their growth is **benign,** not invasive or spreading, or **malignant,** invasive and capable of spreading (Table 20-2).

Benign tumors remain at their site of development. They may grow large, but their growth rate is slower than that of malignant tumors. They usually do not cause death unless their location impairs the function of a vital organ, such as the brain. On the other hand, malignant

TABLE 20-1	CLASSIFICATION OF TUMOR CELLS	
ORIGIN	**MALIGNANT**	**BENIGN**
Skin	Basal cell carcinoma	
	Squamous cell carcinoma	Papilloma
	Malignant melanoma	Nevus (mole)
Epithelium	Adenocarcinoma	Adenoma
Muscle	Myosarcoma	Myoma
Connective tissue		
Fibrous tissue	Fibrosarcoma	Fibroma
Adipose (fatty) tissue	Liposarcoma	Lipoma
Cartilage	Chondrosarcoma	Chondroma
Bone	Osteosarcoma	Osteoma
Nerve tissue	Neurogenic sarcoma	Neuroma
	Neuroblastoma	Ganglioneuroma
	Glioblastoma	Glioma
Bone marrow	Multiple myeloma Leukemia	

tumors grow rapidly and, unless completely removed, are likely to undergo **metastasis** (spreading). Cancer can metastasize by direct extension to adjacent tissues, from lymph vessels into the tissues adjacent to lymphatic vessels, by transport from blood or lymph systems, and by diffusion within a body cavity. The *primary site* is the area where malignant cells first form. The *secondary* or metastatic sites are regions to which cancer cells have spread. Metastasis is one of cancer's most discouraging characteristics because even one malignant cell can give rise to a metastatic lesion in a distant part of the body. Metastatic tumors are treated aggressively when possible

to improve quality of life and lengthen survival time. Cancer is known to spread to the lymph nodes that drain the tumor area. When a malignant tumor is removed, lymph node dissection usually also is done, along with a wide excision of the tumor.

Etiology

Cancer is the second leading cause of death in the United States, where half of all men and one-third of all women will develop cancer during their lives (American Cancer Society, 2001). Lung cancers are the most deadly for both men and women. Common cancers in men include prostate, lung, and colon. Breast, lung, and colon cancer most commonly affect women.

Damage to cellular deoxyribonucleic acid (DNA) causes cancer cells to develop. In many cases, the body repairs such damage; in cancer cells, the DNA remains damaged. Inherited cancers occur when the damaged DNA passes to the next generation. In many instances, however, certain factors and agents contribute to the development of cancer. These factors are called **carcinogens** and include chemical agents, environmental factors, dietary substances, viruses, defective genes, and medically prescribed interventions.

Chemical agents in the environment are believed to account for 85% of all cancers. The effects of tobacco smoke and nicotine are related to cancers of the lung, mouth, throat, neck, esophagus, pancreas, cervix, and bladder. Prolonged exposure to chemicals such as asbestos and coal dust is associated with some cancers. Chemical substances in workplaces can cause cancer. Organs most affected are the lungs, liver, and kidneys because they are involved with biotransformation and excretion of chemicals.

Environmental factors include prolonged exposures to sunlight, radiation, and pollutants. Electromagnetic fields from microwaves, power lines, and cellular phones are

TABLE 20-2	CHARACTERISTICS OF BENIGN AND MALIGNANT TUMORS
BENIGN TUMORS	**MALIGNANT TUMORS**
Usually slow, steady rate of growth	Usually rapid rate of growth; can be unpredictable
Growth remains localized	Invade surrounding tissue and metastasize to other tissues
Usually remain encapsulated	Rarely encapsulated
When palpated, are smooth, easily defined, and movable	When palpated, have irregular borders and are immobile.
Less profuse blood supply	Greater than normal blood supply
Cells resemble the cells of the tissue of origin.	Cells cannot be readily identified as to tissue of origin.
Only destroy normal tissue by compression or obstruction of normal tissue	Invade normal tissue and compete with normal cells for oxygen and nutrients; also destroy by compression and destruction
When removed, recurrence is rare.	When removed, recurrence is more common.
Rarely fatal	Fatal if not treated

other possible carcinogens, although study results related to such factors are conflicting.

Diet is an important variable. What a person fails to consume is as important as what he or she does consume (Box 20-1). Foods high in fat and those smoked or preserved with salts, alcohol, or nitrates are associated with an increased cancer risk. Foods believed to reduce cancer risk are high in fiber, cruciferous (e.g., cabbage, broccoli), and high in carotene (e.g., winter squash, carrots, and cantaloupe). Vitamins A, C, and E also seem to have anticancer value.

Viruses are implicated in many cancers. The cell changes that a virus incorporates into the genetic information may cause cancerous cells to form. An example is Kaposi's sarcoma, which is associated with human immunodeficiency virus (HIV; see Chap. 43).

Defective genes are responsible for diverse cancers. Some types of leukemia, retinoblastoma (an eye tumor in children), and skin cancer are associated with genetic factors. Breast, prostate, and colorectal cancers are also associated with defective genes.

Medically prescribed interventions such as immunosuppressive drugs, hormone replacements, and anticancer drugs have been associated with increased incidence of cancer in people or their offspring exposed in utero.

Assessment

Signs and Symptoms

Cancer is insidious (slow growing). It initially may cause no symptoms or signs or it may be vague. This factor underscores the importance of educating clients about prevention and self-examination so that cancer can be diagnosed as early as possible. Seven warning signals of cancer should be familiar to all:

1. A change in bowel habits or bladder function
2. Sores that do not heal
3. Unusual bleeding or discharge
4. Thickening or lump in breast or other body parts
5. Indigestion or difficulty swallowing
6. A recent change in a wart or mole
7. A nagging cough or hoarseness

Better education has improved awareness of warning signals and factors that may influence cancer development. Public education focuses on periodic physical examinations and cancer screening programs. Healthcare providers must emphasize and teach self-examination of the breasts, testicles, and skin. Avoidance of factors that predispose to cancer and early detection increase the chances of cure. Box 20-2 lists healthy habits that reduce cancer risk.

Diagnostic Findings

A client's history, physical examination, and diagnostic studies contribute to the diagnosis of cancer. In some cases the physical examination findings are unremarkable, but the client's history is suspect. In addition, the client is evaluated for risk factors. Many diagnostic studies are used to establish a diagnosis of cancer. The physician, using information obtained during the history and physical examination, selects tests that help establish a diagnosis.

LABORATORY TESTS

Specific cancers alter the chemical composition of blood and other body fluids. Specialized tests have been developed for *tumor markers,* specific proteins, antigens, hormones, genes, or enzymes that cancer cells release (Table 20-3). Normally, tumor markers are not present in or not found in large quantities in the blood.

Other laboratory tests may be useful in establishing a diagnosis. Although abnormal values do not directly indicate a malignant process, they may help to formulate a total clinical picture. For example, a complete blood count may indicate anemia in a client with possible colon cancer. Occult blood in the stool may indicate colorectal cancer.

BOX 20-1 ● Diet Modifications for Reducing the Risk of Cancer

- Decrease intake of red meat.
- Increase the number of servings of cruciferous vegetables such as broccoli, cabbage, and cauliflower.
- Reduce intake of processed meats that contain nitrites and nitrates as preservatives.
- Increase fiber intake.
- Decrease fat intake to 20%–30% of total daily calories.
- Increase intake of foods rich in vitamins A and C, such as fruits and yellow and leafy green vegetables.
- Reduce alcohol intake to no more than one drink per day.

BOX 20-2 ● Healthy Lifestyle Habits That Reduce the Risk of Cancer

- Learn and regularly practice self-examination techniques.
- See physician or nurse practitioner regularly.
- Include periodic colon examinations, mammograms, Pap smears, testicular examinations, and prostate-specific antigen testing as indicated.
- Eat a healthy diet (see Box 20-1).
- Abstain from smoking or using tobacco products.
- Avoid overexposure to the sun; use sunscreen with SPF of 15 or greater.
- Maintain weight within suggested limits.
- Exercise regularly.
- Practice safety in the workplace to avoid exposure to chemicals and radiation.
- Limit alcohol intake.

TABLE 20-3	SOME SPECIFIC TUMOR MARKERS	
MARKER	NORMAL VALUE	SIGNIFICANCE
Alpha-fetoprotein (α FP)	<12.8 IU/mL	Serum globulin normally secreted by liver cells in embryonic life. High levels seen in carcinomas of testicles, pancreas, and liver but may be elevated in acute viral hepatitis.
Carcinoembryonic antigen (CEA)	0.0–3.4 ng/mL	Glycoprotein found in fetal pancreas, liver, and colon. Increased antibody titers found in serum of persons with breast cancer, pancreatic, liver, kidney, and colon cancer. Also may be elevated in pancreatitis, acute renal failure, pneumonia, ulcerative colitis, cigarette smokers, and for no apparent reason.
Prostate-specific antigen (PSA)	Female: <0.5 ng/mL Male: 0.0–4 ng/mL	Protein tumor-specific antigen expressed from prostatic tissues, markedly increased in prostatic cancer, slightly increased in benign prostatic hyperplasia, prostatitis, prostate surgery.
CA 15-3	0–30 U/mL	Glycoprotein elevated in metastatic breast cancer; a smaller percentage is elevated in primary breast cancer, but the marker may be elevated in benign breast disease and gastrointestinal disease.
CA 19-9	0–37 U/mL	Antibody developed against tumor-associated antigens from gastrointestinal and pancreatic cancers. Shows greater specificity for pancreatic cancers than CEA.
CA 125	0–35 U/mL	Antibody developed against tumor-associated antigen, a glycoprotein found on the surface of ovarian cancer cells; also may be elevated during pregnancy, pelvic inflammatory disease; and in endometriosis.
CA 27, 29	0–32 U/mL	Membrane antigen for breast cancer screening; when associated with other marker tests, positive predictive values improve.
Human chorionic gonadotropin (hCG)	<5 mIU/mL	Glycoprotein used in diagnosis and monitoring of gestational trophoblastic diseases such as hydatidiform mole, invasive mole, and choriocarcinoma.

(From Bullock, B. L. & Henze, R. L. [2000]. *Focus on pathophysiology* [p. 80]. Philadelphia: Lippincott Williams & Wilkins.)

RADIOLOGIC AND IMAGING TESTS

X-Ray Studies. X-ray studies, such as plain films or radiographs using contrast media or specialized equipment, detect tumors in specific organs. A *contrast medium* is a substance that highlights, outlines, or provides more detail than shown in a plain film. A barium enema is an example of a study done with contrast medium.

Computed Tomography. The computed tomography (CT) scan provides three-dimensional cross-sectional views of tissues to determine tumor density, size, and location. CT is useful in diagnosing many types of cancer.

Magnetic Resonance Imaging. Producing detailed sectional images, magnetic resonance imaging (MRI) uses magnetic fields to differentiate diseased tissue from healthy tissue and to study blood flow. It helps to visualize tumors hidden by bone or other structures.

Positron Emission Tomography. The positron emission tomography (PET) scan uses computed cross-sectional images of increased concentrations of radioisotopes in malignant cells. It provides information about the biologic activity of the cells and assists in differentiating benign and malignant processes and responses to treatment. PET is principally used for lung, colon, liver, and pancreatic cancers.

Radioimmunoconjugates. Monoclonal antibodies, labeled with radioisotopes and injected intravenously, accumulate at the tumor site. Scanners may then visualize the tumor. These studies are particularly useful for colorectal, breast, ovarian, head, and neck tumors. They also may be used for lymphomas and melanomas.

Ultrasound. Ultrasound uses high-frequency sound waves to detect abnormalities of a body organ or structure. The sound wave reflections are projected on a screen and may be recorded on film. These studies help differentiate solid and cystic tumors of the abdomen, breasts, pelvis, and heart.

OTHER STUDIES

Biopsy. Tissue samples excised from the body are directly examined microscopically for malignant or premalignant processes. Tissue samples may be obtained during surgery, insertion of a biopsy needle under local anesthesia, or endoscopic procedures. A biopsy provides the most definitive method for diagnosing cancer.

Frozen Section. During some surgeries, when a tumor or node is removed, it is taken to the pathologist for immediate examination. The specimen is quickly frozen and then sliced into very thin pieces so that it may be examined under a microscope. Once the preliminary findings are known, the surgeon decides the type of surgery needed. Healthcare providers make the client aware of the possibilities before surgery.

Endoscopy. Fiberoptic instruments are flexible tubes that contain optical fibers, which enable light to travel in a straight line or at various angles and illuminate the area being examined. Specific body areas can be examined with endoscopy, gastroscopy, bronchoscopy, and colonoscopy. Tissue biopsies may be done if a malignancy is suspected.

Cytology. Microscopic examination of cells from various body areas may be used to diagnose malignant or premalignant disorders. Cells are obtained by needle aspiration, scraping, brushing, or sputum. An example of a cytologic test is the Papanicolaou (Pap) smear used to diagnose changes in the endometrium, cervix, and vagina (see Chap. 59).

Staging of Tumors

Before a client is treated for cancer, the tumor is staged and graded based on how it tends to grow and the cell type of the tumor. The American Joint Committee on Cancer developed a grading system referred to as the TNM classification: *T* indicates the size of the tumor, *N* stands for the involvement of regional lymph nodes, and *M* refers to the presence of metastasis (Table 20-4). Once the TNM descriptions are established, they are grouped together in a simpler set of stages that include tumor size, evidence of metastasis, and lymph node involvement.

- *Stage I:* Malignant cells are confined to the tissue of origin, with no signs of metastasis.
- *Stage II:* Spread of cancer is limited to the local area, usually to area lymph nodes.
- *Stage III:* Tumor is larger, probably has invaded surrounding tissues, or both.
- *Stage IV:* Cancer has invaded or metastasized to other parts of the body.

Grading of tumors involves the differentiation of the malignant cells. Basically there are two classifications: differentiated and undifferentiated. Cancer cells are evaluated in comparison with normal cells. *Well-differentiated* cells are those that most closely resemble the tissue of origin. *Undifferentiated cells* bear little resemblance to the tissue of origin. Cell differentiation is graded from I to IV. The higher the number, the less differentiated is the cell type. Tumors with poorly differentiated cells are graded

TABLE 20-4	TNM STAGING SYSTEM AND CLASSIFICATION
SYMBOL	**MEANING**
T	Tumor
TX	Primary tumor cannot be assessed
T0	No evidence of primary tumor
T1s	Carcinoma in situ
T1, T2, T3, T4	Progressive increase in tumor size and extension
N	Regional lymph nodes
NX	Regional lymph nodes cannot be assessed clinically
N0	No regional lymph node involvement
N1, N2, N3	Increase in regional lymph node involvement
M	Distant metastasis
MX	Cannot be assessed
M0	No distant metastasis
M1	Distant metastasis present
Example: T2, N1, M0	Indicates the primary tumor has grown and spread to regional lymph nodes but is not metastasized
G1	Well-differentiated grade
G2	Moderately well-differentiated grade
G3, G4	Poorly to very poorly differentiated grade

IV. These tumors are very aggressive and unpredictable, and the prognosis usually is poor.

Medical and Surgical Management

Three basic methods are used to treat cancer: (1) surgery, (2) radiation therapy, and (3) chemotherapy. Another method, bone marrow transplantation, is used for selected cancers. Immunotherapy, gene therapy, and other alternative therapies also may be used. Cancer frequently is treated with a combination of therapies using standardized protocols.

Surgery

Surgery may range from tumor excision alone to extensive excision, including removal of the tumor and adjacent structures such as bone, muscle, and lymph nodes. The type and extent of surgery depends on the extent of the disease, actual pathology, client's age and physical condition, and anticipated results. When tumors are confined and have not invaded vital organs, the surgery is more likely to be curative and is referred to as the *primary treatment.* In some cases, the entire tumor cannot be removed but as much of it as possible is removed, which is referred to as *debulking.* Two types of excisions are done. The first is *local excision,* in which the tumor is removed along with a small margin of healthy tissue. The other type is *wide* or *radical excision,* which removes the primary tumor, lymph nodes, any involved adjacent structures, and surrounding tissues that pose a risk for metastasis.

Salvage surgery is done when there is a local recurrence of cancer. It usually is more extensive. For example, a cancerous tumor may be removed from the breast (lumpectomy). If a tumor reappears, a mastectomy most likely will be done.

Prophylactic surgery may be done if the client is at considerable risk for cancer. According to Smeltzer and Bare (2000), prophylactic surgery may be done when there is a family history or genetic predisposition, ability to detect surgery at an early stage, and client acceptance of the postoperative outcome. Examples of prophylactic surgery include mastectomy and hysterectomy. Clients who choose prophylactic surgery require careful preoperative counseling and teaching so that they are fully aware of the consequences of surgery.

Surgery that helps to relieve uncomfortable symptoms or prolong life is considered *palliative.* Some palliative surgeries are used to remove excess fluid and increase comfort, such as *paracentesis* (removal of fluid from the abdominal cavity) and *thoracentesis* (removal of fluid from the chest). Surgical procedures used to relieve pain include nerve blocks, placement of epidural catheters for administration of epidural analgesics, and placement of venous access devices for administration of parenteral analgesics.

Reconstructive or *plastic surgery* may be done after extensive surgery to correct defects caused by the original surgery. Some surgeries are disfiguring or so profound that the client may have difficulty adjusting to body changes. In these cases, radiation therapy may be a better option. Preoperative and postoperative care is discussed in Chapter 25.

Specific surgeries are addressed in separate chapters. Other surgical interventions include the following:

- *Electrosurgery*—uses electric current to destroy tumor cells
- *Laser* (*l*ight *a*mplification by *s*timulated *e*mission of *r*adiation) *surgery*—uses light and energy aimed directly at an exact tissue location and depth to vaporize cancer cells
- *Chemosurgery*—combines topical chemotherapy with layer-by-layer surgical removal of abnormal tissue
- *Cryosurgery*—uses liquid nitrogen to freeze tissue, which destroys cells (Nevidjon & Sowers, 2000; Smeltzer & Bare, 2000).

Radiation Therapy

Radiation therapy uses high-energy ionizing radiation, such as high-energy x-rays, gamma rays, and radioactive particles (alpha and beta particles, neutrons, and protons) to destroy cancer cells (Box 20-3). Cells are destroyed by

---

BOX 20-3 ● New Radiation Therapy Procedures

Stereotactic surgery/stereotactic radiation therapy (SRS) (external)—A linear accelerator called a *gamma knife* delivers large, precise radiation doses to a small tumor area. Although there is no actual surgery, the gamma knife is referred to as "surgery" because of its accuracy. Currently, this type of radiation therapy is used on brain tumors. The head must be immobilized. Angiography, CT, or MRI locates the tumor. It is hoped that this method can be used on other types of cancer.

Three-dimensional conformal radiation therapy (3DCRT) (external)—Special computers precisely map the cancer's location. A plastic mold or cast keeps the body part stabilized so that radiation beams can be more accurately aimed from several directions. It is hoped that radiation damage to normal tissues will decrease while the radiation dose to the cancer increases.

Conformal proton beam radiation therapy (external)—This procedure is similar to 3DCRT but uses protons instead of x-rays. The protons are parts of atoms that pass through tissues without causing much damage but are effective in destroying cells at the end of their path. It is hoped that the proton beam therapy will deliver higher doses of radiation while reducing side effects to adjacent tissue.

Intraoperative radiation therapy (IORT) (external)—Radiation therapy is delivered directly to the tumor during surgery. It usually is used on abdominal and pelvic cancers or those cancers that are most likely to return. IORT reduces damage to normal tissues because they can be moved out of the way during surgery and protected from radiation. The advantage is that higher doses of radiation can be delivered. The disadvantage is that clients must move from the operating room (OR) to the radiation therapy department and then back to the OR to complete the surgery.

(Adapted from American Cancer Society [2001]: What's new in radiation therapy? [On-line.] Available: http://www.cancer.org; and Nevidjon, B. M. & Sowers, K. W. [2000]. *A nurse's guide to cancer care.* Philadelphia: Lippincott Williams & Wilkins.)

---

disruption of cell function and division and alteration of DNA molecules. Cell death can occur immediately or when the cell can no longer reproduce.

The goal of radiation therapy is to destroy malignant, rapidly dividing cells without permanently damaging surrounding healthy tissues. Radiation therapy may destroy both normal and malignant cells, but the more rapidly reproducing malignant cells are more sensitive to radiation because it affects cells undergoing mitosis (cancer cells) more than cells in slower growth cycles (normal cells). Radiation therapy may be applied externally or internally, both with curative and palliative intent. Nearly 60% of all clients with cancer receive some form of radiation; about 60% of those clients are cured (Washington & Leaver, 1997).

EXTERNAL RADIATION THERAPY

External radiation therapy or external beam radiation uses high-energy x-rays aimed at a specific body location. A treatment plan, using beams from multiple directions, is developed and customized for each client. Linear accelerators are machines that deliver external beam radiation.

External radiation therapy enables treatment of large body areas, targeting the tumor and nearby lymph nodes.

Clients usually have daily radiation treatments over several weeks on an outpatient basis. Their skin is marked with a marker or tattoo to identify the reference points for the treatment plan. Clients are instructed not to wash off these markings until the therapy is complete. Clients are not radioactive when receiving external beam radiation therapy.

INTERNAL RADIATION THERAPY

Internal radiation therapy (**brachytherapy**) refers to short-distance therapy. It involves the direct application of a radioactive source on or within a tumor and can deliver a high dose of radiation to a small area. The most common methods include interstitial implants, intracavitary implants, and systemic therapy. Its advantage is that it delivers a high dose of radiation to a specific tumor, applying less radiation to adjacent normal tissues. Brachytherapy may be used alone or combined with surgery, chemotherapy, and external radiation therapy.

Sealed brachytherapy sources include interstitial and intracavitary implants. Needles, seeds, wires, or catheters contain the radioactive source and are implanted directly into the tumor. For intracavitary implants, the radioactive source is placed directly in the body cavity and an applicator holds it in place. When the implants are removed, no radioactivity is left in the body. In some cases seeds are left in permanently, such as with prostate or brain cancer (Nevidjon & Sowers, 2000). The radioactivity of the seeds decays over several weeks or months, depending on the radioactive element's half-life. Clients usually go home if they have permanent implants. Clients must stay away from other people for a few days while the radiation is most active. They must restrict close contact with children or pregnant women to 5 minutes and no closer than 6 feet for 2 months after the implant.

A client must be hospitalized when receiving sealed brachytherapy because he or she will emit radiation during therapy. Specific orders for treatment and precautions to be taken, as well as the type and dosage of the radioactive substance, time and area of insertion, type of applicator used, and when to remove the material are noted in the client's chart. If any orders are unclear, the nurse should contact the radiation oncologist or radiation safety officer. Box 20-4 lists safety measures when a client is receiving radiation therapy. Everyone involved in the client's care must recognize the necessity to limit radiation exposure. The degree of possible hazard depends on the type and amount of radioactive material used. Usually, no special precautions are required when a small amount of a radioactive substance is used for diagnostic studies. If necessary, the radiation oncologist specifies precautions, informs personnel, and posts a radiation sign (Fig. 20-1).

Unsealed radiation sources (radiation in a suspension or solution or radiopharmaceutical therapy), such as iodine 131, may be administered orally, intravenously, or into a body cavity. Various body parts take up these sources in doses sufficient to treat cancer or, if received

---

BOX 20-4 • Safety Measures for Protecting Healthcare Personnel and Visitors From Excessive Exposure to Radiation

Client is placed in private room; some rooms have walls that are lined with lead.

Standardized sign (see Fig. 20-1) is placed on door to designate the room as a radiation room.

Anyone entering the room must have knowledge of the precautions required. Children younger than age 18 and pregnant women are never permitted in the room.

Healthcare personnel limit time spent in the room and limit distance from source of radiation by working as far from the source of radiation as possible.

The physician and radiation safety personnel are notified if the sealed sources become dislodged.

When the client has unsealed sources, gloves must be worn at all times. Policies regarding disposal of body fluids and contaminated articles such as dressings must be adhered to.

---

in small amounts, to diagnose cancer. This type of radiation has systemic effects and is excreted primarily in urine, but also through saliva, sweat, and feces. As an example, the *half-life* (time for 50% of the isotope to lose its radioactivity) for iodine 131 is 8.05 days (Nevidjon & Sowers, 2000). To reduce exposure, clients are asked to:

- Wash hands carefully after going to the bathroom.
- Flush toilet several times after each use.
- Use separate eating utensils and towels.
- Wash laundry separately.
- Drink plenty of fluids to help flush radioactive substances away.
- Avoid kissing and sexual contact.

The National Committee on Radiation Protection publishes guides for radiation safety. The effects of long and short exposures must be considered. The latent period between the exposure and the accumulated biologic effect often is long, and great care is taken to protect occupationally exposed workers from radiation injury that can accumulate over years. Pregnant women should avoid exposure to radioactive substances. Nursing Guidelines 20-1 provide standard interventions for clients re-

CAUTION

RADIATION AREA

FIGURE 20-1 International radiation symbol.

NURSING GUIDELINES 20-1

Managing Clients Receiving Radiation Therapy

- Provide information regarding the safety of radiation: effects on others, effects on tumor, and side effects related to radiation.

- Teach client about the actual procedure of external or internal radiation therapy.

- Explain the need for optimal nutritional intake.

- Protect the skin from irritation.

- Assess skin and mucous membranes for changes, particularly the areas being treated.

- Advise client that effects of radiation on skin include redness, tanning, peeling, itching, hair loss, and decreased perspiration.

- Cleanse with mild soap (be careful not to wash radiation marks) and tepid water. Advise the client to shave with electric razors.

- Moisturize with mild, water-based lubricant lotions.

- Advise client to wear loose cotton clothing and to protect skin from sun exposure, chlorine, and wind. He or she must avoid heat lamps and heating pads and report any blistering (use prescribed creams or ointments).

- Maintain intact oral mucous membranes.

- Teach client to:
  - Report oral burning, pain, open lesions, or problems with swallowing; use nonalcoholic mouthwash.
  - Brush with soft toothbrush and avoid electric toothbrushes.
  - Floss gently; use WaterPik cautiously.
  - Keep lips moist with lip balm.
  - Avoid alcoholic beverages, very hot drinks and foods, highly seasoned foods, acidic foods, and tobacco products.
  - Assess lesions—culture as necessary.

- Monitor client for signs of bone marrow suppression: decreased leukocyte, erythrocyte, and platelet counts.

- Assess for signs of bleeding; assess lesions and culture as necessary.

- Monitor for signs and symptoms related to area of irradiation: cerebral edema, malabsorption, pleural effusion, pneumonitis, esophagitis, cystitis, and urethritis.

- Encourage client to share fears and anxieties related to radiation therapy.

- Inform client that fatigue is a common effect of radiation therapy.

ceiving radiation therapy. When providing information, clients need to know the type and duration of treatment, what is required of the client, possible side effects, skin and mouth care, nutritional and dietary concerns, and precautions needed.

Expected side effects may result from the destruction of normal cells in the area being irradiated and are specific to the anatomic site treated. They include the following:

- **Alopecia** (hair loss)
- Erythema (local redness and inflammation of the skin)
- Desquamation (shedding of epidermis, which can be dry or moist)
- Alterations in oral mucosa, including **stomatitis** (inflammation of the mouth), xerostomia (dryness of the mouth), change or loss in taste, and decreased salivation
- Anorexia (loss of appetite)
- Nausea and vomiting
- Diarrhea
- Cystitis (inflammation of the bladder)
- Pneumonitis (inflammation of the lungs)
- Fatigue
- **Myelosuppression** (depression of bone marrow function) if marrow-producing sites are irradiated, resulting in anemia (decreased red blood cells, hemoglobin, or volume of packed red blood cells), **leukopenia** (decreased white blood cell count), and **thrombocytopenia** (decreased platelet count)

Effects of radiation are cumulative. Often the client experiences chronic or long-term side effects after completing therapy. Many times these effects result from decreased blood supply and normal tissue destruction. The changes are irreversible. Possible effects include fibrosis (abnormal formation of scar tissue) in the small intestine, lungs, and bladder; cataracts; disturbances in blood cell formation; sterility; and new cancers.

When radioisotopes are used to treat cancer, three safety principles must always be kept in mind: time, distance, and shielding (where applicable).

Time. *Time* refers to the length of exposure. The less time spent in the vicinity of a radioactive substance, the less radiation is received. Healthcare personnel must plan carefully and work quickly and efficiently to spend minimal time at the bedside. Careful psychological preparation helps the client accept the limited amount of nursing time.

Distance. *Distance* refers to the length in feet between the person entering the room and the radioactive source (client). The inverse square law applies to radiation exposure. The rate of exposure varies inversely to the square of the distance from the source (client). For example, nurses standing 4 feet from the source of radiation receive 25% of the radiation they would receive if they stood 2 feet from the source.

Shielding. *Shielding* is the use of any type of material to decrease the radiation that reaches an area. The material usually used is lead, such as lead-lined gloves and lead aprons. Other materials, such as concrete walls, are capable of shielding (Client and Family Teaching Box 20-1).

20-1 *Client and Family Teaching* Radiation Therapy

The nurse instructs clients who receive radiation therapy on an outpatient basis as follows:

- Avoid using ointments or creams on the area receiving radiation therapy unless prescribed or instructed to by a physician or radiation therapist.
- Avoid extremes of heat or cold, including heating pads, ultraviolet light, diathermy, whirlpool, sauna, steam baths, or direct sunlight.
- If receiving radiation to the head or scalp, avoid shampooing with harsh shampoos (baby or mild shampoo is acceptable), tinting, permanent waving, hair dryers, curling irons, and any hair products or treatments unless approved by the physician or radiation therapist.
- Bathe carefully. Avoid using soap and friction over the irradiated area. Do *not* wash off skin markings because they serve as guides for setting and adjusting the treatment machine over the area to be radiated.
- Wear loose clothing to avoid irritating the irradiated areas.

Chemotherapy

Chemotherapy uses **antineoplastic** agents to treat cancer cells locally and systemically. These agents may be used alone or combined with other therapies to cure cancer, prevent it from metastasizing, slow its growth, destroy tumor cells that have metastasized, or relieve symptoms.

Antineoplastic agents work by interfering with cellular function and reproduction. They are classified according to their relationship to cell division and reproduction. Healthy and malignant cells follow a cell-cycle pattern, which involves division of the cell and reproduction of two identical daughter cells. There are distinct phases:

- G1 phase—ribonucleic acid (RNA) and protein synthesis take place.
- S phase—RNA synthesis is complete, and DNA synthesis occurs.
- G2 phase—DNA synthesis is complete, and cell mitosis begins.
- M phase—Mitosis or cell division takes place.
- G0 phase—This is a dormant or resting phase, which can occur after mitosis and during the G1 phase.

CELL CYCLE–SPECIFIC DRUGS

Antineoplastic drugs are most effective during cell division. Cell cycle-specific drugs are used to treat rapidly growing tumors because they attack cancer cells when they enter a specific phase of cell reproduction. Most chemotherapeutic agents affect cells in the S phase by interfering with RNA and DNA synthesis. Others are more specific to the M phase. Chemotherapy is administered in multiple, repeated doses to produce a greater cell kill and to halt the growth of tumor cells. Examples of cell cycle–specific agents are topoisomerase I inhibitors, antimetabolites, mitotic spindle poisons, and some of the miscellaneous agents (Drug Therapy Table 20-1).

CELL CYCLE–NONSPECIFIC DRUGS

Cell cycle–nonspecific drugs are effective during any phase of the cell cycle, whether reproducing or resting. They are used for large, slow-growing tumors. The amount of drug given is more important than the frequency. Cell cycle–nonspecific drugs have more prolonged effects on cells, which results in cell damage and destruction. They often are given in combination with cell cycle–specific drugs, and also may be combined with or follow radiation therapy. Examples of cell cycle–nonspecific agents are alkylating agents, antitumor antibiotics, nitrosoureas, hormones, and some of the miscellaneous agents (see Drug Therapy Table 20-1).

ROUTES AND DEVICES FOR ADMINISTRATION OF CHEMOTHERAPY

Chemotherapeutic drugs are administered by several routes. The most common are the oral and intravenous (IV) routes, but they also may be given intramuscularly, intraperitoneally, intra-arterially, intrapleurally, topically, intrathecally, or directly into a cavity. Dosage is based on the client's total body surface area, prior responses to chemotherapy and other therapies, function of the major organs, and the client's health status. IV administration is monitored closely to prevent the drug from leaking into surrounding tissues, referred to as **extravasation.** Most agents can be very irritating. Blistering and tissue necrosis are possible effects of extravasation. If a client complains of burning or pain during the chemotherapy infusion, the drug must be discontinued. **Vesicants** are particularly damaging antineoplastics, in that they cause tissue necrosis of underlying tendons, nerves, and blood vessels. Sloughing and ulceration of the skin may be so severe that the client needs skin grafts. If vesicants are being administered, there are protocols for treating the extravasation (Table 20-5). In addition, there are safety issues for the nurse who administers chemotherapy (Box 20-5).

Various vascular devices are used to administer chemotherapy and are particularly beneficial for long-term chemotherapy. The client does not have to endure repeated venipunctures. In addition, they are beneficial when a client has poor veins. One method used is the insertion of venous access devices, which are special catheters inserted into a peripheral or central vein so that the catheter tip is located in the superior vena cava or right

🔖 **DRUG THERAPY TABLE 20-1**	**ANTINEOPLASTIC AGENTS**

DRUG CATEGORY AND EXAMPLES	MECHANISM OF ACTION	CELL CYCLE SPECIFICITY	SIDE EFFECTS
Alkylating Agents			
busulfan, carboplatin, chlorambucil, cisplatin, cyclophosphamide, dacarbazine, hexamethyl melamine, ifosfamide, melphalan, nitrogen mustard, thiotepa	Alters DNA structure by mis-reading DNA code, initiating breaks in the DNA molecule, cross-linking DNA strands	Cell cycle–nonspecific	Bone marrow suppression, nausea, vomiting, cystitis (cyclophosphamide, ifosfamide), stomatitis, alopecia, gonadal suppression, renal toxicity (cisplatin)
Nitrosoureas			
carmustine (BCNU), lomustine (CCNU), semustine (methyl CCNU), streptozocin	Similar to the alkylating agents; cross the blood–brain barrier	Cell cycle–nonspecific	Delayed and cumulative myelo-suppression, especially thrombo-cytopenia; nausea, vomiting
Topoisomerase I Inhibitors			
irinotecan, topotecan	Induces breaks in the DNA strand by binding to enzyme topo-isomerase I, preventing cells from dividing	Cell cycle–specific	Bone marrow suppression, diarrhea, nausea, vomiting, hepato-toxicity
Antimetabolites			
5-azacytadine, cytarabine, edatrexate fludarabine, 5-fluorouracil (5-FU), FUDR, gemcitabine, hydroxyurea, leustatin, 6-mercaptopurine, methotrexate, pentostatin, 6-thioguanine	Interferes with the biosynthesis of metabolites or nucleic acids necessary for RNA and DNA synthesis	Cell cycle–specific (S phase)	Nausea, vomiting, diarrhea, bone marrow suppression, proctitis, stomatitis, renal toxicity (methotrexate), hepatotoxicity
Antitumor Antibiotics			
bleomycin, dactinomycin, daunorubicin, doxorubicin (Adriamycin), idarubicin, mitomycin, mitoxantrone, plicamycin	Interferes with DNA synthesis by binding DNA; prevent RNA synthesis	Cell cycle–nonspecific	Bone marrow suppression, nausea, vomiting, alopecia, anorexia, cardiac toxicity (daunorubicin, doxorubicin)
Mitotic Spindle Poisons			
Plant alkaloids: etoposide, teniposide, vinblastine, vincristine (VCR), vindesine, vinorelbine	Arrests metaphase by inhibiting mitotic tubular formation (spindle); inhibit DNA and protein synthesis	Cell cycle–specific (M phase)	Bone marrow suppression (mild with VCR), neuropathies (VCR), stomatitis
Taxanes: paclitaxel, docetaxel	Arrests metaphase by inhibiting tubulin depolymerization	Cell cycle–specific (M phase)	Bradycardia, hypersensitivity reactions, bone marrow suppression, alopecia, neuropathies
Hormonal Agents			
androgens and antiandrogens, estrogens and antiestrogens, progestins and anti-progestins, aromatase inhibitors, luteinizing hormone–releasing hormone analogs, steroids	Binds to hormone receptor sites that alter cellular growth; block binding of estrogens to receptor sites (antiestrogens); inhibit RNA synthesis; suppress aromatase of P450 system, which decreases estrogen level	Cell cycle–nonspecific	Hypercalcemia, jaundice, increased appetite, masculinization, feminization, sodium and fluid retention, nausea, vomiting, hot flashes, vaginal dryness
Miscellaneous Agents			
asparaginase, procarbazine	Unknown or too complex to categorize	Varies	Anorexia, nausea, vomiting, bone marrow suppression, hepatotoxicity, anaphylaxis, hypotension, altered glucose metabolism

TABLE 20-5	TREATMENT OF EXTRAVASATION	
GENERAL MEASURES	**SPECIFIC MEASURES**

Stop administration of drug.
Leave needle in place.
Gently aspirate residual drug and blood into tubing or needle.
Inject neutralizing solution such as sodium thiosulfate, hyaluronidase, or sodium bicarbonate to reduce tissue damage. Selection of neutralizing agent depends on vesicant.
	Vesicant:
	  Doxorubicin
	    Elevate and rest extremity.
	    Apply topical cooling for 24 hours.
	    Give hydrocortisone as ordered.
	  Nitrogen mustard
	    Apply cold compresses.
	    Administer thiosulfate as ordered.
	  Vinca alkaloids (vinblastine, vincristine, vindesine)
	    Apply warm compresses.
	    Do not apply ice—increases skin toxicity.
	    Administer hyaluronidase as ordered.
	  Mitomycin
	    Apply ice.
	    Administer dimethylsulfoxide (DMSO) as ordered.

atrium. Examples include peripheral indwelling catheters (PIC lines), peripherally inserted central catheters (PICC lines), and external catheters (Hickman catheters, Broviac catheters). Another type is the implanted vascular access device (IVAC), also referred to as a *port*. A metal or plastic port encloses a self-sealing silicone rubber septum. The port is surgically implanted subcutaneously. A silicone catheter attached to the port is threaded subcutaneously to the right atrium. To access the port, a needle is inserted in the self-sealing septum of the port.

Chemotherapy infusion pumps are used for some cancers. They provide constant infusion of an antineoplastic drug directly into the cancerous organ. A small pump (similar in size to a hockey puck) is surgically implanted subcutaneously in the abdomen or attached externally.

ADVERSE EFFECTS OF CHEMOTHERAPY

Nursing management of the client receiving chemotherapy varies depending on the drug, dose administered, and route used (Nursing Guidelines 20-2). Some clients experience little discomfort or few adverse effects. Others have a wide range of symptoms. The tissues most susceptible to chemotherapy are those with rapidly growing cells, such as epithelial tissue, hair follicles, and bone marrow. Chemotherapy can potentially harm all body systems. Common adverse effects associated with chemotherapy are as follows:

- Nausea and vomiting are common during the first 24 hours after chemotherapy administration; use of concurrent antiemetics helps to reduce the incidence and severity.
- Stomatitis and mouth soreness or ulceration may result from destruction to the epithelial layer.
- Alopecia develops because chemotherapy affects rapidly growing cells of the hair follicles.
- Myelosuppression results from inhibition of the manufacture of red and white blood cells and platelets. Severe anemia, bleeding tendencies, leukopenia, **neutropenia** (decreased neutrophils), and thrombocytopenia are possible if bone marrow depression is profound. Blood transfusions may be necessary, as well as protection of the client from infections.
- Fatigue results from the aforementioned effects, the chemotherapy itself, and the increased metabolic rate that accompanies cell destruction (Client and Family Teaching Box 20-2).

BOX 20-5 ● **Safety Measures When Administering Chemotherapy**

Prepare chemotherapy in designated biologic safety area.
Use gloves when handling chemotherapy drugs and excretions from clients receiving chemotherapy.
Wear disposable long-sleeved gowns when preparing and administering chemotherapy.
Use Luer-lock fittings on IV tubing used in delivering chemotherapy.
Dispose of all equipment used in chemotherapy preparation and administration in designated containers.
Dispose of all chemotherapy wastes as hazardous materials.

Stop, Think, and Respond ● **BOX 20-1**

You are assigned to a client who was recently diagnosed with lung cancer. Surgery is planned, followed by chemotherapy. Your client says that he has heard that large doses of vitamin C would contribute to postoperative healing and also would enhance chemotherapy. He asks if he should begin megadoses of vitamin C. How should you respond?

NURSING GUIDELINES 20-2

Managing Clients Receiving Chemotherapy

- Monitor client for symptoms of anaphylactic reaction: urticaria (hives), pruritus (itching), sensation of lump in throat, shortness of breath, wheezing.

- Assess for electrolyte imbalances (see Chap. 22).

- Teach client and family to report excessive fluid loss or gain, change in level of consciousness, increased weakness or ataxia (lack of muscle coordination), paresthesia (numbness, prickling, or tingling), seizures, persistent headache, muscle cramps or twitching, nausea and vomiting, or diarrhea.

- Prevent extravasation of vesicant drugs. Implement measures to treat extravasation of vesicant medications if it occurs (see Table 20-5).

- Teach client to increase fluid intake to 2500 to 3000 mL/day unless contraindicated.

- Assess for signs of bone marrow depression: decreased white and red blood cell, granulocyte, and platelet counts.

- Assess for signs of bleeding and infection.

- Monitor for signs of renal insufficiency:
  - Elevated urine specific gravity
  - Abnormal electrolyte values
  - Insufficient urine output (<30 mL/hour)
  - Elevated blood pressure, BUN (blood urea nitrogen), and serum creatinine

- Inform client about the reasons for nausea and vomiting.

- Administer antiemetics before and during administration of chemotherapy, or as indicated.

- Encourage the following dietary modifications:
  - Eat small, frequent meals.
  - Eat slowly.
  - Eat cool, bland foods and liquids.
  - Suck on hard candy during chemotherapy if taste alterations occur.
  - Avoid hot or very cold liquids, food with fat and fiber, spicy foods, and caffeine.

- Assess oral mucosa for dryness, redness, swelling, lesions, ulcerations, viscous (sticky) saliva, or white patches.

Bone Marrow Transplantation

Cancers that are very sensitive to high doses of chemotherapy and radiation therapy may be treated with bone marrow transplantation (BMT). The survival rate after BMT for malignant disease is approximately 50%. There are four possible sources for BMT: autologous (client receives BMT from self), allogeneic (BMT is from a histocompatible but unrelated donor), syngeneic (BMT is from an identical twin), or stem cell transplant.

20-2 *Client and Family Teaching* Chemotherapy

The nurse instructs clients receiving chemotherapy on an outpatient basis to:

- Keep all appointments for chemotherapy treatments.
- Follow recommendations of the physician or healthcare personnel regarding diet, oral fluids, and adverse effects to report.
- Purchase a wig, cap, or scarf before therapy begins, if hair loss is anticipated. Hair usually begins to grow again within 4 to 6 months after therapy; new growth may have a slightly different color and texture.
- Have periodic evaluations and examinations as recommended.

AUTOLOGOUS BONE MARROW TRANSPLANTATION

Autologous BMT involves harvesting the client's own bone marrow and storing it in a frozen state. The client then receives intensive chemotherapy (also referred to as *ablative chemotherapy*) and radiation therapy to eliminate any remaining tumor. The client's own bone marrow is then reinfused. The harvested bone marrow also may be treated with chemotherapy to kill any malignant cells. Until the bone marrow is established (a process referred to as **engraftment**), the client is at high risk for infections and bleeding. This type of BMT is done for clients who have cancer affecting the bone marrow but do not have a matched donor, or for clients who have aggressive cancer that has not affected the bone marrow (Smeltzer & Bare, 2000). Clients having autologous BMT do not require immunosuppressant drugs. A risk persists that tumor cells remain in the bone marrow.

ALLOGENEIC BONE MARROW TRANSPLANTATION

Allogeneic BMT is primarily done for clients who have cancer affecting the bone marrow. Bone marrow is obtained from a compatible donor, one who has the same leukocyte antigens as the client. The client receives ablative chemotherapy and often also has total-body irradiation to destroy the cancer cells and bone marrow. The client then receives the donor bone marrow. It takes 2 to 4 weeks for the transplanted marrow to establish itself and to begin producing blood cells. Clients receive immunosuppressant drugs, which may include cyclosporine and azathioprine (Imuran), to prevent rejection of the bone marrow, referred to as *graft-versus-host disease* (GVHD). GVHD occurs with allogeneic BMT because the T lymphocytes in the donor's marrow view the recipient's tissues as "foreign," causing an immune reaction. The first 3 months after allogeneic BMT are the most critical for the client in terms of rejection, infection, hemorrhage, nausea, vomiting, and fatigue.

SYNGENEIC BONE MARROW TRANSPLANTATION

Syngeneic BMT is possible only if the client has an identical twin. The process is the same as for allogeneic BMT. Because the donor is an identical tissue match, however, the recipient needs fewer immunosuppressant drugs because there is no issue with bone marrow rejection.

STEM CELL TRANSPLANTATION

The most recent innovation in BMTs is peripheral *stem cell transplantation.* Clients having this type of BMT receive chemotherapy and hematopoietic growth factors that stimulate the production of hematopoietic stem cells. The stem cells are collected by **apheresis** (process of separating blood into components) for later reinfusion. Stem cells are essentially bone marrow because of their role in engraftment and repopulation of hematopoietic tissue (Smeltzer & Bare, 2000). After collection of stem cells, clients have ablative chemotherapy and possibly radiation therapy. Stem cells are then reinfused. Recovery tends to be faster than with other BMTs.

NURSING MANAGEMENT

Nursing management for the client receiving any form of BMT is crucial. Before the procedure, the nurse thoroughly evaluates the client's physical condition, organ function, nutritional status, complete blood studies (including assessment for past antigen exposure such as HIV, hepatitis, or cytomegalovirus), and psychosocial status.

When clients are ready to receive a BMT, they undergo intensive chemotherapy and possibly whole-body radiation. Because a large amount of tissue is treated, nausea, vomiting, diarrhea, and stomatitis are common. In addition, until the transplanted bone marrow begins to produce blood cells, these clients have no physiologic means to fight infection, which makes them very prone to infection. They are at high risk for dying from sepsis and bleeding before engraftment. Thus, nurses *must* monitor clients closely and take measures to prevent infection. Clients also are at risk for bleeding, renal complications, and liver damage.

After a BMT, the nurse closely monitors the client for at least 3 months because complications related to the transplant are still possible. Infections are common, as is GVHD. The client's immune system is deficient because of the chemotherapy and radiation therapy. Throughout the entire BMT, the nurse assesses the client's psychological status. Clients experience many mood swings and need support and assistance throughout this process. Their families and significant others also require support. See Nursing Guidelines 20-3.

Immunotherapy

Immunotherapy uses biologic response modifiers (BRMs) to stimulate the body's natural immune system to restrict and destroy cancer cells. Many of these treat-

---

> ### NURSING GUIDELINES 20-3
>
> ### *Managing Clients Receiving a Bone Marrow Transplant*
>
> - Assess client's nutritional status.
> - Monitor for signs and symptoms of infection and renal insufficiency (see Nursing Guidelines 20-2).
> - Assess for signs and symptoms of graft-versus-host disease (GVHD): irritability, pulmonary infiltration, hepatitis, enlarged spleen, enlarged lymph nodes, anemia, sepsis, diarrhea, maculopapular rash, and skin desquamation.
> - Implement Standard Precautions and use protective isolation as needed.
> - Assist with thorough hygiene.
> - Review information related to prevention of infection, signs of rejection, importance of adherence to medical regimens and follow-up, medication instructions, and dietary needs.
> - Encourage client to discuss anxieties and fears.
> - Provide ongoing information about recovery phase and status of recuperation.

ments are new and in trial phases. Recent research has demonstrated that the body's natural immunity, a process of surveillance, recognition, and attack on foreign cells, is a defense against cancer (see Chap. 41). Use of BRMs attempts to manipulate the natural immune response by restoring, modifying, stimulating, or augmenting the natural defenses (Smeltzer & Bare, 2000).

Results of immunotherapy vary. Some clients respond well; others have little or no response. Usually, immunotherapy is not instituted until surgery, radiation therapy, and chemotherapy have failed. The three categories of immunotherapy are nonspecific, monoclonal antibody, and cytokines.

NONSPECIFIC IMMUNOTHERAPY

Nonspecific immunotherapy uses nonspecific agents such as bacille Calmette-Guerin (BCG) or *Corynebacterium parvum* to act as antigens to stimulate an immune response. When these agents are injected into a client, the goal is for the stimulated immune system to destroy malignant growths. These agents are useful in treating localized melanoma and localized bladder cancer (Smeltzer & Bare, 2000).

MONOCLONAL ANTIBODY IMMUNOTHERAPY

Monoclonal antibody immunotherapy uses monoclonal antibodies (MoAbs), a form of BRM. Specific tumor cells are injected into mice and act as antigens. The mice produce antibodies, which are found in their spleens. The antibody-producing spleen cells are combined with a cancer cell that then produces more antibodies in a culture medium. These cells are referred to as *hybridomas.* The desired antibodies are harvested from the hybridomas and purified and prepared for use in humans. MoAbs have several uses:

- Diagnostic—radioactive substances are attached to the MoAbs to detect tumors (radioimmuno-detection)
- To purge remaining tumor cells from blood or bone marrow for clients who are having a peripheral stem cell BMT
- Cancer therapy—used directly to destroy tumor cells (still in trial stages)

The goal is for the MoAbs to overwhelm and destroy the tumor cells. Clinical trials for solid tumors and cancers affecting the blood have had limited success. The incidence of allergic reactions, headaches, wheezing, tachycardia, nausea, vomiting, rash, fever, and chills is high.

CYTOKINES

Cytokines are substances that immune system cells produce to enhance the immune system. The four categories of cytokines are interferons, interleukin-2, colony-stimulating factors, and tumor necrosis factor (Table 20-6). In general, they stimulate the immune system or assist in inhibiting tumor growth. Side effects include flu-like symptoms, gastrointestinal (GI) disturbances, alopecia, and low blood counts (Nevidjon & Sowers, 2000).

Hyperthermia

Hyperthermia or thermal therapy uses temperatures greater than 41.5°C (106.7°F) to destroy tumor cells. Heat is in the form of radio waves, ultrasound, microwaves, magnetic waves, hot water baths, or immersion in hot wax. Methods of delivery include extracorporeal circulators, probes, or infusion of heated chemotherapeutic agents into the blood or directly into a cancerous organ. A client also may be immersed in heated water or paraffin. Tumor cells are more sensitive to the harmful effects of high temperatures for several reasons:

- Malignant cells cannot repair themselves.
- Many tumor cells lack sufficient blood supply to provide the increased need for oxygen required during hyperthermia.
- The tumor blood vessels are inadequate for dispersing heat.
- Hyperthermia appears to stimulate the immune system (Smeltzer & Bare, 2000).

Hyperthermia is combined with other therapies. When used with radiation therapy, the tumor cells are more sensitive to the radiation and cannot repair themselves at all. Hyperthermia alters cell membrane permeability so that uptake of chemotherapy is increased. It enhances the function of immunotherapeutic agents. Clients receiving

TABLE 20-6	CYTOKINES*		
CYTOKINES	HOW PRODUCED	FUNCTION	USE
Interferons	Naturally occurring protein molecules produced in response to viral infections	Stimulate immune system, inhibit tumor cell growth, or both	Used to treat hairy cell leukemia, chronic myelogenous leukemia, melanoma, and Kaposi's sarcoma
Interleukins	Produced by lymphocytes and monocytes About 15 types have been identified	Signal and coordinate other cells of the immune system	Interleukin-2 (IL-2) approved for treatment of renal cell cancer Clinical trials with various interleukins in process for treatment of cancer in monotherapy and combined with chemotherapy, and for treatment of myelosuppression after treatment with chemotherapy
Hematopoietic growth factors (colony-stimulating factors)	Hormone-like substances produced by the immune system	Stimulate production of blood cells: neutrophils, lymphocytes, platelets, erythrocytes, monocytes, and macrophages	Do not treat cancers but instead treat the negative effects of cancer treatments on bone marrow Higher doses of chemotherapy may be given with less suppression of bone marrow function.
Tumor necrosis factor (TNF)	Naturally produced by macrophages, lymphocytes, astrocytes, and microglial cells of the brain	Exact mechanism of action not understood—appears to stimulate other cells in the immune response and directly kills tumor cells	Research is being done in the treatment of melanoma and lung and renal cancer.

*Cytokines, substances produced by cells of the immune system, promote the activities of the immune system and may have antiviral, antibacterial, and antitumor effects.

hyperthermia may experience local burns and tissue damage, electrolyte imbalances, fatigue, GI disturbances, and neuropathies.

Gene Therapy

Scientists have theorized that many cancers result from gene alterations. Strategies to confront this problem include **gene therapy,** which involves replacing altered genes with correct genes, inhibiting defective genes, and introducing substances that destroy genes or cancer cells (Smeltzer & Bare, 2000). Scientists predict that gene therapy will play a significant role in the future prediction, diagnosis, and treatment of cancer. It is currently being investigated in the treatment of brain tumors, melanoma, and renal, breast, and colon cancers.

Clinical Trials

Clinical trials provide methods to test new treatments for specific cancers. The trials may involve a new drug, a new combination of existing drugs, or new therapies. The process for new treatments to become accepted practice is lengthy. Before testing on humans, there is testing on laboratory animals to ascertain safety and effectiveness. After animal testing, there are four phases:

1. Phase I—Treatment is given to a small group of people to determine dosing, schedule for treatment, and toxicity. Participants usually are clients for whom standard treatment has been ineffective. Clients are fully aware of the trial's experimental nature.
2. Phase II—Treatment is given to a larger group of clients to further determine effectiveness with specific cancers and to get better information about dosing, side effects, and toxicity. Clients are similar to the clients selected for phase I.
3. Phase III—If the treatment appears effective in phase II, then a larger number of clients are selected and compared with clients receiving accepted treatments for a particular type of cancer. At this point, the new treatment has had significant testing and review.
4. Phase IV—In this phase, there is further testing of newly accepted treatments for other uses, dosing, and toxicity.

Complementary and Alternative Therapy

Complementary and alternative therapy includes imagery, medicinal therapy, special diets, and mystical and spiritual approaches. Alternative therapy also refers to treatments that are not proven to be effective in treating a particular disease, but are used instead of conventional treatments. Examples include hydrogen peroxide therapy, hydrazine sulfate, and Essiac tea (American Cancer Society, 2001). Table 20-7 briefly describes some methods used to treat cancer. It is difficult for healthcare professionals to condone unconventional therapies because many of the methods do not have a scientific foundation. There also are legal and ethical implications if healthcare personnel participate in unaccepted treatments. Information that they provide to clients must be factual and understandable. Although some alternative methods have successfully augmented conventional treatments, many methods have no positive effects, and indeed some actually are harmful.

Nursing Management

Managing the care of clients with cancer is challenging. The diagnosis itself implies multiple problems, and the treatments result in many secondary problems. This care requires a comprehensive plan designed to meet or assist the client and family's needs. In addition to the following discussion, see Nursing Care Plan 20-1.

Pain is a major problem for clients with cancer (see Chap. 21). Sources of pain include bone metastasis; nerve compression; obstructed blood vessels, lymph systems, or

TABLE 20-7	ALTERNATIVE METHODS OF CANCER TREATMENT

METHOD	DESCRIPTION
Imagery, relaxation techniques, stress reduction exercises, yoga, biofeedback, massage, and music therapy	These methods are used to reduce pain, promote relaxation, and enhance conventional treatment methods based on beliefs that there is a link between the immune system and cancer and that these methods boost the immune system's ability to fight the cancer cells.
Medicinal agents	Many "cures" for cancer have been concocted from plants, herbs, flowers, and fluids of humans and animals. Although a few merit scientific investigation, many are considered quackery. The use of vitamins, minerals, proteins, and other ingredients is advocated for treatment of many cancers and prevention of treatment side effects.
Special diets	Many diet regimens are advocated as treatment for certain cancers or as adjuncts to treatment. Examples include organic foods, macrobiotic diets, and particular foods that reportedly kill cancer cells.
Spiritual methods	These methods are derived from powers of faith that people believe will help them to overcome cancer. Examples include faith healing, laying on of hands, and prayer.

Nursing Care Plan 20-1

THE CLIENT WITH CANCER

Assessment

- Assess client's level of understanding about the diagnosis, treatment, and follow-up care.
- Determine the client's strengths, coping mechanisms, response to diagnosis, and emotional and physical support systems.
- Evaluate the family's response to illness.
- Check client's overall physical condition, energy and pain levels, and nutritional and fluid status.

Nursing Diagnosis: **Anxiety** related to diagnosis, prognosis, treatments, changes in health status

Expected Outcome: Client demonstrates decreased anxiety.

Refer to Chapter 14 for nursing interventions.

Evaluation of Expected Outcome: Client and family share anxieties about diagnosis and care.

Nursing Diagnosis: **Fatigue** related to side effects of treatments, weakness from cancer, and physical and psychological stress

Expected Outcomes: (1) Client will participate in daily care as much as possible. (2) Client will identify measures to conserve and improve energy.

Interventions	*Rationales*
Identify energy level by asking client to evaluate it on a scale of 0 (not tired) to 10 (totally exhausted).	Such identification establishes current level of fatigue.
Plan care around energy level and include rest periods.	Rest reduces physical stress and conserves energy.
Encourage adequate protein and calorie intake.	It increases activity tolerance.
Encourage use of relaxation techniques and mental imagery.	They promote relaxation and reduce psychological stress.

Evaluation of Expected Outcomes: (1) Client can participate in care without becoming exhausted. (2) Client can identify need for rest.

Nursing Diagnosis: **Anticipatory Grieving** related to potential loss and altered role status

Expected Outcomes: Client will identify and verbalize feelings. Client will continue to make future-oriented plans, even if one day at a time. Client will verbalize understanding of the dying process.

Refer to Chapter 26 for nursing interventions.

Evaluation of Expected Outcomes: (1) Client expresses feelings of guilt, anger, or sorrow. (2) Client plans for future one day at a time.

Nursing Diagnosis: **Chronic Pain** related to disease, metastasis, effects of surgery and treatments

Expected Outcomes: Client will report pain relief. Client will use relaxation methods and other alternatives to reduce pain and discomfort.

Refer to Chapter 21 for nursing interventions.

Evaluation of Expected Outcomes: Client states that pain medications are effective.

Nursing Diagnosis: **Disturbed Body Image** related to side effects of treatments, weight loss, and changes in appearance

(continued)

Nursing Care Plan 20-1 (Continued)

THE CLIENT WITH CANCER

Expected Outcomes: Client will verbalize understanding of changes in appearance. Client will demonstrate coping methods and adaptation to changes he or she is experiencing.

Interventions	*Rationales*
Explore strengths and resources with client.	Emphasizing strengths promotes a positive self-image.
Discuss possible changes in weight and hair loss. Suggest that the client select a wig before hair loss occurs.	Planning for an event such as weight or hair loss decreases anxiety associated with a change in appearance.
Acknowledge client's anger, sadness, or depression.	Body image changes cause anxiety and other feelings; acknowledging such feelings assists the client to cope.
Refer client to a support group or counseling.	Support groups and counseling allow the client to share feelings and to recognize that he or she is not alone.

Evaluation of Expected Outcomes: Client states acceptance of change or loss and demonstrates ability to adjust.

Nursing Diagnosis: **Imbalanced Nutrition: Less than Body Requirements** related to loss of appetite, difficulty swallowing, side effects of chemotherapy, or obstruction by tumor

Expected Outcomes: Client will increase dietary intake. Client will demonstrate understanding of the need for adequate intake of nutrients and fluids.

Interventions	*Rationales*
Monitor daily food intake.	Such monitoring provides baseline data.
Encourage intake of sufficient calories, nutrients, and fluids (see Nursing Guidelines 20-2), offering small, frequent meals and fluids.	These measures reduce the sensation of fullness and decrease the stimulus to vomit.
Administer antiemetics as ordered before meals.	They are more effective when given before nausea.
Monitor laboratory studies for signs of dehydration, biochemical imbalances, and malnutrition.	Such monitoring reveals evidence of imbalances and assists in making needed interventions.

Evaluation of Expected Outcomes: Client demonstrates minimal weight loss and verbalizes necessity to have adequate intake.

Nursing Diagnoses: **Impaired Skin Integrity** and **Impaired Oral Mucous Membranes** related to immunologic deficits, effects of chemotherapy and radiation therapy, poor nutrition, immobility, and altered oral flora

Expected Outcome: Client will demonstrate measures to prevent complications from skin or tissue impairment or to promote tissue or skin healing.

Refer to Chapter 19 for interventions.

Evaluation of Expected Outcome: Client manages treatment for skin impairment and has minimal impairment of oral mucous membranes.

organs; inflammation; ulceration; infection; or necrosis. Pain ranges from dull and aching to sharp, unrelenting, and throbbing.

Clients with cancer also experience fatigue, which is a frequent side effect of cancer treatments that rest fails to relieve. Fatigued clients are constantly weary, lack energy, and often feel too weak to carry out normal activities. The nurse must assess the client for other stressors that contribute to fatigue, such as pain, nausea, fear, and lack of adequate support. The nurse works with other healthcare team members to treat the client's fatigue.

Another major problem for clients with cancer is infection. Many factors predispose clients with cancer to infection: impaired skin and mucous membranes, chemotherapy, radiation therapy, and other therapies, the malignancy itself, malnutrition, medications, invasive catheters and IV lines, contaminated equipment, age, chronic illness, and prolonged hospitalization (Smeltzer & Bare, 2000). Nurses must provide scrupulous care to clients with cancer and monitor for signs and symptoms of infection, including fever, elevated white blood cell counts, pain, redness, swelling, and drainage.

Psychological Support

The diagnosis of cancer is frightening and frequently overwhelming. Psychological support is as important as medical treatments and physical care. Clients have many reactions, ranging from anxiety, fear, and depression to feelings of guilt related to viewing cancer as a punishment for past actions or failure to practice a healthy lifestyle. They also may express anger related to the diagnosis and their inability to be in control. Clients have the right to know their diagnosis, treatment plan, and prognosis so they can make informed decisions. A client may never accept a cancer diagnosis. When provided with adequate information and supported psychologically, however, clients are more likely to face their diagnosis and be involved with their care and treatment. Families and significant others also require support.

Client and Family Teaching

Clients and their families or significant others require education to understand the diagnostic procedures, make treatment choices, participate in preventing complications, and recognize side effects and other adverse signs. Teaching focuses on:

- Medications, treatments, and procedures
- Adverse effects associated with treatment
- Possible changes in body image or function
- Resources for support
- Follow-up needed after discharge from the hospital

When developing a plan for client and family teaching, the nurse must consider facts such as the type of malignancy, treatment given, proposed treatments, client's condition, and effectiveness of the family support system. These facts will determine the areas to discuss in more detail. The nurse should be aware of any explanations or information that other healthcare providers give to the client and family. He or she also must allow time for clients to express their feelings or discuss home care. Doing so also helps identify issues the client or family does not understand.

The Terminally Ill Client

Nursing management of the terminally ill client can be both physically and emotionally difficult. It must include both client and family. The nurse must carry out tasks gently to reduce the possibility of pain and discomfort and to keep the client as comfortable as possible. He or she pays attention to controlling pain, providing adequate fluid and nutrition, keeping the client warm and dry, and controlling odors (when present). An important part of nursing care is to help the client maintain dignity, despite an illness that often requires dependence on others for activities of daily living. See Chapter 26 for more information on nursing and hospice care.

GENERAL NUTRITIONAL CONSIDERATIONS

Improving the client's nutritional status not only improves quality of life, but may make cancer cells more susceptible to treatment. Good nutrition also promotes rehabilitation, may lessen the effects of treatment, and may increase the chances of survival. Conversely, poor nutritional status may potentiate the toxicity of cancer treatments.

Malnutrition is not an inevitable consequence of cancer; once established, however, it can be difficult to reverse. To prevent malnutrition, it usually is more effective to increase the nutrient density of foods consumed rather than to expect a client to eat more food. Fortifying casseroles, beverages, cereals, and other foods with skim milk powder, whole milk, cheese, cream cheese, peanut butter, eggs, butter, and honey increases density without increasing volume. Small, frequent feedings also are beneficial.

Side effects of cancer and cancer therapies can devastate the client's ability to eat, which may change daily or as often as with each meal. Clients with nausea fare better with low-fat foods and "dry" meals (taking liquids between meals). Clients receiving chemotherapy should avoid eating or drinking for 1 to 2 hours after treatment to avoid nausea.

Clients with anorexia should consume small, frequent meals. Encourage clients to view eating as part of therapy, not a voluntary activity.

Clients with vomiting need to replenish fluids by taking water or flat beverages every 10 to 15 minutes.

Clients who develop taste alterations from chemotherapy often complain that meat tastes "bad" or "rotten." Offer cold protein alternatives: cheese, cottage cheese, protein beverages, and sandwiches. Assure the client that eating meat is not the only way to consume adequate protein.

Sucking on hard candy during chemotherapy infusion may prevent a bitter or metallic taste.

Clients with fatigue should rest before meals and avoid items that require a lot of chewing.

Clients with difficulty swallowing should use gravies and sauces liberally. They may tolerate semisolid foods better than liquids. They should avoid extremely hot foods.

A high fluid intake is necessary to promote excretion of chemotherapeutic drugs. Water, milk, fruit juices, and high-protein beverages are all good choices; clients should avoid beverages containing caffeine and limit soft drinks, which are high in empty calories.

Clients with a sore mouth should avoid highly seasoned foods, acidic juices, salty items, and coarse breads and cereals. They may tolerate cold food and beverages better than warm items.

For clients receiving palliative care, do not force feedings, weigh clients, or use nutritional support.

GENERAL PHARMACOLOGIC CONSIDERATIONS

Monitor the client taking an antineoplastic agent for symptoms of gout, which include increased uric acid levels, joint pain, and edema. Allopurinol may be prescribed to decrease the uric acid level. Encourage the client to increase fluid intake (up to 2000 mL/day) if his or her condition permits.

Anemia may occur as an adverse reaction to antineoplastic agents. Fatigue, dyspnea, or orthostatic hypotension should be reported.

Most antineoplastic agents are teratogenic. Female clients taking these drugs must use birth control measures throughout therapy. If a client suspects pregnancy, she must notify the primary healthcare provider immediately.

Because antineoplastic drugs can depress the immune system, advise clients to avoid crowds (e.g., shopping malls, movie theaters) and people with colds, flu, or other infectious diseases.

If stomatitis occurs, the primary healthcare provider may prescribe topical agents to promote eating. If stomatitis pain is severe, an analgesic may be prescribed.

Antineoplastic drugs are potentially toxic. Nurses must be thoroughly familiar with their adverse effects and toxicity. The dose or length of treatment depends, in some cases, on the client's response to therapy.

Many antineoplastic drugs profoundly affect the bone marrow. Observe clients for signs of bone marrow depression (fever, sore throat, chills), infection, and bleeding (oozing from venipuncture or parenteral injection sites, bleeding from gums, signs of blood in urine or stools).

Intra-arterial or IV administration of antineoplastic agents may lead to thrombophlebitis. Inspect sites daily (including above or below) for tenderness, pain, swelling, or induration.

Therapy may induce nausea, vomiting, and diarrhea. These adverse effects must be reported immediately because dehydration and electrolyte imbalance often ensue rapidly. The client may need antiemetic or antidiarrheal drugs or IV fluid and electrolyte replacement.

Drugs may be ordered for other adverse effects during radiation therapy: aspirin or acetaminophen for fever, antibiotics for infection, and various ointments and creams (applied exactly as prescribed) for skin irritation.

GENERAL GERONTOLOGIC CONSIDERATIONS

Older adults with cancer may have additional problems with nutrition, adequate fluid intake, skin care, and complications related to inactivity.

Older adults often have decreased resistance to infection, which may pose problems if they receive antineoplastic agents that have a depressant effect on bone marrow.

Because of concurrent disease and the effects of aging on the body's tissues and organs, older adults may not receive the same treatments for cancer that younger clients do.

Older adults, faced with long and sometimes rigorous cancer treatment, may refuse treatment. Those who have undergone extensive surgery for cancer require detailed home care planning before discharge from the hospital.

Arthritis, as well as general muscular stiffness, may make lying supine on an x-ray table difficult for older adults. It may be necessary to pad bony prominences and provide support to the back or legs during radiation therapy.

The skin of older adults often is dry. They may experience intense itching and dryness during and after radiation therapy; therefore, additional treatment of skin problems may be necessary. Inspect the skin frequently for signs of breakdown, excessive scratching, and infection.

Older adults are more prone to electrolyte imbalance. Excessive vomiting during or after treatments may result in a serious electrolyte imbalance.

Older adults who receive internal radiation therapy may experience difficulty in lying still until the end of the treatment. Check these clients more frequently for displacement of the applicator.

Critical Thinking Exercise

1. *A client with endometrial cancer has been told that she will be treated with internal radiation therapy. Discuss what information to include in her teaching plan.*

References and Suggested Readings

American Cancer Society. (2001). *Cancer reference information.* [On-line.] Available: http://www.cancer.org.

Bullock, B. L. & Henze, R. L. (2000). *Focus on pathophysiology.* Philadelphia: Lippincott Williams & Wilkins.

Cerrato, P. L. (2000). Preventing cancer. *RN, 63*(11), 38–44.

Eremita, D. (2001). Dolasetron for chemo nausea. *RN, 64*(3), 38–40.

Haylock, P. J. (2000). The universal specialty. *American Journal of Nursing, 100*(4), 9.

Giarelli, E., Pisano, R., & McCorkle, R. (2000). Stable and able. *American Journal of Nursing, 100*(12), 26–31.

Houldin, A. D. (2000). *Patients with cancer: Understanding the psychological pain.* Philadelphia: Lippincott Williams & Wilkins.

Jaquette, S. G. (2000). The octopus and me. *American Journal of Nursing, 100*(4), 23–24.

Mayer, D. K. (2000). Cancer overview. *American Journal of Nursing, 100*(4), 24D–H.

Myers, J. M. (2000). Chemotherapy-induced hypersensitivity reaction. *American Journal of Nursing, 100*(4), 53–54.

Nevidjon, B. M. & Sowers, K. W. (2000). *A nurse's guide to cancer care.* Philadelphia: Lippincott Williams & Wilkins.

Perin, M. L. & Pasero, C. (2000). Corticosteroids for cancer pain. *American Journal of Nursing, 100*(4), 15–16.

Smeltzer, S. C. & Bare, B. G. (2000). *Brunner & Suddarth's textbook of medical–surgical nursing* (9th ed.). Philadelphia: Lippincott Williams & Wilkins.

Starr, J. H. (2000). Radiation is lonely. *RN, 63*(8), 40–42.

Thayler-DeMers, D. (2000). The cancer survival toolbox. *American Journal of Nursing, 100*(4), 87.

Washington, C. M. & Leaver, D. T. (1997). *Principles and practice of radiation therapy: Practical applications.* St. Louis: Mosby.

Wilby, M. L. (1998). Improving the health profile: Decreasing risk for cancer through primary prevention. *Holistic Nursing Practice, 12*(2), 52–61.

Worthington, K. (2000a). Chemotherapy on the unit. *American Journal of Nursing, 100*(4), 88.

Worthington, K. (2000b). Guarding against radiation exposure. *American Journal of Nursing, 100*(5), 104.

Caring for Clients With Pain

Learning Objectives

On completion of this chapter, the reader will:

- Define the term *pain*.
- Name two types of pain classified according to their source and two types classified according to onset, intensity, and duration.
- Compare nociceptive pain with neuropathic pain.
- Give three characteristics distinguishing acute from chronic pain.
- List four phases of pain transmission.
- Differentiate between pain perception, pain threshold, and pain tolerance.
- List seven essential components of pain assessment.
- Explain why assessing pain is difficult.
- Name four tools for assessing the intensity of pain.
- Discuss the Joint Commission on Accreditation of Healthcare Organizations' standards on pain assessment and pain management.
- Explain pain management, and list five techniques commonly used.
- Name two categories of analgesic drugs.
- Identify two surgical procedures performed on clients with intractable pain.
- List at least five examples of noninvasive techniques that nurses can implement independently to manage pain.
- Name two endogenous opiates that block pain transmission.
- Discuss the nursing management of clients with pain.
- List at least three nursing diagnoses, besides Acute Pain and Chronic Pain, that are common among clients with pain.
- Discuss information pertinent to teach clients and family about pain management.

Pain is a privately experienced, unpleasant sensation usually associated with disease or injury. Pain also has an emotional component referred to as *suffering*. Extensive research is being conducted to discover more about various types of pain, pain transmission, and treatment.

TYPES OF PAIN

Pain can be classified into categories according to (1) its source or (2) its onset, intensity, and duration. When using the source of pain as a framework, pain can be categorized as either nociceptive or neuropathic. When using characteristics such as onset, intensity, and duration as criteria, pain can be categorized as either acute or chronic.

Nociceptive Pain

Nociceptive pain is the noxious stimuli that are transmitted in an orderly fashion from the point of cellular injury over peripheral sensory nerves to pathways between the spinal cord and thalamus, and eventually from the thalamus to the cerebral cortex of the brain (Fig. 21-1).

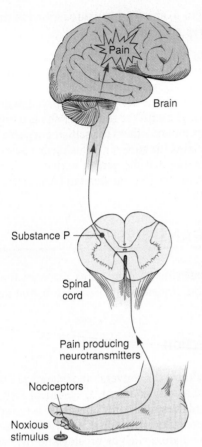

FIGURE 21-1 Pain transmission pathway.

poorly localized, and accompanied by autonomic nervous system symptoms such as nausea, vomiting, pallor, hypotension, and sweating. **Referred pain** is a term used to describe discomfort that is perceived in a general area of the body, but not in the exact site where an organ is anatomically located (Fig. 21-2).

Neuropathic Pain

Neuropathic pain is pain that is processed abnormally by the nervous system (McCaffery & Pasero, 1999). It results from damage to either the pain pathways in peripheral nerves or pain processing centers in the brain. One theory is that activation of receptors for *N*-methyl-D-aspartate (NMDA) sensitizes pain circuits in the spinal cord and brain. An example of neuropathic pain is *phantom limb*

Nociceptive pain is subdivided into somatic and visceral pain.

Somatic Pain

Somatic pain is attributed to mechanical, chemical, thermal, or electrical injuries or disorders affecting bones, joints, muscles, skin, or other structures composed of connective tissue. *Superficial somatic pain,* also known as *cutaneous pain* (like that from the bite of an insect or a paper cut), is perceived as sharp or burning discomfort. *Deeper somatic pain* such as that caused by trauma (e.g., a fracture) produces localized sensations that are sharp, throbbing, and intense. Dull, aching, diffuse discomfort is more common with long-term disorders like arthritis.

Visceral Pain

Visceral pain arises from internal organs like the heart, kidneys, and intestine that are diseased or injured. Causes for visceral pain are varied and include ischemia (reduced arterial blood flow to an organ), compression of an organ (as may be the case from a tumor), intestinal distention with gas, or contraction (spasm), as occurs with gallbladder or kidney stones. Visceral pain usually is diffuse,

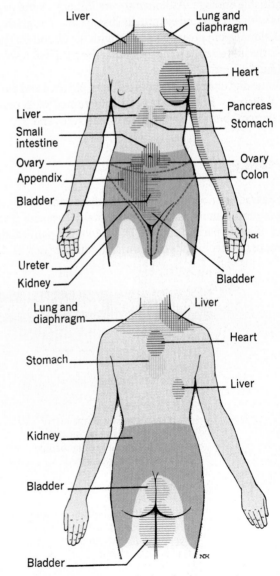

FIGURE 21-2 Common areas of referred pain.

pain or *phantom limb sensation,* in which persons with an amputated arm or leg perceive that the limb still exists and that sensations such as burning, itching, and deep pain are located in tissues that have been surgically removed. Other examples include pain that is experienced by people with spinal cord injuries, strokes, diabetes, and herpes zoster (shingles).

Cancer pain may be either nociceptive or neuropathic. Nociceptive pain occurs when a tumor creates pressure in the organ or on adjacent tissue from its increased size. Neuropathic pain occurs when drugs or radiation used to treat the cancerous tumor cause nerve damage.

Acute Pain

Acute pain is discomfort that has a short duration (from a few seconds to less than 6 months). It is associated with tissue trauma, including surgery, or some other recent identifiable etiology. Although severe initially, acute pain eases with healing and eventually disappears. The gradual reduction in pain promotes coping with the discomfort because there is a reinforcing belief that the pain will resolve in time.

Acute and chronic pain both result in physical and emotional distress. Both also may be interrupted with pain-free periods, but that is where the similarities end.

Chronic Pain

The characteristics of **chronic pain,** discomfort that lasts longer than 6 months, are almost totally opposite from those of acute pain (Table 21-1). The longer pain exists, the more far-reaching its effects on the sufferer (Box 21-1).

Others begin to show negative reactions to the chronic pain sufferer, such as:

- Saying they are tired of hearing about the pain
- Ignoring the sufferer's concerns and complaints
- Getting angry at the sufferer
- Suggesting that the pain has a psychological basis
- Telling the sufferer that he or she is using the pain to manipulate others for selfish purposes
- Criticizing the sufferer for using drugs as a "crutch"
- Suggesting that the person with chronic pain is addicted to analgesic medication (American Pain Society, 1999)

PAIN TRANSMISSION

The transmission of pain takes place in four phases: transduction, transmission, perception, and modulation (Fig. 21-3).

Transduction

Transduction is the conversion of chemical information in the cellular environment to electrical impulses that move toward the spinal cord. This phase is initiated by cellular disruption during which affected cells release various chemical mediators such as prostaglandins, bradykinin, serotonin, histamine, and substance P. The chemicals that are released by the damaged cells stimulate specialized pain receptors located in the free nerve endings of peripheral sensory nerves called **nociceptors.**

Nociceptors carry pain impulses by fast and slow nerve fibers. *A-delta fibers,* which are large and myelinated, carry impulses rapidly at a rate of approximately 5 to 30 meters per second (Porth, 2002). Impulses transmitted by the fast

TABLE 21-1	CHARACTERISTICS OF ACUTE AND CHRONIC PAIN
ACUTE PAIN	**CHRONIC PAIN**
Recent onset	Remote onset
Symptomatic of primary injury or disease	Uncharacteristic of primary injury or disease
Specific and localized	Nonspecific and generalized
Severity associated with the acuity of the injury or disease process	Severity out of proportion to the stage of the injury or disease
Responds favorably to drug therapy	Responds poorly to drug therapy
Requires gradually decreased drug therapy	Requires increasing drug therapy
Diminishes with healing	Persists beyond healing stage
Suffering decreases	Suffering intensifies
Associated with sympathetic nervous system responses such as hypertension, tachycardia, restlessness, anxiety	Absence of autonomic nervous system responses; manifests depression and irritability

BOX 21-1 ● Quality-of-Life Activities Affected by Chronic Pain

Exercising
Working around the house
Sleeping
Enjoying hobbies and leisure time
Socializing
Walking
Concentrating
Having sex
Maintaining relationships with family and friends
Working a full day at employment
Caring for children

pain pathway result in sharp, acute initial sensations like those that are felt when touching a hot iron. The result is that the person withdraws from the pain-provoking stimulus. After the fast transmission, impulses from small un-myelinated fibers known as *C-fibers* carry impulses at a slower rate of 0.5 to 2 meters a second. They are responsible for the throbbing, aching, or burning sensation that persists after the immediate discomfort.

Transmission

Transmission is the phase during which peripheral nerve fibers form synapses with neurons in the spinal cord. The pain impulses move from the spinal cord to sequentially

higher levels in the brain. The impulses ascend to the reticular activating system, the limbic system, the thalamus, and finally the cerebral cortex.

Perception

Perception refers to the phase of impulse transmission during which the brain experiences pain at a conscious level, but many concomitant neural activities occur almost simultaneously. Besides perceiving pain, the brain structures in the pain pathway also help to discriminate the location of the pain, determine its intensity, attach meaningfulness to the event, and provoke emotional responses (Bullock & Henze, 2000).

Pain perception, the conscious experience of discomfort, occurs when the pain threshold is reached. The **pain threshold** is the point at which the pain-transmitting neurochemicals reach the brain, causing conscious awareness. Pain thresholds tend to be the same among healthy persons; however, people tolerate or bear the sensation of pain differently. **Pain tolerance** is the amount of pain a person endures once the threshold has been reached. Learned behaviors that are gender, age, and culture specific often influence a person's pain tolerance.

Modulation

Modulation is the last phase of pain impulse transmission, during which the brain interacts with the spinal nerves in a downward fashion to alter the pain experi-

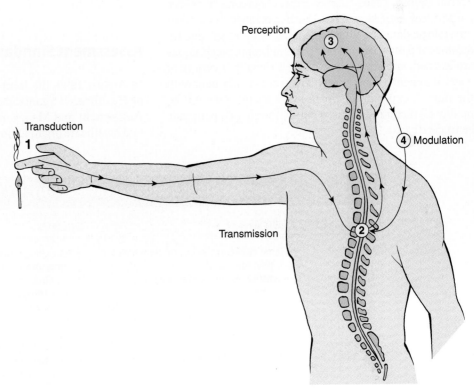

FIGURE 21-3 The phases of pain transmission.

ence. At this point, the painful sensation is reduced with the release of pain-inhibiting neurochemicals such as endogenous opioids, which are discussed later in this chapter, gamma-aminobutyric acid (GABA), and others.

PAIN ASSESSMENT

There is no perfect way to determine if pain exists and how severe it is. Margot McCaffery, a nursing expert on pain, states, "Pain is whatever the person says it is, and exists whenever the person says it does" (McCaffery & Beebe, 1989). A full pain assessment includes the client's description of its onset, quality, intensity, location, and duration (Table 21-2). In addition, nurses assess for accompanying symptoms, such as nausea or dizziness, and what makes the pain better or worse. The American Pain Society has proposed that pain assessment should be considered the fifth vital sign. In other words, the nurse should check and document the client's pain every time he or she assesses the client's temperature, pulse, respirations, and blood pressure.

Assessment Biases

Despite the fact that the client is the only reliable source for quantifying pain, nurses are not consistent in responding to the client's description of pain intensity with pain-relieving interventions. According to McCaffery and Ferrell (1999), "Most nurses expect someone in severe pain to *look* as if he hurts." Neither behavior nor other physiologic data like vital signs, however, are reliable indicators of pain. Responses to pain and coping techniques are learned, and clients may express them in a variety of ways. If a client's expressions of pain are incongruent with the nurse's expectations, pain management may not be readily forthcoming. Consequently, the client's pain may be undertreated.

Assessment Tools

Because there are no reliable objective indicators for pain, assessment tools are necessary. Common assessment tools for quantifying pain intensity include a numeric scale, a word scale, and a linear scale (Fig. 21-4). Clients identify how their pain compares with the choices on the assessment tool. One tool is not better than another. A numeric scale is commonly used when assessing adults. The Wong-Baker FACES scale is best for pediatric, culturally diverse, and mentally challenged clients (Fig. 21-5). It uses pictures and short descriptive phrases. The FACES scale is available in English as well as 10 foreign languages: Spanish, French, German, Italian, Portuguese, Japanese, Chinese, Vietnamese, Romanian, and Bosnian. Children as young as 3 years of age can use the FACES scale.

Stop, Think, and Respond ● BOX 21-1

When assessing the pain of two postoperative clients, each tells the nurse that her incisional pain is a "10" using the numeric scale, in which "0" equals no pain and "10" is the most pain the person has ever felt. One of the clients is laying quietly in bed watching television. The other is restless and has placed both hands over the incisional area. Both have medical orders for 50 to 75 mg of meperidine intramuscularly (IM) every 3 to 4 hours as needed for pain. Both clients received 75 mg of meperidine IM 3 hours ago. What is the best nursing action at this time?

Assessment Standards

In August 1999, the Joint Commission on Accreditation of Healthcare Organizations (JCAHO) established Pain Assessment and Management Standards that all accredited healthcare organizations must comply with beginning

TABLE 21-2	COMPONENTS OF A BRIEF PAIN ASSESSMENT	
CHARACTERISTIC	**DESCRIPTION**	**EXAMPLES**
Onset	Time or circumstances under which the pain appeared	After eating, while shoveling snow, during the night
Quality	Sensory experiences and degree of suffering	Throbbing, crushing, agonizing, annoying
Intensity	Magnitude of the pain, such as moderate, severe; or a quantifying scale, such as from 0 to 10	None, slight, mild; a level of "7"
Location	Anatomic site	Chest, abdomen, jaw
Duration	Time span of the pain	Continuous, intermittent, hours, weeks, months

Pain intensity scales

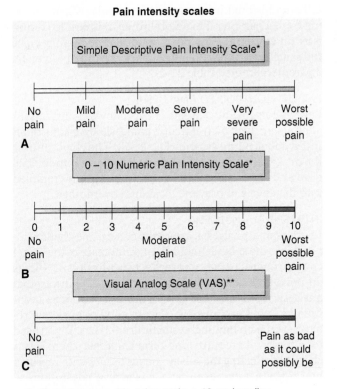

* If used as a graphic rating scale, a 10-cm baseline is recommended.
** A 10-cm baseline is recommended for VAS scales.

FIGURE 21-4 Pain assessment tools: (**A**) word scale, (**B**) numeric scale, and (**C**) linear scale.

TABLE 21-3	JCAHO COMPONENTS OF A COMPREHENSIVE PAIN ASSESSMENT*
COMPONENT	**FOCUS OF ASSESSMENT**
Intensity	Rating for present pain, worst pain, and least pain using a consistent scale
Location	Site of pain or identifying mark on a diagram
Quality	Description in client's own words
Onset	Time the pain began
Duration	Period that pain has existed
Variations	Pain characteristics that change
Patterns	Repetitiveness or lack thereof
Alleviating factors	Techniques or circumstances that reduce or relieve the pain
Aggravating factors	Techniques or circumstances that cause the pain to return or escalate in intensity
Present pain management regimen	Approaches used to control the pain and results and effectiveness
Pain management history	Past medications or interventions and response; manner of expressing pain; personal, cultural, spiritual, or ethnic beliefs that affect pain management
Effects of pain	Alterations in self-care, sleep, dietary intake, thought processes, lifestyle, and relationships
Person's goal for pain control	Expectations for level of pain relief, tolerance, or restoration of functional abilities
Physical examination of pain	Assessment of structures that relate to the site of pain

*If clients have pain in more than one area, assessment data are collected for each.

in 2001. Aspects that are incorporated in the JCAHO standards include the following:

- Everyone cared for in an accredited hospital, long-term care facility, home healthcare agency, outpatient clinic, or managed care organization has the right to assessment and management of pain.
- Pain is assessed using a tool that is appropriate for the person's age, developmental level, health condition, and cultural identity. Refer to Table 21-3 for pain-related information that is included in an initial comprehensive pain assessment.
- Pain is regularly reassessed throughout healthcare delivery.
- Pain is treated in the healthcare agency or the client is referred elsewhere.
- Healthcare workers are educated regarding pain assessment and management.
- Clients and their families are educated about effective pain management as an important part of care.
- The client's choices regarding pain management are respected.

FIGURE 21-5 Wong-Baker FACES Pain Rating Scale. Instructions: Explain to the person that each face is for a person who feels happy because he has no pain (hurt) or sad because he has some or a lot of pain. Face 0 is very happy because he doesn't hurt at all. Face 1 hurts just a little bit. Face 2 hurts a little more. Face 3 hurts even more. Face 4 hurts a whole lot. Face 5 hurts as much as you can imagine, although you don't have to be crying to hurt this bad. Ask the person to choose the face that best describes how he or she is feeling. Rating scale is recommended for persons age 3 years and older. (From Wong, D. L., Hockenberry-Eaton, M., Wilson, D., Winkelstein, M. L., Ahmann, E., & DiVito-Thomas, P. A. [1999]. *Whaley & Wong's nursing care of infants and children* [6th ed., p. 1153]. St. Louis: Mosby. Copyrighted by Mosby-Year Book Inc. Reprinted by permission.)

PAIN MANAGEMENT

Pain management refers to the techniques used to prevent, reduce, or relieve pain. The following are five general techniques for achieving pain management:

1. Blocking brain perception
2. Interrupting pain-transmitting chemicals at the site of injury
3. Combining analgesics with adjuvant drugs
4. Using gate-closing mechanisms
5. Altering pain transmission at the level of the spinal cord

Any one or a combination of these techniques may be used.

Drug Therapy

Drug therapy is the cornerstone for managing pain. The World Health Organization (WHO) recommends following a three-tiered approach, according to the client's pain intensity and response to selected drug therapy (Fig. 21-6). A fourth step being considered for clients with pain associated with cancer may include nerve blocks, analgesics administered *intrathecally* (in the subarachnoid or epidural spaces of the spine), electrical stimulation in the spinal cord, and neurosurgical analgesic techniques (Miguel, 2000). Examples of neurosurgical analgesic techniques are discussed later in this chapter.

Opioid and opiate **analgesics** such as morphine and meperidine (Demerol) are controlled substances referred to as *narcotics.* They interfere with pain perception centrally (at the brain). Nonopioid analgesics are not narcotics; they relieve pain by altering neurotransmission at the peripheral level (site of injury) (Drug Therapy Table 21-1).

Methods of Administration

Analgesic drugs are administered by oral, rectal, transdermal, or parenteral (injected) routes, including a continuous infusion that may be instilled into the spinal canal or self-administered intravenously by clients. When changing from a parenteral to an oral route, it is best to administer an **equianalgesic dose** (an oral dose that provides the same level of pain relief as when the drug is given by a parenteral route; Table 21-4).

PATIENT-CONTROLLED ANALGESIA

Patient-controlled analgesia (PCA) allows clients to self-administer their own narcotic analgesic by means of an intravenous pump system (Fig. 21-7). The client infuses the drug when he or she presses a hand-held button. The dose and time interval between doses are programmed into the device to prevent accidental overdosage.

INTRASPINAL ANALGESIA

In intraspinal analgesia, a narcotic or local anesthetic is infused into the subarachnoid or epidural space of the spinal cord through a catheter inserted by a physician. Nurses do not administer intraspinal analgesia. The intraspinal analgesic is administered several times per day or as a continuous low-dose infusion. This method of analgesia relieves pain with minimal systemic drug effects. When used for clients who require long-term analgesia, there is less chance of affecting the subcutaneous tissues with repeated injections that may eventually lessen drug absorption.

Addiction, Tolerance, Physical Dependence

Addiction refers to a repetitive pattern of drug seeking and drug use to satisfy a craving for a drug's mind-altering or mood-altering effects. Although opioid drugs can result in addiction, fewer than 1% of clients who are in need of drugs for pain relief, even for 6 months or longer, become addicted (McCaffery & Ferrell, 1999). Unfortunately, the fear of addiction causes many clients to refuse or self-limit prescribed drug therapy. It also causes some nurses to administer subtherapeutic doses. Both actions are counterproductive to therapeutic outcomes.

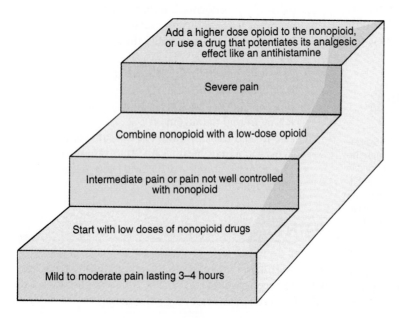

Add a higher dose opioid to the nonopioid, or use a drug that potentiates its analgesic effect like an antihistamine

Severe pain

Combine nonopioid with a low-dose opioid

Intermediate pain or pain not well controlled with nonopioid

Start with low doses of nonopioid drugs

Mild to moderate pain lasting 3–4 hours

FIGURE 21-6 World Health Organization (WHO) analgesic ladder.

DRUG THERAPY TABLE 21-1	ANALGESIC DRUG THERAPY

DRUG CATEGORY AND EXAMPLES/ MECHANISM OF ACTION	SIDE EFFECTS	NURSING CONSIDERATIONS
Opioids Bind with opiate receptors in the central nervous system *morphine sulfate, oxycodone (Roxicodone), hydromorphone (Dilaudid), meperidine (Demerol)*	Sedation, euphoria, nausea, vomiting, constipation, paralytic ileus, respiratory depression, urinary retention, physical dependence, hypotension	Do not administer if respirations are less than 12/minute. Encourage clients to cough and deep breathe to avoid atelectasis. Monitor for excessive sedation. Monitor bowel activity. Maintain safety precautions such as keeping side rails up and call bell within reach. Instruct client to call for assistance before ambulating. Administer before pain is severe to increase effectiveness.
Nonopioids Inhibit the production of prostaglandin that increase sensitivity to pain *Nonsteroidal anti-inflammatory drugs (NSAIDs): ibuprofen (Motrin)*	Headache, dizziness, nausea, gastritis and ulcers, constipation, increased bleeding time, bone marrow depression, tinnitus, dyspnea, anaphylactoid reactions, renal impairment, rash	Administer with food. Inform client of potential side effects, and instruct client to take orally as prescribed. Caution clients not to take more than one NSAID at a time.
aspirin	Nausea, gastritis, dizziness, tinnitus, occult bleeding, increased clotting time	Give with food. Report any side effects, including bleeding gums or bruising easily.
Antidepressants Block the reuptake of serotonin and norepinephrine *Tricyclic antidepressants amitriptyline (Elavil)*	Sedation, confusion, dry mouth, constipation, nausea, orthostatic hypotension, urinary retention, tachycardia, palpitations, bone marrow depression	Give at bedtime if sedation is a problem. Avoid alcohol. Report any side effects. Do not stop drug abruptly.
Corticosteroids Reduce pain with an inflammatory component; control nausea *dexamethasone (Decadron), prednisone (Deltasone)*	Peptic ulcer, weight gain, fluid retention, impaired wound healing, masking of infection, hyperglycemia, fragile skin, redistribution of fat	Monitor weight, vital signs, and serum glucose level. Taper doses when discontinuing.
Anticonvulsants Suppress neuronal firing *carbamazepine (Tegretol), clonazepam (Klonopin), gabapentin (Neurontin)*	Sedation, dizziness, impaired gait, weight gain, nausea, hepatotoxicity, bone marrow suppression, rash	Give with food or milk. Monitor blood counts and liver function tests. Protect from falls and injury. Taper dosage after long-term therapy.
Psychostimulants Counteract sedation; increase activity and appetite *methylphenidate (Ritalin)*	Nervousness, insomnia, tachycardia, hypertension, weight loss, reduced red and white blood cell counts	Give before 6:00 PM to prevent insomnia. Monitor vital signs and weight. Avoid caffeine or other stimulants such as decongestants. Review results of blood tests.

Although addiction rarely develops, tolerance is common. **Tolerance** is a condition in which a client needs larger doses of a drug to achieve the same effect as when the drug was first administered. Although responses to drug therapy differ among individuals, tolerance may not develop until a client has taken an opioid drug regularly for 4 weeks or more (McCaffery & Ferrell, 1999). The development of tolerance is not an indication of addiction. Rather, the client's request for pain-relieving drugs more often is a consequence of poor pain control, not drug-seeking for what some may think is the drug's pleasurable effects. The most appropriate nursing action is to consult

TABLE 21-4	EXAMPLES OF ADULT EQUIANALGESIC DOSES	
DRUG	PARENTERAL DOSE	ORAL DOSE
morphine sulfate	10 mg q 3–4 h	30 mg q 3–4 h
meperidine (Demerol)	100 mg q 3 h	300 mg q 2–3 h
hydromorphone (Dilaudid)	1.5 mg q 3–4 h	7.5 mg q 3–4 h
pentazocine (Talwin)	60 mg q 3–4 h	150 mg q 3–4 h

Adapted from Carr, C. B., Jacox, A. K., Chapman, C. R., et al. (1992; February). *Acute pain management: Operative or medical procedures and trauma. Clinical Practice Guideline No. 1.* (AHCPR Pub. 92-0032). Rockville, MD: Agency for Health Care Policy and Research.

with the physician regarding a need for an increased dose of the drug, not reducing its dosage or frequency of administration. As a rule of thumb, an ineffective dose should be increased by 25% to 50% (McCaffery & Ferrell, 1999).

Stop, Think, and Respond ● BOX 21-2

A medical order states: meperidine hydrochloride 50–100 mg IM q3h prn for pain. If a client does not experience adequate pain relief after receiving 50 mg, what dose may be more effective?

FIGURE 21-7 Patient-controlled analgesia.

Just as tolerance is not a characteristic of addiction, neither is physical dependence. **Physical dependence** means that a person experiences physical discomfort, known as *withdrawal symptoms,* when a drug that he or she has taken routinely for some time is abruptly discontinued (see Chap. 17). To avoid withdrawal symptoms, drugs that are known to cause physical dependence are discontinued gradually. The dosage or the frequency of their administration is lowered over 1 week or longer.

Adjuvant Drug Therapy

Adjuvant drugs are medications that are ordinarily administered for reasons other than treating pain. When adjuvant drugs are combined with opioid and nonopioid analgesics, they may achieve any or all of the following: (1) improvement of analgesic effect without an increased analgesic dosage; (2) control of concurrent symptoms, such as inflammation, that worsen the pain; and (3) moderation of side effects of analgesics, such as nausea or sedation. Examples of adjuvant drugs used to manage pain include tricyclic antidepressants, corticosteroids, anticonvulsants, and psychostimulants (see Drug Therapy Table 21-1).

Nondrug Interventions

Several nondrug interventions can be used to help manage pain (see Chap. 12). Some, like applications of heat and cold, are independent nursing measures or may require collaboration with the client's physician. Others, such as transcutaneous and percutaneous electrical nerve stimulation, acupuncture, and acupressure, are administered by individuals who have specialized training and expertise. The latter interventions are more likely to be used for clients with chronic pain or those in whom acute pain management techniques have been unsuccessful or are contraindicated.

Research is ongoing to determine the mechanism by which nondrug interventions relieve pain. Some question whether their effectiveness is the result of the placebo effect (see Chap. 12) or something more physiologic. McCaffery and Pasero (1999) report that "the brain can accommodate a limited number of sensory signals. When individuals use techniques such as distraction, relaxation, and imagery to control pain, they direct their attention away from the pain sensation" (p. 22). Some believe that these techniques stimulate the visual portion of the brain's cortex in the right hemisphere, where abstract concepts and creative activities take place. In response, the body releases neurotransmitters such as GABA and serotonin that calm the body and promote emotional well-being. This may explain how some adjuvant drugs for pain relief like anticonvulsants and antidepressants effect their actions.

Techniques such as electrical nerve stimulation, acupuncture, and acupressure may work by stimulating sensory nerve fibers that conduct tactile or vibratory sensations over pathways shared for transmitting pain. The result is inhibition of pain transmission. Others speculate that these and other nondrug methods like massage relieve pain by releasing **endogenous opiates** such as endorphins and enkephalins. Endogenous opiates are natural morphine-like substances in the body that modulate pain transmission by blocking receptors for substance P (Fig. 21-8).

Heat and Cold

Applications of heat and cold (thermal therapy) are well-established techniques for relieving pain. Pain associated with injury is best treated initially with cold applications such as an ice bag or chemical pack. The cold reduces localized swelling and decreases vasodilation, which may be used for minor or moderate pain.

Transcutaneous Electrical Stimulation

Transcutaneous electrical nerve stimulation (TENS) is a pain management technique that delivers bursts of electricity to the skin and underlying nerves. It is safe for managing acute and chronic pain, and it does not produce systemic side effects or addiction. The electricity is delivered from a battery-operated unit through electrode patches that are placed at appropriate sites, such as directly over the affected area, at areas along a nerve pathway, or at points distal to the painful area (Fig. 21-9). The client perceives the electrical stimulus as a pleasant tapping, tingling, vibrating, or buzzing sensation. Placement sites, intensity of electrical current, rate of electrical bursts,

and duration can be changed according to the client's response.

Acupuncture and Acupressure

Acupuncture is a pain management technique in which long, thin needles are inserted into the skin. Acupressure uses tissue compression, rather than needles, to reduce pain. The location for needle placement and pressure is based on 2,000-year-old traditions practiced in Chinese medicine (see Chap. 12). Relief of pain, especially chronic pain, is not permanent, and repeated treatments almost are always necessary.

Although both techniques have been demonstrated to prevent or relieve pain, their exact mechanism is not completely understood. Some speculate that the twisting, vibration, or pressure are forms of cutaneous stimuli that close the gates to pain-transmitting neurochemicals. Another theory is that acupuncture and acupressure stimulate the body to release endorphins and enkephalins.

Percutaneous Electrical Nerve Stimulation

One of the newest innovations in acute and chronic pain management is percutaneous electrical nerve stimulation (PENS). It combines the use of acupuncture needles with TENS. The practitioner inserts the needles in soft tissue, and an electrical stimulus is conducted through the needles (see Chap. 12 for a discussion of electroacupuncture). PENS is considered superior to TENS in providing pain relief because the needles are located closer to nerve endings. PENS therapy is administered for 30 minutes three times a week for a total of 3 weeks (White, 1999). The technique has been successful in research trials on clients with low back pain, pain caused by the spread of cancer to bones, shingles (acute herpes zoster viral infection), and migraine headaches.

Other Noninvasive Techniques

Various other techniques are used singly or as adjuncts to more traditional pain management techniques. Some include imagery, biofeedback, humor, breathing exercises and progressive relaxation, and distraction (see Chaps. 12 and 13). In addition, in some situations (e.g., clients with severe burns), hypnosis is used. Hypnosis is a technique in which a person assumes a trancelike state during which perceptions are altered. During hypnosis, a suggestion is made that a person's pain will be eliminated or that the client will experience the sensation in a more pleasant way.

Spinal Surgery Techniques

Intractable pain, pain that does not respond to analgesic medications, noninvasive measures, or nursing management, requires more drastic measures. Neurosurgical pro-

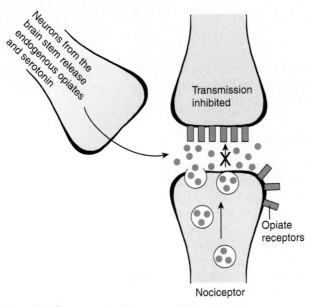

FIGURE 21-8 Action of endogenous opiates.

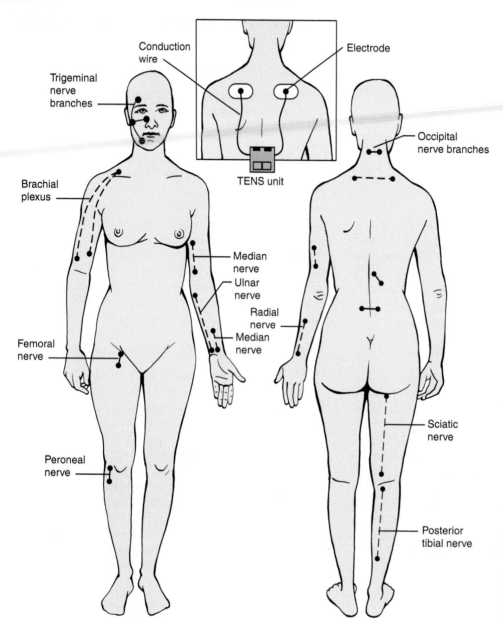

FIGURE 21-9 To activate various sensory nerves, a transcutaneous nerve stimulation (TENS) unit may be placed close to the pain source. The TENS unit floods the gates in the spinal cord, blocking pain perception. Site of placement depends on the pain's location.

cedures that provide pain relief include rhizotomy and cordotomy.

Rhizotomy

A rhizotomy is a surgical procedure on the spine that involves a laminectomy (see Chap. 47) followed by sectioning of the posterior (sensory) nerve root just before it enters the spinal cord. Sectioning a spinal nerve prevents sensory impulses from entering the spinal cord and going to the brain, resulting in a permanent loss of sensation in the area supplied by the sectioned nerve. More than one nerve may need to be sectioned to produce the desired results. Chemical rhizotomy (using chemicals such as alcohol or phenol to destroy the nerve) or percutaneous rhizotomy (use of radiofrequency waves to de-

stroy pain fibers) are alternatives that may provide the same result. Rhizotomy usually is reserved for terminally ill clients.

Cordotomy

A cordotomy is an interruption of pain pathways in the spinal cord. A laminectomy is performed, and sensory nerve tracts in the vertebral column are destroyed, thus preventing sensory nerve impulses from going to the brain. Loss of sensation is permanent. A percutaneous cervical cordotomy is basically the same procedure as a cordotomy but is performed under local anesthesia. It carries less risk and usually is better tolerated by terminally ill clients. Guided by fluoroscopy, the surgeon inserts a needle through the skin (percutaneous) in the neck (cervical) near the mastoid process. Movement of the needle interrupts pain pathways.

Nursing Management

The nurse performs a comprehensive assessment of each client's pain on admission as mandated by JCAHO (see Table 21-3). Regularly thereafter, the nurse determines the onset, quality, intensity, location, and duration of the client's pain. He or she explains the tool for assessing a client's pain so the client understands how to self-report his or her level of pain when the assessment tool is used again. Giving assurance that pain management is a nursing and agency priority is essential throughout the client's care. The nurse informs the client of available pain management techniques and incorporates any preferences or objections to interventions for pain management that the client may have when establishing a plan of care.

The nurse collaborates with each client about his or her goal for a level of pain relief and implements interventions for achieving the goal. The client's description of pain or need for pain relief is never doubted or minimized. If a client's goal for pain relief is not reached, the nurse collaborates with members of the health team for other approaches that may do so. Scheduling the administration of analgesics every 3 hours, rather than on an as-needed (prn) basis, often affords a uniform level of pain relief. Providing a client with equipment to self-administer analgesics, as with a PCA pump, also promotes a more consistent level of pain relief.

When medications are administered, the nurse monitors for and implements measures for managing side effects. Problems that may develop with opioid and opiate therapy include Risk for Impaired Gas Exchange related to respiratory depression, Constipation related to slowed peristalsis, Risk for Injury related to drowsiness and unsteady gait, Risk for Imbalanced Nutrition: Less than Body Requirements related to anorexia and nausea, Risk for Deficient Fluid Volume related to reduced oral intake, and Disturbed Sleep Pattern (excessive or interrupted sleep) related to depression of the central nervous system.

The nurse monitors for the development of side effects to prescribed drugs (see Drug Therapy Table 21-1). Adjuvant drug and nondrug alternatives for pain management are used to potentiate drug therapy or as a substitute when drug side effects jeopardize the client's safety. When planning for the client's discharge from the health agency, the nurse includes interventions for pain relief to facilitate a comfortable transition to the next level of care. An important component of these interventions is client and family teaching (see the accompanying teaching box for more information). See Nursing Care Plan 21-1 for a description of the nursing care of a client with acute pain.

21-1 *Client and Family Teaching* Educating About Pain

The nurse encourages the client and family to:

- Discuss with the physician what to expect from the disorder, injury, or its treatment.
- Talk with the physician about any concerns that relate to drug therapy.
- Share information about what drugs or pain-relieving techniques have and have not been helpful during previous episodes.
- Identify drug allergies to avoid adverse effects.
- Inform the physician about other medications being taken to avoid drug–drug interactions.
- Take prescribed drugs exactly as directed and report untoward effects.
- Avoid taking over-the-counter drugs unless the physician has been consulted; follow label directions for administration.
- Avoid alcohol and sedative drugs if the analgesic causes sedation.
- Keep analgesic drugs out of the reach of children; request childproof caps.
- Never share medications with others or take someone else's medications for pain.

GENERAL NUTRITIONAL CONSIDERATIONS

Painful procedures are performed at times least likely to interfere with meals.

Pain medications administered 30 to 45 minutes before meals may enable the client to consume an adequate intake.

Small, frequent meals may help maximize intake in clients with drug-related or pain-related anorexia. Solicit food preferences.

A high-fiber diet (i.e., whole-grain breads and cereals, fresh fruits and vegetables) along with increased fluids may help ease constipation related to narcotic analgesics.

GENERAL PHARMACOLOGIC CONSIDERATIONS

Analgesic administration is timed to permit maximum client cooperation in care.

Some nonnarcotic analgesics, when used daily over an extended period, can cause undesirable side effects, such as gastrointestinal bleeding and hemorrhagic disorders.

Transdermal fentanyl (Duragesic) may be used to manage chronic pain in clients requiring opioid analgesic therapy. This drug is released into the systemic circulation over 72 hours.

Nursing Care Plan 21-1

THE CLIENT WITH ACUTE PAIN

Assessment

■ Determine the following:

 ■ Source of client's pain; when it began; its intensity, location, characteristics, and related factors such as what makes the pain better or worse

 ■ How client's pain interferes with life, such as diminishing the ability to meet his or her own needs for hygiene, eating, sleep, activity, social interactions, emotional stability, concentration, and so forth

 ■ At what level client can tolerate pain

 ■ Pain-related behaviors such as grimacing, crying, moaning, and assuming a guarded position

■ Measure vital signs.

■ Perform a physical assessment, taking care to gently support and assist client to turn as you examine various structures. Use light palpation in areas that are tender. Show concern when assessment techniques increase client's pain.

■ Postpone nonpriority assessments until client's pain has been reduced.

Nursing Diagnosis: **Acute Pain** related to cellular injury or disease as manifested by stating, "I'm in severe pain"; rating pain at 10 using a numeric scale; pointing to the lower left abdominal quadrant; describing the pain as "continuous, throbbing, and starting this morning" without any known cause

Expected Outcome: Client will rate the pain intensity at his or her tolerable level of "5" within 30 minutes of implementing a pain management technique.

Interventions	*Rationales*
Assess client's pain and its characteristics at least every 2 hours while awake and 30 minutes after implementing a pain management technique.	Quick interventions prevent or minimize pain.
Modify or eliminate factors that contribute to pain such as a full bladder, uncomfortable position, pain-aggravating activity, excessively warm or cool environment, noise, and social isolation.	Multiple stressors decrease pain tolerance.
Determine client's choice for pain relief techniques from among those available.	Encourage and respect client's participation in decision-making.
Administer prescribed analgesics or alternative pain management techniques promptly.	Suffering contributes to the pain experience and can be reduced by eliminating delays in nursing response.
Advocate on client's behalf for higher doses of prescribed analgesics or addition of adjuvant drug therapy if pain is not satisfactorily relieved.	JCAHO standards mandate for nurses and other healthcare workers to facilitate pain relief for clients.
Administer a prescribed analgesic before a procedure or activity that is likely to result in or intensify pain.	Prophylactic interventions facilitate keeping pain at a manageable level.
Plan for periods of rest between activity.	Fatigue and exhaustion interfere with pain tolerance.
Reassure client that there are many ways to modify the pain experience.	Suggesting that there are additional untried options helps alleviate frustration or despair that there is no hope for pain relief.
Assist client to visualize a pleasant experience.	Imaging interrupts pain perception.
Help client focus on deep breathing, relaxing muscles, watching television, putting together a puzzle, or talking to someone on the phone.	Diverting attention to something other than pain reduces pain perception.

(continued)

Nursing Care Plan 21-1 (Continued)

THE CLIENT WITH ACUTE PAIN

Interventions	*Rationales*
Apply warm or cool compresses to a painful sensory site.	Flooding the brain with alternative stimuli closes the spinal gates that transmit pain.
Gently massage a painful area or the same area on the opposite side of the body (contralateral massage).	Massage promotes the release of endorphins and enkephalins that moderate the sensation.
Promote laughter by suggesting that client relate a humorous story or watch a video or comedy of his or her choice.	Laughter releases endorphins and enkephalins that promote a feeling of well-being.

Evaluation of Expected Outcomes

■ Client reports that pain is gone or at a tolerable level of "5" within 30 minutes.

■ Client perceives the pain experience realistically and copes effectively.

■ Client participates in self-care activities without undue pain.

Clients should inform the primary healthcare provider or dentist before any procedure when they use pain medications, especially salicylates or nonsteroidal anti-inflammatory agents, on a regular basis.

Clients should not use an over-the-counter analgesic agent, such as aspirin, ibuprofen, or acetaminophen, consistently to treat chronic pain without first consulting a physician.

⧖ GENERAL GERONTOLOGIC CONSIDERATIONS

Pain perception may be diminished in older adults, causing some acute conditions to go unreported to medical personnel.

Older adults may be reluctant to report pain. They may prefer to describe pain as discomfort, burning, or aching.

Confused older adults may be unable to report pain, but may exhibit other signs such as agitation, behavior changes, or irritability.

Reports from caregivers are valuable when assessing pain in the cognitively impaired older adult.

A reduced dose of analgesics, especially opioid analgesics, may be prescribed for the older adult initially. The nurse carefully assesses the older client for pain relief.

Older adults experience a higher peak effect and longer duration of pain relief from an opioid.

A bowel regimen to prevent constipation should be started when any older adult is treated with the opioids.

Any recurrent or chronic pain may affect the functional ability of the older adult.

Older adults taking nonsteroidal anti-inflammatory drugs are at increased risk for renal toxicity and gastrointestinal problems.

In 1998, the American Geriatric Society recommended no more than 4000 mg of acetaminophen (Tylenol) a day to reduce the risk of liver damage.

Critical Thinking Exercises

1. *What questions should the nurse ask when a client states he or she has pain?*
2. *Discuss how acute pain after surgery is different from pain experienced by a client with chronic back pain.*
3. *Discuss nursing interventions that are appropriate if a client does not experience adequate pain relief from a prescribed analgesic.*

References and Suggested Readings

Acello, B. (2000). Meeting JCAHO standards for pain control. *Nursing, 30*(3), 52–54.

Acello, B. (2000). Controlling pain: Switching to the patch. *Nursing, 30*(8), 72.

Ackerman, C. G. & Turkoski, B. (2000). Using guided imagery to reduce pain and anxiety. *Home Healthcare Nurse, 18*, 524–530.

Agency for Health Care Policy and Research. (1992). *Pain control after surgery, a patient's guide.* Publication No. 92-0021. Silver Spring, MD: Publications Clearinghouse.

American Pain Society. (1999; February 17). New survey of people with chronic pain reveals out-of-control symptoms, impaired daily lives. Glenview, IL: Author.

American Pain Society. (1992). *Principles of analgesic use in treatment of acute pain and cancer pain* (3rd ed.). Skokie, IL: Author.

Arbour, R. (2000). Sedation and pain management in critically ill adults. *Critical Care Nurse, 20*(5), 39–58.

Bullock, B. L. & Henze, R. (2000). *Focus on pathophysiology.* Philadelphia: Lippincott Williams & Wilkins.

Kennedy-Schwarz, J. (2000). Ethical issues: Pain management. *American Journal of Nursing, 100*(8), 49–50.

Kettelman, K. (2000). Controlling pain: What's so bad about meperidine? *Nursing, 30*(10), 20.

Kovach, C. R., et al. (2000). Nurses' perceptions of pain assessment and treatment in the cognitively impaired elderly: It's not a guessing game. *Clinical Nurse Specialist, 14,* 215–220.

Kowal, N. (2000). The Joint Commission mandates pain excellence. *ASPMN Pathways, 9*(2), 3.

Llewellyn, A. (2000). Management perspectives: JCAHO doesn't have time for the pain. *Nursing Spectrum, 13*(2), 24.

McCaffery, M. & Beebe, A. (1989). *Pain, clinical manual for nursing practice.* St. Louis: Mosby.

McCaffery, M. & Ferrell, B. F. (1999). Opioids and pain management: What do nurses know? *Nursing, 29*(3), 48–52.

McCaffery, M. & Pasero, C. (1999). *Pain clinical manual* (2nd ed.). St. Louis: Mosby.

Merboth, M. K., et al. (2000). Managing pain: The fifth vital sign. *Nursing Clinics of North America, 35,* 375–383.

Miguel, R. (2000). Interventional treatment of cancer pain: The fourth step in the World Health Organization analgesic ladder. *Cancer Control, 7,* 149–156.

Miller, C. A. (2000). Advising older adults about pain remedies. *Geriatric Nursing, 21*(1), 55.

Miller, L. L., et al. (2000). Comfort and pain relief in dementia: Awakening a new beneficence. *Journal of Gerontological Nursing, 26*(9), 32–40, 55–56.

Mismanaged pain: Suffering in silence. *Nursing, 30*(10), 84.

Pasero, C., et al. (1999). JCAHO on assessing and managing pain. *American Journal of Nursing, 99*(7), 22.

Pasero, C. (2000). Pain control: Continuous local anesthetics. *American Journal of Nursing, 100*(8), 22.

Pasero, C., & McCaffery, M. (2000). Pain control: When patients can't report pain. *American Journal of Nursing, 100*(9), 22–23.

Porth, C. M. (2002). *Pathophysiology: Concepts of altered health states* (6th ed.) Philadelphia: Lippincott Williams & Wilkins.

Rice, R. (2000) Pain assessment in the home. *Geriatric Nursing, 21*(4), 220–221.

Snyder, D. (2000). Risking failure . . . "Heading off adverse reactions from NSAIDS." *Nursing, 30*(8), 8.

Twycross, A. (2000) Education about pain: A neglected area? *Nurse Education Today, 20*(3), 244–253.

Wentz, J. D. (2000). Practice errors. You've caught the error—now how do you fix it? *American Journal of Nursing, 100*(9), 24.

White, P. F. (1999). Percutaneous electrical nerve stimulation (PENS): A promising alternative approach to pain management. *American Pain Society Bulletin, 9*(2), 1–8.

Caring for Clients With Fluid, Electrolyte, and Acid-Base Imbalances

Words to Know

acidosis	generalized edema
acids	hemoconcentration
active transport	hemodilution
alkalosis	hypervolemia
anion gap	hypovolemia
anions	interstitial fluid
atrial natriuretic peptide	intracellular fluid
baroreceptors	intravascular fluid
bases	ions
bicarbonate–carbonic	osmoreceptors
acid buffer system	osmosis
cation	passive diffusion
Chvostek's sign	pitting edema
circulatory overload	renin-angiotensin-
compensation	aldosterone system
dehydration	serum osmolality
dependent edema	skin tenting
electrolytes	third-spacing
extracellular fluid	thirst
facilitated diffusion	Trousseau's sign
filtration	

Learning Objectives

On completion of this chapter, the reader will:

- Name the two main fluid locations in the human body and two subdivisions.
- Give the average fluid intake per day for adults.
- List four ways in which the body normally loses fluid.
- List three chemical substances that are components of body fluid.
- Name three mechanisms that help regulate fluid and electrolyte balance.
- Identify five processes by which water and dissolved chemicals are relocated.
- List two types of fluid imbalance.
- Explain the difference between hypovolemia and dehydration.
- Explain hemoconcentration and hemodilution.
- Identify at least five assessment findings characteristic of hypovolemia.
- Discuss nursing interventions for fluid volume deficit.
- List and identify the differences in three types of edema.
- Discuss nursing interventions for managing hypervolemia.
- Explain third-spacing and medical techniques for relocating this fluid.
- List at least three factors that contribute to electrolyte loss and excess.
- Name four electrolyte imbalances that pose a major threat to well-being.
- Discuss the nursing management of clients with electrolyte imbalances.
- Discuss the role of acids and bases in body fluid.
- Explain pH and identify the normal range of plasma pH.
- Identify two chemicals and two organs that play major roles in regulating acid-base balance.
- Give the names of two major acid-base imbalances and subdivisions of each.
- List three components of arterial blood gas findings used to determine acid-base imbalances.
- Discuss the nursing management of clients with acid-base imbalances.

About 60% of the adult human body is water (Fig. 22-1). Put another way, for every 100 lb of body weight, approximately 60 lb is water. Most body water is located within cells (**intracellular fluid**). The rest is outside cells (**extracellular fluid**), between cells (**interstitial fluid**), and in the plasma (serum) portion of blood (**intravascular fluid;** Fig. 22-2). The volume of fluid in each location varies with age and sex (Table 22-1). In healthy adults, oral fluid intake averages about 2500 mL/day; however, it can range between 1800 to 3000 mL/day with a similar volume of fluid loss. A standard formula for calculating daily fluid intake is as follows:

- 100 mL/kg for the first 10 kg of weight, plus
- 50 mL/kg for the next 10 kg of weight, plus
- 15 mL/kg per remaining kilograms of weight (Mentes, 2000; Kayser-Jones et al., 1999)

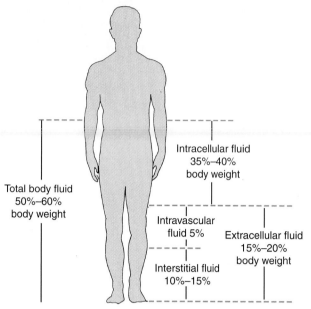

FIGURE 22-1   Total body fluid represents 50% to 60% of body weight in an average adult.

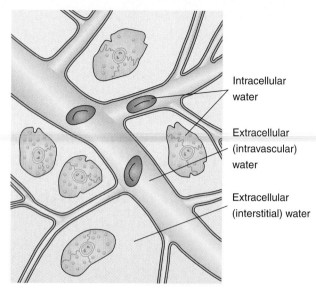

FIGURE 22-2   Distribution of body water.

The primary sources of body fluid are food and liquids. As fluid volume increases, the body loses fluid, primarily through urination, in a proportionate volume to maintain or restore equilibrium. Other mechanisms of fluid loss include bowel elimination, perspiration, and breathing. Losses from sweat and the vapor in exhaled air are referred to as *insensible losses* because they are, for practical purposes, unnoticeable and unmeasurable (Fig. 22-3).

Translocation (movement back and forth) of fluid and exchange of chemicals is continuous in and among all areas where water is located. Some of the chemicals involved are **electrolytes,** substances that when dissolved in fluid carry an electrical charge; **acids,** substances that release hydrogen into fluid; and **bases,** substances that bind with hydrogen. The delicate balance of fluid, electrolytes, acids, and bases is ensured by an adequate intake of water and nutrients, physiologic mechanisms that regulate fluid volume, and chemical processes that buffer the blood to keep its pH nearly neutral.

Stop, Think, and Respond ● BOX 22-1

Using the formula for calculating fluid intake requirements according to weight, how much oral fluid per day is considered adequate for a client who weighs 176 lb?

FLUID AND ELECTROLYTE REGULATION

Under normal conditions, several mechanisms maintain normal fluid volume and electrolyte concentrations. They include those promoted by osmoreceptors (i.e., the release or inhibition of antidiuretic hormone [ADH]), the renin-angiotensin-aldosterone system, and the secretion of atrial natriuretic peptide (ANP).

Osmoreceptors

Fluid volume is regulated primarily by the excretion of water in the form of urine and the promotion of thirst. These processes are in turn regulated by **osmoreceptors**

TABLE 22-1	PERCENTAGES OF BODY FLUID ACCORDING TO AGE AND SEX			
FLUID COMPARTMENT	INFANTS	MALE ADULTS	FEMALE ADULTS	OLDER ADULTS
Intravascular	4%	4%	5%	5%
Interstitial	25%	11%	10%	15%
Intracellular	48%	45%	35%	25%
Total	77%	60%	50%	45%

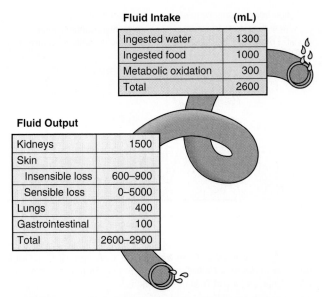

Fluid Intake	(mL)
Ingested water	1300
Ingested food	1000
Metabolic oxidation	300
Total	2600

Fluid Output

Kidneys	1500
Skin	
Insensible loss	600–900
Sensible loss	0–5000
Lungs	400
Gastrointestinal	100
Total	2600–2900

FIGURE 22-3 In the healthy person, fluid intake and output are about equal. The amounts indicated are average daily fluid sources and losses.

in the hypothalamus, specialized neurons that sense the **serum osmolality,** concentration of substances, in blood. When the blood becomes overly concentrated, osmoreceptors stimulate the hypothalamus to synthesize ADH, released by the posterior lobe of the pituitary gland. Release of ADH inhibits urine formation by increasing reabsorption of water from the distal and collecting tubules in the nephrons of the kidneys. The reabsorbed water restores normal serum osmolality, increases circulating blood volume, improves cardiac output, and maintains blood pressure (BP). Osmoreceptors also are sensitive to changes in blood volume and BP through information relayed by baroreceptors. **Baroreceptors** are stretch receptors in the aortic arch and carotid sinus that signal the brain to release ADH when blood volume decreases by 10%, systolic BP falls below 90 mm Hg, or the right atrium is underfilled (Veijo & Nicolaus, 1999). They signal the brain to suppress ADH when blood volume increases, systolic BP rises, or the right atrium is overfilled. Osmoreceptors also trigger **thirst,** a mechanism that promotes increased intake of oral fluid. A person senses thirst when extracellular volume decreases by approximately 700 mL, an amount that equals about 2% of body weight (Edwards, 2001).

Renin-Angiotensin-Aldosterone System

The **renin-angiotensin-aldosterone system** is a chain of chemicals released to increase both BP and blood volume. It is triggered by the *juxtaglomerular apparatus,* a ring of pressure-sensing cells that surround the arterioles leading to each glomerulus in the kidneys. When the volume of arterial blood supplying the glomeruli is reduced, the juxtaglomerular cells release renin. Renin begins the

transformation of angiotensinogen to angiotensin I to angiotensin II. Angiotensin II causes vasoconstriction and raises BP; it also stimulates release of aldosterone from the adrenal cortex. Aldosterone causes the kidneys to reabsorb sodium, which in turn increases blood volume and BP (Fig. 22-4).

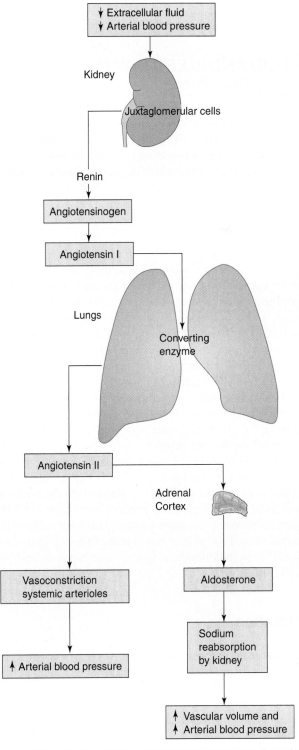

FIGURE 22-4 Control of blood pressure by the renin-angiotensin-aldosterone system.

Atrial Natriuretic Peptide

Atrial natriuretic peptide is a hormone-like substance produced in the heart's atrial muscle. It is released in response to overstretching of the atrial wall. It reduces the increased volume of blood that is filling the heart by inhibiting the release of renin, aldosterone, and ADH; increasing urine production; and directing the kidneys to excrete sodium in urine.

FLUID AND ELECTROLYTE DISTRIBUTION

Once water and electrolytes are absorbed, physiologic processes govern their movement and relocation at the cellular level. These processes include osmosis, filtration, passive and facilitated diffusion, and active transport.

Osmosis

Osmosis is the movement of water through a *semipermeable membrane,* one that allows some but not all substances in a solution to pass through, from a dilute area to a more concentrated area. *Tonicity* refers, in this case, to the quantity (concentration) of substances dissolved in the water. The power to draw water toward an area of greater concentration is referred to as *osmotic pressure. Colloids,* large-sized substances such as serum proteins (e.g., albumin, globulin, fibrinogen) and blood cells, do not readily pass through cell and tissue membranes. They contribute to fluid concentration and act as a force for attracting water—a property referred to as *colloidal osmotic pressure.*

Fluid distribution through osmosis occurs in the following ways. If the concentration is higher in the cell, water is drawn through the membrane into the cell from the interstitial space. The process continues until the concentration is the same (*isotonic*) on both sides of the membrane. The reverse also is true: if the concentration is higher in the interstitial space, water is pulled from the cell (Fig. 22-5).

Filtration

Filtration promotes the movement of fluid and some dissolved substances through a semipermeable membrane according to pressure differences. It relocates water and chemicals from an area of high pressure to an area of lower pressure. For example, fluid is under higher pressure at the arterial end than the venous end of capillaries. Filtration causes the fluid and some dissolved substances (e.g., oxygen) to move to the interstitial space. Most of the water is

FIGURE 22-5 Osmosis. (From Smeltzer, S. C. & Bare, B. G. [2000]. *Brunner & Suddarth's textbook of medical–surgical nursing* [9th ed.]. Philadelphia: Lippincott Williams & Wilkins.)

then reabsorbed at the venous end of the capillaries by colloidal osmotic pressure (Fig. 22-6). Filtration also affects how the kidneys excrete fluid and wastes and then selectively reabsorb water and other chemicals that need to be conserved. The kidneys filter about 180 L of fluid from the blood each day. All but 1 to 1.5 L is reabsorbed.

Diffusion

Passive diffusion is a physiologic process by which dissolved substances (e.g., electrolytes) move from an area of high concentration to an area of lower concentration through a semipermeable membrane. Passive diffusion, like osmosis, remains fairly static (unchanged) once equilibrium occurs. **Facilitated diffusion** is when certain dissolved substances require assistance from a carrier molecule to pass through a semipermeable membrane.

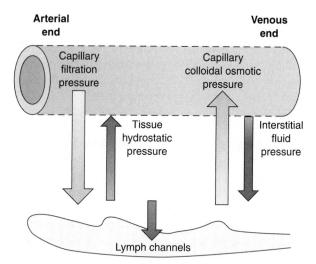

FIGURE 22-6 Fluid exchange at the capillary level.

For example, the carrier substance insulin facilitates the distribution of glucose molecules inside cells.

Active Transport

Active transport requires an energy source, a substance called *adenosine triphosphate* (ATP), to drive dissolved chemicals from an area of low concentration to an area of higher concentration—the opposite of passive diffusion. An example of active transport is the sodium-potassium pump system. Its function is to move potassium from lower concentrations in the extracellular fluid into cells where potassium is highly concentrated. The pump also moves sodium, which is in lower amounts in the cells, to extracellular fluid, where it is more abundant (Fig. 22-7). Metabolic disorders that diminish ATP, such as hypoxia, seriously affect normal cellular functions by impairing the distribution of chemicals in intracellular and extracellular fluid. Any significant change in fluid volume or its distribution can disrupt normal body functioning.

FLUID IMBALANCES

Fluid imbalance is a general term describing any of several conditions in which the body's water is not in the proper volume or location. Common fluid imbalances include hypovolemia, hypervolemia, and third-spacing.

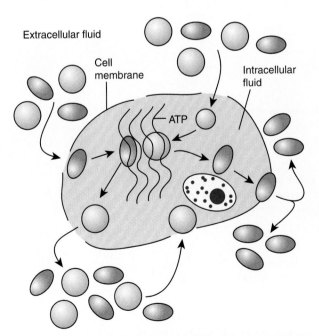

FIGURE 22-7 Active transport. A carrier system (*wavy lines*) +—actively pumps sodium (pink molecules) that diffuses into the cell out through a pore in the cell membrane. Similarly, the carrier system actively replaces potassium (blue molecules) that diffuses from the cell.

● HYPOVOLEMIA

Hypovolemia (fluid volume deficit) refers to a low volume of extracellular fluid. Usually, dissolved chemical substances, such as electrolytes, are similarly depleted. Clients at risk for hypovolemia include those who are lethargic, depressed, or vomiting; have dementia, a fever, difficulty swallowing, or diarrhea; cannot speak to communicate their needs; eat poorly (i.e., less than 50% of their food); require assistance to drink because of weakness, paralysis, or limited range of motion; take diuretics, laxatives, or drugs that inhibit cell hydration (e.g., drugs with anticholinergic properties); or receive tube feedings without additional instillations of water. **Dehydration** results when the volume of body fluid is significantly reduced in both extracellular and intracellular compartments. In dehydration, all fluid compartments have decreased volumes; in hypovolemia, only blood volume is low.

Pathophysiology and Etiology

Factors that contribute to hypovolemia include inadequate fluid intake; fluid loss in excess of fluid intake such as with hemorrhage, prolonged vomiting or diarrhea, wound loss (as with burn injury), or profuse urination or perspiration; and translocation of fluid to compartments where it is trapped, such as the abdominal cavity or interstitial spaces (e.g., third-spacing). When circulatory volume is decreased, the heart compensates by increasing the heart rate to maintain adequate cardiac output (see Chap. 30). BP falls with postural changes, or it may become severely lowered when blood is rapidly lost. **Hemoconcentration,** a high ratio of blood components in relation to watery plasma, increases the potential for blood clots and urinary stones and compromises the kidney's ability to excrete nitrogen wastes. Hypovolemia eventually depletes intracellular fluid, which can affect cellular functions. One example is the change in mentation that usually occurs.

Assessment Findings

One of the earliest symptoms of hypovolemia is thirst. Other signs and symptoms are listed in Table 22-2. Evidence of hemoconcentration is reflected in elevated hematocrit level and blood cell counts, a consequence of water deficiency. Urine specific gravity is high. Serum electrolyte levels tend to remain normal because they are depleted in proportion to the water loss (Bullock & Henze, 2000). Central venous pressure (CVP; see Chap. 30) is below 4 cm H_2O.

TABLE 22-2	SIGNS AND SYMPTOMS OF FLUID VOLUME DEFICIT AND EXCESS	
ASSESSMENT	**FLUID DEFICIT**	**FLUID EXCESS**
Weight	Weight loss ≥2 lb/24 hr	Weight gain ≥2 lb/24 hr
Blood pressure	Low	High
Temperature	Elevated	Normal
Pulse	Rapid, weak, thready	Full, bounding
Respirations	Rapid, shallow	Moist, labored
Urine	Scant, dark yellow	Light yellow
Stool	Dry, small volume	Bulky
Skin	Warm, flushed, dry	Cool, pale, moist
Skin turgor	Poor, tents	Pitting edema
Mucous membranes	Dry, sticky	Moist
Eyes	Sunken	Swollen
Lungs	Clear	Crackles, gurgles
Breathing	Effortless	Dyspnea, orthopnea
Energy	Weak	Fatigues easily
Jugular neck veins	Flat	Distended
Cognition	Reduced	Reduced
Mental state	Sleepy	Anxious

Medical Management

Fluid deficit is restored by treating its etiology, increasing the volume of oral intake, administering intravenous (IV) fluid replacement (see Chap. 24), and controlling fluid losses.

Nursing Management

The nurse gathers assessment data that provide evidence of fluid status (Nursing Care Plan 22-1). If they reflect a fluid deficit, he or she plans measures to restore fluid balance (Nursing Guidelines 22-1) and evaluates the out-

Nursing Care Plan 22-1

THE CLIENT WITH HYPOVOLEMIA

Assessment

■ Look for gross sources of fluid loss: vomiting, diarrhea, bleeding, wound drainage, gastrointestinal (GI) suctioning, and diaphoresis.

■ Weigh client daily at the same time, on the same scale, and dressed similarly. Report a loss of 2 lb (1 kg) or more in 24 hours (a 2-lb loss equals 1 L of body fluid).

■ Note medications. Daily diuretic therapy or chronic laxative use may promote excess fluid losses.

■ Record vital signs regularly; the frequency depends on client's acuity level. Check for postural hypotension (a drop in systolic pressure of 15 mm Hg immediately after client rises from a sitting or recumbent position). Increased insensible losses may cause or result from elevated body temperature.

■ Ask if client is thirsty.

■ Examine skin for dryness. Assess turgor (elasticity) by lifting the skin over the sternum, inner thigh, or forehead each shift. **Skin tenting,** skin that remains elevated and is slow to return to underlying tissue, indicates dehydration.

■ Observe the tongue for furrowing (linear lines), and look for dry oral mucous membranes.

■ Determine cognition by performing a Mini-Mental Status Examination (see Chap. 12).

■ Examine urine. Urine that is dark yellow, has a strong odor, or has a specific gravity of 1.020 or more indicates low fluid volume.

(continued)

Nursing Care Plan 22-1 *(Continued)*

THE CLIENT WITH HYPOVOLEMIA

■ Monitor blood test results for hemoconcentration (high hematocrit level and blood cell counts).

■ Keep a daily record of fluid intake and output. Report output that is less than 500 mL per 24 hours or less than 50 mL if measuring hourly volumes.

■ Observe if client has the strength, ability to swallow, and mental capacity to drink fluid without assistance.

Nursing Diagnosis: Deficient Fluid Volume related to fluid loss greater than intake as manifested by vomiting and diarrhea secondary to gastroenteritis, oral intake of 500 mL, fluid loss of 1700 mL in previous 24 hours, concentrated urine, postural hypotension, tachycardia, and dry mucous membranes

Expected Outcome: Client will have a fluid intake of at least 1500 mL per 24 hours and urine output within 500 mL of oral intake (i.e., at least 1000 mL per 24 hours).

Interventions	*Rationales*
Withhold solid food for 8 hours.	Solid food can irritate gastric mucosa.
Provide dilute mouthwash or weak salt water as an oral rinse after vomiting.	An oral rinse reduces the unpleasant aftertaste of emesis that may trigger additional vomiting.
Empty the emesis basin and change linen soiled with vomitus.	The sight and smell of emesis perpetuate the cycle of vomiting.
Encourage slow, deep breaths when the client experiences waves of nausea.	Breathing distracts the client from the nausea until the reversed peristaltic action passes.
Avoid jarring the bed or activities that require movement on the client's part.	The vestibular center in the ear is sensitive to movement of the head and can stimulate the vomiting center (as in motion sickness).
Administer prescribed antiemetics according to the physician's written orders.	Antiemetics may inhibit the vomiting center directly or help control vomiting by other mechanisms (e.g., slowing GI peristalsis).
Provide sips of liquids like weak tea, flat carbonated soft drinks, and water as often as the client can tolerate them.	Small volumes of fluids that are not strongly flavored or highly carbonated are less likely to cause nausea or distend the stomach.
Progress fluid selection to include gelatin, bouillion, Gatorade, or Pedialyte when the client can tolerate fluids identified earlier.	These products provide glucose, sodium, chloride, and other electrolytes.
Eliminate dairy products if the client is lactose intolerant.	Clients who do not produce lactase, the enzyme that aids in milk digestion, develop cramps and diarrhea when they consume dairy products.
Offer dry crackers or toast if the client retains fluids.	Solid foods in readily digestible carbohydrates are tolerated better than other types of food.
Administer prescribed antidiarrheals as medically ordered.	They reduce the frequency and consistency of watery stools by adsorbing excess liquid from and soothing the bowel and slowing bowel motility.
Increase to a low-residue diet, starting with the BRAT (bananas, rice, applesauce, toast) diet when diarrhea is controlled.	Low-residue foods reduce stool bulk and slow GI transit time; the BRAT diet contains foods that are high in pectin, which helps make stools firm.

Evaluation of Expected Outcomes:

Intake is 1500 mL and output is 1750 mL, 500 mL of which is emesis. Episodes of vomiting and diarrhea are reduced. BP is stable at 110/68 mm Hg in both lying and sitting positions. Urine is medium yellow. Client is tolerating clear fluids, saltines, and dry white toast.

NURSING GUIDELINES 22-1

Managing Fluid Volume Deficit

- Inform client that he or she must increase consumption of oral fluids. Set a target goal for intake per hour, shift, and 24-hour period; a goal of 3000 to 4000 mL is not excessive for dehydrated clients. Schedule the bulk of fluid intake at meals and when the client is awake (i.e., more intake during daytime than throughout the night).

- Offer at least 180 mL of fluid when administering oral medications.

- Implement a "sip n' go" plan by which anyone entering the room offers the client at least 60 mL of fluid (Mentes, 2000).

- Obtain a list of fluids the client prefers; include gelatin, popsicles, ice cream, and sherbet if they are allowed.

- Provide various liquids, replace with a fresh supply periodically, and ensure they are an appropriate temperature.

- Modify fluid containers to accommodate for client's strength and physical skills (e.g., cups with handles, covered cups with an opening for the mouth or insertion of a straw).

- Offer small volumes frequently, rather than expecting the client to consume a large volume at once.

- Thicken watery fluid with a commercial thickener if the client has difficulty swallowing.

- Relieve nausea, vomiting, mouth discomfort, and other problems that interfere with drinking.

- Ensure that clients prone to low fluid volume have fasting tests done expeditiously to reduce the time they are without food or fluids.

- Evaluate goals by recollecting assessment data and analyzing trends, especially in intake and output totals. Report results to the physician, especially if collaborative efforts fall short.

comes of interventions. In addition, the nurse teaches clients who have a potential for hypovolemia and their families to:

- Respond to thirst because it is an early indication of reduced fluid volume.
- Consume at least 8 to 10 glasses of fluid each day, and more during hot, humid weather.
- Drink water as an inexpensive means to meet fluid requirements.
- Avoid beverages with alcohol and caffeine; they increase urination and contribute to fluid deficits.
- Include a moderate amount of table salt or foods containing sodium each day.
- Rise slowly from a sitting or lying position to avoid dizziness and potential injury.

● HYPERVOLEMIA

Hypervolemia (fluid volume excess) means there is a high volume of water in the intravascular fluid compartment.

Pathophysiology and Etiology

Hypervolemia is caused by fluid intake that exceeds fluid loss, such as from excessive oral intake or rapid IV infusion of fluid. It also is a consequence of heart failure (see Chap. 36) when the heart cannot adequately distribute fluid to the kidneys for filtration. It also can result from inadequate fluid elimination, as may accompany kidney disease (see Chap. 64). Fluid retention (reduced fluid loss) also can occur secondary to excessive salt intake (sodium chloride), adrenal gland dysfunction (see Chap. 57), or administration of corticosteroid drugs such as prednisolone (Delta-Cortef).

Hypervolemia can lead to **circulatory overload,** a fluid volume that exceeds what is normal for the intravascular space and can potentially compromise cardiopulmonary function. The excess volume raises BP and causes the heart to increase its force of contraction. As the excess volume is distributed to the interstitial space, **pitting edema,** indentations in the skin after compression, may be noted (see Fig. 22-8). Pitting edema usually does not occur, however, until there is a 3L excess in the intravascular volume.

Assessment Findings

Signs and Symptoms

Early signs of hypervolemia (see Table 22-2) are weight gain, elevated BP, and increased breathing effort. There may be evidence of **dependent edema** (edema in body areas most affected by gravity, such as the feet, ankles, sacrum, or buttocks) in clients confined to bed. Rings, shoes, and stockings may leave marks in the skin. The jugular neck veins may appear prominent when the client sits. Eventually, fluid congestion in the lungs leads to moist breath sounds.

Clients at risk for hypervolemia include those who:

- Have altered cardiac or kidney function
- Have increased ADH production, which sometimes accompanies brain trauma
- Are receiving corticosteroid therapy, large rapid volumes of IV fluid, or IV colloid solutions (e.g., albumin)
- Consume oral fluids to excess, such as clients with schizophrenia who can develop water intoxication
- Ingest highly salted food or foods that contain large amounts of sodium

Diagnostic Findings

The blood cell count and hematocrit level are low as the result of **hemodilution,** a reduced ratio of blood components to watery plasma. Urine specific gravity is also low, reflecting the larger proportion of water. CVP is above 10 cm H_2O.

Medical Management

The condition causing the fluid excess is treated. Oral and parenteral fluid intake is restricted. Diuretics, drugs that promote urinary excretion, are prescribed. Salt and sodium intake is limited.

N U R S I N G   P R O C E S S

● The Client With Hypervolemia

Assessment

The nurse obtains baseline weight and weighs the client daily thereafter on the same scale and at the same time before breakfast, in similar clothing. A 2-lb weight gain in 24 hours indicates that the client is retaining 1L of fluid. The nurse maintains accurate intake and output records and reports significant differences in the two measurements. He or she auscultates the lungs to detect abnormal breath sounds. The nurse determines if an S_3 heart sound is present and inspects the neck veins to assess for disten-

tion (see Chap 30). Regular measurements of BP, heart rate, and respiratory rate are necessary. The nurse notes the client's activity tolerance. To detect pitting edema, he or she gently presses the skin over a bony area, such as the tibia or dorsum of the foot, for up to 5 seconds and observes the results (Fig. 22-8). He or she inspects edematous skin for cracks and breakdown.

Diagnosis, Planning, and Interventions

The nurse implements prescribed interventions such as limiting sodium and water intake and administering ordered medications that promote fluid elimination. Elevating the client's head can relieve labored breathing. The nurse takes measures to prevent skin breakdown in cases of peripheral edema. Reassessment is necessary to determine if planned interventions have restored fluid volume balance. The nurse also performs necessary teaching with the client and family (Client and Family Teaching Box 22-1).

Excess Fluid Volume related to intake that exceeds fluid loss (or reduced fluid loss in relation to intake)

1+ Pitting Edema

- Slight indentation (2mm)
- Normal contours
- Associated with interstitial fluid volume 30% above normal

2+ Pitting Edema

- Deeper pit after pressing (4mm)
- Lasts longer than 1+
- Fairly normal contour

3+ Pitting Edema

- Deep pit (6mm)
- Remains several seconds after pressing
- Skin swelling obvious by general inspection

4+ Pitting Edema

- Deep pit (8mm)
- Remains for a prolonged time after pressing, possibly minutes
- Frank swelling

Brawny Edema

- Fluid can no longer be displaced secondary to excessive interstitial fluid accumulation
- No pitting
- Tissue palpates as firm or hard
- Skin surface shiny, warm, moist

FIGURE 22-8 Grading edema is somewhat subjective; assessment findings may vary depending on the clinician. These criteria are offered to assist in documentation.

Expected Outcome: Fluid status will return to normal as evidenced by weight loss, reduced edema, BP within normal limits, and urine output of at least 2000 mL/day.

- Assess vital signs, daily weight, intake and output, breath sounds, and location and extent of edema as often as necessary. *Focused assessments help determine if interventions are reducing or eliminating the problem.*
- Use guidelines established by the physician for restricting oral fluid. *Limiting fluid intake helps reduce the volume absorbed into the vascular system.*
- Develop a plan with the client for distributing the allotted oral volume over 24 hours. *Involving the client in care promotes compliance and demonstrates that healthcare professionals value and respect the client's preferences.*
- Ration fluid so the client can consume approximately 20% to 25% at times other than meals (Mentes, 2000). *The client should be able to consume some fluid whenever thirsty; restricting fluids to meals only is inappropriate.*
- Collaborate with the dietitian to modify the diet to meet salt/sodium restrictions and to avoid sweet or dry foods. *The higher the concentration of sodium (salt) in the blood, there will be a greater serum osmolality and a proportionate increase in fluid volume. Sweet or dry food increases a client's desire to consume fluid.*
- Administer prescribed diuretics. *They promote sodium excretion and water elimination.*
- Prepare client and assist with medical interventions such as dialysis (see Chap. 64). *Dialysis uses principles of osmosis and filtration to promote fluid elimination from the blood.*

Altered Comfort: Dry Mouth and Thirst related to restricted oral fluid

Expected Outcomes: (1) Client's mouth will be moist despite fluid restrictions. (2) Client will state that thirst is tolerable.

- Provide supplies for frequent oral hygiene. *Keeping the mouth clean and wet reduces discomfort.*
- Substitute ice chips for oral liquids. *The volume of melted ice is half that of solid ice. Holding ice chips in the mouth gives the psychological impression of consuming more fluid. Because melting ice chips stay in the mouth longer than water, they promote the sensation that larger volumes are being ingested.*
- Instruct client to wet the mouth with a measured volume of fluid in a squeezable squirt bottle or spray atomizer. *Squirting or spraying water in the oral cavity moisturizes the surface of the oral mucous membranes with a small volume of fluid and reduces dryness and thirst.*

Risk for Impaired Skin Integrity related to compromised circulation secondary to edema

Expected Outcome: Skin will remain intact.

- Change client's position every 2 hours. *Doing so relieves pressure on capillaries. If capillary pressure falls below 32 mm Hg for more than 2 hours, the skin and underlying tissue are deprived of oxygenated blood, predisposing the client to cell death and skin breakdown.*

- Keep client's legs elevated higher than the heart. *Doing so facilitates return of venous blood to the heart. Improved circulation reduces metabolic waste products and their toxic effects.*
- Encourage ambulation or isometric bed exercises within client's level of tolerance. *Activity increases respiratory and heart rates; muscle contraction promotes venous return to the heart. All these factors improve delivery of oxygenated blood to the skin and other body cells and removal of metabolic wastes.*
- Apply elastic stockings. *They support valves in the veins and prevent fluid from pooling in dependent areas like the feet and ankles.*

Evaluation of Expected Outcomes

Expected outcomes are a daily weight loss of approximately 1 lb, decreased edema from previous assessments, clear lungs, and unlabored respirations. Laboratory values for red blood cells, hematocrit, urine specific gravity, and electrolytes return to normal. Elevations in BP or heart rate resolve. Oral mucous membranes are moist, and the client reports that the distribution of oral fluids controls thirst within a tolerable level. The client shows no evidence of skin breakdown, with reduced or eliminated edema. The toes and feet are warm. Blood returns to the nailbed within 2 to 3 seconds after release of the compressed area.

22-1 *Client and Family Teaching*
Managing Hypervolemia

The nurse educates the client with hypervolemia and his or her family by:

- Showing common containers and indicating the volume that each holds.
- Identifying foods that are high in salt or sodium: processed meats (hot dogs and cold cuts); salted and smoked fish; cheeses, especially processed varieties; peanut butter; powdered cocoa and hot chocolate mixes; canned vegetables; foods preserved in brine (pickles, olives, sauerkraut); tomato and tomato-vegetable juices; canned soup and instant soups or bouillon; boxed casserole mixes; salted snack foods; seasonings—catsup, gravy mixes, soy sauce, monosodium glutamate (MSG), pickle relish, tartar sauce, mustard, horseradish, barbecue sauce, steak sauce.
- Teaching how to read food labels and look for the words *salt, sodium,* and other sources of sodium such as *baking soda* or *baking powder.*
- Providing information concerning diuretic drug therapy.
- Listing ways to determine if fluid excess is recurring or has resolved.

• THIRD-SPACING

Third-spacing describes the translocation of fluid from the intravascular or intercellular space to tissue compartments, where it becomes trapped and useless. It is associated with the loss of colloids, as may accompany *hypoalbuminemia* (low level of albumin in the blood) or burns and severe allergic reactions that alter capillary and cellular membrane permeability. Fluid translocation follows the shift in osmotic pressure to other locations. If the translocation depletes fluid volume in the intravascular area, it can lead to hypotension, shock, and circulatory failure (see Chap. 23).

Assessment Findings

The client manifests signs and symptoms of hypovolemia with the exception of weight loss. Fluid volume remains relatively unchanged, but the percentages in various locations are altered. There may be signs of localized enlargement of organ cavities (like the abdomen) if they fill with fluid, a condition referred to as *ascites* (see Chap. 55). There may be **generalized edema** in all the interstitial spaces, which sometimes is called *brawny edema* or *anasarca*. Results of laboratory blood tests and urine specific gravity are borderline normal or reveal evidence of hemoconcentration. CVP is below normal, as are other hemodynamic measurements (pressure as it relates to intravascular volume, see Chap. 30).

Medical Management

The medical priority is to restore circulatory volume in clients with hypotension and eliminate the trapped fluid. This is done by administering IV solutions—sometimes at rapid rates—and blood products, like albumin, to restore colloidal osmotic pressure. Administration of albumin pulls the trapped fluid back into the intravascular space. When this occurs, clients who were previously hypovolemic can suddenly become hypervolemic. An IV diuretic may be ordered to reduce the potential for circulatory overload.

Nursing Management

Nursing care combines the assessment techniques for detecting both hypovolemia and hypervolemia. Policies and practices vary concerning how much responsibility LPN/LVNs may assume with regard to IV fluid therapy and administration of IV medications (see Chap. 24).

ELECTROLYTE IMBALANCES

Electrolytes are in both intracellular and extracellular water. They include **ions,** positively and negatively charged substances, such as potassium, magnesium, sodium, phosphate, sulfate, calcium, chloride, bicarbonate, protein, and organic acids. Sodium, calcium, and chloride ion concentrations are higher in extracellular fluid, whereas potassium, magnesium, and phosphate concentrations are higher in the cells. These differences are responsible for electrical potentials that develop across cell membranes and perhaps for the degree of cell membrane permeability.

Electrolyte imbalances occur when there is a deficit or an excess of electrolytes or when electrolytes are translocated to any one or more fluid compartments. A loss or gain in fluid usually is accompanied by a similar change in electrolytes. Electrolyte imbalances are identified primarily by measuring their levels in the serum (watery portion of blood).

Electrolyte deficits sometimes result from inadequate intake of food that provides their natural source. Other causes include administering IV solutions that contain none, or only some, needed electrolytes and conditions that deplete water and substances dissolved therein (e.g., vomiting, diarrhea). Administration of certain medications (e.g., diuretics) also depletes electrolytes.

Factors that contribute to excess electrolytes include an overabundance of orally consumed or parenterally administered electrolytes, kidney failure, and endocrine (glandular) dysfunction, especially of the pituitary gland or adrenal cortex. Electrolytes move from within cells into serum when cell membranes are damaged, such as in crushing injuries or burns. Sodium, potassium, calcium, and magnesium deficits or excesses are of particular concern.

• SODIUM IMBALANCES

Sodium (Na^+), the chief **cation** (positively charged electrolyte) in extracellular fluid, is essential for maintaining normal nerve and muscle activity, regulating osmotic pressure, and preserving acid-base balance. The principal role of sodium is to regulate and distribute fluid volume in the body. Normal concentration ranges from 135 to 145 mEq/L. Lower than normal serum sodium level is *hyponatremia;* higher than normal serum sodium level is *hypernatremia.*

HYPONATREMIA

Causes of hyponatremia include profuse diaphoresis, excessive ingestion of plain water or administration of nonelectrolyte IV fluids, profuse diuresis, loss of GI secretions (e.g., in prolonged vomiting, GI suctioning, draining fistulas), and Addison's disease (see Chap. 57).

Assessment Findings

Manifestations include mental confusion, muscular weakness, anorexia, restlessness, elevated body temperature, tachycardia, nausea, vomiting, and personality changes. If the deficit is severe, symptoms are more intense and convulsions or coma can occur. The serum sodium level is below 135 mEq/L.

Medical Management

When possible, the underlying cause is corrected. Treatment of mild deficits includes oral administration of sodium (foods high in sodium, water to which salt has been added, and salt tablets). For severe deficits, administration of IV solutions containing sodium chloride (see Chap. 24) are prescribed.

HYPERNATREMIA

Hypernatremia is excess sodium in the blood. Causes include profuse watery diarrhea, excessive salt intake without sufficient water intake, high fever, decreased water intake (i.e., in elderly, debilitated, unconscious, or developmentally delayed clients), excessive administration of solutions that contain sodium, excessive water loss without an accompanying loss of sodium, and severe burns.

Assessment Findings

Hypernatremia results in thirst; dry, sticky mucous membranes; decreased urine output; fever; a rough, dry tongue; and lethargy, which can progress to coma if the excess is severe. The serum sodium level is above 145 mEq/L.

Medical Management

Treatment depends on the cause and includes oral administration of plain water or IV administration of a hypotonic solution, such as 0.45% sodium chloride or 5% dextrose (see Chap. 24). In mild cases, sodium intake may be restricted until laboratory test results are normal.

NURSING MANAGEMENT FOR SODIUM IMBALANCES

Nursing management includes early detection, especially in those clients at risk for hyponatremia or hypernatremia. The nurse apportions oral fluids according to target volumes, maintains accurate intake and output measurements, assesses vital signs every 1 to 4 hours, and closely monitors the infusion of IV fluids. He or she implements prescribed dietary restrictions or supplements. The nurse gathers data that indicate increased or decreased symptoms and notifies the physician if symptoms worsen or laboratory values show a significant change.

● POTASSIUM IMBALANCES

The potassium cation (K^+) is the chief electrolyte found in intracellular fluid. Potassium has the same functions intracellularly as sodium has extracellularly. A deficit of potassium in the blood is called *hypokalemia;* an excess is called *hyperkalemia.*

HYPOKALEMIA

Potassium-wasting diuretics (e.g., furosemide [Lasix], ethacrynic acid [Edecrin], hydrochlorothiazide [Hydro-Diuril]) contribute to hypokalemia. Loss of fluid from the GI tract (as with severe vomiting or diarrhea, draining intestinal fistulae, or prolonged suctioning) also causes potassium deficit. Large doses of corticosteroids, IV administration of insulin and glucose, and prolonged administration of nonelectrolyte parenteral fluids can deplete potassium.

Assessment Findings

Hypokalemia causes fatigue, weakness, anorexia, nausea, vomiting, cardiac dysrhythmias (abnormal heart rate or rhythm, especially in people receiving cardiac glycosides such as digitalis preparations), leg cramps, muscle weakness, and paresthesias (abnormal sensations). Severe cases result in hypotension, flaccid paralysis, and even death from cardiac or respiratory arrest. Hypokalemia produces characteristic changes in the electrocardiogram (ECG) waveform (Fig. 22-9). The serum potassium level is below 3.5 mEq/L. Symptoms may not develop, however, until the serum potassium level is below 3.0 mEq/L.

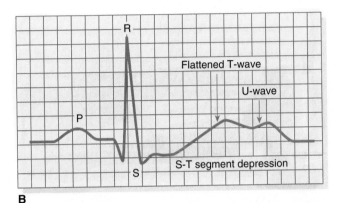

FIGURE 22-9 Effect of potassium on ECG. (**A**) Normal tracing. (**B**) Serum potassium level below normal results in a U wave. (From Smeltzer, S. C. & Bare, B. G. [2000]. *Brunner & Suddarth's textbook of medical–surgical nursing* [9th ed.]. Philadelphia: Lippincott Williams & Wilkins.)

Medical Management

Treatment includes elimination of the cause (when possible). Mild hypokalemia is treated by increasing oral intake of potassium-rich foods or using a prescribed potassium oral replacement such as K-Lor, K-Lyte, or Klorvess. Severe hypokalemia is treated with IV administration of solutions containing a potassium salt, such as potassium chloride.

HYPERKALEMIA

Hyperkalemia can occur with severe renal failure, in which the kidneys cannot excrete potassium; severe burns; administration of potassium-sparing diuretics; overuse of potassium supplements, salt substitutes (which contain potassium instead of sodium), or potassium-rich foods; crushing injuries; Addison's disease; and rapid administration of parenteral potassium salts.

Assessment Findings

Symptoms include diarrhea, nausea, muscle weakness, paresthesias, and cardiac dysrhythmias. The serum potassium level is above 5.5 mEq/L. Hyperkalemia also causes unique changes in ECG waveforms (Fig. 22-10) that can forewarn of sudden cardiac death.

Medical Management

Treatment depends on the cause and severity. Mild hyperkalemia is treated by decreasing the intake of potassium-rich foods or discontinuing oral potassium replacement until laboratory values are normal. Severe hyperkalemia is treated by administering a cation-exchange resin such as Kayexalate or a combination of IV regular insulin and glucose. Peritoneal dialysis or hemodialysis, techniques for removing toxic substances from the blood, also may be used (see Chap. 64).

NURSING MANAGEMENT FOR POTASSIUM IMBALANCES

The nurse assesses clients for conditions with the potential to cause potassium imbalances, identifies signs and symptoms associated with potassium imbalances, monitors laboratory findings measuring serum potassium, administers medications that restore potassium balance, and evaluates the client's response to medical therapy. He or she consults with the physician when a client is receiving prolonged IV fluid therapy without added potassium. If IV potassium is ordered, it must be diluted in an IV solution and administered at a rate below 10 mEq/hour. The nurse observes the infusion frequently to verify it is being administered at the appropriate rate. He or she also

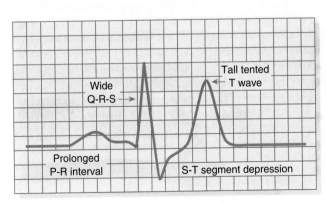

FIGURE 22-10 High potassium on ECG produces a tall T wave. (From Smeltzer, S. C. & Bare, B. G. [2000]. *Brunner & Suddarth's textbook of medical–surgical nursing* [9th ed.]. Philadelphia: Lippincott Williams & Wilkins.)

informs clients at risk for potassium imbalances and their families about:

- Medications that cause urinary excretion of potassium, such as diuretics
- Food sources of potassium: vegetables, dried peas and beans, wheat bran, bananas, oranges, orange juice, melon, prune juice, potatoes, and milk
- Taking oral potassium supplements shortly after meals or with food to avoid GI distress; effervescent tablets or liquids are taken with a full glass of water

● CALCIUM IMBALANCES

Most of the body's calcium (Ca^{++}) is found in the bones and teeth. A small percentage (about 1%) is in the blood. The parathyroid glands regulate the serum calcium level. Calcium is necessary for blood clotting; smooth, skeletal, and cardiac muscle function; and transmission of nerve impulses. Vitamin D is needed for calcium absorption in the intestine. *Hypocalcemia* occurs when the serum calcium level is lower than normal; *hypercalcemia* occurs when the level is higher.

HYPOCALCEMIA

Causes of hypocalcemia include vitamin D deficiency, hypoparathyroidism, severe burns, acute pancreatitis, certain drugs, rapid administration of multiple units of blood that contain an anticalcium additive, intestinal malabsorption disorders, and accidental surgical removal of the parathyroid glands.

Assessment Findings

Hypocalcemia is evidenced by tingling in the extremities and the area around the mouth (*circumoral paresthesia*), muscle and abdominal cramps, carpopedal spasms referred to as **Trousseau's sign** (Fig. 22-11), mental changes, positive **Chvostek's sign** (spasms of the facial muscles when the facial nerve is tapped; Fig. 22-12), laryngeal spasms with airway obstruction, *tetany* (muscle twitching), seizures, bleeding, and cardiac dysrhythmias. The client has hypocalcemia if the total serum calcium level is below 8.8 mg/dl (normal range, 9 to 11 mg/dl) or the ionized calcium level is below 4.4 mg/dl (normal range, 4.4 to 5.4 mg/dl).

Medical Management

Treatment includes administration of oral calcium and vitamin D for mild deficits and IV administration of a calcium salt, such as calcium gluconate, for severe hypocalcemia.

FIGURE 22-11 Trousseau's sign, a characteristic of hypocalcemia, is evidenced by a carpopedal spasm when circulation of blood is occluded in the arm for 3 minutes.

HYPERCALCEMIA

Hypercalcemia is associated with parathyroid gland tumors, multiple fractures, Paget's disease, hyperparathyroidism, excessive doses of vitamin D, prolonged immobilization, some chemotherapeutic agents, and certain malignant diseases (multiple myeloma, acute leukemia, lymphomas).

FIGURE 22-12 Chvostek's sign, unilateral spasm of facial muscles, is elicited in clients with hypocalcemia by tapping over the facial nerve, which lies approximately 2 cm anterior to the earlobe.

Assessment Findings

Hypercalcemia causes deep bone pain, constipation, anorexia, nausea, vomiting, polyuria, thirst, pathologic fractures, and mental changes (usually decreased memory and attention span). Chronic hypercalcemia can promote the formation of kidney stones. The total serum calcium level is above 10 mg/dl, and the ionized calcium level is above 5.4 mg/dl.

Medical Management

Treatment includes determining and correcting the cause when possible. Mild hypercalcemia is treated by increasing oral fluid intake and limiting calcium consumption until laboratory findings are normal. Acute hypercalcemia is treated by administering one or more of the following: IV sodium chloride solution (0.45% or 0.9%) and a diuretic such as furosemide (Lasix) to increase calcium excretion in the urine; oral phosphates; or calcitonin (Cibacalcin), a synthetic hormone for regulating calcium levels. Hypercalcemia associated with cancer or chemotherapy is treated on an individual basis. A decrease in drug dosage or discontinuation of therapy may be necessary. Corticosteroids or plicamycin (Mithracin), an antineoplastic agent, also may be used to treat hypercalcemia of malignant diseases that do not respond to other forms of therapy.

NURSING MANAGEMENT FOR CALCIUM IMBALANCES

The nurse closely monitors the client with hypocalcemia for neurologic manifestations (tetany, seizures, spasms), cardiac dysrhythmias, and airway obstruction because emergency interventions may be necessary. If the deficit is severe, seizure precautions are necessary. Clients with severe muscle cramping remain on bed rest for comfort and to avoid falls. Because a low calcium level interferes with clotting, the nurse routinely checks for signs of bruising or bleeding.

The nurse encourages the client with mild hypercalcemia to drink many oral fluids. He or she collaborates with the dietitian to limit food sources of calcium when calcium is restricted from the diet. Encouraging ambulation as tolerated is important. The nurse provides assistance and instructs the client to wear shoes to avoid falls that may result in pathologic fractures.

A teaching plan for the client with hypocalcemia or hypercalcemia includes the following points:

- Follow the physician's recommendations regarding the addition or restriction of calcium to the diet. Milk and dairy products are rich sources of dietary calcium. Nondairy sources are turnip and mustard greens, collards, kale, broccoli, canned fish with bones, and calcium-fortified orange juice.
- Lactose-free milk and nonprescription lactase enzymes are available for lactose-intolerant clients.
- Take prescribed or physician-recommended drugs as directed; do not exceed or omit a dose.

● MAGNESIUM IMBALANCES

Magnesium (Mg^{++}) is found in bone cells and specialized cells of the heart, liver, and skeletal muscles. Only a small percentage of the total magnesium in the body is found in extracellular fluid. Magnesium is involved in the transmission of nerve impulses and muscle excitability and activates several enzyme systems, including the functioning of B vitamins and use of potassium and calcium. A lower than normal serum level of magnesium is *hypomagnesemia;* higher than normal is *hypermagnesemia.*

HYPOMAGNESEMIA

Conditions that can result in hypomagnesemia include chronic alcoholism, diabetic ketoacidosis, severe renal disease, severe burns, severe malnutrition, toxemia of pregnancy (eclampsia), intestinal malabsorption syndromes, excessive diuresis (drug induced), hyperaldosteronism (see Chap. 57), and prolonged gastric suction.

Assessment Findings

Signs and symptoms include tachycardia and other cardiac dysrhythmias, neuromuscular irritability, paresthesias of the extremities, leg and foot cramps, hypertension, mental changes, positive Chvostek's and Trousseau's signs (see hypocalcemia), dysphagia (difficulty swallowing), and seizures. The serum magnesium level is below 1.3 mEq/L (normal range, 1.3 to 2.1 mEq/L).

Medical Management

Treatment includes administration of oral magnesium salts or the addition of magnesium-rich foods to the diet (see General Nutritional Considerations). A severe magnesium deficit is treated with IV administration of magnesium sulfate.

HYPERMAGNESEMIA

Hypermagnesemia can be a consequence of renal failure, Addison's disease, excessive use of antacids or laxatives that contain magnesium, and hyperparathyroidism.

Assessment Findings

Clients with hypermagnesemia experience flushing, warmth, hypotension, lethargy, drowsiness, *bradycardia* (slow heart rate), muscle weakness, depressed respirations, and coma. The serum magnesium level is above 2.1 mEq/L.

Medical Management

Treatment includes decreasing oral magnesium intake or discontinuing administration of parenteral replacement. In severe hypermagnesemia, hemodialysis may be necessary. If respiratory failure occurs, mechanical ventilation is essential.

NURSING MANAGEMENT FOR MAGNESIUM IMBALANCES

The nurse closely observes clients with hypomagnesemia for dysrhythmias and early signs of neuromuscular irritability, which he or she reports to the physician immediately. If administering IV magnesium sulfate, the nurse checks BP frequently because such administration can produce vasodilation and subsequently hypotension. Calcium gluconate is kept available as an antidote for an adverse reaction during administration of magnesium sulfate. If dysphagia occurs, the nurse consults with the physician and dietitian about alternatives or modifications to dietary management.

Vital signs of clients with actual or potential hypermagnesemia require close monitoring. The nurse notifies the physician immediately of significant changes, especially in respiratory rate, rhythm, or depth.

Teaching points include the following:

- Check with the physician, pharmacist, or nurse concerning antacids or laxatives that contain magnesium.
- If use of an antacid or laxative is allowed, follow the physician's recommendations regarding the frequency of use.

Stop, Think, and Respond ● BOX 22-2

Identify the electrolyte imbalance each client is most likely manifesting:

Client A is nauseous and weak. The ECG shows a U wave.

Client B has muscle twitching and tingling around the mouth. When the nurse applies a BP cuff to the client's arm and occludes blood flow for 3 minutes, the fingers and wrist become flexed.

Client C is thirsty, lethargic, and excreting only scant urine.

ACID-BASE BALANCE

In addition to water and electrolytes, body fluid also contains acids and bases. One of the chief acids is carbonic acid (H_2CO_3). An example of a base, sometimes referred to as an alkaline substance, that neutralizes acids is bicarbonate (HCO_3). Acid and base content influence the pH of body fluid. The symbol *pH* refers to the amount of hydrogen ions in a solution; pH can range from 1, which is highly acidic, to 14, which is highly basic. A pH of 7 is considered neutral. The more hydrogen ions in a solution, the more acidic it is. Acidity is indicated by a pH below 7. The degree of alkalinity is identified by a pH above 7. Normal plasma pH is 7.35 to 7.45, or slightly alkaline. The body maintains the normal plasma pH by two mechanisms: chemical regulation and organ regulation.

Chemical Regulation

Chemical regulation occurs through one or more buffering systems by which hydrogen ions are either added or eliminated. Adding hydrogen ions increases acidity; removing them promotes alkalinity. The major chemical regulator of plasma pH is the **bicarbonate–carbonic acid buffer system.** A ratio of 20 parts bicarbonate to 1 part carbonic acid maintains normal plasma pH (Fig. 22-13).

Oxygen Regulation

The lungs and kidneys facilitate the ratio of bicarbonate to carbonic acid. Carbon dioxide (CO_2) is one of the components of carbonic acid:

$$CO_2 + H_2O \text{ (water)} = H_2CO_3 \text{ (carbonic acid)}$$

The lungs regulate carbonic acid levels by releasing or conserving CO_2 by increasing or decreasing the respi-

FIGURE 22-13 Acid-base balance. Note that *acidosis* is used to describe the condition when pH is between 6.8 and 7.35. When fluid acidity falls below 7, the person is in danger of death.

ratory rate, volume, or both. The kidneys assist in acid-base balance by retaining or excreting bicarbonate ions. If an imbalance in acids or bases occur, these regulatory processes are accelerated, which is referred to as **compensation.**

ACID-BASE IMBALANCES

An imbalance in acids or bases is life-threatening. Death occurs quickly if plasma pH is outside the range of 6.8 to 8.0 (Sherwood, 1995). Arterial blood gas (ABG) results are the main tool for measuring blood pH, CO_2 content ($PaCO_2$), and bicarbonate. An acid-base imbalance may accompany a fluid and electrolyte imbalance.

There are essentially two types of acid-base imbalances: acidosis and alkalosis. **Acidosis** means excessive accumulation of acids or excessive loss of bicarbonate in body fluids. **Alkalosis** means excessive accumulation of bases or loss of acid in body fluids. Either can stem from metabolic or respiratory alterations. There are four subtypes: metabolic acidosis, metabolic alkalosis, respiratory acidosis, and respiratory alkalosis.

● METABOLIC ACIDOSIS

Metabolic acidosis is a condition that results in decreased plasma pH because of increased organic acids (acids other than carbonic acid) or decreased bicarbonate. Organic acids increase during periods of anaerobic metabolism, when cells attempt to produce ATP without oxygen. Anaerobic metabolism is much less efficient than aerobic (with oxygen) metabolism and produces byproducts such as lactic acid. It occurs during shock and cardiac arrest. Acids also increase in starvation and diabetic ketoacidosis (see Chap. 58), as fatty acids accumulate because the body cannot use glucose for energy. Accumulation of acids also may follow renal failure because the kidneys cannot reabsorb bicarbonate to buffer the blood. They also accumulate with aspirin (acetylsalicylic acid) overdosage or profuse diarrhea. Another cause of acid accumulation is loss of intestinal fluid through wound drainage, in which bicarbonate can be lost in disproportionate amounts.

Assessment Findings

Signs and Symptoms

Metabolic acidosis is accompanied by deep and rapid breathing (*Kussmaul's breathing*), a compensatory mechanism to rid the body of CO_2 and thus prevent carbonic acid from forming. The client may experience anorexia, nausea, vomiting, headache, confusion, flushing, lethargy, malaise, drowsiness, abdominal pain or discomfort, and

weakness. Dangerous cardiac dysrhythmias can develop, and the force of cardiac contractions can be weakened. In severe stages, stupor and coma occur, and death may follow shortly.

Diagnostic Findings

The ABG values usually show decreased pH and plasma bicarbonate (HCO_3). Initially, $PaCO_2$ is normal, a condition referred to as an *uncompensated state.* As the rapid and deep breathing becomes effective, $PaCO_2$ decreases. Until pH returns to normal, it is referred to as a *partially compensated state.* When pH returns to normal, it is referred to as a *fully compensated state,* even though HCO_3 and $PaCO_2$ values are abnormal (Table 22-3). In a fully compensated state, regardless of the initial imbalance and current abnormal values, the client is out of danger.

The anion gap also is used to identify metabolic acidosis. The **anion gap** is the difference between sodium and potassium cation (positive ion) concentrations and the sum of chloride and bicarbonate **anions** (negative ions) in the extracellular fluid. The measured cations usually exceed the measured anions; the gap reflects the remaining unmeasured anions, such as phosphates, sulfates, organic acids, and proteins (Porth, 2002). The normal anion gap is 12 ± 4 mEq/L. An anion gap that exceeds 16 mEq/L indicates, but is not absolutely diagnostic for, metabolic acidosis. Low or negative anion gaps are relatively rare (Martin, 1999).

The measurement of all base buffers—sometimes referred to as the base excess or deficit—is used to identify acid-base imbalances. The base buffers include bicarbonate, phosphate, protein, and hemoglobin. To determine if the base is in excess or deficit, the laboratory determines the amount of a fixed acid or base that is necessary to reach a pH of 7.4 in a sample of the client's blood (Porth, 2002). The normal range is ± 3.0 mEq/L. A base deficit indicates metabolic acidosis; a base excess indicates metabolic alkalosis.

Stop, Think, and Respond ● BOX 22-3

Calculate the anion gap using the following measurements, and indicate those that are signs of metabolic acidosis.

Sodium (Na^+): 165 mEq/L
Potassium (K^+): 4.0 mEq/L
Chloride (Cl^-): 112 mEq/L
Bicarbonate (HCO_3): 32 mEq/L

Medical Management

Treatment includes eliminating the cause and replacing fluids and electrolytes that may have been lost. IV bicarbonate is administered for severe metabolic acidosis.

TABLE 22-3	ARTERIAL BLOOD GAS TRENDS IN ACID-BASE IMBALANCES		
CONDITION	pH	HCO_3	$PaCO_2$
Acid-base balance	7.35–7.45	22–26 mEq/L	35–45 mm Hg
Metabolic Acidosis			
Uncompensated	<7.35	<22 mEq/L	Normal
Partially compensated	<7.35	<22 mEq/L	<35 mm Hg
Fully compensated	7.35–7.45	<22 mEq/L	<35 mm Hg
Metabolic Alkalosis			
Uncompensated	>7.45	>26 mEq/L	Normal
Partially compensated	>7.45	>26 mEq/L	>45 mm Hg
Fully compensated	>7.45	>22 mEq/L	>45 mm Hg
Respiratory Acidosis			
Uncompensated	<7.35	Normal	>45 mm Hg
Partially compensated	<7.35	>26 mEq/L	>45 mm Hg
Fully compensated	7.35–7.45	>26 mEq/L	>45 mm Hg
Respiratory Alkalosis			
Uncompensated	7.45	Normal	<35 mm Hg
Partially compensated	7.45	<22 mEq/L	<35 mm Hg
Fully compensated	7.35–7.45	<22 mEq/L	<35 mm Hg

● METABOLIC ALKALOSIS

Metabolic alkalosis results in increased plasma pH because of accumulated base bicarbonate or decreased hydrogen ion concentrations. Factors that increase base bicarbonate include excessive oral or parenteral use of bicarbonate-containing drugs or other alkaline salts, a rapid decrease in extracellular fluid volume (e.g., in diuretic therapy), and loss of hydrogen and chloride ions (e.g., in vomiting, prolonged gastric suctioning, hypokalemia, hyperaldosteronism). The result is retention of sodium bicarbonate and increased base bicarbonate.

Assessment Findings

Clients in metabolic alkalosis can manifest anorexia, nausea, vomiting, circumoral paresthesias, confusion, carpopedal spasm, hypertonic reflexes, and tetany. The respiratory rate and volume decrease in a compensatory effort to produce more carbonic acid to increase and restore the acidic level in the blood. Initially, ABGs show increased pH and HCO_3 and normal $PaCO_2$ levels (see Table 22-3). As compensatory respiratory mechanisms result in slower and more shallow breathing, the $PaCO_2$ level is elevated; eventually, pH may return to normal.

Medical Management

Treatment involves eliminating the cause. It may include prescribing potassium (as a potassium salt) if hypokalemia is present or sodium chloride solutions to correct volume depletion when extracellular fluid volume has decreased rapidly.

● RESPIRATORY ACIDOSIS

Respiratory acidosis, which may be either acute or chronic, is caused by excess carbonic acid, which causes the pH to drop below 7.35. Conditions that predispose to respiratory acidosis include pneumothorax, hemothorax, pulmonary edema, acute bronchial asthma, atelectasis, hyaline membrane disease or other forms of respiratory distress in the newborn, pneumonia (see Chap. 29), some drug overdoses, and head injuries. Chronic respiratory acidosis is associated with disorders such as emphysema, bronchiectasis, bronchial asthma, and cystic fibrosis.

Assessment Findings

Acute respiratory acidosis is associated with extreme respiratory insufficiency. The client may make frantic efforts to breathe, breathe slowly or irregularly, or stop breathing. Expiratory volumes are decreased. Lung sounds may be moist or absent in some lobes. Tachycardia usually is present, and cardiac dysrhythmias can develop. *Cyanosis,* a dusky appearance to the skin, may be evident. The accumulation of CO_2 leads to behavioral changes (mental cloudiness, confusion, disorientation, hallucinations), tremors, muscle twitching, flushed skin, headache, weakness, stupor, and coma. Responses to chronic respiratory acidosis are less prominent and can include an increased breathing effort, lack of energy, reduced activity, dull headache, and weakness.

The ABG values show a decreased pH and an increased $PaCO_2$ above 45 mm Hg. As the kidney attempts to compensate, which may take 2 to 3 days, the HCO_3 rises, followed by a return to normal pH if full compensation occurs (see Table 22-3).

Medical Management

Treatment is individualized, depending on the cause of the imbalance and whether the condition is acute or chronic. Mechanical ventilation may be necessary to support respiratory function. IV sodium bicarbonate is administered when ventilation efforts do not adequately restore a balanced pH. Heart rate and rhythm are monitored to detect sudden cardiac changes. In less acute situations, treatment may include the administration of pharmacologic agents, such as bronchodilators and antibiotics, to improve breathing. Airway suctioning may be necessary if the client is too weak to cough secretions.

● RESPIRATORY ALKALOSIS

Respiratory alkalosis results from a carbonic acid deficit that occurs when rapid breathing releases more CO_2 than necessary with expired air. *Tachypnea* (rapid breathing) may result from acute anxiety, high fever, thyrotoxicosis (overactive thyroid), early salicylate (aspirin) poisoning, *hypoxemia* (low oxygen in the blood), or mechanical ventilation.

Assessment Findings

The most obvious manifestation is an increased respiratory rate. Accompanying symptoms include lightheadedness, numbness and tingling of the fingers and toes, circumoral paresthesias, sweating, panic, dry mouth, and, in severe cases, convulsions. The ABG values indicate a pH above 7.45 and a $PaCO_2$ below 35 mm Hg. If the kidney compensates by excreting bicarbonate ions, the HCO_3 falls below 22 mEq to restore pH (see Table 22-3).

Medical Management

Treatment aims to correct the cause of the rapid breathing. Having the client breathe into a paper bag held over the nose and mouth and rebreathe expired air may be useful temporarily. Sedation may be necessary when extreme anxiety is the cause of tachypnea.

● NURSING MANAGEMENT FOR ACID-BASE IMBALANCES

The nurse carefully documents all presenting signs and symptoms to provide accurate baseline data. He or she monitors laboratory findings; compares ABG findings with previous results (if any); and reports current results to the physician as soon as they are obtained. The same applies to abnormal electrolyte levels. The nurse maintains accurate intake and output records to monitor fluid status. He or she implements prescribed medical therapy, such as administering fluid and electrolyte replacements, suctioning the airway, maintaining mechanical ventilation, and monitoring cardiac rate and rhythm (see Chaps. 29 and 30). The nurse administers cardiopulmonary resuscitation whenever necessary.

GENERAL NUTRITIONAL CONSIDERATIONS

Because salt and sodium compounds are used extensively in food processing and manufacturing, processed and convenience foods are estimated to account for 75% of the sodium in the average American diet. Naturally occurring sources of sodium (milk, meats, certain vegetables) provide 10%. The remaining 15% comes from salt added during cooking and at the table.

The daily value for sodium on the Nutrition Facts food label is 2400 mg/day, far more than the estimated minimum requirement for healthy adults, yet considerably less than most Americans consume. Under normal circumstances, the body maintains sodium balance over a wide range of intakes by regulating urinary sodium excretion.

Magnesium is found in cocoa, chocolate, nuts, soybeans, seafood, dried peas and beans, green leafy vegetables, and whole grains, especially wheat germ and bran. Physical stress or high intake of calcium, protein, vitamin D, or alcohol may increase the need for magnesium.

GENERAL PHARMACOLOGIC CONSIDERATIONS

The dosage of electrolytes is carefully measured and given only as directed by the physician because these agents are potentially dangerous.

Sodium and calcium products are given cautiously to clients with edema, congestive heart failure, or renal dysfunction.

Calcium replacement is given cautiously to clients with kidney stones because high calcium levels in the kidney tubules may contribute to additional stone formation.

Sodium chloride and potassium chloride may be given to help correct metabolic alkalosis.

Clients may experience burning along the vein with IV infusion of potassium. The discomfort is in proportion to the infusion's concentration. If the client can tolerate the fluid, it may be helpful to consult with the physician about possibly diluting the potassium in a larger volume of IV solution.

Clients receiving a digitalis preparation are closely monitored for digitalis toxicity, which can accompany potassium and magnesium deficits.

GENERAL GERONTOLOGIC CONSIDERATIONS

Aging causes skin to lose elasticity. Therefore, assessing skin turgor may be ineffective to detect fluid volume deficit in older adults. If assessing skin turgor in older clients, use the skin of the forehead.

The most common electrolyte imbalance in older adults is dehydration. Older adults tend to drink less water and may incur chronic fluid volume deficit, resulting in electrolyte imbalances.

Hypernatremia is common in older adults; it may be manifested as confusion. In addition, older adults are prone to laxative abuse, which can lead to hypernatremia.

Older adults are at increased risk for hyponatremia related to the kidneys' inability to excrete water and their sluggish renin-angiotensin-aldosterone response.

Use of diuretic medications may deplete fluid volume in older adults, who may be unaware of the problem because a reduced thirst sensation often accompanies aging.

Decreased renal function in older adults can cause an inability to concentrate urine and is associated with fluid and electrolyte imbalance.

A poor appetite, erratic meal patterns, inability to prepare nutritious meals, or financial circumstances may influence nutritional status, resulting in electrolyte imbalances.

Poor respiratory exchange as the result of chronic lung disease, inactivity, or thoracic skeletal changes may lead to chronic respiratory acidosis.

Overuse of sodium bicarbonate (baking soda), an inexpensive substitute for commercial antacids, may lead to metabolic alkalosis.

Critical Thinking Exercises

1. *Describe the relationship of water to imbalances in electrolytes, acids, and bases.*
2. *When assessing a client, discuss data that suggest hypovolemia (fluid volume deficit).*

References and Suggested Readings

Abrams, C. (2000). ADH-associated pathologies: Diabetes insipidus and syndrome of inappropriate ADH. *Medical Laboratory Observer, 32*(2), 24–26, 28, 30, 32–33, 36, 38.

Beck, L. H. (2000). The aging kidney: Defending a delicate balance of fluid and electrolytes. *Geriatrics, 55*(4), 26–28, 31–32.

Bullock, B. L. & Henze, R. L. (2000). *Focus on pathophysiology.* Philadelphia: Lippincott Williams & Wilkins.

Edwards, S. (2001). Regulation of water, sodium and potassium: Implications for practice. *Nursing Standard, 15*(22), 36–42.

Iggulden, H. (1999). Dehydration and electrolyte disturbance. *Elderly Care, 11*(3), 17–23.

Kayser-Jones, J., Schell, E., Porter, E., et al. (1999). Factors contributing to dehydration in nursing homes: Adequate staffing and lack of professional supervision. *Journal of the American Geriatrics Society, 47,* 1187–1194.

Martin, L. (1999). *All you really need to know to interpret arterial blood gases* (2nd ed.). Philadelphia: Lippincott Williams & Wilkins.

Mentes, J. C. (2000). Hydration management protocol. *Journal of Gerontological Nursing, 26*(10), 6–15.

Morrison, C. (2000). Helping patients to maintain a healthy fluid balance. *Nursing Times, 96*(31), NTplus:3–4.

Paradiso, C. (1999). *Fluids and electrolytes.* Philadelphia: Lippincott Williams & Wilkins.

Porth, C. M. (2002). *Pathophysiology: Concepts of altered health states* (6th ed.). Philadelphia: Lippincott Williams & Wilkins.

Rice, V. (2000). Analyzing the anion gap . . . a peek at the past—a look at the future. *CINA: Official Journal of the Canadian Intravenous Nurses Association, 16,* 27–29.

Spangler, A. A. & Chidester, J. C. (1998). Age, dependency, and other factors influencing fluid intake by long term care residents. *Journal of Nutrition for the Elderly, 18*(2), 21–35.

Veijo, A. & Nicolaus, M. J. (1999). Diabetes insipidus: A current perspective. *Critical Care Nurse, 19*(6), 18–31.

c h a p t e r **23**

Caring for Clients in Shock

Words to Know

adrenocorticotropic
  hormone
anaerobic metabolism
anaphylactic shock
antidiuretic hormone
cardiac output
cardiogenic shock
catecholamines
colloid solutions
compensation stage
corticosteroid hormones
crystalloid solutions
decompensation stage
distributive shock
endotoxins

hypovolemic shock
hypoxia
irreversible stage
ischemia
neurogenic shock
obstructive shock
oliguria
positive inotropic
  agents
renin-angiotensin-
  aldosterone system
septic shock
shock
vasopressors

Learning Objectives

On completion of this chapter, the reader will:

- Define shock.
- Name four general categories of shock.
- Identify the subcategories of distributive shock.
- List at least five pathophysiologic consequences of shock.
- Name the three stages of shock.
- Identify three physiologic mechanisms that attempt to compensate for shock.
- Discuss at least eight signs and symptoms manifested by clients in shock.
- Name three diagnostic measurements used when monitoring clients in shock.
- Give three medical approaches for treating shock.
- List at least six complications of shock.
- Discuss the nursing management of clients with shock.

This chapter discusses shock and its various types, pathophysiologic consequences, and assessment findings, which may vary according to type. It also presents the medical and nursing management of clients in shock.

SHOCK

Shock is a life-threatening condition that occurs when arterial blood flow and oxygen delivery to tissues and cells are inadequate. It develops as a consequence of one of three events: (1) blood volume decreases, (2) the heart fails as an effective pump, or (3) peripheral blood vessels massively dilate (Collins, 2000). In some cases, the body implements compensatory mechanisms to counteract the effects of shock. In other cases, shock progresses until therapeutic measures are implemented. If physiologic and therapeutic measures are inadequate, organs are damaged and death may follow.

Types

The four main categories of shock are hypovolemic, distributive, obstructive, and cardiogenic, depending on the cause (Smeltzer & Bare, 2000) (Table 23-1). More than one type of shock can develop simultaneously. Hypovolemic shock is most common, but cardiogenic shock is most lethal (Mower-Wade et al., 2001).

Hypovolemic Shock

In **hypovolemic shock,** the volume of extracellular fluid is significantly diminished, primarily because of lost or reduced blood or plasma (water component; see Chap. 22). Because the intravascular, interstitial, and intracellular fluid volumes are interdependent, a loss from one location results in a similar depletion in the others. Thus, a deficit of intravascular volume (plasma) reduces the net circulating volume. Hypovolemic shock can develop when overall fluid volume is depleted from significant bleeding, such as during surgery, after trauma, or after delivery of

TABLE 23-1	TYPES OF SHOCK	
TYPE	**CAUSE**	**EXAMPLES**
Hypovolemic shock	Decreased blood volume	Hemorrhage (frank and internal) Extreme diuresis Severe diarrhea or vomiting Dehydration Third-spacing
Distributive shock	Redistribution of intravascular fluid from arterial circulation to venous or capillary areas	
Neurogenic		Spinal cord injury
Septic		Toxic reaction to gram-negative bacterial infection
Anaphylactic		Severe allergic reaction
Obstructive shock	Impaired filling of heart with blood	Cardiac tamponade (see Chap. 31) Dissecting aneurysm Tension pneumothorax (see Chap. 29)
Cardiogenic shock	Decreased force of ventricular contraction	Myocardial infarction Cardiac dysrhythmia (see Chaps. 33 and 34)

an infant. It also may result from significant fluid loss, as with burns, large draining wounds, reduced fluid intake, suctioning, or disorders in which fluid losses exceed fluid intake, such as diabetes insipidus (see Chap. 57).

Distributive Shock

Distributive shock sometimes is called *normovolemic shock* because the amount of fluid in the circulatory system is not reduced, yet the fluid circulation does not permit effective tissue perfusion. Vasodilatation, a prominent characteristic of distributive shock, increases the space in the vascular bed. Central blood flow is reduced because peripheral vascular or interstitial areas exceed their usual capacity. Three types of distributive shock are neurogenic, septic, and anaphylactic shock.

NEUROGENIC SHOCK
Neurogenic shock results from an insult to the vasomotor center in the medulla of the brain or to the peripheral nerves that extend from the spinal cord to the blood vessels. Injury to the spinal cord or head or overdoses of opioids, opiates, tranquilizers, or general anesthetics can cause neurogenic shock. The tone of the sympathetic nervous system is impaired, resulting in decreased arterial vascular resistance, vasodilatation, and hypotension. Because blood remains distributed in the periphery, the heart does not fill adequately, cardiac output is reduced, tissue perfusion is compromised, cells are deprived of oxygen and switch to anaerobic metabolism, and metabolic acidosis develops.

SEPTIC SHOCK
Septic shock, also called *toxic shock,* is associated with overwhelming bacterial infections (see Chap. 19). It occurs most commonly in those with gram-negative bacteremia (bacteria in the blood) caused by such pathogens as *Escherichia coli,* species of *Pseudomonas,* and gram-positive

drug-resistant *Staphylococcus aureus* and *Streptococcus.* **Endotoxins,** harmful chemicals released by bacterial cells, are probably the major cause of septic shock. They trigger an immune response in which vasoactive chemicals, such as cytokines (see Chap. 41), dilate the blood vessels and increase capillary permeability, causing vascular fluid to shift to the interstitium. Unlike other forms of shock, clients with septic shock have an elevated leukocyte count and initially manifest a fever accompanied by warm, flushed skin and a rapid, bounding pulse. As septic shock progresses, however, affected clients eventually develop cold, pale or mottled skin and hypotensive symptoms, findings common with other forms of shock.

ANAPHYLACTIC SHOCK
Anaphylactic shock (see Chap. 42) is a severe allergic reaction that follows exposure to a substance to which a person is extremely sensitive. Common allergic substances include bee venom, latex, fish, nuts, and penicillin. The body's immune response to the allergic substance causes mast cells in the connective tissues, bronchi, and gastrointestinal tract to release histamine and other chemicals. The results are vasodilatation, increased capillary permeability accompanied by swelling of the airway and subcutaneous tissues, hypotension, and hives or an itchy rash (Fig. 23-1).

Obstructive Shock

Obstructive shock occurs when the heart or great vessels are compressed. The compression reduces the space available for blood in the heart, compromising the volume of blood that enters and leaves the heart en route to the lungs and tissues. Any condition that fills the thoracic cavity with fluid, air, or tissue can lead to obstructive shock. Examples include increased fluid or blood in the pericardial sac (cardiac tamponade, see Chap. 31); air that accumulates between the layers of pleura (tension pneumothorax,

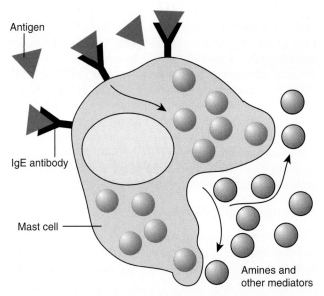

FIGURE 23-1 Vasodilation, increased capillary permeability, smooth muscle contraction, and eosinophilia characterize an anaphylactic reaction. Systemic reactions may involve laryngeal stridor, angioedema, hypotension, and bronchial, gastrointestinal, or uterine spasm. Local reactions are characterized by hives.

see Chap. 29); or abdominal tissue, fluid, or air that crowds the diaphragm, as in an enlarged liver and ascites (see Chap. 55), thus reducing the size of the thorax.

Cardiogenic Shock

In **cardiogenic shock,** heart contraction is ineffective, which reduces **cardiac output,** the volume of blood ejected from the left ventricle per minute. A myocardial infarction (MI) with subsequent heart failure (see Chaps. 34 and 37) is a leading cause of cardiogenic shock.

Stop, Think, and Respond ● BOX 23-1

Indicate the type of shock each client is most likely experiencing:

- *Client A has had an MI and cardiac arrest; paramedics resuscitated him. He is now having difficulty breathing, a rapid heart rate, and chest pain. Urine output is 50 mL in the last 4 hours.*
- *Client B was involved in a motor vehicle collision. Paramedics note a substantial bruise on his right upper thigh, which is much larger than his left upper thigh. Based on assessment findings and a distorted alignment of the right leg, they suspect a fractured pelvis or femur. They also suspect a ruptured spleen because the client has abdominal tenderness. He is hypotensive with pale and cool skin.*
- *Client C was pruning roses when a bee stung her. Within minutes she had difficulty breathing and lost consciousness. Her neighbor called 911. Paramedics note that the client is hypotensive, tachycardic, and barely able to breathe.*

Pathophysiology

Regardless of the type, many complex events accompany shock, which usually progresses through three stages: (1) compensation, (2) decompensation, and (3) irreversible (Fig. 23-2).

Compensation Stage

The **compensation stage** is the first stage of shock, during which several physiologic mechanisms attempt to stabilize the spiraling consequences. If these mechanisms are successful, homeostatic stability potentially can be achieved. If natural or medical means can reverse shock, the chances of uncomplicated recovery are greatly improved. As shock progresses, positive outcomes are less predictable. Compensatory mechanisms include the release of catecholamines; activation of the renin-angiotensin-aldosterone system; and production of anti-

FIGURE 23-2 Stages of shock. *B/P,* blood pressure; *CO,* cardiac output; *HR,* heart rate; *SVR,* systemic vascular resistance; *TPR,* total peripheral resistance.

diuretic and **corticosteroid hormones,** chemicals that promote fluid retention and reabsorption.

CATECHOLAMINES

Catecholamines are neurotransmitters that stimulate responses by the sympathetic nervous system (Table 23-2). To compensate in shock, the sympathetic nervous system releases endogenous catecholamines, epinephrine and norepinephrine into the circulation. The adrenal medulla secretes epinephrine whereas the endings of sympathetic nerve fibers secrete norepinephrine. Epinephrine and norepinephrine increase heart rate and the contractile ability of the myocardium. Venous return to the right atrium subsequently increases, as does blood sent to the lungs. Bronchial dilatation increases the amount of oxygenated air entering the lungs, followed by a more efficient exchange of oxygen and carbon dioxide (CO_2).

RENIN-ANGIOTENSIN-ALDOSTERONE SYSTEM

The **renin-angiotensin-aldosterone system** is a mechanism that restores blood pressure (BP) when circulating volume is diminished. In response to low renal (kidney) blood perfusion, the juxtaglomerular cells release renin, an enzymatic hormone in the nephrons of the kidneys. Release of renin causes a series of chemical reactions that eventually produce angiotensin II, a potent vasoconstrictor that raises BP. Angiotensin II also stimulates the hypothalamus to signal the adrenal cortex to release aldosterone, a mineralocorticoid that promotes reabsorption of sodium and water by the kidney, which serves to increase blood volume.

TABLE 23-2	EFFECTS OF ENDOGENOUS CATECHOLAMINES
EFFECT	**CONSEQUENCES**
Constriction of arterioles of skin, mucous membranes, subcutaneous tissues	Sends blood to larger blood vessels supplying vital organs
Dilatation of arterioles of skeletal muscles	Increases blood supply to skeletal muscles
Dilatation of coronary arteries	Increases oxygen to myocardium
Increased contractile ability of myocardium	Increases amount of blood leaving the left ventricle each time ventricle contracts (cardiac output)
Increased heart rate	Increases blood supply to body, especially vital organs
Bronchial dilatation	Increases amount of air entering the lungs on inspiration
Release of glycogen stored in the liver	Provides energy

ANTIDIURETIC HORMONE AND CORTICOSTEROID HORMONES

Low blood volume also stimulates the pituitary to secrete **antidiuretic hormone** (ADH), also known as *vasopressin,* and **adrenocorticotropic hormone** (ACTH). ADH promotes reabsorption of water that the kidneys would ordinarily excrete. ACTH stimulates the adrenal glands to secrete glucocorticoids and mineralocorticoids. *Glucocorticoids* help the body respond to stress. *Mineralocorticoids,* such as aldosterone, conserve sodium and promote potassium excretion. Thus, they play an active role in controlling sodium and water balance.

Decompensation Stage

The **decompensation stage** occurs as compensatory mechanisms fail. The client's condition spirals into cellular hypoxia, coagulation defects, and cardiovascular changes.

CELLULAR HYPOXIA

Hypoxia refers to decreased oxygen reaching the cells. Hypoxic cells are forced to switch from aerobic metabolism to **anaerobic metabolism,** a less efficient mechanism for meeting energy requirements. As the energy supply falls below the demand, pyruvic and lactic acids increase, causing metabolic acidosis. The structural integrity of cells is impaired because without sufficient adenosine triphosphate (ATP), the energy source for operating the sodium and potassium pumps, sodium and water enter the cell and potassium exits into the extracellular fluid (Fig. 23-3). Eventually, the cells swell and rupture, disrupting their ability to carry out electrochemical processes. Lysosomes, the cellular structure for breaking down cellular waste, leak enzymatic fluid and contribute to further cellular destruction. Gradually, significant numbers of cells are damaged.

COAGULATION DEFECTS

As cells become damaged, an inflammatory response ensues. Platelets become sticky and accumulate in the blood vessels of the volume-depleted client, predisposing him or her to the formation of microemboli. Clots further compromise the ability of the red blood cells (RBCs) to deliver oxygen throughout the body. Cell and organ death is potentiated.

CARDIOVASCULAR CHANGES

Impaired myocardial cells cannot maintain sufficient heart rate and force of contraction to circulate blood efficiently. Subsequently, brain cells in the medulla can no longer sustain the stimulus for vasoconstriction. The blood vessels dilate, blood pools in the periphery or leaks into the interstitium, cardiac output decreases, and BP falls. Clinical signs are more obvious and include bradycardia, hypotension, confusion, lethargy, decreased urine production, cold, pale skin, and reduced peristalsis. Aggressive interventions are necessary to prevent the irreversible stage of shock and ensure the client's survival.

Normal

Effects of shock

FIGURE 23-3 Cellular effects of shock. The cell swells, the cell membrane becomes more permeable, and fluids and electrolytes seep from and into the cell. Mitochondria and lysosomes are damaged, and the cell dies. (From Smeltzer, S. C. & Bare, B. G. [2000]. *Brunner & Suddarth's textbook of medical–surgical nursing* [9th ed., p. 246.]. Philadelphia: Lippincott Williams & Wilkins.)

Irreversible Stage

The **irreversible stage** occurs when significant cells and organs become damaged. The client's condition reaches a "point of no return" despite treatment efforts. The client no longer responds to medical interventions. Multiple systems begin to fail. When the kidneys, heart, lungs, liver, and brain cease to function, death is imminent.

Assessment Findings

Signs and Symptoms

The nurse monitors for evidence that blood volume or circulation is becoming compromised. Although shock can develop quickly, early signs and symptoms are evident during the decompensation stage. Critical assessments include vital signs, characteristics of peripheral pulses, and changes in mentation, skin, and urine output (Table 23-3).

ARTERIAL BLOOD PRESSURE
In shock, both systolic and diastolic arterial BPs fall because cardiac output decreases or the vascular bed size increases. Hypotension may be rapid and sudden or slow and insidious. For the normotensive (normal BP) adult, average systolic BP is 120 mm Hg. Therefore, a systolic BP of 90 to 100 mm Hg indicates impending shock, whereas 80 mm Hg or below indicates shock. If it is difficult to aus-

cultate BP but a peripheral pulse can be palpated, the BP is at least 80 mm Hg (Collins, 2000).

To determine the presence of shock, the client's previous BP must be known. Regardless of the numeric figure, a progressive fall in BP is serious. For example, a BP of 120/82 mm Hg usually is considered normal; however, if an individual with an original BP of 190/112 mm Hg has a BP of 120/82 mm Hg, shock may be developing. The nurse must make the physician aware of any fall in systolic BP below 100 mm Hg, any fall of 20 mm Hg or more below the client's usual systolic BP, or any trend in progressively decreasing BP. Direct BP monitoring (intra-arterial) is more accurate than indirect monitoring—the usual, auscultatory method using a BP cuff (see Chap. 30)—but it is implemented primarily in critical care areas.

PULSE PRESSURE
Pulse pressure is the numeric difference between systolic and diastolic BP. If a client has a BP of 120/80 mm Hg, the pulse pressure is 40 mm Hg. A pulse pressure between 30 and 50 mm Hg is considered normal, with 40 mm Hg being a healthy average. In shock, the pulse pressure tends to narrow (decrease) as the falling systolic pressure nears the diastolic pressure.

PULSE RATE, VOLUME, AND RHYTHM
In hypovolemic shock, healthcare personnel use the pulse rate and other assessment data to identify the severity of shock and estimate the approximate reduction in blood

TABLE 23-3	SHOCK CLASSIFICATION AND ESTIMATED BLOOD LOSS			
ASSESSMENT DATA	CLASS I	CLASS II	CLASS III	CLASS IV
Pulse rate	<100	>100	>120	>140
Pulse pressure	Normal or increased	Decreased	Decreased	Decreased
Blood pressure	Normal	Normal	Decreased	Decreased
Respirations	14–20	20–30	30–40	>35
Urine output/hr	≥30 mL	20–30 mL	5–15 mL	Negligible
Mental status	Slightly anxious	Mildly anxious	Anxious and confused	Confused and lethargic
Blood loss	≤750 mL	750–1000 mL	1500–2000 mL	≥2000 mL
Percentage of total blood volume lost*	≤15%	15%–30%	30%–40%	≥40%

*Estimates are based on an adult male weighing 70 kg.
(Adapted from American College of Surgeons. [1993] *Advanced trauma life support for physicians.* Chicago: Author.)

volume. As cardiac output decreases, compensatory tachycardia initially develops to increase cardiac output. Pulse volume becomes weak and thready as circulating volume diminishes. In the later stages, the pulse may be slow and imperceptible. Pulse rhythm may change from regular to irregular. Hypoxia, especially when it affects heart tissue, is a leading cause of dangerous cardiac dysrhythmias such as ventricular fibrillation (see Chap. 34).

RESPIRATIONS

In shock, tissues receive less oxygen. In response, the body tries to obtain more oxygen by breathing faster. Rapid respirations help move blood in the large veins toward the heart. Respirations are shallow, and the client may be heard grunting. In early stages, the client is hungry for air, but in profound shock as death nears, the respiratory rate decreases.

TEMPERATURE

Heat-regulating mechanisms are depressed in shock, and added diaphoresis increases heat loss. With the possible exception of septic shock, subnormal body temperature is characteristic.

MENTATION

Altered cerebral function often is the first sign of inadequate oxygen delivery to the tissues. Mild anxiety, increasing restlessness, agitation, or confusion accompany shock. As the condition deteriorates, the client becomes listless and stuporous, ultimately losing consciousness.

SKIN

In all but the early stages of septic and neurogenic shock, the skin is cold and clammy. As peripheral blood vessels constrict to direct blood from the skin to more vital organs (heart, kidneys, brain), the skin becomes paler. Eventually the skin may appear mottled (i.e., a mix of pale and cyanotic areas lacking any uniform consistency). Capillary filling longer than 3 seconds and cyanosis, especially of the nailbeds, lips, and earlobes, indicate oxygen deficiency. In clients with highly pigmented skin (such as African-American clients), cyanosis is more accurately detected by inspecting the conjunctiva and oral mucous membranes. Lack of cyanosis, however, does not prove the absence of hypoxia because cyanosis is one of the last signs to appear.

URINE OUTPUT

Reduced cardiac output decreases renal blood flow, which leads to decreased urine output. Vasoconstriction, the physiologic response to shock, also contributes to markedly reduced renal blood flow. In many instances, the rate of urine formation is an important indicator of the status of a client in shock (see Table 23-2). When shock is quickly reversed, urine output usually returns to normal. Continued **oliguria** (decreased urine formation) indicates renal damage, caused by reduced blood flow to the kidney.

Stop, Think, and Respond ● BOX 23-2

Which stage of shock is characterized by the following physiologic changes?

1. *Client is unconscious, with a slow pulse, systolic BP of 85 mm Hg, and mottled skin color.*
2. *Client is alert and oriented, with tachycardia but normal BP and skin color.*
3. *Client is somewhat disoriented, with BP lower than earlier assessment and pale skin.*

Diagnostic Findings

Arterial blood gas (ABG), central venous pressure, and pulmonary artery pressure measurements can support a diagnosis of shock. They also are used to monitor response to treatment.

ARTERIAL BLOOD GAS (ABG) MEASUREMENTS

ABG specimens are drawn from a direct arterial puncture or an indwelling arterial catheter (see Chap. 30). In shock, the partial pressure of oxygen in arterial blood (PaO_2, normally 80 to 100 mm Hg) falls below 60 mm Hg. The partial pressure of CO_2 in arterial blood ($PaCO_2$) may be normal or decreased. A pulse oximeter, sometimes used to monitor oxygenation continuously, measures the amount of oxygen bound to hemoglobin, or the saturated oxygen (SpO_2) level, which normally is 95% to 100%. If the SpO_2 level is above 90%, it can be assumed that the PaO_2 is 60 mm Hg or above.

CENTRAL VENOUS PRESSURE

Central venous pressure (CVP) is the pressure of the blood in the right atrium or venae cavae. It distinguishes relationships among hemodynamic variables in shock: venous return, quality of right ventricular function, and vascular tone. CVP measurements, especially trends in readings, are useful in the management of a client in shock (see Chap. 30). Normal CVP is 4 to 10 cm H_2O. In hypovolemic shock, the CVP is lower than normal; in cardiogenic shock, it usually is above normal. The trend in CVP measurements is more helpful than isolated readings.

PULMONARY ARTERY PRESSURE

Although CVP measurements can indicate the status of right ventricular function, they do not provide information about left ventricular function. Because left ventricular function is more pertinent to circulation than right, knowing fluid pressures on the left side of the heart is more meaningful. To assess left ventricular function, a two-, three-, or four-lumen catheter is inserted into the vena cava and advanced through the right atrium and right ventricle into the pulmonary artery (Fig. 23-4). The catheter is connected to a monitor from which the *pulmonary artery pressure* (PAP) or *pulmonary capillary wedge pressure* (PCWP) is measured (see Chap. 30). Normal PAP ranges from 20 to 30 mm Hg systolic and from 8 to 12 mm Hg diastolic. Normal PCWP ranges from 4 to 12 mm Hg. In shock, PAP measurements usually are low because they reflect the low volume of blood in the arterial system.

Medical Management

Aggressive treatment of conditions that predispose to shock may prevent it. Once shock develops, treatment depends on its type and level and usually includes one or more of the following: intravenous (IV) fluid therapy, vasopressor drug therapy, and mechanical devices that restore blood circulation to cells.

Intravenous Fluid Therapy

IV fluids are prescribed to restore intravascular volume. The total volume, type of solution(s), and rate of administration vary according to the etiology of shock. Usually, a ratio of 3:1 is followed; that is, 3 L of fluid is administered

FIGURE 23-4 Example of a pulmonary artery (PA) pressure monitoring system. The PA catheter is inserted into the internal jugular vein and advanced into the pulmonary artery. (From Dailey, E. [1994]. *Techniques in bedside hemodynamic monitoring* [6th ed.]. St. Louis: Mosby.)

for every 1 L of fluid lost. This amount stabilizes the client, replaces the deficit, and provides a reserve to prevent shock from recurring. Initially, as much as 250 to 500 mL may be infused in 1 hour. Solutions may include **crystalloid solutions,** those containing dissolved substances such as sodium, other electrolytes, or glucose in water; **colloid solutions,** those containing proteins (such as albumin) to increase osmotic pressure; and blood and blood products if blood loss has been major (see Chap. 24).

To ensure oxygenation of tissues, especially in cases of hemorrhage or if the hemoglobin level is 70 g/L or less, administering whole blood or packed RBCs is best. One unit of RBCs can increase an adult's hemoglobin by 10 g/L (Gilcreast et al., 2001). Clients who are alert and capable of making informed decisions but refuse blood transfusions on the basis of religious beliefs (e.g., Jehovah's Witnesses) require bloodless alternatives and measures that conserve blood and its oxygen-carrying capacity. Such measures include the following:

- Drawing the minimum volume of blood for laboratory analysis
- Restricting movement and activity to only that which is essential
- Reinfusing the client's own blood that has been collected in a closed-circuit cell saver

- Using lasers and electrocautery devices to minimize bleeding during surgery
- Administering pharmacologic agents like erythropoietin to stimulate the bone marrow to manufacture RBCs
- Administering cryoprecipitate, factor VIII, and thrombin to promote *hemostasis,* control of bleeding using substances in the body's natural coagulation process

Drug Therapy

Medical management of shock is extremely complex; drugs are carefully titrated and used alone or in combination to improve cardiovascular status (Drug Therapy Table 23-1). Adrenergic drugs are the main medications used to treat shock. **Vasopressors,** drugs with alpha-adrenergic activity, increase peripheral vascular resistance and raise BP. Examples include dopamine (Intropin), norepinephrine (Levophed), and metaraminol (Aramine). They are best administered after fluid therapy increases the intravascular fluid volume; otherwise, the vasoconstrictive qualities further impair cellular circulation, which already is compromised by the effects of angiotensin.

Drugs with beta-adrenergic activity that increase heart rate and improve the force of heart contraction are **posi-**

DRUG THERAPY TABLE 23-1	AGENTS TO TREAT SHOCK		
DRUG CATEGORY AND EXAMPLES	**MECHANISM OF ACTION**	**SIDE EFFECTS**	**NURSING CONSIDERATIONS**
Vasopressor Agents (Alpha-Adrenergic Activity) *norepinephrine (Levophed), metaraminol (Aramine), phenylephrine (Neo-Synephrine)*	Increase peripheral vascular resistance and raise BP	Headaches, restlessness, palpitations, tremors, nausea, vomiting, anxiety, dizziness	Protect from light. Monitor BP closely during administration. Monitor intake and output. Avoid abrupt withdrawal of these medications.
Positive Inotropic Agents (Beta-Adrenergic Activity) *dobutamine (Dobutrex), isoproterenol (Isuprel), milrinone (Primacor), amrinone (Inocor)*	Strengthen cardiac contraction and increase cardiac output	Headache, tremors, nervousness, fatigue, palpitations, nausea, vomiting, anxiety, flushing	Inform client to report anginal pain. Observe for dysrhythmias. Monitor BP, pulse, respirations, intake, output, and weight.
digoxin (Lanoxin)		Visual disturbances, diaphoresis, confusion	Take apical pulse for 1 full minute before giving. Note rate and rhythm. Withhold if pulse is below 60 or above 110 beats/min. Do not administer with an antacid. Monitor serum levels for possible toxicity.
Combined Alpha- and Beta-Adrenergic Activity *epinephrine (Adrenalin), dopamine (Intropin)*	Strengthen myocardial contraction, increase cardiac rate and output	Nervousness, anxiety, tremors, headache, weakness, nausea, vomiting, palpitations	Protect from light. Do not use discolored solutions. Monitor BP, pulse, respirations, intake, and output. Check blood glucose levels, which may increase.

tive inotropic agents (*inotropic* means affecting the force of muscular contraction). Digoxin (Lanoxin), isoproterenol (Isuprel), dobutamine (Dobutrex), milrinone (Primacor), and amrinone (Inocor) are examples.

Many drugs have combined alpha- and beta-adrenergic effects. Epinephrine is an example and is the drug of choice in anaphylactic shock. Dopamine also has combined actions. Anaphylactic shock also may be treated with an antihistamine, ACTH, or adrenal corticosteroids to counter the allergen. Other drug categories, such as antidysrhythmics and drugs that reduce peripheral vascular resistance, like calcium channel blockers, angiotensin-converting enzyme inhibitors, and vasodilators like the nitrates, are appropriate for cardiogenic shock.

Mechanical Devices

Mechanical devices help improve cardiac output or redistribute blood. Those used in the treatment of cardiogenic shock include the intra-aortic balloon pump (IABP) and ventricular assist device (VAD; see Chap. 37). First responders (paramedics) use a pneumatic antishock garment (PASG), also called *military antishock trousers* (MAST), which redistributes blood from the lower extremities to the central circulation. The use of PASGs and MAST, however, is somewhat controversial because (1) incorrect application or removal is life-threatening, (2) poor outcomes have occurred when such garments have been used indiscriminately to manage types of shock other than hypovolemic, and (3) their application lengthens the time between the field treatment of the client and transport to a trauma center (O'Connor & Domeier, 1997). Currently, there are two justifications for their use: (1) to control hemorrhage and hypotension resulting from pelvic fractures, and (2) to compensate for severe hypovolemia after intra-abdominal trauma en route to the operating room (National Association of EMS Physicians, 2000). Consensus is that PASGs are contraindicated in uncontrolled hemorrhage outside the area covered by the garment, pulmonary edema, rupture of the diaphragm, dysfunction of the left ventricle, intrathoracic hemorrhage, and severe injuries of the central nervous system (Cumpston, 1999).

Although there are reservations concerning PASGs and MAST, a new type of antishock garment known as Dyna Med Anti-Shock Trousers (DMAST) has been developed. In contrast to PASGs, the DMAST is noninflatable, uses lower pressures to promote central circulation, and can be applied in less than 60 seconds (Fig. 23-5).

Prognosis and Complications

When shock is treated adequately and promptly, the client usually recovers. Recovery may be tenuous, however, because of secondary complications, which almost always result directly from tissue hypoxia and organ **ischemia,** reduced oxygenation. Life-threatening complications

FIGURE 23-5 Dyna Med Anti-Shock Trousers (DMAST).

include kidney failure, neurologic deficits, bleeding disorders such as disseminated intravascular coagulation, acute respiratory distress syndrome (see Chap. 29), stress ulcers, and sepsis that can lead to multiple organ dysfunction (see Chap. 19).

NURSING PROCESS

● The Client in Shock

Regardless of the cause, prolonged shock is incompatible with life. In few instances is the careful attention to nursing practices and principles more important than in the management of a client in impending or actual shock.

Assessment

The nurse assesses for early signs of shock and reports such findings to the physician immediately. He or she checks vital signs on initial contact and frequently thereafter to monitor closely the client's condition. An automatic BP device may be substituted for manual assessments. The nurse observes skin color and temperature and assesses the rate and quality of radial and peripheral pulses. He or she monitors urine output and determines respiratory rate and effort to detect evidence of dyspnea or airway obstruction resulting from edema, which accompanies anaphylactic shock. The nurse inspects for bleeding or other causes that may explain the developing symptoms of shock. He or she determines level of consciousness and orientation status regularly to detect changes. In cases of suspected cardiogenic shock, the nurse auscultates the chest for abnormal lung and heart sounds. He or she checks laboratory test results for evidence of low RBCs and hemoglobin, findings that correlate with hypovolemic shock. An elevated white blood cell count supports septic shock. Analysis of ABG findings is essential for evidence of hypoxemia and metabolic acidosis. The nurse applies a pulse oximeter to monitor SpO2. He or she monitors the results of coagulation tests such as platelet counts, the international normalized ratio, prothrombin time, and partial thromboplastin time.

Diagnosis, Planning, and Interventions

The nurse implements measures to control bleeding, other fluid losses, or fluid maldistribution, and to promote blood circulation to the brain and vital organs. Support of breathing is necessary to ensure adequate blood oxygenation. The nurse uses measures to maintain normal body temperature and implements medical therapy as directed. Other care includes, but is not limited to, the following:

Decreased Cardiac Output related to (specify) blood loss, impaired fluid distribution, impaired circulation, inadequate heart contraction, massive vasodilatation
Expected Outcome: Cardiac output will be of adequate volume, as evidenced by heart rate between 60 and 120 beats/minute, systolic BP between 90 and 139 mm Hg, urine output greater than 35 to 50 mL/hour, alert mental status, and warm, dry skin.

- Restrict activity to total rest. *Rest decreases cellular oxygen requirements, which already are compromised in shock. Inactivity reduces heart rate, allowing the heart to fill with more blood between contractions. The force of heart contraction, which promotes cardiac output, is related to myocardial stretch as the heart fills with blood.*

- Establish at least one and preferably two IV sites with large-gauge catheters. *Access to the intravascular fluid compartment ensures the speedy replacement of circulating fluid. Cardiac output depends on circulating volume and adequate contraction of heart muscle. Emergency medications usually are administered by the IV route. If the client is volume depleted, IV fluid therapy with or without whole blood or packed cells may be necessary.*

- Administer IV fluids or blood products at the prescribed rate, ensuring patency of the IV catheter(s). *IV fluids replace fluid lost or trapped in the interstitial space. Administration of whole blood or packed cells increases tissue and cellular oxygenation. IV fluids are delivered through a high-volume infusion device at 400 to 700 mL/minute in severe hemorrhage; type O negative blood is transfused until type-specific blood is available (Laskowski-Jones, 1997).*

- Administer prescribed vasopressor or inotropic drugs. *They can raise BP, increase the force of heart contraction, and promote blood circulation to the kidneys to ensure waste excretion.*

- Measure fluid intake and compare with voided urine output; obtain a medical order for insertion of an indwelling catheter if hourly urine output measurements are necessary. *Urine output above 35 to 50 mL/hour or 500 mL/day indicates that kidney perfusion is sufficient to ensure the excretion of toxic wastes. Urinary volume aids in the evaluation of the effectiveness of therapeutic interventions.*

Impaired Tissue Perfusion related to reduced cardiac output secondary to blood loss, heart failure, altered body fluid distribution, vasodilatation, and bradycardia secondary to neurologic trauma or adverse effects from central nervous system depressants
Expected Outcomes: (1) Systolic BP will be at least 90 mm Hg, with hourly urine output 50 mL or greater. (2) Peripheral pulses will be strong. (3) Capillary refill time will be between 2 and 3 seconds. (4) Skin will be warm. (5) Client will be alert and oriented.

- Control frank bleeding by applying direct pressure to the site. *Pressure compresses the area and slows blood loss from the vascular system.*

- Maintain client in a supine position with legs elevated 12 inches (higher than the heart) unless there is head injury, heart failure, increased intracranial pressure, possible spinal cord injury, or dyspnea. *Elevating the legs promotes blood perfusion to heart, lungs, and brain.*

- In cases of shock accompanied by lung congestion, raise client's upper body to approximately 45° and lower extremities approximately 15°. *Elevating the upper body lowers the diaphragm and provides more room for lung expansion and gas exchange. Elevating the head reduces intracranial pressure. Elevating the legs promotes blood perfusion to heart, lungs, and brain.*

- Administer oxygen by the medically prescribed method and percentage. *Administration at higher percentages than in room air increases the oxygen bound to hemoglobin and dissolved in blood so that cells can maintain aerobic metabolism.*

- Collaborate with the physician about alternative techniques to control internal bleeding such as esophageal gastric balloon tamponade with a Sengstaken-Blakemore tube (see Chap. 55) used to manage bleeding esophageal varices. *An internally inflated balloon is used to apply internal pressure to esophageal and gastric areas of venous bleeding that are impossible to reach manually.*

- Monitor PASG pressure (if used), and notify the physician if it is greater than 30 mm Hg for more than 2 hours. *Prolonged pressure can interfere with capillary blood flow as well as circulation of oxygenated blood and tissue perfusion, defeating the purpose of the PASG.*

- Deflate a PASG when the client is stable, starting with the abdominal port or leg section; never remove the entire garment at once. *Gradual deflation facilitates maintenance of BP and ensures adequate blood circulation to vital organs.*

- Increase the rate of IV fluid infusion if BP falls by 5 mm Hg during deflation of the PASG (Laskowski-

Jones, 1997). *Increasing the circulating fluid volume maintains BP.*

- Implement measures to reduce the work of the heart in cardiogenic heart failure, such as administering diuretics, vasodilators, and antidysrhythmics. *A heart in failure is best supported by reducing the volume it must circulate, decreasing the arterial resistance that it must overcome to eject blood, and slowing the heart to reduce its oxygen requirements.*
- Prepare the client in cardiogenic shock for insertion of an IABP or VAD. *Mechanically supporting or enhancing natural heart contractions improves cardiac output and tissue perfusion (see Chap. 36).*
- Immobilize possible spinal injuries and splint fractures. *Reducing complications from trauma can minimize the potential for neurogenic and hypovolemic shock.*

Impaired Gas Exchange related to edema of the airway secondary to a severe allergic reaction leading to anaphylactic shock

Expected Outcomes: (1) SpO_2 level will be at least 90%, PaO_2 will be 80 to 100 mm Hg, and $PaCO_2$ will be 35 to 45 mm Hg. (2) Airway will be patent, respiratory rate will be no more than 24 breaths/minute at rest, and breathing will be quiet and effortless.

- Assist with the insertion of an artificial airway and ventilatory support (see Chap. 28). *Intubation facilitates maintenance of a patent airway; artificial ventilation ensures that respiratory gases enter and leave the lungs.*
- Suction the airway when secretions compromise gas exchange. *Suctioning removes fluid that occupies space in the airways needed for the movement and exchange of gases.*
- Administer prescribed adrenergic, bronchodilating, anti-inflammatory, and antihistamine medications. *Drug therapy helps to improve the potential for gas exchange.*

Hypothermia related to hemorrhage
Expected Outcome: Body temperature will be restored to normal range.

- Keep client dry and covered. *Measures that prevent evaporation and heat loss from radiation interfere with the loss of body heat.*
- Raise the room temperature to approximately 80°F. *Using the physics of convection, warming the environment can raise body temperature.*
- Place client on a warming blanket or direct warming lights to the client's body. *Conduction and radiation transfer heat.*
- Keep client's head covered with a turban made of stockinette or other material. *Body heat is lost in significant amounts from the head; covering the head reduces heat loss.*
- Warm IV solutions and blood products. *Warmed infusions raise the temperature of tissues where they are circulated.*

- Warm the humidified air that is mixed with oxygen during mechanical ventilation. *Inhalation of warmed air increases core body temperature.*

Hyperthermia related to altered temperature regulation secondary to sepsis
Expected Outcome: Body temperature will be reduced to normal range.

- Administer prescribed antipyretics. *They block the production of prostaglandins, which elevate the temperature set point within the hypothalamus.*
- Place client on a cooling mattress. *Contact with a cool surface lowers body temperature.*
- Control shivering. *Shivering increases body heat through the contraction of skeletal and pilomotor muscles in the skin.*
- Administer a tepid sponge bath. *Body temperature is lowered when the heat of the skin vaporizes water.*
- Administer prescribed antibiotics. *They reduce or destroy pathogens responsible for sepsis.*

Evaluation of Expected Outcomes

Vital signs are stable. Tissue perfusion is satisfactory, as evidenced by adequate urine output; strong, palpable peripheral pulses; warm, dry skin; and intact sensorium. Capillary refill is immediate. ABGs are within normal range. Blood pH is between 7.35 and 7.45. The client is normothermic.

 GENERAL NUTRITIONAL CONSIDERATIONS

Because carbohydrate metabolism produces more CO_2 than either fat or protein metabolism, recommendations are for fat intake to increase and carbohydrate intake to decrease to reduce the burden on the lungs in clients with respiratory distress syndrome. Protein should provide approximately 20% of total calories, with the rest divided evenly between carbohydrates and fat.
Avoid overfeeding, which causes overproduction of CO_2.

 GENERAL PHARMACOLOGIC CONSIDERATIONS

Ringer's lactate and 0.9% sodium chloride (isotonic solutions) commonly are used to treat hypovolemic shock.
Morphine sulfate may be administered to decrease anxiety and pain.
Dopamine (Intropin) is used to treat shock resulting from MI, trauma, septicemia, renal failure, and cardiac decompensation. It must be properly diluted and administered by continuous infusion regulated by an infusion pump.
Administration of vasopressors such as dopamine demands constant nursing supervision. Depending on institutional policy, BP is monitored every 5 minutes with an automatic monitoring device. The infusion rate is adjusted to maintain a specific BP.

GENERAL GERONTOLOGIC CONSIDERATIONS

Older adults, particularly those with cardiac disease, are prone to cardiogenic shock. They also have a decreased percentage of body water and are more likely to develop hypovolemic shock.

Critical Thinking Exercises

1. *Which types of shock usually are accompanied by warm skin rather than cool skin?*
2. *In which type of shock does the client manifest a slow rather than a rapid heart rate?*

References and Suggested Readings

Atassi, K. A. & Harris, M. L. (2001). Disseminated intravascular coagulation. *Nursing, 31*(3), 64.

Bullock, B. L. & Henze, R. L. (2000). *Focus on pathophysiology.* Philadelphia: Lippincott Williams & Wilkins.

Collins, T. (2000). Understanding shock. *Nursing Standard, 14*(49), 35–39.

D'Epiro, N. W. (1999). Current thinking on sepsis treatment. *Patient Care, 33*(15), 78–92.

Edwards, D., Taylor, L., & Vorster, K. (2000). Shock. *Journal of PeriAnesthsia Nursing, 15,* 221–223.

Edwards, S. (2001). Shock: Types, classifications and explorations of their physiological effects. *Emergency Nurse, 9*(2), 29–38.

Frank, L. R. (2000). Is MAST in the past? The pros and cons of MAST usage in the field. *Journal of Emergency Medical Services, 25*(2), 38–41, 44–45.

Gilcreast, D. M., Avella, P., Camarillo, E., et al. (2001). Trauma: Treating severe anemia in a trauma patient who is a Jehovah's witness. *Critical Care Nurse, 21*(2), 69–81.

Gordon, L. (1999). The sepsis continuum from systemic inflammatory response syndrome to multiple organ dysfunction syndrome. *Nursing in Critical Care, 4,* 238–244.

Laskowski-Jones, L. (1997). Managing hemorrhage: Taking the right steps to protect your patient. *Nursing, 27*(9), 36–42.

Mattera, C. J. (2000). Heart failure and pulmonary edema: Understanding and correcting problems with the body's amazing pump. *Journal of Emergency Medical Services, 35*(5), 36–39, 41–42, 44–47.

Mayers, I. & Johnson, D. (2000). Septic shock: Treating more than just blood pressure. *Journal of the Canadian Medical Association, 162,* 369–370.

Molitor, L. (2000). Triage decisions. An obtunded elderly woman with tachycardia and tachypnea . . . septic shock. *Journal of Emergency Nursing, 26,* 188–189, 194–198.

Mower-Wade, D. M., Bartley, M. K., & Chiari-Allwein, J. L. (2001). How to respond to shock. *Dimensions of Critical Care Nursing, 20*(2), 22–27.

National Association of EMS Physicians. (2000). *Anthology of Association position papers.* [On-line.] Available: http://www.naemsp.org/Position%20Papers/Contents.html

O'Connor, R. E. & Domeier, R. (1997). Use of the pneumatic antishock garment (PASG). *Prehospital Emergency Care.* [On-line.] Available: http://www.naemsp.org/Position%20Papers/PASG.html.

Putman, H. & May, K. R. (2001). Relief for patients with severe allergies. *RN, 64*(6), 26–31.

Rembacz, J. M. & Abel, C. J. (2000). Pericardial tamponade. *American Journal of Nursing, 100*(9, Suppl.), 10–14, 24–26.

Rowe, P. M. (1999). Septic shock: Finding the way through the maze. *Lancet, 354*(9195), 2058.

Smeltzer, S. C. & Bare, B. G. (2000). *Brunner & Suddarth's textbook of medical–surgical nursing* (9th ed.). Philadelphia: Lippincott Williams & Wilkins.

Snooks, H., Moore, F., & Palmer, Y. (2000). Care of patients with anaphylactic shock. *Pre-hospital Immediate Care, 4*(1), 51.

Stoll, E. H. (2001). Sepsis and septic shock. *Clinical Journal of Oncology Nursing, 5*(2), 71–72.

Tangredi, M. (1998). Septic shock. *American Journal of Nursing, 98*(3), 46–47.

Caring for Clients Requiring Intravenous Therapy

Words to Know

blood products
central venous infusions
colloid solutions
crystalloid solutions
drop factors
drop size
electronic infusion device
emulsion
hypertonic solution
hypotonic solution
infusion pump
in-line filter
intravenous (IV) therapy
isotonic solution
macrodrip tubing
medication lock
microdrip tubing
midclavicular catheter

midline catheter
packed cells
peripheral venous sites
phlebitis
plasma expanders
pressure infusion
    sleeve
primary tubing
secondary tubing
total parenteral
    nutrition
unvented tubing
venipuncture
vented tubing
volumetric controller
whole blood
Y-administration
    tubing

Learning Objectives

On completion of this chapter, the reader will:

- Explain intravenous (IV) therapy, and list three substances commonly infused.
- Differentiate between crystalloid and colloid solutions.
- Describe the difference between isotonic, hypotonic, and hypertonic solutions.
- Discuss the purpose of total parenteral nutrition, and name one solution often administered concurrently.
- Explain the difference between whole blood, packed cells, blood products, and plasma expanders.
- List nursing responsibilities that must be implemented before IV therapy is administered.
- List three types of tubing used to administer IV solutions.
- Name two techniques for infusing IV solutions.
- Explain the difference between an infusion pump and a volumetric controller.
- Give three nursing actions involved in performing a venipuncture.
- Name three venipuncture devices, and identify the one most commonly used.
- Name two general sites used for IV therapy.
- Identify three nursing diagnoses common to clients who require IV therapy.
- Discuss the nursing management of clients receiving IV therapy.
- List three complications of IV therapy and three associated with administering blood.
- Discuss the purpose of a medication lock.

Intravenous (IV) therapy, the parenteral administration of fluids and additives into a vein, is used to maintain or restore fluid balance when oral replacement is inadequate or impossible, maintain or replace electrolytes, administer water-soluble vitamins, provide a source of calories and nutrients, administer drugs (Box 24-1), and replace blood and blood products. IV administration of solutions (e.g., dextrose, plasma expanders, amino acids), whole blood and blood components, and medications demands skillful administration techniques, close obser-

vation of the client, and several specific nursing considerations, all of which are discussed in this chapter.

TYPES OF SOLUTIONS

The two types of IV solutions are crystalloid and colloid solutions. **Crystalloid solutions** consist of water and uniformly dissolved crystals such as salt (sodium chloride) and sugar (glucose, dextrose) (Fig. 24-1). **Colloid solutions** consist of water and molecules of suspended substances such as blood cells and blood products (e.g., albumin).

Crystalloid Solutions

Crystalloid solutions are divided into isotonic, hypotonic, and hypertonic solutions (Table 24-1). These terms refer to the concentration of dissolved substances in relation to the plasma into which they are instilled. When crystalloid solutions are administered to clients, the concentration influences the osmotic distribution of body fluid (Fig. 24-2).

Isotonic Solutions

An **isotonic solution** contains the same concentration of dissolved substances as is normally found in plasma. Isotonic solutions are administered to maintain fluid balance when clients temporarily cannot eat or drink. Because of its equal concentration to plasma, an isotonic solution causes no appreciable redistribution of body fluid on administration.

Hypotonic Solutions

A **hypotonic solution** contains fewer dissolved substances compared with plasma. Hypotonic solutions are effective in rehydrating clients experiencing fluid deficits;

therefore, they are administered to clients experiencing fluid losses in excess of fluid intake, such as those who have diarrhea or are vomiting. Because a hypotonic solution is dilute, the water in the solution passes through the semipermeable membrane of blood cells, causing them to swell. This swelling can temporarily increase blood pressure because it expands the circulating volume. The water also may pass through capillary walls and become distributed in other body cells and the interstitial spaces.

Hypertonic Solutions

A **hypertonic solution** is more concentrated (contains more dissolved substances) than body fluid. Consequently, it draws fluid into the intravascular compartment from the more dilute areas in the cells and interstitial spaces. Hypertonic solutions are not used very frequently except when it is necessary to reduce cerebral (brain) edema, expand circulatory volume rapidly, or administer nutrition parenterally.

Total parenteral nutrition (TPN) is a hypertonic solution consisting of nutrients designed to meet nearly all the caloric and nutritional needs of clients who are severely malnourished or cannot consume food or liquids for a long time (Box 24-2). TPN solutions, which are extremely concentrated, are instilled into the central circulation (see discussion of central venous sites later in this chapter), where they are diluted in a fairly large volume of blood. Because of their immediate dilution, TPN solutions do not dehydrate cells.

An **emulsion** is a mixture of two liquids, one of which is insoluble in the other; when combined, the two are distributed throughout the mixture as small, undissolved droplets. A lipid emulsion, which is sometimes administered intermittently with TPN, is a mixture of water and fats in the form of soybean or safflower oil, egg yolk phospholipids, and glycerin, which looks milky white. It provides additional calories and promotes adequate blood levels of fatty acids.

Colloid Solutions

Colloid solutions are used to replace circulating blood volume because the suspended molecules in the solutions pull fluid from other compartments. Examples include blood (whole blood and packed cells), blood products, and solutions known as plasma expanders.

Blood

Whole blood and packed cells probably are the most commonly administered colloid solutions. One unit of **whole blood** (Fig. 24-3) contains approximately 475 mL of blood cells and plasma, with 60 to 70 mL of preservative and anticoagulant added. Whole blood is administered when clients need fluid restorations as well as blood cells. **Packed cells** have most of the plasma (fluid) removed and

FIGURE 24-1 Crystalloid solution. (Photo © B. Proud.)

TABLE 24-1	TYPES OF CRYSTALLOID SOLUTIONS	
SOLUTION	**COMPONENTS**	**SPECIAL COMMENTS**
Isotonic Solutions		
0.9% Saline, also called normal saline (NS)	0.9 g sodium chloride/100 mL water	Contains sodium and chloride in amounts physiologically equal to those in plasma
5% Dextrose in water, also called D_5W	5 g dextrose (glucose/sugar)/100 mL water	Isotonic when infused, but the glucose is metabolized quickly, leaving a solution of dilute water
Ringer's solution or lactated Ringer's	Water and a mixture of sodium, chloride, calcium, potassium, bicarbonate, and, in some cases, lactate	Replaces electrolytes in amounts similarly found in plasma; lactate, when present, helps maintain acid–base balance
Hypotonic Solutions		
0.45% Sodium chloride, also called half-strength saline	0.45 g sodium chloride/100 mL water	Contains a smaller proportion of sodium and chloride than found in plasma, causing it to be less concentrated in comparison
5% Dextrose in 0.45% saline	5 g dextrose and 0.45 sodium chloride/ 100 mL water	The sugar provides a quick source of energy, leaving a hypotonic salt solution
Hypertonic Solutions		
10% Dextrose in water, also called $D_{10}W$	10 g dextrose/100 mL water	Contains twice the concentration of glucose found in plasma
3% Saline	3 g sodium chloride/100 mL water	The high concentration of salt in the plasma dehydrates cells and tissue
20% Dextrose in water	20 g dextrose/100 mL water	Rapidly increases the concentration of sugar in the blood, causing a fluid shift to the intravascular compartment

are preferred for clients who need cellular replacements but do not need and may be harmed by the administration of additional fluid. Such clients include those who have an inadequate oral intake of fluid and clients at risk for congestive heart failure (see Chap. 36). Whole blood and packed cells are typed and crossmatched in the laboratory before administration to ensure that the donor's and recipient's blood types are compatible (Table 24-2).

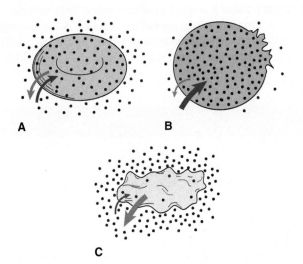

FIGURE 24-2 Osmotic distribution of fluid: (**A**) isotonic fluid, (**B**) hypotonic fluid, and (**C**) hypertonic fluid.

Blood Products

Several types of solutions contain **blood products,** components extracted from blood (Table 24-3). Blood products are administered to clients who need specific blood substances but not all the fluid and cellular components in whole blood.

Plasma Expanders

Plasma expanders are nonblood solutions, such as dextran 40 (Rheomacrodex) and hetastarch (Hespan), that pull fluid into the vascular space. They are used as an economical and virus-free substitute for blood and blood products when treating clients with hypovolemic shock.

BOX 24-2 ● Candidates for Total Parenteral Nutrition

Candidates for TPN include clients:
- Who have not eaten for 5 days and are not likely to eat during the next week
- Who have had a 10% or more loss of body weight
- Exhibiting self-imposed starvation (anorexia nervosa)
- With cancer of the esophagus or stomach
- With postoperative gastrointestinal complications
- With acute inflammatory bowel disease
- With major trauma or burns
- With liver and renal failure

FIGURE 24-3 Unit of whole blood. (Photo © B. Proud.)

TABLE 24-2	BLOOD GROUPS AND COMPATIBLE TYPES	
BLOOD GROUPS	**PERCENTAGE OF POPULATION**	**COMPATIBLE BLOOD TYPES**
A	41%	A and O
B	9%	B and O
O	47%	O
AB	3%	AB, A, B, and O
Rh⁺	85% Whites 95% African Americans	Rh⁺ and Rh⁻
Rh⁻	15% Whites 5% African Americans	Rh⁻ only

ADMINISTERING INTRAVENOUS THERAPY

Selecting and Preparing Equipment

Equipment commonly used when administering IV therapy includes the solution, IV tubing, and an IV pole or infusion device. A fluid warmer may be used to raise the temperature of parenteral solutions when it is beneficial to ensure stable body temperature. The nurse selects and prepares the fluid that will be administered, chooses appropriate tubing, and decides on an infusion technique.

Preparing Intravenous Solutions

Crystalloid solutions are stored in plastic bags containing volumes of 1000, 500, 250, 100, and 50 mL. Only a few solutions are in glass containers. The physician specifies the type of solution, additional additives, and the volume to infuse over a specific period. To reduce the potential for infection, standard practice is to replace IV solutions every 24 hours even if the total volume in a container has not been instilled. Before preparing the solution, the nurse inspects the container and determines that the type of solution is the one prescribed, the solution is clear and transparent, the expiration date has not elapsed, no leaks are apparent, and a separate label is attached identifying the type and amount of drugs added to the original solution.

Choosing Intravenous Tubing

The IV tubing consists of a spike for piercing the container of solution, a drip chamber for holding a small amount of fluid, a length of plastic tubing with one or more ports for instilling IV medications or additional solutions, and a roller or slide clamp for regulating the rate of the infusion (Fig. 24-4). Despite the common components, the nurse selects from various options in the tubing design. The choice depends on four considerations: (1) whether to use primary, secondary, or Y-administration tubing; (2) whether to use vented or unvented tubing; (3) the drop size indicated; and (4) whether a filter is needed.

PRIMARY, SECONDARY, AND Y-ADMINISTRATION TUBING
Primary tubing is used to administer a large volume of IV solution over a long period or a small volume through a medication lock (discussed later). Primary tubing usually is quite long to span the distance from the solution, which

TABLE 24-3	TYPES OF BLOOD PRODUCTS	
BLOOD PRODUCT	**DESCRIPTION**	**PURPOSE FOR ADMINISTRATION**
Platelets	Disk-shaped cellular fragments that promote coagulation of blood	Restores or improves the ability to control bleeding
Granulocytes	Types of white blood cells	Improves the ability to overcome infection
Plasma	Serum without blood cells	Replaces clotting factors or increases intravascular fluid volume by increasing colloidal osmotic pressure
Albumin	Plasma protein	Pulls third-spaced fluid by increasing colloidal osmotic pressure
Cryoprecipitate	Mixture of clotting factors	Treats blood clotting disorders such as hemophilia

FIGURE 24-4 Basic components of intravenous tubing.

FIGURE 24-5 Blood administration set.

hangs several feet above the infusion site, to the site itself. **Secondary tubing,** which is shorter, is used to administer smaller volumes of solution through a port in the primary tubing. **Y-administration tubing** is used to administer whole blood or packed cells (Fig. 24-5). It contains two branches: one for blood and one for isotonic (normal) saline. The two branches extend above a filter that removes blood clots and cellular debris. The normal saline infuses before and after the blood infuses, or during the infusion if a transfusion reaction occurs.

VENTED VERSUS UNVENTED TUBING
IV tubing may be vented or unvented (Fig. 24-6). **Vented tubing** draws air into the container of solution and is used for administering solutions packaged in glass containers to facilitate their flow. **Unvented tubing** does not draw air into the container of solution and is used for solutions packaged in plastic bags.

DROP SIZE
The opening through which fluid passes from the solution container into the drip chamber determines the **drop size.** Tubing manufacturers design the drop size to deliver large-sized drops (**macrodrip tubing**) or small-sized drops (**microdrip tubing**). The nurse determines which to use. When a solution infuses by gravity at a fast rate, it usually is easier to count larger drops than to count smaller ones. When the rate must be infused very precisely or at a slow rate, smaller drops are preferred.

FIGURE 24-6 (*Left*) vented tubing and (*right*) unvented tubing. (Photo © Ken Timby.)

Microdrip tubing, regardless of the manufacturer, delivers a standard volume of 60 drops (gtt)/mL. Macrodrip tubing, however, varies in the drop size. Common **drop factors,** the ratio of drops per milliliter, are 10, 15, and 20 gtt/mL. The nurse determines the drop factor, which is important in calculating the gravity infusion rate, by reading the package label.

FILTERS

An **in-line filter** (Fig. 24-7) is a device that removes air bubbles as well as undissolved drugs, bacteria, and large molecules from the infusing solution. Filtered tubing is used when administering TPN, blood and packed cells, and solutions to immunosuppressed or pediatric clients.

Another factor that may affect the type of tubing selected is the technique that will be used to administer the IV solution.

Deciding on an Infusion Technique

IV solutions are instilled by gravity or with an **electronic infusion device,** a machine that regulates and monitors the administration of IV solutions. In some cases, the use of an electronic infusion device affects the type of tubing used.

The method for calculating the rate of infusion varies depending on the infusion technique (Box 24-3). If the solution is infused by gravity, the rate is calculated in drops per minute. When an electronic infusion device is used, the rate is calculated in milliliters per hour.

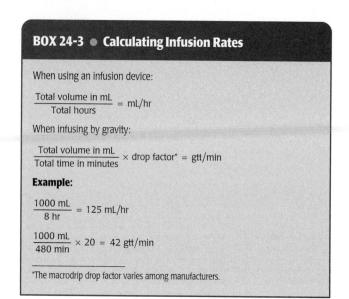

BOX 24-3 • Calculating Infusion Rates

When using an infusion device:

$$\frac{\text{Total volume in mL}}{\text{Total hours}} = \text{mL/hr}$$

When infusing by gravity:

$$\frac{\text{Total volume in mL}}{\text{Total time in minutes}} \times \text{drop factor}^* = \text{gtt/min}$$

Example:

$$\frac{1000 \text{ mL}}{8 \text{ hr}} = 125 \text{ mL/hr}$$

$$\frac{1000 \text{ mL}}{480 \text{ min}} \times 20 = 42 \text{ gtt/min}$$

*The macrodrip drop factor varies among manufacturers.

GRAVITY INFUSION

When IV solutions are infused by gravity, the height of the IV solution in relation to the infusion site influences the rate of flow. To overcome the pressure in the client's vein, which is higher than atmospheric pressure, the nurse must elevate the solution at least 18 to 24 inches (45 to 60 cm) above the infusion site. The higher the solution, the faster it infuses, and vice versa. The nurse uses the roller clamp to adjust the rate of flow. In some cases he or she may apply a **pressure infusion sleeve** around the bag of solution. The sleeve exerts a squeezing action around the solution bag to facilitate rapid infusion.

ELECTRONIC INFUSION DEVICES

The two general types of electronic infusion devices are infusion pumps and volumetric controllers. Both are programmed to deliver a preset volume per hour and sound audible and visual alarms if the infusion is not progressing at the preprogrammed rate. They also produce an audible sound when the infusion container is nearly empty, air is inside the tubing, or an obstruction or resistance to delivering the fluid occurs.

Infusion Pump. An **infusion pump** (Fig. 24-8) is a device that exerts positive pressure to infuse solutions. Infusion pumps usually require special tubing that contains a cassette for creating sufficient pressure to push fluid into the vein. The machine adjusts the pressure according to the resistance it meets. This feature accounts for one of its major disadvantages: if the catheter or needle within the vein becomes displaced, the pump may continue to infuse fluid into the tissue.

Volumetric Controller. A **volumetric controller** (see Fig. 24-8) is a device that infuses IV solutions by gravity by compressing the tubing at a certain frequency to infuse the solution at a precise preset rate. Volumetric con-

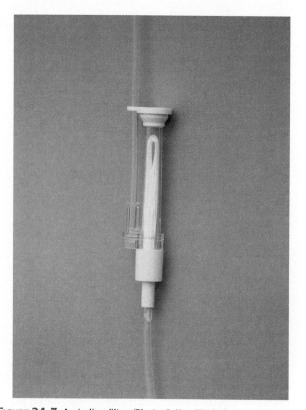

FIGURE 24-7 An in-line filter. (Photo © Ken Timby.)

FIGURE 24-8 (*Left*) An infusion pump requires specialized tubing and cassette. (*Right*) An electronic infusion controller. (Photo © Ken Timby.)

trollers may or may not require special tubing. Some models allow the nurse to program the infusion of more than one solution. In some cases, when one container of fluid finishes infusing, the controller automatically shifts to infuse another.

Stop, Think, and Respond ● BOX 24-1

The physician orders an IV infusion of 1000 mL of 5% dextrose in water that will infuse over 8 hours. The nurse asks you to collect the fluid infusion supplies. What will you assemble?

Preparing the Client for Venipuncture

A **venipuncture** is the method for gaining access to the venous system by piercing a vein with one of a variety of devices. The nurse explains the purpose of the procedure to clients at their level of understanding. It is best to do so before bringing the equipment to the client's room. The nurse tries as much as possible to make the explanation clear, concise, and informative without causing the client undue anxiety. He or she also allows time to answer the client's questions. The nurse may include the following points in the explanation: why the client needs IV therapy, about how long the procedure will take, the site to be used,

the amount of discomfort that normally accompanies insertion of the needle or catheter, and instructions regarding limitation of activities.

Performing a Venipuncture

Venipunctures are performed by nurses who are trained to do so. The nurse assesses the client to detect alterations in fluid volume and implements the physician's orders for IV fluid therapy. While the client undergoes fluid therapy, the nurse monitors to detect an increase, decrease, or rapid shift from one fluid compartment to another. The nurse follows the agency's infection control policies as they relate to IV fluid therapy, uses aseptic techniques when caring for the venipuncture site or changing equipment, and gathers data as they relate to the presence of an infection.

For all venipunctures, the following items are necessary: venipuncture device, gloves, tourniquet, antiseptic swabs to clean the skin, antiseptic ointment, a dressing, tape for securing the catheter or needle, dressing, tubing, and solution. An armboard or splint may be needed to prevent dislodging the venipuncture device.

Venipuncture Devices

Several devices are used for accessing a vein: a butterfly needle, an over-the-needle catheter (most commonly used), or a through-the-needle catheter (Fig. 24-9). Regardless of the design, venipuncture devices come in various diameters or gauges; the larger the gauge number, the smaller the diameter. The diameter of the venipuncture device always should be smaller than the vein into which it will be inserted to reduce the potential for occluding blood flow. The 18-, 20-, or 22-gauge venipuncture devices are the sizes most used for adults.

Venipuncture Sites

IV therapy is administered through peripheral venous sites or central veins. Selection of a vein depends on several factors, such as the client's age, condition of the veins, duration of IV therapy, IV solution ordered, size of venipuncture device, and client cooperation.

PERIPHERAL VENOUS SITES

Short-term **peripheral venous sites** are superficial veins of the arm and hand (antecubital fossa, or inner elbow; dorsum, or back, of the hand; and forearm veins; Fig. 24-10). They are the most common sites for infusing IV fluids. Scalp veins are used in infants. Veins in the foot are avoided because infusions in the lower extremities restrict mobility and increase the risk for forming blood clots.

A **midline catheter** is another type of peripherally inserted venous access device. It is 7 to 8 inches long, but

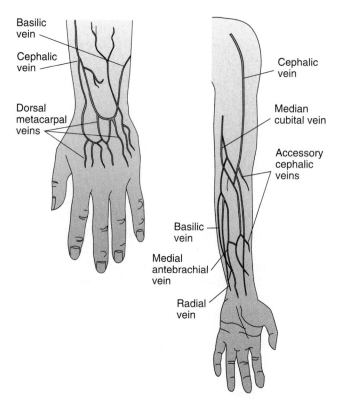

FIGURE 24-9 Venipuncture devices: (**A**) butterfly needle, (**B-1**) over-the-needle catheter, (**B-2**) needle removed, (**C-1**) through-the-needle catheter, (**C-2**) a needle guard covers the tip of the needle, which remains outside the skin.

only 3 to 6 inches of the catheter are inserted from just above or below the antecubital area in the basilic, cephalic, or median cubital vein until the tip rests in the upper arm just short of the axilla (Larouere, 2000b). Midline catheters are best suited for clients who have limited peripheral veins or who require an extended period of IV fluid therapy (Intravenous Nurses Society, 1997). This type of catheter can be used for up to 4 weeks before it requires replacement, which makes it ideal for use in the home healthcare setting.

When a peripherally inserted catheter extends from a superficial vein to the proximal end of the axillary or subclavian vein, it is referred to as a **midclavicular catheter,** which can be used for 2 to 3 months. All three of these types, peripheral, midline, and midclavicular, are considered to be in peripheral venous sites because the tip remains distal to a central vein (i.e., the thoracic vena cava). Therefore, their use is confined to administering IV solutions and medications that would be given through a short-term peripheral venous access device.

Midline and midclavicular sites should not be used to administer antineoplastic (cancer) chemotherapy, TPN (see later discussion), solutions with a pH less than 5 or greater than 9, solutions with an osmolality greater than 500 mOsm/L, rapid, high-volume infusions, or high-pressure bolus injections (Larouere, 2000a).

CENTRAL VENOUS SITES

Central venous infusions are those that deliver solutions into a large central vein, such as the vena cava (Fig. 24-11A). A physician inserts a central venous catheter into the jugular or subclavian vein until the tip is located just above the heart. Specially trained nurses insert a long catheter, called a *peripherally inserted central catheter* (PICC) or a *long line,* peripherally to a similar location (Fig. 24-11B). Central venous catheters are inserted when providing TPN, monitoring central venous pressure, or administering concentrated or irritating IV solutions; when peripheral veins have collapsed; or when long-term IV therapy or thrombophlebitis (inflammation of a vein) and infiltration have reduced the availability of peripheral veins. After insertion of the catheter, a chest radiograph is taken to confirm catheter placement and

FIGURE 24-10 Venipuncture sites.

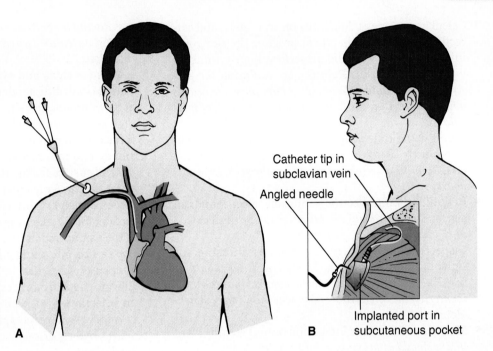

FIGURE 24-11 (A) Placement of triple-lumen nontunneled percutaneous central venous catheter. **(B)** Placement of an implanted port with the tip in the subclavian vein. Angled needle is inserted through skin and rubber septum into port.

A

Catheter tip in subclavian vein

Angled needle

B

Implanted port in subcutaneous pocket

rule out an accidental puncture of the pleural membrane causing a pneumothorax (see Chap. 29).

Stop, Think, and Respond ● BOX 24-2

A client with cancer has a central venous catheter though which he receives antineoplastic drugs. Why is the medication infused through a central venous catheter and filtered tubing?

NURSING PROCESS

● The Client Requiring IV Therapy

Assessment

Before initiating fluid therapy, the nurse gathers clinical data that relate to fluid status (see Chap. 22). Examples include vital signs; body weight; color, volume, and specific gravity of urine; skin turgor; characteristics of oral mucous membranes; respiratory effort; and level of consciousness. The nurse also reviews laboratory test results such as blood cell count and hematocrit and serum electrolyte levels.

The nurse identifies the purpose(s) for administering IV fluid therapy. Before performing the venipuncture, he or she asks the client to identify the nondominant hand. The nondominant hand or forearm is preferred unless there are contraindications to its use such as having had a breast and lymph nodes removed on that side or having had vascular surgery for kidney dialysis. If the client cannot respond, the nurse assumes that the client is right-handed because that is true in most cases. To de-

termine which vein is most appropriate, the nurse first assesses the size and condition of the veins in the hand or wrist area. If they are exceptionally small, tortuous, or traumatized by previous venipunctures, the nurse inspects veins in more proximal areas, trying to avoid the veins in the antecubital fossa where the elbow bends, if at all possible. The nurse reads the label on the IV fluid at least three times to confirm that it is the volume and type of solution the physician has ordered.

After performing the venipuncture, the nurse monitors the IV site for swelling, warmth, pain, and induration. He or she assesses the rate at which fluid is infusing and the client's condition at least hourly. The nurse examines the electronic infusion device, if one is used, to ensure that it is correctly programmed and functioning properly. Throughout fluid therapy, the nurse measures intake and output volumes to determine trends in fluid balance. He or she auscultates lung sounds and heart sounds each shift or more often to evaluate the client's capacity to circulate the infusing fluid without complications. The nurse inspects the venipuncture site at least once a day for signs of inflammation or infection and observes the condition of the dressing, which should be dry and intact.

Diagnosis, Planning, and Interventions

Risk for Imbalanced Fluid Volume related to rate of infusion that exceeds circulatory capacity or a shift in a fluid compartment

Expected Outcomes: (1) Fluid volume will be maintained or restored. (2) Client will not experience cardiopulmonary complications secondary to the IV infusion of fluid.

- Calculate the rate of fluid infusion accurately, and correctly regulate the drip rate or program the electronic infusion device with the prescribed hourly infusion volume. *Errors in calculating or regulating the prescribed rate of fluid infusion can compromise the heart's ability to circulate the fluid or delay restoration of fluid balance.*
- Monitor the time strip on the container of IV solution hourly. *Reading the time strip is a quick method for determining if fluid is infusing at the predetermined hourly rate.*
- Respond when an electronic infusion device sounds an alarm. *Audible alarms call attention to a problem associated with the infusion of IV fluid.*
- Inspect the site where the fluid is infusing for signs of localized edema. *Parenteral fluid should be instilled in the vein; local edema suggests that the fluid is entering the interstitial space, where it is more slowly absorbed.*
- Maintain an accurate intake and output record. *Fluid intake should approximate fluid output.*
- Note the amount of fluids the client takes orally and report when the combined volume of oral and parenteral fluid exceeds 3000 mL in 24 hours. *Normal adult fluid intake generally is 1500 to 3000 mL/24 hours. Volumes that exceed 3000 mL/day may be excessive unless the client is dehydrated or losing large volumes of fluid simultaneously.*
- Reassess fluid status at regular intervals according to the client's acuity level. *Changes in weight (e.g., 2 lbs in 24 hours), elevated blood pressure, dyspnea or adventitious lung sounds, abnormal heart sounds, peripheral edema, intake that significantly exceeds output, distended neck veins, anxiety, or diminished level of consciousness suggest excessive fluid volume.*

Risk for Infection related to disrupted skin integrity secondary to venipuncture and presence of a venous access device

Expected Outcome: Client will remain free of localized or generalized infection.

- Follow agency protocol for changing IV sites and venipuncture devices. *To avoid infection, the standard of care is to change IV sites every 48 to 72 hours. Clients with suppressed immune systems may require the use of tubing with a bacterial filter and more frequent site changes.*
- Check the initial date of use on the IV fluid container and tubing and change equipment according to the agency's infection control policies. *Infection control policies usually advise changing IV solution containers every 24 hours; IV tubing can be used for up to 72 hours provided solution is continuously infusing through it. Nurses change tubing for intermittent infusions more frequently.*
- Use aseptic technique when changing IV site dressings, tubings, and solution containers. *Preventing*

or reducing the entrance of bacteria in the venipuncture site or vascular system decreases the potential for infection.

- Assess for signs and symptoms of infection such as redness, warmth, tenderness, and purulent drainage at the venipuncture site; elevated temperature; and an increased white blood cell count. Discontinue the IV infusion and remove the venipuncture device if signs and symptoms of infection exist. *Removing the venipuncture device enables the impaired skin to heal and restores the barrier to microorganisms.*
- Document and report assessments that relate to an infection; follow agency protocols for obtaining a culture of the wound and its drainage. *Local antimicrobial therapy or systemic antibiotic therapy may be indicated in some cases of infection.*
- Elevate the extremity and apply warm compresses if an infection is suspected. *Elevation promotes venous circulation and reduces swelling. Warmth dilates blood vessels, relieves discomfort, and facilitates a reduction in local edema.*
- Restart the IV infusion in another site, preferably in the opposite upper extremity. *Fluid therapy should not be interrupted if it is still necessary.*

Risk for Imbalanced Nutrition: Less than Body Requirements related to an inadequate nutritional intake from crystalloid solutions without oral nutrition

Expected Outcome: The client will have adequate nutrition to meet needs for growth and repair of tissue.

- Weigh the client daily. *Weight loss indicates imbalanced nutrition.*
- Monitor laboratory test results such as blood cell count and hemoglobin, albumin, and transferrin levels. *A drop in specific laboratory findings indicates insufficient protein to ensure their normal production or replacement.*
- Implement the physician's orders to provide TPN if it becomes necessary (Nursing Guidelines 24-1). *TPN provides the client with protein, vitamins, and minerals as well as glucose and water. Intermittent fat emulsions complete the requirements for adequate nutrition.*

Evaluation of Expected Outcomes

Expected outcomes are that the client's fluid status is improved or maintained within normal, with approximately equal intake and output volumes and normal vital signs. Breathing remains quiet and effortless, with no signs of localized or generalized edema. The IV site is not red, tender, or warm and shows no drainage. The client's body temperature remains within normal range. The client uses the extremity with minimal inconvenience from the IV infusion. He or she maintains preillness weight. Blood cell count and hemoglobin, albumin, and transferrin levels are within normal limits.

NURSING GUIDELINES 24-1

Administering Total Parenteral Nutrition

- Weigh client daily.

- Use tubing that contains a filter; however, bypass the filter when administering lipid emulsions to prevent large fat molecules from obstructing the filter.

- Label the tubing used for TPN to ensure that it is used exclusively for TPN and not IV medications or blood products.

- Change TPN tubings daily.

- Tape all connections in the tubing to prevent accidental separation and the potential for an air embolism.

- Clamp the central catheter whenever separating the tubing from its catheter connection.

- Use an electronic infusion device to administer TPN.

- Infuse initial TPN solutions gradually (e.g., 25–50 mL/hr); increase rate according to the agency's standard of care or the physician's medical orders.

- Monitor blood glucose levels regularly to assess the client's ability to metabolize the concentrated glucose.

- Administer insulin on a sliding scale according to blood glucose levels.

- Wean client from TPN gradually to avoid a sudden drop in blood glucose level.

- Infuse IV lipids three times a week.

- Monitor the following laboratory test results to evaluate the nutritional status of the client receiving TPN and lipids: serum transferrin, serum osmolality, cholesterol, triglycerides, electrolytes, blood urea nitrogen (BUN), and urine creatinine.

Stop, Think, and Respond ● BOX 24-3

Read the following scenario, and answer the questions as they relate to the client.

Client A had surgery 2 days ago, at which time he lost approximately 500 mL of blood. After surgery, he is not allowed to have anything orally because he has a nasogastric tube connected to suction. In the meantime, he has also developed diarrhea, which the physician attributes to being a side effect from the parenteral antibiotic he is receiving. When you assess this client, his blood pressure is 104/62 mm Hg, much lower than his admission blood pressure of 132/86 mm Hg. His skin is dry and tents when you assess turgor; his urine output has been 350 mL in the past 8 hours, and the urine appears dark yellow.

1. *What additional information would you gather to assess the client's fluid status?*
2. *If IV fluids are administered, which type of solution is most appropriate to use, and why?*

COMPLICATIONS OF INTRAVENOUS THERAPY

Several complications are associated with the infusion of IV solutions. Any time the integrity of the skin is compromised with a venous access device like a catheter or needle, the client is at risk for infection. Because the venous access device traumatizes the vein wall and disturbs the flow of blood cells in the vein, there is a potential for **phlebitis,** inflammation of the vein (Fig. 24-12), and thrombus formation, development of a clot. If the clot breaks free, it may travel to the lungs and cause a pulmonary embolism, which can be fatal. A bolus of air traveling through the venous system to the lungs is just as serious. If the venous access device fails to remain in the vein, fluid infiltrates the tissue, causing localized edema. Last, circulatory overload can develop if the volume of infusing solution exceeds the heart's ability to circulate it effectively. Table 24-4 identifies the causes and manifestations of these complications and appropriate nursing actions should they occur.

Complications of Blood Transfusion

Clients who receive blood are at risk for the same complications as those receiving crystalloid fluids. They also face additional risks, however, because blood contains cells, usually from nonautologous donors, and additives and preservatives that enable it to be stored in a refrigerated state for approximately 1 month without clotting. One of the most life-threatening complications is an incompatibility reaction that occurs when the donor and recipient blood types are incorrectly matched. In this instance, the recipient's antibodies destroy the donor cells. Although an incompatibility reaction occurs once in approximately 25,000 blood transfusions, it accounts for more than 50% of reported transfusion-related deaths (Ting, 1999). An

FIGURE 24-12 Checking inflammation surrounding infusion site. (Photo © B. Proud.)

TABLE 24-4	COMPLICATIONS OF INTRAVENOUS THERAPY		
COMPLICATION	SIGNS AND SYMPTOMS	CAUSE(S)	ACTION
Infection	Swelling, discomfort, redness at site, drainage from site	Growth of microorganisms	Change site. Apply antiseptic and dressing to previous site. Report findings.
Circulatory overload	Elevated blood pressure, shortness of breath, bounding pulse, anxiety	Rapid infusion Reduced kidney function Impaired heart contraction	Slow the IV rate. Contact the physician. Elevate the client's head. Give oxygen.
Infiltration (extravasation)	Swelling at the site, discomfort, decrease in infusion rate, cool skin temperature at the site	Displacement of the venipuncture device	Restart the IV. Elevate the arm.
Phlebitis	Redness, warmth, and discomfort along the vein	Administration of irritating fluid Prolonged use of the same vein	Restart the IV. Report the findings. Apply warm compresses.
Thrombus formation	Swelling, discomfort at site, slowed infusion	Stasis of blood at the catheter, needle tip, or vein	Restart the IV. Report the findings. Apply warm compresses.
Pulmonary embolus	Sudden chest pain, shortness of breath, anxiety, rapid heart rate, drop in blood pressure	Movement of previously stationary blood clot	Stay with the client. Call for help. Administer oxygen.
Air embolism	Same as pulmonary embolus	Failure to purge air from the tubing Disconnected tubing from central venous catheter	Same as for pulmonary embolus, but also place the client's head lower than the feet. Position the client on left side.

acute incompatibility reaction occurs within minutes of infusing the donor blood. Milder allergic reactions such as hives and itching or a febrile response may occur if the recipient is sensitive to noncellular substances in the donor blood. Delayed reactions, which are milder than incompatibility reactions, can occur weeks to months after a transfusion. Delayed reactions are more likely the result of an immune response against the antigens of the Rh component of blood cells.

Nonimmune complications also are possible after blood transfusion. Clients may become septic if pathogens have grown and multiplied in the stored blood or during the interim when blood is being infused. A universal standard is to keep the blood refrigerated until just before use and to infuse the blood in 4 hours or less to prevent a septic reaction from bacterial contamination. Some clients have shaking chills and a fever during a septic or febrile reaction. Monitoring the client's temperature before, during, and after a blood transfusion is necessary to determine if chilling is the result of an emerging complication or of infusing cold blood.

Reduced levels of serum calcium can produce symptoms in clients who receive massive transfusions of blood over a very short time. Citrate, which is added to the donor blood, binds with calcium in the recipient's blood, causing hypocalcemia.

Blood-borne infections such as hepatitis A, B, and C and human immunodeficiency virus (HIV) infection also can be transmitted through blood from infected donors. Donors are asked questions about their infection history, foreign travel, and risk behaviors when being screened before donating blood. Donated blood also is tested for hepatitis virus and HIV antibody levels. Although it is impossible to guarantee that all donated blood is free of blood-borne pathogens, the incidence of transmission is much smaller than it was at one time. An overview of potential complications from blood transfusion and specific nursing actions is provided in Table 24-5.

Site Care

Because the venipuncture is a type of wound, inspecting the site routinely and observing for signs of infection, infiltration, phlebitis, and thrombus formation are important interventions (see Table 24-4). The nurse documents site appearance daily in the client's medical record. A common practice is to change the dressing over the venipuncture site every 24 to 72 hours according to the agency's infection control policy or immediately if complications develop.

TABLE 24-5	COMPLICATIONS OF BLOOD TRANSFUSION		
COMPLICATION	**SIGNS AND SYMPTOMS**	**CAUSE(S)**	**ACTION**
Incompatibility reaction	Hypotension, rapid pulse rate, difficulty breathing, back pain, flushing	Mismatch between donor and recipient blood groups	Stop the infusion of blood. Infuse the saline at a rapid rate. Call for assistance. Administer oxygen. Raise the feet higher than the head. Be prepared to administer emergency drugs. Send first urine specimen to laboratory. Save the blood and tubing.
Febrile reaction	Fever, shaking chills, headache, rapid pulse, muscle aches	Allergy to foreign proteins in the donated blood	Stop the blood infusion. Start the saline. Check vital signs. Report findings.
Septic reaction	Fever, chills, hypotension	Infusion of blood that contains microorganisms	Stop the infusion of blood. Start the saline. Report findings. Save the blood and tubing.
Allergic reaction	Rash, itching, flushing, stable vital signs	Minor sensitivity to substances in the donor blood	Slow the rate of infusion. Assess the client. Report findings. Be prepared to give an antihistamine.
Moderate chilling	No fever or other symptoms	Infusion of cold blood	Continue the infusion. Cover and make the client comfortable.
Circulatory overload	Hypertension, difficulty breathing, moist breath sounds, bounding pulse	Large volume or rapid rate of infusion; inadequate cardiac or kidney function	Reduce the rate of infusion. Elevate the head. Give oxygen. Report findings. Be prepared to give a diuretic.
Hypocalcemia (low calcium)	Tingling of fingers, hypotension, muscle cramps, convulsions	Multiple blood transfusions containing anticalcium agents	Stop the blood infusion. Start saline. Report findings. Be prepared to give antidote, calcium chloride.
HIV and hepatitis B virus transmission	Opportunistic infections; elevated antibody titers, abnormal blood cell counts or liver enzyme levels	Blood collected from infected donors that passed screening examinations	Encourage autologous (self) blood collection if possible.

Equipment Replacement

Solutions are replaced when they finish infusing or every 24 hours, whichever comes first. Most IV tubing is changed every 72 hours, but the exact parameters depend on agency policy. Some exceptions include tubing used to administer TPN and intermittent secondary infusions. Y-tubing used to administer blood can be reused one time for a second unit that immediately follows the first. Medication locks (discussed later) and venipuncture devices are replaced every 3 days or immediately if evidence of complications develops. Central catheters remain in the same site indefinitely.

DISCONTINUING INTRAVENOUS THERAPY

IV infusions are discontinued when the solution has infused and no more is scheduled to follow (Nursing Guidelines 24-2). Alternatively, the venipuncture device may be temporarily capped and kept patent with the use of a **medication lock,** which is a sealed chamber that allows intermittent access to a vein (Fig. 24-13). The lock is inserted into the venipuncture device. The vein is kept patent by flushing the lock with saline or heparinized saline. Medication locks are used when the client no

NURSING GUIDELINES 24-2

Discontinuing an Intravenous Infusion

- Wash your hands.
- Clamp the tubing and remove the tape holding the dressing and venipuncture device in place.
- Don clean gloves.
- Gently press a dry, sterile gauze square over the site (use of an alcohol swab interferes with blood clotting).
- Remove the venipuncture device by pulling it out without hesitation, following the course of the vein.
- Continue to apply pressure to the site for 30 to 45 seconds while elevating the forearm to control bleeding.
- Cover the site with a dressing or bandage.
- Remove gloves and wash your hands.
- Record the time the IV infusion was discontinued, the amount of fluid infused, and the appearance of the venipuncture site.

longer needs continuous infusions, needs intermittent IV medication administration, or may need emergency IV fluids or medications.

GENERAL NUTRITIONAL CONSIDERATIONS

When administered parenterally, dextrose provides 3.4 cal/g, not 4 cal/g like carbohydrates consumed orally. Therefore, 1 L of 5% dextrose in water (D_5W), which contains 50 g dextrose, provides a total of 170 calories. Three liters of D_5W infused over 24 hours provides only 510 calories. Because simple IV solutions (i.e., dextrose in water) are nutritionally and calorically inadequate, it is best to avoid maintaining clients on them longer than 1 to 2 days.

The composition of TPN formulas are individualized according to the client's nutritional requirements and medical condition. Because con-

centrations of protein, carbohydrate, and fat are standard in standard volumes, individualization is somewhat limited.

Although IV lipid emulsions offer several advantages (they are isotonic and high in calories and prevent fatty acid deficiency), they are contraindicated in clients with egg allergy, hyperlipidemia, severe liver disease, and acute pancreatitis.

Cyclical TPN, infused over 10 to 16 hours with 8 to 14 hours of "rest," is used most often for clients on home TPN or to supplement clients consuming an inadequate oral diet. Cyclical TPN offers the client more mobility, especially if infused during the night, and has the advantage of allowing enzyme and hormone levels to drop to normal during the "off" periods. To give the body time to adjust to the decreasing glucose load (and prevent rebound hypoglycemia), the infusion should be tapered near the end of each cycle.

GENERAL PHARMACOLOGIC CONSIDERATIONS

Read labels carefully on vials containing flush solutions for medication locks. Deaths have occurred when potassium chloride has been used incorrectly to flush a lock or central venous catheter.

Never add medications to whole blood or to the saline solution used to start the transfusion.

Additive sets and secondary (piggyback) solution bags are used for intermittent IV drug administration and usually administered in 30 minutes to 2 hours.

Drugs given by the IV route have a more rapid effect than when they are given by other routes.

Before adding a drug to an IV solution, read the label on the container carefully. Only drugs labeled for IV use are given by this route.

Check the literature carefully before adding drugs that will be administered by the IV route. Some medications require special dilution or the use of specific diluents or have warnings regarding the maximum dose allowed.

When medications are added to an IV solution, the container is labeled with the name and dose of the medication, the date and time, and the name of the nurse who added the medication.

Some IV medications, such as dopamine (Intropin), can cause severe tissue damage if they infiltrate. Phentolamine (Regitine) is kept available should dopamine infiltrate. Report infiltration to the physician as soon as possible.

Insulin may be added to TPN solutions to facilitate the metabolism of glucose.

GENERAL GERONTOLOGIC CONSIDERATIONS

IV solutions usually are given at a slower rate for older adults because many of these clients have cardiac or renal disorders.

The application of a tourniquet may traumatize an older adult's skin. Placing a hand towel or washcloth or the sleeve of the gown over the area may reduce skin trauma.

Because veins of older adults tend to be rigid, a venipuncture may pose special difficulty. Poor skin turgor may make it difficult to keep the skin taut over the vein when stabilizing the vein during venipuncture.

Observe confused or disoriented clients frequently because excessive movement or pulling on the IV line may dislodge the venipuncture device.

Older adults are more prone to fluid overload; thus, closely observe them for signs and symptoms of this complication.

FIGURE 24-13 Attaching a lock device with extension tubing to the IV catheter hub. (Photo © B. Proud.)

Critical Thinking Exercises

1. *Determine the rate of infusion for 1000 mL of solution ordered to infuse by gravity over 10 hours. You have tubing with a drop factor of 15 gtt/mL. Explain how you determine if the solution is infusing according to the calculated rate.*
2. *Discuss the nursing care of a client receiving IV therapy.*
3. *Describe one complication of IV therapy and blood administration, and identify its cause, signs and symptoms, and appropriate nursing actions.*

References and Suggested Readings

American Nurses Association. (1997). Post-exposure programs in the event of occupational exposure to HIV/HBV. [On-line.] Available: http://ana.org/readroom/position/blood/blpoex. htm.

Atterbury, C. & Wilkinson, J. (2000). Blood transfusion. *Nursing Standard, 14*(34), 47–53.

Bliss, D. Z. & Dysart, M. (1999). Using needleless intravenous access devices for administering total parenteral nutrition (TPN): Practice update. *Nutrition in Clinical Practice, 14,* 299–303.

Brown, M. & Whalen, P. K. (2000). Red blood cell transfusion in critically ill patients: emerging risks and alternatives. *Critical Care Nurse* December:Suppl:1–16.

Charting tips. (2000). Documenting I.V. therapy: Part 2. *Nursing, 30*(3), 83.

Donnelly, K. (2000). Hepatitis and transfusions. *Nephrology Nursing Journal, 27,* 538–538.

Fabian, B. (2000). Intravenous complication: Infiltration. *Journal of Intravenous Nursing, 23,* 229–231.

Godfrey, K. (2000). In the bag . . . serious hazards of transfusion (SHOT) report. *Nursing Times, 96*(14), 26–27.

Gray, S. & Murphy, M. (1999). Guidelines for administering blood and blood components. *Nursing Standard, 14*(13–15), 36–39.

Harrahill, M. & Boshkov, L. (2000). ABO incompatible transfusion: what you need to know. *Journal of Emergency Nursing, 26*(4), 387–389, 394–398.

Huckleberry, Y. (2001). Intravenous fluids: Which solution and why? *Support Line, 23*(1), 12–13.

Infusion equipment. (2000). *Journal of Intravenous Nursing, 23*(6 Suppl.), S32–S37.

Infusion therapies. (2000). *Journal of Intravenous Nursing, 23* (6 Suppl.), S48–S55.

Intravenous Nurses Society. (1997). Position paper: Midlines and midclavicular catheters. *Journal of Intravenous Nursing, 20,* 175–178.

Karadag, A. & Grgl, S. (2000). Devising an intravenous fluid therapy protocol and compliance of nurses with the protocol. *Journal of Intravenous Nursing, 23*(4), 232–238.

Larouere, E. (2000a). Managing a midline catheter. *Nursing, 30*(4), 17.

Larouere, E. (2000b). Placing a midline catheter. *Nursing, 30*(3), 26.

McConnell, E. A. (2000). Clinical do's & don'ts: Infusing packed RBCs. *Nursing, 30*(1), 82–83.

Morrison, A. (2000). Warming up to safe infusions. *Nursing, 30*(7), 78.

Muder, R. R. (2001). Frequency of intravenous administration set changes and bacteremia: Defining the risk. *Infection Control and Hospital Epidemiology, 22*(3), 134–135.

Pearson, M. L. (2001). Guideline for prevention of intravascular device-related infections. Centers for Disease Control and Prevention. [On-line.] Available: http://www.cdc.gov/ncidod/hip/iv/iv.htm.

Powers, F. A. (1999). Your elderly patient needs I.V. therapy. *Nursing, 29*(7), 54–55.

Raad, I., Hanna, A. A., Awad, A., et al. (2001). Optimal frequency of changing intravenous administration sets: Is it safe to prolong use beyond 72 hours? *Infection Control and Hospital Epidemiology, 22*(3), 136–139.

Simcock, L. (2001). The use of central venous catheters for IV therapy. *Nursing Times, 97*(18), 34–35.

Site care and maintenance. (2000). *Journal of Intravenous Nursing, 23*(6 Suppl.), S48–S55.

Smith, S. A. & Andrews, M. (2000). Artificial nutrition and hydration at the end of life. *MEDSURG Nursing, 9*(5), 233–247.

Stovall, C. J. & Nohe, C. (2001). Attorney General's Opinion No. 95-84: Qualifications of licensed practical nurses to administer intravenous fluid therapy. *Kansas Nurse, 76*(1), 5–8.

Ting, P. (1999) Complications of blood transfusion (part 1 of 2). [On-line.] Available: http://anesthesiology.about.com/health/anesthesiology/library/weekly/aa091399.htm.?iam=dpile&terms=%2Bblood=%2Btransfusion=%2Breaction.

Welk, T. A. (1999). Clinical and ethical considerations of fluid and electrolyte management in the terminally ill client. *Journal of Intravenous Nursing, 22*(1), 43–47.

Workman, B. (2000). Peripheral intravenous therapy management. *Emergency Nurse, 7*(9), 31–37.

Young, J. (2000). Transfusion reaction. *Nursing, 30*(12), 33.

Caring for Perioperative Clients

Words to Know

ambulatory surgery
anesthesia
anesthesiologist
anesthetist
conscious sedation
dehiscence
embolus
evisceration
intraoperative
malignant
   hyperthermia
paralytic ileus
perioperative
phlebothrombosis
postoperative
preoperative
surgical asepsis
thrombophlebitis

Learning Objectives

On completion of this chapter, the reader will:

- Identify reasons why surgical procedures may be performed.
- Differentiate the phases of perioperative care.
- Outline the preoperative assessments needed to identify surgical risk factors.
- Develop a preoperative teaching plan.
- Compare the types of anesthesia.
- Describe members of the surgical team and their functions.
- Discuss assessments needed to prevent postoperative complications.
- Describe standards of care, nursing diagnoses, and common interventions for the general surgical client in the later postoperative period.
- Describe the criteria for clients admitted for ambulatory surgery.

Surgery, no matter how minor, causes stress and poses risks for complications. Many variables, such as procedure performed, age of the client, and coexisting medical conditions determine the care a client needs before, during, and after surgery. Nevertheless, administering anesthesia and disrupting physiologic processes (i.e., through creation of the surgical wound and the operation itself) subject all clients undergoing surgery to a common set of problems, which requires standardized, in addition to individualized, assessments and interventions. All clients require thorough preoperative education.

Nursing goals when caring for surgical clients are to minimize clients' anxiety, prepare them for surgery, and assist in their speedy, uncomplicated recovery. Surgical procedures are performed on emergency, nonurgent, and elective bases. Table 25-1 identifies reasons for surgery; Table 25-2 categorizes surgery in terms of urgency.

PERIOPERATIVE CARE

Perioperative is a term used to describe the entire span of surgery, including before and after the actual operation. The three phases of perioperative care are as follows:

1. **Preoperative:** begins with the decision to perform surgery and continues until the client reaches the operating area
2. **Intraoperative:** includes the entire surgical procedure until transfer of the client to the recovery area
3. **Postoperative:** begins with admission to the recovery area and continues until the client receives a follow-up evaluation at home or is discharged to a rehabilitation unit

Each phase requires specific assessments and nursing interventions.

● PREOPERATIVE CARE

Time for preoperative assessment, nursing diagnoses, and evaluation of the nursing management may be limited when a client is admitted for ambulatory surgery or shortly before surgery. Recognition of the client's immediate preoperative needs is important, however, and preparation for surgery still requires the nursing process.

TABLE 25-1	REASONS FOR SURGERY	
TYPE OF SURGERY	**PURPOSE**	**EXAMPLES**
Diagnostic	Removal and study of tissue to make a diagnosis	Breast biopsy Biopsy of skin lesion
Exploratory	More extensive means to diagnose a problem; usually involves exploration of a body cavity or use of scopes inserted through small incisions	Exploration of abdomen for unexplained pain Exploratory laparoscopy
Curative	Removal or replacement of defective tissue to restore function	Cholecystectomy Total hip replacement
Palliative	Relief of symptoms or enhancement of function without cure	Resection of a tumor to relieve pressure and pain
Cosmetic	Correction of defects, improvement of appearance, or change to a physical feature	Rhinoplasty Cleft lip repair Mammoplasty

Assessment

Preoperative care requires a complete assessment of the client. The assessment varies, depending on the urgency of the surgery and whether the client is admitted the same day of surgery or earlier. Even in emergencies, however, the nurse must make every effort to gather as much data as possible. Box 25-1 lists important information when assessing the preoperative client.

On admission, the nurse reviews preoperative instructions, such as diet restrictions and skin preparations, to ensure the client has followed them. If the client has not carried out a specific portion of the instructions, such as withholding foods and fluids, the nurse immediately notifies the surgeon. He or she identifies the client's needs to determine if the client is at risk for complications during or after the surgery. General risk factors are related to age; nutritional status; use of alcohol, tobacco, and other substances; and physical condition (Table 25-3).

When surgery is not an emergency, the nurse performs a thorough history and physical examination. He or she assesses the client's understanding of the surgical procedure, postoperative expectations, and ability to participate in recovery. The nurse also considers cultural needs, specifically as they relate to beliefs about surgery, personal privacy, and presence of family members during the preoperative and postoperative phases (see Chap. 11). The nurse also questions if the client has strong culturally influenced feelings related to the disposal of body parts and blood transfusions.

If the surgical procedure is an emergency, the nurse may have to omit some tasks because of the client's condition or need for rapid preparation. There may not be time to perform a thorough assessment or write a com-

TABLE 25-2	CATEGORIES OF SURGERY BASED ON URGENCY	
CLASSIFICATION	**CONDITIONS**	**EXAMPLES**
Emergency	Immediate; condition is life-threatening, requiring surgery at once	Gunshot wound Severe bleeding Small bowel obstruction
Urgent	Within 24 to 30 hours; client requires prompt attention	Kidney stones Acute gallbladder infection Fractured hip
Required	Planned for a few weeks or months after decision; client requires surgery at some point	Benign prostatic hypertrophy Cataracts Hernia without strangulation
Elective	Client will not be harmed if surgery is not performed but will benefit if it is performed	Revision of scars Vaginal repairs
Optional	Personal preference	Cosmetic surgery

(Adapted from Smeltzer, S. C. & Bare, B. G. [2000]. *Brunner and Suddarth's textbook of medical–surgical nursing* [9th ed., p. 318]. Philadelphia: Lippincott Williams & Wilkins.)

BOX 25-1 ● Preoperative Assessment

REVIEW PREOPERATIVE LABORATORY AND DIAGNOSTIC STUDIES
- Complete blood count
- Blood type and crossmatch
- Serum electrolytes
- Urinalysis
- Chest x-ray
- Electrocardiogram
- Other tests related to procedure or client's medical condition (e.g., prothrombin time, partial thromboplastin time, blood urea nitrogen, creatinine, other radiographic studies)

REVIEW CLIENT'S HEALTH HISTORY AND PREPARATION FOR SURGERY
- History of present illness and reason for surgery
- Past medical history
  Medical conditions—acute and chronic
  Previous hospitalizations and surgeries
  Any past problems with anesthesia
  Allergies
  Present medications
  Substance use: alcohol, tobacco, street drugs
- Review of systems

ASSESS PHYSICAL NEEDS
- Ability to communicate
- Vital signs

- Level of consciousness
  Confusion
  Drowsiness
  Unresponsiveness
- Weight and height
- Skin integrity
- Ability to move/ambulate
- Level of exercise
- Prostheses
- Circulatory status

ASSESS PSYCHOLOGICAL NEEDS
- Emotional state
- Level of understanding of surgical procedure and preoperative and postoperative instructions
- Coping strategies
- Support system
- Roles and responsibilities

ASSESS CULTURAL NEEDS
- Language—need for an interpreter
- Particular customs related to surgery, privacy, disposal of body parts, and blood transfusions

---

plete care plan. Assessment of the surgical client is essential, but the situation dictates the extent of this process.

Stop, Think, and Respond ● BOX 25-1

A client who is admitted for knee replacement surgery is 100 lb overweight. What are the potential postoperative concerns?

Surgical Consent

Before surgery, the client must sign a surgical consent form or operative permit. When signed, this form indicates that the client consents to the procedure and understands its risks and benefits as explained by the surgeon. If the client has not understood the explanations, the nurse notifies the surgeon before the client signs the consent form. Clients must sign a consent form for any invasive procedure that requires anesthesia and has risks of complications.

If an adult client is confused, unconscious, or not mentally competent, a family member or guardian must sign the consent form. If the client is younger than 18 years of age, a parent or legal guardian must sign the consent form. Persons younger than age 18 years of age, living away from home and supporting themselves, are regarded as emancipated minors and sign their own consent forms. In an emergency, the surgeon may have to operate without consent. Healthcare personnel, however, make every effort to obtain consent by telephone, telegram, or fax. Each nurse must be familiar with agency policies and state laws regarding surgical consent forms.

Clients must sign the consent form before receiving any preoperative sedatives. When the client or designated person has signed the permit, an adult witness also signs it to indicate that the client or designee signed voluntarily. This witness usually is a member of the healthcare team or an employee in the admissions department. The nurse is responsible for ensuring that all necessary parties have signed the consent form and that it is in the client's chart before the client goes to the operating room (OR).

Preoperative Teaching

Teaching clients about their surgical procedure and expectations before and after surgery is best done during the preoperative period. Clients are more alert and free of pain at this time. Clients and family members can better participate in recovery if they know what to expect. The nurse adapts instructions and explanations to the client's ability to understand. The teaching plan addresses the client's cognitive abilities. When clients understand what they can do to help themselves recover, they are more likely to follow the preoperative instructions and work with healthcare team members.

Information to include in a preoperative teaching plan varies with the type of surgery and the length of the hos-

TABLE 25-3	SURGICAL RISK FACTORS AND POTENTIAL COMPLICATIONS
VARIABLE	**POTENTIAL COMPLICATION**
Age	
Very young—Immaturity of organ systems and regulatory mechanisms	Respiratory obstruction, fluid overload, dehydration, hypothermia, and infection
Elderly—Multiple organ degeneration and slowed regulatory mechanisms	Decreased metabolism and excretion of anesthetics and pain medications, fluid overload, renal failure, formation of blood clots, delayed wound healing, infection, confusion, and respiratory complications
Nutritional Status	
Malnourished—Low weight and nutrient deficiencies	Fluid and electrolyte imbalances, cardiac dysrhythmias, delayed wound healing, wound infections
Obese—Stressed cardiovascular system, decreased circulation, decreased pulmonary function	Atelectasis, pneumonia, blood clots, delayed wound healing, wound infection, delayed metabolism and excretion of anesthetics and pain medication
Substance Abuse	
Altered respiratory function, nutritional status, or liver function	Atelectasis, pneumonia, altered effectiveness of anesthetics and pain medications, drug interactions, drug withdrawal
Medical Problems	
Immune—Allergies and immunosuppression secondary to corticosteroid therapy, transplants, chemotherapy, or diseases such as AIDS	Adverse reactions to medications, blood transfusions, or latex; infection
Respiratory—Acute and chronic respiratory problems and history of tobacco use	Atelectasis, bronchopneumonia, respiratory failure
Cardiovascular—Hypertension, coronary artery disease, peripheral vascular disease	Hypotension, hypertension, fluid overload, congestive heart failure, shock, dysrhythmias, myocardial infarction, stroke, blood clots
Hepatic—Liver dysfunction	Delayed drug metabolism leading to drug toxicity, disrupted clotting mechanisms leading to excessive bleeding or hemorrhage, confusion, increased risk of infection
Renal—Kidney disease, chronic renal insufficiency, renal failure	Fluid and electrolyte imbalances, congestive heart failure, dysrhythmias, delayed excretion of drugs leading to drug toxicity
Endocrine—Diabetes	Hypoglycemia, hyperglycemia, hypokalemia, infection, delayed wound healing

pitalization. The following are examples of information to include in preoperative teaching:

- Preoperative medications—when they are given and their effects
- Postoperative pain control
- Explanation and description of the postanesthesia recovery room or postsurgical area
- Discussion of the frequency of assessing vital signs and use of monitoring equipment

The nurse also explains and demonstrates deep breathing and coughing exercises, use of incentive spirometry, how to splint the incision for breathing exercises and moving, position changes, and feet and leg exercises.

The nurse also must inform the client about intravenous (IV) fluids and other lines and tubes. Sometimes IV fluids are initiated before surgery, along with indwelling catheters or nasogastric tubes. When clients have received demonstrations, it is important they return the demonstrations to practice these skills and provide an op-

portunity for the nurse to assess whether the client understood the instructions. Preoperative teaching time also gives the client the chance to express any anxieties and fears and for the nurse to provide explanations that will help alleviate those fears.

When clients are admitted for emergency surgery, time for detailed explanations of preoperative preparations and the postoperative period is unavailable. If the client is alert, however, the nurse provides brief explanations. During the postoperative period, explanations will be more complete. Family members require as many preoperative explanations as possible.

The purpose of adequate preoperative teaching/learning is for the client to have an uncomplicated and shorter recovery period. He or she will be more likely to deep breathe and cough, move as directed, and require less pain medication. The client and family members will demonstrate sufficient knowledge of the surgical procedure, preoperative preparations, and postoperative procedures, and can participate fully in the client's care.

Preoperative Preparation

Preparing a client for surgery is an essential element of preoperative care. It includes both physical and psychosocial preparation.

Physical Preparation

Depending on the time of admission to the hospital or surgical facility, the nurse may perform some of the physical preparation, which includes the following:

- *Skin preparation:* Skin preparation depends on the surgical procedure and the policies of the surgeon or institution. The goal is to decrease bacteria without compromising skin integrity. For planned surgery, the client may be asked to cleanse the particular area with detergent germicide soap for several days before surgery. Hair usually is not removed before surgery unless it is likely to interfere with the incision. In that case, the hair is removed with electric clippers at the time of surgery.
- *Elimination:* The nurse may need to insert an indwelling urinary catheter preoperatively for some surgeries, particularly of the lower abdomen. A distended bladder increases the risks of bladder trauma and difficulty in performing the procedure. The catheter keeps the bladder empty during surgery. If a catheter is not inserted, the nurse instructs the client to void immediately before receiving preoperative medication. Enemas or laxatives may be ordered to clean out the lower bowel if the client is having abdominal or pelvic surgery. A clean bowel allows for accurate visualization of the surgical site and prevents trauma to the intestine or accidental contamination by feces to the peritoneum. A cleansing enema or laxative is prescribed the evening before surgery and may be repeated the morning of surgery. If bowel surgery is scheduled, antibiotics also may be prescribed to reduce intestinal flora.
- *Food and fluids:* The physician gives specific instructions about how long before surgery food and fluids are to be withheld, often at least 8 to 10 hours before surgery. After midnight the night before surgery, the client usually is not allowed to have anything by mouth (NPO). Many ambulatory surgical centers, however, allow clear fluids up to 3 or 4 hours before surgery. Before these times, the nurse encourages the client to maintain good nutrition to help meet the body's increased need for nutrients during the healing process. Protein and ascorbic acid (vitamin C) are especially important in wound healing.
- *Care of valuables:* The nurse encourages the client to give valuables to a family member to take home. If this is not possible, however, the nurse itemizes the valuables, places them in an envelope, and locks them in a designated area. The client signs a receipt, and the nurse notes on the client's chart their disposition. If the client is reluctant to remove a wedding band, the nurse may slip gauze under the ring then loop the gauze around the finger and wrist or apply adhesive tape over a plain wedding band. The client also removes eyeglasses and contact lenses, which the nurse places in a safe location or gives to a family member.
- *Attire/grooming:* Usually clients wear a hospital gown and a surgical cap in the OR. Hair ornaments and all makeup and nail polish must be removed. If the client is having minor surgery performed under local anesthesia in a room separate from the general surgical suites, the nurse instructs the client on what clothing and cosmetics to remove and provides appropriate hospital attire. The physician may order thigh-high or knee-high antiembolism stockings or order the client's legs to be wrapped in elastic bandages before surgery to help prevent venous stasis during and after the surgery. Removal of cosmetics assists the surgical team to observe the client's lips, face, and nail beds for cyanosis, pallor, or other signs of decreased oxygenation. If a client has acrylic nails, one usually is removed to attach a pulse oximeter, which measures oxygen saturation (see Chap. 27).
- *Prostheses:* Depending on agency policy and physician preference, the client removes full or partial dentures. Doing so prevents the dentures from becoming dislodged or causing airway obstruction during administration of a general anesthetic. Some anesthesiologists prefer that well-fitting dentures be left in place to preserve facial contours. If dentures are removed, the nurse usually places them in a denture container and leaves them at the client's bedside or places them with the client's belongings. Other prostheses, such as artificial limbs, also are removed, unless otherwise ordered.

Preoperative Medications

The anesthesiologist frequently orders preoperative medications. Common preoperative medications include the following:

- *Anticholinergics,* which decrease respiratory tract secretions, dry mucous membranes, and interrupt vagal stimulation
- *Antianxiety drugs,* which reduce preoperative anxiety, slow motor activity, and promote induction of anesthesia
- *Histamine-2 receptor antagonists,* which decrease gastric acidity and volume
- *Narcotics,* which decrease the amount of anesthesia needed, help reduce anxiety and pain, and promote sleep
- *Sedatives,* which promote sleep, decrease anxiety, and reduce the amount of anesthesia needed

- *Tranquilizers,* which reduce nausea, prevent emesis, and enhance preoperative sedation

Drug Therapy Table 25-1 provides more information about dosages and desired and adverse effects of preoperative medications.

Before administering preoperative medications, the nurse checks the client's identification bracelet, asks about drug allergies, obtains blood pressure (BP) and pulse and respiratory rates, asks the client to void, and makes sure the surgical consent form has been signed. The nurse also reviews with the client what to expect after receiving the medications. Immediately after giving the medications, the nurse instructs the client to remain in bed; he or she places side rails in the up position and ensures that the call button is within easy reach.

Psychosocial Preparation

Preparing the client emotionally and spiritually is as important as doing so physically. Psychosocial preparation should begin as soon as the client is aware that surgery

---

DRUG THERAPY TABLE 25-1 | PREOPERATIVE MEDICATIONS

DRUG CATEGORY AND EXAMPLES	MECHANISM OF ACTION	SIDE EFFECTS	NURSING CONSIDERATIONS
Anticholinergics atropine sulfate, scopolamine, glycopyrrolate (Robinul)	Decreases oral, respiratory, and gastric secretions Prevents laryngospasm and reflex bradycardia	Dry mouth; tachycardia; excessive CNS stimulation (tremor, restlessness, confusion), followed by excessive CNS depression (coma, respiratory depression); constipation; paralytic ileus; urinary retention; ocular effects: mydriasis, blurred vision, photophobia	Inform client that a dry mouth may occur, but to refrain from taking oral fluids. Immediately after administering the medications, instruct client to remain in bed. Place side rails in the up position, and ensure the call button is in easy reach.
Antiemetics droperidol (Inapsine), promethazine (Phenergan)	Reduces nausea, prevents emesis, and enhances preoperative sedation	Dry mouth; urinary retention; hypotension, including orthostatic hypotension; extrapyramidal reactions—dyskinesia, dystonia, akathisia, parkinsonism	Inform client that drowsiness may occur about 20 minutes after administration.
Tranquilizers (hypnotics) diazepam (Valium), flurazepam (Dalmane), lorazepam (Ativan)	Reduces preoperative anxiety and promotes induction of anesthesia	Depression of breathing	Inform client that drowsiness will occur about 20 minutes after administration. Immediately after administering the medication, instruct client to remain in bed. Place side rails in the up position, and ensure the call button is in easy reach.
Sedatives midazolam (Versed), barbiturates: phenobarbital (Nembutal), secobarbital (Seconal)	Promotes sleep, decreases anxiety, and promotes the use of anesthesia	Depression of breathing; may produce coughing, sneezing, and laryngospasm	Inform client that drowsiness will occur about 20 minutes after administration. Immediately after administering the medication, instruct client to remain in bed. Place side rails in the up position, and ensure the call button is in easy reach. Because these drugs require injection, they are not useful for children, who have small veins.
Opioids (narcotics) morphine, meperidine (Demerol)	Reduces anxiety and pain, promotes sleep, and decreases amount of anesthesia needed	May slow rate of respiration, hypotension, dizziness, nausea, vomiting, constipation	Inform client that drowsiness will occur about 20 minutes after administration. Immediately after administering the medication, instruct client to remain in bed. Place side rails in the up position, and ensure the call button is in easy reach.

CNS, central nervous system.

is necessary. Anxiety and fear, if extreme, can affect a client's condition during and after surgery. Anxious clients have a poor response to surgery and are prone to complications. Many clients are fearful because they know little or nothing about what will happen before, during, and after surgery. Careful preoperative teaching can reduce fear and anxiety. Careful listening and explaining by the nurse about what will happen and what to expect can help allay some of these fears and anxieties. The nurse also must assess methods the client uses for coping. Religious faith is a source of strength for many clients; therefore, nurses facilitate contact with a client's clergyperson or the hospital chaplain, if requested.

Preoperative Checklist

Most clients are transported to the OR on a stretcher. To provide privacy, safety, and warmth, the nurse covers the client with a blanket and fastens the restraint straps around the client. Before the client leaves the room, the nurse records all necessary information on the client's chart: vital signs, weight, preoperative medications administered, procedures performed, whether the client has voided, disposition of valuables and dentures, and pertinent observations.

Most hospitals or surgical facilities use a preoperative checklist to ensure that all assessments and procedures for the client are complete before surgery. A checklist usually includes the following:

- *Assessment:* includes the identification and allergy bracelet; identification of allergies; list of current medications; last time the client ate or drank; disposition of valuables, dentures, or prostheses; removal of makeup and nail polish; and wearing of hospital attire
- *Preoperative medications:* includes route and time administered
- *IV:* includes location, type of solution, rate
- *Preoperative preparations:* includes, as appropriate, skin preparation; indwelling urinary catheter or nasogastric tube insertion; time and results of enemas or douches; application of antiembolism stockings or wraps; and time and amount of last voiding
- *Chart:* includes surgical consent signed and on chart; history and physical completed by physician and on chart; old records with chart; and ordered test results on chart (e.g., electrocardiogram, complete blood count, urinalysis, type and screen or type and crossmatch for blood transfusions)
- *Other information:* as required by agency policy
- *Signature(s):* of nurse and other personnel involved with preparing the client for surgery and transporting the client to the OR

When the preoperative checklist is complete, the client is ready to go to the operating suite. Personnel from the OR assist in the transfer of the client to the stretcher and then to the OR or surgical holding area.

NURSING PROCESS

● **Preoperative Care**

Assessment

The nurse assesses the client's physical and psychological status, as described earlier in this section.

Diagnosis, Planning, and Interventions

Anxiety related to upcoming surgery, results of surgery, and postoperative pain
Expected Outcome: Client will express feelings of anxiety.
- Ask what concerns the client has about the upcoming surgery. *Such discussion provides specific information about the client's fears.*
- Provide appropriate explanations for preoperative procedures and postoperative expectations. *Clients will experience less anxiety if they know what to expect.*
- Maintain as much contact as possible with the client. *Being present and approachable encourages communication.*

Deficient Knowledge related to preoperative procedures and postoperative expectations
Expected Outcome: Client will verbalize understanding of preoperative and postoperative procedures.
- Assess client's level of knowledge about the perioperative plans. *Building on a client's knowledge assists in reinforcing instructions and helps to correct false information.*
- Use audiovisual aids to present information. *Verbal reinforcement of other forms of instruction promotes learning.*
- Include family members or significant others in preoperative instructions. *These people help in reinforcing instructions and providing support to the client.*

Evaluation of Expected Outcomes

The client reports minimal anxiety. He or she demonstrates knowledge of the preoperative instructions and demonstrates postoperative exercises.

● INTRAOPERATIVE CARE

The intraoperative period begins when the client is transferred to the operating table. The surgical team is responsible for the client's care during this time.

Anesthesia

Anesthesia is the partial or complete loss of the sensation of pain with or without the loss of consciousness. Surgical procedures are performed with general, regional, or local anesthesia.

General Anesthesia

General anesthesia acts on the central nervous system to produce loss of sensation, reflexes, and consciousness. Vital functions such as breathing, circulation, and temperature control are not regulated physiologically when general anesthetics are used. General anesthetics are administered as IV, intramuscular (IM), inhaled, or rectal medications. Four stages are used to describe the induction of general anesthesia:

1. *Induction or beginning stage:* This short period is crucial for producing unconsciousness. The client experiences dizziness, detachment, a temporary heightened sense of awareness to noises and movements, and a sensation of "heavy" extremities and being unable to move them. Inhaled or IV anesthetics are used to produce this phase. When the client becomes unconscious, his or her airway is secured with an endotracheal tube.

2. *Excitement:* During this stage the client may struggle, shout, talk, sing, laugh, or cry. He or she may make uncontrolled movements, so team members must protect the client from falling or other injury. Quick and smooth administration of anesthesia can prevent this phase.

3. *Surgical anesthesia:* In this stage the client remains unconscious through continuous administration of the anesthetic agent. This level of anesthesia may be maintained for hours with a range of light to deep anesthesia.

4. *Medullary depression:* This stage occurs when the client receives too much anesthesia. The client will have shallow respirations, weak pulse, and widely dilated pupils unresponsive to light. Without prompt intervention, death can occur (Smeltzer & Bare, 2000).

Usually, with smooth administration of general anesthesia, there is no major division between the first three stages, and the fourth stage does not occur. Throughout the duration of and recovery from anesthesia, team members closely monitor the client for effective breathing and oxygenation, effective circulatory status, including BP and pulse within normal ranges, effective regulation of temperature, and adequate fluid balance. When anesthetics are carefully withdrawn at the end of a surgical procedure, the client will wake enough to follow commands and breathe independently. The endotracheal tube used for inhaled anesthetics may be removed before the client leaves the OR. The recovery period can be brief or long. Many effects of general anesthesia take some time for the client to eliminate completely. Usually clients do not remember much about the initial recovery period.

Regional Anesthesia

Regional anesthesia uses local anesthetics to block the conduction of nerve impulses in a specific region (Table 25-4). The client experiences loss of sensation and decreased mobility to the specific anesthetized area. He or she does not lose consciousness. Depending on the surgery, the

TABLE 25-4	REGIONAL ANESTHESIA	
TYPE OF REGIONAL ANESTHESIA	**ANESTHETIC USES AND EFFECTS**	**EXAMPLES**
Local anesthesia	Provides local loss of sensation Used primarily for dental, eye, and minor surgeries Administered topically or by local infiltration when medicine is injected into and under the epidural surface of the area to be treated	procaine (Novocaine) lidocaine (Xylocaine) bupivacaine (Marcaine) dibucaine (Nupercaine)
Spinal anesthesia	Local anesthetic injected into the subarachnoid space of the lumbar area (usually L4 or L5), which contains cerebrospinal fluid Anesthetizes spinal nerves as they exit the spinal cord Used for surgery involving the abdomen, perineum, and lower extremities	procaine (Novocaine) lidocaine (Xylocaine) tetracaine (Pontocaine)
Epidural block	Local anesthetic injected into the extradural space near the spinal cord, anesthetizing several spinal nerves at once Although similar to spinal anesthesia, headache that frequently follows usually not present; greater technical competence, however, is required	Same as above; opioids such as morphine or fentanyl may be added to enhance the anesthetic effect and to provide analgesia when the block has worn off
Peripheral nerve block	Local anesthetic injected in a specific body region and directed at a particular nerve or group of nerves Peripheral nerve blocks named according to region in which anesthetic is injected; examples are brachial plexus block, ulnar nerve block, and sciatic nerve block Requires a high level of technical competence	lidocaine (Xylocaine) mepivacaine (Carbocaine) bupivacaine (Marcaine)

client may be given a sedative before the local anesthetic to promote relaxation and comfort during the procedure. Types of regional anesthesia include local anesthetics, spinal anesthesia, and conduction blocks. Advantages of regional anesthesia include less risk for respiratory, cardiac, or gastrointestinal complications. There may be issues related to allergic responses and toxicity (overdose). Team members must monitor the client for signs of allergic reactions, changes in vital signs, and toxic reactions. In addition, they must protect the anesthetized area from injury while sensation is absent. The client is at risk for injuries and burns.

Surgical Team

The surgical team consists of an anesthesiologist or anesthetist, surgeon and his or her assistants, and intraoperative nurses.

The **anesthesiologist** is a physician who has completed 2 years of residency in anesthesia. This person is responsible for administering anesthesia to the client and for monitoring the client during and after the surgical procedure. The anesthesiologist assesses the client before surgery, writes preoperative medication orders, informs the client of the options for anesthesia, and explains the risks involved.

The **anesthetist** may be a medical doctor who administers anesthesia but has not completed a residency in anesthesia, a dentist who administers limited types of anesthesia, or a registered nurse (RN) who has completed an accredited nurse anesthesia program and passed the certification examination (Certified Registered Nurse Anesthetist [CRNA]). The anesthesiologist supervises the anesthetist. The anesthetist may assess the client before surgery, discuss options for anesthesia, write preoperative medication orders, administer anesthesia, and monitor the client during and after surgery. The anesthesiologist and anesthetist are not sterile members of the surgical team, meaning that they wear OR attire but they do not wear sterile gowns or work within the sterile field.

The *surgeon* heads the surgical team. He or she is a physician, oral surgeon, or podiatrist with specific training and qualifications. The surgeon is responsible for determining the surgical procedure required, obtaining the client's consent, performing the procedure, and following the client after surgery.

Surgical assistants are classified as either first, second, or third assistants. The *first assistant* assists in the surgical procedure and may be involved with the client's preoperative and postoperative care. He or she may be another physician, a surgical resident, or an RN who has appropriate approval and endorsement from the American Operating Room Nurses and the American College of Surgeons. Second or third assistants are RNs, licensed practical or vocational nurses (LPNs/LVNs), or surgical

technologists who assist the surgeon and first assistant. All assistants are sterile members of the surgical team—they wear sterile gloves and gowns over OR attire and work within the sterile field.

Intraoperative nurses include the *scrub nurse* and *circulating nurse*. The scrub nurse wears a sterile gown and gloves and assists the surgical team by handing instruments to the surgeon and assistants, preparing sutures, receiving specimens for laboratory examination, and counting sponges and needles. The circulating nurse wears OR attire but not a sterile gown. Responsibilities include obtaining and opening wrapped sterile equipment and supplies before and during surgery, keeping records, adjusting lights, receiving specimens for laboratory examination, and coordinating activities of other personnel, such as the pathologist and radiology technician.

The Operating Room Environment

The OR or surgical suite environment is physically isolated from other areas of the hospital or surgical clinic. This restricts access to the area, so that only authorized OR personnel and surgical clients are there. In the surgical suite, air is filtered and positive pressure is maintained to reduce the number of possible microbes that can cause infection. There also are separate clean and contaminated areas. Surgical suites are designed to be efficient, in that the needed equipment and supplies are immediately available for use. Usually the furniture is made of stainless steel for easy cleaning and disinfecting. The temperature in the OR is kept below 70°F to provide a cooler environment that does not promote bacterial growth, to offer more comfort for OR personnel working in bright lights and wearing OR attire, and to maintain a temperature that enhances client comfort and safety.

OR personnel wear specific attire that decreases the opportunity for microbial growth. They strictly adhere to rules about where to change clothes and what to wear in the OR, including protective attire. Box 25-2 identifies typical OR attire. In addition, OR personnel must report any symptoms of infection they are experiencing, be-

---

BOX 25-2 ● Operating Room Attire

- *Scrubs* include tops, pants with cuffs, and jackets with cuffs. Changing rooms are located near the OR; personnel change into OR attire before entering the OR and take OR attire off when they leave.
- *Masks* are worn at all times in the OR; personnel change masks between surgical procedures or if masks become wet.
- *Headgear* is worn to cover the hair and hairline. Beards also must be covered.
- *Shoes* should be comfortable. Agencies vary in specific requirements. Shoe covers also are worn over the shoes. The conductive covers provide an electrical ground.

cause colds, sore throats, and skin infections are potential sources of infection to the client.

Nursing Management

Nursing management during the intraoperative period depends on routine tasks performed during surgery as well as on variables such as type of surgery performed, type of anesthesia used, client's age and condition, and any complications. Asepsis in the OR is the responsibility of all OR personnel. **Surgical asepsis** prevents contamination of surgical wounds. The risk of infection is high because of the break in skin integrity from the surgical incision. The client's own pathogens, plus those found in the OR, create an unsafe environment if personnel neglect to uphold strict aseptic technique. Thus, they strictly follow asepsis protocols to protect the client as much as possible.

The client's safety and protection during surgery are essential. Assessment of the client in the OR is based largely on the type or extent of surgery, the client's age, and any pre-existing conditions. Depending on circumstances, assessment before the administration of the anesthetic may include the following:

- BP and pulse and respiratory rates
- Level of consciousness
- General physical condition
- Presence of catheters and tubes
- Review of client's chart, including a signed operative permit, administration of preoperative medications (time, dose, client response), voiding, skin preparation, carrying out other preoperative orders, and laboratory and diagnostic tests

Possible Intraoperative Complications

Nurses who work in the OR assess the client continuously and protect the client from potential complications, including:

- *Infection:* Strict aseptic technique is absolutely necessary before and during surgery. If a nurse notes a break in technique, he or she immediately notifies the surgeon and OR personnel. Clients are also at risk for the retention of foreign objects in the wound. The scrub nurse and circulating nurse count surgical instruments, gauze sponges, and sharps to prevent this problem. The circulating nurse records the counts on the intraoperative record.
- *Fluid volume excess or deficit:* The anesthesiologist usually adds fluids to the IV lines, but the circulating nurse also may perform this function. The circulating nurse is responsible for recording and keeping a running total of IV fluids administered. If the client has an indwelling catheter, the nurse measures urine output during surgery.

- *Injury related to positioning:* The OR staff positions the client on the OR table according to the type of surgery. Careful positioning and monitoring help to prevent interruption of blood supply secondary to prolonged pressure, nerve injury related to prolonged pressure, postoperative hypotension, dependent edema, and joint injury related to poor body alignment.
- *Hypothermia:* During the procedure, the client may be at risk for hypothermia related to the low temperature in the OR, administration of cold IV fluids, inhalation of cool gases, exposure of body surfaces for the surgical procedure, opened incisions/wounds, and prolonged inactivity. For some surgeries, the body temperature is deliberately lowered to make the procedure safer (Smeltzer & Bare, 2000).
- *Malignant hyperthermia:* This inherited disorder occurs when body temperature, muscle metabolism, and heat production increase rapidly, progressively, and uncontrollably in response to stress and some anesthetic agents. Symptoms include tachycardia, tachypnea, cyanosis, fever, muscle rigidity, diaphoresis, mottled skin, hypotension, irregular heart rate, decreased urine output, and cardiac arrest. Prevention of malignant hyperthermia is essential because the mortality rate is high. Clients at risk include "those with bulky, strong muscles, a history of muscle cramps or muscle weakness and unexpected temperature elevation and an unexplained death of a family member during surgery that was accompanied by a febrile response" (Smeltzer & Bare, 2000, p. 343). The circulating nurse closely monitors the client for signs of hyperthermia. If the client's temperature begins to rise rapidly, anesthesia is discontinued and the OR team implements measures to correct physiologic problems, such as fever or dysrhythmias.

● POSTOPERATIVE CARE

The postoperative period designates the time that the client spends recovering from the effects of anesthesia. Factors such as the client's age and nutritional status, pre-existing diseases, type of surgery, and length of anesthesia may affect the duration, type, and extent of nursing management.

Transport of the Client

Immediately after the surgical procedure is complete, the client is transported to the postanesthesia care unit (PACU), also known as the *recovery room*, located near the OR. The nursing staff there is specifically knowledgeable in the care of clients recovering from anesthesia. Specialized equipment is available to monitor and treat the client. Surgical and anesthesia personnel are immediately available for any emergencies.

Nursing Management

Nurses must follow standards of care for postoperative clients. The following material provides commonly used nursing diagnoses and interventions in postoperative care. It does not provide a complete list but contains minimum standards for the general surgical client. Other standards may also apply.

NURSING PROCESS

● **Nursing Standards for Care of the Postsurgical Client**

Standard I: Respiratory function is maintained.

Risk for Altered Respiratory Function and **PC: Atelectasis/Pneumonia** related to immobility, effects of anesthesia and analgesics, and pain
Expected Outcome: Client will have clear lungs and full and unlabored respirations.
- Monitor respiratory rate and characteristics.
- Auscultate lung sounds once a shift or more often if indicated.
- Help client turn and deep breathe every 1 to 2 hours.
- Reinforce use of incentive spirometer.
- Show client how to splint incision before coughing.
- Assess client's ability to mobilize secretions; suction if necessary.
- Administer oxygen as ordered.
- Refrain from administering narcotic analgesics if respiratory rate is less than 12 breaths/minute.
- Encourage early ambulation.

Standard II: Circulatory function is maintained.

PC: Fluid/Electrolyte Imbalance
Expected Outcome: The nurse will manage imbalances in fluid and electrolytes.
- Assess vital signs and monitor laboratory values.
- Ensure that IV fluids are infusing at the prescribed rate and that the IV site is patent.
- Monitor postoperative intake and output for at least 48 hours or until all drains and tubes have been removed, client is tolerating oral intake, and urine output is normal.
- Report discrepancies in intake and output, hypotension, dizziness, palpitations, or abnormal laboratory values. (See Chap. 22 for additional information on management of fluid and electrolyte imbalance.)

PC: Hemorrhage and **Hypovolemic Shock**
Expected Outcome: The nurse will manage and minimize hemorrhage and shock.
- Monitor for signs or symptoms of shock: tachycardia, hypotension, decreased urine output, cold, clammy skin, restlessness.
- Keep head of bed flat unless contraindicated.
- Maintain patent IV line.
- Assess surgical site for excessive external bleeding.
- Reinforce dressing or apply pressure if bleeding is frank.
- Monitor for internal bleeding: peri-incisional hematoma and swelling, abdominal distention if abdominal surgery was performed, excessive bloody output in wound drainage collection devices, falling hemoglobin and hematocrit levels, orthostatic hypotension, and signs of impending shock. (See Chap. 23 for additional information on management of shock.)
- Report findings immediately.

Standard III: Pain and discomfort are recognized and effectively treated.

Pain related to surgical incision and manipulation of body structures
Expected Outcome: Client will experience relief of pain.
- Assess pain level using an established scale (visual or numerical).
- Determine source of pain (e.g., incision, body position, flatus, IV lines or drainage tubes, distended bladder).
- Provide pain medication and evaluate effectiveness 30 minutes after administration.
- Reposition client to improve comfort.
- Teach client nonpharmacologic methods of pain relief: breathing exercises, relaxation techniques, and distraction. (See Chap. 21 for additional information on pain management.)

Altered Comfort (nausea and vomiting) related to effects of anesthesia or side effects of narcotics
Expected Outcome: Client will report increased comfort and relief of nausea and vomiting.
- Encourage client to breathe deeply to help eliminate inhaled anesthetics.
- Help client sit up and turn head to one side while vomiting to avoid aspiration.
- Record intake and output.
- Offer small sips of flat ginger ale or cola, or ice chips if permitted.
- Administer antiemetics as ordered.
- Provide mouth care and fresh linens after vomiting.
- Monitor intake and output and assess for signs or symptoms of dehydration or electrolyte imbalance (see Chap. 22).

Risk for Sleep Pattern Disturbance related to difficulty in assuming comfortable position secondary to surgery, unusual environment, noise, and interruptions

Expected Outcome: Client will report enhanced sleep pattern.
- Identify factors contributing to poor sleep (noise, room temperature, position, daytime sleeping, hospital routines).
- Reduce environmental distractions—use night lights, close door.
- Schedule nursing activities to coincide with client's schedule.
- Teach client progressive relaxation techniques and deep breathing exercises to facilitate sleep.
- Provide back rub.
- Assist with hygiene; provide clean gown and linens.
- Limit daytime sleeping; encourage increased daytime activity.
- Collaborate with physician about sleeping medication if other methods fail.

Standard IV: Client safety is maintained.

Risk for Injury related to decreased alertness secondary to effects of anesthesia and pain medication
Expected Outcome: Client will remain free of injury.
- Place bed in low position and elevate side rails.
- Place call bell in reach.
- Ensure that tubings are long enough or properly secured to allow for movement. Inspect drainage tubes for kinks.
- Ensure that all equipment is functioning properly.
- Provide emesis basin, tissues, ice chips (if allowed), bedpan, and urinal within easy reach.
- Instruct clients to call for assistance with any activity.

Standard V: Wound healing is promoted and wound management is provided.

Risk for Infection related to break in skin integrity (surgical incision, wound drainage devices)
Expected Outcome: Wound healing is uncomplicated, as shown by intact edges, granulation tissue, and lack of induration or swelling at site.
- Inspect surgical site and peri-incisional drain sites for signs or symptoms of infection (redness, warmth, tenderness, separation of wound edges, purulent drainage).
- Wash hands before and after dressing changes; follow aseptic or sterile technique.
- Change wet dressings frequently (surgeon usually does first dressing change).
- Use skin barrier to protect skin and wound from irritating drainage.
- Avoid using excessive tape.
- Keep drainage tube exit sites clean.
- Prevent excess tension on drainage tubes by securing tubes to dressing.
- Empty collection devices frequently to promote drainage; note characteristics of drainage.

- Teach client to splint wound when coughing or changing position.

Standard VI: Complication potential is continuously assessed, and any complications are immediately and effectively treated.

PC: Deep Vein Thrombosis
Expected Outcome: The nurse will manage and minimize risk of phlebitis/thrombosis.
- Reinforce need to perform leg exercises every hour while awake.
- Instruct client not to cross legs or prop pillow under knees.
- Apply compression and antiembolic stockings as ordered.
- Monitor for signs and symptoms of thrombophlebitis: calf pain, tenderness, warmth, or redness; swelling of the extremity, low-grade fever. Notify physician of any such signs or symptoms, and maintain bed rest until client can be further evaluated.
- Ambulate or encourage client to ambulate for a few minutes each hour while awake.
- Help client avoid prolonged sitting and poorly fitting, constrictive antiembolic hose.
- Do not massage calves or thighs.
- Administer anticoagulant medication as ordered; monitor laboratory values for therapeutic levels.

PC: Acute Urinary Retention
Expected Outcome: The nurse will manage and minimize risk of urinary retention.
- Assess for bladder distention, discomfort, and urge to void.
- Encourage client to try to void within the first 4 hours after surgery.
- Assess volume of first voided urine to determine adequacy of output (voiding frequent, small amounts indicates retention of urine with elimination of overflow only).
- If client has difficulty voiding in the bedpan or using the urinal in bed, stand male clients (if allowed) and ambulate female clients to bathroom (if allowed).
- If client cannot void within 8 hours of surgery, consult with physician regarding instituting intermittent catheterization until voluntary voiding returns.

PC: Paralytic Ileus
Expected Outcome: The nurse will manage and minimize risk for developing postoperative paralytic ileus.
- Assess bowel sounds every shift or more often if indicated.
- Assess returning bowel function as evidenced by passage of flatus or stool.
- Maintain NPO status until bowel sounds return.
- Report large amounts of emesis (more than 300 mL).
- Provide client with moistened gauze to wet lips and tongue until oral intake is allowed.
- Assist with passage of nasogastric tube, if ordered.

Standard VII: Gastrointestinal function is maintained.

Risk for Colonic Constipation related to effects of anesthesia, surgery (manipulation of abdominal organs), side effects of narcotics, and decreased intake of fluids and fiber

Expected Outcome: Client will have regular bowel movements.

- Once bowel sounds have returned and client resumes oral intake, encourage intake of sufficient fluids and fiber.
- Encourage ambulation to promote peristalsis.
- Encourage use of bathroom if possible. Provide privacy if client must use bedside commode or bedpan.
- Administer bulk-forming laxatives or stool softeners prophylactically if ordered.
- Notify physician if client has had no bowel movement within 2 to 3 days after surgery.

Standard VIII: Self-care and mobility are encouraged as appropriate.

Activity Intolerance related to decreased mobility and weakness secondary to anesthesia and surgery

Expected Outcome: Client will regain strength and activity tolerance.

- Encourage progressive activity.
- Help client dangle legs over bedside the evening of surgery or the next morning, if allowed, followed by sitting out of bed for 15 minutes (or more if tolerated).
- Progress to ambulation in room and hallway.
- Collaborate with client in establishing goals to increase ambulation.
- Help client with hygiene the evening of surgery; encourage increased self-care as appropriate.
- Schedule regular rest periods.

Standard IX: Psychosocial needs are recognized and effectively managed.

Anxiety related to unfamiliar environment, loss of privacy, threat to biologic integrity, and fear secondary to illness and surgery

Expected Outcome: Client will share anxieties and report increased psychological comfort.

- Ask client to rate anxiety level on a scale of 0 (none) to 10 (unbearable).
- Explore reasons for anxiety (concerns about health, financial status, family coping, effects on independence). Provide information and reassurance.
- Provide referrals if appropriate.
- Encourage client to use anxiety reduction techniques (see Chap. 14).
- Determine how to modify the environment to improve relaxation (e.g., close or open curtains, reduce noise, move client closer to nurses' station).
- Assess anxiety level after interventions.

Standard X: Discharge instructions, including follow-up care and home health services, are provided.

Risk for Ineffective Management of Therapeutic Regimen related to incomplete knowledge of wound care, activity and diet restrictions, medications, reportable signs and symptoms, and follow-up care

Expected Outcome: Client or family will demonstrate ability to provide wound care, restate specific instructions regarding diet and activity, and identify signs and symptoms of complications and needed follow-up care.

- Explain, demonstrate, and provide written instructions about care of surgical wound.
- Observe the client or family performing care.
- Discuss signs and symptoms of wound infection, and instruct client and family to contact healthcare provider if they develop.
- Describe and provide written instructions about activity restrictions and when to resume normal activity.
- Include information on walking, bending, lifting, climbing stairs, bathing, showering, driving, and engaging in sexual activity.
- Explain need for adequate nutrition and fluids and how to manage constipation, which can result from decreased intake, decreased activity, and narcotic pain relievers.
- Review all medications, including dose, route of administration, intended effect, side effects, and duration of prescription.
- Review signs and symptoms of complications such as shortness of breath, fever, productive cough, weakness, new or unusual pain, pain unrelieved by medication, calf tenderness and swelling, and wound drainage.
- Evaluate client and family's understanding of discharge instructions.

(Adapted from Carpenito, L. J. [2001]. *Nursing diagnosis: Application to clinical practice* (9th ed.). Philadelphia: Lippincott, Williams & Wilkins; and Nettina, S. [2000]. *The Lippincott manual of nursing practice* (7th ed.). Philadelphia: Lippincott, Williams & Wilkins.)

Immediate Postoperative Period

The circulating nurse or anesthesiologist reports pertinent information regarding the surgery, including any complications. The most important aspect of nursing management is close observation and monitoring of the client during emergence from anesthesia.

INITIAL ASSESSMENT

Initial postoperative assessments include airway patency; effectiveness of respirations; presence of artificial airways, mechanical ventilation, or supplemental oxygen; circulatory status; vital signs; wound condition, including dressings and drains; fluid balance, including IV fluids, output from catheters and drains, and ability to void; level of consciousness; and pain. The nurse's major responsibilities during the client's PACU stay are to ensure a patent airway; help maintain adequate circulation; prevent or assist with the treatment of shock; maintain proper position and function of drains, tubes, and IV infusions; and monitor for potential complications.

POSTOPERATIVE COMPLICATIONS

Hemorrhage. Hemorrhage can be internal or external. If the client loses a lot of blood, he or she will exhibit signs and symptoms of shock (see Chap. 23). The nurse inspects dressings frequently for signs of bleeding and checks the bedding under the client, because blood may pool under the body and be evident on the bedding. If bleeding is internal, the client may need to return to surgery for ligation of the bleeding vessels. Blood transfusions may be necessary to replace lost blood. When bleeding occurs, the nurse notes the amount and color on the chart. Bright red blood signifies fresh bleeding; dark, brownish blood indicates older blood. The nurse may need to reinforce soiled or saturated dressings. A written order is needed to change dressings. The nurse also must be aware of any wound drains and the type and amount of drainage expected. If such drainage is expected, the nurse explains to the client that the drainage is normal and does not indicate a complication. He or she places incontinence pads under the client if drainage occurs.

Shock. Fluid and electrolyte loss, trauma (both physical and psychological), anesthetics, and preoperative medications all may contribute to shock. Signs and symptoms include pallor, fall in BP, weak and rapid pulse rate, restlessness, and cool, moist skin (see Chap. 23). Shock must be detected early and treated promptly because it can irreversibly damage vital organs such as the brain, kidneys, and heart.

Narcotics are not administered to a client in shock until a physician evaluates the client, who should remain supine. Some physicians advocate elevating the legs to enhance the flow of venous blood to the heart. Treatment of shock varies and depends on the cause, if known. Blood, plasma expanders, parenteral fluids, oxygen, and medications such as adrenergic agonists may be used (see Chap. 23).

Hypoxia. Factors such as residual drug effects or overdose, pain, poor positioning, pooling of secretions in the lungs, or obstructed airway predispose the client to hypoxia (decreased oxygen). Oxygen and suction equipment must be available for immediate use. The nurse observes the client closely for signs of cyanosis and dyspnea. Breathing may be obstructed if the tongue falls back and blocks the nasopharynx. If this occurs, the nurse pulls the lower jaw and inserts an oropharyngeal airway (Fig. 25-1). Positioning the client on his or her side also may relieve nasopharyngeal obstruction. Restlessness, crowing or grunting respirations, diaphoresis, bounding

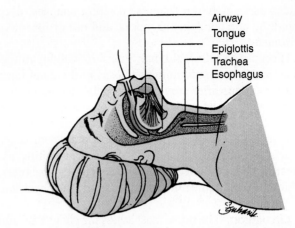

FIGURE 25-1 Oropharygeal airway in place. (From Smeltzer, S. C. & Bare, B. G. [2000]. *Brunner & Suddarth's textbook of medical–surgical nursing* [9th ed.]. Philadelphia: Lippincott Williams & Wilkins.)

pulse, and rising BP may indicate respiratory obstruction. If a client cannot breathe effectively, mechanical ventilation is used.

Aspiration. Danger of aspiration from saliva, mucus, vomitus, or blood exists until the client is fully awake and can swallow without difficulty. Suction equipment must be kept at the client's bedside until the danger of aspiration no longer exists. The nurse closely observes the client for difficulty swallowing or handling of oral secretions. Unless contraindicated, the nurse places the client in a side-lying position until the client can swallow oral secretions.

Later Postoperative Period

The later postoperative period begins when the client arrives in the hospital room or postsurgical care unit. Because nurses can anticipate, prevent, or minimize many postoperative problems, they must approach the care of the client systematically.

ONGOING ASSESSMENTS

Assessment during this period includes respiratory function; general condition; vital signs; cardiovascular function and fluid status; pain level; bowel and urinary elimination; and dressings, tubes, drains, and IV lines.

Respiration. The nurse focuses on promoting gas exchange and preventing atelectasis. Hypoventilation related to anesthesia, postoperative positioning, and pain is a common problem. Preoperative and postoperative instructions include teaching the client to deep breathe and cough and how to splint the incision to minimize pain. Clients who have abdominal or thoracic surgery have greater difficulty taking deep breaths and coughing. Some clients require supplemental oxygen. Nursing management to prevent postoperative respiratory problems includes early mobility, frequent position changes, deep breathing and coughing exercises, and use of incentive spirometer.

Hiccups (*singultus*) also may interfere with breathing. They result from intermittent spasms of the diaphragm and may occur after surgery, especially abdominal surgery. They may be mild and last for only a few minutes. Prolonged hiccups not only are unpleasant but may cause pain or discomfort. They may result in wound dehiscence or evisceration, inability to eat, nausea and vomiting, exhaustion, and fluid, electrolyte, and acid-base imbalances. If hiccups persist, the nurse needs to notify the physician.

Circulation. The nurse must assess the client's BP and circulatory status frequently. Although problems with postoperative bleeding decrease as the recovery time advances, the client is still at risk for bleeding. Some clients experience syncope when moving to an upright position. To prevent this (and the danger of falling), the nurse helps the client slowly move to an upright or standing position.

The client also is at risk for impaired venous circulation related to immobility. When clients lie still for long periods without moving their legs, blood may flow sluggishly through the veins (venous stasis), predisposing the client to venous inflammation and clot formation in the veins (**thrombophlebitis**), or clot formation with minimal or absent inflammation (**phlebothrombosis**). These two conditions are most common in the lower extremities. If the clot travels in the bloodstream (an **embolus**), it may obstruct circulation to a vital organ such as the lungs and cause severe symptoms and possibly death.

To prevent venous stasis and other circulatory complications, the nurse encourages the client to move his or her legs frequently and do leg exercises. The nurse also does not place pillows under the client's knees or calves unless ordered. He or she avoids placing pressure on the client's lower extremities, applies elastic bandages or anti-embolism stockings as ordered, ambulates the client as ordered, and administers low-dose subcutaneous heparin every 12 hours as ordered.

Pain Management. Most clients experience pain after an operation, and a range of postoperative analgesics usually are ordered. The most severe pain occurs during the first 48 hours after surgery. Pain creates varying degrees of anxiety and emotions. If accompanied by great fear, the degree of pain can increase. Clients must receive pain and discomfort relief. When patient-controlled analgesia (PCA) is used, clients administer their own analgesic (see Chap. 21).

The nurse assesses for adverse effects of analgesics, timing of the medication in relation to other activities, effects of other comfort measures, contraindications, and source of the pain. The need for pain medications depends on the type and extent of the surgery, and the client. Pain unrelieved by medication may signal a developing com-

plication, which underscores the need for a thorough assessment of the cause and type of pain (see Chap. 21).

Fluids and Nutrition. IV fluids usually are administered after surgery. Length of administration depends on the type of surgery and the client's ability to take oral fluids. The nurse monitors the IV fluid flow rate and adjusts it as needed. He or she also assesses for signs of fluid excess or deficit (see Chap. 22) and notifies the physician of any such signs.

Many clients complain of thirst in the early postoperative recovery period. Because anesthesia slows peristalsis, ingesting liquids before bowel activity resumes can lead to nausea and vomiting. Pain medications also may cause nausea and vomiting. See Nursing Guidelines 25-1 for factors to consider before resuming oral fluids.

Once peristalsis has returned and the client is tolerating clear liquids, the nurse helps the client to increase dietary intake. Dietary progression (from clear liquids to a full, solid diet) often depends on the type of surgery, the client's progress, and physician preference. IV fluids usually are discontinued when the client can take oral fluids and food and nutritional needs are met.

Skin Integrity/Wound Healing. A surgical incision is a wound or injury to skin integrity. Initially the client may have a wound or incisional drain, which is a tube that exits from the peri-incisional area into either a dressing or

---

NURSING GUIDELINES 25-1

Resuming Oral Fluids After Surgery

Most clients can begin to take fluids within 4 to 24 hours after surgery (except when surgery has involved the gastrointestinal tract). The nurse must check the physician's orders first to ensure that fluids can be given.

- If not allowed oral fluids, the client may use mouth rinses and a cool, wet cloth or ice chips against the lips to relieve dryness.

- Before giving fluids, the nurse assesses that the client has recovered sufficiently from anesthesia to swallow. The nurse asks the client to try swallowing without drinking anything. If the client can do so, the nurse may offer a small sip of water or a few ice chips.

- The nurse gives only a few sips of water or ice chips at a time. He or she introduces fluids slowly and gives them in small amounts to prevent vomiting. The client can take fluids through a straw so he or she does not have to sit up. Once the client can sit up, however, straws are discouraged because clients tend to swallow air as well, which can lead to abdominal distention and gastric discomfort.

- If the client vomits, the nurse reassures him or her that it should cease shortly. The nurse offers mouthwash to remove the taste of anesthetics and vomitus. He or she administers antiemetics as indicated.

portable wound suction device. Figure 25-2 depicts three types of wound devices: Penrose, Hemovac, and Jackson-Pratt drains.

When assessing the wound, the nurse inspects for approximation of the wound edges, intactness of staples or sutures, redness, warmth, swelling, tenderness, discoloration, or drainage. He or she also notes any reactions to the tape or dressings. The first phase of wound healing is the *inflammatory stage,* which is when a blood clot forms, swelling occurs, and phagocytes ingest the debris from damaged tissue and the blood clot. This phase lasts 1 to 4 days. The second phase is the *proliferative phase,* in which collagen is produced and granulation tissue forms. It occurs over 5 to 20 days. The last phase is referred to as the *maturation or remodeling phase* and lasts from 21 days

to several months and even 1 to 2 years. During this phase, the tensile strength of the wound increases through synthesis of collagen by fibroblasts and lysis by collagenase enzymes.

In addition, surgical wounds are formed aseptically, depending on the nature of the incision and the underlying condition. There are three modes of wound healing (Fig. 25-3):

1. *Primary intention:* The wound layers are sutured together so that wound edges are well approximated. This type of incision usually heals in 8 to 10 days, with minimal scarring.
2. *Secondary intention:* Granulating tissue fills in the wound for the healing process. The skin edges are

Safety pin keeps drain from slipping into wound

Drain sponge

A

B

C

FIGURE 25-2 Types of surgical drains. (**A**) Penrose, (**B**) Jackson-Pratt, and (**C**) Hemovac. (From Smeltzer, S. C. & Bare, B. G. [2000]. *Brunner & Suddarth's textbook of medical–surgical nursing* [9th ed.]. Philadelphia: Lippincott Williams & Wilkins.)

Primary Intention

Clean incision   Early suture   Hairline scar

Secondary Intention

Gaping irregular wound   Granulation   Epithelium grows over scar

Tertiary Intention

Wound   Increased granulation   Late suturing with wide scar

FIGURE 25-3 Types of wound healing. (From Smeltzer, S. C. & Bare, B. G. [2000]. *Brunner & Suddarth's textbook of medical-surgical nursing* [9th ed.]. Philadelphia: Lippincott Williams & Wilkins.)

not approximated. This method is used for ulcers and infected wounds. This type of wound healing is slow, although new products have speeded healing.

3. *Tertiary intention:* The approximation of wound edges is delayed secondary to infection. When the wound is drained and cleaned of infection, the wound edges are sutured together. The resulting scar is wider than that with primary intention.

The key to healing is adequate blood flow. Poor blood supply to the wound delays healing, as can excessive tension or pulling on wound edges. The nurse must be alert for signs and symptoms of impaired circulation, such as swelling, coldness, absence of pulse, pallor, or mottling, and report them immediately. Other factors that interfere with healing include malnutrition, impaired inflammatory and immune responses, infection, foreign bodies, and age.

The nurse must be careful when changing dressings to avoid damaging new tissue as well as causing the client unnecessary discomfort. Using normal saline to soak packings and dressings that adhere to the wound bed may ease removal.

The nurse closely monitors for signs and symptoms of wound infection such as increased incisional pain; redness, swelling, and heat around the incision; purulent drainage; fever and chills; headache; and anorexia. Treatment of wound infections includes antibiotics, wound care, and measures to promote healing such as adequate nutrition and rest.

Other complications of wound healing are dehiscence and evisceration. Wound **dehiscence** is the separation of wound edges without the protrusion of organs. **Evisceration** occurs when the wound completely separates and organs protrude. These complications are most likely within 7 to 10 days after surgery. Predisposing factors for wound disruption include malnutrition, particularly insufficient protein and vitamin C; defective suturing; unusual strain on the incision (e.g., from severe coughing or sneezing), prolonged vomiting, dry heaves, and hiccuping; obesity; enlarged abdomen; and abdominal wall weakened by other surgeries.

The client may complain of something "giving way." Pinkish drainage may appear suddenly on the dressing. If wound disruption is suspected, the nurse places the client in a position that puts the least strain on the operative area. If evisceration occurs, the nurse places sterile dressings moistened with normal saline over the protruding organs and tissues. For any wound disruption, the nurse notifies the physician immediately.

Activity. When possible, the client begins ambulatory activities shortly after surgery. Factors such as pain tolerance, response to analgesics, general physical condition, and desire to participate affect the client's ability to be active. Some clients need encouragement. The nurse must emphasize the importance of increasing activities. He or she assists the client to a sitting position at the side of the bed. If the client becomes dizzy longer than momentarily, the nurse returns the client to a supine position. When the client can stand, the nurse assists and supports the client. The nurse continues to assist with ambulation until the client can walk without help. Some clients experience moderate to severe fatigue after surgery. For these clients, the nurse spaces activities such as ambulation and personal care throughout the day.

If the client has received regional anesthesia, activity may initially be restricted. At first, the client experiences numbness and a feeling of heaviness in the anesthetized area. Reassuring the client that the numbness is typical and will subside shortly may be necessary. Unless ordered otherwise, the client who has received spinal anesthesia remains flat for 6 to 12 hours. If permitted, the nurse turns the client from side to side at least every 2 hours. As the anesthesia wears off, the client begins to have a pins-and-needles sensation in the anesthetized parts and to feel pain in the operative area. Clients who develop a headache after spinal anesthesia may have to remain lying flat for a longer period.

Bowel Elimination. Constipation may develop after the client begins to take solid food. Causes of such constipation include inactivity, diet, or narcotic analgesics. Some clients may experience diarrhea as a result of diet, medications such as antibiotics, or the surgical procedure. The nurse maintains a record of bowel movements and notifies the physician of either problem.

Abdominal distention results from the accumulation of gas (flatus) in the intestines because of failure of the intestines to propel gas through the intestinal tract by peristalsis. Contributing factors include manipulation of the intestines during abdominal surgery, inactivity after

surgery, interruption of normal food and fluid intake, swallowing of large quantities of air, and anesthetics and medications given during or after surgery. If the symptoms are mild, they can be treated with nursing measures. The nurse encourages and assists clients who are permitted out of bed to ambulate. Sometimes walking, plus privacy in the bathroom, enables the client to expel the gas. The nurse encourages clients to change position frequently and to eat as normally as possible within the allowed dietary limits. If discomfort is severe or not relieved promptly by nursing measures, the nurse must contact the physician.

Sometimes a serious condition called **paralytic ileus** occurs in which the intestines are paralyzed and, thus, peristalsis is absent. Fluids, solids, and gas do not move through the intestinal tract. Bowel sounds are absent, the abdomen is distended, and abdominal pain often is severe. Vomiting also may occur. If the client complains of severe abdominal pain, assessment includes inspecting the abdomen for distention, palpating for rigidity, and auscultating for bowel sounds. If bowel sounds are absent or abnormal or the abdomen is distended or rigid, the nurse notifies the physician immediately. A nasogastric tube usually is inserted and food and fluids withheld until bowel sounds return.

Acute gastric dilatation, a condition in which the stomach becomes distended with fluids, is a complication similar to paralytic ileus. The client may regurgitate small amounts of liquid, the abdomen appears distended, and, as the condition progresses, symptoms of shock may develop. Treatment includes inserting a nasogastric tube, applying suction, and removing the gas and fluid. Some surgeons routinely use suction of the gastrointestinal tract to prevent paralytic ileus and acute gastric dilatation.

Urinary Elimination. Some clients experience difficulty voiding after surgery, particularly lower abdominal and pelvic surgery. Operative trauma in the region near the bladder may temporarily decrease the voiding sensation. Fear of pain also causes tenseness and difficulty voiding. If the client has an indwelling catheter, the nurse monitors urine output frequently. If the client does not have a catheter, the nurse assesses the client's ability to void and measures urine output. If the client cannot void within 8 hours after surgery, the nurse notifies the physician unless catheterization orders are in place. Signs and symptoms of bladder distention include restlessness, lower abdominal pain, discomfort or distention, and fluid intake without urinary output.

Psychosocial Care. Many clients experience anxiety and fear after surgery, as well as an inability to cope with changes in body image, lifestyle, and other factors. The nurse assesses what the client is experiencing and how the client is dealing with those issues. Many clients need referrals for counseling, support groups, and social services.

The nurse acts as an effective listener, identifies areas of concern, and works with other healthcare professionals to assist the client and family to work through the problems.

CLIENT AND FAMILY TEACHING

Before discharge, the client needs to receive instructions on how to carry out treatments at home. The client and family must understand the prescribed treatment regimen. The nurse evaluates clients to determine their ability to carry out their care and to determine their specific needs, such as the need for:

- Supervised home care (e.g., visiting nurse, other healthcare agencies and personnel)
- Supplies (e.g., dressings, tape, ostomy supplies, crutches)
- Special dietary needs
- Adjustments to the living environment (e.g., special bed, portable commode, wheelchair access)

Client and Family Teaching Box 25-1 presents more information.

AMBULATORY CARE

Many surgeries and procedures that once were complicated or confined to hospitals now are performed in outpatient settings and ambulatory surgical centers. As a

---

25-1 *Client and Family Teaching*
Postoperative Instruction

The nurse develops a teaching plan to meet the client's needs. Points may include the following:

- Follow physician's instructions about cleaning the incision, applying the dressing, bathing, diet, and physical activity.
- Notify physician of any of the following: chills or fever; drainage from the incision (some drainage may be expected in certain cases); foul odor or pus from the incision; redness, streaking, pain, or tenderness around the incision; other symptoms not present at discharge (e.g., vomiting, diarrhea, cough, chest or leg pain)
- Take medications as prescribed. Do not omit or change the dose unless the physician advises to do so.
- Do not take nonprescription medications unless approved by the physician.
- Keep all postoperative appointments.
- Tell the physician about any problems during recovery.

---

result, nurses must become increasingly familiar with ambulatory surgery and conscious sedation.

Ambulatory Surgery

Ambulatory surgery, sometimes referred to as *same-day* or *outpatient surgery,* is defined as surgery that requires fewer than 24 hours of hospitalization. These short-term admissions may be as brief as 1 to 2 hours or extend to overnight. Ambulatory surgical units are located either in a hospital or in a separate building that the hospital owns. Others are freestanding, privately owned facilities not affiliated with a hospital.

The number of ambulatory surgical procedures has dramatically increased since the early 1980s. This is related to advances in surgical techniques and methods of anesthesia, prospective reimbursement, managed care, and changes in Medicare and Medicaid provisions (Smeltzer & Bare, 2000). A client admitted for ambulatory surgery must meet the following criteria:

- The client is not critically ill.
- The surgical procedure is not extensive and does not require many hours of general anesthesia.
- The client has few, if any, coexisting and disabling illnesses.
- Recovery is expected to be quick, with minimal specialized care after surgery.
- The client or family can provide adequate postoperative care.

Usually, clients are discharged from ambulatory surgical units by mid-afternoon or early evening. If a complication develops, the client is transferred to an inpatient hospital unit.

Conscious Sedation

Many diagnostic and short therapeutic procedures formerly performed on an inpatient basis now are performed on an outpatient basis. During these procedures, clients are sedated but not unconscious. *Sedation* refers to a pharmacologically induced state of relaxation and emotional comfort. *Analgesia* is the absence or relief of pain. **Conscious sedation** describes a state in which clients are free of pain, fear, and anxiety and can tolerate unpleasant procedures while maintaining independent cardiorespiratory function and the ability to respond to verbal commands and tactile stimulation. IV anesthesia usually is used to induce conscious sedation. If other routes are used, the client must have venous access for treatment of possible adverse effects, such as anaphylaxis.

Diagnostic and therapeutic procedures that require sedation and analgesia, such as bone marrow biopsy, endoscopy, cardiac catheterization, or magnetic resonance imaging and computed tomography scanning, take place in several settings. Clients often are discharged shortly after the procedure. The responsibility for ensuring client safety and comfort during the sedation process rests with the nurse who is directly involved in the client's care. Although numerous types of equipment for monitoring clients are available, no equipment replaces a nurse's careful observations.

Presedation Evaluation

The presedation evaluation determines which clients are suitable for administration of sedative medications. It is similar to the preoperative evaluation. The nurse considers past adverse reactions to sedative medication. The client's age and weight help determine the amount of medication he or she will need.

Sedative Medications

Nurses who care for clients receiving sedation must be aware of the effects, side effects, and desired doses of sedative medications. Benzodiazepines, opioids, sedative-hypnotics, and barbiturates are the drug classes used in conscious sedation (Drug Therapy Table 25-2). These drugs can cause nausea, dizziness, euphoria or depression, flushed skin, coughing, jerking movements, and unusual eye and tongue movements. Although harmless, such side effects can frighten clients. Because virtually all sedative medications carry a risk of respiratory depression, the nurse also must be prepared for respiratory or cardiopulmonary arrest.

Antagonists, also called *reversal drugs*, reverse the effects of narcotics or benzodiazepines. Drugs from this

DRUG THERAPY TABLE 25-2	AGENTS USED TO SEDATE CLIENTS FOR DIAGNOSTIC AND THERAPEUTIC PROCEDURES	

DRUG CATEGORY AND EXAMPLES	SIDE EFFECTS	NURSING CONSIDERATIONS
Opioids meperidine hydro-chloride (Demerol) morphine sulfate fentanyl (Sublimaze)	Respiratory and CNS depression, hypotension, nausea, vomiting, constipation, histamine release, headache, restlessness, tachycardia, seizures, increased intracranial pressure, decreased urination, rash, hives, pain at injection site, bronchospasm, laryngospasm	Use with caution in clients with asthma, hepatic or renal disorders, or seizure disorders. These drugs are useful for sedation during painful procedures. They may cause hypotension in clients with acute myocardial infarction.
Benzodiazepines midazolam hydro-chloride (Versed) diazepam (Valium) lorazepam (Ativan)	Respiratory depression, cardiac arrest, hypotension, bradycardia, tachycardia, nausea, vomiting, bronchospasm, laryngospasm, blurred vision, diplopia, pain and local reaction at injection site, hiccups, amnesia, paradoxical excitement	Use with caution in clients with hypersensitivity reactions to other opioid agonists. Respiratory depression may persist beyond period of analgesia. Do not use in clients with increased intracranial pressure. Theophylline may antagonize the sedative effects of midazolam. Adverse effects increase when these drugs are administered with narcotics. These drugs cause profound retrograde amnesia and have no analgesic effect.
Sedative-hypnotics chloral hydrate	Respiratory depression, nausea, vomiting, diarrhea, hallucinations, rash, urticaria, paradoxical excitement, fever, headache, confusion	Use with caution in clients with congestive heart failure, renal impairment, pulmonary disease, or hepatic failure. Do not use in clients with narrow-angle glaucoma, hepatic or renal impairment, gastritis, peptic ulcer disease, or severe cardiac disease.
Barbiturates pentobarbital (Nembutal)	Respiratory depression, laryngospasm, cardiac dysrhythmias, bradycardia, hypotension, CNS excitement or depression, pain or thrombophlebitis at injection site, hallucinations	Use can result in false-positive urine glucose with Clinitest method. Do not give to clients with marked liver impairment or porphyria. Use with caution in clients with hypovolemic shock, congestive heart failure, hepatic impairment, or respiratory or renal dysfunction.

CNS, central nervous system.

class should be readily available whenever narcotics or benzodiazepines are used. If reversal drugs are required, the nurse *must* observe the client for an extended period, because the reversal effects nearly always are shorter than the effects of the drugs being reversed. This may result in resedation. Naloxone (Narcan) reverses narcotics; flumazenil (Romazicon) reverses benzodiazepines.

Phases of the Sedation Process

The three phases of the sedation process are as follows:

1. The titration of sedative medications, which is the administration of multiple small doses of medication until the desired drug effect is achieved
2. The performance of the diagnostic or therapeutic procedure
3. The recovery phase

In each phase, the client requires careful monitoring for complications. Levels of sedation range from slight drowsiness to anesthesia. Unpredictable absorption, metabolism, and excretion of medications make the client vulnerable to complications of undersedation or oversedation. Increased vigilance is necessary during titration of medications and recovery. At this time, the client has the greatest potential to become more deeply sedated because there is no painful stimulus. Even when the client does not seem to be sedated at the end of the procedure, late sedation may develop from continued drug uptake, delayed excretion, pharmacodynamics, or lack of stimulation. In addition to monitoring for adverse effects of medications, the nurse monitors for complications of the procedure itself.

Discharge and Teaching

Specific, standardized outcome criteria help determine if the client's condition is stable and if he or she can safely leave the hospital or outpatient setting. These criteria include that the client:

- Has stable cardiovascular function and a patent airway
- Is easily aroused
- Has intact protective reflexes
- Can talk
- Can sit up unaided
- Is adequately hydrated

When the client meets the appropriate discharge criteria, the nurse provides discharge instructions. Because sedative medications affect memory for events surrounding their administration, the nurse must review discharge instructions with an adult who will be responsible for the client after discharge. The nurse conveys the discharge instructions verbally and in writing. He or she instructs the client not to drink alcoholic beverages for a specified

period after the procedure and to resume prescription and nonprescription medications when appropriate. Pain medications may have an additive effect with the sedative medications that were administered, so the nurse must instruct the client about when it is appropriate to begin taking such medications. The nurse also provides dietary instructions and encourages the client to drink plenty of fluids. The client needs specific activity guidelines. In general, the client should temporarily refrain from activities that depend on good physical coordination, such as driving or operating machinery. The nurse also tells the client to telephone the physician with any concerns about untoward effects of the medications or complications of the procedure.

NURSING PROCESS

● The Client Undergoing Conscious Sedation

Assessment

Before sedation, the nurse gathers important client data, records baseline vital signs and oximeter readings, and provides education to clients and their families. Education includes instructions specific to the procedure, preparations for the procedure, likely sensations (pain, discomfort, cramping, gagging, nausea), and common side effects of medications.

During sedation, the nurse continuously evaluates the client. Monitoring during all phases includes assessment of heart rate, respiratory rate, BP, oxygen saturation, and level of consciousness. The nurse monitors cardiac rhythm in clients who are at risk for dysrhythmias or cardiovascular compromise. If vital signs deviate significantly during sedation, the nurse collects additional information to help determine if those deviations are secondary to an adverse reaction to the sedation or to the procedure itself. When the client shows signs of distress (i.e., deviation in vital signs, respiratory compromise), the nurse immediately reports these signs to the physician and provides interventions such as suctioning, gentle tactile stimulation, or administration of oxygen. He or she continues to monitor the client's response until level of consciousness and vital signs are at baseline. The nurse documents these observations at intervals specified by the institution.

Diagnosis, Planning, and Interventions

Risk for Ineffective Breathing Patterns related to effect of sedative medications
Expected Outcome: Client will demonstrate a normal breathing pattern.
- Position client in an upright or semi-Fowler's position. *These positions facilitate lung expansion.*
- Observe for signs and symptoms of distress related to inappropriate head position (stridor, increased respira-

tory effort); reposition head as indicated. *Early intervention prevents further complications.*

● Encourage client to take deep breaths and cough at least every hour. *Deep breathing and coughing improve oxygenation and assist in clearing the effects of anesthesia.*

Risk for Injury related to sedation

Expected Outcome: Client will remain safe and free of injury.

● Provide safety by preventing client from falling out of bed, stretcher, or recliner; assisting with ambulation; and carefully monitoring all activities. *Clients recovering from sedation may have impaired judgment and reflexes; the nurse must protect them from injury.*

● Monitor client for return to presedation level of consciousness. *Until client is fully responsive, he or she continues to be at risk for injury.*

● Discharge client to the care of a person who has received instructions regarding client safety. *Sedative effects may last for several more hours; the client requires continued care after discharge.*

Evaluation of Expected Outcomes

The client has a patent airway and effective breathing patterns. He or she experiences no threats to safety.

GENERAL NUTRITIONAL CONSIDERATIONS

Progress the diet as soon as possible after surgery to promote an adequate oral intake. Encourage clients who are anorectic or nauseated to consume small, frequent feedings. They may tolerate high-protein, low-fat liquids better than traditional meals.

If possible, schedule pain medications enough in advance to allow the client a pain-free mealtime.

Normal weight loss during the early postoperative period is about half a pound daily. Weight gain during this period signifies fluid accumulation.

Protein, calories, vitamins A and C, and zinc are important for wound healing and immune system functioning; actual requirements depend on the client's nutritional status, extent of surgery, and development of complications.

Unlike the stomach, which does not regain motility for 24 to 48 hours after surgery, the small intestine resumes peristalsis and the ability to absorb nutrients within several hours after surgery. If the client is malnourished, hypermetabolic, or not expected to resume an oral intake within a few days, a needle-catheter jejunostomy tube may be inserted during surgery so enteral feedings can be given.

GENERAL PHARMACOLOGIC CONSIDERATIONS

Preoperative medication is given precisely at the time prescribed by the anesthesiologist. If the preoperative medication is given too early, the optimum potency will be reached before it is needed; if the drug is given too late, its action will not begin before the anesthesia is initiated.

Postoperative pain reaches its peak between 12 and 36 hours after surgery and diminishes significantly after 48 hours.

Antiemetics such as promethazine (Phenergan) or prochlorperazine (Compazine) can potentiate the hypotensive effects of opioids.

During the postoperative period, closely monitor the client for adverse reactions to the narcotic analgesics, such as respiratory depression, decreased BP, nausea, excessive drowsiness, agitation, or hallucinations. Naloxone (Narcan) can be given to counteract narcotic-induced respiratory depression.

Some clients experience acute anxiety before surgery. The physician may prescribe a tranquilizer or sedative. Notify the physician if the medication does not appear to be effective.

The evening before surgery, a hypnotic drug may be ordered to ensure rest. Document the effects of the medication on the client's chart.

The use of PCA does not eliminate the need for frequent observation of the client for effectiveness of the analgesic. Monitor BP and pulse and respiratory rates frequently. Bring a decrease in BP or respiratory rate to the physician's attention immediately.

Antibiotics may be ordered before as well as after surgery. The antibiotic must be given at specified intervals to maintain consistent therapeutic blood levels.

GENERAL GERONTOLOGIC CONSIDERATIONS

A major adverse reaction to anesthesia in older adults is decreased mental functioning, which can manifest as delirium.

Medications such as opioids and barbiturates may cause confusion and disorientation in older adults, even when given in standard doses.

The respiratory depressive effects of opioids may be increased in older adults.

Sometimes the risk of surgery is increased for older adults because they may have disorders (e.g., cardiac or renal disease) that interfere with recovery.

A detailed medication history is important because some medications persist in the body and may interfere with administration of anesthetic agents or medications given before, during, or after surgery.

A diminished ability to hear, see, and understand may interfere with preoperative and postoperative teaching. Nurses may need to repeat explanations and demonstrations.

Older adults usually receive smaller doses of preoperative, intraoperative, and postoperative medications, especially those that affect the central nervous, cardiovascular, and renal systems.

Older adults are prone to postoperative complications such as shock, atelectasis, pneumonia, paralytic ileus, gastric dilatation, and venous stasis.

Postoperative ambulatory activities are essential but planned according to the older adult's tolerance, which usually is less than that of a younger person.

The convalescent period usually is longer for older adults. They may require positive reinforcement throughout the postoperative period as well as extensive discharge planning.

If an older adult lives alone or with a spouse who also is older or is ill or infirm, give additional consideration to discharge planning. This client may require the services of relatives or friends, a public health nurse, a visiting nurse, or home healthcare personnel during the convalescent period. In some instances, admitting the client to a skilled nursing facility for convalescent care is necessary.

A loss of subcutaneous tissue and thinning of the skin accompany the aging process. This, in turn, may lead to stress-producing situations, such as poor wound healing, tissue breakdown caused by excessive pressure on a part, or inadequate development of granulation tissue in healing wounds.

Critical Thinking Exercises

1. *The nurse is checking to ensure that a client's surgical consent form is signed and on the chart the evening before surgery. When the nurse assesses this client, he reports that he is uncertain about having the surgery and does not understand what is expected or its long-term consequences. What steps should the nurse take? What must the nurse document?*

2. *A client reports to the nurse that her family has lost several family members unexpectedly during surgery. The client is very scared about her upcoming surgery. What actions should the nurse take? What should the nurse document?*

3. *It is the fifth day of a client's postoperative period (5 days postop). He complains of incisional pain, feeling warm, and nausea. What assessments should the nurse make? What should he or she document?*

References and Suggested Readings

Arsenault, C. (1998). Nurses' guide to general anesthesia: Part 1. *Nursing, 28*(3), 32.

Bullock, B. A. & Henze, R. L. (2000). *Focus on pathophysiology.* Philadelphia: Lippincott Williams & Wilkins.

Carpenito, L. (2001). *Nursing diagnosis: Application to clinical practice* (9th ed.). Philadelphia: Lippincott Williams & Wilkins.

Carroll, P. (2000). A new way to monitor paralyzing drugs. *RN, 63*(5), 62–66.

Dunn, D. (1998). Preoperative assessment criteria and patient teaching for ambulatory surgery patients. *Journal of Perianesthesia Nursing, 13,* 274–291.

Evans, T. (2000). Neuromuscular blockade: When and how. *RN, 63*(5), 56–60.

Holmes, H. N. (Ed.). (1998). *Mastering medical-surgical nursing.* Springhouse, PA: Springhouse Corporation.

Kingsley, C. (2001). Epidural anesthesia: Your role. *RN, 64*(3), 53–57.

Martin, S. (2001). There's what in the wound? *RN, 64*(2), 44–47.

Nettina, S. (2000). *The Lippincott manual of nursing practice* (7th ed.). Philadelphia: Lippincott Williams & Wilkins.

Pasero, C. (2000). Continuous local anesthetics. *American Journal of Nursing, 100*(8), 22–23.

Patel, C. T., Kinsey, G. C., Koperski-Moen, K. J., & Bubgum, L. D. (2000). Vacuum-assisted wound closure. *American Journal of Nursing, 100*(12), 45–48.

Reiff, P. A. & Niziolek, M. M. (2001). Troubleshooting tips for PCA. *RN, 64*(4), 33–37.

Smeltzer, S. C. & Bare, B. G. (2000). *Brunner & Suddarth's textbook of medical–surgical nursing* (9th ed.). Philadelphia: Lippincott Williams & Wilkins.

Caring for Dying Clients

Words to Know

acceptance
anger
anticipatory grieving
bargaining
denial
depression
hospice

near death experience
nearing death
    awareness
palliative treatment
respite care
waiting for permission
    phenomenon

Learning Objectives

On completion of this chapter, the reader will:

- Define attitudes of society and healthcare workers toward death.
- Discuss outcomes of informing a client about a terminal illness.
- Explain how clients and families can maintain hopefulness during a terminal illness.
- Name emotional reactions the dying client experiences.
- Identify how the dying client can ensure that others carry out his or her wishes for terminal care.
- Describe physical phenomena that occur during the dying process.
- Summarize psychological events that dying clients have reported.
- Apply the nursing process to the care of the dying client and the family.

According to DeSpelder and Strickland, "Of all human experiences, none is more overwhelming in its implications than death. Yet, for most of us, death remains a shadowy figure whose presence is only vaguely acknowledged" (2001, p. 5). Earlier in the 20th century, many people died in their homes, surrounded by family and loved ones. Later, it became more common to die in a hospital or nursing home. In the 1970s, the hospice movement began to promote care of dying clients at home or in hospice settings, providing a more dignified and supportive climate.

Increased technology and aggressive treatment have, in some ways, distorted the reality of dying and death for healthcare providers. For some, death signifies a failure to save lives and act as healers. Death, however, is a natural and universal experience, a part of life, and a component of healthcare. Healthcare providers must acknowledge death as the final stage of growth and development (Kübler-Ross, 1975). They also must explore their own mortality and feelings about dying and death. This is the only way that they can then provide care and comfort to dying clients and their families.

Education about death helps healthcare professionals to be better informed about dying and death and to incorporate this knowledge into the care they give clients.

Nurses who care for dying clients share emotional pain with them and their families. Denying death creates a barrier to becoming involved with clients and families and interferes with personal growth.

Death can occur in any healthcare setting; therefore, facing the death of clients is necessary for nurses. It is not partial to a particular age group or population. Death can be slow and tortuous or very sudden and unexpected. Preparing the client and his or her family for an expected death is usually very different from caring for grieving family members after an unexpected death. Recognizing that nursing care always requires sensitivity and compassion for the client, family, and significant others is an essential component of quality care.

THE DYING CLIENT

Although most people recognize that death is inevitable, they do not spend time getting ready until actually faced with the prospect. Factors the nurse needs to consider when caring for the dying client include informing the client, sustaining hope, assisting the client and family with emotional reactions, and recognizing the client's right to make final decisions.

Informing the Dying Client

Nurses honor the dying client's right to know the seriousness of his or her condition. The physician usually is responsible for informing clients of the nature and gravity of their illness. Even though some informed clients react negatively at first, outcomes of being frank include the following:

- The nurse–client relationship is based on honesty rather than on the false pretense that recovery will occur.
- The client's autonomy and right to determine how to spend the rest of her or his life is upheld.
- The client can complete unfinished business—prepare for and arrange legal and personal affairs and complete any remaining tasks or goals.
- The client can use inner resources and determination to survive and prolong life, often referred to as the "will to live."
- Meaningful communication between the client and family is promoted.

All members of the healthcare team must know what the client has been told regarding his or her prognosis. Lack of this knowledge greatly interferes with the nurse–client relationship. For example, the nurse may avoid all but the most superficial topics of conversation out of uncertainty about how to respond if asked, "Am I going to die?" Some nurses feel that, regardless of how others might try to conceal the truth, most clients gradually recognize clues that their illness is terminal. Avoidance alone tends to confirm their suspicions that they are dying. When uninformed clients are given the opportunity, they may give hints of their awareness of approaching death. Some may even indicate they are ready to discuss dying. If a nurse replies to comments by saying, "Don't talk like that," he or she conveys a message that the subject of dying is uncomfortable for the nurse. Often, the client will then avoid the subject in all future interactions.

Sustaining Hope

Nurses must recognize the value of communicating a spirit of hopefulness. Hopefulness means that dying clients have a right to believe that the healthcare team will make their remaining days meaningful, use whatever treatment and comfort measures are appropriate, and dignify the approaching death. Both nurses and clients, however, should not confuse hope with unrealistic optimism. When clients learn that their condition is terminal, they must also understand that the healthcare team remains dedicated to

providing **palliative treatment,** which is treatment that reduces physical discomfort but does not alter a disease's progression (Box 26-1).

Assisting With Emotional Reactions

Although each dying client responds to terminal illness in unique ways, studies show a common emotional pattern. Elisabeth Kübler-Ross, a physician who has studied death and dying extensively, described a series of five reactions—(1) denial, (2) anger, (3) bargaining, (4) depression, and (5) acceptance—that dying clients often demonstrate. Clients do not always follow these stages in order. Some regress, then move forward again. Others may be in several stages at once (e.g., a client who is angry as well as depressed).

The first stage, **denial,** is a psychological defense mechanism (see Chap. 12) in which a person refuses to believe certain information. Dying clients usually first deny that the diagnosis is accurate. A common response is "No, not me; there must be some mistake." They may imagine that test results are erroneous or reports have been confused. Denial of the diagnosis may be followed by a refusal to accept that the condition is actually terminal.

During the second stage, **anger,** clients ask, "Why me?" Clients may say, "I'm still young. My children still need me. Why did I get this disease?" They may displace this anger onto others, such as the physician, nurses, family, or even God. They may express such anger in less obvious ways, such as complaining about their care or blaming anyone and everyone for the slightest aggravation.

BOX 26-1 ● Five Principles of Palliative Care

1. Palliative care respects the goals, likes, and choices of the dying person and his or her loved ones . . . helping them to understand the illness and what can be expected from it, and to figure out what is most important during this time.
2. Palliative care looks after the medical, emotional, social, and spiritual needs of the dying person . . . with a focus on making sure he or she is comfortable, not left alone, and able to look back on his or her life and find peace.
3. Palliative care supports the needs of family members . . . helping them with the responsibilities of caregiving and even supporting them as they grieve.
4. Palliative care helps to gain access to needed healthcare providers and appropriate care settings . . . involving various kinds of trained providers in different settings, tailored to the needs of the patient and his or her family.
5. Palliative care builds ways to provide excellent care at the end of life . . . through education of care providers, appropriate health policies, and adequate funding from insurers and the government.

(Used with permission. The Robert Wood Johnson Foundation, Last Acts Palliative Care Task Force. [1999]. Five Principles of Palliative Care. Special supplement to *Advances, 2,* 3.)

The third stage, **bargaining,** is an attempt to postpone death. Usually the client makes a secret bargain with God or some higher power. Clients attempt to negotiate a delay in dying until after a particularly significant event. They may say, "If I can just live until my daughter graduates from high school, I will accept death when it eventually comes."

The fourth stage is marked by **depression.** As clients realize the reality of their situation, they may mourn their potential losses such as separation from their loved ones, the inability to fulfill their future goals, or loss of control.

In the fifth stage, **acceptance,** dying clients accept their fate and make peace spiritually and with those to whom they are close. Clients may begin to detach themselves from activities and acquaintances and seek to be with only a small circle of relatives or friends.

Stop, Think, and Respond ● BOX 26-1

A client has learned that he has a terminal illness. He pleads with God to allow him to live long enough to see the birth of his first grandchild. What is this stage called? What may have preceded this stage? bargaining

---

Supporting Final Decisions

The nurse presents options of where and how terminal care may be provided, respects the client and family's choices, and facilitates their preferences. As long as the dying client remains competent (retains the ability to understand the consequences of his or her choices), he or she has the right to request or refuse a variety of options. Problems arise when clients become incompetent before indicating their wishes about terminal care. Consequently, dying clients may become victims of decisions they would ordinarily oppose. Therefore, some clients write down their wishes, called *advance directives,* in a living will or legally designate someone to have durable power of attorney (see Chap. 5).

During this emotional turmoil, dying clients often must make some tough decisions. Dying clients or their families control their destiny. Under a federal law called The Patient Self-Determination Act, passed in 1990, all healthcare facilities in the United States funded by Medicare must inform clients on admission of their right to refuse medical treatment and their right to prepare an advance directive. Most agencies supply the necessary forms.

Living Wills

A *living will* is a written or printed statement describing a person's wishes concerning her or his own medical care when death is near (see Fig. 5-4). Usually, a living will describes a desire to avoid being kept alive by artificial means or use of heroic measures. It is not a legal document and, as such, is not binding under the law. Rather,

it serves as an informal directive, which others may or may not feel compelled to follow. Many physicians try to abide by their clients' wishes, however, if they are known or stated in writing.

Durable Power of Attorney

Some states are now encouraging people to appoint someone to have durable power of attorney for their healthcare. This procedure makes it possible for another person whom the client selects to make medical decisions on the client's behalf when the client no longer can do so. It allows competent clients to identify exactly what life-sustaining measures they want implemented, avoided, or withdrawn, and offers reassurance that others will carry out their wishes. The appointee cannot exercise this authority at any other time or in any other matters. For obvious ethical reasons, the client's physician or other healthcare workers may not be designated as durable power of attorney. When a durable power of attorney document exists, the client brings it to the institution at each admission, a photocopy of which is attached to the chart.

CARE OF THE DYING CLIENT

Some terminally ill clients spend their last days in an acute care setting, using the best technology and resources available. Others prefer to be at home, with or without assistance from hospice home care. Others choose a hospice or extended care facility. Regardless of the setting, clients need to know that their symptoms, particularly pain, will be controlled and that they will be a part of the planning process for their care.

Home Care

In the early stages of a terminal illness, the client usually remains at home. Nurses often coordinate community services and secure needed home equipment. Many clients report experiencing greater emotional and physical comfort in their own home. They have greater security and personal integrity in a familiar environment. Family members also may experience fewer feelings of guilt when they are involved in caring for the client. In addition, children can interact more frequently and may be helped to understand death with less fear.

A negative factor of home care is the burden it places on the primary caregiver. If prolonged, the role of primary caregiver can be very isolating and physically exhausting because the responsibility for providing care continues 24 hours a day, day after day. Home care nurses periodically need to assess the toll on the caregiver's physical and emotional health. They may arrange **respite care,** or care for the caregiver, to provide periodic relief.

Hospice Care

In 1967, Dr. Cicely Saunders founded St. Christopher's Hospice in Sydenham, England. This hospice has served as a model for hospice care in the United States. A **hospice** is a facility for the care of the terminally ill clients, who can live out their final days with comfort, dignity, and meaningfulness. Hospice care emphasizes helping clients live however they wish until they die. Clients receive services that relieve their physical symptoms and emotional distress and promote spiritual support. Pain is liberally controlled. In the United States, facilities have implemented the hospice philosophy in various ways. In general, most hospice clients, who usually have 6 months or less to live, receive care in their own homes. A multidisciplinary team of hospice professionals and volunteers provides support to the dying client and caregivers. Services include personal care, homemaking services, companionship, and support programs for family members and significant others, including individual counseling during and after the death of the client (grief counseling).

Institutionally Based Palliative Care

Some institutions provide palliative care to terminally ill clients who cannot maintain independent living. This care also may be referred to as hospice care. These units may be located in hospitals, long-term care facilities, or other, separate facilities. Nurses and other healthcare personnel give 24-hour care. Factors that influence the decision to use institutionally based palliative care include the following:

- The client's weakness or immobility causes him or her to require more assistance than can be provided at home.
- The client cannot manage elimination needs.
- The client has uncontrolled or inadequately controlled pain or nausea.
- The family cannot provide adequate care.
- The client requires too complex and demanding care.
- The caregiver is too exhausted to provide care.

Many of the rules that govern traditional hospital and long-term care are relaxed for palliative care units. Visiting hours and ages of visitors are not restrictive. In addition, the family is encouraged to bring in personal items for the client to enjoy and value.

Acute Care

Hospitals offer acute care with a 24-hour staff of nurses and other medical personnel, readily available resuscitative equipment, and access to a greater variety of medications than those in long-term care. This form of terminal care, however, is probably the most expensive. In this setting, the time and attention afforded to the supportive care of dying clients may be limited.

SIGNS OF APPROACHING DEATH

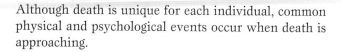

Although death is unique for each individual, common physical and psychological events occur when death is approaching.

Physical Events

Death usually occurs gradually over hours or days. Cells deteriorate from an underlying lack of sufficient oxygen, which leads to multisystem failure. The following are signs of impending death that alert the nurse that the client will die shortly:

- *Cardiac dysfunction.* Failing cardiac function is one of the first signs that a client's condition is worsening. At first, heart rate increases in a futile attempt to deliver oxygen to cells. The apical pulse rate may reach 100 or more beats/minute. Cardiac output, the amount of blood that the heart pumps per minute, may decrease, because a fast heart rate impairs the heart's ability to fill with blood. This may diminish the heart's own oxygen supply, which causes the heart rate to decrease and blood pressure to fall.
- *Peripheral circulation changes.* Reduced cardiac output compromises peripheral circulation, and impaired cellular metabolism produces less heat. The skin becomes pale or mottled, nail beds and lips may appear blue, and the client may feel cold.
- *Pulmonary function impairment.* Failure of the heart's pumping function causes fluid to collect in the pulmonary circulation. Breath sounds become moist. Oxygen does not diffuse very well, and the client cannot exhale carbon dioxide adequately, compounding the state of generalized hypoxia (low oxygenation).
- *Central nervous system alterations.* With hypoxia, the brain is less sensitive to accumulating levels of carbon dioxide; therefore, the client may experience periods of apnea (no breathing). Pain perception may be diminished; the client may stare blankly through partially open eyes; and the senses may become impaired, although hearing tends to remain intact. Eventually, the client becomes insensitive to all but extreme pressure.
- *Renal impairment.* Low cardiac output causes urine volume to diminish and toxic waste products to accumulate.
- *Gastrointestinal disturbances.* Peristalsis slows, causing gas and intestinal contents to accumulate. This

[handwritten: hearing is 1st to return if in coma]

buildup may stimulate the vomiting center, resulting in nausea and vomiting.

- *Musculoskeletal changes.* Reflexes become hypoactive. The client loses urinary and rectal sphincter muscle control, causing incontinence of urine and stool. The jaw and facial muscles also relax. As the tongue falls to the back of the throat, respirations become noisy. The accumulation of secretions in the respiratory tract, coupled with noisy respirations, is referred to as the death rattle. A brief period of restlessness may occur just before death.

Psychological Events

If they have reached the stage of acceptance, some terminally ill clients look forward to dying because it will end their suffering. Some clients, however, seem to forestall dying when they feel that their loved ones are not yet prepared to deal with their death. This has been described as the **waiting for permission phenomenon,** because death often occurs shortly after a significant family member communicates that he or she is strong enough and ready to "let go." Nurses must support family members at this time because they may feel as though they have given up and let their loved one down.

Near death experiences, in which a person almost dies but is resuscitated, have been reported for some time. People who experience near death report similar events, such as:

- Floating above their bodies
- Moving rapidly toward a bright light
- Seeing familiar people who have already died
- Feeling warm and peaceful
- Being told that it is not time yet for them to die
- Regretting having to return to their resuscitated body

Nearing death awareness is a phenomenon characterized by a dying client's premonition of the approximate time or date of death. In addition, just before death, clients may reach out, point, or open their arms as if to embrace someone or call them by name.

NURSING MANAGEMENT *[handwritten: hearing 1st to go]*

Nursing care of dying clients focuses on providing palliative care to the client and supporting family members and significant others. Client comfort is the primary goal, with the major long-term goal being that the client will die with dignity. Other client goals include control of pain, maintenance of basic physiologic functions, relief of fears and anxieties, completion of unfinished business, and acceptance of death. Having the client's family remain cohesive and supportive is another goal, as is providing a safe and secure environment. See Nursing Care Plan 26-1.

Assessment

Initially, nurses focus assessment on the client's basic physical needs, such as pain, breathing, nutrition, hydration, and elimination. They then include the psychosocial needs of the client and family. Nurses must try not to repeat unnecessary assessments so as to allow the client to rest. They can make frequent checks without being physically intrusive. This frequency provides security, so that the client does not feel abandoned.

Pain Control

The primary objective of pain control for dying clients is to block pain without suppressing level of consciousness or breathing. The nurse usually gives pain medications on a routine schedule to avoid causing intense discomfort followed by a period of heavy sedation. Regular dosing sustains a plateau of continuous pain relief and prevents exhausting the client, who must use additional energy to cope with severe pain (see Chap. 21). The nurse also reassures the client that frequent use of narcotic analgesia will not cause addiction. The physician may prescribe other medications such as mild tranquilizers or antidepressants to reduce fear and anxiety. This is important because fear and anxiety can exacerbate pain. Other techniques such as imagery, humor, and progressive relaxation (see Chap. 12) are useful in potentiating the effects of pain medication.

Breathing

The dying client may have difficulty breathing; therefore, placing him or her in a Fowler's position may help ease breathing. If the client cannot cough and raise secretions, the nurse gently suctions the client. Suctioning will not clear the lungs or ease breathing if the client has pulmonary edema (fluid in the lungs from heart failure). In this case, the physician may prescribe a sedative to relieve the anxiety created by the feeling of suffocation. Oxygen eventually may be used.

Food and Fluids

If the client can take oral fluids and food, the nurse offers nourishment frequently in small amounts and serves it at the appropriate temperature. He or she encourages the family to bring in foods that the client likes or have been a tradition in the family's diet.

Impaired Swallowing

Difficulty in swallowing, gastric and intestinal distention, and vomiting create a potential for aspiration of fluids, as well as a decrease in food intake. The nurse administers

Nursing Care Plan 26-1

CARE OF THE DYING CLIENT

Assessment

In addition to performing physical assessments of the dying client:

- Assess feelings of the client and family about losses, isolation, grief, hopelessness, and distress.
- Assess family and client communication and coping patterns, strengths, and supports.
- Assess spiritual and cultural beliefs and practices.
- Assess family's ability to provide care at home.

Nursing Diagnosis: **Anticipatory Grieving** related to functional losses and impending death

Expected Outcome: Client will verbalize grief and identify support systems.

Interventions	Rationales
Provide opportunities for client and family to share feelings.	These opportunities allow client and family to discuss anticipated losses.
Assist dying client to focus on the moment, review assets, and maintain relationships.	Doing so helps client to remain connected to his or her world.
If appropriate, encourage client to take care of any unfinished business.	Doing so assists client to heal spiritually and move on.
Identify support systems. Refer client and family to support groups and other resources.	Contact with such groups and resources promotes positive bereavement experiences.

Evaluation of Expected Outcome: Client and family can grieve and become reconciled to impending death.

Nursing Diagnosis: **Compromised Family Coping** related to client's inability to provide support to family and loved ones

Expected Outcome: Client and family verbalize resources to help deal with the situation.

Interventions	Rationales
Assist family to use coping skills that have been effective in other situations.	Coping skills decrease stress and strengthen use of resources.
Encourage family members to identify strengths and express feelings.	These measures help family members to draw on one another's strengths and share feelings, which increases coping.
Involve client and family in planning care.	Such involvement encourages feelings of control.
Refer family to appropriate resources.	They can help the client deal with stressors such as child care, financial needs, and other needs.

Evaluation of Expected Outcome: Client and family demonstrate use of other resources to increase coping with impending loss.

Nursing Diagnosis: **Fear** related to physical pain and concern that needs will not be met

Expected Outcome: Client will express trust that needs will be met.

(continued)

Nursing Care Plan 26-1 (Continued)

CARE OF THE DYING CLIENT

Interventions	Rationales
Discuss client's fears with client and family.	Such discussion provides an opportunity to empathize with and provide accurate information for the client.
Encourage client to make decisions about care.	Doing so gives client some control and decreases fear that needs will not be met.
Plan care with client and family that addresses fears.	Addressing fears enhances feelings of control.
Discuss pain management program, including adjuncts to medication that promote comfort (see Chap. 21-1).	Information about pain management decreases fear of physical pain.

Evaluation of Expected Outcome: Client participates in decisions about care and expresses confidence that needs will be met.

Nursing Diagnosis: Readiness for Enhanced Spiritual Well-being related to desire to achieve harmony of mind, body, and spirit

Expected Outcome: Client will express feelings of hope.

Interventions	Rationales
Provide client time to meditate, pray, and contemplate changes in health status.	Clients need time to be alone when health needs are changing.
Help client develop and accomplish short-term goals and tasks.	Such accomplishment increases self-esteem and self-worth.
Help client to find reasons to live and look forward.	Doing so promotes positive attitudes and ability to live for the moment.
Provide requested religious materials, books, or music.	They assist client to incorporate reading, music, imagery, or meditation into daily routine and spiritual life.
Provide privacy for client to pray with others or for members of his or her faith to visit.	Doing so demonstrates respect for and sensitivity to the client.

Evaluation of Expected Outcome: Client demonstrates spiritual well-being as evidenced by statements of hope, purpose, and trust in his or her faith.

medications for controlling nausea and vomiting 1 hour or so before meals. The nurse and family should not insist that the client eat or drink if these symptoms cannot be controlled. The nurse reports weight loss and inadequate intake so the team can consider alternative nutritional and fluid administration routes. If drooling occurs, the nurse may elevate and turn the client's head to the side or suction the oral cavity.

Temperature Regulation

Skin temperature drops as death nears; the client may describe feeling cold. The nurse can give the client cotton socks, light blankets, and other light clothing if the client feels chilled. Gentle massaging of the arms and legs also may help because it transfers body heat from the hands to the skin surface and improves circulation. Touch also provides support and communicates personal concern.

Skin and Tissue Integrity

A drop in blood pressure and rapid heart failure lead to poor tissue and organ perfusion. The nurse protects the client's skin from breakdown by changing the client's position at least every 2 hours. He or she must consult with the physician about administering intramuscular injections to clients with poor tissue perfusion; doing so may cause inadequate drug absorption and decreased effectiveness.

Self-Care and Activity

Dying clients may not tolerate physical activity well. The nurse may need to assist with personal hygiene. The client needs to be clean, well groomed, and free of unpleasant odors to promote dignity and self-esteem. The nurse gives oral care and ice chips because mouth breathing makes the oral mucous membranes and lips dry. Petroleum jelly helps keep the lips lubricated. The nurse avoids glycerin applications because they tend to pull fluid from the tissue and eventually accentuate the drying problem.

Sleep

A disturbance in sleep pattern may occur because of anxiety, fear, pain, or other environmental stimuli, such as bright lights and disturbing noise. For this reason, nurses must cluster necessary activities to avoid awakening the client and to protect the client from a steady stream of healthcare workers or visitors. When possible, it is helpful to turn off or dim the lights at night and keep noise to a minimum. The radio, television, or recordings of the client's favorite music may mask the continuous hum of equipment and monitors.

Elimination

The nurse can promote normal elimination by offering a bedpan or assisting the client to the bathroom or bedside commode. Incontinence of the bowel or bladder may occur because of the client's disease process or because the client is near death. The client needs absorbent pads when he or she has lost bowel or bladder control. The nurse assists with thorough cleaning. The client may need an indwelling or external catheter, particularly if skin breakdown is a problem.

Fear, Social Isolation, Hopelessness, and Powerlessness

Because the dying client tends to become isolated from others, the nurse must spend time with him or her apart from when doing so is necessary to provide physical care. It is important for nurses to be flexible and to interrupt physical care if and when the client indicates a need for companionship, support, and communication. During unplanned, spontaneous moments, clients often discuss fears or concerns that nurses should not ignore or rush. The nurse can communicate interest and a willingness to listen by sitting down, leaning forward in the client's direction, and making direct eye contact. Nodding, responsive comments such as "Yes," or brief periods of silence encourage the client to continue verbalizing.

Grieving

Grieving is a painful yet normal reaction that helps clients cope with loss and leads to emotional healing. **Anticipatory grieving** occurs before death, often when the dying client and family begin to consider the impact of their potential loss. People express grief in a variety of ways: some become depressed and cry; some are angry and hostile; and some develop physical symptoms, such as anorexia and insomnia. Family members may withdraw emotionally from the dying client because they find the experience too painful, whereas others draw closer, realizing they have only a short time to be with their loved one. The nurse is responsible for facilitating the grieving process and helping the client and family deal with their emotions. To do this, nurses may empathetically share perceptions of what the client and family is experiencing by saying something like, "It must be a very helpless feeling." Once the client and family sense they can speak freely, the nurse needs to listen in a nonjudgmental manner and avoid criticism or giving advice.

Spiritual Distress

Religious beliefs and cultural customs influence attitudes about death. Clients may find great comfort and support from their religious faith and may want someone associated with their religion to visit. If clients indicate such a desire, the nurse notifies appropriate clergy. If asked, the nurse may pray with clients or assist as indicated. When clients are too ill to express their wishes, the nurse must ask the family about spiritual care.

Family Coping

People often find it difficult to communicate frankly with a dying person. Failure to verbalize feelings, express emotions, and show tenderness for the dying person is often a source of regret for grieving relatives. Therefore, families must feel that they can express their feelings with nurses who are compassionate listeners. If nurses encourage family members and listen to them in their frank communication, family members may feel more prepared to carry on a similarly honest dialogue with the dying client. Once they mutually express feelings and break communication barriers, both relatives and the client often experience comfort in their meaningful relationship.

If possible, the family should have a room where they can talk with other relatives, cry, and rest. For emotional support, the nurse may sit with the family for a short time, express concern for their welfare, and listen to their concerns. The nurse explains measures taken to provide comfort and pain relief for the dying client. Families may find it helpful for the nurse to explain that as death draws near, the dying client may appear to become detached and unaware of those nearby, and may slip into unconsciousness before death. The nurse is likely to be with the dying client and family at the moment of death. Some families may want to remain for a time with the body of the deceased. Therefore, the nurse allows a period of privacy before giving postmortem care. If family members or relatives seem unusually distraught, the nurse remains with them until a clergy member or other family member or friend arrives to be with them.

GENERAL NUTRITIONAL CONSIDERATIONS

Good nutrition becomes a quality-of-life issue for dying clients. Eating favorite foods with a mealtime companion may stimulate appetite and promote a sense of comfort. Loss of appetite and weight, however, may be inevitable. "Force feeding" a dying client orally or through a tube may cause nausea and serves no useful purpose. Assure family members that decreased appetite and altered gastrointestinal function are a normal part of the dying process.

GENERAL PHARMACOLOGIC CONSIDERATIONS

A priority for dying clients is pain control. Pain relief is best achieved by administering the analgesic on a regular, around-the-clock basis, rather than on an as-needed basis. Pain control often is a great challenge (see Chap. 21).

Morphine and meperidine (Demerol) can stimulate the chemoreceptor trigger zone, causing vomiting.

Discuss fears related to the possibility of the client developing a tolerance to pain relief medications with the client, family, and other staff members.

Drugs for raising blood pressure, improving tissue and organ perfusion, and correcting cardiac or circulatory problems may be ordered.

GENERAL GERONTOLOGIC CONSIDERATIONS

Older adults may fear prolonged illness, dependency, and loss of cognitive ability more than death itself.

Older adults are more likely to talk about and express less fear concerning death than are younger adults.

Some terminally ill older adults do not want to be alone and fear abandonment by family, who may have difficulty coping with death.

Older adults may die alone, without support from family members, relatives, and close friends. The nurse may be the only person to give close emotional support during the final hours of life.

Because of their own unresolved fears concerning death, nurses may administer less emotional support to older dying clients, even though they require as much emotional support as do young and middle-aged dying clients.

Critical Thinking Exercises

1. *Describe how nursing care of a young adult dying from acquired immunodeficiency syndrome (AIDS) would differ from the nursing care of an older adult dying from pneumonia.*
2. *A client with treatable cancer expresses a desire to go to Mexico, where they offer coffee enemas and injections with sheep urine as a cure. How would you respond? Would your response change if the client's cancer were untreatable? Why?*
3. *If a client wanted to die at home, how would you help the family prepare for terminal home care?*

References and Suggested Readings

Cyhan, T. (2000). Dying for relief. *American Journal of Nursing, 100*(7), 59.

Davidhizar, R., Bechtel, G. A., & Cosey, E. J. (2000). The spiritual needs of hospitalized patients. *American Journal of Nursing, 100*(7), 24C–24D.

DeSpelder, L. A. & Strickland, A. L. (2001). *The last dance: Encountering death and dying* (6th ed.). Mountain View, CA: Mayfield.

Hooks, F. J. & Daly, B. J. (2000). Hastening death. *American Journal of Nursing, 100*(5), 56–63.

Kennedy-Schwarz, J. (2000). Ethical issues: Pain management—a moral imperative. *American Journal of Nursing, 100*(8), 49–50.

Kübler-Ross, E. (1969). *On death and dying.* New York: Macmillan.

Kübler-Ross, E. (1975). *Death: The final stage of growth.* Englewood Cliffs, NJ: Prentice-Hall.

Powers, P. L., Goldstein, C., Plank, G., Thomas, K., & Conkright, L. (2000). The value of patient- and family-centered care. *American Journal of Nursing, 100*(5), 84–88.

Tammelleo, A. D. (2000). Protecting patients' end-of-life choices. *RN, 63*(8), 75–79.

Wolfe, S. (1998). When is it time to die? *RN, 60*(11), 51.

chapter 27

Introduction to the Respiratory System

Words to Know

adenoids
alveoli (sing. alveolus)
bronchioles
bronchi (sing. bronchus)
carina
cilia
diaphragm
diffusion
epiglottis
ethmoidal sinuses
frontal sinuses
glottis
hilus
interstitium
larynx
lungs
maxillary sinuses
mediastinum
nasal septum
nasopharynx
oropharynx
paranasal sinuses
parietal pleura
perfusion
pharynx
pleura
pleural space
respiration
sphenoidal sinuses
tonsils
trachea
turbinates (conchae)
ventilation
visceral pleura
vocal cords

Learning Objectives

On completion of this chapter, the reader will:

- Describe the structures of the upper and lower airways.
- Explain the normal physiology of the respiratory system.
- Differentiate respiration, ventilation, diffusion, and perfusion.
- Describe oxygen transport.
- Define forces that interfere with breathing, including airway resistance and lung compliance.
- Identify elements of a respiratory assessment.
- List diagnostic tests that may be performed on the respiratory tract.
- Discuss preparation and care of clients having respiratory diagnostic procedures.

The respiratory system provides oxygen for cellular metabolic needs and removes carbon dioxide (CO_2), a waste product of cellular metabolism. Respiratory disorders and diseases are common, ranging from mild to life-threatening. Disorders that interfere with breathing or the ability to obtain sufficient oxygen greatly affect respiratory and overall health status.

RESPIRATORY ANATOMY

The respiratory system is divided into the upper airway (Fig. 27-1) and lower airway. The following sections briefly describe the anatomic structures of both divisions.

Upper Airway

Nose

Nasal bones and cartilage support the external nose. The nares are the external openings of the nose. The internal nose is divided into two cavities separated by the **nasal septum.** Each nasal cavity has three passages created by the projection of turbinates or conchae from the lateral walls. The vascular and ciliated mucous lining of the nasal cavities warms and humidifies inspired air. Mucus secreted from the nasal mucosa traps small particles (e.g., dust, pollen). **Cilia** (fine hairs) move the mucus to the back of the throat. This movement helps prevent irritation to and contamination of the lower airway. The nasal mucosa also contains olfactory sensory cells that are responsible for the sense of smell.

317

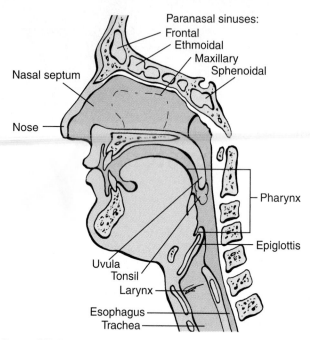

FIGURE 27-1 Major structures of the upper airway.

Paranasal Sinuses

The **paranasal sinuses** are extensions of the nasal cavity located in the surrounding facial bones (see Fig. 27-1). They lighten the weight of the skull and give resonance to the voice. There are four pairs of these bony cavities. The two **frontal sinuses** lie in the frontal bone that extends above the orbital cavities. The ethmoid bone, located between the eyes, contains a honeycomb of small spaces called the **ethmoidal sinuses.** The **sphenoidal sinuses** lie behind the nasal cavity. The **maxillary sinuses** are found on either side of the nose in the maxillary bones. The maxillary sinuses are the largest sinuses and the most accessible to treatment.

The lining of the sinuses is continuous with the mucous-membrane lining of the nasal cavity. Mucus traps particles that cilia sweep toward the pharynx. Immunoglobulin A (IgA) antibodies in the mucus protect the lower respiratory tract from infection.

The olfactory area lies at the roof of the nose. The cribriform plate forms part of the roof of the nose and the floor of the anterior cranial fossa. Trauma or surgery in this area carries the risk of injuring or causing infection in the brain.

Turbinate Bones (Conchae)

The **turbinates** (or **conchae**) are bones that change the flow of inspired air to moisturize and warm it better. As air is inhaled, the turbinates deflect it toward the roof of the nose. They have a large, moist, and warm mucous-membrane surface that can trap almost all dust and microorganisms. They also contain sensitive nerves that detect odors or induce sneezing to remove irritating particles, such as dust or soot.

Pharynx

The **pharynx,** or throat, carries air from the nose to the larynx, and food from the mouth to the esophagus. The pharynx is divided into three continuous areas: the **nasopharynx** (near the nose and above the soft palate), the **oropharynx** (near the mouth), and the *laryngeal pharynx* (near the larynx). The nasopharynx contains the adenoids and openings of the eustachian tubes. The eustachian tubes connect the pharynx to the middle ear and are the means by which upper respiratory infections spread to the middle ear. The oropharynx contains the tongue. The muscular nature of the pharynx allows for closure of the epiglottis during swallowing and relaxation of the epiglottis during respiration.

Tonsils and **adenoids,** which do not contribute to respiration but instead protect against infection, are found in the pharynx. Palatine tonsils consist of two pairs of elliptically shaped bodies of lymphoid tissue. They are located on both sides of the upper oropharynx. Adenoids, or pharyngeal tonsils, also composed of lymphoid tissue, are found in the nasopharynx. Chronic throat infections often lead to removal of the tonsils and adenoids. In adults, adenoids may shrink and become nonfunctional.

Larynx

The **larynx,** or voice box, is a cartilaginous framework between the pharynx and trachea. Its primary function is to produce sound. The larynx also protects the lower airway from foreign objects because it facilitates coughing.

Important structures in the larynx include the **epiglottis,** a cartilaginous valve flap that covers the opening to the larynx during swallowing; the **glottis,** an opening between the vocal cords; and the **vocal cords** themselves, folds of tissue in the larynx that vibrate and produce sound as air passes through (Fig. 27-2). The pharynx, palate, tongue, teeth, and lips mold the sounds made by the vocal cords into speech. Table 27-1 reviews laryngeal structures.

Lower Airway

The lower respiratory airway consists of the trachea, bronchi, bronchioles, lungs, and alveoli (Fig. 27-3). Accessory structures include the diaphragm, rib cage, sternum, spine, muscles, and blood vessels.

Trachea

The **trachea** is a hollow tube composed of smooth muscle and supported by C-shaped cartilage. The cartilaginous rings are incomplete on the posterior surface. The trachea transports air from the laryngeal pharynx to the bronchi and lungs.

Bronchi and Bronchioles

The trachea bifurcates (divides) at the **carina** (lower end of the trachea) to form the left and right **bronchi.** Stim-

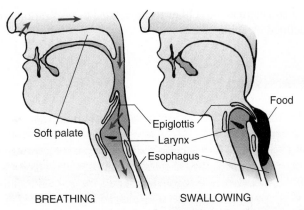

FIGURE 27-2 (A) During swallowing, the soft palate elevates to close off air from the nose. Breathing is interrupted momentarily. **(B)** The larynx rises, and the epiglottis shuts off the laryngeal opening until the food has passed down into the esophagus.

ulation of the carina causes coughing and *bronchospasm* (spasm of the bronchial smooth muscle causing narrowing of the lumen). The right mainstem bronchus is shorter, more vertical, and larger than the left mainstem bronchus. Aspiration of foreign objects is more likely in the right mainstem bronchus and right upper lung. Mucous membrane continues to line this portion of the respiratory tract. Cilia sweep mucus and particles toward the pharynx.

The right and left mainstem bronchi divide into three secondary right bronchi and two secondary left bronchi. Each secondary bronchus supplies air to the three right lobes and two left lobes of the lung. The entrance of the bronchi to the lungs is called the **hilus.** The bronchi branch, enter each lobe, and continue to branch to form smaller bronchi and finally terminal **bronchioles** (smaller subdivisions of bronchi).

Lungs and Alveoli

The **lungs** are paired elastic structures enclosed by the thoracic cage. They contain the **alveoli,** small, clustered sacs that begin where the bronchioles end. Adult lungs contain approximately 300 million alveoli, which form most of the pulmonary mass. Each alveolus consists of a single layer of squamous epithelial cells. Capillaries surround these thin-walled alveoli and are the site of exchange of oxygen and CO_2.

The epithelium of the alveoli consists of the following types of cells:

- Type I cells—line most alveolar surfaces
- Type II cells—produce *surfactant,* a phospholipid that alters the surface tension of alveoli, preventing their collapse during expiration and limiting their expansion during inspiration
- Type III cells—destroy foreign material, such as bacteria

The **interstitium** lies between the alveoli and contains the pulmonary capillaries and elastic connective tissue. Elastic and collagen fibers allow the lungs to have *compliance,* or the ability to expand. Lung expansion creates a negative or subatmospheric pressure, which keeps the lungs inflated. If air gets into the space between the lungs and the thoracic wall, the lungs will collapse.

Accessory Structures

The **diaphragm** separates the thoracic and abdominal cavities. On inspiration, the respiratory muscles contract. The diaphragm also contracts and moves downward, enlarging the thoracic space and creating a partial vacuum. On expiration, the respiratory muscles relax, and the diaphragm returns to its original position. The **mediastinum** is a wall that divides the thoracic cavity into two halves. This wall has two layers of **pleura,** a saclike serous membrane. The **visceral pleura** covers the lung surface, whereas the **parietal pleura** covers the chest wall. Serous fluid within the **pleural space** separates and lubricates the visceral and parietal pleurae. The remaining thoracic structures are located between the two pleural layers.

RESPIRATORY PHYSIOLOGY

The main function of the respiratory system is to exchange oxygen and CO_2 between the atmospheric air and the blood and between the blood and the cells. This process is

TABLE 27-1	STRUCTURES OF THE LARYNX
STRUCTURE	**DESCRIPTION**
Epiglottis	Valve flap of cartilage that covers the opening of the larynx during swallowing
Glottis	Opening between the vocal cords in the larynx
Thyroid cartilage	Largest cartilage in the trachea; part of it forms the Adam's apple
Cricoid cartilage	Only complete cartilaginous ring in the larynx, located below the thyroid cartilage
Arytenoid cartilages	Used in vocal cord movement with the thyroid cartilage
Vocal cords	Ligaments controlled by muscular movement that produce vocal sounds

(Adapted from Smeltzer, S. C. & Bare, B. G. [2000]. *Brunner & Suddarth's textbook of medical–surgical nursing* [9th ed.]. Philadelphia: Lippincott Williams & Wilkins.)

Overview of lower airway

Section of lung enlarged

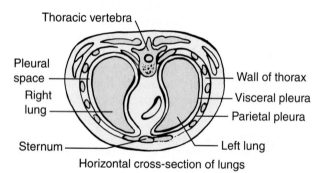

Horizontal cross-section of lungs

FIGURE 27-3 Lower respiratory tract.

called **respiration.** Other terms related to respiration are defined in Table 27-2.

Ventilation

Ventilation is the actual movement of air in and out of the respiratory tract. Air must reach the alveoli for gas to be exchanged. This process requires a patent airway and intact and functioning respiratory muscles. Pressure gradients between atmospheric air and the alveoli enable ventilation. Air flows from an area of higher pressure to an area of lower pressure.

Mechanics of Ventilation

During inspiration, the diaphragm contracts and flattens, which expands the thoracic cage and increases the thoracic cavity. The pressure in the thorax decreases to a level below atmospheric pressure. As a result, air moves into the lungs. When inspiration is complete, the diaphragm relaxes, and the lungs recoil to their original position. The size of the thoracic cavity decreases, increasing the pressure to levels greater than the atmospheric pressure. Air then flows out of the lungs into the atmosphere (Fig. 27-4).

Neurologic Control of Ventilation

Several mechanisms control ventilation. The respiratory centers in the medulla oblongata and pons control rate and depth. Central chemoreceptors in the medulla respond to changes in CO_2 levels and hydrogen ion concentrations (pH) in the cerebrospinal fluid. They convey a message to the lungs to change the depth and rate of ventilation. Peripheral chemoreceptors in the aortic arch and carotid arteries respond to changes in the pH and levels of oxygen and CO_2 in the blood. Table 27-3 describes other neurologic controls of ventilation.

TABLE 27-2	TERMS RELATED TO RESPIRATION
TERM	**DEFINITION**
Ventilation	Movement of air in and out of the lungs sufficient to maintain normal arterial oxygen and carbon dioxide tensions
Inspiration	Movement of oxygen into the lungs
Expiration	Removal of carbon dioxide from the lungs
Diffusion	Transfer of a substance from an area of higher concentration or pressure to an area of lower concentration or pressure; exchange of oxygen and carbon dioxide across the alveolar–capillary membrane and at the cellular level
Perfusion	Flow of blood in the pulmonary circulation
Distribution	Delivery of atmospheric air to the separate gas exchange units in the lungs

is in column one at top.

FIGURE 27-4 The mechanics of ventilation: (From Rosdahl, C. B. [1999]. *Textbook of basic nursing* [7th ed.]. Philadelphia: Lippincott Williams & Wilkins.)

Diffusion

Diffusion is the exchange of oxygen and CO_2 through the alveolar–capillary membrane. Concentration gradients determine the direction of diffusion. During inspiration, the concentration of oxygen is higher in the alveoli than in the capillaries. Therefore, oxygen diffuses from the alveoli to the capillaries, and is carried to the arteries. The concentration of oxygen in the arteries is higher than that in the cells; thus, oxygen diffuses into the cells.

As cellular CO_2 gradients increase, CO_2 diffuses from the cells into the capillaries and then into the venous circulatory system. As CO_2 travels to the pulmonary circulation, its concentration is higher there than in the alveoli. Therefore, CO_2 diffuses into the alveoli.

Alveolar Respiration

Alveolar respiration determines the amount of CO_2 in the body. Increased CO_2, which is present in body fluids primarily as carbonic acid, causes the pH to decrease below the normal 7.4. Decreased CO_2 causes the pH to increase above 7.4. The pH affects the rate of alveolar respiration by a direct action of hydrogen ions on the respiratory center in the medulla oblongata.

The kidneys contribute to maintaining normal pH by excreting excess hydrogen ions, which in turn keep serum bicarbonate levels near normal. The lungs and kidneys combine to maintain the ratio of carbonic acid to bicarbonate at 1 : 20, fixing the pH at approximately 7.4.

In a critically ill client, various homeostatic mechanisms compensate for alterations. In an attempt to maintain normal pH, two mechanisms may occur:

- The lungs eliminate carbonic acid by blowing off more CO_2. They also conserve CO_2 by slowing respiratory volume and reabsorbing bicarbonate (HCO_3).
- The kidneys excrete more bicarbonate.

A client's condition remains compensated if the carbonic acid-to-bicarbonate ratio remains 1 : 20.

Disturbances in pH that involve the lungs are considered respiratory. Disturbances in pH involving other mechanisms are termed *metabolic*. At times, respiratory and metabolic disturbances coexist (see Chap. 22).

Transport of Gases

Oxygen transport occurs in two ways: (1) a small amount is dissolved in water in the plasma, and (2) a greater portion combines with hemoglobin in red blood cells (RBCs; oxyhemoglobin). Dissolved oxygen is the only form that can diffuse across cellular membranes. As this oxygen crosses cellular membranes, oxygen from the hemoglobin rapidly replaces it. Large amounts of oxygen are transported in the blood as oxyhemoglobin. The formula for this process is $O_2 + Hgb \leftrightarrow HgbO_2$.

CO_2 diffuses from the tissue cells to the blood. Bicarbonate ions are then transported to the lungs for excretion. Most of the CO_2 enters the RBCs, although some combines with hemoglobin to form carbaminohemoglobin. Most of the CO_2 combines with water in the cells and exits as bicarbonate ions (HCO_3), which the plasma transports to the kidneys. A small portion remains in the plasma and is called *carbonic acid*. The formation of carbonic acid yields hydrogen ions (H^+). The amount of hydrogen ions determines the pH, which also determines the amount of CO_2 for the lungs to excrete. Refer to Chapter 22 for a

TABLE 27-3	NEUROLOGIC CONTROL OF RESPIRATION
CONTROL	**DESCRIPTION**
Hering-Breuer reflex	Stretch receptors located in the alveoli are activated during inspiration, so that inspiration is inhibited and lungs are not overdistended.
Proprioceptors	Exercise stimulates breathing. Movement activates proprioceptors located in the muscles and joints and increases ventilation.
Baroreceptors	These receptors in the aortic and carotid bodies respond to changes in arterial blood pressure (BP). Elevated arterial BP causes a reflex hypoventilation; lowered BP causes a reflex hyperventilation.

review of acid-base balance. Briefly, acid-base imbalances are compensated in the following ways:

- Respiratory acidosis—kidneys retain more HCO_3 to raise the pH
- Respiratory alkalosis—kidneys excrete more HCO_3 to lower pH
- Metabolic acidosis—lungs "blow off" CO_2 to raise pH
- Metabolic alkalosis—lungs retain CO_2 to lower pH

Pulmonary Perfusion

Perfusion refers to blood supply to the lungs, through which the lungs receive nutrients and oxygen. The two methods of perfusion are the bronchial and pulmonary circulation.

Bronchial Circulation

The bronchial arteries, which supply blood to the trachea and bronchi, arise in the thoracic aorta and intercostal arteries. The bronchial arteries also supply the lungs' supporting tissues, nerves, and outer layers of the pulmonary arteries and veins. This circulation returns either to the left atrium through the pulmonary veins or to the superior vena cava through the bronchial and azygos veins.

The bronchial circulation does not supply the bronchioles or alveoli unless pulmonary circulation is interrupted. In that event, it will supply those areas, but the bronchioles and alveoli cannot perform their function of gas exchange (Bullock & Henze, 2000).

Pulmonary Circulation

The pulmonary artery transports venous blood from the right ventricle to the lungs. It divides into the right and left branches to supply the right and left lungs. The blood circulates through the pulmonary capillary bed, where diffusion of oxygen and CO_2 occurs. The blood then returns to the left atrium through the pulmonary veins.

Pulmonary circulation is referred to as a *low-pressure system* (Smeltzer & Bare, 2000). This means that gravity, alveolar pressure, and pulmonary artery pressure affect pulmonary perfusion. A person in an upright position has less perfusion to the upper lobes. If a person is in a side-lying position, perfusion is greater to the dependent side. In addition, increased alveolar pressure can cause pulmonary capillaries to narrow or collapse, affecting gas exchange. Decreased pulmonary artery pressure results in decreased perfusion to the lungs. Clients with lung and cardiovascular diseases may have decreased pulmonary perfusion.

Problems in Respiratory Physiology

The respiratory system usually has sufficient reserves to maintain the normal partial pressures or tension of oxygen and CO_2 in the blood during times of stress. Respiratory insufficiency develops if there is too much interference with ventilation, diffusion, or perfusion. Abnormalities in these processes can lead to hypoxia, hypoxemia, hypercapnia, and hypocapnia (Table 27-4).

Several factors influence the work of breathing. Pressures needed to overcome the forces interfering with breathing determine the respiratory effort needed. Forces that interfere with breathing include airway resistance and lung compliance.

Airway resistance is related to airway diameter, rate of air flow, and speed of gas flow. As the rate of breathing increases, so does the resistance. A narrowed airway results from increased or thick mucus, bronchospasm, or edema. Conditions that may alter bronchial diameter and affect airway resistance include contraction of bronchial smooth muscle (e.g., asthma); thickening of bronchial mucosa (e.g., chronic bronchitis); airway obstruction by mucus, a tumor, or a foreign body; and loss of lung elasticity (e.g., emphysema).

Decreased surfactant, fibrosis, edema, and atelectasis (alveolar collapse) affect lung compliance. Greater pressure gradients are needed when lungs are stiff.

ASSESSMENT

Assessment of the respiratory system includes obtaining information about physical and functional issues related to breathing. It also means clarifying how these issues may affect the client's quality of life.

History

Often a client seeks medical attention because of respiratory problems related to one or more of the following: dyspnea (labored or difficult breathing), pain on inspiration, increased or more frequent cough, increased sputum production or change in the color/consistency of the mucus, wheezing, or hemoptysis (blood in the sputum). The nurse obtains information about the client's general health history and his or her family history. He or she asks the client about the frequency of respiratory ill-

TABLE 27-4	CONDITIONS RELATED TO ABNORMALITIES IN VENTILATION, PERFUSION, DIFFUSION, AND DISTRIBUTION
CONDITION	**DESCRIPTION**
Hypoxia	Decreased oxygen in inspired air
Hypoxemia	Decreased oxygen in the blood
Hypercapnia	Increased carbon dioxide in the blood
Hypocapnia	Decreased carbon dioxide in the blood

nesses, allergies, smoking history, nature of any cough, sputum production, dyspnea (Box 27-1), and wheezing. Questioning the client about respiratory treatments or medications (prescription and over the counter) is essential. In addition, the nurse inquires about last pulmonary tests (chest radiograph, tuberculosis test). He or she includes questions about occupation, exercise tolerance, pain, and level of fatigue.

Physical Examination

The physical examination begins with a general examination of overall health and condition. Clients with respiratory problems may show signs of shortness of breath when speaking, or they may have a certain posture or position to facilitate breathing. Other observations include skin color; level of consciousness; mental status; respiratory rate, depth, effort, and rhythm; use of accessory muscles; and shape of the chest and symmetry of chest movements.

The nurse inspects the nose for signs of injury, inflammation, symmetry, and lesions. He or she examines the posterior pharynx and tonsils with a tongue blade and light and notes any evidence of swelling, inflammation, or exudate, as well as changes in color of the mucous membranes. The nurse also notes any difficulty with swallowing or hoarseness.

A physician or nurse practitioner inspects the larynx either directly with a laryngoscope or indirectly with a light and laryngeal mirror. Both procedures require a local anesthetic to suppress the gag reflex and reduce discomfort.

The nurse inspects and gently palpates the trachea to assess for placement and deviation from the midline. He or she notes any lymph node enlargement. The nurse also examines the anterior, posterior, and lateral chest walls for lesions, symmetry, deformities, skin color, and evidence of muscle weakness or weight loss. Checking the contour of the chest walls is important. Normally the anteroposterior diameter of the chest wall is half the transverse diameter; however, some pulmonary conditions (e.g., emphysema) change the chest dimensions.

BOX 27-1 ● Questions for the Client With Dyspnea

- What makes you short of breath?
- Do you cough when you are short of breath?
- Do you have other symptoms when you are short of breath?
- Do you get short of breath suddenly or gradually?
- When do you usually have difficulty breathing?
- Can you lie flat in bed?
- Do you get short of breath when you rest? With exercise? Running? Climbing stairs?
- How far can you walk before you get short of breath?

An experienced examiner palpates the chest wall to detect tenderness, masses, swelling, or other abnormalities (Table 27-5). Tactile or vocal *fremitus* (vibrations from the client's voice transmitted to the examiner's fingers) depends on the capacity to feel sound through the fingers and palm placed on the chest wall. The palpable vibrations occur when the client speaks. The examiner uses the palmar surface of the fingers and hands to palpate and asks the client to repeat "99" as the examiner moves his or her hands. If the client is healthy and thin, the fremitus will be highly palpable. Conditions that affect fremitus include a thick or muscular chest wall (decreases fremitus), lung diseases such as emphysema and pneumonia (increase fremitus), and fluid, air, or masses in the pleural space (decrease fremitus).

The experienced examiner performs percussion of the chest wall to assess normal and abnormal sounds. With the client sitting, the examiner places his or her middle finger on the chest wall and taps that finger with the middle finger of the opposite hand. Table 27-6 describes the types of sounds heard with percussion.

The nurse auscultates breath sounds from side to side, moving from the upper to the lower chest (Fig. 27-5). He or she listens anteriorly, laterally, and posteriorly. Normal breath sounds include the following:

- Vesicular sounds—Produced by air movement in bronchioles and alveoli, these sounds are heard over the lung fields; they are quiet and low pitched, with long inspiration and short expiration.

TABLE 27-5	COMMON ABNORMALITIES OF THE CHEST
CONDITION	**DESCRIPTION**
Kyphosis	Exaggerated curvature of the thoracic spine; congenital anomaly or associated with injuries and osteoporosis
Scoliosis	Lateral S-shaped curvature of the thoracic and lumbar spine
Barrel chest	Anteroposterior diameter increases to equal the transverse diameter; chest is rounded; ribs are horizontal; sternum is pulled forward; associated with emphysema and aging
Funnel chest	Also known as *pectus excavatum;* the sternum is depressed from the second intercostal space—more pronounced with inspiration; a congenital anomaly
Pigeon chest	Also known as *pectus carinatum;* the sternum abnormally protrudes; the ribs are sloped backward; a congenital anomaly

TABLE 27-6	SOUNDS HEARD WITH CHEST WALL PERCUSSION	
SOUND	**DESCRIPTION**	**IMPLICATIONS**
Flat	High pitch, little intensity, decreased duration	Heard during percussion of a solid area, such as a mass or pleural effusion
Dull	Medium pitch, medium intensity, medium duration	Heard when no air or fluid is in the lung (e.g., atelectasis, lobar pneumonia)
Tympanic	High pitch, loud intensity, long duration	Normal sounds heard over stomach and bowel; abnormal sounds heard over lungs, such as in a pneumothorax
Resonant	Low pitch, loud intensity, long duration	Normal lung sounds
Hyperresonant	Lower pitch, very loud, longer duration	Abnormal sounds that occur when free air exists in the thoracic cavity (e.g., emphysema, pneumothorax)

- Bronchial sounds—Produced by air movement through the trachea, these sounds are heard over the trachea and are loud with long expiration.
- Bronchovesicular sounds—These normal breath sounds are heard between the trachea and upper lungs; pitch is medium with equal inspiration and expiration.

Adventitious or abnormal breath sounds are categorized as crackles or wheezes. *Crackles* (formerly called *rales*) are discrete sounds that result from the delayed opening of deflated airways. They resemble static or the sound made by rubbing hair strands together near one's ear (Owen, 1998). Sometimes they clear with coughing. They may be present because of inflammation or congestion. Crackles that do not clear with coughing may indicate pulmonary edema or fluid in the alveoli (Owen, 1998).

Sibilant (hissing or whistling) wheezes (formerly called *wheezes*) are continuous musical sounds that can be heard during inspiration and expiration. They result from air passing through narrowed or partially obstructed air passages and are heard in clients with increased secretions. Sonorous wheezes (formerly called *rhonchi*) are lower pitched and are heard in the trachea and bronchi. Friction rubs are heard as crackling or grating sounds on inspiration or expiration. They occur when the pleural surfaces are inflamed and do not change if the client coughs.

Diagnostic Tests

Arterial Blood Gases

Oxygenation of body tissues depends on the amount of oxygen in arterial blood. Arterial blood gases (ABGs) determine the blood's pH, oxygen-carrying capacity, and levels of oxygen, CO_2, and bicarbonate ion. Blood gas samples are obtained through an arterial puncture at the radial, brachial, or femoral artery. A client also may have an indwelling arterial catheter from which arterial samples are obtained.

ABGs frequently are ordered when a client is acutely ill or has a history of respiratory disorders. If the partial pressure of oxygen in arterial blood (PaO_2) is decreased, body tissues do not receive sufficient oxygen. Table 27-7 presents the descriptions and measures of normal ABGs. Clients with respiratory disorders can neither get oxygen into the blood nor get CO_2 out of the blood. Some conditions that affect ABGs are as follows:

- Hyperventilation during collection of ABGs, causing elevated PaO_2
- Hypoventilation with neuromuscular disease, chronic obstructive pulmonary disease (COPD), or insufficient oxygen in the atmosphere, causing decreased PaO_2
- Elevated $PaCO_2$ in clients with COPD, inadequate ventilation with a mechanical ventilator, or decreased respiratory rates
- Decreased $PaCO_2$ in clients who are nervous or anxious or have a condition that causes hyperventilation or a rapid respiratory rate

Pulse oximetry is a noninvasive method that uses a light beam to measure the oxygen content of hemoglobin

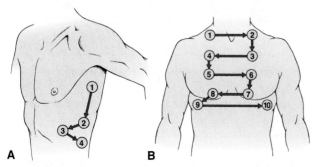

A   **B**

FIGURE 27-5 (**A**) Each side of the chest is auscultated and compared. (**B**) The anterior chest is systematically examined over each lung field.

TABLE 27-7	NORMAL VALUES FOR ARTERIAL BLOOD GASES

BLOOD GAS	NORMAL VALUE
pH, hydrogen ion concentration, acidity or alkalinity of the blood	7.35–7.45
PaO_2, partial pressure of oxygen in arterial blood	80–100 mm Hg
$PaCO_2$, partial pressure of carbon dioxide in arterial blood	35–45 mm Hg
HCO_3, bicarbonate ion concentration in the blood	22–26 mm Hg
SaO_2, arterial oxygen saturation or percentage of the oxygen-carrying capacity of the blood	95%–100%

(SaO_2). The monitoring device is attached to the earlobe or fingertip and connects to the oximeter monitor. Wavelengths of light passing through the earlobe or fingertip are registered by the monitor and used to calculate the arterial oxygen saturation, which is displayed on a readout. Normal values are 95% or higher (Nursing Guidelines 27-1).

Tuberculin Skin Test

The Mantoux test (tuberculin skin test) commonly is done to determine if a client has been infected with *Mycobacterium tuberculosis*. Nurses must remember that this test does not differentiate between active and dormant disease (Nursing Guidelines 27-2).

Pulmonary Function Studies

Pulmonary function studies measure the functional ability of the lungs. Measurements are obtained with a spirometer and include:

- Tidal volume—volume of air inhaled and exhaled with a normal breath
- Inspiratory reserve volume—maximum volume of air that normally can be inspired
- Expiratory reserve volume—maximum volume of air that normally can be exhaled by forced expiration
- Residual volume—volume of air left in the lungs after maximal expiration
- Vital capacity—maximum amount of air that can be expired after maximal inspiration
- Forced vital capacity—amount of air exhaled forcefully and rapidly after maximal inspiration

NURSING GUIDELINES 27-1

Pulse Oximetry

- Explain the procedure to the client.
- Assess potential sensor sites for quality of circulation, edema, tremor, restlessness, nail polish, or artificial nails.
- Review the medical history for data indicating vascular or other pathology (e.g., anemia, carbon monoxide poisoning).
- Check prescribed medications for vasoconstrictive effects.
- Assess client's understanding of pulse oximetry.
- Position the sensor so that the light emission is directly opposite the detector.
- Observe the numeric display, audible sound, or waveform on the oximeter.
- Set the high and low alarms according to the manufacturer's directions.

Pulse oximeter.

NURSING GUIDELINES 27-2

Mantoux Test

- Draw up 0.1 mL of intermediate-strength purified protein derivative (PPD) in a tuberculin syringe ($^1/_2$-inch 26- to 27-gauge needle).
- Prepare the injection site on the inner aspect of the forearm, approximately halfway between the elbow and wrist.
- Hold the syringe bevel up, almost parallel to the forearm.
- Inject the PPD to form a pronounced wheal, which indicates proper intradermal injection.
- Record the site, name of PPD, strength, lot number, and date and time of test.
- Read the test site 48 to 72 hours after injection by palpating the site for induration. If induration is present, measure it at its greatest width. Erythema (redness) without induration is not significant. If erythema is present with induration, read the induration only. Interpret the test results as follows:

  Negative reaction—0- to 4-mm induration; no follow-up needed

  Questionable reaction—5- to 9-mm induration; if the client is aware of contact with someone with active tuberculosis, this reaction is seen as significant

  Positive reaction—10 mm or greater induration

- Inspiratory capacity—maximum amount of air that can be inhaled after normal expiration
- Functional residual capacity—amount of air left in the lungs after a normal expiration
- Total lung capacity—total volume of air in the lungs when maximally inflated

Pulmonary function results vary according to age, sex, weight, and height. The maximum lung capacities and volumes are best achieved when the client is sitting or standing. These studies are done to diagnose pulmonary conditions and to assess preoperative respiratory status. They also may be used to determine the effectiveness of bronchodilators or to screen employees who work in environments that are hazardous to pulmonary health (Nursing Guidelines 27-3).

Sputum Studies

Sputum specimens are examined for pathogenic microorganisms and cancer cells. Culture and sensitivity tests are done to diagnose infections and prescribe antibiotics. Negative results on the examination of sputum smears do not always indicate the absence of disease, so collection of sputum for successive days may be necessary. Sputum is collected by having the client expectorate a specimen, by suctioning the client, or during a bronchoscopy (Nursing Guidelines 27-4).

Radiography

Chest radiographs show the size, shape, and position of the lungs and other structures of the thorax. Physicians use chest radiography to screen for asymptomatic disease and to diagnose tumors, foreign bodies, and other abnormal conditions. Fluoroscopy enables the physician to view the thoracic cavity with all its contents in motion. It more precisely diagnoses the location of a tumor or lesion. Computed tomography scanning or magnetic resonance imaging may be used to produce axial views of the lungs to detect tumors and other lung disorders during early stages.

Pulmonary Angiography

Pulmonary angiography is a radioisotope study that allows the physician to assess the arterial circulation of the lungs, particularly to detect pulmonary emboli. A catheter is introduced into an arm vein and threaded through the right atrium and ventricle into the pulmonary artery. Contrast medium is rapidly injected into the femoral artery, and radiographs are taken to see the distribution of the radiopaque material.

During pulmonary angiography, nurses obtain data about the client's level of anxiety and knowledge of the procedure. They provide explanations and reinforce the client's understanding. They inform the client that he or she will experience a feeling of pressure on catheter insertion. When the contrast medium is infused, the client will sense a warm, flushed feeling and an urge to cough.

Nurses must determine if the client has any allergies, particularly to iodine, shellfish, or contrast dye. During the procedure, they monitor for signs and symptoms of allergic reactions to the contrast medium, such as itching, hives, or difficulty breathing. Infusion of contrast dye is discontinued immediately if the client has an allergic reaction.

After the procedure, nurses inspect the puncture site for swelling, discoloration, bleeding, or hematoma. They assess distal circulation and sensation to ensure that circulation is unimpaired. If bleeding occurs, pressure must be applied to the site. Nurses must notify the physician about diminished or absent distal pulses, cool skin temperature in the affected limb, poor capillary refill, client complaints of numbness or tingling, and bleeding or hematoma. The client remains on bed rest for 2 to 6 hours after the procedure. The pressure dressing, applied after the catheter is removed, remains in place for this period.

NURSING GUIDELINES 27-4

Sputum Specimen

- Explain the procedure to the client.
- Collect a sputum specimen early in the morning or after an aerosol treatment.
- Collect the specimen in a sterile specimen container.
- Instruct the client to rinse the mouth with tap water.
- Instruct the client to take several deep breaths, cough forcefully, and expectorate into the container.
- Collect at least 1 to 3 mL (½ teaspoon).
- Deliver the specimen to the laboratory as soon as possible. The container should be transported in a sealed plastic bag with requisition.

NURSING GUIDELINES 27-3

Pulmonary Function Studies

- Explain the procedure to decrease anxiety and promote cooperation.
- Assure the client that although the spirometry equipment looks complex, the pulmonary function test is simple.
- Explain that the client may be tired after the study.
- Remind the client that the tests should not be performed within 2 hours after a meal.
- Tell the client that bronchodilators may be used during the study.
- Inform the client that he or she will use a nose clip during the study so that air cannot escape through the nose.
- Instruct the client to wear loose-fitting clothing.

Lung Scans

Two types of lung scans may be done for diagnostic purposes: the perfusion scan and the ventilation scan. These procedures may be referred to as a *V-Q scan*. Both require the use of radioisotopes and a scanning machine to detect patterns of blood flow through the lungs and patterns of air movement and distribution in the lungs. V-Q scans are particularly useful in diagnosing pulmonary emboli. They are also used to diagnose lung cancer, COPD, and pulmonary edema.

A radioactive contrast medium is administered intravenously for the perfusion scan and by inhalation as a radioactive gas for the ventilation scan. Before the perfusion scan, nurses must assess the client for allergies to iodine. During the procedure, the radiologist asks the client to change positions. During inhalation, the client may need to hold his or her breath for short periods as scanning images are obtained. The client must receive adequate explanations before the procedure to reduce anxiety. Nurses must reassure the client that the amount of radiation from this procedure is less than that used during a chest radiograph.

Bronchoscopy

Bronchoscopy allows for direct visualization of the larynx, trachea, and bronchi using a flexible fiberoptic bronchoscope. The physician introduces the bronchoscope through the nose or mouth or through a tracheostomy or artificial airway. Bronchoscopy is used to diagnose, treat, or evaluate lung disease; obtain a biopsy of a lesion or tumor; obtain a sputum specimen; perform aggressive pulmonary cleansing; or remove a foreign body.

Bronchoscopy is very frightening to clients, who require thorough explanations throughout the procedure. For at least 6 hours before the bronchoscopy, the client must abstain from food or drink to decrease the risk of aspiration. Risk is increased because the client receives local anesthesia, which suppresses the swallow, cough, and gag reflexes.

The client receives medications before the procedure—usually atropine to dry secretions and a sedative or narcotic to depress the vagus nerve. This consideration is important because if the vagus nerve is stimulated during the bronchoscopy, hypotension, bradycardia, or dysrhythmias may occur. Other potential complications include bronchospasm or laryngospasm secondary to edema, hypoxemia, bleeding, perforation, aspiration, cardiac dysrhythmias, and infection. See Nursing Care Plan 27-1 for more information.

Laryngoscopy

Laryngoscopy provides direct visualization of the larynx using a laryngoscope. It is done to diagnose lesions, evaluate laryngeal function, and determine any inflammation. Physicians also may dilate laryngeal strictures and biopsy lesions. Refer to the preceding section and Nursing Care Plan 27-1 for more information.

Mediastinoscopy

Mediastinoscopy provides visualization of the mediastinum and is done under local or general anesthesia. The physician makes an incision above the sternum and inserts a mediastinoscope. With this procedure, the physician can visualize lymph nodes and obtain biopsy samples. Possible complications include dysrhythmias, myocardial infarction, pneumothorax, and bleeding.

Thoracentesis

A small amount of fluid lies between the visceral and parietal pleurae. When excess fluid or air accumulates, the physician aspirates it from the pleural space by inserting a needle into the chest wall. This procedure, called **thoracentesis,** is performed with local anesthesia. Thoracentesis also may be used to obtain a sample of pleural fluid or a biopsy specimen from the pleural wall for diagnostic purposes, such as a culture and sensitivity or microscopic examination. Bloody fluid usually suggests trauma. Purulent fluid is diagnostic for infection. Serous fluid may be associated with cancer, inflammatory conditions, or heart failure. When thoracentesis is done for therapeutic reasons, 1 to 2 L of fluid may be withdrawn to relieve respiratory distress. Medication may be instilled directly into the pleural space to treat infection.

Thoracentesis is done at the bedside or in a treatment or examining room. The client either sits at the side of the bed or examining table or is in a side-lying position on the unaffected side. If the client is sitting, a pillow is placed on a bedside table, and the client rests her or his arms and head on the pillow. The physician determines the site for aspiration by radiography and percussion. The site is cleaned and anesthetized with local anesthesia. When the procedure is complete, a small pressure dressing is applied. The client remains on bed rest and usually lies on the unaffected side for at least 1 hour to promote expansion of the lung on the affected side. A chest radiograph is done after the procedure to rule out a pneumothorax. See Nursing Guidelines 27-5 for specific measures. Complications that can follow a thoracentesis are pneumothorax, subcutaneous emphysema (air in subcutaneous tissue), infection, pulmonary edema, and cardiac distress.

Stop, Think, and Respond ● BOX 27-1

Your client had a thoracentesis 2 hours ago. He begins to complain of feeling short of breath and is very anxious. What should you assess?

Nursing Care Plan 27-1

THE CLIENT UNDERGOING A BRONCHOSCOPY

Assessment

- Assess level of anxiety and understanding of the procedure.
- Obtain baseline vital signs.
- Assess lung sounds.
- Ask client if he or she wears dentures and when he or she last ate or drank.
- Check record to ensure that the consent form is signed and witnessed.

Nursing Diagnosis: **Fear** related to lack of knowledge about what to expect during and after procedure

Expected Outcome: Client will exhibit coping behaviors and follow instructions.

Interventions	Rationales
Acknowledge client's fear.	Validating fear communicates acceptance.
Provide simple explanations about the procedure after determining what the client knows and his or her misconceptions.	Acknowledging misconceptions provides a starting point. Adults learn more readily when teaching is based on their previous knowledge and experience. Understanding helps to alleviate fear.
Inform client that he or she will receive medications to alleviate anxiety, reduce secretions, and block the vagus nerve.	Information reduces fear and anxiety.
Explain that a tube will be inserted through the nose and throat and into the lungs and that the medication will assist the client.	Thorough explanations reinforce understanding and reduce fear.
Tell client that after the procedure, food and fluids are withheld until the cough reflex returns.	Preoperative sedation and local anesthesia impair the cough reflex and swallowing for several hours.
Inform client that the throat will be irritated and sore for a few days, and that he or she may cough up blood-tinged mucus.	Knowledge about expected signs and symptoms reduces fear after the procedure.

Evaluation of Expected Outcome: Client tolerates procedure without untoward effects, follows instructions, and states that fear is minimal.

Nursing Diagnosis: **Risk for Aspiration** related to diminished gag reflex

Expected Outcomes: (1) Client will maintain a patent airway. (2) Risk of aspiration will decrease.

Interventions	Rationales
Assess cough and gag reflexes.	Depressed cough or gag reflex increases risk of aspiration.
Keep client NPO until the gag reflex returns (usually 2 to 8 hours).	NPO status reduces the risk of aspiration.
Keep suction equipment available.	If the client aspirates, suctioning helps to maintain a patent airway.
Place client in semi-Fowler's position with the head to one side.	Proper positioning decreases the risk of aspiration.
Encourage client to expectorate secretions frequently into an emesis basin.	Expectoration reduces the risk of aspiration.

(continued)

Nursing Care Plan 27-1 (Continued)

THE CLIENT UNDERGOING A BRONCHOSCOPY

Interventions	*Rationales*
After the gag reflex returns, offer sips of water or ice chips initially, then progress the diet to soft foods.	Beginning with sips of water or ice chips ensures that the gag reflex has returned. The client can most easily swallow soft foods.

Evaluation of Expected Outcomes: Airway remains patent. Client does not experience aspiration.

PC: **Pneumothorax:** dysrhythmia, bronchospasm

Expected Outcome: The nurse will manage and minimize potential complications.

Interventions	*Rationales*
Monitor vital signs and respiratory status, comparing against baseline assessment data.	Comparison helps the nurse determine if the client is experiencing any respiratory distress.
Observe for symmetric chest movements.	Decreased or asymmetric chest expansion is a sign of pneumothorax.
Report hemoptysis, stridor, or dyspnea immediately.	These findings indicate respiratory distress and probable pneumothorax.

Evaluation of Expected Outcome: Client experiences no postprocedure complications.

NURSING GUIDELINES 27-5

Thoracentesis

- Explain the procedure to the client.
- Reassure the client that he or she will receive local anesthesia. Explain that the client will still experience a pressure-like pain when the needle pierces the pleura and when fluid is withdrawn.
- Assist client to an appropriate position (sitting with arms and head on padded table or in side-lying position on unaffected side).
- Instruct client not to move during the procedure, including no coughing or deep breathing.
- Provide comfort.
- Inform client about what is happening.
- Maintain asepsis.
- Monitor vital signs during the procedure—also monitor pulse oximetry if client is connected to it.
- During removal of fluid, monitor for respiratory distress, dyspnea, tachypnea, or hypotension.
- Apply small sterile pressure dressing to the site after the procedure.
- Position client on the unaffected side. Instruct client to stay in this position for at least 1 hour and to remain on bed rest for several hours.
- Check that chest radiography is done after the procedure.
- Record the amount, color, and other characteristics of fluid removed.

- Monitor for signs of increased respiratory rate, asymmetry in respiratory movement, syncope or vertigo, chest tightness, uncontrolled cough or cough that produces blood-tinged or frothy mucus (or both), tachycardia, and hypoxemia.

Client positioning for thoracentesis.

NURSING MANAGEMENT

In addition to the nursing management of individual tests, clients require informative and appropriate explanations of any diagnostic procedures they will experience. Nurses must remember that, for many of these clients, breathing may in some way be compromised. Energy levels may be decreased. For that reason, explanations should be brief yet complete and may need to be repeated. The nurse also must help ensure adequate rest periods before and after the procedures. After invasive procedures, the nurse must carefully assess for signs of respiratory distress, chest pain, blood-streaked sputum, and expectoration of blood. He or she needs to repeat postprocedure expectations to help reduce the client's anxiety and to ensure the best possible recovery.

GENERAL PHARMACOLOGIC CONSIDERATIONS

Clients scheduled for diagnostic tests that involve the use of a contrast medium containing iodine are questioned about allergies, especially to seafoods (which contain iodine) and iodine. If the client appears to have an iodine allergy, notify the physician before the test. An allergic reaction to iodine can be serious and sometimes fatal.

GENERAL GERONTOLOGIC CONSIDERATIONS

Although the numbers of alveoli remain stable with age, the alveolar walls become thinner and contain fewer capillaries, resulting in decreased gas exchange. The lungs also lose elasticity and become stiffer. These changes place older adults at increased risk for respiratory disease.

Older clients may have difficulty understanding explanations or directions given by the physician or nurse. Repeating or restating information or directions may be necessary before or during a diagnostic test.

Critical Thinking Exercise

1. *Your client had a thoracentesis today. When he returns to your unit, he begins to complain of pain. What risks are associated with this procedure?*

References and Suggested Readings

Bullock, B. L. & Henze, R. L. (2000). *Focus on pathophysiology.* Philadelphia: Lippincott Williams & Wilkins.

Carpenito, L. J. (2000). *Nursing diagnosis: Application to clinical practice* (8th ed.). Philadelphia: Lippincott Williams & Wilkins.

Faria, S. H. & Taylor, L. J. (1997). Interpretation of arterial blood gases by nurses. *Journal of Vascular Nursing, 15*(4), 128–130.

Fritz, D. J. (1997). Fine tune your physical assessment of the lungs and respiratory system. *Home Care Provider, 2,* 299–302; quiz 303–305.

O'Hanlon-Nichols, T. (1998). Basic assessment series: The adult pulmonary system. *American Journal of Nursing, 98*(2), 39–45.

Owen, A. (1998). Respiratory assessment revisited. [On-line.] Available: http://www.findarticles.com/cf_o/m3231/n4_v28/20512635/print.jhtml.

Smeltzer, S. C. & Bare, B. G. (2000). *Brunner & Suddarth's textbook of medical–surgical nursing* (9th ed.). Philadelphia: Lippincott Williams & Wilkins.

Caring for Clients With Upper Respiratory Disorders

Learning Objectives

On completion of this chapter, the reader will:

- Describe nursing care for clients experiencing infectious or inflammatory upper respiratory disorders.
- Discuss assessment data required to provide nursing care to clients with structural disorders of the upper airway.
- Describe the airway problems a client may experience following trauma or obstruction to the upper airway.
- Identify risk factors that contribute to the development of laryngeal cancer.
- Identify the earliest symptom of laryngeal cancer.
- Discuss treatments for laryngeal cancer.
- Describe measures used to promote alternative methods of communication for clients with a laryngectomy.
- Discuss psychosocial issues that clients may experience following a laryngectomy.
- Relate treatment modalities for clients experiencing short-term or long-term problems with airway management.
- Identify possible reasons for and nursing management of a tracheostomy.
- Explain why a client may require endotracheal intubation.

Disorders of the upper airway range from common colds to cancer. The severity depends on the nature of the disorder and the client's physiologic response. Most people experience common colds and sore throats and find them more inconvenient than serious. For others, even the most common disorders of the upper respiratory airway are of great concern because other physical problems compound their effects.

INFECTIOUS AND INFLAMMATORY DISORDERS

The most common upper airway illnesses are infectious and inflammatory disorders. Although dismissing these illnesses as unimportant is easy, the average person experiences three to five upper respiratory infections (URIs) each year. For some individuals, URIs develop into bronchitis or pneumonia, which involves more serious symptoms and may require antibiotics or other treatments (see Chap. 29).

● RHINITIS

Rhinitis is inflammation of the nasal mucous membranes. It also is referred to as the *common cold*, or **coryza.** Rhinitis may be acute, chronic, or allergic, depending on the cause. The most common cause is the rhinovirus, of which more than 100 strains exist. Colds are rapidly spread by inhalation of droplets and direct contact with contaminated articles (e.g., telephone receivers, doorknobs). Allergic rhinitis is a hypersensitive reaction to allergens, such as pollen, dust, animal dander, or food. Rhinitis is usually not a serious condition; however, it may lead to pneumonia and other more serious illnesses for debilitated, immunosuppressed, or older clients.

Symptoms associated with rhinitis include sneezing, nasal congestion, **rhinorrhea** (clear nasal discharge), sore throat, watery eyes, cough, low-grade fever, headache, aching muscles, and malaise. With the common cold, these symptoms continue for 5 to 14 days. A sustained elevated temperature suggests a bacterial infection or infection in the sinuses or ears. Symptoms of allergic rhinitis will persist as long as the client is exposed to the specific allergen.

For most clients, treatment for rhinitis is minimal (Box 28-1). Unless specific bacteria are identified as the cause of the infection, antibiotics are not used. Clients may be advised to use antipyretics for fever, decongestants for severe nasal congestion, antitussives for prolonged cough, saline gargles for sore throat, or antihistamines for allergic rhinitis. Medications that desensitize or suppress immune responses may also be prescribed for allergic rhinitis.

Teaching clients about URIs helps prevent them and minimizes potential complications. Maintaining a healthy lifestyle of adequate rest and sleep, proper diet, and moderate exercise is the best prevention. Another important preventive factor is frequent handwashing, which greatly reduces the spread of infection.

● SINUSITIS

Sinusitis is inflammation of the sinuses. The maxillary sinus is affected most often. Sinusitis can lead to serious complications, such as infection of the middle ear or brain.

Pathophysiology and Etiology

The principle causes are the spread of an infection from the nasal passages to the sinuses and the blockage of normal sinus drainage (Fig. 28-1). Interference with sinus

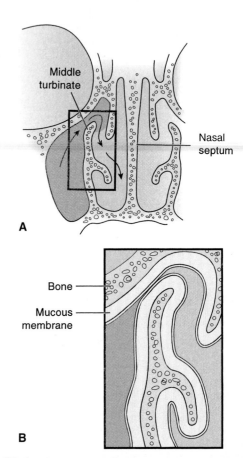

FIGURE 28-1 Edema can obstruct sinus drainage. (**A**) The maxillary sinuses normally drain through the openings that lie under the middle turbinates. The openings for the drainage are near the upper portion of the sinus. (**B**) Edema, which commonly accompanies upper respiratory infections, can obstruct the openings and prevent normal sinus drainage.

drainage predisposes a client to sinusitis because trapped secretions readily become infected. Allergies frequently cause edema of the nasal mucous membranes, leading to obstruction of sinus drainage and sinusitis. Nasal polyps or a deviated septum may also impair sinus drainage. Measures that help reduce the incidence or severity of sinusitis include eating a well-balanced diet, getting plenty of rest, engaging in moderate exercise, avoiding allergens, and seeking medical attention promptly if a cold persists longer than 10 days or nasal discharge is green or dark yellow and foul-smelling.

Assessment Findings

Signs and symptoms depend on which sinus is infected. They include headache, fever, pain over the affected sinus, nasal congestion and discharge, pain and pressure around the eyes, and malaise. A nasal smear or material obtained from irrigation of the sinus for culture and sensitivity testing identifies the infectious microorganism and appropri-

---

BOX 28-1 ● Treating Rhinitis

For all types of rhinitis:
- Rest as much as possible.
- Increase fluid intake to assist in liquefying secretions.
- Use a vaporizer to help liquefy secretions.
- Blow nose with mouth open slightly to equalize pressure.
- Wash hands frequently to avoid spreading infection.
- Use over-the-counter medications as directed; be aware of possible side effects, especially interactions with food and alcohol.

For allergic rhinitis:
- Be tested for allergen sensitivity.
- Avoid specific allergens.
- Use antihistamines and decongestants as ordered.

ate antibiotic therapy. Transillumination and radiographs of the sinuses may show a change in the shape of or fluid in the sinus cavity. A thorough history, including an allergy history, usually confirms the diagnosis.

Medical and Surgical Management

Acute sinusitis frequently responds to conservative treatment designed to help overcome the infection. Saline irrigation of the maxillary sinus may be done to remove accumulated exudate and promote drainage. Such irrigation is accomplished by insertion of a catheter through the normal opening under the middle concha. Antibiotic therapy is necessary for severe infections. Vasoconstrictors, such as phenylephrine nose drops, may be recommended for short-term use to relieve nasal congestion and aid in sinus drainage.

Surgery is often indicated for chronic sinusitis. Endoscopic sinus surgery helps provide an opening in the inferior meatus to promote drainage. More radical procedures, such as the Caldwell-Luc procedure and external sphenoethmoidectomy, are done to remove diseased tissue and provide an opening into the inferior meatus of the nose for adequate drainage.

Nursing Management

If the client is receiving medical treatment, the nurse informs him or her that use of mouthwashes and humidification, as well as increased fluid intake, may loosen secretions and increase comfort. He or she instructs the client to take nasal decongestants and antihistamines as ordered.

If the client has sinus surgery, the nurse institutes standards for postoperative care (see Chap. 25). He or she observes the client for repeated swallowing, a finding that suggests possible hemorrhage. One risk of sinus surgery is damage to the optic nerve. Thus, the nurse assesses postoperative visual acuity by asking the client to identify the number of fingers displayed. The nurse monitors the client's temperature at least every 4 hours. He or she assesses for pain over the involved sinuses, a finding that may indicate postoperative infection or impaired drainage. The nurse administers analgesics as indicated and applies ice compresses to involved sinuses to reduce pain and edema.

The client will have nasal packing and a dressing under the nares ("moustache" dressing or "drip pad"). Because nasal packing forces the client to breathe through the mouth, the nurse encourages oral hygiene and gives ice chips or small sips of fluids frequently. Such measures will alleviate the dryness caused by mouth breathing. The nurse changes the drip pad as needed and reports excessive drainage. Postoperative client and family teaching includes telling the client not to blow the nose, lift objects more than 5 to 10 lbs, or do the Valsalva maneuver for 10 to 14 days postoperatively. The nurse urges the client to remain in a warm environment and to avoid smoky or poorly ventilated areas.

Stop, Think, and Respond ● BOX 28-1

A neighbor tells you that she is taking antibiotics for an acute sinus infection. She states that she has severe pain in her sinuses and wonders what she can do other than take analgesics. What advice might you give?

● PHARYNGITIS

Pharyngitis, inflammation of the throat, is often associated with rhinitis and other URIs (Figure 28-2). Viruses and bacteria cause pharyngitis. The most serious bacteria are the group A streptococci, which cause a condition commonly referred to as *strep throat*. Strep throat can lead to dangerous cardiac complications (endocarditis and rheumatic fever) and harmful renal complications (glomerulonephritis). Pharyngitis is highly contagious and spreads via inhalation of or direct contamination with droplets.

The incubation period for pharyngitis is 2 to 4 days. The first symptom is a sore throat, sometimes severe, with accompanying *dysphagia* (difficulty swallowing), fever, chills, headache, and malaise. Some clients exhibit a white or exudate patch over the tonsillar area and swollen glands. A throat culture reveals the specific causative bacteria. Rapid identification methods, such as the Biostar or the Strep A optical immunoassay (OIA), are available to diagnose group A streptococcal infections. These tests are done in clinics and physician offices. Standard 24-hour throat culture and sensitivity tests identify other organisms.

FIGURE 28-2 Pharyngitis—inflammation without exudate. (From Bickley, L. S. & Hoekelman, R. A. [1999]. *Bates' guide to physical examination and history taking* [7th ed.]. Philadelphia: Lippincott Williams & Wilkins.)

Early antibiotic treatment is the best choice for pharyngitis to treat the infection and help prevent potential complications. Penicillin or its derivatives are generally the antibiotics of choice. Clients sensitive to penicillin receive erythromycin. The antibiotic regimen is 7 to 14 days.

● TONSILLITIS AND ADENOIDITIS

Tonsillitis is inflammation of the tonsils, and **adenoiditis** is inflammation of the adenoids. These conditions generally occur together—the common diagnosis is tonsillitis. Although both disorders are more common in children, they also may be seen in adults.

Pathophysiology and Etiology

The tonsils and adenoids are lymphatic tissues and common sites of infection. Primary infection may occur in the tonsils and adenoids, or the infection can be secondary to other URIs. Chronic tonsillar infection leads to enlargement and partial upper airway obstruction. Chronic adenoidal infection can result in acute or chronic infection in the middle ear (otitis media). If the causative organism is group A streptococcus, prompt treatment is needed to prevent potential cardiac and renal complications.

Assessment Findings

Sore throat, difficulty or pain on swallowing, fever, and malaise are the most common symptoms. Enlarged adenoids may produce nasal obstruction, noisy breathing, snoring, and a nasal quality to the voice. Visual examination reveals enlarged and reddened tonsils. White patches may appear on the tonsils if group A streptococci are the cause. A throat culture and sensitivity test determines the causative microorganism and appropriate antibiotic therapy.

Medical and Surgical Management

Antibiotic therapy, analgesics such as acetaminophen, and saline gargles may be used to treat the infection and associated discomfort. Chronic tonsillitis and adenoiditis may require **tonsillectomy,** operative removal of the tonsils, and **adenoidectomy,** operative removal of the adenoids. The criteria for performing these procedures are repeated episodes of tonsillitis, hypertrophy of the tonsils, enlarged obstructive adenoids, repeated purulent otitis media, hearing loss related to serous otitis media associated with enlarged tonsils and adenoids, and other conditions (e.g., asthma, rheumatic fever) exacerbated by tonsillitis. Tonsillectomy and adenoidectomy are generally done as outpatient procedures.

NURSING PROCESS

● Tonsillectomy and Adenoidectomy

Assessment

The nurse assesses the client's understanding of the procedure and obtains baseline vital signs. He or she asks if the client wears dentures and when the client last had food or drink. The need to pay special attention to hematocrit, platelet count, and clotting time emphasizes the high risk for postoperative hemorrhage. The nurse asks the client about bleeding tendencies and recent use of aspirin, nonsteroidal anti-inflammatory drugs (NSAIDs), or other medications that prolong bleeding time. Some herbal supplements also prolong bleeding, so the nurse must ask about the use of these supplements.

Diagnosis, Planning, and Intervention

Following surgery, the nurse implements the postoperative standards described in Chapter 25. Additional nursing care is discussed as follows and in Client and Family Teaching Box 28-1.

Risk for Aspiration related to impaired swallowing secondary to throat surgery and reduced gag reflex secondary to anesthesia

Expected Outcomes: (1) Client will maintain a patent airway with clear breath sounds. (2) Client will expectorate secretions and vomitus as needed.

- After surgery, position client, until alert, on either side with emesis basin to catch drainage or vomitus. *Retained secretions/vomitus can obstruct airway and cause aspiration.*
- Assess gag reflex and ability to swallow. *A depressed gag reflex and inability to swallow increase the risk for aspiration.*
- Elevate head of bed 45° when client is fully awake. *This position decreases surgical edema and increases lung expansion.*
- Monitor respiratory rate, rhythm, and effort at least every hour. *Increased respiratory rate, decreased breath sounds, or both indicate an increased respiratory effort, possibly related to a partially obstructed airway, aspiration, or both.*
- Auscultate breath sounds for crackles at least every hour. *Aspiration of small amounts may occur without evidence of coughing or respiratory distress.*

- Encourage client to spit secretions/vomitus into the emesis basin. *Removal of secretions/vomitus maintains a clear airway and prevents aspiration.*
- Assess for lethargy, behavior changes, or disorientation. *Decreased level of consciousness indicates poor air exchange.*
- Have oral suction equipment available. *Prompt oral suctioning removes secretions/vomitus from the mouth, preventing aspiration.*

Risk for Impaired Tissue Integrity related to injury to the suture line

Expected Outcome: Client will maintain an intact suture line.

- Monitor client for bloody drainage from mouth or frequent swallowing. *These findings indicate increased bleeding from suture site and require immediate attention.*
- Instruct client not to cough, clear the throat, blow the nose, or use a straw in the first few postoperative days. *These actions increase pressure on the suture line and may cause disruption and bleeding.*
- Instruct client to avoid carbonated fluids and fluids high in citrus content. *Such fluids are caustic to the surgical site and may traumatize tissue, disrupting the suture line.*
- Encourage client to first try ice chips, then small sips of cold fluids, and then popsicles and full liquids as tolerated. *Gradual introduction of increasingly thick fluids provides client with an opportunity to slowly try swallowing, without disrupting the suture line.*
- Add soft food, such as gelatin and sherbet, as tolerated, after the first 24 hours postoperatively. *As the diet advances, small amounts of soft foods are less likely to traumatize the suture line.*

Pain related to the surgical incision in the throat

Expected Outcomes: Client will acknowledge relief from pain medications and demonstrate an improved ability to swallow.

- Anticipate the need for pain relief, medicating client as ordered. *Early treatment of pain assists to decrease its intensity.*
- Apply ice collar as ordered. *Cold reduces swelling and inflammation in the soft tissues surrounding the surgical incision. The ice pack will help to control bleeding, reduce edema and inflammation, and block pain receptors.*
- Encourage client to gently gargle with warm saline three to four times daily. *Gentle gargling cleanses the surgical site and helps reduce inflammation and pain, remove thick mucus, and improve swallowing.*

Evaluation of Expected Outcomes

Client maintains a clear airway and can expectorate secretions and vomitus. He or she experiences minimal postoperative bleeding. The suture line remains in-

28-1 *Client and Family Teaching*
Tonsillectomy and Adenoidectomy

The nurse ensures that the client and family members can manage self-care at home by communicating the following points:

- Report any signs of bleeding to the physician—this is particularly important in the first 12 to 24 hours, and then 7 to 10 days after surgery as the throat heals.
- Gently gargle with warm saline or an alkaline mouthwash to assist in removing thick mucus.
- Maintain a liquid and very soft diet for several days after surgery—avoid spicy foods and rough-textured foods.
- Also, avoid milk and milk products if the client does not tolerate them well.

tact. Client states relief of pain and that he or she can swallow.

● PERITONSILLAR ABSCESS

A **peritonsillar abscess** is an abscess that develops in the connective tissue between the capsule of the tonsil and the constrictor muscle of the pharynx. It may follow a severe streptococcal or staphylococcal tonsillar infection. The client with a peritonsillar abscess experiences difficulty and pain with swallowing, fever, malaise, ear pain, and difficulty talking. On visual examination, the affected side is red and swollen, as is the posterior pharynx. Drainage from the abscess is cultured to identify the microorganism. Sensitivity studies determine the appropriate antibiotic therapy.

Immediate treatment of a peritonsillar abscess is recommended to prevent the spread of the causative microorganism to the bloodstream or adjacent structures. Penicillin or another antibiotic is given immediately after a culture is obtained and before results of the culture and sensitivity tests are known. Surgical incision and drainage of the abscess is done if the abscess partially blocks the oropharynx. A local anesthetic is sprayed or painted on the surface of the abscess, and the contents are evacuated. Repeated episodes may necessitate a tonsillectomy.

Nursing management of the client undergoing drainage of an abscess includes placing the client in a semi-Fowler's position to prevent aspiration. An ice collar may be ordered to reduce swelling and pain. The nurse encourages the client to drink fluids. He or she observes the client for signs of respiratory obstruction (e.g., dyspnea, restlessness, cyanosis) or excessive bleeding.

● LARYNGITIS

Laryngitis is inflammation and swelling of the mucous membrane that lines the larynx. Edema of the vocal cords frequently accompanies laryngeal inflammation. Laryngitis may follow a URI and results from spread of the infection to the larynx. Other causes include excessive or improper use of the voice, allergies, and smoking.

Hoarseness, inability to speak above a whisper, or **aphonia** (complete loss of voice) are the usual symptoms. Clients also complain of throat irritation and a dry, nonproductive cough. The diagnosis is based on the symptoms. If hoarseness persists more than 2 weeks, the larynx is examined (**laryngoscopy**). Persistent hoarseness is a sign of laryngeal cancer and thus merits prompt investigation. Treatment involves voice rest and treatment or removal of the cause. Antibiotic therapy may be used if a bacterial infection is the cause. If smoking is the cause, the nurse encourages smoking cessation and refers the client to a smoking-cessation program.

STRUCTURAL DISORDERS

● EPISTAXIS

Pathophysiology and Etiology

Epistaxis, or nosebleed, is a common occurrence. It is not usually serious but can be frightening. Nosebleeds are the rupture of tiny capillaries in the nasal mucous membrane. They occur most commonly in the anterior septum, referred to as *Kiesselbach's area.* Causes of nosebleed include trauma, rheumatic fever, infection, hypertension, nasal tumors, and blood dyscrasias. Epistaxis that results from hypertension or blood dyscrasias is likely to be severe and difficult to control. Those who abuse cocaine may have frequent nosebleeds. Foreign bodies in the nose and deviated septum contribute to epistaxis, along with forceful nose blowing and frequent or aggressive nose picking.

Assessment Findings

Inspection of the nares, using a nasal speculum and light, reveals the area of bleeding. The examiner uses a tongue blade to check the back of the throat and a laryngeal mirror to view the area above and behind the uvula.

Medical and Surgical Management

The severity and location of the bleeding determine the treatment. One or a combination of the following therapies may be used:

- Direct continuous pressure to the nares for 5 to 10 minutes with the client's head tilted slightly forward
- Application of ice packs to the nose
- Cauterization with silver nitrate, electrocautery, or application of a topical vasoconstrictor such as 1:1000 epinephrine
- Nasal packing with a cotton tampon
- Pressure with a balloon inflated catheter—inserted posteriorly for a minimum of 48 hours

Nursing Management

The nurse monitors vital signs and assesses for signs of continued bleeding. He or she may initiate measures to control bleeding, such as applying pressure and ice packs. Other treatments require a physician's order. The client experiencing epistaxis is usually anxious and requires reassurance. If underlying conditions are the cause, the nurse refers the client for medical follow-up. He or she may also recommend humidification, use of a nasal lubricant to keep the mucous membranes moist, and avoidance of vigorous nose blowing and nose picking, or other nose trauma. Teaching about treatment of severe nosebleed includes the following:

- If epistaxis recurs, apply pressure to nares with two fingers. Breathe through the mouth and sit with the head tipped forward slightly to prevent blood from running down the throat.
- Do not swallow blood; spit out any blood that is oozing from the area. Do not blow the nose.
- If blood has been swallowed, diarrhea and black tarry stools may be seen for a few days.
- Do not attempt to remove nasal packing or to cut the string anchoring the packing.
- Take pain medications as ordered. Do not use aspirin or ibuprofen products until bleeding is controlled.
- Notify the physician if bleeding persists or if any respiratory problems develop.

● NASAL OBSTRUCTION

Obstruction of the nasal passage interferes with air passage. Three primary conditions lead to nasal obstruction: a deviated septum, nasal polyps, and hypertrophied turbinates.

Pathophysiology and Etiology

A **deviated septum** is an irregularity in the septum that results in nasal obstruction. The deviation may be a deflection from the midline in the form of lumps or sharp projections or a curvature in the shape of an "S." Marked deviation can result in complete obstruction of one nostril and interference with sinus drainage. A deviated septum may be congenital, but often it results from trauma.

Nasal polyps are grapelike swellings that arise from the nasal mucous membranes. They probably result from chronic irritation related to infection or allergic rhinitis. They obstruct nasal breathing and sinus drainage, ultimately leading to sinusitis. Most are benign and tend to recur when removed.

Hypertrophied turbinates are enlargements of the nasal concha, three bones that project from the lateral wall of the nasal cavity. The hypertrophy, which results from chronic rhinitis, interferes with air passage and sinus drainage, and eventually leads to sinusitis.

Assessment Findings

Symptoms include a history of sinusitis, difficulty breathing out of one nostril, frequent nosebleeds, and nasal discharge. Clients usually report difficulty breathing through one or both sides of the nose. Inspection with a nasal speculum reveals a left or right deviation of the nasal septum, the number and location of the polyps, or enlarged turbinates.

Medical and Surgical Management

A submucous surgical resection or septoplasty may be necessary to restore normal breathing and to permit adequate sinus drainage for the client with a deviated septum. This procedure involves an incision through the mucous membrane and removal of the portions of the septum that cause obstruction. After this procedure, both sides of the nasal cavity are packed with gauze, which remains in place for 24 to 48 hours. A moustache dressing or drip pad is applied to absorb any drainage.

Rhinoplasty, reconstruction of the nose, may also be done at the same time. This procedure enhances the client's appearance cosmetically and corrects any structural nasal deformities that interfere with air passage. The surgeon makes an incision inside the nostril and restructures the nasal bone and cartilage. As with septoplasty, the nasal cavity is packed with gauze, and the nose is taped. Application of a nasal splint maintains the shape and structure of the nose and reduces edema. The splint remains in place for at least 1 week.

Treatment for polyps includes a steroidal nasal spray to reduce inflammation or direct injection of steroids into the polyps. If nasal obstruction is severe, the surgeon performs a *polypectomy,* the removal of polyps with a nasal snare or laser under local anesthesia. The polyps are examined microscopically to rule out malignant disease.

Hypertrophied turbinates are often treated with the application of astringents or aerosolized corticosteroids to shrink them close to the nose. Occasionally, one of the turbinates may be surgically removed (*turbinectomy*).

Nursing Management

Surgery for correction of nasal obstruction is usually done on an outpatient basis. The nurse provides thorough explanations throughout the procedures to alleviate anxiety. It is particularly important to emphasize that nasal packing will be in place postoperatively, necessitating mouth breathing. The application of an ice pack will reduce pain and swelling.

Placing the client in a semi-Fowler's position promotes drainage, reduces edema, and enhances breathing. The nurse inspects the nasal packing and dressings frequently for bleeding and asks the client to report excessive swallowing, which can indicate bleeding. Ongoing monitoring of vital signs is necessary, as is providing oral hygiene and saline mouth rinses (when permitted) to keep mucous membranes moist. The nurse tells the client that feeling or hearing a sucking noise when swallowing is normal and will resolve when the nasal packing is removed.

Teaching measures include preparing the postoperative client for edema and discoloration around the eyes and nose that will disappear after a few weeks. The nurse also instructs the client in the following measures to prevent bleeding:

- Do not bend over.
- Do not blow nose.
- If sneezing, keep mouth open.
- Avoid contact with nose or surrounding tissue.
- Keep head elevated with an extra pillow when lying down.
- Avoid heavy lifting.
- Do not use aspirin, ibuprofen, alcohol, or tobacco products.

TRAUMA AND OBSTRUCTION OF THE UPPER AIRWAY

● FRACTURES OF THE NOSE

A nasal fracture usually results from direct trauma. It causes swelling and edema of the soft tissues, external and internal bleeding, nasal deformity, and nasal obstruction. In severe nasal fractures, cerebrospinal fluid, which is colorless and clear, may drain from the nares. Drainage of cerebrospinal fluid suggests a fracture in the cribriform plate.

The diagnosis of a nasal fracture may be delayed because of significant swelling and bleeding. As soon as the swelling decreases, the examiner inspects the nose internally to rule out a fracture of the nasal septum or septal hematoma. Both conditions require treatment to prevent destruction of the septal cartilage. If drainage of clear fluid is observed, a Dextrostix is used to determine the presence of glucose, which is diagnostic for cerebrospinal fluid. Radiography studies are done to ascertain any other facial fractures.

Medical and Surgical Management

If the fracture is a lateral displacement, pressure applied to the convex portion of the nose reduces the fracture. Cold compresses control the bleeding. If the fracture is more complex, surgery is done after the swelling subsides, usually after several days. The surgeon applies a splint postoperatively to maintain the alignment.

Nursing Management

Nursing management is similar to that for nasal obstruction. The nurse instructs the client to keep the head elevated and to apply ice four times a day for 20 minutes, to reduce the swelling and pain. He or she gives analgesics as ordered to alleviate pain. Postoperatively, the nurse assesses the client for airway obstruction, respiratory difficulty (i.e., tachypnea, dyspnea), dysphagia, signs of infection, pupillary responses, level of consciousness, and periorbital edema. In addition, the nurse helps reduce the client's anxiety by answering questions and offering reassurance that the bruising and swelling will subside and sense of smell will return.

Stop, Think, and Respond ● BOX 28-2

On your way to class you see a woman suddenly slip on ice and fall on her face. As you approach, she gets to a sitting position. She is wearing a scarf. Blood is pouring from her nose, and your initial impression is that the nose appears deformed. What actions should you take?

● LARYNGEAL TRAUMA AND LARYNGEAL OBSTRUCTION

Pathophysiology and Etiology

Laryngeal trauma occurs during motor vehicle accidents when the neck strikes the steering wheel or other blunt trauma occurs in the neck region. Endoscopic and endo-

tracheal intubation are other possible causes. Although uncommon, a fracture of the thyroid cartilage is also traumatic to the larynx.

Laryngeal obstruction is an extremely serious and often life-threatening condition. Some causes of upper airway obstruction include edema from an allergic reaction, severe head and neck injury, severe inflammation and edema of the throat, and aspiration of foreign bodies.

Assessment Findings

Signs and Symptoms

Laryngeal trauma causes neck swelling, bruising, and tenderness. If the tissues surrounding the larynx are greatly swollen, the client will exhibit **stridor,** a high-pitched, harsh sound during respiration, indicative of airway obstruction. The client also has dysphagia, hoarseness, cyanosis, and possible **hemoptysis** (expectoration of bloody sputum).

Total obstruction prevents the passage of air from the upper to the lower respiratory airway; choking clients will clutch their throats—the universal distress sign for choking. Unless total obstruction is relieved immediately, death occurs from respiratory arrest. Partial obstruction results in difficulty breathing.

Diagnostic Findings

Laryngoscopy reveals the extent of trauma and internal swelling. Radiographs and oxygenation studies will be performed after a patent airway has been established.

Medical and Surgical Management

Maintenance of a patent airway is crucial. If the client has aspirated a foreign body, the Heimlich maneuver is performed to force the object out of the upper respiratory passages (Box 28-2). Allergic reactions resulting in severe inflammation and edema may be treated with epinephrine or a corticosteroid and possibly intubation. Severe obstruction requires an emergency *tracheostomy* (surgical opening into the trachea).

NURSING PROCESS

● Trauma to the Upper Airway

Assessment

The nurse assesses for air movement within the upper respiratory tract. He or she listens to lung sounds, monitors respiratory patterns, and looks for signs of increased nasal swelling and bleeding and symptoms of laryngeal edema. The nurse determines if the airway is obstructed.

BOX 28-2 ● The Heimlich Maneuver for Dislodging an Airway Obstruction

- Ask the person if he or she is choking.
- Assess ability to speak and cough. If the person cannot talk or cough, say that you can help and place your arms around his or her waist.
- Make a fist with one hand and place the thumb toward the victim above the umbilicus.
- Hold your fist with the other hand and thrust upward into the abdomen five times.
- If the object is dislodged and the victim can cough effectively, encourage him or her to do so to eject the object.
- If the object is not ejected or coughed out and the victim loses consciousness, lower the victim to the ground.
- Straddle the victim's body and place the heel of one hand on top of the other. Position the hands midway between the umbilicus and the xiphoid process.
- Deliver five forceful thrusts.
- Open the mouth to assess if the object can be swept out with a hooked finger (do not sweep the mouth in children).
- If the airway remains obstructed, repeat the procedure.

Heimlich maneuver on a conscious victim.

Diagnosis, Planning, and Intervention

Partial or total obstruction of the upper airway requires immediate recognition and intervention. If the nurse is present when a victim aspirates a foreign body, he or she can use the Heimlich maneuver. If this maneuver fails to dislodge the object, a physician may perform an emergency tracheostomy. If edema is the cause of partial upper airway obstruction, oxygen can be given until a physician examines the client. Emergency drugs and a tracheostomy tray are made available for immediate use. Other measures are as follows.

Ineffective Breathing Pattern related to partial obstruction of the upper airway secondary to trauma, nasal packing, bleeding, or edema

Expected Outcomes: (1) Client will maintain a patent airway. (2) Client will demonstrate improved breath sounds.

- Assess airway patency at least every 2 hours. *Maintaining the airway is the highest priority.*
- Auscultate lungs for wheezing or decreased or absent breath sounds every 4 hours. *Wheezing may indicate increased airway resistance. Decreased or absent breath sounds indicate obstruction.*
- Assess respiratory effort, including respiratory rate, depth, nasal flaring, and use of accessory muscles. *Increased respiratory effort indicates respiratory difficulties.*
- Assess vital signs and monitor for changes at least every 4 hours. *Increased work of breathing will increase respiratory rate and heart rate.*
- Monitor arterial blood gases (ABGs). *Increasing $PaCO_2$ and decreasing PaO_2 indicate impending respiratory failure.*
- Position client in semi-Fowler's position. *This position promotes maximum lung expansion and improved air exchange.*
- Apply ice to nasal area four times a day for 20 to 30 minutes. *Ice helps to reduce inflammation and bleeding.*
- Initiate CPR and prepare for possible airway intubation/tracheostomy if airway is completely obstructed. *Preparation for potential emergency assists to maintain the airway.*

Anxiety related to airway obstruction, pain, injury, bleeding, or anticipation of medical or surgical treatments

Expected Outcome: Client will communicate a decreased level of anxiety.

- Assess level of apprehension. *Anxiety increases with respiratory difficulties. Fear can interfere with ability to follow instructions.*
- Monitor for increased respiratory rate and irritability. *These signs indicate increased anxiety.*
- Provide brief explanations. *Increased anxiety impairs ability to focus.*
- Reassure client that he or she is safe—stay with client if necessary. *An anxious client will benefit from the nurse's calm and reassuring presence.*
- Assist client to practice anxiety-reducing methods such as relaxation or positive visualization. *Anxiety-reducing strategies assist client to feel that he or she has control.*

Pain related to injury, surgical incision, or both

Expected Outcome: Client will verbalize relief of or reduced pain.

- Assess nature of pain: quality, severity, location, duration and onset, what precipitated it, and if anything relieves it. *Pain assessment provides a qualitative description of the pain and a baseline of the client's experience.*
- Monitor vital signs, restlessness, or other signs related to pain. *These assessments give additional data for determining level of pain, particularly in clients who deny discomfort.*

- Evaluate response to analgesics and comfort measures such as ice packs and repositioning. *Such evaluation helps determine the need for changes to the treatment regimen.*

Evaluation of Expected Outcomes

The airway is free of obstruction, and breathing patterns improve. Client reports decreased anxiety and that pain has decreased in intensity and duration.

LARYNGEAL CANCER

With early detection, cancer of the larynx has great potential for cure. Preventive health measures focus on early consultation for persistent hoarseness and other changes in voice quality.

Pathophysiology and Etiology

Laryngeal cancer is most common in people 50 to 70 years of age. Men are affected more frequently than are women. The cause of laryngeal cancer is unknown. Carcinogens, such as tobacco, alcohol, and industrial pollutants, are associated with laryngeal cancer. In addition, chronic laryngitis, habitual overuse of the voice, and heredity may contribute. Most laryngeal malignancies are squamous cell carcinomas, that is, a malignancy arising from the epithelial cells lining the larynx. The tumor may be located on the glottis (true vocal cords), above the glottis (supraglottis or false vocal cords), or below the glottis (subglottis).

Assessment Findings

Signs and Symptoms

Persistent hoarseness is usually the earliest symptom. At first the hoarseness is slight, and clients tend to ignore it. Later, the client notes a sensation of swelling or a lump in the throat, followed by dysphagia and pain when talking. The client may also complain of burning in the throat when swallowing hot or citrus liquids. If the malignant tissue is not removed promptly, symptoms of advancing carcinoma, such as dyspnea, weakness, weight loss, enlarged cervical lymph nodes, pain, and anemia develop.

Diagnostic Findings

Visual examination of the larynx (laryngoscopy) and biopsy confirm the diagnosis and identify the type of malignancy. In addition, computed tomography (CT) scanning and chest radiography are used to detect metastasis and to determine tumor size. The physician also assesses the mobility of the vocal cords. Limited mobility indicates that the tumor growth is affecting the surrounding tissue, muscle, and airway.

Medical and Surgical Management

Treatment depends on factors such as the size of the lesion, the client's age, and metastasis. Medical treatment may include chemotherapy, which appears to have only minimal effects, and radiation therapy, either alone or with surgery.

Surgical treatment (Table 28-1) includes laser surgery for early lesions or a partial or total laryngectomy. In more advanced cases, total laryngectomy may be the treatment of choice. If the disease has extended beyond the larynx, a radical neck dissection (removal of the lymph nodes, muscles, and adjacent tissues) is performed. Laser surgery may also be used to relieve obstruction in more advanced cases.

A client with a total laryngectomy has a permanent tracheal *stoma* (opening) because the trachea is no longer connected to the nasopharynx. The larynx is severed from the trachea and removed completely. The only respiratory organs in use are the trachea, bronchi, and lungs. Air enters and leaves through the tracheostomy. The client no longer feels air entering the nose (Fig. 28-3). Because the anterior wall of the esophagus connects with the posterior wall of the larynx, it must be reconstructed. Tube feeding facilitates healing by preventing muscle activity and irritation of the esophagus (see Chap. 52).

Loss of the ability to speak normally is a devastating consequence of laryngeal surgery. Communication with others is a basic need. Clients with a malignancy of the larynx require emotional support before and after surgery and help in understanding and choosing an alternative method of speech. Some methods of alaryngeal speech used after a laryngectomy include the following:

- *Esophageal speech*—requires regurgitation of swallowed air and formation of words with lips
- *Artificial (electric) larynx*—a throat vibrator held against the neck that projects sound into the mouth; words are formed with the mouth
- *Tracheoesophageal puncture (TEP)*—a surgical opening in the posterior wall of the trachea, followed by the insertion of a prosthesis such as a Blom-Singer device (Figure 28-4). Air from the lungs is diverted through the opening in the posterior tracheal wall to the esophagus and out the mouth.

A speech pathologist works with the client to use an artificial speech device, learn esophageal speech, or speak clearly with a prosthesis. Clients having a partial laryngectomy also may require speech therapy.

TABLE 28-1	DESCRIPTIONS OF LARYNGEAL SURGERY		
SURGERY	**DESCRIPTION**	**INDICATION**	**POSTOPERATIVE EXPECTATIONS**
Partial laryngectomy	The affected vocal cord is removed; other structures remain intact	For early-stage laryngeal cancer when only one cord is involved	Voice will be hoarse; intact trachea; no problems with swallowing; high cure rate
Supraglottic laryngectomy	Hyoid bone, glottis, and false cords removed; radical neck dissection done on involved side; remaining structures left intact	For supraglottic tumors	Voice will be hoarse; postoperative tracheostomy until glottic airway functions; nutrition administered through nasogastric tube until surgical sites heal; recurrence is possible
Hemivertical laryngectomy	Thyroid cartilage of trachea is split at midline; one true cord and one false cord are removed along with arytenoid cartilage and half the thyroid cartilage.	When tumor extends beyond the vocal cord but is smaller than 1 cm	Client will have a tracheostomy and nasogastric tube after surgery until healed; voice will be hoarse and diminished; client will have an intact airway and the ability to swallow.
Total laryngectomy	Both vocal cords removed along with the hyoid bone, epiglottis, cricoid cartilage, and two or three rings of the trachea; the tongue, pharyngeal walls, and trachea remain intact; usually a radical neck dissection is done on the affected side.	When the cancer extends beyond the vocal cords	Permanent tracheal stoma; prevents aspiration. No voice but ability to swallow remains. Metastasis to cervical lymph nodes is common.
Radical neck dissection	The neck is opened from the jaw to the clavicle from the midline to the interior border of the trapezius muscle. The following are removed: subcutaneous and soft tissue, sternocleidomastoid muscle, jugular vein, and spinal accessory nerve innervates trapezius muscle—client's shoulder will droop after surgery as the trapezius muscle atrophies). A split-thickness skin graft is applied over the carotid artery.	When cancer has metastasized to cervical lymph nodes	Permanent tracheal stoma. No voice; ability to swallow remains. Client requires physical therapy for neck muscles, along with a prescribed exercise program.

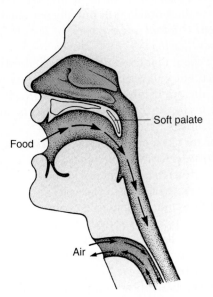

Soft palate

Food

Air

FIGURE 28-3 Air enters and leaves through a permanent tracheal stoma.

NURSING PROCESS

● The Client Undergoing Laryngeal Surgery

Assessment

The nurse determines the client's level of understanding of the diagnosis, reason for surgery, and probable outcome. He or she assesses for hoarseness, sore throat, dyspnea, dysphagia, pain, or burning in the throat. Ascertaining the client's level of anxiety is important, as is identifying coping strategies. The nurse also must assess the client's ability to communicate in ways other than speaking, such as ability to read and write. He or she begins preoperative teaching, allowing the client to express fears about the surgery, diagnosis, and potential loss of voice postoperatively. The nurse discusses alternative methods of communication and identifies which method the client prefers. After surgery, the nurse carefully assesses for a patent airway and effective airway clearance.

Voice prosthesis

Tracheostoma valve

FIGURE 28-4 Schematic representation of TEP. (From Smeltzer, S. C. & Bare, B. G. [2000]. *Brunner & Suddarth's textbook of medical–surgical nursing* [9th ed.]. Philadelphia: Lippincott Williams & Wilkins.)

Diagnosis, Planning, and Interventions

Care centers around preventing postoperative complications, managing pain, preventing wound infection, helping the client communicate, and fostering the client's ability to cope with changes in body image. The nurse provides the client and family with the following postoperative instructions:

- Water should not enter the stoma because it will flow from the trachea to the lungs. Thus, avoid swimming, and take care when bathing. Avoid showers until experienced with care of the stoma, and then use a hand-held shower device if possible.
- Wear a scarf or gauze dressing over the stoma to make the opening less obvious.
- Avoid fabrics or dressings that fray to prevent small fibers from being drawn into the stoma.

In addition to the following diagnoses, outcomes, and interventions, refer to Chapter 25 for general postoperative care.

Ineffective Airway Clearance related to surgical alterations of the airway

Expected Outcome: Client will maintain effective airway clearance as evidenced by clear breath sounds, normal respirations, and effective cough.

- Position client in semi-Fowler's position. *This position provides optimal lung expansion and decreases edema in the surgical site.*
- Auscultate breath sounds and respiratory effort at least every 4 hours. *Initial and ongoing assessments provide a baseline for comparison.*

- Assess effectiveness of client's cough. *An effective cough will promote airway clearance.*
- Encourage deep breathing and coughing every 2 hours while client is awake. *These measures prevent atelectasis and promote effective gas exchange.*
- Monitor for restlessness, dyspnea, anxiety, and increased heart rate. *These signs indicate ineffective airway clearance.*
- Observe level of consciousness for signs of lethargy or disorientation. *These signs indicate poor gas exchange.*

Impaired Verbal Communication related to removal of larynx and postoperative edema

Expected Outcome: Client will communicate effectively with alternative methods.

- Frequently assess client's need to communicate. *Assessments alleviate client's anxiety.*
- Allow client time to communicate needs. *Adequate time promotes acceptance of client and decreases anxiety about ability to communicate.*
- Provide alternative methods of communication: paper and pen, wipe board, or word or picture board. *Having supplies available provides comfort to client.*
- Reinforce instructions regarding use of a voice prosthesis, electrolarynx, or esophageal speech. *Support and instruction help client to become more proficient with alternative speech methods.*

Imbalanced Nutrition: Less than Body Requirements related to swallowing deficits

Expected Outcome: Client will have adequate caloric and fluid intake as evidenced by increase in or maintenance of preoperative weight.

- Instruct client on need for enteral feedings if prescribed. *Enteral feedings are used until the suture line heals, usually 10 to 14 days postoperatively.*
- Provide meticulous mouth care every 4 hours. *Oral care keeps mouth fresh and promotes interest in caloric intake.*
- Introduce thick oral liquids initially and solid foods as tolerated. *Gradual advancement of the diet promotes ease in swallowing.*
- Instruct client that the sense of taste and smell are diminished but will return as client accommodates to airway alterations. *Inhaled air passes directly into the trachea, bypassing the nose. Loss of ability to smell alters taste sensations.*
- Monitor for signs of dysphagia. *Difficulty swallowing will decrease caloric content and lead to weight loss.*

Social Isolation related to change in body image, tracheal stoma, and change in or loss of speech

Expected Outcome: Client will demonstrate evidence of adjustment to changes and resume social interactions.

- Demonstrate acceptance of client's changed appearance. *Acceptance provides a sense of belonging and promotes positive self-esteem.*
- Encourage client to maintain or reestablish social relationships. *Social relationships reduce the sense of isolation and increase feelings of acceptance.*

- Provide time for client to express feelings about changes. *Allowing time for expression of feelings assists the client to cope with changes.*
- Refer client to support services such as the International Association of Laryngectomies, and arrange for visits from clients who have had a laryngectomy. *Rehabilitation is lengthy; support from others has a positive effect.*

Evaluation of Expected Outcomes

The client maintains a clear airway, effectively clearing secretions. He or she demonstrates effective alternative communication methods and maintains adequate caloric and fluid intake. The client maintains or establishes social interactions and copes with changes.

FIGURE 28-5 A cuffed tracheostomy tube with inner cannula. The cuff at the lower end of the outer tracheostomy tube is inflated with air to provide a snug fit in the trachea.

TREATMENT MODALITIES FOR AIRWAY OBSTRUCTION OR AIRWAY MAINTENANCE ●

Clients with serious airway conditions require aggressive treatment to maintain an airway or relieve airway obstruction. This section discusses tracheostomy, tracheotomy, endotracheal intubation, and mechanical ventilation.

● TRACHEOSTOMY AND TRACHEOTOMY

A **tracheotomy** is the surgical procedure that makes an opening into the trachea. A **tracheostomy** is a surgical opening into the trachea into which a tracheostomy or laryngectomy tube is inserted. A tracheostomy may be temporary or permanent. A permanent opening in the trachea is required for certain disorders, such as a laryngectomy for laryngeal cancer.

General Considerations

Tracheostomy tubes come in several sizes and differ from laryngectomy tubes in their length and diameter. A cuffed tracheostomy tube has a cuff on the lower end that is inflated with air to provide a snug fit (Fig. 28-5). The cuff prevents aspiration of liquids or escape of air when a mechanical ventilator is used. The physician specifies the amount of air to be injected into the cuff, usually to achieve a pressure between 20 and 25 mm H$_2$0. The amount of air determines the seating of the cuff in the trachea. The pressure in the cuff requires monitoring with a pressure gauge every 8 hours.

During the immediate postoperative period, the physician may change the tracheostomy tube every 3 to 5 days. Before a tracheostomy tube is inserted into the tracheal opening, the obturator is placed in the tube and then removed as soon as the tube is in place. The outer tube is held snugly in place by tapes inserted in openings on either side of it and tied at the side of the client's neck.

The respiratory passages react to the creation of the new opening with inflammation and excessive mucus secretion. Copious respiratory secretions are life-threatening. The client cannot be left unattended during the immediate postoperative period because the secretions make frequent suctioning necessary. Additionally, inspired air passes directly into the trachea, bronchi, and lungs without becoming warmed and moistened by passing through the nose. Dry secretions can subsequently develop, which easily form crusts and can break off, obstruct the lower airway, and cause serious respiratory problems. Humidification by a mist collar is usually necessary to prevent drying and incrustation of the mucous membrane in the trachea and the main bronchus. The long-term and short-term complications of tracheostomy include infection, bleeding, airway obstruction resulting from hardened secretions, aspiration, injury to the laryngeal nerve, erosion of the trachea, fistula formation between the esophagus and trachea, and penetration of the posterior tracheal wall.

Nursing Management

After surgery, the nurse monitors vital signs and auscultates breath sounds. He or she assesses skin color, level of consciousness, and mental status. The nurse monitors for potential complications and checks airway patency frequently. Secretions can rapidly clog the inner lumen of the tracheostomy tube, resulting in severe respiratory difficulty or death by asphyxiation. If the airway is obstructed, the client becomes cyanotic, restless, and frightened.

To facilitate breathing during the immediate postoperative period, the nurse positions the client as ordered. When the client is fully awake and blood pressure is stable, the nurse elevates the head of the bed to about 45°. This position decreases edema and makes breathing easier.

The nurse inspects the tracheostomy carefully, ensuring that tapes are secure. If the tube is not tied securely, the client can cough it out, a serious occurrence if the edges of the trachea have not been sutured to the skin. This may be the case in a temporary tracheostomy. The nurse keeps a tracheal dilator at the bedside at all times. If the outer tube accidentally comes out, the nurse inserts the dilator to hold the edges of the stoma apart until the physician arrives to insert another tube. A tracheal tube must never be forced back in place. Use of force may compress the client's trachea (by pushing the tube alongside and compressing the trachea, rather than inserting the tube into the stoma). Such action could cause respiratory arrest.

The nurse suctions the client to remove secretions that can obstruct the airway (Nursing Guidelines 28-1). He or she avoids unnecessary suctioning to decrease trauma to the airway. When explaining the procedure, the nurse tells the client that the suction catheter will be inserted for only a few seconds. Keeping an extra tracheostomy tube of the same size at the bedside is essential, because an immediate change may be necessary if the tube becomes blocked with mucus that cannot be removed. The nurse provides routine tracheostomy care (Nursing Guidelines 28-2). He or she places a gauze dressing under the tube to absorb secretions. The hospital gown and bed

---

NURSING GUIDELINES 28-1

Suctioning the Client With a Tracheostomy

- Use sterile equipment (e.g., gloves, suction catheter, normal saline) and aseptic technique for tracheal suctioning.

- Place client in Fowler's position. Preoxygenate client for at least 1 to 2 minutes. Check that suction pressure is at a low setting.

- Open the suction kit, don gloves, lubricate a sterile, 10- to 14-French disposable catheter with sterile saline, and insert it into the lumen of the tube.

- Do not apply suction while the catheter is inserted down the trachea because this irritates the lining of the trachea.

- Begin intermittent suctioning while slowly withdrawing and rotating the catheter. Do not suction for more than 10 seconds at a time.

- Allow client to rest and deep breathe before repeating if more suctioning is necessary.

- Discard the suction catheter after use.

NURSING GUIDELINES 28-2

Tracheostomy Care

- Maintain aseptic technique, washing hands before, during, and after the procedure.

- Position client in a supine or low Fowler's position.

- Using a clean glove, remove the soiled stomal dressing and discard it, glove and all, in appropriate receptacle.

- Open the tracheostomy kit without contaminating the contents. Don sterile gloves—keep the dominant hand sterile. Pour hydrogen peroxide and normal saline into respective containers.

- Unlock the inner cannula by turning it counterclockwise. Remove it and place in hydrogen peroxide. Clean the inside and outside of the cannula with pipe cleaners.

- Rinse the cleaned cannula with normal saline. Tap the cannula and wipe the excess solution with sterile gauze.

- Replace the inner cannula and turn it clockwise within the outer cannula.

- Clean around the stoma with an applicator moistened with normal saline.

- Place a sterile dressing around the tracheostomy tube. Change the tracheostomy ties by placing the new ones on first, and removing the soiled ones last. Tie the new ends securely, but not tightly, at the side of the neck.

Securing a tracheostomy dressing.

---

linens must never cover the opening of the tracheostomy tube. For additional care, see Nursing Care Plan 28-1.

● ENDOTRACHEAL INTUBATION AND MECHANICAL VENTILATION

An endotracheal tube (Fig. 28-6) is inserted through the mouth or nose into the trachea to provide a patent airway for clients who cannot maintain an adequate airway on their own. Examples include those with respiratory difficulty, comatose clients, those undergoing general anesthesia, and clients with extensive edema of upper airway passages.

Nursing Care Plan 28-1

THE CLIENT WITH A TRACHEOSTOMY

Assessment

- Monitor vital signs and auscultate breath sounds.
- Assess skin color, level of consciousness, and mental status.
- Monitor for potential complications.
- Assess frequently for a patent airway.
- Inspect tracheostomy frequently for placement and security of ties.

PC: Hypoxia, Hemorrhage, Displaced Tracheostomy Tube, Accidental Extubation

Expected Outcome: The nurse will prevent or manage complications of the tracheostomy.

Interventions	*Rationales*
Monitor for signs and symptoms of respiratory distress: difficulty breathing, diminished or absent breath sounds, use of accessory muscles, and asymmetric chest wall movements.	Early recognition of signs and symptoms of respiratory distress prevents further complications.
Assess for subcutaneous emphysema (air trapped in tissues) around the stoma, neck, and chest.	Injury or trauma to the airway can cause air to leak into surrounding tissues. Severe subcutaneous emphysema indicates significant leaking and potential airway obstruction.
Provide humidification.	A tracheostomy bypasses the nose; thus, inspired air is not warmed or humidified. Increased warmth and humidity thin and help remove secretions.
Keep tracheostomy ties secure but not too tight (one finger should slip easily under ties).	Ties maintain tube placement without damaging underlying skin or causing discomfort.
Monitor pulse oximetry or arterial blood gas results. Administer oxygen as needed.	Such monitoring ensures adequate oxygenation.

Evaluation of Expected Outcome: The nurse manages the client's care and prevents complications.

Nursing Diagnosis: Risk for Ineffective Airway Clearance related to increased secretions and possible occlusion of the inner cannula

Expected Outcome: Airway and tracheostomy tube will remain clear.

Interventions	*Rationales*
Provide warm, humidified air.	Such air prevents drying and crusting of secretions.
Suction as needed.	Suctioning clears secretions.
Maintain a patent airway. In cases of suspected obstruction: (1) suction the tracheostomy, (2) induce coughing, (3) change the inner cannula, and (4) position client to maximize respiratory effort.	These measures remove thick secretions and possible mucus plugs and promote lung expansion.

Evaluation of Expected Outcome: Client's airway and tracheostomy are patent.

Nursing Diagnosis: Risk for Infection related to loss of upper airway protection

Expected Outcome: Risk for infection will be reduced.

(continued)

Nursing Care Plan 28-1 (Continued)

THE CLIENT WITH A TRACHEOSTOMY

Interventions	*Rationales*
Monitor stoma for erythema, exudate, or odor.	Such findings may indicate infection.
Assess skin around stoma and under tracheostomy ties for signs of breakdown.	Intact skin prevents infection.
Monitor white blood cell (WBC) count.	Elevated WBCs may indicate infection.
Provide routine tracheostomy care every 8 hours and as necessary. Maintain sterile technique.	These measures prevent infection.
Position client so that secretions do not pool around the stoma.	Maintaining a clean and dry stoma prevents infection.

Evaluation of Expected Outcome: Client does not have any signs or symptoms of infection.

Nursing Diagnosis: **Risk for Ineffective Management of Therapeutic Regimen** related to lack of knowledge about tracheostomy care and home support

Expected Outcome: Client or caregiver will demonstrate skills appropriate for tracheostomy care.

Interventions	*Rationales*
Assess client's and caregiver's ability to provide adequate home care.	This assessment provides a baseline for teaching needs and referrals.
Begin teaching skills one at a time.	Step-by-step teaching provides time to absorb information.
Teach client how to suction airway, clean tube, change dressing and ties, provide stoma care, and reinsert tracheostomy tube. Have client demonstrate skills.	Demonstration of skills ensures that client or caregiver has adequate knowledge for home care.
Teach client or caregiver to check for signs and symptoms of infection.	Such measures prevent or enable early treatment of infection.
Refer client and caregiver to support groups and home care services.	Home care needs are planned for before discharge.

Evaluation of Expected Outcome: Client or caregiver demonstrates adequate skill in tracheostomy care and is sufficiently independent for discharge home.

General Considerations

An endotracheal tube can remain in place for up to 2 weeks. The cuff is inflated to provide a tight seal. The endotracheal tube is attached to a ventilator for control of respirations and ventilation of the lungs. Humidification is necessary because air going to the lungs through an endotracheal tube does not pass through the moist mucous membranes of the upper airway.

There are several modes of mechanical ventilation, classified according to the manner in which they support ventilation. Two major classifications are negative-pressure and positive-pressure ventilators (Table 28-2). Positive-pressure ventilators are used more commonly. The major difference between the two types is that negative-pressure ventilators exert negative pressure, a pulling or sucking force, on the external chest, while positive-pressure ventilators inflate the lungs by exerting positive pressure, pushing air into the airway. Negative-pressure ventilators are used for clients with chronic respiratory failure related to neuromuscular disease such as poliomyelitis or myasthenia gravis. Positive-pressure ventilators require intubation and are used for clients with acute respiratory failure and primary lung disease, such as cystic fibrosis, or for clients who are comatose, are under general anesthesia, or have extensive upper airway edema.

FIGURE 28-6 Endotracheal tubes.

Accidental removal of an endotracheal tube must be prevented because this can result in laryngeal edema or **laryngospasm** (spasm of the laryngeal muscles, resulting in narrowing of the larynx) and subsequent respiratory arrest. The inflated cuff and placement of tape around the tube attached to the client's cheek secures the endotracheal tube. The proximal end of the tube is marked for determining if downward displacement has occurred.

The intubated client has the endotracheal tube removed when the vital capacity is adequate and the client can breathe without assistance. Blood gas studies also are used as a guideline for removal. Depending on hospital policy, the removal of an endotracheal tube may be done by the nurse, the respiratory therapist, or the doctor. Before removing the tube, emergency equipment for respiratory support must be available. The pharynx must be suctioned before the cuff is deflated to prevent the aspiration of secretions during extubation. The tube usually is removed with the client in semi-Fowler's position. If laryngospasm occurs, air is administered by positive pressure. Reinsertion of the endotracheal tube by the physician or other trained personnel may be necessary if laryngospasm continues. Possible complications with the use of endotracheal intubation include ulceration and stricture of the trachea or larynx, atelectasis, and pneumonia.

Nursing Management

Major goals for the client with an intubation are to improve respirations, maintain a patent airway, and communicate needs to others. The nurse monitors vital signs periodically, depending on the client's condition and the reason for endotracheal tube insertion. Blood gas studies and pulse oximetry provide methods of ongoing evaluation of the client's respiratory status. The nurse reviews the results of these studies and reports changes to the physician.

The nurse observes the client at frequent intervals for response to respiratory support and complications associated with endotracheal intubation. He or she evaluates

TABLE 28-2	TYPES OF MECHANICAL VENTILATORS
CLASSIFICATION	**HOW USED**
Negative pressure	Exerts negative pressure on chest; decreases intrathoracic pressure during inspiration, allowing air to flow into lungs; does not require intubation
	Used for clients experiencing chronic respiratory failure, such as in poliomyelitis, myasthenia gravis, muscular dystrophy, amyotrophic lateral sclerosis
Drinker respirator tank	Also known as the *iron lung;* a negative-pressure chamber; used extensively in the past for clients with poliomyelitis
Body wrap (pneumowrap) and chest cuirass (tortoise shell)	Requires a rigid cage or shell around the thorax to create a negative-pressure chamber
Positive pressure	Exerts positive pressure on airway to inflate lungs; expiration is passive
	Usually requires endotracheal or tracheal intubation
Pressure-cycled	Inspiration ends when a preset pressure is reached; *cycle* means that ventilator cycles on, delivers flow of air until a certain pressure is reached, and then cycles off
	Designed for short-term use because volume of air varies as client's airway resistance or compliance changes
Time-cycled	Controls respiration after a preset time; length of inspiration and flow rate of air regulate volume the client receives; usually used on newborns and infants
Volume-cycled	Delivers a preset volume of air with each inspiration; once volume is delivered, ventilator cycles off and client expires air passively
	Provides consistent adequate breaths despite airway resistance or changes in compliance; most commonly used ventilator for adults
Noninvasive	Ventilation delivered by face masks or other nasal devices; does not require intubation of any kind; used for clients with sleep-related breathing disorders or other chronic respiratory disorders

any change in mental status. Confusion may result from abnormal blood gas levels or electrolyte imbalances. Sudden restlessness or agitation may indicate obstruction of the endotracheal tube, which can be life-threatening. The nurse auscultates the lungs and observes the symmetrical rise and fall of the chest every 30 to 60 minutes. If he or she cannot detect bilateral breath sounds, the nurse notifies the physician immediately.

Humidification is necessary to keep the inspired air moist. Clients with endotracheal intubation cannot cough, secretions are often thick and tenacious, and swallowing reflexes are depressed. An increase in $PaCO_2$ caused by blockage of the endotracheal tube or malfunctioning of the ventilator may occur secondary to secretions or because the client is biting on the tube. Keeping the airway patent at all times is absolutely necessary, using the same suctioning technique as for a tracheostomy. If the client is biting on the tube, a bite block or oral airway may be used to keep the tube patent.

The nurse changes the client's position every 2 hours to prevent atelectasis. He or she gives oral care as needed to keep the mouth and lips free of crusts and mucus. The nurse suctions the oropharynx and mouth as needed and cleans the teeth with applicators. The nurse inspects the oral cavity frequently and reports any signs of oral bleeding to the physician.

The client may display anxiety or fear because of the tube, inability to speak, suctioning, and dependence on a machine for breathing. Each time suctioning is needed, the nurse reassures the client that the procedure takes only a short time. The client may attempt to remove or pull on the tube if he or she is awake or partially awake. Restraining the client may be necessary. The nurse should contact the physician if he or she notes extreme restlessness on the client's part. Providing a "Magic Slate," wipe board, or pencil and paper to the client enables communication, as does asking questions that the client can answer by shaking the head yes or no.

Once the endotracheal tube is removed, the nurse places the client in a high Fowler's or semi-Fowler's position to promote optimal chest and lung expansion. The posterior pharynx may be dry, and the voice may be hoarse. The nurse observes the client frequently for signs of laryngeal edema and increased respiratory distress. He or she immediately reports any sign of respiratory distress because reinsertion of the endotracheal tube may be necessary.

GENERAL NUTRITIONAL CONSIDERATIONS

Claims that megadoses of vitamin C cure the common cold generate interest and controversy. Well-controlled studies suggest that large doses of vitamin C neither prevent nor cure colds but may help minimize their severity and duration.

Findings from approximately half the studies done on zinc lozenges show that they shorten the duration of colds. Until more conclusive studies are conducted, it is reasonable and safe for clients to use zinc lozenges at the first sign of a cold. Because excess zinc can impair the immune system and lower levels of high-density lipoproteins ("good" cholesterol), long-term or ongoing use of zinc lozenges to prevent colds is not recommended.

A high fluid intake helps thin respiratory secretions.

Enteral feedings are used 10 to 14 days after a laryngectomy to avoid irritation to the sutures and reduce the risk of aspiration. When oral intake resumes, offer small amounts of thick liquids. Advance the diet according to the client's tolerance.

Clients who have difficulty swallowing may be able to maintain oral intake if the texture of the food is altered. The client may need a pureed diet, thickened pureed diet, semisolid diet, or soft diet until he or she can resume regular eating. Thickening liquids may also promote ease of swallowing.

Following a laryngectomy, the client may experience anorexia related to a diminished sense of taste and smell. The appearance of food becomes more important. Attractive food, served in pleasant surroundings and seasoned according to individual taste, may help promote intake. Reassure the client that some sense of taste and smell will return.

GENERAL PHARMACOLOGIC CONSIDERATIONS

In some instances, one or more drugs contained in multiple-ingredient cold preparations may be contraindicated in certain disorders (e.g., glaucoma, heart disease, hypertension, prostatic enlargement). Encourage clients with one or more of these diseases who are taking prescription drugs to consult a physician before using nonprescription drugs to treat a cold.

Aspirin prolongs bleeding time by inhibiting the aggregation (clumping) of platelets. When bleeding time is prolonged, blood takes longer to clot after a cut, surgery, or injury to the skin or mucous membranes.

Some cold tablets contain antihistamines that thicken nasal secretions. Although this action may temporarily decrease the discomfort of profuse nasal secretions, thickened secretions can block the drainage openings of the sinus cavity, lead to failure of the sinuses to drain adequately, and become a focus for continuing infection.

GENERAL GERONTOLOGIC CONSIDERATIONS

If an older adult requires a tracheostomy, be alert to possible confusion after the procedure. If clients are confused or do not understand the purpose of the procedure, they may attempt to pull at the tube or remove it. Restraining measures may be required.

The common cold may be potentially serious for older adults, especially when they have other diseases such as a chronic respiratory disorder or heart disease. Advise older clients to see a physician if cold symptoms are severe or breathing is difficult.

After a laryngectomy older clients may require extra time and instruction to learn esophageal speech, speak with an electric larynx, or use TEP.

Critical Thinking Exercises

1. A client with severe pharyngitis is diagnosed with a group A streptococcal infection. The physician prescribes penicillin. What discharge instructions should you give the client?

2. Mr. Evans has an endotracheal tube. Although critically ill, he is somewhat alert and wants to communicate with his family. An intravenous (IV) line is in his right hand; his position is low Fowler's. What method of communication could you suggest for Mr. Evans and his family?

3. Your client is scheduled for a partial laryngectomy. What information must you share to help prepare her for the postoperative period?

References and Suggested Readings

Carpenito, L. J. (2002). *Nursing diagnosis: Application to clinical practice* (9th ed.). Philadelphia: Lippincott Williams & Wilkins.

Fowler, S. (2000). Know how: Humidification. A guide to humidification. *Nursing Times, 96*(20), 10–11.

Klein, L. (2001). Sinusitis: When to treat and how. *RN, 64*(1), 42–48.

Putnam, H., & May, K. R. (2001). Relief for patients with severe allergies. *RN, 64*(6), 27–30.

Smeltzer, S. C., & Bare, B. G. (2000). *Brunner & Suddarth's textbook of medical–surgical nursing* (9th ed.) Philadelphia: Lippincott Williams & Wilkins.

Caring for Clients With Disorders of the Lower Respiratory Airway

Words to Know

acute bronchitis
asbestosis
asthma
atelectasis
bronchiectasis
chronic bronchitis
chronic obstructive
    pulmonary disease
cystic fibrosis
emphysema
empyema
flail chest
hemoptysis
influenza
lobectomy
lung abscess
orthopnea
pleural effusion
pleurisy
pneumoconiosis

pneumonectomy
pneumonia
pneumothorax
polysomnography
pulmonary contusion
pulmonary edema
pulmonary embolism
pulmonary hypertension
segmental resection
septicemia
silicosis
sleep apnea syndrome
subcutaneous
    emphysema
thoracentesis
thoracotomy
tracheitis
tracheobronchitis
tuberculosis
wedge resection

Learning Objectives

On completion of this chapter, the reader will:

- Describe infectious and inflammatory disorders of the lower respiratory airway.
- Identify critical assessments needed for a client with an infectious disorder of the lower respiratory airway.
- Define disorders classified as obstructive pulmonary disease.
- Discuss strategies for preventing and managing occupational lung diseases.
- Describe the pathophysiology of pulmonary hypertension.
- List risk factors associated with the development of pulmonary embolism.
- Discuss conditions that may lead to acute respiratory distress syndrome.
- Differentiate acute and chronic respiratory failure.
- Explain why lung cancer often is diagnosed after the disease is advanced.
- Describe the nursing assessments required for a client who experiences trauma to the chest.
- Explain the purpose of chest tubes after thoracic surgery.
- Describe the preoperative and postoperative nursing management for clients undergoing thoracic care.

Exchange of gases and ventilation occur in the lower respiratory tract, which is subject to various problems and disorders that compromise its ability to perform its primary functions. If untreated, many of these disorders can lead to respiratory failure. Other disorders become chronic and affect the client's quality of life.

INFECTIOUS AND INFLAMMATORY DISORDERS

Infectious and inflammatory disorders of the lower airway are medically more serious than those of the upper airway. Inflammation and infection in the alveoli and

bronchioles impair gas exchange. In addition, clients may experience greater difficulty in maintaining a clear airway secondary to retained secretions.

• ACUTE BRONCHITIS

Pathophysiology and Etiology

Inflammation of the mucous membranes that line the major bronchi and their branches characterizes **acute bronchitis.** If the inflammatory process involves the trachea, it is referred to as **tracheobronchitis.** Typically, acute bronchitis begins as an upper respiratory infection

(URI); the inflammatory process then extends to the tracheobronchial tree. The secretory cells of the mucosa produce increased mucopurulent sputum.

Viral infections most commonly give rise to acute bronchitis. Clients with viral URIs are more vulnerable to secondary bacterial infections, which then may lead to acute bronchitis. Sputum cultures identify the causative bacterial organisms, the most common of which are *Haemophilus influenzae* and *Mycoplasma pneumoniae.* Chemical irritation from noxious fumes also may induce acute bronchitis. A potential complication is bronchial asthma.

Assessment Findings

Signs and symptoms initially include fever, malaise, and a dry, nonproductive cough that later produces mucopurulent sputum, which may be blood streaked if the airway mucosa becomes irritated with severe tracheobronchitis and coughing. Clients experience paroxysmal attacks of coughing and may report wheezing. Laryngitis and sinusitis complicate the symptoms. Moist inspiratory crackles may be heard on chest auscultation. A sputum sample is collected for culture and sensitivity testing to rule out bacterial infection. A chest film also may be done to detect additional pathology, such as pneumonia.

Medical Management

Acute bronchitis usually is self-limiting, lasting for several days. Treatment is bed rest, antipyretics, expectorants, antitussives, and increased fluids. Humidifiers assist in keeping the mucous membranes moist because dry air aggravates the cough. If secondary bacterial invasion occurs, the previously mild infection becomes serious, accompanied by a persistent cough and thick, purulent sputum. Secondary infections usually subside as the bronchitis subsides, but they may persist for several weeks. When a secondary infection is evident, the physician orders a broad-spectrum antibiotic when sputum culture results are available.

Nursing Management

The nurse auscultates breath sounds and monitors vital signs every 4 hours, especially if the client has a fever. He or she encourages the client to cough and deep breathe every 2 hours while awake and to expectorate rather than swallow sputum. Humidification of surrounding air loosens bronchial secretions. The nurse changes the bedding and the client's clothes if they become damp with perspiration and offers fluids frequently. The nurse instructs in preventing the spread of infection by teaching the client to wash the hands frequently, particularly when handling secretions and soiled tissues; cover the mouth when sneezing and coughing; discard soiled tissues in a plastic bag; and avoid sharing eating utensils and personal articles with others.

● PNEUMONIA

overview

Pneumonia is an inflammatory process affecting the bronchioles and alveoli. Although it usually is associated with an acute infection, pneumonia also can result from radiation therapy, chemical ingestion or inhalation, or aspiration of foreign bodies or gastric contents.

Pathophysiology and Etiology

Pneumonia is classified according to its etiology and presenting symptoms. Bacterial pneumonias are referred to as *typical pneumonias.* Atypical pneumonias (Box 29-1) are those caused by mycoplasmas, *Legionella pneumophila* (the causative agent of Legionnaire's disease), viruses, and fungi. *Mycobacterium tuberculosis* also may cause pneumonia. Viruses are the most common etiology, with type A virus the usual causative organism. Bacterial pneumonias are less common but more serious. Causative bacterial organisms include *Streptococcus pneumoniae, Pneumocystis carinii, Staphylococcus aureus, Klebsiella pneumoniae, Pseudomonas aeruginosa,* and *H. influenzae.*

Radiation pneumonia results from damage to the normal lung mucosa during radiation therapy for breast or lung cancer. Chemical pneumonia results from ingestion

---

BOX 29-1 ● Atypical Pneumonias

Mycoplasma pneumoniae
  Is the most common cause of atypical pneumonia
  Develops gradually, with a prolonged clinical course
  Is rarely fatal
Chlamydia pneumoniae
  Is a common cause of pneumonia and URIs
  Requires long-term treatment with broad-spectrum antibiotics
Chlamydia psittaci
  Causes psittacosis, a flulike disease progressing to irregular consolidation and interstitial pneumonia
  Is transmitted from birds and sheep
Legionella pneumophila
  Was first described at an American Legion convention in Philadelphia, Pennsylvania
  Is a fastidious bacterium that resides in aquatic environments
  Outbreaks traced to air conditioners and humidifiers
  Is rapid growing, causing inflammation and fibrin formation within the alveoli, and often complicated by empyema
  Symptoms include fever, cough, and chest pain, with a mortality rate of 10% to 20%

of kerosene or inhalation of volatile hydrocarbons (kerosene, gasoline, or other chemicals), which can occur in industrial settings. Aspiration pneumonia may occur when a person inhales a foreign body or gastric contents during vomiting or regurgitation. Hypoventilation of lung tissue over a prolonged period can occur when a client is bedridden and breathing with only part of the lungs. Bronchial secretions subsequently accumulate, which may lead to hypostatic pneumonia.

Bronchopneumonia means that the infection is patchy, diffuse, and scattered throughout both lungs. Lobar pneumonia means that the inflammation is confined to one or more lobes of the lung (Fig. 29-1).

Another classification of pneumonia refers to where the client acquired the inflammatory process. Community-acquired pneumonia (CAP) means that the client contracted the illness in a community setting or within 48 hours of admission to a healthcare facility. Hospital-acquired pneumonia (HAP), or nosocomial pneumonia, occurs in a healthcare setting more than 48 hours after admission. HAP is the most dangerous nosocomial infection (Smeltzer & Bare, 2000).

Organisms that cause pneumonia reach the alveoli by inhalation of droplets, aspiration of organisms from the upper airway, or, less commonly, seeding from the bloodstream. When the organisms reach the alveoli, the inflammatory reaction is intense, producing an exudate that impairs gas exchange. Capillaries surrounding the alveoli become engorged and cause the alveoli to collapse (atelectasis), further impairing gas exchange and interfering with ventilation. White blood cells (WBCs) move into the area to destroy the pathogens, filling the interstitial spaces. If untreated, consolidation occurs as the inflammation and exudate increase. Hypoxemia results from the inability of the lungs to oxygenate blood from the heart. Bronchitis, **tracheitis** (inflammation of the trachea), and spots of *necrosis* (death of tissue) in the lung may follow.

In atypical pneumonias, the exudate infiltrates the interstitial spaces rather than the alveoli directly. The pneumonia is more scattered, as described for bronchopneumonia. As the inflammatory process continues, it increasingly interferes with gas exchange between the bloodstream and lungs. Increased carbon dioxide (CO_2) in the blood stimulates the respiratory center, causing more rapid and shallow breathing.

Without an interruption of any type of pneumonia, the client becomes increasingly ill. If the circulatory system cannot compensate for the burden of decreased gas exchange, the client is at risk for heart failure. Death from pneumonia is most common in older adults and those weakened by acute or chronic diseases or disorders (e.g., acquired immunodeficiency syndrome [AIDS], cancer, lung disease) or prolonged periods of inactivity. Complications of pneumonia include congestive heart failure (CHF), **empyema** (collection of pus in the pleural cavity), **pleurisy** (inflammation of the pleura), **septicemia** (infective microorganisms in the blood), atelectasis, hypotension, and shock. In addition, septicemia may lead to a secondary focus of infection, such as endocarditis (inflammation of the endocardium), pericarditis (inflammation of the pericardium), and purulent arthritis. Otitis media (infection of the middle ear), bronchitis, or sinusitis also may complicate recovery, especially from atypical pneumonia.

Assessment Findings

Signs and Symptoms

Symptoms vary for the different types of pneumonia. The onset of bacterial pneumonia is sudden. The client experiences fever, chills, a productive cough, and discomfort in the chest wall muscles from coughing. There also is general malaise. The sputum may be rust colored. Breathing causes pain; thus, the client tries to breathe as shallowly as possible.

Viral pneumonia differs from bacterial pneumonia in that results of blood cultures are sterile, sputum may be more copious, chills are less common, and pulse and respiratory rates are characteristically slow. The course of viral pneumonia usually is less severe than that of bacterial pneumonia. The mortality rate from viral pneumonia is low but rises when bacterial pneumonia occurs as a secondary infection. Many clients with viral pneumonia are weak and ill for a longer period than those with successfully treated bacterial pneumonia.

Diagnostic Findings

Auscultation of the chest reveals wheezing, crackles, and decreased breath sounds. The nail beds, lips, and oral mucosa may be cyanotic. Sputum culture and sensitivity studies can help to identify the infectious microorganism

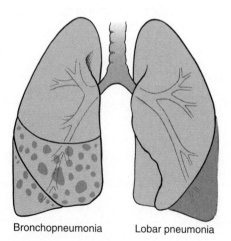

Bronchopneumonia   Lobar pneumonia

FIGURE 29-1 Distribution of lung involvement in bronchopneumonia and lobar pneumonia.

and effective antibiotics for treatment in cases of bacterial pneumonia. A chest film shows areas of infiltrates and consolidation. A complete blood count discloses an elevated WBC count. Blood cultures also may be done to detect any microorganisms in the blood.

Medical Management

Medical management involves prompt initiation of antibiotic therapy for bacterial pneumonia, hydration to thin secretions, supplemental oxygen to alleviate hypoxemia, bed rest, chest physical therapy, bronchodilators, analgesics, antipyretics, and cough expectorants or suppressants, depending on the nature of the client's cough. If a client is hospitalized, treatment is more vigorous, depending on the potential or actual complications. Fluid and electrolyte replacement sometimes is necessary secondary to fever, dehydration, and inadequate nutrition. If the client experiences severe respiratory difficulty and thick, copious secretions, he or she may require intubation along with mechanical ventilation.

Nursing Management

The nurse auscultates lung sounds and monitors the client for signs of respiratory difficulty. He or she checks oxygenation status with pulse oximetry and monitors arterial blood gases (ABGs). Assessments of cough and sputum production also are necessary.

The nurse places the client in semi-Fowler's position to aid breathing and increase the amount of air taken with each breath. Increased fluid intake is important to encourage because it helps to loosen secretions and replace fluids lost through fever and increased respiratory rate. The nurse monitors fluid intake and output, skin turgor, vital signs, and serum electrolytes. He or she administers antipyretics as indicated and ordered.

Identifying clients at risk for pneumonia provides a means to practice preventive nursing care. Nursing Guidelines 29-1 identifies strategies to implement for clients who are at risk for pneumonia. In addition, nurses encourage at-risk and elderly clients to receive vaccination against pneumococcal and influenza infections. Because the nursing care of clients with infectious lung disorders is similar regardless of the etiology, refer to Nursing Process: Tuberculosis for additional interventions.

● PLEURISY

Pleurisy or *pleuritis* refers to acute inflammation of the parietal and visceral pleurae. During the acute phase, the pleurae are inflamed, thick, and swollen, and an exudate forms from fibrin and lymph. Eventually the pleu-

---

NURSING GUIDELINES 29-1

Preventing Pneumonia

- Promote coughing and expectoration of secretions if client experiences increased mucus production.
- Change position frequently if client is immobilized for any reason.
- Encourage deep breathing and coughing exercises at least every 2 hours.
- Administer chest physical therapy as indicated.
- Suction client if he or she cannot expectorate.
- Prevent aspiration in clients at risk.
- Prevent infections.
- Cleanse respiratory equipment on a routine basis.
- Promote frequent oral hygiene.
- Administer sedatives and opioids carefully to avoid respiratory depression.
- Encourage client to stop smoking and reduce alcohol intake.

---

rae become rigid. During inspiration, the inflamed pleurae rub together, causing severe, sharp pain.

Pathophysiology and Etiology

Pleurisy usually is a consequence of a primary condition, such as pneumonia or other pulmonary infections. The inflammatory process spreads from the lungs to the parietal pleura. Pleurisy also may develop with tuberculosis (TB), lung cancer, cardiac and renal disease, systemic infections, or pulmonary embolism.

Assessment Findings

Respirations become shallow secondary to excruciating pain. Pleural fluid accumulates as the inflammatory process worsens. The pain decreases as the fluid increases because the fluid separates the pleura. The client develops a dry cough, fatigues easily, and experiences dyspnea. A *friction rub* (coarse sounds heard during inspiration and early expiration) is heard during auscultation early in the disease process. As fluid accumulates, the pleural friction rub disappears. Decreased ventilation may result in atelectasis, hypoxemia, and hypercapnia.

Chest radiography shows changes in the affected area. Microscopic examination of sputum and a sputum culture may reveal pathogenic microorganisms. If a **thoracentesis** (removal of fluid from the chest) is performed, a pleural fluid specimen is sent to the laboratory for analysis. Occasionally the physician may perform a pleural biopsy.

Medical Management

The underlying condition dictates the treatment. Analgesic and antipyretic drugs provide relief for pain and fever. A nonsteroidal anti-inflammatory drug (NSAID) such as indomethacin (Indocin) provides analgesia and promotes more effective coughing. Severe cases may require a procaine intercostal nerve block.

Nursing Management

The client has considerable pain with inspiration; thus, the nurse instructs the client to take analgesic medications as prescribed. Heat or cold applications may provide some topical comfort. The nurse teaches the client to splint the chest wall by turning onto the affected side. The client also can splint the chest wall with his or her hands or a pillow when coughing. Providing emotional support is essential—the client is very anxious and needs reassurance.

● PLEURAL EFFUSION

Pleural effusion is the collection of fluid between the visceral and parietal pleurae. It may be a complication of pneumonia, lung cancer, TB, pulmonary embolism, and CHF (Fig. 29-2). The amount of accumulated fluid may be so great that the lung partially collapses on the affected side. As a consequence, pressure is placed on the heart and other organs of the mediastinum.

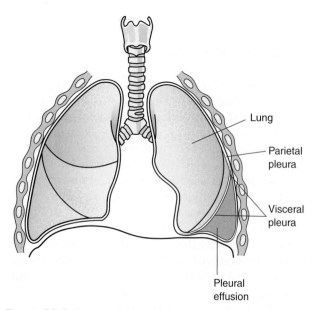

Lung

Parietal pleura

Visceral pleura

Pleural effusion

Figure 29-2 Pleural effusion. (From Smeltzer, S. C. & Bare, B. G. [2000]. *Brunner & Suddarth's textbook of medical–surgical nursing* [9th ed.]. Philadelphia: Lippincott Williams & Wilkins.)

Assessment Findings

Fever, pain, and dyspnea are the most common symptoms. Chest percussion reveals dullness over the involved area. The examiner may note diminished or absent breath sounds over the involved area when auscultating the lungs; he or she also may hear a friction rub. Chest radiography and computed tomography (CT) scan show fluid in the involved area. Thoracentesis sometimes is done to remove pleural fluid for analysis and examination for malignant cells.

Medical Management

The main goal of treatment is to eliminate the cause. Treatment includes antibiotics, analgesics, cardiotonic drugs to control CHF (when present), thoracentesis to remove excess pleural fluid, and surgery for cancer when present.

Nursing Management

If thoracentesis is needed, the nurse prepares the client for this procedure (see Nursing Guidelines 27-5). The client usually is frightened; thus, the nurse must provide support.

● LUNG ABSCESS

A **lung abscess** is a localized area of pus formation in the lung parenchyma. As the abscess increases, the tissue becomes necrotic. Later, the affected area collapses and creates a cavity. The infection can then extend into one or both bronchi and the pleural cavity.

Pathophysiology and Etiology

A lung abscess may develop from aspiration, pneumonia, or mechanical obstruction of the bronchi, such as with a tumor. Other causes include necrosis of lung tissue after an infection and necrotic lesions resulting from inhalation of dust particles. Clients with an impaired cough reflex or altered immune function are at risk for lung abscesses.

Assessment Findings

Signs and symptoms include chills, fever, weight loss, chest pain, and a productive cough. Sputum may be purulent or blood streaked. Finger clubbing may occur in chronic cases. Chest auscultation reveals dull or absent breath sounds in the area of the abscess. Chest radiography and CT scan usually locate the abscess. Results of blood and sputum cultures may be positive for pathogens. Chest percussion detects an area of dullness. In some instances, thoracentesis may be done, with the aspirated fluid sent to the laboratory for culture and sensitivity tests.

Medical and Surgical Management

Postural drainage and antibiotics assist in controlling the infection. Occasionally, a lobectomy is performed to remove the abscess and surrounding lung tissue.

Nursing Management

The nurse monitors the client for possible adverse effects of antibiotics. He or she administers chest physical therapy as indicated and encourages the client to deep breathe and cough frequently. A diet high in protein and calories is pivotal. The nurse provides emotional support, while being honest with the client that the lung abscess may take a long time to resolve.

● EMPYEMA

Empyema is a general term used to denote pus in a body cavity. It usually refers, however, to pus or infected fluid in the pleural cavity (*thoracic empyema*). Empyema may follow chest trauma, such as a stab or gunshot wound, or a pre-existing disease, such as pneumonia or TB. The pus-filled area may become walled off and enclosed by a thick membrane.

Assessment Findings

Fever, chest pain, dyspnea, anorexia, and malaise may accompany empyema. Chest auscultation reveals diminished or absent breath sounds over the affected area. The affected lung area is distinguished on a chest radiograph.

Medical and Surgical Management

Aspiration of purulent fluid by thoracentesis may be necessary to identify the microorganisms, remove pus or fluid, and select appropriate antibiotic therapy. Closed drainage may be used to empty the empyemic cavity. **Thoracotomy** (surgical opening of the thorax) is performed, and one or more large chest tubes are inserted, which are then connected to an underwater-seal drainage bottle. Open drainage, which necessitates the removal of a section of one or more ribs, may be used when pus is thick and the walls of the empyemic cavity are strong enough to keep the lung from collapsing while the chest is opened. One or more tubes may be placed in the opening to promote drainage. The wound is then covered by a large absorbent dressing, which is changed as necessary. The drainage of pus results in a drop in temperature and general symptomatic improvement.

Inadequately treated empyema may become chronic. A thick coating forms over the lung, preventing its expansion. *Decortication* (removal of the coating) and evacuation of the pleural space allow the lung to re-expand.

Nursing Management

Empyema takes a long time to resolve. The client requires emotional support during treatment. The nurse teaches the client to do breathing exercises as prescribed.

● INFLUENZA

Influenza (flu) is an acute respiratory disease of relatively short duration. The major strains of the flu virus are A, B, and C; the strains are related yet distinct from one another. Each virus can mutate and produce variants within the given strain. The variants are called *subtypes*. Viruses that cause influenza are transmitted through the respiratory tract.

Flu chiefly occurs in epidemics, although sporadic cases appear between them. Because the viruses change, antibodies produced by those who have had one case of flu are not effective against new subtypes, and a different antibody must be produced annually or during major epidemics. Most clients recover. Fatalities usually are related to secondary bacterial complications, especially among pregnant women, elderly or debilitated clients, and those with chronic conditions, such as cardiac disease and emphysema.

During a flu epidemic, the death rate from pneumonia and cardiovascular disease rises. Complications include tracheobronchitis, bacterial pneumonia, and cardiovascular disease. Staphylococcal pneumonia is the most serious complication. Table 29-1 lists signs and symptoms of flu, which form the basis for diagnosis. Additional diagnostic studies, such as chest radiography and sputum analysis, may be performed to rule out other diseases.

Nursing management focuses on prevention. Annual flu vaccinations are recommended for healthcare workers and people at high risk for complications or exposed daily to many different people. Each year a new vaccine is developed from three different virus strains that are predicted to be present in the coming flu season.

Clients admitted to the hospital with flu need to be isolated from clients who do not have it. Nurses must maintain airborne transmission precautions when caring for those clients. If a community is experiencing an epidemic,

TABLE 29-1	SIGNS AND SYMPTOMS OF INFLUENZA
Incubation period	1–3 days
Onset	Sudden
	Abrupt onset of fever and chills
	Severe headache
	Muscle aches
Progression	Anorexia
	Weakness, apathy, malaise
	Respiratory symptoms:
	Sneezing
	Sore throat, laryngitis
	Dry cough
	Nasal discharge—rhinitis
	Conjunctival irritation
Duration	Fever may persist for 3 days; other symptoms usually continue for 7–10 days.
	Cough may persist longer.
Period of contagion	2–3 days beginning with onset of symptoms

hospitals and other healthcare facilities usually develop policies regarding visitation and admissions.

● PULMONARY TUBERCULOSIS

Pulmonary **tuberculosis** is a bacterial infectious disease primarily caused by *M. tuberculosis.* TB essentially affects the lungs, but it may also affect the kidneys and other organs. TB continues to be a worldwide health problem. It affects one third of the world's population and is the leading cause of death from infectious diseases and among people with human immunodeficiency virus (HIV) infection (World Health Organization, 2001). In the United States, cases of TB continue to increase, with newer cases found to be resistant to drugs.

Pathophysiology and Etiology

Tubercle bacilli are gram-positive, rod-shaped, acid-fast, and aerobic. Although they can live in the dark for months as spores in particles of dried sputum, exposure to direct sunlight, heat, and ultraviolet light destroys them in a few hours. They are difficult to kill with ordinary disinfectants and are destroyed by pasteurization, a process widely used in milk and milk products to prevent the spread of TB.

TB is transmitted most commonly through the inhalation of droplets produced by coughing, sneezing, and spitting from a person with active disease. Brief contact usually does not result in infection. In contrast to the number of people who have been infected with tubercle bacilli, only a small proportion ever become ill. Many factors predispose a client to the development of TB, including inadequate healthcare, malnutrition, overcrowding, and poor housing.

TB is characterized by stages of early infection (or primary TB), latency, and potential for recurrence after the primary disease (called *secondary TB*). The bacilli may remain dormant for many years and then reactivate, producing clinical symptoms of TB.

Early Infection

Tubercle bacilli, when inhaled, pass through the bronchial system and implant on the bronchioles or alveoli. Initially, the host has no resistance to this infection. *Phagocytes* (neutrophils and macrophages) engulf the bacilli, which continue to multiply. At this time, the bacilli also spread through the lymphatic channels to the regional lymph nodes and subsequently to the circulating blood and distant organs. Eventually, the cellular immune response limits further multiplication and dissemination of the bacilli.

IMMUNE ACTIVATION

When immune activation occurs (usually a full response within 2 weeks), a characteristic tissue reaction results in the formation of a granuloma, referred to as the *Ghon tubercle,* from epithelial cells merging with the macrophages. Lymphocytes surround the Ghon tubercle, of which the central portion undergoes necrosis. This caseous necrosis has a cheesy appearance and may liquefy and slough into the connecting bronchus, producing a cavity. It also may enter the tracheobronchial system, promoting airborne transmission of infectious particles.

HEALING OF THE PRIMARY LESION

Healing of the primary lesion occurs through resolution, fibrosis, and calcification. The granulation tissue of the primary lesion becomes more fibrous and creates a scar around the tubercle. This is referred to as the *Ghon complex* and is visible on radiography.

Latent Period

As the lesion heals, the infection enters a latent period that can persist for many years or even an entire lifetime without producing clinical symptoms. If the immune response has been inadequate, however, the affected person eventually will develop clinical disease. Clients at particular risk are those with HIV infection or diabetes and those on chemotherapy or long-term steroids. Only a small percentage of those infected with TB actually develop clinical symptoms.

Secondary Tuberculosis

Secondary TB usually involves reactivation of the initial infection. The person already has had an immune response, and thus the lesions that form tend to remain in the lungs. The course of this phase usually is as follows:

1. Acute local inflammation and necrosis occur.
2. Infected lung tissue becomes ulcerated.
3. Tubercles cluster together and become surrounded by inflammation.
4. Exudate fills the surrounding alveoli.
5. The client develops bronchopneumonia.
6. TB tissue becomes caseous and ulcerates into the bronchus.
7. Cavities form.
8. Ulcerations heal, with scar tissue left around cavities.
9. Pleurae thicken and retract.

The course of TB becomes a cyclical one of inflammation, bronchopneumonia, ulceration, cavitation, and scarring. The TB gradually spreads throughout the lung fields and into the rest of the respiratory structures, as well as to other organs through the lymph system. A client may experience periods of exacerbation, followed by remissions.

Assessment Findings

Signs and Symptoms

The onset of TB is insidious, and early symptoms vary. An infected person may be asymptomatic until the disease is advanced. As symptoms develop, they often are vague and can be overlooked, particularly because they are systemic. Fatigue, anorexia, weight loss, and a slight, nonproductive cough are all symptoms attributable to overwork, excessive smoking, or poor eating habits. They also, however, are early symptoms of TB. Low-grade fever, particularly in the late afternoon, and night sweats are common as the disease progresses. The cough typically becomes productive of mucopurulent and blood-streaked sputum. Marked weakness, wasting, **hemoptysis** (expectoration of blood or bloody sputum), and dyspnea are characteristics of later stages. Chest pain may result from spread of the infection to the pleurae.

Diagnostic Findings

Diagnostic tests chiefly consist of tuberculin skin tests (see Chap. 27), chest radiography, CT scan, magnetic resonance imaging (MRI), and analysis of sputum and other body fluids. A positive tuberculin skin test result is evidence that a TB infection has existed at some time somewhere in the body, but does not indicate active disease. The chief value of tuberculin skin tests lies in case-finding.

Microscopic examination of sputum and other body fluids identifies the bacilli and is ordered when TB is suspected, during and after a course of drug therapy for TB, and after surgical removal of a diseased lobe of the lung. The client is instructed to cough deeply so that the specimen does not consist mainly of saliva. Most clients find that it is easier to raise sputum when they first awaken. It may be necessary to collect specimens on several consecutive days (see Nursing Guidelines 27-4).

Gastric lavage, gastric aspiration, or bronchoscopy may be used to determine the presence of the tubercle bacilli, particularly when a client has had difficulty raising a sputum specimen for examination. Tubercle bacilli may reach the stomach from the lungs when the client raises sputum but swallows rather than expectorates it. When invasion of other body areas by tubercle bacilli is suspected, specimens are obtained to confirm the diagnosis.

Medical and Surgical Management

In many cases, drugs have speeded recovery and provided a chance to arrest TB in clients with advanced lesions; however, they do not guarantee a cure. Their usefulness lies in their ability to retard the growth and multiplication of tubercle bacilli, thus giving the body a chance to overcome the disease. Two factors make drug therapy less than ideal: drug toxicity and the tendency of the tubercle bacilli to develop drug resistance. Combined therapy with two or more drugs decreases the likelihood of drug resistance, increases the tuberculostatic action of the drugs, and lessens the risk for toxic drug reactions (Drug Therapy Table 29-1).

Resistance of the bacilli to drugs is an important factor in the lack of response to medical treatment. Drug therapy usually is carried out while the client is at home. Regular visits to the physician's office or clinic for follow-up care are necessary for assessment of response to therapy. Culture and sensitivity tests may be performed, and the adverse effects of the drugs are evaluated.

When the disease is located primarily in one section of the lung, that portion may be removed by **segmental resection** (removal of a lobe segment) or **wedge resection** (removal of a wedge of diseased tissue). If the diseased area is larger, **lobectomy** (removal of a lobe) may be performed. In some cases, the lung is so diseased that **pneumonectomy** (removal of an entire lung) is necessary (see Box 29-3).

N U R S I N G   P R O C E S S

● Pulmonary Tuberculosis

Assessment

The nurse assesses breath sounds, breathing patterns, and overall respiratory status. He or she asks the client about any pain or discomfort experienced with breathing. The nurse inspects the client's sputum for color, viscosity, amount, and signs of blood. Clients with primary TB may have complaints related to fatigue, weakness, anorexia, weight loss, or night sweats. Clients with secondary TB may report chest pain and a cough that pro-

DRUG THERAPY TABLE 29-1	DRUG REGIMEN FOR TUBERCULOSIS	
TREATMENT PERIOD	**DRUGS PRESCRIBED**	**LENGTH OF DRUG THERAPY**
Initial treatment	isoniazid (INH) rifampin (RIF) pyrazinamide (PZA) (These three medications now in combination tablet.)	INH, RIF, PZA for 4 months INH and RIF for additional 2 months
Suspected drug resistance	isoniazid (INH) rifampin (RIF) pyrazinamide (PZA) ethambutol (EMB) or streptomycin (SM)	If sensitive, continue INH and RIF for 6 more months. If resistant to INH, use other drugs for 6 months. If resistant to RIF, use other drugs for 12–18 months.
Prophylactic treatment	isoniazid (INH) May use pyridoxine (vitamin B$_6$) to minimize side effects	6–12 months

duces mucopurulent or blood-tinged mucus or blood. They also may report a low-grade fever.

Diagnosis, Planning, and Interventions

Antitubercular drug regimens extend for long periods and without interruption because healing is slow and interrupted treatment increases drug resistance. The primary focus of nursing management is encouraging the client to adhere to the prescribed medication regimen and teaching.

The nurse instructs the client to take medications exactly as prescribed, closely observing the time interval between each dose. Clients must not skip doses or take more than the amount prescribed. Drugs used to treat TB must be taken for a long time. Thus, clients need to complete the entire course of drug therapy to control infection. Continuous therapy is essential because lapses in taking the prescribed drugs can result in reactivation of the infection. Clients should notify the physician if symptoms worsen or sudden chest pain or dyspnea develops. Clients also should drink plenty of fluids, discontinue smoking immediately, and avoid exposure to secondhand smoke. They need to eat a balanced but light diet.

Other nursing care includes the following diagnoses, outcomes, and interventions.

Ineffective Airway Clearance related to pain with coughing, inability to cough, and abnormal respirations
Expected Outcome: Client will effectively clear secretions.

- Assess cough, noting the attributes of the secretions: color, consistency, amount, and presence of blood. *Coughing usually becomes more frequent with increased expectorant; hemoptysis occurs in advanced TB.*
- Encourage client to drink 3 to 4 L/day. *This amount liquefies and thins secretions and facilitates expectoration.*
- Humidify inspired air. *Humidified air maintains moisture to assist in liquefying secretions.*
- Encourage deep breathing and coughing every 2 hours while awake. *These measures promote lung expansion and mobilization of secretions.*

- Place client in semi-Fowler's position. *This position improves breathing and assists client to expectorate mucus.*
- Provide instructions about postural drainage. *Postural drainage facilitates airway drainage and clearance.*

Pain related to chest expansion secondary to lung infection/inflammation
Expected Outcome: Client will manage pain with analgesics and use of splinting techniques when coughing.

- Assess pain level. *This information provides a baseline for treatment and evaluation.*
- Evaluate effectiveness of pain relief measures. *Such evaluation helps the nurse to determine if measures are effective or other therapies are necessary.*
- Administer analgesics as indicated. *Proper pain assessment and appropriate analgesic administration provide more effective pain control.*
- Instruct client in splinting techniques for use during coughing. *Proper splinting decreases pain and facilitates expectoration of secretions.*

Activity Intolerance related to general weakness, respiratory difficulties, fever, and severity of illness
Expected Outcome: Client will demonstrate increased activity tolerance.

- Encourage rest periods, particularly before meals, performing activities of daily living (ADLs), and exercise. *Rest reduces fatigue and spaces activities.*
- Prioritize necessary tasks, eliminating nonessential tasks. *Prioritization of tasks promotes rest.*
- Assist client with activities as required. *Giving assistance reduces client's energy expenditure, but allows him or her choices.*
- Keep equipment (e.g., telephone, tissues, wastebasket, bedside commode) close to client. *Keeping needed items close by reduces energy expenditure.*
- Encourage active range-of-motion (ROM) exercises three times a day. *Active ROM exercises maintain muscle strength and joint ROM.*

PC: Side Effects of Medication Therapy—hepatitis, neurologic changes, gastrointestinal (GI) upset

Expected Outcome: Nurse will assist client to minimize side effects of medications.

- Instruct client to take medication 1 hour before or 2 hours after meals. *Food interferes with medication absorption.*
- Instruct clients taking isoniazid (INH) to avoid foods with tyramine and histamine (e.g., tuna, aged cheese, red wine, soy sauce, yeast extracts). *INH, when combined with these foods, may cause light-headedness, flushing, hypotension, headache, and other symptoms.*
- Ask if client is taking any beta blockers or oral anticoagulants. *Rifampin increases the metabolism of beta blockers and oral anticoagulants. Dosages may need to be adjusted or medications changed.*
- Inform the client who wears contact lenses that rifampin may color them. *The client may prefer to wear glasses while taking rifampin.*
- Monitor for side effects related to medication regimen. For hepatitis, check liver enzymes. For kidney function, check blood urea nitrogen and serum creatinine levels. For neurologic changes, look for hearing loss and neuritis. Also check for skin rash. *Early identification of side effects promotes prompt treatment of side effects and adjustments in medications.*

Evaluation of Expected Outcomes

The client manages secretions with effective coughing, increased fluid intake, and appropriate postural drainage. He or she reports adequate pain relief and can tolerate increased amounts of time out of bed and perform most ADLs. The client adheres to treatment regimen and schedules tests for liver and kidney function.

Stop, Think, and Respond ● BOX 29-1

A client diagnosed with TB lives in a four-room apartment with his wife. What precautions must the couple follow?

OBSTRUCTIVE PULMONARY DISEASE

Obstructive pulmonary disease describes conditions in which airflow in the lungs is obstructed. Resistance to inspiration is decreased, whereas resistance to expiration is increased, so that the expiratory phase of respiration is prolonged (Bullock & Henze, 2000). **Chronic obstructive pulmonary disease** (COPD) is a broad, nonspecific term that describes a group of pulmonary disorders with symptoms of chronic cough and expectoration, dyspnea, and impaired expiratory airflow. Bronchiectasis, atelectasis, chronic bronchitis, and emphysema are categorized as COPDs. Asthma also is an obstructive disorder that is

more episodic and usually more acute than the COPDs. Sleep apnea syndrome also can have obstructive causes. Cystic fibrosis also has obstructive characteristics and is included in this section.

● BRONCHIECTASIS

Bronchiectasis is a COPD characterized by chronic infection and irreversible dilatation of the bronchi and bronchioles. Causes include bronchial obstruction by tumor or foreign body, congenital abnormalities, exposure to toxic gases, and chronic pulmonary infections. When clearance of the airway is impeded, an infection can develop in the walls of the bronchus or bronchioles. The structure of the wall tissue subsequently changes, resulting in the formation of saccular dilatations, which collect purulent material. Airway clearance is further impaired, and the purulent material remains, causing more dilatation, structural damage, and more infection (Fig. 29-3).

Assessment Findings

Clients with bronchiectasis experience a chronic cough with expectoration of copious amounts of purulent sputum and possible hemoptysis. The coughing worsens when the client changes position. The amount of sputum produced during one paroxysm varies with the stage of the disease, but it can be several ounces. When the sputum is collected, it settles into three distinct layers: the top layer is frothy and cloudy, the middle layer is clear saliva, and the bottom layer is heavy, thick, and purulent. Clients also experience fatigue, weight loss, anorexia, and dyspnea.

Chest radiography and bronchoscopy demonstrate the increased size of the bronchioles, possible areas of atelectasis, and changes in the pulmonary tissue. Sputum culture and sensitivity tests identify the causative micro-

FIGURE 29-3 Bronchiectasis, showing abnormal saccular dilatations of the large bronchi that are filled with inflammatory exudate.

organism and effective antibiotics to control the infection. Pulmonary function studies also may be done.

Medical Management

Treatment of bronchiectasis includes drainage of purulent material from the bronchi; antibiotics, bronchodilators, and mucolytics to improve breathing and help raise secretions; humidification to loosen secretions; and surgical removal if bronchiectasis is confined to a small area.

Nursing Management

Nursing management focuses on instructing the client in postural drainage techniques, which help the client mobilize and expectorate secretions. The positions for the

client to assume depend on the site or lobe to be drained. Figure 29-4 shows positions that drain specific segments of all lobes of the lungs. The client remains in each position for 10 to 15 minutes. Chest percussion and vibration may be performed during this time. When complete, the client coughs and expectorates the secretions. This procedure may be repeated. The nurse provides oral hygiene after treatment.

● ATELECTASIS

Atelectasis is the collapse of alveoli (Fig. 29-5). It may involve a small portion of the lung or an entire lobe. When alveoli collapse, they cannot perform their function of gas exchange. Atelectasis occurs secondary to aspiration of food or vomitus, a mucus plug, fluid or air in the thoracic cavity, compression on tissue by tumors, an

FIGURE 29-4 Lung areas to be drained and the best postural drainage positions for them. (From Smeltzer, S. C. & Bare, B. G. [2000]. *Brunner & Suddarth's textbook of medical–surgical nursing* [9th ed.]. Philadelphia: Lippincott Williams & Wilkins.)

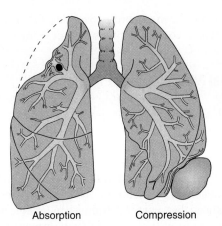

Absorption   Compression

FIGURE 29-5 Atelectasis caused by airway obstruction and absorption of air from the involved lung area on the *left* and by compression of lung tissue on the *right.*

enlarged heart, an aneurysm, or enlarged lymph nodes in the chest. Ill clients may experience atelectasis when on prolonged bed rest, when unable to breathe deeply or cough and raise secretions, or both.

Assessment Findings

The amount of involved lung tissue determines the extent of the symptoms. Small areas of atelectasis may cause few symptoms. With larger areas, cyanosis, fever, pain, dyspnea, increased pulse and respiratory rates, and increased pulmonary secretions may be seen. Although crackling may be auscultated over the affected areas, usually breath sounds are absent. A chest radiograph reveals dense shadows, indicating collapsed lung tissue. Sometimes the radiograph results are inconclusive. ABG and pulse oximetry results may be abnormal.

Medical Management

Treatment includes improving ventilation, suctioning, and deep breathing and coughing to raise secretions. Bronchodilators and humidification assist in loosening and removing secretions. Oxygen is administered for dyspnea. Removal of the cause of atelectasis helps to correct the condition.

Nursing Management

Nursing care focuses on preventing atelectasis, especially when the client is at risk because of failure to aerate the lungs properly. Postoperative deep breathing and coughing can prevent atelectasis. If atelectasis occurs, the nurse encourages the client to take deep breaths and cough at

frequent intervals and instructs the client in the use of an incentive spirometer (Nursing Guidelines 29-2).

● CHRONIC BRONCHITIS

Chronic bronchitis is a prolonged (or extended) inflammation of the bronchi, accompanied by a chronic cough and excessive production of mucus for at least 3 months each year for 2 consecutive years. This serious health problem develops gradually and may go untreated for many years until the disease is well established.

Pathophysiology and Etiology

Chronic bronchitis is characterized by hypersecretion of mucus and recurrent or chronic respiratory tract infections. As the infection progresses, the ability of the cilia that line the airway to propel secretions upward becomes significantly altered. Secretions remain in the lungs and form plugs in the smaller bronchi. These plugs become

NURSING GUIDELINES 29-2

Incentive Spirometer

1. Sit upright unless contraindicated.
2. Mark the goal for inhalation.
3. Exhale normally.
4. Place mouthpiece in mouth, sealing lips around it.
5. Inhale slowly until predetermined volume has been reached.
6. Hold breath for 2 to 6 seconds.
7. Exhale normally.
8. Repeat the exercise 10 to 20 times per hour while awake, or as ordered.
9. Do not rush during the procedure. Slow down if dizziness is experienced.

areas for bacterial growth and chronic infection, which increases mucous secretion and eventually causes areas of focal tissue death. Airway obstruction results from the bronchial inflammation.

Multiple factors are associated with chronic bronchitis. Its development may be insidious or follow a long history of bronchial asthma or an acute respiratory tract infection, such as influenza or pneumonia. Air pollution and smoking are significant factors.

Chronic bronchitis may develop at any age, but it appears most commonly in middle age after years of untreated, low-grade bronchitis. Diagnosis is based on evaluation of the duration of symptoms, determination of how the disease process began, and history of occupational health hazards, pulmonary disease, and smoking.

Stop, Think, and Respond ● BOX 29-2

Your client with acute bronchitis smokes two packs of cigarettes per day. What would you advise this client?

Assessment Findings

Signs and Symptoms

The earliest symptom is a chronic cough productive of thick, white mucus, especially when rising in the morning and in the evening. Bronchospasm may occur during severe bouts of coughing. Acute respiratory infections are frequent during the winter months and may persist for at least several weeks. As the disease progresses, the sputum may become yellow, purulent, copious, and blood streaked after paroxysms of coughing. Expiration is prolonged secondary to obstructed air passages. Cyanosis secondary to hypoxemia may be noted, especially after severe coughing. Dyspnea begins with exertion, but progresses to occurring with minimal activity, and later occurs at rest. Right-sided heart failure results from tachycardia in response to hypoxemia, which causes edema in the extremities.

Diagnostic Findings

The progression and history of symptoms determine the diagnostic studies needed. Initially, results of the physical examination, chest radiography, and pulmonary function tests may be normal. As the disease progresses, these findings become increasingly abnormal. Chest radiography shows signs of fluid overload and consolidation in the lungs.

As right-sided failure develops, the heart enlarges. Pulmonary function test results demonstrate decreased vital capacity and forced expiratory volume and increased residual volume and total lung capacity. Diagnostic studies such as bronchoscopy, microscopic examination of the sputum for malignant cells, and lung scan may be neces-

sary to rule out cancer, bronchiectasis, TB, or other diseases in which cough is a predominant feature.

Medical Management

The goals of treatment are to prevent recurrent irritation of the bronchial mucosa by infection or chemical agents, maintain the function of the bronchioles, and assist in the removal of secretions. Treatment includes smoking cessation, bronchodilators to reduce airway obstruction and bronchospasm, increased fluid intake, maintenance of a well-balanced diet, postural drainage to remove bronchial secretions, steroid therapy if other treatment is ineffective, change in occupation if work involves exposure to dust and chemical irritants, filtration of incoming air to reduce sputum production and cough, and antibiotic therapy.

Nursing Management

Nursing management focuses on educating clients in managing their disease. The nurse helps clients identify ways to eliminate environmental irritants. Such measures include smoking cessation, occupational counseling, monitoring air quality and pollution levels, and avoiding cold air and wind exposure that can cause bronchospasm.

Preventing infection is another important aspect of care. The nurse instructs clients to avoid others with respiratory tract infections and to receive pneumonia and flu immunizations. He or she teaches the client to monitor sputum for signs of infection. The nurse also teaches the proper use of aerosolized bronchodilators and corticosteroids. Nursing Guidelines 29-3 discusses teaching a client how to use a metered-dose inhaler (MDI); nurses must warn clients against overuse of this modality.

The nurse instructs the client in postural drainage techniques and measures to improve overall health, such as eating a well-balanced diet, getting plenty of rest, and engaging in moderate aerobic activity. For clients with lung disease, dyspnea, not heart rate, should determine the amount of aerobic activity. In other words, clients should exercise at the pace and for the length of time they can tolerate without dyspnea. Refer to nursing management of emphysema for nursing diagnoses and additional interventions.

● PULMONARY EMPHYSEMA

Emphysema is a chronic disease characterized by abnormal distention of the alveoli. The alveolar walls and capillary beds also show marked destruction. This process of destruction occurs over a long period. By the time of diagnosis, damage to the lungs usually is permanent. Emphy-

NURSING GUIDELINES 29-3

Metered-Dose Inhaler

1. Attach the stem of the canister into the hole of the mouthpiece so that the inhaler looks like an "L."

2. Shake the canister to distribute the drug in its pressurized chamber.

3. Exhale slowly through pursed lips.

4. Seal lips around the mouthpiece *or* hold inhaler a few inches from mouth and inhale.

5. Compress the canister between thumb and fingers and slowly inhale at the same time.

6. Release the pressure on the canister, but continue inhaling as much as possible.

7. Withdraw the mouthpiece.

8. Hold breath for a few seconds.

9. Exhale slowly through pursed lips.

10. If second dose is required, wait for a few seconds before repeating procedure.

© B. Proud.

sema is a common cause of disability and the most common COPD.

Pathophysiology and Etiology

In emphysema, the alveoli lose elasticity, trapping air that the client normally would expire. On microscopic examination, the alveolar walls have broken down, forming one large sac instead of multiple, small air spaces. The capillary beds, previously located within the alveolar walls, are destroyed, and fibrous scarring replaces much of the tissue. The formation of fibrous tissue and destruction of the alveoli prevent the proper exchange of oxygen and CO_2 during respiration.

As the disease progresses, large air sacs (bullae, blebs) may be seen over the lung surface. These sacs can rupture, allowing air to enter the thorax (**pneumothorax**) with

each respiration. In this case, emergency thoracentesis is performed to remove the air from the thoracic cavity. A chest tube may be inserted to keep additional air from entering. Recurrent episodes of pneumothorax may require surgery to correct the problem (see section on Thoracic Surgery).

Assessment Findings

Signs and Symptoms

Shortness of breath with minimal activity is called *exertional dyspnea* and often is the first symptom of emphysema. As the disease progresses, breathlessness occurs even at rest. A chronic cough invariably is present and productive of mucopurulent sputum. Inspiration is difficult because of the rigid chest cage, and the chest is characteristically barrel shaped (Fig. 29-6).

The client uses the accessory muscles of respiration (muscles in the jaw and neck and intercostal muscles) to maintain normal ventilation. Expiration is prolonged, difficult, and often accompanied by wheezing. In advanced emphysema, respiratory function is markedly impaired.

FIGURE 29-6 Characteristics of chest wall in emphysema. (From Smeltzer, S. C. & Bare, B. G. [2000]. *Brunner & Suddarth's textbook of medical–surgical nursing* [9th ed.]. Philadelphia: Lippincott Williams & Wilkins.)

Clients with advanced emphysema characteristically appear drawn, anxious, and pale. They speak in short, jerky sentences. When sitting up, they often lean slightly forward and are markedly short of breath. The neck veins may distend during expiration.

In advanced emphysema, memory loss, drowsiness, confusion, and loss of judgment may result from the markedly reduced oxygen that reaches the brain and the increased CO_2 in the blood. If the disorder goes untreated, the CO_2 content in the blood may reach toxic levels, resulting in lethargy, stupor, and, eventually, coma. This condition is called *carbon dioxide narcosis.* Lung auscultation reveals decreased breath sounds, wheezing, and crackles. Heart sounds are diminished or muffled. Visual inspection shows a barrel-chested person breathing through pursed lips and using the accessory muscles of respiration.

Diagnostic Findings

Chest radiography and fluoroscopy demonstrate hyperinflated lung fields. Results of pulmonary function studies show a marked decrease in overall function, including increased total lung capacity and residual volume and decreased vital capacity and forced expiratory volume. ABG analysis usually reveals hypoxemia and respiratory acidosis.

Medical Management

The goals of medical management include improving the client's quality of life, slowing the disease progression, and treating the obstructed airways. Treatment includes the following measures:

- Bronchodilators to dilate airways by decreasing edema and spasms and improving gas exchange
- Aerosol therapy with nebulized aerosols for deep inhalation of bronchodilators and mucolytics in the tracheobronchial tree
- Antibiotics
- Corticosteroids on a limited basis to assist with bronchodilation and removal of secretions
- Physical therapy to increase ventilation—deep breathing, coughing, chest percussion, vibration, and postural drainage

If the prescribed treatment regimen does not help the client, progressive loss of sleep, appetite, weight, and physical strength is likely. As the disease progresses, the client may need to curtail physical activities.

Nursing Management

The respiratory center of the brain is sensitive to the level of CO_2 in the blood. If the level increases slightly, respiratory rate and depth increase to eliminate the excess CO_2. If, however, the CO_2 level is chronically elevated, the respiratory center becomes insensitive to CO_2 changes. Under these circumstances, the level of oxygen in the blood becomes a regulatory factor—the hypoxic drive to breathe. As long as the level of oxygen saturation of the blood is low, a client breathes sufficiently to maintain oxygenation. If oxygen is given at or above 32% by mask or other means, the hypoxic drive to breathe is lost and the respiratory rate drops, leading to further retention of CO_2, apnea, and death.

If the client requires oxygen, the safest method of administration is by nasal catheter or cannula, with the oxygen flow rate set at no more than 2 to 3 L/min. If the client's color improves but his or her level of consciousness decreases, the nurse discontinues oxygen administration and notifies the physician; the client may be approaching a state of respiratory arrest.

Therapeutic breathing exercises effectively use the diaphragm, thus relieving the compensatory burden on the muscles of the upper thorax. The nurse teaches the client to let the abdomen rise when taking a deep breath and to contract the abdominal muscles when exhaling. Clients can feel the correct way to do this by placing one hand on the chest and the other on the abdomen: during abdominal breathing, the chest should remain quiet and the abdomen should rise and fall with each breath.

Other exercises include blowing out candles at various distances and blowing a small object, such as a pencil or piece of chalk, along a tabletop. The nurse encourages the client to exhale more completely by taking a deep breath and then bending the body forward at the waist while exhaling as fully as possible. Pursed-lip breathing (i.e., breathing with the lips pursed or puckered on expiration) helps to control the respiratory rate and depth and slows expiration. This maneuver may decrease dyspnea and in turn reduce the anxiety that often is associated with breathing difficulties. See Client and Family Teaching Box 29-1 for additional nursing management.

NURSING PROCESS

● Obstructive Pulmonary Disease

Assessment

The nurse assesses the client's respiratory status, including respiratory effort, rate, and pattern. He or she determines if the client has diminished breath sounds and prolonged expiration. The nurse observes for evidence of dyspnea at rest, as well as accentuated accessory neck muscles and barrel-shaped chest. He or she asks the client about tolerance for activity and checks the characteristics of secretions: consistency, quantity, color, or odor. Other important assessment data are the client's ability to expectorate secretions, signs and symptoms of infection, and what the client does to relieve pulmonary symptoms.

Diagnosis, Planning, and Interventions

Ineffective Airway Clearance related to broncho-constriction, increased mucus production, and ineffective cough

Expected Outcome: Client will maintain a patent airway and adequate airway clearance.

- Auscultate breath sounds at least every 8 hours. *Findings may indicate airway obstruction secondary to mucus plug, increasing airway resistance, or fluid in larger airways.*
- Encourage client to cough and clear secretions; suction as needed. *These measures promote airway clearance and improve ventilation.*
- Perform postural drainage with percussion and vibration twice a day as indicated. *Postural drainage assists in mobilizing secretions for expectoration.*
- Observe for dyspnea, restlessness, increased anxiety, or use of accessory muscles. *Such findings indicate possible airway obstruction or ineffective clearance of secretions.*
- Increase fluid intake to 3 L/day if not contraindicated. (Right-sided or left-sided cardiac failure is a contraindication.) Humidify inspired air. *These measures keep secretions moist and easier to expectorate.*
- Instruct client in early signs of infection: increased sputum production, change in sputum color and consistency, fever, increased coughing, and increased dyspnea. *Early recognition prevents an infection from progressing to a potentially lethal process.*
- Administer bronchodilators by nebulizer or MDI as indicated. *Bronchodilators open airways, facilitating breathing and expectoration of secretions.*
- Teach and encourage the use of diaphragmatic and pursed lip breathing. *These techniques improve ventilation and mobilize secretions.*

Impaired Gas Exchange related to prolonged expiration, loss of lung tissue elasticity, and atelectasis

Expected Outcome: Client will maintain optimal gas exchange.

- Promote more effective breathing patterns through optimal positioning, pursed-lip breathing, and use of abdominal muscles. *High-Fowler's position promotes better lung expansion; turning side-to-side promotes aeration of lung lobes; pursed-lip breathing and other methods open airways and provide for better exhalation.*
- Administer oxygen as prescribed. *Clients with COPD chronically retain CO_2 and depend on hypoxic drive as the stimulus for breathing; accurate oxygen administration is essential for preventing cessation of breathing.*
- Monitor level of consciousness and mental status. *Problems with mentation indicate inadequate oxygenation.*

- Monitor results of ABGs and pulse oximetry. *Changes in these findings indicate respiratory deterioration and provide an opportunity for early interventions.*

PC: Atelectasis

Expected Outcome: Nurse will manage and minimize atelectasis.

- Instruct client to do deep breathing and coughing exercises, incentive spirometry, or both. *These techniques promote lung expansion.*
- Encourage client to use abdominal muscles when breathing. *Diaphragmatic breathing promotes lung expansion.*

Evaluation of Expected Outcomes

The client's airway is free of secretions; breath sounds are clear. ABG and pulse oximetry results are within baseline values, and client remains alert and responsive. The client has no signs or symptoms of atelectasis and demonstrates the ability to do pulmonary exercises and abdominal breathing as instructed by the nurse.

 29-1 *Client and Family Teaching* Emphysema

Education is an important part of therapy aimed at helping clients adjust to their current level of disability and to the potential for increased disability in the future. The primary goal is to prevent or delay the progression of emphysema. The nurse explains strategies to slow the disease progression.

- Emphasize that success depends on strict adherence to the treatment regimen. Motivated clients profit more from available treatments and make the best use of their remaining pulmonary function.
- Take medication exactly as prescribed. Observe the time intervals between medications. Do not skip doses or take more than what is prescribed.
- Maintain close medical supervision.
- Contact the physician if adverse drug effects occur, drugs fail to relieve symptoms, new symptoms appear, symptoms become more severe, or signs or symptoms of respiratory infection develop.
- Drink extra fluids as indicated, unless fluids are restricted.
- Avoid respiratory irritants and people with respiratory infections.
- Eat a well-balanced diet.
- Perform breathing exercises as prescribed.
- Take frequent rests during the day. Space activities to prevent fatigue and shortness of breath.
- Avoid dry-heated areas that can aggravate symptoms.
- Humidify inspired air during the winter months.

● ASTHMA

Asthma is a reversible obstructive disease of the lower airway. Inflammation of the airway and a hyperresponsiveness of the airway to internal or external stimuli characterize asthma. The incidence of asthma is increasing, particularly in children and adolescents. Asthma affects almost one fifth of the population at some time in their lives. Asthma may be fatal, but for most people it causes disruptions in school and work attendance and affects choices in careers and activities.

Pathophysiology and Etiology

There are three types of asthma: *allergic asthma* (extrinsic), which occurs in response to allergens, such as pollen, dust, spores, and animal danders; *idiopathic asthma* (intrinsic) associated with factors such as upper respiratory infections, emotional upsets, and exercise; and *mixed asthma,* which has characteristics of allergic and idiopathic asthma. Mixed asthma is the most common form.

Acute asthma results from increasing airway obstruction caused by bronchospasm and bronchoconstriction, inflammation and edema of the lining of the bronchi and bronchioles, and production of thick mucus that can plug the airway (Fig. 29-7). The airways in people with asthma are hyperreactive in response to stimuli. Allergic asthma causes the immunoglobulin E (IgE) inflammatory response (see Chap. 41). These antibodies attach to mast cells within the lungs. Re-exposure to the antigen causes the antigen to attach to the antibody, releasing mast cell products such as histamine. The manifestations of asthma

become evident as this occurs. Other types of asthma are hyperresponsive to the inflammatory changes.

Because the alveoli cannot expel air, they hyperinflate and trap air in the lungs. The client breathes faster, blowing off excess CO_2. Although the client tries to force the air out, the narrowed airway makes it difficult. Wheezing usually is audible with expiration, resulting from air being forced out of the narrowed airway. Other pathophysiologic changes include interference with gas exchange, poor perfusion, possible atelectasis, and respiratory failure if inadequately treated.

Asthma may develop at any age. There appears to be a significant relationship between bronchiolitis (inflammation of the bronchioles) in the first year of life and development of asthma in early childhood. Asthma may be limited to occasional attacks, with the client symptom free between attacks.

Assessment Findings

Signs and Symptoms

Asthma is typified by paroxysms of shortness of breath, wheezing, and coughing and the production of thick, tenacious sputum. Duration of acute episodes varies; it may be brief (less than 1 day) or extended (lasting for several weeks).

Most clients are aware of the wheezing and report it as one of their symptoms. Every breath becomes an effort. During an acute episode, the work of breathing greatly increases, and the client may suffer from a sensation of suffocation. The client frequently assumes a classic sitting position, with the body leaning slightly forward and the arms at shoulder height. This position facilitates chest expansion and more effective excursions of the diaphragm. Because life depends on the power to breathe, fear and anxiety often accompany and also intensify the symptoms.

Marked prolongation of the expiratory phase of respiration accompanies the effort to move trapped air. Coughing commences with the onset of the attack but is ineffective in the early stage. Only as the attack begins to subside can the client expectorate large quantities of thick, stringy mucus. The skin usually is pale. During a severe attack, the nurse may observe cyanosis of the client's lips and nail beds. Perspiration typically is profuse during an acute attack. After spontaneous or drug-induced remission of the episode, examination of the lungs commonly shows normal findings. Sometimes an acute attack intensifies and progresses to status asthmaticus (persistent state of asthma), which can be life-threatening.

Diagnostic Findings

Chest auscultation reveals expiratory and sometimes inspiratory wheezes and diminished breath sounds. Results of pulmonary function studies, especially of forced

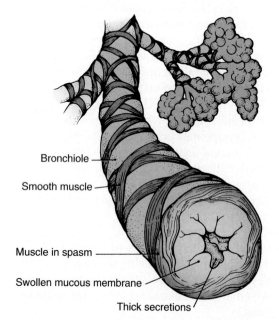

FIGURE 29-7 Bronchial asthma. Muscle spasms, mucosal edema, and thick secretions obstruct the bronchiole on expiration.

Bronchiole

Smooth muscle

Muscle in spasm

Swollen mucous membrane

Thick secretions

expiratory volume, may be abnormal, with total lung capacity and functional residual volume increased secondary to trapped air. The forced expiratory volume and forced vital capacity are decreased. During acute attacks, blood gases show hypoxemia. The partial pressure of carbon dioxide ($PaCO_2$) level may be elevated if the asthma becomes worse, but usually the $PaCO_2$ level is decreased because of the rapid respiratory rate. A normal $PaCO_2$ level in the latter part of an asthma attack may indicate impending respiratory failure.

Medical Management

Symptomatic treatment is given at the time of the attack. Long-term care involves measures to treat as well as prevent further attacks. An effort must be made to determine the cause. If the history and diagnostic tests indicate allergy as a causative factor, treatment includes avoidance of the allergen, desensitization, or antihistamine therapy. Oxygen usually is not necessary during an acute attack because most clients are actively hyperventilating. Oxygen may be necessary if cyanosis occurs.

Pharmacologic management is classified as rescue therapy and maintenance therapy (Eisenbeis, 1996). Rescue therapy medications treat acute episodes of asthma, whereas maintenance therapy is a daily regimen designed to prevent and control symptoms. Many medications are taken through MDIs. Drug Therapy Table 29-2 lists medications used in maintenance therapy.

Humidification of inspired air is valuable because dehydration of the respiratory mucous membrane may lead to asthmatic attacks. Use of steam or cool vapor humidifiers also has proved effective. Liquefaction of the secretions promotes more effective clearing of the airways and a rapid return to normal. Air conditioners may filter offending allergens as well as control temperature and humidity.

Nursing Management

During asthma attacks, clients are extremely anxious. The nurse reassures the client that someone will remain with him or her during the acute phase. The nurse administers oxygen as indicated and puts the client in a sitting posi-

DRUG THERAPY TABLE 29-2	**MAINTENANCE DRUG THERAPY FOR ASTHMA**	
DRUG CATEGORY AND EXAMPLES/ MECHANISM OF ACTION	**SIDE EFFECTS**	**NURSING CONSIDERATIONS**
Beta Agonists *albuterol (Ventolin)* Dilate the smooth muscles of the bronchioles, reduce muscle spasm, and therefore increase the size of the airway	Restlessness, apprehension, anxiety, fear, central nervous system stimulation, nausea, dysrhythmias, sweating, flushing, paradoxical airway resistance with repeated excessive use	Ensure that client understands technique for administering inhalers. Tell client not to exceed recommended dose and to report chest pain, dizziness, irregular heart rate, difficulty breathing, productive cough, or failure to achieve relief.
Anticholinergics *ipratropium bromide (Atrovent)* Decrease vagal tone to airways, resulting in bronchodilation	Nervousness, dizziness, headache, nausea, cough, palpitations, exacerbation of glaucoma and urinary retention	Demonstrate proper use of inhaler. Tell client to report eye pain or visual changes, rash, difficulty voiding.
Corticosteroids *triamcinolone (Azmacort)* Decrease inflammatory response	Inhalants: oral, laryngeal, and pharyngeal irritation and fungal infections*	Tell client not to use during an acute asthma attack and not to use more often than prescribed. If using an aerosolized bronchodilator, administer the bronchodilator first. Tell client not to discontinue medication abruptly.
Mast Cell Inhibitors *Inhaled cromolyn (Intal)* Prevent the release of mast cell products, promoting bronchodilation and decreasing inflammation; ineffective in acute attacks, but very therapeutic if taken regularly	Dizziness, nausea, throat irritation	Tell client not to use during an acute attack, to follow manufacturer's instructions for administration, and not to discontinue abruptly.

*Corticosteroids administered by other routes and in higher dosages are associated with multiple adverse effects.

tion. Rest and adequate fluid intake are important. Increased fluid intake makes secretions less tenacious and replaces the fluids lost through perspiration. Thus, the nurse keeps fluids within easy reach and encourages the client to drink them. He or she checks the intravenous (IV) site frequently for signs of extravasation. This monitoring is especially important during an acute attack because restlessness can result in needle dislodgment. The nurse observes for adverse drug effects, especially when the client is receiving epinephrine or other adrenergic agents, which may cause palpitations, nervousness, trembling, pallor, and insomnia.

After the acute asthma attack subsides, the nurse assesses level of understanding about the disease process, which for many clients may not be clear. He or she asks if the client has a peak flow meter. If the client does not, the nurse obtains one for the client and tells him or her how to use it to monitor the degree of asthma control. Explanations include the following:

- Sit upright in bed or chair or stand and inhale as deeply as possible.
- Form a tight seal around the mouthpiece with lips.
- Exhale forcefully and quickly.
- Note the reading.
- Repeat these steps two more times—write the highest number in the asthma record.
- Explain that best individual peak flows are determined after 2 to 3 weeks of asthma therapy.
- Instruct the client about the zones of peak flow: green—80% to 100% best individual peak flow; yellow—60% to 80%; and red—less than 60%.
- Provide actions for the client to take for each zone.

The client can use the peak flow meter to assess the effectiveness of medication or breathing status. The nurse tells the client to seek care if readings fall below baseline and teaches correct use of inhalers. He or she also helps clients identify triggering events such as dust, smoking, emotional upset, or exposure to irritants such as cleaning fluids or insecticides. The nurse teaches the client relaxation techniques and therapeutic breathing techniques, as discussed previously in the section on nursing management of emphysema.

Stop, Think, and Respond ● BOX 29-3

Your client has asthma caused by extrinsic factors, particularly dust. How can this client reduce asthma attacks?

● SLEEP APNEA SYNDROME

Sleep apnea syndrome is characterized by frequent, brief episodes of respiratory standstill during sleep. It is classified according to respiratory muscle effort:

- Central—air movement is absent secondary to absence of ventilatory efforts.
- Obstructive—air movement is absent secondary to pharyngeal obstruction; chest and abdominal movements are present; this is the most common form of sleep apnea.
- Mixed—combination of central and obstructive sleep apnea in one apneic episode

Pathophysiology and Etiology

Sleep apnea occurs most commonly in older obese men. Cigarette smokers are at increased risk, as are clients with any condition that reduces pharyngeal muscle tone: neuromuscular disease, use of sedative or hypnotic medications, and frequent and heavy intake of alcohol.

Obstructive sleep apnea results from a reduced diameter of the upper airway, which may develop when the upper airway collapses secondary to the normally reduced muscle tone during sleep. The repeated apneic spells have serious effects on the cardiopulmonary system. Clients with sleep apnea often have hypertension and are at greater risk, therefore, of cerebrovascular accident and myocardial infarction (MI) (Smeltzer & Bare, 2000).

Assessment Findings

Clients with obstructive sleep apnea snore loudly during sleep, with cessation of breathing for at least 10 seconds. They awaken suddenly as the partial pressure of oxygen (PaO_2) level drops, usually with a loud snort. These episodes are frequent, from five in 1 hour to several hundred per night (Smeltzer & Bare, 2000). Other symptoms include daytime fatigue, morning headache, sore throat, enuresis, and erectile dysfunction. Partners may report that the client behaves differently and is not the same in terms of affect and personality and that the snoring is progressively worse.

Initial diagnosis is made according to the client's reported symptoms. To determine the nature of the sleep apnea, clients undergo **polysomnography,** which consists of tests that monitor the client's respiratory and cardiac status while he or she is asleep.

Medical and Surgical Management

If the cause is obstructive, surgical procedures are done to relieve the obstruction. The most common surgery is *uvulopalatopharyngoplasty,* a surgical procedure to reconstruct the uvula, palate, and pharynx to relieve obstruction.

If surgery is not an option, clients are advised to lose weight and avoid alcohol and drugs that depress respirations. Additional treatment includes continuous positive airway pressure (CPAP) with supplemental oxygen at night through a nasal cannula or face mask. Clients often have difficulty remaining compliant with CPAP because they must use equipment and oxygen every night, and because CPAP relieves but does not eliminate the problem.

Tracheostomy is a successful treatment. Clients may reject this option, however, because of the trauma, the seemingly barbaric nature of the procedure, and the alteration it creates in appearance. Tracheostomy also may be technically difficult if the client is markedly obese. If a client chooses to have a tracheostomy, he or she may plug it during the day.

Medication sometimes is prescribed for central sleep apnea, and clients take such drugs at bedtime. The goal is to increase the respiratory drive and improve upper airway muscle tone. An example of a medication for this purpose is protriptyline (Vivactil). Clients also may use low-flow oxygen at night to relieve hypoxemia.

Nursing Management

Clients with sleep apnea usually are anxious and require reassurance and adequate instruction about their condition. The nurse provides thorough explanations of the disease process, polysomnography, and treatments. He or she refers clients to self-help groups or appropriate counseling for weight loss or alcohol and substance abuse issues. The nurse collaborates with respiratory therapists to instruct the client in the use of CPAP. He or she furnishes the client with information about sleep apnea and its potential complications if not treated.

● CYSTIC FIBROSIS

Cystic fibrosis (CF) is a multisystem disorder that affects infants, children, and young adults. In the past, children with CF did not survive much beyond adolescence. Although CF remains a serious childhood disease, new treatments and therapies are enabling clients with CF to live longer and are improving their lives in terms of quality and productivity.

Pathophysiology and Etiology

CF results from a defective autosomal recessive gene. A person with CF inherits a defective copy of the CF gene from both parents. When two carriers give birth to a child, the child has a 25% chance of having CF, a 50% chance of being a carrier, and a 25% chance of not being a carrier. The genetic mutation causes dysfunction of the exocrine glands, involving the mucus-secreting and eccrine sweat glands. Resulting major abnormalities include the following:

- Faulty transport of sodium and chloride in cells lining organs, such as the lungs and pancreas, to their outer surfaces
- Production of abnormally thick, sticky mucus in many organs, especially the lungs and pancreas
- Altered electrolyte balance in the sweat glands

The genetic defect causes inadequate synthesis of a protein (CF gene product) referred to as the *CF transmembrane conductance regulator* (CFTR). CFTR molecules are located in the cells lining the ducts of the exocrine glands, particularly the lungs, pancreas, intestine, and sweat ducts. Clients with CF cannot synthesize adequate CFTR to regulate the combination of water and electrolytes with exocrine secretions and mucus. Subsequently, thick, viscous secretions and protein plugs eventually block the ducts of the exocrine glands. Eventually, ducts may become fibrotic and convert into cysts (Bullock & Heinze, 2000).

Assessment Findings

Signs and Symptoms

Clients usually exhibit signs and symptoms in infancy or early childhood. Some individuals, however, do not have signs of the disease until late childhood or adolescence. Clinical manifestations differ related to the degree of organ involvement and the progression of the disease. The three major reasons to suspect CF in children are respiratory symptoms, failure to thrive, and foul-smelling, bulky, greasy stools. In newborns, the first clinical sign may be a meconium ileus (impacted meconium in the intestines). Another sign may be salty-tasting skin.

Respiratory symptoms become very common and include frequent respiratory infections, ranging from URIs with increased cough and purulent sputum to the production of thick, tenacious mucus. Finger clubbing is common. Hemoptysis also may occur as blood vessels are damaged in the lungs, secondary to frequent coughing and constant efforts to clear mucus.

Children also experience malabsorption of fats and fat-soluble vitamins, secondary to impaired pancreatic function. They have difficulty gaining weight. Risk for bowel obstruction, cholecystitis, and cirrhosis is increased.

Diagnostic Findings

The standard and most reliable diagnostic test for CF is the pilocarpine iontophoresis sweat test. Up to 20 years of age, levels higher than 60 mEq/L are diagnostic, and those between 50 and 60 mEq/L are highly suggestive for CF.

Chest radiography demonstrates widespread consolidation, fibrotic changes, and overaerated lungs. Some clients also have areas of collapse. Pulmonary function tests assist in determining current function as well as progression of the disease.

Radiographic studies of the GI system show fibrous abnormalities. In 80% of those with CF, tests for pancreatic enzymes in duodenal contents fail to show evidence of trypsin (Bullock & Henze, 2000). Feces show steatorrhea (fat in stools).

Medical and Surgical Management

Treatment depends on the stage of the disease and the extent of organ involvement; it aims at relieving the symptoms. Respiratory treatment includes promoting the removal of the thick sputum through postural drainage, chest physical therapy with vigorous percussion and vibration, breathing exercises, hydration to help thin secretions, bronchodilator medications, nebulized mist treatments with saline or mucolytic medications, and prompt treatment of lung infections with antibiotics.

When the digestive system is involved, clients take pancreatic enzyme replacements (Pancrease) with meals to aid with digestion and absorption of fats. Clients also take fat-soluble vitamin supplements and follow a high-calorie diet.

Clients with end-stage lung disease sometimes receive a lung transplant. In some cases, clients may receive a liver transplant as well. If successful, the transplants greatly extend the client's life.

Other new treatments are in various stages of implementation and investigation. These include mucus-thinning drugs that reduce lung infections, NSAIDs, inhaled antibiotics, drugs to stimulate cells to secrete chloride and thin mucus, and gene therapy. The potential for clients with CF to live longer increases every year. Current research is focused on treating not only the symptoms but the causes of CF (Cystic Fibrosis Foundation, 2001).

Nursing Management

Nursing care of clients with CF focuses on preventing complications and promoting as normal a lifestyle as possible. The nurse teaches clients to prevent respiratory infections by giving instructions similar to those to prevent pneumonia (see Nursing Guidelines 29-1). Strict adherence to a vigorous pulmonary toilet is essential for the client with CF who has significant respiratory involvement. Components include chest physical therapy (including postural drainage, percussion, and vibration) two to four times daily, deep breathing and coughing exercises, nebulized treatments, and medications.

Clients also need to recognize early signs and symptoms of infection, which include low-grade temperature, increased mucus production, increased cough, and change in color of secretions (white to yellow to greenish). Clients must begin antibiotics as soon as infection occurs to prevent the infection from getting worse. Preventing or minimizing infection prevents or slows lung damage. Some clients are on prophylactic antibiotic therapy to decrease the occurrence of infections. This form of treatment is not common because of the threat of developing antibiotic-resistant infections, which can be deadly for clients with CF. Clients may be taught to administer IV antibiotics at home.

For the client with CF who has significant GI involvement, the nurse must review the client's diet. Collaboration with dietitians can ensure that the client has a diet high in calories, with appropriate amounts of carbohydrates, fats, and proteins. It is essential for the client to take his or her pancreatic enzymes (Cotazym, Creon, or Pancrease), which aid in the digestion of carbohydrates, fats, and proteins. The nurse reminds the client to take the pancreatic enzymes before or during meals.

Young adults with CF usually are very knowledgeable about their condition. Nurses must respect their knowledge and allow them to determine their schedule for treatments and procedures. The nurse provides support for clients' efforts in self-care. He or she refers the client as requested to other healthcare professionals, such as dietitians and respiratory and physical therapists, as needed.

OCCUPATIONAL LUNG DISEASES

Exposure to organic and inorganic dusts and noxious gases over a long period can cause chronic lung disorders. **Pneumoconiosis** refers to a fibrous inflammation or chronic induration of the lungs after prolonged exposure to dust or gases. It specifically refers to diseases caused by the inhalation of silica (**silicosis**), coal dust (black lung disease, miners' disease), or asbestos (**asbestosis**). Although these conditions are not malignant, they may increase the client's risk for development of malignancies. Table 29-2 describes these specific conditions in more detail.

The primary focus is prevention, with frequent examination of those who work in areas of highly concentrated dust or gases. Laws require work areas to be safe in terms of dust control, ventilation, protective masks, hoods, industrial respirators, and other protection. Workers are encouraged to practice healthy behaviors, such as quitting smoking.

Dyspnea and cough are the most common symptoms of occupational lung diseases. Those exposed to coal dust may expectorate black-streaked sputum. The diagnosis is based on the history of exposure to dust or gases in the workplace. A chest radiograph may reveal fibrotic changes in the lungs. The results of pulmonary function studies usually are abnormal.

Treatment typically is conservative because the disease is widespread rather than localized. Surgery seldom is of value. Infections, when they occur, are treated with antibiotics. Other treatment modalities include oxygen therapy if severe dyspnea is present, improved nutrition, and adequate rest. Many people with advanced disease are permanently disabled.

TABLE 29-2	OCCUPATIONAL LUNG DISEASES	
OCCUPATIONAL LUNG DISEASE	**PATHOPHYSIOLOGY AND ETIOLOGY**	**SIGNS AND SYMPTOMS**
Coal worker's pneumoconiosis	Referred to as black lung disease, this condition is caused by inhalation of coal dust and other dusts. Initially, lungs clear particles by phagocytosis and transport out of the lungs. When dust inhalation becomes too great, macrophages collect in the bronchioles, leading to clogging of the airways with dusts, macrophages, and fibroblasts. This results in local emphysema and eventually massive blackened lung lesions. Coal macules eventually form, seen as black dots on radiography.	Chronic cough–sputum production Dyspnea Large amounts of sputum containing black fluid (melanoptysis) Respiratory failure
Silicosis	This illness results from inhalation of silica dust and is seen in workers involved with mining, quarrying, stone-cutting, and tunnel building. Silica particles inhaled into the lungs cause nodular lesions that enlarge and form dense masses over time. The results are loss of lung volume and restrictive and obstructive lung disease.	Shortness of breath Hypoxemia Obstruction of airflow Right-sided heart failure Edema
Asbestosis	This illness results from inhalation of asbestos dust. Laws restrict asbestos use, but old materials still contain asbestos. Asbestos fibers enter the alveoli and cause fibrous tissue to form around them. Pleura also have fibrous changes and plaque formation. Results are restrictive lung disease, decreased lung volume, and decreased gas exchange.	Dyspnea Chest pain Hypoxemia Anorexia and weight loss Respiratory failure

Nursing management of clients with occupational lung diseases is basically the same as for clients with emphysema. Many clients require a great deal of emotional support because these diseases may result in permanent disability at a relatively young age.

PULMONARY CIRCULATORY DISORDERS

● PULMONARY HYPERTENSION

Pulmonary hypertension results from heart disease, lung disease, or both. It does not become clinically apparent until the client is quite ill. Diagnosis is difficult without invasive testing. Clients with pulmonary hypertension experience difficulty breathing and usually present as quite ill.

Pathophysiology and Etiology

Resistance to blood flow in the pulmonary circulation causes pulmonary hypertension. The pressure in the pulmonary arteries increases, which in turn increases the workload of the right ventricle. Normal pulmonary arterial pressure is approximately 25/10 mm Hg. In pulmonary hypertension, the pressure rises above 40/15 mm Hg and can be higher as the disease progresses.

Primary pulmonary hypertension, which exists without evidence of other disease, is a rare condition. Although the cause is not apparent, there appears to be a familial tendency. "It occurs most often in women 20 to 40 years of age and is usually fatal within 5 years of diagnosis" (Smeltzer & Bare, 2000, p. 469). Secondary pulmonary hypertension accompanies other heart and lung conditions, most commonly COPD.

Complex mechanisms cause pulmonary hypertension. In primary pulmonary hypertension, the inner lining of the pulmonary arteries thickens and hypertrophies, followed by increased pressure in the pulmonary arteries and vascular bed (Fig. 29-8). In secondary pulmonary hypertension, alveolar destruction causes increased resistance and pressure in the pulmonary vascular bed. In both types of pulmonary hypertension, the increased resistance and pressure in the pulmonary vascular bed results in pulmonary artery hypertension. Consequently, strain is placed on the right ventricle, resulting in enlargement and possible failure.

Assessment Findings

The most common symptoms of primary and secondary hypertension are dyspnea on exertion and weakness. In clients with secondary pulmonary hypertension, addi-

A. Normal
Pulmonary arteriole is
normally thin and
distensible.

**B. Pulmonary
hypertension (early)**
Mild pulmonary
hypertension is
characterized by
thickening of the
medial (muscular) layer.

**C. Pulmonary
hypertension (late)**
Severe pulmonary
hypertension exhibits
extensive intimal fibrosis
and medial thickening.

FIGURE 29-8 Progression of pulmonary hypertension.

tional symptoms are those of the underlying cardiac or respiratory disease: chest pain, fatigue, weakness, distended neck veins, **orthopnea** (difficulty breathing while lying flat), and peripheral edema.

An electrocardiogram (ECG) may show right ventricular hypertrophy or failure. Results of ABG analysis are abnormal. Cardiac catheterization demonstrates elevated pulmonary arterial pressures. The results of pulmonary function studies show an increased residual volume but a decreased forced expiratory volume. Echocardiography may show various abnormalities, such as left ventricular dysfunction and tricuspid valve insufficiency.

Medical Management

Treatment of primary pulmonary hypertension includes the administration of vasodilators and anticoagulants. Primary pulmonary hypertension has a poor prognosis; therefore, some affected clients are considered candidates for heart–lung transplantation. Treatment of secondary pulmonary hypertension includes management of the underlying cardiac or respiratory disease. Oxygen therapy

commonly is used to increase pulmonary arterial oxygenation. If right-sided failure is present, other treatments include medications such as digitalis to improve cardiac function, rest, and diuretics.

Nursing Management

Nursing management focuses on recognizing signs and symptoms of respiratory distress. The nurse can reduce the body's need for oxygen by preventing fatigue, assisting with ADLs, and administering oxygen, when needed.

● PULMONARY EMBOLISM

Pulmonary embolism involves the obstruction of one of the pulmonary arteries or its branches. The blockage is the result of a thrombus that forms in the venous system or right side of the heart.

Pathophysiology and Etiology

An embolus is any foreign substance, such as a blood clot, air, or particle of fat, that travels in the venous blood flow to the lungs. The clot moves to and occludes one of the pulmonary arteries, causing infarction (necrosis or death) of lung tissue distal to the clot. Scar tissue later replaces the infarcted area.

Clots usually form in the deep veins of the lower extremities or pelvis and become the source for pulmonary emboli. Emboli also may arise from the endocardium of the right ventricle when that side of the heart is the site of an MI or endocarditis. A fat embolus usually occurs after a fracture of a long bone, especially the femur. Other conditions that cause pulmonary emboli include recent surgery, prolonged bed rest, trauma, the postpartum state, and debilitating diseases. Three conditions, referred to as *Virchow's triad,* predispose a person to clot formation: venostasis, disruption of the vessel lining, and hypercoagulability (Bullock & Henze, 2000).

Assessment Findings

When a small area of the lung is involved, signs and symptoms usually are less severe and include pain, tachycardia, and dyspnea. The client also may have fever, cough, and blood-streaked sputum. Larger areas of involvement produce more pronounced signs and symptoms, such as severe dyspnea, severe pain, cyanosis, tachycardia, restlessness, and shock. Sudden death may follow a massive pulmonary infarction when a large embolism occludes a main section of the pulmonary artery.

Serum enzymes typically are markedly elevated. A chest radiograph may show an area of atelectasis. An ECG rules out a cardiac disorder such as MI, which produces some of the same symptoms. In addition, a lung scan, CT scan, or pulmonary angiography may be performed to detect the involved lung tissue.

Medical and Surgical Management

Treatment of a pulmonary embolism depends on the size of the area involved and the client's symptoms. IV heparin may be administered to prevent extension of the thrombus and the development of additional thrombi in veins from which the embolus arose. IV injection of a thrombolytic drug (one that dissolves a thrombus) such as urokinase, streptokinase, or tissue plasminogen activator also may be used (see Chap. 33). Anticoagulants commonly are given after thrombolytic therapy. Other measures used to treat symptoms of pulmonary emboli include complete bed rest, oxygen, and analgesics.

Pulmonary embolectomy, using cardiopulmonary bypass to support circulation while the embolus is removed, may be necessary if the embolus is lodged in a main pulmonary artery. The insertion of an umbrella filter device (Greenfield filter) in the vena cava prevents recurrent episodes of pulmonary embolus. The umbrella filter is inserted by an applicator catheter inserted into the right internal jugular vein and threaded downward to an area below the renal arteries. Another surgical treatment is the placement of Teflon clips on the inferior vena cava. These clips create narrow channels in the vena cava, allowing blood to pass through on its return to the right side of the heart but keeping back large clots.

Nursing Management

The best management of pulmonary emboli is preventing them (Box 29-2). When assessing the client's potential for pulmonary emboli, the nurse tests for a positive Homan's sign (see Chap. 31). The client lies on his or her back, lifts his or her leg, and dorsiflexes his or her foot. If the client reports calf pain (positive Homan's sign) during this maneuver, he or she may have a deep vein thrombosis.

Pulmonary embolism almost always occurs suddenly, and death can follow within 1 hour. Obviously, early recognition of this problem is essential. The nurse starts an IV infusion as soon as possible to establish a patent vein before shock becomes profound. He or she administers vasopressors such as dopamine or dobutamine as ordered to treat hypotension. The nurse provides oxygen for dyspnea and analgesics for pain and apprehension. Close monitoring of vital signs is necessary, as is observing the client at frequent intervals for changes. The nurse institutes continuous ECG monitoring because right ventricular failure is a common problem.

Areas for the nurse to monitor include fluid intake and output, electrolyte determinations, and ABGs. The nurse assesses the client for cyanosis, cough with or without hemoptysis, diaphoresis, and respiratory difficulty. He or she monitors blood coagulation studies (i.e., partial thromboplastin time, prothrombin time) when anticoagulant or thrombolytic therapy is instituted.

The nurse assesses the client for evidence of bleeding and relief of associated symptoms. Because clients with pulmonary emboli are discharged on oral anticoagulants, they require instruction related to checking for signs of occult bleeding, taking medication exactly as prescribed, reporting missed or extra doses, and keeping all appointments for follow-up blood tests and office visits.

Stop, Think, and Respond ● BOX 29-4

A 54-year-old woman recently experienced thrombophlebitis in her left calf, probably related to prolonged bed rest after a motor vehicle collision. The thrombophlebitis resolved without complications. She is no longer taking anticoagulants. She expresses concerns about having clots in the future. What should she do?

● PULMONARY EDEMA

Pulmonary edema is accumulation of fluid in the interstitium and alveoli of the lungs. Pulmonary congestion results when the right side of the heart delivers more blood to the pulmonary circulation than the left side of the heart can handle. The fluid escapes the capillary walls and fills the airways. A client with pulmonary edema experiences dyspnea, breathlessness, and a feeling of suffocation. In addition, he or she exhibits cool, moist, and cyanotic extremities. The overall skin color is cyanotic and gray. The client has a continual cough productive of blood-tinged, frothy fluid. This condition requires emergency treatment. (See Chap. 36 for a discussion of cardiogenic pulmonary edema.)

BOX 29-2 ● **Preventing the Formation of Pulmonary Emboli**

Help client practice active and passive leg exercises.
Instruct client to pump muscles (tense and relax) to improve circulation in lower extremities.
Assist client to ambulate as early as possible after a procedure.
Teach client to:
- Wear support hose/elastic hose as directed
- Avoid constrictive clothing
- Avoid sitting for long periods or with legs crossed
- Drink fluids liberally unless contraindicated
- When traveling, move lower legs and feet while sitting, change positions as able, do not cross legs, and ambulate if able

RESPIRATORY FAILURE

Respiratory failure describes the inability to exchange sufficient amounts of oxygen and CO_2 for the body's needs. Even when the body is at rest, basic respiratory needs cannot be met. The ABG values that define respiratory failure include a PaO_2 less than 50 mm Hg, a $PaCO_2$ greater than 50 mm Hg, and a pH less than 7.25.

Respiratory failure is classified as acute or chronic. Acute respiratory failure occurs suddenly in a client who previously had normal lung function. In chronic respiratory failure, the loss of lung function is progressive, usually irreversible, and associated with chronic lung disease or other disease.

Pathophysiology and Etiology

Table 29-3 describes precipitating factors that can result in respiratory failure. Acute respiratory failure is a life-threatening condition in which alveolar ventilation cannot maintain the body's need for oxygen supply and CO_2

TABLE 29-3	FACTORS THAT PRECIPITATE RESPIRATORY FAILURE
PRECIPITATING FACTOR	**EXAMPLE**
Pulmonary infection— especially with COPD	Bacterial, viral, or fungal pneumonia
Trauma	Motor vehicle collision Gunshot/knife wound Burns
Infection	Sepsis Wound infection
Cardiovascular event	Myocardial infarction Aortic aneurysm Pulmonary embolism
Allergic reaction	Transfusion reaction Drug allergy Bee sting or other venom
Pulmonary aspiration	Vomitus Near drowning
Surgical procedure	Abdominal or thoracic surgery
Drug reaction	Overdose of barbiturates or narcotics Reaction to anesthesia
Mechanical factor	Pneumothorax Pleural effusion Abdominal distention
Iatrogenic factor	Endotracheal intubation Failure to clear tracheo- bronchial secretions
Neuromuscular disorders	Guillain-Barré syndrome Multiple sclerosis Muscular dystrophy

removal. The result is a fall in arterial oxygen (hypoxemia) and a rise in arterial CO_2 (hypercapnia), detected by ABG analysis. Ventilatory failure develops when the alveoli cannot adequately expand, when neurologic control of respirations is impaired, or when traumatic injury to the chest wall occurs.

The most common diseases leading to chronic respiratory failure are COPD and neuromuscular disorders. The underlying disease accounts for the pathology that is seen when the respiratory system fails. Gas exchange dysfunction occurs over a long period. Symptoms of acute respiratory failure are not apparent in chronic respiratory failure because the client experiences chronic respiratory acidosis over a long period. Refer to the section on COPD for discussion of diagnostic findings, medical management, and nursing management of chronic respiratory failure.

Assessment Findings

Apprehension, restlessness, fatigue, headache, dyspnea, wheezing, cyanosis, and use of the accessory muscles of respiration are seen in clients with impending respiratory failure. If the disorder remains untreated, or if treatment fails to relieve respiratory distress, confusion, tachypnea, cyanosis, cardiac dysrhythmias and tachycardia, hypotension, CHF, respiratory acidosis, and respiratory arrest occur.

The client's symptoms, history (e.g., surgery, known neurologic disorder), and ABG results form the basis for a diagnosis of respiratory failure. Additional tests include chest radiography and serum electrolyte determinations.

Medical Management

Treatment of respiratory failure focuses on maintaining a patent airway (in cases of upper respiratory airway obstruction) by inserting an artificial airway, such as an endotracheal or a tracheostomy tube. Additional treatments include administration of humidified oxygen by nasal cannula, Venturi mask, or rebreather masks (Fig. 29-9). Respiratory failure is managed with mechanical ventilation using intermittent positive-pressure ventilation. When possible, the underlying cause of respiratory failure is treated.

Nursing Management

Because symptoms often occur suddenly, recognition is important. The nurse must notify the physician immediately and obtain emergency resuscitative equipment. Assessment and monitoring of respirations and vital signs are necessary at frequent intervals. The nurse must pay

Venturi mask

Nonrebreather mask

Partial rebreather mask

FIGURE 29-9 Types of oxygen masks. (From Smeltzer, S. C. & Bare, B. G. [2000]. *Brunner & Suddarth's textbook of medical–surgical nursing* [9th ed.]. Philadelphia: Lippincott Williams & Wilkins.)

particular attention to respiratory rate and depth, signs of cyanosis, other signs and symptoms of respiratory distress, and the client's response to treatment. He or she monitors ABG results and pulse oximetry findings and implements strategies to prevent respiratory complications, such as turning and ROM exercises. The nurse provides explanations to the client and initiates measures to relieve anxiety.

● ACUTE RESPIRATORY DISTRESS SYNDROME

Acute respiratory distress syndrome (ARDS), previously referred to as *adult respiratory distress syndrome,* is a clinical condition that occurs following other clinical conditions. It is not a primary disease. When it occurs, ARDS can lead to respiratory failure and death. It is referred to as *noncardiogenic pulmonary edema* (pulmonary edema not caused by a cardiac disorder—occurs without left-sided heart failure). Sudden and progressive pulmonary edema, increasing bilateral infiltrates seen on chest radiography, severe hypoxemia, and progressive loss of lung compliance characterize ARDS (Smeltzer & Bare, 2000).

Pathophysiology and Etiology

Factors associated with the development of ARDS include aspiration related to near drowning or vomiting; drug ingestion/overdose; hematologic disorders such as disseminated intravascular coagulation or massive transfusions; direct damage to the lungs through prolonged smoke inhalation or other corrosive substances; localized lung infection; metabolic disorders such as pancreatitis or uremia; shock; trauma such as chest contusions, multiple fractures, or head injury; any major surgery; embolism; and septicemia (Smeltzer & Bare, 2000). The mortality rate with ARDS is high, particularly if the underlying cause cannot be treated or is inadequately treated.

The body responds to injury by reducing blood flow to the lungs, resulting in platelet clumping. The platelets release substances such as histamine, bradykinin, and serotonin, causing localized inflammation of the alveolar membranes. Increased permeability of the alveolar capillary membrane subsequently ensues. Fluid then enters the alveoli and causes pulmonary edema. The excess fluid in the alveoli and decreased blood flow through the capillaries surrounding them cause many of the alveoli to collapse (microatelectasis). Gas exchange decreases, resulting in respiratory and metabolic acidosis. ARDS also causes decreased surfactant production, which contributes to alveolar collapse. The lungs become stiff or noncompliant. Decreased functional residual capacity, severe hypoxia, and hypocapnia result.

Assessment Findings

Severe respiratory distress develops within 8 to 48 hours after the onset of illness or injury. In the early stages, few definite symptoms may be seen. As the condition progresses, the following signs appear: increased respiratory rate; shallow, labored respirations; cyanosis; use of accessory muscles; respiratory distress unrelieved with oxygen administration; anxiety; restlessness; and mental confusion, agitation, and drowsiness with cerebral anoxia.

Diagnosis is made according to the following criteria: evidence of acute respiratory failure, bilateral infiltrates on chest radiography, and hypoxemia as evidenced by PaO_2 less than 50 mm Hg with supplemental oxygen of 50% to 60%. Chest radiographs reveal increased infiltrates bilaterally. There is no evidence of left-sided heart failure (see Chap. 36), such as increased size of the left ventricle.

Medical Management

The initial cause of ARDS must be diagnosed and treated. The client receives humidified oxygen. Insertion of an endotracheal or a tracheostomy tube ensures maintenance of a patent airway. Mechanical ventilation usually is necessary, using positive end-expiratory pressure (PEEP), which provides pressures to the airway that are higher than atmospheric pressures. Mechanical ventilators usually raise airway pressure during inspiration and let it fall to atmospheric or zero pressure during expiration (intermittent positive-pressure ventilation). When PEEP is used, positive airway pressure is maintained on inspiration, expiration, and at the end of expiration (continuous positive-pressure ventilation). The client's pulmonary status, determined by ABG findings and pulse oximetry results, dictates the oxygen concentration and ventilator settings. Complications associated with the use of PEEP include pneumothorax and pneumomediastinum (air in the mediastinal space).

Hypotension results in systemic hypovolemia. Although the client experiences pulmonary edema, the rest of the circulatory volume is decreased. Pulmonary artery pressure monitors the client's fluid status and assists in determining the careful administration of IV fluids. Colloids such as albumin are used to help pull fluids in from the interstitium to the capillaries. Adequate nutritional support is essential. Usually, the first choice is enteral feedings, but total parenteral nutrition may be necessary.

Nursing Management

Nursing management focuses on promotion of oxygenation and ventilation and prevention of complications. Assessing and monitoring a client's respiratory status are essential. Potential complications include deteriorating respiratory status, infection, renal failure, and cardiac complications. The client also is anxious and requires explanations and support. In addition, if the client is on a ventilator, verbal communication is impaired. The nurse provides alternative methods for the client to communicate.

MALIGNANT DISORDERS

Tumors and growths affecting the respiratory system usually are malignant. Malignancies may be primary in that they arise from the lungs or mediastinum, or they can be secondary metastatic growths from other sites. Treatment of these cancers usually does not stop progression of the disease (see Chap. 20). Disability, debilitation, and death are common outcomes from respiratory malignancies.

● LUNG CANCER

Lung cancer is a very common cancer, particularly among cigarette smokers and those regularly exposed to second-hand smoke. It remains the number-one cause of cancer-related deaths among men and women in the United States (American Cancer Society, 2001), with more Americans dying each year from lung cancer than from breast, prostate, and colorectal cancers combined. The incidence of lung cancer has markedly increased since the early 1980s, related to:

- More accurate methods of diagnosis
- The growing population of aging people
- The continued popularity of cigarette smoking
- Increased air pollution
- Increased exposure to industrial pollutants

Lung cancer is more common in men than in women. The rate of women dying from it continues to increase, however, and indeed is greater than the rate of women dying from breast cancer. Most clients are older than 40 years of age when diagnosed with lung cancer.

Pathophysiology and Etiology

The exact mechanism for the development of lung cancer is unknown; however, the link between irritants and lung cancer is well established. Prolonged exposure to carcinogens more than likely will produce cancerous cells. Smokers who quit reduce their risk of lung cancer to that of nonsmokers within 10 to 15 years.

There are four major cell types of lung cancer: the large cell or undifferentiated type, the small cell or oat cell type, the epidermoid or squamous cell type, and adenocarcinoma. Many tumors begin in the bronchus and spread to the lung tissue, regional lymph nodes, and other sites, such as the brain and bone. Many tumors have more than one type of cancer cell. Table 29-4 differentiates the major cell types of lung cancer.

The transformation of an epithelial cell in the airway initiates the growth of a lung cancer lesion. As the tumor grows, it partially obstructs the lumen of an airway or completely obstructs it, resulting in airway collapse distal to the tumor. The tumor may hemorrhage, causing hemoptysis (Bullock & Henze, 2000).

TABLE 29-4	DIFFERENTIATION OF LUNG CANCERS	
CELL TYPE	**PATHOLOGY**	**METASTASIS**
Non-small Cell Carcinomas		
Epidermoid or squamous cell carcinomas (located in the bronchial tubes; 25% to 35% of all lung tumors)	These slow-growing tumors arise from bronchi and bronchioles and spread into the bronchial lumen, causing obstruction.	Well-differentiated epidermoid cells typically metastasize in the thorax, whereas poorly differentiated epidermoid cells metastasize to the small bowel.
Large cell (undifferentiated) carcinomas (found near the bronchial surface; 5% to 20% of all lung tumors)	These arise in peripheral bronchi and do not have well-defined growth patterns. They usually are diagnosed first as a bulky tumor mass.	These metastasize early, usually to the CNS.
Adenocarcinoma (arise from mucous glands; 25% to 35% of all lung tumors)	These occur in the peripheral lung tissue and lead to patchy growth throughout the lung fields. They typically invade the pleura, leading to malignant pleural effusion.	Early metastasis occurs to the brain, other lung tissue, bone, liver, and adrenal glands.
Small Cell Carcinoma		
Oat cell (10% to 25% of lung tumors)	This most malignant form of lung cancer arises from the bronchi. The tumor cells hypersecrete antidiuretic hormone, leading to hyponatremia.	Metastasis is early through the bloodstream and lymphatics to the mediastinum, liver, bone, bone marrow, CNS, adrenal glands, pancreas, and other endocrine organs.

CNS, central nervous system.

Assessment Findings

Signs and Symptoms

The cell type of the lung cancer, size and location of the tumor, and degree and location of metastasis determine the presenting signs and symptoms. A cough productive of mucopurulent or blood-streaked sputum is a cardinal sign of lung cancer. The cough may be slight at first and attributed to smoking or other causes. As the disease advances, the client may report fatigue, anorexia, and weight loss. Dyspnea and chest pain occur late in the disease. Hemoptysis is common.

If pleural effusion occurs from tumor spread to the outside portion of the lungs, the client experiences dyspnea and chest pain. Other indications of tumor spread are symptoms related to pressure on nerves and blood vessels. Symptoms include head and neck edema, pericardial effusion, hoarseness, and vocal cord paralysis.

Diagnostic Findings

Early diagnosis of cancer of the lung is difficult because symptoms often do not appear until the disease is well established. Because diagnosis often is late, the long-term survival rate for victims of lung cancer is low. The sputum is examined for malignant cells. Chest films may or may not show a tumor. A CT scan or MRI is done if results from the chest radiograph are inconclusive, or to further delineate the tumor area.

Bronchoscopy may be done to obtain bronchial washings and a tissue sample for biopsy. Fine-needle aspiration under fluoroscopy or CT guidance may be done to aspirate cells from a specific area that is not accessible by bronchoscopy. A lung scan also may locate the tumor. A bone scan detects metastasis to the bone. The results of a lymph node biopsy may be positive for malignant changes if the lung tumor has metastasized. Mediastinoscopy provides a direct view of the mediastinal area and possible visualization of tumors that extend into the mediastinal space.

Medical and Surgical Management

The client's prognosis is poor unless the tumor is discovered in its early stages and treatment begins immediately. Because lung cancer produces few early symptoms, its mortality rate is high. Metastasis to the mediastinal and cervical lymph nodes, liver, brain, spinal cord, bone, and opposite lung is common.

Treatment depends on several factors. One major consideration is the classification and staging of the tumor. After classification of the tumor, the stage of the disease is determined. Staging refers to the extent and location of the tumor and the absence or presence and extent of metastasis. Other factors that determine treatment are the client's age and physical condition and other diseases or disorders, such as renal disease and CHF.

Surgical removal of the tumor offers the only possibility of cure and usually is successful only in the early stages of the disease. The type of lung resection (Box 29-3) depends on the tumor's size and location.

BOX 29-3 ● Types of Lung Resections

Lobectomy—single lobe of lung removed
Bilobectomy—two lobes of lung removed
Sleeve resection—cancerous lobe(s) removed and a segment of the main bronchus resected
Pneumonectomy—removal of entire lung
Segmentectomy—segment of lung removed
Wedge resection—removal of small, pie-shaped area of the segment
Chest wall resection with removal of cancerous lung tissue—for cancers that have invaded the chest wall

(Adapted from Smeltzer, S. C. & Bare, B. G. [2000]. *Brunner and Suddarth's textbook of medical–surgical nursing* [9th ed.]. Philadelphia: Lippincott Williams & Wilkins.)

Radiation therapy may help to slow the spread of the disease and provide symptomatic relief by reducing tumor size, thus easing the pressure exerted by the tumor on adjacent structures. In turn, pain, cough, dyspnea, and hemoptysis may be relieved. In a small percentage of cases, radiation may be curative, but for most, it is palliative. Complications associated with the use of radiation therapy include esophagitis, fibrosis of lung tissue, and pneumonitis.

Chemotherapy may be used alone or with radiation therapy and surgery. The principal effects of chemotherapy are to slow tumor growth and reduce tumor size and accompanying pressure on adjacent structures. Chemotherapy also is used to treat metastatic lesions. Most chemotherapeutic regimens use a combination of drugs rather than a single agent and, although not curative, often make the client more comfortable.

New treatments in various stages of development include the following:

- New chemotherapy regimens
- Monoclonal antibodies that target specific cancer proteins
- Photodynamic therapy that is a combination treatment with chemicals and light
- Lung cancer vaccines to stimulate effective immune response (Lung Cancer, 2001)

Nursing Management

Management of clients with lung cancer is essentially the same as that for any client with a malignant disease. See Chapter 20 for the nursing management of a client with cancer and Chapter 25 for perioperative care.

● MEDIASTINAL TUMORS

Tumors of the mediastinum in adults often are malignant and metastatic. They are designated as anterior, middle, or posterior, according to their location on the mediastinum. The cause of these tumors is not known. Mediastinal tumors may be asymptomatic initially. When symptoms occur, they include chest pain, chest wall bulging, difficulty swallowing, dyspnea, and orthopnea. Symptoms are related to pressure of the tumor on other chest structures. Chest radiography, CT scan, MRI, mediastinoscopy, and biopsy of the lesion identify the tumor. Malignant tumors of the mediastinum almost always are inoperable but may respond to radiation therapy and chemotherapy. Benign tumors are operable.

Stop, Think, and Respond ● BOX 29-5

Your 65-year-old neighbor tells you that he smoked for 25 years but quit 5 years ago. He has experienced a productive cough for 3 weeks. Occasionally he sees blood in the sputum. What can you advise him?

TRAUMA

All chest injuries are serious or potentially serious. A client with a chest injury must be observed for dyspnea, cyanosis, chest pain, weak and rapid pulse, and hypotension—all signs and symptoms of respiratory distress. Clients with a chest injury need to be examined by a physician as soon as possible.

● FRACTURED RIBS

Fractured ribs are a common injury and may result from a hard fall or a blow to the chest. Fractured ribs usually are not considered serious, unless accompanied by other injuries.

Pathophysiology and Etiology

Automobile and household accidents are frequent causes of fractured ribs. Rib fractures are painful, but not life-threatening. When a client experiences a fractured rib, other structures may be injured as well. For example, the sharp end of the broken rib may tear the lung or thoracic blood vessels. If the injury involves fractured ribs without complications, the client usually may return home after emergency treatment.

Flail chest occurs when two or more adjacent ribs fracture in multiple places (two or more) and the fragments are free-floating (Fig. 29-10). This affects the stability of the chest wall and results in impairment of chest wall movement. A paradoxical movement develops: with inspiration the chest expands, but the free-floating segments move inward instead of outward. On expiration

Inspiration   Expiration

FIGURE 29-10 Flail chest during inspiration and expiration.

the free-floating segments move outward, interfering with exhalation. Consequently, intrathoracic pressures are greatly affected, so that movement of air is greatly decreased. Many pathophysiologic phenomena occur as a result: increased dead space, reduced gas exchange, decreased lung compliance, retained airway secretions, atelectasis, and hypoxemia.

Assessment Findings

Symptoms consist primarily of severe pain on inspiration and expiration and obvious trauma. The client experiences shortness of breath. With flail chest, the client has hypotension and inadequate tissue perfusion secondary to decreased cardiac output. Respiratory acidosis occurs because of increased CO_2. Chest radiographs (usually from several angles) are necessary to confirm the diagnosis.

Medical Management

Supporting the chest with an elastic bandage or a rib belt assists in immobilizing the rib fractures. These measures, however, can lead to decreased lung expansion followed by pulmonary complications such as pneumonia and atelectasis. Therefore, the use of these devices usually is limited to multiple rib fractures. Analgesics such as codeine may be prescribed for pain. Sometimes a regional nerve block is used to relieve pain.

Management of flail chest includes supporting ventilation, clearing lung secretions, and managing pain. Other treatment depends on the severity of the flail chest. If a **pulmonary contusion** (crushing bruise of the lung) also exists, fluids are restricted because of the damage to the pulmonary capillary bed. Antibiotics are given to prevent infection, which is common after this type of injury. Endotracheal intubation and mechanical ventilation may be necessary if a client's respiratory status is greatly compromised.

Nursing Management

With fractured ribs, the nurse may apply the immobilization device after the physician examines the client. In such a case, the nurse instructs the client about the application and removal of the rib belt or elastic bandage. He or she stresses the importance of taking deep breaths every 1 to 2 hours, even though breathing is painful. Nurses plan and implement care of clients with more severe injuries based on respiratory needs. The nurse assesses and monitors the client for signs of respiratory distress, infection, and increased pain.

● BLAST INJURIES

Compression of the chest by an explosion can seriously damage the lungs by rupturing the alveoli. Death often results from hemorrhage and asphyxiation. Severe respiratory distress with outward evidence of chest trauma is apparent. **Subcutaneous emphysema** (air in subcutaneous tissues) is a common finding because the lungs or air passages have sustained an injury. This condition resembles a superficial swelling. When the area is palpated with the fingers, crepitation (a crackling sound) is heard or felt and may be caused by air leaking around the chest wound. Diagnosis is based on symptoms and physical examination. Additional diagnostic tests, such as chest radiography and lung scan, may be necessary to identify foreign objects or air in the chest. Treatment includes complete bed rest and oxygen administration. Thoracentesis to remove air or fluid may be necessary. Some clients may require surgery and the insertion of chest tubes if severe injury to lung tissue has occurred or if pneumothorax is present. When a client has suffered a blast injury, the most important nursing task is immediate recognition of respiratory distress. Victims of a blast injury are closely observed for early signs of respiratory distress.

● PENETRATING WOUNDS

Gunshot and stab wounds are common types of penetrating wounds to the lungs. Penetrating wounds potentially affect cardiopulmonary function and may be life-threatening.

Pathophysiology and Etiology

Penetrating wounds are classified according to the velocity of the cause. Stab wounds usually are low velocity because they involve a small area. Knives and switchblades are the most common weapons that cause stab wounds. Gunshot wounds may be low, medium, or high velocity, depending on the caliber of the gun, the distance from which the gun was fired, and the nature of the ammunition (Smeltzer & Bare, 2000).

Any type of penetrating wound to the chest is serious because of the opening into the thorax. On inspiration, the thorax normally is at negative pressure. The penetrating wound creates continuous and direct communication with the outside, which is at positive pressure. Thus, air enters the thoracic cavity, causing a pneumothorax (Fig. 29-11). If not recognized and treated promptly, death may occur. If the wound is large, a sucking noise may be heard as air enters and leaves the chest cavity. Depending on the size of the wound, it takes seconds to hours before the lung collapses as the pressure in the thorax reaches atmospheric pressure. Many chest injuries involve both pneumothorax and hemothorax. Subcutaneous emphysema also may be present. Other possible trauma includes hemorrhage, lung contusion, damage to surrounding tissues, fractured ribs or other bones, and injury to the heart, blood vessels, or both.

Assessment Findings

Clients exhibit various signs and symptoms, depending on the location and extent of the penetrating wound; dyspnea, pain, and bleeding are common. Clients are at

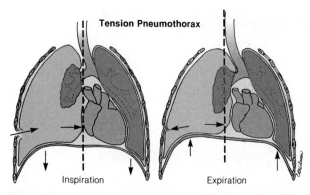

FIGURE 29-11 In open or communicating pneumothorax (*top*), air enters the chest during inspiration and exits during expiration. In tension pneumothorax (*bottom*), air enters but does not leave the chest. As pressure increases, the heart, great vessels, and unaffected lung are compressed, while the mediastinal structures and trachea shift toward the opposite side of the chest.

risk for respiratory distress and shock. It also is important that the client is thoroughly examined to ascertain if other injuries are present, such as more penetrating wounds, particularly in the abdominal area.

Diagnosis is based on the history of injury, physical examination, and auscultation of the lungs. Radiographs show the degree of lung collapse and the amount of air or blood in the thoracic cavity. The client's cardiopulmonary status is assessed through ABG analysis, pulse oximetry, and ECGs. CT scans or MRI may be necessary depending on the extent of the injuries.

Medical and Surgical Management

Airway management is the first concern. Once an airway is established, then other treatment begins. Thoracentesis is done to remove air and blood from the pleural space. A chest tube is inserted and attached to an underwater-seal drainage system. A thoracotomy may be required to repair the injury. Foreign bodies that entered the chest, such as a bullet or a knife, are surgically removed. Their presence in the wound may prevent or slow the entrance of air. Removal before the victim is transported to the hospital may result in continuous sucking of air into the chest, collapse of the lung, compression of the heart and opposite lung, and death. Surgical intervention may be necessary if there is bleeding from the chest tube or indications of injury to other organs or blood vessels.

Emergency treatment of pneumothorax caused by a penetrating wound includes the application of a tight pressure dressing over the injury site to prevent more air from entering the thorax. Immediate evaluation of the client's respiratory status is imperative. Oxygen is given until the physician examines and treats the injury. IV fluids, colloid solutions, or blood are administered to treat or prevent shock. An indwelling catheter is inserted to monitor urine output. A nasogastric tube is placed to prevent aspiration of stomach contents and to decompress the GI tract.

Nursing Management

Care of a client with a penetrating chest wound is similar to that of a client who has thoracic surgery. Refer to the nursing management of a client undergoing thoracic surgery in the next section.

THORACIC SURGERY

A thoracotomy is a surgical opening in the chest wall. It may be done to:

- Remove fluid, blood, or air from the thorax
- Remove tumors of the lung, bronchus, or chest wall

- Remove all or a portion of a lung (see Box 29-3)
- Repair or revise structures contained in the thorax, such as open heart surgery or repair of a thoracic aneurysm
- Repair trauma to the chest or chest wall, such as penetrating chest wounds or crushing chest injuries
- Sample a lesion for biopsy
- Remove foreign objects such as a bullet or metal fragments

A thoracentesis may be done as an emergency procedure to remove blood, fluid, or air from the chest. In some instances, it is necessary to perform a thoracotomy to insert chest tubes (tube thoracotomy) to remove air or fluid from the chest during the preoperative period.

Preoperative Nursing Management

Preparing clients for thoracic surgery includes assessment of vital signs and breath sounds, particularly noting the presence or absence of breath sounds in any area of the chest. The client's condition dictates the extent of the assessment and obtaining a history. If the surgery is an emergency, physical assessment may be limited to a general statement of the client's condition, a list of emergency measures and treatments done, and vital signs (see Chap. 25).

Postoperative Nursing Management

The opening of the thoracic cavity requires special postoperative nursing measures. A significant issue is the interference with normal pressures in the thoracic cavity. When the chest is opened, air from the atmosphere rushes in because of the negative pressure that exists in the thoracic cavity on inspiration. The entrance of air under atmospheric pressure causes the lungs to collapse and no longer expand or contract. The anesthesiologist ventilates the client during surgery.

After thoracic surgery, draining secretions, air, and blood from the thoracic cavity is necessary to allow the lungs to expand. A catheter placed in the pleural space provides a drainage route through a closed or underwaterseal drainage system. Sometimes two chest catheters are placed—one anteriorly and one posteriorly (Fig. 29-12). The anterior catheter (usually the upper one) removes air; the posterior catheter removes fluid.

Chest tubes are securely connected to an underwaterseal system. The tube coming from the client always must be under water. A break in the system, such as from loose or disconnected fittings, allows air to enter the tubing and then the pleural space, further collapsing the lung. When chest tubes are inserted at the end of the surgical procedure, they are connected to an underwater-seal drainage system. All connections are taped carefully to minimize the possibility of air entering the closed system.

When caring for a client with chest tubes, the nurse should be aware of the following:

- Fluctuation of the fluid in the water-seal chamber is initially present with each respiration. Fluctuations cease when the lung re-expands. The time for lung re-expansion varies. Fluctuations also may cease if:
  - The chest tube is clogged.
  - The wall suction unit malfunctions.
  - A kink or dependent loop develops in the tubing.
- Bubbling in the water-seal chamber occurs in the early postoperative period. If bubbling is excessive, the nurse checks the system for leaks. If leaks are not apparent, the nurse notifies the physician.
- Bloody drainage is normal, but drainage should not be bright red or copious.
- The drainage tube(s) must remain patent to allow fluids to escape from the pleural space.
- Clogging of the catheter with clots or kinking causes drainage to stop. The lung cannot expand, and the heart and great vessels may shift (mediastinal shift) to the opposite side. The nurse must be alert to the proper functioning of the drainage system. Malfunctions need immediate correction.
- If a break or major leak occurs in the system, the nurse clamps the chest tube immediately with hemostats kept at the bedside. He or she notifies the physician if this occurs.

Immediate postoperative care includes following the standards outlined in Chapter 25. It also is essential that the nurse check the underwater-seal drainage system, noting the amount and color of drainage and any bubbling or fluctuation. The nurse assesses dressings for drainage and firm adherence to the skin. He or she inspects the skin around the dressings for signs of subcutaneous emphysema. The nurse assesses the client's color, neurologic status, and heart rate and rhythm; monitors respiratory rate, depth, and rhythm; and auscultates the chest for normal and abnormal breath sounds. He or she also assesses levels of pain and anxiety. See Nursing Care Plan 29-1 and Client and Family Teaching Box 29-2 for additional nursing management.

GENERAL NUTRITIONAL CONSIDERATIONS

Malnutrition among clients with emphysema is multifactorial. Shortness of breath and difficulty breathing impair the ability to chew and swallow. Inadequate oxygenation of GI cells causes anorexia and gastric ulceration. Slowed peristalsis and digestion contribute to loss of appetite. Labored breathing increases calorie requirements, and eating is not a priority among clients who are anxious about breathing. To correct malnutrition, a high-protein, high-calorie diet is indicated. Because carbohydrates produce more CO_2 when metabolized than either protein or fat (and thus increase the burden on the lungs), carbohydrates are limited and fat is increased.

FIGURE 29-12 Chest drainage system. (A) Strategic placement of a chest catheter in the pleural space. (B) Three types of mechanical drainage systems. (C) A Pleur-Evac operating system, which is a single unit with three bottles identified as chambers: (1) the collection chamber, (2) the water-seal chamber, and (3) the suction control chamber.

The diet should consist of approximately 40% carbohydrates, 40% fat, and 20% protein for clients with hypercapnia or those on ventilator support. Small, frequent feedings of nutrient-dense and calorie-dense foods help maximize intake and lessen fatigue; concentrated liquid supplements are beneficial. Encourage ample fluid intake. Obese clients with emphysema are encouraged to lose weight to improve breathing.

Encourage clients with asthma to consume adequate calories and protein to optimize health and resist infection. Certain vitamins and minerals are important for immune function, especially vitamins A, C, B_6, and zinc, and should be liberally consumed. Food allergens that may trigger asthma include milk, eggs, seafood, and fish.

Specially designed enteral formulas are available for clients with respiratory failure; they are high in calories and consist of 40% to 55% of calories from fat to reduce CO_2 production. They should be administered continuously and advanced gradually as tolerated.

GENERAL PHARMACOLOGIC CONSIDERATIONS

Antibiotics may be ordered for the client with a respiratory tract infection; a culture and sensitivity test may be performed to identify the causative

microorganisms. Once the microorganisms are identified and their sensitivity to various antibiotics is determined, the appropriate antibiotic is prescribed.

The indiscriminate use of nonprescription cough medicines may cause more harm than good. Coughing is the mechanism the body uses to clear the respiratory passages of mucus; depressing the cough reflex may cause a pooling of secretions and lead to further problems. Clients with respiratory disease are advised to check with their physicians before using nonprescription antitussive preparations (drugs used to prevent coughing).

Bronchodilators are used to manage acute breathing disorders, such as acute asthma attacks or reversible bronchospasm.

Examples of bronchodilators include adrenergic drugs, such as epinephrine, isoproterenol (Isuprel), and terbutaline (Bricanyl), and the xanthine derivatives, such as aminophylline and theophylline.

When theophylline or aminophylline are used to manage attacks of acute bronchial asthma and bronchospasm associated with chronic bronchitis and emphysema, serum theophylline levels should be maintained in the therapeutic range of 10 to 20 micrograms (μg)/mL. Levels over 20 μg/mL are associated with toxicity.

INH is used in combination with other antitubercular drugs and alone as a prophylactic to prevent the spread of TB. For example, INH may be given to household members and close associates of those recently diagnosed with TB.

Nursing Care Plan 29-1

THE CLIENT RECOVERING FROM THORACIC SURGERY

Assessment

- Assess respirations: rate, depth, rhythm, and use of accessory muscles.
- Observe skin color, particularly for signs of cyanosis.
- Auscultate breath sounds at least every 4 hours.
- Evaluate mental status.
- Monitor heart rate and rhythm.
- Monitor results of ABGs, pulse oximetry, and other blood tests.
- Assess dressings and incisions for drainage or adherence.
- Check the chest tube drainage system.
- Assess level of pain.

Nursing Diagnosis: **Impaired Gas Exchange** related to decreased lung expansion, impaired lung function, and surgical procedure

Expected Outcome: Client will maintain optimal gas exchange.

Interventions	Rationales
Monitor vital signs every 15 minutes for at least 2 hours after return from postanesthesia care unit and then less frequently as condition stabilizes.	Such information provides baseline data and early indications of problems.
Reinforce preoperative instructions about deep breathing, coughing, and incentive spirometry. Remind client to do these exercises every 1 to 2 hours.	These exercises expand the alveoli, which prevents atelectasis.
Position client with the head of the bed elevated 30° to 40° initially. When the client can tolerate it, position him or her on operative side.	Such positioning promotes lung expansion and drainage from operative side.

Evaluation of Expected Outcome: Client demonstrates improved gas exchange, as evidenced by results of ABGs and pulse oximetry and improved efforts with incentive spirometry.

Nursing Diagnosis: **Impaired Physical Mobility: Arm on Affected Side** related to incisional pain, edema, and decreased strength

Expected Outcome: Client will demonstrate effective range-of-motion (ROM) on affected side.

Interventions	Rationales
Assess ROM in affected upper extremity within 24 hours by having the client raise arm laterally.	This assessment provides baseline data about ROM. During thoracotomy, chest muscles are incised, making ROM difficult after surgery.
Perform passive ROM exercises on affected arm four times a day.	These exercises increase mobility and promote renewed strength of affected arm.
Encourage client to use affected arm in activities of daily living (ADLs).	Gradual use of arm promotes movement of it.
Instruct client to move arms, slowly increasing movement and exercise as tolerated.	These measures promote mobility and begin to increase strength in affected side.

(continued)

Nursing Care Plan 29-1 (Continued)

THE CLIENT RECOVERING FROM THORACIC SURGERY

Interventions	*Rationales*
Increase exercise level after removal of chest tubes.	Removal of chest tubes decreases discomfort and assists client to move more freely.
Collaborate with physical therapists to plan therapy; reinforce instructions regarding exercise and discharge.	A full exercise plan will help client gain full ROM of affected upper extremity.

Evaluation of Expected Outcome: Client demonstrates increased ROM and better ability to perform ADLs independently.

Nursing Diagnosis: **Deficient Fluid Volume** related to surgical procedure, drains, and pain

Expected Outcome: Client will maintain adequate fluid volume.

Interventions	*Rationales*
Monitor and record intake and output hourly.	Such monitoring provides ongoing information about client's fluid status.
Assess skin turgor and mucous membranes for signs of dehydration.	These assessments provide baseline data about fluid status.
Monitor and document vital signs.	Tachycardia can occur with hypovolemia to maintain adequate cardiac output. Pulse may be weak with hypovolemia. Hypotension occurs with hypovolemia.
Report urine output less than 30 mL/hour for 2 consecutive hours.	Urine output of less than 30 mL/hour for 2 or more hours indicates dehydration.
Monitor serum electrolyte and urine osmolality levels, reporting abnormal values.	Elevated hemoglobin, blood urea nitrogen, and urine specific gravity suggest fluid deficit.
Administer parenteral fluids as ordered, and maintain an accurate record of intravenous intake.	Parenteral fluids prevent dehydration.
Encourage client to drink at least 30 mL every hour.	This amount promotes adequate fluid intake.

Evaluation of Expected Outcome: Client is adequately hydrated as evidenced by urine output greater than 30 mL/hour, stable blood pressure and pulse, and normal skin turgor.

PC: **Blood Loss; Hemorrhage**

Expected Outcome: Nurse will manage and minimize blood loss.

Interventions	*Rationales*
Monitor and record vital signs.	Monitoring vital signs provides baseline data and information about changes in a client's status.
Assess chest tube drainage and dressings for signs of bleeding.	Bloody drainage from chest tubes may occur initially but should decrease. Increased blood in chest tubes, on dressings, or both indicates a bleeding problem that requires immediate intervention.
Anticipate or prepare client for return to surgery if bleeding is secondary to surgical procedure.	These measures are necessary to resolve the problem.
Increase parenteral fluids as ordered.	Increased parenteral fluid maintains an adequate circulating volume until bleeding stops.
Administer blood products as ordered.	Blood products replace lost blood and volume.

Evaluation of Expected Outcome: Nurse ensures the management of bleeding and its complications.

29-2 *Client and Family Teaching* Care After Thoracic Surgery

The nurse develops a teaching plan that includes instructions given by the physician as well as the following guidelines:

■ Continue to perform arm exercises to prevent stiffness and pain.
■ Eat a well-balanced diet, or follow the recommended diet.
■ Take rest periods throughout the day until fatigue decreases.
■ Practice breathing exercises, and take frequent deep breaths.
■ Contact the physician if breathing is difficult; drainage, excessive redness, or pain develops around the incision; fever develops; or pain occurs elsewhere in the body.
■ Avoid infection or irritants.
■ Increase activities slowly and avoid fatigue.
■ Take drugs as prescribed, and do not omit, increase, or decrease doses.

Zafirlukast (Accolate) is one of a new classification of antiasthma drugs, the leukotriene receptor antagonists. The drug is administered to manage asthma symptoms on an ongoing basis. Asthma symptoms should improve within 1 week of beginning therapy. Zafirlukast is *not* beneficial during an acute asthma attack.

When a narcotic is administered to a client who has had thoracic surgery, the respiratory rate is counted before and 20 to 30 minutes after the client receives the medication. If the respiratory rate falls below 10 breaths per minute at either time, the physician must be notified immediately.

GENERAL GERONTOLOGIC CONSIDERATIONS

Older adults are more prone to pneumonia and may be more acutely ill with this infection because of concomitant health problems, such as heart disease and diabetes.

Before the flu season begins, the physician may recommend administration of a vaccine. Older and debilitated clients are more likely to contract the disease and develop complications.

Older adults, who are more subject to falls, may fracture one or more ribs and be more susceptible to pneumonia after a rib fracture.

During the postoperative period, the older client may be confused and attempt to pull out the chest tubes. Notify the physician if confusion in a client is apparent. An order for soft restraints may be needed.

If confusion occurs, the client requires more frequent observation and assessment of needs.

The older client may require more detailed explanation of home care management. Adequate time and repeated demonstrations may be necessary.

When possible, teach a family member postoperative exercises to ensure proper return of function to the muscles on the operative side.

For clients older than 50 years of age, nursing home residents, and debilitated clients, vaccination against pneumococcal pneumonia is recommended.

Critical Thinking Exercises

1. *A male client who underwent cholecystectomy (removal of the gallbladder) 2 days ago presses his call button. As you enter his room, he tells you that he is having trouble breathing and has chest pain. What brief questions would you ask the client before you call the physician?*

2. *A female client has a history of asthma and was admitted to the hospital with uncontrolled diabetes mellitus. What nursing assessments would you make if she experiences respiratory problems?*

3. *A client who has AIDS developed pleurisy. His physician instructs him to perform deep breathing and coughing exercises hourly. What can you do to ease the client's pain and discomfort when he is performing these exercises?*

4. *A client who has bronchiectasis in his left lower lobe attends a pulmonary disease clinic. His physician instructs him to perform postural drainage by lying on the bed, bending at the waist, and lowering his head close to the floor. Two weeks later, the client tells you that he cannot tolerate this postural drainage position. Can you think of another way to perform postural drainage for the left lower lobe that may cause less discomfort?*

References and Suggested Readings

American Cancer Society. (2001). *Cancer facts and figures.* Atlanta, GA: Author.

Bullock, B. & Henze, R. L. (2000). *Focus on pathophysiology.* Philadelphia: Lippincott Williams & Wilkins.

Carroll, P. (2001). How to intervene before asthma turns deadly. *RN, 64*(5), 52–58.

Cystic Fibrosis Foundation. (2001). Cystic fibrosis. [On-line.] Available: http:// www.cff.org/facts.htm.

Dest, V. M. (2000). Oncology today: Lung cancer. *RN, 63*(5), 32–38.

DiTrapano, C. (2001). Antibiotic therapy: Nurses need to remain current about old drugs, new drugs and resistant organisms. *Advances for Nurses, 1*(3), 15–19.

Dunn, N. A. (2001). Keeping COPD patients out of the ED. *RN, 64*(2), 33–37.

Eisenbeis, C. (1996). Full partner in care: Teaching your patient how to manage her asthma. *Nursing96, 26*(1), 48–51.

Lungcancer.org. (2001). It's time to focus on lung cancer. [On-line.] Available: http://www.lungcancer.org.

Smeltzer, S. C. & Bare, B. G. (2000). *Brunner & Suddarth's textbook of medical–surgical nursing* (9th ed.). Philadelphia: Lippincott Williams & Wilkins.

World Health Organization. (2001). Tuberculosis. [On-line.] Available: http://www.who.int.

Introduction to the Cardiovascular System

Words to Know

angiocardiography
aortography
arteriography
automaticity
baroreceptors
cardiac index
cardiac output
central venous pressure
chemoreceptors
conductivity
contractility
depolarization
dysrhythmias
echocardiography
electrocardiography
electron beam computed
    tomography
electrophysiology study
excitability
hemodynamic
    monitoring
isoenzyme
left ventricular
    end-diastolic pressure
nomogram
phonocardiography
polarization
pulmonary capillary
    wedge pressure
refractory period
repolarization
rhythmicity
Starling's law
stroke volume
telemetry
transesophageal
    echocardiography

Learning Objectives

On completion of this chapter, the reader will:

- Describe the normal anatomy and physiology of the cardiovascular system.
- Identify and describe focus assessment criteria when caring for a client with cardiovascular problems.
- List common diagnostic tests used to evaluate the client with suspected heart disease.
- Discuss the nursing management of a client undergoing cardiovascular diagnostic tests.

The function of the cardiovascular system is to supply body cells and tissues with oxygen-rich blood and eliminate carbon dioxide (CO_2) and cellular wastes. Damage to and disease in the cardiovascular system greatly jeopardize a person's health. In fact, heart disease is the leading cause of death for adults in the United States. Many advanced treatments have been and are being created to treat heart disease. Human heart transplantation and the temporary use of an artificial heart are realities. Clinical trials are underway in the United States after the implantation of a permanent, self-contained artificial heart, called the AbioCor, in Kentucky in 2001. Nevertheless, the primary focus remains preserving the natural heart by preventing heart disease.

ANATOMY AND PHYSIOLOGY

The cardiovascular system consists of the heart, the major blood vessels that empty into or exit directly from the heart, and a vast network of smaller peripheral blood vessels. The heart's ability to pump blood is the result of five qualities unique to cardiac tissue:

- **Automaticity**—the ability to initiate electrical stimulus independently
- **Excitability**—the ability to respond to electrical stimulation
- **Conductivity**—the ability to transmit the electrical stimulus from cell to cell in the heart

387

- **Contractility**—the ability to stretch as a single unit and recoil
- **Rhythmicity**—the ability to repeat the cycle with regularity

Heart Chambers

The heart is a four-chambered muscular pump about the size of a fist (Fig. 30-1). The upper chambers, the right and left *atria* (singular, *atrium*), are receiving chambers for blood. The lower chambers, the right and left *ventricles,* are the heart's pumping chambers. A thick *septum,* or wall, separates the right side of the heart from the left side. The right atrium receives deoxygenated blood from the venous system, and the right ventricle pumps that blood to the lungs to be oxygenated. The left atrium receives oxygenated blood from the lungs, and the left ventricle pumps that blood to all the cells and tissues of the body. Therefore, the heart is a double pump—the right side conducts pulmonary circulation, and the left side is responsible for systemic circulation.

The heart lies below and slightly to the left of the midline of the sternum in the mediastinum, a portion of the thoracic cavity that also contains the trachea and blood vessels. The upper portion of the heart is the base, and the tip is the apex. The right ventricle is directly under the sternum, a location that is significant in cardiopulmonary resuscitation. The lower border of the right ventricle rests on the diaphragm and forms a blunt point that angles to the left side of the body (Fig. 30-2).

Cardiac Tissue Layers

Three distinct layers of tissue make up the heart wall. The outer layer is the *epicardium,* which is composed of fibrous and loose connective tissue. The middle layer, the *myocardium,* consists of muscle tissue and is the force be-

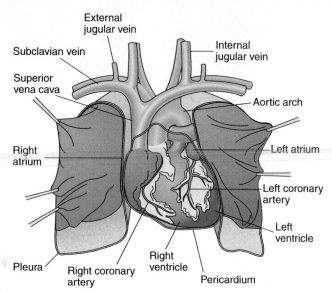

FIGURE 30-2 Anterior view of the heart and great vessels.

hind the heart's pumping action (see previous discussion). The inner layer, the *endocardium,* is composed of a thin, smooth layer of endothelial cells. Folds of endocardium form the heart valves. The endocardium is in direct contact with the blood that passes through the heart.

The *pericardium* is a saclike structure that surrounds and supports the heart. Two membranous layers form the pericardium. The outer, tougher layer is called the *parietal pericardium.* The inner serous layer is called the *visceral pericardium* (also called the *epicardium*), which adheres to the heart itself. The density of the parietal pericardium safeguards the heart from invasion by infectious microorganisms. Serous fluid fills the pericardial space between the two layers, lubricating the heart and reducing friction with each heartbeat (Fig. 30-3).

Heart Valves

The valves of the heart are membranous structures that ensure that blood passes through the heart in a one-way, forward direction. In a normal heart, the valves do not allow blood to backflow, or regurgitate, into the chamber from which it has come.

The two *atrioventricular valves* separate the atria from the ventricles. They prevent blood from returning to the atria when the ventricles contract. These valves are cusped, or leaflike. The valve between the right atrium and right ventricle is the tricuspid valve. The word *tricuspid* signifies that the valve has three cusps. The valve between the left atrium and left ventricle is the bicuspid, or two-cusped, valve. Another name for the bicuspid valve is the *mitral valve.*

Attached to the mitral and tricuspid valves are cord-like structures known as *chordae tendineae,* which in turn attach to two major muscular projections from the ventricles, the *papillary muscles.* When the ventricles

FIGURE 30-1 Layers of the heart, showing the visceral pericardium, the pericardial cavity, and the parietal pericardium. *LA,* left atrium; *LV,* left ventricle; *RA,* right atrium; *RV,* right ventricle.

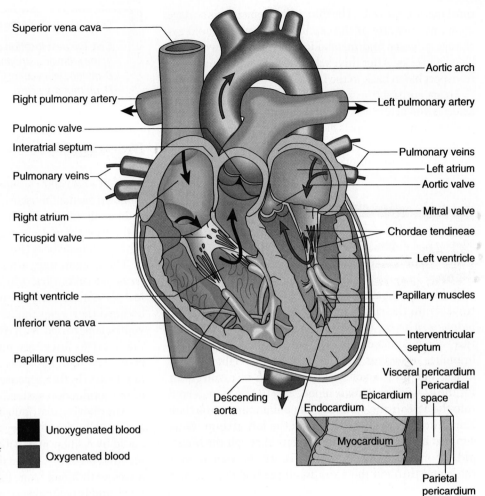

FIGURE 30-3 Structure of the heart. Arrows show the course of blood flow through the heart chambers. (From Smeltzer, S. C. & Bare, B. G. [2000]. *Brunner & Suddarth's textbook of medical–surgical nursing* [9th ed.]. Philadelphia: Lippincott Williams & Wilkins.)

■ Unoxygenated blood

■ Oxygenated blood

contract, the papillary muscles also contract, applying tension to the atrioventricular valves. The contraction of the papillary muscles and the firm support of the chordae tendineae prevent eversion of the valves and regurgitation of blood back into the atria.

The other two valves, called the *semilunar valves* because they resemble portions of the moon, prevent blood from flowing back into the ventricles after the heart contracts. The valves are named for the blood vessel into which the blood is deposited. The valve between the right ventricle and pulmonary artery is called the *pulmonary,* or *pulmonic, valve.* The valve between the left ventricle and aorta is called the *aortic valve.* Contraction of the ventricles forces blood into the pulmonary artery and aorta. Relaxation follows, and the fall in pressure in the ventricles causes the pulmonic and aortic valves to close, preventing backflow into the ventricles.

Stop, Think, and Respond ● BOX 30-1

Where are the following cardiac valves located?—A, mitral valve; B, tricuspid valve; C, pulmonic valve.

Arteries and Veins

Arteries carry oxygenated blood from the heart, and veins return deoxygenated blood to the heart. The smallest arteries are called *arterioles,* and the smallest veins are called *venules.* Arteries and arterioles are elastic and dilate or constrict to accommodate changes in blood flow. Veins have thinner walls than arteries because venous pressure is lower than arterial pressure. Despite being thinner, veins have larger diameters than corresponding arteries (Martini, 1998).

Arteries and veins consist of three layers. The outer layer, the *tunica adventitia,* consists of connective tissue; the middle layer, the *tunica media,* is composed of smooth muscle; and the inner layer, the *tunica intima,* is composed of endothelial cells. The tunica media is thicker in arteries than in veins to accommodate the higher blood pressure (BP) in the arteries.

Arterioles branch into *capillaries,* which are microscopic vessels that form a connecting network between arterioles and venules. Capillaries are one cell layer thick and in direct contact with the cells of all tissues. This complex circulatory network delivers oxygen and metabolic substances to the cells. The thin walls, tremendous surface area, and tiny size of the capillaries allow for rapid exchange of gases and metabolic substances between the blood and cells. After this exchange, the venules and veins transport blood back to the heart.

Heart contraction moves blood from the heart into arteries and arterioles; skeletal muscle contraction compresses veins and propels blood back to the heart. Closure of successive sets of valves in veins keeps the blood from pooling under the influence of gravity.

Cardiopulmonary Circulation

The largest veins, the *inferior* and *superior venae cavae,* bring venous (deoxygenated) blood from all areas of the body into the right atrium. The right atrium fills with blood, and the tricuspid valve opens. Blood then travels into the right ventricle and is pumped into the *pulmonary artery* (the only artery in an adult that carries deoxygenated blood). The pulmonary artery branches to deliver venous blood to the right and left lungs. The lungs exchange the oxygen in inspired air for the CO_2 in the venous blood. The CO_2 is transferred into the alveoli and exhaled. The pulmonary veins then bring the oxygenated blood into the left atrium. Oxygenated blood leaves the left atrium through the bicuspid, or mitral, valve. The left ventricle then pumps the blood through the aorta to all the body's cells and tissues.

Stop, Think, and Respond ● BOX 30-2

Give the next location of blood when it is in the following structures: A, right ventricle; B, inferior vena cava; C, left ventricle; D, pulmonary veins.

Blood Supply to the Heart

The *left and right coronary arteries* supply oxygenated blood to cardiac muscle. The openings to the coronary arteries lie just inside the aorta. Thus, the myocardium is the first tissue to be supplied with oxygenated blood with each heartbeat (Fig. 30-4).

The left coronary artery and its branches, the *left anterior descending artery* and *left circumflex artery,* are critical for maintaining the pumping function of the heart because they keep the left atrium and most of the left ventricle perfused with oxygen, enabling the left side of the heart to forcefully pump oxygen-rich blood to the body. The right coronary artery and its branches maintain heart rhythm because they nourish the nerve tissue of the conduction system.

After having distributed oxygenated blood to the myocardial cells, the coronary veins carry away the CO_2 produced by cellular metabolism. The coronary veins empty into the coronary sinus in the right atrium. The blood then mixes with blood from the inferior and superior venae cavae and is recirculated to the lungs.

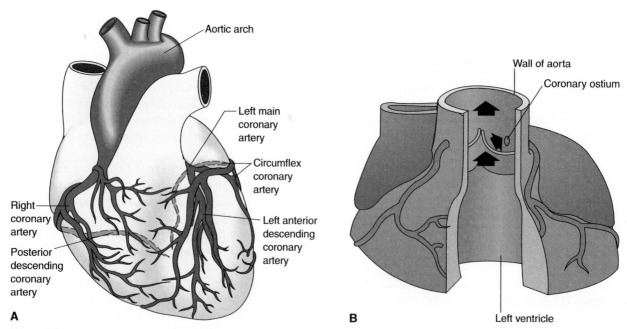

A **B**

FIGURE 30-4 (**A**) Coronary arteries (*red vessels*) arise from the aorta and encircle the heart; coronary veins (*blue vessels*). (**B**) The orifices of the coronary arteries lie just beyond the aortic valve.

| Atrial diastole | Atrial systole / Ventricular diastole | Ventricular systole |

FIGURE 30-5 Pumping cycle of the heart. During atrial diastole, blood from the venae cavae and pulmonary veins fills the atria. During atrial systole, blood is delivered to the ventricles. When the ventricles contract, blood is pumped into the aorta and pulmonary arteries.

Cardiac Cycle

The term *cardiac cycle* refers to the contraction (systole) and relaxation (diastole) of both atria and both ventricles (Fig. 30-5). The atria contract simultaneously; then, as they relax, the ventricles contract and relax. The contraction of the left ventricle can be felt as a wavelike impulse (the pulse) in peripheral arteries. The pause between pulsations is ventricular diastole. The contraction of the atria and then the ventricles can be heard with a stethoscope as the "lub-dub" sounds. The sounds are created when the atrioventricular and semilunar valves alternately snap shut.

Both sides of the heart work in unison to accomplish different goals. Blood enters both atria and as pressure builds from the increasing volume of blood in the atria, the atrioventricular valves open, depositing blood into the ventricles. During atrial systole, the contraction of the upper chambers squeezes the remaining blood into the ventricles. When pressure builds in the ventricles, the atrioventricular valves snap shut.

During ventricular systole, blood is pumped through the semilunar valves into the major vessels exiting the heart. The greater the stretch of the myocardium as the ventricles fill with blood, the stronger is the ventricular contraction. This phenomenon is called **Starling's law.** It can be compared to the effect created by stretching a rubber band: the more the rubber band is stretched, the greater the snap when it is released.

Conduction System

The conduction system sustains the electrical activity of the heart. It consists of the sinoatrial (SA) node, atri-

oventricular (AV) node, bundle of His, bundle branches, and Purkinje fibers.

The *SA node* is an area of nerve tissue located in the posterior wall of the right atrium. The SA node is called the *pacemaker of the heart* because it initiates the electrical impulses that cause the atria and ventricles to contract. Normally, it produces between 60 and 100 impulses per minute; the average is approximately 72 impulses per minute. The SA node initiates impulses faster in response to sympathetic nervous system stimulation and slows impulses in response to parasympathetic stimulation. Other areas in the conduction pathway may initiate an electrical impulse if the SA node malfunctions, but they do so at rates slower than that of the SA node.

In the normal sequence of events, the cardiac impulse starts in the SA node (Fig. 30-6). It spreads throughout

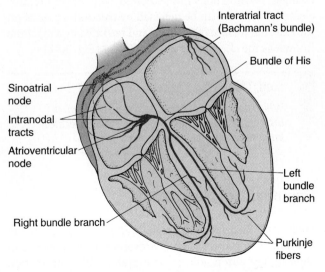

FIGURE 30-6 Electrical conduction system of the heart.

the atria over internodal and interatrial pathways. The waves of stimulation through the heart resemble the rings that a pebble makes when dropped into a pond. Once the cells in the atria are excited, they contract in unison. When the impulse reaches the *AV node,* it is delayed a few hundredths of a second. The impulse then stimulates the ventricles. While the ventricles fill with blood, the impulse travels from the AV node to the *bundle of His,* to the *right and left bundle branches,* and eventually to the *Purkinje fibers.* Then, both ventricles contract.

During diastole, while the myocardial cells are at rest, and before an impulse is generated, the cells are in a polarized state (**polarization**). Positive ions predominate outside myocardial cell membranes; negative ions predominate inside. When an electrical impulse is initiated, it spreads from cell membrane to cell membrane, causing a transfer of ions. The positive ions move inside the myocardial cell membranes, and the negative ions move outside. This process, which corresponds with cardiac muscle contraction, is called **depolarization.** It occurs first in the atria and then in the ventricles. Once depolarization has occurred, the ions realign themselves in their original position and wait for another electrical impulse. This process is called **repolarization.** Another normal cardiac impulse cannot be carried out until the ions are again in polarized alignment. The time during which the cells are resistant to electrical stimulation is called the **refractory period.**

Electrolyte balance is important for the proper functioning of all the cells in the body. Normal ranges of potassium and calcium ions are particularly essential for maintaining heart function (see Chap. 22). Excess potassium ions decrease the heart rate and strength of contraction. Abnormally low potassium levels disturb cardiac rhythm. Excess calcium ions increase and prolong heart contraction. Low serum calcium levels reduce heart function.

Depolarization and repolarization produce electrical changes. Because body tissues conduct current easily, this electrical activity can be detected by electrodes placed on the external surface of the body and recorded by a machine known as the *electrocardiograph (ECG)* (Fig. 30-7).

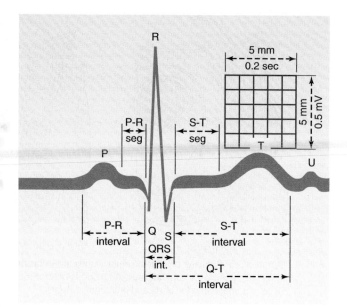

FIGURE 30-7 ECG graph and commonly measured complex components. Each small box represents 0.04 seconds on the horizontal axis and 1 mm or 0.1 millivolt on the vertical axis. The PR interval is measured from the beginning of the P wave to the beginning of the QRS complex; the QRS complex is measured from the beginning of the Q wave to the end of the S wave; the QT interval is measured from the beginning of the Q wave to the end of the T wave. (From Smeltzer, S. C. & Bare, B. G. [2000]. *Brunner & Suddarth's textbook of medical–surgical nursing* [9th ed.]. Philadelphia: Lippincott Williams & Wilkins.)

Stop, Think, and Respond ● BOX 30-3

Which part of the conduction system is known as the natural pacemaker because it initiates electrical impulses in normal heart conduction?

Regulation of Heart Rate

Heart rate fluctuates according to stimulation from the autonomic nervous system, baroreceptors, and chemoreceptors. The autonomic nervous system affects heart rate through sympathetic and parasympathetic nervous system innervation. When released by sympathetic nerve fibers, adrenergic neurotransmitters, such as norepinephrine and epinephrine, excite the SA and AV nodes in the conduction system, increasing heart rate. These same neurotransmitters also stimulate beta$_1$ receptors in the atria and ventricles, increasing the force of myocardial contraction. Conversely, the heart rate slows when parasympathetic nerve fibers from the cardiac branches of the vagus nerve release the cholinergic neurotransmitter, acetylcholine. Parasympathetic neurostimulation, however, usually does not affect the force of contraction.

Responses to **baroreceptors,** pressure-sensitive nerve endings in the walls of the atria and major blood vessels (e.g., vena cava, arch of the aorta, and carotid arteries), also affect the heart rate. The main function of baroreceptors is to sense the pressure from blood as it stretches vascular tissues containing the baroreceptors. If BP decreases in the areas of the baroreceptors, such as when a person rises quickly from a lying or standing position, the baroreceptors send impulses to the brain stem to increase heart rate. An almost immediate reflexive response of accelerated heart contractions follows (Nursing Guidelines 30-1). The heart rate increases to compensate for the drop in BP. When the BP is stabilized, the heart rate returns to within a normal range.

Chemoreceptors, structures that are sensitive to the pH and CO_2 and oxygen levels of blood, are located in the

NURSING GUIDELINES 30-1

Assessing Blood Pressure and Pulse for Postural Changes

- Have the client lie down for at least 3 minutes.
- Take the client's blood pressure and pulse.
- Assist the client to a sitting position.
- Be prepared to steady or assist the client should he or she become dizzy or faint.
- Reassess the blood pressure and pulse within 30 seconds after the client sits.
- Repeat the assessments with the client standing.
- Determine the difference in systolic and diastolic blood pressure in the upright position from that recorded in the previous position.
- Determine the difference in the heart rate from that recorded in the previous position.
- Conclude that the client manifests postural changes if the blood pressure is lower than 10 mm Hg from the previous measurement and the heart rate increases 10% or more from the previous measurement (Bickley & Hoekelman, 1998).

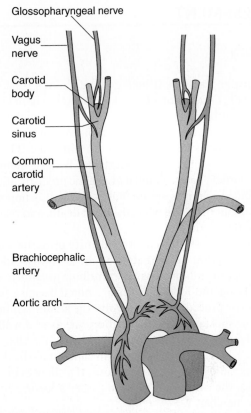

FIGURE 30-8 Location and innervation of the aortic arch and carotid sinus baroreceptors and the carotid body chemoreceptors. (From Chaffee, E. E., & Lytle, I. M. [1980]. *Basic physiology and anatomy* [4th ed.]. Philadelphia: J.B. Lippincott.)

carotid bodies, aortic bodies, and medulla of the brain (Fig. 30-8). They regulate sympathetic stimulation or inhibition (Bullock & Henze, 2000). A fall in pH, rise in CO_2, and decrease in oxygen levels in the blood results in increased heart contraction. The heart rate returns to a more usual parameter when pH and CO_2 levels become normalized. Box 30-1 highlights additional factors that alter heart rate.

Stop, Think, and Respond ● BOX 30-4

What effect will each of the following have on heart rate?—A, anxiety; B, fever; C, hypothyroidism; D, caffeine; E, athletic conditioning.

Cardiac Output

Cardiac output is the amount of blood pumped out of the left ventricle each minute. In a healthy adult, cardiac output ranges from 4 to 8 L/min (the average is approximately 5 L/min). Volume varies according to body size. The heart adjusts cardiac output to the body's changing needs. During active exercise, athletes may have a cardiac output that is five to seven times the normal amount. Cardiac output can be increased in two ways: by increasing the heart rate and by increasing the stroke volume. **Stroke volume** is the amount of blood pumped per contraction of the heart. The stroke volume averages about 65 to 70 mL. The following formula is used to calculate cardiac output:

$$\text{Cardiac output} = \text{heart rate} \times \text{stroke volume}$$

Stop, Think, and Respond ● BOX 30-5

If a person's heart rate is 72 beats per minute (bpm), what is the cardiac output?

BOX 30-1 ● Factors That Alter Heart Rate

Increase Heart Rate	Decrease Heart Rate
Exercise	Rest
Fever	Hypothermia
Hyperthyroidism	Hypothyroidism
Hypoxia	Athletic conditioning
Dehydration	Drugs: Cardiac glycosides (digoxin
Shock and hemorrhage	[Lanoxin]), central nervous sys-
Anxiety	tem depressants (morphine),
Caffeine	calcium channel blockers
Drugs: Central nervous system stim-	(verapamil [Calan], nifedipine
ulants (cocaine, methylphenidate	[Procardia]), beta-adrenergic
[Ritalin], methamphetamine),	blockers (atenolol [Tenormin],
adrenergic drugs (epinephrine,	metoprolol [Lopressor], propra-
isoproterenol [Isuprel]), anti-	nolol [Inderal])
cholinergic drugs (atropine,	
glycopyrrolate [Robinul])	
Alcohol withdrawal	

ASSESSMENT

History

The initial assessment includes the client's (or family member's) description of the symptoms the client experienced before and during admission. A past medical history of angina, myocardial infarction (MI), or any cardiac surgeries also is important to note at this time. The family medical history must be ascertained because many cardiac disorders have a familial or genetic predisposition. If close blood relatives are no longer living, it is important to ask about the cause of death, age at death, and relationship to the client.

The nurse asks the client to identify prescription and nonprescription drugs that he or she is taking. Adverse effects or drug interactions can contribute to cardiac symptoms. Drug and food allergies are noted because future diagnostic procedures may involve the administration of drugs or substances, such as radiopaque dyes. An allergy to seafood may indicate that the client also is allergic to iodine, which commonly is used in contrast media during various radiographic examinations. If a client is in acute distress, the nurse may need to gather a history from a family member.

Physical Examination

General Appearance

An appraisal of the client's general appearance may suggest problems that require further exploration. The client's nonverbal behavior and body position may indicate that he or she is anxious, depressed, in pain, or uncomfortable.

Pain

Poor circulation, a common problem in clients with cardiovascular disorders, causes ischemia (reduced blood supply) to body organs. A classic sign of ischemia is pain, which results from a lack of oxygen in the tissue. Chest pain is a manifestation of ischemia to the heart muscle. Leg pain, especially with activity, can indicate inadequate oxygenation to leg muscles.

When present, the nurse evaluates pain carefully. Obtaining as much information as possible is essential. Rapid treatment of pain is extremely important.

Vital Signs

TEMPERATURE

Fever is characteristic in some types of heart disease. It can accompany the inflammatory response when myocardial cells are damaged after an acute MI (heart attack) or infections such as rheumatic fever and bacterial endocarditis. The nurse must observe agency policy about taking the temperature rectally on clients with a cardiac disorder. In the past, this method was contraindicated because it was thought to stimulate the vagus nerve and cause bradycardia. Many agencies now have abandoned this restriction.

PULSE

When taking a client's pulse, the nurse notes its rate, rhythm, and quality. Pulse rhythm is the pattern of the pulsations and the pauses between them. A normal pulse is felt regularly with a similar length of pause. The pulse quality refers to its palpated volume. Pulse volume is described as feeling full, weak, or thready, meaning barely palpable. The nurse also determines any pulse deficit by counting the heart rate through auscultation at the apex while a second nurse simultaneously palpates and counts the radial pulse for a full minute. The difference, if any, is the pulse deficit.

RESPIRATORY RATE

The nurse counts the respiratory rate for 60 seconds. He or she observes the character of the respirations, noting whether the client's breathing is easy or labored (dyspneic), deep or shallow, noisy or quiet. The use of accessory muscles (neck or abdominal muscles) during respiration is an indication that the client is having difficulty breathing.

BLOOD PRESSURE

Cardiac disorders often are associated with changes in BP. If the client is not acutely ill, the nurse takes the BP with the client in the standing, sitting, and lying positions (orthostatic vital signs). These baseline determinations are necessary to monitor the effects of cardiovascular diseases and drugs that can alter the BP during position changes. To ensure an accurate assessment, the nurse selects the cuff width most appropriate for the diameter of the client's arm.

The nurse takes the BP in both arms on admission and at least once daily thereafter. He or she reports a marked difference in pressure between the left and right arms. When charting, the nurse identifies the arm used to measure the BP and the client's position at the time it was measured. The nurse questions the client about dizziness or light-headedness when changing positions, such as rising from a sitting or lying position. These symptoms may indicate postural (or orthostatic) hypotension.

Cardiac Rhythm

The electrical activity that produces the heart rhythm can be observed continuously with bedside cardiac monitoring. Electrodes are attached to the chest and connected to a machine that displays the cardiac rhythm on an oscilloscope. The components of an ECG are discussed later in the chapter. A paper strip of the cardiac rhythm can be printed and attached to the client's record. Most cardiac monitors sound an alarm and automatically print out tracings of abnormal rhythms, called **dysrhythmias** (or arrhythmias).

A cardiac monitor reveals the heart's electrical but not its mechanical activity. The healthcare provider must palpate a peripheral pulse or auscultate the apical heart rate to obtain this information. Comparing the heart rate and rhythm with the information displayed on the monitor is important because the ECG pattern may appear normal in some clients even when mechanical function is abnormal.

Cardiac **telemetry** sends ECG information over radio waves to a monitor that is distant from the client. Paramedics use telemetry to communicate information to personnel in the hospital emergency department. Telemetry also may be used when a client's condition is stable enough to allow transfer from a critical care unit but still requires continuous monitoring. When telemetry is used, the electrodes are attached to a battery pack, which is secured inside a pocket on the client's hospital gown or clothing.

Heart Sounds

NORMAL HEART SOUNDS

Auscultation of the heart requires familiarization with normal and abnormal heart sounds. The first heart sound ("lub"), referred to as S_1, is the closing of the mitral and tricuspid valves. S_1 is heard loudest over the apex of the heart and occurs nearly simultaneously with the palpated pulse. The second heart sound ("dub"), referred to as S_2, is the closing of the aortic and pulmonic valves. S_2 is heard loudest with the stethoscope at the second intercostal space to the right of the sternum.

ABNORMAL HEART SOUNDS

All other heart sounds are abnormal and take considerable practice to recognize. A sound that follows S_1 and S_2 is called an S_3 heart sound or a ventricular gallop. When the three sounds are heard together, some say the cadence sounds like "Ken-tuck-y" or "lub-dub-dee." An S_3, although normal in children, often is an indication of heart failure in an adult. An extra sound just before S_1 is an S_4 heart sound, or atrial gallop. Some say this sound resembles the word "Ten-nes-see" or "lub-lub-dub." An S_4 sound often is associated with hypertensive heart disease.

In addition to heart sounds, auscultation may reveal other abnormal sounds, such as murmurs and clicks caused by turbulent blood flow through diseased heart valves. A friction rub may cause a rough, grating, or scratchy sound that is indicative of pericarditis (inflammation of the pericardium).

Peripheral Pulses

The nurse palpates the radial arteries and the major arteries of the leg bilaterally during the physical assessment (Fig. 30-9). He or she records the presence or absence of these pulses and their strength.

FIGURE 30-9 Proper placement of the fingers along the radial artery.

Skin

Many clients with cardiac disorders exhibit changes in skin color (e.g., cyanosis, pallor). A good light is necessary when assessing skin color. Cyanosis can be detected by carefully noting color changes in the oral mucous membranes as well as on the lips, earlobes, skin, and nail beds. In light-skinned clients, extreme pallor is easy to detect because the skin appears almost bloodless. In dark-skinned clients, a grayish cast to the skin usually indicates pallor.

During assessment of the skin, noting whether the skin is warm or cold, dry or clammy, is important. If the client has a problem with peripheral circulation, the nurse inspects the arms and legs for variations in skin color and temperature and compares his or her bilateral findings with other areas of the body. Sparse hair growth on the legs and thick toenails can indicate poor circulation. The nurse also notes any varicosities (enlargement of veins).

Peripheral Edema

Edema occurs when blood is not pumped efficiently or plasma protein levels are inadequate to maintain osmotic pressure. When right-sided heart failure occurs, blood accumulates in the great vessels and backs up in peripheral veins. Because it has nowhere else to go, the extra fluid enters the tissues. Particular areas for examination are the dependent parts of the body, such as the feet and ankles. Other areas prone to edema are the fingers, hands, and over the sacrum. To assess for edema, the examiner gently presses his or her fingers into the skin and then quickly releases. If the marks of the fingers remain, the effect is termed *pitting edema*. Edema is evaluated on a scale of +1 to +4, depending on the depth of the pit and the amount of time it takes the pit to disappear (see Chap. 22). The higher the number, the more pronounced is the edema.

Weight

Weight gain can indicate edema. A rapid gain in weight often means that edema is increasing. A 2-lb weight gain in a short period indicates that the client has an additional liter of fluid in the body. Weight loss often reflects the loss of excess fluid from the tissues and is used to evaluate the effectiveness of drug therapy, especially diuretics. If weight is recorded daily, the client is weighed at the same time, with the same amount of clothing, using the same scale, each day. The weight is recorded as accurately as possible.

Jugular Veins

If the right side of the heart fails to pump efficiently, blood becomes congested in the neck veins (Fig. 30-10). With the client sitting at a 45° angle, the client turns his or her head to the left or right so the nurse can inspect the external jugular vein. Distention of this vein usually indicates increased fluid volume and pressure in the right side of the heart (see Chap. 36).

Lung Sounds

If the left side of the heart fails to pump efficiently, blood backs up into the pulmonary veins and lung tissue. The nurse auscultates the lungs for abnormal and normal breath sounds. With left-sided congestive heart failure, auscultation reveals a crackling sound and possibly wheezes and gurgles. Wet lung sounds are accompanied by dyspnea and an effort to sit up to breathe. If uncorrected, left-sided heart failure is followed by right-sided heart failure because the circulatory system is a continuous loop.

Sputum

Clients with cardiac disease may have a productive or nonproductive cough. The nurse notes the type and frequency of the cough and the amount and appearance of

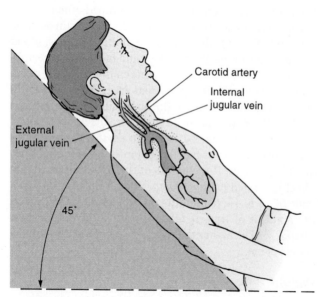

FIGURE 30-10 Jugular vein distention is assessed with the client at a 45° angle.

the sputum. These findings can be important in diagnosing heart failure or other pulmonary complications.

Mental Status

Some clients with cardiac disorders may be alert and oriented; others may be confused and disoriented. Confusion or disorientation can result from a decrease in the oxygen supply to the brain (cerebral ischemia) as a result of poor circulation. Chest pain and impaired breathing can create anxiety. The nurse reports extremes of emotion or disturbances in thought processes to the physician because such effects could interfere with the client's safety, diagnostic testing, and prescribed therapy.

Diagnostic Tests

Laboratory Tests

Various general laboratory tests are used in the diagnosis of heart disease and in monitoring the client's progress. Laboratory tests may be performed daily or every few days. They may be used to monitor the results of therapy.

BLOOD CHEMISTRY

Blood chemistries, such as fasting blood glucose and serum electrolyte, cholesterol, and triglyceride levels, may be used as part of the diagnostic analysis. Hyperglycemia (elevated blood glucose) and hypertriglyceridemia (elevated triglyceride level) indicate undiagnosed or unsuccessful control of diabetes mellitus. Diabetes mellitus (see Chap. 58) is associated with accelerated pathologic changes leading to coronary artery disease. Elevated serum sodium is associated with fluid retention and hypertension; abnormal sodium, potassium, calcium, and magnesium levels may cause dysrhythmias. A total serum cholesterol level above 200 mg/dL, a low-density lipoprotein level above 130 mg/dL, or a high-density lipoprotein level below 30 mg/dL suggests the propensity for development of atherosclerotic heart disease.

SERUM ENZYMES AND ISOENZYMES

Enzymes are complex proteins produced by living cells that function as catalysts, substances capable of producing chemical changes without being changed themselves. An **isoenzyme** is one of several forms of the same enzyme that may exist in cells and is capable of being identified separately from others.

When tissues and cells break down, are damaged, or die, great quantities of certain enzymes are released into the bloodstream. The following enzymes are important in cardiac disease:

- Troponin, an enzyme in myocardial contractile tissue
- Creatine kinase (CK), formerly creatine phosphokinase, and its isoenzymes

- Lactate dehydrogenase (LDH) and its isoenzymes
- Aspartate aminotransferase (AST), formerly serum glutamic oxaloacetic transaminase

Troponin is present only in myocardial tissue; therefore, it is specific for determining heart damage in the early stages of an MI (see Chap. 33). The other enzymes can be elevated in response to cardiac or other organ damage. Therefore, the isoenzymes CK-MB, LDH$_1$, and LDH$_2$ are evaluated for their cardiac specificity.

Electron Beam Computed Tomography

Electron beam computed tomography (EBCT) is a radiologic test that produces x-rays of the coronary arteries using an electron beam. This noninvasive test can scan the heart in 1/20 of a second using 10 times less exposure to radiation than that of mechanical computed tomography (CT) machines. EBCT also produces much clearer images for diagnostic purposes. The advantage of EBCT is that it can detect and quantify calcified plaque (Table 30-1) in the coronary arteries before clients who do not fit the usual cardiac risk profile are symptomatic. There is a high degree of correlation between the amount of calcium plaque identified by EBCT and the future risk of MI. If the test results demonstrate the existence of heart disease, treatment interventions are instituted earlier than with conventional diagnostic regimens. The efficacy of treatment or the need to modify it is evaluated by repeating the test at 1-year or longer intervals.

Radiography and Radionuclide Studies

Chest radiography and fluoroscopy are used to determine the size and position of the heart and condition of the lungs. These studies also are used to guide the insertion and confirm the placement of cardiac catheters and pacemaker wires. CT scanning and magnetic resonance imaging are used to determine heart size and detect lung involvement.

TABLE 30-1	OUTCOMES OF ELECTRON BEAM COMPUTED TOMOGRAPHY
CORONARY ARTERY CALCIUM PLAQUE SCORE	**INTERPRETATION**
0	No identifiable atherosclerotic plaque
1–10	Minimal plaque burden
11–100	Mild plaque burden
101–400	Moderate plaque burden
>400	Extensive plaque burden

(Adapted from Heart Check America. [2002]. [On-line.] Available: http://www.heartcheck.com/cas_more.htm.)

Radionuclides are radioactive chemical elements that are injected into and travel through the bloodstream. Their use sometimes is referred to as *nuclear cardiology.* The radionuclide technetium 99m is used to detect areas of myocardial damage. The radionuclide thallium 201 is used to diagnose ischemic heart disease during a stress test.

Echocardiography

Echocardiography uses ultrasound waves to determine the functioning of the left ventricle and to detect cardiac tumors, congenital defects, and changes in the tissue layers of the heart. High-frequency sound waves, which the human ear cannot hear, pass through the chest wall (transthoracic) and are displayed on an oscilloscope. The image is recorded and kept as a permanent record.

A second ultrasound technique is **transesophageal echocardiography** (TEE), which, as the name implies, involves passing a tube with a small transducer internally from the mouth to the esophagus (Fig. 30-11). When the transducer is located in the esophagus, which lies behind the heart, images of the posterior heart and its internal structures are obtained. TEE is an alternative to standard transthoracic echocardiography and provides superior

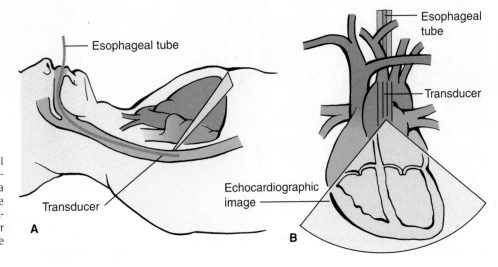

FIGURE 30-11 Transesophageal echocardiography. (**A**) An ultrasound transducer mounted on a flexible tube is passed into the esophagus. (**B**) When the transducer is at the level of the posterior heart, it transmits an image of the heart and its internal structures.

views that are not possible using the conventional technique. It also is an adjunct for assessing intraoperative complications in the heart during cardiothoracic surgery. Clients whose chests are rotund or who are obese are candidates for TEE. Because the throat is anesthetized locally, the nurse cautions the client to avoid eating or drinking until sensation and the gag reflex return, which may take 1 hour or longer after removal of the tube containing the transducer.

Phonocardiography

Phonocardiography is the graphic representation of normal and abnormal heart sounds. It is used in the diagnosis of valvular and other cardiac disorders. Microphones placed on the chest pick up heart sounds, which then are amplified and converted to electrical impulses. These impulses are relayed to a recorder, which produces a graph of the heart sounds.

Electrocardiography

Electrocardiography is the graphic recording of the electrical currents generated by the heart muscle. This method is especially helpful in identifying cardiac dysrhythmias and detecting myocardial damage. Color-coded electrodes matched to corresponding lead wires connect the client to the recording machine. The electrodes are coated with conductive gel and applied to the skin surface of the wrists, ankles, and chest (Fig. 30-12). Computerized ECG machines immediately interpret the tracings, or rhythm strips, which serve as screening devices. A physician later interprets the rhythm strips. He or she uses the 12-lead ECG to aid in diagnosing heart disease. The nurse can continuously monitor a client's cardiac activity by observing one or more leads.

The ECG pattern consists of waves, intervals, segments, and complexes (see Fig. 30-7). The P wave represents the initiation of the electrical impulse that causes depolarization of the atria. The PR interval is the time it takes for the impulse to travel from its point of initiation, through the atrial conduction pathways, to the AV node. The QRS complex, the collective term for the Q, R, and S waves, is the measurement of time that it takes for the impulse to spread throughout the ventricles from the AV node to the Purkinje fibers, causing its subsequent depolarization. The ST segment represents early repolarization of the ventricular muscle, which ends after the T wave. The ST segment is a particularly sensitive indicator of ischemia and myocardial damage. Ischemia causes the ST segment to sag below the baseline (isoelectric line). An elevated ST segment indicates muscle injury. The QT interval represents ventricular depolarization and repolarization.

AMBULATORY ELECTROCARDIOGRAPHY

Ambulatory ECG, or Holter monitoring, is the recording of an ambulatory client's cardiac rate and rhythm over 24 to 48 hours as the client performs daily activities. The Holter monitor, which is worn on a belt or carried on a shoulder strap, consists of a tape recorder connected to ECG leads attached to the client's chest (Fig. 30-13). During the test period, the client keeps a diary of activities and associated symptoms. At the end of the recording

FIGURE 30-12 The nurse attaches electrodes to the client's chest and limbs before an ECG.

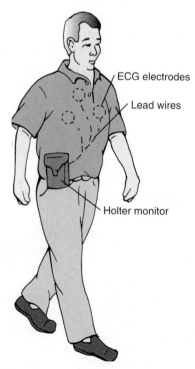

FIGURE 30-13 Ambulatory electrocardiography.

period, the monitor is returned to the hospital or physician and the tape is analyzed. The client's written notes are compared with the recorded information. Ambulatory ECG helps to detect dysrhythmias and myocardial ischemia that occur sporadically during activity or rest.

EXERCISE-INDUCED STRESS TESTING

Stress testing is done to evaluate how the heart functions during exercise. The electrical activity of the heart is assessed with an ECG monitor while the client walks on a treadmill, pedals a stationary bicycle, or climbs up and down stairs.

A resting ECG is taken as a baseline before the test is started. During the test, the speed of the treadmill, the force required to pedal the bicycle, or the pace of stair climbing is gradually increased. The goal is to increase the heart's workload until a predetermined target heart rate is reached. The client's heart rate and rhythm are monitored continuously, and ECG waveforms are recorded periodically. The client's BP and respiratory rate also are assessed. The client is instructed to report the onset of chest pain, dizziness, leg cramps, or weakness. A radionuclide such as thallium may be injected intravenously (IV) during the test, followed by a heart scan.

The stress test is aborted if the client develops chest pain, severe dyspnea, elevated BP, confusion, or dysrhythmias. The physician interprets ECG tracings obtained during the test. Radionuclides also may be used during a stress test to provide additional information.

DRUG-INDUCED STRESS TESTING

Drugs may be used to stress the heart for clients with sedentary lifestyles or those with a physical disability, such as severe arthritis, that interferes with exercise testing. Drugs such as adenosine (Adenocard), dipyridamole (Persantine), or dobutamine (Dobutrex) may be administered singularly or in combination by the IV route. The drugs dilate the coronary arteries, similar to the vasodilation that occurs when a person exercises to increase the heart muscle's blood supply. When thallium, a radionuclide, is injected a few minutes later, a scan of the heart can detect compromised blood flow, which indicates coronary artery disease, or evidence of well-perfused heart muscle.

Cardiac Catheterization

Cardiac catheterization provides a means for measuring fluid pressures in the chambers of the heart and collecting blood samples to analyze the oxygen and CO_2 content. A long, flexible catheter is inserted from a peripheral blood vessel in the groin, arm, or neck into one of the great vessels and then into the heart. Cardiac catheterization may be carried out on the left side of the heart by way of an artery or on the right side by way of a vein.

The usual length of stay is at least 5 to 9 hours or overnight. The client needs to consult the physician about which prescribed medications to take or omit the day of the cardiac catheterization. Food and fluids usually are withheld; however, if the test is late in the day, light food may be permitted. Allergies must be identified; those of primary concern before a cardiac catheterization are iodine, shellfish, radiographic dye, and latex. IV fluids are administered before the test to maintain hydration and to administer any necessary medications. A sedative is administered before the test, but anesthesia is not necessary.

While the client lies on the examination table, the site where the catheter is inserted, usually the groin or arm, is scrubbed and covered with a sterile cloth. Electrode patches with wires are attached to the chest to monitor heart rhythm. The physician injects local anesthesia at the insertion site and threads a catheter while watching its progress toward the heart on an imaging screen that also is visible to the client. Dye is instilled when the catheter reaches its destination. The client feels a brief warm sensation as the dye is administered. He or she must report chest discomfort, nausea, or difficulty breathing. Several images are taken for future evaluation. The catheter is removed and the site is covered with a pressure dressing to control bleeding; sometimes sutures also are used.

After the test, the nurse should discuss the following with the client and family:

- Keeping the extremity straight for several hours and avoiding movement are important.
- BP and pulse are monitored frequently to detect complications.
- The dressing over the insertion site is checked frequently for signs of bleeding.
- The pulse is palpated in various locations and the color and temperature in the extremity are checked to confirm that blood is circulating well.
- Report any warm, wet feeling that may indicate oozing blood, numbness, tingling, or sharp pain in the extremity.
- Drink a large volume of fluid to relieve thirst and promote the excretion of the dye.
- Follow discharge instructions (Box 30-2) for home care.

BOX 30-2 ● **Discharge Instructions for Clients Having Cardiac Catheterization**

- Rest for the next 3 days, and avoid heavy lifting, strenuous activity, or sports during this time.
- Do not drive or climb stairs for the next 24 hours.
- Do not take a tub bath until the puncture site is healed.
- Change the bandage in 24 hours; continue changing the bandage until a crust or scab forms over the puncture site.
- You may experience some soreness at the puncture site; however, if it becomes worse, notify your physician.
- If pain or swelling of the puncture site occurs, notify your physician.
- If the puncture site begins to bleed, hold pressure over the site and call 911 or another emergency services number.

Electrophysiology Studies

Clients who experience dysrhythmias may be candidates for electrophysiology studies. An **electrophysiology study** is a procedure that enables the physician to examine the electrical activity of the heart, produce actual dysrhythmias by stimulating structures in the conduction pathway, determine the best method for preventing further dysrhythmic episodes, and, in some cases, eradicate the precise location in the heart that is producing the dysrhythmia.

The test is performed by passing three flexible wire electrode catheters into veins in the neck and groin. The catheters are then advanced into the heart in each of the following locations: right atrium, bundle of His, and right ventricle (Fig. 30-14). The electrode catheters monitor and record the heart's rhythm. The physician can use these same catheters to reproduce the abnormal heart rhythm that the client usually experiences by stimulating areas in the conduction system. When the dysrhythmia is produced, the physician uses several drugs to evaluate each one's efficacy at restoring normal heart rhythm. The outcome of the trial drugs helps determine how to relieve the client's symptoms medically. The normal heart rhythm also may be restored with electrical shocks. With the catheters in place, the physician may use the opportunity to prevent the dysrhythmia from ever reoccurring by delivering electricity to the area that originates the dysrhythmia. The electricity destroys the pathogenic tissue (see discussion of radiofrequency catheter ablation, Chap. 34).

Preparation, management, and recovery for the client undergoing an electrophysiology study are similar to those for a client undergoing a heart catheterization. Usually, the client is monitored for a full day and discharged the following day if no bleeding or vascular complications occur.

Arteriography

CORONARY ARTERIOGRAPHY

The most common use of a left-sided cardiac catheterization is to determine the degree of blockage of the coronary arteries by performing arteriography while the catheter is in place. An **arteriography** is a diagnostic procedure that involves instilling dye, referred to as *contrast medium,* into an artery. In this case, it is instilled into the catheter and deposited into each coronary artery. Occlusive heart disease is indicated if one or more coronary arteries appear narrow or do not fill. Clients with coronary artery disease who are considered candidates for invasive treatment procedures must undergo cardiac catheterization and coronary arteriography.

After removal of the catheter, the nurse inspects the insertion site for bleeding, tenderness, hematoma formation, and inflammation. The client remains on bed rest for the rest of the day. He or she must avoid flexion, or bending, of the arm or leg used for catheter insertion. Vascular assessments distal to the insertion site continue at frequent intervals. Absent distal peripheral pulses, cool toes, and pale or cyanotic arms and legs indicate arterial occlusion, usually from a blood clot. These signs as well as a rapid or irregular pulse rate indicate a medical emergency that the nurse must report immediately to the physician.

ANGIOCARDIOGRAPHY

In **angiocardiography,** a radiopaque dye is injected into a vein, and its course through the heart is recorded by a series of radiographic pictures taken in rapid succession. The pictures reveal the size and shape of the heart chambers and great vessels and the sequence and time of their filling with dye. Angiocardiography is used particularly to diagnose congenital abnormalities of the heart and great vessels. It usually is performed when simpler diagnostic measures fail to provide the necessary information. The client fasts for at least 3 hours before the test. A sedative and an antihistaminic medication usually are administered before the client is taken to the radiography department.

AORTOGRAPHY

Aortography detects aortic abnormalities such as aneurysms (abnormal dilatation of a blood vessel wall) and arterial occlusions. When aortography is performed, contrast medium is injected and radiographic films are taken of the abdominal aorta and major arteries in the legs. Distribution of the contrast medium also may be observed as it circulates to other vessels, such as the renal arteries.

PERIPHERAL ARTERIOGRAPHY

Peripheral arteriography is used to diagnose occlusive arterial disease in smaller arteries. Contrast medium is

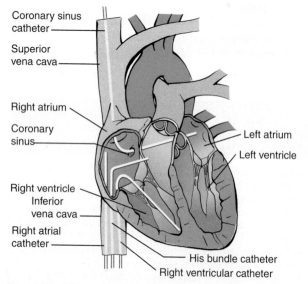

Coronary sinus catheter

Superior vena cava

Right atrium

Coronary sinus

Left atrium

Left ventricle

Right ventricle

Inferior vena cava

Right atrial catheter

His bundle catheter

Right ventricular catheter

FIGURE 30-14 During an electrophysiology test, flexible wires are advanced from a site in the groin to record the natural heart rhythm and allow electrical stimulation to provoke a dysrhythmia.

injected into an artery, and radiographic films are taken. After the procedure, the chance for bleeding is greater than after a venipuncture; therefore, a pressure dressing is applied and client activity is restricted for about 12 hours. The nurse observes the client for bleeding and cardiac dysrhythmias and assesses the adequacy of peripheral circulation by frequently checking the peripheral pulses.

Hemodynamic Monitoring

Hemodynamic monitoring is used to assess the volume and pressure of blood in the heart and vascular system by means of a surgically inserted catheter. Such monitoring is used to assess cardiac function and circulatory status, detect fluid imbalances, adjust fluid infusion rates, and evaluate the client's response to therapeutic measures, such as drug therapy. Methods for hemodynamic monitoring include direct BP monitoring, central venous pressure (CVP) monitoring, and pulmonary artery pressure monitoring.

DIRECT BLOOD PRESSURE MONITORING

Direct BP monitoring requires the placement of a catheter in a peripheral artery. The artery most commonly used is the radial artery. The brachial and femoral arteries also may be used. The catheter tip contains a sensor that measures and transmits the fluid pressure to a transducer, which electronically converts the data to a visual waveform. A monitor continuously displays the waveform and indicates the client's systolic, diastolic, and mean arterial pressures. This type of equipment eliminates the need to auscultate the BP. Direct BP monitoring may be used in clients with severe and sustained hypertension or hypotension, and during and after surgery in clients who have undergone cardiac surgery. A three-way stopcock can be attached to the tubing to allow the nurse periodically to draw arterial blood samples for blood gas analysis.

CENTRAL VENOUS PRESSURE MONITORING

Right atrial pressure, or **central venous pressure,** is the pressure produced by venous blood in the right atrium. Normal CVP is 2 to 7 mm Hg or 4 to 10 cm H_2O. This measurement is used to detect an excess or a deficit in venous blood volume.

To monitor CVP, a catheter is inserted into a large vein, usually the jugular or subclavian vein in the neck, and advanced into the superior vena cava. The catheter's proximal end is connected to a three-way stopcock, which controls the direction in which IV fluid flows. The stopcock may be mounted on a calibrated tube, called a *manometer* (or the catheter may be attached to a transducer that connects to a computer used to analyze hemodynamic data). The manometer is used periodically to measure fluid pressure. The nurse must be familiar with the type of CVP manometer being used.

When measuring CVP, the nurse makes sure that the zero mark on the manometer is at the level of the client's right atrium; otherwise, an incorrect reading is obtained. The client is positioned supine or with the head slightly elevated but in exactly the same position as during previous measurements. The stopcock is rotated so that the manometer is partially filled with IV solution. The fluid in the manometer is then allowed to flow into the client. The fluid stops flowing when the pressure in the manometer equals the pressure in the right atrium. The CVP measurement is obtained by noting the calibrated mark on the manometer that corresponds with the top of the fluid column (Fig. 30-15). The stopcock is then repositioned to resume the infusion of IV fluid. Between CVP measurements, the head of the bed can be raised or lowered. The physician orders the frequency of CVP measurements; however, the nurse may obtain measurements any time he or she suspects a change in the client's fluid status.

PULMONARY ARTERY MONITORING

By inserting a catheter into the pulmonary artery, pressures and cardiac output can be measured to assess left ventricular function. When in place, the pulmonary artery

FIGURE 30-15 Central venous pressure (CVP) measured by a water manometer. The arrow points to the zero mark, which must be at the level of the client's right atrium. (**A**) Stopcock position for filling the manometer. (**B**) Position for measuring CVP. (**C**) Position for allowing IV solution to flow through the tubing to the client, keeping the CVP line patent.

catheter, a multilumen catheter, can measure both pulmonary artery pressure and right atrial pressure or CVP. Pulmonary artery pressure monitoring aids in the early treatment of fluid imbalances, prevents left-sided congestive heart failure or promotes its early correction, and helps monitor the client's response to treatment.

The pulmonary artery catheter is inserted into a large peripheral vein and advanced through the right side of the heart until the distal tip rests in the right or left pulmonary artery. When the small balloon at the tip of the catheter is inflated, the balloon floats forward, eventually wedging in a pulmonary capillary (Fig. 30-16). As the balloon blocks the flow of blood through the capillary, the catheter tip that protrudes from the inflated balloon senses the fluid pressure ahead of it. **Pulmonary capillary wedge pressure** is the retrograde pressure from the fluid on the left side of the heart at the end of left ventricular diastole. Sometimes this is abbreviated LVEDP, for **left ventricular end-diastolic pressure.** The balloon must be deflated immediately after the pressure is measured to avoid pulmonary infarction from prolonged blockage of capillary blood flow.

To measure cardiac output, a syringe with 5 to 10 mL of 5% dextrose in water solution (D_5W) is pushed through a port of the catheter. In the past, iced injectate was used, but with the newer computers, injectate at room temperature may be used. A computerized probe measures the temperature change as the fluid exits the catheter in the heart. The computer then calculates the rate of temperature change with the speed at which the fluid traveled through the heart. A solution that is quite warm after its instillation indicates impairment of the heart's pump function. If the solution remains close to the instillation temperature, the heart's pump function is working optimally. The computer converts the electronic data into numerical equivalents for cardiac output. The nurse repeats the assessment three to four times in succession and takes the average of the data. Using a formula, the nurse can calculate the **cardiac index,** which reflects the cardiac output in relation to the particular client's body size. The cardiac index is computed by dividing the cardiac output by the client's body surface area. Body surface area is obtained from a **nomogram,** a chart based on height and weight.

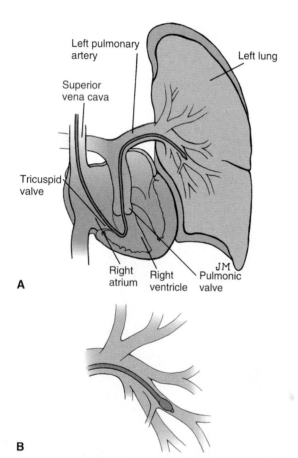

FIGURE 30-16 Fluid status can be monitored with a pulmonary artery catheter. (**A**) Location of the catheter in the heart. The catheter enters the right atrium through the superior vena cava. The balloon is then inflated, allowing the catheter to follow the blood flow through the tricuspid valve, right ventricle, pulmonic valve, and main pulmonary artery. Waveform and pressure readings are noted during insertion to identify the location of the catheter within the heart. The balloon is deflated once the catheter is in the pulmonary artery and properly secured. (**B**) Pulmonary capillary wedge pressure (PCWP). The catheter floats into a distal branch of the pulmonary artery when the balloon is inflated and becomes "wedged." The wedged catheter occludes blood flow from behind, and the tip of the lumen records pressures in front of the catheter. The balloon is then deflated, allowing the catheter to float back into the main pulmonary artery.

NURSING PROCESS

● **Diagnostic Procedures of the Cardiovascular System**

Assessment

For both outpatients and inpatients, the nurse performs a thorough initial assessment of clients undergoing diagnostic testing to establish accurate baseline data for use before, during, and after the procedure. The nurse weighs the client and measures vital signs. He or she may measure BP in both arms and compare findings. The nurse assesses apical and radial pulses, noting rate, quality, and rhythm. He or she checks peripheral pulses in the lower extremities.

The nurse asks the client to describe any symptoms. If the client is experiencing chest pain, a history of its location, frequency, and duration is necessary, as is a description of the pain, if it radiates to a particular area, what precipitates its onset, and what brings relief. Another important area of questioning is whether the client is experiencing pressure, fluttering, or palpitations in the chest. The nurse asks if the client has episodes of dyspnea, dizziness, or fainting. He or she assesses the lower extremities for edema and toes for color and temperature.

The nurse auscultates heart and lung sounds and obtains family history of heart disease or other chronic diseases that are related to cardiovascular disorders such as diabetes mellitus. Another important area is the identification of current prescribed medications, herbal preparations, and over-the-counter drugs used for self-treatment. The nurse also determines the client's anxiety and knowledge level about the procedure.

Diagnosis, Planning, and Interventions

Anxiety related to insecurity

Expected Outcome: Anxiety will be reduced to whatever the client identifies as tolerable using a scale from 0 to 10.

- Greet client by name and introduce personnel involved in care. *Introductions are a common courtesy, promote personal involvement, and eliminate the feeling of being cared for by strangers.*
- Promote a relaxed environment by sitting during the interview, reducing unnecessary noise and activity, and giving client time to think and respond to questions. *A relaxed nurse promotes relaxation in the client. Rushing or exposing the client to sensory stimulation is likely to communicate and heighten anxiety.*
- Orient client to surroundings. *Familiarity with the testing area and equipment that will be used reduces fears that may be highly exaggerated.*
- Tell client when the test will begin and how long it will take. *Giving the client a time frame reduces anticipatory anxiety.*
- Keep client informed of unexpected delays. *Providing information decreases anxiety.*
- Remain in view of the client or establish some other means of contact for assistance such as a signal light. *Knowing that he or she can summon the nurse for questions or assistance is reassuring to the client.*

Deficient Knowledge related to the test's purpose, performance, and after-care

Expected Outcome: Client and family will demonstrate sufficient knowledge from which to provide informed consent and perform self-care afterward.

- Assess client's and family's knowledge of the diagnostic procedure. *Clarifying any misconceptions or misinformation and building on what is already known are important interventions.*
- Provide both verbal and written information concerning the test's purpose, procedure, and after-care. *Written information enables the client to further process the verbal information and serves as a basis for recalling verbal instructions.*
- Use language that the client can easily understand. *Medical terminology that is not part of the client's vocabulary may heighten anxiety and intimidate the client to the extent that he or she may not ask further questions.*
- Ask client, family, or both to paraphrase information. *The ability to paraphrase provides evidence as to whether they understood information the nurse provided.*

Pain and **Activity Intolerance** related to ischemia

Expected Outcomes: (1) Pain will be relieved or controlled within a tolerable level during the diagnostic procedure. (2) Activity will be limited to that which avoids dyspnea or tachycardia.

- Assess pain level (see Chap. 21) frequently before, during, and after the diagnostic procedure. *Pain is a subjective symptom that the nurse can reliably assess only by asking the client to rate and describe it.*
- Allow for rest periods. *Rest reduces heart rate and demand for increased oxygenated blood.*
- Stop the procedure, assess vital signs, give a short-acting prescribed vasodilator such as nitroglycerin, and administer oxygen if chest pain occurs. *Monitoring and treating chest pain with prescribed interventions that improve blood flow to the heart are within the interdependent nursing domain.*
- Notify the physician if rest, oxygen, or prescribed medications do not provide relief. *Sustained chest pain may require medical assessment and additional interventions.*

Risk for Injury related to untoward reactions during or after diagnostic tests

Expected Outcome: The client's condition will remain stable during and after diagnostic tests.

- Assess for dyspnea, hypotension or hypertension, cardiac dysrhythmias, mental changes, pain or discomfort, and cyanosis. *Post-test findings that differ significantly from pretest results are highly suggestive of a cause-and-effect relationship between the test's physiologic requirements and the client's response.*
- Implement nursing measures to stabilize the client, such as ensuring a patent IV access and administering oxygen and prescribed medications. *The nurse's role includes independent, interdependent, and dependent nursing actions.*
- Collaborate with the physician to restore client to a stable condition. *The physician's role is to manage complications medically; the nurse assists the physician.*

Evaluation of Expected Outcomes

The client is relaxed and feels secure. The test is performed uneventfully or the client is stabilized when complications are managed successfully. The client and family have an accurate understanding of the diagnostic testing process and discharge instructions.

GENERAL NUTRITIONAL CONSIDERATIONS

Food and fluid are withheld before invasive diagnostic procedures and are not resumed until the client is stable and free of nausea and vomiting.

GENERAL PHARMACOLOGIC CONSIDERATIONS

Medications can affect BP and pulse rate and rhythm. When conducting a medication history, obtaining a list of all prescription and nonprescription medications and medicinal herbs from the client or a family member is very important.

When a contrast medium is used during a cardiac catheterization or arteriogram, the client may feel an intense flushed feeling and the need to void when the dye is injected. Inform the client that these feelings will pass soon (30 to 60 seconds).

Assess the client for iodine or seafood allergy before beginning any diagnostic test requiring an iodinated contrast. Usually, a hypoallergenic nonionic contrast may be used if an allergy is suspected.

GENERAL GERONTOLOGIC CONSIDERATIONS

Older clients are more likely to experience confusion and disorientation because of advanced arteriosclerotic and atherosclerotic age-related changes that cause decreased perfusion to the brain. Repeated explanations and reassurances throughout all phases of the nursing process are indicated.

The aging heart is less able to meet the demands placed on it during times of stress and requires more time to return to baseline levels after stress. This inability to handle stress results from decreased cardiac output and contractile strength and delayed conduction in the heart.

The older adult who has renal impairment or is chronically dehydrated is at increased risk for complications during and after diagnostic studies requiring the use of a dye because the iodinated contrast is nephrotoxic.

The incidence of cardiac dysrhythmias increases with age because of anatomic changes that accompany aging. Dysrhythmias also are more serious and difficult to treat in the older adult because organs that already are impaired by aging can be further compromised by the lack of adequate blood supply caused by the dysrhythmia.

Critical Thinking Exercises

1. *An outpatient client is scheduled to have a cardiac catheterization. The client's spouse asks you what the catheter is for and what will happen once it is placed. How will you respond?*
2. *You are assisting a client who is undergoing an exercise-induced stress test. What assessments would indicate that the client is responding adversely to the exercise?*

References and Suggested Readings

American Heart Association. (2001). Calcium scan predicts heart attack risk in physically fit people. [On-line.] Available: http://www.americanheart.org/presenter.jhtml?identifier=3292.

Beattie, S. (1999). Cut the risks for cardiac cath patients. *RN, 62*(1), 50–55.

Bickley, L. S. & Hoekelman, R. A. (1998). *Bates' guide to physical examination and history taking* (7th ed.). Philadelphia: Lippincott Williams & Wilkins.

Brown, K. A., Rosman, D. R., & Dave, R. M. (2000). Stress nuclear myocardial perfusion imaging versus stress echocardiography: prognostic comparisons. *Progress in Cardiovascular Diseases, 45*, 231–244.

Budoff, M. J. & Raggi, P. (2001). Coronary artery disease progression assessed by electron-beam computed tomography. *American Journal of Cardiology, 88*(2-1), 46-E–50-E.

Bullock, B. L. & Henze, R. L. (2000). *Focus on pathophysiology.* Philadelphia: Lippincott Williams & Wilkins.

Dabbs, A. D., Walsh, R. M., Beck, J., et al. (1999). Nursing assessment of patient readiness for ambulation after cardiac catheterization. *MEDSURG Nursing, 8*, 309–314.

Gauss, A., Ruhm, H., & Schduffelen, A. (2001). Electrocardiographic exercise testing for cardiac risk assessment in patients undergoing noncardiac surgery. *Anesthesiology, 94*, 38–46.

Gottdiener, J. S. (2001). Overview of stress echocardiography: Uses, advantages, and limitations. *Progress in Cardiovascular Diseases, 43*, 315–334.

He, Z., Hedrick, T. D., Pratt, C. M., et al. (2000). Severity of coronary artery calcification by electron beam computed tomography predicts silent myocardial ischemia. [On-line.] Available: http://circ.ahajournals.org/cgi/content/abstract/101/3/244.

Ide, B. & Drew, B. (2001). EKG clinical questions: How a rhythm strip aids in clinical diagnosis. *Progress in Cardiovascular Nursing, 16*(2), 88.

Karras, D. J. & Kane, D. L. (2001). Serum markers in the emergency department diagnosis of acute myocardial infarction. *Emergency Medicine Clinics of North America, 19*, 321–337.

Kleinpell, R. M. (1999). New cardiac catheterization technology shortens hospital stays, reduces patient discomfort. *Nursing Spectrum, 9*(25), 26–27.

Khorovets, A. (2000). What is an electrocardiogram (ECG)? *Internet Journal of Advanced Nursing Practice, 4*(2), 6.

Marolf, G. A., Kuhn, A., & White, R. D. (2001). Exercise testing in special populations: Athletes, women, and the elderly. *Primary Care: Clinics in Office Practice, 28*(1), 55–72.

Martini, F. H. (1998). *Fundamentals of anatomy and physiology.* Englewood Cliffs, NJ: Prentice-Hall.

Ott, K., Johnson, K., & Ahrens, T. (2001). New technologies in the assessment of hemodynamic parameters. *Journal of Cardiovascular Nursing, 15*(2), 41–55.

Rogers, G. P. & Winters, W. L. (2000). American College of Cardiology/American Heart Association clinical competence statement on stress testing. *Circulation, 102*, 1726–1738.

Schickel, S. I., Adkisson, P., Miracle, V., et al. (1999). Achieving femoral artery hemostasis after cardiac catheterization: A comparison of methods. *American Journal of Critical Care, 8*, 406–409.

Stein, R. A., Chaitman, R. R., Balady, G. J., et al. (2000). AHA science advisory. Safety and utility of exercise testing in emergency room chest pain centers: An advisory from the Committee on Exercise, Rehabilitation, and Prevention, Council on Clinical Cardiology, American Heart Association. *Circulation, 102*, 1463–1467.

Tasota, F. J. & Tate, J. (2000). Eye on diagnostics: Understanding transesophageal echocardiography. *Nursing, 30*(8), 26.

Way, S., Redeker, N. S., Moreyra, A. E., et al. (2001). Comparison of comfort and local complications after cardiac catheterization. *Clinical Nursing Research, 10*(1), 29–39.

White, R. D. & Evans, C. H. (2001). Performing the exercise test. *Primary Care: Clinics in Office Practice, 28*(1), 29–53.

Caring for Clients With Infectious and Inflammatory Disorders of the Heart and Blood Vessels

Words to Know

cardiac tamponade
cardiomyopathy
decortication
deep vein thrombosis
effusion
emboli
Homans' sign
impedance
    plethysmography
infective endocarditis
intermittent claudication
murmur
myocardial disarray
myocarditis
myofibrils
pericardiectomy
pericardiocentesis
pericardiostomy
pericarditis
petechiae

polyarthritis
postphlebitic syndrome
precordial pain
pulmonary embolus
pulsus paradoxus
rheumatic carditis
splinter hemorrhages
sympathectomy
syncope
thrombectomy
thromboangiitis
    obliterans
thrombophlebitis
vegetations
vena caval filter
vena caval plication
    procedure
venography
ventriculomyomectomy
Virchow's triad

Learning Objectives

On completion of this chapter, the reader will:

- List four inflammatory conditions of the heart.
- Identify three organisms that cause infectious conditions of the heart.
- Describe treatment for inflammatory and infectious heart disorders.
- Discuss the nursing management of clients with infectious or inflammatory heart disorders.
- Name three types of cardiomyopathy.
- Differentiate between thrombophlebitis and thromboangiitis obliterans.
- List three interventions that reduce the risk of thrombophlebitis.
- Discuss the nursing management of clients with inflammatory disorders of peripheral blood vessels.

The body uses many defense mechanisms to combat the effects of trauma, disease, and microorganisms. The inflammatory response, skin and mucous membranes, and immune system work together to protect the body's cardiovascular system. Despite these protective mechanisms, infectious and inflammatory disorders may compromise the heart and blood vessels.

INFECTIOUS AND INFLAMMATORY DISORDERS OF THE HEART

● RHEUMATIC FEVER AND RHEUMATIC CARDITIS

Rheumatic fever is a systemic inflammatory disease that sometimes follows group A streptococcal infection of the throat. **Rheumatic carditis** refers to the inflammatory cardiac manifestations of rheumatic fever in either the acute or later stage. Cardiac structures that usually are affected include (1) heart valves, particularly the mitral valve; (2) endocardium; (3) myocardium; and (4) pericardium.

Pathophysiology and Etiology

The inflammatory symptoms of rheumatic carditis are believed to be induced by antibodies originally formed to destroy the group A beta-hemolytic streptococcal microorganisms. The antibodies, however, "mistakenly" cross-react against the proteins in the connective tissue of the heart, joints, skin, and nervous system (Fig. 31-1). This cross-reaction causes valvular damage and *pancarditis,*

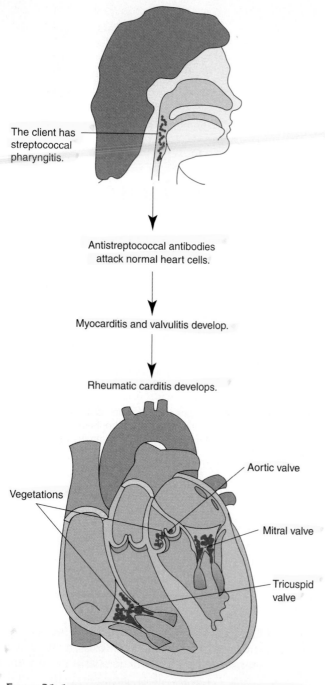

The client has streptococcal pharyngitis.

↓

Antistreptococcal antibodies attack normal heart cells.

↓

Myocarditis and valvulitis develop.

↓

Rheumatic carditis develops.

Vegetations

Aortic valve

Mitral valve

Tricuspid valve

FIGURE 31-1 Rheumatic carditis after group A streptococcal pharyngitis.

inflammation of all layers of the heart (endocardium, myocardium, and pericardium).

As the antibody response ensues, white blood cells (WBCs) migrate to the endocardium, causing inflammatory debris to accumulate as **vegetations** around the valve leaflets. When the inflammatory process is relieved, fibrinous tissue that fuses or thickens valve leaflets and shortens the chordae tendineae replaces the damaged areas. The valves may subsequently lose their ability to

open fully or close tightly (see Chap. 32). The fibrinous replacements also cause surface irregularities around the valves, making them prone to future colonization by blood-borne bacteria.

The antibodies also attack cardiac myosin, the muscle protein in myocardial tissue. Because myosin is instrumental in cardiac muscle contraction, rheumatic carditis may cause weakened heart contractions and heart failure (see Chap. 36). If the pericardium is involved, it becomes tough and leathery from accumulated fibrinous fluid that interferes with the heart's ability to stretch and fill with blood. Tachydysrhythmias, fast abnormal heart rhythms, develop to compensate for the decreased cardiac output, the volume of blood ejected from the left ventricle per minute. After the acute episode, most clients recover, but valvular changes remain.

Assessment Findings

Signs and Symptoms

Acute rheumatic fever is most common in children 2 to 3 weeks after a streptococcal infection. Carditis (inflammation of the layers of the heart), **polyarthritis** (inflammation of more than one joint), rash, subcutaneous nodules, and chorea characterized by involuntary grimacing and an inability to use skeletal muscles in a coordinated manner are the classic symptoms. Adults do not exhibit the same degree and range of symptoms as young children.

A mild fever, if untreated, continues for several weeks. The heart rate is rapid and rhythms may be abnormal. A red, spotty rash appears on the trunk but disappears rapidly, with irregular circles on the skin remaining. Several joints, most commonly the knees, ankles, hips, and shoulders, become swollen, warm, red, and painful. The involvement migrates across joints. Sometimes marble-sized nodules appear around the joints. Central nervous system manifestations result in chorea. Cardiac complications may develop: a heart murmur suggests valve damage; a pericardial friction rub indicates pericarditis; and congestive heart failure (CHF) develops if the myocardium fails to compensate for functional demands.

Diagnostic Findings

No laboratory test is specific for the diagnosis of rheumatic fever. The results of laboratory tests such as an antistreptolysin O titer, erythrocyte sedimentation rate (ESR), and C-reactive protein are elevated, indicating an inflammatory process involving the streptococcal organism. Specific cardiac tests, such as electrocardiography (ECG) and echocardiography, may show structural changes in the valves, size of the heart, and the heart's ability to contract.

Medical and Surgical Management

Intravenous (IV) antibiotics are given. Penicillin is the drug of choice for group A streptococci, unless contraindicated because of an allergy. For clients who are allergic to the penicillin family of antibiotics, another antibiotic such as azithromycin (Zithromax), clindamycin (Cleocin), or vancomycin (Vancocin) may be prescribed. Cephalosporins such as cephalexin (Keflex) or cefadroxil (Duricef) may be prescribed if the client has not had a previous severe allergic reaction to penicillin. Bed rest may be indicated depending on the client's condition. Aspirin is used to control the formation of blood clots around heart valves. Steroids are used to suppress the inflammatory response.

Concurrent treatment of rheumatic carditis depends on the extent of heart involvement. If minor, no treatment may be given; if heart failure or life-threatening dysrhythmias occur, extensive treatment is necessary. Surgery may be required to treat constrictive pericarditis and damage to heart valves. Prophylactic antibiotic therapy is recommended before future procedures that are associated with the dissemination of microorganisms that can lead to bacteremia and recurrence of endocarditis (Box 31-1).

Nursing Management

The nurse administers prescribed drug therapy and monitors for therapeutic and adverse effects. He or she plans diversional activities that require minimal activity, such

as reading and putting puzzles together, to reduce the work of the myocardium and counteract the boredom of weeks of bed rest. Focused cardiac assessments help to track the progression or improvement of heart involvement. Clients with a history of rheumatic fever are susceptible to infective endocarditis (discussed next) and are told to take prophylactic antibiotics before any invasive procedure, including dental work. Additional nursing management depends on assessment data.

Stop, Think, and Respond ● BOX 31-1

What information is important to provide parents whose children develop a severe sore throat?

● INFECTIVE ENDOCARDITIS

Infective endocarditis (formerly called *bacterial endocarditis*) is inflammation of the inner layer of heart tissue as a result of an infectious microorganism. Although clients with rheumatic carditis do develop endocarditis, it is initially considered an autoimmune response—not an infection—because no microorganism can be isolated from blood or other cultured specimens. Subsequent to the initial rheumatic carditis, however, the valvular changes increase the client's susceptibility to endocardial colonization by pathogens. In addition to clients who have recovered from rheumatic carditis, other susceptible clients include those who have nonrheumatic valve disease or artificial heart valves, repaired congenital heart defects, a prolapsed mitral valve, or hypertrophic cardiomyopathy (discussed later); IV drug users; and immunosuppressed clients with central venous catheters.

Pathophysiology and Etiology

The microorganisms that cause infective endocarditis include bacteria and fungi (Box 31-2). *Streptococcus viridans* and *Staphylococcus aureus* are the bacteria most frequently responsible for this disorder. They are found abundantly on the skin and mucous membranes of the mouth, nose, throat, and other cavities.

Most pathogens find their way into the bloodstream through trauma caused by invasive procedures involving mucous membranes or other tissues that harbor microorganisms. Although anyone can contract endocarditis, clients with a history of rheumatic carditis are especially susceptible. Prolonged IV therapy, insertion of cardiac pacemakers, cardiac catheterization, tracheal intubation, cardiac surgery, genitourinary instrumentation (Foley catheters and cystoscopy), and IV drug abuse create portals of entry for the causative microorganisms. Once the

---

BOX 31-1 ● High-Risk Procedures for Clients With a History of Rheumatic Carditis or Infective Endocarditis

Prophylactic antibiotic therapy is recommended before:

- Dental procedures associated with significant bleeding from hard or soft tissues, including tooth extraction, dental implant and reimplantation, teeth cleaning, scaling, periodontal surgery, root canal instrumentation, orthodontic band placement (initial), and intraligamentary local anesthetic injections
- Gastrointestinal procedures associated with a high rate of transient bacteremia, such as dilation of esophageal stricture, sclerotherapy of esophageal varices, biliary tract surgery or instrumentation (e.g., endoscopic retrograde cholangiography), and operative procedures involving the intestinal mucosa
- Genitourinary surgery, instrumentation, or diagnostic procedures, especially in the presence of a urinary tract infection, such as transurethral resection of the prostate, cystoscopy, urethral dilation, and urethral catheterization
- Respiratory tract procedures that involve bronchoscopy with a rigid endoscope or surgery involving respiratory mucosa such as a tonsillectomy and adenoidectomy

Adapted from Dajani, A. S., Tauber, K. A., & Wilson, W. [1997]. Prevention of bacterial endocarditis: Recommendations by the American Heart Association. [On-line.] Available: http://www.americanheart.org/Scientific/statements/1997/079701.html.

BOX 31-2 ● Microorganisms That Cause Endocarditis

Streptococci	Account for 55% of cases of endocarditis
Group A beta-hemolytic	Attack normal or damaged heart valves and may cause rapid destruction
S. bovis	Related to GI malignancy
S. viridans	Tend to affect previously damaged heart valves
Staphylococci	Cause 30% of cases of endocarditis
S. aureus	Virulent strain with high mortality rate
S. epidermidis	Associated with dental procedures and valve replacements
S. faecalis	Cause both acute and subacute infections
	Associated with urologic instrumentation in men, bacteremia, respiratory tract infections, pneumonia, sinusitis, otitis media, and epiglotitis
Enterococci	Normal inhabitants of the GI tract, anterior urethra, and occasionally the mouth
E. faecalis and E. faecium	Relatively resistant to single antibiotics; require combination of antibiotic therapy for a minimum of 4 weeks
HACEK Group	Slow-growing gram-negative bacilli
Haemophilus parainfluenzae and Haemophilus aphrophilus	Require culture for 2 weeks or longer when initial culture is negative
	Cause subacute presentations
Actinobacillus actinomycetemcomitans	Associated with very large vegetations
Cardiobacterium hominis	
Eikenella corrodens	
Kingella kingae	
Fungi	Increased incidence in IV drug users
Candida	Risk increased with improper use of antibiotics and steroids
Gram-negative bacteria	May travel from GI or genitourinary tracts
Escherichia coli	
Klebsiella	Increased risk in older adults
Pseudomonas	

GI, gastrointestinal.

FIGURE 31-2 Bacterial endocarditis. The mitral valve shows destructive vegetations. (Rubin E., & Farber J. L. [1999]. *Pathology* [3rd ed., p. 572]. Philadelphia: Lippincott Williams & Wilkins.)

ciency as a pump. Heart failure often is a consequence. The vegetations can break off to form **emboli,** mobile masses of fibrin and clusters of platelets that circulate in the bloodstream. Emboli may occlude small blood vessels and interfere with an organ's blood supply.

Assessment Findings

Signs and Symptoms

Infective endocarditis can have an acute onset (less than 1 week) from a previously healthy state. The client presents with fever, chills, muscle aches in the lower back and thighs, and joint pain. Subacute infections progress more insidiously over weeks to months with more vague manifestations like headache, malaise, fatigue, and sleep disturbances. As the condition advances, purplish, painful nodules may appear on the pads of the fingers and toes. Black longitudinal lines, called **splinter hemorrhages,** can be seen in the nails. The spleen may be enlarged, and tenderness may be noted on abdominal palpation. A heart murmur may be present from malfunctioning valves. **Petechiae,** tiny, reddish hemorrhagic spots on the skin and mucous membranes, are signs of embolization. Pronounced weakness, anorexia, and weight loss are common. Symptoms can change suddenly if embolization or heart failure occurs. Emboli to the brain cause cerebrovascular accidents (see Chap. 46); emboli to the kidneys cause flank pain and renal failure (see Chap. 64); pulmonary emboli result in sudden chest pain and dyspnea (see Chap. 29). Clients with heart failure present with dyspnea, hypotension, and peripheral or pulmonary edema.

Diagnostic Findings

Anemia and slight leukocytosis are common findings. A series of three blood cultures collected over 1 to 24 hours

microorganisms migrate to the endocardial surface, they attach themselves to the vegetations composed of fibrin and platelets surrounding the heart valves, chordae tendineae, and papillary muscles (Fig. 31-2). The microorganisms bury themselves in the vegetative mass, making them difficult to destroy with natural defenses or antibiotic therapy. The cycle continues with layer upon layer of imbedded microorganisms and fibrin/platelet deposits.

The endocardium on the left side of the heart is affected more often than on the right. The mitral valve is the most common location of vegetations and microbial deposits. If the valve leaflets erode and slough, blood leaks between the heart chambers, diminishing the heart's effiusually identifies the microorganism circulating in the blood. Some cultured specimens require incubation for 3 weeks or more to identify accurately the infecting species. Occasionally the vegetations also can be cultured. Transesophageal echocardiography is more likely than transthoracic echocardiography to reveal the vegetations, altered valvular function, and impaired pumping quality of the ventricles. ECG may reveal abnormalities in heart rhythm if the vegetations involve a valve close to conduction tissue.

Medical and Surgical Management

High doses of an IV antibiotic to which the organism is susceptible are prescribed initially (Drug Therapy Table 31-1). Antibiotic therapy extends at least 2 to 6 weeks. It is resumed if the infection recurs after discontinuation of the drug. Bed rest is ordered initially. When the client begins to improve, bathroom privileges and increased activity are allowed. If a heart valve has been severely damaged and drug therapy does not adequately support the

DRUG THERAPY TABLE 31-1	**AGENTS USED TO TREAT ENDOCARDITIS**		
DRUG	MECHANISM OF ACTION	SIDE EFFECTS	NURSING CONSIDERATIONS
penicillin G (Pfizerpen, Pentids, Wycillin, Bicillin)	Inhibits cell wall synthesis of organisms sensitive to penicillin G, killing the organisms	Allergic reaction: rash, fever, wheezing; possibly anaphylaxis and death Nausea, vomiting, diarrhea, abdominal pain, glossitis, stomatitis, gastritis, furry tongue	Be sure to check client's allergy history before administering. In acute care settings, retrieve the antibiotic from the refrigerator 15 minutes before administration. Evaluate the IV site for phlebitis before and after administration. Administer IM penicillin deep into the muscle mass.
nafcillin (Unipen)	Inhibits cell wall synthesis of organisms sensitive to nafcillin, killing the organisms	Lethargy, hallucinations, seizures, glossitis, stomatitis, gastritis, furry tongue, anemia, nephritis	Use cautiously in clients with renal disorders. If giving IM, alternate sites. Repeated use of the same site can result in atrophy. Be sure to administer oral forms 1 hour before or 2 hours after meals. Do not administer with soft drinks or fruit juices.
gentamicin (Garamycin, Gentacidin)	Inhibits protein synthesis in gram-negative, susceptible strains Appears to disrupt function of bacterial cell membranes, killing the bacteria	Tinnitus, dizziness, vertigo, nausea, vomiting, palpitations, purpura, rash, fever, apnea, irreversible ototoxicity, nephrotoxicity	Give by IM route if possible. Ensure that the client receives adequate hydration throughout therapy. Monitor results of renal function tests, complete blood counts, and serum drug levels.
ceftriaxone (Rocephin)	Inhibits cell wall synthesis of bacteria sensitive to ceftriaxone, killing the organisms	Nausea, vomiting, diarrhea, anorexia, abdominal pain, flatulence, rash, fever, pain, superinfections	Advise clients to avoid alcohol and substances that contain alcohol to prevent a disulfiram-like reaction. Protect the drug from exposure to light. For clients with renal or hepatic impairment, monitor blood levels of the drug to prevent toxicity.
vancomycin (Vancocin)	Inhibits cell wall synthesis of bacteria sensitive to vancomycin, killing the organisms	Ototoxicity, nausea, nephrotoxicity, urticaria (hives)	When clients are receiving long-term therapy, continually monitor results of renal function tests. Advise the client not to discontinue the drug without notifying the physician.
rifampin (Rifradin)	Inhibits RNA polymerase activity in sensitive bacterial cells	Headache, drowsiness, fatigue, dizziness, heartburn, epigastric distress, eosinophilia, thrombocytopenia, rash, "flulike syndrome"	Administer this drug to a client with an empty stomach 1 hour before or 2 hours after meals. Advise client that this drug will color body fluids orange-red. Tell the client to report fever, chills, muscle and bone pain, fatigue, anorexia, yellow skin or eye, or unusual bruising, bleeding, rash, or itching.

heart in failure, valve replacement may be necessary (see Chaps. 32 and 37).

Nursing Management

Many clients cannot appreciate the danger of the disease without seeing external signs of the damage. The nurse gently but firmly reminds the client to limit activity. He or she continually assesses for changes in weight and pulse rate and rhythm and notes and reports new symptoms. The nurse administers prescribed antibiotics around the clock to sustain therapeutic blood levels of the medication at all times. He or she informs clients that periodic antibiotic therapy is a lifelong necessity because they will be vulnerable to the disease for the rest of their lives.

Stop, Think, and Respond ● BOX 31-2

If a client asks why he or she has been advised to take an antibiotic such as penicillin before having dental work done, what information is appropriate to provide?

● MYOCARDITIS

Pathophysiology and Etiology

Myocarditis is an inflammation of the myocardium (the muscle layer of the heart). A viral, bacterial, fungal, or parasitic infection causes most cases; a viral origin is most common in the United States. The usual viral agents are coxsackie virus A and B, influenza A and B, measles, adenovirus, mumps, rubella, rubeola, Epstein-Barr virus, and cytomegalovirus (Lewandowski, 1999). The myocardium also can become inflamed from the toxins of microorganisms, chronic alcohol and cocaine abuse, radiation therapy, or autoimmune disorders.

Whatever the damaging agent, an inflammatory response causes the cardiac muscle tissue to swell, which interferes with the myocardium's ability to stretch and recoil. Cardiac output is reduced and blood circulation is impaired, predisposing the client to CHF (see Chap. 36). The myocardium becomes ischemic from a reduced supply of oxygenated blood, predisposing the client to tachycardia and dysrhythmias. Cardiomyopathy, evidenced as atypical changes in the myocardial wall, may develop as a complication of myocarditis and other disorders.

Assessment Findings

Signs and Symptoms

Clients may complain of general chest discomfort relieved by sitting up, low-grade fever, tachycardia, dysrhythmias, dyspnea, malaise, fatigue, and anorexia. The skin may be pale or cyanotic. If the heart's pumping activity becomes impaired, neck vein distention, ascites, and peripheral edema may be noted, indicating right-sided heart failure. Crackles may be heard in the lungs if the left side fails. An S_3 galloping rhythm or a pericardial friction rub may be heard.

Diagnostic Findings

Serum electrolyte levels and thyroid function studies help rule out other causes for the client's symptoms. The WBC count is slightly elevated. C-reactive protein, a nonspecific antigen–antibody test, is elevated in inflammatory conditions. Cardiac isoenzyme levels are elevated, and the results of ECG may be abnormal. Chest radiography shows overall heart enlargement and fluid infiltration in the lungs. Echocardiography demonstrates structural and functional abnormalities in the ventricles such as impaired motion of the ventricular wall and reduced ejection of blood from the heart. Radionuclide studies reveal areas where the myocardial wall is enlarged, thickened, or scarred. A myocardial biopsy may be done to obtain a definitive diagnosis.

Medical and Surgical Management

Management aims at treating the underlying cause and preventing complications. Antibiotics are prescribed if the infecting microorganism is bacterial. Bed rest, a sodium-restricted diet, and cardiotonic drugs (digitalis and related drugs) are prescribed to prevent or treat heart failure. In severe cases of cardiomyopathy, a heart transplant is necessary.

Nursing Management

The nurse monitors the client's cardiopulmonary status to assess for possible complications such as CHF or dysrhythmias. Assessments include vital signs, daily weights, intake and output, heart and lung sounds, pulse oximetry measurements, and dependent edema. The nurse also maintains the client on bed rest to reduce cardiac workload and promote healing. If the client has a fever, the nurse administers a prescribed antipyretic along with independent nursing measures like minimizing layers of bed linen, promoting air circulation and evaporation of perspiration, and offering oral fluids. He or she administers supplemental oxygen to relieve tachycardia that may develop from hypoxemia. The nurse elevates the client's head to promote maximal breathing potential. He or she uses a bedside cardiac monitor or telemetry unit to assess heart rhythm. The nurse uses cardiac rhythm analyses to determine if and when antidysrhythmic medications are necessary, or the client's response to their use.

● CARDIOMYOPATHY

Cardiomyopathy is a chronic condition characterized by structural changes in the heart muscle. The three major types of cardiomyopathies are (1) dilated cardiomyopathy, (2) hypertrophic cardiomyopathy, and (3) restrictive cardiomyopathy (Table 31-1; Fig. 31-3). The International Society and Federation of Cardiology and the World Health Organization added two other types of cardiomyopathy to the list in 1989: arrhythmogenic right ventricular cardiomyopathy, which is inherited, and peripartum cardiomyopathy, which develops in women shortly before or after giving birth (Porth, 2002). The focus of the following discussion is on dilated, hypertrophic, and restrictive cardiomyopathies.

Pathophysiology and Etiology

In some cases, there is no explanation for the development of cardiomyopathy. In others, cardiomyopathy accompanies or follows another medical problem, such as myocarditis, connective tissue disorders like systemic lupus erythematosus, muscular dystrophy, chronic alcoholism, or cancer chemotherapy. Regardless of the cause, the heart muscle loses its ability to pump blood efficiently. When a client's medical history includes disorders that are bacterial or viral in origin, a family history of early cardiac deaths, or any of several other conditions that correlate with heart involvement, the possibility of cardiomyopathy is considered. For some affected clients, their condition remains stable for a long period before disabling symptoms develop; others may be unaware of their condition until they experience a potentially fatal cardiac event like a sudden dysrhythmia or heart failure.

Assessment Findings

Signs and Symptoms

The manifestations of cardiomyopathy vary slightly according to the type that develops:

- *Dilated cardiomyopathy,* the most common type, is accompanied by dyspnea on exertion and when lying down. The client feels fatigued and his or her legs swell. He or she may experience palpitations and chest pain.
- *Hypertrophic cardiomyopathy* is associated with **syncope** (sudden loss of consciousness) or near-syncopal episodes, which the client may describe as "graying out." Clients also may feel fatigued, become short of breath, and develop chest pain. Many are asymptomatic, however, and the disorder is not discovered until the affected person dies or becomes acutely ill after strenuous exercise.

TABLE 31-1	TYPES OF CARDIOMYOPATHY		
TYPE	CAUSES	DESCRIPTION	TREATMENT
Dilated	Viral myocarditis Autoimmune response Chemicals (e.g., chronic alcohol ingestion)	The cavity of the heart is stretched (dilated).	Drug therapy to minimize symptoms and prevent complications Abstinence from alcohol Salt restriction Weight loss Possible heart transplantation
Hypertrophic	Hereditary Unknown	The muscle of the left ventricle and septum thickens, causing heart enlargement.	Drug therapy to reduce heart rate and force of contraction Antidysrhythmic drugs Artificial pacemaker Alcohol ablation: injection of alcohol into an artery supplying the extra tissue to destroy excess heart muscle (currently experimental) Ventriculomyotomy, a surgical procedure to reduce muscle tissue
Restrictive	Deposits of amyloid Scleroderma, a connective tissue disorder Granulomatous tumors Hemochromatosis, iron stores in tissue Scar tissue that forms after a myocardial infarction	Heart muscle stiffens, which interferes with its ability to stretch and fill with blood.	No specific treatment; drugs such as diuretics and antihypertensives used to control symptoms

FIGURE 31-3 The various types of cardiomyopathies compared with the normal heart. AO, aortic valve; LV, left ventricle; LA, left atrium. (Roberts W. C. & Ferrans V. J. [1975]. Pathologic anatomy of the cardiomyopathies. *Human Pathology, 6,* 289.)

FIGURE 31-4 (**A**) Normal muscle structure. (**B**) Myocardial disarray.

show the heart muscle's inability to contract efficiently when stressed during exercise.

Medical and Surgical Management

Treatment depends on the type of cardiomyopathy (see Table 31-1). In general, diuretics, cardiac glycosides like digitalis, and antihypertensives are prescribed to promote effective heart contraction and adequate cardiac output. Antidysrhythmics are used to manage abnormally conducted heart impulses. Anticoagulants are administered to prevent the formation of blood clots that may develop when blood pools in the heart chambers. Anti-inflammatory agents such as corticosteroids are used in selected clients to control cardiomyopathy caused by autoimmune connective tissue disorders. Dietary sodium is restricted to reduce fluid retention.

Drug therapy sometimes is accompanied by placement of an artificial pacemaker or implanted automatic defibrillator (see Chap. 34). Clients with hypertrophic cardiomyopathy may experience relief of symptoms when a **ventriculomyomectomy,** removal of thickened myocardial muscle from the septum, is performed. This surgical procedure enlarges the left ventricular chamber and allows a greater ejection of blood with each heart contraction. The mitral valve also may be replaced at the same time as the ventriculomyomectomy to correct the leakage of blood from the left atrium into the left ventricle (see Chap. 32). When there are no other alternatives for supporting the heart's pumping function, the client may become a candidate for heart transplantation (see Chap. 37). If current clinical trials of a permanent artificial heart pump are successful, candidates for heart transplantation may be treated with this alternative.

Nursing Management

The nurse obtains a comprehensive medical and family history and asks the client to describe any symptoms. Outpatients may be attached to an ambulatory cardiac monitor; nurses teach such clients to keep a journal of their symptoms. The nurse performs a physical examination that includes taking vital signs, auscultating heart and lung sounds, and checking for peripheral edema and abdominal enlargement. He or she is especially alert for an irregular pulse, tachycardia, or reduced levels of oxygen saturation (SpO_2) on pulse oximetry, which may occur during pos-

- *Restrictive cardiomyopathy,* which is the least common type in the United States but more common in tropical locales of Africa, India, South and Central America, and Asia, has symptoms of exertional dyspnea, dependent edema in the legs, ascites (fluid in the abdomen), and hepatomegaly (enlarged liver).

A heart **murmur,** which is an atypical heart sound, may be the first abnormal sign detected. Forceful heart contractions may be palpated over the left chest wall.

Diagnostic Findings

Cardiomyopathy sometimes is detected among asymptomatic clients during other diagnostic tests. For example, chest radiography may show heart enlargement. An exercise, chemical, or ambulatory ECG provides evidence of abnormal cardiac rhythm. Definitive diagnosis is determined by performing an echocardiogram and cardiac catheterization. During cardiac catheterization, elevated pressures are detected in the ventricles of the heart. In some cases, an endomyocardial biopsy is performed to obtain a specimen of heart tissue for microscopic examination. The biopsy may reveal **myocardial disarray** (Fig. 31-4), an alteration in the usual alignment of **myofibrils,** the contractile component of muscle tissue. The result is a lack of coordination during systole (ventricular contraction) and impaired diastole, the period of ventricular relaxation (Porth, 2002). Radionuclide studies tural changes or exercise. The nurse advocates for cardiac monitoring either at the bedside or by telemetry.

Oxygen is administered either continuously or when dyspnea or dysrhythmias develop. The nurse administers prescribed medications and collects data to evaluate their effectiveness. For example, if the client receives a diuretic, the nurse monitors intake and output, assesses weight, and checks for dependent edema regularly. He or she ensures that the client's activity level is reduced and sequences any activity that is slightly exertional between periods of rest.

The nurse supports the client emotionally as he or she copes with a chronic, perhaps life-threatening illness. The nurse helps the client identify realistic limitations, yet avoid becoming a self-restricted invalid as a consequence of fear. Depending on the type of cardiomyopathy, the nurse may encourage family members to undergo diagnostic testing to determine if they also have the same disorder. A teaching plan includes the following components:

- Achieve a healthy weight by following dietary instructions, limiting sodium to reduce fluid retention, and avoiding beverages containing caffeine, which contributes to tachycardia.
- Stop using tobacco products because nicotine is a vasoconstrictor and cardiac stimulant.
- Stay within your level of exercise tolerance or stop activity immediately if dyspnea or chest pain develops.
- Restrict driving or operating equipment if syncope is a common symptom.
- Keep appointments for medical follow-up to evaluate the status of the disease and symptom control.
- Receive the pneumonia vaccine and yearly influenza vaccinations to avoid pulmonary complications that may compromise cardiopulmonary function.
- For female clients, seek co-consultation with a cardiologist and an obstetrician if pregnancy is desired.

● PERICARDITIS

Pericarditis, inflammation of the pericardium, can be a primary condition (develops independently of any other condition) or a secondary condition (develops because of another condition). The inflammation can occur with or without **effusion,** the accumulation of fluid between two layers of tissue.

Pathophysiology and Etiology

Pericarditis usually is secondary to endocarditis, myocarditis, chest trauma, or myocardial infarction (MI; heart attack) or develops after cardiac surgery. Other contributing causes include tuberculosis, malignant tumors, uremia, and connective tissue disorders. When the pericardial cells become inflamed, their membranes become more permeable and intracellular fluid leaks into the interstitial spaces (Fig. 31-5). The exudate or effusion can be serous, resembling clear serum; fibrinous, like thick, congealed liquid; purulent, containing pus; or sanguineous, containing blood.

Pericardial fluid accumulation results in **cardiac tamponade,** acute compression of the heart. The pericardial fluid occupies space the heart needs to accommodate for filling with blood (Fig. 31-6). The impaired filling is reflected by a condition called *pulsus paradoxus* or *paradoxical pulse*. **Pulsus paradoxus** is a difference of 10 mm Hg or more between the first Korotkoff sound heralding systolic blood pressure (BP) heard during expiration and the first that is heard during inspiration. Normally, the difference between the two is 4 to 5 mm Hg. The technique for detecting pulsus paradoxus is described in Nursing Guidelines 31-1. Pulsus paradoxus develops because the reduction in the volume capacity of the left ventricle during inspiration is greater, combined with an impaired ability of the left ventricle to expand because of the rigid pericardium. The smaller capacity reduces the stroke volume from the left ventricle. As cardiac tamponade progresses, stroke volume is diminished, cardiac output is compromised, and death may result if the condition continues uncorrected.

Assessment Findings

Signs and Symptoms

The typical signs and symptoms that accompany an inflammatory response, such as fever and malaise, are present. The client is dyspneic or complains of heaviness in

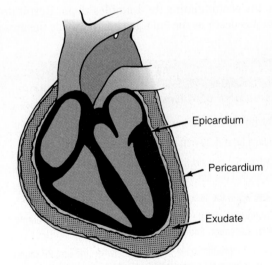

FIGURE 31-5 Pericarditis. Normally, the epicardium and pericardium slide over each other easily. They are lubricated by a small amount of fluid, which thicker material replaces in pericarditis.

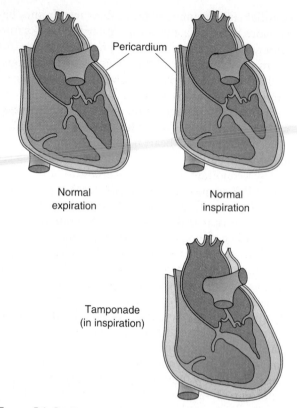

FIGURE 31-6 Effects of respiration and cardiac tamponade on ventricular filling and cardiac output.

Normal expiration

Normal inspiration

Tamponade (in inspiration)

Pericardium

the chest. One chief characteristic is **precordial pain** (pain in the anterior chest overlying the heart). It may be slight or severe and can be mistaken for esophagitis, indigestion, pleurisy, or MI. Moving and breathing deeply worsen the pain; sitting upright and leaning forward relieve it. In contrast, the pain of acute MI remains unchanged regardless of position, movement, or breathing. A pericardial friction rub, a scratchy, high-pitched sound, is a diagnostic sign. Heart sounds are difficult to hear because the accumulating fluid muffles them. Respiratory symptoms occur as the enlarged heart crowds the airway

passages and lung tissue and respirations become rapid and labored. Hypotension is severe, and pulse quality is weak.

Diagnostic Findings

The ST segment of the ECG is elevated, but cardiac isoenzyme levels are normal. The heart may appear enlarged on chest radiography. Echocardiography demonstrates a wide gap between the pericardium and epicardium, indicating that the space is filled with fluid. Hemodynamic monitoring values are abnormal. Pericardial fluid may be cultured, but if the cause of the pericarditis is nonbacterial, the test results often are nondiagnostic. Because of the inflammatory nature of pericarditis, the WBC count and ESR often are elevated.

Medical and Surgical Management

MI (see Chap. 33) must be ruled out. Treatment of pericarditis depends on the underlying cause. Rest, analgesics, antipyretics, nonsteroidal anti-inflammatory drugs, and sometimes corticosteroids are prescribed. **Pericardiocentesis,** needle aspiration of fluid from between the visceral and parietal pericardium, may be necessary when cardiac output is severely reduced. A small drainage catheter can be left in place. Needle aspiration is hazardous because the needle can puncture the myocardium, a branch of a coronary artery, or the pleura.

When pericardiocentesis and catheter drainage are inadequate, a **pericardiostomy,** a surgical opening or window, is made in the pericardium to allow the fluid to drain. Constrictive pericarditis is treated surgically by removing the pericardium (**pericardiectomy** or **decortication**) to allow more adequate filling and contraction of the heart chambers.

N U R S I N G   P R O C E S S

● **The Client With Pericarditis**

Assessment

The nurse asks the client about the incidence and nature of the pain and what worsens or relieves it. He or she assesses for a pericardial friction rub by asking the client to briefly hold his or her breath while the nurse auscultates heart sounds; a pericardial friction rub does not disappear when the client holds the breath. The nurse notes additional signs and symptoms that may further suggest cardiac tamponade and decreased cardiac output (Fig. 31-7), such as muffled heart sounds, pulsus paradoxus, jugular neck vein distention, persistent cough, dyspnea, fainting or near-fainting, anxiety, and changes in pulmonary function.

NURSING GUIDELINES 31-1

Assessment of Pulsus Paradoxus

- Advise client to breathe normally throughout the assessment.
- Inflate BP cuff 20 mm Hg above systolic pressure.
- Deflate the cuff slowly, noting that sounds are audible during expiration but not inspiration.
- Note when the first BP sound (Korotkoff's) is heard.
- Continue to deflate the cuff until BP sounds are heard during both inspiration and expiration.
- Measure the difference in mm Hg between the first BP sound heard during expiration and the first BP sound heard during both inspiration and expiration.

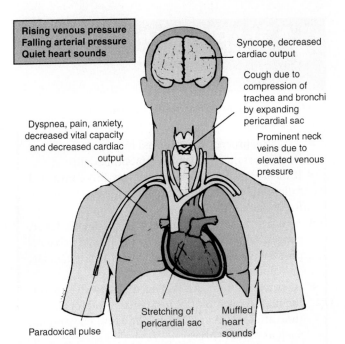

Rising venous pressure
Falling arterial pressure
Quiet heart sounds

Syncope, decreased cardiac output

Cough due to compression of trachea and bronchi by expanding pericardial sac

Prominent neck veins due to elevated venous pressure

Dyspnea, pain, anxiety, decreased vital capacity and decreased cardiac output

Stretching of pericardial sac

Muffled heart sounds

Paradoxical pulse

FIGURE 31-7 Signs and symptoms of cardiac tamponade. (From Smeltzer, S. C. & Bare, B. G. [2000]. *Brunner & Suddarth's textbook of medical–surgical nursing* [9th ed.]. Philadelphia: Lippincott Williams & Wilkins.)

Diagnosis, Planning, and Interventions

Pain related to pericardial inflammation and decreased myocardial perfusion

Expected Outcome: Client will be free of pain or pain will be tolerable 30 minutes after a nursing intervention.

- Assess pain status as often as vital signs. *Pain is considered the fifth vital sign. Whenever pain exists, the nurse must implement interventions targeted for its relief.*
- Assist client to a position of comfort such as sitting upright and leaning forward. *Only the outer layer of the lower parietal pericardium is sensitive to pain (Porth, 2002); some of the pain of pericarditis results from inflammation of surrounding structures. Sitting up and leaning forward positions the stretched pericardium away from the pleura, which relieves discomfort.*
- Administer anti-inflammatory drugs and analgesics as prescribed. *Reduced inflammation and pain transmission promote comfort.*
- Reassure the client that pericardial pain does not indicate an MI. *Anxiety increases heart rate and force of heart contraction, which contribute to pain. Clarifying the reality and significance of the pain may reduce the workload of the heart and acuity of discomfort.*

Decreased Cardiac Output related to inability of the heart muscle to stretch completely, fill with appropriate amount of blood, and eject a sufficient volume during ventricular systole

Expected Outcome: Client will (1) maintain normal arterial BP, (2) remain alert, (3) be free of chest pain, and (4) eliminate at least 35 mL of urine per hour.

- Monitor vital signs every 4 hours and as needed. *Hypotension and tachycardia are signs of decreased cardiac output.*
- Measure urine output every hour unless output is greater than 35 mL/hour. *The kidneys cannot form urine when the renal artery blood supply is reduced secondary to decreased cardiac output. An output of at least 35 mL/hour is necessary to eliminate nitrogen wastes and other toxic substances.*
- Monitor for cardiac dysrhythmias. *Hypoxemia is a leading cause of dysrhythmias. Inadequate cardiac output creates a potential for myocardial ischemia and disturbances in electrical conduction.*
- Assess orientation. *Confusion and disorientation are signs of compromised cerebral arterial blood flow secondary to decreased cardiac output.*
- Instruct the client to report chest pain. *It is a consequence of inadequate blood supply to the myocardium.*
- Maintain bed rest. *Activity increases the demand for myocardial oxygenation, which depends on cardiac output.*
- Administer supplemental oxygen as prescribed. *Giving more than the 20% oxygen that is present in room air helps to reduce hypoxemia that results from inadequate cardiac output.*
- Provide six small meals a day; avoid gas-forming foods. *Abdominal distention crowds the thoracic cavity and compresses the space the heart needs to fill with blood and the lungs need to fill with air.*
- Restrict caffeine and sodium. *Caffeine increases heart rate and sodium increases circulating blood volume, both of which increase myocardial work and the need for cardiac output.*
- Collaborate with the physician regarding a stool softener. *Bearing down during bowel movements interferes with cardiac filling and output. Stool softeners promote ease of eliminating stool.*
- Administer prescribed medications such as sedatives, anxiolytics, vasodilators, diuretics, antidysrhythmics. *Reducing anxiety, keeping the client calm and quiet, reducing BP and volume, and facilitating normal heart conduction help avoid exceeding the heart's ability to eject an adequate cardiac output.*

PC: Cardiac Tamponade

Expected Outcome: The nurse will manage and minimize cardiac tamponade.

- Monitor for tachycardia, pulsus paradoxus, neck vein distension, cough, syncope, and muffled heart sounds every 4 hours and as needed. *This cluster of signs and symptoms accompanies cardiac tamponade, which interferes with filling volumes. Blood that cannot enter the heart accumulates in both venous and pulmonary circulation.*
- Have an emergency pericardiocentesis tray available. *Removing fluid from between the parietal and visceral pericardium relieves cardiac tamponade.*

- Reinforce the physician's explanation of a pericardiocentesis and witness the client's signature on a consent form. *Pericardiocentesis is an invasive procedure that requires informed consent from the client if he or she is alert or from whomever has durable power of attorney for healthcare.*
- Obtain baseline vital signs before pericardiocentesis. *They are used for comparison during and after the pericardiocentesis.*
- Measure, describe, and record the amount of pericardial fluid removed. *Documentation is a record of the client's care and outcomes of treatment.*
- Label all specimens for laboratory analysis and send them promptly to the laboratory. *Accurate information and prompt delivery facilitate diagnosis and appropriate treatment.*
- Cover the site of the pericardiocentesis with a sterile dressing and inspect the dressing for bleeding or leaking fluid. *Compromising the skin and underlying tissue creates a potential for blood and fluid loss as well as providing an entry site for microorganisms.*
- Reinforce the dressing if it becomes moist. *Moist gauze acts as a wick and pulls microorganisms from the skin surface toward the puncture wound and deeper tissue.*
- Continue to monitor vital signs until they are stable. *Continued assessments help identify complications so they can be treated early or validate a favorable response to therapy.*

Evaluation of Expected Outcomes

The client states pain is relieved. Vital signs are stable, and cardiac rhythm is normal. The client is alert and oriented. Urine output exceeds 35 mL/hour. Cardiac tamponade is managed (see Client and Family Teaching Box 31-1).

Stop, Think, and Respond ● BOX 31-3

While caring for a client with pericarditis, you measure the client's BP and hear the first Korotkoff sound during expiration at 110 mm Hg. The sounds continue throughout auscultation, and you note that when the manometer is at 98 mm Hg, you hear sounds during both inspiration and expiration. Is this client manifesting pulsus paradoxus?

INFLAMMATORY DISORDERS OF THE PERIPHERAL BLOOD VESSELS

● THROMBOPHLEBITIS

Thrombophlebitis is an inflammation of a vein accompanied by clot or thrombus formation. Although clots can form in any blood vessel, the veins deep in the lower

---

31-1 *Client and Family Teaching*
Infectious and Inflammatory Heart Disorders

The nurse performs the following teaching components:

- Explains procedures required during therapy and the importance of each treatment modality
- Informs clients of the necessity for continued follow-up care because they will always be at risk for endocarditis
- Advises those with a history of rheumatic fever, congenital valve disorders, or prosthetic valve replacements to see their physician if fever, malaise, or other symptoms of infection occur
- Instructs clients with damaged heart valves about the need for antibiotics just before, and for a short time after, an event that might cause bacteremia, such as dental surgery
- Ensures that clients who are prescribed antibiotics understand that they must take the full dose for the full time because noncompliance with the drug regimen can hinder the complete destruction of the pathogen
- Explains how to take medications, potential adverse effects, and signs to report
- Provides written instructions or pamphlets explaining the prescribed drugs if they are written in language the layperson can understand
- Finds discreet ways to quiz the client, such as asking, "How often must you take this drug?" to evaluate if the client has understood the instructions
- Documents information that has been provided and evidence of the client's understanding

---

extremities are most commonly affected. In such cases, the condition is referred to as **deep vein thrombosis** (DVT). Thrombi that form in or above the popliteal vein of the leg are at high risk for migration toward the pulmonary circulation; these cases are referred to as a **pulmonary embolus** (PE).

Pathophysiology and Etiology

When the inner lining of a vein is irritated or injured, platelets clump together, forming a clot. The clot interferes with blood flow, causing congestion of venous blood distal to the blood clot. Sometimes collateral vessels recirculate the blood blocked by the clot. Accumulated waste products in the blocked vessel irritate the vein wall, initiating an inflammatory response. The increased permeability of cells and the convergence of leukocytes and lymphocytes cause the area to swell, redden, and feel warm and tender.

The development of a PE may complicate thrombophlebitis if the clot in the extremity becomes mobile and moves in the venous circulation to the lungs (see Chap. 29). Despite appropriate and successful treatment of thrombophlebitis, some clients experience a vascular complication referred to as **postphlebitic syndrome** for up to 5 years after the initial episode (Church, 2000). For example, valvular impairment in the affected vein may follow the original thrombotic event. The incompetent valves are less efficient at returning venous blood to the heart. When venous pressure increases because of pooled blood, some fluid leaks from capillaries into subcutaneous tissue, causing leg ulcers.

Venous stasis (slowed circulation), altered blood coagulation, and trauma to the vein, referred to as **Virchow's triad,** predispose clients to thrombosis and thrombophlebitis. Factors that contribute to clot formation include inactivity, reduced cardiac output, compression of the veins in the pelvis or legs, and injury. Some IV drugs and chemicals also irritate the vein. Thrombi are prone to form in arm, subclavian, or jugular veins cannulated for extended IV use. Older adults with heart and blood vessel disease are susceptible to thrombophlebitis because of impaired mobility, reduced activity, and compromised circulation. Risk for clot formation is increased among women who take oral contraceptives, although the exact trigger is not known. Women who take oral contraceptives and smoke are at even higher risk.

Assessment Findings

Clients with thrombophlebitis frequently complain of discomfort in the affected extremity. Calf pain that increases on dorsiflexion of the foot is referred to as a positive **Homans' sign.** Heat, redness, and swelling develop along the length of the affected vein. Capillary refill takes less than 2 seconds because of venous congestion. The client often has a fever, malaise, fatigue, and anorexia.

Most cases of thrombophlebitis are diagnosed according to clinical findings alone. **Venography,** using radiopaque dye instilled into the venous system, indicates a filling defect in the area of the clot. Doppler ultrasound may detect an area of venous obstruction. The results of Doppler ultrasound sometimes are difficult to interpret because there are so many collateral vessels, and deep veins are especially difficult to assess. **Impedance plethysmography** (IPG) is the preferred test for diagnosing clots in deep veins. During IPG, a sensor records blood volume in the arm or leg before and after inflating a BP cuff to stop venous blood flow. If a clot is present, the blood volumes are nearly the same because the clot impairs venous return.

Medical and Surgical Management

Complete rest of the arm or leg is essential to prevent the thrombus from breaking free and floating in the circulation (embolus). Anticoagulant therapy with heparin, oral anticoagulants, or drugs that prevent platelet aggregation (clustering) are prescribed to decrease the incidence of future clot formation (Drug Therapy Table 31-2). With the advent of low–molecular-weight heparins such as enoxaparin (Lovenox), some clients with thrombophlebitis in which the thrombi are small are not hospitalized, but rather treated at home. People with repeated episodes may be placed on oral anticoagulant therapy for 3 to 6 months.

Continuous warm, wet packs are ordered to improve circulation, ease pain, and decrease inflammation. Surgical intervention may be necessary when a clot occludes a large vein or the danger of a PE arises. **Thrombectomy,** the surgical removal of a clot, is performed if the clot interferes with venous drainage from a large vein such as the femoral vein. With danger of PE, surgery on the inferior vena cava may be necessary to reduce the possibility of a clot traveling from the legs to the lungs. Several surgical procedures may be performed on the vena cava: ligation, insertion of an umbrella-like **vena caval filter** (Fig. 31-8) to trap emboli before they reach the heart and lungs, or plication. A **vena caval plication procedure** changes the lumen of the vena cava from a single channel to several small channels through the use of a suture or Teflon clip.

NURSING PROCESS

● **The Client With Thrombophlebitis**

Assessment

The nurse determines if the client has a history of blood clots or other risk factors that predispose to thrombus formation, such as cardiovascular disorders or recent surgery, especially repair of a hip fracture or hip joint replacement; self-imposed inactivity as a result of obesity or sedentary lifestyle; immobility from a medical condition, pain, or treatment regimen; current use of an oral contraceptive; use of tobacco products; dehydration that may decrease the fluid volume of blood; or recent trauma to an extremity. The nurse assesses for Homans' sign by asking the client whether he or she experiences pain or tenderness in the calf of the affected extremity when dorsiflexing the foot, or if movement causes or aggravates pain. The nurse inspects the color, temperature, and capillary refill of extremities and measures the circumference of the leg (or arm) at various areas and compares the findings with the unaffected extremity. He or she regularly checks for a low-grade fever. The nurse consults with the client about chest pain and dyspnea, which are

DRUG THERAPY TABLE 31-2 | ANTICOAGULANTS

DRUG	MECHANISM OF ACTION	SIDE EFFECTS	NURSING CONSIDERATIONS
heparin sodium (Hepalean)	Inhibits thrombus and clot formation by blocking the conversion of prothrombin to thrombin and fibrinogen to fibrin	Hemorrhage, bruising, thrombocytopenia, alopecia, chills, fever Chance of hemorrhage increases with oral anticoagulants	Monitor PTT test range between 1½ to 2½ times normal. Apply pressure to all IM injection sites. Monitor for epistaxis and other forms of bleeding. Have protamine sulfate readily available in case of overdose.
low–molecular-weight heparin *enoxaparin (Lovenox), dalteparin (Fragmin), ardeparin (Normiflo)*	Inhibits thrombus and clot formation by blocking factors Xa and IIa	Bruising, hemorrhage, fever, pain, local irritation	Note that laboratory monitoring is not done. Provide devices like a soft toothbrush and electric razor to protect against bleeding. Ensure the availability of protamine sulfate in case of overdose. Ensure that the client avoids foods with vitamin K.
warfarin (Coumadin)	Interferes with the hepatic synthesis of vitamin K–dependent clotting factors	Nausea, alopecia, urticaria, dermatitis, prolonged bleeding	Monitor PT ratio or INR regularly to adjust dosage. Evaluate client regularly for signs of blood loss—petechiae, dark stools and urine, bruises, bleeding gums. Keep vitamin K on hand in case of overdose. Monitor WBC count before and during therapy to assess for neutropenia.
ticlopidine (Ticlid)	Inhibits binding of fibrinogen and interactions of platelets	Diarrhea, nausea, vomiting, abdominal pain, neutropenia, phlebitis	Administer with food. Give with food.
aspirin	Inhibits platelet aggregation	Nausea, epigastric pain, occult blood loss, anaphylaxis, tinnitus, dizziness, increased risk of bleeding, especially with other anticoagulants	Advise client not to crush or chew enteric-coated or sustained-release tablets.
glycoprotein IIb/IIIa inhibitors *tirofiban (Aggrastat)*	Binds to the platelet receptor glycoprotein, preventing fibrinogen from binding	Dizziness, weakness, bleeding, hypotension	Use in conjunction with heparin. Assess complete blood count, PT, aPTT, and active clotting time before and periodically during therapy.

hallmarks of PE, a complication of thrombophlebitis. If drug therapy is prescribed, the nurse monitors the laboratory test results associated with anticoagulant therapy.

Diagnosis, Planning, and Interventions

An important role is to prevent venous stasis and thrombophlebitis by promoting activity and exercise for at-risk clients. Ankle-pumping exercises are imperative for clients on bed rest (Fig. 31-9). For inactive clients, the nurse applies knee- or thigh-high elastic stockings or uses a pneumatic venous compression device that alternately inflates and deflates to support vein walls and promote venous circulation (Fig. 31-10). He or she assists the client to change positions frequently and avoid restricting venous blood flow from prolonged sitting or gatching the bed at the knees (see Client and Family Teaching Box 31-2).

Additional nursing management includes the following measures.

Pain related to venous inflammation

Expected Outcome: Discomfort will be relieved or reduced to a tolerable level.

- Administer prescribed non-narcotic analgesics and anti-inflammatory agents. *Non-narcotic agents inhibit prostaglandin, a chemical that sensitizes nerve receptors that transmit pain. Relief of inflammation interferes with the release of cellular chemicals that contribute to pain and localized swelling.*
- Support and handle the extremity gently. *Movement and muscle contraction increase pain.*

Ineffective Tissue Perfusion related to localized swelling secondary to the inflammatory response and impaired venous circulation

FIGURE 31-8 A permanently implanted vena caval filter allows blood to circulate to the lungs but traps blood clots before they enter the pulmonary circulation.

FIGURE 31-10 Pneumatic compression device.

Expected Outcomes: Client's venous circulation will be adequate as evidenced by (1) reduced localized edema, (2) capillary refill less than 3 seconds in the toes of the affected extremity, (3) skin color in affected extremity that is similar to that of the unaffected extremity.

- Elevate the affected extremity 20° or more in a straight plane on pillows (do not bend the knees). *Elevation relieves swelling and promotes venous circulation; bending the knees interferes with venous circulation and may increase the size of the existing clot or contribute to the formation of additional thrombi.*

- Apply warm, moist compresses to the area of discomfort or apply an aquathermia pad over protected skin at a setting of approximately 105°F (40.5°C). Remove compresses and reapply after 20 minutes or sooner if cooling occurs. Remove the aquathermia pad every 2 hours for 20 minutes to assess the skin. *Warmth dilates blood vessels, improves circulation, and relieves*

FIGURE 31-9 Leg exercises help prevent thrombophlebitis. (**A**) Have client bend knee, raise the foot, and hold for 3 seconds. Repeat with each leg five times each hour. (**B**) Have client trace circles five times with each foot every hour.

31-2 *Client and Family Teaching* **Thrombophlebitis**

The nurse teaches clients with thrombophlebitis and their families the following:

- Methods to prevent recurrences: avoiding prolonged sitting and crossing the legs at the knee, performing active movement, elevating the legs periodically, wearing support hose, and drinking fluids liberally

- The importance of taking long-term anticoagulant therapy exactly as prescribed and keeping appointments for the ordered laboratory tests to determine the effectiveness of therapy

- Signs that indicate impaired clotting: nosebleeds, bleeding gums, rectal bleeding, easy bruising, and prolonged oozing from minor cuts *swelling, all of which relieve discomfort. Moist heat is more comforting than dry heat. Skin assessments are standard care to avoid injury.*

- Promote a liberal intake (2000 to 2500 mL/24 hours) of oral fluid unless contraindicated. *Adequate fluid volume dilutes blood cells in plasma and reduces the risk for platelet aggregation.*

PC: Pulmonary Embolus

Expected Outcome: The nurse manages and minimizes complications such as a PE.

- Maintain bed rest after the diagnosis of thrombophlebitis for approximately 1 week or until the physician discontinues activity restriction. *Restricting activity helps stabilize the blood clot to the vein wall and decreases the risk of its conversion to an embolus.*
- Administer prescribed anticoagulant therapy. *Depending on the prescribed drugs, medications that alter clotting factors or interfere with platelet aggregation prevent additional thrombi and subsequent emboli.*
- Instruct client to perform active leg exercises with the unaffected extremity at least five times each waking hour. *Exercise prevents venous stasis by promoting venous circulation toward the heart. Promoting venous blood flow prevents the formation of thrombi and subsequent potential for emboli in the unaffected extremity.*
- Apply elastic stockings to extremities if prescribed by the physician. *Elastic stockings support the valves in veins and reduce the potential for venous stasis and clot formation.*
- Monitor for dyspnea, tachypnea, cough, hypotension, abnormal lung sounds, or chest pain. *Abnormal results of focus assessments indicate cardiopulmonary complications such as a PE.*
- Elevate the head if dyspnea develops. *Head elevation lowers abdominal organs away from the diaphragm and facilitates increased inspiration of higher lung volumes to compensate for impaired oxygenation in the pulmonary circulation.*
- Prepare to administer oxygen by cannula or mask if dyspnea and chest pain occur. *Raising oxygen levels above 20% compensates for impaired oxygenation at the alveolar–capillary level.*
- Prepare to start an IV and administer parenteral narcotic analgesia and emergency medications by the IV route. *Drug therapy helps relieve severe chest pain and improve BP.*

PC: Bleeding

Expected Outcome: The nurse will manage and minimize blood loss.

- Monitor laboratory test findings that reflect coagulation status such as partial thromboplastin time (PTT), prothrombin time (PT), and international normalized ratio (INR); report values that exceed therapeutic levels. *With the exception of low–molecular-weight heparin, doses of anticoagulant drug therapy are adjusted according to laboratory test results.*

- Calculate dosages of anticoagulants carefully and administer drug therapy as prescribed. *Unfractionated heparin may be administered by IV infusion; the dose often is titrated according to PTT and may require periodic rate adjustments during the infusion. Oral and subcutaneous dosages of anticoagulants (except low–molecular-weight heparin) may be changed daily.*
- Keep antidotes for overdose of anticoagulants (protamine sulfate for unfractionated heparin and vitamin K for warfarin) available. *In extreme cases, it may be prudent quickly to reverse the effects of anticoagulant therapy.*
- Inspect the skin for signs of bruising. *Tendency to bruise suggests that the client could easily bleed internally.*
- Provide the client with a soft-bristled toothbrush for oral hygiene; advise using an electric razor for shaving. *Reducing the potential for skin and soft tissue trauma decreases the possibility of bleeding.*
- Test stools, emesis, urine, and nasogastric drainage for blood. *Hemoccult testing may detect blood that is not obvious to the naked eye.*
- Protect the client from falls or other trauma. *An injury, even though ordinarily minor, may precipitate excessive or prolonged bleeding if the client is receiving anticoagulant therapy.*
- Perform neurologic assessments every 1 to 2 hours if the client experiences a head injury (see Chap. 47). *Changes in level of consciousness, size and response of pupils to light, and verbal responses suggest intracranial bleeding.*
- Apply direct pressure to the site of external bleeding. *Pressure compresses vascular walls and decreases blood flow, providing time for an initial clot to form.*
- Place an ice pack at the site of prolonged oozing of blood. *Ice causes vasoconstriction and decreases the volume of blood loss.*
- Be prepared to administer IV fluid, blood, or blood products. *Parenteral fluids replace lost fluid volume; blood and blood products replace cells and fluid.*

Evaluation of Expected Outcomes

Expected outcomes include reduced or eliminated pain. Venous circulation improves and adequate blood flow to the heart is maintained; both extremities are comparable in size, temperature, and color. Homans' sign is negative; a PE does not develop, or if it does, it is managed successfully. Bleeding is prevented or controlled.

THROMBOANGIITIS OBLITERANS (BUERGER'S DISEASE)

Thromboangiitis obliterans is inflammation of blood vessels associated with clot formation and fibrosis of the blood vessel wall. It affects primarily the small arteries and veins of the legs. It occasionally involves the arms.

Pathophysiology and Etiology

The cause of thromboangiitis obliterans has not been established. It is far more common in men than in women, and the onset usually is during young adulthood. Cigarette smoking aggravates the condition. The affected arteries are prone to spasms that constrict the arterial lumen. Inflammatory lesions are found in isolated segments intermixed among healthy areas of the same vessel. The lesions occlude blood flow through the vessel during exercise and at rest. Skin and soft tissue cells experience degrees of hypoxia and anoxia. Some cells die. The necrotic (dead) tissues slough, forming ulcerations. The extent may be so severe that gangrene results. Thrombophlebitis also may be present.

Assessment Findings

The client notes that one or both feet are always cold and may report numbness, burning, and tingling in some areas of the feet. **Intermittent claudication,** leg cramps after exercise, is a common symptom. Pain occurs at rest when circulation has been seriously impaired. The symptoms usually fluctuate in severity; remissions often follow attacks of acute distress.

Cyanosis and redness of the feet and legs sometimes occur. The skin frequently is a mottled purplish-red and appears thin and shiny, with sparse hair growth. Shallow, dry leg ulcers in various stages of healing may be seen. Black gangrenous areas may develop on the toes and heels. The nails are thick. Peripheral pulses are present during rest but diminish or disappear with activity. Capillary refill is prolonged. Doppler ultrasound, IPG, and angiography help to evaluate the location and extent of vessel destruction.

Medical Management

Tobacco in any form is restricted. Buerger-Allen exercises are ordered to stimulate and promote collateral circulation (Nursing Guidelines 31-2). Walking and active foot exercises are allowed as long as they do not cause pain. Analgesics are prescribed to ease discomfort. If leg ulcers develop, treatment may include moist dressings that are changed when the gauze becomes damp (i.e., wet-to-dry dressings) and topical antiseptics or antibiotic ointments.

Surgical Management

Sympathectomy, the interruption or suppression of some portion of the sympathetic nerve pathway, is performed to relieve vasospasm. If ulcerations occur, wound debridement (removal of necrotic tissue) and skin graft-

---

> **NURSING GUIDELINES 31-2**
>
> *Buerger-Allen Exercises*
>
> Tell the client to:
>
> 1. Lie flat in bed with both legs elevated above the level of the heart for 2 or 3 minutes.
> 2. Sit on the edge of the bed with the legs dependent for 3 minutes.
> 3. Exercise the feet and toes by moving them up, down, inward, and outward.
> 4. Return to the first position and hold it for about 5 minutes.
>
> The client should repeat the exercises several times during one exercise period and perform them periodically throughout the day.

---

ing may be required. If circulation becomes so impaired that gangrene results, amputation is necessary.

Nursing Management

The nurse takes a thorough history, including a smoking history and a review of symptoms and how long they have been present. He or she records the client's description of the type and degree of pain and factors that increase or decrease it. The nurse examines the affected areas for redness, swelling, and other color changes, such as cyanosis and mottling. He or she inspects the nails and skin for changes and notes the skin temperature above and below the affected area. The nurse also monitors the presence and quality of peripheral pulses and assesses capillary refill time.

The nurse instructs and supervises the client about Buerger-Allen leg exercises (see Nursing Guidelines 31-2). When the client is not performing exercises, he or she must keep the legs horizontal or dependent. Elevating the legs increases ischemia and, therefore, contributes to pain. The nurse carries out meticulous wound care if leg or foot ulcers exist.

Hospitalization for acute problems or complications may occur, but the client must carry out most care at home. The nurse teaches the client self-care techniques and stresses the importance of smoking cessation and performing prescribed exercises consistently. He or she instructs clients to avoid caffeine, tobacco products, and over-the-counter drugs that cause vasoconstriction, such as nasal decongestants. The nurse advises the client to inspect the fingernails, toenails, and skin on the arms and legs daily. He or she teaches the client to clean the arms and legs daily; prevent trauma to the extremities; wear properly fitting shoes and stockings (or socks); and avoid prolonged exposure to the cold. When cold weather is unavoidable, the nurse advises the client to wear thick socks or insulated boots and gloves to protect against exposure to low temperatures.

GENERAL NUTRITIONAL CONSIDERATIONS

A full liquid diet is used in the initial treatment of rheumatic heart disease and is progressed as tolerated. Sodium is restricted if the client has edema or is treated with steroids.

Anorexia and weight loss are common side effects of infections; increase calories and protein as needed to replenish losses. Fever increases fluid requirements. Encourage small, frequent feedings to maximize intake.

Encourage weight loss in obese clients with thrombophlebitis.

GENERAL PHARMACOLOGIC CONSIDERATIONS

Most clients with peripheral vascular disease have pain, for which non-narcotic analgesics, such as salicylates, may be used.

Pentoxifylline (Trental) may be used to improve (but not cure) intermittent claudication. This drug decreases blood viscosity and improves blood flow. Common adverse reactions include nausea, dizziness, headache, and dyspepsia.

Oral anticoagulants (e.g., warfarin sodium [Coumadin]) may be prescribed as part of the long-term management of venous thrombosis. Frequent monitoring of PT is important for clients taking warfarin; PT should be 1.5 to 2.5 times the control value (12 to 15 seconds) to achieve the therapeutic effect of anticoagulant therapy. When PT is reported as an INR factor, the normal range is 2.0 to 3.0.

Vitamin K (phytonadione, Aqua-Mephyton) is given as an antidote for overdose of Coumadin. Heparin therapy may be instituted for a client with thrombophlebitis. Heparin, an anticoagulant, prevents extension of the thrombus and the development of additional thrombi.

Heparin is measured in units and the dosage is regulated by venous clotting time determinations, such as PTT or activated partial thromboplastin time (aPTT). Optimum drug effect is reached when PTT and aPTT are 1.5 to 2.5 times normal.

Clients receiving an anticoagulant must be observed for signs of bleeding tendency (blood in the urine or stool, easy bruising, bleeding gums, excessive bleeding from minor cuts or scratches).

GENERAL GERONTOLOGIC CONSIDERATIONS

Older adults are at increased risk for infectious or inflammatory disorders of the cardiovascular system. A decreased inflammatory and immune response may prolong recovery.

Discourage older adults from using electric heating devices because of decreased temperature perception resulting from impaired circulation. Burns are more likely to occur. Thermal underwear and blankets are alternatives to electric blankets and heating pads.

Encourage older clients who are inactive to move every hour during the day to promote circulation. Such movement is especially important during long automobile or airplane trips.

Rheumatic heart disease may occur in the older adult who had rheumatic fever at an earlier age, or an acute episode may develop later in life.

Joint inflammation is more disabling in the older adult who may have some joint deformity or damage from chronic disorders such as osteoarthritis.

Many older adults have peripheral vascular insufficiency that is manifested in weak or absent pedal pulses; cold, clammy feet; thickened toenails; and shiny skin on the lower extremities.

The risk of hemorrhage during heparin therapy is greater in clients 60 years of age or older.

Critical Thinking Exercises

1. *A client complains of intermittent claudication, pain when the legs are elevated, and cold, numb feet. The nurse notes several dry ulcerations of the feet. Does the client suffer from venous or arterial insufficiency? What additional assessment data must the nurse collect? What lifestyle habits might predispose the client to this disorder?*

2. *What health teaching is important for a client with a history of thrombophlebitis?*

References and Suggested Readings

Alderman, L. M. (2000). At risk: Adolescents and adults with congenital heart disease. *Dimensions in Critical Care Nursing, 19*(1), 2–14.

Allen, J. K. (2000). Genetics and cardiovascular disease. *Nursing Clinics of North America, 35,* 653–662.

Benton, L. (2000). A question of practice: DVT prevention . . . deep vein thrombosis. *American Journal of Nursing, 100* (2), 84.

Breen, P. (2000). DVT: What every nurse should know . . . deep vein thrombosis. *RN, 63*(4), 58–63.

Brenner, Z. R. (2000). Preventing postoperative complications: What's old, what's new, what's tried-and-true. *Nursing Management, 31*(12), 17–23.

Bryant, J. L. & Turkoski, B. B. (1999a). Critical care extra. New drugs. Cilostazol (Pletal): New treatment for intermittent claudication. *American Journal of Nursing, 99*(6), 24 NN.

Bryant, J. L. & Turkoski, B. B. (1999b). Relieving intermittent claudication: A nursing approach. *Journal of Vascular Nursing, 17*(4), 81–85.

Carroll, P. (2000). Treating deep venous thrombosis at home with molecular weight heparin. *Home Healthcare Nurse,* (January Suppl.), 3–15.

Church, V. (2000). Staying on guard for DVT and PE. *Nursing, 30*(2), 34–42.

Dajani, A. S., Taubert, K. A., Wilson, W., et al. (1997). Prevention of bacterial endocarditis; recommendations by the American Heart Association. *Journal of the American Medical Association, 277*(22), 1794–1801.

Epley, D. (2000). Pulmonary emboli risk reduction. *Journal of Vascular Nursing, 18*(2), 61–70.

Gargiulo, J. (2000). Critical care extra. Hypertrophic cardiomyopathy: Preventing tragic endings. *American Journal of Nursing, 100*(8), 24JJ, 24LL.

Gorski, L. A. (2000). A clinical pathway for deep vein thrombosis. *Home Healthcare Nurse, 18,* 451–462.

Guglielmo, B. J. (1999). Use of antimicrobial agents in patients with cardiovascular disease. *Journal of Cardiovascular Nursing, 13*(2), 23–30.

Harris, G. D. & Steimle, J. (2000). Compiling the identifying features of bacterial endocarditis. [On-line.] Available: http://www.postgradmed.com/issues/2000/01_00/harris.htm

Lewandowski, D. M. (1999). Clinical snapshot: Myocarditis. *American Journal of Nursing, 99*(8), 44–45.

Lynch, L. I. (1999). A teaching module: Promoting awareness of effective bacterial endocarditis prophylaxis in children. *Pediatric Nursing, 25,* 621–626.

Molitor, L. (2000). Triage decisions: A 64-year-old woman with a swollen and painful leg . . . deep vein thrombosis. *Journal of Emergency Nursing, 26,* 278–279.

Oliver-McNeil, S. (2001). Treating hypertrophic cardiomyopathy without surgery. *Nursing, 31*(2), Critical Care, 32cc1–32cc2, 32cc4.

Piano, M. R. (1999). Familial hypertrophic cardiomyopathy. *Journal of Cardiovascular Nursing, 13*(4), 46–58.

Porth, C. M. (2002). *Pathophysiology: Concepts of altered states* (6th ed.). Philadelphia: Lippincott Williams & Wilkins.

Rydberg, E. J., Westfall, J. M., & Nicholas, R. A. (1999). Low-molecular weight heparin in preventing and treating DVT. *American Family Physician.* [On-line.] Available: http://www.findarticles.com/cf_dls/m3225/6_59/54129418/p1/article.jhtml?term = Low-molecular + weight + heparin + in + preventing + and + treating + DVT.

Schell, H. M. (1999). The immunocompromised host and risk for cardiovascular infection. *Journal of Cardiovascular Nursing, 13*(2), 31–48.

Sparacino, P. S. A. (1999). Cardiac infections: Medical and surgical therapies. *Journal of Cardiovascular Nursing, 13*(2), 49–65.

Wackel, J. (2000). Altered coagulation: A diagnosis for the problem of deep vein thrombosis. *Nursing Diagnosis, 11*(2), 69–79.

Wallis, M. & Autar, R. (2001). Deep vein thrombosis: Clinical nursing management. *Nursing Standard, 15*(18), 47–54.

chapter **32**

Caring for Clients With Valvular Disorders of the Heart

Words to Know

annuloplasty
aortic regurgitation
aortic stenosis
balloon valvuloplasty
commissures
mitral regurgitation
mitral stenosis
mitral valve prolapse
mitral valve prolapse
  syndrome

point of maximum
  impulse
pulmonary hyper-
  tension
sequela
valvular incompetence
valvular regurgitation
water-hammer pulse

Learning Objectives

On completion of this chapter, the reader will:

● List five disorders that commonly affect heart valves.
● Discuss assessment findings common among clients with valvular disorders.
● Name three diagnostic tests used to confirm valvular disorders.
● Identify consequences of valvular disorders.
● Name five categories of drugs used to treat valvular disorders.
● Give two examples of treatments other than drug therapy to correct valvular disorders.
● Discuss nursing management of clients with valvular disorders.

Each heart structure helps to maintain normal cardiac function. The four cardiac valves—aortic, mitral, tricuspid, and pulmonic—promote the forward circulation of blood to sustain adequate cardiac output (Fig. 32-1). Malformations at birth, inflammatory and infectious disorders (see Chap. 31), age-related degeneration, structural damage after myocardial infarction (MI), or injury during an intracardiac procedure can alter the structure and function of cardiac valves. The aortic and mitral valves, located on the left side of the heart, where fluid pressures are higher than on the right side, are most commonly affected. Less common are disorders involving the pulmonic and tricuspid valves.

DISORDERS OF THE AORTIC VALVE

The aortic valve has three cusps, or leaflets, and is described as a *semilunar* valve because each cusp appears like a half-moon (Fig. 32-2). The left ventricle pumps blood from the heart through the aortic valve. When a nondiseased aortic valve opens during contraction of the left ventricle, it facilitates the unrestricted passage of oxygenated blood into the arterial vascular system. The coronary arteries supplying the myocardium are the first blood vessels perfused. After ejection of left ventricular blood, the aortic valve closes tightly to prevent backflow of blood. Two valvular conditions interfere with unidirectional blood flow from the left side of the heart: aortic stenosis and aortic regurgitation.

● AORTIC STENOSIS

Stenosis means *narrowing*. **Aortic stenosis** describes narrowing of the opening in the aortic valve when the valve cusps become stiff and rigid.

Pathophysiology and Etiology

In older adults without predisposing cardiac conditions, narrowing of the aortic valve is an age-related degenerative change from progressive calcium deposits in valve

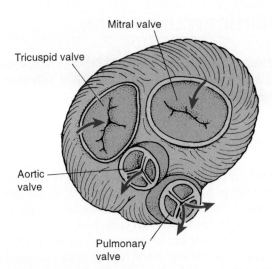

FIGURE 32-1 The tricuspid and mitral valves, located between the atria and ventricles, prevent blood from returning to the atria during ventricular contraction. The aortic and pulmonary valves, referred to as semilunar valves, open as blood is ejected from the ventricles.

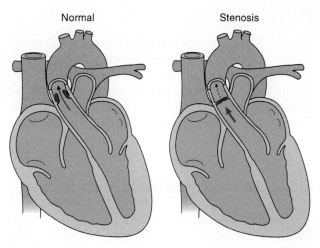

FIGURE 32-3 Aortic stenosis. Blood pools in the left ventricle, and cardiac output is reduced because the blood cannot completely pass through the narrowed valve opening.

cells. In young adults, aortic stenosis usually is a later consequence of a congenital defect in which the valve has two instead of three cusps. At birth and throughout childhood, this defect does not produce symptoms. Symptoms appear after several decades, when the same calcification process that affects older adults causes the valves to harden. In others, aortic stenosis results directly from valvular damage related to rheumatic carditis and infective endocarditis (see Chap. 31).

The stiff, calcified valve cannot open properly and needs more force to push blood through its narrowed opening (Fig. 32-3). The muscular wall of the left ventricle enlarges and thickens (*hypertrophies*) in response. The blood volume passing through the narrowed valve eventually becomes insufficient to nourish the myocardium and other organs. Exercise or any circumstance that increases heart rate can cause myocardial ischemia, affect-

ing the heart's ability to contract effectively. Left-sided heart failure (see Chap. 36) may develop because the heart cannot fully empty during systole and becomes more fatigued as it tries to overcome the resistance created by the narrowed valve. Should the adult with aortic stenosis develop coronary artery disease (CAD) and MI (see Chap. 33), the infarct may enlarge. Risk of mortality thus increases because of the valve's compromised ability to perfuse the myocardium with oxygen.

Assessment Findings

Signs and Symptoms

A client with aortic stenosis may be asymptomatic for several decades. When symptoms develop, they include dizziness, fainting, and angina because of insufficient cardiac output. At first, the client experiences dyspnea and fatigue during activity. With ventricular enlargement, heart pulsations are displaced laterally or distally on the chest wall from the usual **point of maximum impulse** (PMI) at the fifth intercostal space medial to the left midclavicular line. The carotid pulse feels weak because of a low stroke volume.

The S_2 heart sound is split; that is, there is a definite separation between the sounds of the aortic valve and pulmonic valve closing. Usually, these sounds occur in unison or are so closely timed that they seem as one. While listening at the second intercostal space to the right and left of the sternum, the S_1 and split S_2 sounds like "lub-t-dub." The split persists throughout inspiration and expiration and does not disappear when the client sits up during auscultation. This finding distinguishes the split S_2 from a normal, physiologic splitting. Sometimes auscultation identifies other abnormal sounds (e.g., systolic murmur, click).

FIGURE 32-2 The aortic valve has three cusps or leaflets. (From Smeltzer, S. C. & Bare, B. G. [2000]. *Brunner & Suddarth's textbook of medical–surgical nursing* [9th ed.]. Philadelphia: Lippincott Williams & Wilkins.)

Diagnostic Findings

Ventricular enlargement is evident on a chest radiograph. An echocardiogram validates ventricular thickening and diminished transvalvular size. The height of the R wave on the electrocardiogram (ECG) may be increased, reflecting the large mass and force of contracting muscle. During left-sided cardiac catheterization, the pressure of blood in the left ventricle is higher than usual.

Medical and Surgical Management

Medical treatment may begin while the client is asymptomatic and focuses on maintaining adequate cardiac output by supporting the heart's pumping activity. Digitalis, an antihypertensive, antidysrhythmic drug particularly for atrial fibrillation with rapid ventricular response (see Chap. 34) and a diuretic may be prescribed. Sodium is restricted. Antibiotics are prescribed to prevent recurrences of infective endocarditis, which compound valvular damage. Nitrates or beta-adrenergic blockers are beneficial for relieving chest pain.

Additional treatment eventually becomes critical because average survival is 2 to 3 years once symptoms develop (Bonow et al., 1998). **Balloon valvuloplasty** is an invasive, nonsurgical procedure to enlarge a narrowed valve opening. A catheter with a deflated balloon is threaded through a peripheral blood vessel into the heart until the tip is located in the stenotic valve. When in position, the balloon is inflated to stretch the opening. Balloon valvuloplasty is considered temporary for clients whose conditions are too unstable for immediate surgery, yet whose symptoms cannot be adequately controlled more conservatively. The stretched valve opening tends to narrow again within 6 to 12 months (Bonow et al., 1998). Surgical aortic valve replacement eventually becomes necessary. Ideally, aortic valve replacement is performed before the client reaches the late stages of heart failure (see Chap. 36). A coronary arteriogram is performed to identify CAD; if present, valve replacement and surgical measures to improve vascular supply to the myocardium may be performed at the same time.

Nursing Management

The nurse monitors subjective and objective symptoms and explains the purposes and techniques of diagnostic tests. He or she administers prescribed medications and monitors for therapeutic or adverse responses. The nurse institutes measures to ensure adequate cardiac output and tissue oxygenation. He or she assists the client to comply with dietary modifications to reduce fluid volumes and the work placed on the heart (Nursing Care Plan 32-1).

● AORTIC REGURGITATION

Aortic regurgitation occurs when the aortic valve does not close tightly, a condition called **valvular incompetence.**

Pathophysiology and Etiology

Valvular incompetence can result from damage to the valve cusps or papillary muscles. It may be a consequence of various disorders such as rheumatic carditis, endocarditis, syphilis, age-related stretching of the proximal aorta, and systemic inflammatory conditions. In 1997, the incidence of aortic and mitral regurgitation increased as a result of the use of fenfluramine (Pondimin) with phentermine (known as FenPhen), fenfluramine alone, and dexfenfluramine (Redux) alone for weight loss. Various researchers identified that 29% to 36% of clients who took these drugs developed valvular disorders (Bonow et al., 1998).

When blood is pumped through the incompetent aortic valve, some leaks backward (**valvular regurgitation**) into the left ventricle. This backflow reduces cardiac output and causes fluid overload in the left ventricle, which becomes chronically stretched, hindering its ability to pump effectively (see Chap. 36). High fluid pressure in the left ventricle causes the mitral valve to shut early, which interferes with left atrial emptying. The blood in the left atrium backs up into the pulmonary circulation. Left ventricular enlargement increases the heart's need for oxygen. When the coronary arteries cannot supply the heart muscle with enough oxygen because of decreased cardiac output, the myocardium becomes ischemic and the client experiences angina. Dizziness, confusion, and left ventricular failure may develop.

Assessment Findings

Signs and Symptoms

The client remains asymptomatic as long as the left ventricle can sustain adequate circulation. Tachycardia is one of the first signs. When valve damage affects the left ventricle, the client becomes aware of forceful heart contractions (palpitations). At first, palpitations occur only when lying flat or on the left side. In later stages, the client experiences dyspnea and chest pain.

During physical examination, skin may be flushed and moist, especially in the upper body. The radial pulse may be very strong, with quick, sharp beats followed by a sudden collapse of force, a characteristic called a **water-hammer pulse** or *Corrigan's pulse.* Often, pulse pressure is wide because systolic blood pressure (BP) tends to be extremely high, whereas diastolic BP usually remains low

Nursing Care Plan 32-1

THE CLIENT WITH A VALVULAR DISORDER

Assessment

Determine the following:

- Vital signs, noting tachycardia, rapid respirations, dyspnea, hypotension, or hypertension
- Any episodes of dizziness or fainting with or without confusion
- Chest pain and its characteristics
- Normal or abnormal lung and heart sounds
- Fluid intake and output
- Current weight and fluctuations during treatment
- Level of activity tolerance
- Social aspects (e.g., occupational activities) as they relate to physical energy requirements
- Knowledge of medical condition and current and future treatment protocols

Nursing Diagnosis: **Risk for Decreased Cardiac Output** related to diminished cardiac muscle contractility, tachycardia, and hypertension

Expected Outcome: Cardiac output will be adequate as evidenced by no chest pain, hypotension, or dizziness.

Interventions	Rationales
Monitor cardiac rhythm and rate.	Heart rate affects and tachydysrhythmias compromise cardiac output.
Measure urine output every 8 hours or more often if less than 500 mL/day.	Renal output reflects the heart's ability to perfuse the renal arteries.
Maintain client on bed rest.	Rest lowers heart rate, which increases diastolic filling volume.
Reduce anxiety by responding to requests for attention or assistance.	Relief of anxiety reduces tachycardia and hypertension.
Provide substitutes for dietary sources of caffeine and sodium.	Caffeine increases heart rate and promotes vasoconstriction; sodium contributes to fluid retention.
Promote ease in eliminating stool through such measures as increasing fiber and administering a prescribed stool softener.	Bearing down to eliminate stool interferes with cardiac filling; reduced cardiac filling decreases cardiac output.
Reduce any fever by changing to lighter or fewer bed linens, assisting with tepid sponge baths, or administering prescribed antipyretics.	Increased heart rate accompanies fever and adds to the heart's workload, which may compromise cardiac output.

Evaluation of Expected Outcome: Client is pain free; heart rate, BP, and urine output are within normal ranges. The client's sensorium is clear.

Nursing Diagnosis: **Activity Intolerance** related to decreased cardiac output

Expected Outcome: Client will tolerate activity without dyspnea or heart rate above 100 beats/min.

Interventions	Rationales
Provide complete or partial assistance with activities of daily living.	Activity taxes endurance and results in increased heart rate and blood pressure.

(continued)

Nursing Care Plan 32-1 (Continued)

THE CLIENT WITH A VALVULAR DISORDER

Interventions	Rationales
Allow adequate time for client to perform self-care.	Activity that is done without urgency is less physically demanding.
Intersperse periods of activity with rest.	Rest helps the heart recover from demands that increase its rate or force of contraction.

Evaluation of Expected Outcome: Client manages self-care and moderate activity without becoming breathless, hypotensive, or tachycardic.

Nursing Diagnosis: **Pain** related to myocardial ischemia

Expected Outcome: Pain will be reduced to client's self-described tolerance level within 30 minutes of a nursing intervention.

Interventions	Rationales
Provide rest immediately.	Rest slows the heart rate and decreases the myocardium's need for oxygen.
Administer oxygen temporarily.	Increasing inhaled oxygen concentration promotes myocardial cellular oxygenation.
Give prescribed short-acting nitrate or analgesic.	Nitrates cause vasodilatation and increase blood flow from the coronary arteries to the myocardium; analgesics block the transmission or perception of pain.
Assist clients with mitral valve prolapse to lie flat and elevate the legs 90° for 3 to 5 minutes.	Elevating the legs facilitates volume changes in the heart.

Evaluation of Expected Outcome: Client is free of pain.

Nursing Diagnosis: **Risk for Infection** related to increased susceptibility secondary to previous endocardial inflammatory or infectious disorders

Expected Outcome: Client will remain free of infection as evidenced by normal temperature and white blood cell count.

Interventions	Rationales
Reassign care of client if designated caregiver has infectious symptoms, or have caregiver don protective garments (e.g., face mask) and change them frequently.	Reducing exposure to microorganisms associated with infective endocarditis minimizes the potential for infection and repeated valvular damage.
Perform conscientious handwashing.	Handwashing is the single most effective method to reduce infectious microorganisms.
Follow aseptic principles when changing dressings covering impaired skin and vascular insertion sites.	Impaired skin is an entrance site for microorganisms that may lead to bacteremia and repeated valvular damage.

Evaluation of Expected Outcome: Client does not acquire a nosocomial infection.

PC: **Congestive Heart Failure**

Expected Outcome: The nurse will monitor for, manage, and minimize heart failure.

Interventions	Rationales
Auscultate lung and heart sounds at least once per shift or more often if abnormal sounds are evident.	Crackles, rhonchi (gurgles), and an S_3 heart sound are signs of cardiopulmonary complications such as left-sided congestive heart failure.

(continued)

Nursing Care Plan 32-1 (Continued)

THE CLIENT WITH A VALVULAR DISORDER

Interventions	*Rationales*
Weigh client daily at the same time, with similar clothing, on the same scale.	A weight gain of 2 lb or more in 24 hours suggests fluid retention equal to 1 L.
Support compliance with prescribed sodium and fluid restrictions.	Such restrictions decrease the work and sustain the ability of the heart to contract efficiently.

Evaluation of Expected Outcome: The nurse documents appropriate assessment findings, reports critical information to the physician, and implements prescribed interventions.

Nursing Diagnosis: **Risk for Ineffective Management of Therapeutic Regimen** related to insufficient knowledge of self-care

Expected Outcome: Client will accurately describe discharge instructions.

Interventions	*Rationales*
Completely explain all treatments.	Client cannot implement interventions that are not explained.
Advise client to consult the physician about prophylactic antibiotic therapy before dental or invasive treatments.	Prophylactic antibiotics reduce the potential for recurrent endocarditis and additional valvular damage.
Caution against lifting heavy objects or straining at stool.	Bearing down with forced expiration through a closed glottis (Valsalva maneuver) increases BP, which predisposes client to heart failure.
Teach client to recognize signs and symptoms of heart failure (see Chap. 36) and to report them immediately.	Early intervention facilitates an improved prognosis if a complication develops.
Advise client to avoid caffeine and over-the-counter medications that contain cardiac stimulants (e.g., decongestants).	They cause tachycardia and vasoconstriction, increasing the risk for myocardial ischemia, tachydysrhythmias, and heart failure.
Instruct client to avoid strenuous exercise and competitive sports.	Activity beyond tolerance and competition increase heart rate, BP, and cardiac risks.

Evaluation of Expected Outcome: Client accurately describes his or her disorder, methods for controlling symptoms, and precautions that reduce the risk for complications.

or normal. The enlarged heart displaces the PMI. The chest may heave or rock from the forceful contractions of the enlarged left ventricle. A heart murmur, caused by the turbulence of blood falling back through the dilated aortic valve, also may be heard.

Diagnostic Findings

Cardiac catheterization reveals high left ventricular pressure and backward movement of blood. A chest radiograph reveals heart enlargement, and the aortic valve appears dilated. The ECG presents with tall R waves; depressed ST segments indicate myocardial ischemia (see Chap. 30). A radionuclide scan comparing blood flow through the heart at rest and during exercise reveals the severity of the disease. Standard or transesophageal echocardiography provides images of atypical valvular and myocardial function. A computed tomography or magnetic resonance imaging scan may be performed if the echocardiographic images are inconclusive.

Medical and Surgical Management

Because aortic regurgitation is mild and only slowly progressive in most people, clients are sustained with cardiac glycosides (Drug Therapy Table 32-1) or beta blockers and diuretics. When taken appropriately, prophylactic antibiotics prevent recurrences of infective endocarditis. Clients are advised to modify their lifestyles to avoid excessive demands on the heart, such as those that may result from strenuous exercise and emotional stress. When a client becomes symptomatic, replacement of the dis-

DRUG THERAPY TABLE 32-1	AGENTS TO TREAT VALVULAR HEART DISORDERS		
DRUG CATEGORY AND EXAMPLES	**MECHANISM OF ACTION**	**SIDE EFFECTS**	**NURSING CONSIDERATIONS**
Antibiotics penicillin G potassium (Pfizerpen)	Inhibit cell wall synthesis in susceptible organisms, causing cell death	Anaphylaxis, glossitis, gastritis, sore mouth, nausea, vomiting, diarrhea, rash, fever, superinfection, phlebitis	Ascertain if client is allergic to penicillin before administering. After administering first parenteral dose, monitor client's response for 30 minutes. Assess IV site for pain and signs and symptoms of phlebitis. Administer oral doses with a full glass of water to a client on an empty stomach.
Anticoagulants warfarin sodium (Coumadin)	Prevent thrombi Prolong clotting times by interfering with vitamin K–dependent clotting factors	Increased bleeding, nausea, leukopenia, alopecia, dermatitis, fever, rash	Monitor complete blood counts, PT, and INR frequently. Advise client to wear a Medic Alert tag. Instruct client to report any unusual or excessive bleeding.
Cardiac Glycosides digoxin (Lanoxin)	Increase cardiac output by slowing heart rate (negative chronotropic action) and increasing force of contraction (positive iotropic action)	Fatigue, generalized muscle weakness, agitation, hallucinations (toxic effects on heart may be life-threatening and require immediate attention), yellow-green halos around images, blurred vision, anorexia	Assess pulse rate before each dose. Withhold administration if pulse is <60 or >120 beats/min. Monitor serum potassium levels; ensure intake of potassium. Administer before meals to promote absorption.
Antiplatelets ticlopidine hydrochloride (Ticlid)	Decrease clot production by interfering with platelet aggregation	Dizziness, diarrhea, nausea, abdominal pain, neutropenia, bleeding, rash	Administer with food or meals. Monitor white blood cell count, and assess for excessive bleeding. Relate need for regular, follow-up laboratory tests.
Antidysrhythmics quinidine (Quinaglute)	Alter the action potential of cardiac cells and interfere with heart's electrical excitability	Nausea, vomiting, diplopia, new dysrhythmias, hemolytic anemia, rash, tinnitus, headache	Monitor for new or worse dysrhythmias. Ensure reduced dosage in clients with hepatic or renal failure. Monitor blood counts during prolonged therapy.

eased aortic valve is considered (see Chap. 37). The less heart damage that occurs before surgery, the better the outcome. If the aorta is diseased, the procedure is more involved because repair involves a vascular graft.

Nursing Management

The nurse prepares the client for diagnostic procedures and monitors responses. He or she reports changes in heart rate and rhythm, dyspnea, chest pain, and loss of consciousness to the physician immediately. The nurse administers prescribed medications and evaluates the client's response. Ensuring that physical activity is balanced according to the client's tolerance is important. Before discharge, the nurse explains the need for antibiotic therapy before medical and dental procedures and teaches how to assess BP regularly as well as methods to control hypertension. See Nursing Care Plan 32-1 for more information.

Stop, Think, and Respond ● BOX 32-1

A client with an aortic valvular disorder experiences chest pain while performing bathing and hygiene. What nursing actions are appropriate?

DISORDERS OF THE MITRAL VALVE

The mitral valve, which lies between the left atrium and left ventricle, is a bicuspid valve. The two cusps are attached on the ventricular surface to strands of fibrous tissue called *chordae tendineae,* which are projections from papillary muscles (Fig. 32-4). The papillary muscles contract in unison with the ventricle, pull on the chordae tendineae, and prevent the cusps from ballooning into the left atrium. The functions of the mitral valve are to open widely to allow oxygenated blood to fill the left ventricle and close tightly to prevent blood from re-entering the left atrium after the left ventricle is filled. As long as the mitral valve remains structurally sound, blood exits the left ventricle through the aortic valve, where the aorta receives a 50- to 70-mL bolus of oxygenated blood, referred to as the *stroke volume.* The valve may become rigid (stenotic), incompetent (inadequate closure), or prolapsed (floppy). Mitral valve prolapse is the most common valvular disorder.

• MITRAL STENOSIS

Pathophysiology and Etiology

Mitral stenosis means that the valve does not open properly to facilitate filling of the left ventricle (Fig. 32-5). It is primarily a **sequela** (a condition that follows a disease) of rheumatic carditis (see Chap. 31). Mitral stenosis worsens with each recurrence of endocarditis. The inflammation causes the cusps to stick together and form a thick, rigid, calcified scar at the **commissures,** the area where the

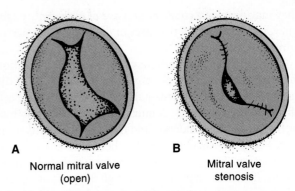

A Normal mitral valve (open) **B** Mitral valve stenosis

FIGURE 32-5 (**A**) The normal mitral valve opens widely to allow blood to pass from the left atrium to the left ventricle. (**B**) Following what is generally an infectious process, the mitral valve leaflets become fused with scar tissue, causing a partially obstructed pathway for the passage of blood.

cusps contact each other, and the chordae tendineae fuse and shorten. The mitral valve cannot open completely, leading to incomplete emptying of the left atrium. Pooled blood from incomplete emptying contributes to clot formation, which puts the client at risk for arterial emboli. The left atrium enlarges because it has to contract more forcibly to empty. Pressure from overfilling is conveyed backward through the blood vessels to the lungs, creating **pulmonary hypertension** and the potential for pulmonary edema (see Chap. 36). Pulmonary hypertension increases the work of the right ventricle as it pumps against the high pressure in the pulmonary vascular system.

Because blood flows in a circuit, the disease on the left side of the heart eventually affects the right side. The right ventricle may enlarge in response to its increased workload. When the contraction of the right ventricle can no longer overcome the pulmonary resistance, right-sided heart failure develops. Excess blood accumulates in the venous circulation, the liver becomes congested, and edema occurs in the legs.

Assessment Findings

Signs and Symptoms

It may take 20 to 40 years for a client who has had rheumatic fever to develop mitral stenosis. The normal valve opening is 4 to 5 cm²; symptoms develop when the valve area is less than 2.5 cm² (Bonow et al., 1998). At that time, clients report fatigue and dyspnea after slight exertion. Symptoms become disabling approximately 10 years after onset; they are accentuated when unusual demands are placed on the heart (e.g., fever, emotional stress, pregnancy). Later, clients experience heart palpitations caused by *tachydysrhythmias* (rapid dysrhythmias). With the onset of pulmonary hypertension, clients may become more dyspneic at night and must sleep in a sitting position.

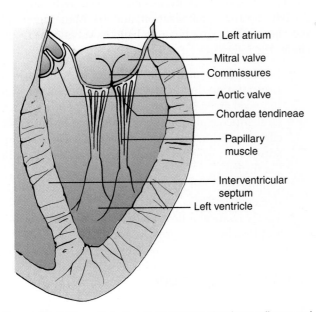

Left atrium

Mitral valve

Commissures

Aortic valve

Chordae tendineae

Papillary muscle

Interventricular septum

Left ventricle

FIGURE 32-4 The mitral valve is attached to chordae tendineae and papillary muscles.

They may develop a cough productive of pink, frothy sputum. Crackles heard in the bases of the lungs are a sign of pulmonary congestion.

Changes in heart sounds may be the earliest indication of mitral valve stenosis. S_1 may be extremely loud if the cusps are fused, or muffled or absent if the cusps have calcified and are immobile. A murmur, described as sounding like a rumbling underground train, can be heard at the heart's apex, especially when the client assumes a left lateral position. The systolic BP is low from reduced cardiac output. If backward pressure through the pulmonary circulation is sufficient to affect the right ventricle, the client's face is flushed; neck vein distention is evident; the liver is enlarged; and there is peripheral edema.

Diagnostic Findings

A chest radiograph reveals an enlarged left atrium and mitral valve calcification. In advanced stages, evidence of fluid congestion in the lungs (pulmonary edema) is found. A standard or esophageal echocardiogram demonstrates decreased movement of the mitral valve cusps and changes in the size of the atrial chamber. On ECG, the P wave is notched, showing that the left atrium takes longer to depolarize than the right atrium because of its increased size.

Medical and Surgical Management

Antibiotic therapy is prescribed to prevent future episodes of infective endocarditis. Preventing or relieving the symptoms of heart failure is essential. A daily aspirin, dipyridamole (Persantine), or other oral anticoagulant may be ordered to avoid clot formation. Dysrhythmias, such as *atrial fibrillation* (quivering of the atrial muscle with insufficient force to pump blood), are treated with drugs or cardioversion. Cardioversion stops the heart momentarily to allow the sinoatrial node to re-establish itself as the pacemaker.

Not all clients with mitral stenosis are suitable candidates for surgery. Those whose condition is so slight that it does not cause symptoms or so severe or of such long duration that profound changes in the heart and lungs have occurred usually are excluded. The earlier surgery is performed, the greater is the likelihood that it will relieve the symptoms.

Percutaneous balloon valvuloplasty, also called *valvotomy,* is a nonsurgical alternative to *commissurotomy,* a surgical technique to separate the fused leaflets (see Chap. 37). When percutaneous balloon valvuloplasty is performed, a catheter with an uninflated balloon is passed through the femoral vein and threaded into the right atrium. The septum is then punctured between the right and left atria. When the catheter is in the mitral valve, it is inflated (Fig. 32-6). Clients often are discharged on the same day as the procedure. The atrial puncture allows

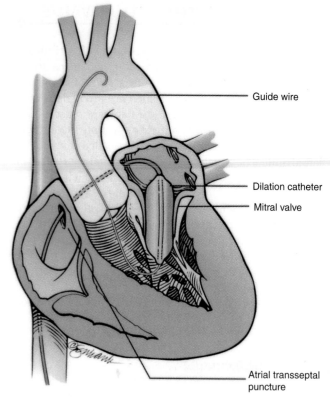

Figure 32-6 Balloon valvuloplasty cross-section of heart illustrating dilation catheter placed through an atrial transseptal puncture and across the mitral valve. The guide wire extends from the aortic valve into the aorta for catheter support. (From Smeltzer, S. C. & Bare, B. G. [2000]. *Brunner & Suddarth's textbook of medical–surgical nursing* [9th ed.]. Philadelphia: Lippincott Williams & Wilkins.)

Labels on figure: Guide wire; Dilation catheter; Mitral valve; Atrial transseptal puncture

some blood to shunt from the left atrium to the right, but the opening usually closes within 6 months. Complications, although rare, include mitral regurgitation (discussed next), residual atrial-septal defect, perforation of the left ventricle, embolization, and MI. Management of the client after percutaneous balloon valvuloplasty includes the following:

- Echocardiogram within 72 hours to detect mitral regurgitation, left ventricular dysfunction, or pronounced atrial-septal defect
- Oral anticoagulation therapy within 1 to 2 days for clients who have a history of atrial fibrillation or instituted for others if atrial fibrillation develops in the future
- Prophylactic antibiotic protocols to prevent infective endocarditis
- Yearly medical follow-up that includes echocardiography, chest radiography, and ECG

Nursing Management

The nurse monitors the client's physical condition, prepares him or her for diagnostic testing, and provides post-treatment care. Discharge teaching includes information regarding drug therapy, activity modification, signs and symptoms of complications, and when to contact the physician. See Nursing Care Plan 32-1 for additional discussion.

● MITRAL REGURGITATION (INSUFFICIENCY)

Mitral regurgitation, sometimes referred to as *mitral insufficiency,* occurs when the mitral valve does not close completely (Fig. 32-7). Some clients present with severe acute symptoms; others, whose heart muscle increases in size to compensate, remain asymptomatic or develop symptoms gradually over many years.

Pathophysiology and Etiology

Mitral regurgitation is associated with rheumatic carditis and mitral valve prolapse (discussed next). It also is linked with damage to the papillary muscles, impaired myocardial function after MI, connective tissue disorders, stretching of the valve opening from an enlarged left ventricle, and malfunction of a replaced valve. It also can develop after balloon valvuloplasty. Use of the anorectic drugs identified in the discussion of aortic regurgitation also has been associated with mitral valve regurgitation.

When the mitral valve becomes incompetent (i.e., does not close completely), blood flows backward into the left atrium during ventricular systole and leaks into the left ventricle during atrial diastole. The heart usually can compensate for a small amount of blood that is regurgitated backward and forward by increasing the

size of the left ventricle and left atria. The larger size facilitates ejection of blood from the heart, in which case pulmonary congestion does not occur. If the regurgitation occurs rapidly, however, the heart is less able to compensate. Forward output from the left ventricle is diminished, and the client develops signs of shock. Accumulation of blood in the left atrium results in pulmonary congestion.

Assessment Findings

Signs and Symptoms

The client typically experiences chronic fatigue and dyspnea on exertion. He or she may notice heart palpitations caused by the forceful contraction of the left ventricle as it attempts to empty the excess blood from its chamber. The S_1 heart sound is diminished because of incomplete closure of the mitral valve. An S_3 heart sound, if heard, is an early sign of impending heart failure. Hypertension may develop when reduced cardiac output triggers the renin-angiotensin-aldosterone cycle. Tachycardia is a compensatory mechanism when stroke volume decreases. A loud, blowing murmur often is heard throughout ventricular systole at the heart's apex. If pulmonary congestion occurs, the client develops shortness of breath and moist lung sounds typical of left ventricular failure (see Chap. 36).

Diagnostic Findings

Standard transthoracic or transesophageal echocardiography is the best technique to identify structural changes in the mitral valve. Chest radiography shows enlarged chambers on the left side of the heart. Radionuclide angiography provides information on the volume of regurgitated blood. ECG reflects cardiac enlargement, papillary muscle or chordae tendineae dysfunction, and various associated dysrhythmias (e.g., atrial fibrillation).

Medical and Surgical Management

Asymptomatic clients are monitored through physical examination and annual echocardiograms. Exercise is not limited until mild symptoms develop. An angiotensin-converting enzyme inhibitor like quinapril (Accupril) reduces afterload, preserving the left ventricle's ability to eject blood effectively. Digitalis, calcium channel blockers, beta blockers, or other antidysrhythmic drugs control tachycardia. Some clients are given drugs to prevent intracardiac thrombi, a common complication of blood stasis that accompanies atrial fibrillation. Prophylactic antibiotics are prescribed to prevent recurrences of infective endocarditis. An intra-aortic balloon pump, which pro-

FIGURE 32-7 Mitral insufficiency. The incompetent atrioventricular valve allows blood to return to the left atrium.

vides counterpulsation to the contraction of the left ventricle, can be used in an emergency to stabilize a client in left ventricular failure (see Chap. 36).

Surgery to correct mitral regurgitation includes **annuloplasty,** repair of the valve leaflets and their fibrous ring. The implantation of a biologic or prosthetic valve to restore unidirectional blood flow may accompany annuloplasty (see Chap. 37).

Nursing Management

The nurse closely monitors BP, heart rate and rhythm, heart sounds, and lung sounds. He or she weighs the client to determine changes in fluid balance. If sodium is restricted, the nurse works with the client and dietitian to find palatable seasonings and foods. He or she administers medications to treat symptoms and reports signs of left- or right-sided heart failure immediately. The nurse emphasizes the need for prophylactic antibiotics and periodic health assessments. Refer to Nursing Care Plan 32-1 for more specific interventions.

● MITRAL VALVE PROLAPSE

In **mitral valve prolapse,** the valve cusps enlarge, become floppy, and bulge backward into the left atrium (Fig. 32-8). Mitral regurgitation may occur, but not in all cases. Besides being the most common valvular disorder, mitral valve prolapse is the leading cause of mitral re-

gurgitation. It is more common in young women than men. Despite its high incidence, it is considered to be a benign disease for most people affected (Joy, 1996).

Pathophysiology and Etiology

The cause of mitral valve prolapse is not completely understood, and it often is classified as idiopathic (having no known cause). It also has been suggested that the tissue changes result from an inherited connective tissue disorder that affects the mitral valve and other connective tissues in the body. It has been observed that some clients develop mitral valve prolapse in association with CAD, although there is speculation that no etiologic relationship actually exists. There is, however, strong evidence that mitral valve prolapse accompanies the valvular changes of rheumatic carditis, and structural changes predispose the valve to further damage if infective endocarditis develops.

Some people develop **mitral valve prolapse syndrome,** symptoms that cannot be attributed to valvular disease alone (Joy, 1996). It is associated with autonomic nervous system dysfunction. This association may explain why some clients have increased levels of catecholamines (i.e., epinephrine, norepinephrine), abnormal catecholamine regulation, and decreased intravascular volume, which causes symptoms that mimic severe anxiety (tachycardia, palpitations, breathlessness, dizziness). Decreased circulatory volume may contribute to the client's symptomatology by triggering an abnormal renin-angiotensin-aldosterone response (see Chap. 23). Changes in the mitral

Normal mitral
valve closed

Prolapsed valve
leaflet

FIGURE 32-8 In mitral valve prolapse, the floppy valve leaflets allow blood to regurgitate, or move in retrograde fashion, from the left ventricle to the left atria.

valve tissue layers cause the cusps to distend. The billowing cusps stretch the papillary muscles as they balloon backward into the left atrium. The stretching of the papillary muscles causes local ischemia and atypical chest pain. As the papillary muscles provide less support to the mitral valve, valvular incompetence occurs. The left atrium and ventricle eventually may enlarge and subsequently progress to congestive heart failure.

Assessment Findings

Many clients with mitral valve prolapse are asymptomatic. When symptoms are present, they include chest pain, palpitations, and fatigue. The chest pain differs from that of angina: its onset does not correlate with physical exertion, its duration is prolonged, and it is not easily relieved. Some clients also experience symptoms that resemble anxiety or panic, such as a rapid and irregular heart rate, shortness of breath, light-headedness, difficulty concentrating, and fear that the symptoms indicate impending death. Auscultation of heart sounds reveals a characteristic "click" during ventricular systole caused by tightening of the chordae tendineae. A systolic murmur is associated with mitral regurgitation. The presumptive diagnosis of mitral valve prolapse is strong if the murmur disappears or diminishes when the client squats during auscultation. Additional symptoms of mitral regurgitation also may be manifested.

Echocardiography shows abnormal movement of one or more mitral valve leaflets during systole. The ECG (resting, exercise, chemical, or ambulatory) is essentially normal, eliminating MI as a cause for the chest pain. ECG, however, may detect other causes.

Medical and Surgical Management

Many clients with mitral valve prolapse require no treatment except periodic antibiotic therapy before invasive procedures. Such drugs as digitalis, beta blockers, and calcium channel blockers control tachydysrhythmias; all but digitalis also control hypertension. Medications to reduce platelet aggregation (e.g., a single daily aspirin, ticlopidine [Ticlid]) are prescribed to prevent thrombus formation. If symptoms become severe, valve replacement is indicated.

Antianxiety medication may be prescribed to prevent symptoms related to the sympathetic nervous system among those with mitral valve prolapse syndrome. Such clients also are advised to avoid caffeine to prevent tachycardia and heart palpitations. To compensate for symptoms associated with hypovolemia, liberal fluid and adequate sodium intake are recommended. Because alcohol can suppress antidiuretic hormone, leading to loss of extracellular fluid, clients with mitral valve prolapse syndrome are advised to restrict or eliminate its use.

Nursing Management

One measure to relieve chest pain is to have the client lie flat with the legs elevated and supported against a wall or couch at a 90° angle for 3 to 5 minutes to facilitate volume changes in the heart. Other recommendations include increasing activity when tachycardia occurs to eliminate the initiation of extra, ineffective beats, make up for reduced cardiac output, and lower levels of catecholamines. To relax or decrease shortness of breath, the nurse instructs the client to breathe deeply and slowly and then exhale through pursed lips. He or she advises the client to avoid caffeinated beverages and over-the-counter medications that contain stimulating chemicals to avoid contributing to an already rapid heart rate. If hypertension is not a problem, the nurse encourages the client to drink adequate fluid and continue moderate use of salt to maintain intravascular fluid volume. He or she discourages the use of alcohol because of its dehydrating effects and because withdrawal after chronic use can cause cardiac stimulation. The nurse warns clients who are prescribed minor tranquilizers not to stop the medication abruptly or they may experience stimulating withdrawal symptoms. Additional nursing management depends on other assessment data. See Nursing Care Plan 32-1.

> ### Stop, Think, and Respond ● BOX 32-2
> *Explain why clients with valvular disorders may need exercise modifications.*

GENERAL NUTRITIONAL CONSIDERATIONS

Because approximately 75% of sodium in the typical American diet comes from processed foods, encourage clients who must limit their sodium intake to substitute homemade foods for mixes and prepared items. Foods to avoid include canned fish, meat, poultry, soup, vegetables, and vegetable juices; smoked and processed meats; sauerkraut; commercial mixes; instant rice and pasta mixes; casserole mixes; instant and quick-cooking cereals; condiments such as catsup, relish, pickles, barbecue sauce, soy sauce, and Worcestershire sauce; and seasoning salts.

Salt substitutes replace sodium with potassium or other minerals and may taste bitter. Low-sodium salt substitutes may contain up to half as much sodium as regular table salt. Clients should not use either type without a physician's approval.

Foods that liquefy at room temperature (ice cream, ice milk, gelatin, ice pops, sherbet) are counted as liquids when fluid intake is restricted.

GENERAL PHARMACOLOGIC CONSIDERATIONS

Closely monitor clients receiving oral anticoagulants for episodes of bleeding, melena (blood in stool), easy bruising, and oozing from superficial injuries, such as cuts from shaving or bleeding from the gums after brushing the teeth. Oral anticoagulant therapy requires close monitoring of prothrombin time (PT). Therapeutic PT levels are 1.5 to 2.5 times the control value. When the PT is reported as an international normalized ratio, the normal range is 2.0 to 3.0.

Nonselective beta blockers can aggravate chronic obstructive pulmonary disease and contribute to hypoglycemia in insulin-dependent adults. Some diuretics deplete potassium, causing hypokalemia.

Before administering beta blockers, take the client's apical pulse. If the heart rate is less than 60 beats/minute, withhold the drug and notify the primary healthcare provider.

Closely monitor clients taking beta blockers for signs and symptoms of overdosage: bradycardia, severe dizziness, drowsiness, and bluish discoloration of the palms, fingernails, or both. Notify the primary care provider immediately if these symptoms appear.

When administering quinidine observe the client for symptoms of cinchonism (quinidine toxicity), which include ringing of the ears, headache, nausea, dizziness, and fever.

GENERAL GERONTOLOGIC CONSIDERATIONS

Older adults may require lower doses of cardiac glycosides than younger clients because of age-related metabolic changes. The more medications older adults take, the more likely they are to have dangerous interactions. Monitor the heart rate and BP of older adults taking beta blockers closely; the adverse effects of bradycardia and hypotension can cause confusion and falls.

Fluid and electrolyte imbalances resulting from diuretic therapy can cause fatigue and weakness, which older adults may confuse as a worsening of the symptoms related to valvular disease.

Calcification of heart structures, especially valvular tissue and the proximal aorta, increases with aging, putting older adults at increased risk for dangerous dysrhythmias and heart failure with subsequent alterations in cardiac output.

Syncope and falls resulting from decreased cardiac output occur more often in older adults.

Critical Thinking Exercises

1. *Compare and contrast stenosis and regurgitation of the aortic and mitral valves.*

2. *You are assisting a newly admitted client with a diagnosis of mitral stenosis into his hospital room. The individual in the next bed is diagnosed with tracheobronchitis, has a humidifier at the bedside, and receives frequent aerosol breathing treatments. What is the potential problem? What measures are appropriate to correct it?*

References and Suggested Readings

Baptiste, M. M. (2001). Aortic valve replacement. *RN, 64*(1), 58–64.

Bonow, R. O., Carabellow, B., DeLeon, A. C., et al. (1998). ACC/AHA guidelines for the management of patients with valvular heart disease. *Journal of American College of Cardiology, 32*, 1486–1588.

Joy, E. (1996). Mitral valve prolapse in active patients: Recognition, treatment, and exercise recommendations. [Online.] Available: http:www.physsportsmed.com/issues/jul_96/joy.htm.

Linden, B. (2000). Systems and diseases: The heart, part seven. Valvular heart disease. *Nursing Times, 96*(4), 49–52.

Linden, B. (2000). Systems and diseases: The heart, part eight. Valvular heart disease. *Nursing Times, 96*(8), 49–52.

Sutaria, N., Elder, A., & Shaw, T. (2000). Mitral balloon valvotomy for the treatment of mitral stenosis in octogenarians. *Journal of the American Geriatrics Society, 48*, 971–974.

Caring for Clients With Disorders of Coronary and Peripheral Blood Vessels

Words to Know

aneurysm
angina pectoris
apolipoproteins
arteriosclerosis
atherectomy
atheroma
atherosclerosis
bruit
cardiac rehabilitation
cholesterol
collateral circulation
coronary artery
  bypass graft
coronary artery disease
coronary occlusion
coronary stent
coronary thrombosis
embolus
enhanced external
  counterpulsation
high-density lipoprotein
homocysteine
hyperlipidemia
infarct
ischemia
laser angioplasty

low-density lipoprotein
neoangiogenesis
percutaneous
  transluminal coronary
  angioplasty
peripheral vascular
  disease
phlebothrombosis
phytoestrogens
plaque
subendocardial
  infarction
thrombolytic agents
thrombosis
thrombus
topical hyperbaric
  oxygen
transmural infarction
transmyocardial
  revascularization
varicose veins
vein ligation
vein stripping
venous insufficiency
venous reflux
venous stasis ulcer

Learning Objectives

On completion of this chapter, the reader will:

● Distinguish between arteriosclerosis and atherosclerosis.
● List risk factors associated with coronary artery disease, and discuss which can be modified.
● Discuss the symptoms, diagnosis, treatment, and nursing management of myocardial infarction.
● Discuss the symptoms, diagnosis, and treatment of Raynaud's disease, thrombosis, phlebothrombosis, and embolism.
● Describe nursing management of clients with an occlusive disorder of peripheral blood vessels.
● Discuss the symptoms, diagnosis, and treatment of varicose veins.
● Describe nursing management of clients undergoing surgery for varicose veins.
● Discuss the symptoms, diagnosis, treatment, and nursing management of clients with an aortic aneurysm.

Uninterrupted blood flow is essential to cells and tissues. Cardiovascular disease is the leading cause of death in the United States. Occlusive disorders of the coronary arteries and resulting complications are largely responsible. Occlusive disorders of peripheral blood vessels also affect many. The most common causes of occlusive vascular diseases are atherosclerosis, arteriosclerosis, clot formation, and vascular spasm. Venous insufficiency and valvular incompetence also contribute to peripheral vascular disorders.

ARTERIOSCLEROSIS AND ATHEROSCLEROSIS

Arteriosclerosis refers to the loss of elasticity or hardening of the arteries. **Atherosclerosis** is a condition in which the lumen of the artery fills with fatty deposits (chiefly composed of cholesterol) called **plaque.** Arteriosclerosis and atherosclerosis affect many blood vessels that supply body organs and tissues (i.e., heart, brain, kidneys, extremities). Consequently, these two conditions contribute to several disorders (myocardial infarction [MI], cerebrovascular accidents, renal failure).

To some degree, arteriosclerosis and atherosclerosis normally accompany the aging process. The rate at which arterial changes occur varies. Many factors affect the rate of onset and overall severity of these conditions. As cells in arterial tissue layers degenerate with aging, calcium is deposited in the cytoplasm. The calcium causes the arteries to lose elasticity. As the left ventricle contracts, sending oxygenated blood from the heart, the rigid arterial vessels fail to stretch. The potential result is a reduced volume of oxygenated blood delivered to organs.

Hyperlipidemia, or high levels of blood fat, triggers atherosclerotic changes. Factors such as sex, heredity, diet, and activity individually or collectively contribute to hyperlipidemia. For example, some clients inherit genetic codes that replicate cells with reduced numbers of receptors for binding with cholesterol; therefore, they are more likely to develop high lipid levels. Clients who consume a high-fat diet may saturate all available cholesterol receptors, which also results in hyperlipidemia. Above-normal cholesterol levels have been linked to a byproduct of methionine, an amino acid present in meat, called **homocysteine.** High levels of homocysteine also are implicated in thickening, narrowing, and scarring of arterial walls.

A current hypothesis is that atherosclerosis is linked with prior infections with *Chlamydia pneumoniae,* a bacterium that commonly causes respiratory infections (Fong, 2000; Ross, 1999). Research has shown that *C. pneumoniae* can infect smooth muscle and endothelial cells of arterial walls. Some evidence suggests that *C. pneumoniae* either accelerates the atherosclerotic process or destabilizes one that already exists, leading to an area of local inflammation. Scientists support their hypothesis with the finding that *C. pneumoniae* has been cultured from the **atheroma** (fatty mass) in the arterial wall. Furthermore, results of blood tests such as C-reactive protein levels and white blood cell (WBC) counts, which reflect inflammation and infection, are elevated among clients hospital-

ized for coronary events. The National Heart, Lung, and Blood Institute, a division of the National Institutes of Health, began funding a national clinical trial in 1999 at the University of Washington and 27 cardiac treatment centers nationwide to determine if administering an antibiotic to clients with coronary artery disease has positive outcomes. Currently, it is safe to assume that multiple factors contribute to arterial disease. A client with elevated lipid levels who also has other risk factors (cigarette smoking, stressful lifestyle, diabetes mellitus, hypertension, or a previous infection with *C. pneumoniae* or other microorganisms) is predisposed to the accelerated accumulation of fatty plaque beneath the intimal layer of the arteries.

The body responds to microscopic injury in arterial walls by activating the inflammatory response. Monocytes migrate to the site of injury and deposit themselves under the endothelial cells of the tunica intima. The monocytes then attract and accumulate lipid (fatty) material. The enlarging lesion elevates the endothelium of the artery wall and narrows the lumen (Fig. 33-1). Atherosclerotic vessels cannot produce endothelial-derived relaxing factors, which impairs the ability of the artery to dilate. As the subendothelial atheroma enlarges, the intimal layer may split and expose the lesion. As blood flows through the vessel, platelets become trapped in the roughened wall and initiate the clotting cascade. When this occurs in a coronary artery, the resulting mass is called a *coronary thrombosis.*

OCCLUSIVE DISORDERS OF CORONARY BLOOD VESSELS

Coronary occlusion is the closing of a coronary artery, which reduces or totally interrupts blood supply to the distal muscle area. Coronary artery disease precedes coronary occlusion, which, untreated, leads to MI. Symptoms usually do not occur until at least 60% of the arterial lumen is occluded.

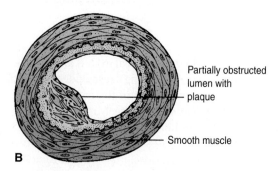

FIGURE 33-1 (**A**) Cross-section of a normal artery in which the lumen is fully patent, or open. (**B**) Cross-section of an atherosclerotic artery. (From Smeltzer, S. C. & Bare, B. G. [2000]. *Brunner & Suddarth's textbook of medical–surgical nursing* [9th ed.]. Philadelphia: Lippincott Williams & Wilkins.)

● CORONARY ARTERY DISEASE

Coronary artery disease (CAD) refers to arteriosclerotic and atherosclerotic changes in the coronary arteries supplying the myocardium. It may not be diagnosed until clients are in late middle age or older, but the vascular changes most likely begin much earlier. CAD occurs 10 to 15 years earlier in men than in women (Halm & Penque, 1999).

Pathophysiology and Etiology

CAD results from many factors rather than a single cause. Several inherited and behavioral risk factors contribute to the development of CAD (Box 33-1). Although men are affected earlier than women, the incidence rises in postmenopausal women and becomes similar to that in men thereafter.

At rest, ample blood flow may be maintained despite considerable CAD. The condition may go unrecognized, particularly among those with a sedentary lifestyle. During situations that increase myocardial oxygen demand (i.e., exercise, emotional stress), however, the compromised coronary arteries cannot adequately oxygenate the myocardium. When the myocardial tissue becomes *ischemic* (deprived of oxygen), clinical manifestations of CAD, such as **angina pectoris** (chest pain of cardiac origin) occur. Death of heart muscle does not accompany angina.

Assessment Findings

Signs and Symptoms

In mild CAD, clients are asymptomatic or complain of fatigue. The classic symptom is chest pain (angina) or discomfort during activity or stress. Such pain or discomfort typically is manifested as sudden pain or pressure that may be centered over the heart (precordial) or under the sternum (substernal). The pain may radiate to the shoulders and arms, especially on the left side, or to the jaw,

neck, or teeth (Fig. 33-2). Some clients describe discomfort other than pain, such as indigestion or a burning, squeezing, or crushing tightness in the upper chest or throat. Table 33-1 highlights various types of angina.

Some clients present with signs suggesting hyperlipidemia. They may be obese and hypertensive. An obese person with an apple-shaped body (carries most weight in the abdomen) is at higher risk for CAD than one with a pear-shaped body (carries most weight below the hips). The pulse may be high at rest and become irregular with exercise. An opaque white ring about the periphery of the cornea, called *arcus senilis* (Fig. 33-3), results from a deposit of fat granules but may be apparent only in older adults. *Xanthelasma,* a raised yellow plaque on the skin of the upper and lower eyelids (Fig. 33-4), suggests lipid accumulation. Although research is ongoing, some cardiologists indicate a relationship between a diagonal crease in the earlobe and the risk for CAD (Motamed & Pelekoudas, 1998).

Diagnostic Findings

The level of total serum **cholesterol,** a fatty (lipid) substance, is elevated; sometimes the level of triglycerides, which are chains of fatty acids, is increased as well. Proteins transport lipids (cholesterol) in the blood. **Low-density lipoprotein** (LDL) has a higher ratio of cholesterol than protein; **high-density lipoprotein** (HDL) is just the opposite—it has more protein than cholesterol. In clients with CAD, the level of LDL, which sometimes is referred to as "bad cholesterol" because it sticks to arteries, exceeds recommended amounts. The level of HDL, or "good cholesterol" because it carries cholesterol to the liver for removal, is lower than desirable (Table 33-2). Cardiac risk can be estimated by dividing the total serum cholesterol level by the HDL level; a result greater than 5 suggests a potential for CAD.

Apolipoproteins are proteins on the surface of cholesterol molecules that bind to enzymes that direct cholesterol to sites for metabolism. They often are low or absent among clients genetically prone to hyperlipidemia. They also are considered better direct indicators of CAD in women than are other standard blood fat profile measurements (HeartCenter Online, 2001). In 1998, the American Heart Association suggested measuring two apolipoprotein levels during routine cholesterol screenings: apolipoprotein B100 (Apo-B) and apolipoprotein C-II (Apo-C-II).

Exercise electrocardiogram (ECG) or stress testing may reveal ST segment depression, dysrhythmias, or exercise-induced hypertension. Narrowing of one or more coronary arteries is documented during coronary arteriography. Electron-beam computed tomography detects calcified plaque in one or more coronary arteries in asymptomatic clients.

BOX 33-1 ● Risk Factors for Coronary Artery Disease

Inherited	Behavioral
Middle age or older	Smoking
Male sex	Sedentary lifestyle
Diabetes mellitus	Obesity
Increased lipid levels	Competitive, aggressive personality
Genetic predisposition	High-fat diet
Hypertension	

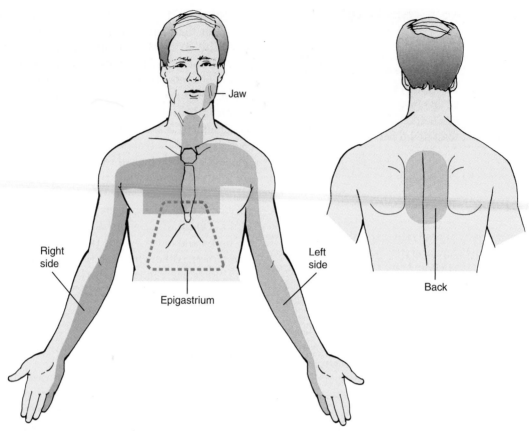

Jaw

Right
side

Epigastrium

Left
side

Back

FIGURE 33-2 Pain patterns with myocardial ischemia. Blue indicates usual distribution of pain with myocardial ischemia.

TABLE 33-1	TYPES OF ANGINA			
	STABLE ANGINA	**UNSTABLE ANGINA**	**VARIANT (PRINZMETAL'S) ANGINA**	**MICROVASCULAR ANGINA (CARDIAC SYNDROME X)**
Causes	75% Coronary occlusion that accompanies exertion Elevated heart rate or BP Eating a large meal	Progressive worsening of stable angina, with more than 90% coronary occlusion	Arterial spasm in normal or diseased coronary arteries	Constriction of myocardial capillaries too small for standard cardiac tests to detect
Symptoms	Chest pain that lasts 15 minutes or less and may radiate Similar pain severity, frequency, and duration with each episode	Chest pain of increased frequency, severity, and duration poorly relieved by rest or oral nitrates Client at risk of MI within 18 months of angina's onset	Chest pain that occurs at rest (usually between 12 and 8 AM), is sporadic over 3 to 6 months, and diminishes over time ST elevation rather than depression on ECG	Prolonged chest pain that accompanies exercise and is not always relieved by medication
Treatment	Rest, sublingual nitrates, antihypertensives, lifestyle changes	Sedation, IV nitroglycerin, oxygen, antihypertensives, anticoagulant or antiplatelet therapy, revascularization procedures	Nitrates or calcium channel blockers	Heart-healthy habits and trials with medications like a nitrate, beta blocker, or calcium channel blocker

FIGURE 33-3 Arcus senilis, an opaque ring in the periphery of the cornea, is a sign of systemic fat deposits. (Courtesy of Patrick J. Saine, CRA.)

Stop, Think, and Respond ● BOX 33-1

Although the recommended total cholesterol level is below 200 mg/dL, determine which client has the lowest cardiac risk by dividing total cholesterol level by HDL level and explain your answer.

Client A: Total cholesterol level is 224 mg/dL; HDL level is 38 mg/dL.
Client B: Total cholesterol level is 198 mg/dL; HDL level is 35 mg/dL.
Client C: Total cholesterol level is 210 mg/dL; HDL level is 55 mg/dL.

Medical and Surgical Management

The first line of defense is lifestyle changes such as smoking cessation, weight loss, stress management, and exercise. When these are inadequate, drug therapy and other noninvasive, nonsurgical, or surgical interventions are indicated.

FIGURE 33-4 Xanthelasma, yellowish plaques about the eyelids, is a sign of lipid accumulation. (Courtesy of Patrick J. Saine, CRA.)

TABLE 33-2	CARDIAC RISK ASSOCIATED WITH BLOOD FAT LEVELS*	
SUBSTANCE	**VALUE**	**INTERPRETATION**
Total cholesterol	<200 mg/dL	Desirable
	200–239 mg/dL	Borderline high
	240 mg/dL or greater	High
Low-density lipoprotein (LDL)	<100 mg/dL	Optimal
	100–129 mg/dL	Near optimal
	130–159 mg/dL	Borderline high
	160–189 mg/dL	High
	190 mg/dL or more	Very high
High-density lipoprotein (HDL)	<40 mg/dL	Low
	40–59 mg/dL	Acceptable
	60 mg/dL or more	Optimal
Apolipoproteins		
Apo-B	40–125 mg/dL	Normal
Apo-C-II	Absent or low	Familial hyper-lipidemia
Triglycerides	Present	Normal
	<150 mg/dL	Acceptable
	150–199 mg/dL	Borderline high
	200 mg/dL or more	High

*Adult Treatment Panel (ATPIII). (2001). Clinical guidelines for cholesterol testing and management. The National Cholesterol Education Program, a division of the National Heart, Lung, Blood Institute. [On-line.] Available: http://www.mhbi.gov/guidelines/cholesterol/dskref.html.

Drug therapy includes medications that produce arterial vasodilation, such as nitrates (e.g., nitroglycerin, isosorbide dinitrate). Beta-adrenergic blocking agents, which decrease consumption of myocardial oxygen by reducing heart rate, also are used. Calcium channel blocking agents may be used as well, although research has shown that they may be less beneficial than beta-adrenergic blocking agents. A clinical trial known as the Cardiac Events Study is underway; it is testing if antibiotic therapy such as azithromycin (Zithromax) should be used to treat CAD (McHale, 1998). Drugs such as angiotensin-converting enzyme inhibitors and diuretics, as well as stress management, are used to control hypertension. Nicotinic acid (niacin) in pharmacologic doses (e.g., not the dosage in multivitamins) helps increase HDL and lower LDL. Daily intake of food sources or supplements of folate or folic acid, vitamin B_6 (pyridoxine), and vitamin B_{12} (cyanocobalamin) reduce homocysteine levels.

Blood glucose is kept regulated, and weight loss is encouraged. Prevention of further plaque formation is attempted by lowering elevated cholesterol and triglyceride levels through diet, exercise, and, in extreme cases, lipid-lowering drugs such as HMG-CoA reductase inhibitors, known as *statins,* and bile acid sequestrants. Some physicians advise taking one aspirin tablet (325 mg or less) daily to prevent thrombi from developing. Because soy products are classified as **phytoestrogens,** plant sources of estrogen, some clients are increasing consumption of soy as a cardioprotective strategy.

Enhanced External Counterpulsation

Enhanced external counterpulsation (EECP) may be used as an adjunct to drug therapy and lifestyle modifications. This fairly new, noninvasive and nonsurgical approach helps relieve angina. It requires 1- to 2-hour sessions in the physician's office, 5 days a week for approximately 7 weeks. During EECP, the client dons a pressure suit with pneumatic cuffs at the upper and lower thighs and calves. The cuffs are connected to a cardiac monitor and are sequentially inflated in a wavelike fashion from the calves to the upper thighs during ventricular diastole (resting; Fig. 33-5). The cuff pulsation, which has been compared to a "strong hug," moves blood toward the heart. Because the coronary arteries fill during ventricular diastole when the aortic valve closes, cuff inflation increases perfusion of the coronary arteries with oxygenated blood. When the cuffs deflate during ventricular systole (contraction), the left ventricle's work is reduced because there

is less resistance. Some believe that EECP is a form of passive exercise that promotes the development of **collateral circulation,** accessory vascular pathways for blood.

Although the mechanism by which EECP relieves symptoms is not well understood, research has shown that the therapeutic results are more than a placebo effect (Lawson & Hui, 2000). Advantages are that it reduces the frequency of angina and improves exercise tolerance. Disadvantages are that EECP is time-consuming and few physicians offer or refer clients for it. Some believe that lack of interest from medical personnel is related to the fact that third-party payers can better reimburse physicians for other, less time-consuming treatment modalities.

Invasive Perfusion Techniques

Invasive nonsurgical procedures can reopen narrowed coronary arteries and include percutaneous transluminal coronary angioplasty, coronary stent, and atherectomy. Surgical procedures include coronary artery bypass graft and transmyocardial revascularization.

PERCUTANEOUS TRANSLUMINAL CORONARY ANGIOPLASTY

For clients who fit specific criteria, **percutaneous transluminal coronary angioplasty** (PTCA), sometimes referred to as *balloon angioplasty,* is performed. In PTCA, which uses sedation and local anesthesia, a balloon-tipped catheter is inserted through the skin and threaded from a peripheral artery into the diseased coronary artery (Fig.

Step 1	Step 2	Step 3	Step 4
Inflation initiates retrograde pulse wave	Inflation of lower thigh cuffs 50 milliseconds later	Inflation of upper thigh cuffs 50 milliseconds later	Deflation facilitates cardiac unloading

FIGURE 33-5 Inflation and deflation sequence of enhanced external counterpulsation.

33-6). While passage of the catheter is monitored under fluoroscopy, the catheter is positioned in the area of stenosis and the balloon is inflated with carbon dioxide (CO_2) from several seconds to several minutes. Inflation of the balloon compresses the atherosclerotic plaque against the arterial wall, increasing the diameter of the artery. Arterial rupture, MI, and abrupt reclosure are complications of PTCA. Repeating PTCA often is necessary because the artery tends to reocclude in 40% to 50% of clients who undergo the procedure. Clients who have not had an accompanying MI but have had PTCA or any procedure that uses a percutaneous catheter are provided with the following discharge instructions for self-care:

- Avoid lifting more than 10 lbs for at least 3 days if the groin was used for catheter insertion. Avoid lifting more than 1 lb for at least 3 days if a site in the upper extremity was used.
- Refrain from riding a bicycle, driving a vehicle, or mowing the lawn for at least 3 days.
- Refrain from sexual activity for 1 week.
- Shower rather than bathe until the cutaneous catheterization site heals.
- Clean the site with soap and water; eliminate any dressing.
- Relieve discomfort at the site with a mild analgesic like acetaminophen (Tylenol); numbness at the site is temporary and not unusual.
- Expect to see a bruise, which may last 1 to 3 weeks, at the catheter insertion site.

- Report any signs of infection or impaired circulation: fever, swelling, redness, drainage, acute pain in the extremity, cold or pale skin.
- Notify the cardiologist immediately if there is pain or tightness in the chest, which could indicate obstructed blood flow through the coronary artery.

CORONARY STENT

A **coronary stent** is a small metal coil with meshlike openings placed in the coronary artery during PTCA (Fig. 33-7). The stent prevents the coronary artery from collapsing shortly after the procedure and keeps the lumen open for a longer period than traditional PTCA alone. The stent remains permanently in the enlarged artery, and endothelial tissue is incorporated into the mesh within 4 to 6 weeks. Restenosis usually is a problem even with placement of a stent. Restenosis does not necessarily result from an accelerated atherosclerotic process, but from an overgrowth of cells accompanying the inflammation caused by the local trauma to the tissue. A newly developed stent known as *Cypher,* however, which is coated with an anti-inflammatory/antibiotic substance called sirolimus (Rapamune), has shown spectacular results in current clinical trials. Not one person in the research group experienced coronary artery restenosis 6 months after insertion (Associated Press, 2001).

ATHERECTOMY

Clients whose atherosclerotic plaque is no longer soft and pliable may benefit from an **atherectomy,** removal of

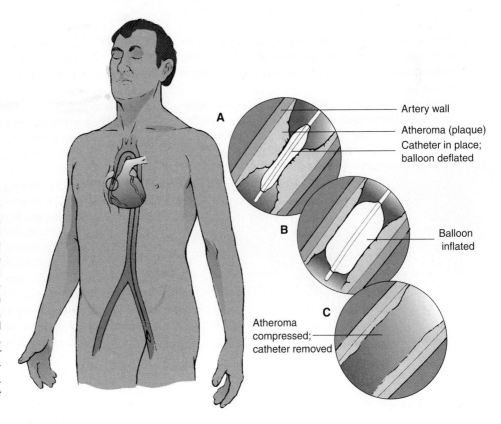

FIGURE 33-6 Percutaneous transluminal coronary angioplasty. (**A**) A balloon-tipped catheter is passed into the affected coronary artery and placed within the area of the atheroma (plaque). (**B**) The balloon is then rapidly inflated and deflated with controlled pressure. (**C**) After the atheroma is compressed, the catheter is removed, and blood flow improves. (From Smeltzer, S. C. & Bare, B. G. [2000]. *Brunner & Suddarth's textbook of medical–surgical nursing* [9th ed.]. Philadelphia: Lippincott Williams & Wilkins.)

Artery wall
Atheroma (plaque)
Catheter in place; balloon deflated
Balloon inflated
Atheroma compressed; catheter removed

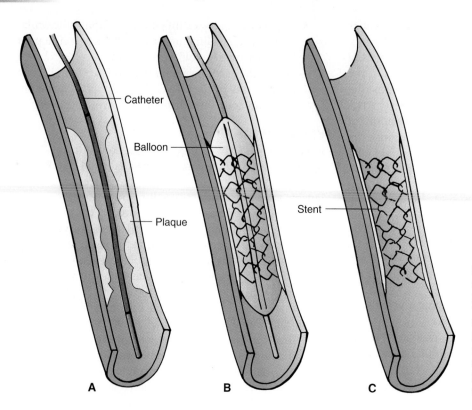

FIGURE **33-7** Insertion of a cardiac stent. (**A**) The stent is collapsed and placed over a balloon-tipped catheter. The catheter is threaded through a blood vessel in the groin and into the artery. (**B**) The balloon is inflated, and the stent expands. (**C**) The stent locks and forms a scaffold to keep the artery open. The balloon is deflated, and the catheter is withdrawn.

fatty plaque. The plaque is removed by either inserting a cardiac catheter with a cutting tool at the tip (Fig. 33-8) or performing laser angioplasty. The following describes four atherectomy options:

1. *Directional coronary atherectomy* shaves the plaque from the arterial wall and stores the particles in the catheter.
2. *Transluminal extraction* uses a cardiac catheter with a spinning blade to separate plaque from the arterial wall and removes the debris with a vacuum attachment.
3. *Percutaneous transluminal catheter* rotational ablation uses a rotating bur that spins at 200,000 revolutions per minute. Because the particles of freed plaque are smaller than red blood cells, phagocytes and the lymphatic system remove them.

FIGURE **33-8** An atherectomy catheter removes plaque with either a circular blade or an abrasive material. A balloon catheter opens the coronary artery by compressing soft plaque.

4. **Laser angioplasty** uses short pulses of light that vaporize plaque without creating heat that is intense enough to damage the arterial wall.

Atherectomy usually is followed by PTCA and placement of a stent.

CORONARY ARTERY BYPASS GRAFT SURGERY

Coronary artery bypass graft (CABG) surgery (see Chap. 37) is a technique for revascularizing the myocardium. A section from a healthy leg vein or chest artery is used to reroute the flow of oxygenated blood from the aorta or a chest artery to below the obstruction in the diseased coronary artery. More than one graft may be necessary if several coronary arteries are occluded. The procedure is performed through a 10- to 12-inch midsternal incision, which is closed with wire, staples, or sutures. The heart is stopped during CABG surgery, but blood is circulated through a heart–lung machine so that oxygen continues to be delivered to cells, tissues, and organs while CO_2 is removed. When the vascular reconnections are completed, heart function is restored. The client remains on a ventilator for approximately 24 hours. It may be several weeks before the client can return to work. Results after CABG surgery tend to last longer than PTCA, stenting, or atherectomy. Refer to Chapter 37 for information about minimally invasive direct coronary artery bypass, a recent modification in CABG surgery.

TRANSMYOCARDIAL REVASCULARIZATION

A **transmyocardial revascularization** (TMR) laser procedure, which improves oxygenation of myocardial tissue, may improve quality of life for clients with chest pain that does not respond to medication and who are not candidates for CABG surgery. TMR may be performed for the following reasons:

- The occluded coronary arteries are too narrow or distal to permit catheter insertion.
- There are so many occlusions that risks from a lengthy surgical procedure are unreasonable.
- The client has end-stage (seriously advanced) CAD, which increases the potential for life-threatening complications or death.

To access the heart, a thoracotomy incision is made between ribs on the left side of the chest. While the heart is visualized with transesophageal echocardiography, the laser probe is aimed at the beating heart. The probe makes 15 to 40 channels that are 1 mm deep and 1 cm apart from the epicardium, through the ischemic myocardium, to the endocardium. The channels that the laser creates allow the ischemic myocardium to absorb the oxygenated blood that seeps into the area. Therefore, the myocardium receives oxygen not from a coronary artery, but from the blood that seeps into the space between the cells. There are other hypotheses for the mechanism by which TMR relieves the client's symptoms. Some believe that it disrupts the myocardial nerve supply, which suppresses the ability to perceive anginal pain. Others suggest that the trauma stimulates **neoangiogenesis,** new growth of blood vessels, which results in additional collateral blood supply to the heart muscle.

Clients remain in the hospital for up to 1 week. Activity is restricted for several weeks to allow a safe period of healing. Because TMR relieves symptoms only, cardiac rehabilitation requires clients to continue to modify risk factors that caused CAD. Such modification means the client must eliminate smoking, follow a heart healthy diet, and incorporate regular, moderate exercise. Variations in TMR also are being implemented. Sometimes TMR is performed with a percutaneously inserted catheter.

Nursing Management

The nurse assesses the characteristics of chest pain and administers prescribed drugs that dilate the coronary arteries or reduce the work of the heart. He or she encourages rest and administers oxygen to improve the available oxygen supply to the heart muscle. If drugs, rest, and oxygen do not relieve the pain, the nurse notifies the physician.

The nurse helps clients learn how to reduce modifiable CAD risk factors, which can improve not only cardiac health but overall well-being. He or she explains that a low-fat diet and regular aerobic exercise (e.g., walking, swimming) can significantly reduce risks. The nurse arranges a consultation with a dietitian and provides written material about a heart healthy diet (see General Nutritional Considerations). He or she refers clients to smoking cessation programs and discusses medications that can help (see Chaps. 7 and 17).

The nurse teaches about the administration and side effects of antianginal drugs (Client and Family Teaching Box 33-1). He or she emphasizes that severe, unrelieved chest pain indicates a need to be examined by a physician without delay. The nurse advises the client to report changes in the usual pattern of angina, like increased frequency or severity or occurrence with rest or during sleep.

The nurse informs clients about diagnostic tests or treatment procedures. The nurse who prepares the client for invasive, nonsurgical procedures performed with a percutaneous catheter cleanses and removes hair from skin insertion sites (one for the coronary catheter and the other for an arterial line through which blood pressure [BP] will be directly monitored). He or she withholds anticoagulant therapy before the procedure to decrease the chance of hemorrhage. The nurse monitors all vascular sites for bleeding after a procedure and assesses distal pulses. He or she observes mental status because cerebral emboli can occur. The nurse monitors urine output and administers analgesics for discomfort. He or she reports any of the following data immediately: severe chest pain, abnormal heart rate or rhythm, mental confusion or loss of consciousness, hypotension, urine output less than 30 to 50 mL/hour, or a cold, pulseless extremity.

• MYOCARDIAL INFARCTION

An **infarct** is an area of tissue that dies (*necrosis*) from inadequate oxygenation. An MI or heart attack occurs when there is prolonged total occlusion of coronary arterial blood flow. The larger the necrotic area is, the more serious the damage. An infarct that extends through the full thickness of the myocardial wall is called a **transmural infarction** or Q-wave MI. A partial-thickness infarct is called a **subendocardial infarction** or a non–Q-wave MI. Each coronary artery supplies oxygenated blood to a different area of the myocardium. The location of the infarction depends on the area where the blood supply to the myocardium is interrupted by the respective occluded coronary artery (Fig. 33-9).

Pathophysiology and Etiology

The most common cause of MI is a **coronary thrombosis,** a blood clot within a coronary artery. Thrombosis usually is secondary to arteriosclerotic and atherosclerotic changes. Arterial spasms also may cause an MI. Once an area of the myocardium has been damaged and destroyed, the cells in that area lose their special functions of automaticity, excitability, conductivity, contractility, and rhythmicity. Thus, dysrhythmias and heart failure are common consequences (see Chaps. 34 and 36).

Injury to the myocardium triggers the inflammatory response. Proinflammatory chemicals disrupt the perme-

33-1 *Client and Family Teaching*
Use of Short-Acting Nitroglycerin

The nurse discusses the following points with clients who are prescribed short-acting nitroglycerin and their families.

For sublingual nitroglycerin:

- Sit down and rest before self-administering nitroglycerin. Decreased activity may relieve chest pain; sitting will prevent injury should the nitroglycerin lower BP and cause fainting.
- Place one nitroglycerin tablet under the tongue if 2 to 3 minutes of rest fails to relieve pain.
- Expect to feel dizzy or flushed or to develop a headache.
- Let the tablet dissolve slowly; there should be slight tingling or burning under the tongue.
- Take a second nitroglycerin tablet in 5 minutes if chest pain is still present.
- Take a third nitroglycerin tablet in 5 more minutes if chest pain is still present.
- Call 911 if chest pain continues; do not drive to an emergency department. Discuss the chest pain with the physician if self-management relieved it or its usual characteristics changed.
- Keep a few nitroglycerin tablets in a dark, dry container with you at all times; consult with the pharmacist about a sealed metal container that you can wear around the neck.

- Do not place other medications in the container with the nitroglycerin.
- Replace nitroglycerin tablets every 6 months or after any container has been opened six times.

For nitroglycerin spray:

- Assume a sitting position.
- Hold the cannister upright.
- Spray the nitroglycerin onto the tongue without inhaling.
- Close the mouth immediately afterward.
- Expect to feel dizzy or flushed or to develop a headache.
- Repeat spraying every 5 minutes for a second and third time if chest pain is unrelieved.
- Call 911 if chest pain continues.
- Discuss the chest pain with the physician if self-management relieved it or its usual characteristics changed.
- Expect a new cannister of nitroglycerin to deliver approximately 200 doses.
- Check the amount of nitroglycerin in the cannister by floating it in a bowl of water; the higher the cannister floats, the less medication it contains. Obtain a reserve cannister when the present cannister shows signs of becoming empty.

---

ability of cell membranes (see Chap. 19). The damaged cells release serum cardiac markers (intracellular enzymes) and electrolytes into the extracellular fluid. Loss of intracellular potassium and accumulation of lactic acid from anaerobic cellular metabolism affect depolarization and repolarization of myocardial cells. Dangerous dysrhythmias can develop during this time because the affected areas are electrically unstable.

The infarction process can take up to 6 hours. There are three zones of tissue damage:

1. The first zone consists of a central area of necrotic—dead—myocardial cells.
2. A second zone of injured cells, which may live if blood supply to the area is restored, surrounds the first zone.
3. The third zone is the ischemic area that will probably survive.

Thrombolytic drugs (clot busters) are given during this 6-hour window of opportunity to re-establish blood flow and save as much myocardial tissue as possible.

Leukocytosis and slightly elevated body temperature follow in 3 to 7 days. New capillaries begin to grow to es-

tablish collateral circulation to the infarcted area; however, it takes 2 or 3 weeks before such flow is significant. A "cardiac patch" of collagen fibers begins to form within the first 2 weeks of the infarct, but it takes as long as 3 months for the scar to grow firm. The scar tissue is less effective than the myocardium it is replacing; it does not stretch and contract like the original tissue. Lack of resiliency impairs the heart's ability to pump effectively. Consequently, cardiomyopathy (see Chap. 31) and heart failure (see Chap. 36) are always lifelong, potential complications.

Complications

Dysrhythmias

Any number of dysrhythmias (see Chap. 34) may occur during the acute phase. More than 50% of deaths from MI occur within 72 hours for this reason. Some abnormal rhythms can be fatal within a few minutes. Early detection and treatment of them reduce the fatality rate.

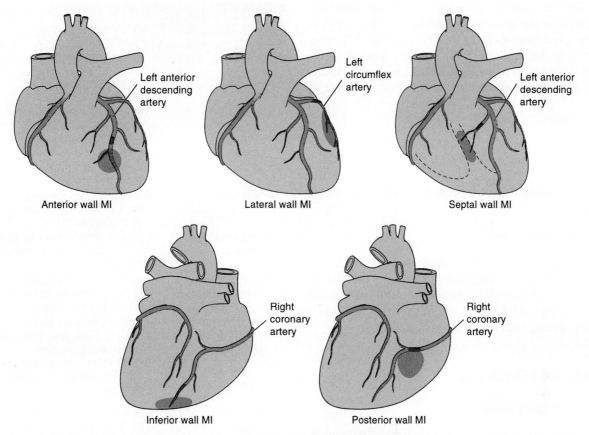

FIGURE 33-9 Zones of myocardial infarction based on the artery that becomes occluded.

Cardiogenic Shock

Cardiogenic shock, which has a high mortality rate, occurs when 40% of the left ventricle has lost the ability to pump effectively (see Chap. 23). The onset may be sudden, or the condition may develop over hours or days. The sooner shock is detected (monitoring with a pulmonary artery catheter) and treatment is instituted, the better are the client's chances of survival. This complication has been successfully treated with medications, ventricular assist devices, and an intra-aortic balloon pump (see Chap. 36).

Ventricular Rupture

Ventricular rupture occurs when a soft necrotic area from a transmural or interventricular septal MI ruptures. Dyspnea, rapid right-sided heart failure, and shock result. *Hemopericardium* (blood in the pericardium) and cardiac tamponade follow. The prognosis is poor, although survival is possible.

Ventricular Aneurysm

A ventricular aneurysm is a bulging of the portion of the heart affected by the MI. This area of poorly contractile tissue predisposes the heart to failure. Blood trapped in the projection tends to form thrombi, which may be released into the arterial circulation. The aneurysm may burst, resulting in hemorrhage and death.

Arterial Embolism

Clots can form in the cavity of the ventricular aneurysm (mural thrombi), or tissue debris can break free. If clots enter the systemic arterial circulation, they may occlude a peripheral artery. Symptoms depend on the location of the affected artery. Arteriotomy (opening of an artery) and embolectomy (removal of an embolus) may be necessary; a client who has recently had an MI, however, is a poor surgical risk.

Venous Thrombosis

Venous thrombosis arises mostly in the veins of the lower extremities and pelvis. The use of antiembolism stockings and regular performance of foot and leg exercises help to prevent thrombus formation. Antiplatelet medications and anticoagulants also are given.

Pulmonary Embolism

Most pulmonary emboli arise from venous thrombi in the lower extremities and pelvis (see Chap. 29). They also may arise from the right ventricle after an MI. The onset of a pulmonary embolism usually is sudden, with chest pain, dyspnea, and cyanosis being the first symptoms. The sputum may be tinged with blood. Treatment depends on the size of the infarcted pulmonary area, the age and condition of the client, and the seriousness (or extent) of the MI.

Pericarditis

Pericarditis may be mild or severe. The mild form may not require treatment (see Chap. 31). If pericardial effusion develops, the client is observed closely for signs of cardiac tamponade; pericardiocentesis is done to remove excess fluid.

Mitral Insufficiency

If the papillary muscles are involved in an MI and the mitral valve leaflets are compromised, mitral regurgitation may occur. In this condition, blood not only flows forward into the aorta but backward into the left atrium through an incompetent mitral valve (see Chap. 32).

Assessment Findings

Signs and Symptoms

Symptoms vary but typically include sudden, severe chest pain, which usually is substernal and may radiate to the shoulder, arm, teeth, jaw, or throat. Most clients are aware of its seriousness and are apprehensive. The pain is more severe and lasts longer than anginal pain. Some clients describe it as squeezing or crushing. Unlike anginal pain, rest and sublingual nitrates do not relieve MI pain. If untreated, it may last for several hours or 1 or 2 days. Finally, it becomes sore or achy before disappearing entirely. A few clients experience little or no pain and may never know that they had an MI until an ECG detects it weeks, months, or years later. Clients appear pale and diaphoretic. They may experience nausea and vomiting or be hypotensive and faint. Pulse is rapid and weak and may be irregular. Signs of left-sided heart failure (dyspnea, cyanosis, cough) may appear if left ventricular pumping is sufficiently impaired.

Diagnostic Findings

Laboratory tests include a series of serum cardiac markers, substances that damaged myocardial cells release during an infarct (Table 33-3). They include myoglobin and cardiospecific troponin subunits known as troponin T and troponin I. The subunit troponin C is the same for cardiac and skeletal muscle and therefore is not measured. Fractions or isoforms of cardiac enzymes such as creatine kinase and lactate dehydrogenase are measured initially and every 8 hours for 24 hours to determine elevated levels. The WBC count, C-reactive protein, and erythrocyte sed-

TABLE 33-3	SERUM CARDIAC MARKERS AFTER AN ACUTE MYOCARDIAL INFARCTION
CARDIAC MARKER	**CHARACTERISTICS**
Myoglobin	Present as early as 2 hours after MI; peaks in 3 to 15 hours; returns to normal in 20 to 24 hours
Troponin T	Rises 3 to 4 hours after MI; peaks in 4 to 6 hours; returns to normal in several weeks
Troponin I	Rises 4 to 6 hours after MI; peaks in 14 to 18 hours; returns to normal in 6 to 7 days
CK-MB (creatine kinase)	Rises 4 to 12 hours after MI; peaks in 24 hours; returns to normal in 3 to 4 days
AST (aspartate aminotransferase)	Increases 6 to 12 hours after MI; peaks in 36 hours; returns to normal in 3 to 4 days
LDH_1 and LDH_2 (lactate dehydrogenase)	Rises 24 to 48 hours after MI; peaks in 3 to 6 days; returns to normal in 7 to 14 days. An LDH_1–LDH_2 ratio greater than 1.0 indicates myocardial damage.

imentation rate increase on about the third day because of the inflammatory response that the injured myocardial cells triggered. Blood glucose level may be elevated in clients with diabetes (and those without) because of the body's response to a major stressor. After an MI, characteristic changes appear on the ECG within 2 to 12 hours. They may, however, take as long as 3 days to develop. These changes include ST segment elevation, T-wave inversion, and a Q wave (Fig. 33-10).

Medical Management

Treatment is directed toward reducing tissue hypoxia, relieving pain, treating shock (if present), and alleviating dysrhythmias if they occur.

Thrombolytic Therapy

If the client is seen within 6 hours of the onset of the occlusion, re-establishing coronary artery blood flow can reduce the zone of necrosis. Treatment may include the administration of **thrombolytic agents,** drugs that dissolve blood clots, unless the client is disqualified on the following bases:

- BP greater than 180/110 mm Hg
- History of a hemorrhagic stroke
- History of cerebral thrombotic stroke within 1 year

FIGURE 33-10 (**A**) Normal QRS complex. (**B**) A pathologic Q wave indicates a transmural myocardial infarction.

- Head trauma within past 2 to 4 weeks
- Known bleeding disorder; does not include menses
- Active internal bleeding in the past 2 weeks; active peptic ulcer
- Noncompressible vascular punctures

- Traumatic or prolonged (> 10 minutes) cardiopulmonary resuscitation in past 2 to 4 weeks
- Surgery or trauma within the past 2 to 4 weeks
- Pregnancy
- Terminal illness
- Jaundice, hepatitis, kidney failure
- Use of anticoagulants in therapeutic doses

Drugs such as streptokinase, urokinase, and recombinant tissue plasminogen activator dissolve the thrombus occluding the coronary artery, thus restoring the circulation of oxygenated blood to the myocardium. Depending on how stable the client's condition is, PTCA or CABG may follow thrombolytic therapy after the risk for bleeding has been reduced. Clients who are not candidates for thrombolytic therapy should undergo PTCA within 1 to 2 hours of admission or within 12 hours from the onset of symptoms (American College of Cardiology [ACC] and American Heart Association [AHA], 1999).

Symptomatic Treatment

An intravenous (IV) infusion is initiated to provide fluid while eating is restricted. The IV route also is used to administer parenteral medications. Drug therapy includes analgesics for pain, nitrates or other vasodilating drugs to improve blood flow, diuretics to reduce circulating blood volume, sedatives to promote rest and reduce anxiety, anticoagulants to prevent additional thrombus formation, and drugs to treat dysrhythmias (Drug Therapy Table 33-1).

DRUG THERAPY TABLE 33-1	AGENTS USED TO TREAT MYOCARDIAL INFARCTION		
DRUG CATEGORY AND EXAMPLES	**MECHANISM OF ACTION**	**SIDE EFFECTS**	**NURSING CONSIDERATIONS**
Vasodilators nitroglycerin	Relieve chest pain by dilating coronary arteries Reestablish blood flow around thrombi	Headache, dizziness, orthostatic hypotension, tachycardia, flushing, nausea	Assess for hypotension. Monitor for pain relief, headache, and flushed skin.
Beta-Adrenergic Blockers propranolol (Inderal)	Prevent or inhibit sympathetic stimulation, decreasing myocardial oxygen demand Are used to prevent anginal attacks	Hypotension, bradycardia, bronchospasm, CHF, depression, erectile dysfunction, hypoglycemia	Administer with meals. Advise client not to discontinue medication abruptly. Monitor for fluid retention, rash, and difficulty breathing. Monitor blood glucose level in clients with diabetes.
Thrombolytics alteplase (Activase); recombinant tissue plasminogen activator (r-TPA)	Reestablish blood flow to ischemic areas by dissolving thrombi Are contraindicated in clients with history of cerebrovascular accident or bleeding tendencies	Cardiac dysrhythmias, hypotension, bleeding at venous or arterial access sites, nausea, vomiting	Use caution when administering with heparin because of increased risk for hemorrhage. Monitor PT and PTT. Apply pressure to control superficial bleeding.

(continued)

DRUG THERAPY TABLE 33-1	AGENTS USED TO TREAT MYOCARDIAL INFARCTION (Continued)		
DRUG CATEGORY AND EXAMPLES	**MECHANISM OF ACTION**	**SIDE EFFECTS**	**NURSING CONSIDERATIONS**
Anticoagulants heparin sodium (Hepalean)	Inhibit thrombus and clot formation by blocking conversion of prothrombin to thrombin and fibrinogen to fibrin	Hemorrhage, bruising, thrombocytopenia, alopecia, chills, fever	Monitor closely for bleeding or hemorrhage when combined with oral anticoagulants. Give subcutaneously or IV. Apply pressure to all intramuscular injection sites. Monitor for epistaxis and other bleeding. Ensure protamine sulfate is on the unit in case of overdose.
Calcium Channel Blockers diltiazem (Cardizem)	Relieve angina by dilating arteries, which improves blood supply to myocardium and reduces myocardial oxygen demand by decreasing myocardial contractility and heart rate Reduce dysrhythmias	Hypotension, dizziness, CHF, pulmonary edema, nausea	Check BP and heart rate before each dose. Withhold drug in the presence of hypotension. Observe for signs and symptoms of CHF and fluid overload.
Diuretics furosemide (Lasix)	Decrease work of heart by promoting excretion of sodium and water, thus reducing circulating blood volume	Dizziness, dehydration, nausea, diarrhea, nocturia, polyuria, orthostatic hypotension, hypokalemia	Weigh client daily. Measure intake and output. Monitor serum potassium level, and replace potassium with bananas, orange juice, or prescribed supplement.

CHF, congestive heart failure; PT, prothrombin time; PTT, partial thromboplastin time.

Oxygen is ordered to treat or prevent hypoxemia. Complete bed rest is prescribed initially but not recommended for uncomplicated MIs after the first 12 hours. Activity is adjusted according to the extent of the MI, complications, and response to therapy. When chest pain is controlled, a clear liquid diet is allowed and progressed to a heart-healthy diet thereafter (see General Nutritional Considerations). Clients who regularly consumed caffeine before an MI are allowed up to 400 mg/day, which equals two to four cups of coffee, without danger of increasing BP (ACC/AHA, 1999). A stool softener is prescribed to prevent increased BP from straining with the passage of stool. Permanent smoking cessation is imperative. The intra-aortic balloon pump may be used for clients who develop severe left ventricular failure (see Chap. 36).

Surgical Management

CABG surgery (see Chap. 37) is done to revascularize the myocardium surgically. In clients who are experiencing cardiogenic shock, a ventricular assist device may be im-planted, or cardiomyoplasty, a new procedure for grafting skeletal muscle to replace a dysfunctional area of myocardium, may be used (see Chap. 36).

Cardiac Rehabilitation

After a significant cardiac event like an MI or heart surgery, clients are encouraged to participate in a medically supervised **cardiac rehabilitation** program, which combines exercise and educational activities to speed recovery and reduce or prevent recurring episodes. Cardiac rehabilitation usually begins before discharge but continues on an outpatient basis. The plan is designed according to the client's unique needs. Some clients may achieve the goals of therapy by meeting two to three times a week for 1 hour or more over a few weeks. Other clients may require therapy for 3 to 4 months. Activities and educational topics include the following:

- Gradual exercise that increases according to the client's tolerance

- Establishment of physical limitations such as the maximum amount the client can lift
- Recognition and management of depression
- Medication regimen: importance of drug therapy, dose, time taken, adverse drug effects
- Smoking cessation
- When and how to resume sexual activity (Box 33-2)
- Diet modifications, how to read food labels, what food labels indicate
- How to monitor pulse rate and BP
- Symptoms to report to a physician as soon as possible
- How to avoid or minimize stressors
- Importance of continued medical supervision

Nursing Management

The detailed nursing management of a client experiencing an acute MI is discussed in Nursing Care Plan 33-1.

OCCLUSIVE DISORDERS OF PERIPHERAL BLOOD VESSELS

Peripheral vascular disease is a term for disorders that affect blood vessels distant from the large central blood vessels supplying the myocardium or that circulate blood directly in and out of the heart. Common peripheral vascular disorders, which occlude blood flow by various mechanisms, include Raynaud's disease, thrombosis, phlebothrombosis, and embolism.

● RAYNAUD'S DISEASE

Raynaud's disease is characterized by periodic constriction of the arteries that supply the extremities. The disorder is most common in young women.

BOX 33-2 ● Sexual Guidelines After Myocardial Infarction

- Check with physician before resuming sexual activity.
- Avoid sex with anyone other than your usual partner.
- Avoid positions that require supporting your own weight.
- Get adequate rest before sexual intercourse.
- Have sex in the same environment as before the MI.
- Postpone sex for 2 to 3 hours after eating a heavy meal or consuming alcohol.
- Use a short-acting nitrate, if the physician approves, before intercourse.
- Begin with moderate sexual foreplay.
- Use medium water temperatures when bathing or showering before or after sexual activity.

Pathophysiology and Etiology

Raynaud's disease is characterized by brief spasms of the arteries and arterioles in the fingers (most common site), toes, nose, ears, or chin. The spasms last approximately 15 minutes and cause temporary **ischemia** (impaired oxygenation) to the tissues. The vessels then dilate widely, apparently to compensate for the restriction. Patchy areas of necrosis occur with prolonged ischemia.

The underlying cause of Raynaud's disease is not entirely clear. In some clients, it seems *idiopathic* (no explainable reason); in others, it is secondary to connective tissue diseases, such as scleroderma, systemic lupus erythematosus, or rheumatoid arthritis (see Chap. 67).

The anatomy of the arteries and arterioles is normal. One theory explaining the vasospasms is impaired release of *prostaglandins* (chemicals stored in cellular membranes). Some prostaglandins cause vasoconstriction; others cause vasodilation. The type that accompanies an inflammatory response causes vasodilation.

Assessment Findings

Signs and Symptoms

Attacks are intermittent and of varying frequency but are especially common after exposure to cold. When the condition occurs in the hands, they become cold, blanched, and wet with perspiration. Numbness and tingling also may occur. The client may note awkwardness and fumbling, especially when attempting fine movements. After the initial pallor, the hands, especially the fingers, become deeply cyanotic and begin to ache. The hallmark symptoms of arterial insufficiency include ischemia, pain, and paresthesia. Placing the affected part in warm water or going to a warm area can relieve an attack. Eventually the vasospasm is relieved, and blood rushes to the affected part. The skin in the deprived areas becomes flushed, swollen, and warm, and the person has a sensation of throbbing pain.

In the early stages of the disease, the hands usually appear normal between attacks. The disease does not necessarily progress to cause severe disability. Symptoms often are mild and may even improve spontaneously. When the disease is severe and of long standing, cyanosis of the fingers persists between attacks and skin changes gradually develop. Painful ulcers and superficial gangrene may appear at the fingertips. The fingers are especially vulnerable to infection. Healing of even minor lesions often is slow and uncertain.

Diagnostic Findings

No specific laboratory studies can confirm Raynaud's disease. Diagnosis is made by a history of the symptoms and examination of the involved part. Laboratory blood tests

Nursing Care Plan 33-1

THE CLIENT WITH ACUTE MYOCARDIAL INFARCTION

Assessment

Determine the following:

■ Client's description of pain: location, type, duration, intensity using a scale of 0 to 10, and whether it radiates to other areas

■ Vital signs every 30 minutes until stable and then every 4 hours and as needed (prn)

■ Presence of nausea, vomiting, diaphoresis, anxiety

■ Oxygen saturation level with pulse oximeter

■ Cardiac rhythm via cardiac monitor or ECG

■ Heart and lung sounds

■ Presence and quality of peripheral pulses

■ Results of serum cardiac markers

■ A thorough history to establish baseline data about disorders such as diabetes mellitus, hypertension, recent streptococcal infection or allergic reaction to streptokinase and findings that may disqualify the client from thrombolytic therapy

■ Drug history for prescribed, over-the-counter, and herbal products

Nursing Diagnosis: Acute Pain related to diminished myocardial oxygenation

Expected Outcome: Pain will be within client's identified comfort level within 30 minutes.

Interventions	Rationales
Administer prescribed sublingual or spray nitroglycerin every 5 minutes, up to three doses, if pain is unrelieved.	Nitroglycerin dilates blood vessels, improving blood flow through coronary arteries, and lowers BP, which decreases cardiac afterload.
Administer prescribed IV morphine sulfate.	Morphine reduces pain perception and anxiety. Reduced anxiety decreases heart rate and BP, alleviating the heart's demand for oxygenation.
Administer oxygen at 2 L/minute by nasal cannula or as prescribed.	Supplemental oxygen raises hemoglobin saturation and oxygen in plasma. Adequate myocardial oxygen diminishes angina.

Evaluation of Expected Outcome: Pain is eliminated or reduced to a tolerable level.

Nursing Diagnosis: Anxiety or **Fear** related to perception of impending doom, concern over actual/potential lifestyle changes, worry concerning family situation

Expected Outcome: Client will report decreased anxiety and fear.

Interventions	Rationales
Allow client to express fears and anxiety.	Sharing feelings with a supportive person tends to relieve or reduce emotional distress.
Explain all procedures before performing them.	Information eliminates the element of surprise or misinterpretation of nursing activities.
Carry out procedures in a calm, relaxed manner.	A client who senses confidence in the nurse may experience less apprehension.

(continued)

Nursing Care Plan 33-1 (Continued)

THE CLIENT WITH ACUTE MYOCARDIAL INFARCTION

Interventions	Rationales
Promote uninterrupted blocks of time for rest, sleep, or visits with family members.	Physical rest and support from others promote the ability to cope.
Check client frequently, and answer call lights promptly.	Knowing that help is quickly available can relieve fear.
Acknowledge grief over perceived or actual changes in lifestyle.	Dealing with reality facilitates grieving.
Administer prescribed sedatives and anxiolytic drugs as indicated.	They block sympathetic nervous system responses, which reduces anxiety and fear.

Evaluation of Expected Outcome: Anxiety is reduced as evidenced by normal heart rate and BP, no nervous activity, and self-reported tolerance of stressors.

PC: Hemorrhage related to thrombolytic therapy

Expected Outcome: The nurse will monitor to detect, manage, and minimize bleeding.

Interventions	Rationales
Observe closely for bleeding during thrombolytic therapy and until sufficient half-lives reduce pharmacodynamic effects.	The client is at risk for bleeding when thrombolytic drugs change plasminogen to plasmin.
Check for blood in stool or urine, bruising, epistaxis, abdominal pain, or altered neurologic status.	Thrombolytic drugs dissolve blood clots and interfere with their formation.
Avoid intramuscular, IV, and arterial punctures during therapy and until the risk for excessive bleeding has subsided.	Controlling bleeding may be difficult while an active level of thrombolytic drug remains in the bloodstream.
Keep client on bed rest; pad the side rails if agency policy mandates.	Trauma can cause excessive blood loss.
Have aminocaproic acid (Amicar) available as an antidote for bleeding.	Aminocaproic acid is an antiplasmin agent that inhibits plasminogen activator.

Evaluation of Expected Outcome: Client shows no evidence of bleeding.

PC: Dysrhythmias related to reperfusion of myocardium with thrombolytic therapy and instability of the conduction system

Expected Outcome: The nurse will monitor to detect, manage, and minimize dysrhythmias.

Interventions	Rationales
Place client on a cardiac monitor and closely observe for dangerous dysrhythmias.	A cardiac monitor continuously displays heart rate and rhythm; it sounds an alarm to call attention to a dysrhythmic event.
Be prepared to perform CPR if a life-threatening dysrhythmia or asystole occurs.	CPR provides basic life support (Nursing Guidelines 33-1).
Assist with endotracheal intubation, defibrillation, and administration of antidysrhythmic drugs.	Advanced cardiac life support may resuscitate a client.

Evaluation of Expected Outcome: Dysrhythmias are controlled.

NURSING GUIDELINES 33-1

Performing Cardiopulmonary Resuscitation

- Attempt to arouse client by shaking and calling his or her name.
- Notify emergency personnel if client does not respond.
- Open airway with head-tilt, chin-lift.
- Remove objects or emesis from the mouth.
- Ascertain whether client is breathing by looking and listening for air.
- If client is not breathing, pinch his or her nose shut and give two rescue breaths through the mouth, using a one-way valve pocket mask, if available.
- Feel for a carotid pulse. If absent, administer cardiac compressions at a rate of 15 compressions to 2 breaths for both one- and two-rescuer resuscitation. Give 100 compressions per minute for adults in cardiac arrest.
- Check effectiveness of CPR after 4 cycles of 15 compressions to 2 breaths (pupils responding to light, pulse at carotid artery, improved skin color).
- Use an automatic electronic defibrillator (AED) if available.
- Continue with CPR between or in lieu of defibrillation if an AED is not available.
- Do not interrupt CPR for more than 6 to 7 seconds.

(Adapted from Part I: Introduction to the international guidelines 2000 for CPR and ECC: A consensus on science. [2000]. *Circulation, 102*[8, Suppl.], I1–I11.)

are ordered to confirm or rule out an accompanying connective tissue disorder (see Chap 67).

Medical and Surgical Management

Treatment involves avoiding factors that precipitate attacks. Smoking is contraindicated because it causes vasoconstriction. Drug therapy with peripheral vasodilators, such as isoxsuprine (Vasodilan), may be attempted, but results usually are less favorable than desired. Other drugs, such as nifedipine (Procardia), are being used investigationally. An IV infusion of prostaglandin E may provide temporary relief. *Sympathectomy* (cutting peripheral sympathetic nerves) may be performed; however, because of disappointing results, the procedure is performed less frequently than in the past. Gangrenous areas are amputated.

Nursing Management

Once an episode of pain occurs, there are several ways that the attack can be aborted. If warming the hands in water is impossible, the nurse encourages the client to imagine warming them in some way such as holding them

near a roaring fire. The mind can alter the physiology of blood flow. Another technique is to teach clients to imitate the exercise snow skiers use called the McIntyre maneuver: while standing, clients swing their arms behind and then in front of their bodies at a rate of about 180 times per minute. The swinging motion distributes blood to the distal areas of the fingers.

Teaching for clients with Raynaud's disease and their family members is important. The nurse instructs clients to avoid situations that contribute to ischemic episodes. He or she explains that injuries may heal slowly. If clients smoke, they must stop because nicotine causes vasoconstriction and increases the frequency of episodes. The nurse advises clients to wear wool socks and mittens during cold weather. Clients should avoid over-the-counter decongestants, cold remedies, and drugs for symptomatic relief of hay fever because of their vasoconstrictive qualities. The nurse advises clients to wear work gloves during household chores like gardening and washing dishes to prevent accidental injury. He or she informs clients how to perform nail care to avoid injury, like soaking the hands or feet before trimming nails, trimming nails straight across, and seeing a podiatrist for the treatment of corns or calluses. If a sympathectomy is done, the nurse emphasizes that the areas of altered sympathetic stimuli no longer perspire. He or she instructs the client that applying cream to prevent excessive skin dryness may be helpful.

● THROMBOSIS, PHLEBOTHROMBOSIS, AND EMBOLISM

A **thrombus** is a stationary clot. **Thrombosis** is a state in which a clot has formed in a blood vessel. **Phlebothrombosis** is the development of a clot within a vein without inflammation. Phlebothrombosis and thrombophlebitis have similar symptoms and treatment (see Chap. 31). An **embolus** is a moving mass (clot) of particles, either solid or gas, in the bloodstream.

Pathophysiology and Etiology

Thrombosis in the venous system most often occurs in the lower extremities and usually is associated with disorders or circumstances that cause venous stasis (inactivity, immobility, or trauma to a blood vessel). Orthopedic surgical procedures increase the incidence of deep vein thrombosis (DVT) of the lower extremities. Atherosclerosis, endocarditis, pooling of blood in a ventricular aneurysm, and dysrhythmias like atrial fibrillation can precipitate arterial thrombosis and subsequent embolization. When a thrombus forms or an embolus reaches a blood vessel too small to permit its passage, blood flow is partly or totally occluded.

Assessment Findings

Signs and Symptoms

When an arterial clot is present, symptoms arise from ischemia to the tissues that depend on the obstructed vessel for their oxygenated blood supply. With total occlusion, the extremity suddenly becomes white, cold, and extremely painful. Arterial pulsations are absent below the obstructed area. Numbness, tingling, or cramping also may be present, and surrounding blood vessels spasm. Loss of sensation and ability to move the part follows. Symptoms of shock frequently result if a large vessel is obstructed. When a small vessel is occluded, symptoms of ischemia, such as pallor and coldness, occur but are less severe. Unless blood flow is restored, gangrene develops (Fig. 33-11).

Clients with phlebothrombosis may have few, if any, symptoms because inflammation is absent. Signs and symptoms of DVT usually include mild fever and pain, swelling, and tenderness of the affected extremity. A positive *Homans' sign,* pain on dorsiflexion of the foot, may be present. A thrombus may become a mobile embolus and lodge in a distal blood vessel, like the pulmonary capillaries, causing symptoms related to the organ to which circulation has become impaired. (See discussions of pulmonary embolism in Chap. 29 and cerebral embolism in Chap. 46.)

Diagnostic Findings

Arteriography or venography (also called *phlebography*) using a contrast dye identifies the point of obstruction. Doppler ultrasonography is used to detect abnormalities in peripheral blood flow. Plethysmography measures volume changes in the venous or arterial system.

FIGURE 33-11 Gangrene of the toes from severe arterial ischemia. (From Smeltzer, S. C. & Bare, B. G. [2000]. *Brunner & Suddarth's textbook of medical–surgical nursing* [9th ed.]. Philadelphia: Lippincott Williams & Wilkins.)

Medical and Surgical Treatment

Treatment depends on whether an artery or a vein is occluded and the degree of occlusion (partial or complete).

Arterial Occlusive Disease

If an artery is completely occluded, treatment cannot be delayed. The physician may order an immediate IV injection of heparin to prevent the development of further clots or the extension of those already present. An attempt may be made to improve circulation by administering vasodilating drugs. A sympathetic nerve block (injection of a local anesthetic into the sympathetic ganglia) may relieve vasospasm. Narcotics may relieve pain and ease the client's apprehension. A thrombolytic agent may be prescribed if the client has experienced a pulmonary embolism or the embolus is occluding a large arterial vessel. If circulation to the extremity cannot be restored, a thrombectomy, embolectomy, *endarterectomy* (removal of the lining of an artery), or CABG is necessary. Nursing management of thrombectomy, embolectomy, endarterectomy, and bypass grafting is discussed in Chapter 37.

Venous Occlusive Disease

Venous thrombosis is treated with bed rest, elevation of the extremity, local heat, analgesics for pain, and intermittent subcutaneous injections or continuous IV heparin therapy, followed by oral anticoagulants once the heparin has achieved a therapeutic effect. DVT may necessitate surgical removal of the clot (*thrombectomy*).

Nursing Management

The nurse obtains a history of symptoms and identifies characteristics of the pain. He or she assesses for Homans' sign by having the client dorsiflex each foot. The nurse examines the extremities and compares skin color, temperature, capillary refill time, and tissue integrity; he or she also measures each calf. The nurse palpates peripheral pulses or uses a Doppler ultrasound device if pulses cannot be palpated. He or she marks the location of each peripheral artery with a soft-tipped pen to facilitate its relocation. The nurse immediately reports any change in the quality of a peripheral pulse or its sudden absence. Outlining any color change (line of demarcation) above or below the occluded area with a soft-tipped pen is useful to establish a baseline for future comparison.

The nurse monitors the client's response to anticoagulation therapy. If heparin is administered, the nurse assesses IV infusions hourly. He or she monitors partial thromboplastin time (PTT), prothrombin time (PT), and international normalized ratio (INR) when concurrent oral anticoagulation is prescribed. These values help determine therapeutic response and daily dosage. The nurse is alert for signs of bleeding and keeps protamine sulfate on hand for reversing heparin and vitamin K on hand for reversing oral anticoagulants. Additional nursing management is directed at increasing arterial or venous blood flow, relieving pain, and preventing complications.

Thorough teaching before discharge is essential. To prevent a recurrence of thrombosis, phlebothrombosis, or embolism, the nurse informs clients to avoid prolonged periods of inactivity (especially sitting), elevate the legs periodically, and walk or do isometric leg exercises frequently if sitting is unavoidable. He or she recommends wearing antiembolism stockings to prevent venous stasis (especially if the client has venous leg ulcers). The nurse instructs the client to apply these stockings before assuming a dependent position or after elevating the extremities for several minutes. The client needs to remove and reapply antiembolism stockings twice a day or as recommended by the physician. The nurse informs those who must take continued anticoagulants to observe for signs of unusual bleeding and keep appointments for laboratory tests.

● VENOUS INSUFFICIENCY

Venous insufficiency is a peripheral vascular disorder in which the flow of venous blood is impaired through deep or superficial veins (or both). The condition usually affects the lower extremities, most often the medial aspect of the leg or around the ankle.

Pathophysiology and Etiology

Venous insufficiency may be a consequence of varicose veins (discussed later) or valvular damage from a previous venous thrombosis. When the forward movement of venous blood is affected, venous congestion develops from the accumulating blood volume. Increased hydrostatic fluid pressure causes fluid to leave the veins and enter interstitial spaces. Localized edema is evident; the skin becomes shiny and hard. The fluid-filled space acts as a barrier between the cells in the surrounding tissue and their capillary blood supply. Consequently, cells are subjected to accumulating amounts of CO_2. As unoxygenated cells die, they release inflammatory chemicals that cause *dermatitis,* inflammation of the dermis layer of skin. The skin becomes red and "hot." Hemoglobin from blood cells also escapes into the extravascular space, causing the tissue to appear dark brown, deep purple, or black. Serous fluid oozes from the skin when there is no outlet for vascular or lymphatic circulation. Eventually the skin becomes impaired. A lesion referred to as a **venous stasis ulcer** forms (Fig. 33-12). Without adequate circulation, healing is retarded. Some ulcers may be present for years. The skin is fragile and easily retraumatized in the pro-

FIGURE 33-12 Ulcer from venous stasis. (From Smeltzer, S. C. & Bare, B. G. [2000]. *Brunner & Suddarth's textbook of medical–surgical nursing* [9th ed.]. Philadelphia: Lippincott Williams & Wilkins.)

cess of healing. Secondary infections often occur in the ulceration.

Assessment Findings

Signs and Symptoms

The foot or feet appear swollen. Testing for pitting is difficult because the congested fluid cannot be displaced. Superficial veins are dilated and obvious during inspection. Skin color is not uniform; there usually is a red or darkly pigmented area. If a lesion is present, its margin usually is irregular. Serous fluid may have collected in a pocket beneath the skin, or the area has beads of fluid on its surface that return after being wiped away. If an infection is present the drainage may change from clear to opaque. Most clients report moderate pain. Pedal and tibial pulses may be difficult to palpate because of the congestion of venous fluid.

Diagnostic Findings

Doppler ultrasound demonstrates a reversed direction of blood flow, indicating valvular incompetence in superficial or deep veins. *Photoplethysmography,* a diagnostic test for venous pathology, measures light that is not absorbed by hemoglobin and consequently is reflected back to the machine. When clients with venous insufficiency undergo photoplethysmography during exercise and rest, light reflection is greater during rest, showing that the client has decreased oxygen-bound hemoglobin and an increased volume of **venous reflux** (downward flow of venous blood). Air plethysmography measures venous pressure by filling a cuff with air after it is applied to the calf while the client is supine with the legs elevated. When the client stands, the pressure is measured again and venous pressure increases, indicating an increased volume of venous reflux.

Medical and Surgical Management

A major goal of therapy is to promote venous circulation. This is accomplished by applying elastic compression stockings such as *Jobst* stockings that maintain venous pressure at 40 mm Hg. The client wears the stockings at all times except when lying down. Because older adults have difficulty applying elastic compression stockings, the physician may apply a nonelastic gauze dressing soaked in zinc paste and glycerine known as an *Unna boot.* Pneumatic compression pump therapy, similar to EECP, also may be implemented. The compression pump promotes venous blood flow more efficiently than compression stockings but is more expensive and time-consuming. Furthermore, it interferes with performance of daily activities during its use. Mild analgesics are recommended for pain. Vascular surgery can be performed in which the valves in larger veins are repaired or incompetent valves are bypassed using a length of vein with healthy valves from elsewhere in the body.

A stasis ulcer is managed by keeping the skin and ulcer clean with soap and water or a diluted solution of a disinfectant like Hibiclens. Necrotic tissue is debrided. Any infection is treated by applying Silvadene, an antibacterial cream, or an antibiotic ointment. The wound is covered with an occlusive transparent dressing like *Tegaderm* that traps moisture, which speeds healing. Chronic, nonhealing skin lesions also are treated with **topical hyperbaric oxygen** (THBO) therapy. This approach delivers oxygen above atmospheric pressure directly to the wound rather than to the full body as with other disorders like carbon monoxide poisoning. Oxygen accelerates the healing process. THBO is applied by covering the area with an inflatable boot that confines the oxygen at low hyperbaric pressure at the wound site. The boot remains in place for approximately 90 minutes a day for 4 consecutive days. The treatment is repeated after 3 days of nontreatment in a cycle over 8 to 10 weeks.

Nursing Management

The nurse assesses the appearance of the extremities and quality of circulation. If an ulcer is present, he or she measures it and describes its appearance. The nurse asks the client to rate his or her pain and administers an analgesic if warranted. He or she measures the diameter of the calf and ankle and the length of the leg from heel to knee to obtain accurately fitting compression stockings. The nurse helps apply the stockings each morning before the client lowers the legs to the floor. He or she implements wound care according to physician directives.

The nurse teaches the client to do the following:

- Purchase more than one pair of compression stockings so one pair is worn while the other pair is laundered.
- Dry elastic stockings by laying them flat rather than hanging them, which stretches elastic.
- Lose weight if necessary.
- Elevate the legs periodically for at least 15 to 20 minutes.
- Walk or do isometric calf muscle pumps hourly to promote venous circulation.
- Raise the foot of the bed to promote venous drainage during sleep.
- Avoid morning showers or sitting in front of a fire because heat dilates blood vessels and contributes to venous congestion.
- Wear shoes with laces rather than slippers or sandals to reduce pooling of blood in the feet.

DISORDERS OF BLOOD VESSEL WALLS

● VARICOSE VEINS

Varicose veins or varicosities are dilated, tortuous veins. Both sexes suffer equally from this disorder. The saphenous leg veins commonly are affected because they lack support from surrounding muscles. Varicose veins also may occur in other body parts, such as the rectum (hemorrhoids) and esophagus (esophageal varices).

Pathophysiology and Etiology

Varicose veins have a familial tendency. The valves of the veins become incompetent in early adulthood, resulting in varicosities. In others, anything that constricts or interferes with venous return contributes to the formation of varicose veins. Prolonged standing compromises venous return as blood pools distally with gravity. Obesity and pressure on blood vessels from an enlarging fetus, liver, or abdominal tumor contribute to venous congestion. Thrombophlebitis may lead to varicose veins because the inflammatory process may damage vein valves.

Normally, the action of leg muscles during movement and exercise aids venous return (Fig. 33-13). When valves in veins become incompetent, blood accumulates rather than being propelled efficiently to the heart. The congestion stretches the veins. Over time, they cannot recoil and remain chronically distended. Venous hypertension then forces some fluid to move into the interstitial spaces of surrounding tissue. Venous congestion and local edema may diminish arterial blood flow, impairing cellular nutrition. Even minor skin or soft tissue injuries easily become in-

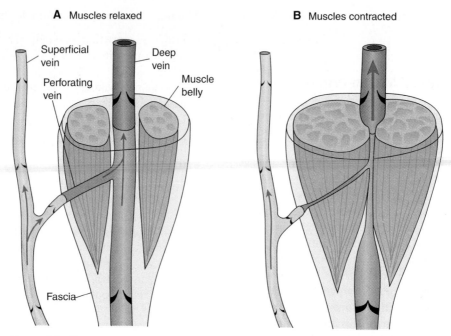

A Muscles relaxed

B Muscles contracted

Superficial vein
Deep vein
Perforating vein
Muscle belly
Fascia

FIGURE 33-13 The skeletal muscle pumps and promotes blood flow in the deep and superficial calf vessels. Most perforating veins lie below the knee. When the calf muscle is relaxed (**A**), blood moves from the superficial to the deep veins. Muscle contraction (**B**) propels blood in the deep veins toward the heart; closure of the venous valves prevents backflow. (Margolis, D. J. [1992]. Management of venous ulcerations. *Hospital Practice, 27*(5), 37. © 1992, The McGraw-Hill Companies.)

fected and ulcerated. The healing of such lesions is slow and uncertain.

Assessment Findings

Signs and Symptoms

Often the condition first manifests itself when other factors impair venous return. The legs feel heavy and tired, particularly after prolonged standing. The client may say that activity or elevation of the legs relieves the discomfort. The leg veins look distended and torturous and can be seen under the skin as dark blue or purple, snakelike elevations. The feet, ankles, and legs may appear swollen. The skin may be slightly darker in the areas of impaired circulation. There may be signs of skin ulcerations in various stages of healing. Capillary refill may be abnormal.

Diagnostic Findings

The Brodie-Trendelenburg test is performed for diagnostic purposes. The client lies flat and elevates the affected leg to empty the veins. A tourniquet is then applied to the upper thigh, and the client is asked to stand. If blood flows from the upper part of the leg into the superficial veins when the tourniquet is released, the valves of the superficial veins are considered incompetent. Ultrasonography and venography also are used to detect impaired blood flow.

Medical Management

Treatment of mild varicose veins includes exercising (walking, swimming), losing weight (if needed), wearing elastic support stockings, and avoiding prolonged periods of sitting or standing. The defective vein may be sclerosed or occluded by injecting a chemical that sets up an inflammation in the vein wall. Eventually adhesions form, and blood flow must find an alternate route through collateral veins.

Surgical Management

Surgical treatment for severe or multiple varicose veins consists of vein ligation with or without vein stripping. A **vein ligation** is a procedure in which the affected veins are ligated (tied off) above and below the area of incompetent valves, but the dysfunctional vein remains. For better results, a **vein stripping** is performed; in this procedure the ligated veins are severed and removed (Fig. 33-14). The entire great saphenous vein, which extends from the groin to the ankle, or the small saphenous vein may be removed.

Nursing Management

The nurse assesses the skin, distal circulation, and peripheral edema. He or she asks the client to rate the level of discomfort and ability to do active and isometric leg

FIGURE 33-14 Ligation and stripping of the great and small saphenous veins. (**A**) The tributaries of the saphenous vein have been ligated, and the saphenous vein has been ligated at the saphenofemoral junction. (**B**) The vein stripper has been inserted from the ankle superiorly to the groin. The vein is stripped from above downward. Several alternate incisions may be needed to remove separate varicose masses. (**C**) The small saphenous vein is stripped from its junction with the peripheral vein to a point posterior to the lateral malleolus. (From Smeltzer, S. C. & Bare, B. G. [2000]. *Brunner & Suddarth's textbook of medical–surgical nursing* [9th ed.]. Philadelphia: Lippincott Williams & Wilkins.)

exercises. Refer to Chapter 25 for routine perioperative care.

When the client returns from surgery with a gauze dressing covered by elastic roller bandages on the operative leg, the nurse monitors for swelling in the operative leg(s) and its effect on circulation. He or she removes and rewraps the roller bandage to facilitate blood flow. The nurse inspects the dressing for signs of active bleeding. In the immediate postoperative period, the nurse elevates the foot of the bed to aid venous circulation to the heart and reminds the client to alternately contract and relax the lower leg muscles. If active exercise is inadequate, the nurse consults with the physician about using pneumatic venous compression stockings, which cover the leg from foot to thigh and periodically inflate and release air, simulating isometric muscle contraction. The nurse helps the client ambulate as soon as possible to promote venous circulation, reduce edema, and prevent venous thrombosis. When bleeding is no longer a problem, the nurse applies elastic antiembolism stockings in place of the elastic roller bandage. He or she provides adequate fluid to decrease potential thrombosis.

When teaching the client and family, the nurse identifies factors that impair venous circulation: wearing elastic girdles or tight belts, using round garters or rolling and twisting nylon stockings, standing or sitting for prolonged periods, and sitting with the knees crossed. He or she describes appropriate foot and nail care to facilitate tissue integrity. The nurse explains that any open areas on the feet or lower legs require examination and treatment by the physician. He or she recommends active or isometric exercises and elevation of the extremities frequently during the day. The nurse demonstrates how to apply and remove elastic support stockings. He or she refers the client to the dietitian if weight loss is indicated.

● ANEURYSMS

An **aneurysm** is stretching and bulging of an arterial wall. Aneurysms of the aorta (aortic arch, thoracic, abdominal) are the most common, but aneurysms can be found in other arteries, such as those in the leg and brain.

Pathophysiology and Etiology

Arteriosclerosis, hypertension, trauma, or a congenital weakness can affect the elasticity of the *tunica media* (middle layer of the artery wall), causing part of the vessel to bulge. Once formed, some aneurysms lay down layers of clots, blocking the vessel until blood flow stops. Most aneurysms enlarge until they rupture. Loss of a large volume of arterial blood leads to shock and death if not controlled. Some aneurysms tear and leak blood into surrounding cavities, like the thorax or abdomen. Blood in a dissecting aneurysm is unavailable to arteries that branch off the aorta. When blood flow decreases or stops, tissue necrosis occurs.

Assessment Findings

Signs and Symptoms

Many aneurysms go unnoticed until found during physical examination or the client has a massive hemorrhage. Some cause pain, discomfort, and symptoms related to pressure on nearby structures. For example, a thoracic aortic aneurysm can cause bronchial obstruction, *dysphagia* (difficulty swallowing), and dyspnea. An abdominal aortic aneurysm can produce nausea and vomiting from pressure exerted on the intestines, or it may cause back pain from pressure on the vertebrae or spinal nerves. Most clients are hypertensive. A pulsating mass may be felt or even seen around the umbilicus or to the left of midline over the abdomen. A **bruit** (purring or blowing sound) can be auscultated over the mass. Circulation to tissue may be impaired.

Symptoms of a dissecting aneurysm vary and depend on whether a branching artery has been occluded or a tear has occurred in the aortic wall. Many clients become suddenly and acutely ill. Difference in the BPs of the left and right arms may be marked, or the BPs of the left and right legs may be unequal. Severe pain and signs of shock usually are present, but symptoms can be less severe in some instances. Because symptoms vary, diagnosis may be difficult.

Diagnostic Findings

Radiographs can demonstrate aneurysms when the arterial wall contains calcium deposits. Aortography identifies the size and exact location of the aneurysm.

Medical and Surgical Management

Medical treatment includes administering antihypertensive drugs to keep BP within normal range. Aneurysms are treated surgically whenever possible; no other cure exists. They are repaired by bypass or replacement grafting. A dissecting or ruptured aneurysm is a surgical emergency.

Nursing Management

The nurse helps control hypertension by keeping activity and stress to a minimum. The client should avoid straining during bowel movements, coughing, and holding the breath while changing positions. The nurse monitors BP, pulse, hourly urine output, skin color, level of consciousness, and characteristics of pain for signs of hemorrhage or dissection. He or she prepares the client for diagnostic testing and operative interventions. Afterward, the nurse monitors for shock and adequate tissue perfusion. See Chapter 37 for nursing management of a client undergoing cardiovascular surgery.

 GENERAL NUTRITIONAL CONSIDERATIONS

Total serum cholesterol is a measure of all cholesterol. Its value as a screening tool is limited because it does not distinguish between "bad" and "good" cholesterol. LDL cholesterol increases the risk of CAD. High LDL level is associated with obesity and excessive intake of calories, saturated fat, total fat, and cholesterol. HDL is inversely correlated with CAD. Smoking cessation, weight loss, exercise, and small amounts of alcohol increase HDL levels.

The National Cholesterol Education Program urges all Americans older than 2 years to follow a Step One Diet to reduce their risk of heart disease. The Step One Diet also is the initial treatment for clients with hypercholesterolemia who have not yet modified their diets. Recommended food choices include the following:

- Consume 6 oz or less per day of lean meat, fish, and skinless poultry. Limit red meat to three to four times per week, and remove all visible fat. Dried peas and beans are recommended as a low-fat protein source for meatless meals.
- Eat three egg yolks or fewer per week; use egg whites freely.
- Use 1% or skim milk, yogurt, and cheeses.
- Consume 6 teaspoons or less of added fats per day (margarine, oils, salad dressings), including that used in cooking. Avoid hydrogenated fats—the softer the margarine, the better. Olive and canola oils are preferred because they are highest in monounsaturated fats.
- Add more fruits and vegetables to the diet.
- Choose whole-grain breads and cereals.
- Select low-fat desserts such as gelatin, sherbet, angel-food cake, and fruit.

Clients who fail to achieve desired cholesterol levels after 3 months of good compliance with the Step One Diet are progressed to the Step Two Diet, which limits saturated fat and cholesterol more severely. A heart-healthy diet limits complex carbohydrates to 50% to 55% of calories, allows no more than 30% of calories from monounsaturated and unsaturated fat, and includes foods high in potassium, magnesium, and fiber.

Weight reduction lowers LDL levels, increases HDL levels, reduces cardiac workload, and has the added benefits of reducing triglyceride levels, lowering BP, and reducing the risk for diabetes. Eating less fat enhances weight loss.

Antioxidants like vitamin E and beta carotene may help prevent the oxidation of cholesterol in the artery wall and the subsequent events that lead to plaque formation. Relatively newly recognized antioxidant phytochemicals such as flavonoids in citrus fruit and resveratrol in red wine show promise in protecting against heart disease. Because researchers are only beginning to identify and understand how phytochemicals function, the best advice for now is to eat more fruits and vegetables—the greater variety the better.

Omega-3 fatty acids, abundant in fish oils, lower serum triglyceride levels and decrease platelet aggregation. Populations that eat fish frequently have a decreased incidence of heart disease; however, fish oil supplements have not been demonstrated to be either safe or effective.

Soluble fiber, most abundant in oats, various brans, citrus fruits, carrots, and dried peas and beans, helps decrease serum cholesterol by promoting cholesterol excretion. Rich fiber sources also are low in fat and high in vitamins, minerals, and phytochemicals.

Folic acid is being investigated for its role in preventing heart disease through its effect on homocysteine metabolism. Foods high in folic acid include enriched cereals, brewer's yeast, dried peas and beans, orange juice, and asparagus.

Although moderate alcohol consumption increases HDL cholesterol, it also raises BP, impedes weight loss, and appears to increase the risk of breast cancer in women. Men who drink alcohol should limit their intake to two drinks or less per day; women who drink should consume less than one drink per day.

GENERAL PHARMACOLOGIC CONSIDERATIONS

Physicians may recommend aspirin, one tablet (325 mg) daily, for clients with CAD. Aspirin inhibits platelet aggregation, thereby decreasing the blood's ability to clot. It may slightly prolong the PTT.

When the client with CAD requires rest and reduced anxiety, sedatives or tranquilizers may be prescribed. Notify the physician if the client becomes somnolent and no longer initiates deep breathing, leg exercises, or moving in bed.

All nitroglycerin preparations are stored in their original container and never placed in a container with other drugs. Each time the tablet, capsule, or ointment is used, the cover or cap must be tightly closed.

The sustained-release form of nitroglycerin is used for prevention (prophylaxis) rather than relief of anginal attacks. The transdermal systems are pads or disks applied to the skin that slowly release nitroglycerin over time. With the topical ointment, a measured amount (in inches) is squeezed from a tube, applied in a uniform layer on the skin, and covered with a plastic wrap.

Nitroglycerin can cause a throbbing headache, flushing, and nausea; decreasing the dose usually minimizes these effects. A client not accustomed to taking nitroglycerin should remain seated for a few minutes after taking the medication; some people experience faintness.

Use of oral and topical nitrate preparations on a continuous basis can diminish their vasodilating effects. Removing the transdermal patch at night and reapplying it in the morning or giving the oral preparation three times a day may prevent a diminished effect.

Before administering thrombolytic agents such as anistreplase or streptokinase, question the client about recent streptococcal infections. Such infections may decrease the effectiveness of anistreplase or streptokinase.

Treatment with a thrombolytic agent must begin within 2 to 6 hours of the onset of symptoms for an MI or within 7 days of other type of thrombi (e.g., DVT).

Administration of a thrombolytic agent with heparin increases risk of bleeding. The primary healthcare provider usually discontinues the heparin until thrombolytic treatment is completed. An antidote for overdosage of thrombolytic therapy is aminocaproic acid (Amicar).

GENERAL GERONTOLOGIC CONSIDERATIONS

Incidence of arteriosclerosis and other vascular disorders rises with age.

Older clients who take medication can ask their pharmacists to dispense the drug in a container without a childproof cap. This cap usually is difficult to remove when the client has arthritis or limited vision.

General physiologic changes of aging predispose clients to vascular occlusive disorders, especially as a result of atherosclerotic plaque formation. In addition, the heart's pumping ability decreases with age, increasing the risk of heart failure after an MI.

CAD is the most common cause of death in older adults. Less than 50% of older adults report chest pain with acute MI, whereas approximately 80% of younger adults report chest pain. Older adults are more likely to have nonspecific symptoms such as dyspnea, confusion, and syncope.

Use of calcium channel blockers, such as nifedipine and verapamil, to treat angina causes a peripheral vasodilating effect. Therefore, they are given cautiously to older adults who are at increased risk for hypotension.

Older adults are more sensitive to the hypotensive effects of nitrates, probably because of impaired venous valves, diminished baroreceptor reflex, and decreased vascular volume.

Critical Thinking Exercises

1. *A client presents in the emergency department complaining of substernal chest pain. He has a history of angina. What assessment criteria will help you differentiate between an anginal attack and an MI? What diagnostic tests will confirm an MI?*
2. *A client with Raynaud's disease relates that she has difficulty reducing attacks during the winter. What client teaching is indicated? How can the client reduce the ischemic episodes?*
3. *A client who has had a ligation of varicose veins returns to her room after surgery. What assessments are a priority? How can you teach the client to reduce the incidence of further varicose vein formation?*

References and Suggested Readings

American College of Cardiology and American Heart Association. (1999). 1999 Update: ACC/AHA guidelines for the management of patients with acute myocardial infarction. [On-line.] Available: http://www.acc.org/clinical/guidelines/nov96/1999/index.htm.

Anderson, J. J. (2000). Transmyocardial laser revascularization. *Progress in Cardiovascular Nursing, 15*(3), 76–81.

Anderson, L. A. (2001). Abdominal aortic aneurysm. *Journal of Cardiovascular Nursing, 15*(4), 1–14.

Associated Press. (2001). Drug-coated stent hailed by doctors. [On-line.] Available: http://www.msnbc.com/news/623923.asp?cp1=1.

Breen, P. (2000). DVT: What every nurse should know . . . deep vein thrombosis. *RN, 63*(4), 58–63.

Church, V. (2000). Staying on guard for DVT & PE . . . deep vein thrombosis . . . pulmonary embolism. *Nursing, 30*(2), 34–44.

Dorn, B. R., Dunn, W. A. Jr., & Progulske-Fox, A. (1999). Invasion of human coronary artery cells by periodontal pathogens. *Infection and Immunity, 67*, 5792–5798.

Fong, I. W. (2000). Emerging relations between infectious diseases and coronary artery disease and atherosclerosis. *Canadian Medical Association Journal, 163*, 49–56.

Halm, M. A. & Penque, S. (1999). Heart disease in women. *American Journal of Nursing, 99*(4), 26–32.

HeartCenterOnline. (2001). Women and cholesterol. [On-line.] Available: http://www.heartcenteronline.com.

Kunimoto, B., Cooling, M., Gulliver, W., et al. (2001). Best practices for the prevention and treatment of venous leg ulcers. *Ostomy/Wound Management, 47*(2), 34–44.

Lawson, W. E. & Hui, J. C. K. (2000). Enhanced external counterpulsation for chronic myocardial ischemia: How to use nonpharmacologic, noninvasive treatment for patients with angina. *Journal of Critical Illness, 15,* 629–636.

McHale, L. (1998). Clinical trial to test effectiveness of antibiotic treatment for coronary artery disease. [On-line.] Available: http://www.depts.washington.edu/hsnews/news/antibiotics.html.

Motamed, M. & Pelekoudas, N. (1998). The predictive value of diagonal ear-lobe crease sign. *International Journal of Clinical Practice, 52,* 305–306.

Part I: Introduction to the international guidelines 2000 for CPR and ECC: A consensus on science. *Circulation, 102*(8, Suppl.), I1–I11.

Patterson, S. (1999). Percutaneous myocardial revascularization: New treatment option for patients with angina. *Critical Care Nurse, 19*(5), 27–33, 35–36.

Platek, Y. M. (1999). PTMR . . . percutaneous transluminal myocardial revascularization. *American Journal of Nursing, 99*(7), 64–66.

Ross, R. (1999). Mechanisms of disease: atherosclerosis: An inflammatory disease. *New England Journal of Medicine, 340,* 115–126.

Rudolph, D. (2001). Standards of care for venous leg ulcers; compression therapy and moist wound healing. *Journal of Vascular Nursing, 19*(1), 20–27.

Ryan, D. (2000). Is it an MI? A lab primer. *RN, 63*(1), 26–31.

Stapleton, E. R. (2001). International guidelines 2000 for CPR and ECC: What do they mean for you? *Emergency Medical Services, 30*(9), 45–48.

Sullivan, C. (2000). Easing severe angina with laser surgery. *Nursing, 30*(4), Crit Care 32cc1–32cc2, 32cc4.

The cholesterol connection: Homocysteine: the cholesterol for the 21st century. *National Women's Health Report, 22*(4), 7.

Title, L. M., Cummings, P. M., Giddens, K., et al. (2000). Effect of folic acid and antioxidant vitamins on endothelial dysfunction in patients with coronary artery disease. *Journal of the American College of Cardiology, 36,* 758–765.

Vermuelen, E. G. J., Stehouwer, C. D. A., Twisk, J. W. R., et al. (2000). Effect of homocysteine-lowering treatment with folic acid plus vitamin B6 on progression of subclinical atherosclerosis: A randomised placebo-controlled trial. *Lancet, 355,* 517–522.

Wackel, J. (2000). Altered coagulation: A diagnosis for the problem of deep vein thrombosis. *Nursing Diagnosis, 11*(2), 17–23.

Wald, D. S., Bishop, L., & Wald, N. J. (2001). Randomized trial of folic acid supplementation and serum homocysteine levels. *Archives of Internal Medicine, 162,* 695–700, 779–777, 780.

Wigley, F. M. (1999). Raynaud's phenomenon: How to give cold comfort this winter. *Consultant, 39*(2), 540–542.

Caring for Clients With Cardiac Dysrhythmias

Words to Know

asystole
atrial fibrillation
atrial flutter
automatic implanted
    cardiac defibrillator
bigeminy
bradydysrhythmia
chemical cardioversion
couplets
defibrillation
demand (or synchronous)
    mode pacemaker
dysrhythmia
ectopic site
elective electrical
    cardioversion
fixed-rate (or
    asynchronous)
    mode pacemaker
heart block
implanted pacemaker

Maze procedure
multifocal PVCs
pacemaker
premature atrial
    contraction
premature ventricular
    contraction
radiofrequency catheter
    ablation
R on T phenomenon
sinus bradycardia
sinus tachycardia
supraventricular
    tachycardia
tachydysrhythmias
transcutaneous
    pacemaker
transvenous pacemaker
ventricular fibrillation
ventricular tachycardia

Learning Objectives

On completion of this chapter, the reader will:

- Name and describe six common dysrhythmias.
- Identify four medications to control or eliminate dysrhythmias.
- Explain the purpose and two advantages of elective cardioversion.
- Explain when defibrillation is used to treat dysrhythmias.
- Discuss the purpose for implanting an automatic internal cardiac defibrillator.
- Name various types of artificial pacemakers and the purpose for their use.
- Describe nursing management of the client with a dysrhythmia treated by drug therapy, elective cardioversion, defibrillation, or pacemaker insertion.

Cardiac rhythm refers to the pattern (or pace) of the heartbeat. The conduction system of the heart and the inherent rhythmicity of cardiac muscle produce a rhythm pattern, which greatly influences the heart's ability to pump blood effectively. Cardiac conduction and electrocardiogram (ECG) waveforms are discussed in Chapter 30. The usual cardiac rhythm is called *normal sinus rhythm* (Box 34-1; Fig. 34-1).

A **dysrhythmia** (also called an *arrhythmia*) is a conduction disorder that results in an abnormally slow or rapid heart rate or one that does not proceed through the conduction system in the usual manner. Some dysrhythmias do not require treatment; others require immediate intervention because they are potentially fatal. The most common cause of dysrhythmias is ischemic heart disease (see Chap. 33). Drug therapy, electrolyte distur-

---

BOX 34-1 ● Characteristics of Normal Sinus Rhythm

- Heart rate is between 60 and 100 beats/minute.
- The SA node initiates the impulse (upright P wave before each QRS complex).
- Impulse travels to the AV node in 0.12 to 0.2 second (the PR interval).
- The ventricles depolarize in 0.12 second or less (the QRS complex).
- Each impulse occurs regularly (evenly spaced).

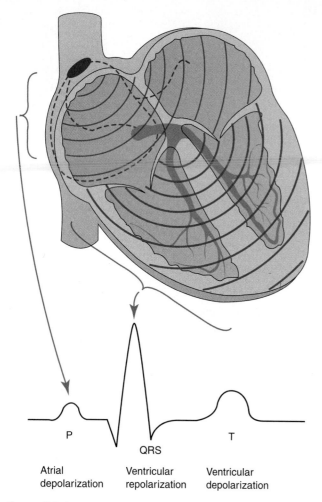

FIGURE 34-1 Normal conduction and ECG waveforms.

P — Atrial depolarization

QRS — Ventricular repolarization

T — Ventricular depolarization

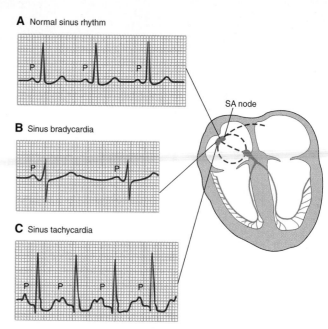

A Normal sinus rhythm

B Sinus bradycardia

C Sinus tachycardia

SA node

FIGURE 34-2 (**A**) In sinus rhythm, the SA node initiates impulses (P waves) 60 to 100 times/min. (**B**) In sinus bradycardia, the SA node initiates impulses at 40 to 60 times/min. (**C**) In sinus tachycardia, the SA node initiates impulses at 100 to 150 times/min.

bances, metabolic acidosis, hypothermia, and degenerative age-related changes are other conditions that cause dysrhythmias.

Stop, Think, and Respond ● **BOX 34-1**

Describe the characteristics of normal sinus rhythm.

CARDIAC DYSRHYTHMIAS

Dysrhythmias Originating in the Sinoatrial Node

Sinus Bradycardia

Sinus bradycardia is a dysrhythmia that proceeds normally through the conduction pathway but at a slower than usual rate (≤60 beats/minute; Fig. 34-2). Healthy athletes and others who are physically fit often have heart rates below 60 beats/minute; however, this finding reflects a well-toned heart conditioned through regular exercise. Such a heart rate is pathologic in clients with heart disorders, increased intracranial pressure, hypothyroidism, or digitalis toxicity. The danger in sinus bradycardia is that the slow rate may be insufficient to maintain cardiac output. Atropine sulfate is given intravenously (IV) to increase a dangerously slow heart rate.

Sinus Tachycardia

Sinus tachycardia is a dysrhythmia that proceeds normally through the conduction pathway but at a faster than usual rate (100 to 150 beats/minute; see Fig. 34-2). It occurs in clients with healthy hearts as a physiologic response to strenuous exercise, anxiety and fear, pain, fever, hyperthyroidism, hemorrhage, shock, or hypoxemia.

Premature Atrial Contractions

Occasionally, neural tissue in the atrial conduction system initiates an early electrical impulse called a **premature atrial contraction** (PAC), which is identified by an irregularity in the underlying rhythm (Fig. 34-3). The P wave of the waveform may look similar to other conducted impulses or may differ slightly because it is initiated somewhere in the atria other than the sinoatrial (SA) node. PACs can occur for various reasons: consumption of caffeine, use of nicotine or other sympathetic nervous system stimulants, or in response to heart disease or metabolic disorders like hyperthyroidism. When PACs are isolated or infrequent, there is no cause for alarm. Elimi-

FIGURE 34-3 Normal sinus rhythm with 1 PAC.

nating the cause usually controls PACs. Occasionally, the **ectopic site,** one that initiates an electrical impulse independently of the SA node, can lead to more serious dysrhythmias like supraventricular tachycardia.

Supraventricular Tachycardia

Supraventricular tachycardia (SVT) is a dysrhythmia in which the heart rate is dangerously high (≥150 beats/minute). Diastole is shortened and the heart does not have sufficient time to fill. Cardiac output drops dangerously low and heart failure can occur, especially in clients with pre-existing heart disease or damage. Clients with coronary artery disease (CAD) and SVT can develop chest pain because coronary blood flow cannot meet the increased need of the myocardium imposed by the fast rate. Besides tachycardia and angina, hypotension, syncope, and reduced renal output are signs and symptoms of low cardiac output and impending heart failure. Digitalis, adrenergic blockers, and calcium channel blockers are used to slow the heart rate.

Atrial Flutter

Atrial flutter (Fig. 34-4) is a disorder in which a single atrial impulse outside the SA node causes the atria to contract at an exceedingly rapid rate (200 to 400 contractions/minute). The atrioventricular (AV) node conducts only some impulses to the ventricle, resulting in a ventricular rate that is slower than the atrial rate. The

atrial waves in atrial flutter have a characteristic sawtooth pattern.

Atrial Fibrillation

In **atrial fibrillation,** several areas in the right atrium initiate impulses resulting in disorganized, rapid activity. The atria quiver rather than contract (Fig. 34-5). The ventricles respond to the atrial stimulus randomly, causing an irregular ventricular heart rate, which may be too infrequent to maintain adequate cardiac output. Ibutilide (Corvert) is an antidysrhythmic drug used to convert new-onset atrial fibrillation into sinus rhythm; flecainide (Tambocor) and propafenone (Rythmol) also are used to treat and prevent atrial fibrillation. Use of drugs to eliminate a dysrhythmia is referred to as **chemical cardioversion.** Atrial fibrillation also is treated with elective cardioversion (discussed later) or digitalis if the ventricular rate is not too slow. Clients who are not candidates for cardioversion and fail to respond to conventional measures may be candidates for a surgical intervention referred to as the **Maze procedure.** During the Maze procedure, the surgeon creates a new conduction pathway that eliminates the rapid firing of ectopic pacemaker sites in the atria. Some individuals with atrial fibrillation continue to experience chronic atrial fibrillation or episodic events.

Dysrhythmia Originating in the Atrioventricular Node: Heart Block

Heart block refers to disorders in the conduction pathway that interfere with the transmission of impulses from the SA node through the AV node to the ventricles. Heart block may be first degree, second degree, or third degree (also called *complete*). In first- and second-degree heart block, the impulse is delayed. In complete heart block (Fig. 34-6), the atrial impulse never gets through, and the ventricles develop their own rhythm independent of the atrial rhythm. The ventricular rate usually is slow (30 to 40 beats/minute). Pacemaker insertion (discussed later) is the treatment for complete heart block.

FIGURE 34-4 Atrial flutter produces sawtooth flutter waves. Most of the atrial impulses are not conducted to the ventricles.

Flutter waves

200-400/min

Fibrillatory waves

FIGURE 34-5 There are no identifiable P waves in atrial fibrillation. The atrial impulses look like a fine, undulating line.

Dysrhythmias Originating in the Ventricles

Premature Ventricular Contractions

Premature ventricular contraction (PVC) is a ventricular contraction that occurs early and independently in the cardiac cycle before the SA node initiates an electrical impulse. No P wave precedes the wide, bizarre-looking QRS complex (Fig. 34-7). If the heart rate is very slow, the ventricles can repolarize after a PVC in sufficient time to receive the atrial stimulus precisely when it is due. PVCs often cause a flip-flop sensation in the chest, sometimes described as "fluttering." Associated signs and symptoms include pallor, nervousness, sweating, and faintness. Many people experience occasional PVCs, which usually are harmless. They may be related to anxiety, stress, fatigue, alcohol withdrawal, or tobacco use. Although PVCs normally are not associated with a specific heart disorder, those whom they frequently trouble should consult a physician. A thorough examination is important to ensure no heart disease exists.

In the presence of acute heart injury, such as after surgery or with acute myocardial infarction (MI), PVCs in certain patterns suggest myocardial irritability and are precursors of lethal dysrhythmias (Fig. 34-8):

- Six or more PVCs per minute
- Runs of **bigeminy** (every other beat is a PVC)
- Two PVCs in a row (**couplets**)
- Runs of PVCs (three or more in a row)
- **Multifocal PVCs** (originating from more than one location)
- A PVC whose R wave falls on the T wave of the preceding complex (**R on T phenomenon**)

When dangerous PVCs occur, the client is given an IV bolus of lidocaine, followed by an IV infusion of the drug.

Ventricular Tachycardia

Ventricular tachycardia is caused by a single, irritable focus in the ventricle that initiates the heartbeat (see Fig. 34-7). The ventricles beat very fast (150 to 250 beats/minute), and cardiac output is decreased. Depending on how long the dysrhythmia is present, the client may lose consciousness and become pulseless. Ventricular tachycardia sometimes ends abruptly without intervention but often requires defibrillation. It may progress to ventricular fibrillation.

Ventricular Fibrillation

Ventricular fibrillation (Fig. 34-9) is the rhythm of a dying heart. PVCs or ventricular tachycardia can precipitate it. The ventricles do not contract effectively and there is no cardiac output. Ventricular fibrillation is an indication for cardiopulmonary resuscitation (CPR) and immediate defibrillation.

FIGURE 34-6 In heart block, SA-initiated impulses are delayed at the AV node or fail to progress altogether. In this example of complete heart block, the ventricles are beating independently of the atria.

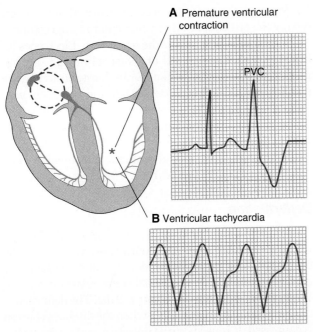

A Premature ventricular contraction

PVC

B Ventricular tachycardia

FIGURE 34-7 (**A**) An area outside the normal conduction pathway in the ventricles initiates a PVC. (**B**) Continuous generation of impulses results in ventricular tachycardia.

Pathophysiology and Etiology of Cardiac Dysrhythmias

Many clinical states predispose clients to dysrhythmias. One of the most common causes of serious dysrhythmias is myocardial ischemia, lack of oxygenated blood to the heart muscle, which can occur secondary to CAD, congestive heart failure, inadequate ventilation, and shock. The conduction system also is susceptible to disturbances from anxiety, pain, endocrine disorders, electrolyte imbalances, valvular heart disease, placement of invasive catheters in the heart, and drug effects. Because of the altered rate and rhythm, all dysrhythmias affect the heart's pumping action and cardiac output to some degree.

Assessment Findings

A client whose dysrhythmia causes decreased cardiac output is likely to feel weak and tired, experience anginal pain, or faint. Some clients with **tachydysrhythmias** (abnormally fast rhythms) describe palpitations or flutterings in their chest. Blood pressure (BP) usually is low. Pulse is irregular or difficult to palpate; the rate is unusually fast or slow. The apical and radial pulse rates may differ. The skin may be pale and cool. The client may be disoriented and confused if the brain is not adequately oxygenated, or there may be loss of consciousness and even clinical death. A monitor rhythm strip or 12-lead ECG can identify dysrhythmias. Electrophysiology studies can locate their origin.

A

B

C

D

E

FIGURE 34-8 Dangerous forms of PVCs: (**A**) bigeminal, (**B**) couplets, (**C**) run, (**D**) multifocal, and (**E**) R on T phenomenon.

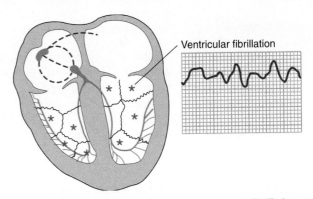

Ventricular fibrillation

FIGURE 34-9 The ventricles quiver during ventricular fibrillation, as shown by a wavy line.

Medical and Surgical Management

Some dysrhythmias are not life-threatening and may not require treatment. Many are treated with drug therapy and electrical modalities such as elective electrical cardioversion, defibrillation, or temporary or permanent pacing (Table 34-1).

Drug Therapy

Oral and IV antidysrhythmic drugs are used to treat clients with dysrhythmias; however, not all clients require medication. Usually, long-term antidysrhythmic drug therapy is based on the degree of hemodynamic compromise and the potential for the client to develop a life-threatening dysrhythmia. During resuscitation efforts, one or more of the various drugs used in cardiac emergencies is administered (Drug Therapy Table 34-1).

Elective Electrical Cardioversion

Elective electrical cardioversion is a nonemergency procedure done by a physician to stop rapid atrial, but not necessarily life-threatening, dysrhythmias. It is similar to defibrillation (Table 34-2). One difference is that the machine that delivers the electrical stimulation waits to discharge until it senses the appearance of an R wave.

By doing so, the machine prevents disrupting the heart during the critical period of ventricular repolarization.

The client is sedated for the procedure. Electrodes lubricated with a special gel or moist saline pads are applied to the chest wall. When the discharge button on the paddles (Fig. 34-10) is depressed and the heart is in ventricular depolarization, the electrical energy is released. The electric current completely depolarizes the entire myocardium. As the heart repolarizes, the normal pacemaker regains control and restores continued normal conduction through the heart.

Defibrillation

The only treatment for a life-threatening ventricular dysrhythmia is immediate **defibrillation,** which has the exact same effect as cardioversion except defibrillation is used when there is no functional ventricular contraction. Without defibrillation, the client will die. The defibrillator discharges its electrical energy when the discharge button is depressed. It is used during pulseless ventricular tachycardia, ventricular fibrillation, and **asystole** (cardiac arrest) when no identifiable R wave is present. The American Heart Association currently recommends public access defibrillation—that is, that automatic electrical defibrillators (AEDs) be located in public places such as worksites and locations where large numbers of people

TABLE 34-1	CHARACTERISTICS AND TREATMENT OF SELECTED DYSRHYTHMIAS			
DYSRHYTHMIA	RHYTHM	ATRIAL RATE (BEATS/MIN)	VENTRICULAR RATE (BEATS/MIN)	TREATMENT
Sinus bradycardia	Regular	<60	<60	None unless symptomatic; atropine
Sinus tachycardia	Regular	100–150	100–150	None unless symptomatic; treat underlying disease
Premature atrial contraction	Irregular	60–100	60–100	None or treat underlying cause, if known
Supraventricular tachycardia	Regular	150–250	150–250	Valsalva maneuver, unilateral carotid massage, immersion of face in ice water, administration of IV adenosine, cardioversion, radiofrequency ablation
Atrial flutter	Usually regular	250–350	75–175	Cardioversion, digitalis, quinidine, propranolol, verapamil
Atrial fibrillation	Grossly irregular	400–600	100–160	Digitalis, quinidine, cardioversion, verapamil, ibutilide, flecainide, amiodarone, anticoagulant
First-degree AV block	Regular	60–100	30–100	None unless symptomatic
Second-degree AV block	Regular	60–100	30–100	Pacemaker
Complete heart block	Regular	60–100	<40	Pacemaker
Ventricular tachycardia	Regular	60–100*	150–300	Lidocaine, procainamide, bretylium, cardioversion, defibrillation if pulseless
Ventricular fibrillation	Chaotic	60–100*	400–600	Defibrillation preceded by or followed with epinephrine

*Rate may not be distinguishable.
(Adapted from Kelley, W. N. [1996]. *Textbook of internal medicine* [3rd ed.]. Philadelphia: Lippincott-Raven.)

DRUG THERAPY TABLE 34-1	ANTIDYSRHYTHMICS		
DRUG CATEGORY AND EXAMPLES	**MECHANISM OF ACTION**	**SIDE EFFECTS**	**NURSING CONSIDERATIONS**
Class I Antidysrhythmics lidocaine hydrochloride (Xylocaine)	Suppress ventricular dysrhythmias by decreasing ventricular excitability	Dizziness, fatigue, drowsiness, nausea, vomiting, vision changes, seizures, hypotension	Monitor cardiac rhythm and vital signs. Keep life support equipment available.
procainamide hydrochloride (Pronestyl)	Slow electrical conduction, suppressing ventricular dysrhythmias	Hypotension, rash	Monitor cardiac rhythm and BP frequently.
Class III Antidysrhythmic bretylium tosylate (Bretylol)	Inhibit the release of norepinephrine Used for ventricular dysrhythmias resistant to other antidysrhythmic agents	Nausea, vomiting, hypotension, pain at IV site	Monitor cardiac rhythm and BP continuously. Keep client recumbent.
Class IV Antidysrhythmics verapamil hydrochloride (Calan)	Suppress tachydysrhythmias by inhibiting the movement of calcium across cell membranes	Dizziness, headache, bradycardia, hypotension, heart block	Monitor BP, heart rate, rhythm, and output. Keep client flat for 1 hr after administration. Have equipment for cardioversion and pacing available.
adenosine (Adenocard)	Slow rapid conduction through the AV node, restoring sinus rhythm	Headache, dizziness, nausea, other dysrhythmias, facial flushing, dyspnea, chest pain	Monitor BP and cardiac rhythm continuously, and have emergency equipment nearby. Monitor client frequently, especially those with underlying asthma or chronic obstructive pulmonary disease.
Vasopressors epinephrine hydrochloride (Adrenalin)	Increase heart rate, force of contraction, and BP Used in asystole	Hypertension, dysrhythmias, pallor, oliguria	Administer every 5 min during cardiac resuscitation. Monitor vital signs and cardiac rhythm.
Cholinergic Antagonists atropine sulfate	Block the effects of vagus nerve stimulation Increase heart rate Used for bradydysrhythmias	Palpitations, tachycardia, urinary retention	Monitor for therapeutic and adverse effects. Document heart rate before and after administration.
Other calcium chloride	Increase cardiac contraction in cases of cardiac standstill Improve weak or ineffective myocardial contractions when epinephrine fails	Slowed heart rate, tingling, hypotension with rapid IV administration	Give intravenously. Avoid extravasation. Monitor cardiac response.

gather. AEDs currently are carried on some airplanes and police cars. Nontraditional rescuers, those other than emergency medical technicians and paramedics, are encouraged to take the Heartsaver AED Course to learn how to provide defibrillation in out-of-hospital locations as soon as possible after a person becomes unresponsive. If defibrillation is performed within the first 5 minutes of ventricular fibrillation or cardiac arrest, the potential for survival is 50%; after 10 minutes without defibrillation, the chance for resuscitation is unlikely (American Heart Association, 2000).

AUTOMATIC IMPLANTED CARDIAC DEFIBRILLATOR

The **automatic implanted cardiac defibrillator** (AICD) is an internal electrical device used for selected clients with recurrent life-threatening tachydysrhythmias. Can-

TABLE 34-2	COMPARISON OF CARDIOVERSION AND DEFIBRILLATION
CARDIOVERSION	**DEFIBRILLATION**
Scheduled procedure 1 to several days in advance	Emergency procedure performed during resuscitation
Used to eliminate atrial dysrhythmias (e.g., atrial flutter, atrial fibrillation, supraventricular tachycardia)	Used to eliminate ventricular dysrhythmias (e.g., ventricular fibrillation, asystole)
Client sedated before procedure	Client not sedated but unresponsive
Uses less electrical energy (50–100 joules) than defibrillation, but higher levels can be administered if initial outcome is unsuccessful	Uses more electrical energy (200–360 joules) than cardioversion
Delivers electrical energy when the machine senses the R wave of the ECG	Delivers electrical energy whenever the buttons on the paddles are pressed

didates for an AICD include those who (1) have survived at least one episode of cardiac arrest from a ventricular dysrhythmia, (2) experience recurrent episodes of ventricular tachycardia, or (3) are at risk for sudden cardiac death because of structural heart disease like cardiomyopathy (see Chap. 31) with poor ventricular function.

An AICD consists of a generator with a battery and one (sometimes two) electrical lead that resembles a wire (Fig. 34-11). The generator is placed in a pocket under the skin near the clavicle, and the lead wire is inserted transvenously through the subclavian or cephalic vein to the apex or septum of the right ventricle. The lead senses the cardiac rhythm, which it transmits to the generator. The generator, which is programmed for various responses depending on the sensed rhythm, delivers an electrical shock through the lead to restore a life-sustaining cardiac rhythm, records the data, and then resets itself. A conscious client perceives the defibrillating shock as a thump or "kick" to the chest. AICDs also can pace the heart to obliterate a tachydysrhythmia and perform low-energy cardioversion. Various studies conducted by the National Institutes of Health have confirmed that AICDs

significantly reduce death rates among at-risk clients far better than drug therapy alone (Groh et al., 1998; Wolfe et al., 1998).

The AICD is checked every 3 to 4 months. The stored information can be retrieved by passing a electromagnetic wand over the implanted generator. The AICD can be reprogrammed in the same way. AICDs can deliver approximately 200 to 250 discharges and last for approximately 3 to 6 years before the battery requires replacement. Although AICDs are highly safe, some forms of electrical interference may adversely affect their function. Clients are instructed to avoid devices with a magnetic field. Examples include magnetic resonance imaging devices, extracorporeal shock wave lithotripsy machines (see Chap. 64), electrocautery and diathermy devices, peripheral nerve stimulators, large industrial electrical motors, and arc welding equipment. Analog cellular telephones are safe, but electrical signals from digital cellular telephones can mimic an abnormal heart rhythm, activating the AICD.

FIGURE 34-10 Standard paddle placement for defibrillation.

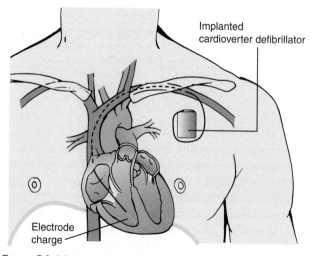

FIGURE 34-11 The automatic implanted cardiac defibrillator (AICD).

Most power tools and microwave ovens have shields or are grounded, making them safe. Occasionally, however, electric razors and remote-controlled toy cars have affected AICDs (Groh et al., 1998). A hand search is preferable to a scan with a metal detector at airports. Placing a donut magnet over the generator deactivates the device and should be done only if equipment is available to use an external defibrillator.

Clients with AICDs are advised to carry information about the device on their person, including the names of physicians involved in their care. Driving usually is restricted for at least 6 months. Furthermore, clients are told to report episodes in which they sense AICD activity. If the AICD discharges repeatedly or the client is symptomatic, immediate assessment by a cardiologist or electrophysiologist is warranted. The AICD may need to be reprogrammed, additional therapy with antidysrhythmic drugs may be initiated, or current medications may be adjusted.

Stop, Think, and Respond ● BOX 34-2

Explain why ventricular dysrhythmias are more serious than most atrial dysrhythmias.

Pacemakers

A **pacemaker** provides an electrical stimulus to the heart muscle to treat an ineffective **bradydysrhythmia** (slow abnormal rhythm). Pacemakers can be categorized into two broad divisions: temporary or permanent. The three types of temporary pacemakers are transcutaneous, transthoracic, and transvenous. An internal pacemaker is totally implanted and designed for permanent use.

Temporary pacing is done under urgent or emergency circumstances. Transcutaneous pacemakers are applied and transvenous pacemakers may be inserted at the bedside. The leads of a transthoracic pacemaker are inserted during open heart surgery. They extend from the chest incision. If the client requires cardiac pacing, the leads are connected to a temporary pacing unit. An internally implanted pacemaker is used when the client has a chronic bradydysrhythmia that requires long-term electrical support.

Pacemakers function in either a demand (synchronous) or fixed-rate (asynchronous) mode. **Demand (synchronous) mode pacemakers** self-activate when the client's pulse falls below a certain level. Thus, if the pacemaker is set at 72 beats/minute, it will not activate until the client's natural heart rate falls below 72 beats/minute. **Fixed-rate (asynchronous) mode pacemakers** produce an electrical stimulus at a preset rate (usually 72 to 80 beats/minute) despite the client's natural rhythm. This type is used less frequently than the demand (synchronous) mode pacemaker.

TRANSCUTANEOUS PACEMAKER

An external **transcutaneous pacemaker** is an emergency measure for maintaining adequate heart rate. It uses disposable, self-adhering leads attached to the chest wall (transcutaneous; Fig. 34-12). The heart rate is paced from an external generator. Use of a transcutaneous pacemaker is temporary until either a transvenous or permanent pacemaker can be placed, or the client is stabilized with medication.

TRANSVENOUS PACEMAKER

A **transvenous pacemaker** is a temporary pulse-generating device that sometimes is necessary to manage transient bradydysrhythmias such as those that occur during acute MIs or after coronary artery bypass graft surgery, or to override tachydysrhythmias. The electrical lead is introduced through the subclavian, external or internal jugular, or cephalic vein and threaded first into the right atrium, then into the right ventricle (Fig. 34-13). Fluoroscopy and a cardiac monitor are used to determine the correct placement of the tip of the pacemaker lead.

IMPLANTED PACEMAKER

An **implanted pacemaker** is an electrical device used to manage a chronic bradydysrhythmia. The most frequent indication for inserting a permanent pacemaker is complete or second-degree heart block accompanied by a slow ventricular rate. Occasionally, permanent pacing is used to treat certain tachydysrhythmias that do not respond to treatment or whose treatment results in bradycardia.

The lead of an implanted pacemaker is inserted transvenously, and the pacing threshold, voltage, and rate are set. One type of pacemaker has leads in both the right atrium and right ventricle (dual chamber); the lead of a single-chamber pacemaker is in either the right atrium or

FIGURE 34-12 Transcutaneous pacemaker with electrode pads connected to the anterior and posterior chest walls.

FIGURE 34-13 A transvenous pacemaker.

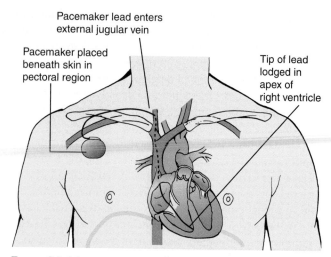

Pacemaker lead enters external jugular vein

Pacemaker placed beneath skin in pectoral region

Tip of lead lodged in apex of right ventricle

FIGURE 34-14 Implanted transvenous pacing electrode and pacemaker generator.

right ventricle. The implantable pacemaker generator, which is about the size of a half-dollar coin and three times as thick, is then positioned under the skin (Fig. 34-14) below the right or left clavicle. The small incision is closed with sutures. PVCs are more frequent during the early postimplantation period, and drug therapy may be ordered to suppress this dysrhythmia.

Power for the pacemaker is provided by mercury, lithium, or nuclear-powered (plutonium) batteries. The mercury battery has the shortest life (5 to 7 years); the nuclear-powered has the longest (8 to 10 years). Externally charged batteries also are used. Pacemaker batteries do not fail suddenly. The physician regularly monitors the status of their power. When the battery is nearing its end, the entire generator is replaced and the leads are connected to the new generator. After the pacemaker is inserted, the client is reassessed in 3 months and every 6 months thereafter. If the client redevelops original symptoms or suddenly shows dyspnea, vertigo, syncope, unexplained fatigue, edema in upper or lower extremities, muscle twitching, or extended hiccupping develop in the interim, the pacemaker is checked over the telephone. Routine telephone checks are scheduled every 2 to 4 months for the first 3 years and every month after. If a problem develops, the pacemaker is reprogrammed with an external wand just like the AICD.

Radiofrequency Catheter Ablation

Radiofrequency catheter ablation is a procedure in which a heated catheter tip destroys dysrhythmia-producing tissue. A catheter is threaded transvenously into the heart, initially for electrophysiology studies (see Chap. 30). Once the location of the dysrhythmia-generating tissue is identified, electrical energy is sent to the catheter tip (Fig. 34-15). The heat destroys the errant tissue, allowing impulse conduction to travel over appropriate pathways. Accompanying risks include bleeding from the insertion site, perforation of the catheterized vein, and vascular complications like thrombus formation. When the cath-

eter is in the heart itself, it may pierce the myocardium, leading to pericardial tamponade. Or the heated tip may obliterate normal conductive tissue, requiring a permanent pacemaker to ensure heart contraction.

Nursing Management

Clients with symptomatic dysrhythmias require careful monitoring and documentation of symptoms. Clients with serious dysrhythmias are potentially unstable, making frequent rhythm analyses important. Administering and monitoring the effects of antidysrhythmic drugs are key nursing responsibilities. Drugs given to restore or control cardiac rhythm are powerful, and their therapeutic levels often are close to toxic levels. Many of these drugs cause unwanted side effects and are contraindicated in certain conditions. The nurse assists with medical procedures that help to restore normal sinus rhythm and manages postprocedural care. He or she provides health teaching that promotes the client's ability to maintain safe self-management after discharge.

Elective Electrical Cardioversion

The nurse prepares the client for electrical cardioversion similarly to preparing a client for a surgical procedure. He or she verifies that a consent form has been signed. Food and oral fluids are restricted. The nurse ensures a patent IV line. He or she consults the physician to determine if scheduled drugs are to be temporarily withheld or additional drugs to decrease anxiety are to be administered. The physician may order a sedative 30 to 60 minutes before the procedure. Digitalis and diuretics are withheld for 24 to 72 hours before cardioversion; it is believed that the presence of these drugs in myocardial cells

FIGURE 34-15 A catheter is guided to the heart, and radiofrequency ablation destroys the defective conducting tissue.

Ablation catheter

decreases the ability to restore normal conduction and increases the chances of a fatal dysrhythmia developing after cardioversion.

The nurse places the cardioverter in the client's room. He or she checks that emergency equipment, such as an oral airway, oxygen, suction, and emergency drugs are on hand. Just before the procedure, the nurse assists the client with bladder or bowel elimination. He or she administers an IV tranquilizer, usually diazepam (Valium) or midazolam (Versed), as prescribed and inserts an oral airway once the client is sedated. The desired response to elective cardioversion is a normal sinus rhythm, normal or adequate BP, and strong peripheral pulses in all extremities. After cardioversion, the nurse monitors vital signs every 15 minutes for the first 1 or 2 hours and then as ordered. He or she observes the cardiac monitor to evaluate heart rate and rhythm continuously and compares ECG changes with those before the procedure.

Defibrillation

Defibrillation is instituted as soon as possible after a dangerous dysrhythmia is detected. Until such time, the nurse administers CPR to maintain oxygenation and circulation of blood. Defibrillation is performed by a nurse or some other health team member who is trained in the use of the defibrillator (Nursing Guidelines 34-1).

After successful defibrillation, the nurse frequently monitors level of consciousness, ECG pattern, BP, and

---

NURSING GUIDELINES 34-1

Steps in Defibrillation

When performing defibrillation, the nurse:

- Determines that there is no breathing or pulse
- Checks the ECG rhythm
- Facilitates CPR until the client is prepared for defibrillation
- Applies gel or saline pads to the skin of the upper right chest near the sternum and apical area
- Charges the paddles to 200 joules of energy while stating "Charging"
- Selects the nonsynchronized mode on the defibrillator (the synchronized mode is used for cardioversion)
- Places the paddles on the chest over the gel or pads with firm pressure
- Shouts "All clear" to ensure that no one is in contact with the client or the bed
- Presses the discharge buttons on each paddle with the thumbs while stating "Shocking now"
- Evaluates the postdefibrillation cardiac rhythm
- Repeats defibrillation using 200 joules one more time and 360 joules for subsequent defibrillation attempts if there is no improvement in the cardiac rhythm
- Continues CPR as IV medications are administered and between defibrillation attempts

pulse and respiratory rates. He or she reviews laboratory results, such as arterial blood gas analyses and serum electrolyte levels. The nurse checks the paddle application sites for redness and impaired skin integrity. The defibrillator is kept on standby because repeat defibrillation may be necessary. Even when cardiac activity is restored, the possibility remains that oxygen deprivation has affected one or more organs. The nurse monitors urine output to detect kidney failure and assesses for motor weakness or paralysis, memory impairment, and level of consciousness to detect for possible effects from cerebral anoxia.

Pacemakers

TRANSCUTANEOUS PACEMAKER

When initiating the use of a transcutaneous pacemaker, the nurse:

- Attaches the anterior electrode patch to the left side of the chest, halfway between the xiphoid process to below the left nipple
- Adheres the posterior electrode patch to the left posterior chest beneath the scapula and lateral to the spine
- Adjusts the rate knob beginning at 40 beats/minute in increments of 10 until reaching the rate prescribed by the physician or established by agency policy
- Regulates the current knob, which has a capacity starting at zero and advancing to 120 milliamps until capturing is observed—that is, a QRS complex follows each spike of the pacemaker; capturing usually occurs between 50 to 100 milliamps
- Selects the demand mode, which programs the pacemaker to produce an electrical stimulus whenever the heart rate falls below a preset rate but remains inactive when the client's heart beats naturally at an adequate rate
- Palpates the pulse and observes the client's response

TRANSVENOUS PACEMAKER

The nurse keeps resuscitation equipment close by because the tip of the pacemaker lead can mechanically provoke ventricular fibrillation. Once the pacemaker lead is inserted, the nurse attaches the external end to the external pacemaker unit, which is held securely to the client's forearm by means of tape or other anchoring device. The nurse positions the unit so that no tension is on the pacemaker lead. He or she checks the connection several times each day because an improper connection or displacement of the wire from the terminal results in pacemaker malfunction. If the client is confused or restless and movement disturbs the external pacemaker or its lead, the nurse notifies the physician. Only grounded electrical equipment is used in the room. This means that all electrical plugs must have three prongs.

If the client is on a cardiac monitor, an alarm sounds if the client's heart rate drops below the lowest level set on the alarm system. The drop in heart rate may result from battery failure, internal dislodgment of the pacemaker lead, or a break in the pacemaker lead. The battery of an external pacemaker is easily replaced; the nurse keeps one or more spare batteries readily available. The nurse reports dislodgment of the pacemaker lead or a broken wire to the physician immediately so that the pacemaker can be repositioned or replaced by a new one.

PERMANENT PACEMAKER

The nurse places the client with an internal pacemaker on a cardiac monitor and examines the rhythm strip for the pacemaker's characteristic electrical artifact or "spike," identified by a thin, straight stroke. Absence of the spike with a demand pacemaker setting means that the natural pacemaker, the SA node, initiates the impulse. With a fixed-rate pacemaker, there is a spike each time the heart is stimulated. The location of the spike in the series of waveforms is important to note. The nurse reports any deviation from the expected pattern. Absence of the spike in a fixed-rate pacemaker may mean faulty monitoring equipment or, more seriously, failure to pace. Other complications include infection, perforation of the ventricular myocardium by the tip of the pacemaker lead, and development of dysrhythmias. Postimplantation instructions for the client include the following:

- Avoid strenuous movement especially of the arm on the side where the pacemaker is inserted.
- Keep the arm on the side of the pacemaker lower than the head except for brief moments when dressing or performing hygiene.
- Delay for at least 8 weeks such activities as swimming, bowling, playing tennis, vacuum cleaning, carrying heavy objects, chopping wood, mowing or raking, and shoveling snow.
- Avoid sources of electrical interference similar to those problematic for people with AICDs.

Client and Family Teaching Box 34-1 highlights maintenance and care instructions for clients with permanent pacemakers.

NURSING PROCESS

● The Client With a Dysrhythmia

Assessment

The nurse reviews the client's medical history, including allergy and drug history. In addition to performing a general cardiovascular assessment (see Chap. 30), the nurse notes trends in heart rate, cardiac rhythm, BP, level of consciousness, urinary output, and physiologic changes in response to activity. If hemodynamic monitoring devices like an arterial line, central venous pressure manometer, or pulmonary artery catheter are used, the nurse analyzes the results of pressure readings and measurements of cardiac output. He or she records any symptoms the client reports, such as dizziness, fainting, or chest pain. The nurse determines the level of the client's knowledge about drug therapy or other supportive treatment measures such as elective cardioversion or use of an AICD or a pacemaker.

Diagnosis, Planning, and Interventions

Decreased Cardiac Output related to ineffective heart contraction secondary to dysrhythmia or ineffective response to treatment measures

Expected Outcome: Client will maintain adequate cardiac output as evidenced by stable vital signs; no chest pain, dizziness, or syncope; and urinary output of at least 1500 mL per 24 hours.

- Maintain physical and emotional rest. *Rest reduces tachycardia and may relieve the consequences of a tachy-dysrhythmia.*
- Provide supplemental oxygen for dyspnea, chest pain, or syncope. *Supplemental oxygen by inhalation diffuses at the alveolar-capillary level and increases oxygen concentration in the blood, making more oxygen available for cellular metabolism.*

PC: Life-Threatening Dysrhythmia

Expected Outcome: The nurse will monitor to detect dysrhythmias and manage and minimize any that occur.

- Monitor cardiac rhythm continuously. *Cardiac monitors display real-time heart rate and rhythm and alert the nurse to potentially life-threatening dysrhythmias.*
- Ensure a patent IV access. *Emergency medications are usually given by the IV route.*
- Administer antidysrhythmic drugs as prescribed. *They restore normal sinus rhythm by interfering with ectopic pacemaker sites.*
- Prepare client for elective cardioversion or use of a temporary pacemaker (see earlier discussion). *An alert client will be less anxious when given an explanation of the purpose and techniques for measures to restore normal cardiac rhythm.*
- Summon the team who will provide advanced cardiac life support measures such as defibrillation, and administer CPR. *CPR provides supportive breathing and circulates blood by heart compression to facilitate resuscitation. Advanced cardiac life support provides endotracheal intubation, positive pressure ventilation, and electrical defibrillation to enhance the potential for resuscitation (see earlier discussion for specifics on defibrillation).*

Risk for Ineffective Management of Therapeutic Regimen related to unfamiliarity with treatment measures

Expected Outcome: Client will describe ways to manage self-care before discharge.

- Explain the action, side effects, dosage, route, administration, and importance of medications used to control the dysrhythmia. *Thorough understanding promotes safety and adherence.*

- Teach client the technique for palpating and counting the radial pulse. *An accurate pulse assessment helps the client evaluate his or her response to treatment measures.*
- Identify the guidelines for withholding specific drugs and reporting symptoms to the physician. *Communication enhances early intervention when complications develop.*
- Provide information about the precautions required with an AICD or a pacemaker. *Electrical interference and magnetization can impair the function of these devices.*
- Stress the importance of continued medical follow-up. *Regular medical consultations ensure that the client's condition remains stable or facilitate early modifications to treatment.*

Evaluation of Expected Outcomes

Expected outcomes are the restoration and maintenance of adequate cardiac output. Any life-threatening dysrhythmias are effectively treated. The client and family accurately relate the treatment plan and postdischarge care.

34-1 *Client and Family Teaching* Permanent Pacemakers

The nurse instructs clients with permanent pacemakers and their families as follows:

- Maintain follow-up care.
- Report if the suture line becomes inflamed or sore.
- Avoid injury to the area where the pacemaker is inserted.
- Follow the physician's advice regarding lifting, sports, and exercise.
- Palpate the pulse and count the rate for a full minute daily or when feeling ill.
- Obtain and wear a Medic Alert bracelet or tag identifying that a pacemaker is implanted.
- Be cautious of situations that can cause pacemaker malfunction: gravitational force during airplane departures or landings, bumpy car rides, high-tension wires, short-wave radio transmissions, telephone transformers, and nuclear magnetic resonance imaging. Move to another location and check the pulse rate if dizziness or palpitations occur.
- Request hand scanning during airport security checks; some pacemakers trigger alarms.
- Maintain at least 6 inches between a cellular phone and the pacemaker generator or 12 inches if the cellular phone transmits over 3 watts.
- Check with the physician concerning transtelephonic pacemaker checks or when a pacemaker battery change will be necessary in the future.

GENERAL NUTRITIONAL CONSIDERATIONS

During alcohol withdrawal, catecholamines are released and may cause dangerous dysrhythmias. Clients with cardiac risk factors should avoid drinking more than 6 oz of beer or wine per day.

GENERAL PHARMACOLOGIC CONSIDERATIONS

Administration of lidocaine can have serious adverse effects, including convulsions and cardiac arrest. An airway should be readily available. If hypotension or additional dysrhythmias occur during administration, adjust the IV infusion to the slowest possible rate until the physician can examine the client.

Drug toxicity can occur even when normal doses of digitalis and cardiac glycosides are administered. Signs of toxicity include anorexia; nausea; vomiting; visual disturbances (e.g., halos around dark objects, objects appear green or yellow); diarrhea; abdominal discomfort; and such dysrhythmias as bradycardia, tachycardia, and bigeminal pulse. Withhold the drug and notify the physician if the heart rate is less than 60 beats/minute.

Digitalis toxicity usually is treated by discontinuing the preparation. Digitalis levels usually return to normal within a short time. Severe digitalis toxicity resulting in life-threatening overdosage may be treated with digoxin immune Fab (Digibind) as an antidote for digoxin or digitoxin. Most life-threatening states can be treated with 800 mg digoxin immune Fab given IV over 30 minutes.

The cholinergic blocking agent atropine is used to treat the severe bradycardia of complete heart block. A dose of 0.5 to 1 mg may be given every 1 to 2 hours. A maximum of 2 mg is given IV. Isoproterenol (Isuprel) also is used to treat severe bradycardia. When either drug is administered, closely monitor the pulse rate for drug response.

GENERAL GERONTOLOGIC CONSIDERATIONS

Age increases the risk for dysrhythmias because of several degenerative changes. The cells in the SA node of older adults continue to decrease and accumulate fat and calcium.

In older adults, stress, exercise, or illness may cause dysrhythmias and other cardiac disorders, such as congestive heart failure and myocardial ischemia.

Sinus bradycardia and heart block are common dysrhythmias in older clients.

Critical Thinking Exercises

1. *A client for whom an antidysrhythmic drug has been prescribed returns for a follow-up examination. How would you determine if the client has followed the drug therapy regimen?*

2. *What information is essential to document when helping to resuscitate a client who has experienced a cardiac arrest?*

References and Suggested Readings

American Heart Association. (2000). Early defibrillation. [On-line.] Available: http://216.185.112.5/presenter.jhtml?identifier=7252.

Dhala, A., Sra, J., Blanck, Z., et al. (1999). Ventricular arrhythmias, electrophysiologic studies, and devices. *Critical Care Nursing Clinics of North America, 11,* 375–382.

Docherty, B. & Roe, J. (2001). Cardiac arrhythmias: Recognition and care. *Professional Nurse, 16,* 1492–1496.

Dwyer, D. (2000). Pacing your patients. *Nursing, 30*(3), 82.

Gollob, M. H. & Seger, J. J. (2001). Current status of the implantable cardioverter-defibrillator. *Chest, 119,* 1210–1221.

Groh, W. J., Foreman, L. D., & Zipes, D. P. (1998). Advances in the treatment of arrhythmias: Implantable cardioverter-defibrillators. *American Family Physician, 57,* 297–307, 310–312.

Hatchett, R., Arundale, K., & Francis-Reeme, L. (1999). Systems and diseases. The heart, part four: Basic cardiac arrhythmias. *Nursing Times, 95*(43), 44–47.

Moss, A. J., Fadl, Y., & Zareba, W. (2001). Survival benefit with an implanted defibrillator in relation to mortality risk in chronic coronary heart disease. *American Journal of Cardiology, 88,* 516–520.

Sims, J. M. & Miracle, V. A. (2001). Fast facts about supraventricular tachycardia. *Nursing, 31*(6), 44–45.

Teplitz, L. (2000). Treating tachyarrhythmias with radiofrequency catheter ablation. *Dimensions of Critical Care Nursing, 19*(3), 28–31.

Teplitz, L. (2000). Zapping tachyarrhythmias with radiofrequency catheter ablation. *Nursing, 30*(2), Crit Care: 32cc1–32cc2, 32cc4, 32cc6.

Thomas, S. A., Friedmann, E., & Kelley, F. J. (2001). Living with an implantable cardioverter–defibrillator: A review of the current literature related to psychosocial factors. *AACN Clinical Issues: Advanced Practice in Acute and Critical Care, 12*(1), 156–163.

Wolbrette, D. L. & Naccarelli, G. V. (2001). Management of implantable cardioverter defibrillator patients: Role of predischarge electrophysiologic testing and proper patient instruction before hospital discharge. *Current Opinion in Cardiology, 16,* 72–75.

Wolfe, D. A., Kosinski, D., & Grubb, B. P. (1998). Update on implantable cardioverter-defibrillators. *Postgraduate Medicine, 103,* 115–116, 119–123, 129–130.

Woods, A. (2001). Calling all pacemakers. *Nursing, 31*(7), 46–47.

Wooten, J. M., Earnest, J., & Reyes, J. (2000). Review of common adverse effects of selected antiarrhythmic drugs. *Critical Care Nursing Quarterly, 22*(4), 23–38.

Caring for Clients With Hypertension

Words to Know

accelerated hypertension
diastolic blood pressure
essential hypertension
hypernatremia
hypertension
hypertensive
   cardiovascular disease
hypertensive heart
   disease

hypertensive vascular
   disease
malignant hypertension
natriuretic factor
papilledema
secondary hypertension
systolic blood pressure
white-coat hypertension

Learning Objectives

On completion of this chapter, the reader will:

- Identify the two physiologic components that create blood pressure.
- List factors that influence blood pressure.
- List three structures that physiologically control arterial pressure.
- Explain systolic and diastolic arterial pressure.
- Define hypertension and identify two groups at risk for it.
- Differentiate essential and secondary hypertension.
- Identify at least four causes of secondary hypertension.
- List three consequences of chronic hypertension.
- Discuss the assessment findings and treatment of hypertension.
- Discuss the nursing management of clients with hypertension.
- Differentiate between accelerated and malignant hypertension.
- Identify at least four potential complications of uncontrolled malignant hypertension.
- Discuss the medical and nursing management of the client with malignant hypertension.

Blood pressure (BP) is the force produced by the volume of blood in arterial walls. It is represented by the formula:

BP = CO (cardiac output) × PR (peripheral resistance)

The measured BP reflects the ability of the arteries to stretch and fill with blood, the efficiency of the heart as a pump, and the volume of circulating blood. Blood pressure is affected by age, body size, diet, activity, emotions, pain, position, gender, time of day, and disease states. Studies of healthy persons show that BP can fluctuate within a wide range and remain normal. Thus, obtaining several measurements for comparison is important.

ARTERIAL BLOOD PRESSURE

The autonomic nervous system, the kidneys, and various endocrine glands regulate arterial pressure. When measured, the pressure during systole and diastole is ex-

pressed as a fraction. The top number is the systolic BP; the bottom number is the diastolic BP. Normal BP for adults ranges from 100/60 to 139/89 mm Hg. BP tends to increase with age, most likely from arteriosclerotic and atherosclerotic changes in blood vessels or other effects of chronic diseases. Screening of BP is an important method for identifying people at risk for heart failure, renal failure, and stroke. Those at highest risk are older adults, African Americans, and clients with diabetes mellitus.

Systolic Blood Pressure

Systolic blood pressure is determined by the force and volume of blood that the left ventricle ejects during systole and the ability of the arterial system to distend at the time of ventricular contraction. The arterial walls are normally elastic and yield to the force and volume of ventricular contraction. In older clients, systolic BP may be elevated because of loss of arterial elasticity (arteriosclerosis). Narrowing of the arterioles, either from arteriosclerosis or some other mechanism causing vasoconstriction, increases peripheral resistance, which in turn increases systolic BP. This resistance can be compared to the narrowing of a tube, such as a drinking straw. The narrower the lumen is, the greater the pressure needed to move air or liquid through it.

Diastolic Blood Pressure

Diastolic blood pressure reflects arterial pressure during ventricular relaxation. It depends on the resistance of the arterioles and the diastolic filling times. If arterioles are resistant (constricted), blood is under greater pressure.

HYPERTENSIVE DISEASE

The term **hypertension** refers to a sustained elevation of systolic arterial BP of 140 mm Hg or higher, a sustained diastolic arterial BP of 90 mm Hg or higher, or both. The Joint National Committee on Detection, Evaluation, and Treatment of High Blood Pressure (1997) has identified three stages of hypertension (Table 35-1). When elevated BP causes a cardiac abnormality, the term **hypertensive heart disease** is used. When vascular damage is present without heart involvement, the term **hypertensive vascular disease** is used. When both heart disease and vascular damage accompany hypertension, the appropriate term is **hypertensive cardiovascular disease.**

● ESSENTIAL AND SECONDARY HYPERTENSION

Hypertension is divided into two main categories: essential (primary) and secondary. **Essential hypertension,** about 95% of cases, is sustained elevated BP with no known cause. **Secondary hypertension** is elevated BP that results from or is secondary to some other disorder.

Some people experience **white-coat hypertension,** a term describing elevated BP that develops during evaluation by medical personnel, who traditionally have worn a "white coat." This hypertension most likely results from anxiety. To confirm or exclude this phenomenon, the BP is measured a second time before the client leaves the agency. In cases of white-coat hypertension, this subsequent measurement is likely to be normal. If the client remains hypertensive, he or she is advised to check BP regularly, either at home with the help of a family member or at a public-service location in the community (e.g., pharmacy). The client should bring the BP measurements to his or her next medical appointment.

Pathophysiology and Etiology

The exact cause of essential hypertension is unknown. BP often increases with age; hypertension may run in families. Essential hypertension affects African Americans at a higher rate than it does other ethnic groups. Obesity, inactivity, smoking, excessive alcohol intake, and ineffective stress management are risk factors.

Research into specific factors that contribute to the development of essential hypertension continues. For instance, it is well documented that **hypernatremia** (elevated serum sodium level) increases blood volume, which raises BP. A low serum potassium level, however, actually may cause sodium retention as the kidneys try to maintain a balanced number of cations (positively charged electrolytes) in body fluid. Scientists are also investigating the role of calcium in hypertension because serum calcium levels are low in some hypertensive clients.

Essential hypertension also may develop from alterations in other body chemicals. Defects in BP regulation may result from an impairment in the renin-angiotensin-aldosterone mechanism (see Chap. 22). Renin is a chem-

TABLE 35-1	RECOMMENDATIONS FOR BLOOD PRESSURE FOLLOW-UP*		
CATEGORY	SYSTOLIC (mm Hg)	DIASTOLIC (mm Hg)	RECOMMENDED FOLLOW-UP
Optimal†	<120 and	<80	Recheck in 2 years.
Normal	<130 and	<85	Recheck in 2 years.
High normal	130–139 or	85–89	Recheck in 1 year.
Hypertension			
Stage 1 (mild)	140–159 or	90–99	Confirm within 2 months.
Stage 2 (moderate)	160–179 or	100–109	Evaluate within 1 month.
Stage 3 (severe)	≥180 or	≥110	Evaluate immediately or within 1 week, depending on clinical situation.

*Classification of BP for adults 18 years of age or older, with recommended follow-up.
†Optimal blood pressure with respect to cardiovascular risk is <120/80 mm Hg; however, unusually low readings should be evaluated for clinical significance.
(From Joint National Committee on Detection, Evaluation, and Treatment of High Blood Pressure. [1997]. The Sixth Report of the Joint National Committee on Detection, Evaluation, and Treatment of High Blood Pressure. *Archives of Internal Medicine, 157,* 2413–2446.)

ical that the kidneys release to raise BP and increase vascular fluid volume. For those with a heightened stress response, hypertension may be correlated with a higher than usual release of catecholamines, such as epinephrine and norepinephrine, which elevate BP. Last, some researchers theorize that a deficiency of **natriuretic factor,** a hormone produced by the heart, causes arteries and arterioles to remain in a state of sustained vasoconstriction (see Chap. 22).

Secondary hypertension may accompany any primary condition that affects fluid volume or renal function or causes arterial vasoconstriction. Predisposing conditions include kidney disease, pheochromocytoma (a tumor of the adrenal medulla), hyperaldosteronism, atherosclerosis, use of cocaine or other cardiac stimulants (e.g., weight control drugs, caffeine), and use of oral contraceptives.

Regardless of whether a person has essential or secondary hypertension, the accompanying organ damage and complications are the same. Hypertension causes the heart to work harder to pump against the increased resistance. Consequently, the size of the heart muscle increases. When the heart no longer can pump adequately to meet the body's metabolic needs, heart failure occurs (see Chap. 36). The extra work and the greater mass increase the heart's need for oxygen. If the myocardium does not receive sufficient oxygenated blood, myocardial ischemia occurs and the client experiences angina.

In addition to its direct effects on the heart, high BP damages the arterial vascular system. It accelerates atherosclerosis. Furthermore, the increased resistance of the arterioles to the flow of blood causes serious complications in other body organs, including the eyes, brain, heart, and kidneys. Hemorrhage of tiny arteries in the retina may cause marked visual disturbances or blindness. A cerebrovascular accident may result from hemorrhage or occlusion of a blood vessel in the brain. Myocardial infarction (MI) may result from occlusion of a branch of a coronary artery. Impaired circulation to the kidneys may result in renal failure.

Assessment Findings

Signs and Symptoms

Clients with hypertension may be asymptomatic. The onset of hypertension, considered "the silent killer," often is gradual. It can exist for years but be discovered only during a routine physical examination or when the client experiences a major complication. As the BP becomes elevated, clients may identify symptoms such as a throbbing or pounding headache, dizziness, fatigue, insomnia, nervousness, nosebleeds, and blurred vision. Angina or dyspnea may be the first clue to hypertensive heart disease.

The most obvious finding during a physical assessment is a sustained elevation of one or both BP measurements. The pulse may feel bounding from the force of ventricular contraction. Clients may be overweight. They may have a flushed face from engorgement of superficial blood vessels. Peripheral edema may be present. An ophthalmic examination may reveal vascular changes in the eyes, retinal hemorrhages, or edema of the optic nerve, known as **papilledema.**

Diagnostic Findings

Diagnostic tests are performed to determine the extent of organ damage. Electrocardiography, echocardiography, and chest radiography may reveal an enlarged left ventricle. Blood tests may show elevated blood urea nitrogen and serum creatinine levels, indicating impaired renal function, findings that excretory urography (intravenous [IV] pyelography) may further validate. Fluorescein angiography, an ophthalmologic test using IV dye, often reveals leaking retinal blood vessels.

If the cause of hypertension is a renal vascular problem, renal arteriography demonstrates narrowing of the renal artery. If the cause is related to dysfunction of the adrenal gland, a 24-hour collected urine specimen detects elevated catecholamines. Blood studies reveal elevated cholesterol and triglyceride levels, indicating that atherosclerosis is an underlying factor.

Medical Management

The primary objective of therapy for either type of hypertension is to lower the BP and prevent major complications. Recommended follow-up is based on BP measurements (see Table 35-1). Initial management depends on the stage of hypertension; however, nonpharmacologic interventions usually are used first. For mild elevations, weight reduction, decreased sodium intake (Box 35-1), moderate exercise, and reduced contributing factors (e.g., smoking, alcohol use) may return the BP to normal levels. A diet low in saturated fats is recommended if cholesterol and triglyceride levels are high.

Depending on the client's response to nonpharmacologic therapy, one of several drugs may be prescribed (Drug Therapy Table 35-1). If the BP remains elevated, the dosage may be increased or a second, third, or fourth antihypertensive agent may be added (Fig. 35-1). Secondary hypertension often resolves by treating its cause.

NURSING PROCESS

● **The Client With Hypertension**

Assessment

The nurse initially takes BP in both arms with the client in a standing, sitting, and then supine position, using an appropriately sized cuff (Table 35-2). Thereafter, the nurse uses the same arm and places the client in the same position each time he or she takes a reading. The nurse asks questions to determine if the client is following the

---

BOX 35-1 ● Recommendations for Limiting Sodium

■ Consume no more than 2.4 g (2400 mg) of sodium per day in the form of salt (sodium chloride) or other compounds such as monosodium glutamate (MSG) or sodium bicarbonate. One teaspoon of table salt contains 2300 mg of sodium.
■ Read food labels to determine the sodium content per serving.
■ Prepare fresh rather than canned products, or buy those that are labeled as "unsalted, no salt, sodium-free, low sodium, or reduced sodium."
■ Prepare food from "scratch" without adding salt, as opposed to purchasing premade entrées, which usually are highly salted.
■ Drain and rinse canned foods.
■ Avoid or limit consumption of frankfurters, ham, bacon, and processed meat products, which often contain sodium nitrate as a preservative.
■ Substitute healthy snacks like fresh or dried fruit for those that are salted.
■ Experiment with seasonings like lemon, garlic, and onion powder as alternatives to salt.
■ Eliminate or restrict items that contain significant sodium like pickles, green olives, sauerkraut, mustard, catsup, barbecue sauce, pizza sauce, canned soup, and packaged mixes.

(Adapted from U.S. Department of Agriculture and U.S. Department of Health and Human Services. [1995]. Dietary guidelines for Americans. [On-line.] Available: http://www.nalusda.gov/fnic/dga95/cover.html.)

---

treatment regimen. He or she performs additional cardiac assessments (see Chap. 30) depending on the client's medical history and current symptoms. The nurse teaches about nonpharmacologic and pharmacologic methods for restoring and maintaining BP below hypertensive levels, as well as techniques for self-management (Client and Family Teaching Box 35-1). He or she collaborates with a dietitian to provide information on dietary modifications such as Dietary Approaches to Stop Hypertension (see DASH diet in General Nutritional Considerations).

Diagnosis, Planning, and Interventions

Risk for Decreased Cardiac Output related to excessive or prolonged systemic vascular resistance
Expected Outcome: Client will maintain an adequate cardiac output as evidenced by reduced BP to normal or near-normal levels, heart rate between 60 and 100 beats/minute, effortless breathing, clear lung sounds, alert mental status, and urine output that approximates or slightly exceeds intake.

● Promote physical rest. *Rest decreases BP and reduces the resistance that the heart must overcome to eject blood.*
● Relieve emotional stress. *Reduced stress decreases production of neurotransmitters that constrict peripheral arterioles.*
● Instruct client to avoid bearing down against a closed glottis (Valsalva maneuver). *Straining or bearing down against a closed glottis momentarily increases BP.*
● Encourage compliance with salt/sodium restrictions. *Doing so decreases blood volume and improves the potential for greater cardiac output.*

● Recommend smoking cessation. *Nicotine raises heart rate, constricts arterioles, and reduces the heart's ability to eject blood.*
● Enforce prescribed fluid restrictions. *Reduced oral fluid ultimately decreases circulating blood volume and systemic vascular resistance.*
● Help client reduce or eliminate caffeine. *Caffeine increases heart rate and causes vasoconstriction.*
● Administer prescribed antihypertensives. *They use various mechanisms to control BP, including increasing urine elimination, blocking production of angiotensin, and dilating blood vessels.*

Risk for Injury related to syncope and dizziness secondary to antihypertensive drugs
Expected Outcome: The client will be injury free.

● Monitor postural changes in BP by assessing client while he or she is lying, sitting, and standing. *BP usually falls when assuming an upright position. Assessment validates whether the drop in BP is significant.*
● As appropriate, ensure the signal cord is in the client's reach and advise him or her to use it whenever getting out of bed. *Nursing personnel can prevent injury if they assist clients.*
● Encourage client to rise slowly from a sitting or lying position. *Gradual changes in position provide time for the heart to increase its rate of contraction to resupply oxygen to the brain.*
● Help client to sit or lie down if he or she is dizzy. *The support of a chair or bed reduces the potential for falling.*

Evaluation of Expected Outcomes

Expected outcomes are that adequate cardiac output is maintained or improved when systolic and diastolic BP are reduced. The client does not experience syncope or fall from postural changes in BP.

Stop, Think, and Respond ● BOX 35-1

A neighbor asks you to take her BP. The measurement is 160/90 mm Hg. What questions will you ask? What recommendations will you make for follow-up?

●ACCELERATED AND MALIGNANT HYPERTENSION

Accelerated and malignant hypertension are more serious forms of elevated BP that develop in clients with either essential or secondary hypertension. **Accelerated hypertension** describes markedly elevated BP, accompanied by hemorrhages and exudates in the eyes. If untreated, accelerated hypertension may progress to **malignant hypertension,** which describes dangerously elevated BP accompanied by papilledema.

DRUG THERAPY TABLE 35-1 | **ANTIHYPERTENSIVE AGENTS**

DRUG CATEGORY AND EXAMPLES	MECHANISM OF ACTION	SIDE EFFECTS	NURSING CONSIDERATIONS
Alpha-Adrenergic Blockers prazosin (Minipress)	Relax vascular smooth muscle by blocking alpha1 receptor sites for epinephrine and norepinephrine	Hypotension, dizziness, drowsiness, nausea, palpitations	Administer first dose just before bedtime to reduce potential for syncope. Monitor client for postural hypotension. Caution client to change positions slowly.
Beta-Adrenergic Blockers propranolol (Inderal)	Blocks $beta_1$ and $beta_2$ adrenergic receptors Decrease renin levels	Hypotension, bradycardia, bronchospasm, CHF, depression, erectile dysfunction, hypoglycemia	Administer with meals. Advise client not to discontinue medication abruptly. Monitor for fluid retention, rash, and difficulty breathing. Monitor blood glucose level in clients with diabetes. These drugs are contraindicated in clients with chronic respiratory disorders.
Alpha-Beta Blockers labetalol (Normodyne)	Block alpha-, beta-, and $beta_2$-adrenergic receptors	Dizziness, GI symptoms, dyspnea, cough, erectile dysfunction, decreased libido	Administer with meals. Caution client to avoid discontinuing drug therapy abruptly and to inform anesthesiologist of use before surgery to avoid drug–drug interaction.
Diuretics furosemide (Lasix)	Promote sodium and water excretion, thus reducing circulating blood volume	Dizziness, dehydration, blurred vision, anorexia, diarrhea, nocturia, polyuria, thrombocytopenia, orthostatic hypotension, hypokalemia	Weigh client daily. Measure intake and output. Monitor serum potassium level. Advise client to replace lost potassium with bananas, orange juice, or prescribed supplement.
ACE Inhibitors captopril (Capoten)	Block ACE from converting angiotensin I to angiotensin II (a potent vasoconstrictor) Promote fluid and sodium loss and decrease peripheral vascular resistance	Tachycardia, hypotension, GI irritation, pancytopenia, proteinuria, rash, cough, dry mouth, hyperkalemia	Excretion is reduced in clients with renal failure. First-dose hypotension is common in older adults. Administer 1 hour before or 2 hours after meals. Monitor serum potassium blood urea nitrogen and creatinine.
Angiotensin II Receptor Antagonists losartan (Cozaar)	Block effects of angiotensin II Relax vascular smooth muscle Increase salt and water excretion Reduce plasma volume	Orthostatic hypotension; GI disturbances; hyperkalemia; respiratory congestion; swelling of face, lips, eyelids, tongue in hypersensitive persons	Assess BP for postural changes. Monitor serum potassium levels. Observe for allergic reactions when drug therapy begins.
Calcium Channel Blockers nifedipine (Procardia XL)	Decrease BP by dilating coronary and peripheral arteries	Hypotension, dizziness, CHF, edema, atrioventricular block, nausea	Check BP and heart rate before each dose. Withhold drug in cases of hypotension. Observe for signs and symptoms of CHF and fluid overload.

ACE, angiotensin-converting enzyme; *BP,* blood pressure; *CHF,* congestive heart failure; *GI,* gastrointestinal.

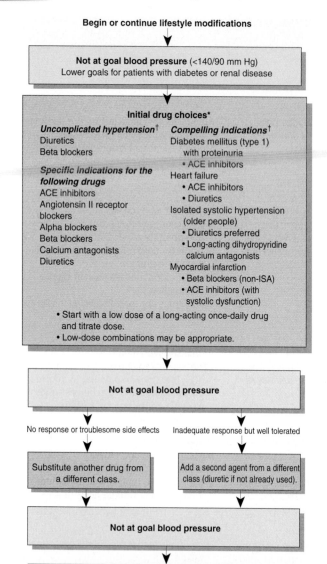

Begin or continue lifestyle modifications

↓

Not at goal blood pressure (<140/90 mm Hg)
Lower goals for patients with diabetes or renal disease

↓

Initial drug choices*

Uncomplicated hypertension†
Diuretics
Beta blockers

Specific indications for the following drugs
ACE inhibitors
Angiotensin II receptor blockers
Alpha blockers
Beta blockers
Calcium antagonists
Diuretics

Compelling indications†
Diabetes mellitus (type 1)
  with proteinuria
  • ACE inhibitors
Heart failure
  • ACE inhibitors
  • Diuretics
Isolated systolic hypertension
  (older people)
  • Diuretics preferred
  • Long-acting dihydropyridine
    calcium antagonists
Myocardial infarction
  • Beta blockers (non-ISA)
  • ACE inhibitors (with
    systolic dysfunction)

• Start with a low dose of a long-acting once-daily drug
  and titrate dose.
• Low-dose combinations may be appropriate.

↓

Not at goal blood pressure

↓   ↓

No response or troublesome side effects   Inadequate response but well tolerated

↓   ↓

Substitute another drug from
a different class.

Add a second agent from a different
class (diuretic if not already used).

↓   ↓

Not at goal blood pressure

↓

Continue adding agents from other classes.
Consider referral to a hypertension specialist.

* Unless contraindicated.
  ACE, angiotensin-converting enzyme; ISA, intrinsic sympathomimetic activity.
† Based on randomized controlled trials.

FIGURE 35-1 Individualized step care therapy for hypertension (NIH Publication No. 98-4080, November 1997).

35-1 *Client and Family Teaching* Hypertension

The nurse instructs as follows:

- Adhere to the treatment regimen even if you have few, if any, symptoms and feel well. Hypertension is a chronic condition requiring lifelong management and treatment.
- Learn to regularly monitor BP using a home sphygmomanometer or arrange for monitoring by a community agency that provides this service at no or low cost.
- Keep a log of BP measurements for follow-up visits.
- Comply with the treatment regimen involving diet, exercise, and drug therapy.
- Consult cookbooks published or endorsed by the American Heart Association, American Diabetes Association, or other reliable sources for "heart smart" recipes.
- Follow directions for medications; never increase, decrease, or omit a prescribed drug unless first conferring with the primary care provider.
- Report adverse effects from medications to the prescribing provider. Get medical approval before taking nonprescription drugs. Inform all physicians and dentists of medications that you are taking.
- Avoid tobacco and beverages containing caffeine or alcohol, unless permitted by the provider.

Pathophysiology and Etiology

Accelerated and malignant hypertension occur in clients with undiagnosed hypertension or in those who fail to maintain follow-up or comply with medical therapy. Accelerated and malignant hypertension usually have an abrupt onset; if untreated, severe symptoms and complications follow rapidly. Malignant hypertension is fatal unless BP is quickly reduced. Even with intensive treat-

TABLE 35-2	RECOMMENDED BLADDER DIMENSIONS FOR BLOOD PRESSURE CUFFS		
ARM CIRCUMFERENCE AT MIDPOINT* (cm)	**CUFF NAME**	**BLADDER WIDTH (cm)**	**BLADDER LENGTH (cm)**
27–34	Adult	13	30
35–44	Wide adult	16	38
45–52	Thigh	20	42

*Midpoint of arm is defined as half the distance from the acromion to the olecranon processes. (American Heart Association. [1993]. Human blood pressure determined by sphygmomanometry. [On-line]. Available: http://www.216.185.112.5/presenter.jhtml?identifier=3000894.

ment, the kidneys, brain, and heart may be permanently damaged.

Consequences are life-threatening when the BP in the vascular system becomes extremely elevated. Some arterial blood vessels already may have ruptured or will soon. Retinal hemorrhages can lead to blindness. A stroke occurs if vessels in the brain rupture and bleed. If an aneurysm has developed in the aorta from chronic hypertension, it may burst and cause hemorrhage and shock. Cardiac effects include left ventricular failure with pulmonary edema or MI. Renal failure also may be forthcoming if the pressure is not reduced.

Assessment Findings

Signs and Symptoms

Some clients may present with confusion, headache, visual disturbances, seizures, and, possibly, coma. The sudden, marked rise in BP may cause chest pain, dyspnea, and moist lung sounds. Renal failure is evidenced by less than 30 mL/hour of urine. The onset of sudden, severe back pain accompanied by hypotension (abnormally low BP) indicates that an aortic aneurysm is dissecting or has ruptured (see Chap. 33).

Systolic BP is 160 mm Hg or higher, diastolic BP is 115 mm Hg or higher, or both. The optic disk (nerve) appears to bulge forward into the posterior chamber from swelling of the brain. The retinal blood vessels are obscured where they radiate from the bulging disk, making identification of their continuous pathway difficult. The retinas may show flame-shaped hemorrhages or fluffy white exudates.

Diagnostic Findings

Diagnostic studies that may reveal abnormalities include computed tomographic scan, positron emission tomography scan, and magnetic resonance imaging. Reduced BP is a priority, and these neurologic tests may be postponed while emergency treatment measures are instituted.

Medical Management

In true hypertensive emergencies, the goal is to lower the BP within 1 to 2 hours by using potent IV drugs, such as diazoxide (Hyperstat IV), nitroprusside (Nitropress), nitroglycerin, or labetalol (Normodyne). If the client's condition is not extremely critical, other alternative antihypertensive drugs, such as nifedipine (Procardia), verapamil (Isoptin), captopril (Capoten), and prazosin (Minipress), are prescribed for oral administration. Oxygen is ordered to reduce hypoxia-induced tachycardia.

Nursing Management

The nurse implements medical orders promptly to ensure that BP is lowered as quickly and safely as possible. He or she mixes drugs with IV solution after carefully calculating the dosage and follows the five rights of medication administration. The nurse administers the medicated solution with an infusion pump or controller and titrates the rate of infusion according to the client's response and the parameters set by the physician. He or she checks the site and progress of the infusion at least hourly. The nurse applies an automatic BP recording machine to the arm to measure the BP every few minutes, or assesses the BP directly if using an arterial catheter. The nurse reports a systolic BP of 160 mm Hg or higher or a diastolic BP of 115 mm Hg or higher immediately. While awaiting medical orders, the nurse restricts client activity and monitors the client closely for neurologic, cardiac, and renal complications. He or she keeps emergency equipment and drugs ready in case complications develop. See Nursing Process: The Client With Hypertension for additional nursing management.

 GENERAL NUTRITIONAL CONSIDERATIONS

For years, standard interventions to control hypertension have been to reduce sodium intake, lose weight if overweight, exercise, and limit alcohol to two or fewer drinks per day. For many clients with essential hypertension, these measures eliminate the need for drug therapy.

Numerous studies show that lowering sodium intake can lower BP. Although some researchers argue that only a small percentage of the population is sensitive to sodium, its restriction usually is accepted as a lifelong component of treatment. All Americans—those with hypertension and those who wish to prevent it—are urged to lower sodium intake to 2400 mg/day.

Losing weight without reducing sodium intake lowers BP, even if the client does not attain ideal weight and regardless of the degree of excess weight. Weight reduction is recommended as the initial step in treating overweight clients with mild to moderate hypertension.

In addition to the preceding recommendations, results of a new study called DASH (Dietary Approaches to Stop Hypertension) show that eating the right foods can lower BP. Although the study does not identify which dietary components do so, it clearly demonstrates that a high intake of fruit, vegetables, and low-fat dairy products, combined with a low intake of total and saturated fat, lowers BP as effectively as drug therapy. In hypertensive clients, the "DASH combination diet" (high in fruits and vegetables combined with fat restriction) lowered systolic BP 11.4 mm Hg and diastolic BP 5.5 mm Hg. It includes the following elements:

- 7 to 8 servings of grains
- 4 to 5 servings of vegetables
- 4 to 5 servings of fruit
- 2 to 3 servings of low-fat or nonfat dairy products
- 2 or fewer servings of meat
- 4 to 5 servings of nuts per week

• 2 to 3 servings of added fat per day, and 5 snacks and sweets per week

Estimates are that a population-wide decrease in BP as seen in DASH would reduce the incidence of stroke by 27% and coronary heart disease by 15%.

GENERAL PHARMACOLOGIC CONSIDERATIONS

Drug therapy may include potent antihypertensive agents with many possible adverse effects. All antihypertensive drugs can cause postural hypotension, which can lead to falls. Teaching should include tips for managing syncope and dizziness.

Medication controls but does not cure hypertension. Clients with hypertension must control body weight, restrict dietary sodium, and learn ways to manage stress appropriately.

Monitor ACE inhibitors cautiously in clients with renal or hepatic impairment and older adults. A sudden drop in BP may occur during the first 1 to 3 hours after the initial dose of an ACE inhibitor. The administration of IV normal saline may manage the hypotensive episode. This type of hypotensive episode is not an indication to discontinue the drug.

ACE inhibitors may cause a persistent cough until the medication is discontinued.

GENERAL GERONTOLOGIC CONSIDERATIONS

Hypertension caused by arteriosclerosis or atherosclerosis is not uncommon in older adults. It may go undiagnosed unless the client sees a physician regularly. Encourage older adults to have their BP checked at least every 6 months. Older adult centers and pharmacies frequently offer free BP monitoring.

Because postural hypotension is common in older adults, correct BP measurement is particularly important. Measurements are obtained while the older person is supine or sitting, and immediately after he or she stands.

Older adults are at increased risk for development of hypokalemia from diuretic drugs. Lower doses of hydrochlorothiazide or chlorthalidone can control hypertension and minimize the risk of hypokalemia.

Critical Thinking Exercises

1. *On admission, a client's BP is 210/112 mm Hg in a supine position. What additional data would be pertinent to collect before reporting the finding to the nurse in charge and physician?*
2. *To which community resources in your locale would you refer a client with hypertension for support or care after discharge?*

References and Suggested Readings

Avvampato, C. S. (2001). Effect of one leg crossed over the other at the knee on blood pressure in hypertensive patients. *Nephrology Nursing Journal, 28,* 325–328.

Baldwin, C. M., Bevan, C., & Beshalske, A. (2000). At-risk minority populations in a church-based clinic: Communicating basic needs. *Journal of Multicultural Nursing and Health, 6*(2), 26–28.

Bisognano, J. D. & Weder, A. B. (1999). Considerations in drug therapy: Effective treatment of severe hypertension. *Progress in Cardiovascular Nursing, 14*(4), 150–152.

Bruni, K. R. (2001). Renovascular hypertension. *Journal of Cardiovascular Nursing, 15*(4), 78–90.

Buijs, R. & Olson, J. (2001). Parish nurses influencing determinants of health. *Journal of Community Health Nursing, 18*(1), 13–23.

Barker, E. (2001). What's your patient's stroke risk? *Nursing, 31*(4), Hospital Nursing: 32hn1, 32hn4–32hn5.

Clark, M. J., Curran, C., & Noji, A. (2000). The effects of community health nurse monitoring on hypertension identification and control. *Public Health Nursing, 17,* 452–459.

Daly, G. (2000). A protocol for patients with hypertension. *Practice Nurse, 20*(2), 80, 83, 86.

Denton, E. (1999). Treating hypertension in elderly people. *Journal of Community Nursing, 13*(9), 10, 12, 15–16.

Feather, C. (2001). Blood pressure measurement. *Nursing Times, 97*(4), 33–34.

Fleury, J. & Keller, C. (2000). Cardiovascular risk assessment in elderly individuals. *Journal of Gerontological Nursing, 26*(5), 30–37.

Frazier, L. (2000). Factors influencing blood pressure: Development of a risk model. *Journal of Cardiovascular Nursing, 15*(1), 62–79.

Gassianos, G. (2000). Managing hypertension. *Practice Nurse, 20,* 514, 516–519.

Gibson, B. & Pittard, J. (1999). A fresh look at blood pressure guidelines. *Practice Nurse, 18,* 653–654.

Graham-Garcia, J., Raines, T. L., Andrews, J. O., et al. (2001). Race, ethnicity, and geography: disparities in heart disease in women of color. *Journal of Transcultural Nursing, 12*(1), 56–67.

Halm, M. A. & Penque, S. (2000). Heart failure in women. *Progress in Cardiovascular Nursing, 15*(4), 121–133.

Joint National Committee on Prevention, Detection, Evaluation, and Treatment of High Blood Pressure. (1997). The sixth report of the Joint National Committee on Prevention, Detection, Evaluation, and Treatment of High Blood Pressure. *Archives of Internal Medicine, 157,* 2413–2446.

Karch, A. M. & Karch, F. E. (2000). Practice errors: When a blood pressure isn't routine. *American Journal of Nursing, 100*(3), 23.

Kozuh, J. L. (2000). NSAIDs and antihypertensives: An unhappy union. *American Journal of Nursing, 100*(6), 40–43.

Lahdenper, T. S. & Kyngs, H. A. (2000). Compliance and its evaluation in patients with hypertension. *Journal of Clinical Nursing, 9,* 826–833.

Mansfield, J. & Daley, K. (2000). Hypertensive emergencies. *American Journal of Nursing, 100*(9, Suppl.), 20–26.

Mulrow, C. D., Chiquette, E., Angel, L., et al. (2001). Dieting to reduce body weight for controlling hypertension in adults. *Nursing Times, 97*(20), 42.

Murphy, M. (2000). Your patient may be at risk for isolated systolic hypertension. *Home Healthcare Nurse, 18,* 606–614.

Nunnelee, J. D. & Spaner, S. D. (2000). Assessment and nursing management of hypertension in the perioperative period. *Journal of PeriAnesthesia Nursing, 15*(3), 163–168.

Perry, M. (2001). Systolic hypertension. *Practice Nurse, 21*(3), 18, 20, 22.

Peters, R. M. & Flack, J. M. (2000). Salt sensitivity and hypertension in African Americans: Implications for cardiovascular nurses. *Progress in Cardiovascular Nursing, 15*(4), 138–144.

Reeder, S. J. & Hoffmann, R. L. (2001). Beta-blocker therapy for hypertension. *Dimensions of Critical Care Nursing, 20*(2), 2–12.

Reifsteck, S. W. & Roberts, F. (2001). The parish nurse movement. *Viewpoint, 23*(1), 19–21.

Robinson, A. W. & Sloan, H. L. (2000). Healthy people 2000: Heart health and older women. *Journal of Gerontological Nursing, 26*(5), 38–45.

Sherif, K. (2000). Considerations in drug therapy: The effects of hormone replacement therapy and oral contraceptive pills on blood pressure. *Progress in Cardiovascular Nursing, 15*(1), 21–23, 28.

Swinney, J., Anson-Wonkka, C., & Maki, E. (2001). Community assessment: A church community and the parish nurse. *Public Health Nursing, 18*(1), 40–44.

Weiss, D., Matheus, R., & Schank, M. J. (2001). The aging spirit: Research shows how parish nursing improves elders' care. *Aging Today, 22*(2), 13.

Woods, A. D. (2001). Improving the odds against hypertension. *Nursing, 31*(8), 36–42.

Yucha, C. B., Clark, L., Smith, M., et al. (2001). The effect of biofeedback in hypertension. *Applied Nursing Research, 14*(1), 29–35.

Yung, P., French, P., & Leung, B. (2001). Relaxation training as complementary therapy for mild hypertension. *Complementary Therapies in Nursing and Midwifery, 7*(2), 59–65.

Caring for Clients With Heart Failure

The heart is a double pump: the right side pumps deoxygenated blood to the lungs for oxygenation, and the left side pumps oxygen-rich blood into the systemic circulation (Fig. 36-1). This process provides a continuous supply of oxygen and nutrients for cellular metabolism and a mechanism to eliminate carbon dioxide (CO_2) and metabolic wastes. Disturbances in one part of the heart, if they are severe or last long enough, eventually affect the entire circulation.

HEART FAILURE

Heart failure is the inability of the heart to pump sufficient blood to meet the body's metabolic needs. The term **congestive heart failure** (CHF) describes the accumulation of blood and fluid in organs and tissues from impaired circulation.

Types

One way to classify heart failure is by how it develops: acute or chronic. Another way to classify it is by location: right-sided or left-sided. The New York Heart Association classifies heart failure based on the amount of activity restriction it imposes (Table 36-1). Many cardiologists use this classification as well.

Acute and Chronic Heart Failure

Acute heart failure is a sudden change in the heart's ability to contract. It can cause life-threatening symptoms and pulmonary edema (discussed later). **Chronic heart failure** occurs when some other chronic disorder gradually compromises the heart's ability to pump effectively.

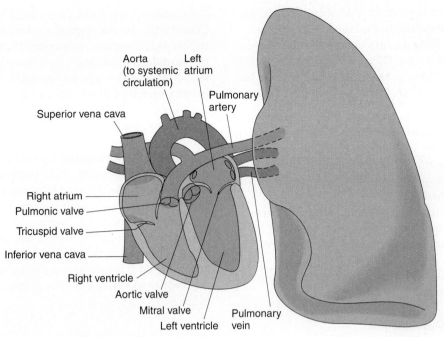

FIGURE 36-1 Right and left cardiac pumps.

Left-Sided and Right-Sided Heart Failure

Because the heart is a double pump, it is possible for either the left or right ventricle (or both) to become impaired. The terms *left-sided* (left ventricular) heart failure and *right-sided* (right ventricular) heart failure describe the location of the pumping dysfunction. **Left-sided heart failure** results from various conditions that impair the left ventricle's ability to eject blood into the aorta. **Right-sided heart failure** occurs when the right ventricle fails to eject its total diastolic filling volume into the pulmonary artery, causing congestion of blood in the venous vascular system. The major cause of right-sided heart failure is left-sided heart failure.

Pathophysiology and Etiology

Two mechanisms can cause heart failure. The primary reason for failure of either the left or right ventricle is inability of the heart muscle to contract because of direct damage to the muscular wall. Myocardial infarction (MI) usually affects the pumping ability of the left or right ventricle and frequently contributes to acute heart failure. Acute heart failure may immediately follow an MI or develop some time after the initial episode. The second mechanism occurs when the pumping chambers enlarge and weaken, as in cardiomyopathy (see Chap. 31), making it impossible for the ventricles to eject all the blood they receive.

Left-Sided Heart Failure

When the left ventricle fails, the heart muscle cannot contract forcefully enough to expel blood into the systemic circulation (cardiac output). Blood subsequently becomes congested in the left ventricle, left atrium, and finally the pulmonary vasculature. The fluid accumulates and creates congestion in the **pulmonary vascular bed** (the capillary network surrounding the alveoli). Increased pulmonary vascular bed pressure causes fluid to move from the pulmonary capillaries into the alveoli. Gas exchange is im-

TABLE 36-1	NEW YORK HEART ASSOCIATION FUNCTIONAL CLASSIFICATION OF HEART FAILURE
CLASS	**LIMITATIONS**
I	No symptoms and no limitation in ordinary physical activity
II	Mild symptoms and slight limitation during ordinary activity; comfortable at rest
III	Marked limitation in activity from symptoms, even during less-than-ordinary activity; comfortable only at rest
IV	Severe limitations; symptoms even while at rest

paired, cells become hypoxic (a state of insufficient oxygen), and CO_2 accumulates in the blood.

Hypertension, tachydysrhythmias, valvular disease, cardiomyopathy, and renal failure can contribute to chronic heart failure. These conditions reduce cardiac output by:

1. Increasing afterload or systemic vascular resistance. **Afterload**, the force that the ventricle must overcome to empty its diastolic volume, increases with arterial hypertension, aortic stenosis, pulmonary hypertension, or excessive blood volume from renal failure.
2. Reducing ventricular ejection volume because diastole, during which the ventricle fills with blood (**preload**), is shortened as a result of a tachydysrhythmia
3. Causing a loss of elasticity in the muscle as a result of cardiomyopathy

Right-Sided Heart Failure

When right ventricular failure develops, the right ventricle cannot forcefully contract and push the blood into the pulmonary artery. As a result, congestion of blood and backflow accumulate first in the right ventricle, then in the right atrium, the superior and inferior vena cava, and subsequently the venous vasculature. MIs that affect the

right ventricle also can cause right ventricular failure. Clients with chronic respiratory disorders tend to develop right-sided failure as a consequence of cor pulmonale. **Cor pulmonale** is a condition in which the heart (*cor*) is affected by lung damage (*pulmonale*). Pulmonary disease impairs exchange of oxygen and CO_2 in the alveoli, leading to increased CO_2 in the blood. By some unknown mechanism, pulmonary arterial vasoconstriction occurs. Prolonged pulmonary arterial vasoconstriction results in **pulmonary hypertension** (elevated pressure in the pulmonary arterial system). With pulmonary hypertension, the right ventricle is forced to pump against a high pressure gradient. Subsequently, the right ventricle enlarges and weakens under the increased workload, leading to failure. When the right ventricle fails to empty completely, blood is trapped in the venous vascular system. Eventually, the fluid is forced to move in retrograde fashion into the interstitial spaces and cells of other organs and tissues of the body.

Compensatory Mechanisms

The body can compensate for changes in heart function that occur over time (Fig. 36-2). When cardiac output falls, the body uses certain compensatory mechanisms designed to increase stroke volume and maintain blood pressure (BP). These compensatory mechanisms can tem-

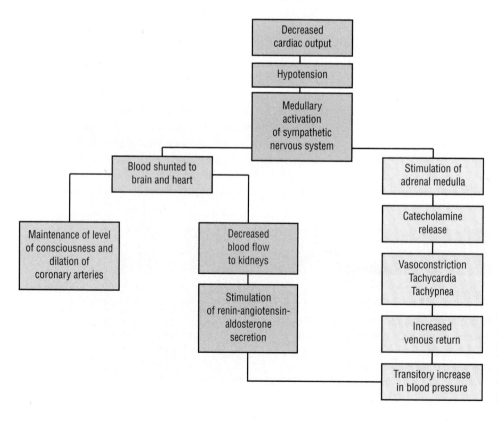

FIGURE 36-2 Compensatory mechanisms of the sympathetic nervous system. Decreased cardiac output triggers a series of compensatory mechanisms in the body in an effort to maintain level of consciousness and blood pressure.

porarily improve the client's cardiac output but ultimately fail when contractility is further compromised.

As cardiac output falls, the client becomes hypotensive. The low BP stimulates the sympathetic nervous system to release catecholamines (e.g., epinephrine, norepinephrine) to raise heart rate and BP. The increased force and contraction of the heart maintain the client's BP but increase **myocardial oxygen demand** (the amount of oxygen the heart needs to perform its work). Epinephrine also causes blood vessels to constrict in an effort to raise BP. As the sympathetic nervous system is stimulated, the body shunts more blood to the vital organs of the brain and heart, decreasing blood supply to the kidneys. The kidneys secrete renin in response to decreased blood flow, which initiates the renin-angiotensin-aldosterone mechanism. Renin activates angiotensin. Angiotensin causes vasoconstriction and increases BP. Angiotensin also stimulates the adrenal gland to secrete **aldosterone,** a hormone that causes retention of sodium and water to increase BP by increasing the amount of blood returning to the heart.

Ultimately, these compensatory mechanisms further compromise the client's status by increasing the amount of blood volume the heart must pump and the resistance it must overcome from arterial constriction. If cardiac output continues to fall, the body's cells become deprived of oxygen and switch from aerobic metabolism to the less efficient anaerobic metabolism. Anaerobic metabolism results in an accumulation of lactic acid, which lowers blood pH and can eventually cause metabolic acidosis.

Assessment Findings

Signs and Symptoms

The severity of symptoms depends on the body's ability to adjust to the decreased cardiac output. Initial signs and symptoms reflect the ventricle of the heart that is experiencing dysfunction. Usually when a client has chronic heart failure, he or she develops signs and symptoms of both right-sided and left-sided heart failure. Table 36-2 highlights the clinical differences between left ventricular and right ventricular heart failure.

LEFT-SIDED HEART FAILURE

Left-sided heart failure produces hypoxemia as a result of reduced cardiac output of arterial blood and respiratory symptoms. Many clients notice unusual fatigue with activity. Some find **exertional dyspnea** (effort at breathing when active) to be the first symptom. Inability to breathe unless sitting upright (**orthopnea**) or being awakened by breathlessness (**paroxysmal nocturnal dyspnea**) may prompt the client to use several pillows in bed or to sleep in a chair or recliner. Pulse may be rapid or irregular. BP may be elevated from sympathetic nervous system stimulation. A cough, **hemoptysis** (blood-streaked sputum), and moist crackles on auscultation are typical respiratory

TABLE 36-2	SIGNS AND SYMPTOMS OF LEFT AND RIGHT VENTRICULAR FAILURE
LEFT VENTRICULAR FAILURE	**RIGHT VENTRICULAR FAILURE**
Fatigue	Weakness
Paroxysmal nocturnal dyspnea	Ascites
Orthopnea	Weight gain
Hypoxia	Nausea, vomiting
Crackles	Dysrhythmias
Cyanosis	Elevated central venous pressure
S_3 heart sound	Jugular vein distention
Cough with pink, frothy sputum	
Elevated pulmonary capillary wedge pressure	

findings. Urine output is diminished. If acute left-sided heart failure with pulmonary edema develops, the client suddenly becomes hypoxic, restless, and confused.

RIGHT-SIDED HEART FAILURE

The client with right-sided heart failure may have a history of gradual unexplained weight gain from fluid retention. Dependent **pitting edema** (Fig. 36-3) in the feet and ankles can be observed. This type of edema may seem to disappear overnight but really is temporarily redistributed by gravity to other tissues, such as the sacral area. Fluid may distend the abdomen (ascites), and the liver may be enlarged (hepatomegaly). Jugular veins often are distended from increased central venous pressure (Nursing Guide-

FIGURE 36-3 Example of pitting edema.

lines 36-1). Enlarged abdominal organs often restrict ventilation, creating dyspnea. Clients may observe that rings, shoes, or clothing have become tight. Accumulation of blood in abdominal organs may cause anorexia, nausea, and flatulence.

Stop, Think, and Respond ● BOX 36-1

Which type of heart failure is evidenced by the following assessment findings?

Client A has swollen ankles. His clothes fit poorly, and he has purchased larger pants and shirts. When he is weighed, he remarks that he has gained 10 lb in the last month, but his diet has not changed. He says he feels "full," can't eat as much as usual, and "works hard" to breathe.

Client B becomes breathless while changing into a gown before the assessment. She reports sleeping better when sitting up in a recliner. Her cough is "wet." She is tachycardic and says she has noticed less frequent urination.

Diagnostic Findings

LEFT-SIDED HEART FAILURE

Chest radiography shows cardiac enlargement and fluid accumulation in the lungs. An echocardiogram can reveal the increased size of the left ventricle and ineffective pumping of the heart. At first, arterial blood gas (ABG) analysis may reveal respiratory alkalosis as a result of rapid, shallow breathing. Later, there is a shift to metabolic acidosis as gas exchange becomes more impaired. Serum sodium levels may be elevated. Elevated blood urea nitrogen indicates impaired renal perfusion. If the client is seriously ill, a pulmonary artery catheter may be inserted for hemodynamic monitoring. Cardiac output can be measured by the pulmonary artery catheter. Cardiac output is diminished in left-sided heart failure, and pulmonary artery pressure and pulmonary capillary wedge pressure measurements are elevated.

RIGHT-SIDED HEART FAILURE

A chest radiograph, electrocardiogram (ECG), and echocardiography reveal right ventricular enlargement. A lung scan and pulmonary arteriography can confirm cor pulmonale. Liver enzymes are elevated if the liver is impaired.

Medical Management

Medical management of both left-sided and right-sided heart failure is directed at reducing the heart's workload and improving cardiac output, primarily through dietary

---

NURSING GUIDELINES 36-1

Estimating Central Venous Pressure (CVP)

The nurse estimates CVP by measuring the height of jugular vein distention.

1. Obtain a centimeter ruler.

2. Help client to lie flat.

3. Slowly elevate head of bed to 45°.

4. Locate the sternal angle by placing two fingers at the sternal notch and sliding them down the sternum until they reach a bony prominence.

5. Estimate venous pressure by measuring the vertical distance from the sternal angle (0 cm) to the level of jugular vein distention (cm above 0).

6. Add 5 cm to the ruler measurement to estimate CVP. CVP is elevated more than 12 to 15 cm H_2O in clients who have right ventricular heart failure. A more accurate measurement of CVP is obtained by using a central venous catheter.

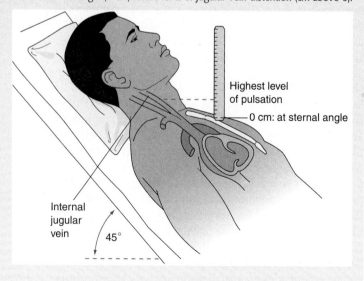

modifications, drug therapy, and lifestyle changes. A low-sodium diet is prescribed, and fluids may be restricted. Activity is limited according to the condition's severity. Sedatives or tranquilizers reduce dyspnea and relieve anxiety. In acute or worsening heart failure, a device for re-synchronizing the heart's contraction or an intra-aortic balloon pump may be used to support left ventricular function.

Drug Therapy

Drug therapy with one or more medications aims at improving cardiac output (Drug Therapy Table 36-1). Digoxin is the primary drug used to slow and strengthen the heart. The method of giving large doses of digoxin at the beginning of therapy to build up therapeutic blood levels of the drug is termed **digitalization.** The apical heart rate is assessed for a full minute before every administration and is documented in the medication administration record. Digitalis drugs are withheld if heart rate is less than 60 or more than 120 beats/minute until a physician is consulted. In acute heart failure or pulmonary edema

(discussed later), the physician may prescribe a potent inotropic agent, one that increases the force of contraction, thereby improving stroke volume. Examples include dopamine (Intropin) and dobutamine (Dobutrex).

Diuretic therapy helps reduce the heart's work by decreasing the exertion required to overcome afterload. Loop diuretics like furosemide (Lasix) or thiazide diuretics like chlorothiazide (Diuril) commonly are prescribed. These drugs increase sodium and therefore water excretion, but they also increase potassium excretion. Digitalis toxicity evidenced by loss of appetite; nausea or vomiting; rapid, slow, or irregular heart rate; or sudden disturbance in color vision is more likely if a client becomes hypokalemic. Low serum potassium levels and signs of digitalis toxicity must be reported to the physician. The blood level of digitalis is measured if there is a question concerning its concentration.

Vasodilators also reduce afterload. Clients with a history of heart failure may receive a drug like an angiotensin-converting enzyme (ACE) inhibitor (captopril [Capoten]) or some other category of drug that causes vasodilatation.

DRUG THERAPY TABLE 36-1	**HEART FAILURE AGENTS**		
DRUG CATEGORY AND EXAMPLES	**MECHANISM OF ACTION**	**SIDE EFFECTS**	**NURSING CONSIDERATIONS**
Cardiac Glycosides digoxin (Lanoxin)	Increase cardiac output by slowing heart rate (negative chronotropic action) and increasing force of contraction (positive chronotropic action)	Fatigue, generalized muscle weakness, anorexia, nausea, vomiting, yellow-green halos around visual images, dysrhythmias	Monitor pulse rate before each dose. Withhold if pulse is <60 or >120 beats/min. Provide dietary sources of potassium.
Diuretics furosemide (Lasix)	Promote sodium and water excretion, thus reducing circulating blood volume and decreasing heart's workload	Dizziness, dehydration, blurred vision, anorexia, diarrhea, nocturia, polyuria, thrombocytopenia, orthostatic hypotension, hypokalemia	Weigh client daily. Measure intake and output. Monitor serum potassium levels. Replace lost potassium with bananas, orange juice, or prescribed supplement.
Vasodilators nitroglycerin	Improve stroke volume by reducing afterload; reduce preload by dilating veins and arteries	Headache, dizziness, orthostatic hypotension, tachycardia, flushing, nausea, hypersensitivity	Assess for hypotension. Monitor for headache and flushed skin.
ACE Inhibitors captopril (Capoten)	Block ACE from converting angiotensin I to angiotensin II (a potent vasoconstrictor); promote fluid and sodium loss and decrease peripheral vascular resistance	Tachycardia, hypotension, GI irritation, pancytopenia, proteinuria, rash, cough, dry mouth, hyperkalemia, increased BUN and creatinine	Excretion is reduced in clients with renal failure. First-dose hypotension is common in older adults. Administer 1 hr before or 2 hr after meals.
Nonglycoside Inotropic Agents dobutamine (Dobutrex)	Relieve cardiogenic shock by strengthening force of myocardial contraction and increasing cardiac output	Headache, hypertension, tachycardia, angina, nausea	Monitor for increased heart rate, elevated BP, and dysrhythmias.

ACE, angiotensin-converting enzyme; *BP*, blood pressure; *BUN*, blood urea nitrogen; *GI*, gastrointestinal.

A new synthetic peptide compound, chrysalin, is undergoing clinical trials. If successful, it will be used to promote **angiogenesis,** regeneration of myocardial blood vessels. Its developers envision that it will be used to improve the prognosis for clients in early stages of heart failure or in combination with a ventricular assist device (VAD; see later discussion) in later-stage heart failure.

Stop, Think, and Respond ● BOX 36-2

A client with a possible bowel obstruction has a history of chronic heart failure. He has been taking digoxin (Lanoxin) at home. What nursing actions are appropriate?

Cardiac Resynchronization Therapy

Cardiac resynchronization therapy (CRT) is a new technique that restores synchrony in the contractions of the right and left ventricles. CRT is used primarily for clients whose heart failure is caused by dilated cardiomyopathy (see Chap. 31). It is achieved with a biventricular pacemaker, which was approved by the U.S. Food and Drug Administration in July 2001 after a series of successful clinical trials in Europe and the United States. The biventricular pacemaker is inserted transvenously similarly to a traditional pacemaker, with electrical leads in the right atrium and right ventricle and the battery placed beneath the skin of the chest. It has an additional internal third lead, however, that is placed outside the left ventricle. The dual ventricular leads stimulate the right and left ventricles to contract at the same time. When the ventricles contract simultaneously, the force of contraction improves and more blood is ejected with each heartbeat.

Intra-Aortic Balloon Pump

If cardiogenic shock accompanies acute left ventricular heart failure (see Chap. 23), an **intra-aortic balloon pump** (IABP) may be used. An IABP acts as a temporary, secondary pump to supplement the ineffectual contraction of the left ventricle. It is inserted as a catheter into the left femoral artery and threaded up to the descending aortic arch (Fig. 36-4). The IABP is connected to a machine that inflates the balloon portion during ventricular diastole and deflates during systole, a process known as *counterpulsation.* Inflation of the IABP increases coronary artery, renal artery, and myocardial perfusion. Deflation actually keeps the aorta distended so that cardiac output is improved; the work of the left ventricle is decreased, and peripheral organs are more adequately perfused with oxygenated blood. The IABP is intended only for a few days' use.

Surgical Management

When medical treatment alone is unsuccessful, clients may require surgical treatment options such as the in-

Diastole   Systole

FIGURE 36-4 The intra-aortic balloon pump (IABP).

sertion of a VAD, cardiomyoplasty, or an implantable artificial heart. Human heart transplantation is discussed in Chapter 37.

Ventricular Assist Device

Some clients awaiting heart transplants are treated with a **ventricular assist device,** which is an auxiliary heart pump that supplements the heart's ability to eject blood. If the VAD supports left ventricular function, it is referred to as a *left ventricular assist device* or LVAD, which is designed to be used for weeks to months. Some clients have relied on LVADs for more than 1 year. The natural heart remains in place and continues to function at whatever capacity is possible. Some LVADs are currently available, whereas others are presently in clinical trials. Examples include the Heartmate II, Jarvik 2000 Flowmaker, and the MicroMed DeBakey VAD. Most LVADs use an outflow and inflow cannula to carry blood from the left ventricle into the aorta (Fig. 36-5). They are battery operated through an external power source worn about the waist. By assisting the weak, ineffective left ventricle, LVADs maintain cardiac output at normal volumes. Because the trend is to develop miniaturized devices such as the MicroMed DeBakey VAD, which internally measures

1 × 3 inches and weighs less than 4 ounces, clients can easily manage the newest models, making it possible for some to return home until heart transplantation. The Thoratec VAD is a double-assist device that can be used for left-sided, right-sided, or biventricular heart failure. A large external driver powers this device, however, necessitating continuous hospitalization for its use.

Cardiomyoplasty

Cardiomyoplasty is a surgical procedure in which the client's own chest muscle (latissimus dorsi) is grafted to the aorta and wrapped around the heart. An electrical stimulator placed in a subcutaneous pouch triggers skeletal muscle contraction (Fig. 36-6). The contraction acts as a counterpulsation mechanism similar to the IABP. It augments the ineffective myocardial muscle contraction.

Although another surgical procedure known as a *partial left ventriculectomy,* the surgical excision of a wedge-shaped portion of the left ventricle from the apex to below the mitral valve, has been performed for clients who have cardiomyopathy, results have been disappointing. The hypothesis is that reducing the radius of the myocardial tissue in the left ventricle will increase ventricular wall tension. Statistics have shown, however that only approximately 25% of those receiving this surgical treatment improved; the remainder deteriorated immediately or shortly thereafter (Abe et al., 2001; Schreuder et al., 2000).

Artificial Heart

Adults younger than 55 years are candidates for heart transplantation when medical treatment is unsuccessful

FIGURE 36-6 In cardiomyoplasty, the latissimus dorsi muscle is dissected and wrapped around the heart itself.

(see Chap. 37). An artificial heart may be used while the client awaits a donor organ compatible with his or her tissue and blood type. Until recently, hopes for long-term use of artificial mechanical hearts were disappointing. Early attempts at their use resulted in multiple complications, including malfunction of artificial valves, formation of emboli, and stroke. The complications and need for recipients to be tethered to a large, noisy air compressor raised ethical questions about quality of life. In 2001, however, several individuals received the AbioCor, an experimental, softball-sized artificial heart made of plastic and titanium. The device is attached to the great vessels of the heart and powered by a small battery pack that clients wear on a belt outside the body (Fig. 36-7). The AbioCor has two improvements over previous models: (1) it replaces the entire diseased heart, and (2) is self-contained within the body and does not require a tethering system to a large power-generating console. If use of the AbioCor is successful, it may well become an alternative to human heart transplantation. The first two U.S. recipients of the AbioCor, however, have died.

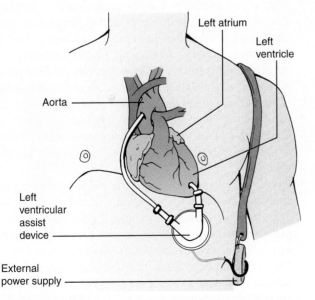

Left atrium

Left ventricle

Aorta

Left ventricular assist device

External power supply

FIGURE 36-5 The LVAD pump weighs 1.5 lb. It is implanted below the diaphragm; its battery pack is carried outside the body. Tubes connect the pump to the left ventricle and aorta.

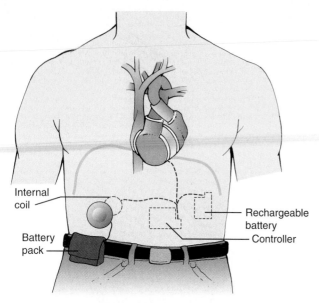

FIGURE 36-7 The newest artificial heart fits inside the chest with no external wires or tubes. An external battery pack transmits power to the internal coil and keeps the backup battery charged.

Nursing Management

Most clients can manage chronic heart failure at home. Many medications, lifestyle changes, and diet restrictions are involved to control heart failure. During times of acute illness, usual methods may not control symptoms, and the client may require hospitalization for additional treatment. The home health nurse, the nurse in an extended or intermediate care facility, as well as nurses in acute care settings administer prescribed medications and monitor for therapeutic and adverse effects. They implement interventions that promote the heart's ability to eject as much blood as possible, monitor for signs of excess fluid volume and evidence of electrolyte imbalance, promote oxygenation, balance activity according to the client's tolerance, and support family members who may be the usual primary caregivers (Client and Family Teaching Box 36-1).

N U R S I N G   P R O C E S S

● **The Client With Congestive Heart Failure**

Assessment

The nurse elicits the client's history of symptoms and medications. He or she performs an initial physical assessment to establish baseline data. During a head-to-toe assessment, the nurse observes for dyspnea, auscultates apical heart rate and counts radial heart rate, measures BP, observes for distended neck veins, and notes any signs of peripheral edema, lethargy, or confusion. He or she ob-

tains an admission weight and thereafter weighs the client daily on the same scale, at about the same time of day, with the client wearing similar clothing. The nurse notes laboratory test results of serum electrolytes because drug therapy with certain diuretics depletes potassium blood levels. He or she initiates intake and output measurements and evaluates fluid volumes at least every 8 hours. The nurse may measure abdominal girth to determine if the client is developing ascites or responding to therapeutic measures. He or she notes respiratory difficulties during activity and rest. The nurse questions the client about nocturnal dyspnea (asking how many pillows the client normally uses for sleep) and listens for crackles on auscultation of lungs. While auscultating the chest, the nurse listens for additional heart sounds. He or she monitors oxygenation status with pulse oximetry or reviews the results of ABG studies.

Diagnosis, Planning, and Interventions

Decreased Cardiac Output related to ineffective ventricular contraction, tachycardia, reduced stroke volume, hypertension, and increased vascular volume

Expected Outcome: Client will have increased cardiac output as evidenced by heart rate between 60 to 100 beats/minute, urinary output between 1500 to 3000 mL/day, systolic BP below 140 mm Hg, diastolic BP below 90 mm Hg, and no mental confusion.

- Assess apical heart rate before administering a cardiac glycoside (digitalis) or other drug that slows heart rate. *Cardiac output is related to heart rate and stroke volume. Withhold a cardiac glycoside until the physician is consulted when the heart rate is less than 60 or more than 120 beats/minute.*

- Administer prescribed medications such as cardiac glycosides (digitalis), diuretics, and antihypertensives. *Cardiac glycosides slow heart rate and increase force of contraction. Diuretics decrease afterload by reducing circulating fluid volume. Antihypertensives promote vasodilatation, thus reducing afterload. One or a combination of these drugs reduces the workload of the left ventricle.*

- Promote rest. *Rest reduces heart contraction (ventricular work). Increasing diastole helps increase the volume in the ventricles (preload) and the ejected volume (stroke volume).*

- Avoid activities that engage the Valsalva maneuver, such as straining with bowel elimination or using the arms to pull and reposition oneself. *The Valsalva maneuver increases intrathoracic pressure, reduces right atrial filling, triggers tachycardia, and increases BP.*

- Prepare client or assist with procedures that improve cardiac output, such as the insertion of a biventricular pacemaker, cardiomyoplasty, LVAD, IABP, or artificial mechanical heart. *Improving the heart's force of contraction or stroke volume improves cardiac output.*

Excess Fluid Volume related to reduced renal function secondary to increased antidiuretic hormone and aldosterone production and reduced cardiac output

Expected Outcome: Fluid volume will be reduced as evidenced by reduced weight and peripheral edema, normal BP measurements, increased urine output, and no adventitious lung sounds.

- Administer prescribed diuretic. *Diuretics promote the excretion of sodium and water.*
- Provide sodium-restricted diet as prescribed. *Sodium attracts water; reduced sodium decreases water retention.*
- Apportion oral fluid according to prescribed limitations. *Limiting oral fluid intake reduces circulating volume.*

Risk for Impaired Gas Exchange related to pulmonary congestion secondary to left ventricular dysfunction

Expected Outcome: Client will maintain adequate gas exchange as evidenced by clear lung sounds, decreased work of breathing, pulse oximeter reading above 90%, partial pressure of arterial oxygen (PaO_2) between 80 to 100 mm Hg, partial pressure of arterial CO_2 ($PaCO_2$) between 35 to 45 mm Hg, and blood pH between 7.35 to 7.45.

- Maintain client in a high Fowler's, semi-Fowler's, or orthopneic position. *Elevating the upper body maximizes lung expansion by decreasing pressure on the diaphragm.*
- Administer supplemental oxygen therapy as prescribed to maintain the pulse oximetry level (SpO_2) at or above 90%. *If SpO_2 is at or above 90%, PaO_2 usually is high enough to maintain plasma levels of oxygen in less than critical ranges.*
- Avoid gas-forming foods. *Gas that accumulates in the intestine increases the volume in the abdominal cavity. Expansion of the intestine can crowd the diaphragm and interfere with inspired volumes of air.*
- Offer small, frequent feedings. *Preventing stomach distention increases the space in the thoracic cavity for lung expansion.*
- Limit physical activity. *Activity requires increased oxygen for cellular metabolism.*

Activity Intolerance related to hypoxemia secondary to decreased cardiac output

Expected Outcome: Client will tolerate activity associated with daily living without becoming breathless, hypertensive, or tachycardic.

- Space activities of daily living (ADLs) between periods of rest. *Rest reduces oxygen deficits.*
- Keep personal items within easy reach. *Reduced exertion decreases oxygen expenditure.*
- Gradually increase activity and self-care as condition improves. *Tolerance for activity increases after a therapeutic response to the treatment regimen.*

PC: Hypokalemia related to excretion of potassium secondary to diuretic therapy

Expected Outcome: The nurse will monitor for evidence of hypokalemia and prevent or manage low serum potassium levels.

- Monitor for clinical signs of hypokalemia: fatigue, muscle weakness, and abnormal sensations like tingling or numbness. *Potassium is necessary for normal nerve and muscle activity; neuromuscular changes, anorexia, nausea, and vomiting are signs of a low potassium level.*
- Observe the ECG, cardiac monitor, or cardiac rhythm strip for a U wave or cardiac dysrhythmia. *A U wave is associated with hypokalemia. The heart is a muscle that may develop a dysrhythmia if the potassium level is not within normal range.*
- Provide foods and beverages that are good sources of potassium, like bananas and orange juice, within the client's dietary and fluid restrictions. *Dietary intake of foods and beverages that are rich in potassium affect serum potassium levels (Box 36-1).*
- Administer a prescribed potassium supplement. *They ensure potassium replacement.*

Evaluation of Expected Outcomes

Expected outcomes are that BP and heart rate return to baseline, with no evidence of excess fluid. Respirations are unlabored, and lungs are clear. Fluid intake approximates output. The client can participate in ADLs within his or her level of tolerance. Serum potassium level remains within or is restored to normal range.

 36-1 *Client and Family Teaching*
Heart Failure

The nurse instructs about the disease process, meaning of the term failure, *signs and symptoms of impending CHF (weight gain, ankle swelling, fatigue, dyspnea), and importance of taking all medications regularly. He or she also covers the following points:*

- Measure pulse and blood pressure daily.
- Check weight at the same time each day using the same scale; consult a physician if you gain more than 2 lb in 24 hours.
- Schedule rest periods to reduce or eliminate fatigue and dyspnea.
- Increase activities such as walking when able to do so without dyspnea or fatigue.
- Identify and avoid occasions that produce stress.
- Elevate the legs while sitting.
- Follow the diet prescribed by the physician.
- Avoid extreme heat, cold, or humidity.
- Report a heart rate less than 60 or more than 120 beats/minute before taking digitalis.
- Contact the physician if symptoms return or swelling in the legs, ankles, or feet suddenly increases.
- Maintain follow-up care.

BOX 36-1 • Potassium-Rich Foods

Potatoes, sweet potatoes, winter squash, tomatoes, tomato juice
Milk, yogurt
Dates, bananas, cantaloupes, orange juice, prunes, raisins, prune juice
Dry beans, peas, lentils
Peanut butter
Bran cereals

PULMONARY EDEMA

Pulmonary edema is fluid accumulation in the lungs, which interferes with gas exchange in the alveoli. It represents an acute emergency and is a frequent complication of left-sided heart failure. Cardiac dysrhythmias and cardiac or respiratory arrest are associated complications. Noncardiogenic pulmonary edema, also referred to as *acute respiratory distress syndrome,* develops when a pulmonary embolism, infection, or blast injury alters the pulmonary capillary membrane (see Chap. 29). The following discussion focuses on cardiogenic pulmonary edema.

Pathophysiology and Etiology

In cardiogenic pulmonary edema, the left ventricle becomes incapable of maintaining sufficient output of blood with each contraction. The right ventricle continues to pump blood toward the lungs, however, and the left ventricle has difficulty emptying. There is retrograde fluid accumulation in the left atrium and pulmonary veins. The pulmonary capillaries and alveoli become engorged with blood. The lungs rapidly fill with fluid, and acute respiratory distress develops. As CO_2 accumulates, respiratory rate and depth increase. Without treatment, hyperventilation becomes insufficient to prevent respiratory acidosis. Metabolic acidosis follows.

Assessment Findings

Clients with acute pulmonary edema exhibit sudden dyspnea, wheezing, orthopnea, restlessness, cough (often productive of pink, frothy sputum), cyanosis, tachycardia, and severe apprehension. Respirations sound moist or gurgling. If a pulmonary artery catheter is in place, the pulmonary artery and pulmonary capillary wedge pressures are elevated, and cardiac output is reduced. While the body responds with arterial vasoconstriction, it may temporarily sustain adequate BP; however, the client eventually becomes hypotensive and peripheral pulses disappear. Chest radiographs show pulmonary infiltration with fluid. ABGs indicate severe hypoxemia (low PaO_2), hypercapnia (high $PaCO_2$), and a pH below 7.35.

Medical Management

Every effort is made to relieve lung congestion as quickly as possible because pulmonary edema can be fatal. Inotropic medications, which improve myocardial contractility, are administered to relieve symptoms. Supplemental oxygen or mechanical ventilation is used to support breathing. If the cause of heart failure and pulmonary edema can be corrected surgically (e.g., a mitral valve disorder), the client is supported medically while being prepared for surgery.

Drug Therapy

Inotropic agents, such as dopamine (Intropin), dobutamine (Dobutrex), and amrinone (Inocor), or digitalis are administered IV to improve the force of ventricular contraction. To reduce myocardial oxygen consumption, drugs that reduce venous return to the heart (diuretics) and promote vasodilatation (nitrates, ACE inhibitors, calcium channel blockers), are prescribed. IV morphine sulfate often is given to lessen anxiety. Morphine seems to help relieve respiratory symptoms by depressing higher cerebral centers, thus relieving anxiety and slowing respiratory rate. Morphine also promotes muscle relaxation and reduces the work of breathing.

Oxygenation

To facilitate gas exchange, oxygen is administered. A mask rather than nasal cannula is needed to deliver the maximum percentages of oxygen. If respiratory failure occurs, the client is intubated and oxygen is administered under continuous positive airway pressure or with mechanical ventilation with positive end-expiratory pressure.

Invasive Measures

If the client does not respond to drug therapy and oxygenation, additional interventions such as the insertion of an IABP, biventricular pacemaker, or LVAD are used to sustain life. Cardiomyoplasty, use of an artificial heart, and subsequent heart transplantation are further treatments.

Nursing Management

Effective resolution of pulmonary edema requires both medical and nursing management. The nursing diagnoses, interventions, and expected outcomes for clients with pulmonary edema are similar to those for clients experiencing CHF. Clients with pulmonary edema need close assessment in an intensive care unit.

The nurse establishes an IV line immediately (if one is not already in place) for medication administration. Because of the severity of symptoms and respiratory compromise, he or she administers IV diuretics and inotropic agents. The nurse monitors the therapeutic and adverse effects of medication therapy. Bedside ECG monitoring is standard, as are continuous pulse oximetry and automatic BP and pulse measurements approximately every 15 to 30 minutes. Critically ill clients may have a pulmonary artery catheter inserted to measure the pressure readings in the heart chambers and to estimate cardiac output. A urinary catheter is inserted to evaluate response to diuretics. The nurse assesses for proper placement/adherence of electrodes and ascertains that electronic monitoring equipment is functioning properly. The client receives oxygenation to maintain normal blood gases. If the client requires mechanical ventilation, the nurse suctions the airway as needed, provides frequent mouth care, and establishes an alternative method for verbal communication.

GENERAL NUTRITIONAL CONSIDERATIONS

Until edema resolves, severe heart failure requires restriction of sodium to 500 to 1000 mg/day. Daily food choices of sodium are limited to 6 oz of meat, 8 oz of milk, specially prepared low-sodium breads, low-sodium cereals and grains, distilled water for drinking and cooking, and low-sodium margarine and salad dressings. Processed and commercially prepared foods are eliminated, as are vegetables with natural sodium (e.g., beets, carrots, "greens"). Fresh, frozen, and canned fruit and fruit juices are not restricted.

Clients with mild heart failure may tolerate up to 3000 mg of sodium daily. The amount can remain below this number by not adding salt to food and avoiding processed food.

Encourage overweight clients to lose weight to reduce cardiac workload. Edema can mask clinical signs of malnutrition; weight is not a reliable indicator of nutritional status.

Dyspnea and nausea related to enlarged abdominal organs interfere with appetite and intake. Provide five to six small meals of soft or easily chewed foods. Encourage the client to rest after eating and to avoid spicy, gas-forming, and high-fiber foods to lessen heartburn and flatulence.

GENERAL PHARMACOLOGIC CONSIDERATIONS

Thiazide diuretics such as hydrochlorothiazide (HydroDIURIL) or chlorthalidone (Hygroton) can manage many cases of mild heart failure. Severe heart failure usually requires a loop diuretic such as furosemide (Lasix).

ACE inhibitors such as captopril (Capoten), fosinopril (Monopril), enalapril (Vasotec), and ramipril (Altace) may be used to treat heart failure in clients who have not responded to digitalis and diuretics.

Digitalis preparations are potent and may cause various toxic effects. The margin between a therapeutic and toxic effect is narrow. Thus, observe client for signs of digitalis toxicity, not just during the initial period of therapy but throughout care management. Instructions for clients taking diuretics should include a discussion of the signs and symptoms of electrolyte and water loss and the importance of adhering to the prescribed medication schedule. Also instruct the client to eat foods high in potassium.

Observe the effectiveness of drug therapy and any adverse effects in clients who are receiving emergency drug therapy for acute pulmonary edema. Many medications given for this disorder are IV drugs and occasionally are administered in large doses (hence the importance of client observation). Common drugs are morphine, aminophylline, digoxin (or other digitalis preparations), and vasopressors for hypotension.

GENERAL GERONTOLOGIC CONSIDERATIONS

Dyspnea on exertion is the earliest symptom of heart failure in many older clients. They also may experience a change in mental status, particularly confusion.

The heart is not exempt from aging. Cardiac reserve is lessened, and the heart becomes less able to withstand the effects of injury or disease.

Vascular changes can lead to heart failure by interfering with the blood supply to the heart muscle and causing the heart to pump blood through vessels that have become narrowed and inflexible.

A thorough drug history from a new client or the family is essential because many older adults take digitalis preparations for cardiac disorders. Age-related changes in the gastrointestinal, renal, and hepatic systems necessitate careful monitoring for therapeutic effects and adverse reactions. Older adults are at increased risk for toxicity because of the decreased ability of the kidneys to excrete the drug.

If limited finances prevent a client from preparing or purchasing special foods and needed medications, contact a social service worker or other community agent for assistance.

Critical Thinking Exercises

1. *Discuss how the care of a client with right-sided heart failure differs from the care of a client with left-sided heart failure.*
2. *A client diagnosed with heart failure presents with the following assessment data: temperature 99.1°F, pulse 100 beats/minute, respirations 42 breaths/minute, BP 110/50 mm Hg; crackles in both lung bases; nausea; pulse oximeter reading of 89%; enlarged, soft abdomen. Which assessment findings need immediate attention? Why?*

References and Suggested Readings

Abe, T., Fukada, J., & Morishita, K. (2001). The Batista procedure: Fact, fiction and its role in the management of heart failure. *Heart Failure Reviews, 6,* 195–199.

Abraham, W. T. (2000). Rationale and design of a randomized clinical trial to assess the safety and efficacy of cardiac resynchronization therapy in patients with advanced heart failure: The Multicenter InSync Randomized Clinical Evaluation (MIRACLE). *Journal of Cardiac Failure, 6,* 369–389.

Artrip, J. H., Oz, M. C., & Burkhoff, D. (2001). Left ventricular volume reduction surgery for heart failure: A physiologic perspective. *Journal of Thoracic and Cardiovascular Surgery, 122,* 775–782.

Barold, S. S. (2001). What is resynchronization therapy? *The American Journal of Medicine, 111,* 224–232.

Beattie, S. (2000). Heart failure with preserved LV function: Pathophysiology, clinical presentation, treatment, and nursing implications. *Journal of Cardiovascular Nursing, 14*(4), 24–37.

Bhat, G. & Dowling, R. D. (2001). Evaluation of predictors of clinical outcome after partial left ventriculectomy. *Annals of Thoracic Surgery, 72,* 91–95.

Bradley, C. (2000). Drug therapy review. Spironolactone in heart failure: A revived role for an old drug. *Intensive and Critical Care Nursing, 16,* 403–404.

Chamoun, A. J., Lenihan, D. J., McCulloch, M., et al. (2001). Resynchronization therapy in dilated cardiomyopathy: Confirmation of hemodynamic improvement with real-time three-dimensional echocardiography. *Circulation, 103*(19), E98–E108.

Christensen, D. M. (2000). The ventricular assist device: an overview. *Nursing Clinics of North America, 35,* 945–959.

DeWald, T., Gaulden, L., Beyler, M., et al. (2000). Current trends in the management of heart failure. *Nursing Clinics of North America, 35,* 855–875.

Franco-Cereceda, A., McCarthy, P. M., Blackstone, E. H., et al. (2001). Partial left ventriculectomy for dilated cardiomyopathy: Is this an alternative to transplantation? *Journal of Thoracic and Cardiovascular Surgery, 121,* 879–893.

Henrick, A. (2001). Cost-effective outpatient management of persons with heart failure. *Progress in Cardiovascular Nursing, 16*(2), 50–56.

Lazzara, D. (2001). Respiratory distress: Loosening the grip. *Nursing, 31*(6), 58–64.

Lucchese, F. A., Frota, F., Blacher, C., et al. (2000). Partial left ventriculectomy: Overall and late results in 44 class IV patients with 4-year follow-up. *Journal of Cardiac Surgery, 15,* 179–185.

MacKlin, M. (2001). Managing heart failure: A case study approach. *Critical Care Nurse, 21*(2), 36–38, 40–46, 48, 50–51.

Martens, K. H. (2000). Home care nursing for persons with congestive heart failure: Description and relationship to hospital readmission. *Home Healthcare Nurse, 18,* 404–409.

Mendzef, S. D. (2000). Neurohormonal factors in heart failure. *Nursing Clinics of North America, 35,* 841–853.

Nelson, G. S., Berger, R. D., Fetics, B. J., et al. (2000). Left ventricular or biventricular pacing improves cardiac function at diminished energy cost in patients with dilated cardiomyopathy and left bundle-branch block. *Circulation, 102,* 3053–3059.

Parsons, C. L., Sole, M. L., & Byers, J. F. (2000). Noninvasive positive-pressure ventilation: Averting intubation of the heart failure patient. *Dimensions of Critical Care Nursing, 19*(6), 18–24.

Pugh, L. C., Havens D. S., Xie, S., et al. (2001). Case management for elderly persons with heart failure: The quality of life and cost outcomes. *MEDSURG Nursing, 10*(2), 71–78.

Schreuder, J. J., Steendijk, P., van der Veen, F. H., et al. (2000). Acute and short-term effects of partial left ventriculectomy in dilated cardiomyopathy: Assessment by pressure-volume loops. *Journal of the American College of Cardiology, 36,* 2104–2114.

Tedesco, C., Reigle, J., & Bergin, J. (2000). Sudden cardiac death in heart failure. *Journal of Cardiovascular Nursing, 14*(4), 38–56.

Toussaint, J. F., Lavergne. T., Ollitraut, J., et al. (2000). Biventricular pacing in severe heart failure patients reverses electromechanical dyssynchronization from apex to base. *Pacing and Clinical Electrophysiology, 23,* 1731–1734.

Caring for Clients Undergoing Cardiovascular Surgery

Words to Know

annuloplasty
cardioplegia
cardiopulmonary bypass
commissurotomy
coronary artery
  bypass graft
embolectomy
endarterectomy
extracorporeal
  circulation
myocardial
  revascularization
thrombectomy
valvuloplasty

Learning Objectives

On completion of this chapter, the reader will:

- Identify the purpose of cardiopulmonary bypass.
- List several disadvantages of cardiopulmonary bypass.
- Name five indications for cardiac surgery.
- Describe how coronary artery blood flow is surgically restored.
- Name four surgical procedures for revascularizing the myocardium.
- Identify three techniques to correct valvular disorders.
- Describe two methods for controlling bleeding from heart trauma.
- List five problems associated with heart transplantation.
- Discuss the preoperative preparation of a client undergoing cardiovascular surgery.
- Discuss the nursing management of clients undergoing cardiac surgery.
- List three types of surgery performed on central or peripheral blood vessels.
- Discuss the nursing management of clients undergoing vascular surgery.

Before the 1950s, few attempts at cardiac surgery were made. Initially, hypothermia and crude mechanisms for oxygenating blood outside the body were used. In the 1960s, the technique for mechanically circulating and oxygenating blood outside the body, called **extracorporeal circulation** or **cardiopulmonary bypass** (Fig. 37-1), was developed. Removing blood from the venae cavae, circulating it through an oxygenator, and returning it to the aorta or femoral artery provides a nearly bloodless area while the beating heart is stopped.

Although most forms of cardiac surgery use cardiopulmonary bypass, some new surgical techniques have eliminated its use. Surgery on the beating heart without cardiopulmonary bypass reduces the potential for negative "pump" consequences (Box 37-1).

CARDIAC SURGICAL PROCEDURES

Cardiac surgery is used to correct and treat various cardiac disorders. It is done to revascularize the myocardium, repair or replace cardiac valves, repair ventricular aneurysm, remove heart tumors, manage heart trauma, and replace the heart with one from a human donor.

Myocardial Revascularization

Myocardial revascularization refers to surgical techniques that improve the delivery of oxygenated blood to the myocardium for clients who have coronary artery disease (CAD). It is accomplished by performing one or more

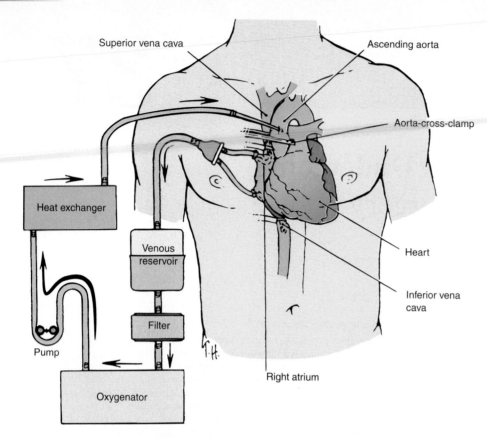

Superior vena cava

Ascending aorta

Aorta-cross-clamp

Heat exchanger

Venous reservoir

Heart

Filter

Pump

Inferior vena cava

Oxygenator

Right atrium

FIGURE 37-1 The cardiopulmonary bypass system. Cannulae are placed into the superior and inferior vena cava to divert blood from the body and into the bypass system. The pump creates a vacuum and pulls blood into the venous reservoir. The filter clears the blood of air bubbles, clots, and particulates. The blood then passes through the oxygenator, to the pump, and to the heat exchanger, which regulates the blood's temperature. The blood is then returned to the body. (From Smeltzer, S. C. & Bare, B. G. [2000]. *Brunner & Suddarth's textbook of medical–surgical nursing* [9th ed.]. Philadelphia: Lippincott Williams & Wilkins.)

coronary artery bypass grafts. A **coronary artery bypass graft** (CABG) improves myocardial oxygenation by bypassing or detouring around the occluded portion of one or more coronary arteries with a relocated blood vessel. The saphenous vein in the leg is the vessel most often used for grafting. It is harvested by making a long incision on the medial aspect of the leg or by removing the vein endoscopically through one to three small (1-inch) leg incisions (Fig. 37-2). An endoscopically removed vein results in less muscle and tissue damage, decreased pain, and reduced scarring. Alternative graft vessels include the following:

- The basilic and cephalic veins in the arm
- The internal mammary and internal thoracic arteries in the chest
- The radial artery in the arm
- In some cases, the gastroepiploic artery from the stomach.

CABG is reserved for clients with CAD who are not candidates for less invasive procedures like percutaneous coronary angioplasty and atherectomy. CABG is performed when (1) the client has multiple coronary artery

BOX 37-1 ● Disadvantages of Cardiopulmonary Bypass

- Long operative period (6 hours)
- Necessity for anticoagulation
- Hypotension
- Need for postoperative blood replacement
- Overall decline in mental function, perhaps because of an inflammatory response triggered by blood circulating through plastic tubing or gaseous bubbles in the circulated blood
- Risk for stroke, dysrhythmias, and renal failure

FIGURE 37-2 Two methods for harvesting the saphenous vein. (**A**) Traditional surgery requires a long incision in the leg. (**B**) Endoscopic removal involves one to three 1-inch incisions.

occlusions, (2) the atheromas are calcified and non-compressible, or (3) the anatomic location of the occlusion(s) interferes with the safe insertion of a coronary artery catheter.

The most conventional technique for performing CABG involves a long (approximately 12-inch) mid-chest incision, use of a cardiopulmonary bypass machine, and **cardioplegia** (stopping the heart) during surgery. Three other techniques for surgically revascularizing the myocardium are (1) off-pump coronary artery bypass (OPCAB), (2) minimally invasive coronary bypass (MIDCAB), and (3) port access coronary artery bypass (PACAB). Table 37-1 compares the various methods for performing myocardial revascularization.

Conventional Coronary Artery Bypass Graft

A CABG procedure involves attaching one end of a vessel such as a harvested portion of the saphenous vein or other distant vessel to the aorta and the other end below the occlusion in the coronary artery. One or several occluded areas can be bypassed during the surgical procedure, which is referred to as a *double, triple,* or *quadruple* bypass depending on the number of vessels that are grafted.

As an alternative, the distal end of the internal mammary or internal thoracic artery can be reattached below the occlusion on the anterior surface of the heart while leaving the proximal end in its natural location (Fig. 37-3). The advantage of using chest arteries is that doing so avoids making a second operative incision elsewhere on

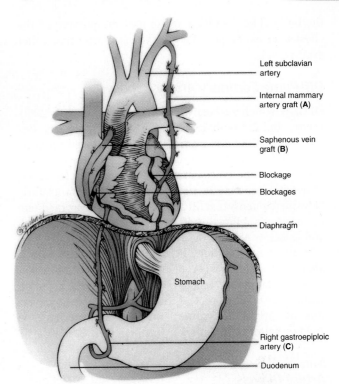

FIGURE 37-3 Three coronary artery bypass grafts in the (**A**) internal mammary artery, (**B**) saphenous vein, and (**C**) right gastroepiploic artery. (From Smeltzer, S. C. & Bare, B. G. [2000]. *Brunner & Suddarth's textbook of medical–surgical nursing* [9th ed.]. Philadelphia: Lippincott Williams & Wilkins.)

TABLE 37-1	COMPARISON OF SURGICAL MYOCARDIAL REVASCULARIZATION TECHNIQUES			
	CONVENTIONAL CABG	MIDCAB	PACAB	OPCAB
Length of incision	12″	4″	(3) ⅓″ (1) 1″	8–12″
Duration of hospitalization	7–10 days	4–6 days	3–4 days	6–10 days
Time for full recovery	6–10 weeks	2–4 weeks	2–3 weeks	4–6 weeks
Maximum number of grafted arteries	5	1–2	4	4
Years in clinical practice*	38 years	4 years	5 years	1 year
Cost	$35–45,000	~40% less than conventional CABG	~15% less than conventional CABG	~25% less than conventional CABG
Operation on beating heart	No	Yes	No	Yes
Use of cardiopulmonary bypass	Yes	No	Yes	No
Time in surgery	3–6 hours	2–3 hours	2 hours	2–5 hours
Operative mortality rate	2.9%	1.5%	1.0%	0.8%

*Since 2001.
(Source: Biomedical Department, Brown University, Providence, Rhode Island, 2001.)

the body. The disadvantage is that the portion of the chest arteries available for graft use is shorter than other graft vessels.

Off-Pump Coronary Artery Bypass

OPCAB, which has been performed only since early 2000, is very similar to conventional CABG except that the surgeon keeps the heart beating at a slow rate, eliminating the need for use of the cardiopulmonary bypass machine. The OPCAB chest incision is approximately 8 to 10 inches, somewhat less than in a conventional CABG procedure. New instruments that lift and stabilize the heart facilitate the surgeon's ability to graft vessels on the anterior, lateral, and posterior walls of the beating heart.

Advocates note that OPCAB reduces the risks associated with using the coronary bypass machine and decreases postoperative recovery time spent in the hospital. Until more OPCAB procedures are performed, however, it is too early to determine if the long-term success is as good or better than with conventional CABG.

Minimally Invasive Direct Coronary Artery Bypass

A MIDCAB is another example of a "beating heart" procedure. It is called *minimally invasive* because the incision, which is made between the ribs, is only about 3 to 5 inches long. Because the incision is small, the surgeon uses an endoscope to view the heart while grafting the vessels. Some surgeons are learning to use a robotic instrument inside the chest cavity rather than their hands.

This type of procedure is limited to grafting only one or two vessels on the anterior surface of the heart in clients who are not obese or whose coronary arteries are not heavily calcified. Despite these limitations, the MIDCAB procedure shortens the surgical time and postoperative recovery period, eliminates the risks of cardiopulmonary bypass, and is cosmetically more acceptable because of the smaller scar.

Port Access Coronary Artery Bypass

PACAB is a coronary artery bypass technique that uses the cardiopulmonary bypass machine, yet eliminates the long sternal incision common in conventional CABG. The surgeon gains access to the heart through several small incisions (Fig. 37-4). The small incisions on the left lateral chest near the axilla facilitate the insertion of metal tubes approximately the diameter of a pencil. It is through these tubes, or ports, that surgical instruments are inserted. A fourth and slightly larger incision in the chest permits the insertion of a video camera attached to an endoscope called a *thorascope*. The surgeon uses the image from the video camera and transesophageal echocardiography to visualize the operative area after the heart is stopped. A robotic hand, which is activated by the surgeon's voice command,

Thoracic incision

FIGURE 37-4 In a PACAB technique, the surgeon makes three small incisions in the chest near the axilla. He or she inserts surgical instruments through the ports and an endoscope through a larger incision. The surgeon then views the surgical field.

manipulates the surgical instruments that are inserted through the ports (Fogoros, 2001).

PACAB has shortened the operative procedure from 3 to 6 hours to 2 hours and reduced mortality rates from complications. Clients stay in the hospital only 2 to 3 days after the procedure, compared with 7 to 10 days after conventional CABG. Full recovery is much faster as well.

Valvular Repairs

Heart valves need surgical repair or replacement if they become narrowed (stenosed) or stretched (incompetent) (see Chap. 32). One method of repair is **commissurotomy** (opening adhesions in the valve cusps), which is done without direct visualization of the valve. This procedure is performed by means of a thoracotomy (chest incision). The surgeon places a purse-string suture in the wall of the heart, makes an incision, and inserts his or her finger or a metal dilator into the narrowed valve, stretching its opening. The surgeon then pulls the pursestring suture tight to prevent blood from escaping. Cardiopulmonary bypass is not required but usually is kept available for immediate use if complications develop or direct visualization is required to repair the valve. **Valvuloplasty** (valve repair) and **annuloplasty** (repair of the fibrous ring that encircles the valve) tighten an incompetent valve (Fig. 37-5). The diseased valve also can be excised and replaced with a mechanical valve or a bioprosthetic valve (Fig. 37-6 and Table 37-2).

Surgeons also are using minimally invasive approaches when replacing heart valves. Some of these approaches

FIGURE 37-5 Annuloplasty ring insertion. (**A**) Mitral valve regurgitation; leaflets do not close. (**B**) Insertion of an annuloplasty ring. (**C**) Completed valvuloplasty; leaflets close.

are performed through a mini-sternotomy, or parasternal incision, or a port access approach. Although cardio-pulmonary bypass is required, proponents of the minimally invasive approaches to valve replacement cite the following advantages:

- Less surgical trauma
- Decreased blood loss
- Less mechanical ventilation
- Reduced postoperative pain
- Faster mobility

FIGURE 37-6 Common mechanical and biologic valve replacements. (**A**) Caged ball valve (Starr-Edwards, mechanical). (**B**) Tilting-disk valve (Medtronic-Hall, mechanical). (**C**) Porcine heterograft valve (Carpenter-Edwards, biologic).

- Shortened hospital stay
- Reduced perioperative costs
- Improved cosmetic appearance

Repair of Ventricular Aneurysm

An aneurysm of the ventricular wall develops when an infarcted area of myocardium balloons outward. Thrombi commonly form in the crater of the bulging tissue. A ventricular aneurysm is the most lethal complication among clients who survive the acute stage of a myocardial infarction (MI). Because the motion of the myocardium may rupture the aneurysm, an emergency procedure may be performed to suture the weakened area (Fig. 37-7). If waiting is possible, the stretched tissue is excised 4 to 8 weeks after the MI when scar tissue has formed. If surgery is performed too early, it is difficult to differentiate healthy from necrotic tissue, and sutures placed in necrotic tissue usually are not retained.

Removal of Heart Tumors

Primary tumors of the heart, both benign and malignant, are rare. The clinical course and operative procedure depend on the type of tumor and its location in the heart. Benign tumors typically extend from a pedicle or stem, making their removal uncomplicated. Malignant tumors are more difficult to remove, and the prognosis is extremely poor.

TABLE 37-2	TYPES OF HEART VALVES		
TYPE	MATERIAL	ADVANTAGES	DISADVANTAGES
Mechanical	Man-made from carbon, stainless steel, Dacron	Durable Last 20 years Life-long	Risk for thrombi and emboli Anticoagulation necessary Risk for bleeding Sudden malfunction
Bioprosthetic	Natural tissue mounted on a metallic or polymer stent or unstented	Low potential for thrombi No anticoagulation necessary Gradual malfunction	Xenografts less durable than allografts Prone to deterioration and calcification
Xenograft	Porcine (pig) valve or bovine (cow) pericardium	Highly available Less expensive	Last 7–10 years
Allograft (also known as *homograft*)	Human cadaver	Last 10–15 years Better blood flow characteristics	Less available Expensive
Autograft	Tissue from patient's own pulmonic valve or pulmonary artery	Viable for 20+ years	More difficult to insert surgically

Repair of Heart Trauma

A nonpenetrating injury of the chest, such as being crushed against a steering wheel, may cause bruising and bleeding of the heart. Because the pericardium encloses the heart, blood accumulates in the pericardial space, resulting in cardiac tamponade. Sometimes traumatic cardiac tamponade is treated conservatively with bed rest. The inactivity and increased pressure from blood in the pericardium may stop the bleeding. The client may need to have the blood aspirated from the pericardial sac, in which case pericardiocentesis is performed (see Chap. 31). One aspiration is sufficient in most cases, but if bleeding continues, open thoracotomy is indicated to control blood loss.

A penetrating injury, such as a stab wound, also causes blood to leak into the pericardium. A pericardial tear often seals with a clot, whereas a myocardial tear continues to bleed. Large tears necessitate surgery. If the wound is severe enough to cause immediate shock from hemorrhage, the prognosis is poor.

Heart Transplantation

In adults, heart transplantation is indicated for cardiomyopathy (see Chap. 31) and end-stage coronary artery disease (see Chap 33). In newborns and infants, heart transplantation is indicated for a severe congenital car-

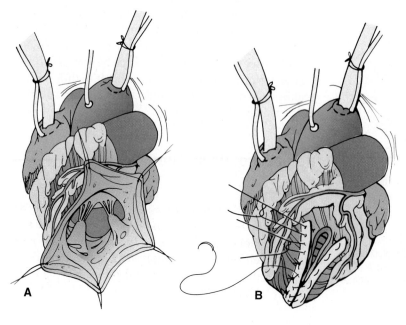

FIGURE 37-7 Surgical repair of a ventricular aneurysm. (**A**) The ventricle is opened and the nonfunctioning tissue from the aneurysm is differentiated from normal myocardium. (**B**) Healthy tissue from the endocardium through the epicardium is approximated.

diac defect. It is performed only when other treatment modalities fail. At almost any given time, almost 3500 to 4000 people are waiting for a heart or heart–lung transplant. Approximately 2300 transplantations are performed each year in the United States; 50% of recipients live at least 3 years after the surgery (National Heart, Lung, and Blood Institute, 1997).

The National Organ Transplant Act, which Congress passed in 1984, outlaws the sale of human organs. The United Network for Organ Sharing (UNOS) is the organization that maintains a computerized database with which to match organs with recipients (Box 37-2).

Once a client is certified as a candidate for transplantation, his or her name and tissue type are placed on a computerized recipient list. Tissue typing is necessary to match the recipient with a donor. Many problems are associated with heart transplantation, including the scarcity of donor organs, tissue rejection, postoperative infection, postoperative psychosis, and cost.

When a donor heart becomes available, it must be removed from the donor and transplanted within 6 hours of being harvested. There are two methods of heart transplantation. The most common method is an orthotopic heart transplant, in which the recipient's failing heart is removed and the donor heart is sutured onto the native great vessels of the heart. Recipients are given immunosuppressive drugs such as cyclosporine (Sandimmune), azathioprine (Imuran), and prednisone (Meticorten) to prevent organ rejection. The client is closely observed for signs of organ rejection (e.g., elevated white blood cell count, electrocardiographic [ECG] changes, fever), and is placed in protective isolation because an infection can be life-threatening. Throughout the client's lifetime, a heart biopsy in which cardiac tissue is obtained by an instrument attached to a venous catheter inserted into the heart is performed to detect rejection. Heart biopsies are performed every week for the first 3 to 6 weeks after surgery, then every 3 months for 1 year, and every year thereafter (National Heart, Lung, and Blood Institute, 1997). When signs of rejection occur, the dose or number of immunosuppressives is increased. The UNOS estimates that it costs more than $200,000 for transplant-related expenses the first year after a heart transplantation and approximately $15,000 per year thereafter. Insurance carriers, Medicare, or Medicaid assume most of this financial burden.

The transplanted heart beats faster than the client's natural heart, averaging about 100 to 110 beats/minute, because nerves that affect heart rate have been severed. The new heart also takes longer to increase the heart rate in response to exercise. CAD is a common problem among heart transplant recipients; however, they do not experience angina because the transplanted heart's nerve supply is no longer intact.

CENTRAL OR PERIPHERAL VASCULAR SURGICAL PROCEDURES

Vascular Grafts

Just as grafts are used to bypass a diseased section of a coronary blood vessel, vascular grafts are used to bypass or replace diseased sections of major systemic blood vessels such as the aorta or femoral arteries. The replacement graft may be made of synthetic fiber, such as Dacron or Teflon, or may be human tissue harvested from cadavers. A clamp is placed above and below the affected area, and the diseased blood vessel is removed. The replacement graft is then sewn in place, and the clamps are removed (Fig. 37-8). Depending on the area involved, cardiopulmonary bypass may be necessary.

Embolectomy and Thrombectomy

When thrombi or emboli occlude a major vessel, a **thrombectomy** (removal of a thrombus) or **embolectomy** (removal of an embolus) is performed. The vessel is opened above the clot, the clot is removed, and the vessel is sutured closed. This type of surgery may be an emergency because complete occlusion results in loss of blood supply to an area.

BOX 37-2 ● **UNOS Criteria for Thoracic Organ Distribution**

When a thoracic organ becomes available, it will be allocated according to the following criteria:

- Potential recipients must be classified as Status 1A, which means that within the past 1 to 14 days, they have required
  - Mechanical circulatory support such as implanted left or right ventricular assist device for 30 days or less, total artificial heart, intra-aortic balloon pump, or
  - Extracorporeal membrane oxygenator (ECMO), or
  - Mechanical circulatory support for more than 30 days with evidence of device-related complications, or
  - Mechanical ventilation, or
  - Continuous infusion of a single high-dose intravenous inotrope (e.g., dobutamine)
- In the absence of the preceding, potential recipients must have a life expectancy of less than 7 days without a heart transplant.
- Potential recipients must be tissue-compatible with the donor organ.
- Potential recipients must live within the locale (500 miles) of the available organ; thereafter, preference is given to someone 500 but not more than 1000 miles from the available organ, and last, someone who lives beyond 1000 miles from the available organ will be considered.
- Potential recipients must be medically recertified every 7 to 14 days to remain at Status 1A.

(Adapted from United Network of Organ Sharing. [2001]. Policy 3.7 Allocation of Thoracic Organs. [On-line.] Available: http://www.unos.org/About/policy_policies03_07.htm.)

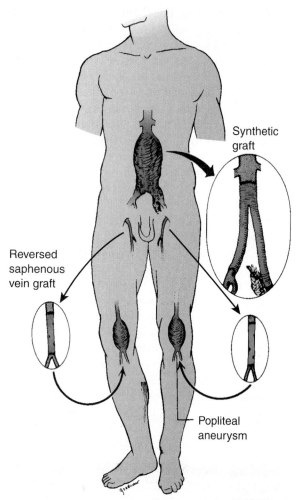

FIGURE 37-8 Surgical repair of an abdominal aneurysm and bilateral popliteal aneurysms. (From Smeltzer, S. C. & Bare, B. G. [2000]. *Brunner & Suddarth's textbook of medical–surgical nursing* [9th ed.]. Philadelphia: Lippincott Williams & Wilkins.)

Endarterectomy

Endarterectomy is the resection and removal of the lining of an artery (see Chap. 46). This type of surgery is performed to remove obstructive atherosclerotic plaques from the carotid, femoral, or popliteal arteries (Fig. 37-9).

NURSING PROCESS

● The Client Undergoing Cardiac or Vascular Surgery

The nurse manages the care of the client undergoing cardiac surgery throughout the perioperative and rehabilitation phases. Clients who undergo cardiovascular surgery are cared for in an intensive care unit during the immediate postoperative period because of their unstable condition and the need for nurses with expertise in managing complex monitoring equipment (Fig. 37-10).

Assessment

The nurse obtains the client's medical and surgical history and performs a physical examination (see Chap. 30). He or she obtains a drug history and determines if the client has any drug allergies. The nurse weighs the client, records vital signs regularly, and measures intake and output. He or she prepares the client for extensive diagnostic assessment tests such as chest radiography, ECG, exercise ECG (stress test), pulmonary function studies, echocardiography, laboratory blood tests, and coronary arteriography, and carefully checks the results.

The nurse takes time to assess the client's understanding of the scheduled procedure. After open heart surgery, the anesthetist and other members of the operating team send many clients directly from the operat-

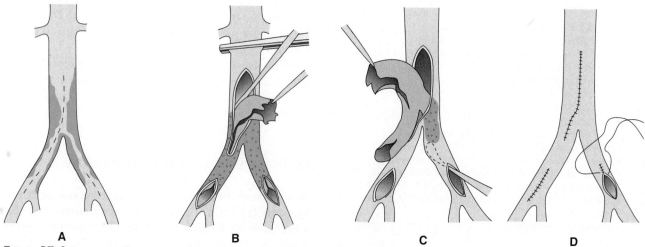

    A   **B**   **C**   **D**

FIGURE 37-9 In an aortoiliac endarterectomy, the vascular surgeon (**A**) identifies the diseased area, (**B**) clamps off blood supply to the vessel, (**C**) removes the plaque, and (**D**) sutures the vessel shut, after which blood flow is restored. (Adapted with permission from Rutherford, R. B. [1995]. *Vascular surgery* [4th ed., Vols. I and II]. Philadelphia: W. B. Saunders.)

Nasogastric tube to decompress stomach.

Endotracheal tube for providing mechanical ventilation, ventilatory assistance, suctioning, and use of end-tidal CO_2 monitor.

Swan-Ganz catheter for monitoring central venous pressure, pulmonary artery and pulmonary artery wedge pressures, temperature, $S\bar{v}O_2$. Can be used for determining cardiac output, for venous and pulmonary artery blood sampling, and for medication administration. Venous lines can be used for fluid administration.
Fluid intake is monitored.

ECG electrodes for monitoring heart rate and rhythm.

SpO_2 monitor for measuring arterial oxygen saturation.

Assess peripheral pulses: radial, popliteal, posterior tibial, dorsalis pedis.

Neurological assessment;
levels of responsiveness
hand grasp
pupils
pain

Assess skin color and temperature, color of lips, and color and capillary refill of nail beds.

Epicardial pacing electrodes to temporarily pace the heart.

Mediastinal and pleural chest tubes attached to suction; drainage and wound healing are monitored.

Radial arterial line with wrist armboard; used for monitoring arterial blood pressure and for blood sampling.

Indwelling catheter to closed drainage system for accurate measurement of urine output; a temperature probe may be part of the indwelling catheter.

FIGURE 37-10 Postoperative care of the client undergoing cardiac surgery. (From Smeltzer, S. C. & Bare, B. G. [2000]. *Brunner & Suddarth's textbook of medical–surgical nursing* [9th ed.]. Philadelphia: Lippincott Williams & Wilkins.)

ing room to the intensive care unit. The nurse obtains a comprehensive surgical report from the anesthetist or anesthesiologist and checks all invasive monitoring devices. He or she thoroughly and systematically assesses for signs and symptoms of potential complications, such as hemorrhage and shock, thrombus or embolus formation, cerebral anoxia, cardiac dysrhythmias, fluid overload, electrolyte imbalance, respiratory failure, and cardiac tamponade.

The nurse palpates the peripheral pulses or uses a Doppler ultrasound device if the pulses are not palpable.

He or she checks for inadequate tissue perfusion, such as a weak or absent pulse, cold or cyanotic extremity, or skin mottling. The nurse assesses blood pressure (BP) and pulse rate in both arms after thoracic surgery. He or she inspects intravenous (IV) sites and monitors the rates of infusing solutions. The nurse calculates urine output and other fluid intake hourly. He or she performs a neurologic assessment every 30 minutes, including evaluation of level of consciousness, size of pupils and their reaction to light, movement in both arms and legs, verbal response, and status of orientation.

Diagnosis, Planning, and Interventions

Deficient Knowledge related to unfamiliarity with diagnostic tests, preoperative preparations, and postoperative care

Expected Outcome: Client and family will understand the purpose, preparation, and after-care of tests and surgery.

- Assess client and family's knowledge concerning procedures. *Teaching builds on their foundation of knowledge.*
- Provide both verbal and written information concerning the surgical procedure and after-care, using language the client can understand. *Using terms the client can easily understand and giving both auditory and visual information enhance the learning process.*
- Ask the client or family member to explain the surgical procedure before signing the consent form. *The ability to paraphrase information validates that the client understands and is capable of giving informed consent.*
- Explain coughing, deep breathing, and leg exercises. Teach the use of an incentive spirometer and splinting the incision to cough. *The standard of care for all clients undergoing general anesthesia is to preoperatively teach techniques that prevent postoperative pneumonia and stasis of venous circulation.*
- Promote a relaxed environment conducive to asking questions. *Demonstrating personal interest and encouraging verbal interaction promotes free communication.*
- Clarify misconceptions concerning surgery. *The nurse is obligated to ensure that the client's knowledge and perceptions are accurate.*

Anxiety related to fear of surgery

Expected Outcome: Client will develop realistic expectations concerning surgery.

- Provide clear information about the surgical procedure and after-care in short, simple explanations. *Anxiety interferes with the ability to attend to, concentrate on, and process information, especially if it is extensive or complex.*
- Acknowledge emotions and expressions of fear. *Empathetic acceptance of fears decreases anxiety.*
- Demonstrate competence when performing skills. *Sensing that the nurse is knowledgeable and competent relieves the client's insecurity.*

Acute Pain related to surgical trauma to skin and operative tissue

Expected Outcome: Pain will be reduced to a tolerable level within 30 minutes of a nursing intervention.

- Assess the location, intensity, and quality of pain when assessing vital signs. *Pain assessment is the fifth vital sign. Pain beyond the client's tolerance requires immediate intervention.*
- Demonstrate how to self-administer narcotic analgesia with a patient-controlled analgesia (PCA) pump. *Small, frequent self-administrations of an opioid drug control acute pain within consistently tolerable levels.*

- Administer narcotic analgesics promptly as prescribed if PCA is not used. *Pain is more easily controlled by giving analgesic medication before the pain becomes severe.*
- Administer non-narcotic analgesics between prescribed doses of narcotic analgesics. *Non-narcotics have a different mechanism of action and are not likely to cause respiratory depression or depressed level of consciousness if given concurrently with narcotics.*

Risk for Ineffective Airway Clearance related to ineffective cough secondary to pain and accumulated secretions in response to artificial airway

Expected Outcome: Client will have a patent airway as evidenced by noiseless respirations and clear lung sounds.

- Assess lung sounds every 4 hours or as often as indicated by the client's condition. *Early detection of problems allows for swift intervention.*
- Suction when respirations are noisy and an endotracheal tube is in place; promote deep breathing and coughing every hour while the client is awake after extubation. *Suctioning uses negative pressure to remove mucus from the airway. Coughing is a natural method for clearing the airway.*
- Administer prescribed analgesics. *Analgesia relieves incisional pain and facilitates deep breathing and coughing.*
- Instruct client to press a pillow against the chest when deep breathing, coughing, and performing active exercise. *Splinting promotes comfort and decreases the potential for dehiscence.*
- Encourage oral fluids to the extent allowed when extubated; humidify oxygen. *Hydration and humidification liquefy mucous secretions, making them easier to expectorate.*

Risk for Impaired Gas Exchange related to retained secretions, hypoventilation secondary to pain, displacement of chest tubes

Expected Outcome: Client maintains adequate gas exchange as evidenced by arterial blood gases (ABGs) within normal limits and no dyspnea or tachycardia.

- Assess lung sounds, heart rate, level of consciousness, pulse oximetry, and ABG results as often as necessary. *Any abnormal findings are indicators of developing hypoxemia.*
- Notify physician if oxygen saturation falls below 90%. *This finding indicates that the client requires supplemental oxygenation.*
- Administer oxygen as prescribed. *Supplemental oxygen prevents hypoxemia or relieves oxygen deficits.*
- Elevate head of bed as much as possible. *Elevation of the head facilitates maximum chest/lung expansion, promotes comfort, and decreases the work of breathing.*
- Hyperoxygenate with 100% oxygen before suctioning; do not suction for more than 10 to 15 seconds. *Suctioning removes oxygen and can cause hypoxemia, myocardial ischemia, and dysrhythmias. Hyperoxygenation saturates the blood and hemoglobin to compensate for temporary removal during suctioning.*

- Promote rest and administer prescribed sedatives. *Rest reduces oxygen consumption; sedatives promote rest and are sympathetic antagonists.*
- Inspect chest tubes frequently to ensure that they are not kinked or compressed. *Obstructed chest tubes interfere with removal of air from the pleura, which interferes with lung expansion.*

Risk for Decreased Cardiac Output related to impaired ventricular contraction.

Expected Outcome: Client will maintain an adequate cardiac output as evidenced by stable vital signs, alertness, adequate urine output, and no dysrhythmias, chest pain, dyspnea, confusion, or dizziness. Cardiac output readings are within normal limits.

- Assess hemodynamics with direct BP monitoring by arterial line, pulmonary artery catheter and cardiac output measurements, vital signs, heart and lung sounds, intake and output, pulse rhythm and quality, mental status, and signs of peripheral edema as often as necessary. *Focused assessments that reflect the heart's ability to circulate intravascular fluid are an indication of an adequate or inadequate cardiac output.*
- Administer IV fluids and blood replacement at the rate prescribed. *Parenteral fluids increase the intravascular volume to facilitate an adequate cardiac output.*
- Administer prescribed inotropic medications. *They increase the force of heart contraction.*
- Administer prescribed vasodilators or diuretics. *They decrease afterload and promote optimum cardiac output.*
- Administer prescribed antidysrhythmics. *They promote normal conduction, depolarization, and repolarization of myocardial tissue to ensure normal cardiac output.*
- Be prepared to use a transcutaneous or transvenous pacemaker. *A temporary pacemaker ensures a heart rate that is compatible with life.*

Risk for Infection related to impaired skin

Expected Outcome: Client will remain free of infection.

- Assess incisions for redness, warmth, swelling, or purulent drainage. *Focused assessments that reflect the inflammatory process signify a possible infection.*
- Practice conscientious handwashing. *Handwashing is the single most important method for preventing infection.*
- Change moist or loose dressings. Use aseptic technique when changing dressings, IV tubing, bags, or other equipment. *Sterile technique prevents the transmission of microorganisms to impaired tissue. Dry, intact dressings are a barrier to microorganisms in the environment.*
- Administer prescribed antibiotic therapy. *Antibiotics are administered prophylactically and must be given on time to maintain therapeutic blood levels.*
- Implement infection control precautions for the immunosuppressed client. *They reduce the potential for exposing such clients to infectious microorganisms.*

PC: Hemorrhage

Expected Outcome: The nurse will monitor for, manage, and minimize hemorrhage.

- Assess incisional drainage; sites used for cardiopulmonary bypass cannulation; volume and color of chest tube drainage; BP and pulse rate; urinary output; mental status; partial thromboplastin time, prothrombin time, and international normalized ratio; presence of occult blood in stool; bruising; bleeding gums; and hemodynamic measurements as often as necessary. *Abnormal findings of such focused assessments are indicators of bleeding.*
- Report to the physician a cluster of symptoms that suggest significant blood loss. *The nurse works collaboratively to manage complications.*
- Be prepared to administer parenteral fluids, blood replacement, fresh frozen plasma, or antidotes for anticoagulants. *Fluids, blood, and blood products increase blood volume. Fresh frozen plasma replaces clotting factors. Antagonists of anticoagulants restore endogenous clotting mechanisms.*
- Apply direct pressure to bleeding sites. *Pressure promotes stasis of blood.*

Risk for Ineffective Tissue Perfusion: Peripheral related to compromised collateral circulation in extremity used to harvest donor vein, cannulation of peripheral artery and vein for cardiopulmonary bypass, venous stasis secondary to inactivity

Expected Outcome: Client's donor extremities will be adequately perfused with oxygenated blood; venous blood circulation will be adequate.

- Assess peripheral pulses, dependent edema, capillary refill, skin color and temperature, urinary output, mental status, and Homans' sign as often as necessary. *Focused assessment of these data reflects the status of peripheral blood flow.*
- Position extremity above level of heart. *Gravity promotes venous return to the heart. Reducing edema facilitates potential space for arterial circulation.*
- Encourage leg exercises every hour while awake. *Contraction of skeletal leg muscles propels venous blood toward the heart.*
- Apply elastic stockings or use a mechanical compression device. *Elastic stockings support valves in the leg veins to prevent venous stasis. Mechanical compression devices apply pressure to the tissues of the legs to propel venous blood.*
- Assist the client to ambulate several times a day. *Walking contracts leg muscles that promote venous blood return.*
- Ensure the client avoids prolonged sitting or crossing the legs at the knee. *Gravity and pressure contribute to venous stasis.*
- Encourage oral fluids within prescribed limits. *Adequate fluid volume decreases the potential for hemoconcentration and thrombus formation.*

PC: Paralytic Ileus related to intestinal handling during repair of abdominal aortic aneurysm, effects of narcotics and other medications

Expected Outcome: The nurse will monitor for, manage, and minimize atony of the bowel.

- Assess bowel sounds, abdominal distention, vomiting or color and amount of nasogastric tube drainage, and bowel elimination pattern as often as necessary. *Such focused assessments help determine the absence of peristalsis in the gastrointestinal tract.*
- Relieve pain with medications other than narcotic analgesics. *Narcotics slow peristalsis.*
- Withhold oral food and fluid. *Keeping the client NPO (nothing by mouth) decreases nausea and vomiting.*
- Ensure that the nasogastric tube remains patent. *A patent nasogastric tube provides an outlet for accumulating secretions and intestinal gas.*

Evaluation of Expected Outcomes

Expected outcomes for the client undergoing cardiac surgery are that he or she understands the treatment and recovery regimen and can cope with the fears created by the change in health status and surgical experience. Pain is controlled or eliminated; the airway is patent. The client ventilates adequately to maintain adequate gas diffusion; cardiac output is sufficient to maintain vital signs and renal output within normal ranges. There is no evidence of wound infection, and no significant bleeding develops. The extremities are warm and nonedematous, reflecting adequate arterial and venous circulation; bowel sounds are active.

Stop, Think, and Respond ● BOX 37-1

Mr. Jones has been in the intensive care unit for the past 4 days after CABG surgery. Normally alert and oriented, he is very confused, restless, and agitated. What could be possible reasons for this new-onset confusion? What other data will you need to collect? What can you do to help Mr. Jones right now?

 GENERAL NUTRITIONAL CONSIDERATIONS

Clients with atherosclerosis and elevated serum cholesterol and triglyceride levels should follow a low-fat, low–saturated-fat, or low-cholesterol diet (see General Nutritional Considerations in Chap. 33); additional diet modifications may be necessary to control other risk factors, such as hypertension, diabetes, and obesity.

 GENERAL PHARMACOLOGIC CONSIDERATIONS

Narcotic analgesics may be used before surgery to lessen anxiety and sedate the client. Clients who are relaxed and sedated when anesthesia

 37-1 *Client and Family Teaching* **Discharge Instructions After Cardiac Surgery**

The nurse teaches the following points:

- It may take several weeks for a normal appetite to return.
- Increase fruits, fiber, and liquids to relieve constipation, or use an occasional mild laxative.
- Depression is normal and temporary.
- You may have some slight problem with memory, but it should not be severe.
- A painless lump, if felt at the top of the chest incision, will disappear given time.
- There may be an occasional "grating" sound in the chest until the sternum heals.
- There may be some numbness in the chest if the internal mammary artery was used as a graft.
- After 1 week, the adhesive strips that cross the incision can be removed.
- Wait to take a tub bath until all incisions are healed; take showers until then.
- Report any redness, drainage, or tenderness from any incision.
- Loose, nonconstricting clothing promotes comfort and avoids interfering with circulation.
- Refrain from lifting, pushing, or pulling anything that weighs more than 10 lb until the physician relieves the restriction (approximately 6 weeks).
- Sexual relations usually can be resumed in 2 to 4 weeks depending on your comfort level and tolerance for activity; climbing two flights of stairs without dyspnea or chest pain is a common guideline.
- Perform exercises as taught; report if swelling of the legs increases.
- Continue to wear support hose or elastic stockings during the day and remove them at night.
- Check your weight daily and report if you gain more than 2 lb in 24 hours.
- Count your pulse rate at the wrist or neck and report a rate that exceeds 150 beats/minute.
- Contact the physician if you have difficulty breathing without a logical reason.
- If chest pain develops, rest; if the chest pain is unrelieved, take nitroglycerin as prescribed, and report the event to the physician regardless of whether it was relieved.
- Avoid crowds if you are taking an immunosuppressive drug.

(Portions adapted from The Society of Thoracic Surgeons [2001]. What to expect after your heart surgery. [On-line]. Available: http://www.sts.org/doc/3563.)

is given require a smaller dose of anesthetic. If the client is taking digitalis to improve myocardial contractility, the drug may be discontinued before surgery to decrease the risk of digitalis-induced dysrhythmias.

Anticoagulant drugs may be discontinued several days before cardiac surgery to allow the re-establishment of normal clotting patterns.

Many types of drugs may be administered before and after cardiac or vascular surgery (e.g., antibiotics, anticoagulants, vasopressors, diuretics, electrolytes, cardiotonics). Review the dose, route of administration, and adverse effects of each prescribed drug because many of these drugs have narrow margins of safety.

 ## GENERAL GERONTOLOGIC CONSIDERATIONS

Narcotics must be given with caution in older adults because the respiratory system of the older adult is more sensitive to the depressant effect of narcotic analgesics. Anticholinergic drugs such as atropine and scopolamine are used cautiously (if at all) in older adults because they are at greater risk for adverse reactions.

The older adult is prone to postoperative confusion. This confusion may manifest as disorientation, paranoia, aggression, or visual hallucinations.

Many older adults are poor surgical risks and have other concurrent medical problems, such as diabetes, heart failure, cardiac dysrhythmias, hypertension, and poor renal function. These clients require close observation during the postoperative period.

Critical Thinking Exercises

1. *What information would you offer to a person with CAD who says the physician has advised myocardial revascularization but the thought of a long midchest incision and leg incision are very frightening?*

2. *While caring for a client who is recovering from CABG surgery, you gather the following data: the client has leg pain, which he rates as 8 on a scale of 1 to 10; his respiratory rate is 30 breaths/minute at rest; there is dried blood on the thoracic dressing; the client's throat is sore after being weaned from mechanical ventilation; and he is concerned because he has not had a bowel movement in 3 days. Which assessment finding should be the major concern at this time?*

3. *What teaching would you do on seeing a client with a conventional CABG using a saphenous vein graft sitting in a chair with his or her legs crossed at the knee?*

References and Suggested Readings

Akpinar, B., Guden, M., Sanisoglu, I., et al. (2001). Does off-pump coronary artery bypass surgery reduce mortality in high risk patients? *Heart Surgery Forum, 4*, 231–237.

Allen, S. (2000). Off-pump bypass technique gets high praise from patients. *Nursing Spectrum* (Greater Chicago/NE Illinois & NW Indiana Edition), *13*(23), 14–15.

Augustine, S. M. (2000). Heart transplantation: Long-term management related to immunosuppression, complications, and psychosocial adjustments. *Critical Nursing Clinics of North America, 12*, 69–77.

Baptiste, M. M. (2001). Aortic valve replacement. *RN, 64*(1), 58–64.

Becker, C. & Petlin, A. (1999). Heart transplantation. *American Journal of Nursing, 99*(5, Suppl.), 8–14, 50–52.

Blank-Reid, C. (2001). What can we learn from famous traumas? . . . Princess Grace of Monaco . . . Diana, Princess of Wales . . . Rev. Dr. Martin Luther King, Jr. *Nursing, 31*(4), Critical Care: 32cc1–32cc2, 32cc4.

Bogan, L. M., Rosson, M. W., & Petersen, F. F. (2000). Organ procurement and the donor family. *Critical Care Nursing Clinics of North America, 12*, 23–33.

Brown, K. K. (1998). Minimally invasive valve surgery . . . port-access mitral valve repair or replacement. *Critical Care Nursing Quarterly, 20*(4), 40–52.

Cleveland, J. C. Jr., Shroyer, A. L., Chen, A. Y., et al. (2001). Off-pump coronary artery bypass grafting decreases risk-adjusted mortality and morbidity. *Annals of Thoracic Surgery, 72*, 1282–1288.

Cope, S. & Hawley, R. (2001). Needs of the older patient in the intensive care unit following heart surgery. *Progress in Cardiovascular Nursing, 16*(2), 44–48.

Dewey, T. M., Magee, M. J., Edgerton, J. R., et al. (2001). Off-pump bypass grafting is safe in patients with left main coronary disease. *Annals of Thoracic Surgery, 72*, 788–791.

Drug Watch. (1999). Post-transplant immunosuppression. *American Journal of Nursing, 99*(2), 14.

Filsoufi, F., Aklog, L., & Adams, D. H. (2001). Minimally invasive CABG. *Current Opinion in Cardiology, 16*, 306–309.

Fitzgerald, C. A. (1998). Minimally invasive cardiac valve surgery. *Critical Care Nursing Quarterly, 21*(1), 41–47.

Fogoros, R. (2001). Robotic heart surgery—a status report. [On-line.] Available: http://heartdisease.about.com/library/weekly/aa060401a.htm.

Holmquist, M., Chabalewski, F., Blount, T., et al. (1999). A critical pathway: Guiding care for organ donors. *Critical Care Nurse, 19*(2), 84–88, 90–100.

Kaba, E., Thompson, D. R., & Burnard, P. (2000). Coping after heart transplantation: A descriptive study of heart transplant recipients' methods of coping. *Journal of Advanced Nursing, 32*, 930–936.

Kappert, U., Cichon, R., Schneider, J., et al. (2001). Technique of closed chest coronary artery surgery on the beating heart. *European Journal of Cardio-thoracic Surgery, 20*, 765–769.

Kavarana, M. N., Asher, A. S., Barbone A., et al. (2001). A comparison of consecutive off-pump versus conventional coronary artery bypass. *Heart Surgery Forum, 4*, 160–165.

Lewis, D. D. & Valerius, W. (1999). Organs from non-heart-beating donors: An answer to the organ shortage. *Critical Care Nurse, 19*(2), 70–74.

Ley, S. J. (2001). Keeping pace. Cardiac surgery 2001: What's hot, what's not. *Progress in Cardiovascular Nursing, 16*(3), 132–133.

Mann, D. (2001). Moving toward better bypass surgery: Surgeons report better results when they operate on beating hearts. [On-line.] Available: http://www.my.webmd.com/content/article/1728.72285

Mason, V. F. & Miller, K. H. (2001). Optimizing outcomes: Nurses caring for patients after cardiac surgery can promote early transfers. *American Journal of Nursing, 101*(5, Suppl.), 13–15, 48–50.

Morse, C. J. (2001). Advance practice nursing in heart transplantation. *Progress in Cardiovascular Nursing, 16*(1), 21–24, 38.

National Heart, Lung, and Blood Institute. (1997). Facts about heart and heart-lung transplants. [On-line.] Available: http://www.nhlbi.nih.gov/health/public/heart/other/hrt_lung.htm.

Patetsios, P., Priovolos, S., Slesinger, T. L., et al. (2000). Lacerations of the left ventricle from rib fractures after blunt trauma. *Journal of Trauma: Injury, Infection, and Critical Care, 49,* 771–773.

Popernack, M. L. (2000). Are we overlooking a hidden source of organs? *Nursing, 30*(1), 44–47.

Prescott, L. M. (1998). Minimally invasive port-access cardiac surgery. *Surgical Technologist, 30*(6), 10–15.

Quigley, R. L., Weiss, S. J., Highbloom, R. Y., et al. (2001). Creative arterial bypass grafting can be performed on the beating heart. *Annals of Thoracic Surgery, 72,* 793–797.

Rembacz, J. M. & Abel, C. J. (2000). Pericardial tamponade. *American Journal of Nursing, 100*(9, Suppl.), 10–14.

Rogers, J. P., Novchich, T. M., Pearce, G. L., et al. (1998). Port-access cardiac surgery protocols and early outcomes. *Critical Care Nursing Clinics of North America, 10*(1), 61–73.

Steeves, S. A. (2000). New technique avoids heart-lung machine. [On-line.] Available: http://www.my.webmd.com/content/article/2793.189.

van Dijk, D., Nierich, A. P., Jansen, E. W., et al. (2001). Early outcome after off-pump coronary bypass surgery: Results from a randomized study. *Circulation, 104,* 1761–1766.

Vlassov, G. P., Deyneka, C. S., Travine, N. O., et al. (2001). Acute myocardial infarction: OPCAB is an alternative approach for treatment. *Heart Surgery Forum, 4,* 147.

c h a p t e r

38

Introduction to the Hematopoietic and Lymphatic Systems

Words to Know

agranulocytes
basophils
eosinophils
erythrocytes
erythropoietin
granulocytes
hematopoiesis
hemoglobin
leukocytes
leukocytosis
leukopenia
lymph
lymphatics
lymph nodes
lymphocytes
neutrophils
phagocytosis
plasma
platelets
pluripotential stem
  cells

Learning Objectives

On completion of this chapter, the reader will

- Explain hematopoiesis and name two structures involved in it.
- Name three types of blood cells produced by bone marrow, and discuss the function of each.
- List at least five components of plasma.
- Name three plasma proteins and explain the function of each.
- Identify the four blood groups and discuss the importance of transfusing compatible types.
- Explain the function of the lymphatic system and its role in hematopoiesis.
- Discuss the pertinent assessments of the hematopoietic and lymphatic systems when obtaining a health history and conducting a physical examination.
- Name at least five laboratory and diagnostic tests for disorders of the hematopoietic and lymphatic systems.
- Discuss the nursing management of clients with hematopoietic or lymphatic disorders.

Hematopoiesis is the manufacture and development of blood cells. The hematopoietic system consists of bone marrow, where most blood cells are produced, and the lymphatic system, which includes the thymus gland and spleen.

Bone marrow is the substance in the interior of the long bones and spongy bones of the skeleton. The two types of bone marrow are (1) red marrow and (2) yellow marrow. Red marrow is primarily found in the ribs, sternum, skull, clavicle, vertebrae, proximal ends of the long bones, and iliac crest. It manufactures blood cells and hemoglobin. Yellow marrow consists primarily of fat cells and connective tissue. It does not participate in the manufacture of blood cells; however, yellow bone marrow can form blood cells under conditions involving intense stimulation, such as after significant blood loss (hemor-

rhage). Lymphoid tissue, which includes the thymus gland and spleen, also plays a role in hematopoiesis.

HEMATOPOIETIC SYSTEM

● ANATOMY AND PHYSIOLOGY

Blood consists of cells suspended in a fluid called plasma (Fig. 38-1). All blood cells are produced from undifferentiated precursors called **pluripotential stem cells** in the bone marrow (Fig. 38-2). Myeloid stem cells are converted to (1) **erythrocytes,** which are red blood cells (RBCs); (2) several types of **leukocytes,** or white blood cells (WBCs), and (3) **platelets,** also known as *thrombo-*

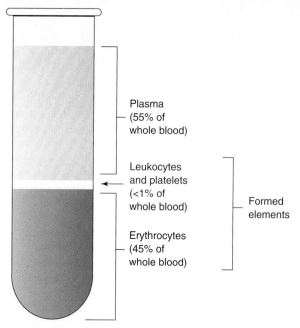

Plasma
(55% of
whole blood)

Leukocytes
and platelets
(<1% of
whole blood)

Formed
elements

Erythrocytes
(45% of
whole blood)

FIGURE 38-1 Components of blood.

cytes because they help control bleeding by forming a loose blood clot.

Lymphoid stem cells are converted to **lymphocytes,** WBCs with immune functions. Each component of blood has specialized functions (Table 38-1).

Erythrocytes

Erythrocytes are flexible, anuclear (lacking a nucleus), biconcave disks covered by a thin membrane through which oxygen and carbon dioxide (CO_2) pass freely. The flexibility of erythrocytes allows them to change shape as they travel through capillaries. Their major function is to transport oxygen to and remove CO_2 from the tissues.

The production of erythrocytes is called *erythropoiesis.* The rate of erythrocyte production is regulated by **erythropoietin,** a hormone released by the kidneys. Erythrocytes arise from myeloid stem cells, which also require iron and B vitamins such as B_{12}, B_6, and folic acid to mature properly. Immature erythrocytes, known collectively as *erythroblasts,* go through several intermediary stages of maturation before being released into the blood. In their immature state, erythroblasts contain a nucleus; the mature erythrocyte has no nucleus.

The normal number of erythrocytes varies with age, sex, and altitude but is between 3.6 and 5.4 million/μL. Infants have more erythrocytes than adults; women have fewer erythrocytes than men. People who live at high altitudes or engage in strenuous activity have an increased number of erythrocytes.

The red color of blood is caused by **hemoglobin,** an iron-containing pigment attached to erythrocytes. The heme portion of the molecule freely binds with oxygen,

forming a substance called *oxyhemoglobin.* Hemoglobin carries oxygen to the cells of the body. In adults, the normal amount of hemoglobin is 12 to 17.4 g/dl. As erythrocytes pass through the lungs, the hemoglobin picks up oxygen and releases CO_2. Oxygenated blood is bright red and carried by arteries, arterioles, and capillaries to all body tissues. After hemoglobin releases oxygen for use by the tissues, the hemoglobin is called *reduced* (or *deoxygenated*) *hemoglobin.* The blood becomes dark red and returns by way of the veins to the heart and lungs, where CO_2 is released and the blood is reoxygenated.

Erythrocytes circulate in the blood for about 120 days, after which the spleen removes them; the liver removes severely damaged erythrocytes. When erythrocytes are destroyed, the iron component of hemoglobin is returned to the red marrow and reused. The residual pigment is stored in the liver as bilirubin and excreted in bile.

Leukocytes

Leukocytes are divided into two categories: **granulocytes,** which contain cytoplasmic granules, and **agranulocytes,** which do not contain granules (Fig. 38-3). Leukocytes perform various protective functions such as engulfing invading microorganisms and cellular debris, and manufacturing antibodies (see Chap. 41). They circulate in blood but also migrate from the blood into body tissues to search for and destroy potentially harmful substances.

The normal leukocyte count is between 5000 and 10,000/mm³. An increased number of leukocytes is called **leukocytosis;** a decreased number is called **leukopenia.** Table 38-2 shows the differential leukocyte count. The life span of leukocytes is only 1 to 2 days; consequently, the demand for the production of WBCs is continuous. The need is even greater with an infection.

Granulocytes

Granulocytes, also called *polymorphonuclear leukocytes,* are divided into three subgroups: neutrophils, basophils, and eosinophils. **Neutrophils** are a major component of the inflammatory response and defense against bacterial infection. Also called *microphages,* they protect the body by **phagocytosis,** the ingestion and digestion of bacteria and foreign substances (Fig. 38-4). Immature neutrophils, called *band cells,* circulate in peripheral blood.

Basophils are also capable of phagocytosis; they are active in allergic contact dermatitis (immediate hypersensitivity) and some delayed hypersensitivity reactions. **Eosinophils** phagocytize foreign material. Their numbers increase in allergies, some dermatologic disorders, and parasitic infections.

Agranulocytes

Agranulocytes are divided into two groups: *lymphocytes* and *monocytes.* Lymphocytes are divided into *B lympho-*

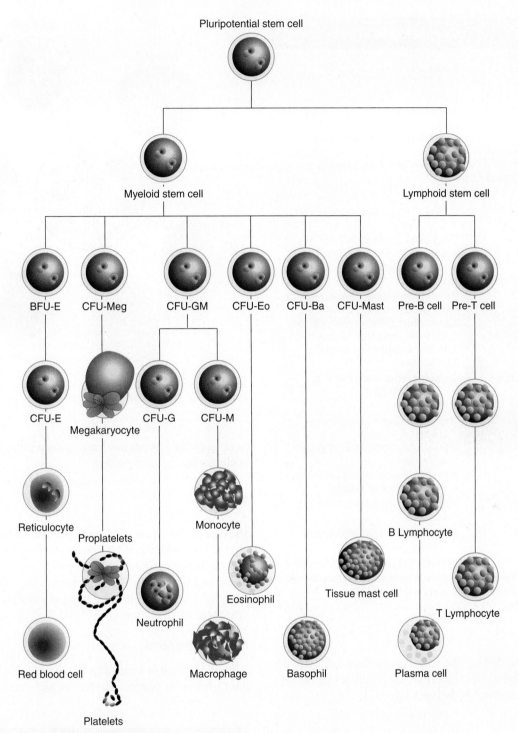

FIGURE 38-2 Hematopoiesis. (From Smeltzer, S. C. & Bare, B. G. [2000]. *Brunner & Suddarth's textbook of medical–surgical nursing* [9th ed.]. Philadelphia: Lippincott Williams & Wilkins.)

cytes (or B cells), which provide humoral immunity by producing antibodies (immunoglobulins), and *T lymphocytes* (or T cells), which provide cellular immunity (or cell-mediated response). B lymphocytes produce antibodies against foreign antigens, and T lymphocytes interact with foreign cells and release a substance called *lymphokine*, which enhances the actions of phagocytic cells. Some lym-

phoid stem cells mature in the bone marrow, whereas others migrate to peripheral lymphoid tissue to complete their maturation.

Monocytes, also known as *macrophages* because they phagocytize large-sized debris, help to combat severe infections and contribute to the immune response. They are antigen-presentation cells, which engulf microbial

TABLE 38-1	COMPONENTS OF BLOOD
COMPONENT	FUNCTION
Blood Cells	
Erythrocytes (red blood cells)	Transport oxygen
Leukocytes (white blood cells)	Protect against infection
Platelets (thrombocytes)	Participate in clotting blood
Plasma	
Water	Circulates blood cells and noncellular components
	Contributes to blood pressure
	Relocates to other fluid compartments as needed
Plasma proteins	
Albumin	Affects intravascular osmotic pressure
Fibrinogen	Participates in clotting blood
Globulin	Carries other protein substances, for example, those that are involved in inflammatory and immune responses
Clotting factors	Convert a loose blood clot to a stabilized blood clot
Nutrients	
Glucose	Provides of source of immediate energy
Amino acids	Provide components for cell growth and repair
Lipids	Provide a reserve for cellular energy in the absence of glucose
Vitamins	Participate in essential physiologic functions
Electrolytes	Facilitate a variety of biochemical actions
Hormones	Perform multiple endocrine functions
Wastes (carbon dioxide, drug metabolites)	Prevent toxicity when biotransformed and excreted

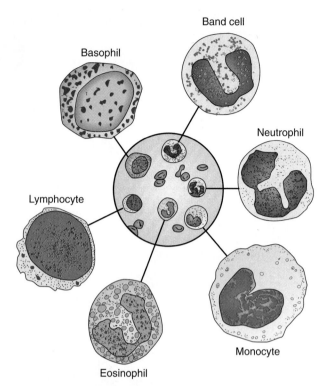

FIGURE 38-3 White blood cells.

here (platelet aggregation) and form a plug, or clot, that occludes the injured vessel.

Plasma

Plasma is the liquid, or serum, portion of blood. It consists of 90% water and 10% proteins. Besides blood cells, plasma contains and transports proteins (albumin, globulins, and fibrinogen), clotting factors like prothrombin, pigments, vitamins, glucose, lipids, electrolytes, minerals, enzymes, and hormones.

Plasma Proteins

Albumin, which is formed in the liver, is the most abundant protein in plasma. Under normal conditions, albu-

invaders and display the antigenic surface to T lymphocytes. T lymphocytes then engage B lymphocytes to make the appropriate antibody (see Chap. 41).

Platelets

Platelets (*thrombocytes*) are disklike, non-nucleated cell fragments with a life span of approximately 7.5 days. They are manufactured in the red bone marrow. Approximately two thirds of the total 150,000 to 350,000/mm³ platelets circulate in the blood and contribute to hemostasis. The remaining one third are sequestered in the spleen, where they remain unless needed in cases of significant bleeding. When a blood vessel is injured, platelets migrate to the injury site. The platelets release a substance known as glycoprotein IIb/IIIa, which causes the platelets to ad-

TABLE 38-2	DIFFERENTIAL WHITE BLOOD CELL COUNT	
	PERCENT OF TOTAL WBCs	NUMERIC RANGE (mL)
Neutrophils	60–70	3000–7000
Basophils	1–4	50–400
Eosinophils	0.5–1	25–100
Lymphocytes	20–40	1000–4000
Monocytes	2–6	100–600

leukocyte   capillary   bacteria

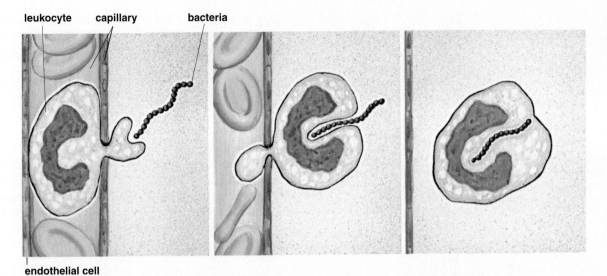

endothelial cell

FIGURE 38-4 Phagocytosis. The cell membrane of the neutrophil surrounds and pinches off the bacteria or dead tissue. Enzymes within the cell destroy the foreign material. (From Smeltzer, S. C. & Bare, B. G. [2000]. *Brunner & Suddarth's textbook of medical–surgical nursing* [9th ed.]. Philadelphia: Lippincott Williams & Wilkins.)

min cannot pass through a capillary wall. Consequently, albumin helps maintain the osmotic pressure that retains fluid in the vascular compartment.

Globulins are divided into three groups: alpha, beta, and gamma. The gamma globulins are also called *immunoglobulins*. Globulins function primarily as immunologic agents; they prevent or modify some types of infectious diseases. Like albumin, they help maintain osmotic pressure in the vascular compartment.

Fibrinogen, the largest plasma protein, plays a key role in forming blood clots. It can be transformed from a liquid to fibrin, a solid that controls bleeding.

Blood Groups

There are four blood groups or types, A, B, AB, and O, which are determined by heredity. Blood type is ascertained by identifying the protein, or *antigen,* on the red cell membranes. Group A has A antigen, group B has B antigen, group AB has A and B antigen, and group O has no antigen. *Antibodies,* immunoglobulins in plasma that inactivate any substance that is nonself, react with incompatible RBC antigens. Therefore, people with type O blood are universal donors because they do not have antigens on the red cell membrane. People with type AB blood are universal recipients because they are compatible with blood types A, B, and O (see Chap. 24 and Table 24-2).

The Rh factor is a specific protein on the RBC membrane. If the protein is present, the person is Rh positive. If the protein is absent, the person is Rh negative. When blood is transfused, donor blood must be type and Rh compatible with the recipient's blood. The donor's blood is typed and labeled at the time of donation. When a blood transfusion is needed, the recipient's blood is typed and crossmatched (matched for compatibility with donor blood). Donor and recipient blood are considered compatible if there is no clumping or *hemolysis* (destruction of erythrocytes) when both samples are mixed in the laboratory. In an emergency, type O blood can be given to recipients with type A, B, AB, or O. People with Rh-positive blood can receive Rh-positive or Rh-negative blood because Rh negative indicates the Rh factor is missing; those with Rh-negative blood, however, must never receive Rh-positive blood regardless of whether the blood type is compatible. Chapter 24 discusses various types of transfusion reactions.

Stop, Think, and Respond ● BOX 38-1

When you go to the hospital's blood bank to obtain a unit of blood for a client with blood type A, Rh-positive blood, you receive a unit of blood that is blood type A, Rh negative. Is this unit of blood compatible? Explain your answer.

LYMPHATIC SYSTEM

● ANATOMY AND PHYSIOLOGY

The lymphatic system includes the thymus gland, spleen, and a network of lymphatic vessels, lymph nodes, and lymph. This system of **lymphatics** circulates interstitial fluid and carries it to the veins (Fig. 38-5). Along the pathway, the lymphatic system filters and destroys pathogens and removes other potentially harmful substances.

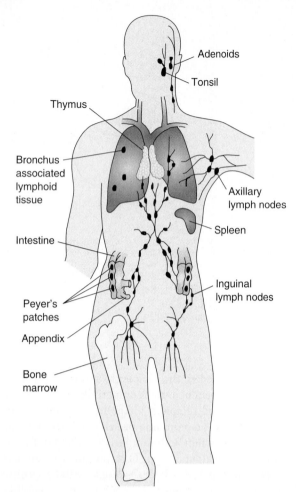

FIGURE 38-5 Central and peripheral lymphoid organs and tissues.

Thymus Gland

The thymus gland is lymphatic tissue in the upper chest that contains undifferentiated stem cells released from bone marrow. Once the undifferentiated cells migrate to the thymus gland, they develop into *T lymphocytes* because they are thymus derived (Fig. 38-6).

Spleen

The spleen is the largest lymphatic structure. It lies in the abdomen beneath the diaphragm and behind the stomach. The spleen is a reservoir of blood and contains phagocytes that engulf damaged erythrocytes and foreign substances.

Lymph Nodes

Lymph nodes, glandular tissue along the lymphatic network, are clustered in the axilla, groin, neck, and large vessels of the thorax and abdomen. Lymphatic ducts, through which lymph flows, connect the nodes. The nodes contain

both T and B lymphocytes (released from the bone marrow but do not reach the thymus gland) in the smaller nodules of each lymph node.

Lymph

Lymph is fluid with a similar composition to plasma. It flows through lymphatics by contraction of skeletal muscles. Lymph enters each node by way of the afferent lymph duct, passes through the node, and leaves by the efferent lymph duct (Fig. 38-7). As lymph passes through the node, macrophages attack and engulf foreign substances like bacteria and viruses, abnormal body cells, and other debris.

ASSESSMENT

The nurse collects data by taking a health history, examining the client, and monitoring the results of laboratory tests.

History

The health history includes the client's description of signs and symptoms. If abnormalities are present, the nurse determines when the signs or symptoms began, their severity, and frequency. In relation to the hematopoietic and lymphatic systems, it is especially important to establish if the client:

- Experiences prolonged bleeding from an obvious injury
- Has unexplained blood loss as in rectal bleeding, nosebleeds, bleeding gums, or vomiting blood
- Feels fatigued with normal activities
- Becomes dizzy or faints
- Bruises easily
- Is easily chilled
- Has frequent infections
- Feels discomfort in the axilla, groin, or neck
- Has difficulty swallowing with localized throat tenderness
- Has had surgery with lymph node removal or splenectomy, is undergoing treatment for cancer, or has renal failure—all of which may affect blood cell volume or lymphatic circulation

The nurse takes a drug history of prescribed and nonprescribed medications. Some antibiotics and cancer drugs contribute to hematopoietic dysfunction. Aspirin and anticoagulants can contribute to bleeding and interfere with clot formation. Because industrial materials, environmental toxins, and household products also can affect

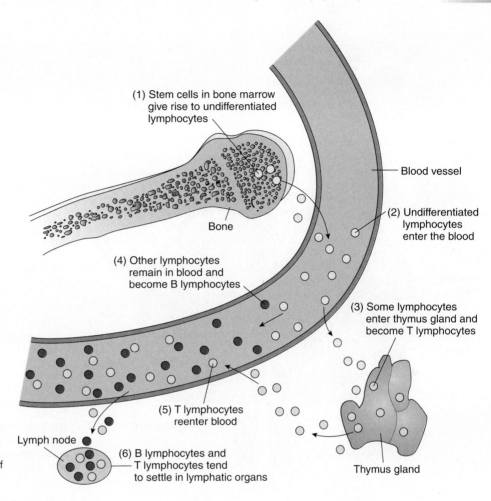

FIGURE 38-6 Transformation of T and B lymphocytes.

(1) Stem cells in bone marrow give rise to undifferentiated lymphocytes

Bone

Blood vessel

(2) Undifferentiated lymphocytes enter the blood

(4) Other lymphocytes remain in blood and become B lymphocytes

(3) Some lymphocytes enter thymus gland and become T lymphocytes

(5) T lymphocytes reenter blood

Lymph node

(6) B lymphocytes and T lymphocytes tend to settle in lymphatic organs

Thymus gland

blood-forming organs, the nurse explores any exposure to these agents. He or she asks about foreign travel to countries where malaria or parasitic roundworms are common. The infectious agent that causes malaria invades erythrocytes and causes anemia. Filariasis is a consequence of a roundworm infection in which the lymphatic vessels become occluded. The nurse obtains a dietary history because compromised nutrition interferes with the production of blood cells and hemoglobin.

Physical Examination

Physical examination includes inspection of the skin with particular attention to color (e.g., normal, extreme redness, pallor), temperature, and ecchymosis or other lesions. A rapid pulse rate can indicate reduced erythrocytes or inadequate hemoglobin levels.

The nurse palpates the lymph nodes in the neck for tenderness or swelling and notes the size, location, and characteristics of symptomatic lymph nodes. He or she examines the skin adjacent to the node for redness, streaking, and swelling. The nurse inspects the tonsils for size and appearance. He or she examines the extremities

to determine if they are of similar size—obstruction of lymphatic circulation can cause unilateral enlargement.

Diagnostic Tests

The nurse obtains blood samples from a vein, finger, or earlobe. Laboratory tests include a complete blood count and tests that reflect the clients blood clotting status such as prothrombin time, fibrinogen level, activated partial thromboplastin time, D-dimer test for fibrin, fibrin degradation products, and factor assays.

A bone marrow aspiration, a procedure in which bone marrow is removed under local anesthesia, is performed to determine the status of blood cell formation. The marrow is examined for the types and percentage of immature and maturing blood cells. The nurse assists the physician, supports the client during a bone marrow aspiration, and monitors his or her status afterward (Nursing Guidelines 38-1).

The Schilling test is performed to diagnose pernicious anemia, macrocytic anemia, and malabsorption syndromes. Radioactive vitamin B_{12} is given orally, followed in 1 hour by an injection of nonradioactive B_{12}. All urine

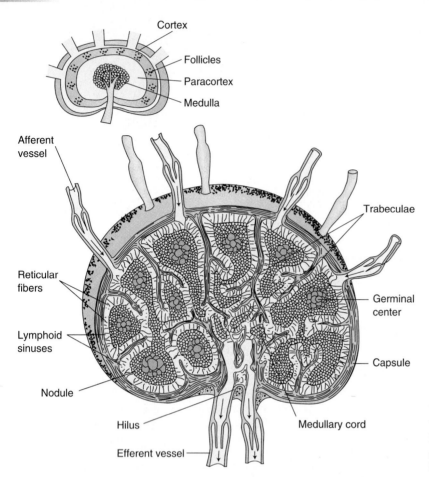

FIGURE 38-7 Structural features of a lymph node. The lymph filters out bacteria that gain entry to the body. (From Chaffee, E. E., & Lytle, I. M. [1980]. *Basic physiology and anatomy* [4th ed., p. 356]. Philadelphia: J. B. Lippincott.)

is collected for 24 to 48 hours after the client receives the nonradioactive B_{12}. Little or no vitamin B_{12} in the urine indicates absence of the intrinsic factor or defective absorption of vitamin B_{12} from the intestinal tract.

Lymphatic disorders are diagnosed using procedures such as lymph node biopsy, ultrasound of the spleen or selected lymph nodes, and lymphangiography (radio-graphic examination using contrast media). Additional diagnostic tests include radiography, computed tomography, bone scan, and magnetic resonance imaging. Although they are not specific for hematologic or lymphatic disorders, they are used to rule out other disorders or note changes in organs that have a direct or indirect relationship to a hematologic or lymphatic disorder.

NURSING GUIDELINES 38-1

Assisting With a Bone Marrow Aspiration

- Inform the client of the plan and approximate time for the bone marrow aspiration. Allow time to answer questions.

- Witness the client's signature on a consent form.

- Check the client's medical record for history of allergies, especially to local anesthetics or latex.

- Obtain a sterile bone marrow aspiration tray and add the type and strength of local anesthetic according to the physician's orders.

- Determine the site from which the physician intends to obtain the sample of bone marrow.

- Position the client on his or her back or side to facilitate access to the aspiration site.

- Suggest distraction techniques to avoid focusing on the pressure or discomfort associated with puncturing the bone.

- Label the specimen and ensure its delivery to the laboratory.

- Follow Standard Precautions when there is a potential for contact with blood from the client, equipment, and bedside environment.

- Limit the client's activity for approximately 30 minutes after the procedure.

- Monitor the puncture site frequently for continued bleeding; change or reinforce the dressing as needed.

- Report prolonged bleeding, unusual pain at the site, and signs of an infection.

NURSING MANAGEMENT

The nurse collects appropriate data to assist the physician in diagnosing hematologic or lymphatic disorders and the client's response to treatment. Before any diagnostic testing, the nurse determines the client's knowledge of the procedure and offers a description of the test routine, what tasks are necessary to participate in the test, and what discomfort is likely.

The nurse wears gloves when collecting specimens. After collection, he or she checks the specimen for the correct label and immediately takes it to the laboratory. When the test involves a puncture, the nurse assesses the area for excessive bleeding and applies pressure or a pressure dressing to the site as needed. The nurse monitors vital signs to assess the client's recovery, notifies the physician regarding adverse responses, and analyzes and reports test results promptly.

GENERAL NUTRITIONAL CONSIDERATIONS

In addition to iron, vitamin B_{12}, and folic acid, several other nutrients are involved in erythrocyte production. Vitamin C enhances the absorption of folic acid and iron. Vitamin B_6 serves as a coenzyme in hemoglobin formation, and copper is involved in the transfer of iron from storage to plasma. Hemoglobin is made from protein, as are the enzymes involved in RBC production. The exact roles of vitamins A and E are not clear.

GENERAL PHARMACOLOGIC CONSIDERATIONS

Many pharmacologic agents affect the hematopoietic system, causing a decrease in various blood components.

Closely monitor clients taking medications that depress the hematopoietic system, particularly thrombocytes and leukocytes, for signs of leukopenia (fever, sore throat, chills) and thrombocytopenia (unusual or easy bleeding, oozing from injection sites, bleeding gums, dark, tarry stools).

The drug epoetin alfa (Epogen) can be used to stimulate the production of RBCs. Filgrastim (Neupogen) promotes proliferation of neutrophils.

GENERAL GERONTOLOGIC CONSIDERATIONS

The components of blood change only slightly with age. RBCs become slightly less flexible and fewer in number.

With age, lymphocytes decrease in number, causing a decreased resistance to infection.

The Schilling test may pose a problem in older adults if proper collection of the 24-hour specimen is not possible as a result of cognitive problems or urinary incontinence.

Critical Thinking Exercises

1. *Describe the process of blood cell formation.*
2. *Describe the nurse's responsibilities when assisting with bone marrow aspiration.*
3. *Three clients have the following blood count values:*
   Client A = 80,000 platelets
   Client B = 2,400,000 RBCs
   Client C = 24,500 WBCs.
   After notifying the physician, what precautions are appropriate to institute?

References and Suggested Readings

Abramson, N. & Melton, B. (2000). Leukocytosis: Basics of clinical assessment. *American Family Physician, 62,* 2053–2060.

Bell, S. G. (1999). Back to basics: An introduction to hemoglobin physiology. *Neonatal Network: Journal of Neonatal Nursing, 18*(2), 9–15, 49–52.

Call-Schmidt, T. (2001). Interpreting lab results: A primer. *MEDSURG Nursing, 10,* 179–184.

Cohen, B. J. & Wood, D. L. (1999). *Memmler's the human body in health and disease* (9th ed.). Philadelphia: Lippincott Williams & Wilkins.

Fischbach, F. T. (1999). *A manual of laboratory and diagnostic tests* (6th ed.). Philadelphia: Lippincott Williams & Wilkins.

Kushida, T., Inaba, M., Ikebukuro, K., et al. (2000). A new method for bone marrow cell harvesting. *Stem Cells, 18,* 453–456.

Malloy, B. J. (2000). Hematopoiesis, stem cells, and transplantation: What have we learned for the new millennium? *Journal of Intravenous Nursing, 23,* 298–303.

Martini, F. H. (2001). *Fundamentals of anatomy and physiology* (5th ed.). Englewood Cliffs, NJ: Prentice Hall.

McConnell, E. A. (2000). Clinical do's and dont's: Infusing packed RBCs. *Nursing, 30*(2), 17.

Noerr, B. (1996). Pointers in practical pharmacology: Recombinant erythropoietin. *Neonatal Network: Journal of Neonatal Nursing, 15*(6), 51–59.

Porth, C. M. (2002). *Pathophysiology: Concepts of altered health states* (6th ed.). Philadelphia: Lippincott Williams & Wilkins.

Stock, W. & Hoffman, R. (2000). White blood cells 1: Nonmalignant disorders. *Lancet, 355,* 1351–1357.

Wolf, S. (1999). Evolutions/revolutions: Another source of stem cells. *RN, 62*(9), 30–34.

Caring for Clients With Disorders of the Hematopoietic System

Learning Objectives

On completion of this chapter, the reader will:

- List at least five types of anemia, including two examples of inherited types.
- Identify nutritional deficiencies that can lead to anemia.
- Discuss clinical problems that clients with any type of anemia experience.
- Discuss factors that cause sickling of erythrocytes and related adverse effects.
- List five activities a person with sickle cell disease can do to reduce the potential for a sickle cell crisis.
- Explain the term *erythrocytosis,* give one example of a characteristic disease, and list three possible complications.
- Explain how forms of leukemia are classified.
- List clinical problems or nursing diagnoses common among clients with leukemia.
- Explain the term *pancytopenia* and give one example of a disorder that represents this condition.
- Discuss the meaning of *coagulopathy* and name two coagulopathies.
- Discuss nursing responsibilities when managing the care of clients with coagulopathies.

This chapter discusses common **blood dyscrasias,** abnormalities in the numbers and types of blood cells, and **coagulopathies,** bleeding disorders that involve platelets or clotting factors. These disorders develop from various pathologic processes, some of which are life-threatening. Despite their differences, many blood disorders have similar symptoms and require similar diagnostic tests.

ANEMIA

Erythrocytes are mature red blood cells (RBCs) to which hemoglobin is attached. Their function is to carry oxygen to cells and transport carbon dioxide (CO_2) to the lungs. **Anemia** is a term that refers to a deficiency of either erythrocytes or hemoglobin. Various terms are used to

differentiate the features of erythrocytes and describe pathogenesis related to them (Table 39-1).

Most anemias result from (1) blood loss, (2) inadequate or abnormal erythrocyte production, or (3) destruction of normally formed RBCs. The most common types include hypovolemic anemia, iron deficiency anemia, pernicious anemia, folic acid deficiency anemia, sickle cell anemia, and hemolytic anemias. Although each form of anemia has unique manifestations, all share a common core of symptoms (Fig. 39-1).

● HYPOVOLEMIC ANEMIA

Hypovolemia is caused by a loss of blood volume, which results in fewer blood cells. Because erythrocytes are the

TABLE 39-1	TERMS USED TO DESCRIBE ERYTHROCYTES AND ERYTHROCYTE PATHOLOGY
DESCRIPTOR	**MEANING**
Normocytic	Normal cell size
Microcytic	Small cell size
Macrocytic	Large cell size
Megaloblastic	Large immature cell
Normochromic	Normal hemoglobin concentration
Hypochromic	Low hemoglobin concentration
Hyperchromic	High hemoglobin concentration
Aplastic	Decreased cell production
Hemolytic	Premature destruction
Pernicious	Potentially injurious

most abundant type of blood cell, one consequence of blood loss is *hypovolemic anemia.*

Pathophysiology and Etiology

A sudden loss of a large volume of blood or a gradual, chronic loss of small amounts of blood causes hypovolemic anemia. An example of the former is trauma, such as a gunshot wound; an example of the latter is gastric bleeding from a peptic ulcer. When blood is lost, the bone marrow responds by increasing its number of erythrocytes. As a result, the cells are smaller and contain less **heme,** the pigmented, iron-containing portion of hemoglobin. Consequently, the RBCs are microcytic and hypochromic (see Table 39-1). If the formation of new RBCs cannot compensate for the loss, cellular function is compromised from an inadequate oxygen supply and accumulated CO_2.

Assessment Findings

Acute hypovolemic anemia from severe blood loss is evidenced by signs and symptoms of hypovolemic shock: extreme pallor, tachycardia, hypotension, reduced urine output, and altered consciousness (see Chap. 23). Symptoms of chronic hypovolemic anemia include pallor, fatigue, chills, postural hypotension, and rapid heart and respiratory rates.

Laboratory confirmation of acute or chronic hypovolemic anemia is detected through a complete blood count (CBC), which demonstrates decreased erythrocytes, increased *reticulocytes* (erythrocytes in the process of maturation), and low hemoglobin and hematocrit levels (Table 39-2). Mean cell volume is lower than normal as a result of the smaller size of the erythrocytes. The mean cell hemoglobin concentration is below normal, reflecting the reduced hemoglobin level.

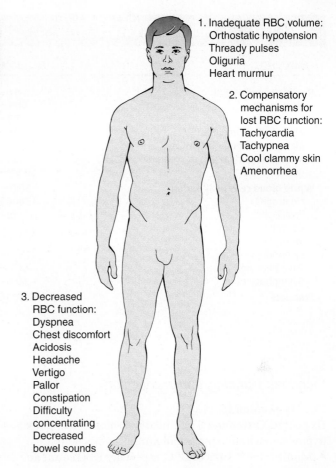

1. Inadequate RBC volume:
   Orthostatic hypotension
   Thready pulses
   Oliguria
   Heart murmur

2. Compensatory mechanisms for lost RBC function:
   Tachycardia
   Tachypnea
   Cool clammy skin
   Amenorrhea

3. Decreased RBC function:
   Dyspnea
   Chest discomfort
   Acidosis
   Headache
   Vertigo
   Pallor
   Constipation
   Difficulty concentrating
   Decreased bowel sounds

FIGURE 39-1 Clinical manifestations of anemia.

Medical Management

Treatment of sudden, severe bleeding involves replacement of blood by transfusions. If blood loss is chronic (e.g., from bleeding uterine tumors, peptic ulcer disease, hemorrhoids), the underlying condition is treated. Depending on how much blood is lost, treatment includes blood transfusion or administration of oral, intravenous (IV), or intramuscular (IM) iron to help the body compensate for the lost hemoglobin. Oxygen therapy sometimes is necessary if the anemia is severe.

NURSING PROCESS

● **The Client With Hypovolemic Anemia**

Assessment

The nurse questions the client to determine possible reasons for the presenting symptoms, obtains vital signs, reviews laboratory test results, prepares the client for diagnostic tests such as endoscopic examination, performs a physical examination to detect bleeding.

TABLE 39-2	NORMAL CBC VALUES	
COMPONENT	**ADULT MALES**	**ADULT FEMALES**
Red blood cells (erythrocytes)	4.6–6.2 million/mm³	4.2–5.4 million/mm³
Hematocrit	40%–54%	38%–47%
Hemoglobin	13.5–18 g/dl	12–16 g/dl
Mean cell volume (MCV)	80–94 µg/m³	81–99 µg/m³
Mean cell hemoglobin (MCH)	27–31 picograms/cell	27–31 picograms/cell
Mean cell hemoglobin concentration (MCHC)	32–36 g/dl	32–36 g/dl
Reticulocytes	0.5%–2.0% of RBCs	Slightly higher in females
White blood cells (leukocytes)	5000–13,000/mm³	5000–10,000/mm³
Neutrophils	3000–7500/mm³	3000–7500/mm³
Eosinophils	50–400/mm³	50–400/mm³
Basophils	25–100/mm³	25–100/mm³
Monocytes	100–500/mm³	100–500/mm³
Lymphocytes	1500–4500/mm³	1500–4500/mm³
T lymphocytes	60%–80% of lymphocytes	60%–80% of lymphocytes
B lymphocytes	10%–20% of lymphocytes	10%–20% of lymphocytes
Platelets	150,000–450,000/mm³	150,000–450,000/mm³

Diagnosis, Planning, and Interventions

PC: Hypovolemia

Expected Outcome: The nurse will monitor to detect hypovolemia and manage and minimize blood loss.

- Monitor the results of CBC, especially RBC count and hematocrit and hemoglobin levels. *Lower than normal RBCs and hemoglobin level reflect blood cell loss. The hematocrit level indicates the percentage of RBCs in the volume of whole blood.*
- Assess vital signs every 2 to 4 hours or more often if indicated. *Hypotension and tachycardia are signs of hypovolemia.*
- Report systolic blood pressure (BP) below 90 mm Hg and heart rate above 100 beats/minute (bpm). *The average adult systolic BP is 120 mm Hg. Tachycardia is a heart rate above 100 bpm.*
- Monitor intake and output accurately each shift or every hour. *Urine output is one indication of the circulating blood volume.*
- Report urine output less than 30 to 50 mL/hour. *Low urine volume reflects inadequate renal perfusion. The kidneys must excrete 30 to 50 mL/hour or 500 mL/24 hours to eliminate wastes sufficiently.*
- Use Standard Precautions to examine and test stool and body fluids for evidence of blood. *Blood may be occult (hidden) rather than obvious. Nurses commonly perform tests to detect blood in stool and body fluids.*
- In cases of hemorrhage, apply direct pressure to the bleeding site. Alternatively, apply pressure to a proximal artery. *Compression of blood vessels decreases blood loss.*
- If an IV solution is infusing, increase the rate of flow if the client is bleeding profusely. *A temporary increase in IV fluid administration compensates briefly for rapid blood loss.*
- Place the client in a modified Trendelenburg position if hypovolemic shock develops. *This position facilitates blood flow to the brain.*
- Notify the physician and be prepared to administer blood or blood products. *Crystalloid solutions do not contain blood cells (see Chap. 24). The most definitive management of hypovolemic anemia is to replace lost blood cells.*
- Supplement parenteral fluids with oral fluids, if possible. *Oral fluids contribute to intravascular fluid replacement.*

PC: Hypoxemia

Expected Outcome: The nurse will monitor to detect hypoxemia and manage and minimize inadequate oxygenation.

- Monitor oxygen saturation continually with a pulse oximeter. *It measures the percentage of oxygen bound to hemoglobin.*
- Report a sustained oxygen saturation value below 90%. *Normal oxygen saturation is 95% to 100%; clients become compromised when oxygen saturation falls below 90%.*
- Give oxygen per nasal cannula or simple mask to maintain oxygen saturation at or above 90%. *Supplemental oxygen delivers more than the 21% oxygen of room air.*

Activity Intolerance related to reduced cellular capacity to carry oxygen

Expected Outcomes: The client will (1) tolerate essential activity as evidenced by a heart rate below 100 bpm and (2) have a respiratory rate less than 28 breaths/minute.

- Limit the client's nonessential activities. *Demands for cellular oxygenation are controlled according to the available supply.*

- Distribute essential tasks over a long period. *Minimizing exertion promotes endurance.*
- Provide periods of rest. *Rest prevents acute hypoxemia.*
- Administer supplemental oxygen during periods of rapid breathing or tachycardia. *Short-term, periodic oxygen administration relieves brief episodes of hypoxemia.*

Risk for Imbalanced Body Temperature related to reduced oxygen for aerobic metabolism

Expected Outcome: Temperature will remain at 98.6°F plus or minus 1°F.

- Prevent drafts. *Air circulating over the body promotes heat loss by convection.*
- Provide additional layers of clothing or cover with warmed blankets. *Covering the client in layers of fabric keeps body heat from escaping.*
- Increase the room temperature and add humidity. *Warming the environment decreases heat loss from convection or conduction. The heat index increases when air contains moisture. Increasing environmental humidity reduces heat loss through evaporation.*
- Offer warm oral fluids. *They maintain or promote an increase in core body temperature.*

Evaluation of Expected Outcomes

Blood volume loss is minimized, RBC count and hematocrit level are within normal ranges. The client has 90% or greater saturation of hemoglobin. The client's BP and heart rate are within normal target ranges before, during, and after performing activities of daily living (ADLs). Body temperature is within 98°F to 99.5°F.

● IRON DEFICIENCY ANEMIA

Pathophysiology and Etiology

Iron deficiency anemia develops when iron is insufficient to produce hemoglobin. Examples include when (1) heme cannot be recycled because of blood loss, (2) dietary intake of iron is insufficient, (3) absorption of iron from food is inadequate, and (4) the need for iron exceeds the reserves. Even when a person consumes a healthy diet, he or she absorbs less than 10% of the iron in food. Clients whose nutrition is compromised by unhealthy dieting, or who cannot afford to eat a healthy diet, lack knowledge about nutrition, or have malabsorption disorders are at great risk for iron deficiency anemia. The need for iron increases during periods of rapid growth, pregnancy, and the female reproductive years when intermittent blood loss accompanies menses.

When iron deficiency develops, the iron stores in the body are depleted first, followed by reduced hemoglobin. The result is smaller (microcytic) and fewer RBCs, which leads to manifestations of anemia. Reduced hemoglobin, for whatever reason, compromises the oxygen-carrying capacity of RBCs. Without sufficient oxygen, cells must switch to anaerobic metabolism, which is less efficient than aerobic metabolism at producing energy and sustaining functions at the cellular level.

Assessment Findings

Most clients with iron deficiency anemia have reduced energy, feel cold all the time, and experience fatigue and dyspnea with minor physical exertion. The heart rate usually is rapid even at rest. The CBC and hemoglobin, hematocrit, and serum iron levels are decreased. A blood smear reveals erythrocytes that are *microcytic* (smaller than normal) and *hypochromic* (lighter in color than normal). Other laboratory and diagnostic tests (e.g., stool examination for occult blood) reveal the source of blood loss.

Medical Management

Treatment aims at determining the cause and, when possible, eliminating it. Correction of a faulty diet by adding foods high in iron is an important aspect of treatment (see General Nutritional Considerations). In some instances, an oral supplement or parenteral administration of iron is prescribed. In severe cases, a blood transfusion is necessary.

Nursing Management

The nurse focuses on improving the client's nutritional intake of iron. The nurse takes a dietary history and collaborates with the dietitian to resolve dietary deficiencies (see Chap. 16 and the General Nutritional Considerations at the end of this chapter). He or she implements medical treatment that involves oral or parenteral iron supplementation. If a client is taking an oral iron supplement, the nurse instructs as follows:

- Dilute liquid preparations of iron with another liquid such as juice and drink with a straw to avoid staining the teeth.
- Take iron with or immediately after meals to avoid gastric distress.
- Avoid taking iron simultaneously with an antacid, which interferes with iron absorption.
- Check with the physician or pharmacist about combining iron with other prescribed or over-the-counter medications to determine appropriate absorption of each.
- Drink orange juice or take other forms of vitamin C with iron to promote its absorption.
- Expect iron to color stool dark green or black.
- Consult the prescribing physician if constipation or diarrhea develops.

- Keep medications containing iron out of the reach of small children, for whom an accidental poisoning may be fatal.

The nurse uses the Z-track technique to administer IM iron (Nursing Guidelines 39-1). For a review of blood transfusion, see Chapter 24. Discharge instructions include pacing activities to minimize fatigue and providing information about oral medications and medical follow-up to determine if the client's hemoglobin level stabilizes within normal limits.

Stop, Think, and Respond ● **BOX 39-1**

Why does the nurse use the Z-track method to administer parenteral iron?

● SICKLE CELL ANEMIA

Sickle cell anemia is so named because erythrocytes become sickle- or crescent-shaped when oxygen supply in the blood is inadequate (Fig. 39-2).

Pathophysiology and Etiology

Hemoglobin A (HbA) normally replaces fetal hemoglobin (HbF) about 6 months after birth. In those with sickle cell anemia, however, an abnormal form of hemoglobin, hemoglobin S (HbS), replaces HbF. HbS causes RBCs to assume a sickled shape under hypoxic conditions.

Sickle cell disease is a hereditary disease found primarily in African Americans but also in people from Mediter-

---

NURSING GUIDELINES 39-1

Administering an Intramuscular Injection by Z-Track Technique

1. Check the medical orders. Read and compare the label on the drug container with the medical order or medication administration record at least three times.

2. Check the client's identity using the identification bracelet.

3. Determine the client's understanding of the purpose and technique for the procedure.

4. Inspect the dorsogluteal site.

5. Obtain the necessary equipment.

6. Wash your hands.

7. Fill the syringe with the prescribed amount of drug and change the needle.

8. Draw up an additional 0.2 mL of air in the syringe.

9. Attach a needle that is at least 1½ to 2 inches long.

10. Don gloves.

11. Position the client on the abdomen or side depending on which injection site you use.

12. Using the side of your hand, pull the tissue laterally about 1 inch (2.5 cm) until it is taut (see Figure A). Swab the site with an alcohol pledget.

13. Insert the needle at a 90° angle while continuing to hold the tissue laterally (see Figure B).

14. Steady the barrel of the syringe with the fingers and use the thumb to manipulate the plunger.

15. Aspirate for a blood return.

16. Instill the medication by depressing the plunger with the thumb.

17. Wait 10 seconds with the needle in place and the skin still held taut.

18. Withdraw the needle and immediately release the taut skin (see Figure C).

19. Apply direct pressure to the injection site with a gauze square, but do not rub it.

20. Cover the injection site with a bandage or gauze square and tape.

21. Discard the syringe without recapping the needle.

22. Remove your gloves and wash your hands.

23. Document the medication administration.

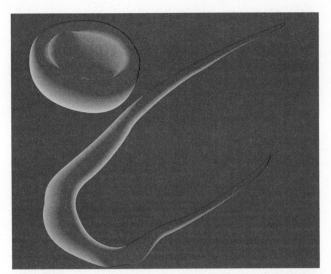

FIGURE 39-2 A normal spherical red blood cell and a sickled cell. (From Smeltzer, S. C. & Bare, B. G. [2000]. *Brunner & Suddarth's textbook of medical–surgical nursing* [9th ed.]. Philadelphia: Lippincott Williams & Wilkins.)

ranean and Middle Eastern countries. To manifest sickle cell disease, a person must inherit two defective genes, one from each parent, in which case all the hemoglobin is inherently abnormal. If the person inherits only one gene, he or she carries sickle cell trait. The hemoglobin of those who have sickle cell trait is about 40% affected. Consequently, these people are at less risk for developing signs and symptoms than their counterparts who have sickle cell disease. Many more people have sickle cell trait than have sickle cell disease.

The person with sickle cell anemia suffers from two problems: (1) episodes of *sickle cell crisis* from vascular occlusion, which develops rapidly under hypoxic conditions; and (2) chronic hemolytic anemia. During a sickle cell crisis, the sickle-shaped cells lodge in small blood vessels, where they block the flow of blood and oxygen to the affected tissue. The vascular occlusion induces severe pain in the ischemic tissue. Stroke is a common complication, even in young children.

The anemia is from the defective HbS molecule, which shortens the life span of affected erythrocytes and causes them to become hemolyzed (destroyed) prematurely. The spleen becomes obstructed and infarcted with the excess dead erythrocytes. Once the spleen is damaged, risk for infection, especially pneumonia, increases. The bone marrow enlarges to compensate for the continuous need to produce more erythrocytes. The persistent anemia causes tachycardia, dyspnea, cardiomegaly (enlargement of the heart), and dysrhythmias.

Assessment Findings

Signs and Symptoms

Evidence of the accelerated rate of erythrocyte destruction is manifested by jaundice caused by *hyperbilirubinemia* (excess bilirubin pigment in the blood; Fig. 39-3). Secondary consequences include gall stones (see Chap. 55) or a predisposition to infection when the spleen becomes dysfunctional. Anaerobic metabolism compromises growth. Chronic leg ulcers develop from the blockage of the small blood vessels of the legs. Priapism (prolonged erection)

FIGURE 39-3 Hemolysis of RBCs causes the release of heme, which becomes unconjugated bilirubin and must be conjugated in the liver for excretion into the bile. Increased amounts of bilirubin lead to bilirubinemia and jaundice.

occurs from delayed emptying of thick blood from the penis (see Chap. 61). Signs and symptoms of anemia also are present.

The reduced blood flow during sickle cell crisis leads to localized ischemia, severe pain, and possible tissue infarction (necrosis) if the oxygen supply is inadequate. Fever, pain, and swelling of one or more joints are common. Other symptoms depend on the blood vessels involved. Sickle cell crisis can lead to cerebrovascular accident, pulmonary infarction, shock, and renal failure.

Diagnostic Findings

A sickle cell screening test called the *Sickledex test* determines the presence of abnormal HbS. Hemoglobin electrophoresis determines whether the person has sickle cell disease or carries the sickle cell trait. Hemoglobin levels tend to range between 7 to 10 g/dl in those with sickle cell disease. An increase in secretory phospholipase A is a predictor of **acute chest syndrome,** a type of pneumonia triggered by decreased hemoglobin and infiltrates in the lungs.

Medical Management

Treatment is supportive rather than curative. Regular blood transfusions decrease the risk for stroke and other complications of infarction. Transfused blood, however, increases blood viscosity (thickness), which can potentially do more harm than good. It also can result in sensitization to minor antigens in donor blood—especially when the source of the donor blood is from someone of different ethnic origin than the recipient. Treatment with hydroxyurea (Hydrea, Droxia), an anticancer agent, shows evidence that it decreases sickling (Day, 2001; Porth, 2002). Hydroxyurea is toxic to RBCs with defective hemoglobin. Consequently, the body uses a yet-unknown alternative method of hematopoiesis to produce RBCs with HbF (fetal hemoglobin), present during intrauterine development through 6 months of age. Drug-induced formation of HbF, which has a high affinity for oxygen, has several benefits: it induces a milder form of the disease, decreases organ damage, protects against vaso-occlusion, and reduces early mortality (Day & Wynn, 2000).

Bone marrow transplantation has cured sickle cell disease in a few people. Researchers continue to investigate the possibility of curing sickle cell disease with gene replacement therapy, but practical application of the technique is remote at this time. Clients with sickle cell disease are subject to potentially life-threatening infections. Continuous antibiotic therapy is prescribed for some; every infection, no matter how minor, is treated promptly with antibiotics. Folic acid is prescribed to facilitate the replacement of hemolyzed erythrocytes.

During sickle cell crisis, clients are given narcotic analgesia on a scheduled basis or can self-administer it using an IV pump. Oxygen is given to relieve hypoxemia. The client must remain on complete bed rest, be hydrated with IV fluids, and may be given blood transfusions. An iron-chelating agent, such as deferoxamine (Desferal), is used to remove excess iron associated with multiple blood transfusions and erythrocyte destruction.

Stop, Think, and Respond ● BOX 39-2

What is the correlation between sickle cell anemia and stroke (cerebrovascular accident)?

N U R S I N G   P R O C E S S

● The Client With Sickle Cell Anemia

Assessment

The nurse obtains a health history focusing on previous episodes of sickle cell crisis and related complications, which may have had their onset as early as age 1 or 2 years. He or she assesses vital signs to detect evidence of infection such as fever and tachycardia. During the physical examination, the nurse observes the client's appearance, looking for evidence of dehydration, which may have triggered a sickle cell crisis (Smeltzer & Bare, 2000). He or she auscultates the lungs and heart to detect abnormal sounds suggestive of pneumonia, acute chest syndrome, and heart failure. The nurse questions the client about pain, which may be localized in the joints, bones, or abdomen, and asks the client whether the pain is similar to or different from previous events. He or she inspects the skin and sclera for jaundice and examines the extremities for ulcerations. The nurse also observes the joints for signs of swelling and collects a urine specimen, which may be concentrated and contain blood cells as a result of renal damage. He or she assesses mental status, verbal ability, and motor strength to detect stroke-related signs and symptoms. The nurse asks the client to identify the therapeutic regimen that the client has used to control or relieve symptoms to determine if the client is experiencing an exacerbation from lack of compliance, or drug toxicity if compliance is verified.

Diagnosis, Planning, and Interventions

Pain related to obstructed blood flow
Expected Outcome: Pain will be reduced or eliminated as evidenced by the client rating the pain at the low end of a numeric scale.

- Administer prescribed analgesics according to the client's level of pain (i.e., use a non-narcotic analgesic for mild or moderate pain and a narcotic analgesic for severe pain). *Categories of analgesics are efficacious for various levels of pain; the nurse selects the best drug from among those prescribed to manage the client's symptoms.*
- Handle painful joints carefully by supporting the extremity. *Aggressive and unsupported movement escalates pain.*

- Elevate swollen joints. *Elevation relieves edema through increased gravity flow.*
- Provide at least 3000 mL of fluid per day either orally or combined with parenteral solutions. *Hydration dilutes blood cells and promotes blood circulation to ischemic tissues.*
- Keep the skin warm with prewarmed or layered blankets. *Warmth promotes vasodilation.*
- Give oxygen according to the physician's orders. *Supplemental oxygen relieves hypoxemia and reduces the potential for sickling and organ infarction.*
- Use nonpharmacologic methods to relieve pain such as imagery and distraction. *Diverting attention and helping the client concentrate on something pleasant or unrelated to the pain can blunt pain perception.*
- Be prepared to administer whole blood if prescribed. *Donated blood provides RBCs with normal hemoglobin, which improves oxygenation of tissues and relieves ischemic pain.*
- Administer prescribed doses of hydroxyurea. *Hydroxyurea switches production of HbS to HbF.*

Risk for Infection related to increased susceptibility to pathogens secondary to dysfunction of the spleen
Expected Outcome: Client will be free of infection.

- Perform conscientious handwashing. *It is one of the best measures to prevent spread of pathogens.*
- Advise visitors who are ill or have a respiratory infection to delay visiting the client. *Pathogens are transmitted by direct contact, droplets, or air transmission.*
- Recommend influenza and pneumococcal vaccines when the client's health improves. *Immunizations reduce the potential for pulmonary infections.*
- Teach the client aseptic techniques for managing open skin lesions. *Impaired skin provides an opportunity for colonization by infectious microorganisms.*

Evaluation of Expected Outcomes

Pain is absent or controlled within a level that facilitates ADLs. The client's temperature and white blood cell (WBC) count support that the client is free of infection. There is no evidence of cough, respiratory distress, or purulent drainage from skin lesions.

Stop, Think, and Respond ● **BOX 39-3**

What are the differences between HbF, HbA, and HbS?

● HEMOLYTIC ANEMIA

The term *hemolytic anemia* refers to the consequence of a widely diverse group of conditions, some acquired, some hereditary, and some idiopathic, in which there is chronic premature destruction of erythrocytes.

39-1 *Client and Family Teaching*
Sickle Cell Anemia

The nurse teaches clients with sickle cell anemia and their families as follows:

- Keep all medical appointments to determine the best drugs and dosages and to detect any developing drug toxicities.
- Never exceed the recommended dosages of analgesics, especially narcotic analgesics, and avoid self-medicating with illegal substances.
- Consume a liberal amount of fluids.
- Dress warmly in cold temperatures.
- Avoid vigorous physical exercise and leg positions or clothing that cause vasoconstriction.
- Stop smoking or other use of nicotine.
- Avoid travel to places with high altitudes.
- Obtain immunizations for pneumococcal pneumonia and influenza caused by *Haemophilus influenzae*.
- See a physician at the first sign of infection.
- Be aware that pregnancy creates risks for maternal and fetal complications. Obtain genetic testing and counseling before conceiving children.

Pathophysiology and Etiology

Some examples of conditions that can produce hemolytic anemia are the use of cardiopulmonary bypass during surgery; arsenic or lead poisoning; invasion of erythrocytes by the malaria parasite, infectious agents; or toxins and exposure to hazardous chemicals. Other causes include the production of antibodies that destroy erythrocytes. Antibodies can be produced against antigens from another person, such as is seen in blood transfusion reactions, as well as against the body's own erythrocytes. As the number of destroyed blood cells increases, the potential for hyperbilirubinemia (excess bilirubin) and jaundice also increases.

Assessment Findings

Symptoms are similar to those associated with hypovolemic anemia. In more severe forms of hemolytic anemia, the client is jaundiced and the spleen is enlarged. In some cases, hemolysis is so extensive that it causes shock.

Microscopic examination reveals erythrocyte fragments. When an erythrocyte survival study is performed using radioactive chromium, the life span of erythrocytes is 10 days or less. Reaction on a direct Coombs' test (direct antiglobulin test) is positive when the hemolytic anemia results from a transfusion reaction, use of certain drugs, or production of antibodies against the erythrocytes.

Medical and Surgical Management

Treatment includes removing the cause (when possible) and administering corticosteroids. In some cases the steroid dose can be reduced and then discontinued after several weeks. Blood transfusions often are necessary. Splenectomy is performed if the client fails to respond to medical treatment.

Nursing Management

The nurse obtains a comprehensive health history to help determine the cause of the hemolysis. Until the cause is determined, the nurse provides supportive care to help the client meet basic needs. When the diagnosis is confirmed, he or she implements the medical regimen for treatment and prepares the client for discharge by teaching measures for self-care. The nurse arranges the plan for follow-up evaluations and shares the information with the client.

● THALASSEMIAS

Thalassemias are hereditary hemolytic anemias. They are divided into two major groups: alpha-thalassemias and beta-thalassemias. Alpha-thalassemias are found in people from Southeast Asia and Africa; beta-thalassemias are found in people from Mediterranean islands and the Po Valley in Italy.

Assessment Findings

Clients with alpha-thalassemias typically are asymptomatic, as are those with minor forms of beta-thalassemia. Clients with Cooley's anemia, a severe form of beta-thalassemia, exhibit symptoms of severe anemia and a bronzing of the skin caused by hemolysis of erythrocytes. Diagnosis is based on symptoms and the results of hemoglobin electrophoresis.

Medical Management

Treatment of the various forms of thalassemia is symptomatic. Clients usually require frequent transfusions. Those with Cooley's anemia require iron chelation therapy because of the iron deposits in the skin.

Nursing Management

When anemia is severe, the nurse places the client on bed rest and protects him or her from contact with those who have infections. When transfusions are necessary, the nurse closely monitors the rate of administration.

● PERNICIOUS ANEMIA

Pernicious anemia develops when a client lacks intrinsic factor, which normally is present in stomach secretions. Intrinsic factor is necessary for absorption of vitamin B_{12}. Vitamin B_{12}, the extrinsic factor in blood, is required for the maturation of erythrocytes.

Pathophysiology and Etiology

The production of intrinsic factor decreases with aging and gastric mucosal atrophy. It also decreases secondary to surgical removal of the stomach or small bowel resection, in which the ileum (site for vitamin B_{12} absorption) is removed. Without adequate vitamin B_{12}, erythrocytes remain in an immature form. If the condition is not recognized and treated promptly, degenerative changes in the nervous system develop. Sometimes permanent damage occurs before treatment begins.

Assessment Findings

Signs and Symptoms

In addition to the usual symptoms of anemia, some clients with pernicious anemia develop stomatitis (inflammation of the mouth) and glossitis (inflammation of the tongue), digestive disturbances, and diarrhea. Anemia may be so severe that dyspnea occurs with minimal exertion. Jaundice, irritability, confusion, and depression are present when the disease is severe. Mental changes usually disappear with treatment. Numbness and tingling in the arms and legs and ataxia are common signs of neurologic involvement. Some affected clients lose vibratory and position senses.

Diagnostic Findings

Diagnosis is established by the client's history, symptoms, and blood and bone marrow studies. The Schilling test is used to confirm the diagnosis. Microscopic examination of a blood smear reveals many large, immature erythrocytes.

Medical Management

Vitamin B_{12} is given IM in a dose adequate to control the disease. Therapy must continue for life. No toxic effects have been noted from the use of vitamin B_{12}. Oral vitamin B_{12} seldom is effective, except for short intervals. Iron therapy seldom is needed because mature erythrocytes are manufactured and the hemoglobin level is normal when the condition is corrected. Clients with permanent neurologic deficits benefit from physical therapy.

Nursing Management

If glossitis and stomatitis are present, a soft, bland diet relieves the discomfort associated with eating. Most clients better tolerate small, frequent meals than three large meals. Meticulous oral care after eating is essential to remove particles of food that may irritate the mucosal lining and increase soreness.

If a permanent neurologic deficit has occurred, the nurse encourages the client to move about as much as possible to prevent complications associated with immobility, such as contractures and pressure ulcer formation. Assistance with ambulation is necessary because some clients have difficulty walking and are prone to falling. If behavioral changes occur, close supervision is necessary. The nurse emphasizes the importance of lifelong administration of vitamin B_{12}. He or she teaches a family member of the client how to administer vitamin B_{12} injections or refers the client to a home health nursing service.

● FOLIC ACID DEFICIENCY ANEMIA

Folic acid deficiency causes anemia that is characterized by immature erythrocytes.

Pathophysiology and Etiology

A folic acid deficiency commonly is related to an insufficient dietary intake of folic acid (vitamin B_9). Older adults and clients with alcoholism, intestinal disorders that affect food absorption, malignant disorders, and chronic illnesses often have a folic acid deficiency because of poor nutrition. Certain drugs, such as anticonvulsants and methotrexate, are folic acid antagonists and interfere with folic acid absorption. Because pregnant women and clients with chronic hemolytic anemias have increased folic acid requirements, they can experience a folic acid deficiency even when they follow a normal diet. Prolonged IV therapy and total parenteral nutrition also can result in a folic acid deficiency.

Assessment Findings

Severe fatigue, a sore and beefy-red tongue, dyspnea, nausea, anorexia, headaches, weakness, and lightheadedness occur. Blood test results reveal low hemoglobin and hematocrit levels. The serum folate level is decreased. A Schilling test differentiates pernicious anemia and anemia caused by a folic acid deficiency.

Medical Management

Oral or parenteral folic acid supplements are provided. Parenteral administration is required for clients with an intestinal malabsorption disorder. A well-balanced diet that includes foods high in folic acid content such as beef liver, peanut butter, red beans, oatmeal, asparagus, and broccoli is recommended.

Nursing Management

The nurse encourages the client to eat foods high in folic acid. He or she encourages eating soft, bland foods and performing good oral hygiene. If fatigue is a prominent symptom, the nurse plans adequate rest periods between activities.

ERYTHROCYTOSIS

● POLYCYTHEMIA VERA

There are some conditions in which one of the primary characteristics is **erythrocytosis,** an increase in circulating erythrocytes. One of these conditions is *polycythemia vera,* which is characterized by a greater than normal number of erythrocytes, leukocytes, and platelets. For people who live at high altitudes, erythrocytosis is a normal phenomenon and usually requires no treatment.

Pathophysiology and Etiology

Polycythemia vera is associated with a rapid proliferation of blood cells produced by the bone marrow. The cause of this accelerated production is unknown. Polycythemia vera usually has an insidious onset and a prolonged course. Despite the abundance of erythrocytes, their life span is shorter. The dead erythrocytes release intracellular potassium, which can cause hyperkalemia, and uric acid, which causes goutlike joint symptoms. The oxygen-combining capacity of the erythrocytes is impaired, which compromises cellular oxygenation. The increased number of erythrocytes makes the blood more viscous than normal and increases the likelihood for the development of thrombi in small blood vessels. Complications include hypertension, congestive heart failure, stroke, areas of infarction, and hemorrhage.

Assessment Findings

Signs and Symptoms

The face and lips are reddish-purple. Fatigue, weakness, headache, pruritus, exertional dyspnea, and dizziness are common. Excessive bleeding after minor injuries, perhaps because of the engorgement of the capillaries and veins, occurs. Hemorrhoids develop. Splenomegaly (enlargement of the spleen) is common. The joints become swollen and painful because of elevated uric acid levels.

Diagnostic Findings

The blood cell count, especially erythrocytes, is elevated, with a similar rise in hemoglobin and hematocrit levels. The platelet and WBC counts are increased. Levels of serum potassium and uric acid are above normal.

Medical Management

Treatment involves measures to reduce the volume of circulating blood, lessen its viscosity, and curb the excessive production of erythrocytes. A phlebotomy (opening a vein to withdraw blood) is done several times a week; 500 mL of blood is removed each time. Anticoagulants are prescribed to reduce the potential for forming clots. Radiophosphorus and radiation therapy can be used to decrease the production of erythrocytes in the bone marrow. Antineoplastic drugs such as mechlorethamine (Mustargen) are given to curb excessive bone marrow activity.

Nursing Management

The nurse observes the client for complications and provides information about drug therapy and techniques to promote circulation and reduce potential thrombi formation. The plan of care includes the following measures:

- Advise drinking 3 quarts (L) of fluid per day. *Adequate hydration promotes venous return and ensures sufficient urine production.*
- Teach the client to avoid crossing the legs at the knee and wearing tight clothing. *Restricting blood circulation increases the risk for thrombus formation.*
- Encourage the client to be physically active, change positions frequently, and elevate the lower extremities as much as possible. *Movement and leg elevation promotes the circulation of venous blood.*

- Teach the client how to perform isometric exercises such as contracting and relaxing the quadriceps and gluteal muscles during periods of inactivity. *Contraction of skeletal muscles compresses the walls of veins and increases the circulation of venous blood as it returns to the heart.*
- Help the client don thromboembolic stockings or support hose during waking hours. *Compression of veins promotes venous circulation and prevents the formation of thrombi.*
- Tell the client to rest immediately if chest pain develops. *Chest pain indicates myocardial ischemia. Rest reduces the work of the heart and restores sufficient oxygenated blood flow to overcome the temporary deficiency.*

LEUKOCYTOSIS

Leukocytosis is an increased number of leukocytes above normal limits. Contrary to wound healing, when increased leukocytes serve as a protective mechanism, in some disease conditions such as leukemia the proliferation of leukocytes is detrimental.

● LEUKEMIA

Leukemia refers to any malignant blood disorder in which proliferation of leukocytes, usually in an immature form, is unregulated. There often is an accompanying decrease in production of erythrocytes and platelets. There are four general types of leukemia, classified according to the bone marrow stem cell line that is dysfunctional (Table 39-3). Acute and chronic lymphocytic leukemias result from bone marrow dysfunction that affects lymphoid stem cells; the primary marrow dysfunction in acute and chronic myelocytic leukemia is in myeloid stem cells (Fig. 39-4).

TABLE 39-3	TYPES OF LEUKEMIA		
TYPE	**CELLULAR CHARACTERISTICS**		**AGE OF ONSET (YR)**
Acute lymphocytic (ALL)	Increased immature lymphocytes Normal or decreased granulocytes Decreased erythrocytes Decreased platelets		Younger than 5; uncommon after 15
Chronic lymphocytic (CLL)	Same as above, but erythrocyte and platelet counts may be normal or low		Older than 40; most common type in adults
Acute myelogenous (AML)	Decrease in all myeloid formed cells: monocytes, granulocytes, erythrocytes, and platelets		Occurs in all age ranges
Chronic myelogenous (CML)	Same as above, but greater number of normal cells than in acute form		Older than 20, but incidence increases with age; genetic link in 90% to 95% of cases

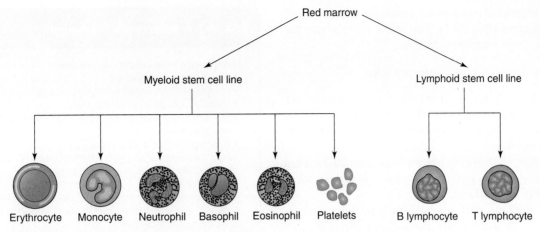

FIGURE 39-4 Maturation of myeloid and lymphoid stem cells.

Pathophysiology and Etiology

The cause of leukemia is unknown, although exposures to toxic chemicals and radiation, viruses, and certain drugs are known to precipitate the disorder. In some cases there is a genetic correlation. Although the increase in leukocytes is rampant, there are many more immature than mature cells. Because of their immaturity, the leukocytes are ineffective at fighting infections. The rapid proliferation of leukocytes results in a decreased production of erythrocytes and platelets. The client eventually develops severe anemia, and the reduction in platelets leads to bleeding. The excessive leukocytes infiltrate the spleen, liver, lymph nodes, and brain if unchecked.

Assessment Findings

Infections, fatigue from anemia, and easy bruising are hallmarks of leukemia. At the onset of leukemia, particularly in acute lymphocytic leukemia (ALL), a fever is present, the spleen and lymph nodes enlarge, and internal or external bleeding develops. Common sites of bleeding include the nose, mouth, and gastrointestinal tract. The leukocyte count is low, normal, or high, but the number of normal leukocytes is decreased. Consequently, the number of erythrocytes and platelets decreases as well.

Medical Management

Drug therapy is the primary weapon for arresting leukemia. Years of research have led to the development of successful drug protocols using one or combinations of antineoplastic drugs. The type of drug or combination of drugs depends on the form of leukemia.

Erythrocyte and platelet transfusions are necessary to treat the anemia and decreased platelets. Antibiotics are given when secondary infections develop.

Bone marrow transplantation and stem cell transplantation have increased survival for some clients. Their source is either *autologous* (from oneself) or *allogenic* (from another; see Chap. 20). Stem cells are harvested by removing them from peripheral blood, obtaining bone marrow, or collecting cord blood from a newborn. Malignant stem cells are removed from an autologous specimen before transplantation. Toxic drugs or radiation are administered before transplantation, which renders the client extremely susceptible to infection. The client remains hospitalized for several weeks to observe if normal blood cells are eventually produced, to detect signs of *graft-versus-host disease,* in which the foreign donor cells destroy the recipient's tissues and organs, and to protect the client who is immunosuppressed from acquiring a life-threatening infection (see Chap. 20).

NURSING PROCESS

● The Client With Leukemia

Assessment

The nurse begins the initial assessment by obtaining a history of symptoms. He or she looks for a cluster of symptoms that includes weakness and fatigue, frequent infections, nosebleeds or other prolonged bleeding events, and joint pain. The nurse also looks for symptoms associated with leukocyte infiltration of the central nervous system, such as headache and confusion.

The nurse examines the client's body, looking for evidence of bruising. He or she palpates the abdomen to detect enlargement and tenderness over the liver and spleen. The nurse reviews laboratory test results, noting the numbers and types of blood cells. He or she may calculate the absolute neutrophil count to determine the client's potential for infection (Box 39-1). The nurse also assesses the outcome of bone marrow aspiration.

Diagnosis, Planning, and Interventions

Risk for Infection related to compromised immunity. **Expected Outcome:** Client will be free of infection as evidenced by normal temperature and no signs of an infectious disorder.

- Implement neutropenic precautions (Box 39-2). *They reduce exposure to pathogens that are dangerous when immunity is suppressed.*
- Ensure that any staff person, family member, or visitor who is ill temporarily discontinues direct contact with the client. *Eliminating direct contact with others who are infectious reduces the potential for transmitting microorganisms to the client.*
- Monitor temperature at lease once per shift and continually assess for signs of infection, such as swelling and tenderness, which can appear in any area or organ of the body. *Progressive hyperthermia occurs in some types of infections, and fever (unrelated to drugs or blood products) occurs in most clients with leukemia. Early intervention is essential to prevent sepsis/septicemia in immunosuppressed persons. (Note: Septicemia may occur without fever.)*

PC: Hemorrhage
Expected Outcome: The nurse will monitor for hemorrhage; if bleeding is detected, the nurse will manage and minimize it.

- Monitor the platelet count. *Suppression of bone marrow and platelet production places the client at risk for spontaneous and uncontrolled bleeding.*
- Inspect the skin for signs of bruising and petechiae; report melena, hematuria, or epistaxis (nosebleeds). *Fragile tissues and altered clotting mechanisms can result in hemorrhage after even minor trauma.*
- Handle client gently when assisting with care and encourage use of electric razors. *Trauma and microabrasions from razors can contribute to anemia from bleeding.*
- Apply prolonged pressure to needle sites or other sources of external bleeding. *Reduced platelet production results in a delayed clotting process.*

BOX 39-1 ● Calculating the Absolute Neutrophil Count

Step 1: Use the formula:

$$ANC = \frac{\% \text{ Neutrophils} + \% \text{ Bands}}{100} \times \text{Total white blood cell count}$$

Step 2: Interpret results:

ANC of 999 to 500 = risk for infection
ANC of 499 to 100 = high risk for infection
ANC of 99 or less = almost certain development of infection

BOX 39-2 ● Neutropenic Precautions

To help prevent infection in clients with neutropenia:
- Place the client in a private room.
- Always wash hands before touching the client; encourage client to remind all staff and visitors to wash hands.
- Tell client to wash his or her hands before and after eating and after using the bathroom.
- Encourage the client to shower daily.
- Place a mask over client's mouth and nose if leaving the room; minimize time client spends in crowded areas.
- Ensure that no raw fruits or vegetables are served.
- Minimize invasive procedures (schedule all blood work to be drawn at one time of the day; discontinue invasive lines as soon as possible).
- Tell client not to handle flowers.

39-2 *Client and Family Teaching* Leukemia

If the client is to take medication at home, the nurse explains the dosage schedule because compliance is essential to treat the disease successfully. If untoward effects occur, the healthcare team will make every effort to control the symptoms while continuing chemotherapy. The nurse includes the following points in a teaching plan:

- Frequent examinations of the blood and sometimes the bone marrow are necessary to monitor the results of therapy. (The nurse emphasizes the importance of these examinations to promote wellness rather than focusing on possible complications from drug therapy.)
- Take precautions to avoid physical injury.
- Avoid exposure to people who have infections (e.g., colds).
- Seek medical care promptly if excessive bleeding or bruising or symptoms of illness or infection occur.
- Obtain sufficient rest and eat an adequate diet to prevent secondary infections.
- When feeling well, continue usual activities unless the physician instructs otherwise.
- If sores in the mouth occur, contact the physician as soon as possible. Do not self-treat this problem.
- Contact the physician immediately about any of the following: severe nausea with prolonged vomiting, severe diarrhea, fever, chills, excessive bleeding or bruising, cough, chest pain, cloudy urine, rash, blood in the stool or urine, severe headache, extreme fatigue, increased respiratory rate or difficulty breathing, and rapid pulse rate.
- Follow the physician's recommendations to monitor temperature and weight.
- Keep all clinic or office appointments.

- Implement physician orders for transfusions of blood and platelets. *Transfusion restores and normalizes the cell count and oxygen-carrying capacity of RBCs to correct anemia and prevent and treat hemorrhage.*

Activity Intolerance related to hypoxia

Expected Outcomes: The client will (1) tolerate essential activity as evidenced by a heart rate below 100 bpm and (2) have a respiratory rate less than 28 breaths/minute.

For interventions, see the discussion that accompanies anemia.

Risk for Disturbed Body Image related to hair loss secondary to chemotherapy

Expected Outcome: Client will cope with hair loss and changing body image.

- Provide opportunity for client to express feelings about hair loss and changing body image; offer suggestions such as scarves, turbans, baseball caps, or wigs. *Head coverings may increase self-esteem and foster more interactions with others.*

Anxiety and Fear related to unfamiliar experiences and unknown prognosis

Expected Outcome: Anxiety and fear will be relieved as evidenced by the client's report of emotional comfort.

- Acknowledge your awareness of the client's anxieties and fears. *Open communication validates and communicates acceptance of the client's feelings.*

- Encourage the client to talk about the disorder and its potential and actual effects. *Vocalizing inner feelings helps identify each client's specific emotional response to the disease and treatment.*

- Explain the plan of care and all treatment procedures. *Explaining the purpose, goal, and plan of care promotes confidence that the healthcare team is dedicated to resolving the illness.*

- Give encouragement and emotional support, and foster hope without implying unrealistic expectations. *A positive attitude sends a message of caring and optimism. Fostering unrealistic hope is not helpful and may significantly decrease the trust that the client places in the healthcare provider.*

Evaluation of Expected Outcomes

Expected outcomes include that the client does not acquire an infection and experiences no or minimal blood loss. He or she tolerates activity between periods of rest. The client adapts to changes in body image and copes with anxiety and fears.

MULTIPLE MYELOMA

Multiple myeloma is a malignancy involving plasma cells, which are B-lymphocyte cells in bone marrow. The prognosis is poor, with an estimated survival of 1 to 5 years after diagnosis.

Pathophysiology and Etiology

The exact triggering mechanism for the disorder is unknown. Multiple myeloma is associated with aging, recurrent infections, drug allergies, and exposure to occupational toxins and radiation (Porth, 2002). Onset is rare before age 40 years. The abnormal plasma cells proliferate in the bone marrow, where they release osteoclast activating factor. This in turn causes osteoclasts to break down bone cells, resulting in increased blood calcium and pathologic fractures. The plasma cells also form single or multiple *osteolytic* (bone-destroying) tumors that produce a "punched-out" or "honeycombed" appearance in bones such as the spine, ribs, skull, pelvis, femurs, clavicles, and scapulae. Weakened vertebrae lead to compression of the spine accompanied by significant pain.

The malignant plasma cells release two types of abnormal proteins. In the process of being excreted by the kidneys, Bence Jones proteins impair renal tubules, causing renal failure. The other protein, called *M-type globulin*, compromises production of functional immunoglobulins (also known as *antibodies*), thus interfering with an optimal immune response (see Chap. 41). The excess production of plasma cells reduces the formation of erythrocytes and platelets, causing anemia and increasing the risk for bleeding. In addition to infection, which may cause death, those with multiple myeloma experience thrombotic complications such as clot formation in the deep veins of the legs, pulmonary embolism, and stroke caused by increased viscosity of the blood.

Assessment Findings

Signs and Symptoms

The first symptom usually is vague pain in the pelvis, spine, or ribs. As the disease progresses, the pain becomes more severe and localized. The pain intensifies with activity and is relieved by rest. When tumors replace bone marrow, pathologic fractures develop. The client may have an unusually high incidence of infection, especially pneumonia, caused by decreased production of appropriate antibodies. The client may experience symptoms typically associated with anemia: weakness, fatigue, and chills. Bruising and nosebleeds are evidence of decreased platelets. Renal calculi (stones) may develop from hypercalcemia and renal failure.

Diagnostic Findings

Skeletal radiographic studies reveal characteristic bone lesions (Fig. 39-5). Blood cell counts are abnormally low. Serum calcium levels are elevated from bone destruction. Urine samples are positive for Bence Jones protein. Bone marrow aspiration demonstrates increased atypical plasma cells. The uric acid level is elevated from cellular destruction.

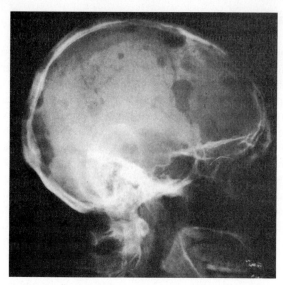

FIGURE 39-5 Multiple myeloma. A radiograph of the skull shows numerous "punched out" radiolucent areas (From Rubin, E. & Farber, J. L. [1999]. *Pathology* [3rd ed.]. Philadelphia: Lippincott Williams & Wilkins.)

Medical Management

Steroids and anticancer drugs, like melphalan (Alkeran) and cyclophosphamide (Cytoxan), and radiation are used to decrease the tumor mass and lessen bone pain. Remission occurs in approximately 60% of clients (Copstead & Banasik, 1999). Analgesics control pain; stronger narcotic analgesics are reserved for the terminal stages of the disease. Allopurinol (Zyloprim) is used to prevent uric acid crystallization and subsequent renal calculus formation. See Chapter 64 for a discussion of the management of renal failure.

Anemia is treated with blood transfusions, and infections are managed with antibiotics. Back braces are necessary when the spine is involved, and body casts are used when involvement is extensive and causes pathologic fractures.

Autologous bone marrow and peripheral stem cell transplants are now considered standard care for clients with multiple myeloma. Since October 2000, Medicare payment for transplants has been approved for those who are newly diagnosed, are younger than 78 years, and have not responded to prior therapy (International Myeloma Foundation, 2000). Research shows that those who receive a bone marrow or stem cell transplant early in the disease have approximately 39 months of disease-free survival.

Nursing Management

The nurse assesses the client frequently for pain, signs of infection, excessive fatigue, bleeding, thrombus formation, and changes in the quantity or quality of urine production. He or she administers prescribed analgesics for effective pain management. The nurse assists the client with ambulation because immobility can worsen loss of calcium from the bone. He or she provides up to 4000 mL of fluid to prevent renal damage from hypercalcemia and precipitation of protein in the renal tubules. The nurse documents and reports signs suggestive of calculus formation in the kidney, ureters, or bladder (see Chaps. 64 and 65).

Safety is paramount because any injury, no matter how slight, can result in a fracture. When pain is severe, the nurse delays position changes and bathing until an administered analgesic has reached its peak concentration level and the client is experiencing maximum pain relief. The nurse takes measures to reduce the potential for infection.

AGRANULOCYTOSIS

Agranulocytosis refers specifically to a decreased production of granulocytes, including neutrophils, basophils, and eosinophils. This is opposed to **leukopenia,** which is a general reduction in all WBCs. Decreased granulocytes place the client at risk for infection.

Pathophysiology and Etiology

The most common cause of agranulocytosis is toxicity from drugs such as sulfonamides, chloramphenicol (Chloromycetin), antineoplastics, and some psychotropic medications.

Assessment Findings

Fatigue, fever, chills, headache, and opportunistic infections in the mouth, throat, nose, rectum, or vagina can develop.

Medical Management

Treatment includes removal of the cause, such as discontinuing the drug that is producing agranulocytosis. The prognosis is related to the condition's cause and severity. When the cause can be determined and promptly removed, the client usually recovers. Some clients improve after receiving filgrastim (Neupogen), a drug that supplies human granulocyte colony-stimulating factor.

Nursing Management

The nurse determines the names of all drugs (prescription and nonprescription) the client has used in the past 6 to 12 months. Protective isolation is necessary if the leukocyte count is extremely low. Visitors or staff with any type of an infection are restricted from close client contact until the infection has cleared.

PANCYTOPENIA

Pancytopenia refers to conditions such as aplastic anemia in which numbers of all marrow-produced blood cells are reduced.

● APLASTIC ANEMIA

Aplastic anemia is more than just a deficiency of erythrocytes, although rarely that is the case. Its name is derived from the word **aplasia,** which means "failure to develop." Usually it is manifested by insufficient numbers of erythrocytes, leukocytes, and platelets, collectively described as *pancytopenia.*

Pathophysiology and Etiology

Aplastic anemia is a consequence of inadequate stem cell production in the bone marrow. In some cases, the cause of the disorder is never determined, but it may be autoimmune (self-destroying) in nature (see Chap. 42). In many cases, the bone marrow becomes dysfunctional from exposure to toxic chemicals, radiation, and drug therapy with anticancer drugs and some antibiotics. Clients with aplastic anemia are very ill, and the death rate is high if the bone marrow has been severely damaged.

Assessment Findings

Clients with aplastic anemia experience all the typical characteristics of anemia (weakness and fatigue). In addition, they have frequent opportunistic infections plus coagulation abnormalities that are manifested by unusual bleeding, small skin hemorrhages called *petechiae,* and *ecchymoses* (bruises). The spleen becomes enlarged with an accumulation of the client's blood cells destroyed by lymphocytes that failed to recognize them as normal cells, or with an accumulation of dead transfused blood cells. The blood cell count shows insufficient numbers of blood cells. A bone marrow aspiration confirms that the production of stem cells is suppressed.

Medical Management

In some instances, withdrawal of the causative agent allows the bone marrow to regenerate and assume normal function. Transfusions of whole blood, packed cells, and platelets are given to boost circulating blood cells. Antibiotics are administered to prevent or treat infection. High doses of corticosteroids that suppress the immune system are given in cases of an autoimmune connection. Bone marrow transplantation is considered if a matching donor can be found; otherwise, stem cell transplantation is an alternative.

Nursing Management

The nurse assesses for signs of severe anemia, infection, and bleeding tendencies. He or she makes every effort to prevent infection. If the leukocyte count is extremely low, the nurse implements special isolation procedures, such as restricting visitors and using a laminar airflow room.

The nurse includes soft foods in the diet and modifies oral hygiene techniques to prevent bleeding from the gums. He or she collaborates with the physician concerning alternative routes for drugs administered parenterally. If that is not possible, the nurse applies additional pressure to any punctures from injections or sites where IV fluids are administered and discontinued. The nurse monitors the client closely during blood transfusions because the risk for a reaction increases with the repeated introduction of foreign cells from multiple blood donors.

COAGULOPATHIES

The term *coagulopathy* refers to conditions in which a component that is necessary to control bleeding (Fig. 39-6) is missing or inadequate. Two common examples are thrombocytopenia and hemophilia. For information on disseminated intravascular coagulation, a condition in which hypercoagulation (excessive clot formation) is followed by diffuse bleeding as clotting factors are exhausted, refer to texts on trauma and critical care nursing.

● THROMBOCYTOPENIA

Thrombocytopenia is a lower than normal number of platelets or thrombocytes.

Pathophysiology and Etiology

Thrombocytopenia occurs when platelet manufacture by the bone marrow is decreased or platelet destruction by the spleen is increased. It accompanies leukemia and other malignant blood diseases and is caused by severe infections and certain drugs. Idiopathic thrombocytopenic purpura is thrombocytopenia without a known cause.

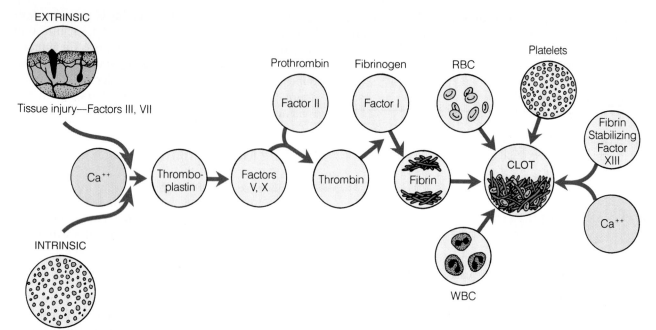

Figure 39-6 The process of clot formation. Clotting factors are identified by name and Roman numeral or by Roman numeral alone.

Assessment Findings

Thrombocytopenia is evidenced by *purpura,* small hemorrhages in the skin, mucous membranes, or subcutaneous tissues. Bleeding from other parts of the body, such as the nose, oral mucous membrane, and the gastrointestinal tract, also occurs. Internal hemorrhage, which can be severe and even fatal, is possible.

Diagnosis is based on symptoms, a low platelet count, and abnormal bleeding and clotting times. In some instances bone marrow aspiration is performed. A health history sometimes reveals agents that are associated with drug-induced thrombocytopenia.

Medical and Surgical Management

When possible, the cause is eliminated. Corticosteroids provide symptomatic relief until the platelet count returns to normal. Transfusions of platelets or whole blood are given in a hemorrhagic emergency. If spontaneous recovery does not occur, splenectomy is necessary to stop destruction of platelets in the spleen. Removal of the spleen results in a rise in the platelet count and relief of symptoms.

Clients with idiopathic thrombocytopenia often recover spontaneously. If the cause can be removed or treated, the prognosis is good. Thrombocytopenia in conjunction with illnesses such as leukemia has a poor prognosis.

Nursing Management

Refer to nursing interventions for managing and minimizing bleeding and hemorrhage discussed with leukemia. If instituting corticosteroid therapy, the nurse observes the client for adverse drug effects. He or she gradually tapers the dose and frequency of steroid medication before discontinuing it to avoid adrenal insufficiency or crisis (see Chap. 57).

● HEMOPHILIA

Hemophilia is a disorder involving clotting factors. The three types of hemophilia are hemophilia A, B, and C. Hemophilia A, the most common type, results from a deficiency of factor VIII (see Fig. 39-6). In a less serious form of hemophilia A, *von Willebrand's disease,* the amount and quality of factor VIII is diminished. Hemophilia B, or Christmas disease, is a deficiency of factor IX. Hemophilia C, also known as *Rosenthal's disease,* is a milder form of factor IX deficiency.

Pathophysiology and Etiology

Hemophilia is inherited from mother to son as a sex-linked recessive characteristic. Daughters can inherit the trait but seldom develop the disease. Women with the trait, however, can transmit it to male offspring.

The severity of hemophilia depends on the type inherited. Bleeding typically is noted in infancy and childhood. Milder forms can go unrecognized for years. The disease considerably shortens life expectancy; many clients with hemophilia do not reach adulthood. Those with mild hemophilia may lead full and productive lives despite the illness. Human immunodeficiency virus and hepatitis virus have been transmitted to clients with hemophilia through transfusion of blood and blood products. The testing of donated blood has markedly reduced the risk for acquiring blood-borne pathogens.

Assessment Findings

Persistent oozing and sometimes severe bleeding that occurs spontaneously or after an injury are manifestations of the disease. Bleeding in joints eventually damages the joints and leads to deformity and limitation of motion. Diagnosis is based on the history of symptoms and laboratory tests such as coagulant factor assay, which shows a deficiency of factor VIII or IX.

Medical Management

Treatment includes transfusions of fresh blood, frozen plasma, factor VIII concentrate, and anti-inhibitor coagulant complex for hemophilia A, factor IX concentrate for hemophilia B, and the application of thrombin to the bleeding area. Other measures used to help control bleeding are direct pressure over the bleeding site and cold compresses or ice packs.

Relatively minor surgical procedures, such as tooth extraction, carry considerable risk and are best performed in a hospital. Transfusions usually are necessary even when minor surgery is performed.

Nursing Management

The nurse obtains a comprehensive health history that includes current symptoms and treatment for the bleeding disorder. He or she questions the client about when the last episode occurred, its location (e.g., mouth, rectum, skin), duration, and what treatments, if any, were necessary. The nurse assesses the joints and mobility and inspects the skin for purpura or hemorrhagic areas. Before taking a blood pressure, the nurse asks the client if the use of a blood pressure cuff ever produced bleeding under the skin or in the arm joints. The nurse takes the temperature tympanically to avoid oral or rectal injuries. He or she checks the urine and stools for signs of bleeding.

Overall care includes preventing trauma, managing and minimizing bleeding episodes, reducing pain or discomfort, conserving energy, and helping the client learn ways to prevent further bleeding episodes. When the client requires transfusion of products such as whole blood, plasma, or antihemophilic factor for bleeding episodes, the nurse closely observes for signs that bleeding has been controlled. He or she keeps the physician informed of the client's progress because additional treatment modalities often are necessary.

The nurse explains the treatment regimen and educates the client and family as follows:

- Eliminate aspirin because this drug can increase bleeding tendencies.
- Avoid activities that can result in injury.
- Wear a Medic Alert bracelet and inform the dentist and others, when appropriate, of the condition.
- Notify the physician promptly if pain, discomfort, or obvious bleeding from the nose, rectum, in vomitus, or elsewhere occurs. Bleeding in internal organs or structures initially produces only vague symptoms.
- Use a soft toothbrush and rinse the mouth with warm water between and after meals.
- Support painful joints on pillows.

GENERAL NUTRITIONAL CONSIDERATIONS

Meat, egg yolks, oysters, shellfish, and the dark meat of poultry are sources of heme iron; its absorption is influenced by body need only. Nonheme iron found in plants represents the most common type of dietary iron. Good sources include enriched and whole-grain breads, iron-fortified cereals, legumes, nuts, greens, and brewer's yeast. Vitamin C (citrus fruits and juices, strawberries, green peppers, tomatoes), heme iron, certain animal proteins, and gastric acidity enhance the absorption of nonheme iron. Tea and coffee and various binding agents like bran in whole grains and phosphates in legumes inhibit the absorption of nonheme iron. To maximize nonheme iron absorption, the client should consume a rich source of vitamin C at every meal and avoid coffee and tea around and during mealtime.

Foods rich in folic acid include enriched breads, fortified cereals, organ meats, broccoli, green leafy vegetables, asparagus, milk, eggs, orange juice, and dried peas and beans. Vitamin C helps convert folic acid to its active form. Folic acid can reverse anemia and the gastrointestinal symptoms of B$_{12}$ deficiency; however, neurologic symptoms continue and, if untreated, can be irreversible. Ascertaining the correct cause of megaloblastic anemia before treatment begins is imperative.

GENERAL PHARMACOLOGIC CONSIDERATIONS

Because some drugs (e.g., antacids, tetracyclines, vitamin C) interact with oral iron, the client should consult the physician before taking other drugs. Absorption of oral iron decreases when a client takes the drug with coffee, tea, eggs, or milk.

Avoid the use of meperidine (Demerol) when treating pain in clients with sickle cell crisis. The liver converts meperidine to normeperidine, which is toxic. Grand mal seizures can result.

Antineoplastic agents produce many serious adverse effects. Be thoroughly familiar with the dose, administration, and adverse effects to accurately administer these drugs and competently assess the client for untoward reactions.

For folic acid anemia, therapy usually is 1 mg oral folic acid daily. An injectable form is available if absorption is a problem.

To correct iron deficiency anemia, 200 mg ferrous sulfate is given three times per day, 1 hour before meals. Therapeutic response is monitored through periodic hemoglobin and hematocrit counts.

Liquid iron preparations are available if the client cannot swallow tablets.

Transfusion is the most expensive and potentially dangerous method for replacing iron.

Pernicious anemia is treated with 100 g vitamin B$_{12}$ IM daily for 2 weeks, then 100 g IM monthly.

GENERAL GERONTOLOGIC CONSIDERATIONS

Iron deficiency anemia is unusual in older adults. Normally, the body does not eliminate excessive iron, causing total body iron stores to increase with age. If an older adult is anemic, blood loss from the gastrointestinal or genitourinary tract is suspected.

Although rare, iron deficiency anemia can develop in older adults for many reasons: living on a fixed income, being unable to shop for food, and lacking energy or motivation to prepare complete meals. These clients require a thorough evaluation of their dietary habits and education in the methods of preventing iron deficiency anemia.

Although treatments have the most success in young clients, acute leukemia is primarily a disease of older adults. ALL occurs at a rate four times higher in older adults than in children.

Pernicious anemia (vitamin B$_{12}$ deficiency) accounts for approximately 9% of all anemias in older adults. Because neurologic damage and dementia may occur before any hematologic changes are found, early detection is critical. Be sure to assess the older adult with neurologic decline or dementia for pernicious anemia.

Older adults are particularly susceptible to drug-induced hemolytic anemia because they often take more drugs than young people. Discontinuing the offending drug usually corrects the anemia.

Because older adults could forget to take medicine or could take more than prescribed, instruction or supervision in drug taking is important.

Critical Thinking Exercises

1. *List hematopoietic disorders associated with anemia and an etiology of each.*
2. *Discuss the problems that clients with anemia, leukemia, or thrombocytopenia share. What interventions can nurses use regardless of the particular disorder?*

References and Suggested Readings

Abramson, N. & Melton, B. (2000). Leukocytosis: Basics of clinical assessment. *American Family Physician, 62,* 1957–1959, 2053–2060, 2154.

Baik, H. W. & Russell, R. M. (1999). Vitamin B$_{12}$ deficiency in the elderly. *Annual Review of Nutrition, 19,* 357–377.

Bell, S. G. (1999). Back to basics: An introduction to hemoglobin physiology. *Neonatal Network: Journal of Neonatal Nursing, 18*(2), 9–15, 49–52.

Bullock, B. A. & Henze, R. L. (2000). *Focus on pathophysiology.* Philadelphia: Lippincott Williams & Wilkins.

Call-Schmidt, T. (2001). Interpreting lab results: A primer. *MEDSURG Nursing, 10*(4), 179–184.

Conley, K. & Letizia, M. (1999). Heparin-induced thrombocytopenia. *MEDSURG Nursing, 8,* 355–357.

Cook, L. S. (2000). A simple case of anemia: Pathophysiology of a common symptom. *Journal of Intravenous Nursing, 23,* 271–281.

Copstead, L. C. & Banasik, J. L. (1999). *Pathophysiology: Biological and behavioral perspectives.* Philadelphia: W.B. Saunders.

Coyne, M. A. & Lusher, J. (2000). Guidelines for emergency care of patients with hemophilia. *Emergency Medicine, 32*(4), 69–70, 73–77.

Day, M. (2001). Action stat: Sickle-cell crisis. *Nursing, 31*(5), 88.

Day, S. W. & Wynn, L. W. (2000). Sickle cell pain and hydroxyurea. *American Journal of Nursing, 100*(11), 34–39.

Derivan, M. & Ferrante, C. (2001). Clinical focus: Aplastic anemia. *Clinical Journal of Oncology Nursing, 5,* 227–229.

Fukuyama, S. N. & Itano, I. (1999). Thrombocytopenia secondary to myelosuppression. *American Journal of Nursing,* April Suppl., 5–8, 34–36.

Goldman, D. (2000). Test your knowledge: Chronic lymphocytic leukemia and its impact on the immune system. *Clinical Journal of Oncology Nursing, 4,* 233–234, 236.

Hays, K. & McCartney, S. (1998). Nursing care of the patient with chronic lymphocytic leukemia. *Seminars in Oncology, 25,* 75–79.

Held-Warmkessel, J. (1998). Chemotherapy complications. *Nursing, 28*(4), 41–46.

Holcomb, S. S. (2001). Anemia: Pointing the way to a deeper problem. *Nursing, 31*(7), 36–43.

Horrell, C. J. & Rothman, J. (2001). The etiology of thrombocytopenia. *Dimensions of Critical Care Nursing, 20*(4), 10–16.

International Myeloma Foundation. (2000). Medicare breakthrough for patients seeking a transplant for myeloma. *Blood and Marrow Transplant Newsletter, 11*(3), 1–3.

Johns, A. (1998). Overview of bone marrow and stem cell transplantation. *Journal of Intravenous Nursing, 21,* 356–360.

Loney, M. & Chernecky, C. (2000). Anemia. *Oncology Nursing Forum, 27,* 951–966.

Mackey, H. T. & Klemm, P. (2000). Leukemia: Aggressive therapies predispose patients to a host of side effects. *American Journal of Nursing,* April Suppl., 27–31, 52–54.

Maloy, B. J. (2000). Hematopoiesis, stem cells, and transplantation: What have we learned for the new millennium? *Journal of Intravenous Nursing, 23,* 298–303.

McDaniel, P. (2000). Focus on (clotting) factors. *Journal of Intravenous Nursing, 23,* 282–289.

Medoff, E. (2000). Oncology today: New horizons. Leukemia. *RN, 63*(9), 42–46, 49–50.

Onega, T. (2000). Sorting out the common anemias. *Journal of the American Academy of Physician Assistants, 13*(9), 30–32, 35–36, 39–42+.

Petersen, K. L. (1999). Diagnosing polycythemia vera. *Journal of the American Academy of Nurse Practitioners, 11,* 485–495.

Porth, C. M. (2002). *Pathophysiology: Concepts of altered health states* (6th ed.). Philadelphia: Lippincott Williams & Wilkins.

Smeltzer, S. C. & Bare, B. G. (2000). *Brunner & Suddarth's textbook of medical–surgical nursing* (9th ed.). Philadelphia: Lippincott Williams & Wilkins.

Smith, D. L. (2000). Anemia in the elderly. *American Family Physician, 62,* 1485–1487, 1565–1572, 1708.

Sobrero, A., Puglisi, F., Guglielmi, A., et al. (2001). Fatigue: A main component of anemia symptomatology. *Seminars in Oncology, 28*(2, Suppl. 8), 15–18.

Steefel, L. (2000). Easing the pain of sickle cell anemia. *Nursing Spectrum (Florida Edition), 10*(4), 25.

Stover, B. (2000). Training the client in self-management of hemophilia. *Journal of Intravenous Nursing, 23,* 304–309.

Tasota, F. J. & Tate, J. (2001). Eye on diagnostics: Interpreting the highs and lows of platelet counts. *Nursing, 31*(2), 25.

Wharton, B. (2001). Iron deficiency: What does it mean? *Professional Care of Mother and Child, 11*(1), Family Healthcare Bulletin, 6.

Wolf, S. (1999). Evolutions/revolutions: Another source of stem cells. *RN, 62*(9), 30–34.

Wright, S. M. & Finical, J. (2000). Beyond leeches: Therapeutic phlebotomy today. *American Journal of Nursing, 100*(7), 55–56, 58–59, 61+.

Yale, S. H., Nagib, N., & Guthrie, T. (2000). Approach to the vaso-occlusive crisis in adults with sickle cell disease. *American Family Physician, 61,* 1243–1246, 1349–1356, 1363–1364.

Caring for Clients With Disorders of the Lymphatic System

Words to Know

Epstein-Barr virus
Hodgkin's disease
infectious mononucleosis
lymph
lymphadenitis
lymphangitis
lymphatics
lymphedema
lymph nodes
lymphoma
non-Hodgkin's
  lymphomas
Reed-Sternberg cells

Learning Objectives

On completion of this chapter, the reader will:

- Explain the cause and characteristics of lymphedema.
- Discuss the role of the nurse when managing the care of clients with lymphedema.
- Describe nursing interventions that promote the resolution of lymphangitis and lymphadenitis.
- Explain the nature and transmission of infectious mononucleosis.
- List suggestions the nurse can offer to those who acquire infectious mononucleosis.
- Define the term *lymphoma* and name two types.
- Name the type of malignant cell diagnostic of Hodgkin's disease.
- List three forms of treatment used to cure or promote remission of lymphomas.
- Name at least four problems that nurses address when caring for clients with Hodgkin's disease and non-Hodgkin's lymphoma.

The lymphatic system is a network of vessels, known as **lymphatics,** that transport **lymph,** the watery fluid derived from plasma that exits the walls of capillaries and enters interstitial spaces. The lymphatic vessels carry the lymph to and through **lymph nodes,** clusters of bean-sized structures located primarily in the neck, axilla, chest, abdomen, pelvis, and groin. The lymph nodes contain lymphocytes and macrophages, specialized immune defensive cells, that trap, destroy, and remove infectious microorganisms, cellular debris, and cancer cells. The tonsils, thymus gland, and spleen are accessory lymphatic structures.

Most lymphatic fluid circulates with the help of skeletal muscle contraction and is returned to venous circulation through one of two ducts. The *thoracic duct,* located in the posterior abdominal cavity, collects lymph from all body areas except that which circulates above the right diaphragm and deposits the fluid into the left subclavian vein. The *right lymphatic duct* returns lymph from the right side of the head, neck, chest, and right arm and empties it into the right subclavian vein (Fig. 40-1).

Occlusive, inflammatory, infectious, or malignant disorders of the lymphatic system result in fluid distribution problems, tender and painful lymph node enlargement, compromised immune functions, or a combination of these. This chapter discusses such disorders.

Right lymphatic duct
Axillary lymph nodes
Mammary lymph vessels
Right subclavian vein
Left subclavian vein
Thoracic duct
Mesenteric lymph nodes
Cubital lymph nodes
Lumbar lymph nodes
Cisterna chyli
Iliac lymph nodes
Iliac vessels
Inguinal lymph nodes
Inguinal lymph nodes
Femoral vessels
Popliteal lymph nodes
Tibial lymph vessels

Lymph nodes and vessels of the head

Occipital lymph nodes
Cervical lymph nodes
Mandibular lymph nodes
Parotid lymph glands

The lymphatic system is made up of vessels, nodes, and ducts.

☐ The right lymphatic duct drains lymph from the upper right side of the body.
☐ The thoracic duct drains lymph from the rest of the body.

FIGURE 40-1 Lymphatic system.

OCCLUSIVE, INFLAMMATORY, AND INFECTIOUS DISORDERS ●

● LYMPHEDEMA

Pathophysiology and Etiology

Lymphedema is a condition that results from obstructed lymph circulation. Primary lymphedema usually is congenitally acquired, although manifestations usually do not appear until adolescence or early adulthood. It affects women more often than men. Secondary lymphedema develops (1) as a complication of other disorders such as repeated bouts of phlebitis and streptococcal infection,

burns, or elephantiasis (an obstructive lymphatic disorder caused by a parasite); or (2) as a consequence of treatment such as mastectomy (see Chap. 60) or radiation for cancer. The causative disorder leads to an occlusion of affected lymphatic vessels, which impairs lymph circulation and causes lymph to accumulate in the lymphatic system. The resulting edema, when massive, results in chronic deformity in locations such as the arms, legs, and genitalia, with subsequent poor nutrition to tissues.

Assessment Findings

The skin in the affected area swells, especially in a dependent position. Pitting is evident, but the tissue remains soft in the early stages. The skin eventually becomes firm, tight, and shiny. Eventually, elevation does not diminish the swelling. The skin also appears thickened, rough, and discolored. Because tissue nutrition is impaired from the stagnation of lymph fluid, ulcers and infection can develop in the edematous area. The area can appear red and feel warm and painful. *Lymphangiography* (a special examination in which an intravenous [IV] dye and radiography are used to detect lymph node involvement in certain diseases or conditions) reveals the degree and extent of blockage in the lymph system.

Medical and Surgical Management

Treatment usually is symptomatic. The affected part is elevated to promote lymphatic drainage. The client wears an elastic stocking or sleeve when the leg or arm is in a dependent position. Massage starting at the toes or fingers and moving toward the body and active exercises are helpful. A mechanical pulsating compression device is applied to the arm or leg at prescribed intervals. The alternating filling and emptying "milk" the lymph toward the duct, leading to venous drainage.

Sometimes surgery relieves the obstruction of lymphatics. Congenital lymphedema responds poorly to surgical intervention. In some cases, lymphedema persists despite treatment.

Nursing Management

The nurse inspects and measures the affected area to assess the extent of enlargement and assess the condition of the skin. He or she encourages the client to move and exercise the affected arm or leg to enhance the flow of lymph from the affected area. The nurse instructs the client to elevate affected extremities when sitting and teaches how to apply and use elastic garments and mechanical devices.

Extensive emotional support is necessary when the edema is severe. The client's self-esteem often is decreased, which can lead to social withdrawal. The nurse supports the client's self-image by suggesting certain styles of clothing that conceal abnormal enlargement of an arm or leg. For information on client teaching, see the discussion that follows nursing management for clients after a mastectomy in Chapter 60.

> ### Stop, Think, and Respond ● BOX 40-1
> *Why is a client at an increased risk for lymphedema after a mastectomy?*

● LYMPHANGITIS AND LYMPHADENITIS

Lymphangitis is inflammation of lymphatic vessels. When such inflammation affects the lymph nodes near the lymphatics, the condition is called **lymphadenitis.**

Pathophysiology and Etiology

An infectious agent, commonly streptococcal microorganisms, usually causes both lymphangitis and lymphadenitis. The lymph nodes and lymph vessels manifest typical signs of inflammation: redness, swelling, discomfort, and compromised function.

Assessment Findings

Red streaks follow the course of the lymph channels and extend up the arm or leg. Fever also may be present. When lymphadenitis is present, the lymph nodes along the lymphatic channels are enlarged and tender on palpation. Diagnosis is made by visual inspection and palpation.

Medical Management

A broad-spectrum antibiotic commonly is ordered.

Nursing Management

The nurse inspects the area two to three times daily and notes the client's response to antibiotic therapy. He or she gives assistance if the discomfort interferes with activities of daily living. Elevation reduces the swelling. Warmth promotes comfort and enhances circulation. The nurse notifies the physician if the affected area appears to enlarge, additional lymph nodes become involved, or the temperature remains elevated. In severe cases with persistent swelling, the nurse teaches the client how to apply an elastic sleeve or stocking.

● INFECTIOUS MONONUCLEOSIS

Infectious mononucleosis is a viral disease that affects lymphoid tissues such as the tonsils and spleen. It can involve other organs such as the brain, meninges, and liver as well.

Pathophysiology and Etiology

The **Epstein-Barr virus** causes infectious mononucleosis. This contagious disorder spreads by direct contact with saliva and pharyngeal secretions from an infected person. It is transmitted at the time of kissing; through oral spray during coughing, talking, or sneezing; or through sharing food, cigarettes, or other items containing oral secretions. The incubation period can be as long as 30 to 50 days. The virus most commonly affects young adults, especially those in close living quarters, such as the armed services and college dormitories.

At the time of infection, macrophages engulf the virus, resulting in a display of the antigen on the cell surface. Active production of T lymphocytes follows. The T lymphocytes trigger the production of B-cell lymphocytes and antibodies. They also infiltrate tissue, particularly the spleen, causing it to enlarge. Force to the abdomen can cause the spleen to rupture when it is enlarged.

The symptoms resolve in approximately 1 to 2 weeks unless complications develop. One episode of infectious mononucleosis produces subsequent immunity; however, the virus remains in the body for the person's lifetime. The Epstein-Barr virus is believed to trigger Hodgkin's lymphoma (discussed later in the chapter) in approximately 40% of people with this disease.

Assessment Findings

Signs and Symptoms

Fatigue, fever, sore throat, headache, and cervical lymph node enlargement typically occur. The tonsils ooze white or greenish gray exudate. Pharyngeal swelling can compromise swallowing and breathing. Some clients develop a faint red rash on their hands or abdomen. The liver and spleen become enlarged. The symptoms persist for several weeks.

Diagnostic Findings

The leukocyte and differential cell counts demonstrate lymphocytosis. A positive slide agglutination test (Monospot, Mono-Test, Monosticon) is presumptive evidence that the Epstein-Barr virus is causing the symptoms. A rise in the Epstein-Barr virus antibody titer and a heterophil agglutination test result of 1:224 or greater is conclusive for infectious mononucleosis.

Medical Management

The infection usually is self-limiting. Bed rest, analgesic and antipyretic therapy, and increased fluid intake are recommended. Corticosteroid therapy is prescribed if complications such as hepatic involvement occur. If a bacterial infection such as sinusitis or streptococcal pharyngitis accompanies mononucleosis, an antibiotic is prescribed.

Nursing Management

The nurse inspects the client's throat for the extent of inflammation or edema. He or she gently palpates the lymph nodes to detect swelling and encourages fluids.

The nurse advises the client to rest as much as possible. If the client expresses concern over prolonged time off from work or school, the nurse listens and helps the client cope with the anxiety. He or she advises the client to withhold donating blood for at least 6 months after recovering from the illness.

LYMPHOMAS

The term **lymphoma** applies to a group of cancers that affect the lymphatic system. The types of lymphoma are classified by the microscopic appearance of the malignant cells and how quickly the malignancy spreads. Two of the most common forms of lymphoma are Hodgkin's disease and non-Hodgkin's lymphoma (Table 40-1). Acquired immunodeficiency syndrome–related lymphoma occurs in those who have been infected with the human immunodeficiency virus.

● HODGKIN'S DISEASE

Hodgkin's disease is a malignancy that produces enlargement of lymphoid tissue, the spleen, and the liver, with invasion of other tissues such as the bone marrow and lungs. It may appear in several forms: acute, localized, latent with relapsing pyrexia (elevated temperature), splenomegaly (enlarged spleen), and as lymphogranulo-

TABLE 40-1	COMPARISON OF LYMPHOMAS
HODGKIN'S	**NON-HODGKIN'S**
Four subtypes	Thirty subtypes
Two peaks of onset: ages 15 to 40 and older than age 55 years	Peaks after age 50 years
Reed-Sternberg cells	No Reed-Sternberg cells
Forty percent of affected clients test positive for Epstein-Barr virus	More common in industrial countries; common among clients with immunosuppression
B-cell origin	B- and T-cell origin
Usually starts in lymph nodes above the clavicle, commonly in the neck and chest; 15% are below the diaphragm; spreads downward from initial site	Common in abdomen, tonsils; can develop in areas other than lymph nodes (e.g., brain, nasal passages)
More orderly growth from one node to adjacent nodes	Less predictable growth; spreads to extranodal sites
More curable	Less curable

matosis (multiple granular tumors or growths composed of lymphoid cells).

Pathophysiology and Etiology

Although the exact cause of Hodgkin's disease is unknown, it appears that a virus, particularly the Epstein-Barr virus (the etiologic agent of infectious mononucleosis), causes mutations in some, but not all lymphocytes, creating a malignant cell type known as **Reed-Sternberg cells.** Reed-Sternberg cells are nearly immortal, continue to reproduce prolifically, and perhaps because of their altered form, are somehow shielded from being destroyed by killer T cells. The virus also is believed to inactivate the immune system's ability to suppress tumor growth. The malignant cells release chemicals known as *cytokines* (see Chap. 41), causing inflammatory symptoms such as pain and fever. Some clients develop generalized itching and a skin rash because of the release of histamine from an atypical allergic/immune response.

The disease is more common in men than in women and most frequently occurs during late adolescence and young adulthood. Some clients survive 10 or more years; others die in 4 to 5 years. A cure is possible when the disease is localized to one section of the body. Clients who receive treatment usually have remissions that last for months or even years. Death results from respiratory obstruction, cachexia (state of ill health, malnutrition, and wasting), or secondary infections.

Assessment Findings

Signs and Symptoms

Early symptoms of Hodgkin's disease include painless enlargement of one or more lymph nodes. The cervical lymph nodes are the first to be affected. As the nodes enlarge, they press on adjacent structures, such as the esophagus or bronchi. As retroperitoneal nodes enlarge, there is a sense of fullness in the stomach and epigastric pain. Marked weight loss, anorexia, fatigue, and weakness occur. Low-grade fever, pruritus, and night sweats are common. Sometimes marked anemia and thrombocytopenia develop, causing a tendency to bleed. Resistance to infection is poor, and staphylococcal skin infections and respiratory tract infections often complicate the illness.

Diagnostic Findings

A complete blood count demonstrates low red blood cell count, elevated leukocytes, and a paradoxical decrease in lymphocytes. The Reed-Sternberg cells, characterized as giant multinucleated B lymphocytes, are microscopically identifiable in lymph node biopsies. Results of blood chemistry tests such as erythrocyte sedimentation rate are

elevated, suggesting a current inflammatory process. Liver enzymes such as alkaline phosphatase are elevated. Lymphangiography, chest radiography, computed tomography, magnetic resonance imaging, or a laparotomy to obtain abdominal nodes for biopsy demonstrate the size of lymph nodes and the spread of the disease in the thorax, abdomen, or pelvis. A bone marrow aspiration and biopsy indicate abnormalities of other blood cells. After diagnosis, the disease is staged from stage I to IV, based on the number of positive lymph nodes and the involvement of other organs (Table 40-2). Staging helps determine treatment.

Stages I, II, III, and IV adult Hodgkin's disease are subclassified into A and B categories: B for those with defined general symptoms and A for those without B symptoms. The B designation is given to clients with any of the following symptoms*:

- Unexplained loss of more than 10% of body weight in the 6 months before diagnosis
- Unexplained fever with temperatures above 38°C
- Drenching night sweats

(*Note: The most significant B symptoms are fever and weight loss. Night sweats alone do not confer an adverse prognosis.) Careful staging and treatment planning by a multidisciplinary team of cancer specialists is required to determine optimal treatment of patients with this disease.

Medical Management

Treatment of Hodgkin's disease includes localized radiation to affected lymph nodes and chemotherapy with combinations of antineoplastic drugs (Table 40-3). Antibiotics are given to fight secondary infections. Transfusions are prescribed to control anemia. If resistance to treatment develops, autologous bone marrow or peripheral stem cells are harvested, followed by high doses of chemotherapy that destroy the bone marrow (see Chaps. 20 and 39). A transplant is performed after separating the normal stem cells from the malignant cells in the harvested specimen.

TABLE 40-2	STAGES OF HODGKIN'S DISEASE
STAGE	**INVOLVEMENT**
I	Single lymph node region
II	Two or more lymph node regions on one side of the diaphragm
III	Lymph node regions on both sides of the diaphragm but extension is limited to the spleen
IV	Bilateral lymph nodes affected and extension includes spleen plus one or more of the following: bones, bone marrow, lungs, liver, skin, gastrointestinal structures, or other sites

TABLE 40-3	CHEMOTHERAPY REGIMENS FOR HODGKIN'S DISEASE
REGIMEN	**DRUGS**
ABVD	doxorubicin (Adriamycin), bleomycin (Blenoxane), vinblastine (Velban), dacarbazine (DTIC)
MOPP	mechlorethamine (Mustargen), vincristine (Oncovin), prednisone (Meticorten), procarbazine (Matulane)
MOPP/ABVD	Alternation of drugs from both regimens
For partial remission or relapse within 1 year	
CBV	cyclophosphamide (Cytoxan), carmustine (BiCNU), Veposid (etoposide)
BEAM	carmustine (BiCNU), etoposide (Veposid), cytosine arabinoside-e (Cytosar-U), melphalan (Alkeran)

NURSING PROCESS

● The Client With Hodgkin's Disease

Assessment

The nurse looks for a history of infectious mononucleosis or symptoms resembling this disorder. He or she assesses for location, size, and characteristics of enlarged lymph nodes, such as whether they are fixed or mobile. The nurse asks how long the client has noticed the enlarged lymph nodes and checks for the presence and extent of tenderness in the area of lymph node enlargement. He or she asks about fever, chills, or night sweats. The nurse checks the client's current weight and deviation from usual weight, enlargement of the liver and spleen, and level of energy and appetite. He or she inspects the appearance of the skin, asks about any itching, and discusses any additional symptoms caused by lymph node enlargement (e.g., coughing, breathlessness, nausea, vomiting).

Diagnosis, Planning, and Interventions

Client and Family Teaching Box 40-1 describes instructions for nurses to communicate to clients with Hodgkin's disease. Other nursing care includes, but is not limited to, the following.

Risk for Ineffective Airway Clearance and **Risk for Impaired Gas Exchange** related to compression of trachea secondary to enlarged cervical lymph nodes
Expected Outcome: Breathing will remain adequate to maintain blood oxygen saturation of 90% or greater.

● Assess respiratory status each shift and prn. Note quality, rate, pattern, depth, flaring of nostrils, dyspnea on exertion, evidence of splinting, use of accessory muscles, and position for breathing. *Any deviation from quiet, effortless breathing indicates compromised ventilation.*

● Keep the neck in midline and place the client in high Fowler's position if respiratory distress develops. *Avoiding unnecessary pressure on the trachea and positioning for increased lung expansion improve air exchange.*

● Administer oxygen per physician's orders if blood saturation is consistently less than 90%. *Increasing the percentage of inhaled oxygen beyond 21% in the atmosphere reduces deficits in the blood oxygen level.*

● Place an endotracheal tube, laryngoscope, and bag–valve mask at the bedside for intubation. *Anticipation of the need for airway management ensures that medical intervention and emergency assistance are not delayed.*

Risk for Infection related to immunosuppression secondary to impaired lymphocytes and drug or radiation therapy
Expected Outcome: Client will remain free of infection as evidenced by no fever and symptoms of secondary infection.

● Restrict visitors or personnel with infections from contact with the client. *Reducing the number of organisms in the environment and restricting visitors and personnel with an infection reduces the transmission of pathogens to the client.*

● Practice conscientious handwashing and follow other principles of medical and surgical asepsis. *Washing hands and using aseptic techniques reduce the risk of transmitting pathogens from one location to another.*

40-1 *Client and Family Teaching* Hodgkin's Disease

The nurse instructs the client as follows:

■ Keep appointments for medical follow-up.
■ Take prescribed medications as directed. Report side effects to the physician.
■ Avoid crowds or people who have infectious diseases.
■ Wash hands frequently.
■ Avoid oral contact with germ-laden objects.
■ Contact the physician if breathing becomes labored.
■ Eat small amounts frequently or include a liquid nutritional supplement between meals and at bedtime.
■ Reduce work schedule to avoid exhaustion. If that is not possible, rest frequently.
■ Consult with an employer about sick-leave considerations or a representative from the Social Security Administration about unemployment benefits and disability payments.
■ Obtain a disability sticker to facilitate easy access to public buildings to lessen fatigue.

- Institute infectious disease precautions if normal white blood cells are suppressed to dangerous limits. *Protective isolation techniques provide an environmental barrier against pathogens while a client is highly susceptible to disease.*

Risk for Impaired Skin Integrity related to pruritus, inadequate nutrition, and inactivity

Expected Outcome: Client's skin will remain intact throughout care.

- Use mild soap for bathing, rinse well, and pat dry. *Mild soap prevents excessive drying of the skin; patting instead of rubbing dry helps prevent friction, which can damage skin.*
- Apply ice to the skin for brief periods, cool sponge baths, or cotton gloves if itching is intolerable. An oral or topical antipruritic medication often is necessary. *Cooling the skin reduces the sensation of itching; cotton gloves reduce skin trauma from scratching with sharp fingernails; antipruritic medications block the release of histamine.*
- Trim nails short to avoid scratching when itching occurs. *Trimming fingernails short prevents abrading the skin and providing an entrance for pathogens.*
- Change bedding as soon as possible if night sweats occur. *Wet bedding contributes to skin maceration.*
- Lift rather than pull client across sheets when changing positions. *Lifting the client prevents shearing forces on the skin.*
- Support and protect bony prominences. *Areas where skin is stretched tautly over bony prominences creates ischemia as a result of compressing skin capillaries between a hard surface (mattress) and the bone.*
- Collaborate with physician to avoid drugs administered by the parenteral route. *Any breaks in skin integrity can provide an open route for the entrance of pathogens.*

Activity Intolerance and **Self-Care Deficit** related to anemia and generalized weakness from disease

Expected Outcome: Client will tolerate essential activities as evidenced by heart and respiratory rates within normal limits.

- Divide care into manageable amounts. *Proportioning activities reduces energy expenditures.*
- Provide rest periods between activities. *Rest allows the body time to recover before the next demand for energy.*
- Perform priority activities first. *Client completes most important or necessary activities while energy levels are highest.*
- Assist client with whatever activities of daily living are independently unmanageable. *Assistance reduces the client's energy expenditure.*

Evaluation of Expected Outcomes

Breathing is noiseless and effortless. The client shows no signs or symptoms of infection, and his or her skin remains intact. He or she can perform essential activities.

● NON-HODGKIN'S LYMPHOMAS

Non-Hodgkin's lymphomas are a group of 30 subclassifications of malignant diseases that originate in lymph glands and other lymphoid tissue. Examples include lymphosarcoma, Burkitt's lymphoma, and reticulum cell sarcoma. The incidence of non-Hodgkin's lymphomas is six to seven times that of Hodgkin's disease, and the number of cases continues to rise.

Pathophysiology and Etiology

No single definitive cause for non-Hodgkin's lymphomas has been found, although a genetic link is strongly implicated in some types. An environmental "trigger," such as a viral agent, chemical herbicides, pesticides, or hair dye, could induce the disease. The administration of immunosuppressive drugs to prevent transplant rejection also has been correlated with cases of non-Hodgkin's lymphoma.

In non-Hodgkin's lymphoma, chromosomal changes occur in the affected lymphocytes, and lymphoid tissue enlarges to accommodate the proliferative production of malignant cells. Non-Hodgkin's lymphoma is classified as either (1) *indolent,* meaning the client is relatively asymptomatic at diagnosis and the disorder is relatively responsive to radiation and chemotherapy; or (2) *aggressive* because the condition has a shorter onset with acute symptoms. Nevertheless, 30% to 60% of aggressive forms of non-Hodgkin's lymphoma are curable with intensive treatment.

Assessment Findings

Symptoms of non-Hodgkin's lymphoma depend on the site of lymph node involvement. Lymph node enlargement, which usually is diffuse rather than localized, occurs in cervical, axillary, and inguinal regions. The diagnosis and differentiation of the subtypes of non-Hodgkin's lymphoma from Hodgkin's disease depend on microscopic examination of lymphoid tissue biopsies. Additional tests are performed to determine the stage of the lymphoma.

Medical Management

Non-Hodgkin's lymphoma is treated with radiation, chemotherapy, or both. The physician may adopt a "watch and wait" approach for clients with indolent forms of non-Hodgkin's lymphoma, choosing to treat the client once the disease accelerates. Immunotherapy with monoclonal antibodies (MABs) and bone marrow transplants also is being used to cure lymphomas or extend the lives of clients with these diseases.

Monoclonal Antibody Therapy

Research continues on the use of biologic therapy (immunotherapy) with MABs to eliminate malignant cells and induce remission. With MABs, human cancer cells are injected into laboratory animals such as mice (see Chap. 20). The mice make lymphocytes that produce antibodies against the cancer cells. The mouse lymphocytes are harvested and fused with a laboratory-grown cell, creating clones that, when administered to a client with cancer, continue to produce tumor-fighting antibodies. The MABs are used alone or are bound to a chemotherapeutic or radioactive agent. The advantage of combining MABs with drugs or radiation is that they target and destroy cancer cells while sparing normal cells. One MAB drug, rituximab (Rituxan), is now approved for treating non-Hodgkin's lymphoma. Three others (Zevalin, Bexxar, and Oncolym) are in clinical trials.

Bone Marrow Transplant

Bone marrow and stem cell transplants are considered a potential treatment modality when others are ineffective. Autologous (self-donated) bone marrow and peripheral blood stem cells are removed from the client with cancer and frozen. The donor cells are then infused with high doses of drugs and sometimes radiated to destroy all cancer cells. The same is done to the client, thus destroying most remaining bone marrow and stem cells. The frozen marrow and cells are thawed and transplanted into the client's vein, whereupon they recolonize the marrow with normal blood cells.

Instead of autologous transplants, some clients receive allogenic bone marrow transplants (i.e., marrow from a human donor), sometimes referred to as *mini-bone marrow transplants* (mini-BMTs). During a mini-BMT, the client is treated with moderate doses of drugs or mild total-body radiation to destroy as many cancer cells as possible and suppress the immune system to reduce the potential for destroying the donor cells. Consequently, when the client undergoes a mini-BMT, the possibility for rejection still exists. The phenomenon is referred to as *graft-versus-host disease* (GVHD) (see Chap. 20). Despite GVHD, allogenic BMTs have two advantages: (1) relapses of lymphoma are less frequent than with autologous transplants, and (2) they induce remissions when a relapse occurs.

Nursing Management

Nursing care is similar for all clients with lymphoma, whether they have non-Hodgkin's lymphoma or Hodgkin's disease. Because chemotherapy and radiation kill many cells, the nurse encourages clients to drink extra fluids (≥2500 mL/day) to facilitate excretion of the cells destroyed by therapy.

GENERAL NUTRITIONAL CONSIDERATIONS

Soft, bland foods and cool liquids are best for clients with ulcerations of the oral mucosa.

Nausea and vomiting often accompany radiation therapy. Clients must maintain food and fluid intake. Offer clear liquids such as carbonated beverages and water, ice pops, and flavored gelatin until nausea subsides. Thereafter, small, frequent, low-fat meals help prevent nausea.

GENERAL PHARMACOLOGIC CONSIDERATIONS

The incidence of Hodgkin's and non-Hodgkin's lymphoma is increased in those taking the hydantoin drugs, such as phenytoin (Dilantin).

Supportive measures are necessary for clients experiencing toxic effects of chemotherapeutic agents. Bone marrow depression, gastrointestinal disturbances, and alopecia (hair loss) are common toxic effects.

Recognizing and treating adverse drug reactions can help optimize response to therapy.

Clients with Hodgkin's disease are extremely susceptible to toxic effects of medication and to secondary infection from the combination of treatments (i.e., radiation and chemotherapy) plus a weakened immune system from the disease.

GENERAL GERONTOLOGIC CONSIDERATIONS

Risk of malignancies (e.g., lymphoma) is increased in older adults primarily because of the immunologic changes of aging and prolonged exposure to carcinogens.

Older adults do not tolerate doxorubicin and methotrexate well because these drugs have toxic effects on the kidney.

Older adults respond less well to chemotherapy than younger persons because older clients cannot tolerate maximum doses.

The benefits of chemotherapy must be weighed against the adverse reactions that occur in older adults. Treatment modalities, however, are not based on age alone.

Critical Thinking Exercises

1. *List the differences between lymphedema and lymphoma.*
2. *What teaching is indicated for a person diagnosed with lymphedema?*

References and Suggested Readings

Anand, S., Lal, H., & Dhaon, B. K. (1998). Lymphedema of the lower extremity as a complication of local burns. *Burns, 24,* 767–769.

Barnes, L. (2000). Non-Hodgkin's lymphoma. *Rehabilitation Oncology, 18*(2), 14–16.

Boyle, D. A. & Angert, V. J. (1998). Lymphoma at the extremes of age. *Seminars in Oncology Nursing, 14,* 302–311.

Buren, J. M. & Linton, C. (2000). The role of exercise in treating lymphedema. *Rehabilitation Management: The Interdisciplinary Journal of Rehabilitation, 13*(6), 26, 28, 30–31.

Capriotti, T. (2001). Monoclonal antibodies: drugs that combine pharmacology and biotechnology. *MEDSURG Nursing, 10*(2), 89–95.

Davis, B. S. (2001). Lymphedema after breast cancer treatment. *American Journal of Nursing, 101*(4), Continuing Care Extra, 24AAAA–DDDD.

Dillman, R. O. (2001). Monoclonal antibody therapy for lymphoma: An update. *Cancer Practice: A Multidisciplinary Journal of Cancer Care, 9*(2), 71–80.

Goldenberg, D., Golz, A., Netzer, A., et al. (2001). Epstein-Barr virus and cancers of the head and neck. *American Journal of Otolaryngology, 22,* 197–205.

Habermann, T. M. (1999). Non-Hodgkin's lymphoma: Present status and future prospects. *Hospital Practice, 34*(13), 81–84, 87–88.

Kotsits, C. & Callaghan, M. (2000). Rituximab: A new monoclonal antibody therapy for non-Hodgkin's lymphoma. *Oncology Nursing Forum, 17*(1), 51–59.

Labson, L. H. (1999). Current approaches to the lymphomas. *Patient Care, 33*(8), 65–66, 69–70, 72+.

McGarvey, C. L. (1998). Pneumatic compression devices for lymphedema. *Rehabilitation Oncology, 16*(3), 28.

Neese, P. Y. (2000). Management of lymphedema. *Lippincott's Primary Care Practice, 4,* 390–399.

Paskett, E. D. & Stark, N. (2000). Lymphedema: Knowledge, treatment, and impact among breast cancer survivors. *Breast Journal, 6,* 373–378.

Pichler, R., Berg, J., Hengstschlager, A., et al. (2001). Recurrent infectious mononucleosis caused by Epstein-Barr virus with persistent splenomegaly. *Military Medicine, 166,* 733–734.

Radina, M. E. & Armer, J. M. (2001). Post-breast cancer lymphedema and the family: A qualitative investigation of families coping with chronic illness. *Journal of Family Nursing, 7,* 281–299.

Roberts, G. H. (1999). The kissing disease. *Journal of Continuing Education Topics and Issues, 1*(3), 127–131.

Rothwell, S. & McAuley, D. (2001). Spontaneous splenic rupture in infectious mononucleosis. *Emergency Medicine, 13,* 364–366.

Ruffer, U., Sieber, M., Josting, A., et al. (1999). Modern treatment strategies in Hodgkin's disease. *Home Health Care Consultant, 6*(9), Oncology, 1A–5A.

Samdani, S., Lachmann, E., & Nagler, W. (2001). Unilateral extremity swelling in female patients with cancer. *Journal of Women's Health and Gender-Based Medicine, 10,* 319–326.

Stremick, K. & Gallagher, E. (2000). Malignant lymphomas: Hodgkin's disease and non-Hodgkin's lymphoma. *American Journal of Nursing,* (April Suppl.), 18–22, 52–54.

Thompson, K. A. (1999). Detecting Hodgkin's disease. *American Journal of Nursing, 99*(5), 61–64.

Whitman, M. (2000). Controlling lymphedema-related swelling. *Clinical Journal of Oncology Nursing, 4,* 101–102.

World Health Organization. (2001). Lymphatic filariasis. *Weekly Epidemiological Record, 76*(20), 149–154.

chapter 41

Introduction to the Immune System

Words to Know

anergy
antibodies
antigens
artificially acquired
    active immunity
cell-mediated response
colony-stimulating
    factors
complement system
cytokines
cytotoxic T cells
effector T cells
helper T cells
humoral response
immune response
immunoglobulins
interferons
interleukins
lymphokines
macrophages
memory cells
microphages
monocytes
natural killer cells
naturally acquired
    active immunity
neutrophils
passive immunity
phagocytes
phagocytosis
plasma cells
regulator T cells
stem cells
suppressor T cells
tumor necrosis factor

Learning Objectives

On completion of this chapter, the reader will:

- Explain the meaning of an immune response.
- List two general components of the immune system.
- Discuss the role of T-cell and B-cell lymphocytes.
- Differentiate between an antigen and an antibody.
- Name examples of lymphoid tissue.
- List some cells and chemicals that enhance the function of the immune system.
- Name three types of immunity, describing how each develops.
- Discuss techniques for detecting immune disorders.
- Describe the role of the nurse when caring for a client with an immune disorder.

Although all humans have the same types of cells, each person's cells are unique and different from those of all others. Everyone's body cells are coded with distinct histocompatibility (tissue cell) markers. These markers act as a "fingerprint" that enables the immune system to differentiate "self" from "nonself." When it detects a nonself substance, the immune system sets about to protect, defend, and destroy what it perceives as atypical or abnormal. The immune system primarily targets infectious, foreign, or cancerous cells. The **immune response,** a target-specific system of defense, is carried out primarily by lymphocytes, specialized cells that are located in blood and lymphoid tissue. Hyperactivity of the immune system, as in allergic or autoimmune disorders (see Chap. 42), or a decrease in its function, as in acquired immunodeficiency syndrome (AIDS; see Chap. 43), can be life-threatening.

STRUCTURES OF THE IMMUNE SYSTEM

The immune system actually is a collection of specialized white blood cells and lymphoid tissues that cooperate to protect a person from external invaders and the body's own altered cells. The function of these structures is assisted and supported by the activities of natural killer (NK) cells, antibodies, and nonantibody proteins like cytokines and the complement system (Fig. 41-1).

White Blood Cells

White blood cells (leukocytes) are produced in the bone marrow. Initially all blood cells are nonspecific **stem cells** that later differentiate into various types of cells including

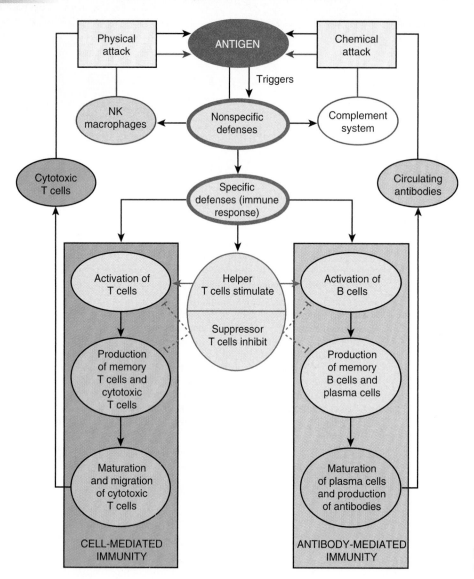

FIGURE 41-1 Schematic representation of the immune response.

lymphocytes, neutrophils, and monocytes. Figure 41-2 shows the development of various types of blood cells.

Lymphocytes

Lymphocytes, which are either T-cell or B-cell lymphocytes, comprise 20% to 30% of all leukocytes. T-cell and B-cell lymphocytes are the primary participants in the immune response. They distinguish harmful substances and ignore those natural and unique to the individual. Table 41-1 identifies various types of lymphocytes and the role they play in the immune response.

T-CELL LYMPHOCYTES

The T-cell lymphocytes are manufactured in the bone marrow and travel to the thymus gland, where they mature to become either regulator T cells or effector T cells. **Regulator T cells** are made up of helper and suppressor cells; **effector T cells** are killer (cytotoxic) cells. **Helper T cells** are especially important in fighting infection. They

recognize **antigens,** protein markers on cells, and form additional T-cell clones that stimulate B-cell lymphocytes to produce antibodies against foreign antigens. **Antibodies** are chemical substances that destroy foreign agents such as microorganisms. Helper T cells also are called T4 cells or CD4 cells. **Cytotoxic T cells** bind to invading cells, destroy the targeted invader by altering their cellular membrane and intracellular environment, and release chemicals called lymphokines. **Lymphokines,** a type of cytokine (discussed later in this chapter), attract neutrophils and monocytes to remove the debris. They also promote the maturation of more T cells when they detect antigens and direct B-cell lymphocytes to multiply and mature. **Suppressor T cells** limit or turn off the immune response in the absence of continued antigenic stimulation. Because the surface molecules of suppressor and killer T cells differ from those of helper T cells, they sometimes are referred to as T8 or CD8 cells.

The immune response that T-cell lymphocytes perform is called a *cell-mediated response*. A **cell-mediated re-**

FIGURE 41-2 Origin of blood cells.

sponse occurs when T cells survey proteins in the body, actively analyze the surface features, and respond to those that differ from the host by directly attacking the invading antigen. An example of a cell-mediated response is one that occurs when an organ is transplanted.

TABLE 41-1	TYPE AND FUNCTIONS OF LYMPHOCYTES
TYPE	**FUNCTION**
T Cells	
Regulator T cells	
Helper T cells	Recognize antigens; stimulate B cells to produce antibodies
Suppressor T cells	Turn off the immune response
Effector cells	
Cytotoxic cells	Bind to and destroy invader cells; stimulate the release of lymphokines
B Cells	
Plasma cells	Produce antibodies
Memory cells	Convert to plasma cells that will produce antibodies when re-exposed to an antigen

B-CELL LYMPHOCYTES

The B-cell lymphocytes mature in the bone marrow and migrate to the spleen and other lymphoid tissues such as the lymph nodes. When stimulated by T cells, the B cells become either plasma or memory cells. **Plasma cells** produce antibodies. Formation of antibodies is called a **humoral response.**

Memory cells convert to plasma cells on re-exposure to a specific antigen. When activated, B cells accumulate in lymphoid tissues, which explains the phenomena of swollen and tender lymph nodes that accompany infectious disorders and an enlarged spleen in various immune disorders.

Stop, Think, and Respond ● BOX 41-1

Explain the difference between a cell-mediated response and a humoral response.

Neutrophils and Monocytes

Neutrophils and **monocytes** are **phagocytes,** cells that perform phagocytosis. **Phagocytosis** is the process of engulfing and digesting bacteria and foreign material. Phagocytes are stationary (fixed) or mobile. Neutrophils, also called **microphages** because they are small, are present in blood and migrate to tissue as necessary. Monocytes, also called **macrophages** because they are large, are present in tissues such as the lungs, liver, lymph nodes, spleen, and peritoneum (Fig. 41-3). They also migrate after a cell-mediated response. The mononuclear phagocyte system was formerly known as the *reticuloendothelial system.*

Lymphoid Tissues

Lymphoid tissues (Fig. 41-4), such as the thymus gland, tonsils and adenoids, spleen, and lymph nodes, play a role in the immune response and prevention of infection (see Chap. 38). Lymphoid tissue also is found on the surface of the mucous membranes of the intestine, on alveolar membranes in the lungs, and in the lining of the sinusoids of the liver. Bone marrow sometimes is included as a component of the immune system because it produces undifferentiated stem cells.

Thymus Gland

The thymus gland is located in the neck below the thyroid gland. It extends into the thorax behind the top of the sternum. The thymus gland produces lymphocytes during fetal development. It may be the embryonic origin of other lymphoid structures such as the spleen and lymph nodes. After birth, the thymus gland programs T lymphocytes to become regulator or effector T cells. The thymus gland becomes smaller during adolescence but retains some activity throughout the life cycle.

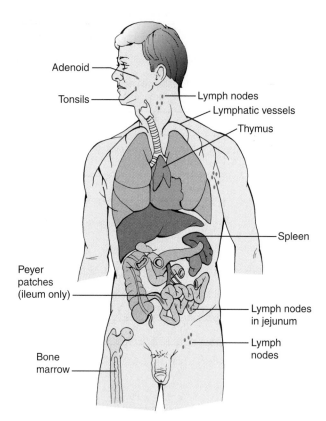

FIGURE 41-4 Lymphoid tissues.

Tonsils and Adenoids

The tonsils are located on either side of the soft palate of the oropharynx. The adenoids are located behind the nose on the posterior wall of the nasopharynx. These tissues filter bacteria from tissue fluid. Because they are exposed to pathogens in the oral and nasal passages, they can become infected and locally inflamed.

Spleen

The spleen has both hematopoietic and immune functions. It acts as an emergency reservoir of blood and filters the blood as well. Macrophages in the spleen remove bacteria and old, dead, or damaged blood cells from circulation.

Lymph Nodes

The lymphatic system consists of vessels similar to capillaries that drain tissue fluid, called *lymph.* At various areas in the body, the lymphatics converge and drain into larger structures called *lymph nodes.* The lymph nodes contain B lymphocytes and T lymphocytes and remove bacteria and other foreign particles from the lymph. Superficial lymph nodes in the axilla, groin, and neck are palpable when enlarged.

Natural Killer Cells

Natural killer (NK) cells are lymphocyte-like cells that circulate throughout the body looking for virus-infected

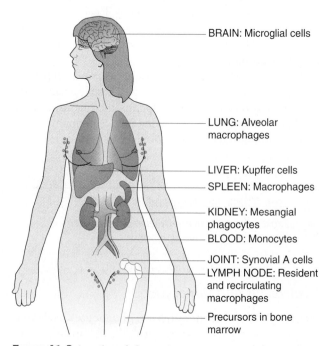

FIGURE 41-3 Location of phagocytes.

cells and cancer cells. NK cells can identify atypical markers on the membranes of these cells without the help of T or B cell lymphocytes. Once identified, NK cells release potent chemicals that lethally alter the target cell's membrane, leading to its demise. Unfortunately, cancer cells can escape NK cell surveillance, which explains how cancer is able to become established and spread beyond its primary site.

Antibodies

Antibodies, proteins produced by B lymphocyte plasma cells, are more correctly referred to as **immunoglobulins** (Ig). There are five classes of immunoglobulins: IgA, IgD, IgE, IgG, and IgM. Each immunoglobulin has a separate role in ensuring the maintenance of a healthy state (Table 41-2).

Immunoglobulins bind with antigens and promote the destruction of invading cells in one of two ways. First, they may hinder antigens physically by (1) neutralizing their toxins; (2) linking antigens together in a process called *agglutination;* and (3) causing antigens to precipitate, or become soluble. Second, antibodies can facilitate the destruction of antigens with other mechanisms such as those performed by nonantibody proteins like the complement system and cytokines.

Nonantibody Proteins

Nonantibody proteins provide additional methods for disabling antigens and further protecting the body. There are two groups of nonantibody proteins. One group is referred to as the *complement system,* and the other is known collectively as *cytokines.*

Complement System

The **complement system** is made up of many different proteins that are activated in a chain reaction when an antibody binds with an antigen. Collectively, the proteins cooperate with antibodies to attract phagocytes, coat antigens to make them more recognizable for phagocytosis (a process known as *opsonization,*) and stimulate inflammation through the release of histamine from mast cells and basophils.

Cytokines

Cytokines are chemical messengers released by lymphocytes, monocytes, and macrophages. There are many subgroups of cytokines, including interleukins, interferons, tumor necrosis factor, and colony-stimulating factors.

INTERLEUKINS
Interleukins carry messages between leukocytes and tissues that form blood cells. Some interleukins enhance the immune response, whereas others suppress it (Martini, 1998). Examples of interleukin activity include the following:

- Promotion of inflammation and fever
- Formation of scar tissue by fibroblasts
- Growth and activation of NK cells and additional T cells
- Production of mast cells

TABLE 41-2	TYPES OF IMMUNOGLOBULINS		
TYPE	**PERCENTAGE OF TOTAL**	**LOCATION**	**FUNCTION**
IgG	75%	Intravascular and intercellular fluid	Neutralizes bacterial toxins; accelerates phagocytosis
IgA	15%	Body secretions such as saliva, sweat, tears, mucus, bile, colostrum	Interferes with entry of pathogens through exposed structures or pathways
IgM	10%	Intravascular serum	Agglutinates (clusters) antigens and lyses (dissolves) cell walls
IgD	0.2%	Surface of lymphocytes	Binds to antigens; promotes secretion of other immunoglobulins
IgE	0.004%	Surface of basophils and mast (connective tissue) cells	Promotes release of vasoactive chemicals such as histamine and bradykinin in allergic, hypersensitivity, and inflammatory reactions

- Growth of B cells, formation of plasma cells, and production of antibodies
- Formation of new blood vessels known as *angiogenesis*
- Stimulation of the anterior pituitary gland to secrete corticotropin

INTERFERONS

Interferons are chemicals that primarily protect cells from viral invasion. They enable cells to resist viral infection and slow viral replication. They have been used as adjunctive therapy in the treatment of AIDS. Interferons also have been used to treat some forms of cancer like leukemia because they stimulate NK cell activity.

TUMOR NECROSIS FACTOR

When **tumor necrosis factor** (TNF), a type of cytokine, was first discovered, it showed promise as a means of shrinking tumors. Although TNF reduced tumors in laboratory animals, it caused toxic effects among humans. Experiments continue to determine if the antitumor effect can be achieved and the toxic side effects limited by injecting TNF directly into the tumor rather than administering it by a route through which it is systemically absorbed and distributed.

Research has found that TNF helps in cellular repair when administered in small doses. Excess amounts destroy healthy tissue. Consequently, TNF is being used to regulate various autoimmune (see Chap. 42) and inflammatory disorders (see General Pharmacologic Considerations).

COLONY-STIMULATING FACTORS

Colony-stimulating factors (CSFs) are cytokines that regulate the production, maturation, and function of blood cells (Nevidjon & Sowers, 2000). Growth factors enable stem cells in bone marrow to differentiate into specific types of cells such as leukocytes, erythrocytes, and platelets. Pharmacologic preparations of cytokines, such as epoetin alfa (Epogen), filgrastim (Neupogen), and sargramostim (Leukine), are used to promote the natural production of blood cells in people whose own hematopoietic functions have become compromised. Consequently, clients with cancer who are receiving antineoplastic drugs may avoid interrupting treatment by reducing their risk for infection. Persons who have undergone bone marrow transplantation may recover sooner, and individuals with chronic renal failure can avoid repeated blood transfusions to compensate for their anemia.

TYPES OF IMMUNITY

The three types of immunity are naturally acquired active immunity, artificially acquired active immunity, and passive immunity (Fig. 41-5). Both forms of active immunity require the individual's own production of plasma and memory cells. Passive immunity occurs when ready-made antibodies are provided.

Naturally Acquired Active Immunity

Naturally acquired active immunity occurs as a direct result of infection by a specific microorganism. An example is the immunity to measles that develops after the initial infection. Not all invading microorganisms produce a response that gives lifelong immunity.

Artificially Acquired Active Immunity

Artificially acquired active immunity results from the administration of a killed or weakened microorganism or toxoid (attenuated toxin). The memory cells manufactured by the B lymphocytes "remember" the killed or weakened antigen and recognize it if a future invasion occurs. Refer to Chapter 19 for a recommended schedule for childhood immunizations. Immunizations that are not administered or completed during childhood are recommended for adults. Some immunizations, such as those for tetanus and influenza, require readministration to maintain adequate immunity.

Passive Immunity

Passive immunity develops when ready-made antibodies are given to a susceptible individual. The antibodies provide immediate but short-lived protection from the invading antigen. No memory cells are produced, and the level of the injected antibodies diminishes over a period of several weeks to a few months.

Ready-made antibodies are obtained from the serum of another organism, either animal or human. Immune serum globulin, also called *gamma globulin* or *immunoglobulin,* is recovered from pooled human plasma. Because the pool comprises plasma from more than one donor, the serum is likely to contain a variety of specific antibodies. Human immune serum is used for passive immunization against measles (rubella), pertussis (whooping cough), hepatitis B, chickenpox (varicella), and tetanus.

Newborns receive passive immunity to some diseases for which their mothers have manufactured antibodies. The circulating maternal antibodies cross the placental barrier. As with other forms of passive immunity, infants are protected for only a few months after birth.

Stop, Think, and Respond ● BOX 41-2

Identify the type of immunity that develops from (1) receiving a vaccine for hepatitis B, (2) having chickenpox, and (3) receiving an injection of gamma globulin.

NATURALLY ACQUIRED
ACTIVE IMMUNITY

Invading viruses
and bacteria act
as antigen

ARTIFICIALLY
ACQUIRED
ACTIVE IMMUNITY

Killed or atten-
uated (weak-
ened) viruses
act as antigen

PASSIVE IMMUNITY

Animal or
human is ex-
posed to antigen

Antigen stimu-
lates formation
of immune anti-
bodies in body

Antibodies
neutralize future
invasion of
same antigen—
disease
resistance

Antibodies are
recovered by
special purifica-
tion procedures

Antibodies are
injected into
susceptible
person

Borrowed anti-
bodies immedi-
ately attack
invading
organisms

FIGURE 41-5 Active and passive immunity.

ASSESSMENT

History

The nurse obtains a history of immunizations, recent and past infectious diseases, and recent exposure to infectious diseases. He or she reviews the client's drug history because certain drugs (e.g., corticosteroids) suppress the inflammatory and immune responses. The nurse investigates the client's allergy history and questions the client about practices that put him or her at risk for AIDS (see Chap. 43).

Physical Examination

The beginning of the physical examination is a general appraisal of the client's health. The nurse notes whether the client appears healthy, acutely or mildly ill, malnourished, extremely tired, or listless. He or she records vital signs and weight. The nurse then performs the following:

- Examines the skin for rashes or lesions
- Assesses the abdomen for an enlarged liver or spleen

- Inspects the pharynx for large, red tonsils and purulent drainage
- Palpates the lymph nodes in the neck, axilla, and groin for enlargement and tenderness

Diagnostic Tests

Laboratory tests are used to identify immune system disorders. They usually include a complete blood count with differential. Protein electrophoresis screens for diseases associated with a deficiency or excess of immunoglobulins. T-cell and B-cell assays (or counts) and the enzyme-linked immunosorbent assay (see Chap. 43) may be performed. Additional tests are performed when an autoimmune or genetic immune disorder is suspected (see Chap. 42).

Skin tests may be administered. Disease-specific antigens, such as purified protein derivative of the tuberculin toxin, are injected intradermally on the inner aspect of the forearm. The injection area swells if the client has developed antibodies against the antigen in the past (see Chap. 29). The client is not necessarily actively infectious if the test results are positive (see Chap. 29). Skin tests using various common disease antigens like mumps are administered if anergy is suspected. **Anergy** is the inability to mount an immune response. It is a common finding among clients who have AIDS or are immuno-suppressed for other reasons.

NURSING MANAGEMENT

Clear identification of any substances to which the client is allergic is essential. The nurse must consult drug references to verify that prescribed medications do not contain substances to which the client is hypersensitive. He or she explains all diagnostic skin testing procedures to the client and informs the client when to return for interpretation of the results. The nurse ensures that a written consent is obtained before testing for human immunodeficiency virus (HIV) and keeps the results of HIV testing confidential. Standard Precautions (see Chap. 19) are required whenever there is the potential for contact with blood or body fluids. The nurse should follow agency guidelines for controlling infectious diseases or protecting the client who is immunosuppressed. Client teaching includes information about immunizations and instructions regarding drug therapy prescribed for disorders involving the immune system.

GENERAL NUTRITIONAL CONSIDERATIONS

Nutrients important in immune system functioning include amino acids such as arginine and glutamine; essential fatty acids and omega-3 fatty acids; the B vitamins, especially vitamin B_6 and folacin; vitamins A, C, and E; and the minerals zinc, iron, copper, magnesium, and selenium. Singly or combined, nutrient deficiencies have the potential to affect almost all aspects of immune system functioning. Excesses of certain nutrients, namely iron, zinc, vitamin E, and polyunsaturated fatty acids, also can impair immune function. The exact amounts and proportions of nutrients needed for optimal immune system function in healthy people, however, are not yet known. Newer studies clearly indicate that the availability of one nutrient may impair or enhance the action of another nutrient in immune system functioning; nutrient supplements may enhance or suppress immune function through the effects of that supplement on other nutrients. Until more is known about nutrient interactions, the best dietary advice to maximize immune function in healthy people is to eat a moderate diet that is balanced and varied.

Several immune-enhancing tube feeding formulas are available, such as Immune-Aid, Impact, Osmolite HN, Peractive, Replete, and Vivonex TEN. These formulas contain standard formula ingredients and glutamine, arginine, omega-3 fatty acids, and nucleotides. These added ingredients enhance the production of lymphocytes and NK cells, resulting in increased cell-mediated immunity.

GENERAL PHARMACOLOGIC CONSIDERATIONS

Some drugs can suppress immune system function. Examples of these drugs are certain antibiotics, corticosteroids, some of the nonsteroidal anti-inflammatory drugs, and many drugs used in the treatment of cancer.

Intentional suppression of the immune system is used after organ transplantation. Azathioprine (Imuran), cyclosporine (Sandimmune), and muromonab-CD3 (Orthoclone OKT3) are immunosuppressive drugs.

When taking drugs to suppress the immune system, the client has no defense against disease and is at increased risk for development of infection, especially in the respiratory or urinary system. Observe such clients for signs and symptoms of infection such as fever, sore throat, productive cough, and dysuria.

Interferon is administered parenterally because digestive enzymes destroy its protein structure.

Cytokines used as biologic response modifiers are known to cause flulike side effects, including fever, chills, muscle aches, and fatigue. The incidence of serious side effects usually is dose related and can include neurologic toxicity manifested by depression, memory impairment, and coma. Dysrhythmias and blood pressure changes are examples of cardiovascular side effects. Other body systems also are subject to toxic effects.

Two new drugs, infliximab (Remicade) and etanercept (Enbrel), block tumor necrosis factor. These drugs are being used therapeutically to minimize inflammation. They are administered to clients with rheumatoid arthritis (see Chap. 67) and Crohn's disease (see Chap. 53).

Aldesleukin (rIL-2) is a genetically engineered form of human interleukin-2. It is being used as biologic therapy for clients who have not responded to conventional cancer treatment to stimulate the immune system's ability to target tumor cells.

GENERAL GERONTOLOGIC CONSIDERATIONS

The older client is more likely to have problems related to the immune system because the activity of the immune system declines with the natural aging process.

Older adults with chronic diseases such as respiratory disorders or cardiac disease should have an annual influenza vaccine and a one-time pneumococcal vaccine.

Although vaccination against viral disorders is recommended for older adults, vaccines are less effective in an older adult than in a younger adult, probably because of the decreased immune response that occurs with age.

Critical Thinking Exercises

1. *How would you respond to a friend who tells you that her sister has an immune disorder and asks what this means?*
2. *Discuss the benefit of obtaining immunizations for common childhood diseases.*

References and Suggested Readings

Alcoser, P. W. & Burchett, S. (1999). Bone marrow transplantation: Immune system suppression and reconstitution. *American Journal of Nursing, 99*(6), 26–32.

Bliss, D. Z. & Lehmann, S. (1999). Tube feeding: immune-boosting formulas. *RN, 62*(8), 26–28, 32.

Bullock, B. & Henze, R. L. (1999). *Focus on pathophysiology.* Philadelphia: Lippincott Williams & Wilkins.

Cohen, B. J. (1999). *Memmler's the human body in health and disease* (9th ed.). Philadelphia: Lippincott Williams & Wilkins.

Copstead, L. C. & Banasik, J. L. (1999). *Pathophysiology: Biological and behavioral perspectives* (2nd ed.). Philadelphia: W. B. Saunders.

Decker, G. M. (2000). Integrated care. Pharmacologic and biologic therapies in cancer care: Part II. *Clinical Journal of Oncology Nursing, 4,* 283–284, 287.

Dudek, S. G. (2001). *Nutrition handbook for nursing practice* (4th ed.). Philadelphia: Lippincott Williams & Wilkins.

Fischbach, F. T. (1999). *A manual of laboratory diagnostic tests* (6th ed.). Philadelphia: Lippincott Williams & Wilkins.

Gonzalez, Z. A. (2000). Practical aspects of nutritional modulation of the cytokines response. *Nutrition in Clinical Practice, 15*(1), 45–47.

Kaye, J. (2000). Stress, depression, and psychoneuroimmunology. *Journal of Neuroscience Nursing, 32*(2), 93–100.

Martini, F. (1998). *Fundamentals of anatomy and physiology* (4th ed.). Englewood Cliffs, NJ: Prentice Hall.

Moldawer, N. & Carr, E. (2000). The promise of recombinant interleukin-2. *American Journal of Nursing, 100*(5), 35–40.

Nevidjon, B. M. & Sowers, K. (2000). *A nurse's guide to cancer care.* Philadelphia: Lippincott Williams & Wilkins.

Pace, B. (2000). Suppressing the immune system for organ transplants. *Journal of the American Medical Association, 283*(18), 2484.

Smeltzer, S. C. & Bare, B. G. (1999). *Brunner and Suddarth's textbook of medical-surgical nursing* (9th ed.). Philadelphia: Lippincott Williams & Wilkins.

Caring for Clients With Immune-Mediated Disorders

Words to Know

allergen
allergic disorder
alloimmunity
anaphylaxis
angioneurotic edema
autoantibodies
autoimmune disorder
chemotaxis
chronic fatigue syndrome
desensitization
exacerbation

fibromyalgia
histocompatible cells
mast cells
neurally mediated
    hypotension
remission
sensitization
tilt-table test
urticaria

Learning Objectives

On completion of this chapter, the reader will:

- Describe an allergic disorder.
- List five examples of allergic signs and symptoms.
- Name four categories of allergens, and give an example of each.
- Give four examples of allergic reactions, including two that are potentially life-threatening.
- Describe diagnostic skin testing.
- Name three methods for treating allergies.
- Discuss the nursing management of a client with an allergic disorder.
- Explain the meaning of autoimmune disorder, and give at least three examples of related diseases.
- Discuss at least one theory that explains the development of an autoimmune disorder.
- Name three categories of drugs used in the treatment of autoimmune disorders.
- Discuss the nursing management of a client with an autoimmune disorder.
- Give two explanations for how chronic fatigue syndrome develops.
- List common symptoms experienced by people with chronic fatigue syndrome.
- Name three common nursing diagnoses, desired outcomes, and related nursing interventions for clients who have chronic fatigue syndrome.

The immune system sometimes responds aggressively and destructively to substances that may not always be potentially harmful. Two examples of such a response include allergic and autoimmune disorders. This chapter discusses allergic and autoimmune disorders and appropriate nursing care for clients who have them. It also explores chronic fatigue syndrome, which is a consequence of an immune-mediated disorder, and nursing management of this condition.

ALLERGIC DISORDERS

An **allergic disorder** is characterized by a hyperimmune response to weak antigens that usually are harmless (Table 42-1). The antigens that can cause an allergic response are called **allergens.** Allergens have a protein component and gain entry to the host from the environment. Allergies can occur at any age, and the pattern of allergic response can vary in the same person during his

TABLE 42-1	COMMON ALLERGENS	
TYPE OF ALLERGEN	**EXAMPLES**	**COMMON REACTION**
Ingestants	Food, drugs (especially penicillin)	Gastroenteropathy, dermatitis, asthma, anaphylaxis, urticaria, angioedema, serum sickness
Inhalants	House dust and mites, insect excrement, animal products (dander, saliva, urine), pollens, spores	Allergic asthma, rhinitis, hypersensitivity pneumonitis
Contactants	Plant oils, topical medications, occupational chemicals, cosmetics, metals in jewelry and clothing fasteners, hair dyes, latex	Contact dermatitis, urticaria or anaphylaxis (rare)
Injectants	Drugs, bee venom	Anaphylaxis, angioedema, acute urticaria

or her life. For example, a person may suddenly develop an allergic reaction to a substance like latex, even though he or she has had multiple prior contacts with latex and no past problems. On the other hand, an allergic response to one agent may gradually disappear or be replaced by sensitivity to another substance. The reason for these changes is unclear.

Types of Allergies

An allergic disorder is manifested in a variety of ways depending on the manner in which the allergen gains entry to the body and the intensity of the response. Organs and structures that are primarily involved in allergic reactions include the skin, respiratory passageways, gastrointestinal tract, blood, and vascular system (Table 42-2). Some types of allergic manifestations cause temporary, localized discomfort, whereas others are life-threatening.

Stop, Think, and Respond ● BOX 42-1

List substances to which you or others you know are allergic.

Pathophysiology and Etiology

Approximately 10% to 15% of the population develop allergies. The tendency can be inherited. Although members of the same family may have allergies, they may not all be sensitive to the same allergens. Allergy-prone individuals may react to more than one type of antigen. For example, the same person may be sensitive to ragweed pollen and eggs.

The first exposure to an allergen does not produce symptoms; rather, it causes sensitization. **Sensitization** is the process by which cellular and chemical events follow during a second or subsequent exposure to an allergen.

TABLE 42-2	TYPES OF ALLERGIES	
ALLERGY TYPE	**SIGNS AND SYMPTOMS**	**MEDICAL MANAGEMENT**
Allergic rhinitis	Sneezing, itching, nasal congestion, watery nasal discharge, itching and redness of the eyes	Antihistamines, nasal decongestants, corticosteroid nasal spray, immunotherapy, allergen avoidance, eye drops
Contact dermatitis	Itching, burning, redness, rash on contact with substance	Allergen avoidance, wearing gloves, topical or oral antihistamines and corticosteroids
Dermatitis medicamentosa	Sudden generalized bright red rash, itching, fever, malaise, headache, arthralgias	Discontinuation of drug, antihistamines and topical corticosteroids
Food allergy	Nausea, vomiting, diarrhea, abdominal cramping, malaise, itching, wheezing, rash, cough	Identification and avoidance of allergenic food
Urticaria	Itching, swelling, redness, wheals of superficial skin layers	Topical or oral antihistamines and corticosteroids
Angioedema	Itching, swelling, redness of deeper tissues and mucous membranes	Intubation, subcutaneous epinephrine, aminophylline

Once sensitization occurs, the hypersensitivity reaction can be immediate or delayed depending on the time it takes for the immune system to mount a response.

An *immediate hypersensitivity response* occurs rapidly. **Anaphylaxis,** a rapid and profound allergic response characterized by shock, laryngeal edema, wheezing, stridor, tachycardia, and generalized itching, can occur seconds to minutes after exposure to the sensitizing allergen (see Chap. 23). The more common immediate hypersensitivity responses result from activation of B-cell lymphocytes and their subsequent production of immunoglobulin E (IgE) antibodies. IgE antibodies attach to basophils or mast cells. **Mast cells** are constituents of connective tissue that contain granules of heparin, serotonin, bradykinin, and histamine (the most potent chemical of this group). With subsequent exposures to the allergen, mast cells and basophils release their vasoactive granules, causing various allergic and inflammatory manifestations (Fig. 42-1). Localized reactions can include watery eyes, increased nasal and bronchial secretions, sneezing, vomiting, and diarrhea. Additional symptoms include hives (called **urticaria**), itching, and localized redness (e.g., in the conjunctiva of the eyes). A massive release of histamine causes vasodilation; increased capillary permeability; **angioneurotic edema** (acute swelling of the face, neck, lips, larynx, hands, feet, genitals, and internal organs); hypotension; and bronchoconstriction (Fig. 42-2).

A *delayed hypersensitivity response* may develop over several hours or reach maximum severity days after exposure. Examples of a delayed hypersensitivity response include a blood transfusion reaction that occurs days to weeks after blood administration, rejection of transplanted tissues, and reaction to a tuberculin skin test. T-cell lymphocytes mediate delayed hypersensitivity reactions.

The body suppresses the allergic response through various mechanisms. One method involves the release of *eosinophil chemotactic factor* (ECF), a chemical mediator from mast cells. **Chemotaxis** refers to a process of attracting migratory cells to a particular area in the body. ECF attracts eosinophils, whose role is to suppress inflammation by degrading histamine and the other vaso-

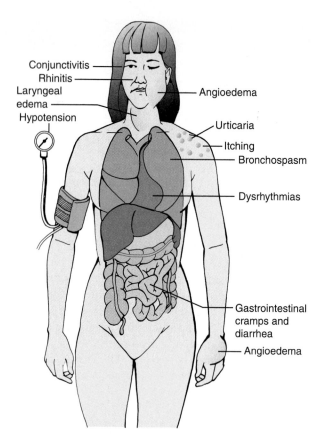

FIGURE 42-2 Manifestations of allergic reactions.

active chemicals. Epinephrine, a neurotransmitter, interferes with the release of vasoactive chemicals from mast cells. Corticosteroids, anti-inflammatory hormones produced by the adrenal cortex, block the synthesis of leukotrienes, also known as *slow-reactive substance of anaphylaxis,* and prostaglandins, both of which contribute to vascular permeability and smooth muscle contraction.

Stop, Think, and Respond ● BOX 42-2

Look up the following medications in a drug reference or pharmacology text: diphenhydramine (Benadryl), epinephrine hydrochloride (Adrenalin chloride), prednisone (Meticorten), montelukast (Singulair), and cromolyn (Intal, Crolom). Correlate their mechanisms of action with events that occur in an allergic reaction.

Assessment Findings

Signs and Symptoms

Clients often identify a cause-and-effect relationship between particular substances and their allergic symptoms. Clinical manifestations often correlate with the manner in

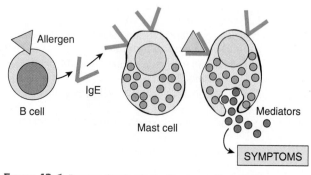

FIGURE 42-1 Process that leads to allergic manifestations.

which the allergen enters the body. For example, inhaled allergens usually cause respiratory symptoms, including nasal congestion, runny nose, sneezing, coughing, dyspnea, and wheezing. Inhaled allergens often trigger asthma (see Chap. 29). Contactants cause skin reactions such as hives, which appear as vesicles filled with clear fluid surrounded by a margin of redness; rash; and localized itching. Cramping, vomiting, and diarrhea are associated with ingested food allergens. Injectants, such as bee venom, and some other allergens can produce systemic and potentially fatal effects, including shock and airway obstruction caused by laryngeal swelling. Clients exhibit the same reaction with each exposure to the allergen.

Diagnostic Findings

Diagnosis of an allergy may be simple and clear-cut or may require multiple tests and extensive history-taking. Diagnosis becomes difficult when a client is allergic to more than one substance or when symptoms vary with fatigue, emotional stress, or the seasons.

Various abnormalities in blood test results suggest an allergic disorder. For example, the eosinophil count may be elevated. The radioallergosorbent blood test (RAST) measures IgE. On a scale of 0 to 5, a score of 2 or greater is a significant indication for an allergic disorder. The RAST does not identify which, if any, substances to which a person is allergic. It only validates that the person is potentially hypersensitive to antigenic substances.

Specific allergens can be identified by skin testing with extracts of various substances (antigens), such as pollens, animal danders, food, dust, and stinging insects. The three methods of skin testing are the scratch or prick test, the patch test, and the intradermal injection test.

The *scratch* or *prick test* involves scratching the skin and applying a small amount of the liquid test antigen to the scratch. The tester applies one allergen per scratch over the client's forearm, upper arm, or back. The back is more sensitive than the arms. It also provides a larger area for testing because each substance being tested should be distributed at least 3 cm and preferably up to 5 cm (slightly more than 1 to 2 inches) from one another. Results from a scratch test are identifiable in as little as 20 minutes. If a raised wheal or localized erythema appears, the tester measures its length and width in millimeters. The larger the reaction, the greater the likelihood that the tested allergen causes symptoms in the tested individual.

The *patch test* is used to identify the offending substance in allergic contact dermatitis. The tester applies a concentrated form of the substance to the skin and covers the area with an occlusive dressing. After 48 hours, the tester removes the dressing and examines the area for erythema, edema, and vesicles.

In the *intradermal injection test,* which usually is performed only when results of a scratch test are negative

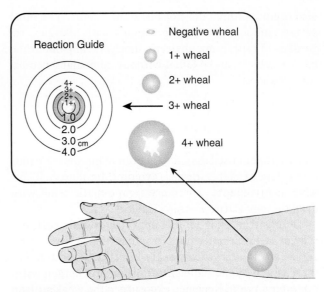

FIGURE 42-3 The wheal that forms after an intradermal skin test is measured to interpret the allergic response. The following scale is used: Negative = soft wheal and minimal redness; 1+ = 5–8 mm wheal and redness; 2+ = 7–20 mm wheal and redness; 3+ = 9–15 mm asymmetric wheal and redness; 4+ = >12 mm asymmetric wheal and diffuse redness.

for allergies, the tester injects a dilute solution of an antigen intradermally. A positive reaction is based on the size of a raised wheal and localized erythema (redness) that forms where the antigen was injected (Fig. 42-3).

To identify food allergens, the client fasts for 1 to 2 days, consuming only distilled water. He or she is then monitored for symptoms as new foods are added to the diet. Nursing Guidelines 42-1 explains the process of identifying food allergens in more detail.

Complications

Clients with inhalant allergies such as seasonal or allergic rhinitis (also known as *hay fever*) may develop nasal polyps from the chronic inflammation. They also are prone to sinus infections related to chronic nasal congestion. Secondary pulmonary infections such as bronchitis

---

NURSING GUIDELINES 42-1

Identifying Food Allergens

- Have the client fast for 1 to 2 days, drinking only distilled water.
- Introduce hypoallergenic foods (e.g., rice, tapioca) one at a time.
- Introduce allergenic foods (e.g., wheat, peanuts) one at a time in small quantities.
- Observe client for allergic symptoms after introducing each new food.

also occur. Asthma develops in some clients. The most severe complication among persons with allergies, regardless of type, is anaphylactic shock and angioneurotic edema, which can be lethal without immediate medical interventions.

Medical Management

The treatment used to relieve allergic symptoms depends on the type of allergy. Besides avoiding the allergen if possible, many clients experience symptomatic relief with drug therapy (Drug Therapy Table 42-1).

Desensitization is another option. **Desensitization** is a form of immunotherapy in which the individual receives weekly or twice-weekly injections of dilute but increasingly higher concentrations of an allergen without interruption. Repeated exposure to the weak antigen promotes the production of IgG, an antibody that blocks IgE so it cannot stimulate mast cells. When the maximum dose is achieved after 2 to 4 months of treatment, maintenance injections are administered at longer intervals, usually every 2 to 4 weeks. It may take several years before a person treated with desensitization experiences significant relief. After a desensitization injection, the client is observed for 30 minutes to assess for allergic symptoms. Epinephrine (Adrenalin) is administered if a severe reaction occurs.

Stop, Think, and Respond ● BOX 42-3

List signs and symptoms that suggest a person who is undergoing desensitization needs epinephrine.

Clients with severe allergies to bee venom are advised to carry an emergency kit that contains a premeasured dose of injectable epinephrine. The syringe autoinjects the epinephrine when pressed to the skin. The lateral thigh is the site most commonly used for injection (Fig. 42-4).

Nursing Management

Throughout the client's care, the nurse observes for signs of an allergic reaction, especially when administering medications, applying substances like tape or adhesive patches to the skin, or caring for a client receiving contrast media for diagnostic testing. If the nurse suspects a mild allergic reaction, he or she removes or withholds the offending substance and notifies the physician. If a client has an anaphylactic reaction, the nurse acts immediately to stop the client's exposure to the allergen and provides life support while summoning the code team or calling the 911 operator.

Occasionally, the nurse needs to remove a ring from a swelling finger. If applying soap or oil to the finger proves unsuccessful, the nurse may wrap the finger with twine (Fig. 42-5). Once the tissue is compressed, the ring slides off the finger by pulling on the free end of the twine. This technique is preferable to damaging the ring with a metal cutter. If nothing else facilitates ring removal, however, cutting still is a better option than allowing tissue damage from ischemia to develop.

The nurse instructs clients who will undergo diagnostic skin testing to avoid taking prescribed or over-the-counter antihistamine or cold preparations for at least 48 to 72 hours before testing. Doing so reduces the potential for false-negative test results. Clients must temporarily discontinue some medications for even longer (see General Pharmacologic Considerations). The nurse assists the provider who performs diagnostic testing and helps to document findings. Once the test is completed, the nurse monitors the client's response until it is safe for the person to return home.

For clients who elect to undergo desensitization, the nurse administers the serial doses and monitors the client for 30 minutes after administration. He or she teaches clients who are being desensitized and those who choose drug therapy for relief of their allergy symptoms how to self-administer prescribed medications, especially those that are delivered by metered dose or dry powder inhalers, because many people use these devices incorrectly. The nurse must make clients aware of possible side effects and when medical follow-up is necessary.

Techniques for avoiding or reducing exposure in the client's home and work environment are nursing areas for health teaching. Some examples include the following:

- Insisting that the environment be "smoke free" when a person manifests inhalant allergies or respiratory symptoms
- Keeping pets outdoors or at least in one confined area of the home
- Bathing pets weekly or at frequent intervals
- Covering the mattress and box springs with an impervious material to reduce dust mites
- Eliminating area rugs
- Contracting with an exterminator if cockroaches or other vermin are present
- Cleaning humidifiers and heating and cooling ducts to remove mold spores

For other health teaching information, see Client and Family Teaching Box 42-1.

Stop, Think, and Respond ● BOX 42-4

Discuss ways to avoid inhaled and ingested allergens.

DRUG THERAPY TABLE 42-1 | **ALLERGIC DISORDERS**

DRUG CATEGORY AND EXAMPLES	MECHANISM OF ACTION	SIDE EFFECTS	NURSING CONSIDERATIONS
Antihistamines diphenhydramine (Benadryl), hydroxyzine (Atarax), fexofenadine (Allegra), astemizole (Hismanal), loratidine (Claritin), cetirizine (Zyrtec)	Block histamine (H₁) receptors	Sedation, dryness of mucous membranes; rare: heart dysrhythmias	Caution client not to drive or operate machinery until sedative effects of medication are known.
Nasal Decongestant Agents flunisolide (Nasalide), oxymetazoline hydrochloride (Afrin)	Vasoconstrict nasal membranes	Headache, transient nasal burning, nasal congestion, sneezing, epistaxis, rebound nasal congestion	Advise client to pump spray three to four times before first use and one to two times before each daily use to prime. Caution clients using Afrin to avoid using for longer than 3 to 5 days in a row or rebound nasal congestion may occur.
Nasal Steroid Spray and Inhalant beclomethasone dipropionate (Beconase), fluticasone propionate (Flonase), fluticasone propionate (Flovent)	Anti-inflammatory	Headache, fungal infection, nasal irritation, cough, flulike illness	Examine nares. Avoid contact with the eyes. Several weeks of therapy may be necessary for full benefit. Report sore throat or signs of oral fungal infection.
Oral Corticosteroids dexamethasone (Decadron), hydrocortisone (Cortef), methylprednisolone (Medrol)	Regulate immune response; control inflammatory response	Euphoria, insomnia, gastrointestinal irritation, increased appetite, weight gain, hyperglycemia	Taper doses when discontinuing; abrupt discontinuation may lead to acute adrenal insufficiency. Give doses in the morning with food. Monitor blood sugar levels. Assess for peripheral edema.
Oral Decongestant Agents pseudoephedrine hydrochloride (Sudafed), albuterol (Proventil), metaproterenol (Alupent), ipratropium (Atrovent), terbutaline (Brethine)	Vasoconstrict nasal membranes (sympathomimetics)	Anxiety, nervousness, palpitations, headache, dizziness, tremors, sleeplessness, hypertension	Use cautiously in clients with severe hypertension, diabetes, glaucoma, hyperthyroidism, prostatic hyperplasia, coronary artery disease, those taking monoamine oxidase inhibitors, and women who are breast-feeding. Avoid taking within 2 hours of bedtime. Brethine interferes with labor and delivery.
Bronchodilating Inhaled Agents epinephrine (Primatene Mist)	Stimulate adrenergic receptors or block cholinergic receptors	Nervousness, tremor, euphoria, palpitations, hypertension, dysrhythmias, headache	Monitor blood pressure and heart rate. Use caution in those with hypertension, heart disease, diabetes, cirrhosis, or those using digitalis glycosides. Teach proper technique for using inhaler.
Oral or Parenteral Sympathomimetic Agents epinephrine (Adrenalin chloride), theophylline (Theo-Dur, Elixophyllin), theophyllin (Aminophyllin)	Act on alpha or beta receptors	Nausea, anxiety, restlessness, headache, trembling, tachycardia, hypertension, increased urination, increased gastric secretions	Use cautiously in clients with gastritis or peptic ulcer disease, congestive heart failure, hyperthyroidism, or seizure disorders. Monitor vital signs regularly. Give oral drugs with food to decrease gastric irritation.
Leukotriene Antagonists montelukast (Singulair), zileuton (Zyflo)	Block receptors for leukotreines (slow-reacting substance of anaphylaxis)	Headache, nausea, abdominal upset, flulike symptoms such as fatigue, hepatotoxicity	Avoid if breast-feeding. Monitor for infections. Administer on an empty stomach.

1. Carefully uncap the Epipen device, holding it so that the injecting end is upright.

2. Position the device at the middle portion of the thigh.

3. Push the device into the thigh as far as possible. The Epipen device will autoinject a premeasured dose of epinephrine into the subcutaneous tissue.

FIGURE 42-4 To avoid an anaphylactic reaction, a premeasured dose of epinephrine is autoinjected into subcutaneous tissue.

FIGURE 42-5 Technique for ring removal.

42-1 *Client and Family Teaching*
Allergies

The nurse teaches clients who have allergic disorders and their family members the following guidelines:

- Never begin smoking or quit if you are currently smoking if your allergy causes respiratory symptoms.
- Treatment for chronic allergic disorders, such as allergic rhinitis and food allergies, may extend over several years.
- Follow the medical regimen as instructed by the physician.
- Do not overuse nose drops or sprays for nasal congestion. Use only prescribed or recommended drugs and only in the dosage suggested by the physician.
- Keep a record of symptoms or lack of symptoms. Bring the record to the physician's office or clinic. The record will help the physician determine therapy.
- Keep a record of symptoms or absence of symptoms each time you add a new food to the diet. Add new foods to the diet slowly and one at a time.
- Avoid environmental substances that cause allergic reactions.
- Seek immediate medical attention if symptoms worsen or new symptoms occur.
- Carry identification, such as a Medic-Alert card or bracelet, to inform medical personnel of allergies, especially if you have a history of anaphylactic reactions.
- Do not miss an immunotherapy appointment; missed appointments may necessitate restarting the series of injections.
- Check prefilled syringes that contain epinephrine for an expiration date. You must refill the prescription and discard the old prescription on or immediately before this date. Keep the directions for use with the product.

NURSING PROCESS

● The Client With an Allergic Disorder

Assessment

The nurse obtains a thorough history from the client with an actual or suspected allergic disorder. He or she gathers data about the client's diet history, paying particular attention to foods that cause problems. Determining if others in the family have allergies is important. The nurse records the client's description of allergic symptoms and the factors that appear to increase or decrease symptoms (e.g., exposures, time of year) in detail. Many clients say they are "allergic" to substances, but their descriptions of manifestations do not always support that conclusion. The nurse identifies all prescription and nonprescription drugs that the client takes and has reacted to in the past. He or she must be especially alert to allergic manifestations caused by contact with products that contain latex (Box 42-1). The nurse examines the skin and describes any rashes or eruptions.

Close observation of a client with allergies is essential each time a new drug is added to the therapeutic regimen. This includes drugs given by the nurse and drugs used for diagnostic studies, such as radiopaque dyes. Continual monitoring of the client is necessary when a second dose of a new drug is given because reactions may follow the first sensitizing dose.

Diagnosis, Planning, and Interventions

Altered Comfort: Itching related to histamine release
Expected Outcome: The client will have reduced itching and intact skin.

- Remove clothing and wash the skin with soap and flowing water after exposure to contact allergens (e.g., poison ivy, poison oak, poison sumac). *Reducing the source and duration of contact limits the severity of an allergic skin reaction.*
- Advise the client to limit the frequency of bathing with conventional bar soap and to use superfatted or castile soap. *Conventional bar soap contains lye, which dries the skin and predisposes it to itching and flaking. Superfatted soap uses less lye (sodium hydroxide, caustic soda). Castile soap contains a greater proportion of vegetable (e.g., olive, coconut, soybean, castor) oils.*
- Recommend bathing with tepid, rather than hot, water when hygiene is necessary and patting the skin dry rather than rubbing a towel vigorously over the skin. *Heat and rubbing intensify itching.*
- Advise the client to avoid scratching the skin. *Scratching releases additional histamine from cells, which leads to a self-stimulating cycle of itching–scratching–more itching.*

BOX 42-1 ● **Products that Contain Latex**

Household	Medical
Carpet backing	Gloves
Feeding nipples	Face masks
Pacifiers	Mattresses
Elastic in clothing	Patient-controlled analgesia syringes
Sports equipment	Ambu bags
Balloons	Stethoscope
Erasers	Blood pressure cuff tubing
Toys	Dental devices
Shoe soles	Urinary catheters
Condoms/diaphragms	Tourniquets
Computer mouse pads	Electrode pads
Buttons on electronic equipment	Bulb syringes
Food handled with powdered latex gloves	Syringe stoppers and medication vial stoppers
Handles on racquets, tools, and similar items	Adhesive tape
	Bandages
	Injection ports
	Wound drains

- Encourage the client to keep fingernails short or to wear cotton gloves, especially during sleep. *Impaired skin integrity predisposes the client to secondary bacterial infection. Short nails prevent skin trauma should the client be unable to resist scratching.*
- Apply a skin lubricant or emollient frequently. *Lubricants or emollients act as barriers on the skin that prevent loss of moisture. Moist skin is less vulnerable to trauma and itching.*
- Suggest using distracting techniques like doing a crossword puzzle or handicraft during periods of itching. *Flooding the brain with alternate stimuli removes the focus from itching.*
- Tell the client to dress in cotton garments rather than those made of rough or synthetic fibers. *Natural fibers facilitate escape of heat from the skin surface, reducing vasodilation and intensification of itching. Rough fabrics irritate the skin, which exacerbates itching.*
- Humidify the environment. *Adding moisture to the environment reduces the potential for dry, itchy skin.*
- Administer prescribed topical, inhaled, oral, or intravenous (IV) drugs. *Antihistamines block histamine receptors, and corticosteroids interfere with release of chemicals from mast cells, thereby relieving itching, redness, rash, and localized swelling.*

Impaired Home Maintenance related to an environment that produces moderate to severe allergic symptoms
Expected Outcome: The client will modify the home environment, subsequently reducing allergic symptoms.

- Explore ways to avoid the offending allergen. *Preventing contact with the allergen is the first step in avoiding an allergic reaction.*
- Propose using air conditioning during summer months and special furnace filters or electrostatic cleaners for

home heating and cooling. *Limiting allergen sources in inhaled air reduces allergic symptoms.*

- Recommend using hypoallergenic products and wearing rubber or vinyl gloves (avoid latex) when using cleaning chemicals. *Hypoallergenic products contain ingredients that do not commonly cause reactions in sensitive people. Gloves act as a barrier between a person's skin and the offending allergen.*

PC: Anaphylaxis and Angioedema

Expected Outcome: The nurse will manage and minimize manifestations of a severe allergic reaction.

- Closely monitor the client's blood pressure, pulse rate and quality, respiratory effort, and urine output. *Vasodilation and increased capillary permeability affect circulating volume. Hypotension, tachycardia, thready pulse, and oliguria are evidence of reduced circulating volume. Respiratory distress is associated with contraction of smooth muscles in the bronchi or swelling of tissues in the airway.*
- Place the client in mid- or high-Fowler's position if respiratory distress is evident. *An upright position allows greater lung expansion by lowering abdominal organs away from the diaphragm.*
- Maintain an open airway and administer high-flow rates of oxygen. *Cells and organs die when they are deprived of oxygen.*
- Initiate the system for obtaining advanced cardiac life support (ACLS) either through a 911 system in the community or by announcing a "Code Blue" and its location in a healthcare agency. *Implementation of ACLS measures enhances resuscitation efforts.*
- In the healthcare facility, delegate someone to bring the emergency cart to the client's bedside. *When the code team arrives, emergency drugs, an endotracheal tube, bag-valve mask, and defibrillator may be needed. Saving time improves the outcome for the client.*
- Administer cardiopulmonary resuscitation with the client on a hard surface if cardiac or respiratory arrest occurs. *Pulmonary resuscitation, preferably with a resuscitation mouthpiece, promotes alveolar capillary diffusion of oxygen. Chest compressions squeeze the heart between the sternum and vertebrae, increasing cardiac output and blood supply to vital organs.*
- Seek the assistance of a registered nurse to insert an IV line as soon as possible if one is not already in place. *Decreased blood pressure reduces the ability to distend and cannulate a vein. Emergency medications usually are administered by the IV route.*
- Report assessment findings as the code team arrives. *Problem-solving and definitive treatment depend on analyzing current data.*
- Assist the code team in delegated activities or intervene in crowd control. *The code team has preassigned responsibilities, but they may need assistance in contacting the laboratory or radiology department for specific requests. Curious spectators or concerned family may interfere with resuscitation efforts.*

Evaluation of Expected Outcomes

The client reports relief of itching. He or she shows no evidence of rash. Skin is smooth and uniform in color. The client makes necessary changes in the home to reduce allergies (e.g., client removes area throw rugs; a friend adopts the family pet; the client contacts a heating and cooling specialist to discuss modifications to present system). Vital signs are stable. Breathing is effortless.

AUTOIMMUNE DISORDERS

Autoimmune disorders are those in which killer T cells and autoantibodies attack or destroy natural cells—those cells that are "self." **Autoantibodies,** antibodies against self-antigens, are immunoglobulins. They target **histocompatible cells,** cells whose antigens match the individual's own genetic code. Diseases are considered autoimmune disorders when they are characterized by unrelenting, progressive tissue damage without any verifiable etiology. Various specific disorders classified as autoimmune are discussed throughout this text. Refer to Chapter 45 for information on multiple sclerosis, Chapter 64 for discussion of acute glomerulonephritis, and Chapter 67 for coverage of rheumatoid arthritis and systemic lupus erythematosus.

The term **alloimmunity** is used to describe an immune response that is waged against transplanted organs and tissues that carry nonself antigens. See Chapters 37 and 64 for more information.

Pathophysiology and Etiology

Several theories have been proposed to explain the cause of autoimmune disorders (Table 42-3). None appears to explain autoimmunity completely, which suggests that more than one mechanism is responsible.

In many autoimmune disorders, there tends to be a triggering event, such as an infection, trauma, or introduction of a drug that integrates itself into the membranes of the host's cells. One hypothesis is that the triggering event upsets the immune system's tolerance or recognition of self-antigens. A cause-and-effect relationship exists between some viral and bacterial infections (e.g., measles) and the development of a blood disorder called *thrombocytopenic purpura* (see Chap. 39). Another cause-and-effect relationship is found between streptococcal infections and disorders like rheumatic heart disease (see Chap. 31). Despite such relationships, no scientific evidence has been found to support the hypothesis. It may be that the antigenic surface of the microorganism so closely resembles the person's histocompatible cell markers that the antibodies cannot differentiate between host and invader.

TABLE 42-3	AUTOIMMUNITY THEORIES
THEORY	**HYPOTHESIS**
Cross-antigen theory	Self-antigens that resemble foreign antigens cause T cells to misidentify natural cells and mount an immune attack.
Tissue injury theory	Infection, trauma, drugs, and radiation alter natural cells. Consequently, they no longer resemble self-antigens.
Viral mutation theory	Viruses alter T-cell receptors that are used to differentiate self from nonself.
Sequestered antigen theory	Some cells, like those of the thyroid, brain, and lens of the eye, are separated from lymphocytes during fetal development. When these cells enter circulation later because of trauma or infection, T cells do not recognize them as "self."
Diminished T-suppressor theory	Reduced numbers of suppressor cells or a shortened life span because of aging and atrophy of the thymus gland alters immunoregulation.
Genetic instruction theory	Genetic coding for antibody production is altered, which explains the familial pattern to some autoimmune disorders.

Some believe that certain individuals are genetically predisposed to autoimmune disorders. Theorists have proposed that the histocompatible markers, which are genetically inherited, act as receptors for disease-causing microorganisms, making certain cells more vulnerable than others. Another possibility is that some people inherit a trait for suppressor T-cell dysfunction. The role of suppressor T cells is to mediate immune responses. Without adequate suppressor T-cell function, killer T cells can destroy healthy cells, tissues, and organs without restraint. Consequently, genetic factors may also be a link in explaining why autoimmune disorders have a tendency to occur among blood relatives.

Another interesting phenomenon supports the sequestered antigen theory. Evidence has shown that when a person experiences trauma followed by inflammation to the iris, ciliary body, and choroid layer of one eye, the vision in the untraumatized eye also becomes affected. The term for this phenomenon is *sympathetic uveitis.* The explanation may be related to the fact that during fetal development, the cells and tissues of the eye are not exposed to the lymphatic drainage system. Therefore, the lymphocytes have never learned to recognize the ocular cells as having self-antigens. When trauma occurs and these cells are no longer sequestered, or hidden, from the lymphocytes, the immune system attacks what it perceives to be foreign.

Regardless of whether one or all of these theoretical etiologies is valid, the outcome is clear. The immune system fails to recognize histocompatible cells. Consequently, T and B cells mount a cell-mediated or humoral response (see Chap. 41). The attack may be localized to one organ or type of tissue or it may be systemic (Box 42-2). Cells, tissues, and organs under attack are damaged or destroyed.

Assessment Findings

Signs and Symptoms

Autoimmune disorders produce various signs and symptoms depending on the tissues and organs affected. The symptoms are characteristic of an acute inflammatory response. They develop as antibodies attack normal tissue mistakenly identified as nonself. In some cases, the inflammatory symptoms are episodic. Periods of acute flare-ups (known as **exacerbations**) alternate with periods of **remission** (asymptomatic periods). The duration of these periods is completely unpredictable. During acute exacerbations, clients often experience a low-grade fever, malaise, or fatigue. They also may lose weight.

Stop, Think, and Respond ● BOX 42-5
What could explain why autoimmune disorders have periods of remission and exacerbation?

Diagnostic Findings

Diagnostic testing varies depending on the autoimmune disorder. Overall, elevated circulating antibodies are the hallmark findings for autoimmune disorders. Some examples include elevated erythrocyte sedimentation rate, antistreptolysin-O titer, antinuclear antibody titer, and rheumatoid factor.

BOX 42-2 ● Examples of Autoimmune Disorders

ORGAN SPECIFIC
Blood
  Hemolytic anemia
  Thrombocytopenia purpura
Central nervous system
  Multiple sclerosis
  Guillain-Barré syndrome
Heart
  Endocarditis
Muscles
  Myasthenia gravis
Endocrine
  Hashimoto's thyroiditis
  Type 1 diabetes mellitus

Eye
  Uveitis
Joint
  Ankylosing spondylitis
Gastrointestinal
  Ulcerative colitis
Renal
  Glomerulonephritis

SYSTEMIC
Systemic lupus erythematosus
Scleroderma
Rheumatoid arthritis
Sjögren's syndrome

Medical Management

Autoimmune disorders are rarely cured. The goal of therapy is to induce a remission or slow the immune system's destruction. Drug therapy using anti-inflammatory and immunosuppressive agents is the mainstay for alleviating symptoms (Drug Therapy Table 42-2).

Some antineoplastic (cancer) drugs also are used for their immunosuppressant effects. Controlling or limiting side effects of the drugs, one of which is increased susceptibility to infection, is a major concern. Even with remission, most people must continue taking prescribed medications to avoid another acute exacerbation.

DRUG THERAPY TABLE 42-2	IMMUNOSUPPRESSIVE DRUGS		
DRUG CATEGORY AND EXAMPLES	**MECHANISM OF ACTION**	**SIDE EFFECTS**	**NURSING CONSIDERATIONS**
Corticosteroids			
prednisone (Meticorten) methylprednisolone (Medrol)	Initiates many immuno-suppressive and anti-inflammatory cellular responses	Euphoria, insomnia, gastrointestinal irritation, increased appetite, weight gain	Dose must be tapered. Abrupt withdrawal may cause acute adrenal insufficiency.
Cytotoxic Drugs			
azathioprine (Immuran)	Suppresses cell-mediated hypersensitivity and alters antibody production	Oral ulceration, nausea, vomiting, pancreatitis, leukopenia, bone marrow suppression, hepatotoxicity, immunosuppression, thrombocytopenia, rash, hair thinning	Follow facility policy on administration of cytotoxic drugs. Instruct clients not to take aspirin. Warn client to report signs of infection and to use effective birth control during treatment and for 4 months after.
cyclophosphamide (Cytoxan)	Interferes with replication of lymphocytes	Cardiotoxicity, anorexia, nausea, vomiting, oral ulceration, hemorrhagic cystitis, leukopenia, thrombocytopenia, anemia, pulmonary fibrosis, reversible alopecia	Advise clients to void every 1 to 2 hours while awake and to drink at least 3 L of fluid per day to reduce risk of cystitis. Do not give drug at bedtime.
methotrexate (Folex-PFS, Mexate-AQ, Rheumatrex)	Inhibits cellular replication	Stomatitis, diarrhea, nausea, vomiting, tubular necrosis, anemia, leukopenia, thrombocytopenia, hepatotoxicity, pulmonary fibrosis, urticaria, photosensitivity, alopecia	Follow facility policy on administration of cytotoxic drugs. Advise client to use birth control while on medication and to report signs of infection immediately.
Immunosuppressives			
cyclosporine (Sandimmune)	Inhibits lymphocytes; exact mechanism of action unknown	Tremor, gum hyperplasia, nausea, vomiting, diarrhea, nephrotoxicity, leukopenia, thrombocytopenia, hepatotoxicity	Warn client to report signs of infection, take drug at same time every day, take with meals if it causes nausea, avoid pregnancy, and not to stop medication without physician approval. Risk for anaphylaxis is high with injection form. Advise clients to report signs of infection immediately.
tacrolimus (Prograf)	Inhibits T-cell activation; exact mechanism of action unknown	Hypersensitivity, headache, tremor, insomnia, hypertension, diarrhea, nausea, abnormal renal function, anemia, leukocytosis, thrombocytopenia, hyperkalemia, hyperglycemia, hypomagnesemia, pleural effusion, pain, fever, asthenia	Monitor for anaphylaxis for 30 minutes after starting an infusion and frequently thereafter. Have epinephrine (1:1000) and oxygen available at the bedside. Check blood cell counts for suppression. Inform client of an increased risk for cancer. Store diluted solution in glass or polyethylene (not polyvinyl chloride) containers and discard if unused after 24 hours.

42-2 *Client and Family Teaching*
Autoimmune Disorders

The nurse teaches clients who have autoimmune disorders and their family members the following guidelines:

- Notify a healthcare practitioner of any sign of infection such as cough, fever, severe diarrhea, mouth lesions, or sore throat.
- Notify a healthcare practitioner of any new side effects to prescribed medications.
- Do not stop taking any medications abruptly.
- Avoid crowds or people with infections if you are taking an immunosuppressant drug.
- Limit stress and use stress reduction techniques such as progressive relaxation or breathing exercises.
- Maintain close follow-up with a physician.

NURSING PROCESS

● The Client With an Autoimmune Disorder

Assessment

During the initial interview with the client, the nurse obtains a family history and is alert to information about family members who have had chronic diseases with an inflammatory component that involve cardiac, urinary, neurologic, or connective tissues. During acute exacerbations, the client is quite ill. Vital signs may reveal elevated temperature, a finding supporting an infectious or inflammatory process. The nurse examines the client for signs of localized inflammation and compromised body functions such as changes in the skin, joints, gait, heart, and renal function. He or she asks about the client's level of energy because fatigue is common. The nurse reviews laboratory test findings for evidence that correlates with an inflammatory process or immunologic changes typical of one of many autoimmune disorders. Teaching points for those with autoimmune disorders are discussed in Client and Family Teaching Box 42-2.

Diagnosis, Planning, and Interventions

Activity Intolerance related to joint pain secondary to inflammation, malaise, and fatigue
Expected Outcome: The client will perform activities of daily living (ADLs) without extreme fatigue or discomfort.

- Encourage rest during periods of severe exacerbation and regular exercise during periods of remission. *Activity levels within a client's level of endurance*

promote well-being. Endurance is related to the frequency, duration, and intensity of activity (Carpenito, 2000).

- Provide nonpharmacologic and pharmacologic pain management as ordered by the physician. *Nonpainful stimuli (e.g., massage, activity, heat, cold, imagery, pleasant sounds) can reduce or relieve pain. Analgesic anti-inflammatory medications block neurotransmitters that carry pain stimuli to the brain; narcotic analgesics dull the brain, making it less perceptive to pain transmission; corticosteroids suppress the immune response.*

Risk for Infection related to immunosuppression secondary to drug therapy for the autoimmune disorder and generally poor physical condition
Expected Outcome: The client will be free of infection.

- Instruct the client about signs and symptoms of and the increased risk for infection. *Access to knowledge facilitates an active role in restoring health.*
- Instruct the client to report signs and symptoms of infection (e.g., cough, dyspnea, diarrhea, fever) immediately to the physician. *Early treatment promotes a shorter duration of illness and reduced complications.*
- Tell the client to avoid high-risk activities, such as being in crowds, during periods of immunosuppression. *Risk for infection increases with exposure to others who may have infectious disorders or whose handwashing and hygiene measures are less than adequate.*

Disturbed Personal Identity related to coping with chronic illness and physical changes associated with autoimmune disorders
Expected Outcome: The client will maintain a positive self-concept.

- Interact with and frequently show genuine interest in the client. *A person's concept of "self" is determined to a great extent by the response of others. The client may interpret lack of interest and avoidance as rejection and being unworthy of attention.*
- Refer the client to community organizations and support groups. *Sharing problems and experiences with others who are similarly affected dispels the idea that a person's symptoms and feelings are unique. A person can more easily resolve and tolerate problems when he or she shares the burden with others.*

Evaluation of Expected Outcomes

The client participates in self-care and ADLs without overwhelming fatigue. There is no evidence of *iatrogenic* (treatment-caused) infection. The client perceives himself or herself realistically with more positive attributes than negative.

CHRONIC FATIGUE SYNDROME

Chronic fatigue syndrome (CFS), also called *chronic fatigue* and *immune dysfunction syndrome*, is a complex of symptoms primarily characterized by profound fatigue with no identifiable cause. The fatigue worsens with physical activity and does not improve with rest. The term *chronic* refers to the fact that the duration of fatigue has been unrelenting for 6 or more months. Some believe that CFS is associated with **fibromyalgia**, pain in fibrous tissues of the body such as muscles, ligaments, and tendons, because both conditions share many symptoms.

Since beginning to collect surveillance data in 1989, the Centers for Disease Control and Prevention estimates that as many as 500,000 people in the United States have symptoms that correspond with CFS (National Center for Infectious Diseases, 2001). Most of those who seek treatment for their symptoms are white women 20 to 50 years of age. CFS also occurs in men and among other races. Some clients experience improvement, but not a cure, after 1 year of treatment; most suffer with their symptoms for years and may feel worse. When the duration of symptoms is lengthy, the prognosis is less optimistic.

Pathophysiology and Etiology

A cause for CFS has not yet been established. Some believe that the disorder results from immune system dysregulation, in which the immune system remains activated for an extended period after an infectious triggering event. Although researchers have attempted to find a link between CFS and viral diseases (like infectious mononucleosis caused by the Epstein-Barr virus and enteroviruses), fungal and mycoplasmal infections, or others, no single causal relationship has been found. Some hypothesize that T cells are activated initially in response to a virus and that levels of proinflammatory cytokines, like various interleukins and tumor necrosis factor, remain elevated (see Chap. 41). It is well documented that cytokines produce achy, flulike symptoms accompanied by fever and malaise during the early stages of infections. People with CFS experience these same symptoms. The difference is that during infections the symptoms are brief, but in CFS they are relentlessly prolonged.

The fact that serum cortisol levels are low among those with CSF symptoms leads to a second hypothesis. Some believe that CSF is a consequence of impaired activation of three neuroendocrine structures: the hypothalamus, pituitary gland, and adrenal glands. Collectively, these structures are sometimes referred to as the *HPA axis*. When the HPA axis functions normally, it is stimulated to release hormones during periods of physical stress, like an infection, or emotional stress. The hypothalamus secretes corticotropin-releasing factor, which tells the pituitary to release adrenocorticotropic hormone (ACTH). When ACTH stimulates the adrenal glands, they make corticosterone (cortisol). Cortisol suppresses inflammation and immune activity. Down-regulation of the HPA axis interferes with immune suppression and allows the hyperfunctioning immune processes to continue unabated.

Down-regulation of the HPA axis also helps to explain why those with CFS experience **neurally mediated hypotension** (NMH). NMH is a condition in which individuals experience hypotension accompanied by fatigue after standing for more than 10 minutes. Some attribute the symptoms to pooling of blood in the lower limbs, resulting in decreased cerebral oxygenation. Because corticosteroids are associated with fluid retention, reduced cortisol levels may cause the hypotension.

Assessment Findings

Signs and Symptoms

Many clients with CFS report having had a recent illness with flulike symptoms or an upper respiratory infection. Despite having been uncomfortable, most clients do not describe their initial symptoms as being extraordinarily severe. In fact, the opposite is true. Thereafter, however, severe, ongoing fatigue has lasted for at least 6 months without any explanation. Even though the fatigue is constant, it worsens after physical activity. The fatigue is so debilitating that it usually interferes with a person's ability to work in or outside the home.

In addition to fatigue, the client exhibits at least four or more of the following:

- Low-grade fever
- Sore throat
- Tender cervical or axillary lymph nodes
- Muscle weakness
- Myalgia (muscle pain)
- Headaches
- Migrating joint pain without any accompanying swelling or redness
- Unrefreshing sleep
- Neurologic symptoms like photophobia, defects in the visual field, irritability, forgetfulness, confusion, difficulty concentrating, and depression

---

Stop, Think, and Respond ● BOX 42-6

Discuss possible consequences among people who suffer unrelenting fatigue and pain.

Diagnostic Findings

Findings of the medical history and physical examination are unremarkable. Although the client may have other physical or psychological conditions, they are unrelated to the client's presenting symptoms. Results from a battery of blood tests specific for diagnosing diseases associated with fatigue such as alkaline phosphatase; blood urea nitrogen; serum calcium, glucose, and thyroid-stimulating hormone levels; and tests for antinuclear antibodies all fail to reveal an explanation for the client's symptoms. The exhaustive medical workup excludes all diagnoses except CFS.

A **tilt-table test,** one in which the client lays horizontally on a table whose incline is elevated to approximately 70 degrees for 45 minutes, may be done. During the test, the blood pressure and pulse are monitored. The test tends to provoke hypotension in 96% of those eventually diagnosed with CFS (National Center for Infectious Diseases, 2001).

Medical Management

Treatment focuses on relieving the client's symptoms because nothing, as yet, holds promise for a cure. One drug, polyl:polyC12U (Ampligen), is producing modest improvement among individuals with CFS. This drug is a synthetic nucleic acid that stimulates the production of interferons, which have antiviral functions and modify the immune response. Ampligen has been used in the adjunctive treatment of cancer and AIDS, but results have not been extraordinarily promising. Manufacturers of nicotinamide adenine dinucleotide (NADH), a nutritional supplement known as Enada, claim it stimulates the production of adenosine triphosphate, which provides cellular energy. Approximately one third of participants with CFS using Enada in clinical trials report more endurance and less fatigue.

Without any definitive drug treatment, the client is advised to balance activity with rest. An employed client may need to resign from his or her job or negotiate for a less physically demanding position. The physician may prescribe a modest exercise program under the supervision of a physical therapist to avoid muscle atrophy that contributes to weakness. The client is to avoid overexertion at all costs.

Mild pain and fever are treated with aspirin, acetaminophen (Tylenol), or nonsteroidal anti-inflammatory agents like ibuprofen (Motrin, Advil) or naproxen sodium (Naprosyn, Aleve). Even low doses of tricyclic antidepressants like amitriptyline (Elavil), doxepin (Sinequan), or nortriptyline (Pamelor) can relieve pain and improve sleep.

Clients who experience hypotension are advised to increase salt and water intake as long as doing so is not contraindicated by cardiac or renal disease. Some clients also experience greater blood pressure stability when fludrocortisone (Florinef), a corticosteroid, is prescribed. An antihypotensive agent like midodrine (ProAmatine) may be prescribed to increase vascular tone and elevate blood pressure.

Several adjunct and alternative therapies are suggested to treat clients with CFS holistically. Some benefit from cognitive therapy, a form of psychotherapy in which persons learn skills to change distorted thoughts about themselves. For example, cognitive therapy may help a person with CFS who believes that he or she is a helpless victim of the disease to perceive himself or herself as capable of dealing with the fatigue. Some promote the use of acupuncture, Eastern exercise and meditation techniques like yoga and tai chi, and phototherapy (see Chaps. 12 and 15) to contribute to well-being. Until more information is known about CFS, however, clients may fall victim to herbal and dietary claims that promise a cure. As long as the alternative therapy is not dangerous, the client's right to incorporate unproven or unstandardized methods is not challenged.

Nursing Management

The nurse educates the client about his or her disease process and the limitations that it requires (see Client and Family Teaching Box 42-3 and Nursing Care Plan 42-1).

42-3 *Client and Family Teaching* Chronic Fatigue Syndrome

The nurse teaches clients who have CFS and their family members the following guidelines:

- When using over-the-counter analgesics, follow the recommended dosages and frequency for administration. Excess use can lead to increased potential for bleeding, liver, and kidney damage.
- Herbal products also have potential side effects and toxic effects; therefore, consult with the physician and keep him or her informed of any alternative therapeutic approaches you are using.
- Many companies make herbal and health-related supplements, but there is no standard among them for safe, effective dosages. Read and compare labels and ask the physician for his or her opinion on a product's efficacy.
- No scientific evidence has shown that vitamins or minerals alter the course of CFS; however, they are not harmful taken in recommended dosages.
- When searching for a support group, be wary of organizations that
  - Promise a cure for CFS
  - Use meetings as an opportunity to criticize specific physicians or treatment programs
  - Advise abandoning standard treatment regimens
  - Recommend an untested, unresearched, unscientific approach for managing CFS
  - Press participants to discuss information of a personal nature
  - Charge unreasonable fees for membership
  - Do not tolerate differences of opinion among group participants
  - Sell health-related items for a profit
- A strong network of family and supportive friends is an important factor in coping with the chronicity of CFS.

Nursing Care Plan 42-1

THE CLIENT WITH CHRONIC FATIGUE SYNDROME

Assessment

- Ask client to rate his or her energy level using a scale of 0 to 10, with 10 being the highest level. Have the client keep an energy diary to track periods during the day when energy levels are highest and lowest to determine any predictable pattern.
- Assess blood pressure and pulse in resting and sitting positions to detect postural changes.
- Have client report his or her estimation of the quality of sleep.
- Determine client's pain level and location of discomfort.

Nursing Diagnosis: **Fatigue** related to chronic immune response secondary to CFS

Expected Outcome: Client's fatigue will be reduced sufficiently so that he or she can manage ADLs.

Nursing Intervention	Rationale
Have client identify ADLs of high priority.	Setting limits keeps physical and mental stress manageable.
Determine ADLs that the client can delegate.	Delegation ensures completion of ADLs without the client expending personal energy.
Help client perform one or more priority ADLs during a period of peak energy.	Matching periods of activity with peaks in energy minimizes fatigue and avoids overexertion, which contributes to a relapse.
Schedule 5- to 10-minute rest periods every hour or more.	Relaxation can be more restorative than long naps.
Assist client to perform gentle stretching exercises in a chair followed by low-grade active exercises recommended by the physician or physical therapist for 2 to 5 minutes daily.	Stretching exercises promote blood circulation to muscles and ease the response to exercise.
Increase exercise periods by ½ to 1 minute every 2 to 3 weeks according to client's response.	Conditioning increases endurance.

Evaluation of Expected Outcome: Client performs hygiene and essential ADLs between periods of rest.

Nursing Diagnosis: **Chronic Pain** related to unknown etiology

Expected Outcome: Client's pain will be reduced to a tolerable level.

Nursing Intervention	Rationale
Apply a covered hot or cold pack to joints or muscles for 20 minutes; reapply after allowing the skin some recovery time.	Heat improves circulation and relieves muscle spasm and pain. Cold prevents swelling, numbs sensation, and relieves pain.
Encourage client to float in a pool or tub of tepid water (85°F) for 15 minutes as desired.	Cool temperatures reduce metabolic processes, including the immune response. Submersion in water results in buoyancy, a feeling of weightlessness, and relaxation. Movement and exercise are easier to perform in water.
Massage painful areas gently.	Massage releases endorphins and enkephalins that inhibit neurotransmission of pain.
Administer prescribed analgesics, corticosteroids, and antidepressants.	Medications relieve pain through several physiologic mechanisms.

(continued)

Nursing Care Plan 42-1 (Continued)

THE CLIENT WITH CHRONIC FATIGUE SYNDROME

Evaluation of Expected Outcome: The client's pain is reduced to a level of 5, which is within the client's tolerable range.

Nursing Diagnosis: **Risk for Injury** related to neurally mediated hypotension

Expected Outcome: The client will remain injury free.

Nursing Intervention	*Rationale*
Advise client to salt food liberally and to consume at least eight full glasses of fluid per day.	Sodium attracts water. An adequate amount of fluid maintains circulating blood volume, reducing the potential for hypotension.
Keep the signal for assistance within reach, and advise client to use it before attempting to ambulate.	A nursing staff member may support the client in such a way as to break his or her fall and reduce or eliminate injury.
Apply elastic stockings or thigh-high support hose before client lowers legs below the level of the heart.	Elastic fibers compress vein walls and prevent pooling of blood in the extremities.
Have client dangle and flex his or her lower limbs before getting out of bed.	Muscle contraction promotes circulation of blood from distal body areas to the heart and brain. Adequate blood flow to the brain reduces hypotensive episodes.
Instruct client to use a shower chair and avoid hot water when performing hygiene.	Remaining seated reduces the potential for injury from a fall. Hot water causes vasodilation and a drop in blood pressure.
Administer prescribed antihypotensive or corticosteroid medications.	Raising vascular tone and promoting sodium and water retention reduce the potential for low blood pressure.

Evaluation of Expected Outcome: Client's blood pressure is within normal limits and no fainting or injuries have occurred.

GENERAL NUTRITIONAL CONSIDERATIONS

Proteins in milk, egg whites, peanuts, wheat, and soybeans trigger approximately 90% of food allergies. Other common allergens are fish, shellfish, nuts, corn, and strawberries.

Meticulous record-keeping of symptoms and a food diary listing all food and beverages consumed provide a basis for diagnosing food allergies. Skin testing and a blood test for IgE antibodies provide more objective data. Elimination diets try to establish cause-and-effect relationships: the client completely avoids suspected foods for 1 to 2 weeks and then adds them back to the diet one at a time and in small amounts so if symptoms develop, the offending food can be identified. Because this is not a blind study, clients may experience symptoms based on their expectations, not from a true allergy. Clients who have experienced severe allergic reactions should not use elimination diets.

Food allergies are more common among infants and children. Many infants outgrow food allergies. Food allergies may develop in adults with no history of food allergies.

Food intolerances often produce symptoms similar to those of food allergies, such as nausea, vomiting, diarrhea, and cramping. The difference, however, is that an immune response is not involved. With food intolerances (e.g., lactose intolerance caused by a deficiency of the digestive enzyme lactase), most people can eat a small amount of the offending food without adverse effects. With true food allergies, even a tiny amount of a food allergen produces symptoms.

Food oils such as peanut or soybean oils are highly refined and therefore do not contain allergenic proteins. Cold pressed or flavored oils, such as various nut oils, may contain allergenic proteins that are capable of producing allergic reactions in sensitive clients.

Some studies suggest that people with chronic fatigue syndrome may be marginally deficient in various nutrients, including B vitamins, vitamin C, magnesium, zinc, and essential fatty acids. It is not known, however, whether nutrient deficiencies precede CFS or are a consequence of the illness process. Because the potential benefits outweigh potential risks, a multivitamin and mineral supplement may be prudent.

An omega-3 fatty acid known as *eicosapentaenoic acid* (EPA) is thought to block the release of cytokines and prostaglandins and therefore may prevent or reduce inflammation and pain experienced with CFS and other inflammatory autoimmune disorders. Fish oils provide the only dietary source of EPA. Fatty fish, such as mackerel, sardines, herring, salmon, and tuna, are the best sources. Fish oil supplements usually are not recommended because no clearly prescribed guidelines on the optimal dose are available. Also, fish oil supplements have the potential to cause gastrointestinal upset, increased bleeding time, vitamin A and D toxicity, and decreased levels of various immune system components, the significance of which is uncertain.

GENERAL PHARMACOLOGIC CONSIDERATIONS

Most antihistamines cause drowsiness. Advise the client not to drive a car, operate machinery, or perform tasks that require alertness when taking antihistamines. Some newer antihistamines are less likely to cause drowsiness.

Advise clients taking antihistamines not to take them with alcohol or other central nervous system depressants because additive sedative effects can occur.

Antihistamines are not administered to clients with disorders of the lower respiratory tract. If, for example, these drugs are administered for asthma, a drying effect may occur, making secretions thicker and more difficult to expectorate.

Clients should avoid the use of nonprescription eye preparations to reduce redness. An ophthalmologist should evaluate and treat itching and redness of the eyes because the symptoms may or may not be caused by an allergy.

Some antihistamines are more likely than others to interfere with results of skin testing. Those taking hydroxyzine (Atarax, Vistaril) or cetirizine (Zyrtec) should cease administration for 5 days before skin testing.

Metered-dose inhalers that deliver medications using propellant gases are being phased out because they are sources of environmental pollutants of the ozone layer. Dry powder inhalers are now being substituted.

To protect against poison ivy, the client can apply a new barrier cream called Ivy Block or bentoquatam 5% to the skin before to exposure. The cream forms a protective layer on top of the skin. The drug Trental may decrease the rash slightly, but the client must take it before exposure. Immunization for poison ivy, oak, or sumac currently is unavailable.

GENERAL GERONTOLOGIC CONSIDERATIONS

T-cell lymphocytes decrease with age, which may be the result of gradual degeneration of the thymus gland.

With age, the body's autoimmune response increases, which subsequently raises the risk for the older adult to develop autoimmune disorders, such as food or environmental allergies or rheumatoid arthritis.

Antihistamines are used cautiously in older men with prostatic hypertrophy because these clients may experience difficulty voiding while taking an antihistamine.

Adverse reactions to antihistamines, such as dizziness, sedation, and confusion, are more common in older adults. Careful monitoring of the older adult by the nurse or, if an outpatient, by a family member may be necessary.

When an older adult reports chronic fatigue, evaluate the client for depression.

Critical Thinking Exercises

1. *A client complains about being delayed from going home for 30 minutes after receiving a desensitizing injection to control his allergies. How would you respond?*
2. *Explain why allergies, autoimmune diseases, and CFS are classified as immune-mediated disorders.*

References and Suggested Readings

Advice from your allergist . . . house-dust allergies. (1999). *Annals of Allergy, Asthma, and Immunology, 82*(4), 335–338.

Advice from your allergist . . . pet allergies. (1999). *Annals of Allergy, Asthma, and Immunology, 82*(5), 429–430.

Bowyer, R. V. S. (1999). Latex allergy: How to identify it and the people at risk. *Journal of Clinical Nursing, 8*(2), 144–149.

Carpenito, L. J. (2000). *Nursing diagnosis, application to clinical practice* (8th ed.). Philadelphia: Lippincott Williams & Wilkins.

Carroll, P. (1999). Latex allergy: What you need to know. *RN, 62*(9), 40–42, 45–46.

Castillo, B. (2000). Overcoming fatigue . . . "Chronic fatigue syndrome: Do you know what it means?" *American Journal of Nursing, 100*(1), 14.

Cui, D. J. (2000). Better care for patients with an allergic disorder. *Journal of the American Academy of Physician Assistants, 13*(3), 46–48, 51–52, 58.

Food allergy: Current knowledge and future directions. (1999). *Immunology and Allergy Clinics of North America, 19,* 463–646.

Gehring, L. L. & Ring, P. (1999). Latex allergy: creating a safe environment. *MEDSURG Nursing, 8*(6), 358–362.

Khouzam, H. R. (2000). Chronic fatigue syndrome: Update on diagnosis and treatment. *Consultant, 40,* 1441–1443, 1447–1450.

Mendoza, T. R. & Wang, X. S. (1999). The rapid assessment of fatigue severity in cancer patients: Use of the Brief Fatigue Inventory. *Cancer, 85*(5), 1186–1196.

National Center for Infectious Diseases. (2001). Chronic fatigue syndrome, demographics. [On-line.] Available: http://www.cdc.gov/ncidod/diseases/cfs/demographics.htm.

Shute, N. (2000). Allergy epidemic. *U.S. News & World Report, 128*(18), 46–50, 52–53.

Caring for Clients With AIDS

Words to Know

acquired immuno-
deficiency syndrome
acute retroviral
syndrome
AIDS dementia
complex
AIDS drug assistance
program
autologous blood
candidiasis
capsid
codon
directed donor blood
distal sensory
polyneuropathy
drug cross-resistance
drug resistance
enzyme-linked
immunosorbent assay
epidemic
genotype testing
highly active anti-
retroviral therapy

human immuno-
deficiency virus
integrase
Kaposi's sarcoma
mortality
opportunistic infection
p24 antigen test
pandemic
phenotype testing
Pneumocystis
pneumonia
polymerase chain
reaction
protease
protease inhibitor
reverse transcriptase
reverse transcriptase
inhibitor
reverse transcription
safer sex practices
viatical settlement
Western blot

Learning Objectives

On completion of this chapter, the reader will:

- Explain the term *acquired immunodeficiency syndrome (AIDS)*.
- Identify the virus that causes AIDS.
- Discuss the characteristics of a retrovirus.
- Explain how human immunodeficiency virus (HIV) is transmitted.
- Name at least four methods for preventing transmission of HIV.
- List three criteria for diagnosing AIDS.
- Discuss the pathophysiologic process of AIDS.
- List at least five manifestations characteristic of acute retroviral syndrome.
- Name two laboratory tests used to screen for HIV antibodies and one that confirms a diagnosis of AIDS.
- Name two laboratory tests used to measure viral load, and give two purposes for their use.
- Identify two categories of drugs that are used to treat individuals infected with HIV, and give an example of a specific drug in each category.
- Give the criterion for successful drug therapy.
- Discuss the nursing management of a client with AIDS.
- Give examples of information to provide clients infected with HIV.
- Describe techniques for preventing HIV infection among healthcare workers who care for infected clients.
- Discuss two ethical issues that affect healthcare workers in relation to HIV infection.

Acquired immunodeficiency syndrome (AIDS) is an infectious and eventually fatal disorder that profoundly weakens the immune system. AIDS is acquired from a pathogen known as the **human immunodeficiency virus** (HIV). People can remain well, sometimes up to 10 years or longer, despite being infected with HIV before the initial infection develops into AIDS (Fig. 43-1). In the asymptomatic interim, the infected person can infect others.

The U.S. Public Health Service and the World Health Organization agree that HIV/AIDS is more than an **epidemic,** a rapidly spreading disease in a particular region. HIV/AIDS is a **pandemic,** meaning that it is a disease infecting large numbers of people throughout the world.

Based on statistics compiled at the end of 1999 by the Joint United Nations Programme on HIV/AIDS, the Centers for Disease Control and Prevention (CDC) estimates that 33.6 million people are infected with HIV worldwide (National Center for Health Statistics, 2000). Of that number, 95% live in underdeveloped countries.

In the early history of the disease in developed countries, HIV occurred more often among homosexual men and intravenous (IV) drug users, but that exclusivity is no longer the case. Increasing numbers of heterosexual women are being infected, which, in turn, leads to transmission of HIV to newborns. To date, nurses are the largest group of healthcare workers to have occupationally acquired HIV infection (CDC, 1999).

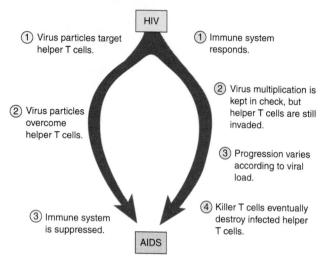

① Virus particles target helper T cells.

② Virus particles overcome helper T cells.

③ Immune system is suppressed.

① Immune system responds.

② Virus multiplication is kept in check, but helper T cells are still invaded.

③ Progression varies according to viral load.

④ Killer T cells eventually destroy infected helper T cells.

FIGURE 43-1 Cycle of HIV infection and development of AIDS.

Globally, 2.8 million deaths were due to AIDS in 1999 (AIDS Education and Research Trust, 2000). This figure represents the highest **mortality** or death rate from AIDS since AIDS statistics have been compiled. AIDS continues to be a major public health problem in the United States. Currently, it is the leading cause of death among African-American men aged 25 to 44 years and the fifth leading cause of death among people of all races and both sexes in this same age range (National Center for Health Statistics, 1999).

HUMAN IMMUNODEFICIENCY VIRUS

It is speculated that HIV is an altered genetic form of simian (monkey) immunodeficiency virus (SIV). It is believed that the transformation facilitated viral transmission from chimpanzees to humans.

Subtypes

Two HIV subtypes have been identified: HIV-1 and HIV-2. HIV-1 mutates easily and frequently, producing multiple substrains that are identified by letters from A through O. HIV-2 is less transmittable, and the interval between initial infection with HIV-2 and development of AIDS is longer. HIV-1 is more prevalent in the United States, where approximately 650,000 to 900,000 people are infected with it. Fewer than 100 Americans are known to be infected with HIV-2. Western Africa is the primary site of infection with HIV-2.

Structural Characteristics

Viruses require a living host cell for survival and duplication. Like all viruses, HIV is genetically incomplete. A

double layer of lipid material surrounds the incomplete HIV, referred to as a **capsid.** Surface-binding proteins, called gp120, project in all directions from the lipid bilayer. Inside the capsid are three important enzymes, reverse transcriptase, integrase, and protease, and strands of RNA (Fig. 43-2).

When HIV encounters a helper T-cell lymphocyte, one of the binding proteins fuses with the T cell's receptor, called a *CD4 receptor.* The fusion provides a means by which the capsid can insert its contents into the helper T cell.

Stop, Think, and Respond ● BOX 43-1

What is the role of helper T cells in the immune response?

Replication

To replicate, which means to produce more copies, HIV becomes a parasite of helper T cells (also known as *T4* or *CD4 cells* because of their CD4 receptor; see Chap. 41). HIV alters the T cell's genetic code to make more viral particles. To do this, the enzyme **reverse transcriptase** copies the RNA into DNA, a process called **reverse transcription.** A second viral enzyme, **integrase,** incorporates the reprogrammed DNA with its new viral code into the host cell's DNA.

The altered DNA tells the cell how to assemble amino acids to form protein substances, like the virus. The transformed DNA provides the blueprint or cookbook for making clones of HIV along with the enzymes the virus needs to continue reinfecting additional cells.

The cell follows the DNA's directions and forms long chains of viral particles enclosed within its membrane.

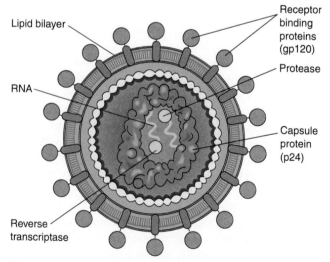

Lipid bilayer

Receptor binding proteins (gp120)

Protease

RNA

Capsule protein (p24)

Reverse transcriptase

FIGURE 43-2 Structure of a retrovirus.

Protease, the third viral enzyme, cuts the long chains, freeing the replicated viral particles into the cytoplasm of the cell. Some migrate to the cell wall and form buds. When the buds rupture, they release many copies of the virus, which reinfect other helper T cells (Fig. 43-3).

More than 10 billion viral particles are released daily. Mutations occur frequently, complicating drug therapy and making production of a vaccine nearly impossible.

Transmission

Human immunodeficiency virus is not transmitted by casual contact. There are only four known body fluids through which HIV is transmitted: blood, semen, vaginal secretions, and breast milk. HIV may be present in saliva, tears, and conjunctival secretions, but transmission of

HIV through these fluids has not been implicated. HIV is not found in urine, stool, vomit, or sweat.

> ### Stop, Think, and Respond ● BOX 43-2
>
> *How would you respond to those who avoid drinking from a common cup, such as those used in Christian church services, because they fear acquiring AIDS?*

Certain behaviors increase the risk for acquiring HIV from infectious body fluids (Box 43-1). Obviously, unprotected sexual intercourse and multiple sexual partners increase the risk for HIV infection and other sexually transmitted diseases. Using a condom is one of the most effective ways to reduce the risk of HIV infection. Condoms are available for both men and women (Fig. 43-4).

Blood and blood products were a major source of transmission before 1984. Since then, an HIV screening test is performed on donated blood. Although screening donated blood for HIV antibodies reduces the risk of transfusion-related infection with HIV, it is not flawless. Antibody screening cannot identify infected blood from donors who have yet to produce significant antibodies. The window of time between infection (entrance of HIV into the body) and production of antibodies varies from 1 to 6 weeks. Thus, a recently infected person with HIV could donate blood containing the virus, even though the screening test results are negative for HIV. Other potential methods of transmission include receiving infected semen from a sperm bank or infected organs or tissues for transplantation.

ACQUIRED IMMUNODEFICIENCY SYNDROME

Acquired immunodeficiency syndrome is the end stage of HIV infection. Certain events establish the conversion of HIV infection to AIDS: (1) a markedly decreased T4 cell count from a normal level of 800 to 1200/mm^3; and

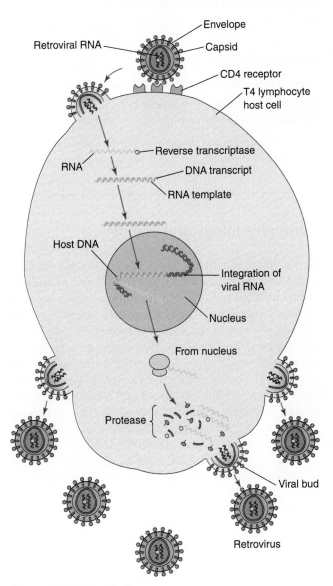

FIGURE 43-3 HIV replication.

> ### BOX 43-1 ● High-Risk Factors for HIV Infection
>
> - Unprotected vaginal, anal, or oral sex
> - Contact with blood and infectious body fluids during medical, surgical, dental, or nursing procedures
> - Sharing intravenous needles or syringes
> - Receiving nonautologous transfusions of blood or blood products
> - Receiving plasma or clotting factors that have not been heat treated
> - Contact with infected blood on body-piercing, tattoo, and dental equipment
> - Transmission from infected mothers to infants during pregnancy, birth, or breast-feeding

43-1 *Client and Family Teaching* Using a Condom

The nurse teaches clients the following points:

MEN	WOMEN
Purchase latex condoms, or vinyl if sensitive to latex.	Make sure that the purchased condom is labeled for female use; one brand available in the United States is called "Reality."
Select a strong condom, and use lubricant liberally for anal intercourse.	Distribute the coated lubricant over the outside by rubbing the outer surface.
Do not store condoms where they are exposed to heat or light.	Observe that a reinforced ring is at the open end and at the bottom.
Use a new condom each time you engage in sexual intercourse.	Compress the bottom ring to form an oval shape.
Apply the condom after the penis is erect and before making any sexual contact with a partner.	Insert the compressed ring with the index finger into the vagina as far as the finger can reach.
Leave a half inch between the tip of the penis and the bottom of the condom.	Ensure that the condom is not twisted and that the ring at the open end is externally visible.
Unroll the condom to the base of the penis.	Guide the penis into the condom.
Expel any air bubbles that have formed.	Remain horizontal after intercourse.
On withdrawal, hold the base of the condom and withdraw the penis before it becomes limp.	Remove the condom by squeezing the lower ring and twisting the polyurethane sheath.
When removing the condom, knot the open end, and discard it in a lined waste container.	Knot the opening and dispose of the condom in a lined waste container; do not flush the condom in the toilet.

(2) the development of certain cancers and **opportunistic infections,** those infections that usually do not occur in individuals with a healthy immune system. In 1993, the CDC devised a classification system involving two categories that constitute an AIDS diagnosis: (1) Category 1, 2, or 3, and (2) Category A, B, or C (Table 43-1).

Stop, Think, and Respond ● BOX 43-3

What classification would be assigned to an HIV-positive person with a T4 cell count of 350/mm³ who develops Pneumocystis carinii *pneumonia?*

A   B

FIGURE 43-4 Applied condoms (**A**) male and (**B**) female.

Pathophysiology and Etiology

Acquired immunodeficiency syndrome is acquired from direct contact with the blood or body fluids of an individual infected with HIV or from indirect contact with infected blood or body fluids. When HIV infection occurs, it gradually impairs the ability of infected T4 cells to recognize foreign antigens (e.g., disease pathogens) and stimulate B-cell lymphocytes. While massive numbers of viral particles are being released, infected T4 cells are destroyed by HIV itself and by killer T8-cell lymphocytes that no longer recognize the altered T4 cell's membrane as being "self." Although new T4 cells are produced, the process is never as fast as replication of the virus. Eventually, T4 cells become significantly depleted, and immunodeficiency develops. The infected person ultimately dies from an opportunistic infection.

The rate of progression from HIV infection to AIDS is related to the concentration of virus in the blood. For some, the process may take 10 years or more. Although most people infected with HIV die of their disease, a few are long-term survivors. Some explanations for long-term survival include the following:

TABLE 43-1	CLASSIFICATION FOR HIV INFECTION

CATEGORY 1	CATEGORY 2	CATEGORY 3
T4 cell count ≥500/mm³	T4 cell count 200–499/mm³	T4 cell count <200/mm³
CATEGORY A	CATEGORY B	CATEGORY C
HIV positive with one or more of the following: • Asymptomatic • Persistent generalized **lymphadenopathy** (swollen lymph nodes) • Symptoms formerly known as *AIDS-related complex* (ARC), such as anorexia, weight loss, fever, night sweats, rash, fatigue, lowered resistance to infection, diarrhea	HIV positive with conditions attributed to or complicated by HIV infection such as: • Bacillary angiomatosis • Candidiasis (oral, vulvovaginal) unresponsive to treatment • Cervical dysplasia or carcinoma • Fever or diarrhea for more than 1 month • Hairy leukoplakia • Herpes zoster (at least two episodes) • Idiopathic thrombocytopenic-purpura • Listeriosis • Pelvic inflammatory disease/tubo-ovarian abscess • Peripheral neuropathy • Toxoplasmosis of the brain • Wasting syndrome	HIV positive with one or more of the following: • Candidiasis (bronchial, tracheal, lungs, or esophagus) • Cervical cancer (invasive) • Coccidiomycosis (disseminated or extrapulmonary) • Cryptococcosis (extrapulmonary) • Cryptosporidiosis for less than 1 month • Cytomegalovirus (other than liver, spleen, or nodes) • Encephalopathy (HIV-related) • Herpes simplex (<1 month) or bronchitis, pneumonitis, esophagitis • Histoplasmosis (disseminated or extrapulmonary) • Isosporiosis (<1 month) • Kaposi's sarcoma • Lymphoma, Burkitt's (or equivalent), immunoblastic (or equivalent), brain (primary) • *Mycobacterium avium* complex or *Mycobacterium kansasii*, disseminated or extrapulmonary • *Mycobacterium tuberculosis*, any site, pulmonary or extrapulmonary • *Mycobacterium*, other species • *Pneumocystis carinii* pneumonia • Pneumonia, recurrent • Progressive multifocal leukoencephalopathy • *Salmonella* septicemia, recurrent

From Centers for Disease Control and Prevention. (1992). 1993 Revised classification system for HIV infection and expanded surveillance case definition for AIDS among adolescents and adults. *Morbidity and Mortality Weekly Report, 41*(51), 961–962.

• The infectious HIV is a weak strain.
• The amount of virus is kept low with stronger-than-normal killer T8 cells.
• The combination of drugs used for treatment is effective.

Prevention Strategies

The transmission of HIV is reduced or eliminated by adhering to the following guidelines:

• Abstain from sexual intercourse.
• Have mutually monogamous sex with an uninfected partner.
• Avoid casual sex with multiple partners.
• Use a condom and spermicide that contains non-oxynol-9 during sexual intercourse.
• Abstain from using IV drugs.
• Use a new needle and syringe each time IV drugs are injected.

• Refrain from donating blood if engaged in high-risk behaviors.
• Bank **autologous blood** (self-donated) or **directed donor blood** (specified blood donors among relatives and friends) when preparing for nonemergency surgical procedures (Table 43-2).

Some authorities believe that directed blood is no safer than blood collected from public donors. Those who support this belief say that directed donors may not reveal their high-risk behaviors that put the potential recipient at risk for blood-borne pathogens like HIV.

Nurses and other healthcare workers use Standard Precautions (see Chap. 19) when caring for all clients whose infectious status is unknown. Because postexposure protocols can reduce the risk of HIV infection if initiated promptly, nurses must immediately report any needlestick or sharp injury to a supervisor. Infected healthcare workers can continue to practice; however, they usually are restricted from performing procedures in which they may exchange blood with clients.

TABLE 43-2	GUIDELINES FOR AUTOLOGOUS AND DIRECTED BLOOD DONATION
AUTOLOGOUS DONATION	**DIRECTED DONATION**
Donor must weigh 95 lb.	Donor must weigh 110 lb.
Donor must be at least 14 years of age.	Donor must be at least 17 years of age.
Exceptions may be made in medical history.	Donor must meet volunteer donor medical history criteria.
Blood is used only for transfusion to donor.	Client's physician must be informed of directed donation.
Blood type does not need to be known at time of donation.	Blood may be transfused to others if not needed by client.
Units that test positive for a disease (other than HIV) will be issued.	Donors should know blood type of client.
Donation frequency may be greater than 1 unit every 56 days.	Units that test positive for HIV or hepatitis will not be used.
Additional fee to hospital or recipient may be charged for holding blood on reserve.	Additional fees may be charged to the recipient.

Assessment Findings

Signs and Symptoms

At the time of primary HIV infection, one third to more than one half of those infected develop **acute retroviral syndrome** (viremia), which often is mistaken for "flu" or some other common illness. Some manifestations include fever; swollen and tender lymph nodes; pharyngitis; rash about the face, trunk, palms, and soles; muscle and joint pain; headache; nausea; vomiting; and diarrhea. In addition, there may be enlargement of the liver and spleen, weight loss, and neurologic symptoms like visual changes or cognitive and motor involvement. Admission of risk behaviors for HIV, however, narrows the differential diagnosis. Although viral replication is rapid at this time, antibody tests cannot detect the infection.

Eventually, individuals infected with HIV present with a form of cancer that is atypical for the person's age and health history, or an opportunistic infection. For example, **Kaposi's sarcoma,** a type of connective tissue cancer common among those with AIDS, may be noted (Fig. 43-5). Others who acquire *Pneumocystis* pneumonia (discussed later) have an unproductive cough and shortness of breath. In women, gynecologic problems may be the focus of the chief complaint. Abnormal results of Papanicolaou tests, genital warts, pelvic inflammatory disease, and persistent vaginitis (see Chaps. 62 and 65) also may correlate with HIV infection.

Diagnostic Findings

The **enzyme-linked immunosorbent assay** (ELISA) test, an initial HIV screening test, is positive when there are sufficient HIV antibodies; it also is positive when there are antibodies from other infectious diseases. The test is repeated if results are positive. If results of a second ELISA test are positive, the **Western blot** is performed. A positive result on Western blot confirms the diagnosis; however, false-positive and false-negative results on both tests are possible. Written consent must be obtained before an ELISA or Western blot test is performed. The results of the tests require strict confidentiality.

FIGURE 43-5 Kaposi's sarcoma (**A**) single lesion and (**B**) multiple lesions.

A total T-cell count, T4 and T8 count, and T4/T8 ratio determine the status of T lymphocytes. A T4-cell count of less than 500 mm³ indicates immune suppression; a T4-cell count of 200/mm³ or less is an indicator of AIDS.

It now is possible to measure a person's viral load, the number of viral particles in the blood. **The p24 antigen test** and **polymerase chain reaction** test measure viral loads. They are used to guide drug therapy and follow the progression of the disease. Viral load tests and T4-cell counts may be performed every 2 to 3 months once it is determined that a person is HIV positive.

Other general laboratory and diagnostic tests are prescribed when opportunistic infections are involved. In addition, cancer screenings, especially Papanicolaou cervical tests for women (see Chap. 59), are recommended for those infected with HIV. Immunosuppression tends to facilitate the development of cancer and accelerate its progression.

Medical Management

People with HIV and AIDS are treated with antiretroviral drugs, adjunct drug therapy to boost the immune response, and supportive care during opportunistic infections. It usually is recommended that clients infected with HIV receive pneumococcal, hepatitis B, and yearly influenza vaccines. Additional medical management includes treating anorexia, diarrhea, and weight loss.

Vaccines that may prevent HIV infection are in clinical trials. Although clients who already are HIV positive cannot benefit from a preventive vaccine, the need to control the global spread of HIV is pressing. Currently, one experimental AIDS vaccine, AIDSVAX, has reached Phase III of clinical trials. This phase of testing may last 2 to 10 years and involves human test subjects. AIDSVAX contains only a subunit or part of HIV. The portion used in AIDSVAX is the gp120 protein. The hope is that the immune system will recognize the foreign gp120 protein, develop memory cells, and speedily destroy the complete virus should it enter the body in the future.

> ### Stop, Think, and Respond ● BOX 43-4
> *What is the role of the gp120 component of HIV?*

Antiretroviral Drug Therapy

The physician decides when and which antiretroviral drugs to prescribe based on the client's T4-cell and viral load counts, potential compliance, medication side effect profiles, cost, and interactions of each drug. Antiretroviral medications are very expensive—as much as $10,000 to $15,000 per year in the United States. Some social agencies and pharmaceutical companies have compassionate need programs through which antiretroviral drugs are supplied to individuals who cannot afford them.

Opinions vary as to when to initiate drug therapy. The development of **drug resistance,** ineffectual response to a prescribed drug because of the survival and duplication of exceptionally virulent mutations (Fig. 43-6), and **drug cross-resistance,** diminished drug response to similar HIV drugs, are common. Because drug resistance limits future treatment options, some physicians believe that delaying drug therapy is justified. One guideline is to wait until the client's viral load is greater than 30,000 copies/ mL or the T4-cell count is less than 350 mm³. Therefore, it is critical that clients with HIV comply with regular appointments for laboratory blood tests.

When drug therapy is begun, clients are started on a combination of generally three antiretroviral drugs: two **reverse transcriptase inhibitors,** drugs that interfere with the virus's ability to make a genetic blueprint, and one **protease inhibitor,** a drug that inhibits the ability

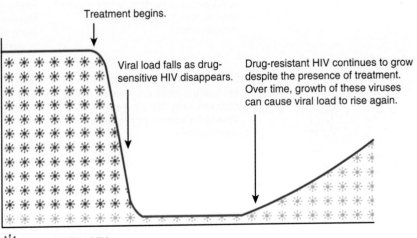

FIGURE 43-6 The development of drug-resistant strains of HIV.

of virus particles to leave the host cell (Drug Therapy Table 43-1). Combination therapy, sometimes referred to as a *drug cocktail* or **highly active antiretroviral therapy,** has several benefits:

- The combination of drugs suppresses replication of the virus using different mechanisms.
- The drugs lower the viral load more quickly—sometimes to undetectable levels. Doing so ultimately slows the rate of disease progression, prevents opportunistic infections, and, in turn, lengthens survival.
- Combination therapy diminishes the rate of viral mutations and prolongs drug effectiveness.

- Using two or more drugs simultaneously reduces the chance that the virus will develop resistance or cross-resistance.

The goal of antiretroviral therapy is to bring the viral load to an "undetectable" level. This level is no more than 500 or 50 copies, depending on the sensitivity of the selected viral load test.

DRUG RESISTANCE

Clients who neglect to take antiretroviral drugs as prescribed (i.e., every dose, at its designated time, with or without food as directed) risk development of drug re-

DRUG THERAPY TABLE 43-1	**EXAMPLES OF DRUGS USED IN HIV THERAPY**	
DRUG CATEGORY AND EXAMPLES	**SIDE EFFECTS**	**NURSING CONSIDERATIONS**
Reverse Transcriptase Inhibitors		
Nucleoside reverse transcriptase inhibitors (NRTIs)		
zidovudine (AZT, Retrovir)	Anemia, nausea, gastrointestinal pain, diarrhea, myositis, headaches, fever, rash	Monitor T4 cell counts. Administer drug every 4 hours around the clock. Tell client to report extreme fatigue, nausea, vomiting, or rash.
didanosine (ddl, Videx)	Pancreatitis, nausea, vomiting, abdominal pain, hepatotoxicity, bone marrow suppression, insomnia	Administer on an empty stomach, 1 hour before or 2 hours after eating. Advise client to chew tablets thoroughly or crush tablets and dissolve in at least 1 ounce of water.
Nonnucleoside reverse transcriptase inhibitors (NNRTIs)		
nevirapine (Viramune, Vistide)	Rash, hepatotoxicity, headache nausea, vomiting, diarrhea	Use is contraindicated during pregnancy or breast-feeding. Avoid combining with protease inhibitors or oral contraceptives. Monitor hepatic and renal function. Consult physician if severe rash occurs.
efavirenz (Sustiva)	Rash, dizziness, fatigue, unusual dreams, confusion, impaired thinking, amnesia, agitation, hallucinations, hepatotoxicity, false-positive test results for cannabinoids	Control intake of fatty foods, which can elevate drug levels. Assess mental status. Monitor liver function. Warn that drug test results may be falsely positive for marijuana.
Protease Inhibitors		
indinavir (Crixivan)	Nephrolithiasis, gastrointestinal intolerance, headache, blurred vision, dizziness, rash, metallic taste, thrombocytopenia, hyperglycemia, lipodystrophy	Monitor for kidney stones. Increase fluid intake to help prevent formation of kidney stones. Wait 1 hour between administration of indinavir and ddl. Give drug 1 hour before or 2 hours after a meal with skim or low-fat milk. Give hard candies to help mask metallic taste. Check blood glucose levels regularly. Observe for signs of bruising or bleeding. Warn that this drug causes a redistribution of body fat.
saquinavir (Invirase, Fortase)	Headache, weakness, muscle aches, nausea, abdominal discomfort, diarrhea, elevated level of creatinine phosphokinase	Administer with or within 2 hours of a full meal. Protect from injury, which may result from weakness. Report alterations in stool or urine color, which may indicate liver dysfunction.

sistance. When drug levels are not adequately maintained, viral replication and mutations increase (Fig. 43-7). In other words, noncompliant clients are one cause of antiretroviral drug failure.

It is possible to detect drug resistance with two different blood tests. When **genotype testing** is done, the blood is examined for genetic changes in circulating HIV particles. Scientists now know to look for points on HIV genes, called **codons,** where mutations occur. With **phenotype testing,** a measured amount of antiviral drug is mixed with the virus until there is a quantity that prevents the virus from reproducing. The higher the dose of drug that eventually inhibits viral growth, the greater is the viral drug resistance.

REVERSE TRANSCRIPTASE INHIBITORS

There are two approved categories of reverse transcriptase inhibitors: nucleoside analogue reverse transcriptase inhibitors (NRTIs) and non-nucleoside reverse transcriptase inhibitors (NNRTIs). Nucleoside is a building block of DNA and RNA. By binding to viral DNA, NRTIs abort the terminal completion of gene copying.

Non-nucleoside drugs are molecularly similar to nucleoside analogues; however, NNRTIs bind directly to the reverse transcriptase enzyme, thus preventing transcription. They are effective only against HIV-1. The potent combination of drugs from these two classes cripples the virus's ability to copy itself. Unfortunately, drug resistance develops very quickly if the client does not take the NNRTI as prescribed. If drug resistance develops to one NNRTI,

cross-resistance usually develops to all others in this same class.

A third group of drugs called *nucleotide analogues* is being developed. Nucleotides are compounds that are part of a chain of substances in nucleic acids (i.e., DNA and RNA). This group of drugs may add yet another weapon to the arsenal being used to extend the lives of those with AIDS.

PROTEASE INHIBITORS

One or two protease inhibitors usually are used in combination with both NRTIs and NNRTIs. Protease inhibitors interfere with the maturation of the viral copies. If viral copies do manage to escape from the host T4 cell, they usually are too immature to invade healthy T4 cells. Because protease inhibitors and reverse transcriptase inhibitors affect totally separate processes in the viral life cycle, the combination is most likely to control the virus.

Stop, Think, and Respond ● BOX 43-5

Explain the concept of antiretroviral drug resistance and cross-resistance and techniques for reducing its potential.

Adjunct Drug Therapy

Other drugs may be used with antiretroviral drug therapy in an overall effort to halt the progression of AIDS.

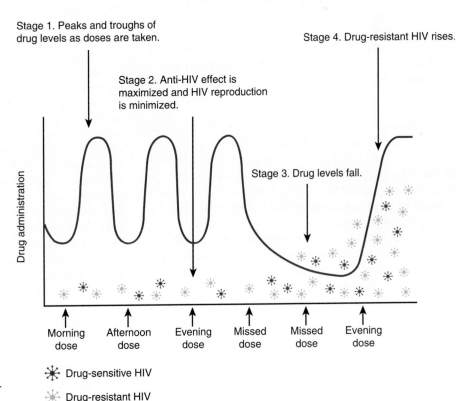

FIGURE 43-7 The effect of noncompliance on drug resistance.

One such drug is hydroxyurea (Hydrea), which usually is used to treat cancer. Hydroxyurea inhibits an enzyme that functions in DNA synthesis, thereby inhibiting or slowing the reproduction of tumor cells. When combined with antiretrovirals, hydroxyurea interferes with viral replication, increasing anti-HIV effects.

The immune system naturally produces interleukin-2 (IL-2), a chemical substance called a *cytokine*. The function of IL-2 is to stimulate the production of lymphocytes. The pharmaceutical counterpart of IL-2 is used to increase the numbers of T4 helper and natural killer lymphocytes. Natural killer lymphocytes specifically target viral infected cells and cancer cells. The use of IL-2 boosts the body's immune defenses against HIV.

Supportive Care of Opportunistic Infections

Clients with AIDS acquire many infectious disorders, any one of which can cause death. These infectious disorders and their comparative severity are uncommon in populations of relatively healthy people. The management of some common infectious conditions follows.

PNEUMOCYSTIS PNEUMONIA

Clients infected with HIV are at particular risk for acquiring a type of pneumonia caused by an organism called *P. carinii*. This form of pneumonia is rare among individuals with an intact immune system. The pneumonia can become so severe as to result in respiratory failure. Mechanical ventilation may be necessary to sustain adequate pulmonary function. Aerosol therapy and deep suctioning after the instillation of saline often are necessary to clear the lungs of thick sputum. To prevent and treat **Pneumocystis pneumonia,** trimethoprim-sulfamethoxazole (Bactrim, Septra) is prescribed. Monthly aerosolized pentamidine isethionate (NebuPent) also is effective.

CANDIDIASIS

Candidiasis is a yeast infection caused by the *Candida albicans* microorganism. Candidiasis may develop in the oral, pharyngeal, esophageal, or vaginal cavities or in folds of the skin. It often is called *thrush* when located in the mouth. Inspection of the mouth, throat, or vagina reveals areas of white plaque that may bleed when mobilized with a cotton-tipped swab.

When candidiasis affects structures in the mouth and throat, it can lead to problems with eating and subsequent weight loss. Topical antifungals, such as nystatin (Mycostatin) oral suspension that is swished in the mouth and then swallowed or taken in an alternate lozenge form, are useful for treating oral candidiasis. Clotrimazole (Gyne-Lotrimin, Mycelex) and miconazole (Monistat) cream, vaginal tablets, and suppositories are used to treat vaginitis. Sometimes systemic antifungals like amphotericin B (Fungizone) or fluconazole (Diflucan) are required to control candidiasis.

CYTOMEGALOVIRUS INFECTION

Opportunistic infections caused by the cytomegalovirus (CMV) affect immunosuppressed people such as clients with AIDS. CMV can infect the choroid and retinal layers of the eye, leading to blindness. It also can cause ulcers in the esophagus, colitis and diarrhea, pneumonia, and encephalitis. Foscarnet (Foscavir), cidofovir (Vistide), and ganciclovir (Cytovene) are used in combination aggressively to treat acute CMV infections. Maintenance drug therapy follows to reduce the potential for future viral activation.

CRYPTOSPORIDIOSIS

Immunosuppressed clients may develop serious diarrhea as a result of infection with a protozoan called *Cryptosporidium*. The organism is spread by the fecal–oral route from contaminated water, food, or human or animal wastes. Those infected can lose up to 20 L of fluid per day (Lisanti & Zwolski, 1997). Losing this magnitude of fluid quickly leads to dehydration and electrolyte imbalances. When diarrhea is accompanied by anorexia, nausea, and vomiting, weight is difficult to maintain.

Definitive diagnosis is made by examining the stool for ova and parasites and other cytologic examinations. Antibiotic therapy is then implemented. The macrolide family of antibiotics, such as azithromycin (Zithromax) or clarithromycin (Biaxin), or an antiprotozoal agent such as paromomycin (Humatin), is used.

Management of AIDS-Related Complications

Besides AIDS-related cancers and opportunistic infections, clients may develop **AIDS dementia complex** (ADC). ADC, a neurologic condition, causes degeneration of the brain, especially in areas that affect mood, cognition, and motor functions. According to Lisanti and Zwolski (1997), clients exhibit forgetfulness, limited attention span, decreased ability to concentrate, and delusional thinking. Moods range from irritability to euphoria. Possible motor dysfunction is manifested by staggering gait and muscle incoordination, slowing of all movements, or paraplegia, which may be accompanied by incontinence.

Antiretroviral therapy can delay or prevent ADC. Other drugs, some of which are in clinical trials, may slow the progression of ADC once it manifests. One such drug is memantine. It is believed that memantine, which has been used in Germany for more than 10 years to treat various forms of dementia, performs a neuroprotective function. This drug blocks N-methyl-D-aspartate (NMDA) receptors in the brain from being overexcited by a neurotransmitter called *glutamate*. Normal concentrations of glutamate enhance memory and learning; too much glutamate is lethal to brain cells. Memantine awaits approval by the U. S. Food and Drug Administration. Research also continues on CPI-1189, an agent that is an antagonist of cytokines like tumor necrosis factor (see Chap. 41), which are produced during gp120-induced inflammation of brain cells. Until these drugs and others are approved, antiretroviral therapy may be combined with selegiline (Eldepryl), an anti-Parkinson's drug, to treat motor and cognitive impairments of ADC, and psychiatric drugs to moderate mood and activity levels.

Still others may develop **distal sensory polyneuropathy** (DSP), which is characterized by abnormal sensations, such as burning and numbness, in the feet and later in the hands. Because neuropathy is a side effect of several antiretroviral drugs, it is difficult to determine if the cause is actually destruction of the sensory peripheral nerves or drug therapy (Lisanti & Zwolski, 1997). DSP responds less well to drug therapy than do neuropathies associated with other primary disorders such as diabetes mellitus (see Chap. 58). Nevertheless, an effort is made to preserve and promote nerve function using vitamin B_{12} and thiamine supplementation. Neuropathic pain also may be amenable to treatment with tricyclic antidepressants like amitriptyline (Elavil) and nortriptyline (Pamelor) or anticonvulsants such as gabapentin (Neurontin) and carbamazepine (Tegretol).

Nursing Management

The role of the nurse involves health teaching and counseling of high-risk populations. Areas of emphasis include HIV prevention strategies such as sexual abstinence and **safer sex practices,** sexual activities in which body fluids are not exchanged. The nurse encourages diagnostic screening for those whose behaviors place them at risk for HIV infection. He or she helps to interpret the results of diagnostic tests and monitors the need for continued follow-up in the months after potential exposure.

For those with an established HIV status, the nurse explains the action of each antiretroviral drug and develops a schedule for the client's self-administration. This includes strong precautions about rigidly adhering to the dosage, time, and frequency of drug administration to avoid resistance. Describing the side effects of drug therapy is essential, with the admonition to refrain from discontinuing any of the prescribed drugs without first consulting the prescribing physician. The nurse makes appointments for laboratory tests for monitoring the effects of drug therapy.

A very important nursing intervention is referral of HIV-positive clients to support groups and resources for information about new HIV drug development, clinical drug trials, **AIDS drug assistance programs** (state-based programs partially funded by Title II of the Ryan White CARE Act), and progress on vaccine development (see Additional Resources). See Nursing Care Plan 43-1 for additional nursing management.

Reducing Occupational Risks

The nurse must observe Standard Precautions whenever there is a risk of exposure to blood and body fluids. He or

she must follow the nursing guidelines for safe handling of needles and sharp instruments (Nursing Guidelines 43-1). The Occupational Safety and Health Administration (OSHA) also recommends the following when caring for all clients regardless of their infectious status:

- Transport specimens of body fluids in leakproof containers.
- Clean and disinfect utility gloves used for cleaning.
- Remove barrier garments (e.g., face shields, glasses) as soon as possible after leaving a client's room.

If exposed to the blood of any client, the nurse should report the incident to the person in charge of employee health immediately. The nurse will be tested for HIV at regular intervals and treated with antiretrovirals depending on the results of tests or the potential for infection. While awaiting the results of diagnostic tests, the nurse must follow the same sexual precautions as someone who has been diagnosed with AIDS.

Client Teaching

For clients who are healthy enough to continue as outpatients, the nurse develops a teaching plan that includes the following guidelines:

- Follow the medication schedule; do not omit or increase the dose without physician approval.
- Comply with the timing of antiviral medications around meals.
- Eat small, frequent, well-balanced meals; try to maintain or gain weight. Drink plenty of water.
- Check weight weekly. Report progressive weight loss or loss of appetite to the physician.
- Avoid exposure to people with infections, including colds, sore throats, upper respiratory tract infections, and childhood diseases (e.g., mumps, chickenpox), and those who have recently been vaccinated. Avoid crowds.
- Notify the physician if signs of infection, such as fever, sore throat, diarrhea, respiratory distress, and cough occur, or if signs of a skin, rectal, vaginal, or oral infection appear.
- Wear gloves and a mask when disposing of animal excreta, such as kitty litter, bird cage liners, and hamster shavings; wash hands thoroughly afterward.
- Wash all food before cooking; do not eat raw meat, fish, or vegetables or food that has not been completely cooked.
- Wash bedding and clothes in hot water and separate from the laundry of others, especially if the bedding and clothes are soiled with body secretions.
- Avoid smoking or exposure to secondhand smoke.
- Personal cleanliness is a must. Bathe or shower daily, wash hands before and after preparing food,

(text continued on page 591)

Nursing Care Plan 43-1

THE CLIENT WITH AIDS

Assessment

■ *Obtain a thorough history,* including risk factors for HIV infection. List all symptoms, exploring each thoroughly. Determine the client's past and current treatment medications. Inspect the oral mucous membranes and all skin surfaces for rashes, skin breakdown, and opportunistic infections such as herpes lesions. Look for Kaposi's sarcoma, which appear as dark purple lesions that may be painful. Examine the arms and legs for edema. Auscultate the lungs for breath sounds. Question the client about coughing, sputum production, dyspnea, and orthopnea. Palpate the lymph nodes and abdomen for organ enlargement. Gather additional data based on the client's complaints or symptoms. Review results of recent laboratory and diagnostic tests.

■ *Obtain vital signs and weight.* Question the client about weight loss and weight before he or she became symptomatic. Explore past and current dietary intake. Ask about factors that interfere with eating, such as difficulty swallowing, diarrhea, and oral discomfort.

■ *Assess the client's mental status (see Chap. 12) and perform a neurologic assessment (see Chap. 44).* Look for peripheral neuropathies (sensation changes in extremities), which may be side effects of antiretroviral medications. Ask about any visual changes (e.g., floaters, spots, loss of peripheral vision).

■ *Evaluate emotional status,* looking for signs of depression or anxiety.

■ *Observe for signs of dehydration.* Examine the skin and mucous membranes for dryness. Evaluate skin turgor. Note additional findings like decreased urine output, hypotension, and slow filling of hand veins. Look for indications of electrolyte deficit(s) such as excessive thirst, muscle weakness, cramping, nausea, vomiting, cardiac dysrhythmia, shallow respirations, and headache.

Nursing Diagnosis: Risk for Infection (opportunistic) related to immunodeficiency

Expected Outcome: Client will experience no secondary infections.

Interventions	Rationales
Follow practices of medical and surgical asepsis.	Aseptic practices break the infection cycle by decreasing or eliminating infectious agents, their reservoirs, and vehicles for transmission.
Place client in protective isolation if T4 cell count is ≤500 mm³.	Keeping the immunosuppressed client in a separate environment and using precautions to limit the introduction of pathogens in that environment reduce the potential for transmission of a nosocomial infection.
Promote hygiene especially before meals and after elimination.	The fecal–oral route is a common mechanism for transfer of endogenous microorganisms from one body site to another, where they can become pathogenic. Handwashing is the best technique for reducing transmission of microorganisms.
Facilitate adequate sleep and nutrition.	Adequate sleep and nutrition reduce fatigue, stabilize mood, increase protein synthesis, maintain disease-fighting mechanisms of the immune system, promote cellular growth and repair, and improve capacity for learning and memory storage.
Prohibit ill visitors and staff from contact with client.	Microorganisms are transferred by one of three routes: airborne, droplet, and contact.

Evaluation of Expected Outcome: Client is free from secondary infections.

PC: *Pneumocystis* Pneumonia

Expected Outcome: Nurse will manage and minimize pneumonia.

(continued)

Nursing Care Plan 43-1 *(Continued)*

THE CLIENT WITH AIDS

Interventions	Rationales
Auscultate the lungs every 4 hours; monitor oxygen saturation at least once per shift.	Diminished or wet lung sounds and arterial oxygen saturation (SpO$_2$) ≤90% indicate poor ventilation and oxygen diffusion.
Assist with measures to clear respiratory secretions such as coughing, pharyngeal suctioning, aerosol treatments, and chest percussion.	Clearing the airway promotes gas exchange.
Give oxygen as medically prescribed if SpO$_2$ is ≤90%.	Keeping SpO$_2$ above 90% ensures that oxygen in plasma (PaO$_2$) is between 80 to 100 mm Hg.
Provide mechanical ventilation for acute respiratory failure (PaO$_2$ ≤50 mm Hg or PaCO$_2$ ≥50 mm Hg).	Mechanical ventilation provides a prescribed rate of respiration, tidal volume, and supplemental oxygen when normal breathing is inadequate.
Administer prescribed antimicrobials.	Antimicrobials exert either bactericidal or bacteriostatic functions.

Evaluation of Expected Outcome: Nurse ensures management of pneumonia and control of complications.

Nursing Diagnosis: **Risk for Deficient Fluid Volume** related to diarrhea secondary to viremia, opportunistic infection, and side effects of medication

Expected Outcome: Client's fluid intake and output will be balanced.

Interventions	Rationales
Keep a record of intake and output, measuring liquid feces.	Measurements provide an objective account of fluid status.
Offer oral fluids every hour while client is awake.	Oral intake increases when the nurse encourages it.
Withhold foods, especially caffeine, that are irritating until bowel function improves.	Fibrous foods increase peristalsis and diarrhea; caffeine is a bowel stimulant and diuretic.
Administer prescribed antidiarrheals.	Antidiarrheals slow peristalsis, adsorbing gastrointestinal irritants and water.
Report evidence of dehydration or electrolyte imbalance.	Parenteral fluids and electrolyte additives are alternate ways to restore fluid and electrolyte balance when the oral route is inadequate.

Evaluation of Expected Outcome: Client's fluid intake and output is 1500 mL/24 hours.

Nursing Diagnoses: **Risk for Activity Intolerance, Impaired Physical Mobility,** and **Deficient Self-Care** related to fatigue, weakness, and neurologic complications

Expected Outcome: Client will tolerate ADLs, maintain mobility, and perform self-care.

Interventions	Rationales
Prevent fatigue by spacing activities between periods of rest.	Aerobic metabolism, which provides greater energy yield than anaerobic metabolism, depends on cellular oxygen.
Assist with ADLs.	Assistance reduces energy expenditure.
Place a commode at the bedside.	Shortening distance between client and toilet conserves energy.
Provide a walker for ambulatory assistance.	Ambulatory aids promote movement and reduce the risk for injury.

(continued)

Nursing Care Plan 43-1 (Continued)

THE CLIENT WITH AIDS

Evaluation of Expected Outcome: Client performs ADLs and self-care and maintains mobility.

Nursing Diagnosis: **Risk for Impaired Skin Integrity** related to impaired capillary blood flow secondary to immobility, skin infection, and rash

Expected Outcome: Client's skin will remain intact.

Interventions	Rationales
Change position every 2 hours.	Relief of pressure ensures that capillary blood flow remains >32 mm Hg to keep tissues oxygenated.
Keep skin clean and dry.	Moist, soiled skin leads to maceration and bacterial growth.
Apply skin moisturizer.	Lubricated skin is more pliable and less likely to break down.
Gently massage intact skin over bony prominences.	Massage increases circulation and delivery of oxygen to tissues.
Clean and dry perineal area after elimination.	Ammonia from urine and stool debris erode skin. Organisms in stool transmit yeast infections.
Use lubricated wipes or a soft washcloth for cleansing.	Rough textures injure skin.

Evaluation of Expected Outcome: Client's skin is intact.

Nursing Diagnosis: **Impaired Oral Mucous Membranes** related to inflammation secondary to opportunistic infections

Expected Outcome: Client's mucous membranes will be pink, moist, and intact.

Interventions	Rationales
Provide meticulous oral care after and between meals.	Oral hygiene removes bacteria and yeast from mouth.
Avoid using mouthwashes that contain alcohol.	Alcohol irritates inflamed tissue.
Use mouth rinses with warm (not hot) plain water, normal saline solution, or water and hydrogen peroxide.	Warmth increases circulation and promotes healing. Water, saline, and dilute peroxide do not irritate oral tissues.
Use a soft toothbrush or foam swabs for oral care.	Soft textures protect gums from injury and infection.

Evaluation of Expected Outcome: Client's mucous membranes are normal.

Nursing Diagnoses: **Powerlessness** and **Hopelessness** related to poor prognosis

Expected Outcomes: Client will control his or her time, make other personal choices, and develop a realistic perception of the immediate future.

Interventions	Rationales
Give client choices whenever possible.	Making choices reaffirms a sense of control.
Help client formulate and achieve short-term goals to enjoy more frequent small successes.	Accomplishment of goals enhances hope.
Discourage client from abandoning traditional treatment for therapies that lack any evidence of effectiveness.	Desperate clients may turn to unsubstantiated claims of a cure for AIDS.

Evaluation of Expected Outcome: Client makes personal choices that give a sense of control without further damaging health, and realistically perceives his or her future.

(continued)

Nursing Care Plan 43-1 (Continued)

THE CLIENT WITH AIDS

Nursing Diagnosis: **Anticipatory Grieving** related to potential for early death; **Social Isolation** related to rejection by others or death of infected friends; **Interrupted Family Processes** related to abandonment; **Ineffective Coping** related to stress of contending with an incurable disease

Expected Outcome: Client will work through grief, maintain social contacts with family and friends, and cope effectively with crises.

Interventions	*Rationales*
Be a role model of acceptance for family and friends.	Learning occurs by example.
Make an effort to touch the client.	Touching demonstrates that casual contact does not transmit the disease.
Avoid wearing gloves and other barrier garments unless absolutely necessary.	Unnecessary use of barrier garments implies that the client is unfit to touch.
Refer client to an AIDS support group.	Groups confer acceptance, calm fear, and decrease isolation.

Evaluation of Expected Outcome: Client deals with grief and crises with support of family and friends.

---

clean the anal and perineal areas well after each bowel movement, and wash the hands after voiding or defecating.
- When possible, avoid dry and dusty areas, excessive humidity, and extreme heat or cold. Wear clothing appropriate to the weather and temperature.
- Take frequent rest periods, and space activities to prevent fatigue.
- Do not share IV needles, and do not donate blood.
- Inform healthcare personnel of HIV-positive status.

NURSING GUIDELINES 43-1

Safe Handling of Needles and Sharp Instruments

■ Do not become distracted when handling needles and sharp instruments. Concentrate on the task being performed.

■ Use a clean tray to pass used or contaminated needles and sharp instruments to another person.

■ Keep the container for disposal of needles and sharp instruments close by. When necessary, carry the container to the bedside.

■ If a client is uncooperative, ask for assistance when obtaining blood specimens, handling body fluids and secretions, giving injections, or starting IV therapy.

■ Do not leave uncapped or used needles unattended. Properly dispose of contaminated sharp instruments and needles as soon as they are used.

UNDERSTANDING FINANCIAL AND INSURANCE IMPLICATIONS

Despite HIV-specific confidentiality laws, clients infected with AIDS fear that disclosure of their condition will affect employment, health insurance coverage, and even housing. An employer cannot cancel a client's currently active health insurance policy on the basis of AIDS. Employers are more apt to dismiss a worker with a known HIV-positive status from employment, however, to reduce future insurance premiums and death payments. The dismissal often is attributed to some reason not associated with HIV to avoid being charged with discrimination under the Americans With Disabilities Act.

Unemployed persons can apply for a continuation of the employer's health plan for 18 months at self-pay. Thereafter, they can extend their insurance for 11 more months if they meet the Social Security Administration's criteria for being disabled. Eventually, the person infected with HIV may need to obtain private health insurance, which is very expensive. Private insurers often exclude individuals with a pre-existing condition or require a long waiting period before the policy takes effect. An AIDS caseworker often can help an HIV-positive person with health insurance questions.

DISCUSSING VIATICAL SETTLEMENTS

A **viatical settlement** is an arrangement in which a terminally ill individual agrees to name a person as beneficiary to his or her life insurance in exchange for immediate cash. It is best to advise a person who is considering this option to work through an attorney or licensed insurance broker who will negotiate the value of the insurance policy with the potential purchaser. Other factors that the client must consider are whether the cash will cancel eligibility for food stamps or other forms of public assistance and that the cash will be considered earned income for tax purposes.

GENERAL NUTRITION CONSIDERATIONS

Because malnutrition may hasten the progression from HIV infection to frank AIDS, interventions to attain or maintain optimal nutritional status should begin as soon as HIV infection is diagnosed.

A high-protein, high-calorie, nutritionally dense diet that contains an adequate level of all nutrients may help to preserve lean body mass and avoid potentiating depressed immunocompetence.

Nutritional intervention may help to alleviate symptoms that interfere with intake or nutrient use. Clients with anorexia should be encouraged to eat small, frequent meals of easily digested food and liquids even when not hungry. Clients with nausea and vomiting may tolerate a low-fat, high-carbohydrate, soft or liquid diet better than large, high-fat meals. Diarrhea and malabsorption may improve when clients avoid residue, lactose, fat, and caffeine. Gluten and sucrose may need to be restricted in some clients with malabsorption. Liquids should be encouraged to replace fluid and electrolyte losses. Although eating may seem to trigger diarrhea, clients must understand that limiting food intake to control diarrhea only exacerbates wasting. Gravies, sauces, and broth added to soft, nonirritating foods may promote ease of swallowing in clients with oral or esophageal ulcerations. Some clients may require a blenderized or liquid diet. Because temperature extremes (very hot or very cold) can irritate the mucosa, room-temperature foods and liquids are recommended for clients with a sore mouth.

Vitamin and mineral requirements for clients with HIV/AIDS are unknown, but poor intake and altered nutrient absorption and metabolism place the client at high risk for nutrient deficiencies. It is recommended that fat-soluble vitamins be taken at Recommended Dietary Allowance (RDA) levels and that water-soluble vitamins be taken in amounts two to five times the RDA. Trace element and antioxidant supplements may be prescribed. Advise clients to avoid large doses of iron and zinc because they can impair immune function.

Clients unable to consume an adequate oral diet may require a tube feeding for supplemental or complete nutrition. Because many formulas have the potential to cause diarrhea, closely monitor the client's tolerance. Advera and Impact are commercial formulas designed for clients with impaired immune function.

GENERAL PHARMACOLOGIC CONSIDERATIONS

The most common adverse effects associated with the administration of zidovudine are anemia and granulocytopenia.

Foscarnet is used to treat CMV retinitis and is given by controlled IV infusion. Alterations in renal function, fever, nausea, anemia, numbness in extremities, and diarrhea are the most common adverse effects of this drug.

Didanosine administration may result in pancreatitis and peripheral neuropathy.

The major adverse effect associated with zalcitabine administration is peripheral neuropathy. Pancreatitis also may be seen.

Clients receiving antiviral drugs are informed that these drugs do not cure AIDS but may slow its progression.

GENERAL GERONTOLOGIC CONSIDERATIONS

According to the CDC, approximately 10% of reported AIDS cases involve those older than 50 years of age.

Stereotyping older adults as asexual may cause the nurse to neglect to question the older adult about sexual matters, resulting in an inaccurate sexual history.

The period between initial infection with HIV and the onset of AIDS-related symptoms is shorter for older adults than others, and death usually occurs earlier in this age group.

The dementia caused by AIDS may be mistaken for other dementias commonly associated with older adults.

Older adults with AIDS may lack an adequate support system and feel lonely, anxious, and isolated.

Older adults in general are less informed about AIDS than younger people. Education campaigns target the younger at-risk population and fail to address the possibility or needs of older adults contracting the disease.

Critical Thinking Exercises

1. *What advice would you give adolescents to reduce their risk for becoming infected with HIV?*
2. *A nurse on a medical unit sustains a needlestick injury. What actions should the nurse take? What are the responsibilities of the employing agency?*

References and Suggested Readings

A scourge beyond imagining. (2000; December 18). *U.S. News and World Report, 129*(24), 34.

AIDS Education and Research Trust. (2000; December 20). United States HIV and AIDS Statistics. [On-line.] Available: http://www.avert.org/usastato.htm.

Barroso, J. (1999). A review of fatigue in people with HIV infection. *Journal of the Association of Nurses in AIDS Care, 10*(5), 42–49.

Bormann, J. & Kelly, A. (1999). HIV and AIDS: Are you biased? *American Journal of Nursing, 99*(9), 38–39.

Centers for Disease Control and Prevention, U.S. Department of Health and Human Services, Public Health Service. (1999). *HIV/AIDS Surveillance Report, 11*(2).

Cochran, A. & Wilson, B. A. (1999). Current management of AIDS and related opportunistic infections. *MEDSURG Nursing, 8*(4), 257–264, 266.

Facing facts and AIDS. (2000, July 24). *U.S. News and World Report, 129*(4), 24.

Joint United Nations Programme on HIV/AIDS (UNAIDS). (1999; December). AIDS epidemic update. [On-line.] Available: http://www.unaids.org/.

Lisanti, P. & Zwolski, K. (1997). Understanding the devastation of AIDS. *American Journal of Nursing, 97*(7), 26–34.

Muma, D. J., et al. (1999). *HIV manual for health care professionals.* New York: McGraw-Hill.

National Center for Health Statistics, Centers for Disease Control and Prevention. (2000). Mortality data from the National Vital Statistics System. [On-line]. http://www.cdc.gov/nchs.

Oestreicher, A. & Kane, B. (2000). HIV/AIDS: Updated recommendations for antiretroviral treatments in adults. *Journal of Care Management, 6*(3) *Disease Management Digest*: 10–11, 14–15.

Introduction to the Nervous System

Words to Know

acetylcholine	meninges
acetylcholinesterase	midbrain
arachnoid	myelin
axon	neurilemma
brain stem	neuron
cauda equina	neurotransmitters
central nervous system	norepinephrine
cerebellum	parasympathetic
cerebrum	nervous system
corpus callosum	peripheral nervous
decerebrate posturing	system
decorticate posturing	pia mater
dendrites	pons
dopamine	pyramidal
dura mater	subarachnoid space
epinephrine	sympathetic nervous
extrapyramidal	system
flaccidity	synapses
medulla oblongata	ventricles

Learning Objectives

On completion of this chapter, the reader will:

- Name the two anatomic divisions of the nervous system.
- Name the three parts of the brain.
- List the four lobes of the cerebrum.
- Give two functions of the spinal cord.
- Name and describe the function of the two parts of the autonomic nervous system.
- Describe methods used to assess motor and sensory function.
- List six diagnostic procedures performed to detect neurologic disorders.
- Discuss the nursing management of the client undergoing neurologic diagnostic testing.

The nervous system consists of the brain, spinal cord, and peripheral nerves. It is responsible for coordinating body functions and responding to changes in or stimuli from the internal and external environment. Changes in the functioning of the nervous system can profoundly affect the entire body.

ANATOMY AND PHYSIOLOGY

The nervous system is divided into two anatomic divisions: the **central nervous system** (CNS) and the **peripheral nervous system** (PNS). The basic structure of the nervous system is the nerve cell or **neuron** (Fig. 44-1). Neurons are either sensory or motor. *Sensory neurons* transmit impulses to the CNS; *motor neurons* transmit impulses from the CNS.

A neuron is composed of a cell body, a nucleus, and threadlike projections or fibers called **dendrites.** Dendrites conduct impulses to the cell body and are called *afferent* ("to" or "toward") nerve fibers. An **axon** is a nerve fiber that projects and conducts impulses away from the cell body. It is therefore called an *efferent* ("away from") nerve fiber. The axon usually is larger than the dendrites.

Neurons are separate units and not directly connected to one another. Impulses travel along neurons, moving from one neuron to the next by means of **synapses,** junctions between the axon of one neuron to the dendrite of another. Substances called **neurotransmitters** (or neurohormones) accomplish the transmission of an impulse from one neuron to the next (see Chap. 12).

A fatty substance called **myelin** covers some axons in the CNS and PNS. Such axons are called *myelinated,* or white, nerve fibers. A sheath called the **neurilemma**

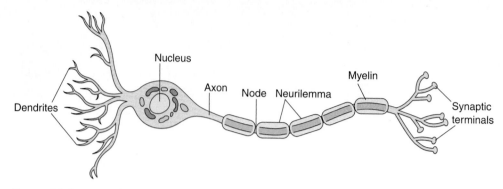

FIGURE 44-1 Neuron. (Adapted from Willis, M. C. [1996]. *Medical terminology: The language of healthcare.* Baltimore: Williams & Wilkins.)

covers the myelin. Myelin serves as an insulating substance for the axon. Axons without myelin are called *unmyelinated,* or gray, nerve fibers.

Central Nervous System

The CNS consists of the brain and spinal cord.

Brain

The brain is divided into three parts: the cerebrum, cerebellum, and brain stem. The **cerebrum** consists of two hemispheres connected by the **corpus callosum,** a band of white fibers that acts as a bridge for transmitting impulses between the left and right hemispheres. Each hemisphere has four lobes: frontal, parietal, temporal, and occipital (Fig. 44-2). The cerebral cortex is the surface of the cerebrum. It contains motor neurons, which

are responsible for movement, and sensory neurons, which receive impulses from peripheral sensory neurons located throughout the body.

Motor tracts are **pyramidal** or **extrapyramidal.** Pyramidal motor pathways originate in the motor cortex of the cerebrum, cross over at the level of the medulla, and end in the brain stem and spinal cord. Extrapyramidal fibers originate in the motor cortex and project to the cerebellum and basal ganglia. They do not cross over as they connect to motor neurons in the spinal cord.

The **cerebellum,** which is located behind and below the cerebrum, controls and coordinates muscle movement. The **brain stem** consists of the midbrain, pons, and medulla oblongata. The **midbrain** forms the forward part of the brain stem and connects the pons and cerebellum with the two cerebral hemispheres. The **pons** is located between the midbrain and medulla and connects the two hemispheres of the cerebellum with the brain stem, spinal

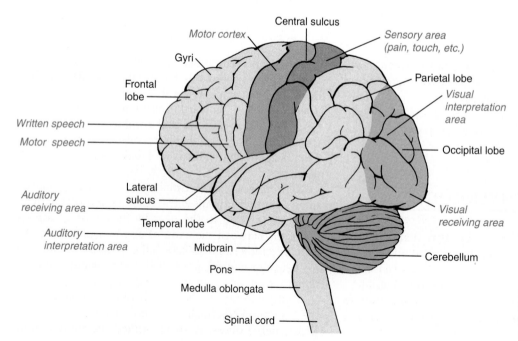

FIGURE 44-2 Structure of the brain. Shaded areas show the region responsible for different functions.

FIGURE 44-3 Schematic diagram of the three connective tissue membranes (pia, arachnoid, and dura) constituting the meninges of the CNS. (From Cormack, D. H. [1987]. *Ham's histology* [9th ed.]. Philadelphia: J. B. Lippincott.)

cord, and cerebrum. The **medulla oblongata** lies below the pons and transmits motor impulses from the brain to the spinal cord and sensory impulses from peripheral sensory neurons to the brain. The medulla contains vital centers concerned with respiration, heartbeat, and vasomotor activity (the control of smooth muscle activity in blood vessel walls).

The brain is protected by the rigid bones of the skull and covered by three membranes or **meninges:** (1) the **dura mater,** the tough, outermost covering; (2) the **arachnoid,** or middle membrane lying directly below the dura; and (3) the **pia mater,** a delicate layer that adheres to the brain and spinal cord. The **subarachnoid space** is between the pia mater and the arachnoid membrane (Fig. 44-3).

Within the brain are four hollow structures called **ventricles** (Fig. 44-4). The ventricles manufacture and absorb cerebrospinal fluid (CSF), which constantly circulates in the subarachnoid space of the brain and spinal cord. CSF produced in the ventricles passes down into the subarachnoid space of the spinal cord, then up through the basilar cisterns and over the cerebral hemispheres to the region of the dural venous sinuses, where most of the absorption occurs. Acting as a cushion, the CSF protects these structures and helps maintain relatively constant intracranial pressure.

Stop, Think, and Respond ● BOX 44-1

Name the three layers of meninges, starting below the skull and proceeding toward the surface of the brain.

Spinal Cord

The spinal cord, which is covered by the meninges, is a direct continuation of the medulla and is surrounded and

protected by the *vertebrae* (or vertebral column). The spinal cord ends between the first and second lumbar vertebrae, where it divides into smaller sections called the **cauda equina.**

The spinal cord functions as a passageway for ascending sensory and descending motor neurons. Its two main functions are to provide centers for reflex action (Fig. 44-5) and to serve as a pathway for impulses to and from the brain. The sensory fibers enter the posterior (dorsal) portion of the cord; the nerve fibers that transmit motor impulses run outward to the peripheral nerves from the anterior (ventral) portion of the cord.

Peripheral Nervous System

The PNS consists of all nerves outside the CNS.

FIGURE 44-4 Ventricles of the brain seen from a lateral view.

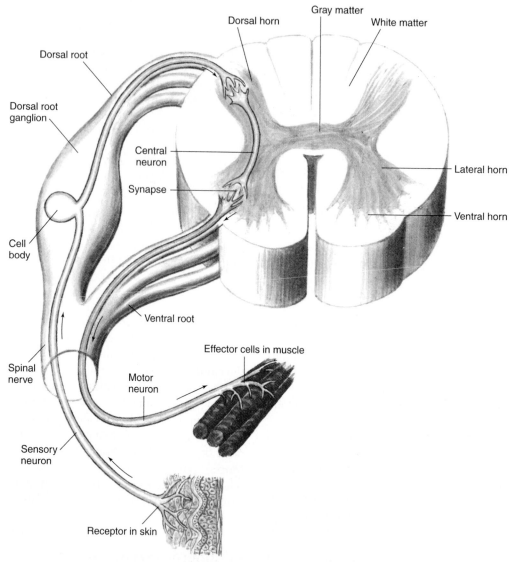

FIGURE 44-5 Reflex arc showing the pathway of impulses and cross-section of the spinal cord.

Cranial Nerves

The 12 pairs of cranial nerves, identified by Roman numerals, are as follows:

- *I*—Olfactory nerve: sense of smell
- *II*—Optic nerve: sight
- *III*—Oculomotor nerve: contraction of iris and eye muscles
- *IV*—Trochlear nerve: eye movement
- *V*—Trigeminal nerve: sensory nerve to face, chewing
- *VI*—Abducens nerve: eye movement
- *VII*—Facial nerve: facial expression, taste, secretions of salivary and lacrimal glands
- *VIII*—Vestibulocochlear (or auditory) nerve: hearing, balance
- *IX*—Glossopharyngeal nerve: taste, sensory fibers of pharynx and tongue, swallowing, secretions of parotid gland

- *X*—Vagus nerve: motor fibers to glands producing digestive enzymes, heart rate, muscles of speech, gastrointestinal motility, respiration, swallowing, coughing, vomiting reflex
- *XI*—Accessory (or spinal accessory) nerve: head and shoulder movement
- *XII*—Hypoglossal nerve: movement of the tongue

Spinal Nerves

There are 31 pairs of spinal nerves: 8 cervical, 12 thoracic, 5 lumbar, 5 sacral, and 1 coccygeal. Spinal nerves have two roots: dorsal and ventral. Dorsal nerve fibers are sensory, and ventral nerve fibers are motor. Peripheral sensory nerve fibers in various areas of the body transmit impulses to the spinal nerves, which transmit impulses up the spinal cord to the brain. Motor impulses traveling from the brain and down the spinal cord leave by the ventral root and travel to areas of the body. Each spinal nerve root innervates a specific area or *dermatome* of the body surface (Fig. 44-6). Knowledge of the distribution of dermatomes is useful for the nurse's assessment and evaluation.

Autonomic Nervous System

The autonomic nervous system consists of the **sympathetic nervous system** and the **parasympathetic nervous system.** It is concerned with functions essential to the survival of the organism.

SYMPATHETIC NERVOUS SYSTEM

This division of the autonomic nervous system regulates the expenditure of energy. The neurotransmitters of the sympathetic nervous system, collectively known as *catecholamines,* are **epinephrine, norepinephrine,** and **dopamine.** The adrenal medulla produces and secretes epinephrine and norepinephrine. Norepinephrine also is produced at sympathetic nerve endings. Dopamine is a precursor (a substance that precedes another) of norepinephrine. Norepinephrine then becomes epinephrine.

Stressful situations such as danger, intense emotion, and severe illness result in the release of catecholamines.

PARASYMPATHETIC NERVOUS SYSTEM

This division of the autonomic nervous system works to conserve body energy and is partly responsible for slowing heart rate, digesting food, and eliminating body wastes. **Acetylcholine** is a neurotransmitter released at the nerve endings of parasympathetic nerve fibers, at some nerve endings in the sympathetic nervous system, and at nerve endings of skeletal muscles. Release of this neurotransmitter allows passage of a nerve impulse from the nerve fiber to the effector organ or structure, where the enzyme **acetylcholinesterase** inactivates acetylcholine.

ASSESSMENT

A neurologic assessment is performed to identify and locate disorders of the nervous system. The scope and extent of the neurologic examination often depend on the symptoms and the probable or actual diagnosis.

FIGURE 44-6 Dermatome distribution.

History

A thorough history is essential. The nurse explores all symptoms and asks questions to clarify each symptom. The history must include a record of trauma (no matter how slight) to the head or body within the past 6 to 12 months, a drug history, an allergy history, and a family medical history. The nurse observes the client's speech pattern, mental status, intellectual functioning, reasoning ability, and movement or lack of movement of all extremities.

Physical Examination

The physical examination consists of assessment of the cerebral, motor, and sensory areas. The nurse usually assesses intellectual function and speech pattern during the history by noting responses to questions. Additional testing of intellectual function includes asking various questions that require mental tasks (see discussion of Mini-Mental State Examination in Chap. 12).

The nurse evaluates the client's body posture and any abnormal position of the head, neck, trunk, or extremities. If head trauma has occurred, the nurse examines the ears and nose for evidence of bleeding or other drainage. He or she carefully examines the head for bleeding, swelling, or wounds. The nurse does not move or manipulate the client's head during this part of the assessment, especially if there is a recent history of trauma.

Cranial Nerves

The experienced examiner evaluates all or some of the 12 cranial nerves (Table 44-1).

Motor Function

Assessment of motor function includes muscle movement, size, tone, strength, and coordination. The nurse inspects large muscle areas for evidence of atrophy and assesses opposing muscles for equality of size and strength. He or she asks the client to perform tasks such as:

- Pushing the palm or sole against the examiner's palm
- Picking small and large objects between the thumb and forefinger
- Grasping objects firmly
- Resisting removal of an object from the fist or fingers

To assess gait, movement, and balance, the nurse asks the client to walk away from the examiner, turn, and walk back. Other tests include climbing a small set of stairs, walking and turning abruptly, and walking heel to toe. In the Romberg test, the client stands with feet close together and eyes closed. If the client sways and tends to fall, this is considered a positive Romberg test, indicating a problem with equilibrium. The examiner stands fairly close to the client during this test in case the client loses balance.

Tests that evaluate motor and cerebral function include doing the finger-to-nose test with eyes closed, writing words, and identifying common objects. The choice of tests depends on the original complaints and the findings of diagnostic tests.

The nurse evaluates motor response in the comatose or unconscious client by administering a painful stimulus to determine if the client makes an appropriate response by reaching toward or withdrawing from the stimulus (Fig. 44-7A and B). Those with impaired cerebral function manifest **decorticate posturing** (decorticate rigidity), **decerebrate posturing** (decerebrate rigidity), or **flaccidity** (see Fig. 44-7C–E). Decerebrate posturing is more serious than decorticate posturing; flaccidity is even more ominous.

Stop, Think, and Respond ● BOX 44-2

Which type of posturing is evidenced by (A) flexion of the arms, (B) extension of the arms, and (C) no movement of any extremities?

Sensory Function

The nurse evaluates the extremities for sensitivity to heat, cold, touch, and pain. He or she can use various objects such as cotton balls, tubes filled with hot or cold water, and sharp objects (that do not pierce the skin) to check sensation in the extremities.

Level of Consciousness

Depending on the client's symptoms, evaluation of the level of consciousness (LOC) is often necessary. The following classification of LOC applies to altered consciousness from any cause. Differentiating between each level can be difficult; some clients show characteristics of two or more levels:

- *Conscious:* The client responds immediately, fully, and appropriately to visual, auditory, and other stimulation.
- *Somnolent or lethargic:* The client is drowsy or sleepy at inappropriate times but can be aroused, only to fall asleep again. Responses to questions are delayed or inappropriate. Speech is incoherent. The client responds slowly to verbal commands. He or she responds to painful stimuli.
- *Stuporous:* The client is aroused only by vigorous and continuous stimulation, usually by manipulation or strong auditory or visual stimuli. Stimulation results in one- or two-word answers or in motor activity or purposeful behavior directed toward avoiding further stimulation.
- *Semicomatose:* The client is unresponsive except to superficial, relatively mild painful stimuli to which

TABLE 44-1	CRANIAL NERVE ASSESSMENT	
CRANIAL NERVE	**ASSESSMENT TECHNIQUE**	**NORMAL FINDINGS**
I—Olfactory	Ask client to occlude each nostril separately and close the eyes. Present familiar odors, such as vinegar, lemon, coffee, and ammonia.	Client identifies odors correctly.
II—Optic	Help client cover each eye separately; test visual acuity using a Snellen chart (see Chap. 49) or newspaper.	Client names letters or reads words accurately.
	Client and examiner cover an eye, and examiner moves an object from the periphery toward client's nose from superior, inferior, medial, and lateral positions while both fix their gaze straight ahead. Examiner then tests opposite eye. Inspect optic nerve with an ophthalmoscope.	Client and examiner see object at the same time in the visual field. Optic nerve appears round and lighter than surrounding retina.
III—Oculomotor	In a darkened room, shine a bright light in each pupil; ask client to look at a near and far object (see Chap. 49).	Pupil constricts briskly in response to light and dilates when looking far away.
	Ask client to follow an object you move in horizontal, vertical, and oblique directions (see Chap. 49).	Eye movement is coordinated in all directions.
IV—Trochlear	See assessment for motor function of oculomotor nerve.	Eyes move inferiorly and medially.
V—Trigeminal	Observe for jaw symmetry while client opens mouth.	Appearance is symmetrical.
	Instruct client to clamp jaws tightly together.	The muscles contract bilaterally.
	Stroke forehead, cheeks, and jaw with a wisp of cotton, sharp object (e.g., pin), cold and warm objects, and a vibrating tuning fork.	Client shows bilateral sensitivity and correctly identifies sensory experience.
	Touch each cornea with a wisp of cotton.	Client blinks.
	Tap center of chin with a reflex hammer while client slightly opens the mouth.	Jaw closes suddenly and slightly.
VI—Abducens	See assessment for motor function of oculomotor nerve.	Client moves eyes in lateral directions.
VII—Facial	Ask client to wrinkle the forehead, smile, frown, raise eyebrows, look at ceiling, and whistle.	Facial movements are symmetrical.
	Instruct client to close eyelids and resist examiner's efforts to open them.	Both eyes equally resist movements to open them.
	Apply sweet, sour, salty, and bitter flavors to both sides of the anterior tongue.	Client accurately identifies tastes.
VIII—Vestibulocochlear	Test hearing acuity and perform the Rinne and Weber tests with a tuning fork (see Chap. 50).	Client repeats whispered words correctly; sound is lateralized equally and heard longer by air than by bone conduction.
	Have client stand with both feet close together; note for swaying with eyes open and then shut.	Client maintains balance or sways slightly.
IX—Glossopharyngeal	Touch palate with a tongue blade.	Blade elicits a gag response.
	Ask client to say "ah."	Uvula remains in midline.
X—Vagus	Have client say "la, la, la."	Client speaks clearly and distinctly, with no hoarseness.
XI—Spinal-accessory	Instruct client to shrug the shoulders as you apply resistance.	Clients raises shoulders.
XII—Hypoglossal	Tell client to stick out the tongue.	Tongue remains in midline with no lateral deviation.

the client makes some purposeful motor response (movement) to evade stimulation. Spontaneous motion is uncommon, but the client may groan or mutter.

- *Comatose:* The client responds only to very painful stimuli by fragmentary, delayed reflex withdrawal; in deeper stages, he or she loses all responsiveness. There is no spontaneous movement, and the respiratory rate is irregular.

The nurse assesses LOC at frequent intervals after injury to the head or neck, cranial surgery, a cerebrovascu-

(A) Localizes to painful stimulus

(B) Withdraws from painful stimulus

(C) Decorticate posturing; one or both arms are fully flexed on the chest

(D) Decerebrate posturing; one or both arms are stiffly extended

(E) Flaccid; no motor response

FIGURE 44-7 Responses to pain and posturing.

lar accident (acute phase), a ruptured cerebral aneurysm, and other neurologic disorders. He or she makes this assessment hourly unless the physician orders otherwise or a change occurs in the client's condition.

The Glasgow Coma Scale (Fig. 44-8) is a measure of the LOC. It consists of three parts: eye opening response, best verbal response, and best motor response. To evaluate responses correctly, several verbal and motor responses are elicited, and the best response is recorded. The eye opening response is determined by talking to the client and calling his or her name. If no response is noted (i.e., the eyes do not open spontaneously), a painful stimulus is introduced and the response noted. The verbal response is evaluated by a verbal reply to questions. The motor response is the ability of the client to follow commands, such as "wiggle your toes" or "move your left hand." If there is no response, a painful stimulus is introduced and the response noted. The responses are assigned numbers and the numbers are totaled. A normal response is 15. A score of 7 or less is considered coma. The evaluations

are recorded on a graphic sheet; connecting lines show an increase or decrease in the LOC.

The Rancho Los Amigos Scale (Box 44-1) is another tool for assessing LOC. Some rehabilitation centers prefer this scale because it is a more flexible assessment tool for identifying the client's status.

Pupils

The size and equality of the pupils and their reaction to light are an assessment of the third cranial (oculomotor) nerve (see Table 44-1). Pupil size (normal, pinpoint, dilated), equality (equal, unequal in size), and reaction to a bright light (normal, sluggish, no reaction, fixed) are noted (see Chap. 49). When the pupils are examined, any abnormal movement or position of one or both eyes is noted.

Unequal pupils (one pupil larger than the other), dilated or pinpoint pupils, and failure of the pupils to respond quickly to light are, in most instances, abnormal findings. Any sudden change in pupil size, equality, or

The Glasgow Coma Scale is a tool for assessing a client's response to stimuli. A score of 10 or less indicates a need for emergency attention: a score of 7 or less is generally interpreted as coma.

Eye opening response	Spontaneous	4
	To voice	3
	To pain	2
	None	1
Best verbal response	Oriented	5
	Confused	4
	Inappropriate words	3
	Incomprehensible Sounds	2
	None	1
Best motor response	Obeys command	6
	Localizes pain	5
	Withdraws (pain)	4
	Flexion (pain)	3
	Extension (pain)	2
	None	1
Total		3 to 15

Figure 44-8 Glasgow Coma Scale.

reaction to light is an important neurologic finding and is reported to the physician at once.

Neck

The neck is examined for stiffness or abnormal position. The presence of rigidity is checked by moving the head and chin toward the chest. Do not perform this maneuver if a head or neck injury is suspected or known or trauma to any part of the body is evident.

Vital Signs

The blood pressure, pulse and respiratory rates, and temperature are closely monitored on all clients with a potential or actual neurologic disorder. The temperature often needs to be monitored every hour because CNS disorders can affect the temperature-regulating ability of the hypothalamus. A sudden increase or decrease in any of the vital signs indicates a change in the neurologic status, and the physician is notified immediately.

Diagnostic Tests

Imaging Procedures

Imaging procedures such as computed tomography (CT), magnetic resonance imaging (MRI), positron emission tomography (PET), and single-photon emission computed tomography are used in the diagnosis of neurologic disorders. Imaging procedures are particularly useful in the diagnosis of neurologic disorders such as brain tumors, Alzheimer's disease, intracranial bleeding or hemorrhage, and cerebral infections. A radiopaque dye is used during a CT scan to emphasize or highlight a certain area. Use of a radiopaque dye decreases the safety of the procedure.

Computed Tomography

CT scanning uses x-rays and computer analysis to produce three-dimensional views of thin cross-sections, or "slices," of the body. A narrow x-ray beam rotates around the client and the results are analyzed by a computer. CT is extremely sensitive to differences in tissue densities, allowing differentiation between intracranial tumors, cysts, edema, and hemorrhage. The client is exposed to the same amount of radiation as in a conventional x-ray.

Magnetic Resonance Imaging

An MRI is based on the magnetic behavior of protons in body tissue. This imaging procedure uses radiofrequency waves to produce images of tissues of high fat and water content such as soft tissue, veins, arteries, the brain, and spinal cord. Images are produced without contrast dye or radiation.

The client lies motionless on a stretcher enclosed in a tunnel containing a powerful magnet (Fig. 44-9). The MRI lasts 15 to 90 minutes. Claustrophobia commonly is experienced. A call button and an intercom are available for two-way communication. The MRI cannot be used for clients with metal implants such as a hip or knee replacement or cardiac pacemaker because metal interferes with the magnetic field.

BOX 44-1 ● Rancho Los Amigos Scales

Level I   No response to stimuli. Appears in deep sleep.

Level II   Generalized response. First reaction may be to deep pain. Has delayed, inconsistent responses.

Level III   Localized response. Inconsistent responses, but reacts in a more specific manner to stimulus. Might follow simple command "squeeze my hand."

Level IV   Confused. Agitated. Reacts to own inner confusion, fear, disorientation. Excitable behavior, may be abusive.

Level V   Nonagitated. Confused. Inappropriate. Usually disoriented. Follows tasks for 2 to 3 minutes, but easily distracted by environment, frustrated.

Level VI   Confused appropriate. Follows simple directions consistently. Memory and attention increasing. Self-care tasks performed without help.

Level VII   Automatic appropriate. If physically able, can carry out routine activities. Appears normal. Needs supervision for safety.

Level VIII   Purposeful. Alert. Oriented. May have decreased abilities relative to premorbid state.

FIGURE 44-9 A technician discusses what the client should expect during MRI. (From Smeltzer, S. C. & Bare, B. G. [2000]. *Brunner & Suddarth's textbook of medical–surgical nursing* [9th ed.]. Philadelphia: Lippincott Williams & Wilkins.)

A

B

FIGURE 44-10 (**A**) Positioning of the client for lumbar puncture. (**B**) Insertion of the spinal needle into the subarachnoid space. (From Smeltzer, S. C. & Bare, B. G. [2000]. *Brunner & Suddarth's textbook of medical–surgical nursing* [9th ed.]. Philadelphia: Lippincott Williams & Wilkins.)

Positron Emission Tomography

PET uses radioactive substances to examine metabolic activity of body structures. The client either inhales or is injected with a radioactive substance with positively charged particles that combine with negatively charged particles found normally in the body. The energy emitted when these combine is converted into color-coded images indicating metabolic activity of the organ involved. The radioactive substances are short-lived, resulting in minimal radiation exposure. PET is used less frequently than CT or MRI because the equipment is available only in major medical research centers.

Lumbar Puncture

Changes in CSF occur in many neurologic disorders. A lumbar puncture (spinal tap) is performed to obtain samples of CSF from the subarachnoid space for laboratory examination and to measure CSF pressure (Fig. 44-10). Bacteriologic tests on specimens of CSF reveal the presence of pathogenic microorganisms. Strict aseptic technique is required during the procedure. The CSF normally is clear and colorless with a pressure of 80 to 180 mm H_2O; a pressure over 200 mm H_2O is considered abnormal. A lumbar puncture also is performed to inject a drug into the subarachnoid space (intrathecal injection), to administer a spinal anesthetic, to withdraw CSF for the relief of intracranial pressure, or to inject air, gas, or dye for a neurologic diagnostic procedure.

Sometimes a cisternal puncture is performed to remove CSF. The back of the neck is shaved, the skin washed with an antiseptic, and a needle inserted just below the occipital bone of the skull. This procedure is performed more commonly on children. Headache appears to occur less frequently with cisternal puncture than with lumbar puncture.

Contrast Studies

Contrast studies include cerebral angiography, which detects distortion of cerebral arteries and veins, indicating an aneurysm, a tumor, or other vascular abnormality. A radiopaque dye is injected into the right or left carotid artery, the brachial artery, or the femoral artery. A rapid sequence of radiographs is taken as the dye circulates through the cerebral arteries and veins.

For a myelogram, a radiopaque substance is injected into the spinal canal by means of a lumbar puncture. Radiographs are taken to demonstrate abnormalities of the spinal canal such as tumors or a ruptured intervertebral disk.

Electroencephalogram

An electroencephalogram (EEG) records the electrical impulses generated by the brain. Electrodes are placed on the scalp and electrical activity is recorded on a graph.

Brain Scan

A brain scan identifies tumors, hematomas in or around the brain, cerebral abscesses, cerebral infarctions, or displaced ventricles. A radioactive material is injected before the procedure. The length of this procedure varies from a few minutes to 1 hour. CT scans and MRI are replacing this procedure.

Electromyography

Electromyography (EMG) studies the changes in the electrical potential of muscles and the nerves supplying the muscles. Needle electrodes are placed into one or more skeletal muscles and the results recorded on an oscilloscope. This test is useful in determining the presence of neuromuscular disorders.

Nerve Conduction Studies

Nerve conduction studies measure the speed with which nerve impulses travel along a peripheral nerve fiber when a specific nerve is electrically stimulated. This test aids diagnosis of nerve injury and compression or neurologic disorders affecting peripheral nerves.

Echoencephalography

An echoencephalogram is an ultrasound examination of the structures of the brain. This procedure is performed to detect abnormalities in the ventricles and the location of intracranial bleeding.

NURSING PROCESS

● The Client Undergoing Neurologic Testing

Assessment

The nurse determines the client's understanding of the diagnostic procedures and answers remaining questions. He or she checks that a consent form has been signed and witnessed. Because some contrast media contain iodine, the nurse checks the client's history for previous allergic reactions to radiographic dyes, iodine, or seafood. He or she obtains the client's weight, baseline vital signs, and neurologic data such as LOC, pupil response, and muscle strength in all four extremities. The nurse uses the assessment findings for comparison when monitoring the client's condition during and after diagnostic testing. He or she closely observes the client for any mental or physical deviations from the baseline assessments.

Diagnosis, Planning, and Interventions

The nurse prepares the client for neurologic diagnostic tests following agency policies. If the diagnostic test is performed at the bedside, the nurse brings necessary equipment to the room. He or she assists the physician and supports the client during a test performed on the nursing unit. During and after the diagnostic test, the nurse monitors for adverse consequences and promotes recovery

after the test. Diagnoses, expected outcomes, and interventions include, but are not limited to, the following.

Deficient Knowledge related to unfamiliarity with diagnostic testing process

Expected Outcome: Client will accurately describe the preparation, procedure, and aftercare that the scheduled diagnostic test involves.

- Clarify the physician's explanation. *Some clients have questions after the physician leaves the nursing unit or healthcare agency.*
- Answer the client's questions. *Clients have the right to information about their plan of care.*
- Describe the procedure to the client as well as what the procedure requires, such as positions to assume or the need to lie still during the procedure. *Specific information decreases anxiety and increases the client's trust and confidence in the nurse.*
- Discuss the preparation for the diagnostic test, which may include temporarily eliminating CNS depressants, such as barbiturates and minor tranquilizers, and CNS stimulants, such as caffeine, for 24 to 48 hours in the case of an EEG. *Drugs that affect neurologic function sometimes are withheld to ensure that factors other than the client's physiology do not affect test results.*
- Explain that hair will be shampooed before an EEG. *Removing scalp and hair oil ensures that electrodes will remain in place until the EEG is completed.*
- Inform the client that he or she will be able to shampoo the hair again after an EEG. *A second shampoo facilitates removing the paste used to secure the electrodes to the scalp.*
- Tell the client to expect some discomfort when undergoing a lumbar puncture, myelogram, EMG, or nerve conduction studies. *Without giving the client information about expected discomfort, the client may assume that he or she is having an adverse reaction.*

PC: Allergic Reaction to contrast dye

Expected Outcome: The nurse will monitor to detect, manage, and minimize an allergic reaction.

- Report the allergy history to the physician. *Reporting helps the physician decide to cancel or modify the diagnostic test by administering a pretest antihistamine or substituting an alternative dye.*
- Identify allergy information prominently on the client's chart. *Documenting allergies on the chart provides a means for communicating the information to all healthcare workers.*
- Attach an allergy band to the client's wrist when that is the agency's policy. *Some healthcare agencies require a second wrist band that is a different color than the client identification band to alert personnel that the client has a history of one or more allergies.*
- Administer pretest antihistamines according to the physician's medical order. *Antihistamines block histamine receptors and reduce the manifestations of an allergic reaction.*

- Monitor client for severe hypotension, tachycardia, profuse diaphoresis, sudden change in LOC, dyspnea, and hives or itching. Notify the physician immediately of any such findings. *The most serious allergic reaction is anaphylaxis.*
- Obtain the emergency cart that contains drugs and resuscitation equipment; follow instructions for administering oxygen, intravenous fluids, drugs, and airway management depending on the client's symptoms. *Emergency measures are required to relieve anaphylaxis and other serious allergic reactions.*

PC: Meningeal Irritation or **CNS Changes**

Expected Outcome: The nurse will monitor to detect, manage, and minimize abnormal neurologic changes.

- Observe closely for any neurologic abnormalities such as diminished LOC, weakness, numbness, paralysis in an extremity, unequal or unresponsive pupil reflexes, posturing, and speech disturbance. *Diagnostic tests pose potential risks for neurologic complications, which are characterized by changes in neurologic functions.*
- Assess for changes in vital signs, restlessness, vomiting, and mental changes in orientation and thought processes. *Rising intracranial pressure affects vital signs, stimulates the vomiting center in the brain, and alters the sensorium and cognition.*
- Report the onset of a headache and sudden or severe pain in any area of the body to the physician immediately. *Headache often accompanies increased intracranial pressure; pain of any kind requires further investigation and pain management.*
- Inspect injection sites, especially those made during a lumbar puncture, for signs of a hematoma (collection of blood). *Trauma at an injection site can result in bleeding; bloody drainage also may contain CSF.*
- Position the client flat for at least 3 hours or as directed by the physician after a lumbar puncture or myelogram. *Keeping the client in a recumbent position provides time for CSF to form and replace what has been lost and reduces the potential for a headache.*
- Encourage a liberal fluid intake. *A generous fluid intake helps to restore the volume of CSF.*
- Keep the room dark and quiet after a lumbar puncture or myelogram. *Sensory stimulation tends to magnify discomfort.*
- Administer a prescribed analgesic if the client develops a headache. *An analgesic reduces the transmission or perception of pain stimuli.*

Evaluation of Expected Outcomes

Expected outcomes for the client are that he or she understands the preparation and performance involved in the neurologic procedure or diagnostic test and aftercare. The nurse gathers data concerning the client's allergy history, communicates the information appropriately, assesses the client for allergic symptoms, and implements interventions that control any allergic reaction. The nurse assesses the client for complications associated with the diagnostic test, uses measures to reduce the manifestation of complications, and carries out prescribed interventions to relieve discomfort.

GENERAL NUTRITIONAL CONSIDERATIONS

Clients who are allergic to iodine cannot receive radiopaque dyes that contain this substance. A thorough allergy history is an essential part of the neurologic examination. Seafood allergies suggest an allergy to iodine.

GENERAL PHARMACOLOGIC CONSIDERATIONS

Morphine and other narcotic depressants for pain affect the response of the pupils to light, making them pinpoint in size. This drug, not a neurologic disorder, causes this problem.

The use of morphine, heroin, or other narcotic or CNS depressants shortly before a neurologic examination affects the results of a neurologic examination.

GENERAL GERONTOLOGIC CONSIDERATIONS

Diseases that are more common in older adults (e.g., dementia) often make it difficult to perform a neurologic assessment.

With age, brain weight and the number of brain cells decrease. Older adults experience short-term memory loss and a slower reaction time.

Pupillary response is more sluggish in the older adult. When cataracts are present, there may be no pupillary response.

The possibility of drug toxicity always should be considered when an elderly person has a change in mental status.

Older adults who have difficulty following directions during a neurologic examination or diagnostic procedure need brief instructions given one step at a time during the examination or procedure.

Obtain facts necessary for a health history from a family member or friend of an older adult who has difficulty remembering recent or past events, symptoms, drug and medical history, and other facts necessary for a history.

Critical Thinking Exercises

1. *Discuss appropriate nursing assessments when managing the care of clients with neurologic disorders.*
2. *Name two potential complications of neurologic testing procedures. How can the nurse prevent, manage, and minimize them?*

References and Suggested Readings

A quick check of the neurologic system. (1999). *Nursing, 29*(6), Crit Care, 32cc10–32cc11.

Addison, C. & Crawford, B. (1999). Not bad, just misunderstood . . . Glasgow Coma Scale. *Nursing Times, 95*(43), 52–53.

Agostino, P. (2001). Cranial nerve assessment in the unconscious patient. *Nursing Spectrum (New York/New Jersey Metro Edition), 13A*(3), NJ15.

Alverzo, J. P. & Galski, T. (1999). Nurses' assessment of patients' cognitive orientation in a rehabilitation setting. *Rehabilitation Nursing, 24*(1), 7–12, 23, 43.

Barry, C. B. (1998). Assessing the older adult in the home. *Home Healthcare Nurse, 16*(8), 518–530.

Beckerman, B. A. (2000). Nervous energy: Conducting a neurologic assessment in the field. *Emergency Medical Services, 29*(8), 45–46, 48, 50.

Cohen, B. J. & Wood, D. L. (1999). *Memmler's the human body in health and disease* (9th ed.). Philadelphia: Lippincott Williams & Wilkins.

Fischer, J. (2001). The history of the Glasgow Coma Scale: Implications for practice. *Critical Care Nursing Quarterly, 23*(4), 52–58.

Fuller, J. & Schaller-Ayers, J. (2000). *Health assessment: A nursing approach* (3rd ed.). Philadelphia: Lippincott Williams & Wilkins.

Jacobus, C. H. (2000). Neuro assessment: Step-by-step neurological evaluation techniques for EMS providers. *Journal of Emergency Medical Services, 25*(1), 56–58, 60–62, 64.

Jagoda, A. & Riggio, S. (1999). The rapid neurologic examination, part 1: History, mental status, cranial nerves: An orderly search identifies problems requiring immediate care. *Journal of Critical Illness, 14,* 325–331.

Lewis, A. M. (1999). Neurologic emergency! *Nursing, 29*(10), 54–56.

Lynch, W. J. (2000). Tests, measurement, and technology. Brief neurocognitive batteries: A review and preview. *Journal of Head Trauma Rehabilitation, 15,* 1172–1178.

McCrea, M. (2001). Standardized mental status assessment of sports concussion. *Clinical Journal of Sports Medicine, 11,* 176–181.

Neal, L. J. (1998). Functional assessment of the home health client. *Home Healthcare Nurse, 16,* 670–678.

Neatherlin, J. S. (1999). Foundation for practice: Neuroassessment for neuroscience nurses. *Nursing Clinics of North America, 34,* 573–592.

O'Hanlon-Nichols, T. (1999). Neurologic assessment. *American Journal of Nursing, 99*(6), 44–50.

Peters, J. (1999). Dedicated follower of neurological trends . . . neurological assessment. *Nursing Times, 95*(27), 19.

Price, T., Miller, L., & deScossa, M. (2000). The Glasgow Coma Scale in intensive care. *Nursing in Critical Care, 5,* 170–173.

Shah, S. (1999). Neurological assessment. *Nursing Standard, 13*(22), 49–56.

Shpritz, D. W. (1999). Neurodiagnostic studies. *Nursing Clinics of North America, 34,* 593–606.

Watson, R. (2000). Assessing neurological functioning in older people. *Elderly Care, 12*(4), 25–27.

Caring for Clients With Central and Peripheral Nervous System Disorders

Words to Know

aura
automatisms
bradykinesia
Brudzinski's sign
Cheyne-Stokes
  respirations
choreiform movements
convulsion
Cushing's triad
demyelinating disease
diplopia
epilepsy
fasciculations

foramen magnum
Kernig's sign
neuralgia
nuchal rigidity
nystagmus
opisthotonos
papilledema
parkinsonism
photophobia
preictal phase
ptosis
seizure
status epilepticus

Learning Objectives

On completion of this chapter, the reader will:

● Discuss at least four signs and symptoms and nursing care of the client with increased intracranial pressure.
● Name four infectious or inflammatory diseases that affect the central or peripheral nervous system.
● Discuss three neuromuscular disorders, common related problems, and nursing management.
● Discuss the nursing management of clients with a cranial nerve disorder.
● List the signs and symptoms of Parkinson's disease.
● Discuss the purpose of drug therapy and drugs commonly prescribed for Parkinson's disease.
● Discuss the pathophysiology of seizure disorders and different types of seizures.
● Discuss the nursing management of clients with seizure disorders.

Acute disorders of the central nervous system (CNS) and peripheral nervous system (PNS) are potentially life-threatening. Chronic neurologic disorders, although not imminently fatal, profoundly affect a person's quality of life. When any part of the CNS or PNS is damaged, removed, or destroyed, a permanent neurologic deficit can occur.

INCREASED INTRACRANIAL PRESSURE

Inside the cranium, there is (1) brain tissue, (2) blood, and (3) cerebrospinal fluid (CSF). If one or more of these increases significantly without a decrease in either of the other two, intracranial pressure becomes elevated.

Pathophysiology and Etiology

Many conditions cause increased intracranial pressure (IICP), including brain tumors, head injury, and infectious and inflammatory disorders of the brain such as encephalitis. As pressure increases, cerebral blood flow decreases. This is followed by an increase in $PaCO_2$ (carbon dioxide level in the blood) and a decrease in the blood pH and PaO_2 (oxygen level in the blood). These changes result in cerebral edema, which further increases intracranial pressure (ICP).

If IICP goes unrecognized or untreated, the contents of the cranium are compressed further. Unrelieved pressure causes brain tissue to herniate or shift from normal locations intracranially and extracranially (Fig. 45-1). The **foramen magnum,** the opening in the lower part of the skull through which the upper part of the spinal cord

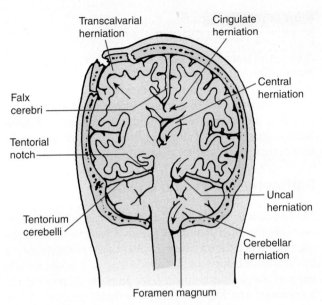

FIGURE 45-1 Major types of intracranial herniations.

connects with the brain, provides the only extracranial exit for brain tissue. If the brain stem herniates through the foramen magnum, respiration, heart rate, blood pressure (BP), and the functions of descending and ascending nerve fibers are affected. As the condition progresses, vital functions ultimately may cease.

Assessment Findings

Signs and Symptoms

The signs and symptoms of IICP (Box 45-1) develop rapidly or slowly. When IICP develops slowly, subtle changes can be overlooked.

Decreasing level of consciousness (LOC) is one of the earliest signs of IICP. Clients may slip from alert and oriented to lethargic, stuporous, semicomatose, and, finally, comatose (see Chap. 44). Confusion, restlessness, and periodic disorientation often accompany decreasing LOC.

Headache is another symptom of IICP. Pain typically is intermittent and increases with activities that elevate ICP, such as coughing, sneezing, or straining at stool. Rest

---

BOX 45-1 ● Signs of Increased Intracranial Pressure

- Altered level of consciousness
- Headache
- Vomiting
- Papilledema
- Change in vital signs
- Unequal pupils and abnormal response to light
- Posturing

---

or elevation of the head relieves the pain. A constant headache is a grave sign.

Vomiting when associated with a neurologic condition also suggests increasing ICP. Emesis commonly occurs without any forewarning of nausea.

Papilledema (swelling of the optic nerve) is caused by interference with venous drainage from the eyeball and is observed through examination with an ophthalmoscope. Pressure on the oculomotor nerve usually accompanies IICP and affects pupillary response to light. Normal pupil response to strong light is rapid constriction. In IICP, the response is sluggish or nonexistent (fixed).

Changes in ICP also influence vital signs. Body temperature may rise or fall depending on the etiology of the IICP or because of its effect on the temperature-regulating center. The pulse increases initially but then decreases, systolic BP rises, and pulse pressure (the difference between the systolic and diastolic measurement) widens—three signs called **Cushing's triad.** Cushing's triad occurs late in IICP. The respiratory rate is irregular. Later, **Cheyne-Stokes respirations** occur, consisting of shallow, rapid breathing followed by a period of apnea.

Decorticate or decerebrate posturing (see Chap. 44) develops spontaneously or in response to a painful stimulus when ICP is increased.

Diagnostic Findings

Diagnostic tests that determine the underlying cause of IICP include skull radiography, computed tomography (CT), magnetic resonance imaging (MRI), lumbar puncture, and cerebral angiography.

Medical and Surgical Management

Immediate treatment aims at relieving the cause, if possible. Monitoring devices (Fig. 45-2) are inserted to measure ICP and in some cases to withdraw CSF. These devices are connected to a transducer and a monitor that display the pressure and a waveform to detect the status of ICP. Normal ICP in the ventricles is 1 to 15 mm Hg; moderate elevation ranges from 15 to 40 mm Hg; high levels exceed 40 mm Hg. Although the ICP varies, a rise of 2 mm Hg from a previous measurement is cause for concern.

Osmotic diuretics such as mannitol (Osmitrol), glycerin (Osmoglyn), or urea (Ureaphil), and corticosteroids such as dexamethasone (Decadron) are given to reduce cerebral edema. Other treatment includes restriction of oral and intravenous (IV) fluids and hyperventilation therapy by means of mechanical ventilation. Hyperventilation produces vasoconstriction of the cerebral arteries, followed by decreased cerebral blood volume and reduced ICP. An anticonvulsant may be ordered to prevent seizures, which elevate intracranial pressure.

Depending on the degree and cause of IICP, the physician may order the insertion of an indwelling catheter, a

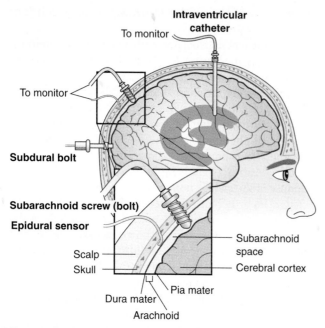

FIGURE 45-2 Technique for monitoring intracranial pressure.

nasogastric tube for gastric decompression or to provide tube feedings, a stool softener to prevent straining at stool, and a histamine antagonist such as famotidine (Pepcid) to prevent stress ulcers. Persistent hyperthermia caused by altered functioning of the hypothalamus requires hypothermic measures such as a cooling blanket if the temperature does not respond to antipyretic drugs.

Emergency surgery is done to remove a blood clot if IICP results from a head injury with bleeding above or below the dura (see Chap 47). Surgery also is performed to relieve pressure caused by a brain tumor.

Nursing Management

Nursing care of the client with IICP is presented in Nursing Care Plan 45-1.

> ### Stop, Think, and Respond ● BOX 45-1
> *What assessment findings suggest that ICP is increasing beyond the compensatory changes that result from autoregulation?*

INFECTIOUS AND INFLAMMATORY DISORDERS OF THE NERVOUS SYSTEM

Four neurologic conditions have an infectious or inflammatory cause: meningitis, encephalitis, Guillain-Barré syndrome, and brain abscess (Fig. 45-3).

● MENINGITIS

Meningitis is an inflammation of the meninges. The inflammation often extends to the cerebral cortex. The client's condition rapidly becomes critical, and death occurs without immediate intervention. Most adults with bacterial meningitis recover without permanent neurologic damage or dysfunction. When complications do occur, they usually are serious.

Pathophysiology and Etiology

Meningococci, streptococci, staphylococci, and pneumococci are the most common causative bacteria of meningitis. They reach the meninges by way of the bloodstream or by direct extension from infected areas such as the middle ear and the paranasal sinuses. Meningococcal meningitis, a common and highly contagious form, usually affects school-aged children and young adults. Viruses such as herpes simplex virus, mumps virus, and enteroviruses can cause viral meningitis, usually in children.

The inflammatory process can advance to cerebral edema, irreversible coma, seizure disorders, brain abscess, and neurologic changes. *Vasculitis,* inflammation of a blood vessel, may be present, and cerebral blood flow may be decreased. Neurologic complications include damage to the cranial nerves that facilitate vision and hearing.

Assessment Findings

Signs and Symptoms

Symptoms include fever, **nuchal rigidity** (pain and stiffness of the neck, inability to place the chin on the chest), nausea, vomiting, **photophobia** (aversion to light), headache, restlessness, irritability, and seizures. Severe irritation of the meninges causes **opisthotonos,** an extreme hyperextension of the head and arching of the back. A positive **Kernig's sign** (inability to extend the leg when the thigh is flexed on the abdomen) and a positive **Brudzinski's sign** (flexion of the neck produces flexion of the knees and hips) are seen (Fig. 45-4). The client with meningococcal meningitis may have multiple, small to large petechiae on the body.

Diagnostic Findings

A lumbar puncture is done and samples of CSF obtained. If the meningitis is bacterial, the CSF appears cloudy. The CSF pressure is elevated, glucose concentration is decreased, protein levels are elevated, and white blood cell (WBC) and red blood cell counts are elevated. Culture and sensitivity studies are done to identify the specific causative bacteria. If meningitis is viral, the results of culture and sensitivity studies are negative. A CT scan, blood culture, complete blood cell count, and other laboratory tests are used to rule out other possible disorders.

(text continued on page 612)

Nursing Care Plan 45-1

THE CLIENT WITH INCREASED INTRACRANIAL PRESSURE (IICP)

Assessment

- Gather from client or a witness, paramedic, or emergency medical technician the history of circumstances surrounding the altered neurologic state. Also gather past medical history, concurrent health problems being treated, current medications, and allergy history.
- Assess level of consciousness (LOC) and vital signs.
- Assist with a head-to-toe physical examination.
- Perform complete neurologic assessments, including the Glasgow Coma Scale (GCS) or Ranchos Los Amigos Scale (see Chap. 44). Repeat these assessments every 30 to 60 minutes.
- Measure current and daily weights and intake and output measurements.
- Study laboratory findings such as serum electrolyte and arterial blood gas levels.
- Evaluate the presence of bowel sounds and bowel elimination.
- Note evidence of any seizures.

Nursing Diagnosis: **Ineffective Tissue Perfusion (cerebral)** related to IICP as evidenced by decreased LOC, sluggish pupil response, papilledema, and posturing

Expected Outcome: ICP will be between 1 and 15 mm Hg, and the GCS will be 9 or greater.

Interventions	*Rationales*
Keep head of bed slightly elevated and the head in midline (straight). For clients with a basal skull fracture, keep bed flat.	Head elevation promotes drainage of venous blood and cerebrospinal fluid from the cranium.
Limit movement, space essential nursing tasks, and reduce or eliminate environmental stimuli (e.g., loud noise, bright lights).	Activities that increase BP, use the Valsalva maneuver, impair blood circulation, or decrease oxygenation raise ICP (Box 45-2).
Avoid extreme hip flexion.	It compresses femoral blood vessels and interferes with circulation.
Keep client quiet. Change position with assistance and use a turning sheet. Avoid range-of-motion (ROM) exercises until ICP approaches normal unless ordered otherwise by the physician.	Activity increases ICP by raising BP. IICP predisposes to cerebral ischemia and cell damage.
Administer reduced fluid volumes at an even rate for 24 hours. Give diuretics and corticosteroids as prescribed; note client's response to therapy.	Reduced fluid volume is one way to decrease the volume in the brain. Corticosteroids stabilize cell membranes, which helps prevent fluid shifts from intracellular to extracellular spaces.
Hyperventilate the mechanically ventilated client according to medical orders.	When CO_2 rises in the blood, cerebral blood vessels dilate as an autoregulatory mechanism to prevent cerebral ischemia; however, vasodilation increases volume in an already overloaded cranium. Hyperventilation reduces the potential for increasing intracerebral blood volume.
Suction the airway only when necessary.	Suctioning stimulates coughing, which raises ICP.
Give 100% oxygen before and after suctioning when it is required.	Preoxygenation reduces the potential for hypoxemia; postoxygenation relieves any oxygen deficit. Keeping blood well oxygenated prevents cerebral ischemia.
Keep suctioning brief, without exceeding 10 to 15 seconds per pass of the catheter.	Prolonged suctioning contributes to hypoxemia and cerebral vasodilation.

(continued)

Nursing Care Plan 45-1 (Continued)

THE CLIENT WITH INCREASED INTRACRANIAL PRESSURE (IICP)

Interventions	*Rationales*
Administer a prescribed stool softener.	It increases moisture in stool, making stool easy to pass and reducing the potential for the Valsalva maneuver.
Ensure that a gastric tube used for decompression or nourishment remains patent.	An obstructed gastric tube can contribute to gastric distention and vomiting. Elevated BP and ICP accompany vomiting.
Administer prescribed medications if vomiting or persistent coughing occur.	Suppressing vomiting and coughing reduces the potential for IICP and cerebral ischemia.

Evaluation of Expected Outcome: ICP returns to normal, and cerebral perfusion is restored.

Nursing Diagnoses: **Risk for Ineffective Breathing Pattern** and **Ineffective Airway Clearance** related to diminished LOC and herniation of the brain stem secondary to IICP

Expected Outcomes: (1) Respiratory rate will be sufficient to maintain the SpO_2 above 90% and PO_2 above 80 mm Hg. (2) Airway will be patent.

Interventions	*Rationales*
Attach a pulse oximeter to the finger, earlobe, bridge of the nose, or toe.	A pulse oximeter measures the percentage of oxygen bound to hemoglobin.
Insert an oral airway if client is comatose.	It prevents the tongue from occluding the natural airway.
Administer prescribed oxygen.	Supplemental oxygen provides a greater percentage of oxygen than in room air.
For mechanically ventilated clients, ensure that the ventilator delivers the prescribed tidal volume at the ordered rate.	A mechanical ventilator supplements or controls the client's breathing.
Suction when necessary to clear tracheal secretions or keep endotracheal tube patent.	Artificial airways increase secretions, which reduce the volume of air within the airway.

Evaluation of Expected Outcomes: Respirations are normal, airway is free of secretions, and lungs are clear to auscultation.

Nursing Diagnosis: **Risk for Imbalanced Nutrition: Less than Body Requirements** related to inability to consume food orally secondary to decreased LOC or endotracheal intubation

Expected Outcome: Body weight will remain within 2 lb of preadmission.

Interventions	*Rationales*
Administer nutritional supplements by gastric tube or total parenteral nutrition (TPN) through a central venous catheter as medically prescribed.	The enteral or parenteral route facilitates a means of providing essential nutrients and fluids.

Evaluation of Expected Outcome: Nutritional needs are met with no evidence of aspiration.

Nursing Diagnosis: **Risk for Infection** related to impaired skin and tissue integrity secondary to surgery, invasive diagnostic or monitoring procedures, or original head injury

Expected Outcome: Client will be free of infection as evidenced by no fever, no purulent drainage from open areas of skin, and white blood cell count within normal limits.

(continued)

Nursing Care Plan 45-1 (Continued)

THE CLIENT WITH INCREASED INTRACRANIAL PRESSURE (IICP)

Interventions	Rationales
Keep wounds clean and dry.	Medical asepsis reduces transient pathogens.
Use aseptic technique when handling any part of the intracranial monitoring device or changing a dressing applied after surgery.	Surgical asepsis ensures that supplies and equipment are not contaminated with pathogens.
Administer antibiotic therapy, if prescribed.	Antibiotics inhibit the growth of or destroy susceptible microorganisms.

Evaluation of Expected Outcome: Temperature is normal with no sign of infection.

PC: **Hyperglycemia** related to corticosteroid therapy or administration of TPN

Expected Outcome: The nurse will monitor to detect, manage, and minimize elevated blood glucose level.

Interventions	Rationales
Assess capillary blood glucose levels three times daily and at bedtime.	Capillary blood glucose is a convenient bedside assessment that provides reliable measurements of current blood glucose level.
Follow medical orders for administering insulin according to a sliding scale.	Insulin helps lower blood sugar by facilitating its movement into body cells.

Evaluation of Expected Outcome: Blood glucose level is within normal range or lowered with insulin therapy.

PC: **Stress Ulcer** related to hyperacidity secondary to stress response

Expected Outcome: The nurse will monitor to detect, manage, and minimize the development of a peptic ulcer.

Interventions	Rationales
Check the pH of gastric secretions per shift.	Obtaining a sample of gastric secretions and using chemical strip for pH provides a quick means for monitoring the acidity of the stomach.
Report a pH of less than 3.	A pH above 3 helps to suppress the release of pepsin, which adds to the gastric pH created by hydrochloric acid.
Administer prescribed drugs that protect the gastric mucosa, reduce histamine secretion, suppress the release of gastric secretions, or neutralize stomach acids.	There are a variety of drugs whose mechanisms of action reduce the potential for developing a peptic ulcer.

Evaluation of Expected Outcome: Gastric mucosa is intact.

Nursing Diagnosis: **Risk for Impaired Skin Integrity** related to low capillary blood flow secondary to pressure and inactivity

Expected Outcome: Skin will remain intact.

Interventions	Rationales
Tilt or turn client from side to side every 2 hours.	Maintaining intracapillary pressure above 32 mm Hg ensures that tissue can exchange oxygen and CO_2 at the cellular level.

(continued)

Nursing Care Plan 45-1 (Continued)

THE CLIENT WITH INCREASED INTRACRANIAL PRESSURE (IICP)

Interventions	Rationales
Avoid friction by using a lift sheet.	Friction causes abrasions that impair skin integrity.
Use a pressure-relieving mattress or mechanical bed for clients whose position cannot be readily changed.	Specialty mattresses and beds are designed to intermittently reduce pressure on skin throughout the time a client is confined to bed.
Keep skin clean and dry.	Clean, dry skin prevents softening and erosion of epidermal cells.

Evaluation of Expected Outcome: Skin is intact.

Nursing Diagnosis: **Self-Care Deficit (total or specify type)** related to diminished LOC as manifested by inability to follow directions and impaired neuromuscular function

Expected Outcome: Client's basic needs will be met.

Interventions	Rationales
Give client complete care, including bathing, oral care, nutrition, and elimination, until ICP is normal and client can resume these activities independently.	The nurse manages needs that a client cannot perform until neurologic function returns.

Evaluation of Expected Outcome: Basic needs are managed.

Nursing Diagnosis: **Impaired Verbal Communication** related to decreased LOC or endotracheal intubation as evidenced by an inability to speak

Expected Outcome: Client will communicate using body language, pantomime, or writing.

Interventions	Rationales
Look for grimacing or moaning.	Sounds of distress are universal.
Correct problems that may be causing discomfort, such as a wrinkled sheet or an object pressing on the skin.	Astute assessment may determine the cause of discomfort and facilitate prompt intervention.
Provide paper and pencil or a magic slate if client is alert but intubated.	Written communication is an alternative to oral communication.

Evaluation of Expected Outcome: Client communicates needs to others when conscious.

For additional suggestions for nursing management of a client undergoing surgery or who develops a neurologic deficit, see Chapter 48.

Medical Management

IV fluids and antimicrobial therapy are started immediately. The appropriate antibiotic is determined when the causative microorganism is identified from the results of the sensitivity tests. Drug therapy is continued after the acute phase of the illness to prevent recurrence. Anticonvulsants are necessary if seizures occur. People who have had recent contact with a person with meningococcal meningitis are placed on prophylactic oral rifampin (Rifadin). The local public health department is notified of all cases.

NURSING PROCESS

● **Care of the Client With a Neurologic Infectious or Inflammatory Disorder**

Assessment

The nurse obtains a health history. Because the client is acutely ill, the nurse interviews a family member to obtain information if the client cannot participate in the data-gathering process. The nurse measures vital signs and performs a neurologic examination. After gathering the

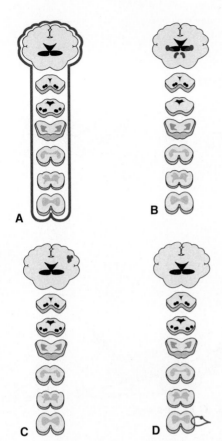

FIGURE 45-3 Sites of infectious and inflammatory disorders. (**A**) Meningitis, (**B**) encephalitis, (**C**) Guillain-Barré syndrome, (**D**) brain abscess.

initial data, he or she initiates an assessment flow sheet for ongoing comparisons. The nurse observes the rate and characteristics of respirations and auscultates the lungs every 4 to 8 hours. He or she evaluates the client's ability to swallow and clear the airway of secretions. The nurse provides for intake and output measurements. He or she records bowel elimination to ensure that constipation does not develop. The nurse asks the client to indicate the severity of a headache, when present. If a seizure occurs, the nurse notes its duration, physical manifestations, and whether it involved only one side of the body or started in one site and spread elsewhere.

BOX 45-2 ● Activities That Increase Intracranial Pressure

- Coughing
- Range-of-motion exercises
- Sneezing
- Hip flexion of 90° or greater
- Vomiting
- Suctioning
- Straining to have a bowel movement (Valsalva maneuver)
- Holding breath
- Digging heels into bed to help in repositioning
- Turning in bed without help

Diagnosis, Planning, and Interventions

Risk for Impaired Gas Exchange related to ineffective breathing, ineffective airway clearance, and aspiration
Expected Outcomes: (1) Blood gases will be within normal ranges. (2) Breathing will be sufficient to maintain the blood oxygen saturation (SpO_2) above 90%. (3) The airway will be free of oral or gastric secretions.

- Keep an oral airway at the bedside; insert it immediately if respiratory distress develops. *An oral airway holds the tongue forward so it does not occlude the pharynx.*
- Administer oxygen as prescribed. *Supplemental oxygen increases the percentage of oxygen in inhaled gas higher than that in room air.*
- Report respiratory difficulty, which may require emergency intubation. *Respiratory distress that is unrelieved by repositioning the head, inserting an oral airway, and administering oxygen may require medical interventions to prevent hypoxemia.*
- Elevate the head of the bed. *Head elevation lowers abdominal organs away from the diaphragm, which facilitates inhalation of a greater volume of air.*
- Hyperoxygenate and hyperventilate before and after tracheal suctioning. *Suctioning removes oxygen as well as secretions from the respiratory passages.*
- Use caution when giving oral fluids, food, or medications to a lethargic client. *A client who is not fully alert may aspirate food, fluids, and oral medications.*

Hyperthermia related to fever-producing mechanisms secondary to microbial infection
Expected Outcome: Body temperature will be controlled below 101°F (38.3°C).

- Administer prescribed antipyretics. *They alter the setpoint in the hypothalamus.*
- Remove unnecessary clothing and blankets. *Layers of fabric trap body heat and prevent its convection into the environment.*
- Administer tepid sponge baths. *Applying moisture to the body's surface promotes heat loss through evaporation.*
- Apply a cooling blanket beneath the client. *It promotes heat loss by conduction.*
- Maintain adequate hydration. *Adequate fluid volume compensates for fluid loss from perspiration and ensures fluid is available to continue this heat-regulating process.*

Acute Pain (headache) related to meningeal irritation, cerebral edema as manifested by client's description of head discomfort
Expected Outcome: Client's discomfort will be relieved or reduced to a tolerable level within 30 minutes of a nursing measure.

- Assess the location and intensity of discomfort whenever you assess vital signs. *Gathering data about pain is considered the fifth vital sign.*
- Report a continuous headache or one that is unrelieved. *An intense or unrelieved headache suggests rising ICP from acute meningeal irritation.*

FIGURE 45-4 Signs of meningeal irritation. (**A**) Nuchal rigidity, (**B**) opisthotonos, (**C**) Kernig's sign, (**D**) Brudzinski's sign.

- Give a prescribed mild analgesic that does not affect pupil size or reaction. *Opioids cause the pupils to constrict, which interferes with accurate neurologic assessment.*
- Facilitate rest and reduced environmental stimuli. *Reduced activity and sensory stimulation help increase pain tolerance.*

PC: Seizures related to meningeal irritation, high fever, or IICP

Expected Outcome: The nurse will monitor to detect, manage, and minimize seizures.

- Raise and pad side rails with soft material. *Modifying the environment helps reduce the potential for injuries during a seizure (Fig. 45-5).*
- Stay with the client if a seizure develops and call for assistance. *A client is defenseless during a seizure. The airway can become obstructed or aspiration can occur if a client is alone during a seizure.*
- Turn client to the side during a seizure. *A lateral position reduces the potential for aspiration of saliva or stomach contents.*
- Do not restrain client's movements. *Doing so during a seizure can cause fractures or other musculoskeletal injuries.*
- Provide privacy. *Privacy protects the client's dignity.*

- Insert a padded tongue blade in the mouth only if the teeth are not tightly shut. *Protecting the tongue and teeth with soft material is dangerous once a seizure begins; if the client experiences an aura before a seizure, there may be time to protect the mouth.*
- Suction client's mouth and pharynx after the seizure. *Suctioning clears accumulated secretions from the airway.*
- Provide oxygen during and after the seizure. *Hypoxemia develops when the client's diaphragm contracts and breathing is irregular throughout the seizure.*
- Reorient client to the surroundings and provide rest after the seizure. *Commonly, clients are sleepy and confused after a seizure.*
- Check for injuries. *A client who experiences a seizure may have oral injuries or contusions to the skin.*
- Administer prescribed anticonvulsants. *They decrease the excitability of neurons in the brain and reduce the potential for additional seizures.*

Evaluation of Expected Outcomes

Oxygenation is adequate throughout care. Temperature is within normal range, and vital signs are stable. The client reports no pain or headache or relief to within a tolerable level. He or she is protected during seizure ac-

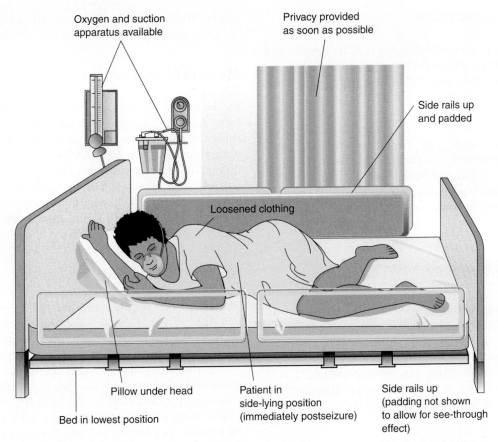

FIGURE 45-5 Environmental modifications for seizure precautions.

tivity and receives medications that reduce their recurrence. If IICP develops, the nurse follows the care described in Nursing Care Plan 45-1.

● ENCEPHALITIS

Encephalitis is an infectious disease of the CNS characterized by pathologic changes in both the white matter and the gray matter of the spinal cord and brain.

Pathophysiology and Etiology

Bacteria, fungi, or viruses cause encephalitis. The disease can follow a viral infection elsewhere in the body, such as measles, or vaccination. Viruses identified as causing encephalitis include the St. Louis, Western equine, and Eastern equine. Ticks or mosquitoes transmit some viruses. Poisoning by drugs and chemicals, such as lead, arsenic, or carbon monoxide, may closely resemble encephalitis clinically.

Severe, diffuse inflammation of the brain occurs. Nerve cell destruction can be extensive. Cerebral edema, neurologic deficits such as paralysis and speech changes, IICP, respiratory failure, seizure disorders, and shock can occur.

Assessment Findings

Sudden fever, severe headache, stiff neck, vomiting, and drowsiness signal the onset of viral encephalitis. Other symptoms include tremors, seizures, spastic or flaccid paralysis, irritability, and muscle weakness. Lethargy, delirium, or coma develop. Incontinence and visual disturbances such as photophobia, involuntary eye movements, and double or blurred vision occur.

A lumbar puncture is performed. CSF pressure is elevated, but the fluid is clear. In some types of encephalitis, serologic studies show a rise in viral antibodies. Electroencephalography (EEG) reveals slow waveforms.

Medical Management

Because no specific antiviral measure has been developed, treatment of encephalitis is supportive.

Nursing Management

The nurse monitors vital signs and LOC frequently and compares findings with previous assessments. If urinary retention or urinary incontinence develops, the nurse consults the physician to discuss whether an indwelling urethral catheter is appropriate. The nurse measures fluid intake and output to detect signs of fluid volume deficit and electrolyte imbalances. He or she assesses bowel elimination to determine if the client needs an enema or a stool softener. For additional nursing management, refer to the Nursing Process discussion on caring for a client with an infectious or inflammatory neurologic disorder.

● GUILLAIN-BARRÉ SYNDROME

Guillain-Barré syndrome (acute postinfectious polyneuro-pathy, polyradiculoneuritis) affects the peripheral nerves and the spinal nerve roots. Most clients begin to show signs of recovery about 1 month after the progression of symptoms ceases. Recovery may be slow and take 1 year or more. Death can occur from complications of immobility, such as pneumonia and infection.

Pathophysiology and Etiology

Although the exact cause of the disorder is unknown, Guillain-Barré syndrome is believed to be an autoimmune reaction (see Chap. 42) that follows a primary disorder, especially one that is infectious. Many clients have a history of a recent viral infection, particularly of the respiratory tract. Others have a history of recent surgery or recent vaccination for a viral disease like influenza. The syndrome also occurs in clients with malignant diseases and lupus erythematosus.

The affected nerves become inflamed and edematous. Myelin is lost. Mild to severe ascending muscle weakness or paralysis develops. Overactivity or underactivity of the sympathetic or parasympathetic nervous system is evidenced by changes in BP and in heart rate and rhythm.

Assessment Findings

Although symptoms vary, weakness, numbness, and tingling in the arms and legs often are the first symptoms. The weakness is progressive and moves to upper areas of the body and affects the muscles of respiration. Paralysis may follow muscle weakness. If cranial nerve involvement develops, chewing, talking, and swallowing become difficult.

A lumbar puncture reveals elevated CSF protein levels and pressure. The results of electrophysiologic testing show marked slowing in the conduction of nerve impulses. Additional neurologic tests are performed to rule out other possible CNS disorders with similar symptoms.

Medical Management

Plasmapheresis, removal of plasma from the blood and re-infusion of the cellular components with saline, has been shown to shorten the course of the disease if performed within the first 2 weeks. Otherwise, treatment is primarily supportive. If the respiratory muscles are involved, endotracheal intubation and mechanical ventilation become necessary. Difficulty chewing and swallowing necessitate the administration of IV fluids, gastric tube feedings, or total parenteral nutrition (TPN).

Nursing Management

The nurse observes the client closely for signs of respiratory distress. He or she uses a spirometer to evaluate the client's ventilation capacity. To assess for pneumonia, the nurse checks vital signs and lung sounds frequently.

Because immobility incapacitates the client, the nurse provides meticulous skin care and changes the client's position every 2 hours. He or she helps the client perform passive range-of-motion (ROM) exercises to prevent muscle atrophy. For further aspects of nursing management, see the Nursing Process section for managing the care of a client with an infectious or inflammatory neurologic disorder.

● BRAIN ABSCESS

A brain abscess is a collection of purulent material in the brain. If untreated, it can be fatal.

Pathophysiology and Etiology

A brain abscess occurs from an infection in nearby structures such as the middle ear, sinuses, or teeth, or from an infection in other organs. A brain abscess can develop after intracranial surgery or head trauma. It can be secondary to such disorders as bacterial endocarditis, bacteremia, and pulmonary or abdominal infections.

A brain abscess produces neurologic changes according to its location. Because it occupies space in the cranium, IICP can develop. Complications include paralysis, mental deterioration, seizure disorder, and visual disturbances.

Assessment Findings

Manifestations of a brain abscess include signs of IICP, fever, headache, and neurologic changes such as paralysis, seizures, muscle weakness, and lethargy.

Laboratory tests show an elevated WBC count. Analysis of CSF obtained by lumbar puncture helps confirm the diagnosis, but this procedure has a risk of herniation of the brain stem. A CT scan, MRI, and skull radiographs are safer techniques for diagnosing and locating the abscess.

Medical and Surgical Management

Antimicrobial therapy begins once the diagnosis is confirmed. A craniotomy, discussed later in this chapter, typically is performed to drain the abscess. Cerebral edema and seizures are treated with drug therapy. Additional treatment includes control of fever, mechanical ventilation, IV fluids, and nutritional support.

Nursing Management

The nurse assesses frequently for altered LOC, changes in sensory and motor functions, and signs of IICP. He or she monitors vital signs frequently. The nurse measures fluid intake and output because overhydration can lead to cerebral edema. See the Nursing Process section for the care of a client with an infectious or inflammatory neurologic disorder for more detailed discussions.

NEUROMUSCULAR DISORDERS

A neuromuscular disorder involves the nervous system and indirectly affects the muscles. Some examples include multiple sclerosis (MS), myasthenia gravis, and amyotrophic lateral sclerosis (ALS)—all of which are chronic and progressively debilitating.

● MULTIPLE SCLEROSIS *autoimmune*

Multiple sclerosis is a chronic, progressive disease of the peripheral nerves. Its onset is in young adulthood and early middle age. The highest incidence is between 20 and 40 years of age, and it affects men and women approximately equally. The disease is more common in northern temperate zones than in warm climates.

Pathophysiology and Etiology

The cause of MS is unknown, but it is considered an autoimmune disorder. It is characterized as a **demyelinating disease** because it causes permanent degeneration and destruction of myelin. Myelin acts as an insulator, enabling nerve impulses to pass along a nerve fiber. Loss of myelin and subsequent degeneration and atrophy of nerve axons interrupt transmission of impulses along these fibers (Fig. 45-6).

FIGURE 45-6 The process of demyelination. **A** and **B** depict a normal nerve cell and axon with myelin. **C** and **D** show the slow disintegration of myelin, which disrupts axon function. (From Smeltzer, S. C., & Bare, B. G. [2000]. *Brunner & Suddarth's textbook of medical–surgical nursing* [9th ed.]. Philadelphia: Lippincott Williams & Wilkins.)

Many clients experience gradual and continuous worsening of their symptoms. A few have the disease in a mild form and do not experience increased severity of symptoms. For some, the symptoms subside during early phases of the illness (remission), and the client seems healthy for several months or even years. With each reappearance (exacerbation), however, the symptoms become more severe and last longer. Infections and emotional upsets precipitate exacerbations. Some people live a long time with MS; survival for 20 years after the diagnosis is not unusual.

As the disease progresses, many complications such as pressure ulcers, cachexia, deformities, and contractures develop. Pneumonia, brought about by limited activity, shallow breathing, and general debility, often is the immediate cause of death.

Assessment Findings

Signs and Symptoms

Many clients first dismiss minor symptoms as a result of fatigue or strain. When they no longer can ignore symptoms, clients with MS report blurred vision, **diplopia** (double vision), **nystagmus** (involuntary movement of the eyeball), weakness, clumsiness, and numbness and tingling of an arm or a leg. An intention tremor and slurred, hesitant speech (scanning speech) may develop. Mood swings (emotional lability) are common.

Weakness of an arm or a leg progresses to ataxia (motor incoordination) or paraplegia (paralysis of both legs). Occasional bowel and bladder incontinence leads to total incontinence. Slight visual disturbances end in blindness. The illness impairs intellectual functioning late in its course. Loss of memory, difficulty concentrating, and impaired judgment occur.

Diagnostic Findings

Early diagnosis is difficult because symptoms are vague and in some cases temporary. A lumbar puncture and CSF analysis reveal an increased WBC count. Electrophoresis of the CSF, a technique for electrically separating and identifying proteins, demonstrates abnormal immunoglobulin G bands, described as oligoclonal bands. The bands appear separated rather than homogeneous, which is the normal finding. A CT scan and MRI may or may not disclose lesions in the brain's white matter.

Medical Management

There is no cure for MS, nor is there any single treatment that relieves all symptoms. The primary aim of treatment is to keep the client functional as long as possible.

Drugs used to treat symptoms include baclofen (Lioresal) and dantrolene (Dantrium) for muscle spasticity and rigidity, antibiotics for infection, and tranquilizers to alleviate mood swings. Oxybutynin (Ditropan) is used to treat urinary incontinence, and bethanechol (Urecholine) to relieve urine retention. The anti-inflammatory action of corticosteroids relieves symptoms and hastens remissions.

N U R S I N G   P R O C E S S

● The Client With a Neuromuscular Disorder

Assessment

The nurse performs a thorough neurologic assessment. He or she evaluates pulmonary function, including respiratory rate, depth, and lung sounds, to determine the client's ability to ventilate. To detect early signs of infection, the nurse takes the client's temperature regularly. He or she notes the client's ability to chew and swallow effectively and observes for drooling, choking when swallowing liquids, and regurgitating fluids through the nose. The nurse assesses muscle strength and coordination as well as the client's response to physical activity. To evaluate fluid status, the nurse measures intake and output.

He or she monitor's the client's elimination patterns. As data accumulate, the nurse analyzes the trends, using the initial baseline for comparisons. In addition, he or she monitors the client's and caregivers' ability to cope with the progressively debilitating nature of the disorder.

Diagnosis, Planning, and Interventions

Risk for Ineffective Breathing Pattern related to weakening of the muscles for respiration
Expected Outcome: Ventilation will be sufficient to maintain the SpO_2 above 90% and PaO_2 above 80 mm Hg.
- Place client in a Fowler's position and support the arms on pillows. *An upright position with the arms supported facilitates maximum chest expansion.*
- Eliminate foods that form intestinal gas or promote the expulsion of gas with a rectal tube. *Intestinal gas rises in the abdomen and places pressure on the diaphragm, which limits the volume of air that the client can inhale.*
- Encourage client to deep breathe several times an hour. *Frequent deep breaths increase tidal volumes, fill alveoli with air, and enhance gas exchange.*
- Notify the physician immediately if the client experiences inadequate ventilation. *Breathing is essential for life; medical interventions may be necessary.*

Risk for Ineffective Airway Clearance related to weak or ineffective cough, **Impaired Swallowing, Risk for Imbalanced Nutrition: Less than Body Requirements,** and **Risk for Aspiration** related to muscular weakness
Expected Outcomes: (1) Airway will be patent. (2) Client will swallow food and fluids without aspiration. (3) Nutritional needs will be met.
- Help client to cough and raise respiratory secretions. *Coughing is a natural protective mechanism for clearing the airway.*
- Suction the oral cavity and airway. *If coughing is ineffective, applying negative pressure with a suction catheter can help clear secretions from the airway.*
- Offer liquids frequently in small amounts. *The client may be able to manage small volumes of liquids, but large volumes increase the risk for aspiration.*
- Consult with the dietitian on techniques for modifying the texture and consistency of foods. *Clients can best swallow smooth foods with texture. Commercial substances are available to thicken liquids to promote swallowing.*
- Provide rest before meals. *The client is more likely to have optimum energy to chew and swallow after rest. Fatigue interferes with attention and coordination.*
- Help client to sit upright when eating. *Sitting is the natural position for eating. It promotes movement of food from the mouth to the esophagus and stomach and reduces the potential for aspiration.*
- Place food in the posterior of the client's mouth. Flex the client's chin toward the chest when swallowing to facilitate passage of food into the esophagus. *Locating*

food posteriorly facilitates swallowing. Flexing the chin diverts food into the esophagus rather than the airway.

- Feed client slowly. Wait to place more food in the client's mouth until he or she has swallowed the previous bolus. *Rushing or overloading the client's mouth increases the risk for airway obstruction or aspiration.*
- Consult with the physician about a plan for tube feedings or TPN. *These forms of nourishment may be necessary if oral nutritional intake becomes inadequate or dangerous.*

Impaired Physical Mobility, Self-Care Deficit (specify type), and **Risk for Impaired Skin Integrity** related to diminished muscle strength and inactivity

Expected Outcomes: (1) Client will be mobile and use muscles to the maximum extent possible. (2) Basic needs will be met. (3) Skin will remain intact.

- Encourage client to participate in self-care. *Attending to personal needs fosters self-image.*
- Provide rest between bathing, shaving, performing oral care, eating, ambulating, toileting, and participating in diversional activities. *Rest provides time to recover from an activity. It builds stamina and endurance to proceed with additional tasks.*
- Complete whatever tasks the client cannot perform. *The nurse relieves the client of further efforts at self-care when he or she becomes fatigued or weak.*
- Change body position every 2 hours. *Changing position relieves pressure on capillaries that traverse over bony prominences. Relief of pressure reduces the potential for skin breakdown.*
- Perform ROM exercises every 8 hours. *ROM exercises promote joint flexibility and muscle tone. They supplement or complement musculoskeletal activities the client actively performs.*
- Use a foot board and trochanter rolls to promote a neutral body position. *A neutral position keeps the body in good alignment and reduces the potential for contractures.*
- Consult with a physical or occupational therapist on techniques to facilitate client's independence and self-care. *They are experts in maintaining and regaining functional activities.*
- Use pressure-relieving devices when client is in bed or a wheelchair. *Relieving pressure prevents skin breakdown.*
- Keep bed dry and free of wrinkles. *Moisture softens the epidermis, making it vulnerable to breaking down. Wrinkles create pressure that interferes with blood circulation to cells and tissues.*
- Wash and dry the skin well. *Clean, dry skin decreases risk factors that can alter its integrity.*

Constipation related to inactivity and abdominal muscle weakness, **Urinary Incontinence** (specify type, such as Total, Functional, or Reflex) related to neuromuscular degeneration

Expected Outcomes: (1) Stool will be soft and bowel elimination will occur at least every 3 days. (2) Urine elimination will be controlled.

- Consult with the physician about a regularly prescribed stool softener, bulk-forming laxative, or suppository. *Medications facilitate bowel elimination through various physical and chemical mechanisms.*
- Include soft fruit or fruit puree in the daily menu. *Fruits are a source of fructose; sugar (fructose) is a natural laxative. Fiber adds bulk to the stool and attracts moisture, making the stool softer and more easy to pass.*
- Assist client to move as much as possible. *Activity promotes peristalsis, which propels stool toward the rectum.*
- Place client on a toilet or commode after meals, especially breakfast, or near the time of the client's usual bowel movement. *The gastrocolic reflex is more active after a meal. Most people have a bowel movement at about the same time each day.*
- Help client select clothing that facilitates toileting. *Clients are less likely to be incontinent if they can manipulate clothing to facilitate using a toilet or commode.*
- Assist client to the toilet regularly and frequently. *Clients can maintain continence if they receive some assistance getting to the bathroom and using toilet facilities.*
- Help client use incontinence garments or consult with the physician when client needs an indwelling or external catheter. *When efforts to maintain continence have been exhausted, measures to unobtrusively collect urine can maintain the client's dignity and reduce the potential for skin breakdown.*

Ineffective Coping related to feelings of helplessness secondary to chronic illness

Expected Outcome: Client will cope effectively with situational stressors.

- Suggest joining a support group of people with a similar disorder or subscribing to the support group's newsletter. *Knowing that others experience similar problems facilitates coping. Clients acquire new coping strategies when others share their problem-solving approaches in person or in written communications.*
- Encourage client to express feelings. *Expressing frustration and other emotions relieves the client's personal emotional burden and fosters support.*
- Provide opportunities in which the client can make choices. *Making choices promotes a feeling of control, which fosters the ability to cope.*
- Facilitate client's network of social support, such as with family, neighbors, coworkers, and church members, through personal visits, telephone conversations, cards, and letters. *A network of supportive others decreases the burden of coping with an illness as an isolated individual.*
- Provide diversional activities that foster feelings of personal accomplishment. *Feeling useful, purposeful, and capable helps a client persevere in coping with adversity.*

Risk for Caregiver Role Strain related to unrelenting responsibility for client's care

Expected Outcome: Primary caregiver will cope with long-term care of client.

- Listen empathetically while caregiver expresses feelings about caring for the client. *Caregiver is likely to feel less guilty if he or she feels comfortable discussing the stressors involved with someone other than the client or another family member.*
- Help caregiver develop a list of surrogates who may provide regular periods of relief. *The caregiver's dedication will be prolonged if he or she experiences intermittent periods when total responsibility is relieved.*
- Give caregiver permission to meet his or her own needs. *Unless encouraged to do so, caregivers suppress their own needs in deference to those for whom they care.*
- Identify available community resources and offer to facilitate a referral. *The caregiver may be unaware of service organizations whose missions are to provide help and support to clients and caregivers with particular disorders.*

Evaluation of Expected Outcomes

Respirations are of normal rate and depth. The airway is clear, and breathing is effortless. Nutrition is adequate to maintain body weight. The client regains mobility and attends to ADLs with minimal or no assistance. Skin is intact with no evidence of breakdown. Bowel elimination is regular; urinary incontinence is minimized or controlled. The client demonstrates effective coping skills. The caregiver continues his or her responsibilities but implements a plan for periodic relief or assistance.

● MYASTHENIA GRAVIS

Myasthenia gravis is a neuromuscular disorder characterized by severe weakness of one or more groups of skeletal muscles.

Pathophysiology and Etiology

Although its exact cause is unknown, the disease is believed to be autoimmune and to develop when blood cells and thymus gland antibodies destroy the nerve ending receptor sites of skeletal muscles. The symptoms develop because acetylcholine cannot stimulate receptors on skeletal muscles (Fig. 45-7). The outcome is extreme muscle weakness.

Assessment Findings

Muscle weakness varies depending on the muscles affected. The most common manifestations are **ptosis** (drooping) of the eyelids (Fig. 45-8), difficulty chewing and swallowing, diplopia, voice weakness, masklike facial expression, and weakness of the extremities. The

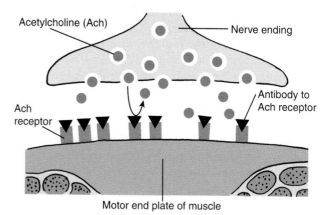

FIGURE 45-7 Inhibition of synaptic transmission of Ach in myasthenia gravis leads to profound muscle weakness. (From Rubin, E. & Farber, J. L. [1999]. *Pathology* [3rd ed.]. Philadelphia: Lippincott Williams & Wilkins.)

respiratory system also is affected. During a myasthenic crisis, the client experiences increased muscle weakness, respiratory distress, decreased tidal volume, and difficulty talking, swallowing, and chewing.

Diagnostic confirmation is made by IV administration of edrophonium (Tensilon), which relieves symptoms in a few seconds. Chest radiography may show a tumor of the thymus (thymoma). Electromyography measures the electrical potential of muscles.

Medical and Surgical Management

Treatment involves facilitating normal neurotransmission with administration of an anticholinesterase drug, such as pyridostigmine bromide (Mestinon) or ambenonium chloride (Mytelase). The therapeutic effect prolongs the action of acetylcholine, which sustains muscle contraction. The dose of the drug is adjusted according to the client's response to therapy.

Other treatments include surgical removal of the thymus gland, prednisone, and plasmapheresis for clients who do not respond to other methods of therapy. If myas-

FIGURE 45-8 Ptosis of the eyelids.

thenic crisis with severe respiratory distress occurs, the client requires intubation and mechanical ventilation.

Nursing Management

The nurse observes the effects of drug therapy, especially when first initiated or at times of stress. He or she must administer medications at the exact intervals ordered to maintain therapeutic blood levels and prevent symptoms from returning. The nurse observes for signs of drug overdose, such as abdominal cramps, clenched jaws, and muscle rigidity, which indicate that the dose is excessive. For more information, see Nursing Process: The Client With a Neuromuscular Disorder.

● AMYOTROPHIC LATERAL SCLEROSIS

Amyotrophic lateral sclerosis (ALS), also known as *Lou Gehrig's disease,* is a progressive, fatal neurologic disorder. The disease is more common in men than in women.

Pathophysiology and Etiology

The cause of ALS is unknown. The disease is characterized by degeneration of the motor neurons of the spinal cord and brain stem, which results in muscle weakness and wasting.

Assessment Findings

Progressive muscle weakness and wasting of the arms, legs, and trunk develop. The client experiences episodes of muscle **fasciculations** (twitching). If ALS affects the brain stem, speaking and swallowing become difficult. The client may display periods of inappropriate laughter and crying. Respiratory failure and total paralysis are seen in the terminal stage.

The disorder is difficult to diagnose in the early stages because no specific diagnostic tests are available for this disease. Electromyography validates weakness in the affected muscles.

Medical Management

There is no specific treatment, and death occurs several years after diagnosis in many cases. The client is encouraged to remain active as long as possible. Death usually results from respiratory arrest or overwhelming respiratory infection. Mechanical ventilation is necessary when ALS affects the muscles of respiration.

Nursing Management

The nurse performs a comprehensive assessment and develops a plan of care based on the client's identified problems. During the early stages of ALS, the nurse provides assistance with walking, bathing, shaving, and dressing. As ALS progresses, the client becomes totally dependent on the family or healthcare personnel for care. The nurse teaches family members required skills, such as suctioning techniques, how to administer tube feedings, and catheter care. Client and Family Teaching Box 45-1 provides more information, as does Nursing Process: The Client With a Neuromuscular Disorder. Additional discussion on caring for clients with a neurologic deficit is covered in Chapter 48. Review Chapter 26 for the care of clients in the terminal phase of ALS or other diseases.

CRANIAL NERVE DISORDERS

● TRIGEMINAL NEURALGIA (TIC DOULOUREUX)

Trigeminal neuralgia is a painful condition that involves the fifth cranial nerve (the trigeminal nerve), which has three major branches: mandibular, maxillary, and ophthalmic (Fig. 45-9). This sensory and motor nerve is important to chewing, facial movement, and sensation.

Pathophysiology and Etiology

The cause of the disorder is unknown. It has been suggested that it is related to compression of the trigeminal nerve root. For reasons not fully understood, the client experiences **neuralgia** (nerve pain) in one or more branches of the trigeminal nerve. The slightest stimulus (e.g., vibration of music, passing breeze, temperature change) over trigger spots (or areas that provoke the pain) can initiate

45-1 *Client and Family Teaching*
Amyotrophic Lateral Sclerosis

The nurse reviews the following components with the client and family:

■ Medication schedule, adverse effects of medications
■ Dietary and feeding suggestions
■ Agencies that can help with or give home care
■ Sources of financial assistance
■ Exercises to prevent muscle atrophy
■ Positioning and good skin care
■ Techniques for preventing skin breakdown

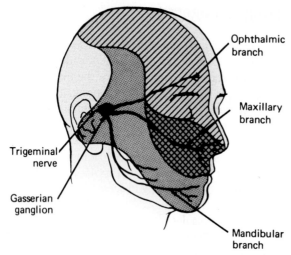

FIGURE 45-9 Areas innervated by the three branches of the trigeminal nerve. These are the areas that become painful in trigeminal neuralgia.

an attack. The forehead over the eyebrow is a common trigger spot when the ophthalmic branch of the nerve is affected.

Assessment Findings

The client describes the pain as sudden, severe, and burning. The pain ends as quickly as it begins, usually lasting a few seconds to several minutes. The cycle repeats many times each day. During a spasm, the face twitches and the eyes tear.

Skull radiography, MRI, or CT are performed to rule out other pathologies, such as a brain tumor and intracranial bleeding. Ultimately, the diagnosis is based on the symptoms.

Medical Management

Medical treatment is primarily supportive and symptomatic rather than curative. Narcotic analgesics are necessary. Anticonvulsants such as phenytoin (Dilantin) and carbamazepine (Tegretol) are used to reduce pain, but are not always successful. The client is referred to a dentist because correction of dental malocclusion has relieved some cases of trigeminal neuralgia.

Surgical Management

If medical management is unsatisfactory, surgical intervention is an option. Surgical division of the sensory root of the trigeminal nerve provides permanent relief; however, some permanent loss of sensation accompanies this

procedure. If the mandibular branch is severed, eating becomes a problem. The client may bite the tongue without realizing it, food may get caught in the mouth, and the jaw will deviate toward the operative side. Until the client adjusts to the altered sensation, swallowing is difficult.

NURSING PROCESS

● The Client With Trigeminal Neuralgia

Assessment

The nurse obtains a complete history, then carefully and gently examines the affected area. He or she asks the client to identify the location, pattern, and events associated with pain and documents the information. The nurse inspects the oral cavity for signs of injury. He or she weighs the client and assesses the client's ability to eat food.

Diagnosis, Planning, and Interventions

Acute Pain related to nerve compression as evidenced by client's description of localized discomfort
Expected Outcome: Pain will be relieved or reduced to a tolerable level.

* Use a scale from 0 to 10 to help client quantify the severity and intensity of pain, both before and after nursing intervention. *Using a scaled range of numbers is the standard for assessing pain. Pain is assessed before and at least 30 minutes after a nursing intervention.*
* Ask what level the client can tolerate pain. *Pain may not be totally relieved, but asking the client to identify his or her tolerance level provides a realistic goal for achievement.*
* Administer prescribed drugs. *Medications relieve pain by various mechanisms.*
* Observe and record client's response. *If an intervention does not reduce pain to the client's level of tolerance, the nurse pursues additional measures and collaborates with the physician when nursing measures are unsuccessful.*
* Avoid drafts in the room. *Even slight stimulation of the trigeminal nerve can trigger pain.*
* Place a sign on the client's bed stating not to jar the bed or touch client's face in any way. *Sudden, unexpected movement can trigger pain.*
* Advise client to use protective measures such as shielding the face from wind and cold and avoiding shaving and situations or activities that cause pain. *The client can implement lifestyle changes to reduce or prevent pain from recurring.*

Evaluation of Expected Outcomes

Pain is alleviated or reduced to a level such that the client can continue functioning. The client cooperates with measures to avoid stimuli that trigger episodes of pain. See Client and Family Teaching Box 45-2 for more information.

● BELL'S PALSY

Bell's palsy involves the seventh cranial nerve, which is responsible for movement of the facial muscles.

Pathophysiology and Etiology

The cause of Bell's palsy is unknown, but a viral link is suspected. Inflammation occurs around the nerve, blocking motor impulses to facial muscles. Inflammation or ischemia resulting from nerve compression leads to impaired nerve function. As a result, there is weakness and paralysis of facial muscles, including the muscles of the eyelids, on one side of the face. Most clients who recover begin to show improvement in a few weeks. Those whose paralysis is permanent fail to show improvement after 3 months or more.

Assessment Findings

Symptoms develop in a few hours or over 1 to 2 days. Facial pain, pain behind the ear, numbness, diminished blink reflex, ptosis of the eyelid, and tearing on the affected side occur. Speaking and chewing become difficult.

There are no specific diagnostic tests for this disorder; diagnosis is based on symptoms and visual examination of the face. In some instances it is necessary to rule out other neurologic problems such as brain tumor and stroke, which have comparable symptoms.

45-2 *Client and Family Teaching*
Trigeminal Neuralgia

The nurse instructs the client as follows:

- Inspect the mouth daily for breaks in the mucous membrane.
- Take small sips or bites of food and concentrate on chewing and swallowing if surgery has been performed.
- Chew on the opposite side.
- Avoid eating hot foods.
- Use mouth rinses after eating.
- Keep regular dental appointments because the warning pain of a cavity, abscess, or other dental problem may be mistaken for neuralgia.

Medical Management

Short-term corticosteroid therapy with prednisone (Deltasone, Meticorten) is prescribed to reduce nerve inflammation and edema. Analgesics are prescribed for pain. Electrotherapy or a facial sling helps to prevent atrophy of the facial muscles on the affected side. Once the diagnosis is confirmed, the client is assured that a more serious problem (e.g., stroke, tumor) has not occurred.

N U R S I N G   P R O C E S S

● The Client With Bell's Palsy

Assessment

The nurse obtains the client's history, noting any recent illness that suggests a viral infection. He or she performs a physical examination to determine which side of the face is involved and the appearance of affected structures. The nurse notes if the client has any speech impairment and observes the client's ability to chew and swallow food.

Diagnosis, Planning, and Interventions

Risk for (Ophthalmic) Infection related to diminished blink reflex
Expected Outcome: The eye will remain free of infection as evidenced by no redness or purulent drainage.
- Cover the eye with an eye patch. *An eye patch keeps the eyelid closed and protects the eye surface from environmental debris.*
- Apply a protective eye shield at night. *An eye shield ensures that the client does not scratch or injure the eye during sleep.*
- Inspect the eye daily for signs of inflammation and infection. *Early treatment facilitates a quick resolution and minimizes potential impairment of vision.*
- Irrigate the eye with normal saline, especially after surgery has been performed. *An irrigation flushes debris and microorganisms from the surface and conjunctival folds.*
- Instill prescribed antibiotic ophthalmic ointment. *Antibiotic therapy inhibits the growth of or destroys pathogens.*

Impaired Oral Mucous Membranes related to loss of sensation in the mouth, paralysis of chewing muscles as manifested by trauma to the cheeks, gums, teeth, or tongue
Expected Outcome: Oral mucous membrane and structures in the mouth will heal.
- Provide supplies for oral hygiene before and after meals. *Keeping the mouth clean promotes healing.*
- Check client's mouth after eating. *The client may be unaware that oral trauma has occurred.*
- Remove food particles that remain by using mouth rinses, cotton-tipped applicators, or a pulsating oral irrigator. *Physical measures are necessary in some cases*

to clear the cheek, buccal areas, and teeth of food residue. Retained food interferes with healing.

- Ensure that food and beverages are not too hot to avoid burning oral mucous membranes. *Extremes in temperatures contribute to thermal injury in the mouth.*
- Encourage biannual dental examinations. *A client with residual paralysis requires regular dental examinations and care to ensure optimum oral health.*

Impaired Verbal Communication related to hemiparalysis of facial muscles and pain

Expected Outcome: Client will communicate verbally and understandably.

- Instruct client to speak slowly and in short sentences. *Slowing the rate of speech enables the client to coordinate the use of his or her teeth, tongue, and lips while speaking.*
- Provide a pad of paper and a pencil to facilitate communication during severe pain. *Written communication is an acceptable substitute for temporarily impaired oral communication.*

Evaluation of Expected Outcomes

Client understands the techniques for instilling ophthalmic ointment and applying an eye patch and eye shield. The affected eye appears similar to the unaffected eye; there is no redness, swelling of orbital tissue, or drainage that suggests an infection. Vision in the affected eye remains unaffected. The client's mouth is free of retained debris. The soft tissue structures in the mouth are pink, moist, and intact. Teeth are in good repair. The client satisfactorily communicates with spoken words.

● TEMPOROMANDIBULAR DISORDER

Temporomandibular disorder (TMD) is a cluster of symptoms localized near the jaw.

Pathophysiology and Etiology

Causes of TMD include degenerative arthritis of the mandibular joint, malocclusion of the teeth, bruxism (grinding of the teeth), and dislocation of the jaw during endotracheal intubation.

TMD occurs when the meniscus, or cartilaginous disk, between the condyle (end of the mandible) and the temporal bone becomes displaced from the fossa (socket) of the temporal bone (Fig. 45-10). Because facial muscles like the masseter and temporalis muscles move this gliding joint, the client develops jaw pain from muscle spasms. If the cartilage wears away, there is a grating sensation when opening and closing the jaw; the client may hear a clicking sound when the joint moves. The joint may even lock periodically. Sometimes nerves and arteries in the area are compressed. The disorder can be confused with trigeminal neuralgia and migraine headache.

Assessment Findings

Symptoms include jaw pain, pronounced muscle spasm, and tenderness of the masseter and temporalis muscles. Headache, tinnitus (ringing in the ears), and ear pain accompany the localized discomfort. The client experiences clicking of the jaw when moving the joint, or the jaw can lock, which interferes with opening the mouth. Special dental radiographs often reveal evidence of joint displacement.

Medical and Surgical Management

Treatment is referral to a dentist who has experience managing clients with TMD. Analgesics are prescribed or recommended; the client wears a custom-fitted mouth guard during sleep. Transcutaneous electrical nerve stim-

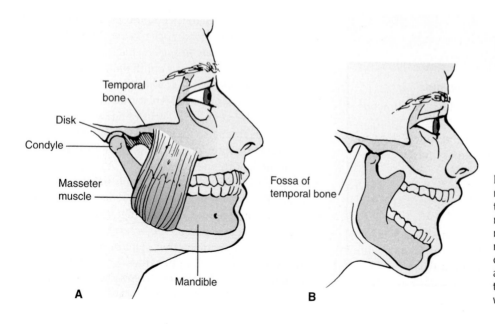

FIGURE 45-10 (**A**) The temporomandibular joint is located between the two bones for which it is named: the temporal bone and mandible. (**B**) The condyle of the mandible, which is covered by a cartilaginous disk, moves forward and backward within the fossa of the temporal bone of the skull, which is located in front of the ear.

ulation, injection of a local anesthetic to relieve muscle spasm, and oral irrigations with ice water also are used to reduce and relieve discomfort. Reconstructive surgery of the temporomandibular joint is available if conservative treatment is ineffective.

Nursing Management

The nurse monitors the client's weight and ability to consume food. If indicated, the nurse obtains a nutritional consultation with the dietitian. With the help of the dietitian, the nurse modifies the diet to include soft rather than coarse food, which is difficult to chew. He or she provides nutritional liquid supplements and assists the client to acquire skills that control pain, such as using a bite guard during sleep.

EXTRAPYRAMIDAL DISORDERS

Extrapyramidal disorders have their origin in the motor cortex and surrounding areas of the cerebellum and basal ganglia. Two common extrapyramidal disorders are Parkinson's disease and Huntington's disease. One of their primary characteristics is abnormal movement.

● PARKINSON'S DISEASE

Parkinson's disease usually begins after 50 years of age. It primarily affects the basal ganglia and connections in the substantia nigra and corpus striatum (Fig. 45-11). The term **parkinsonism** is used to describe the cluster of Parkinson's-like symptoms that develop from several etiologies.

Pathophysiology and Etiology

Parkinson's disease and parkinsonism result from a deficiency of the neurotransmitter dopamine. Depletion of dopamine in affected areas of the brain upsets the balance between dopamine and acetylcholine, which results in movement disorders.

In most cases of Parkinson's disease, no cause can be found for dopamine depletion. The symptoms of parkinsonism are associated with exposure to environmental toxins such as insecticides and herbicides and self-administration of an illegal synthetic form of heroin known as MPTP, and can occur as a sequela of head injuries and encephalitis. Phenothiazine, a category of antipsychotic drugs and other antipsychotic drugs used to treat schizophrenia, also produce parkinsonism, but the symptoms are reversible when the drug is discontinued.

Manifestations of the disorder progress so slowly that years may elapse between the first symptom and diagno-

FIGURE 45-11 Nuclei in the substantia nigra protect fibers to the corpus striatum, where the nerve fibers carry dopamine. Loss of dopamine from nerve cells is thought to cause symptoms of Parkinson's disease. (From Smeltzer, S. C. & Bare, B. G. [2000]. *Brunner & Suddarth's textbook of medical–surgical nursing* [9th ed.]. Philadelphia: Lippincott Williams & Wilkins.)

sis. The symptoms initially are unilateral, but eventually, whether quickly or slowly, become bilateral.

Assessment Findings

Signs and Symptoms

Early signs include stiffness, referred to as *rigidity,* and tremors of one or both hands, described as *pill-rolling* (a rhythmic motion of the thumb against the fingers). The hand tremor is obvious at rest and typically decreases when movement is voluntary, such as picking up an object.

Bradykinesia, slowness in performing spontaneous movements, develops. Clients have a masklike expression, stooped posture, monotonous speech, and difficulty swallowing saliva. Weight loss occurs. A shuffling gait is apparent, and the client has difficulty turning or redirecting forward motion. Arms are rigid while walking (Fig. 45-12).

In late stages, the disease affects the jaw, tongue, and larynx; speech is slurred; and chewing and swallowing become difficult. Rigidity can lead to contractures. Salivation increases, accompanied by drooling. In a small percentage of clients, the eyes roll upward or downward and stay there involuntarily (oculogyric crises) for several hours or even a few days.

Diagnostic Findings

Diagnosis is based on typical symptoms and a neurologic examination. There are no specific tests for this disorder.

Tremor

Masklike facial expression

Arms flexed at elbows and wrists

Stooped posture

Rigidity

Hips and knees slightly flexed

Tremor

Short, shuffling steps

FIGURE 45-12 Typical manifestations of Parkinson's disease.

Medical Management

Treatment aims at prolonging independence. Drugs such as selegiline (Eldepryl), which has neuroprotective properties, dopaminergics such as levodopa (Larodopa) or levodopa-carbidopa (Sinemet), amantadine (Symmetrel), dopamine agonists such as bromocriptine (Parlodel), and anticholinergics such as benztropine (Cogentin) are prescribed (Drug Therapy Table 45-1). Their sequence of use is based on the stage of the disorder and the dwindling effectiveness of the medication initially prescribed. Rehabilitation measures, such as physical therapy, occupational therapy, client and family education, and counseling, are used concurrently with drug therapy.

Surgical Management

Surgery (stereotaxic pallidotomy) is performed in selected cases (Fig. 45-13). The procedure destroys part of the thalamus so that excessive muscle contraction is decreased.

Dopamine-secreting brain cells from pigs have been transplanted into clients with Parkinson's disease with some success. Some fear, however, that viruses unique to pigs could jump species and infect humans, similar to the manner in which the human immunodeficiency virus transferred from primates to humans. Consequently, this approach to treatment is not actively pursued. Some success has been reported outside the United States with human fetal tissue transplantation, in which brain tissue containing the basal ganglia and dopamine-secreting cells is extracted from an aborted fetus and transplanted into the recipient's brain. This procedure is considered unethical and currently is not approved in the United States. Autotransplantation of cells from the client's own adrenal medulla into the brain also has been used with limited success. There is current interest in transplanting human stem cells as a means of curing Parkinson's disease, but this is only in early experimental stages. Cell transplantation requires craniotomy.

Some clients with Parkinson's disease have obtained relief of symptoms through implantation of a brain pacemaker (Fig. 45-14). The pacemaker blocks the tremor with tiny electrical shocks directed at the thalamus and immediately eliminates the tremor in approximately 65% of people in whom it has been used.

Nursing Management

Clients with parkinsonism are admitted to the hospital because of the debilitating effects of the disease. Others are cared for in extended care facilities when they can no longer be managed at home in a chronic state. One of the biggest nursing challenges is managing the client's drug

DRUG THERAPY TABLE 45-1	ANTIPARKINSON AGENTS		
DRUG CATEGORY AND EXAMPLES	MECHANISM OF ACTION	SIDE EFFECTS	NURSING CONSIDERATIONS
Monoamine Oxidase B Inhibitor (MAOI) selegiline (Eldepryl)	Increases dopaminergic activity Slows Parkinson's disease	Dizziness, light-headedness, confusion, nausea, vomiting, diarrhea, dry mouth, palpitations	Never give narcotic analgesics with an MAOI. Administer twice daily with breakfast and lunch. Use ice chips and sugarless candy for dry mouth.
Dopaminergics levodopa (Larodopa, Sinemet)	Dopamine replacement to decrease symptoms	Nausea, vomiting, orthostatic hypotension, dry mouth, constipation, dizziness, cardiac dysrhythmias, sleep disturbance	Do not give with MAOIs. Give with meals. Avoid multivitamins with pyridoxine.
Antiparkinsonism amantadine (Symmetrel)	May increase dopamine release to relieve symptoms	Mood changes, drowsiness, blurred vision, insomnia, nausea, orthostatic hypotension, urinary retention	Do not discontinue abruptly to avoid parkinsonian crisis. Report swelling of fingers, ankles, shortness of breath, difficulty urinating, tremors, slurred speech.
Anticholinergics benztropine (Cogentin) trihexphenidyl (Artane)	Decreases rigidity, akinesia, tremor, and drooling	Dry mouth, constipation, urinary retention, blurred vision, skin rash, flushing, increased temperature, decreased sweating	Decrease or discontinue dosage if dry mouth interferes with eating. Client must use caution in hot weather. Give with meals. Avoid alcohol and sedatives.
Dopamine Agonists bromocriptine (Parlodel)	Mimics effects of dopamine; may be effective when levodopa has decreased efficacy	Hallucinations, confusion, dizziness, drowsiness, nausea, vomiting, constipation, hypotension, shortness of breath	Give with food. Taper dosage before discontinuing. Monitor mental status.

therapy. Levodopa is associated with periods of "breakthrough" in which symptoms are exacerbated when a consistent level is not maintained. The nurse must administer the drugs closely to the schedule the client previously established at home. Drugs administered for parkinsonism can cause a wide variety of adverse effects, which requires careful observation of the client. See Nursing Care Plan 45-2 for more discussion of management of the client with an extrapyramidal disorder such as Parkinson's or Huntington's disease.

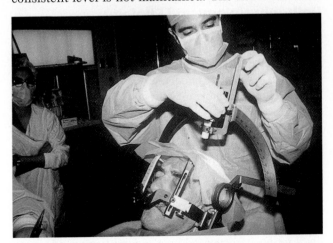

FIGURE 45-13 Client being prepared for pallidotomy. (From Smeltzer, S. C. & Bare, B. G. [2000]. *Brunner & Suddarth's textbook of medical–surgical nursing* [9th ed.]. Philadelphia: Lippincott Williams & Wilkins.)

● HUNTINGTON'S DISEASE

Huntington's disease (Huntington's chorea, hereditary chorea) is a hereditary disorder of the CNS.

Pathophysiology and Etiology

Huntington's chorea is an extrapyramidal disorder that is transmitted genetically and inherited by both sexes. The basal ganglia and portions of the cerebral cortex

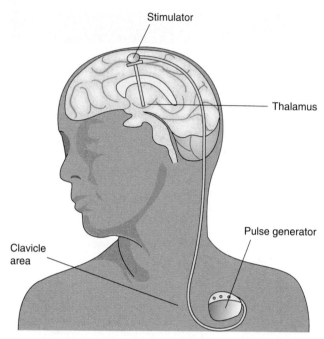

FIGURE 45-14 Deep brain stimulation with the use of a pulse generator. (From Smeltzer, S. C., & Bare, B. G. [2000]. *Brunner & Suddarth's textbook of medical–surgical nursing* [9th ed.]. Philadelphia: Lippincott Williams & Wilkins.)

degenerate. In the early stages, the client can participate in most physical activities. As the disease progresses, however, hallucinations, delusions, impaired judgment, and increased intensity of abnormal movements develop.

Assessment Findings

Symptoms develop slowly and include mental apathy and emotional disturbances, **choreiform movements** (uncontrollable writhing and twisting of the body), grimacing, difficulty chewing and swallowing, speech difficulty, intellectual decline, and loss of bowel and bladder control. Severe depression is common and can lead to suicide.

Diagnosis is based on symptoms as well as a family history of the disorder. Positron emission tomography shows CNS changes, but there is no specific diagnostic test for the disorder. Genetic testing can predict which offspring will develop the disease, but not all individuals choose to undergo testing.

Medical Management

Treatment is supportive because there is no specific therapy or cure. Tranquilizers and antiparkinson drugs re-

lieve the choreiform movements in some clients. No drugs are available to halt the mental deterioration. Because this disorder is inherited, genetic counseling before a pregnancy is advised.

Nursing Management

Nursing management aims at meeting client and family needs, such as preventing complications as well as encouraging counseling. The stage of the disease determines the scope of nursing care. The client eventually becomes totally dependent on others. Pneumonia, contractures, infections, aspiration of food or fluids, falls, and pressure ulcers are complications. The nurse prevents them by assessing the client frequently and updating the plan of care (see Nursing Care Plan 45-2).

The nurse encourages the client to lead as normal a life as possible. He or she emphasizes the importance of exercise and self-care and explains the medical regimen to the client and family. The nurse demonstrates how to facilitate tasks such as using both hands to hold a drinking glass, using a straw to drink, and wearing slip-on shoes.

SEIZURE DISORDERS

The terms *seizure disorder* and *convulsive disorder* are used interchangeably, but they are not necessarily synonymous. A **seizure** is a brief episode of abnormal electrical activity in the brain. A **convulsion,** one manifestation of a seizure, is characterized by spasmodic contractions of muscles. **Epilepsy** is a chronic recurrent pattern of seizures.

Pathophysiology and Etiology

Seizure disorders are classified as idiopathic (no known cause) or acquired. Causes of acquired seizures include high fever, electrolyte imbalances, uremia, hypoglycemia, hypoxia, brain tumor, and drug withdrawal. Once the cause is removed, the seizures cease. The known causes of epilepsy include brain injury at birth, head injuries, and inborn errors of metabolism. In some clients, the cause of epilepsy is never determined.

Seizures represent abnormal motor, sensory, or psychic neural activity. The abnormal neural activity occurs alone or in combination from discharges in one or more specific areas of the cerebral cortex. Each type of seizure disorder is characterized by a specific pattern of events (Box 45-3).

Nursing Care Plan 45-2

THE CLIENT WITH AN EXTRAPYRAMIDAL DISORDER

Assessment

Determine the following:

- Year of current diagnosis
- Concurrent medical disorders
- Weight and vital signs
- Any unilateral or bilateral hand tremor
- Gait and balance
- Use of assistive ambulatory devices
- Ability to swallow
- Quality of speech
- Bowel and urinary elimination patterns
- Mental and emotional status
- Drug therapy, time and frequency of medication administration

Nursing Diagnoses: **Impaired Physical Mobility** and **Self-Care Deficit** (specify type) related to muscle rigidity, tremors, choreiform movements, and dementia as evidenced by inability to complete all or some activities of daily living (ADLs)

Expected Outcomes: (1) Client will be physically active. (2) Client will perform self-care to the level at which he or she is capable.

Interventions	*Rationales*
Assist client with walking and physical activities.	Client is at risk for falls and injuries if activities are not assisted or supervised.
Increase the type and amount of activity gradually.	Client will have more strength and coordination once response to medications has improved.
Minimize fatigue by providing rest periods.	Rest relieves fatigue and restores stamina and endurance.
Promote involvement in self-care activities within the client's individual capacity.	Matching self-care involvement to client's functional level promotes dignity and improves self-image.
Allow ample time to perform ADLs.	Given sufficient time, client is more likely to pace himself or herself to complete ADLs semi-independently.
Modify clothing and self-care supplies to promote independence.	Clothing that is easily put on and taken off and aids for holding a toothbrush, fork, and so forth facilitate ability to perform self-care.
Assist client, but only when client cannot perform certain tasks.	Too much assistance cultivates dependence on the nurse.

Evaluation of Expected Outcomes:

- Client is active in his or her immediate environment and uses assistive devices as necessary.
- Client attends to self-care as much as symptoms allow.

Nursing Diagnoses: **Impaired Swallowing** and **Risk for Aspiration**

Expected Outcomes: (1) Client will swallow food and liquids taken in orally. (2) Client's airway will be free of food or liquids.

(continued)

Nursing Care Plan 45-2 *(Continued)*

THE CLIENT WITH AN EXTRAPYRAMIDAL DISORDER

Interventions	*Rationales*
Place client in a sitting position.	Sitting, the natural position for eating and drinking, helps propel food toward the stomach.
Keep suction equipment at the bedside; use it when the client chokes.	Mechanical suctioning uses negative pressure to pull liquids and solids from the airway.
Decrease environmental distractions.	Reducing distractions helps client focus attention on chewing and swallowing.
Cut food into small pieces. Incorporate mashed potatoes or other pasty foods.	A large bolus of food is more likely to cause a complete obstruction if aspirated. Foods like mashed potatoes bind in a soft bolus that is swallowed more easily.
Thicken liquids with gelatin, cornstarch, applesauce, mashed bananas, ice cream, or a commercial thickener.	Thickeners provide a consistency that the tongue can easily manipulate against the palate.
Position client's chin on the chest during swallowing.	This position decreases the potential for food to enter the airway.
Stroke client's throat as he or she swallows or instruct client to swallow several times in a row.	Stimulating swallowing with stroking or repeated swallowing efforts moves food from the oropharynx to the esophagus.

Evaluation of Expected Outcomes:

- Client can swallow food and fluids without choking.
- Client's lungs remain clear of food and liquids.

Nursing Diagnosis: **Impaired Verbal Communication** related to soft voice or inability to articulate words

Expected Outcome: Client will communicate needs, feelings, and ideas.

Interventions	*Rationales*
Reduce environmental noise.	A quiet environment helps others hear what the client says.
Listen closely to what the client tries to say.	Attention and patience facilitate understanding.
Ask client to speak slowly.	Altering the rate of speech improves clarity.
Anticipate client's needs.	Doing so reduces client's frustration with having to ask for help.

Evaluation of Expected Outcome: Client's verbalizations are heard and understood.

Nursing Diagnoses: **Anxiety** and **Ineffective Coping** related to awareness of diminished physical and mental capacities as manifested by periods of agitation, frustration, emotional irritability, and anger

Expected Outcomes: (1) Client will relax and feel secure. (2) Client will accept the gradual loss of physical or mental attributes and will allow others to help without opposition.

Interventions	*Rationales*
Help client to realistically determine tasks that are feasible and those that are not.	A sense of control reduces anxiety.
Suggest taking a break when the client cannot accomplish an activity.	A break can help the client to regather physical and emotional resources to complete the task successfully.

(continued)

Nursing Care Plan 45-2 (Continued)

THE CLIENT WITH AN EXTRAPYRAMIDAL DISORDER

Interventions	*Rationales*
Offer support and encouragement when client succeeds.	Deserved praise elevates self-esteem and encourages client to persevere.
Help client focus on remaining strengths rather than deficits.	Focusing on strengths promotes a more positive attitude.
Provide information about support groups whose mission is to provide assistance to clients with similar problems.	Clients are more likely to cope when they have an available network of support.

Evaluation of Expected Outcomes:

■ Client feels relaxed and in control.

■ Client implements strategies that facilitate coping with his or her disability.

Nursing Diagnosis: **Risk for Loneliness** related to depression and perceived potential for rejection secondary to altered physical appearance or cognitive function

Expected Outcome: Client will maintain social contacts.

Interventions	*Rationales*
Have client identify persons whose company he or she enjoys and activities they share.	Naming or listing specific people reinforces that the client has a circle of friends.
Encourage client to interact with a few of the designated people for short periods in a place where the client feels secure and comfortable, such as his or her home.	Taking the initiative for contacting friends promotes reestablishing social relationships. Visiting at home shields the client from potential unwanted attention from strangers.
Encourage client to participate in social activities outside the home.	When the client feels more accepted, he or she may extend socialization beyond the home.
Refer client to and encourage joining a support group.	Such groups promote bonding with new acquaintances.

Evaluation of Expected Outcome: Client reestablishes social contacts with previous friends and develops friendships with new acquaintances.

Types of Seizures

Seizures are divided into two general categories: partial and generalized.

Partial Seizures

Partial, or focal, seizures begin in a specific area of the cerebral cortex. They can progress to generalized seizures. The two subcategories of partial seizures are those with elementary (or simple) symptoms and those with complex symptoms. A client who has a partial seizure with elementary symptoms usually does not lose consciousness, and the seizure lasts less than 1 minute. Partial elementary seizures with motor symptoms are accompanied by uncontrolled jerking movements of a body part, such as a finger, mouth, hand, or foot. Partial elementary seizures with sensory symptoms are accompanied by hallucina-

tory sights, sounds, and odors; mumbling; and the use of nonsense words. The terms *jacksonian, focal motor,* and *focal sensory* describe partial elementary seizures.

A client who has a partial seizure with complex symptoms may have several sensory or motor manifestations, which also last less than 1 minute. After the seizure, the client often is confused. Complex partial seizures are manifested by automatic repetitive movements (**automatisms**) that are not appropriate, such as lip smacking and picking at clothing or objects. The terms *psychomotor* and *psychosensory* are used to describe complex partial seizures.

Generalized Seizures

Generalized seizures involve the entire brain. The client loses consciousness, and the seizure may last from several seconds to several minutes. Types of generalized seizures

BOX 45-3 ● International Classification of Seizures

I. Partial (Focal) Seizures
A. Partial seizures (no loss of consciousness)
1. Motor symptoms
2. Special sensory symptoms
3. Autonomic symptoms
4. Psychic symptoms
B. Complex partial seizures (with loss of consciousness)
1. Begins as a partial seizure and progresses to complex partial with loss of consciousness.
2. Loss of consciousness at onset of seizure

II. Generalized Seizures
A. Absence seizures
B. Myoclonic seizures
C. Clonic seizures
D. Tonic seizures
E. Tonic-clonic seizures
F. Atonic seizures

III. Unclassified Seizures
All seizures that do not fit into other classifications

include absence seizures, myoclonic seizures, and tonic-clonic seizures.

ABSENCE SEIZURES

Absence seizures, formerly referred to as *petit mal seizures,* are more common in children. They are characterized by a brief loss of consciousness, during which physical activity ceases. The person stares blankly, the eyelids flutter, the lips move, and slight movement of the head, arms, and legs occurs. These seizures typically last for a few seconds, and the person seldom falls to the ground. Because of their brief duration and relative lack of prominent movements, these seizures often go unnoticed. People with absence seizures can have them many times a day.

MYOCLONIC SEIZURES

These seizures are characterized by sudden, excessive jerking of the arms, legs, or entire body. In some instances, the muscle activity is so severe that the client falls to the ground. These seizures are brief.

TONIC-CLONIC SEIZURES

Formerly referred to as *grand mal seizures,* tonic-clonic seizures are characterized by a sequence of events that begins with a preictal (or prodromal) phase. The **pre-ictal phase** is the time immediately before a seizure and consists of vague emotional changes, such as depression, anxiety, and nervousness. This phase lasts for minutes or hours and is followed by an **aura,** a sensation that occurs immediately before the seizure. The aura is sensory (i.e., a hallucinatory odor or sound) or a sensation of weakness or numbness. In clients who experience an aura, the aura almost always is the same.

The aura is followed by the epileptic cry, which is caused by spasm of the respiratory muscles and muscles of the throat and glottis. This cry immediately precedes loss of consciousness and the ensuing tonic and clonic phases of the seizure. In the tonic phase, the muscles contract rigidly; in the clonic phase, the muscles alternate between contraction and relaxation, resulting in jerking movements and thrashing of the arms and legs. The skin becomes cyanotic, and breathing is spasmodic. Saliva mixes with air, resulting in frothing at the mouth. The jaws are tightly clenched and biting of the tongue and inner cheek occurs. Urinary or fecal incontinence is common. The clonic phase lasts for 1 minute or more, gradually subsides, and is followed by the postictal phase. The manifestations of this phase include headache, fatigue, deep sleep, confusion, nausea, and muscle soreness. Many people fall into a deep sleep for several hours.

Status epilepticus is marked by a series of tonic-clonic seizures in which the client does not regain consciousness between seizures. If this extremely dangerous condition is not terminated, death can occur. Status epilepticus occurs spontaneously in acute neurologic disorders or for no known reason; it can be precipitated by the abrupt discontinuation of anticonvulsant medication.

Other Seizure Types

Atonic (loss of muscle tone) seizures affect the muscles. The person loses consciousness briefly and falls to the ground. Recovery is rapid. An akinetic (loss of movement) seizure is similar because muscle tone is lost briefly. The client may or may not fall, and recovery is rapid.

Assessment Findings

The client's motor, sensory, and neurologic functions are normal except at the time of a seizure. Identification of seizure activity and type of seizure often depends on a witness's description of the client's actions during the seizure.

A neurologic examination and EEG are performed. Other laboratory or diagnostic studies, such as a CT scan, MRI, serology, and serum electrolyte levels, are used to confirm the diagnosis and to determine the cause of the seizure disorder. When epilepsy is suspected, a series of EEGs is required if the first results are normal.

Medical Management

Once a diagnosis of a seizure disorder is confirmed, one or more anticonvulsant drugs are used to control the seizures. Examples of anticonvulsants are phenytoin (Dilantin), phenobarbital, carbamazepine (Tegretol), ethosuximide (Zarontin), valproic acid (Depakene), felbamate (Felbatol), and fosphenytoin injection (Cerebyx) (Drug Therapy Table 45-2). IV barbiturates or diazepam (Valium) are administered to terminate status epilepticus.

Drug therapy controls the seizures or reduces their frequency or severity. The dose is adjusted over a period of several weeks. The drug is changed or another drug is added to the regimen to obtain optimum control. Blood levels of some anticonvulsant drugs are monitored for accurate dose adjustment and to prevent toxicity (Table 45-1). Serum levels also identify clients who are not taking the drug as ordered.

TABLE 45-1	ANTICONVULSANT DRUG MONITORING	
DRUG	**THERAPEUTIC LEVEL**	**TOXIC LEVEL**
carbamazepine	5–12 µg/mL	>12 µg/mL
ethosuximide	40–100 µg/mL	>100 µg/mL
phenobarbital	10–30 µg/mL	>40 µg/mL
phenytoin	10–20 µg/mL	>30 µg/mL
valproic acid	50–100 µg/mL	>100 µg/mL

(From Pagana, K. D. & Pagana, T. J. [1995]. *Mosby's diagnostic and laboratory test reference* [2nd ed.]. St. Louis: Mosby.)

DRUG THERAPY TABLE 45-2	AGENTS TO CONTROL SEIZURES		
DRUG CATEGORY AND EXAMPLES	**MECHANISM OF ACTION**	**SIDE EFFECTS**	**NURSING CONSIDERATIONS**
Anticonvulsants phenytoin (Dilantin)	Stabilizes neuronal membranes Limits spread of seizure activity Controls grand mal seizures	Nystagmus, rash, sedation, gingival hyperplasia, liver toxicity, pancytopenia	Evaluate regular serum levels. Evaluate liver function tests, complete blood count and differential. Assess skin daily. Give oral dose with food. Taper dose gradually; never discontinue abruptly. Instruct client to wear Medic Alert bracelet and have regular dental care.
carbamazepine (Tegretol)	Controls partial seizures with complex symptoms, also grand mal seizures	Dizziness, ataxia, nystagmus, rash, nausea, vomiting, liver toxicity, bone marrow suppression	Same as above
ethosuximide (Zarontin)	Reduces frequency of absence (petit mal) seizures	Drowsiness, rash, headache, nausea and vomiting	Same as above
valproic acid (Depakene, Depakote)	Adjunct treatment for multiple seizure types	Nausea and vomiting, drowsiness, diarrhea, liver toxicity	Avoid alcohol intake. Monitor bruising, bleeding gums. See above nursing considerations.
Barbiturates phenobarbital (Luminal)	Anticonvulsant activity	Sedation, rash, hyperactivity, ataxia, respiratory depression	Take oral dose at bedtime. Monitor vital signs, especially respiratory rate. Administer IM dose in deep muscle mass. Taper dosage before drug is discontinued. Periodic laboratory tests are required.
Benzodiazepines diazepam (Valium)	Skeletal muscle relaxation; adjunct anticonvulsant treatment	Respiratory depression, hypotension, sedation	Monitor BP, pulse, and respiration. Evaluate liver, kidney function, and blood studies. Taper dose before drug is discontinued. Instruct client to wear Medic Alert bracelet.

Surgical Management

Seizures that are caused by brain tumor, brain abscess, or other disorders often require surgical intervention. Surgery for epilepsy is not considered unless the client does not respond to drug therapy and seizures are frequent and severe. The area of the brain in which abnormal electrical discharges are present is identified (mapped). The surgeon must consider if removal of the involved area would result in permanent neurologic dysfunction such as paralysis or loss of speech.

NURSING PROCESS

● The Client With a Seizure Disorder

Assessment

The nurse obtains a complete history, including drug, allergy, and family history. He or she questions the client regarding events or symptoms before and after the seizure. The nurse acquires a description of the client's seizure(s) from an observer. He or she obtains information about any past head injury, neurologic infection like meningitis, previous treatment for a seizure disorder, and whether the client takes medication as prescribed.

The nurse notes the characteristics of seizures if they occur while under his or her care. If the client's history is inconclusive and the type of seizure is unknown, it is important to provide a full, detailed description of the seizure (Box 45-4).

Diagnosis, Planning, and Interventions

The newly diagnosed client with seizures needs information about the specific type of disorder, the medications needed to control the seizures, and the precautions, if any, to take. In addition, the nurse teaches the client as follows:

- Take anticonvulsant medication as prescribed.
- Recognize adverse effects of the medication.
- Keep routine follow-up visits and laboratory appointments for blood level tests.
- Operate a motor vehicle or perform dangerous tasks only when seizures are controlled for at least 6 months.

BOX 45-4 ● Seizure Assessment Data

- Onset—sudden or preceded by an aura
- Duration of seizure
- Behavior immediately before and after
- Type of body movements
- Loss of consciousness, for how long
- Incontinence or not
- Seizure awareness afterward

- Wear a Medic Alert bracelet, tag, or other medical identification.
- Avoid situations known to trigger seizures, such as repetitively flashing or blinking lights, stress, or lack of sleep.

Other nursing care includes, but is not limited to, the following diagnoses, expected outcomes, and interventions.

Risk for Injury related to uncontrolled movements and altered consciousness during seizure; **Risk for Impaired Oral Mucous Membranes** related to oral injury during a seizure and side effects of phenytoin drug therapy

Expected Outcomes: (1) Client will be free of injuries. (2) Oral mucous membranes will remain unaltered.

- Refer to the Nursing Process section on caring for clients with infectious and inflammatory disorders. *Nursing interventions are similar regardless of the cause of a seizure.*
- Use padded head gear on clients with atonic or akinetic seizures. *Loss of consciousness and falls are common with these types of seizures, increasing the potential for head injury.*
- Pad side rails with soft material. *Padding cushions the force on the client's skin and soft tissue when contact with metal side rails occurs during a seizure.*
- Protect client at the onset of the seizure by assisting the client to the floor or moving objects away from the client. *The nurse reduces the risk for serious injuries by modifying the environment and the client's location in the environment.*
- Loosen clothing about the neck. *Tight clothing can impair breathing.*
- Never forcibly restrain the client. *Physically restraining a client during a seizure increases the potential for injuries such as fractures.*
- Inspect the oral cavity and teeth after a generalized seizure. *The nurse assesses the mouth for signs of injury and reports injuries to the physician.*
- Apply ice to bleeding areas; if broken teeth are noted, notify the client's dentist. *Ice constricts blood vessels and reduces bleeding. The client's dentist may be able to reimplant broken teeth or minimize the outcome of the trauma with early interventions.*
- Promote oral hygiene after each meal and recommend dental checkups every 3 to 6 months. *Phenytoin (Dilantin) causes gingival hyperplasia (overgrowth of gum tissue); regular and frequent dental examinations facilitate the maintenance or restoration of teeth and gums.*

Anxiety related to unpredictability of seizures and social stigma as evidenced by uneasiness about resuming previous lifestyle activities with social acquaintances

Expected Outcome: Anxiety will be reduced as evidenced by a resumption of social interactions.

- Help the client understand the disorder and treatment options. *Knowledge about the disorder and making choices promotes a sense of control.*

- Explain that a variety of drugs are available that can successfully reduce or control seizures. *Drug therapy prevents or reduces seizure activity.*
- Encourage the client to share information about the disorder with others. *Providing accurate information dispels fears and helps eliminate the misconception that people with seizure disorders have subnormal intelligence.*
- Suggest contacting the Epilepsy Foundation of America. *The Epilepsy Foundation of America provides counseling, low-cost prescription services, and referrals to agencies for vocational rehabilitation, job opportunities, personal and genetic counseling, and sheltered workshops.*

Evaluation of Expected Outcomes

Expected outcomes for the client are that there are fewer seizures or that they are completely controlled. The client remains safe from injury. The client's mouth and teeth are intact. The client who takes phenytoin understands the importance of regular dental examinations because of the potential for gingival hyperplasia. The client's anxiety is reduced to a tolerable level on a scale of 0 to 10. The client is resolved to maintain social relationships and participate in leisure activities. The client is aware of the services provided by the Epilepsy Foundation of America and how to contact this organization.

BRAIN TUMORS

A brain tumor is a growth of abnormal cells within the cranium. Brain tumors occur in all age groups. Some types are more common in people younger than 20 years of age; others more frequently affect older people. About 50% of all brain tumors are malignant. A brain tumor, whether malignant or benign, can result in death.

Pathophysiology and Etiology

The cause of brain tumors, which occur in various areas of the brain (Fig. 45-15), remains unknown. A small percentage are congenital, such as hemangioblastomas.

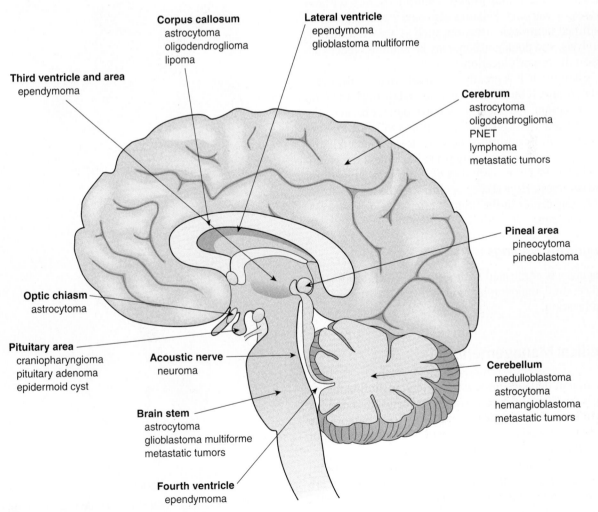

Corpus callosum
astrocytoma
oligodendroglioma
lipoma

Lateral ventricle
ependymoma
glioblastoma multiforme

Third ventricle and area
ependymoma

Cerebrum
astrocytoma
oligodendroglioma
PNET
lymphoma
metastatic tumors

Pineal area
pineocytoma
pineoblastoma

Optic chiasm
astrocytoma

Pituitary area
craniopharyngioma
pituitary adenoma
epidermoid cyst

Acoustic nerve
neuroma

Cerebellum
medulloblastoma
astrocytoma
hemangioblastoma
metastatic tumors

Brain stem
astrocytoma
glioblastoma multiforme
metastatic tumors

Fourth ventricle
ependymoma

FIGURE 45-15 Common sites for a brain tumor.

Genetic factors are associated with two types of brain tumors, *astrocytoma,* a tumor in the frontal lobe, and *neurofibromatosis.* Other causative factors include viral infection, exposure to radiation, head trauma, and immunosuppression. The brain also is the site of metastatic lesions from primary tumors, especially those of the lung and breast.

Tumors that arise from cerebral tissue, such as malignant gliomas and glioblastomas, and angiomas that involve cerebral blood vessels, expand in the confines of the skull and encroach on brain tissue that is vital for life. Extracerebral tumors, such as meningiomas (tumors of the meninges), press on the brain tissue from without.

Assessment Findings

Signs and Symptoms

Because tumors take up space and block the flow and absorption of CSF, symptoms associated with IICP occur. The classic triad of headache, vomiting, and papilledema is common. Headache is most common early in the morning. It becomes increasingly severe and occurs more frequently as the tumor grows. Vomiting occurs without nausea or warning. Seizures also develop. Symptoms of disturbed neurologic function, such as speech difficulty, paralysis, and double vision, may be manifested depending on the tumor's location.

When the ICP is greatly increased, areas of the brain can herniate. If the brain stem is forced through the foramen magnum, the client is in grave danger because the vital centers that control respiration and heart rate are compressed. Respirations become deeper, labored, and noisy and then slow to only periodic. Unless the condition is relieved, the client dies of respiratory failure and cardiac arrest. Hyperthermia occurs as the temperature-regulating center in the brain is affected. Coma progressively deepens.

Diagnostic Findings

Diagnosis is confirmed with CT scan, MRI, brain scan, and cerebral angiography, which reveal the tumor's size and location.

Medical Management

Treatment depends on several factors, including the tumor's location and type (primary or metastatic) and the client's age and physical condition. Brain tumors are treated by surgery, radiation therapy, chemotherapy, or a combination of these methods.

Metastatic tumors and some primary tumors are inoperable, and radiation therapy and chemotherapy are the only treatment choices. Clients who cannot withstand surgery, chemotherapy, or radiation therapy are kept as comfortable and free from pain as possible. Intra-arterial or intrathecal administration of antineoplastic drugs is used to destroy the tumor or slow tumor growth. Symptomatic drug therapy includes corticosteroids and osmotic diuretics to reduce cerebral edema, analgesics, anticonvulsants, and antibiotics.

Complications, such as IICP, paralysis, mental changes, infection, seizures, and prolonged immobility, are treated symptomatically.

Surgical Management

Surgery for an operable brain tumor involves a craniotomy (incision through the skull) or craniectomy (excision of part of the skull). A section of bone (bone flap) is removed to reach the brain (Fig. 45-16). After the tumor is removed, the dura is reapproximated (the cut edges are

A

Craniotomy

B

Craniectomy

FIGURE 45-16 Neurosurgical techniques. (**A**) Craniotomy, (**B**) craniectomy.

lined up and sewn together), the bone flap replaced, and the skin sutured. The bone flap is not reinserted when increasing ICP or tumor growth is expected.

The client's postoperative symptoms are determined by the location and function of any damaged or removed brain tissue. Brain tissue does not regenerate.

Another method of removing brain tumors uses a laser beam directed at the tumor site. This surgical technique enables the physician to reach tumors that previously were considered inoperable. Radioisotopes also are surgically inserted into the tumor. The cure rate for this procedure, however, is about the same as for external radiation therapy.

Nursing Management

Nursing management depends on the area of the brain affected, tumor type, treatment approach, and the client's signs and symptoms. If the tumor is inoperable or has expanded despite treatment, IICP is a major threat (see Nursing Care Plan 45-1). See Chapter 47 for the care of the client undergoing intracranial surgery. Clients who receive chemotherapy and radiation are supported through the adverse effects associated with antineoplastic drug administration (see Chap. 20). The nurse clarifies the client's and family's questions concerning treatment modalities. He or she directs the client to appropriate professionals to discuss treatment alternatives. The nurse explains hospice care and services to clients with brain tumors that no longer are at a stage where they can be cured.

Before the client is discharged, the nurse evaluates the client's and family's immediate and long-term needs. The nurse develops an individualized teaching plan that addresses the following components:

- Medication regimen
- Appointments for chemotherapy or radiation therapy
- Adverse effects of chemotherapy or radiation and techniques for managing them
- Nutritional support
- Home care considerations
- Rehabilitation (exercises, physical therapy)
- Referrals to support services for physical, emotional, and financial assistance

N U R S I N G   P R O C E S S

● The Client With a Brain Tumor

Assessment

The nurse identifies affected areas after a thorough history and neurologic examination. He or she performs a physical assessment and records the abnormal findings.

Diagnosis, Planning, and Interventions

Depending on the stage of the disease and the selected method(s) of treatment, the nurse's role includes but is not limited to the following.

Acute Pain related to IICP secondary to expansion of the tumor or a sequela of surgery
Expected Outcome: Pain will be controlled within client's level of tolerance.

- Assess and monitor characteristics of pain every time you measure vital signs. *Pain assessment is the fifth vital sign.*
- Administer prescribed analgesia and monitor for respiratory depression. *Narcotic analgesics relieve pain, but tolerance develops. High doses of narcotic analgesics depress the respiratory center in the brain.*
- Give analgesia on a scheduled rather than an as-needed basis. *Regular administration of analgesia is most effective at controlling pain.*
- Advocate for patient-controlled analgesia or transdermal analgesic patch. *Methods that facilitate frequent administration of small doses of IV analgesia or continuous absorption through the skin provide more continuous pain relief.*

Imbalanced Nutrition: Less than Body Requirements related to nausea and vomiting or altered LOC
Expected Outcome: Nutritional and fluid needs are met as evidenced by maintenance of weight and intake above 2000 mL.

- Administer prescribed antiemetics before meals. *A client is likely to consume adequate food without nausea or vomiting.*
- Determine client's food preferences and supply them. *Catering to likes and dislikes promotes a greater intake of food.*
- Give small, frequent servings of food or nourishing beverages. *Large servings tend to overwhelm a client. He or she may consume more food overall if smaller amounts are served several times a day. Liquid nutritional supplements provide extra calories and nutrients in an easily consumed form.*
- Collaborate with the physician concerning gastric tube feedings or TPN. *Enteral and parenteral routes for nutrition may be used when the oral route is no longer adequate.*

Impaired Oral Mucous Membranes related to fluid volume deficit, tissue damage secondary to chemotherapy or radiation as manifested by xerostomia (oral lesions)
Expected Outcome: Oral mucous membranes will be pink, moist, and intact.

- Relieve discomfort with a prescribed topical anesthetic. *It blocks sensory nerves and relieves local discomfort.*
- Provide meticulous mouth care. *The mouth contains many microorganisms that thrive on particles of food and sugar clinging to teeth. Increased microbial growth fosters the potential for dental decay and impaired tissue.*

- Offer mouth rinses of tap water or medicated solutions frequently. *Liquids keep the mouth moist and flush debris from the oral cavity.*

Anticipatory Grieving related to uncertain future, physical and social losses

Expected Outcome: Client will express feelings and deal with potential losses while working through acceptance of the diagnosis.

- Give the opportunity to express feelings privately. *A person is more likely to be open and frank in an environment where others will not overhear intimate feelings.*
- Remain with client when emotions are overwhelming. *A supportive other helps client endure emotional pain and cope more effectively.*
- Help clarify any and all questions the client may have. *Honest and accurate information facilitates the client's right to self-determination.*
- Reassure client that he or she will not be abandoned and that comfort and preservation of dignity are priorities of nursing care. *Most clients fear that they will be left alone when dying and will experience extreme pain or discomfort.*
- Assist client to complete unfinished business however he or she defines it. *Taking care of tasks, accomplishing specific goals, or communicating feelings to significant others helps clients die more peacefully.*
- Refer client and family to the local hospice organization if the client is in the terminal stage. *Hospice organizations help client and family meet their physical and emotional needs.*

Evaluation of Expected Outcomes

Client reports that pain is relieved or resolved to a tolerable level. Nutritional intake is sufficient to maintain body weight. Oral mucosa is intact. Client and family progress through the grieving process and implement a plan for postdischarge care.

GENERAL NUTRITIONAL CONSIDERATIONS

General nutritional goals are to maintain healthy weight, prevent or correct malnutrition, reduce the risk of aspiration, and prevent constipation. Adjust calories to prevent weight gain (e.g., clients with multiple sclerosis) or weight loss (e.g., clients with Guillain-Barré syndrome); small, frequent feedings of nutrient-dense and calorie-dense foods help maximize intake and reduce fatigue. Clients with muscle wasting benefit from an increased protein intake; commercial supplements (e.g., thickened liquids, fortified puddings, fortified gelatins) are tasty and easy options. Semisolid foods like puddings and mashed potatoes are easier to swallow than thin liquids or a regular diet. Gastrostomy feedings usually are the best route for clients who require long-term enteral nutritional support. Foods high in fiber, such as whole-wheat bread and cereals, bran cereal, and fiber-fortified supplements, help prevent constipation when consumed with adequate fluids. Prunes and prune juice stimulate peristalsis.

Diet modifications minimize drug–nutrient interactions and side effects of drug therapy. Clients taking levodopa should avoid high intakes of protein (meat, fish, poultry, and dairy foods) and vitamin B$_6$ (legumes, sweet potatoes, avocado, fortified cereal, bran, wheat germ, pork, tuna), because they decrease its effectiveness. Limit daily sodium intake to 2000 mg in clients receiving corticosteroids; if hyperglycemia develops, the client must follow a diabetic diet. Anticonvulsants impair vitamin D metabolism, leading to calcium imbalance, rickets, or osteomalacia if supplemental vitamin D is not given.

A high-fat diet, called the *ketogenic diet,* is used as part of treatment for seizures in children. The high fat content simulates starvation, except that the fat burned for energy comes from food, not stored body fat. Mild dehydration helps concentrate blood ketones; it is not known how or why ketosis affects seizure activity. Grams of fat to grams of protein and carbohydrate start with a 4:1 ratio; simulated starvation results in more efficient use of protein, so needs for growth can be met with 1.0 g protein/kg of body weight. Fruits and vegetables are preferred as the major sources of carbohydrate because they are rich in other nutrients. The diet is inadequate in many vitamins and minerals, so carbohydrate-free supplements are needed. The diet is difficult to follow and unpalatable, but highly motivated families have overcome these obstacles and benefited from this low-risk, noninvasive therapy.

GENERAL PHARMACOLOGIC CONSIDERATIONS

Carbamazepine, a drug used to treat trigeminal neuralgia, is taken with meals. The dose is gradually increased until relief is obtained. The effectiveness of carbamazepine may decrease over time.

Phenytoin, also used to treat trigeminal neuralgia, requires periodic laboratory evaluation to detect bone marrow depression. This drug also has been implicated in birth defects; therefore, pregnant women or those planning to become pregnant must not take it.

Phenytoin may discolor the urine pink or reddish-brown. This color change is not clinically significant.

Clients taking anticonvulsant therapy should carry a Medic Alert bracelet identifying the current medications and disease condition.

Abrupt withdrawal of any anticonvulsant drug may trigger status epilepticus (continuous seizure activity). The drug must be withdrawn gradually.

Corticosteroid administration may produce hyperglycemia, gastrointestinal bleeding, or gastric ulcer. Check the blood for glucose every 4 hours, and check the stools for blood. To decrease the risk for gastric ulcers, an antacid may be prescribed.

Narcotic analgesics depress the respiratory center and raise CSF pressure. Their use is contraindicated in clients with head trauma or increased ICP, unless administration is necessary.

In addition to parkinsonism, tardive dyskinesia, characterized by rhythmic and involuntary movement of the tongue, jaw, neck, arm, and legs as well as grimacing, may be seen with the administration of the phenothiazines and other psychotropic medicines such as haloperidol (Haldol).

GENERAL GERONTOLOGIC CONSIDERATIONS

Older adults are more susceptible to the complications of prolonged bed rest and immobility. Watch these clients closely for such problems as hypostatic pneumonia, pressure ulcers, contractures, and deformities.

Older adults may not exhibit the typical signs and symptoms of meningitis; rather, they may display a change in mental status, slight to no fever, and no nuchal rigidity or headache.

Mortality rates are high in older adults with meningitis. Contributing factors to death from meningitis are chronic illness and delays in diagnosis (partly because of the atypical signs and symptoms).

The incidence of brain tumor decreases with age. Headache and papilledema are less common symptoms of a brain tumor in the older adult.

Critical Thinking Exercises

1. *When caring for a client with a seizure disorder, what nursing interventions are indicated?*
2. *What information can the nurse provide to a person who recently has been diagnosed with multiple sclerosis?*
3. *What discharge teaching is appropriate when discussing home care with the spouse of a client in the deteriorating stages of Parkinson's disease?*

References and Suggested Readings

Arbour, R. (1998). Aggressive management of intracranial dynamics. *Critical Care Nurse, 18*(3), 30–42.

Armstrong, T., Hancock, G., & Gilbert, M. (2000). Symptom management of the patient with a brain tumor at the end of life. *Oncology Nursing Forum, 27*(4), 616.

Armstrong, T. S. & Gilbert, M. R. (2000). Metastatic brain tumors: Diagnosis, treatment, and nursing interventions. *Clinical Journal of Oncology Nursing, 4*, 217–225, 231–232.

Backer, J. H. (2000). Stressors, social support, coping, and health dysfunction in individuals with Parkinson's disease. *Journal of Gerontological Nursing, 26*(11), 6–16.

Buelow, J. M. (2001). Epilepsy management. *Journal of Neuroscience Nursing, 33*, 260–269.

Campbell, J. M., Linc, L. G., & Mutersbaugh, K. (1998). Viral encephalitis: A challenging diagnosis in an ICU. *Critical Care Nurse, 18*(3), 58–65.

Charles, T., Swash, M. (2001). Amyotrophic lateral sclerosis: Current understanding. *Journal of Neuroscience Nursing, 33*, 245–253.

Costa, M. E. (1998). Clinical snapshot: Trigeminal neuralgias. *American Journal of Nursing, 98*(6), 42–43.

Cunning, S. (2000). When the Dx is myasthenia gravis. *RN, 63*(4), 26–31.

Cunning, S. N. (1999). Unraveling the mysteries of Guillain-Barré syndrome. *Nursing Spectrum (Greater Chicago/NE Illinois & NW Indiana Edition), 12*(15), 22–23.

Goldsmith, C. (1999). Clinical snapshot: Parkinson's disease. *American Journal of Nursing, 99*(2), 46–47.

Hatcher, D. (1999). Inheritance and ignorance . . . Huntington's disease. *Nursing Times, 95*(45), 45–49.

Hilton, G. (2000). Cerebral oxygenation in the traumatically brain-injured patient: Are ICP and CPP enough? *Journal of Neuroscience Nursing, 32*, 278–283.

Hofmann, N. (1999). Understanding the neuropsychiatric symptoms of Huntington's disease. *Journal of Neuroscience Nursing, 31*, 309–313.

Holcomb, S. S. (1999). Reviewing bacterial meningitis. *Nursing, 29*(8), Crit Care: 32cc6–32cc7.

Holland, N. (2000). Multiple sclerosis: New options for care. *Nursing Spectrum (Greater Philadelphia/Tri-State Edition), 9*(18), 15–18.

Jastremski, C. (1998). Trauma! Head injuries. *RN, 61*(12), 40–42, 44.

Johnson, L. (1999). Factors known to raise intracranial pressure and the associated implications for nursing management. *Nursing in Critical Care, 4*(3), 117–120.

King, D. S. (1999). Central nervous system infections: Basic concepts. *Nursing Clinics of North America, 34*, 761–771.

Lisak, D. (2001). Overview of symptomatic management of multiple sclerosis. *Journal of Neuroscience Nursing, 33*, 224–230.

Love, R. M. K. (1999). Bell's palsy isn't fatal, but patients need special attention. *RN, 62*(2), 12.

March, K. (2000). Intracranial pressure monitoring and assessing intracranial compliance in brain injury. *Critical Care Nursing Clinics of North America, 12*, 429–436.

McConnell, E. A. (2001). Clinical do's & don'ts: Preventing transient increases in ICP. *Nursing, 31*(3), 17.

Mitsumoto, H., Shockely, L. (1998). Amyotrophic lateral sclerosis: Continuum of care from diagnosis through hospice. *Home Healthcare Consultant, 5*(6), 20, 23–29.

Mosiman, W. (2001). Controlling pain: Taking the sting out of trigeminal neuralgia. *Nursing, 31*(3), 86.

Myers, F. (2000). Meningitis: The fears, the facts. *RN, 63*(11), 52–58.

Parini, S. M. (2001). 8 faces of meningitis: How to tell which type your patient has. *Nursing, 31*(8), 51–53.

Ross, A. P. (1999). Neurologic degenerative disorders. *Nursing Clinics of North America, 34*, 725–742.

Roth, P., Farls, K. (2000). Pathophysiology of traumatic brain injury. *Critical Care Quarterly, 22*(3), 14–25.

Stewart, K. B. (1998). Action stat: Myasthenia gravis cholinergic crisis. *Nursing, 28*(12), 33.

Suddes, M. (1999). Common nursing problems in Parkinson's disease. *Elderly Care, 11*(4), 31–34.

Tait, D. (2000). Coping with Bell's palsy. *Nursing Spectrum (Washington, DC/Baltimore Metro Edition), 10*(19), 28.

Wulf, J. A. (2000). Evaluation of seizure observation and documentation. *Journal of Neuroscience Nursing, 32*(1), 27–36.

Yanko, J. R. & Mitcho, K. (2001). Acute management of severe traumatic brain injuries. *Critical Care Nursing Quarterly, 23*(4), 1–23.

Caring for Clients With Cerebrovascular Disorders

Words to Know

aneurysm
bruit
cephalalgia
cerebral infarction
cerebrovascular accident
collateral circulation
endarterectomy

expressive aphasia
hemianopia
hemiplegia
receptive aphasia
transient ischemic
    attack

Learning Objectives

On completion of this chapter, the reader will:

- Identify three common types of headaches and their characteristics.
- List three nursing techniques that supplement drug therapy in reducing or relieving headaches.
- Name three types of cerebrovascular disorders and their usual causes.
- Explain the significance of a transient ischemic attack.
- Discuss medical and surgical techniques used to reduce the potential for a cerebrovascular accident.
- Identify five manifestations of a cerebrovascular accident; discuss those that are unique to right-sided and left-sided infarctions.
- Identify at least five nursing diagnoses common to the care of a client with a cerebrovascular accident and interventions for them.
- Describe a cerebral aneurysm and the danger it presents.
- Discuss appropriate nursing interventions when caring for a client with a cerebral aneurysm.

Cerebrovascular disorders are major medical problems that affect adults. Some, such as headaches, can disrupt a client's lifestyle, causing tremendous discomfort and anxiety. Others, such as cerebrovascular accident and transient ischemic attacks, are life-threatening.

HEADACHE

Aching in the head is referred to as **cephalalgia.** This symptom accompanies many disorders such as meningitis, increased intracranial pressure (IICP), brain tumors, and sinusitis. When the duration is relatively brief, a headache is considered transient and benign. Although there are many types of headaches, tension, migraine, and cluster headaches are the most common (Table 46-1). It is possible to experience more than one type of headache.

● TENSION HEADACHE

Tension headache is the most common type of headache, accounting for 90% of all cases.

Pathophysiology and Etiology

Neither the skull nor the brain itself contains sensory nerves. A vast network of sensory and motor nerves, however, are distributed throughout the scalp and facial muscles. During stressful conditions, people tend to contract muscles about the neck, face, and scalp. Those with temporomandibular joint disorder may awaken with a tension headache from clenching the jaw and grinding the teeth during sleep. A tension headache also can develop, however, when a person contracts the neck and facial muscles for a prolonged period. Examples include holding

TABLE 46-1	FEATURES OF COMMON HEADACHES		
FEATURE	**CLUSTER HEADACHE**	**MIGRAINE HEADACHE**	**TENSION HEADACHE**
Client sex	Usually male	Usually female	Equally male/female
Age at onset	20–50 yr	10–40 yr	Any age
Frequency of attacks	1–8/day	1–8/month	Almost daily
Duration of attacks	30 min to 4 hr	4 to 72 hr	Gradual onset, steady
Intensity of pain	Excruciatingly relentless	Moderate to severe	Constant dull ache
Location of pain	Strictly unilateral	Unilateral or bilateral	Bilateral
Nasal congestion	70%	None	None
Droopy, teary eye	Common	Uncommon	Uncommon
Incidence of associated nausea and vomiting	Rare	Common	Rare
Incidence of attacks awakening client from sleep	Common	Rare	Rare
Characteristic behavior	Client cannot remain still during severe attack	Client prefers hibernation	Client prefers hibernation
Family history	7%	90%	Associated with stress
Treatment	Refer to physician	Refer to physician	Refer to physician

the head at a particular angle during a work-related task (e.g., looking at a computer screen) or suffering a consequence of limited range of motion from arthritis in the cervical spine. When the tensed muscles sensitize *nociceptors*, pain-relaying nerves, in the head, the nociceptors transmit neurochemicals such as prostaglandin and substance P to the brain, which registers the presence and location of discomfort (see Chap. 21).

Assessment Findings

People who experience tension headaches describe the discomfort as pressure or steady constriction on both sides of the head. Symptoms vary from a mild ache to severe, disabling pain. Some correlate the onset of the headache with anxiety or emotional conflict. Persistent headache requires tests such as computed tomography (CT) scan, brain scan, head and neck radiographs, and angiography to rule out a brain tumor or intracerebral hemorrhage, cervical spondylitis, or infected sinuses.

Medical Management

Transient tension headaches usually are relieved by rest, a mild analgesic, and stress management techniques like relaxation or imaging (see Chap. 12). Treatment for severe, recurrent tension headaches starts with removing or correcting factors or situations that cause them. If muscle contraction is a reaction to anxiety, counseling and psychotherapy may help clients deal with their emotional stressors in healthier ways. Treatment with antidepressants also helps some people who experience tension headaches.

● MIGRAINE HEADACHES

The term *migraine headache* includes several different patterns of headaches that all have a vascular origin. Subcategories include the following:

- *Basilar artery migraine,* in which dizziness, diplopia, and impaired coordination accompany the headache; it occurs primarily in young women
- *Hemiplegic migraine,* in which headache and temporary unilateral paralysis occur
- *Ophthalmoplegic migraine,* characterized by head pain, droopy eyelid, double vision, and distortion of the visual field
- *Exertional migraine,* brought about by running, lifting, coughing, sneezing, or bending
- *Status migrainosus,* a severe migraine headache and nausea that is sustained for 3 or more days (National Institute of Neurological Disorders and Stroke, 2002)

Migraine headaches are more common in women, although men are affected almost equally. Most affected people experience their first episode during childhood to middle age. It is not unusual that other blood relatives also have migraines. Migraine headaches usually are recurrent and severe. Symptoms usually last for 1 day or more.

Pathophysiology and Etiology

Researchers are getting closer to finding what causes migraine headaches. Currently, they have targeted three sequential contributing cofactors: (1) changes in particular serotonin receptors that promote (2) dilation of cerebral blood vessels, and pain intensification from (3) neurochemicals released from the trigeminal nerve (Fig. 46-1).

Some hypothesize that a faulty inherited mechanism causes transient changes in cranial blood vessels. Others believe that an etiologic association exists, with fluctuations in reproductive hormones. It also has been suggested that chemicals in certain foods trigger vascular changes, or the headache results from a food-related allergy.

Although the triggering mechanism remains elusive, the pathophysiologic changes have not. Initially, spasms in arteries in the scalp and neck occur. Platelets that flow through the arteries that supply the brain become trapped in the narrowed passageway. They, in turn, release serotonin, which alters blood flow. Accessory arteries dilate widely. Subsequently, pain-transmitting neurochemicals are released, which stimulate nociceptors. The outcome is a relentless, excruciating headache.

Assessment Findings

Signs and Symptoms

Those who have "classic" migraines experience an *aura,* a sensory phenomenon that precedes the headache by about 10 to 30 minutes. Some have visual disturbances such as flashing lights or wavy lines; some develop weakness or tingling in an extremity; others become confused or have difficulty speaking. For others with the more "common" form of migraine, the prodromal period before the headache is marked by a change in mood, difficulty concentrating, or unusual fatigue. The headache usually starts on one side in the forehead, temple, ear, eye, or jaw; however, it can involve the entire head before the attack is over. The client describes the pain as "throbbing" or "bursting." Nausea and vomiting, vertigo, sensitivity to light, irritability, and fatigue accompany the headache.

Diagnostic Findings

The pattern of headache development and the signs and symptoms are typical of migraine headaches. CT scan, angiography, brain scan, and radiographs are used to rule out other neurologic disorders.

Medical Management

Rest and drug therapy are the mainstays of treatment for migraine headaches. Mild analgesics usually are ineffective. New drugs that affect serotonin levels like methysergide (Sansert) and sumatriptan (Imitrex) are prescribed. Antiemetics also are prescribed if nausea and vomiting become acute during an attack. Some clients learn to shorten or abort migraines with biofeedback techniques (see Chap. 12).

Nursing Management

The nurse reinforces the drug therapy regimen and instructs the client on self-administration of medications. To abort the migraine headache, the nurse stresses the importance of taking medication as soon as symptoms of the

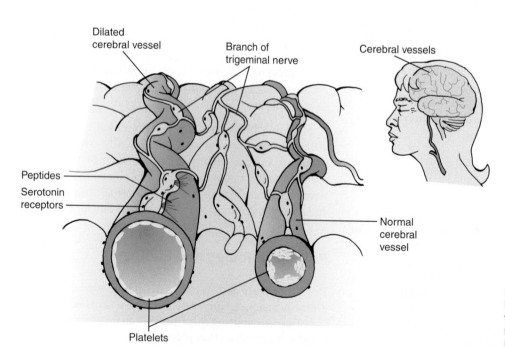

FIGURE 46-1 Chemical developments in migraine headaches. Cerebral blood vessels dilate in response to serotonin from platelets. Peptides released from the trigeminal nerve intensify pain.

migraine begin. He or she encourages the client to lie in bed in a dark room and minimize noise and other stimuli (Client and Family Teaching Box 46-1).

● CLUSTER HEADACHE

The term *cluster* is used to describe episodic headaches in which attacks of head pain last 30 minutes to 2 hours and continually repeat, with brief periods of recovery between attacks. The closely spaced attacks occur over 6 to 8 weeks, with 2 to 10 headaches per day. Each headache quickly escalates in severity, with very little time between the discomfort at onset and the point of maximum pain. The severity tends to diminish when the cycle of episodes begins to terminate. Clients can be headache free from 6 months to 5 years; however, chronic sufferers have attacks much more frequently.

Men and boys experience cluster headaches more commonly than women and girls. In contrast to migraine headaches, family members usually do not have similar headaches.

Pathophysiology and Etiology

The cause of cluster headaches is unknown, but there is a seasonal relationship, suggesting a correlation with physiologic biorhythms. Some suggest that lower-than-normal levels of the neurotransmitter serotonin may disturb the hypothalamus, which regulates autonomic nervous system activities and biologic responses to circadian rhythms. This theory may explain the mechanism by which serotonin-enhancing drugs help to relieve cluster headaches.

Some believe that cluster headaches are a variant of migraine headaches. The headaches can be triggered by vasodilating agents such as nitroglycerin, histamine, and

alcoholic beverages, but smoking, which causes vasoconstriction, also is considered a precipitating factor. The tearing and nasal stuffiness that accompany cluster headaches suggest that acetylcholine, a parasympathetic neurotransmitter, also plays a role in cluster headache symptomatology.

Assessment Findings

A person with a cluster headache has pain on one side of the head, usually behind the eye, accompanied by nasal congestion, *rhinorrhea* (watery discharge from the nose), and tearing and redness of the eye (Fig. 46-2). The pain is so severe that the person is not likely to lie still; rather, he or she paces or thrashes about. The pain may awaken the person from deep sleep.

The diagnosis is based on the history and signs and symptoms that the client discusses and by ruling out other neurovascular causes. In research studies using thermography, a device for measuring heat, when clients experience a cluster headache there tends to be a "cold spot" about the eye, indicating reduced blood flow in that area.

Medical Management

Symptoms are controlled with the administration of various drugs such as an ergotamine derivative like dihydroergotamine (Migranal) or methysergide (Sansert). Some respond to corticosteroids like triamcinolone (Aristocort) and prednisone (Deltasone), lithium carbonate (Eskalith), vasoconstricting drugs in the "triptan" group like sumatriptan (Imitrex) and zolmitriptan (Zomig), anticonvulsants like gabapentin (Neurontin) and divalproex

 46-1 *Client and Family Teaching*
Migraine Headaches

The nurse includes the following instructions:

■ Follow the indications and dosage regimen for medication, and notify the physician of any adverse drug effects.
■ Identify and avoid factors that precipitate or intensify an attack.
■ Keep a record of the attacks, including activities before the attack, and environmental or emotional circumstances that appear to bring on the attack.
■ Lie down in a darkened room, and avoid noise and movement when an attack occurs, if that is possible.

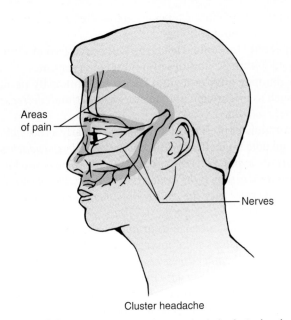

Areas
of pain

Nerves

Cluster headache

FIGURE 46-2 Affected nerves and areas of pain in cluster headache.

(Depakote), and beta-adrenergic blockers like atenolol (Tenormin) and propranolol (Inderal). Inhaled or injected drugs are preferred because they are absorbed more rapidly than those administered by the oral route (Drug Therapy Table 46-1). The client may take a drug daily to prevent the development of a headache and take another to abort a headache when it occurs. Oxygen may be used during a headache to reduce the vasodilating compensatory response occurring in the brain. For clients who do not respond to pharmacologic interventions, neurosurgical techniques such as rhizotomy may be the only hope for relief (see Chap 21).

NURSING PROCESS

● The Client With a Headache

Assessment

The nurse asks the client questions about the location, type of pain, and past history of the same type of headache because another disorder or problem may be occurring. He or she determines if the pain is in one area or over the entire head; factors that appear to bring on, worsen, or relieve the headache; how long the pain lasts; and symptoms such as tearing, nasal congestion, nausea or vomiting, or sensitivity to light.

When assessing clients with chronic headaches or headaches that cause various symptoms, the nurse obtains a complete medical, allergy, and family history, as well as a record of frequency and description of the pain, including its numeric intensity during an attack. The nurse measures vital signs to use as a baseline for comparison.

Diagnosis, Planning, and Interventions

Pain related to muscle tension, changes in cerebral blood flow, or unknown etiology
Expected Outcome: Headache will be reduced or eliminated within 30 minutes of nursing intervention.

- Eliminate environmental factors that intensify pain, such as bright light and noise. *Sensory stimuli decrease pain tolerance.*
- Administer prescribed medications as early as possible and note their effect. *Medications that relieve headaches are in many different categories with various mechanisms of action. If the medication is ineffective, the nurse collaborates with the physician to modify the method of treatment.*
- Offer a back massage to promote muscle relaxation. *Massage relaxes tense muscles, causes local dilation of blood vessels, and relieves headache. This approach is not likely to help a client with migraine or cluster headache.*
- Apply warm (or cool) cloths to the forehead or back of the neck. *Warmth promotes vasodilation; cool stimuli reduce blood flow.*

- Provide distraction with soft, soothing music, or suggest using a relaxation tape or one that provides guided imagery. *Reduced anxiety can relieve a tension headache; clients with migraine or cluster headaches are not receptive to this approach.*

Evaluation of Expected Outcome

Head pain is reduced or eliminated. The client demonstrates understanding of the medication regimen and possible side effects. He or she identifies ways to modify behavior to minimize pain.

CEREBROVASCULAR DISORDERS

Three million people in the United States each year experience temporary or prolonged deprivation of oxygen to the brain either from a transient ischemic attack (TIA) or cerebrovascular accident (CVA), also known as a *stroke*. A stroke develops in one third of those who experience a TIA. Stroke is the third leading cause of death among adult Americans. Each year, approximately 500,000 Americans have a stroke. About one third die; most survivors have permanent disabilities.

● TRANSIENT ISCHEMIC ATTACKS

Transient ischemic attacks are sudden, brief attacks of neurologic impairment caused by a temporary interruption in cerebral blood flow. Symptoms may disappear within 1 hour; some continue for as long as 1 day. When the symptoms terminate, the client resumes his or her presymptomatic state. A TIA is a warning that a CVA can occur in the near future.

Pathophysiology and Etiology

TIAs result from impaired blood circulation in the brain. Common causes of impaired cerebral blood flow include atherosclerosis and arteriosclerosis, cardiac disease, and diabetes (see Chaps. 33, 35, and 58). Circulation is impaired by atherosclerosis (buildup of fatty plaque) in cerebral blood vessels and the formation of thrombi and microemboli. The inelastic arterial system affected by arteriosclerosis restricts the volume of blood circulating through blood vessels. Dysrhythmias and ineffective heart contraction are the catalysts for thrombi that can travel to cerebral vessels. Hypertension, which is associated with some of the previously mentioned etiologies, reduces the blood traveling to the brain and increases the potential for ruptured cerebral vessels from the elevated pressure. Smoking and other forms of tobacco use aggravate hypertension. Some medications, such as estrogens used for hormone replacement therapy and oral contraceptives, are

DRUG THERAPY TABLE 46-1	AGENTS FOR MANAGING HEADACHES

DRUG CATEGORY AND EXAMPLES/ MECHANISM OF ACTION	SIDE EFFECTS	NURSING CONSIDERATIONS
Beta Blockers		
propranolol (Inderal) Prevents vasodilation, drug of choice for prophylaxis	Bradycardia, fatigue, lethargy, depression, GI complaints, orthostatic hypotension	Do not discontinue drug abruptly. Give with food to facilitate absorption. Report difficulty breathing, slow pulse, confusion, depression.
Non-Narcotic Analgesics		
aspirin (Bayer) Analgesic effect early in the attack	Bleeding disorder, GI distress	Monitor for overuse. Give with food to decrease GI upset. Report unusual bleeding.
acetaminophen (Tylenol) Analgesic effect early in the attack	GI, liver, renal effects	Monitor liver and renal function tests. Avoid with use of other over-the-counter preparations.
Nonsteroidal Anti-Inflammatory Drugs (NSAIDs)		
ibuprofen (Advil) *naproxen (Naprosyn)* Analgesic for mild to moderate pain	Headache, dizziness, somnolence, nausea, GI upset, constipation	Better tolerated than ASA. Assess allergy to other NSAIDs. Give with food to reduce GI upset.
Narcotic Analgesics		
codeine For severe headache unrelieved by non-narcotics	Sedation, confusion, constipation	Addictive, use with caution. Report severe nausea, vomiting, palpitations, shortness of breath or difficulty breathing.
meperidine (Demerol) As above	Same as above	Never give to clients taking monoamine oxidase inhibitors. Reassure client that most people who receive opiates for medical reasons do not develop dependency. Avoid alcohol, antihistamines, sedatives, tranquilizers and over-the-counter drugs. Report severe nausea, vomiting, constipation, shortness of breath, or difficulty breathing.
butorphanol (Stadol) Relief of severe migraine headache pain (nasal spray)	Sedation, nausea, sweating, vertigo, lethargy, confusion	Very addictive, must be used cautiously. Report severe nausea, vomiting, palpitations, shortness of breath or difficulty breathing, nasal lesions or discomfort.
Ergots		
ergotamine tartrate (Ergostat) Prevents or aborts vascular headaches such as migraine and cluster	Nausea, ergotism: numbness and tingling of fingers and toes, muscle pain and weakness	Administer at first sign of attack. Need to premedicate with antiemetic. Use sparingly to prevent ergotism.
dihydroergotamine (DHE) Rapid control of vascular headaches, parenteral treatment for established headache	Nausea and vomiting, ergotism: numbness, tingling of fingers and toes, muscle pain and weakness	Premedicate with antiemetic. Administer as soon as possible after first sign of attack. Use sparingly to prevent ergotism.
Antiemetics		
promethazine (Phenergan) Controls nausea early in attack	Drowsiness, dizziness, confusion, hypotension, insomnia, vertigo	Give 15–30 min before meperidine or DHE. Avoid alcohol. Avoid sun exposure. Maintain fluid intake. Report sore throat, fever, unusual bleeding, rash, weakness.
prochlorperazine (Compazine) Control of severe nausea and vomiting	Same as above	Same as above.
Other		
sumatriptan (Imitrex) Antimigraine agent for acute attacks	Dizziness, vertigo, weakness, myalgia, blood pressure alterations	Give as soon as possible after first sign of attack. Monitor blood pressure. Report chest pain or pressure, flushing, facial swelling.

GI, gastrointestinal.

thrombogenic. During the ischemic period, motor, sensory, and cognitive functions are temporarily affected.

Assessment Findings

Symptoms of a TIA include temporary light-headedness, confusion, speech disturbances, loss of vision, diplopia, variable changes in consciousness, and numbness, weakness, impaired muscle coordination, or paralysis on one side. The symptoms are short-lived.

A neurologic examination during an attack reveals neurologic deficits. Auscultation of the carotid artery may reveal a **bruit** (abnormal sound caused by blood flowing over the rough surface of one or both carotid arteries). Ultrasound examination of the carotid artery shows an irregular shape to the artery lining caused by atherosclerotic plaques. A carotid arteriogram shows narrowing of the carotid artery. A CT scan or magnetic resonance imaging (MRI) is used to rule out other neurologic disorders with similar manifestations, such as a brain tumor.

Medical and Surgical Management

Antiplatelet and anticoagulant therapy with aspirin, dipyridamole (Persantine), ticlopidine (Ticlid), and warfarin (Coumadin) are prescribed. Hypertension is controlled with drug and diet therapy (see Chap. 35). If narrowing of the carotid artery by atherosclerotic plaques is the cause, a carotid **endarterectomy** (surgical removal of atherosclerotic plaque) is a treatment option (Fig. 46-3). A balloon angioplasty, a procedure similar to a percutaneous transluminal coronary artery angioplasty (see Chap. 33), is performed to dilate the carotid artery and increase blood flow to the brain.

Nursing Management

The nurse obtains a complete history of symptoms and medical, drug, and allergy histories. He or she weighs the client because obesity, hyperlipidemia, and atherosclerosis are related to cerebrovascular disease. The nurse checks the client's capillary blood sugar to help identify hyperglycemia associated with undiagnosed or uncontrolled diabetes mellitus. He or she measures vital signs and notes if blood pressure (BP) is 140/90 mm Hg or greater. The nurse asks the client about smoking habits. Although symptoms of a TIA usually are not permanent, the nurse performs a neurologic examination to identify the client's current status and establish a baseline for future comparisons. He or she documents and reports even subtle changes.

If the client undergoes carotid artery surgery, the nurse performs frequent neurologic checks to detect paralysis, confusion, facial asymmetry, or aphasia. He or she moni-

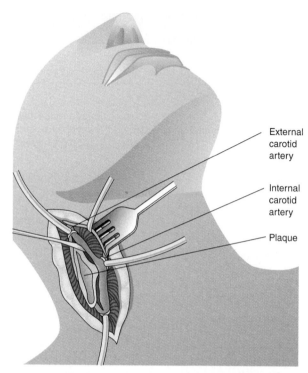

External carotid artery

Internal carotid artery

Plaque

FIGURE 46-3 Plaque is a potential source of emboli in TIAs and CVAs. It is surgically removed from the carotid artery. (From Smeltzer, S. C. & Bare, B. G. [2000]. *Brunner & Suddarth's textbook of medical–surgical nursing* [9th ed.]. Philadelphia: Lippincott Williams & Wilkins.)

tors the heart rhythm because dysrhythmias (see Chap. 34) can alter blood flow to the brain as well. Because it is possible for the neck to swell after surgery, the nurse observes the client closely for difficulty breathing or swallowing and hoarseness. The nurse places an airway at the bedside and is prepared for endotracheal intubation if an airway obstruction occurs.

The nurse teaches the client to:

- Maintain hydration by drinking the equivalent of eight glasses of fluid a day, unless contraindicated.
- Follow directions for drug therapy, including medications for controlling hypertension and diabetes.
- Monitor for signs of bruising or bleeding if antiplatelet or anticoagulant drugs are prescribed.
- Keep appointments for laboratory tests and medical follow-up to monitor the effectiveness of therapy.
- Report any future instances of sensory or motor impairment, or call 911 for emergency assistance.

● CEREBROVASCULAR ACCIDENT (STROKE)

A **cerebrovascular accident,** or stroke, is a prolonged interruption in the flow of blood through one of the arteries supplying the brain (Fig. 46-4). Brain and cerebral nerve cells are extremely sensitive to a lack of oxygen; if the brain

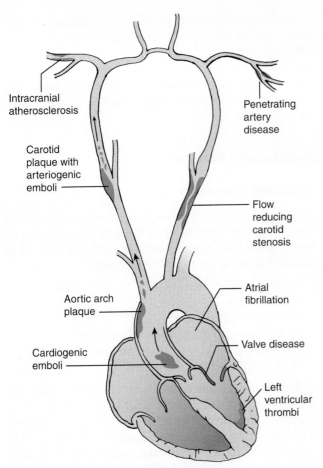

FIGURE 46-4 The most frequent sites of arterial and cardiac abnormalities causing ischemic stroke. (From Albers, G. W., Easton, D., Sacco, R. L., & Teal, P. [1999]. Antithrombotic and thrombotic therapy for ischemic stroke. *Chest, 114* [5] 684S.)

Pathophysiology and Etiology

There are two types of stroke: *ischemic strokes* and *hemorrhagic strokes.* Ischemic strokes occur when a thrombus or embolus obstructs an artery carrying blood to the brain; about 80% of strokes are the ischemic variety (Fig. 46-5). Hemorrhagic strokes occur when a cerebral blood vessel ruptures and blood is released in brain tissue (Fig. 46-6).

When ischemic strokes occur, glucose and oxygen to brain cells are reduced. The reduced glucose quickly depletes the stores of adenosine triphosphate (ATP), resulting in anaerobic cellular metabolism and the accumulation of toxic by-products such as lactic acid. Although some

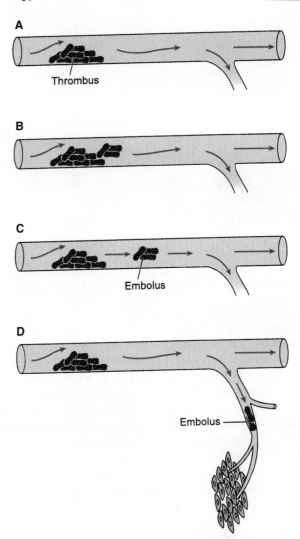

FIGURE 46-5 Evolving thrombotic CVA. (**A**) A thrombus forms in a vessel. (**B**) The force of the flowing blood over the clot helps to break off a piece from it. (**C**) The embolus is loose in the bloodstream and travels to any tissue fed by connecting blood vessels. (**D**) The embolus is pushed into a small terminal vessel, completely occluding it and causing anoxia of the tissue served by the occluded vessel.

is deprived of oxygenated blood for 3 to 7 minutes, both the brain and nerve cells begin to die. Once these cells are destroyed, the outcome is irreversible. Although the site of the cellular damage is located in the brain, the consequences are widespread. Permanent neurologic deficits have a profound physical, emotional, and financial effect on the client and the family.

brain cells die from anoxia, the lack of oxygen destroys additional brain cells by a secondary mechanism. Oxygen depletion triggers the release of glutamate, an excitatory neurotransmitter that activates neuronal receptors known as *N*-methyl-D-aspartate (NMDA) receptors (see Chap 21). The receptors allow large amounts of calcium followed by glutamate to enter the cells. Once glutamate is inside the brain cells, it literally overexcites them, causing disordered enzyme activities that release toxic free radicals, which destroy the cells (Fig. 46-7). This secondary assault extends the zone of **cerebral infarction** (death of brain tissue).

When a hemorrhagic stroke occurs, blood leaks from intracerebral arteries. The collection of blood adds volume to the intracranial contents, resulting in elevated pressure (see Chap. 45). Hemorrhagic strokes are more common in particular areas of the brain such as the cerebellum, the

FIGURE 46-6 Postmortem specimen of a cerebral hemorrhage of the right temporal lobe. (Courtesy of P. S. Milley, MD. Photograph by D. Atkinson)

R   L

structure that facilitates balance and coordination, and brain stem, which controls breathing, BP, and heart rate.

Various factors increase the risk for a CVA. Some are controllable and some are uncontrollable (Box 46-1).

Atherosclerosis and arteriosclerosis are major contributors to the formation of thromboemboli and subsequent CVAs. Common causes of cerebral hemorrhage are rupture of cerebral vessels (discussed later in this chapter), hemorrhagic disorders such as leukemia and aplastic anemia, severe hypertension, and brain tumors.

Clinical manifestations are highly variable and depend on the area of the cerebral cortex and the affected hemisphere (Table 46-2), the degree of blockage (total, partial), and the presence or absence of adequate collateral circulation. **Collateral circulation** is circulation formed by smaller blood vessels branching off from or near larger occluded vessels.

Assessment Findings

Signs and Symptoms

In some instances, clients experience one or more TIAs days, weeks, or years before a CVA, or there may be no warning and the symptoms develop suddenly. Signs of an impending stroke include the following:

- Numbness or weakness of one side of the face, an arm, or leg
- Mental confusion
- Difficulty speaking or understanding
- Impaired walking or coordination
- Severe headache

Immediately after a large cerebral hemorrhage, the client is unconscious. Breathing is noisy and labored. The cheek on the side of the CVA blows out on exhalation. The eyes deviate toward the affected side of the brain. The pulse is slow, full, and bounding. Initially, BP is elevated. Temperature is elevated during the acute phase and persists for several days. The level of consciousness (LOC)

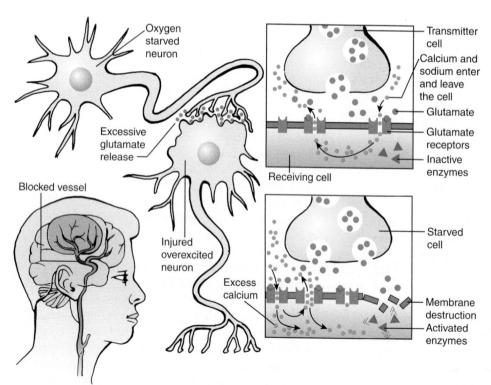

FIGURE 46-7 During stroke, oxygen is depleted, which causes release of glutamate. Glutamate activates NMDA receptors and overexcites brain cells, leading to the release of toxic free radicals, which destroy the cells.

BOX 46-1 ● Risk Factors for Cerebrovascular Accident

UNCONTROLLABLE

Age—Risk of CVA increases with each decade beyond age 55 years.

Sex—Men have a slightly higher risk than women.

Race—African Americans experience more CVAs than do other groups.

Genetics—Those whose blood relatives have had a CVA are at increased risk.

CONTROLLABLE

Hypertension—Forty percent to 90% of clients with CVA have previous hypertension.

Atrial fibrillation—Fifteen percent of those with atrial fibrillation, a dysrhythmia associated with thromboembolic complications, develop a CVA.

Hyperlipidemia—High blood cholesterol and low-density lipoprotein (LDL) levels increase the risk for atherosclerosis and CVA.

Diabetes—Elevated blood glucose level increases triglycerides and accelerates their conversion to LDLs.

History of TIA or CVA—Thirty-five percent of clients who already have had such an episode will have a CVA within 5 years; after one CVA, 42% of men and 24% of women have another.

Smoking—Nicotine is a vasoconstrictor.

Obesity—It contributes to hypertension, hyperlipidemia, and diabetes.

Thrombogenic substances—Stimulants such as herbal products derived from *Ephedra* plants, estrogens, and oral contraceptives increase risk.

Valvular disease or replacement—Thrombi and emboli form and break free from vegetations or valve replacements.

TABLE 46-2	SIGNS AND SYMPTOMS OF RIGHT-SIDED VERSUS LEFT-SIDED HEMIPLEGIA	
RIGHT-SIDED HEMIPLEGIA (STROKE ON LEFT SIDE OF BRAIN)	**LEFT-SIDED HEMIPLEGIA (STROKE ON RIGHT SIDE OF BRAIN)**	
Expressive aphasia	Spatial–perceptual defects	
Receptive aphasia	Denial; the deficits of the affected side require special safety considerations	
Global aphasia	Tendency to distractibility	
Intellectual impairment	Impulsive behavior; unaware of deficits	
Slow and cautious behavior	Poor judgment	
Defects in right visual fields	Defects in left visual fields	
Short retention of information	Misjudge distances	
Require frequent reminding to complete tasks	Difficulty distinguishing upside-down and right-side-up	
Difficulty with new learning	Impairment of short-term memory	
Problems with abstract thinking, such as conceptualizing and generalizing	Neglect left side of body; objects and people on left side	

---

ranges from lethargy and mental confusion to deep coma, which can persist for days or even weeks. The longer the coma, the poorer the prognosis and the less likely that consciousness will return.

A common neurologic result of a CVA in the motor area of the cerebrum is **hemiplegia** (paralysis on one side of the body). Hemiplegia occurs on the side opposite the area of the brain that is affected because motor nerves cross over (decussate) at the level of the neck. For example, when the motor area on the right side of the brain incurs a CVA, hemiplegia develops on the left side of the body: There is left-sided hemiplegia when the CVA occurs in the right hemisphere of the brain. Immediately after the CVA, the affected side is flaccid. This progresses to spastic limbs. The arm typically is more severely affected than the leg.

Expressive aphasia, the inability to speak, or **receptive aphasia,** the inability to understand spoken and written language, can result depending on where the client's speech center is located in the brain. For most, the speech center is in the dominant hemisphere (i.e., if a person is right handed, the speech center is in the left hemisphere). A right-handed person who has a CVA in the left brain usually develops aphasia, and vice versa for a left-handed person.

Hemianopia on the affected side is another potential consequence. **Hemianopia** is the ability to see only half of the normal visual field (Fig. 46-8). When looking straight ahead, the client cannot see to the right or left with either eye. This condition is caused by damage to the visual area of the cerebral cortex or its connections to the brain stem

(optic radiations). This deficit, like other deficits that result from a CVA, may subside completely, partially, or not at all. Confusion and emotional lability also are characteristic symptoms of a CVA.

Diagnostic Findings

A CT scan or MRI differentiates a CVA from other disorders, such as a brain tumor or cerebral edema, and shows the size and location of the infarcted area. Transcranial Doppler ultrasonography determines the size of intracranial vessels and the direction of blood flow, and locates the obstructed cerebral vessel. Single-photon emission CT also determines cerebral blood flow. An electroencephalogram reveals reduced electrical activity in the involved area, but is not a specific diagnostic test for a CVA. A lumbar puncture often is performed. If subarachnoid bleeding has occurred, the cerebrospinal fluid will be bloody. Cerebral angiography shows displacement or blockage of cerebral vessels.

Medical and Surgical Management

CVAs are prevented by reducing certain risk factors such as hypertension, overweight, cardiac dysrhythmias (especially atrial fibrillation), and high blood cholesterol levels. Prevention measures include prophylactic anticoagulant or antiplatelet therapy (including daily aspirin) in selected

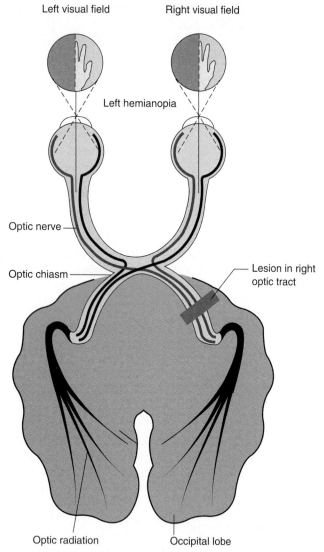

FIGURE 46-8 Hemianopia is a visual-field defect in which a person experiences an inability to see the left or right half of an image. It develops when a stroke involves the visual pathway.

TABLE 46-3	INCLUSION AND EXCLUSION CRITERIA FOR THERAPY WITH TISSUE PLASMINOGEN ACTIVATOR

INCLUSION CRITERIA	EXCLUSION CRITERIA
Clinical evidence of an ischemic attack	Stroke or serious head trauma in past 3 mo
Age >18 yr	Major surgery or invasive procedure within past 14 days
Signed consent, if possible	
Onset of stroke within 3 hr of initiation of therapy (or from time client was last seen as "normal")	Gastrointestinal or urinary bleeding within past 21 days
	Puncture of noncompressible artery or biopsy of internal organ within past 7 days
Normal prothrombin and partial thromboplastin times	Seizure preceding or during stroke
	History of intracranial hemorrhage or known history of cerebral vascular malformations
	Pericarditis, endocarditis, septic emboli, recent pregnancy, or active inflammatory bowel disease

In many cases, treatment is supportive because medical or surgical interventions cannot repair damaged brain tissue. The best treatment available involves an intensive medical program aimed at rehabilitation and the prevention of future CVAs.

Nursing Management

Detailed nursing management for the client with a CVA is discussed in Nursing Care Plan 46-1. Client and family teaching also is essential and focuses on the following points:

- Administer medications as directed and understand the potential side and adverse effects.
- Implement eating and swallowing techniques that reduce the potential for aspiration.
- Perform the Heimlich maneuver to clear the airway if the client cannot speak or breathe after swallowing food (see Chap. 28).
- Continue follow-up care with the speech pathologist and dietitian.
- Contact community resources such as medical supply companies that rent or sell special care devices such as a hospital bed, bedside commode, walker, or tripod cane.
- Remove throw rugs, clutter, and electrical cords from the client's home environment to reduce the potential for falls.

people and management of medical disorders, such as diabetes mellitus and cardiovascular disease.

When a CVA occurs, it is a medical emergency. Treatment varies and is directed toward relieving the cause, if known. Tissue plasminogen activator (TPA), a thrombolytic agent, has been found to limit neurologic deficits when given within 3 to 6 hours after the onset of the CVA (Table 46-3). It is contraindicated in hemorrhagic CVAs, as is anticoagulant therapy. Several neuroprotective agents, such as NMDA receptor blockers, calcium and glutamate antagonists, and antioxidants, are nearing completion in clinical trials. Hypothermia also is being used to protect damaged cells by reducing their metabolic need for oxygen.

If atherosclerosis of the carotid artery is the cause, a carotid endarterectomy is considered. A ruptured cerebral aneurysm is treated surgically.

(text continued on page 654)

Nursing Care Plan 46-1

THE CLIENT WITH A CEREBROVASCULAR ACCIDENT

Assessment

Determine the following:

- Time symptoms began
- Medical, drug, and allergy history from the family (or client if he or she can report)
- Vital signs and LOC
- Any musculoskeletal weakness or paralysis
- Capacity to speak or understand spoken language
- Changes in visual field
- Ability to swallow
- Any alteration in bladder or bowel control
- Integrity of the skin; evidence of soft tissue injury as a consequence of falling

Nursing Diagnoses: **Impaired Swallowing** related to hemiplegia; **Risk for Aspiration** related to impaired swallowing; **Risk for Deficient Fluid Volume** related to impaired swallowing; **Risk for Imbalanced Nutrition: Less than Body Requirements** related to impaired swallowing

Expected Outcomes: (1) Client will swallow without aspiration. (2) Fluid intake will be at least 2000 mL/24 hours. (3) Client will consume sufficient calories to maintain admission weight.

Interventions	Rationales
Elevate client's head for eating or drinking; position client on his or her side at other times.	Sitting and facing food or liquids raises client's awareness and attention; a side-lying position prevents aspiration if vomiting occurs or saliva accumulates in the mouth.
Keep a suction machine at the bedside.	Mechanical suctioning facilitates clearing the airway of saliva, food, and fluids.
Limit distractions (e.g., turn off the television when the client eats or drinks).	The client can better concentrate and follow nursing instructions when distracting stimuli are reduced.
Use a thickening agent for watery substances; request viscous or pureed food from the dietary department.	The tongue can more easily manipulate thickened liquids against the palate and oral pharynx.
Request small, frequent nourishment from the dietary department rather than three large meals.	Eating small amounts is less tiring, and the client may consume more on a daily basis.
Offer or remind client to load the fork or spoon with a small amount of food.	A small amount is easier to manage in the mouth and less likely to cause a complete airway obstruction.
Place thickened liquids or pureed food on the unaffected side of the mouth.	The client can feel and use the unaffected side of the mouth for chewing and swallowing.
Lower client's chin to his or her chest when swallowing.	Lowering the chin helps close the laryngopharynx and reduces the potential for aspiration.
Encourage client to swallow several times.	Several efforts at swallowing may be necessary to move food to the esophagus.

(continued)

Nursing Care Plan 46-1 (Continued)

THE CLIENT WITH A CEREBROVASCULAR ACCIDENT

Interventions	Rationales
Check the mouth for pocketed food before offering more.	The client may be unaware of food that remains unswallowed.
Instruct client to use the tongue to relocate pocketed food or apply gentle pressure on the cheek to reposition food. Collaborate with the physician concerning gastric or enteral tube feedings if oral intake is inadequate.	Physical manipulation helps reposition trapped food.

Evaluation of Expected Outcomes: The airway remains patent, and lungs are clear to auscultation.

Nursing Diagnoses: **Total Urinary Incontinence; Bowel Incontinence** or **Risk for Constipation** related to diminished LOC, confusion, and immobility

Expected Outcome: Urinary and bowel elimination will be controlled independently or with minimal assistance.

Interventions	Rationales
Maintain a record of bowel elimination.	It provides data that can indicate if the client requires a stool softener, laxative, suppository, or enema.
Place an elevated seat over the toilet.	An elevated seat reduces the work of transferring to the toilet seat and back to a wheelchair.
Assist client to the toilet every 2 hours while he or she is awake and after each meal.	Positioning and environmental cues may help stimulate the client to eliminate. The gastrocolic reflex that promotes bowel evacuation is stronger soon after eating.
Dress client in unrestricted clothing that facilitates elimination needs.	Clothing that is easy to undo or lower reduces the potential for incontinence.
Avoid negative comments if incontinence occurs; acknowledge client's success when he or she eliminates while on the toilet or commode.	Criticism lowers self-confidence and self-esteem; praise encourages client to continue efforts at controlling elimination.
Apply incontinence garments or place absorbent pads beneath client.	Concealment of urine or stool preserves client's dignity.
Collaborate with the physician concerning the insertion of an external or indwelling catheter.	An external catheter is less likely to predispose to a urinary tract infection; a catheter helps keep the skin dry and reduces embarrassment of incontinence.
Administer a prescribed suppository or low-volume enema when necessary.	Chemical or mechanical stimulation increases intestinal contraction, which helps to evacuate the bowel.

Evaluation of Expected Outcome: Bowel and urinary elimination are managed at the highest level the client can achieve.

Nursing Diagnoses: **Self-Care Deficit** related to hemiplegia; **Unilateral Neglect** related to hemianopia; **Impaired Mobility: Physical** related to hemiplegia

Expected Outcomes: (1) Client will resume independent activities of daily living (ADLs). (2) Client will identify and care for paralyzed body parts. (3) Client will use assistive devices to achieve mobility.

(continued)

Nursing Care Plan 46-1 *(Continued)*

THE CLIENT WITH A CEREBROVASCULAR ACCIDENT

Interventions	Rationales
Approach and place objects within client's field of vision.	Client is likely to ignore objects and people that are located in areas where the visual field is impaired.
Help reintegrate the weak side by reminding the client to look at it.	Calling attention to the neglected side of the body helps the client recognize and accept that it exists.
Set realistic goals for self-care.	Unrealistic goals lead to frustration and discouragement.
Consult with an occupational therapist (OT) or physical therapist (PT) regarding modifications in clothing, utensils, and assistive devices.	Therapists have expertise in measures to accommodate for neurologic deficits.
Attach a trapeze above the bed.	Client can use a trapeze with one hand to independently facilitate position changes.
Perform range-of-motion (ROM) exercises at least once each shift.	ROM exercises maintain joint mobility and muscle tone.
Support the affected arm in a sling when the client is upright.	An arm sling improves posture and reduces musculo-skeletal changes in the shoulder joint.
Position client to avoid contractures (e.g., use a foot board, trochanter roll at the hip, rolled cloth in the paralyzed hand).	Skeletal muscles tend to become permanently shorted unless efforts are made to maintain normal anatomic position.
Consult the PT about devices to assist ambulation, such as a leg brace and walker.	A brace promotes stability when standing and walking. A walker supports the client and facilitates ambulation.

Evaluation of Expected Outcomes: Client performs ADLs alone or with assistance and learns to use assistive devices.

Nursing Diagnosis: **Risk for Impaired Skin Integrity** related to pressure over bony prominences secondary to immobility

Expected Outcome: Skin will remain intact.

Interventions	Rationales
Keep skin clean and dry.	Cleaning the skin removes transient bacteria. Drying the skin prevents maceration, a process in which skin is softened and easily eroded.
Use a turning sheet and get assistance when changing client's position.	A turning sheet prevents shearing, the movement of a layer of tissue in one direction as another moves in opposition.
Massage skin areas that blanch when pressure is relieved.	Massage improves blood flow to tissue, but it is contra-indicated if tissue is already damaged as evidenced by a sustained lack of color when pressure is relieved.
Use pressure-relieving devices or a therapeutic bed that alternately distributes the client's body weight.	Tissue damage occurs unless intracapillary pressure is maintained at 32 mm Hg or more; relief of pressure at least every 2 hours reduces tissue hypoxia.

Evaluation of Expected Outcome: Skin is intact; there is no evidence of pressure sores.

Nursing Diagnosis: **Impaired Verbal Communication** related to expressive aphasia

Expected Outcome: Client will make needs understood either verbally or nonverbally.

(continued)

Nursing Care Plan 46-1 (Continued)

THE CLIENT WITH A CEREBROVASCULAR ACCIDENT

Interventions	Rationales
Ask questions requiring a "yes" or "no," and suggest the client respond by nodding the head.	Nodding the head is a form of body language that communicates agreement or disagreement.
Instruct client to speak slowly when attempting to communicate orally.	If unpressured to quickly respond, the client may be able to formulate words and sentences more easily.
Have client point to or write key words or phrases.	Some clients retain the ability to read written language although they may not be able to express themselves orally.
Support and practice techniques used in speech therapy.	Practicing new techniques helps to promote mastery.

Evaluation of Expected Outcome: Client can communicate either orally, in writing, or with techniques that facilitate nonverbal communication.

Nursing Diagnoses: **Risk for Ineffective Coping** and **Risk for Compromised Family Coping** related to diminished psychosocial resources to deal with multiple stressors
Expected Outcome: Client and family will cope with illness and changes in lifestyle.

Interventions	Rationales
Listen and try to identify clues to client's or family's future concerns.	Identifying problems that require actions facilitates coping.
Acknowledge personal strengths.	Recognition of strengths promotes confidence in the ability to overcome current problems.
Encourage individuals in the client's social network to collaborate on problem-solving.	Successful outcomes are more likely when there is a team effort.
Refer client and family to a discharge planner, social worker, or community social services for arranging extended care, home care, and respite care.	The health team includes persons with expertise in assisting clients and their families with postdischarge issues.

Evaluation of Expected Outcome:

■ Client and family cope with the client's neurologic deficits; referrals are made to services or facilities that can assist with long-term recovery.

■ The family pursues a plan for postdischarge management.

● Perform regular exercises, change the client's position frequently, and apply braces or splints designed to maintain extremities in proper anatomic position.

Stop, Think, and Respond ● BOX 46-1

When a client with an evolving CVA arrives in the emergency department, her speech is difficult to understand, the left side of her face has a drooped appearance, and she cannot move her left arm and leg. Before this client becomes a candidate for TPA, what other information is important to gather?

● CEREBRAL ANEURYSMS

An **aneurysm** is a weakening in the wall of a blood vessel. Most aneurysms occur in arteries, where blood flow is under high pressure. Cerebral aneurysms usually occur in the circle of Willis, a ring of arteries that supply the brain (Fig. 46-9).

Pathophysiology and Etiology

Aneurysms develop at the site of a weakened area in the blood vessel wall. The defect is congenital or secondary to hypertension and atherosclerosis.

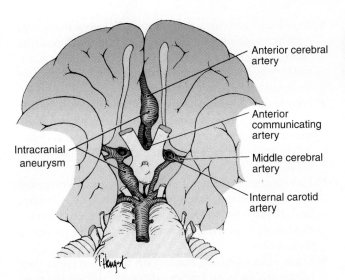

FIGURE 46-9 Intracranial aneurysm within circle of Willis.

TABLE 46-4	THE HUNT-HESS SCALE FOR GRADING A CLIENT WITH A CEREBRAL ANEURYSM
CLASSIFICATION	**CLINICAL CRITERIA**
Grade I	Alert, oriented, asymptomatic
Grade II	Alert, oriented, headache, stiff neck
Grade III	Lethargic or confused, minor focal deficits such as hemiparesis (weakness on one side)
Grade IV	Stupor, moderate to severe focal deficits such as hemiplegia
Grade V	Comatose, severe neurologic deficits such as posturing (see Chap. 47)

(Adapted from Hickey, J. V. [2002]. *The clinical practice of neurological and neurosurgical nursing* [5th ed.]. Philadelphia: Lippincott Williams & Wilkins.)

An aneurysm can affect cranial nerve function (see Chap. 44) as the aneurysm presses on these structures. For many, there is no prior warning that an aneurysm exists. Berry aneurysms, a type of congenital cerebral aneurysm, can rupture at any time without prior symptoms. The sudden cerebral hemorrhage causes immediate neurologic changes from IICP, interruption of oxygenated blood flow to the surrounding cells and tissues, and blood collecting in the subarachnoid space. Occasionally, there is a slow leakage of blood from an aneurysm, in which case symptoms are less severe.

Assessment Findings

Symptoms include sudden and severe headache, dizziness, nausea, and vomiting, usually followed by a rapid loss of consciousness. If the ruptured aneurysm produces a slow leak, a stiff neck, headache, visual disturbances, and intermittent nausea develop.

Cerebral angiography can reveal an unruptured aneurysm. The procedure is done with caution because the added fluid pressure can increase the risk of rupturing the blood vessel, dislodge plaque-formed emboli, and cause ischemia from vasospasm. A CT scan and MRI are safer for locating the site of the aneurysm and determining the amount of blood in the subarachnoid space. A lumbar puncture reveals grossly bloody cerebrospinal fluid when an aneurysm ruptures. The physician may identify the status and prognosis of the client based on criteria in the Hunt-Hess classification system (Table 46-4). As the grade increases, the prognosis becomes less optimistic.

Medical Management

Conservative management is attempted until a decision is made regarding surgical repair of the aneurysm. Some aneurysms are considered inoperable because of anatomic location, and only medical treatment is possible.

Complete bed rest, the prevention of rebleeding at the rupture site, and treatment of complications are primary goals. Absolute bed rest in a quiet area, preferably a private room, is essential. Visitors are restricted except for family members. The head of the bed is elevated to reduce ICP and cerebral edema. Hypertension is treated with antihypertensive agents. Anticonvulsants are given to prevent seizures. Tranquilizers or barbiturates are used to keep the conscious client relaxed and quiet. IICP is managed with osmotic diuretics and corticosteroids (see Chap. 45).

Mechanical ventilation is necessary to support respirations and provide oxygenation if the client is unconscious. Aminocaproic acid (Amicar) is used to delay lysis (breaking up) of the blood clot because lysis results in rebleeding.

Surgical Management

Surgical repair is attempted after the initial hemorrhage because the danger of further hemorrhage from the weakened aneurysm is great. The operation is not without hazard; manipulation of the small cerebral vessels can result in increased vasospasm or thrombosis and cerebral infarction. The risks of surgery are less serious than the dangers of recurrent hemorrhage from the aneurysm. Surgical approaches with a craniotomy include wrapping or clipping the aneurysm in an attempt to control further bleeding (Fig. 46-10).

An alternative to direct repair of the aneurysm by a craniotomy approach is ligation of or application of a clamp to one of the carotid arteries. This is an extracranial (outside the cranium) procedure because the surgical approach is below the jaw. The purpose of this approach is

FIGURE 46-10 An aneurysm is clamped to prevent rupture. Wrapping the aneurysm with supportive material is another alternative.

to obstruct blood flow to the vessel that has an aneurysm, thus reducing the pressure in the aneurysm and preventing rupture or further bleeding. Collateral circulation in the cerebral vessels must be adequate for success.

NURSING PROCESS

● The Client With an Aneurysm

Assessment

The nurse performs a neurologic examination, taking care to avoid disturbing the client. The nurse measures vital signs frequently. If the client is conscious, the nurse asks only essential questions while gathering the client's history, limiting it primarily to the current onset of symptoms. He or she obtains a more complete history from the family.

Diagnosis, Planning, and Interventions

PC: Increased Intracranial Pressure related to bleeding in the brain

Expected Outcome: The nurse will monitor for, manage, and minimize IICP.

- Use the Glasgow Coma Scale (GCS) to assess neurologic status at least every hour (see Chap. 47). *The GCS is a systematic assessment tool for documenting neurologic function and identifying early clinical changes.*
- Report neurologic changes as soon as a trend indicates worsening of the client's condition. *Early collaboration with the physician facilitates implementing medically prescribed interventions that will reduce or eliminate more serious complications.*
- Keep client calm and physically still. *Activity or emotional distress elevates BP and ICP, which could cause or contribute to more bleeding.*

- Avoid any activities that cause a Valsalva maneuver such as coughing, straining at stool, and rough position changes. *Bearing down raises BP and increases the potential for rupture of the aneurysm or increased bleeding if the aneurysm has already ruptured.*
- Follow the physician's orders for fluid restrictions and drug therapy for reducing hypertension, potential seizures, restlessness, and anxiety. *Interventions that reduce BP, large motor movements, and emotional stress help to reduce ICP.*
- Elevate client's head or follow the physician's directive for body position (some prefer that the client remain flat). *Head elevation helps venous blood and cerebrospinal fluid drain from cerebral areas and reduces the volume in the cranium.*
- Limit visitors to the immediate family; suggest they take turns and stay briefly. *Although visitors' and family members' desire to interact with the client are well intentioned, the stimulation can increase ICP or trigger a seizure.*

PC: Seizures related to IICP

Expected Outcome: The nurse will monitor to detect, manage, and minimize seizures.

- Institute seizure precautions (see Chap. 45). *Seizure precautions are used to prevent or minimize seizure-related injuries.*
- Implement anticonvulsant drug therapy as prescribed. *Anticonvulsants reduce excitation of neurons in the brain that result in seizure activity.*

Pain (headache) related to IICP

Expected Outcome: Pain will be reduced or eliminated.

- Avoid administering opioid analgesics, except codeine. *Opioids interfere with accurate assessment of neurologic function because they constrict the pupils and depress LOC.*
- Reduce environmental stimuli, and use nursing interventions such as distraction, guided imagery, and soothing music. *Nonpharmacologic techniques for pain relief are based on blocking the brain's awareness of pain by substituting another form of sensory or cognitive stimulus.*
- Take care not to jar the bed or cause unnecessary activity. *Unexpected movement and physical activity tend to intensify the pain experience.*

Self-Care Deficit related to imposed rest and decreased LOC

Expected Outcome: Client's basic needs will be met.

- Perform only those activities of daily living for the client that are absolutely necessary. *Keeping the client quiet, which reduces the risk for life-threatening complications, takes greater precedence over bathing, ambulating, and the like.*
- Provide rest between necessary nursing tasks. *Limiting tasks to brief moments prevents overstimulating the client.*
- Feed client calorie-dense foods in small amounts at frequent intervals. *In this way, the client's hunger is managed without requiring a large intake of food at any one time.*

Risk for Ineffective Peripheral Tissue Perfusion and **Risk for Impaired Skin Integrity** related to imposed inactivity

Expected Outcomes: (1) Peripheral circulation will be maintained. (2) Skin will remain intact.

• Apply elastic stockings to lower extremities or use a pneumatic compression device. *Intermittent compression passively moves venous blood toward the heart in a way similar to active skeletal muscle contraction. Elastic stockings support the valves of veins in the lower extremities to prevent venous stasis.*

• Use pressure-relieving pads or a similar type of mattress. *Relieving pressure promotes the circulation of oxygenated blood through the capillary to peripheral cells and tissues and facilitates venous blood return.*

Evaluation of Expected Outcomes

The ICP is maintained within a safe range. The client does not manifest seizures. His or her level of discomfort is tolerable. Essential needs for nutrition, hydration, ventilation, and elimination are met. Peripheral circulation is adequate; there are no signs of skin breakdown. For the client who undergoes a craniotomy, refer to Chapter 45.

Discharge teaching depends on the method of treatment and the recommendations of the physician. Usually, the nurse instructs clients to avoid:

• Heavy lifting
• Straining at stool
• Extreme emotional situations
• Other work-related activities that could raise BP and increase ICP

When the client must restrict his or her lifestyle, the changes are likely to cause financial, physical, and social hardships for the client and family. Referrals to a social service worker, counselor, or social service agency are appropriate.

GENERAL NUTRITIONAL CONSIDERATIONS

When the client can resume oral intake after a CVA, individualize the diet according to his or her ability to chew and swallow. Semisolid and medium-consistency foods such as pudding, scrambled eggs, cooked cereals, and thickened liquids are easiest to swallow. The client should avoid foods most likely to cause choking: peanut butter, bread, tart foods, dry or crisp foods, and chewy meats. Progress the texture as swallowing ability improves.

Cold foods stimulate swallowing; avoid tepid foods, because they are more difficult to locate in the mouth, and extremely hot foods, which can cause overreaction.

Clients with decreased salivation benefit from added gravies and sauces. Thinking of a specific food before eating stimulates salivation, as do eating dill pickles and sucking on lemon slices.

To minimize the volume of food needed, provide nutritionally dense foods such as thickened commercial beverages, fortified puddings, fortified cooked cereals, and scrambled eggs.

When a normal oral diet is resumed, encourage the client to eat "heart healthy"—less total fat and saturated fat and more fruits, vegetables, and whole grains. Encourage overweight clients to lose weight to reduce cardiac workload. Sodium restriction is appropriate for clients with hypertension.

GENERAL PHARMACOLOGIC CONSIDERATIONS

Anticoagulant therapy with heparin is given parenterally or with an oral anticoagulant for some clients who have had a CVA.

If the client is receiving heparin, the dose is ordered after each clotting time determination.

If heparin is administered by the subcutaneous route, do not massage the site of injection before or after giving the drug. There is no need to aspirate before injecting the heparin. The recommended site for subcutaneous injection is the abdomen. Rotate injection sites; avoid areas within 2 inches of the umbilicus.

The most notable adverse effect of heparin is hemorrhage. Keep protamine sulfate available if it becomes necessary to counteract the effects of heparin.

Aspirin (1 to 1.3 g/day orally) may be given prophylactically for TIAs. Aspirin prolongs the bleeding time and inhibits platelet aggregation. If gastric upset occurs, the drug may be given with food, with an antacid, or in an enterically coated form.

If the client is receiving an oral anticoagulant, adjust the dose according to laboratory findings. Optimum therapeutic results are obtained when prothrombin levels are 1.5 to 2.5 times the normal control value, or the international normalized ratio value is 2.0 to 3.0.

Bleeding can occur at any time, even when the prothrombin level appears to be within safe limits. Observe the client for evidence of bleeding such as easy bruising, nosebleeds, excessive bleeding from small cuts, and blood in the urine or stool. Keep the antidote for oral anticoagulants, parenteral vitamin K, available.

GENERAL GERONTOLOGIC CONSIDERATIONS

Older adults who experience TIAs may ignore the symptoms, thinking that they are part of the normal aging process, because symptoms usually subside shortly.

One major risk factor for stroke is hypertension. At times, the older adult with hypertension may become noncompliant with his or her medication regimen, thus increasing the risk of CVA. Client education is important to foster compliance.

The rehabilitation of the elderly client with a CVA is difficult and subject to more complications than with a younger adult. The family may be unable to provide the care needed in the home setting, and the client may need to go to a rehabilitation center or a nursing home for rehabilitation.

The older adult client is more susceptible to the complications of prolonged bed rest and inactivity. Because the rehabilitation period after a CVA often is prolonged, closely observe the elderly client for problems such as hypostatic pneumonia, pressure ulcers, and contractures.

Older clients with moderate to severe neurologic deficits may place a financial and physical burden on their spouse or children. The nurse must work closely with the family and social service agencies to help the family assume the care of their family member to the extent possible.

Critical Thinking Exercises

1. *What suggestions could you give to someone who has migraine headaches to help reduce their severity?*
2. *When assigned to care for a client with a leaking cerebral aneurysm, what nursing interventions are appropriate for reducing the potential for a serious intracranial bleed?*

References and Suggested Readings

Bader, M. K. (1998). Case presentations of neuroradiologic interventions for acute cerebrovascular disease. *Journal of Cardiovascular Nursing, 13*(1), 1–16.

Bacoka, J. (2000). Action stat: Aortic dissection—act fast to intervene and prevent stroke, renal failure, or death. *Nursing, 30*(8), 33.

Bell, T. E., Kongable, G. L., & Steinberg, G. K. (1998). Mild hypothermia: An alternative to deep hypothermia for achieving neuroprotection. *Journal of Cardiovascular Nursing, 13*(1), 33–44.

Bostwick, J. & Sneade, M. (2001). Subarachnoid haemorrhage, managing complications. *Nursing Times, 97*(35), 28–29.

Braimah, J., Kongable, G., Rapp, K., et al. (1997). Nursing care of acute stroke patients after receiving rt-PA therapy. *Journal of Neuroscience Nursing, 29,* 393–414.

Evans, V. & Barr, J. (1998). Case study: Nursing care of the patient with vertebral artery aneurysm treated by endovascular stenting and coil implantation. *Journal of Neuroscience Nursing, 30,* 279–282.

Gendreau-Webb, R. (2001). Action stat: Acute ischemic stroke. *Nursing, 31*(9), 120.

Hock, N. H. (1999). Brain attack: The stroke continuum. *Nursing Clinics of North America, 34,* 689–725.

Hock, N. H. (1998). Neuroprotective and thrombolytic agents: Advances in stroke treatment. *Journal of Neuroscience Nursing, 30,* 175–185.

Kunkel, R. S. (2000). Managing primary headache syndromes. *Patient Care, 34*(2), 100–103, 107–110, 115–117+.

Linsey, J. (2000). Implementing a stroke risk assessment program in a community setting. *Journal of Neuroscience Nursing, 32,* 266–271.

Mathers, D. (2001). Kernig's sign . . . Protecting a patient with ruptured cerebral aneurysm. *Nursing, 31*(8), 8.

Meyer, J. S., Thornby, J., Crawford, K., et al. (2000). Reversible cognitive decline accompanies migraine and cluster headaches. *Headache, 40,* 638–646.

Mower-Wade, D., Cavanaugh, M. C., & Bush, D. (2001). Protecting a patient with ruptured cerebral aneurysm. *Nursing, 31*(2), 52–58.

National Institute of Neurological Disorders and Stroke. (2002). Headache—hope through research. [On-line.] Available: http://www.ninds.nih.gov_andmedical/pubs/headache_htr.htm.

Orr, P. (1998). No way home . . . cerebral hemorrhage. *Nursing Times, 94*(22), 40–41.

Pfohman, M. & Criddle, L. M. (2001). Epidemiology of intracranial aneurysm and subarachnoid hemorrhage. *Journal of Neuroscience Nursing, 33,* 39–41.

Pope, W. & Morrison, S. R. (2001). Coiled for success: The endovascular treatment of cerebral aneurysms. *Nursing Spectrum (Greater Philadelphia/Tri-State Edition), 10*(6), 26–27.

Schretzman, D. (2001). Acute ischemic stroke. *Dimensions of Critical Care Nursing, 20*(2), 14–22.

Spilker, J., Kongable, G., Rapp, K., et al. (1997). Using the NIH stroke scale to assess stroke patients. *Journal of Neuroscience Nursing, 29,* 384–393.

Vance, D. L. (2001). Treating acute ischemic stroke with intravenous Alteplase. *Critical Care Nurse, 21*(4), 25–35.

Ward, T. N. (2000). Providing relief from headache: Current options for acute and prophylactic therapy. *Postgraduate Medicine, 108*(3), 121–128.

Weiss, J. (2001). Assessing and managing the patient with headaches. *Dimensions of Critical Care Nursing, 20*(3), 15–23.

Westergren, A., Karlsson, S., Andersson, P., et al. (2001). Eating difficulties, need for assisted eating, nutritional status and pressure ulcers in patients admitted for stroke rehabilitation. *Journal of Clinical Nursing, 10,* 257–269.

Westergren, A., Ohlsson, O., & Hallberg, I. R. (2001). Eating difficulties, complications and nursing interventions during the first three months after a stroke. *Journal of Advanced Nursing, 35,* 416–426.

Willoughby, D. F., Saunders, L., & Privette, A. (2001). The impact of a stroke screening program. *Public Health Nursing, 18,* 418–423.

Caring for Clients With Head and Spinal Cord Trauma

Words to Know

autonomic dysreflexia
autoregulation
Battle's sign
cerebral hematoma
chemonucleolysis
closed head injury
concussion
contrecoup injury
contusion
coup injury
craniectomy
cranioplasty
craniotomy
diskectomy
epidural hematoma
extramedullary
halo sign
infratentorial

intracerebral
  hematoma
intramedullary
laminectomy
open head injury
otorrhea
paraplegia
paresthesia
periorbital ecchymosis
poikilothermia
rhinorrhea
spinal fusion
spinal shock
subdural hematoma
supratentorial
tentorium
tetraplegia
uncal herniation

Learning Objectives

On completion of this chapter, the reader will:

- Differentiate a concussion from a contusion.
- Explain the differences between epidural, subdural, and intracerebral hematomas.
- Discuss the nursing management of a client with a head injury.
- Discuss the nursing management of a client undergoing intracranial surgery.
- Explain spinal shock, listing four symptoms.
- Discuss autonomic dysreflexia and at least five manifestations.
- Describe the nursing management of a client with a spinal cord injury.

Head and spinal cord trauma can result in permanent disability and dysfunction. This chapter discusses head injuries, which include lacerations, skull fractures, internal bleeding, and edema of the brain and surrounding tissues. It also discusses spinal disorders caused by trauma and mechanical injury.

HEAD INJURIES

Injury to the head can cause concussions, contusions, hematomas, or skull fracture.

• CONCUSSION

Pathophysiology and Etiology

A **concussion** results from a blow to the head that jars the brain. It usually is a consequence of falling, striking the head against a hard surface like a windshield, colliding with another person (e.g., between athletes), battering during boxing, or being a victim of violence. A concussion results in diffuse and microscopic injury to the brain. The force of the blow causes temporary neurologic impairment but no serious damage to cerebral tissue. Recovery is complete and usually within a short time. In older adults, however, recovery may take longer.

Assessment Findings

The client may experience a brief lapse of consciousness, with temporary disorientation, headache, blurred or double vision, emotional irritability, and dizziness commonly following. Skull radiography, computed tomography (CT) scan, and magnetic resonance imaging (MRI) rule out a more serious head injury (e.g., skull fracture, intracranial bleeding).

Medical Management

The client's activity is temporarily halted until the seriousness of the injury is determined. Mild analgesia (usually acetaminophen) relieves the headache. The client is observed for neurologic complications.

Nursing Management

The nurse performs a neurologic assessment (see Chap. 44). If findings are normal and the client does not require hospitalization, the nurse instructs the family to watch the client closely for signs of increased intracranial pressure (IICP). Common signs of IICP include behavioral alterations, sleepiness, personality changes, vomiting, and speech or gait disturbances (see Chap. 45). The nurse instructs the client and family to contact a physician or return to the emergency department (ED) if any of these symptoms occur.

● CONTUSION

Pathophysiology and Etiology

A **contusion** is more serious than a concussion and leads to gross structural injury to the brain. Contusions result in bruising and, sometimes, hemorrhage of superficial cerebral tissue. When the head is struck directly, the injury to the brain is called a **coup injury.** Dual bruising can result if the force is strong enough to send the brain ricocheting to the opposite side of the skull, which is called a **contrecoup injury** (Fig. 47-1). Edema develops at the site of or in areas opposite to the injury. A skull fracture can accompany a contusion.

Assessment Findings

Signs and symptoms vary depending on the severity of the blow and the degree of head velocity. Clients exhibit hypotension, rapid and weak pulse, shallow respirations, loss of consciousness, and pale, clammy skin. While un-

FIGURE 47-1 Coup and contrecoup injuries occur at the point of contact and when the brain rebounds from the opposite direction.

conscious, they usually respond to strong stimuli, such as pressure applied to base of the nail (Fig. 47-2). On awakening, clients often have temporary *amnesia* (loss of memory) for recent events. Permanent brain damage can impair intellect and gait and cause speech difficulty, seizures, and paralysis.

Skull radiography is performed to rule out or confirm skull fracture. CT or MRI detects bleeding or small hemorrhages in brain tissue, a shift in brain tissue, and edema at the injury site.

Medical Management

The unstable client's vital functions are supported with drug therapy and mechanical ventilation if necessary.

Nursing Management

The nurse observes the client closely for changes in level of consciousness (LOC), signs of IICP (see Chap. 45), neu-

FIGURE 47-2 The nurse tests the client's motor response by assessing response to a painful stimulus. (Photo © B. Proud.)

rologic changes, respiratory distress, and changes in vital signs every 1 to 2 hours. If symptoms develop, the nurse reports them to the physician.

Prevention of health problems is a major component of nursing care. To reduce the potential for both minor and life-threatening head injuries, the nurse stresses:

- Using seatbelts for all passengers in automobiles
- Restraining infants in approved car seats located in the rear seats of automobiles
- Wearing protective head gear while riding bicycles or motorcycles and participating in contact sports like hockey, baseball, or softball
- Raising neck restraints on the backs of car seats
- Not driving under the influence of alcohol or drugs

● CEREBRAL HEMATOMAS

A **cerebral hematoma** is bleeding within the skull, which forms an expanding lesion. People at high risk for cerebral hematomas are those receiving anticoagulant therapy or those with an underlying bleeding disorder, such as hemophilia, thrombocytopenia, leukemia, and aplastic anemia (see Chap. 39).

Pathophysiology and Etiology

Most hematomas result from head trauma or cerebral vascular disorders. The types are epidural hematoma, subdural hematoma, and intracerebral hematoma (Fig. 47-3). An **epidural hematoma** stems from arterial bleeding, usually from the middle meningeal artery, and blood accumulation above the dura. It is characterized by rapidly progressive neurologic deterioration. A **subdural hematoma** results from venous bleeding, with blood gradually accumulating in the space below the dura. Subdural hematomas are classified as acute, subacute, and chronic according to the rate of neurologic changes. Symptoms progressively worsen in a client with an acute subdural hematoma within the first 24 hours of the head injury. Clients with subacute and chronic subdural hematomas become symptomatic after 24 hours and up to 1 week later. An **intracerebral hematoma** is bleeding within the brain that results from an open or closed head injury or from a cerebrovascular condition such as a ruptured cerebral aneurysm (see Chap. 46).

Bleeding increases the volume of brain contents and intracranial pressure (ICP), which disrupts blood flow and causes the brain to become ischemic and hypoxic. Unrelieved IICP also causes the brain to shift to the lateral side (**uncal herniation**) or herniate downward through the foramen magnum. These developments affect the vital centers for respiration, heart rate, and blood pressure as well as cranial nerve functions. Death occurs if the symptoms are not recognized and the bleeding is not stopped.

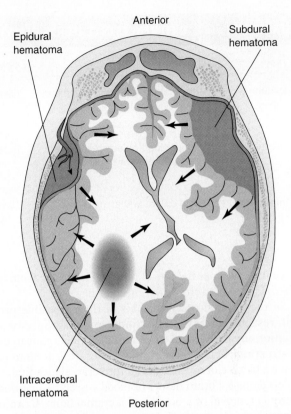

FIGURE 47-3 Location of epidural, subdural, and intracerebral hematomas.

Assessment Findings

The rapidity and severity of neurologic changes (Table 47-1) depend on the location, the rate of bleeding and size of the hematoma, and the effectiveness of **autoregulation,** the brain's ability to provide sufficient arterial blood flow despite rising ICP. MRI and CT scan show densities that indicate the location of the hematoma and shifts in cerebral tissue. ICP monitoring (see Chap. 45) provides direct and continuous data for evaluating the extent to which the lesion is expanding or responding to treatment.

Medical Management

In some cases, the body walls off and absorbs a subdural hematoma with no treatment. A rapid change in LOC and signs of uncontrolled IICP, however, indicate a surgical emergency.

Surgical Management

Surgery consists of drilling holes (*burr holes*) in the skull to relieve pressure, removing the clot, and stopping the bleeding (Fig. 47-4). If the source of bleeding cannot be located by means of burr holes, more invasive surgery is performed. Epidural hematomas require more prompt in-

TABLE 47-1	DIFFERENCES IN CEREBRAL HEMATOMAS	
TYPE	**LOCATION**	**SIGNS AND SYMPTOMS**
Epidural	Arterial blood collects between the skull and dura.	Client may be alert after initial unconsciousness, but then becomes increasingly lethargic before lapsing into coma. Common symptoms are headache, ipsilateral (same side as injury) pupil changes, and contra-lateral (opposite side to injury) hemiparesis (weakness or paralysis).
Subdural	Venous blood collects between the dura and subarachnoid layers.	Deterioration in LOC is progressive. There are ipsilateral pupil changes, decreased extraocular muscle movement, and contralateral hemi-paresis, with periodic episodes of memory lapse, confusion, drowsiness, and personality changes.
Intracerebral	Blood collects within the brain.	Client shows classic signs of IICP: headache, vomiting, seizures, posturing, hyperthermia, irregular breathing.

tervention because the rate of bleeding is greater from an arterial bleed than from a venous bleed.

Intracranial surgery consists of three possible procedures: craniotomy, craniectomy, and cranioplasty. A **craniotomy** is a surgical opening of the skull to gain access to structures beneath the cranial bones. It is done to remove a blood clot or tumor, stop intracranial bleeding, or repair damaged brain tissues or blood vessels. A **craniectomy** is removal of a portion of a cranial bone. **Cranioplasty** is the repair of a defect in a cranial bone (see Chap. 45). A metal or plastic plate or wire mesh is used to replace the removed bone or to reinforce a defect in a cranial bone.

One of two surgical approaches is used to enter the brain above or below the **tentorium,** a double fold of dura mater that separates the cerebrum from the cerebellum (Fig. 47-5). A **supratentorial** (above the tentorium) approach is made through a scalp incision at the site where a particular cerebral lobe requires surgical access. The **infratentorial** (below the tentorium) approach provides an opening to the midbrain and structures of the brainstem. The incision is made at the back of the head with the client in a sitting position.

In cranial surgery, several burr holes are first made in the skull. A saw is then used to cut a section of bone (bone flap). The bone flap is removed to provide a visual field for surgery. After surgery is completed, the bone flap usually is replaced. In some instances, such as with an inoperable tumor, the bone flap is not replaced, allowing the tumor to expand and, thus, preventing IICP. Complications associated with intracranial surgery include cerebral edema, infection, neurogenic shock (see Chap. 23), fluid and electrolyte imbalances, venous thrombosis (especially in the arms and legs), IICP, seizures,

FIGURE 47-4 Neurosurgical procedures may require the use of burr holes to make a bone flap in the skull, aspirate a brain abscess, or evacuate a hematoma. (From Smeltzer, S. C. & Bare, B. G. [2000]. *Brunner & Suddarth's textbook of medical–surgical nursing* [9th ed.]. Philadelphia: Lippincott Williams & Wilkins.)

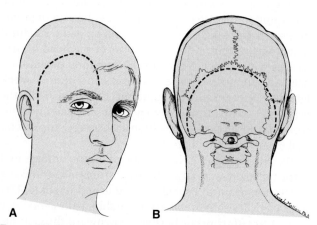

A   B

FIGURE 47-5 (**A**) A supratentorial incision is made behind the hairline on the side of pathology. (**B**) An infratentorial incision is a horseshoe-shaped incision around the occipital lobe. (From Smeltzer, S. C. & Bare, B. G. [2000]. *Brunner & Suddarth's textbook of medical–surgical nursing* [9th ed.]. Philadelphia: Lippincott Williams & Wilkins.)

leakage of cerebrospinal fluid (CSF), and stress ulcers and hemorrhage.

Nursing Management

The nurse regards a head injury, no matter how mild it appears, as an emergency. He or she obtains a history of the injury and performs a neurologic examination, paying particular attention to vital signs, LOC, presence or absence of movement in the arms and legs, and pupil size, equality, and reaction to light. If trauma caused the head injury, the nurse examines the head for bleeding, abrasions, and lacerations. He or she evaluates respiratory status, paying particular attention to the client's ability to maintain adequate oxygenation. The nurse reports neurologic changes immediately. See Chapter 45 for nursing care of a client with IICP that is treated medically.

Preoperative Nursing Care

The nurse prepares the client for surgery once the physician determines the need for an operative intervention. He or she uses electric hair clippers to remove hair where burr holes will be drilled or an incision will be made (sometimes this is deferred until the client is in the operating room). The nurse takes vital signs and maintains a record of continuing neurologic assessment findings. He or she administers prescribed medications, such as the anticonvulsant phenytoin (Dilantin) to reduce the risk of seizures before and after surgery, an osmotic diuretic, and corticosteroids. Preoperative sedation usually is omitted. Before surgery, the nurse restricts fluids to avoid intraoperative complications, reduce cerebral edema, and prevent postoperative vomiting. If indicated, the nurse inserts an indwelling urethral catheter and intravenous (IV) line. To prevent thrombophlebitis and deep vein thrombosis, which may develop from prolonged inactivity during neurosurgery, the nurse applies antiembolism stockings.

Postoperative Nursing Care

After surgery, the nurse places the client in either a supine position with the head slightly elevated or a side-lying position on the unaffected side. He or she performs postoperative and neurologic assessments every 15 to 30 minutes. The nurse maintains a neurologic flow sheet to compare trends in assessment findings. Edema around the eyes (periorbital edema) may make examination of the pupils difficult during the immediate postoperative period. Ecchymosis also can be present. The nurse removes antiembolism stockings briefly every 8 hours and reapplies them to reduce the risk of thrombus or embolus.

The nurse observes the client closely for IICP. He or she administers corticosteroids (when prescribed) and restricts fluids to control cerebral edema and to increase cerebral perfusion. For more information, see Nursing Care Plan 47-1 and Client and Family Teaching Box 47-1.

Nursing Care Plan 47-1

CARE OF THE CLIENT UNDERGOING INTRACRANIAL SURGERY

Assessment

- Assess vital signs, LOC, verbal response, and understanding of oral communication.
- Determine the type and level of discomfort (e.g., headache, sensitivity to light).
- Assess level of pain tolerance using a scale of 0 to 10.
- Evaluate orientation to person, place, and time.
- Check cognitive function by determining ability to follow simple instructions or perform basic mathematical calculations.
- Check pupil size, equality, and response to light. Look for changes in visual field, blurred vision, or diplopia.
- Assess symmetry in facial appearance.
- Test mobility and strength in all four extremities.
- If client is unconscious, look for restlessness.
- Check appropriateness of mood.
- Ask about nausea, and look for evidence of vomiting.
- Monitor seizure activity and status of corneal blink and gag reflexes.
- Monitor urine production, and evaluate the sensation of thirst.

(continued)

Nursing Care Plan 47-1 *(Continued)*

CARE OF THE CLIENT UNDERGOING INTRACRANIAL SURGERY

Nursing Diagnosis: **Risk for Ineffective Breathing Pattern** related to depressive effects of anesthesia and compression of medulla secondary to edema of the brain

Expected Outcome: Breathing will be sufficient to maintain an SPO_2 of at least 90% and a PaO_2 of at least 80 mm Hg.

Interventions	*Rationales*
Monitor SpO_2 with a pulse oximeter.	SpO_2 of at least 90% indicates PaO_2 is at least 80 mm Hg.
Maintain a patent airway by keeping the head erect and in midline, inserting an oral or nasopharyngeal airway if necessary, and suctioning secretions.	Neck flexion or rotation can compromise the diameter of the natural airway; an oral or pharyngeal airway prevents the tongue from obstructing the airway; suction removes secretions that reduce air exchange.
Encourage client to deep breathe at least 10 times each hour or to use a bedside spirometer.	Gas exchange depends on moving atmospheric air to the level of the alveoli and exhaling to remove CO_2.
Avoid administering narcotic analgesia.	Narcotics depress respirations.
Elevate the head of the bed.	Elevating the head lowers abdominal organs away from the diaphragm, which helps improve inspired volume and reduce intracranial swelling.
Report signs of hypoxemia; be prepared to administer supplemental oxygen or provide mechanical ventilation.	Delivering oxygen at a greater concentration than room air increases oxygenation of blood; mechanical ventilation assists breathing.

Evaluation of Expected Outcome: Client's airway is patent, and respirations are normal.

Nursing Diagnosis: **Risk for Ineffective Tissue Perfusion (Cerebral)** related to cerebral edema and bleeding within the cranium

Expected Outcome: ICP will be adequate to perfuse the brain as evidenced by normal neurologic signs and symptoms.

Refer to Nursing Care Plan: The Client With Increased Intracranial Pressure in Chapter 45.

Evaluation of Expected Outcome: Client shows neurologic stability.

Nursing Diagnosis: **Pain** related to chemicals released from traumatized tissue, swelling of cerebral tissue, irritation of meninges

Expected Outcome: Pain will be reduced to client's preidentified level of tolerance within 30 minutes of intervention.

Interventions	*Rationales*
Assess presence, type, and level of pain whenever you assess vital signs and as needed.	Pain assessment is the fifth vital sign.
Reduce bright lights and noise.	Annoying and disturbing sensory stimuli lower the pain threshold.
Minimize activity when pain is acute.	Movement and disturbed rest intensify pain.
Administer prescribed analgesia.	Non-narcotic analgesia is preferred because it does not interfere with neurologic assessment findings.

Evaluation of Expected Outcome: Client reports no pain.

PC: **Seizures**

Expected Outcome: The nurse will monitor to detect, manage, and minimize seizure activity.

(continued)

Nursing Care Plan 47-1 (Continued)

CARE OF THE CLIENT UNDERGOING INTRACRANIAL SURGERY

Interventions	Rationales
Observe client for changes in consciousness and involuntary muscle contraction.	Seizures are categorized as generalized or partial; manifestations vary (see Chap. 45).
Pad side rails; keep the bed in low position.	Padding reduces the potential for trauma.
	Serious injury is less likely if a client falls from a bed in low position.
Stay with the client if a seizure occurs; protect him or her from injury, suction secretions, and promote adequate ventilation.	During a seizure, a client cannot protect himself or herself. Secretions accumulate, increasing the risk for aspiration. Contraction of the diaphragm and intercostal muscles can lead to hypoxia.
Administer prescribed anticonvulsants.	They decrease excitation of brain neurons.

Evaluation of Expected Outcome: The nurse detects seizures and implements interventions to minimize their consequences.

Nursing Diagnosis: **Risk for Infection** related to impaired skin integrity and suppressed inflammatory response secondary to steroid drug therapy

Expected Outcome: Client will remain free of infection.

Interventions	Rationales
Assess temperature, pulse rate, lung sounds, and characteristics of urine. Note the presence of a cough.	Body temperature and pulse rate rise in response to infection. Pneumonia and urinary tract infections are common after surgery because of retained pulmonary secretions, urine stasis, or bacteria entering the urinary tract from the anus.
Inspect the dressing and wound for evidence of purulent drainage.	Impaired skin provides an entrance for microorganisms. Purulent drainage is characteristic of infection.
Follow principles of asepsis when assessing the incision and changing the dressing.	Asepsis reduces or eliminates pathogens.
Administer prescribed antibiotics.	They interfere with the growth and reproduction of pathogens.

Evaluation of Expected Outcome: The surgical site remains free of infection; no other evidence of infection develops.

Nursing Diagnosis: **Risk for Hyperthermia** related to hypothalamic dysfunction or infection

Expected Outcome: Client will maintain body temperature within normal range.

Interventions	Rationales
Measure body temperature every 4 hours.	Routine assessment of body temperature provides early indications of changes in client's thermoregulation.
Help client maintain an adequate oral fluid intake.	Perspiration assists with heat loss through evaporation.
Remove heavy blankets if client develops a fever. Place client on an electrical cooling blanket to reduce fever.	Blankets trap body heat and interfere with convection. A cooling blanket reduces body temperature through conduction.

(continued)

Nursing Care Plan 47-1 (Continued)

CARE OF THE CLIENT UNDERGOING INTRACRANIAL SURGERY

Interventions	Rationales
Administer a prescribed antipyretic when fever does not respond to heat reduction methods.	Antipyretics lower the set-point for body temperature in the hypothalamus.

Evaluation of Expected Outcome: Temperature does not exceed 99.8°F.

Nursing Diagnosis: Disturbed Thought Processes related to cognitive deficits secondary to structural changes in brain tissue and physiology

Expected Outcomes: Client will be oriented to person, place, and time.

Interventions	Rationales
Orient client at frequent intervals.	Until cognition and sensorium return to normal, client may not recall his or her location and the reasons for medical care.
Provide environmental clues such as a calendar with large numbers.	An easy-to-read calendar within client's vision helps reorient the client to time.
Investigate contributing causes of disorientation and restlessness (e.g., full bladder, pain) and intervene as appropriate.	Clients may sense that they are uncomfortable but be unable to identify specifics of their distress.
Share current events, and turn on newsworthy television or radio programs.	Sensory stimulation and communication tend to elevate cognitive functions.
Repeat explanations or answers to questions as needed.	Repetition reinforces information and promotes storage of memory.

Evaluation of Expected Outcome: Client is oriented to person, place, and time.

Nursing Diagnosis: Risk for Injury related to confusion and poor judgment

Expected Outcome: Client will remain free of injuries.

Interventions	Rationales
Locate client near nursing station.	Placing the client in an optimal site for nursing observation increases the nurses' ability to assist the client when necessary.
Place a signal cord within the client's reach; remind client to use it when he or she needs assistance.	The signal cord can help prevent injuries if the client cannot make his or her needs known.
Place a bed/chair alarm that sounds if the client attempts to get out of bed without assistance.	Such an alarm calls attention to the need for assessment and assistance.

Evaluation of Expected Outcome: No injuries occur.

Nursing Diagnosis: Risk for Ineffective Coping related to multiple stressors involving physical losses, lengthy rehabilitation, and compromised finances

Expected Outcome: Client and family will cope with neurologic deficits, participate fully in rehabilitation, and seek assistance from social agencies.

Interventions	Rationale
Consult with the physician about the client's prognosis.	Giving false reassurance is nontherapeutic; offering encouragement promotes motivation.

(continued)

Nursing Care Plan 47-1 (Continued)

CARE OF THE CLIENT UNDERGOING INTRACRANIAL SURGERY

Interventions	*Rationales*
Concur with physician's explanations if client or family raises questions.	Giving consistent responses reinforces that the client has received the same information as other members of the healthcare team.
Keep client and family informed of progress or changes as they occur.	It is easier to cope with and adapt to small changes. Problem-solving is more effective when client and family are provided with facts.
Accept client's and family's behavior under stress in a nonjudgmental manner.	Responses to stress vary. Intolerance of a person's response interferes with a therapeutic alliance between the nurse, client, and family.
Encourage problem-solving techniques and acknowledge positive outcomes.	Unity and cohesiveness develop when client and family resolve problems collaboratively.
Refer client and family to a social worker, discharge planner, or home health agency.	Such providers can assist client and family with the transition from the hospital to other options for care.

Evaluation of Expected Outcomes: Client and family effectively cope with the stress of surgery and possibility of long-term disability.

Stop, Think, and Respond ● BOX 47-1

You are caring for two clients with head injuries. Client A lost consciousness at the time of his head injury. He was alert and oriented on arrival in the ED, but 2 hours later he does not respond even when you press on his nailbeds. Client B has been hospitalized for 1 day. He has not been fully alert since admission and continues to be lethargic. He requires more and more stimulation to give a response. Which client's condition is more serious? Explain your choice.

● SKULL FRACTURES

A skull fracture is a break in the continuity of the cranium. The most common types are simple, depressed, or comminuted fractures (Table 47-2).

Pathophysiology and Etiology

A skull fracture results from a blow to the head. It can be associated with an **open head injury,** in which the scalp, bony cranium, and dura mater (the outer meningeal layer) are exposed, or it may be a **closed head injury,** in which an intact layer of scalp covers the fractured skull.

Open head injuries create a potential for infection because they expose internal brain structures to the environ-ment. They are less likely to produce rapid IICP because the opening gives the brain some room to expand as pressure increases.

Basilar skull fractures are located at the base of the skull. Trauma in this location is especially dangerous because it can cause edema of the brain near the origin of the spinal cord (*foramen magnum*), interfere with circulation of CSF, injure nerves that pass into the spinal cord, or create a pathway for infection between the brain and middle ear (Fig. 47-6), which can result in meningitis.

Assessment Findings

Signs and Symptoms

Simple skull fractures produce few, if any, symptoms and heal without complications. The client may complain of

TABLE 47-2	TYPES OF SKULL FRACTURES
TYPE	**DESCRIPTION**
Simple	Linear crack without any displacement of the pieces
Depressed	Broken bone pushed inward toward the brain
Comminuted	Bone splintered into fragments

47-1 *Client and Family Teaching* Care After Intracranial Surgery

If the client is discharged directly home, the nurse must provide the following verbal and written instructions:

- Signs of intracranial bleeding and infection (expect swelling around the eye and below the incision)
- Purposes for prescribed medications (e.g., anti-convulsants, anti-inflammatory drugs, drugs to control gastric acidity), schedule for administration, and side effects to report
- Expected sensory changes such as hearing a "clicking" sound around the bone flap, which will disappear as healing takes place; headaches also are common, but the client must notify the surgeon if a mild analgesic like acetaminophen (Tylenol) fails to relieve them
- Care for the surgical site as directed by the physician; some recommendations include keep the incision clean, avoid scrubbing it, secure remaining hair away from the incision, resume shampooing the hair when the staples or sutures are removed, and wear a hat when outside to avoid sunburn until hair growth resumes
- Safety precautions to maintain at home, including ambulating only with assistance and ensuring well-lit and clutter-free rooms; driving privileges are temporarily restricted until the risk for seizures has been eliminated
- Exercises that promote strength and endurance
- Techniques to ensure bowel and bladder elimination (see Chap. 48)
- Feeding or nutritional suggestions
- Follow-up appointments for measuring anticonvulsant blood levels, electroencephalograms, and continued medical care and evaluation

FIGURE 47-6 Basilar fractures allow cerebrospinal fluid to leak from the nose and ears. (Adapted from Hickey, J. V. [1997]. *The clinical practice of neurological and neurosurgical nursing* [4th ed.]. Philadelphia: Lippincott-Raven.)

a localized headache. A bump, bruise, or laceration may be visible on the scalp.

Symptoms depend on the area of the brain that has been injured. For example, a large bone fragment that is pressing on the motor area can cause hemiparesis. In any type of skull fracture, shock can develop from injury to the skull or some other area of the body.

Because basilar skull fractures tend to tear the dura, **rhinorrhea,** leaking of CSF from the nose, or **otorrhea,** leakage of CSF from the ear, may occur. In some cases **periorbital ecchymosis,** referred to as *raccoon eyes,* or bruising of the mastoid process behind the ear, called **Battle's sign,** can be present (Fig. 47-7). Conjunctival hemorrhages can occur as well. Injury to the brain tissue may result in seizures. Epilepsy can develop as a sequela of head injury.

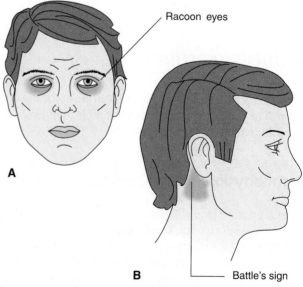

FIGURE 47-7 (A) Periorbital ecchymosis, called *racoon eyes,* and **(B)** periauricular ecchymosis, called *Battle's sign.*

Diagnostic Findings

Skull radiographs, CT scan, or MRI show brain tissue injuries such as a fracture line or embedded skull fragments (compound skull fracture), cerebral edema, or a subdural or epidural hematoma.

Medical and Surgical Management

Simple skull fractures require bed rest and close observation for signs of IICP. If the scalp is lacerated, the wound is cleaned, debrided, and sutured.

Depressed skull fractures require a craniotomy to remove bone fragments and control bleeding, elevation of the depressed fracture, and repair of damaged tissues. A piece of mesh is inserted to replace the bone fragments that are removed. Additional treatment includes antibiotics to control infection, an osmotic diuretic or corticosteroids to prevent or treat cerebral edema, and an anticonvulsant to prevent or treat seizures.

Nursing Management

Most clients are hospitalized for at least 24 hours after a significant head injury. The nurse examines the client to identify signs of head trauma and tests drainage from the nose or ear (Nursing Guidelines 47-1). To detect any CSF drainage, the nurse looks for a **halo sign** (Fig. 47-8). If drainage is present, the nurse allows it to flow freely onto porous gauze and avoids tightly plugging the orifice.

The nurse performs neurologic assessments, which include an hourly evaluation of LOC and of pupil, motor, and sensory status, even if the injury appears mild. It is possible for a hematoma to accompany a skull fracture. The nurse obtains vital signs every 15 to 30 minutes and prepares for the possibility of seizures. See Chapter 45 for additional nursing care.

NURSING GUIDELINES 47-1

Detecting Cerebrospinal Fluid in Drainage

Method #1

1. Wet a Dextrostick or Testape strip with drainage from the nose or ear.

2. Observe if the color change indicates the presence of glucose.

3. Use method #2 if the test is positive, because blood also contains glucose and can result in false results.

Method #2

1. Collect droplets of drainage on a white absorbent pad.

2. Observe the wet area after a few minutes for a halo sign.

3. Note if a yellow ring encircles a central ring that is red: the red ring indicates blood; the yellow ring suggests CSF.

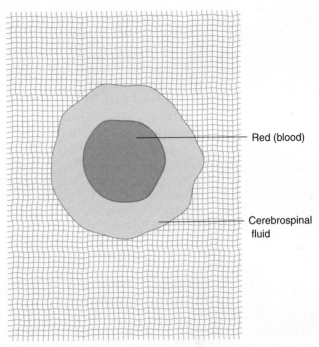

FIGURE 47-8 Halo sign. Clear drainage that separates from bloody drainage suggests the presence of cerebrospinal fluid.

SPINAL CORD INJURIES

Spinal cord trauma is serious and sometimes fatal. The cervical and lumbar vertebrae are the most common sites of injury. Correct emergency management at the time of injury is crucial because moving the client incorrectly can permanently damage the spinal cord.

Pathophysiology and Etiology

Common causes of spinal cord injury include accidents and violence. Vehicular accidents are the leading cause, followed by violence, falls, sports, and miscellaneous injuries.

Trauma to the back can fracture or collapse one or more vertebrae, causing a portion of bone to injure the spinal cord and interfere with the transmission of nerve impulses (Fig. 47-9). Even with no fracture, edema may lead to cord compression, which may permanently damage the cord.

Spinal cord injury also can lead to bleeding within the cord. Because the blood has no place to drain, it forms a hematoma that occupies space and compresses the nerve roots. Injury to the cord also can completely or partially sever spinal cord nerve fibers. With such an injury, the client experiences various consequences of motor and sensory dysfunction below the site of the injury (Table 47-3).

Tetraplegia (a term that replaces *quadriplegia*) results in paralysis of all extremities when there is a high cervical

FIGURE 47-9 Structures affected by spinal nerves.

spine injury. **Paraplegia,** paralysis of both legs, occurs with injuries at the thoracic level. When the tracts of the spinal nerves are severed, no effective nerve regeneration occurs. Muscle spasms occur spontaneously, but they are not evidence that the client is regaining motor function. Many paraplegics return home, live independently, and,

in some instances, resume work. Tetraplegics may return home but require extensive physical care.

Respiratory arrest and spinal shock are immediate complications of spinal cord injury. Long-term complications include autonomic dysreflexia, pressure ulcers, contractures, respiratory and urinary tract infections, calcium loss from bones, and renal calculus formation.

Spinal Shock (Areflexia)

Spinal shock is a loss of sympathetic reflex activity below the level of injury within 30 to 60 minutes of a spinal injury. It is characterized by immediate loss of all cord functions below the point of injury. In addition to paralysis, manifestations include pronounced hypotension, bradycardia, and warm, dry skin. If the level of injury is in the cervical or upper thoracic region, respiratory failure can occur. Bowel and bladder distention develops. The client does not perspire below the level of injury, which impairs temperature control. The client manifests **poikilothermia,** body temperature of the environment. Spinal shock may persist for 1 week to months until the body adjusts to the damage imposed by the injury. Until then, vital functions require medical support.

Autonomic Dysreflexia (Hyperreflexia)

Autonomic dysreflexia is an exaggerated sympathetic nervous system response among those with a spinal cord injury above T6. It can occur suddenly at any time after spinal shock subsides. Box 47-1 lists factors that precipitate autonomic dysreflexia. Characteristics of this acute emergency are as follows:

- Severe hypertension
- Slow heart rate

TABLE 47-3	CONSEQUENCES OF SPINAL CORD INJURIES	
LEVEL OF INJURY	**COMMON MOTOR EFFECTS**	**COMMON SENSORY EFFECTS**
C1, C2, C3	Paralysis below neck; impaired breathing; bowel and bladder incontinence; sexual dysfunction	No sensation below neck
C4, C5	Shoulder elevation possible; ventilation support required	No sensation below clavicle
C6, C7, C8	Some elbow, upper arm, and wrist movement; can do diaphragmatic breathing	Some sensation in arms and thumb; sensation in chest impaired
T1–T6	Paralysis below waist; control of hands; abdominal breathing	No sensation below midchest
T7–T12	Varying degrees of trunk and abdominal control	Varying degrees of sensation below waist
L1–L2	Hip adduction impaired	No sensation below lower abdomen; some sensation in inner thighs
L3–L5	Knee and ankle movement impaired	No sensation below upper thighs
S1–S5	Varying degrees of bowel/bladder control and sexual function	No sensation in perineum

C, cervical; T, thoracic; L, lumbar; S, sacral.

BOX 47-1 ● Common Causes of Autonomic Dysreflexia

- Full bladder
- Abdominal distention
- Impacted feces
- Skin pressure or breakdown
- Overstretched muscles
- Sexual intercourse
- Labor and delivery
- Sunburn below the cord injury
- Infected ingrown toenail
- Exposure to hot or cold environmental temperature
- Taking over-the-counter decongestants

- Pounding headache
- Nausea
- Blurred vision
- Flushed skin
- Sweating
- Goosebumps (erection of pilomotor muscles in the skin)
- Nasal stuffiness
- Anxiety

Uncontrolled autonomic dysreflexia can lead to seizures, stroke, and death. Prevention is the best treatment, but additional measures such as administering antihypertensive drug therapy with nifedipine (Procardia), nitroglycerin ointment, phentolamine (Regitine), hydralazine (Apresoline), or diazoxide (Hyperstat); raising the client's head; and relieving the precipitating cause are necessary once it develops.

Assessment Findings

The degree and location of the injury determine the immediate symptoms. There is pain in the affected area, difficulty breathing, numbness, and paralysis. If the injury is high in the cervical region, respiratory failure and death occur because the diaphragm is paralyzed. When the cord is completely severed, the client permanently loses function below the level of the injury. He or she maintains some function if damage to the cord is minimal.

A neurologic examination reveals the level of spinal cord injury. Radiography, myelography, MRI, and CT scan show evidence of fracture or compression of one or more vertebrae, edema, or a hematoma.

Medical Management

Initially, the head and back are immobilized mechanically with a cervical collar and back support. An IV line is inserted to provide access to a vein if shock develops. Vital signs are stabilized. Corticosteroids may be given to reduce spinal cord edema.

After the client is stabilized, the injured portion of the spine is further immobilized using a cast or brace or surgical intervention. Traction with weights and pulleys is applied to provide correct vertebral alignment and to increase the space between the vertebrae. Additional weight is added over the next few days to increase the space between the vertebrae and to move them into correct alignment. A turning frame is used to change the client's position without altering the alignment of the spine (Fig. 47-10).

Surgical Management

Depending on the extent of the injury, it may be necessary surgically to remove bone fragments, repair dislocated vertebrae, and stabilize the spine. The vertebrae are fused with bone obtained from the iliac crest or stabilized with a steel rod. External immobilization with a brace or cast often is necessary.

NURSING PROCESS

● Care of the Client With Spinal Trauma

Assessment

On the client's arrival in the ED, the nurse obtains information about the injury and treatment given at the scene from family, witnesses, or those who transported the client to the hospital. After gathering such facts, the nurse performs a neurologic assessment, taking care to document findings on a flow sheet to provide a database for future comparison. He or she assesses vital signs, paying particular attention to respiratory status. During the acute phase, the nurse repeats neurologic assessments frequently. He or she determines if the client has movement and sensation below the level of injury, looks to see

FIGURE 47-10 The nurse frequently turns a client on the Stryker frame to relieve pressure. (From Smeltzer, S. C. & Bare, B. G. [2000]. *Brunner & Suddarth's textbook of medical–surgical nursing* [9th ed.]. Philadelphia: Lippincott Williams & Wilkins.)

if neurologic damage is worsening, and observes for signs of respiratory distress and spinal shock.

Diagnosis, Planning, and Interventions

The nurse keeps the client's body and head aligned and limits all movement. If directed by the physician, the nurse inserts a urinary retention catheter. He or she assists with immobilization of the injured spine (Fig. 47-11). Burr holes in the skull are required for inserting the pointed ends of traction tongs or the halo traction apparatus. When applying traction, the nurse checks that the weights hang free. He or she instructs others on the nursing team never to lift or remove the weights or increase or decrease the amount of prescribed weight. The use of external stabilizing devices like the halo vest facilitates early discharge from the acute care facility. To ensure the client's safety and prevent complications, see Nursing Guidelines 47-2.

Besides monitoring for and intervening in cases of spinal shock and autonomic dysreflexia, the nurse's role may include the following.

FIGURE 47-11 (A) Traction for cervical fractures may be applied with tongs. **(B)** A halo vest may be used to maintain alignment in cervical injuries. (From Smeltzer, S. C. & Bare, B. G. [2000]. *Brunner & Suddarth's textbook of medical–surgical nursing* [9th ed.]. Philadelphia: Lippincott Williams & Wilkins.)

NURSING GUIDELINES 47-2

Instructing Clients in Halo Vest Management

Teach client as follows:

■ Turn your whole body rather than trying to turn your head; you will not be able to look down.

■ Do not drive a car.

■ Walk only on level surfaces until you become accustomed to the vest; avoid stairs, curbs, and uneven terrain unless assistance is available.

■ Take care getting in and out of vehicles to avoid bumping the halo and loosening the pins.

■ Use a mirror to inspect the pin sites and as a guide while cleaning them.

■ Clean the pin sites two to three times a day with cotton-tipped applicators saturated with hydrogen peroxide; remove loose crusts.

■ Use a clean applicator after making a full circle around the pin site.

■ Clip the hair that grows around the pin sites.

■ Report pain, redness, drainage from pin sites, fever, or neck tingling or pain to the physician.

■ Never independently adjust the vest if it becomes tight or loose; consult the physician.

■ Pad the vest if it causes pressure or friction.

■ Take sponge baths to maintain hygiene; seek assistance for areas you cannot reach such as around the anus.

■ Use a dry shampoo or consult physician on how to shampoo hair without wetting the vest.

■ Use pillows for support and comfort when sleeping.

■ Wear loose-fitting clothing with wide necklines for ease in dressing.

■ Wear shoes with flat heels that are easy to slip on and off.

Ineffective Breathing Pattern, Ineffective Airway Clearance, and **Risk for Impaired Gas Exchange** related to paralysis of respiratory, chest, and abdominal muscles

Expected Outcomes: (1) Client will breathe independently at a rate of 16 to 20 breaths/minute. (2) The airway will be free of secretions. (3) The client's blood oxygen saturation (SpO$_2$) will be 90% or higher.

● Maintain a patent airway. *A patent airway maximizes passage of air in and out of the lungs.*

● Be prepared for endotracheal intubation and mechanical ventilation if respiratory failure occurs. *An endotracheal tube provides an airway from the nose or mouth to an area above the mainstem bronchi. Mechanical ventilation provides a means to regulate respiratory rate, volume of air, and percentage of oxygen when a client cannot breathe independently.*

- Suction the airway to remove secretions. *A client with spinal trauma may not be able to cough effectively. An artificial airway increases the production of respiratory secretions.*
- Administer oxygen as prescribed. *To prevent hypoxemia, the client may require more oxygen than available in room air.*

PC: Neuropathic Pain related to irritated nerve root and soft tissue injury

Expected Outcome: The nurse will monitor to detect, manage, and minimize neuropathic pain.

- Administer prescribed analgesia intravenously. *IV administration of an analgesic avoids administration of injections into tissues where absorption is compromised.*
- Assist the physician with nerve block procedures if analgesia is ineffective. *A nerve block is a form of regional anesthesia in which an anesthetic agent is injected close to the nerve that is transmitting pain impulses.*

Impaired Physical Mobility and **Risk for Disuse Syndrome** related to loss of motor function

Expected Outcome: (1) Client's ability to be mobile will be maintained. (2) Client will use assistive devices to move and perform activities of daily living. (3) Client will not experience complications associated with inactivity and immobility.

- Position client to avoid joint contractures and foot drop. *Mobility depends on preventing permanent changes to the musculoskeletal system. Inactivity causes joints to assume a position of flexion.*
- Help client perform exercises identified by the physical therapist. *Active and passive exercise maintains joint flexibility and reduces muscle atrophy and atony. For exercises to be effective, clients must perform them several times a day.*
- Apply leg braces when ambulation is possible. *Braces support joints, allowing the client to ambulate independently or with a walker or crutches.*
- Maintain skin integrity by changing client's position at least every 2 hours, using pressure-relieving devices, massaging bony prominences, and keeping skin clean and dry. *Position changes and pressure-relieving devices ensure that capillary pressure stays above 32 mm Hg, thus providing oxygenated blood to cells for their continued survival. Massage increases blood flow to temporarily deprived areas. Keeping skin clean and dry prevents maceration and decreases the potential for bacterial growth.*
- Facilitate urine elimination and keep the bowel evacuated. *Urinary retention and stasis may contribute to autonomic dysreflexia and formation of renal calculi. Infrequent bowel evacuation leads to constipation and impaction.*
- Keep client hydrated. *Adequate hydration reduces potential for formation of thrombi and renal calculi.*
- Provide oral or enteral nutrition. *A well-balanced diet provides nutrients and elements necessary for energy and to sustain cellular growth and repair.*

Anxiety and **Risk for Ineffective Coping** related to prognosis of neurologic deficits

Expected Outcome: (1) Anxiety will be relieved. (2) Client will cope effectively with stressors.

- Discuss information about prognosis with the physician. *Communication facilitates mutual understanding of client's potential for recovery and rehabilitation.*
- Tell client and family that determining the severity of deficits immediately after a spinal cord injury is difficult. Explain that the outcome varies depending on the specific injury and client's response to rehabilitation. *Until the initial trauma and swelling have resolved, any assumptions about the client's outcome are premature. Successful rehabilitation depends on the level of the cord injury, development of complications, client's motivation and perseverance, and intervention of the healthcare team.*
- Be a good listener, and offer encouragement as the client makes progress. *Such encouragement can contribute to the client's resolve to put forth continued effort.*

Evaluation of Expected Outcomes

Breathing is adequate to maintain oxygenation. Pain is relieved or reduced to a tolerable level. The client regains mobility using minimal assistive devices. Complications from inactivity are prevented or reduced. The client's level of anxiety is mild, and he or she begins to cope with the effects of the injury and the challenge of rehabilitation. The client and family demonstrate understanding of postdischarge home care.

SPINAL NERVE ROOT COMPRESSION

There are two basic types of spinal nerve root compression: **intramedullary** lesions that involve the spinal cord and **extramedullary** lesions that involve the tissues surrounding the spinal cord. The most common site of nerve root compression is at the level of the three lower lumbar disks; however, nerve root compression also occurs in the cervical spine.

Pathophysiology and Etiology

Pressure on spinal nerve roots results from trauma, herniated intervertebral disks, and tumors of the spinal cord and surrounding structures (Fig. 47-12). Stress caused by poor body mechanics, age, or disease weakens an area in the vertebra, causing the spongy center of the vertebrae, the *nucleus pulposus,* to swell and herniate. This condition is commonly called a *slipped disk;* the displacement puts pressure on the nearby nerves.

Pain along the distribution of the nerve root is common. Actions that increase pressure intensify the pain.

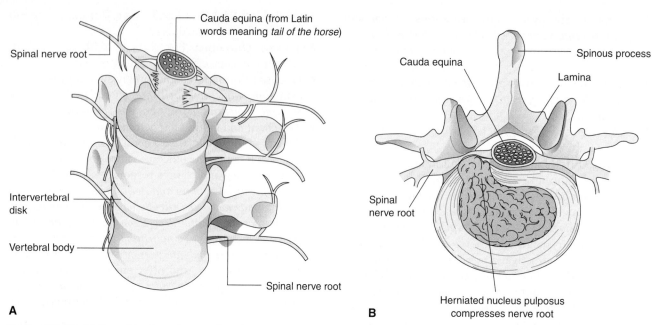

FIGURE 47-12 (**A**) Normal lumbar spine vertebrae, intervertebral disks, and spinal nerve root. (**B**) Ruptured vertebral disk. (From Smeltzer, S. C. & Bare, B. G. [2000]. *Brunner & Suddarth's textbook of medical-surgical nursing* [9th ed.]. Philadelphia: Lippincott Williams & Wilkins.)

Weakness and changes in sensation occur. The symptoms intensify with increasing nerve root compression.

Assessment Findings

Symptoms vary depending on the cause of compression and level involved. They usually include weakness, paralysis, pain, and **paresthesia** (numbness, tingling). When a herniated disk in the lumbar region compresses the sciatic nerve, the client describes feeling pain down the buttocks and into the posterior thigh and leg. Physical examination reveals weakness or paralysis of the extremity innervated by the compressed nerve. If a nerve in the lumbar or sacral area is affected, the client experiences pain when lying supine and lifting the leg without bending the knee. The pain increases when straining, coughing, or lifting a heavy object. Walking and sitting become difficult. Spinal radiography, CT, MRI, myelography, and electromyography show displacement or herniation of an intervertebral disk, tumor, or bleeding around the nerve root.

Medical Management

When a client has a herniated intervertebral disk, conservative therapy is tried first. Metastatic spinal cord tumors also are treated conservatively because removal is not feasible.

A herniated cervical disk is treated by immobilizing the cervical spine with a cervical collar or brace. Later, as inflammation subsides, the client wears the collar or brace intermittently when walking or sitting. Bed rest with a firm mattress and bed board is used for clients with a lumbar herniated disk.

Skin traction, which can be applied in the home, is used to decrease severe muscle spasm as well as increase the distance between adjacent vertebrae, keep the vertebrae correctly aligned, and, in many instances, relieve pain. Treatment relieves symptoms for an extended period.

Hot moist packs are used to treat muscle spasm. Skeletal muscle relaxants, such as carisoprodol (Rela) and chlorzoxazone (Paraflex), help clients with a herniated intervertebral disk. Diazepam (Valium), a tranquilizer with skeletal muscle-relaxing action, is used for its twofold effect: to reduce anxiety associated with the pain of a herniated disk and to relax the skeletal muscle. Drugs such as aspirin, phenylbutazone (Butazolidin), and corticosteroids are used to treat inflammation. Reducing inflammation and muscle spasm helps ease pain, but additional analgesics are given to control pain. Clients with an inoperable spinal cord tumor are given analgesics to maintain comfort.

Surgical Management

If conservative therapy fails to relieve symptoms of a herniated disk with spinal nerve root compression, surgery is considered. Procedures for relieving spinal nerve root compression include the following:

- **Diskectomy**—removal of the ruptured disk
- **Laminectomy**—removal of the posterior arch of a vertebra to expose the spinal cord. The surgeon can

remove whatever lesion is causing compression: a herniated disk, tumor, blood clot, bone spur, or broken bone fragment.

- Diskectomy with **spinal fusion**—removal of the ruptured disk followed by grafting a piece of bone taken from another area, such as the iliac crest, onto the vertebra to fuse the vertebral spinous process. Bone also may be obtained from a bone bank.
- **Chemonucleolysis**—injection of the enzyme chymopapain into the nucleus pulposus to shrink or dissolve the disc, which then relieves pressure on spinal nerve roots

Spinal fusion stabilizes the vertebrae weakened by degenerative joint changes, such as osteoarthritis, and by laminectomy. It results in a firm union; the client loses mobility and must become accustomed to a permanent area of stiffness. When a portion of the lumbar spine is fused, the client usually does not feel the stiffness after a short time because motion increases in the joints above the fusion. Motion is more limited when the area of fusion is in the cervical spine. Spinal fusion also is performed for spinal cord tumors, fractures and dislocations of the spine, and Pott's disease (tuberculosis of the spine).

Nursing Management

The nurse performs a neurologic examination and notes any limitation of motion and the type of movement that causes pain. For nursing responsibilities unique to various types of spinal surgery, see Nursing Guidelines 47-3. For clients being treated conservatively, the nurse uses a firm mattress or applies a bedboard because a firm surface supports the spine and promotes alignment. He or she maintains the client on bed rest, placing him or her in Williams' position with the knees and head slightly elevated to relieve lumbosacral pain. The nurse applies halo vest traction following the guidelines in Box 47-2. For intermittent pelvic or cervical skin traction, he or she attaches the skin device to the client, supports the weights, and lowers them gently to avoid a sudden and strong pull. The nurse reminds the client to roll from side to side without twisting the spine. When the client gets out of bed, the nurse reinforces the use of proper body mechanics. He or she advises clients with cervical nerve root compression to

BOX 47-2 ● Maintaining Traction

For proper application and use of traction:
- The prescribed amount of weight must be used.
- Traction weights must hang above the floor.
- Ropes must move freely through the pulley grooves.
- The client's position must be in line with the pull of the traction apparatus.

NURSING GUIDELINES 47-3

Nursing Care After Specific Spinal Surgeries

Postcervical Diskectomy

- Keep a cervical collar in place at all times; do not remove without a physician's order.
- Instruct client to keep the neck straight in midline position until healing occurs.
- Support client's head, neck, and upper shoulders when moving from a lying to sitting to standing position or when getting into and out of a chair.
- Observe for Horner's syndrome, a complication following anterior cervical diskectomy from cervical sympathetic nerve damage. Manifestations are lid ptosis (drooping), constricted pupil, regression of eye in the orbit, and lack of perspiration on one side of the face.

Postlumbar Laminectomy or Diskectomy With Spinal Fusion

- Logroll when turning client every 2 hours; maintain alignment at all times.

- Caution client to avoid turning self.
- Teach client to avoid twisting or jerking the back; sitting during the first week and prolonged sitting thereafter (client should use a straight-backed chair and not slump); bending from the waist (client should bend from the knees and hips).

avoid extreme hyperextension of the neck and side-to-side rotation of the head. The nurse administers prescribed muscle relaxants and analgesics. He or she applies moist heat for no longer than 20 minutes, but repeats several times a day.

The nurse periodically evaluates the client's response to conservative therapy. It is important to note the activities and positions that increase pain and the gain or loss in motion or sensation since the previous observation. Comparison of current symptoms with those first exhibited provides an evaluation of response to therapy. It is important to note a change in symptoms when the client is removed from traction.

Nursing interventions after spinal surgery are as follows:

- Monitor vital signs.
- Assist client to perform hourly deep breathing exercises while awake but avoid forced coughing because it increases pressure within the spinal canal.
- Examine the dressing for CSF leakage or bleeding.
- Assess neurovascular status (color, temperature, mobility, sensation) in extremities below the area of surgery, which may result from edema or hemorrhage at the operative site.
- Report an inability to void or an output of less than 240 mL in 8 hours.
- Use a fracture bed pan.

GENERAL NUTRITIONAL CONSIDERATIONS

Extended immobility accelerates calcium loss from bone, leading to hypercalcemia. Symptoms include nausea, vomiting, anorexia, abdominal pain, constipation, polyuria, polydipsia, calcium renal stones, headache, and lethargy. Diet interventions help relieve symptoms but cannot prevent or treat the altered calcium metabolism. For instance, a high fluid intake (up to 3 L/day) helps dilute urine to prevent the precipitation of calcium renal stones.

Thirst may not be a valid indicator of need in immobilized clients, and clients following a bladder rehabilitation program may be reluctant to drink liquids, fearing "accidents." Counsel the client on the importance of adequate fluid taken at regular, specified intervals. Likewise, assure clients participating in bowel training that a high-fiber diet (whole grains, legumes, fruits, vegetables) aids in normalizing bowel movements.

Tetraplegics and paraplegics have lower calorie requirements because their energy expenditure is reduced; adjust calorie intake to avoid excessive weight gain. Nutrient needs, however, are stable or higher, depending on the development of complications. For instance, prolonged immobility promotes nitrogen excretion, resulting in an increased protein requirement. Clients with skin breakdown have increased requirements for protein (meat, milk, supplements), vitamin C (citrus fruit and juices, strawberries, "greens," tomatoes), and zinc (meat, seafood, milk, egg yolks, legumes, and whole grains) to promote healing.

GENERAL PHARMACOLOGIC CONSIDERATIONS

An osmotic diuretic such as mannitol may be prescribed to reduce ICP after intracranial surgery. Inspect the mannitol vial before use. If the solution contains crystals, warm the container in hot water and shake it vigorously. Do not administer the drug if crystals are in the solution.

Because respiratory depressant effects are less likely with codeine, it may be prescribed for postoperative pain after intracranial surgery.

Monitor the client's body temperature closely after intracranial surgery. Elevated temperature must be relieved with an antipyretic and other measures because hyperthermia increases brain metabolism, increasing the potential for brain damage.

Clients given a skeletal muscle relaxant or tranquilizer for a herniated intervertebral disk, back strain, or spasms of the back muscles may experience drowsiness and dizziness. They require assistance with ambulatory activities and should not drive or operate equipment.

Clients with impaired swallowing may have difficulty taking pills or capsules. Whenever possible, give medications in liquid form.

GENERAL GERONTOLOGIC CONSIDERATIONS

Older adults often respond less favorably to therapies for a neurologic deficit.

Older adults tend to drink less water and, therefore, may incur a chronic fluid volume deficit. Encourage a fluid intake of 1500 to 2000 mL/day (if physical condition permits).

Critical Thinking Exercises

1. *A man involved in a motor vehicle accident is brought to the ED. You are told that he was not wearing a seat belt and struck his head on the steering wheel. What neurologic assessments would you make? Why?*
2. *You are caring for a paraplegic client. What signs and symptoms suggest that the client is experiencing autonomic dysreflexia? What nursing measures are appropriate?*

References and Suggested Readings

Bryant, G. A. (2000). When spinal cord injury affects the bowel. *RN, 63*(2), 26–30.

Calhoun, K. H. (2000). In consultation. Evaluating patients with nasal fracture: When to suspect more serious injury. *Journal of Critical Illness, 15,* 528.

Carrigan, T. D., Walker, E., & Barnes, S. (2000). Domestic violence: The shaken adult syndrome. *Journal of Accident and Emergency Medicine, 17,* 138–139.

Danis, D. (2001). Clinical decisions. Interdisciplinary practice: Spinal cord injury. *International Journal of Trauma Nursing, 7*(2), 64–66.

Dominique, D. S. & Jallo, J. (1998). Complications of brain and spinal cord injuries. *Trauma Quarterly, 14*(1), 43–59.

Goldberg, G. (2001). Mild traumatic brain injury and concussion. *Physical Medicine and Rehabilitation: State of the Art Reviews, 15,* 363–398.

Guin, P. R. (2001). Advances in spinal cord injury care. *Critical Care Nursing Clinics of North America, 13,* 399–409.

Herbert, C. (2001). Use of morphine for pain after intracranial surgery. *Professional Nurse, 16,* 1029–1033.

Hilton, G. (2001). Emergency. Acute head injury: Distinguishing subdural from epidural hematoma. *American Journal of Nursing, 101*(9), 51–52.

Hoeck, B., Shephard, T., O'Brien, E., et al. (1999). Global views. Postoperative pain control after craniotomy. *Journal of Neuroscience Nursing, 31,* 47–49.

Inamasu, J., Hori, S., Aoki, K., et al. (2000). CT scans essential after posttraumatic loss of consciousness. *American Journal of Emergency Medicine, 18,* 810–811.

Karlet, M. C. (2001). Acute management of the patient with spinal cord injury. *International Journal of Trauma Nursing, 7*(2), 43–48.

Kavchak-Keyes, M. A. (2000). Autonomic dysreflexia. *Rehabilitation Nursing, 25*(1), 31–35.

Keely, R. R. (1998). Preventing complications. Recognition and treatment of autonomic dysreflexia. *Dimensions of Critical Care Nursing, 17,* 170–176.

Leith, B. (1998). Pharmacological management of pain after intracranial surgery. *Journal of Neuroscience Nursing, 30,* 220–224.

Lewis, A. M. (1999). Neurologic emergency. *Nursing, 29*(10), 54–56.

McIlvoy, L., Meyer, K., & Vitaz, T. (2000). Use of an acute spinal cord injury clinical pathway. *Critical Care Clinics of North America, 12,* 521–530.

Mitcho, K. & Yanko, J. R. (1999). Acute care management of spinal cord injuries. *Critical Care Nursing, 22*(2), 60–79.

Robinson, R. & Peacock, J. E. (2000). Law and the emergency nurse. Just "sleeping it off." *Journal of Emergency Nursing, 26,* 249–250.

Roth, P. & Farls, K. (2000). Pathophysiology of traumatic brain injury. *Critical Care Nursing Quarterly, 23*(3), 14–25.

Silver, J. R. (2000). Early autonomic dysreflexia. *Spinal Cord, 38,* 229–233.

Suyama, T., Takahashi, K., Shibuta, H., et al. (2001). Pain and rehabilitation in patients with spinal cord injury. *Journal of Physical Therapy Science, 13*(1), 59–64.

Teasell, R. W., Arnold, J. M. O., Krassioukov, A., et al. (2000). Cardiovascular consequences of loss of supraspinal control of the sympathetic nervous system after spinal cord injury. *Archives of Physical Medicine and Rehabilitation, 81,* 506–516.

Tipton, K. D. (1998). Action stat. Autonomic dysreflexia. *Nursing, 28*(11), 33.

Travers, P. L. (1999). Autonomic dysreflexia: A clinical rehabilitation problem. *Rehabilitation Nursing, 24*(1), 19–23, 43.

Valadka, A. B., Gopinath, S. P., & Peterson, C. S. (2000). Midline shift after severe head injury: Pathophysiologic implications. *Journal of Trauma: Injury, Infection, and Critical Care, 49,* 1–10.

Walshaw, L. K. (2000). Assessment of head injuries in a minor injuries unit. *Accident and Emergency Nursing, 8,* 210–213.

Warbel, A., Lewicki, L., & Lupica, K. (1999). Venous thrombosis: Risk factors in the craniotomy patient population. *Journal of Neuroscience Nursing, 31,* 180–186.

Caring for Clients With Neurologic Deficits

Words to Know

Credé's maneuver
cutaneous triggering
neurologic deficit
reflex incontinence

Learning Objectives

On completion of this chapter, the reader will:

- Define *neurologic deficit*.
- Describe the three phases of a neurologic deficit.
- Give the primary aims of medical treatment of a neurologic deficit.
- Name six members of the healthcare team involved with the management of a client with a neurologic deficit.
- Describe nursing management of a client with a neurologic deficit.

A **neurologic deficit** is when one or more functions of the central and peripheral nervous systems are decreased, impaired, or absent. Examples include paralysis, muscle weakness, impaired speech, inability to recognize objects, abnormal gait or difficulty walking, impaired memory, impaired swallowing, or abnormal bowel and bladder elimination. The client with a neurologic deficit faces many problems. Often, the deficit affects more than one body system. The client may be unable to walk, talk, do simple tasks like feeding and bathing, or recognize family members.

Many members of the healthcare team are involved with the complex management of the client with a temporary or permanent neurologic deficit: the physician, nurse, nursing assistant, social worker, physical therapist, occupational therapist, speech therapist, prosthetist, psychotherapist, dietitian, pharmacist, and vocational counselor. With intensive therapy and a coordinated approach by all team members, many clients have the potential to return to normal or near-normal function or successfully adapt to the changes in function.

PHASES OF A NEUROLOGIC DEFICIT

Neurologic deficits are divided into three phases: acute, recovery, and chronic. Not all clients with a neurologic deficit experience all three phases. Some clients have deficits that begin with an acute phase and move into a recovery phase or into a lifelong chronic phase.

● ACUTE PHASE

The acute phase follows a sudden neurologic event, such as a cerebrovascular accident (CVA) or a head or spinal cord injury. During the acute phase, the client usually is critically ill, with many signs and symptoms such as altered level of consciousness (LOC), hypertension or hypotension, fever, difficulty breathing, or paralysis.

Medical and Surgical Management

The focus of management during the acute phase is to stabilize the client and prevent further neurologic damage. The client with a CVA may require management of hypertension or hypotension through drug therapy or respiratory support through mechanical ventilation. Clients with a head or spinal cord injury may require surgical intervention to stabilize the injured area or remove bone fragments, blood clots, or foreign objects. Sometimes, surgery is postponed until the client is stabilized and the acute phase has passed. For others, surgery is performed during the acute phase as a lifesaving measure.

Nursing Management

The nurse performs frequent and thorough neurologic assessments to evaluate the client's status, need for additional medical or surgical interventions, and response to treatment. He or she uses the Glasgow Coma Scale (see Chap. 44) or other neurologic assessment tools like the Mini-Mental Status Examination (see Chap. 12) to record observations. When significant changes occur, the nurse immediately reports them to the physician. The nurse assesses vital signs as often as necessary and maintains the blood pressure (BP) to ensure adequate cerebral oxygenation. He or she measures intake and output and observes for signs of electrolyte imbalances and dehydration. The nurse reports a urinary output of less than 500 mL/day or urinary or bowel incontinence.

Beginning basic rehabilitation during the acute phase is an important nursing function. Measures such as position changes and prevention of skin breakdown and contractures are essential aspects of care during the early phase of rehabilitation. The nursing goal is to prevent complications that may interfere with the client's potential to recover function. (See this chapter's Nursing Process section for additional nursing management.)

● RECOVERY PHASE

The recovery phase begins when the client's condition is stabilized. It starts several days or weeks after the initial event and lasts weeks or months.

Medical and Surgical Management

Medical management during the recovery phase aims at keeping the client stable and preventing or treating complications, such as pneumonia, and further neurologic impairment.

Nursing Management

During recovery, the nurse works with team members to plan a rehabilitation program in several domains according to the client's abilities and limitations (Table 48-1). Various assessment tools can help identify a client's level of functioning and potential for improvement with a rehabilitation program, including:

- The National Institute for Health Stroke Scale
- The American Heart Association's Stroke Outcome Classification
- The Barthel Index (Table 48-2)

Rehabilitation is designed to meet the client's immediate and long-term needs. To do so, environmental

TABLE 48-1	DOMAINS OF NEUROLOGIC IMPAIRMENT
DOMAIN	**DESCRIPTION**
Motor	A single deficit, or combination of deficits, involving the face, arms, and legs, which affects speech, swallowing, muscle tone and strength, gait, coordination, and ability to use objects for their intended purpose
Sensory	Altered sensation (e.g., numbness, tingling, exaggerated sensation), or altered perception (e.g., inability to identify objects by touch, loss of writing ability)
Vision	Loss of vision in one eye or in the temporal or nasal fields; blindness
Language	Disturbances in comprehension, naming, repeating, clarity of speech, reading
Cognition	Changes in memory, attention, orientation, calculation, and construction
Affect	Altered mood, lability of mood

changes may be necessary to help the client adapt to the disability and fully use any remaining functions. Even though deficits can be temporary, a prolonged period and enrollment in a rehabilitation program often are necessary before a client regains partial or full function. Besides nurses and physicians, a successful rehabilitation program includes several other providers, such as physical therapists, occupational therapists, speech therapists, and enterostomal therapists, all of whom recommend devices or procedures to prevent complications and enhance the client's remaining abilities.

With continuous assessment and identification of the client's needs, the nurse plays an important role in rehabilitation. Devices that help a client walk, eat, groom, and perform other motor skills are recommended or devised to suit particular needs. Flotation pads for wheelchairs, walkers, sheepskin boots, and range-of-motion (ROM) exercises are examples of the many appliances and procedures used in rehabilitation. (See this chapter's Nursing Process section for additional nursing management.)

● CHRONIC PHASE

For some clients (e.g., those with multiple sclerosis or Alzheimer's disease), a neurologic deficit results in a prolonged or lifelong chronic phase. In this phase, the client shows little or no improvement, remains stationary, or progressively worsens. Physical and psychological rehabilitation continues in the chronic phase to prevent complications such as pressure ulcers and muscle contractures.

TABLE 48-2	MODIFIED BARTHEL INDEX				
ITEM	UNABLE TO PERFORM TASK	SUBSTANTIAL HELP REQUIRED	MODERATE HELP REQUIRED	MINIMAL HELP REQUIRED	FULLY INDEPENDENT
Personal hygiene	0	1	3	4	5
Bathing self	0	1	3	4	5
Feeding	0	2	5	8	10
Toilet	0	2	5	8	10
Stair climbing	0	2	5	8	10
Dressing	0	2	5	8	10
Bowel control	0	2	5	8	10
Bladder control	0	2	5	8	10
Ambulation	0	3	8	12	15
or wheelchair*	0	1	3	4	5
Chair/bed transfer	0	3	8	12	15

*Score only if client is unable to ambulate and is trained in wheelchair management.

DEPENDENCY NEEDS

Categories	MBI Total Scores	Dependency Level	Hours of Help Required per Week (Maximum)
1	0–24	Total	27.0
2	25–49	Severe	23.5
3	50–74	Moderate	20.0
4	75–90	Mild	13.0
5	91–99	Minimal	<10.0

Medical and Surgical Management

Medical management continues throughout the chronic phase and uses a wide range of therapies and treatments, such as control of BP, physical therapy, dietary management, and treatment of complications related to disuse and immobility. In some cases, surgery is performed to correct deformities or problems that have developed. Examples include muscle and skin grafts to close a pressure ulcer, surgery to correct a contracture deformity, or removal of a kidney stone (a complication of prolonged immobility).

Stop, Think, and Respond ● BOX 48-1

You have been caring for a client with a head injury who is being transferred to an extended care facility for rehabilitation. What information is important to include to help nurses at the new facility plan the client's care?

Nursing Management

Clients in the chronic phase often are admitted to a hospital for treatment of complications. They also are transferred to a skilled nursing facility or long-term care facility when family members no longer can manage their care, or

when the disease has progressively worsened so that skilled care is mandatory. Nursing management focuses on preventing physical and psychological complications. Therapy in a rehabilitation center may include retraining in skills such as using the telephone, handling money, shopping, using public transportation, maintaining a household, and vocational training.

PSYCHOSOCIAL ISSUES AND HOME MANAGEMENT

Overview

Leaving the inpatient setting, where the daily, intensive support of the healthcare team is readily available, and returning home with life-altering changes can be tremendously frightening. The client and family need additional support to adapt to a new lifestyle. Although many clients recover sufficiently to assume responsibility for some aspects of their own care, others do not. The burden of care often falls on the spouse, who may have physical problems as well, or the adult children, who may not be available or willing to share this responsibility.

Financial resources are strained during a lengthy hospitalization, which may continue after discharge. Adapting the home to accommodate a wheelchair or special bed can be costly. Wide doorways, ramps instead of stairs, and special fixtures in the bathroom for bathing and toileting are examples of changes that often are necessary. The client may have been the major wage earner. Some clients can enter training programs that allow them to find employment outside the home, whereas others learn skills that enable them to be employed at home. Others, because of age or extreme physical disability, cannot be gainfully employed.

Nursing Management

The nurse listens and is alert to subtle hints about the client's and family's adaptation to the client's change in functional status. The nurse asks direct questions to identify problems and needs. He or she evaluates the client's ability to perform self-care, resume his or her role in the family, and call on a support system. The nurse takes appropriate steps to help the client and family attain and maintain a home life as near normal as possible. For example, the nurse assesses available facilities, the family support system, physical aids required (e.g., a wheelchair, cane, walker), and the amount of assistance the client requires with activities of daily living. He or she encourages the family to help plan for the client's return home, to ask questions about care, and to seek assistance from those agencies that can provide emotional, physical, and financial support.

Coping

The nurse addresses each client individually. He or she offers reassurance and emotional support and displays empathetic understanding of the multiple problems the client is facing. Many clients have difficulty coping with their disability. Crises such as being unable to move, having limited movement, being unable to attend to one's most basic needs, and having to totally depend on others for housing, clothing, mobility, and food create strong emotional responses. Some clients eventually accept their disability; others do not. The nurse provides encouragement and praise throughout rehabilitation and shows personal interest and pleasure in each accomplishment, no matter how small, to help clients accept what they cannot or never will be able to do.

The nurse gives clients time to talk about their problems, fears, and concerns. Once needs are identified, he or she encourages the client to set attainable goals, which may help maintain independence as long as possible. The nurse works with the client and family to develop solutions and possible alternatives. This helps the client and family meet each problem as it arises, understand the limitations, establish goals, and work toward a solution.

With rehabilitation comes the client's awareness of progress or lack thereof. At times, improvement is slow and barely noticeable. A client often has difficulty coping. Discouragement, depression, withdrawal, and anger are not unusual. The nurse suggests available support groups for those with neurologic deficits for emotional, physical, and social support.

Socialization

As soon as clients can respond to those around them, the nurse encourages socialization with others. At first, socialization can be limited to health team members and family. The nurse encourages the family to talk to the client, discuss current events, and motivate the client to respond. Those with speech difficulties tend to become withdrawn and depressed. The nurse encourages visitors to talk to the client, include the client in their conversations, and ask the client questions. The nurse suggests that family members use patience when trying to understand what a client with aphasia is trying to communicate.

Occupational and recreational therapies are part of the rehabilitation program and require a team effort. In the beginning, occupational therapy is designed to help strengthen muscles that are under voluntary control. Later, certain tasks are learned or relearned to help the client interact with others. Participation in these therapies increases socialization time and helps the client interact with others.

Family Processes

The nurse recognizes that the family faces many disruptions because of the permanent disability of a family member. Lifestyles are altered, financial resources are strained, conflicts arise, and people must accept new responsibilities. The nurse allows the family time to deal with and accept these changes. The nurse provides the family with opportunities to talk and openly express their anger, fears, guilt, and helplessness. Although no single perfect solution to any problem exists, the following suggestions may help the family adjust to present and future changes:

- Include the family in the client's rehabilitation.
- Give encouragement and praise when a family member is able to help with a part of home care or shows interest in becoming involved in the client's care.
- Explain the purpose of each segment of rehabilitation (e.g., ROM exercises, positioning).
- When the family expresses a desire to assume responsibility for certain procedures to be performed at home, teach each procedure or task slowly and give the family time to practice under supervision.
- Prepare a list of public or private agencies that may assist with home care, transportation, and financial and emotional support.

Client and Family Teaching

The nurse develops a teaching plan for home care management that incorporates the therapies prescribed by the physician and other members of the team. The client and family usually have many questions. The nurse must begin teaching long before discharge so that the client and family have sufficient time to learn and understand home care management. The individualized teaching plan includes discussion of one or more of the topics presented in Client and Family Teaching Box 48-1.

N U R S I N G   P R O C E S S

● The Client With a Neurologic Deficit

Assessment

The nurse obtains a thorough history (including drugs and allergies) from the client or family. He or she as-

---

48-1 *Client and Family Teaching*
Home Care for the Client With a Neurologic Deficit

A teaching plan for the client and family addresses the following key areas and points:

SKIN CARE

- Explain that the client may not feel discomfort caused by a beginning pressure ulcer.
- Demonstrate how to inspect and care for the skin.
- Recommend a change in position at least every 2 hours to relieve pressure on bony prominences.
- Tell the client to contact a healthcare provider immediately if skin is reddened, warm, or disrupted.

BODY ALIGNMENT

- Explain the importance of good body alignment.
- Demonstrate how to put joints through a full ROM. Explain that the client must perform ROM exercises several times per day or as ordered by the physician or physical therapist.
- Demonstrate how the client can use various devices, such as rolled blankets or pillows, to support or align areas of the body, such as the back, hips, and legs. Explain the use of a footboard or other device to prevent footdrop.

NUTRITION AND FLUIDS

- Discuss the importance of a high fluid intake to prevent urinary tract complications. Recommend taking fluids frequently.
- Discuss the importance of a balanced diet in maintaining optimal health.
- Emphasize that the client may better tolerate small meals and between-meal snacks than three large meals.
- Explain that the client who must be fed needs time to chew the food and take fluids.

BOWEL AND BLADDER

- Stress the importance of continuing a bowel and bladder training program.
- Demonstrate clean rather than sterile technique for irrigating, changing, or inserting catheters at home.

- Advise inspecting the urine for cloudiness (which may indicate a urinary tract infection).
- Recommend contacting the physician if chills and fever occur or if the urine is bloody, cloudy, or has an offensive odor.
- Describe skin care of the genitalia and perineum. Emphasize and demonstrate the special care that must be given to the anal area and the genitalia after defecation. If an external urinary sheath is used for the male client, demonstrate its application and how to clean the penis daily to remove urine and dried secretions.

ACTIVITY

- Stress the importance of social contacts, hobbies, and changes in the daily routine to relieve boredom.
- Emphasize the importance of avoiding fatigue and exposure to infection.
- Discuss the importance of having the client take deep breaths every 1 or 2 hours while awake and to cough to raise secretions.

THERAPIES, COMMUNITY SERVICES, AND EQUIPMENT

- Discuss the importance of working with the therapists and of following their advice about performance or practice of the therapies.
- Make the client and family aware of services available for home care.
- Discuss and list the specific types of equipment that will be necessary for home care.
- Provide the names of agencies or retail stores from which the equipment may be purchased, rented, or borrowed.
- Recommend a consultation with a social service worker for information regarding financial assistance or the availability of loan closets that allow people who need certain types of equipment to borrow these materials.

sesses vital signs and level of comfort. The nurse weighs the client for future comparisons. He or she performs a general neurologic assessment and uses a standardized assessment tool (see Table 48-2) to note the extent of neurologic deficits related to swallowing, vision, weakness or paralysis of extremities, speech, and understanding of language. The nurse asks about any seizures and for a description of those that have occurred. He or she evaluates airway, breathing, circulation, and LOC. The nurse inspects the skin, auscultates the abdomen for bowel sounds, palpates the bladder for distention, and determines the client's ability to control bowel and bladder. He or she explores the client's emotional and mental status such as stability of mood, evidence of depression, and motivation for rehabilitation.

Diagnosis, Planning, and Interventions

In addition to the diagnoses discussed in the following, many nursing diagnoses may apply for the client and family facing a neurologic deficit (Boxes 48-1 and 48-2).

Risk for Impaired Skin or Tissue Integrity related to immobility, incontinence, or other factors (specify)
Expected Outcome: Skin will remain intact and free from infection.

- Inspect all pressure points daily; keep skin clean and dry at all times. *Assessment enables identification of problems. Clean, dry skin reduces bacteria and the moisture that promotes their reproduction.*
- Massage bony prominences that blanch when pressure is relieved. *Massage increases circulation to the tissues, bringing oxygen and removing carbon dioxide and cellular wastes. Massage is contraindicated if the skin is*

already impaired, as evidenced by areas that remain reddened with relief of pressure.

- Use a flotation mattress, sheepskin pads, and other devices to relieve pressure when client is lying and sitting (Fig. 48-1). *The integument becomes impaired when capillary pressure falls below 32 mm Hg.*
- Change client's position every 2 hours. *Doing so relieves pressure over bony prominences and maintains sufficient capillary pressure to keep integument intact.*

Risk for Disuse Syndrome related to musculoskeletal inactivity and neuromuscular impairment
Expected Outcome: Client will maintain ROM in all joints.

- Keep extremities aligned with pillows, trochanter rolls, and splints. *A neutral position facilitates functional use of the limbs.*
- Perform passive ROM exercises with the weak or paralyzed extremity. *ROM maintains joint flexibility and prevents permanent contractures (Fig. 48-2).*

BOX 48-2 ● Family and Home Management Nursing Diagnoses

- **Impaired Home Maintenance** related to inability to care for self, inadequacies such as housing, care, financial resources (specify)
- **Impaired Adjustment** related to inability to accept the physical changes and impaired cognition
- **Impaired Social Interaction** related to aphasia, immobility
- **Social Isolation** related to immobility, lack of transportation, other (specify)
- **Interrupted Family Processes** related to changes in health status, disability of family member
- **Compromised Family Coping** related to exhaustion of supportive capacity

---

BOX 48-1 ● Additional Nursing Diagnoses for the Client With a Neurologic Deficit

- **Deficient Knowledge** (specify) related to cognitive limitation, lack of recall, misinterpretation of information
- **Impaired Memory** related to neurologic disturbances
- **Relocation Stress Syndrome** related to losses involved in decision to move, feeling of powerlessness
- **Ineffective Role Performance** related to change in ability to resume role
- **Caregiver Role Strain** related to complexity or amount of care needed
- **Chronic Confusion** related to cognitive changes
- **Powerlessness** related to inability to control situation, dependence on others
- **Hopelessness** related to feeling overwhelmed by prognosis
- **Ineffective Coping** related to chronic stress
- **Deficient Diversional Activity** related to immobility, depression, withdrawal, inability to participate in social activities, monotonous environment
- **Ineffective Therapeutic Regimen Management** related to insufficient knowledge of tests, treatments, home care management, other (specify)

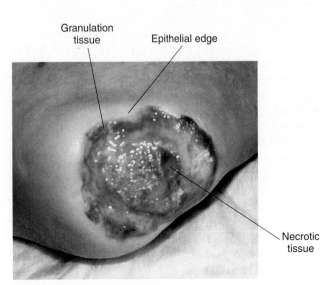

Granulation tissue | Epithelial edge | Necrotic tissue

FIGURE 48-1 Pressure ulcer of the elbow in a client with a cerebrovascular accident cared for at home. This client was admitted to the hospital for treatment of multiple pressure ulcers.

FIGURE 48-2 Contracture of the right leg in a client cared for at home after a cerebrovascular accident. (Photograph by D. Atkinson)

- Prevent footdrop with a footboard. *A footboard positions the foot and ankle in such a way as to prevent plantar flexion.*
- Remove and reapply elastic stockings at least twice a day. *Elastic stockings support vein walls, reduce hemostasis, and decrease the potential for thrombophlebitis.*

Constipation or **Diarrhea (specify)** related to prolonged immobility, tube feedings, decreased fluid intake, effect of disease or injury on the spinal cord nerves

Expected Outcome: Client will have regular bowel movements at least every 3 days.

- Keep a daily record of all bowel movements. *A database helps identify problems.*
- Administer a prescribed stool softener daily. *Stool softeners moisturize the feces, which facilitates passage of stool without straining.*
- Increase client's daily fluid intake. *Oral fluids contribute to moisture in stool.*
- Institute a bowel training program (Nursing Guidelines 48-1). *Bowel training promotes bowel continence.*
- Perform a digital examination of the rectum if there is no bowel elimination in 3 days or if client passes liquid stools. *A digital examination helps determine if hard stool is in the rectum; passage of liquid stool may accompany fecal impaction.*
- Add high-fiber foods to the diet. *Fiber increases fecal bulk and pulls water into the feces, promoting regular bowel elimination.*

NURSING GUIDELINES 48-1

Implementing a Bowel Training Program

Some clients can achieve self-controlled emptying of the bowel provided they and those who care for them exert the persistent effort required. Bowel control typically is easier to achieve than bladder control.

For a bowel training program:

- Keep a record of bowel movements over several weeks. Doing so helps determine the time of day the client is most likely to have a bowel movement.
- Encourage liquids throughout the day. Include foods that produce bulk, such as fresh fruits and vegetables, in the diet. Eliminate foods that cause loose stools.
- Assist client to the bathroom at a certain time each day. The physical activity involved in getting out of bed often increases peristalsis and encourages defecation.
- Administer a low-volume enema or suppository each day at the same time to stimulate a bowel movement. Later, bowel function will become regulated so that the client can have a bowel movement at this time without these aids.

Steps:

1. Tape the paralyzed client's buttocks together to keep a suppository in place. Remove the tape at the time the suppository is expected to work.
2. Give enemas slowly, about 1 to 2 oz followed by a waiting period, to clients with tetraplegia or paraplegia who can retain sufficient enema solution.
3. Check the temperature of the enema solution immediately before administration. Insert the rectal tube gently, especially for clients who cannot feel, because they are vulnerable to trauma.
4. Allow the client privacy and sufficient time to have a bowel movement.

- Discuss persistent diarrhea with physician. *Bacterial growth in warm enteral formula, contamination of tube feeding equipment, and low-fiber formulas can cause enteritis and diarrhea.*

Total Urinary Incontinence or **Urinary Retention** related to effects of disease or injury to the nervous system or spinal cord nerves, loss of bladder tone

Expected Outcome: Client will void, the bladder will empty with no urinary retention, or both.

- Use an indwelling catheter or intermittent catheterization. *Some neurologic deficits are permanent; urinary elimination and continence may require a catheter.*
- Measure intake and output when client has an indwelling urethral catheter and takes fluids poorly and when first removing an indwelling urethral catheter. *Measuring intake and output helps identify whether fluid volume is within normal expectations.*
- Palpate the lower abdomen for bladder distention; notify the physician if client cannot void. *The bladder is*

not palpable unless it becomes distended. The urge to void occurs when the bladder contains 150 to 300 mL; urination needs to occur several times a day to avoid overdistention.

- Ensure client uses incontinence pads or absorbent underwear. *Disposable, porous pads and underwear wick urine away and keep bedding dry.*
- Institute a bladder training program as soon as possible (Nursing Guidelines 48-2). *Bladder training promotes urinary continence.*

Impaired Physical Mobility related to muscle weakness and paralysis

Expected Outcome: Client will tolerate increased physical mobility as demonstrated by use of devices for mobility and remain free of contractures.

- Perform active or passive ROM exercises on the affected and unaffected extremities or encourage client to perform ROM exercises independently (Figs. 48-3 and 48-4). *ROM exercises prevent contractures and muscle atrophy.*
- Regularly position clients with paraplegia or tetraplegia in an upright posture. *An upright posture helps the client*

FIGURE 48-3 Exercises of the affected hand and arm that hemiplegic clients can learn to do themselves. (**A–C**) The affected arm is grasped at the wrist by the unaffected hand and is raised over the head. (**D** and **E**) The unaffected hand is slipped into the spastic hand, and each finger is extended slowly in turn.

NURSING GUIDELINES 48-2

Implementing a Bladder Training Program

- Record the times the client voids over several weeks to help establish voiding patterns.

- Plan a voiding schedule that is similar to the assessed voiding patterns.

- Encourage increased fluid intake; clients who remain relatively immobile for the rest of their lives are subject to bladder infections and calculus (stone) formation in the urinary tract.

- Advise client to note any sensation (chilliness, lower abdominal discomfort, restlessness) that precedes voiding. Doing so helps the client identify when he or she needs to void.

- Encourage client to void every 30 minutes to 2 hours while awake. If the client can use the bedpan or urinal, keep these readily available, and answer the call light promptly when the client requires assistance.

- Instruct client to bend at the waist or press inward and downward over the bladder, a technique referred to as **Credé's maneuver.** It increases abdominal pressure and facilitates emptying the bladder.

- Use other measures to stimulate voiding, such as running water and placing a hand in a basin of water.

- Propose that paralyzed clients with **reflex incontinence**, which occurs spontaneously when the bladder is full, lightly massage or tap the skin above the pubic area, a method known as **cutaneous triggering** that stimulates relaxation of the urinary sphincter.

FIGURE 48-4 Range-of-motion exercises for the affected foot in hemiplegia. The motions should be conducted slowly and smoothly, with a momentary pause when spasticity causes resistance. As soon as the client has movement, these exercises can be done actively rather than passively.

take in the immediate environment and helps promote circulation through regulation of baroreceptors.

- Apply an abdominal binder and elastic stockings before the client gets up. *An abdominal binder and elastic stockings decrease pooling of blood in distal areas, thereby preventing dizziness and faintness.*
- Suggest using parallel bars or a walker (Fig. 48-5). *Before ambulating independently, clients can learn to support body weight and move forward with a variety of ambulatory aids.*

Risk for Sexual Dysfunction related to disturbance or loss of nerve function to genitalia

Expected Outcome: Client will explore sexual alternatives.

- Be alert to subtle references to sexual dysfunction or problems. *Most clients are hesitant to discuss sexuality openly and frankly.*
- Allow client time to talk or ask questions. *Most clients refrain from sexual discussions if they sense the nurse is unreceptive or pressed for time.*
- Convey acceptance; recommend that the client and sexual partner speak with a physician or sexual therapist. *Medical and behavioral approaches may provide alternatives to former sexual activities.*
- Explain to paralyzed men that spontaneous erections may occur when the bladder is full. *Spontaneous erections are unpredictable and sometimes circumstantially inconvenient.*
- Offer information about penile implants (see Chap. 61). *A penile implant provides temporary or permanent penile erection, which facilitates vaginal penetration during intercourse.*
- Inform paralyzed men that ejaculation is rare, which reduces the potential for fathering children. *Clients*

with paraplegia or tetraplegia have the right to information about their potential for fertility.

- Suggest that having intercourse on a water bed may facilitate sexual activity. *The buoyancy of a water bed promotes pelvic movement.*
- Share that some couples use mutual masturbation or electronic vibrators during sexual activity. *Orgasmic arousal can be achieved using alternatives.*
- Instruct female clients that they are still fertile and may need contraception if a pregnancy is undesired. *Motor paralysis does not affect ovulation.*

Risk for Injury related to muscle weakness, paralysis, seizure disorder, loss of calcium from bone, other (specify)

Expected Outcome: Client remains free from injury.

- Use caution when moving and lifting a client who has been immobile. *Prolonged immobility results in calcium loss from bones and increased susceptibility to fractures.*
- Use a mechanical lift to safely transfer client (Fig. 48-6). *It uses principles of physics to raise, lift, and lower clients with minimal exertion on the part of caregivers.*
- Implement seizure precautions for clients with head injuries or brain tumors (see Chap. 45, Nursing Process: The Client With a Seizure Disorder, for specific interventions). *Client is at risk for injury during a seizure because he or she cannot implement self-protective interventions.*

Risk for Situational Low Self-Esteem related to effects of disability on perception of self-worth

Expected Outcome: Client will maintain positive self-regard, accept changes in body function, express feelings about the disability, and participate in rehabilitation.

- Assess for signs of negative responses, such as refusal to discuss loss, lack of participation in care, and increased isolation. *Nonverbal cues provide more reliable feedback about self-regard than do verbalizations.*

FIGURE 48-5 Ambulatory training in the physical therapy department starts as soon as the client can stand.

FIGURE 48-6 A mechanical lift may be used to transfer a client to and from the bed, wheelchair, or shower.

- Convey respect and hope; encourage verbalization of feelings. *Remaining nonjudgmental and giving the client an opportunity to express feelings help relieve stressors.*
- Help client identify his or her positive attributes and strengths from past experiences. *Focusing on successes rather than failures helps decrease feelings of helplessness and hopelessness.*
- Identify ways to support client's independence and role in the family. *Helping the client maintain his or her previous level of functioning maintains self-esteem.*

Risk for Dysfunctional Grieving related to loss of body function

Expected Outcome: Client will adaptively progress through various stages of grieving.

- Convey support and acceptance of client's feelings. *Grief is a normal response to loss; suppressing grief delays emotional healing.*
- Explain that grieving involves a sequence of emotions. *The grief process is a universal experience that begins with shock and progresses through anger, depression, bargaining, and eventually acceptance.*
- Support grief work: explain denial; promote hope during depression; encourage adaptive outlets for anger; encourage decision-making in all aspects of self-care; focus on present and future goals. *Grief work promotes acceptance of losses.*

Evaluation of Expected Outcomes

Expected outcomes vary, depending on the original goals and nursing diagnoses. The client has no evidence of skin breakdown. Complications associated with inactivity and immobility do not develop. The client works through the grieving process and accepts altered abilities. Defecation and urinary elimination are managed. The client is physically active, as demonstrated by use of trapeze, wheelchair, and other methods for mobility. The client continues sexual activities or learns about sexual alternatives. No injuries occur. The client participates in decision-making regarding daily activities, social outlets, vocational options, and applicable therapies.

 GENERAL NUTRITIONAL CONSIDERATIONS

Clients following a bladder rehabilitation program may be reluctant to drink liquids, fearing "accidents." Counsel them on the importance of adequate fluid to maintain normal urine output and to help prevent the formation of renal stones.

Participants in bowel training programs may avoid dietary fiber to decrease stools. Assure them that adding fiber will aid in normalizing bowel movements.

Clients with paraplegia or tetraplegia have decreased energy expenditures and, therefore, must consume fewer calories to avoid excessive weight gain. Most nutrient requirements are not lowered. It is important that the diet contain nutrient-dense foods to be nutritionally adequate.

To help prevent or heal pressure ulcers, the diet should be high in protein (meat, fish, poultry, dairy products, eggs, commercial supplements), vitamin C (citrus fruits and juices, strawberries, "greens," broccoli, tomatoes), and zinc (meat, seafood, milk, egg yolks, legumes, and whole grains).

 GENERAL PHARMACOLOGIC CONSIDERATIONS

Examples of suppositories used for a bowel training program are glycerin suppositories, which soften the stool in the lower rectum, and bisacodyl (Dulcolax), which stimulates peristalsis in the terminal section of the colon. Enemas used in a bowel training program may be plain water, glycerin, and Fleet brand enema.

Clients with impaired swallowing often have difficulty taking pills or capsules. Whenever possible, give them medications in liquid form.

If a client must take solid medications at home, advise family members to check with their physician or pharmacist before crushing or breaking tablets or opening capsules; some medications must not be crushed or opened.

GENERAL GERONTOLOGIC CONSIDERATIONS

Older adults with a neurologic deficit may lack an adequate support system once they are discharged from the hospital. Involve social services and other agencies to assist these clients and their caregivers with rehabilitation.

Functional problems that accompany aging may complicate recovery for a client with a neurologic deficit. For example, an age-related delay in the relaxation of the internal bladder sphincter can make bladder training more difficult.

Older adults cannot perform activities or answer as quickly as younger adults. Therefore, they may become frustrated, irritable, or depressed when they cannot respond quickly. To prevent frustration and depression, allow extra time for older adults to answer questions, perform activities, and so forth.

Regularly palpate the bladder of an older adult for distention. A behavior change or irritability may be the only sign of urinary retention in older adults with a neurologic deficit.

Critical Thinking Exercises

1. *Discuss methods to help clients achieve success in a bowel and bladder training program.*
2. *A client had a CVA 6 months ago and is paralyzed on his right side. He cannot speak and shows signs of mental changes. He now appears agitated and is making motions with his left hand to various areas of his body, mainly his abdomen. What assessments could you make to determine the possible cause of his agitation?*
3. *A 22-year-old client had a spinal cord injury at T11 and is paraplegic. During a conference, team members mention his*

depression and withdrawal. What other members of the health-care team and services may be helpful in this client's care?

References and Suggested Readings

Al-Khawaja, I., Wade, D. T., & Turner, F. (1997). The Barthel Index and its relationship to nursing dependency in rehabilitation. *Clinical Rehabilitation, 11,* 335–337.

Booth, J., Davidson, I., Winstanley, J., et al. (2001). Observing washing and dressing of stroke patients: Nursing intervention compared with occupational therapists. What is the difference? *Journal of Advanced Nursing, 33,* 98–105.

Chemerinski, E., Robinson, R. G., & Kosier, J. T. (2001). Improved recovery in activities of daily living associated with remission of poststroke depression. *Stroke, 32*(1), 113–117.

Green, J., Forster, A., & Young, J. (2001). A test-retest reliability study of the Barthel Index, the Rivermead Mobility Index, the Nottingham Extended Activities of Daily Living Scale and the Frenchay Activities Index in stroke patients. *Disability and Rehabilitation, 23,* 670–676.

Hobart, J. C., Lamping, D. L., Freeman, J. A., et al. (2001). Evidence-based measurement: Which disability scale for neurologic rehabilitation? *Neurology, 57,* 639–644.

Hobart, J. C. & Thompson, A. J. (2001). The five item Barthel Index. *Journal of Neurology, Neurosurgery, and Psychiatry, 71,* 258–261.

Hickey, J. V. (2002). *The clinical practice of neurological and neurosurgical nursing* (5th ed.). Philadelphia: Lippincott Williams & Wilkins.

Hill, M. C. & Johnson, J. (1999). An exploratory study of nurses' perceptions of their role in neurological rehabilitation. *Rehabilitation Nursing, 24*(4), 152–157.

McNaughton, H., Weatherall, M., Taylor, W., et al. (2001). Factors influencing rate of Barthel Index change in hospital following stroke. *Clinical Rehabilitation, 15,* 422–427.

Thorn, S. (2000). Neurological rehabilitation nursing: A review of the research. *Journal of Advanced Nursing, 31,* 1029–1038.

Timby, B. K. (2001). *Fundamental skills and concepts in patient care* (7th ed.). Philadelphia: Lippincott Williams & Wilkins.

chapter

49

Caring for Clients With Eye Disorders

Words to Know

accommodation	myopia
astigmatism	near point
cataract	nystagmus
central vision	ophthalmoscopy
conjunctivitis	photophobia
corneal transplantation	presbyopia
corneal trephine	proptosis
diplopia	ptosis
emmetropia	refraction
endophthalmitis	retinal detachment
enucleation	tonometry
glaucoma	trabeculoplasty
hordeolum	uveitis
hyperopia	visual acuity
intraocular lens implant	visual field
iridectomy	examination
keratitis	visually impaired
keratoplasty	

Learning Objectives

On completion of this chapter, the reader will:

- Describe the basic anatomy and physiology of the eyes.
- Explain the different types of refractive errors.
- Differentiate between the terms *blindness* and *visually impaired.*
- Identify appropriate nursing interventions for a blind client.
- Discuss the nursing management of clients with eye trauma.
- Describe the technique for instilling ophthalmic medications.
- Explain how different infectious and inflammatory eye disorders are acquired.
- Specify the visual changes that result from delayed or unsuccessful treatment of macular degeneration.
- Differentiate between open-angle and angle-closure glaucoma.
- Distinguish categories and mechanisms of actions of medications used to control intraocular pressure.
- Identify a category of drugs contraindicated in clients with glaucoma.
- Name activities clients with glaucoma should avoid because they elevate intraocular pressure.
- Describe methods for improving vision after a cataract is removed.
- Discuss postoperative measures that help prevent complications after a cataract extraction.
- Give classic symptoms associated with a retinal detachment.
- Discuss the care and cleaning of an eye prosthesis.

This chapter presents the structure and function of the eyes. It also discusses the most important disorders that can affect the eyes, as well as accompanying treatment and nursing care measures.

ANATOMY AND PHYSIOLOGY

The *eyeballs* are globes located in a protective bony cavity or *orbit* of the skull. The frontal, maxillary, zygomatic, sphenoid, ethmoid, lacrimal, and palatine bones form the walls of the orbit. Fat and muscle protect the posterior, superior, inferior, and lateral aspects of each eyeball.

The muscles that permit movement include the superior and inferior rectus (move eye up and down), the medial and lateral rectus (move eye toward the nose and the temple), and the superior and inferior oblique muscles (move eye to the left and right). Six cranial nerves innervate the eye, ocular muscles, and lacrimal apparatus: the optic, oculomotor, trochlear, trigeminal, abducens, and facial cranial nerves.

Extraocular Structures

The eyelids, eyelashes, and tears protect the anterior or exposed surface of the eye. The upper and lower eyelids are folds of skin that meet at an angle referred to as the *canthus.* The outer or lateral canthus is the outer angle, and the inner or medial canthus is at the inner aspect of the eye. The line between the lateral and medial canthus usually is horizontal. Children with Down syndrome have a line that slants upward and outward. People of Asian descent have an epicanthal fold, which is a fold of skin that covers the inner canthus.

The eyelids protect against foreign bodies and adjust the amount of light that enters the eye. The eyelashes trap foreign debris. Periodic blinking clears dust and particles from the surface of the eyes. The eyelids also spread tears over the surface of the eye. The eyelids have multiple glands, including sebaceous, sweat, and accessory lacrimal glands. They are lined with a sensitive, transparent mucous membrane called *conjunctiva.* This membrane extends from the lid margins and meets the *cornea* (the transparent domelike structure that covers most of the anterior portion of the eyeball) at the *limbus,* which is the outermost edge of the iris. The lacrimal *caruncle* is a small, reddish elevation on the conjunctiva located at the inner canthus.

Tears, composed of water, sodium chloride, and lysozyme, an antibacterial enzyme, are produced by *lacrimal (tear) glands* found beneath the bony orbital ridge. The *lacrimal apparatus* includes the lacrimal glands, *punctum, lacrimal canals, lacrimal sac,* and *nasolacrimal ducts.* Tears flow across the eyes, continually bathing and lubricating the surface. The tears drain through the punctum into the lacrimal canals and lacrimal sac to the nasolacrimal ducts, tiny openings at the junction of the upper and lower lids, and then into the nose (Fig. 49-1).

Intraocular Structures

Three layers form the intraocular structures. The first layer is the *sclera,* commonly referred to as the "white of the eye." It is composed of tough connective tissue. The sclera protects structures in the eye. It connects directly to the cornea, anterior chamber, iris, and pupil.

The middle layer is the *uvea,* or vascular coat of the eye, located immediately under the sclera. The uvea includes the *choroid* (contains blood vessels and darkly pigmented cells that prevent light from scattering inside the eye) and the *iris* (the highly vascular, pigmented portion of the eye surrounding the pupil). The *pupil* is an opening that dilates and constricts in response to light. The choroid gives rise to the *ciliary body,* composed of *ciliary processes* and the *ciliary muscle.* The ciliary processes produce *aqueous humor,* a nutrient-rich liquid that nourishes eye structures. The ciliary muscle helps change the shape of the lens when adjusting to near or far vision. The *anterior chamber,* behind the cornea, is filled with clear aqueous humor, which provides nourishment to the cornea. The lens lies behind the pupil and iris.

The *posterior chamber* is a small space behind the lens. Aqueous fluid, produced in the posterior chamber by the

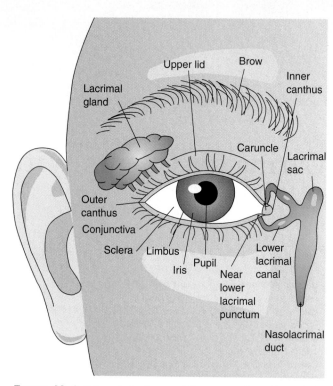

FIGURE 49-1 External structures of the eye and position of the lacrimal structures. (From Smeltzer, S. C. & Bare, B. G. [2000]. *Brunner & Suddarth's textbook of medical–surgical nursing* [9th ed.]. Philadelphia: Lippincott Williams & Wilkins.)

ciliary processes, flows from the posterior chamber to the anterior chamber. It then drains into the *canal of Schlemm.*

Vitreous humor is thick, gelatinous material that maintains the spherical shape of the eyeball. It also maintains the placement of the retina (Fig. 49-2). The *retina,* the innermost layer of the eye, is composed of a pigmented outer layer and an inner neurosensory layer. Light stimulates this neurosensory layer, which contains nerve cells called *rods* and *cones.* Rods function in night or dim light and assist in distinguishing black and white. Cones function in bright light and are sensitive to color. The nerve cells of the retina extend from the optic nerve.

The *macula lutea,* or the "yellow spot," is composed entirely of cones and allows for detailed vision. It lies in the center of the retina. The *fovea centralis* or *foveola* is at the center of the macula. The blood vessels are displaced from the fovea centralis, allowing light to pass to the cones. The density of the cones decreases away from the fovea centralis, as the number of rods increases in the periphery of the retina. The *optic disc,* the anterior surface of the optic nerve, is easily distinguished from the macula because of the vasculature that radiates from the optic disc. No blood vessels radiate directly from the macula (Fig. 49-3). The macula is the area of the eye that provides **central vision,** the ability to discriminate letters, words, and the details of any image. If the macula degenerates or is damaged, only the ability to see movement and gross objects in the peripheral fields of vision remains.

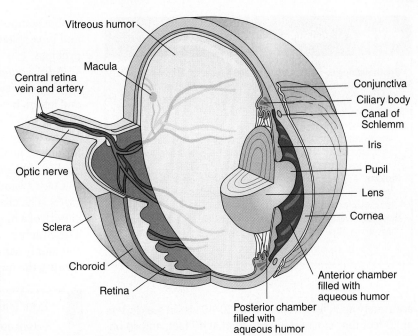

FIGURE 49-2 Three-dimensional cross-section of the eye. (From Smeltzer, S. C. & Bare, B. G. [2000]. *Brunner & Suddarth's textbook of medical–surgical nursing* [9th ed.]. Philadelphia: Lippincott Williams & Wilkins.)

Visual Function

The primary function of the eyeball is to "transform light energy into nerve signals that can be transmitted to the cerebral cortex for interpretation" (Porth, 2002, p. 1242). Every object reflects light. For a person to see it clearly, the reflected light must pass through the intraocular structures—the cornea, anterior chamber, pupil, lens, and vitreous humor. These structures cause **refraction,** which means that the light rays bend and change speed. The lens focuses the light into an upside-down and reversed image on the retina. The rods and cones in the retina send nerve impulses by way of the optic nerve and optic tract to the visual cortex of the occipital lobe. This is where the image is interpreted.

The lens is more convex on the posterior side and can change shape, a process known as **accommodation.** The ciliary muscles contract or relax to focus an image onto the retina, which allows the person to clearly see distant or near objects. For viewing distant objects, the ciliary muscles relax and the lens flattens. The opposite occurs to view objects that are closer. The closest point a person can clearly focus on an object is called the **near point.** Aging results in loss of lens elasticity and makes the use of reading glasses for near vision necessary. When the lens becomes opaque, as when a cataract forms, light is blocked from reaching the macula and the visual image becomes blurred or cloudy.

ASSESSMENT

The ophthalmic assessment provides information about a client's eye health. Nurses usually examine the client's external eye appearance, pupil responses, and eye movements, as well as obtain information about the client's ophthalmic condition. For more complex examinations, nurses need additional education or training. Ongoing eye examinations and treatment require the care of specialists. Box 49-1 provides a list of specialists and technicians who provide eye care and treatment.

Visual Screening Tests

The *Snellen eye chart* (Fig. 49-4) is a simple screening tool for determining **visual acuity,** the ability to see far images clearly. With the chart 20 feet away, the examiner asks the client to identify letters of decreasing size. Results are expressed as a fraction that compares the client's vision with standard norms. If a client has 20/20 vision, it means that he or she sees letters at 20 feet that others see clearly and

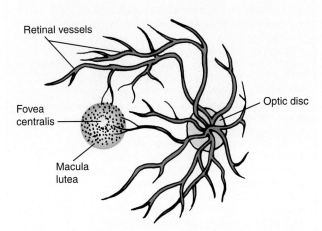

FIGURE 49-3 Structures of the optic disc, including the macular region.

BOX 49-1 ● **Vision Specialists**

Ophthalmologist—A physician (MD) who specializes in the medical and surgical treatment of eye diseases; licensed to diagnose and treat eye disorders, prescribe medications, perform surgery, and prescribe corrective lenses, including contact lenses.

Optometrist—A specialist who earns a Doctor of Optometry (OD) after undergraduate and graduate education. Optometrists test vision, examine eyes, prescribe corrective lenses and contact lenses, and in some states treat limited eye diseases, including prescribing medications.

Optician—A specialist who makes eyeglass or contact lenses based on prescriptions from ophthalmologists and optometrists. The optician also ensures that corrective lenses fit properly.

Ophthalmic technician—Assistants who are certified by the Joint Commission on Allied Health Personnel to assist in selected eye tests and procedures.

with a computerized refractor that records the strength and type of lenses necessary to correct the client's visual problem.

A *Jaeger chart* or *Rosenbaum Pocket Vision Screener* evaluates near vision. These charts contain words, numbers, and letters in various print sizes. The examiner instructs the client to hold the chart approximately 14 inches away and read the smallest print that he or she can see comfortably. The size of the print the client reads indicates the quality of his or her near vision.

Color vision is assessed with *Ishihara polychromatic plates.* The client receives a series of cards on which the pattern of a number is embedded in a circle of colored dots. The numbers are in colors that color-blind individuals commonly cannot see. Clients with normal vision readily identify the numbers.

accurately at 20 feet; a client with 20/40 vision sees letters at 20 feet that most others can read at 40 feet, and so on. If the client cannot identify even the largest letters on the chart, the examiner asks him or her to count the number of fingers that the examiner holds up. If the finger count is inaccurate, the examiner tests the client's ability to distinguish light from dark. Visual acuity also is measured

Stop, Think, and Respond ● **BOX 49-1**

A client asks you what 20/200 visual acuity means. What is the best explanation?

Nursing Assessment

The objective of obtaining a history is to identify any specific problems that the client is experiencing and possible causes. Box 49-2 lists questions that nurses may ask when taking an ocular history. The nurse gathers information related to eye problems: past and current ability to see; any discomfort, pain, or other symptoms; how long the client has experienced problems; any treatments and medications; and other illnesses that may affect eye health.

FIGURE 49-4 The Snellen chart is used to assess far vision.

BOX 49-2 ● **Questions to Ask During an Eye Assessment**

- Are you having any problems with your eyes?
- Do you have any problems with your vision? Do you wear glasses or contact lenses?
- Have you experienced blurred, double, or distorted vision?
- Do you have any pain? Is it sharp or dull? Is it worse when you blink?
- Do you have any itching or feeling that something is in your eye?
- Is there any discharge? What does it look like?
- Are both eyes affected?
- How long have you had this problem?
- Has this happened before?
- What have you done to treat the problem?
- Does anything make the problem better or worse?
- What medications have you used to treat the eye problem?
- Do you have any other diseases or conditions?
- What medications are you taking?
- Have you ever had eye surgery? What? When?
- Do any family members have any eye conditions?

The nurse in the acute care, outpatient, or home setting performs a basic assessment of ocular health by obtaining:

- Client's description of vision changes, any visual or eye discomfort
- Use of glasses or contacts
- Use of prescription and nonprescription eye medication
- Previous eye trauma, ophthalmic and medical diseases, and surgery
- Family history of inherited eye diseases such as glaucoma
- Allergy history associated with seasonal **conjunctivitis** (inflammation of the conjunctiva) that often accompanies hay fever

After the interview, the nurse inspects the eyes for symmetry. He or she also observes the lid margins for signs of inflammation, exudate, or loss of eyelashes. The nurse determines the pupil size, and their change and response to light. Normal pupils are round, of equal size, and constrict simultaneously when stimulated (Fig. 49-5). The nurse

checks the extraocular muscles by asking the client to keep his or her head still while following an object moved up, down, left, and right (Fig. 49-6). Other observations include looking for:

- **Ptosis**—drooping upper eyelid
- **Proptosis**—an extended or protruded upper eyelid that delays closing or remains partially open
- **Nystagmus**—uncontrolled oscillating movement of the eyeball

Diagnostic Studies

Ophthalmoscopy

Direct **ophthalmoscopy** is examination of the fundus or interior of the eye. This examination is done with a direct ophthalmoscope, an instrument that illuminates the internal surface of the eyes and allows the examiner to see the lens, retina, retinal blood vessels, and the optic disc under magnification (Fig. 49-7).

Indirect ophthalmoscopy uses an instrument that produces a bright, intense light. The ophthalmologist uses this instrument in conjunction with an ophthalmoscope to see larger areas of the retina, although no magnification is involved.

Retinoscopy

Use of a *retinoscope* and trial lenses determines the focusing power of each eye. A retinoscope is a hand-held instrument that produces a line of light. The light appears distorted in the eyes of clients with refractive errors. Trial lenses of varying refractive powers are then placed in front of the eye until the light streak does not deviate in any direction.

Tonometry

Tonometry measures intraocular pressure (IOP). It is done by using a tonometer to indent or flatten (applanate) the surface of the eye. The principle is that a soft eye indents more than a hard eye. The force that produces indentation is measured and converted to a pressure reading. Normal IOP is 10 to 21 mm Hg. High readings indicate high IOP; low readings indicate low pressure (Smeltzer & Bare, 2000).

There are various methods for performing tonometry. *Applanation tonometry* provides the greatest accuracy, but the *indentation* method may be used because it is smaller and more portable. Before either is used, a topical anesthetic solution is instilled in the lower conjunctival sac. Anesthesia begins almost immediately and lasts a few minutes. The client does not feel the tonometer while the eye is anesthetized. A *noncontact* tonometer, although less accurate, blows a puff of air against the cornea, and no local anesthetic is required.

FIGURE 49-5 Assessing pupil response to light.

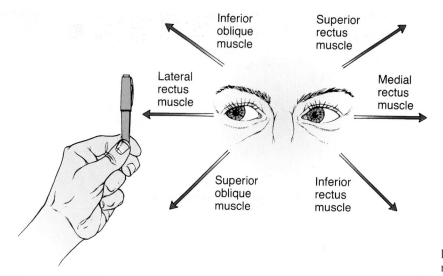

FIGURE 49-6 Assessing extraocular movements.

Visual Field Examination

A **visual field examination** measures peripheral vision and detects gaps in the visual field. The client fixes his or her gaze on a stationary point straight ahead. A light or white object is moved from a point on the side, where it cannot be seen, toward the center. The client indicates the point at which he or she sees the stimulus without directly looking at it. Certain disorders, such as glaucoma, stroke, brain tumor, or retinal detachment, are associated with changes in the visual field.

Slit-Lamp Examination

A *slit lamp* is a binocular microscope that magnifies the surface of the eye. A beam of light, narrowed to a slit, is directed at the cornea, facilitating an examination of structures and fluid in the anterior segment of the eye. This examination is used to identify disorders such as corneal abrasions, iritis, conjunctivitis, and cataracts.

FIGURE 49-7 A nurse examines the interior of the eye with a direct ophthalmoscope.

Retinal Angiography

Retinal angiography is used to detect vascular changes and blood flow through the retinal vessels. Sodium fluorescein, a water-soluble dye, is injected into a peripheral vein. The examiner uses a special camera to photograph the appearance and distribution of the dye in the retinal arteries, capillaries, and veins at 1-second intervals. The photographs provide a record of vascular filling and emptying defects. Many conditions affect retinal circulation, such as diabetes mellitus, hypertension, drug toxicity, tumors, and acquired immunodeficiency syndrome. Intravenous fluorescein causes skin to yellow slightly for 6 to 8 hours. The urine also turns bright yellow, but the color becomes less noticeable over the following 24 to 36 hours as the dye is excreted.

Ultrasonography

Ultrasonography is used when pathologic changes such as an opaque lens, cloudy cornea, or bloody vitreous make it difficult to look directly at the posterior of the eye. Using sound waves, the contour and shape of contents in the eye are imaged and recorded. After instillation of anesthetic ophthalmic drops, an ultrasound probe is placed on the cornea and a recording is made on an oscilloscope. This technique is helpful in detecting eye lesions and measuring for an intraocular lens implant before extracting a cataract.

Retinal Imaging

A new ophthalmologic screening tool uses a *retinal imaging* system to produce a high-resolution image of almost the entire retina without having to dilate the pupil. The Panoramic 200 Non-mydriatic Scanning Laser Ophthalmoscope (Optos, Dunfermline, Scotland) can detect retinal disorders such as diabetic retinopathy, and provides an excellent baseline screening test (Scerra, 2000).

IMPAIRED VISION

● REFRACTIVE ERRORS

Emmetropia, or normal vision, means that light rays are bent to focus images precisely on the retina. In refractive errors, vision is impaired because light rays are not sharply focused on the retina (Fig. 49-8). Refractive errors include myopia, hyperopia, presbyopia, and astigmatism.

Myopia is nearsightedness. People who are myopic hold things close to their eyes to see them well. **Hyperopia** is farsightedness. People who are hyperopic see objects that are far away better than objects that are close. **Presbyopia** is associated with aging and results in difficulty with near vision. People with presbyopia hold reading material or handwork at a distance to see it more clearly. **Astigmatism** is visual distortion caused by an irregularly shaped cornea. Many people have both astigmatism and myopia or hyperopia (Box 49-3).

Pathophysiology and Etiology

Refractive errors are inherited or occur as a result of surgical treatment of disorders of the cornea or lens. Presbyopia occurs because of degenerative changes.

Myopia occurs in people with elongated eyeballs. Because of the excessive length of the eye, light rays focus in the vitreous body before they reach the retina. Hyperopia results when the eyeball is shorter than normal, causing the light rays to focus at a theoretical point behind the retina. Astigmatism results from unequal curvatures in

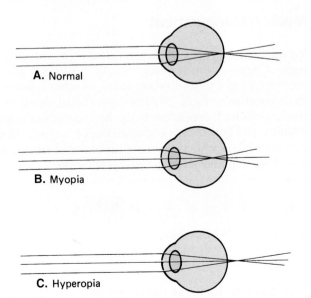

A. Normal

B. Myopia

C. Hyperopia

FIGURE 49-8 Ocular focusing of parallel light rays.

> **BOX 49-3 ● Alterations in Refraction**
>
> **Emmetropia (normal refraction)**—Parallel light rays are focused on the retina. Nearby vision requires contraction of ciliary muscle to bring object into focus. Vision defects are present if light rays converge in front of or behind the retina or if the eyeball is shaped abnormally.
>
> **Myopia (nearsightedness)**—Parallel light rays are focused in front of the retina as a result of increased anteroposterior diameter of the eyeball. Myopic persons cannot focus sharply on a distant object. As the individual moves closer to the object, the rays become more focused, and the focal point finally falls on the retina.
>
> **Hyperopia (farsightedness)**—The eyeball is abnormally short. Parallel light rays are focused beyond the retina. Focus on distant objects occurs through accommodation. As objects move closer to the eye, accommodation can no longer compensate, and images become blurred. The near point is abnormally distant.
>
> **Astigmatism (defect of the curvature of the cornea and lens producing refractive errors)**—Parallel rays are imperfectly focused on the retina. Light striking peripheral areas is bent at different angles and not focused on a single point on the retina.

the shape of the cornea. Presbyopia is caused by the gradual loss of elasticity of the lens, which leads to decreased ability to accommodate, or focus, for near vision. The loss of accommodation progresses gradually.

Assessment Findings

People with refractive errors experience blurred vision. Some seek help for recurrent headaches caused by straining to see clearly.

Refractive errors are detected with the Snellen and Jaeger charts. During retinoscopy, the vision of myopes improves when concave trial lenses correct the focusing power of the eyes. Hyperopes experience improvement when convex lenses are used. The amount of power needed to improve visual acuity indicates the degree of refractive error. The refractive error is not always the same in both eyes.

Medical Management

Refractive errors usually are corrected with eyeglasses or contact lenses. The lenses bend light rays to compensate for the refractive error. Not everyone can wear contact lenses; people with a history of recurrent eye infections, low tear production, or severe allergic reactions are more likely to have trouble with them.

Surgical Management

Incisional radial keratotomy (RK) is a surgical procedure used to correct refractive disorders. Under local anesthesia, the cornea is reshaped by making incisions. It is made flatter for clients with myopia and more cone-shaped for clients with hyperopia, enabling light rays to converge directly at the back of the retina. This procedure is not always successful. Complications include infection and increased glare from microscarring of the cornea. Some clients report a worsening of their vision after surgery. When successful, clients no longer need to wear corrective lenses.

Two newer procedures are similar but use laser to achieve the desired results:

- *Laser-assisted in situ keratomileusis (LASIK)*—The eye surgeon uses a surgical instrument to create a corneal flap, which is gently folded back to expose the inner cornea. A cool-beam laser then resculpts the cornea and the flap is returned to its original position.
- *Photorefractive keratectomy (PRK)*—This procedure involves the removal of the epithelial layer (top surface) of the cornea, exposing the inner cornea. This allows a computer-assisted laser to resculpt the curvature of the eye.

Both procedures potentially provide complete correction of refractive errors, but can result in overcorrection or undercorrection. Other complications include decentered ablation, dry eye syndrome, epithelial abrasion, or infection. With LASIK, complications include wrinkles in the flap, debris under the flap, a displaced flap, or infection or inflammation of the flap.

Nursing Management

Nurses, especially those in pediatric offices, industrial sites, community school systems, and public health clinics, perform screening examinations and refer clients to eye specialists. They are instrumental in teaching clients how to care for their corrective lenses and remove and clean contact lenses (Nursing Guidelines 49-1). In addition, nurses provide preoperative and postoperative care and teach clients about postoperative care at home. Nursing Guidelines 49-2 provides some postoperative teaching points for clients having LASIK or PRK.

• BLINDNESS

Blindness is a legal term for visual acuity of 20/200 or less even with corrective lenses. The term **visually impaired** is used to describe visual acuity between 20/70 and 20/200 in the better eye with the use of glasses. Many who are considered blind perceive light and motion. People with severe loss of visual field also are referred to as blind. Blindness can be congenital or caused by injury, a high fever that damages the optic nerve, or disorders such as cataracts, glaucoma, retinal detachment, macular degeneration, and tumors. Table 49-1 further defines impaired vision.

NURSING GUIDELINES 49-1

Care of Eyeglasses and Contact Lenses

For Eyeglasses

- Clean eyeglasses daily or more often if needed with warm water and soap or detergent, or use a commercial glass cleaner.
- Rinse the glasses well; dry them with a soft, clean cloth.
- Do not use paper tissues—the wood pulp from which they are made can scratch the lenses.

For Contact Lenses

- Use a container that identifies the compartments for the right and left lenses.
- Remove a soft lens by sliding it onto the sclera and grasping it between thumb and forefinger.
- Remove a hard lens by stretching the eyelid at the outer margin and blinking. Clients who cannot master this technique can remove the lens with a suction cup.
- Pour a small amount of cleaning solution into the palm, and rub the solution over the contact lens for 30 seconds on each side.
- Rinse and store the lens in a soaking solution.
- When replacing the lenses, wash hands and rinse the lens in normal saline solution.
- Drop wetting solution in the cup of a hard lens.
- Position the lens on the tip of the index finger and place the lens to the eye.
- To position a hard lens, gently close the eyelids or move the lens by manipulating it beneath the closed lid. To help center a soft lens, blink after its insertion.
- Wash soaking containers for hard lenses daily and allow them to drain dry. Once a day, usually in the evening, sterilize soft lenses in a heating unit. Also clean soft lenses weekly with an enzyme to remove protein deposits.

Medical Management

Vision is improved to its maximum extent with corrective lenses. Clients who are severely visually impaired or blind are referred to a rehabilitation center or other resource for supportive services. Blind or nearly blind clients are taught skills for independent living, how to use a cane for mobility, and how to read and write Braille, a system that uses raised dots to form letters of the alphabet and numbers. Some individuals use trained guide dogs.

NURSING   PROCESS

• The Client Who Is Blind

Assessment

In addition to assessing the degree of the client's impairment, the nurse asks questions about how the client is coping with his or her visual problems. Grief is a nor-

NURSING GUIDELINES 49-2

Postoperative Teaching for Clients Having LASIK or PRK

LASIK

- Stitches are not needed—the corneal flap remains in place through natural eye pressure.

- Antibiotic eyedrops are ordered for up to 1 week to prevent infection.

- The client may resume normal activity within 3 days but must avoid strenuous exercise for 1 week.

- Avoid rubbing eyes for about 1 week.

- Healing occurs within 1 week, but it may take 1 to 3 months for vision to fully stabilize.

- Clients may initially experience discomfort for 5 to 6 hours after the procedure. They may use nonsteroidal anti-inflammatory drugs for relief.

PRK

- Antibiotic and anti-inflammatory eye medications are ordered for 2 to 5 days after surgery.

- Clear contact lenses are placed on each eye for 2 to 5 days to prevent infection.

- The epithelial layer begins to regenerate in 2 to 5 days, but complete healing takes 3 to 4 months.

- Avoid rubbing eyes for at least several weeks.

- Avoid strenuous exercise for 1 week.

- Clients may require pain medication for 1 to 2 days after surgery because of pain fibers located on the surface of the cornea.

TABLE 49-1	VISUAL IMPAIRMENTS: INTERNATIONAL CLASSIFICATION FROM THE WORLD HEALTH ORGANIZATION

INTERNATIONAL CLASSIFICATION OF DISEASES ICD 10 DEFINITION

Category of Visual Impairments	Maximum Less than	Minimum Equal to or Better than
1	6/18	6/60
	3/10	1/10
	20/70	20/200
2	6/60	3/60
	1/10	1/20
	20/200	20/400
3	3/60	1/60
	1/20	1/50
	20/400	5/300
4	1/60	Light
	1/50	perception
	5/300	
5	No light perception	
9	Undetermined or unspecified	

A visual field between 5° and 10° (compared with a normal visual field of about 120°) goes into category 3; less than 5° into category 4, even if the tiny spot of central vision is perfect.
(From World Health Organization. [1994]. *International classifications of diseases and related health problems* [10th ed.]. [On-line.] Available: http://www.who.int/pbd/pbl/img/icd10.gif.)

Disturbed Sensory Perception: Visual related to impaired vision

Expected Outcome: Client will independently complete activities of daily living (ADLs).

- Ask client's preference for where to store hygiene articles and other objects needed for self-care. *Involving the client promotes his or her control over the environment.*

- Keep personal care items in the same location at all times. *Doing so provides client with the ability to locate toiletries easily.*

- Move food items from the tray to a larger surface area. *Doing so facilitates locating food and eating utensils without accidental spilling or dropping.*

- At mealtimes, describe where food is on the plate using the positions on the face of a clock. *This measure assists the client to identify location of food.*

- Offer to open containers, butter bread, and so forth. *Allowing the client a choice facilitates independence.*

Risk for Injury related to compromised vision

Expected Outcome: The client will remain free of trauma.

- Orient client to the physical environment. *Orientation assists the client to remain familiar with the environment and to avoid injury.*

- Indicate the location of the signal cord for obtaining nursing assistance. *Doing so facilitates the client's ability to get help.*

- Keep doors fully open rather than ajar. *This measure helps maintain a safe environment.*

---

mal response to being newly blind or having severely compromised vision. Anger or sadness are typical reactions as clients face their disability. The nurse helps and supports clients during depression. It is therapeutic to acknowledge the grief rather than attempt to cheer clients. Another helpful approach is to express confidence that the client has the inner resources to deal with the adversity.

Diagnosis, Planning, and Interventions

One of the nurse's most important roles is to help the visually impaired client achieve independence. Whether the condition is temporary because both eyes are patched, or permanent, the following measures are appropriate:

- Introduce yourself each time you enter the room because many voices sound similar.

- Call the client by name during group conversations because the blind client cannot see to whom questions or comments are directed.

- Speak before touching the client.

- Tell the client when you are leaving the room.

In addition, the care of a client who is blind or whose vision is severely impaired includes, but is not limited to, the following:

- Help client to feel where the door to the bathroom is located. *This intervention promotes independence and prevents injury.*
- Remove chairs or objects that are in the client's walking pathway. *Doing so maintains a safe environment.*
- Instruct client to grasp your elbow and walk slightly behind and to the side when ambulating. *This positioning helps the client to feel secure and ensures safety.*

Risk for Impaired Home Maintenance related to decreased vision.

Expected Outcome: The client will resume independent living.

- Discuss client's network of support who can help with shopping, banking, and transportation. *This discussion assists the client to plan for meeting needs outside the home.*
- Offer a home health nursing referral for the purpose of assessing the client's needs for a home aide. *Home care nurses can provide assistance with household tasks.*

Situational Low Self-Esteem related to impaired adjustment to loss of vision

Expected Outcome: The client will redevelop a positive self-image.

- Call attention to tasks the client successfully performs without assistance if the client focuses on self-pity. *Encouragement promotes positive feelings about ability to care for self.*
- Help client clarify those activities that are essential and then develop a plan for mastering each one. *A plan reduces frustration and systematically helps client achieve short-term goals.*
- Review progress to nurture self-confidence, self-reliance, and improved self-image. *Reminding the client of progress promotes a positive self-image.*

Interrupted Family Processes related to conflict in reversed roles

Expected Outcome: The family will remain cohesive and supportive.

- Encourage client and family members to verbalize their feelings. *Acknowledging feelings provides them with validation for what they are feeling and experiencing.*
- Promote a discussion of other life changes that were difficult but to which they eventually adjusted. *This discussion provides information that can help to form a plan of care.*
- Have each person share a list of inner strengths of the other to promote insight that, regardless of roles, what each brings to the relationship remains unchanged. *Listing strengths gives information that family members can refer to for positive feedback.*

Deficient Diversional Activity related to transition from sighted to nonsighted

Expected Outcome: The client will develop interests in activities that contribute to the enjoyment and enrichment of life.

- Refer the partially sighted client to the public library where large-print editions of books and magazines are available, as well as "talking books" (recordings of printed books). *Diversional activities must be tailored to the client's abilities.*
- Suggest that the partially sighted client use a magnifying lens to read. *This measure enables the client to enhance his or her sight.*
- Contact or refer clients who can read Braille to special agencies for books, Braille typewriters, and other assistive devices. *Appropriate referrals assist the client to reach maximum potential.*
- Inform client about the availability of optical scanners that use synthesized voice. *Scanners make it possible for the client to "read" printed materials.*
- Tell client that telephone companies exempt visually impaired customers from directory assistance charges and offer a "talking" yellow pages information service. *Providing clients with information about available resources assists them to achieve more independence.*
- Instruct client that laws prohibit the exclusion of patrons with guide dogs from public restaurants, public transportation, schools, and places for entertainment. *Possessing accurate knowledge assists clients to make informed decisions.*

Evaluation of Expected Outcomes

The client can perform self-care activities. He or she remains free of injury and demonstrates an ability to arrange for outside support to meet needs. The client expresses more positive feelings about ability to meet needs independently. The family provides positive support, as evidenced by sharing, planning activities, and relying on one another. The client begins to access resources that provide diversional activities and support.

● EYE TRAUMA

Trauma or injury to the eye and surrounding structures can result in decreased or total loss of vision.

Pathophysiology and Etiology

Children and adults are subject to eye injuries from wind, sun, chemical sprays, direct blows to the eye, lacerations, and penetrating objects, such as fish hooks and bits of metal or wood. Cell and tissue injury causes an inflammatory response. Secondary infections may follow the initial injury. When trauma involves the cornea, scar tissue may affect the refraction of light. If the capsule that contains the lens is damaged, aqueous fluid and vitreous penetrate the lens, causing it to become an opaque cataract. Penetrating trauma can lead to **endophthalmitis,** a condition in which all three layers of the eye and the vitreous are inflamed; removal of the eye may be necessary.

Assessment Findings

Signs and Symptoms

The injured eye is painful or described as feeling "gritty." There is tearing, and the client usually tries to relieve discomfort by squeezing the eyelids closed. The effort helps to control eye movement and reduces the light entering the eye. Vision may be blurred. If the bony orbit is fractured, the eyes may appear asymmetric and the client has **diplopia** (double vision).

A blow to or near the eye results in swelling and bleeding into soft tissues with ultimate discoloration (black eye) of the area. On inspection, hemorrhage may be observed in the subconjunctival tissue. The eye may appear to recede into the orbit, and there may be a change in the normal size or shape of the iris or pupil. Adjacent lid structures may be lacerated, bloody, and swollen (Fig. 49-9). Shining a penlight obliquely across the eye detects an obvious or obscured foreign body. Sometimes the upper lid must be everted to detect an object trapped beneath (Fig. 49-10). If treatment has been delayed, there may be purulent drainage in the conjunctival sac. A rust ring is seen in retained foreign bodies that contain iron.

Diagnostic Findings

Staining the surface with fluorescein dye identifies a minute foreign body or abrasion to the cornea. A slit-lamp examination provides magnification and light to visualize structures in the anterior and posterior segments. Radiog-

FIGURE 49-10 To evert the eyelid, the client looks down, and the eyelash is grasped and pulled up as a cotton-tipped applicator is pressed gently above the eyelid fold. The eyelid resumes its normal position when the client looks upward or the eyelash is pulled gently forward.

raphy and computed tomography help find a penetrating foreign body. A radiograph confirms an orbital fracture.

Medical and Surgical Management

After emergency first aid is performed, the eye is anesthetized to ease examination. Antibiotic ointment or drops are instilled, and the eye is patched. Clients with blunt trauma are hospitalized to reduce the danger of intraocular complications. To repair a laceration of the eyelid, the physician injects a local anesthetic and the lid margins are approximated with sutures. A cut on the eyeball, especially the cornea, is serious and requires immediate treatment. Surgery is performed if internal eye structures are damaged.

N U R S I N G   P R O C E S S

● **The Client With Eye Trauma**

Assessment

If the trauma does not involve gross injury, the nurse gently inspects the eye. He or she darkens the room and directs a penlight at the eye to inspect for the presence of a

FIGURE 49-9 Severe eye lacerations. (Courtesy of Kalamazoo Ophthalmology, PC).

foreign body. If the nurse sees none, he or she everts the lower lid and instructs the client to look up. The nurse inspects the inferior conjunctival sac using direct vision or magnification. If this fails to locate a foreign body, the nurse everts the upper lid and directs the client to look down. If possible, the nurse performs a gross vision assessment.

Diagnosis, Planning, and Interventions

The nurse prevents eye trauma by recommending the use of glasses with shatter-resistant lenses or safety goggles while working with substances that can injure the eyes. When eye trauma occurs, the nurse obtains a brief history of the type or cause of injury from the client or a family member. If eye pain is severe, or if the client cannot or is unwilling to permit an initial examination, the nurse loosely patches both eyes and refers the client immediately for medical treatment. If a foreign body is present, pressure on the eye may push the object into the tissues of the eyeball.

Include the following instructions for home care and instilling eye medications:

- Wash hands thoroughly.
- Wipe the lids and lashes in a direction away from the nose with a moistened, soft gauze pad, paper tissue, or cotton ball. Use a separate item for each wipe.
- Pull the tissue near the cheek downward, forming a sac in the lower lid (Fig. 49-11).
- Tilt the head slightly backward and toward the eye in which the medication is to be instilled.
- Do not allow the tip of the container to touch the eye.

- Instill the prescribed number of drops into the conjunctival pocket, or apply a thin ribbon of ointment directly into the conjunctival pocket, beginning at the inner corner and moving outward.
- Close the eye gently.
- Wipe away excess medication that falls into the skin.
- Secure dressing to the face with tape and use an eye shield for additional protection, especially at night.
- Do not rub the eye, and visit an ophthalmologist or return to the emergency department if it is not completely comfortable within a short time.
- Keep all follow-up visits to check the condition of the eye and surrounding structures.

The care of a client with eye trauma includes, but is not limited to, the following:

Pain related to trauma of the eye or surrounding structures

Expected Outcome: The client's eye discomfort will be reduced to a tolerable level.

- Implement emergency measures, such as irrigating the eye, dimming bright lights, and closing and patching both eyes. *Measures neutralize chemical burns and reduce pain from glare and movement.*
- Instill anesthetic eyedrops under the direction or standing orders of a physician. *Anesthetic eyedrops reduce pain. They must not be given repeatedly after corneal injury because of the risk for masking injury, delaying healing, and causing corneal scarring (Smeltzer & Bare, 2000).*
- Apply cool compresses or an ice pack for the first 24 hours, followed thereafter by warm compresses. *Cold reduces swelling.*

A   **B**

FIGURE 49-11 (**A**) When eye drops are instilled, the client looks up. The lower lid is pulled down, and the drop is placed just inside the conjunctival sac. (**B**) Eye ointment is applied as a thin ribbon onto the margin of the lower lid.

Impaired Tissue Integrity related to physical or chemical injury to the epithelium

Expected Outcome: The tissue of the eye will not be permanently damaged.

- For a chemical splash, take the client to the nearest sink or water fountain, instruct him or her to hold the eyes open, and flush the eyes with running water. *Running water removes chemicals and reduces the potential for chemical burn.*
- Tilt client's head to the side, and direct the flow of solution from the nasal area outward. *Doing so prevents the solution from flowing into the other eye and causing damage.*
- Continue flushing the eye(s) for 10 to 15 minutes. *Flushing removes the chemical, neutralizes the effects of the chemical, and prevents tissue ulceration.*
- After irrigation, instill an antibiotic if prescribed. *Antibiotics prevent infection.*
- Apply an eye pad after irrigation. Instruct the client to close the eye while the eye pad is applied over the lid, and secure the pad with tape. *These measures prevent further injury and reduce eyelid movement.*

Risk for Infection related to disruption of corneal and conjunctival tissue

Expected Outcome: The client will not acquire a secondary ophthalmic infection.

- Wash hands before examining the eyes or performing any procedures about the face. *Handwashing prevents infection.*
- Use sterile solutions to irrigate the eye in nonemergency situations. *Sterile solutions reduce the introduction of microbes.*
- Instill antibiotic ointment or drops as prescribed. *Antibiotics prevent infection.*
- Do not use a container of ophthalmic medication for anyone other than the client. *This measure prevents cross-contamination.*
- Avoid contaminating the medication dropper or tube by holding the tip above the eye and adjacent tissue. *This position reduces the risk of infection.*
- Change gauze eye dressings on a regular basis using aseptic technique. *Maintaining asepsis prevents the introduction and transmission of infection.*

Evaluation of Expected Outcomes

Pain is reduced or eliminated. Trauma is minimized by immediate first aid measures. No purulent exudate is noted.

Stop, Think, and Respond ● BOX 49-2

You are accompanying a group of 10-year-olds on a field trip. One of the boys runs into a tree branch and immediately starts crying and holding his eye, stating that something is stuck in it. What action should you take?

INFECTIOUS AND INFLAMMATORY EYE DISORDERS

● CONJUNCTIVITIS

Conjunctivitis is an inflammation of the conjunctiva. It commonly is called *pinkeye* because of hemorrhage of the subconjunctival blood vessels, which cause the pink appearance. Some forms are highly contagious.

Pathophysiology and Etiology

Conjunctivitis results from a bacterial, viral, or rickettsial infection. The microorganisms most often are introduced by air transmission, direct contact with sources on the fingers, a contaminated face towel or washcloth, or transmission from infected lesions near the eye. Allergic reactions, trauma from chemicals, or foreign bodies in the eye also cause conjunctivitis. A local inflammatory response follows damage to the tissue. Untreated conjunctivitis, especially when caused by *Neisseria gonorrhoeae* and *Chlamydia trachomatis,* can lead to blindness.

Assessment Findings

Symptoms include redness, excessive tearing, swelling, pain, burning or itching, and, possibly, purulent drainage from one or both eyes. In infections with the herpes simplex virus, lesions appear on or near the lid margins. In severe cases, lymph nodes in the neck or throat area are enlarged.

Although cultures identify the causative microorganism, more often than not, the disorder is diagnosed by visual inspection and a history of exposure to someone with similar symptoms.

Medical Management

Treatment includes antibiotic or antiviral ointment or drops. Warm soaks or sterile saline irrigations are used to remove purulent drainage, reduce swelling, and relieve pain or itching. If an allergen causes the conjunctivitis, antihistamines and decongestants are prescribed.

Nursing Management

The nurse cleans the eye and instills or applies the prescribed medication. He or she provides health teaching so that the client can assume the necessary care independently. Because many forms of this condition are infectious, the nurse identifies methods for preventing its spread.

● UVEITIS

Uveitis is an inflammation of the uveal tract, which consists of the iris, ciliary body, and choroid.

Pathophysiology and Etiology

The cause of uveitis is unknown, but it definitely produces inflammatory changes. Pathogens seldom are identified. Although the disorder occurs randomly, it is detected with some frequency among clients with juvenile rheumatoid arthritis, ankylosing spondylitis, tuberculosis, toxoplasmosis, histoplasmosis, and herpes zoster infection. Because some of these diseases are autoimmune disorders, uveitis may be an atypical antigen–antibody phenomenon (see Chap. 41). Complications such as glaucoma, cataracts, and retinal detachment are known to occur secondary to uveitis.

Assessment Findings

Symptoms include blurred vision and **photophobia,** a sensitivity to light. Eye pain is experienced in varying degrees. The eye appears red and congested and the pupil reacts poorly to light.

Uveitis is confirmed by its clinical appearance during slit-lamp examination. Skin tests for primary disorders, such as tuberculosis, are performed to confirm or rule out this etiology.

Medical Management

Treatment includes oral and topical corticosteroids, mydriatic (dilating) eyedrops such as atropine, and antibiotic eyedrops. Analgesics are prescribed for pain. Sunglasses reduce the discomfort of photophobia.

Nursing Management

The nurse instructs the client on the medication regimen and drug administration technique and stresses compliance with therapy. Failure to follow the medication regimen can result in serious complications. The nurse also emphasizes the importance of close follow-up during treatment.

● KERATITIS AND CORNEAL ULCER

Keratitis is an inflammation of the cornea. A corneal ulcer is an erosion in the corneal tissue.

Pathophysiology and Etiology

Trauma to the cornea (e.g., wearing hard contact lenses for an extended period) and infectious agents (e.g., bacteria, fungi, viruses) cause keratitis. Secondary infections are common once the epithelium is damaged. Most clients experience severe pain because of the abundance of nerve endings in the cornea. Inflammation and disruption of the tissue interfere with the transparency and smoothness of the cornea, temporarily impairing vision. When and if scar tissue forms, visual impairment is permanent. The degree of visual change depends on the size and density of the corneal scar tissue.

Assessment Findings

Keratitis is associated with localized pain or sensation that a foreign body is present. Blinking increases the discomfort. Photophobia, blurred vision, tearing, purulent discharge, and redness develop.

In addition to flashlight illumination and slit-lamp examination, fluorescein drops or strips provide evidence of corneal tissue erosion.

Medical and Surgical Management

Treatment is begun promptly to avoid permanent loss of vision. Keratitis is treated with topical anesthetics, mydriatics, and local and systemic antibiotics. Dark glasses are recommended to relieve photophobia. Treatment in the early stages of a corneal ulcer is the same as for keratitis. Once corneal scar tissue has formed, the only treatment is **corneal transplantation (keratoplasty).**

Nursing Management

The nurse removes exudate that harbors microbes and instills antibiotic eye medication. He or she follows aseptic principles to avoid transferring microorganisms to the injured corneal tissues. The nurse advises the client who wears contact lenses to stop wearing them temporarily.

● BLEPHARITIS

Blepharitis is an inflammation of the lid margins.

Pathophysiology and Etiology

One form of blepharitis is associated with hypersecretion from sebaceous glands, which causes greasy scales to form. This type often occurs in conjunction with dandruff of the scalp or seborrheic dermatitis found about the ears and eyebrows. Infectious agents such as staphylococci cause other cases. Some cases are combinations of both. Blepharitis can coexist with conjunctivitis and lead to the development of hordeola and chalazions, which are discussed later.

Assessment Findings

The lid margins appear inflamed. Patchy flakes cling to the eyelashes and are readily visible about the lids. Eyelashes may be missing. Purulent drainage may be present.

The condition is definitively diagnosed by scraping the lid margins and examining the scales microscopically, although that usually is not necessary.

Medical Management

A topical antibiotic ointment is prescribed. The condition also improves with cleaning of the eyelids once or twice daily. Because seborrhea (excessive oiliness of the skin) of the face and scalp is associated with blepharitis, frequent washing of the face and hair is recommended.

Nursing Management

The nurse reinforces the instructions for conscientious performance of hygiene measures. Many clients become discouraged because the condition takes some time to improve. Noncompliance contributes to the chronicity of the condition.

● HORDEOLUM (STY)

A **hordeolum** or sty is an inflammation and infection of the Zeis or Moll gland, a type of oil gland at the edge of the eyelid.

Pathophysiology and Etiology

Staphylococcus aureus is the most common causative pathogen. The microorganisms multiply in the oil gland, which initiates an inflammatory response. A collection of purulent exudate accompanies the inflammation in the channel of the gland. As debris accumulates, it causes swelling and localized discomfort. Sties are common in clients with diabetes mellitus because their glucose-rich blood readily supports microbial growth.

Assessment Findings

A sty appears as a tender, swollen, red pustule in the internal or external tissue of the eyelid. A culture of the exudate, although seldom done, identifies bacterial pathogens.

Medical and Surgical Management

Treatment of a sty includes warm soaks of the area and a topical antibiotic. Severe cases require incision and drainage.

Nursing Management

The nurse assures the client that treatment provides relief from pain and discomfort. He or she explains how to avoid transferring microorganisms from the sty to areas of the body by cleaning the unaffected eye first and changing the washcloth, towel, and water after contact with the affected eye. The nurse also instructs the client to use separate fresh tissues, cotton balls, or gauze for each wiping stroke when cleaning exudate from the eye.

● CHALAZION

A *chalazion* is a cyst of one or more meibomian glands, a type of sebaceous gland in the inner surface of the eyelid at the junction of the conjunctiva and lid margin.

Pathophysiology and Etiology

A chalazion forms when the meibomian gland becomes obstructed and the release of sebaceous secretions is blocked. Consequently, the meibomian gland becomes inflamed and enlarged.

Assessment Findings

A chalazion appears similar to a sty, but the swelling in the upper or lower eyelid is not tender. As the chalazion matures, it feels hard. The enlargement within the eyelid causes clients to feel self-conscious about their appearance and affects their visual acuity.

If a chalazion grows large enough to obscure the pupil or compress corneal tissue, the distortion of vision is similar to that caused by astigmatism.

Medical and Surgical Management

Treatment of a chalazion is not necessary if the cyst is small and does not interfere with vision. Warm soaks and massage of the surrounding area are prescribed to promote spontaneous drainage. If the cyst is firm, becomes infected, or interferes with closure of the eyelid, it is surgically excised.

Nursing Management

The nurse prepares the client for examination and treatment by a physician. He or she gives instructions on methods for carrying out the treatment measures. Some points to include when teaching clients with infectious and inflammatory eye disorders are as follows:

- Comply with the full course of prescribed drugs to achieve satisfactory results.
- Wash hands thoroughly before cleaning the eyelids, instilling eyedrops, or applying eye ointment.
- Do not rub the eyes, and keep hands away from the eyes.
- Use a separate washcloth or towel if the disorder is infectious.
- Do not use nonprescription eye products during or after treatment unless approved by the physician.
- Eliminate the use of eye cosmetics or use hypoallergenic products and replace them frequently to avoid harboring microorganisms.
- Keep all follow-up appointments.

MACULAR DEGENERATION

Macular degeneration is the breakdown of or damage to the macula, the point on the retina where light rays converge for the most acute visual perception. The disorder usually occurs in both eyes, but the vision in one eye tends to deteriorate more rapidly.

Pathophysiology and Etiology

Macular degeneration is more common in aging adults. The underlying problem seems to stem from an opening between one of the membranous layers of the retina and the choroid. Serous fluid seeps into the separation, like a blister, and elevates an area of the retina. One or more blood vessels grows into the defect and produce a subretinal hemorrhage. After the bleed, scar tissue forms. The damage almost always is confined to the macular area.

Assessment Findings

Blurred or distorted vision is the first symptom of macular degeneration. Other symptoms include color vision disturbance (colors become dim), difficulty reading and doing close work, and distortion of objects (especially those with lines). When the macula becomes irreparably damaged, clients compare their vision to a target in which the bull's-eye area of the image is absent (Fig. 49-12). The peripheral field, or side vision, is unaffected, but the client cannot see images by looking at them directly.

Fluorescein angiography shows pooling of the dye in the blister area.

FIGURE 49-12 Visual loss associated with macular degeneration. (From Smeltzer, S. C., & Bare, B. G. [2000]. *Brunner & Suddarth's textbook of medical–surgical nursing* [9th ed.]. Philadelphia: Lippincott Williams & Wilkins.)

Medical Management

A laser procedure called *photocoagulation* is done to seal the serous leak and destroy the encroachment of blood vessels in the area. It must be done early to prevent progression of the disorder. For many clients, the diagnosis is made too late and laser treatment no longer is an option. The client is then provided with suggestions for coping with the visual impairment. Aids, such as magnifying glasses, may be of value, and high-intensity reading lamps have helped some people. The ophthalmologist may refer the client to a specialized center for evaluation and selection of assistive devices.

Nursing Management

The nurse helps the client cope with loss of vision. For additional nursing management of the client with permanent visual impairment, review the information that accompanies the previous discussion of blindness.

GLAUCOMA

Glaucoma, the second most common cause of blindness in the United States, is caused by an imbalance between the production and drainage of aqueous fluid. When the drainage system is obstructed, the anterior chamber becomes congested with fluid and IOP rises.

Glaucoma is classified as either open-angle or angle-closure. *Open-angle glaucoma,* formerly called *chronic* or *simple glaucoma,* is the most common form. Its onset is slow, and the client may not experience noticeable symptoms for several years. *Angle-closure glaucoma* is less common, but acute angle closure requires immediate recognition and treatment to prevent blindness.

Pathophysiology and Etiology

Glaucoma occurs congenitally; secondary to other eye disorders such as ocular trauma, ophthalmic infections, and cataract surgery; or as a primary disease among adults older than 40 years of age. It is more prevalent among those who have a family history of the disorder. The incidence is higher among African Americans, who are four to eight times more likely to develop blindness from glaucoma than are other ethnic groups.

Open-angle glaucoma occurs when structures in the drainage system (i.e., trabecular meshwork and canal of Schlemm) degenerate and the exit channels for aqueous fluid become blocked. As the IOP rises, it causes edema of the cornea, atrophy of nerve fibers in the peripheral areas of the retina, and degeneration of the optic nerve.

Angle-closure glaucoma occurs among people who have an anatomically narrow angle at the junction where the iris meets the cornea (Fig. 49-13). This deviation makes them vulnerable to angle closure when nearby

structures protrude into the anterior chamber and occlude the drainage pathway. For example, an attack can be precipitated when the iris thickens in response to a mydriatic drug, by pupil dilation while sitting in the dark, or when the lens enlarges with age and bulges forward. A delay in treatment may result in partial or total loss of vision in the affected eye.

Assessment Findings

Signs and Symptoms

Many clients experience no symptoms with open-angle glaucoma and the condition may not be discovered until the client has a routine ophthalmologic examination. When symptoms do occur, they often are ignored because they are not dramatic. Clients may complain of eye discomfort, occasional and temporary blurred vision, the appearance of halos around lights, reduced peripheral vision, and the feeling that their eyeglass prescription needs to be changed (Fig. 49-14). Clients with acute angle-closure glaucoma become symptomatic quite suddenly. The eyes are rock hard, painful, and sightless. Nausea and vomiting may occur. The conjunctiva is red; the cornea becomes cloudy and commonly is described as appearing "steamy." The attack is self-limiting, but with each subsequent attack, vision becomes more impaired.

Diagnostic Findings

The optic disc, when visualized directly with an ophthalmoscope or with retinal angiographic photographs, shows a cupping effect (widening and deepening of the optic disc). When the anterior chamber of the eye of a client with angle-closure glaucoma is inspected with a penlight or slit lamp, the angle between the iris and cornea is found to be narrow. Tonometry reveals elevated IOP and reduced aqueous outflow. The visual field examination demonstrates a loss of peripheral vision; nasal and superior areas usually are impaired first.

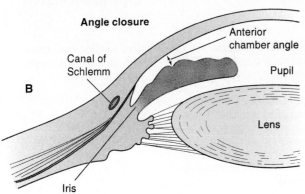

FIGURE 49-13 In the normal eye (**A**), the pathway to the canal of Schlemm is wide and unobstructed. In angle-closure glaucoma (**B**), the movement of fluid is impaired because of the narrowed approach to the canal of Schlemm.

Medical Management

Clients with either type of glaucoma are treated initially with medications (Drug Therapy Table 49-1). IOP can be controlled with miotics such as carbachol (Miostat) and pilocarpine (Pilocar), which constrict the pupil. Miotics pull the iris away from the drainage channels so that the aqueous fluid can escape. Other eye medications that are used for lowering IOP include echothiophate iodide (Phospholine Iodide), epinephrine, dipivefrin (Propine), and timolol maleate (Timoptic). Acetazolamide (Diamox) and methazolamide (Neptazane), which are carbonic anhydrase inhibitors, are given to slow the production of aqueous fluid. In an acute attack of angle-closure glau-

FIGURE 49-14 Gradual loss of vision from glaucoma.

DRUG THERAPY TABLE 49-1	MEDICATIONS USED IN MANAGING GLAUCOMA		
DRUG CATEGORY AND EXAMPLES	**MECHANISM OF ACTION**	**SIDE EFFECTS**	**NURSING CONSIDERATIONS**
Cholinergics (Miotics) *pilocarpine (Pilocar), carbachol (Miostat)*	Increases aqueous fluid outflow by contracting the ciliary muscle and causing miosis (constriction of the pupil) and opening of trabecular meshwork	Periorbital pain, blurry vision, difficulty seeing in the dark	Warn clients about diminished vision in dimly lit areas.
Adrenergic Agonists *dipivefrin (Propine), epinephrine (Epirin)*	Reduces production of aqueous humor and increases outflow	Eye redness and burning; can have systemic effects, including palpitations, elevated blood pressure, tremor, headaches, and anxiety	Teach clients punctal occlusion to limit systemic effects.
Beta-Adrenergic Blockers *betaxolol (Betoptic), timolol (Timoptic)*	Decreases aqueous humor production	Can have systemic effects, including bradycardia, exacerbation of pulmonary disease, and hypotension	Contraindicated in clients with asthma, chronic obstructive pulmonary disease, second- or third-degree heart block, bradycardia, or cardiac failure; teach patients punctal occlusion to limit systemic effects.
Alpha-Adrenergic Agonists *apraclonidine (Iopidine), brimonidine (Alphagan)*	Decreases aqueous humor production	Eye redness, dry mouth and nasal passages	Teach clients punctal occlusion to limit systemic effects.
Carbonic Anhydrase Inhibitors *acetazolamide (Diamox), methazolamide (Neptazane), dorzolamide (TruSopt)*	Decreases aqueous humor production	Oral medications (acetazolamide and methazolamide) associated with serious side effects, including anaphylactic reactions, electrolyte loss, depression, lethargy, gastrointestinal upset, impotence, and weight loss; topical form (dorzolamide) side effects include topical allergy	Do not administer to clients with sulfa allergies; monitor electrolyte levels.
Prostaglandin Analogs *latanoprost (Xalatan)*	Increases uveoscleral outflow	Darkening of the iris, conjunctival redness, possible rash	Instruct clients to report any side effects.

coma, analgesics are given to relieve pain, and the client is kept at complete rest.

Surgical Management

When compliance is poor (e.g., client fails to instill eyedrops as directed) or drug therapy no longer is effective, or if the client develops severe adverse reactions to the medication, more aggressive treatment becomes necessary to preserve vision. One of several procedures that create accessory drainage channels can be performed. These procedures include laser or surgical **iridectomy,** laser **trabeculoplasty,** and **corneal trephine.**

Laser iridectomy, in which holes are burned into the iris to increase areas for drainage, is performed first. If this procedure is unsuccessful, it is followed by a standard surgical iridectomy in which a section of the iris is removed. Either a peripheral or sector iridectomy is used. In a peripheral iridectomy, a small section of iris is removed at the outer margin of the iris. In a sector or keyhole iridectomy, a larger segment of the iris is removed in the direction of the pupil (Fig. 49-15). A laser trabeculoplasty is an alternative to a surgical iridectomy. In this procedure, the laser beam is directed at the trabecular network, which lies near the canal of Schlemm, creating multiple openings for drainage. A corneal trephine is similar to a trabeculoplasty in that it produces a small hole at the junction of the cornea and sclera to provide an outlet for aqueous fluid. The opening is then covered by a flap of the conjunctiva.

Nursing Management

The nurse determines the client's history of symptoms, if the client is already on medication, the medications that have been prescribed, and whether the client is adhering to the prescribed medication schedule. It also is important to ask when the client was first diagnosed with glaucoma.

Acute angle-closure glaucoma is an emergency. The nurse refers the client for medical treatment immediately because vision can be permanently lost in 1 to 2 days. Severe pain requires analgesics. To promote the maximum effect from analgesic drug therapy, it is essential to limit sensory stimulation, such as loud noise, activity, and movement. The nurse informs the physician immediately if the client states that the pain has worsened despite treatment. While clients are incapacitated by their pain or if the disease results in loss of vision, the nurse assists with meeting basic needs. Mydriatics (drugs that dilate the pupil) must never be administered to clients with glaucoma. The nurse consults the physician if drugs with anticholinergic properties, such as atropine sulfate, are prescribed because dilation of the pupil can further obstruct drainage of aqueous fluid, raise IOP, and damage whatever vision remains.

Because glaucoma tends to run in families, the nurse advises adults to be examined regularly. Early diagnosis and treatment are essential for preventing loss of vision. Clients who already are diagnosed with glaucoma are encouraged to maintain close follow-up and comply with the medication regimen. The nurse explains drug instillation techniques. Besides eyedrops, some clients insert an ocular therapeutic system under the upper lid. An *ocular therapeutic system* is a small, thin film that contains eye medication. The film, which is replaced weekly, continuously releases the medication and eliminates the need for frequent eyedrop instillation.

If a client has difficulty remembering when to take the medication, the nurse recommends a watch with a timer. For the client who does not understand the chronic and progressive nature of the disease, it is important to stress that glaucoma has no cure but can be controlled, and that blindness caused by glaucoma usually is preventable.

Other general instructions include the following:

● Obtain assistance from a family member, relative, or friend if you have trouble instilling eyedrops.
● Avoid all drugs that contain atropine. Check with physician or pharmacist before using any nonprescription drug; preparations for cold or allergy symptoms may contain an atropine-like drug.
● Maintain regular bowel habits; straining at stool can raise IOP.
● Avoid heavy lifting and emotional upsets (especially crying) because they increase IOP.
● Limit activities that strain or tire the eyes.
● Keep an extra supply of prescribed drugs on hand for vacations, holidays, or in case some is lost or spilled.
● Seek medical attention immediately if pain or a visual disturbance occurs.
● Tell all physicians that you have this disorder and the treatment prescribed by the ophthalmologist.

FIGURE 49-15 (**A**) Appearance of the eye after peripheral iridectomy. (**B**) Appearance of eye after keyhole (sector) iridectomy.

Carry identification stating that you have glaucoma in case of illness or injury.

Stop, Think, and Respond ● BOX 49-3

What is appropriate advice for a person with a family history of glaucoma?

CATARACTS

A **cataract** is a condition in which the lens of the eye becomes opaque. One or both eyes may be affected.

Pathophysiology and Etiology

Cataracts occur as a result of the aging process or are congenitally acquired, caused by injury to the lens, or secondary to other eye diseases. When cataracts occur in response to injury, they usually develop quickly. Most cataracts result from degenerative changes associated with aging and develop slowly. A high incidence of cataracts occurs among people with diabetes and those with a family history. Prolonged exposure to ultraviolet rays (e.g., sunlight, tanning lamps), radiation, or certain drugs (e.g., corticosteroids) has been associated with cataract formation. In all cases, vision decreases because light no longer has a transparent pathway to the retina.

Assessment Findings

One of the earliest symptoms is seeing a halo around lights. Other symptoms include difficulty reading, changes in color vision, glaring of objects in bright light, and distortion of objects. As the cataract worsens, visual acuity is so severely reduced that the client can read only the largest letter on a Snellen chart, count fingers, and distinguish movement. On inspection, a white or gray spot is visible behind the pupil (Fig. 49-16).

Under ophthalmoscopic and slit-lamp examination, the lens appears in varying stages of opacity. Some lenses are so cloudy that the examiner cannot see through the cataract to the posterior of the eye. Tonometry determines whether the cataract is raising the IOP.

Surgical Management

Cataracts cannot be treated medically and are surgically removed. Surgery often is performed under local anesthesia. A tranquilizer is given before and during surgery to relax the client. Occasionally general anesthesia is used and has certain advantages, especially with an apprehensive client.

FIGURE 49-16 A cataract is a cloudy or opaque lens that appears gray or milky. (From Rubin, E., & Farber, J. L. [1999]. *Pathology* [3rd ed.]. Philadelphia: Lippincott Williams & Wilkins.)

The lens is removed by *intracapsular extraction* (removal of the lens within its capsule) or *extracapsular extraction* (removal of the lens, leaving the posterior portion of its capsule in position).

Phacoemulsification, which uses ultrasound to break the lens into minute particles that are then removed by aspiration, is a technique that may accompany the extracapsular method. When phacoemulsification is used, a smaller incision is required and most clients return to full activity sooner than after the other methods.

After surgery, vision is restored with one of three methods: corrective eyeglasses, a contact lens, or an **intraocular lens** (IOL) **implant.** When cataract eyeglasses are prescribed, the correcting lens for the *aphakic eye* (the eye without a lens) causes the client to see objects about one third larger than normal. These lenses also distort peripheral vision, and the client must learn to turn his or her head to see objects that are not in the center of vision. If only one lens is removed, the client must use one eye or the other to avoid seeing a distorted image. A coating usually is applied to the eyeglasses so that only the aphakic eye with a corrective lens is used.

A contact lens also can restore vision after cataract extraction. Advantages of the contact lens are that peripheral vision is not lost and objects appear about their actual size. A disadvantage is that the lens must be removed at night, cleaned, and reinserted daily, which can be difficult for an older client who has poor manual dexterity or a cataract in the other eye.

A third method for improving vision is the insertion of an IOL at the time of cataract surgery. IOLs most commonly are inserted behind the iris (Fig. 49-17). Candidates for IOLs are those who are 60 years of age or older and at risk for experiencing difficulty with a contact lens or cataract glasses. Ultrasonography is performed before surgery to determine the size and prescription of the IOL. When an IOL is implanted, vision is blurred for a week or more. Reading glasses still are required for optimum vision.

Complications after cataract surgery include infection, loss of vitreous, intraocular hemorrhage, retinal detach-

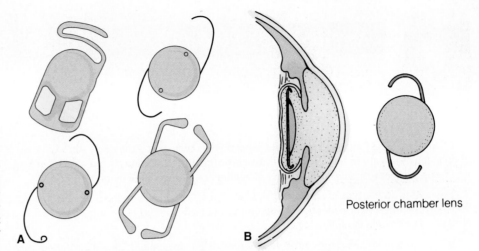

FIGURE 49-17 (A) Intraocular implants are designed to be held in place by various wing-like attachments that center and support the lens. **(B)** The intraocular lens implant is placed in the lens capsule after cataract extraction.

Posterior chamber lens

ment, clouding of the lens capsule, and displacement of the IOL implant. Loss of vitreous is serious because the vitreous body does not regenerate. Its loss, as well as hemorrhage, seriously damages the eye.

Nursing Management

If outpatient surgery is planned, the nurse explains and provides a written list of preoperative preparations that the client is to perform. The nurse is responsible for providing preoperative and postoperative care of the surgical client as well as discharge instructions (Nursing Care Plan 49-1). In addition, the nurse helps the client to take the following postoperative measures to prevent complications and to keep the IOP from rising:

- Tell the client to avoid coughing or sneezing.
- Give antiemetics if nausea occurs.
- Patch both eyes and give dilating drugs to keep the client from squinting.
- Tell the client to avoid lying on the operative side, bending, and lifting.
- Administer stool softeners to prevent straining.

Positioning depends on the type of cataract surgery performed. If an air bubble is instilled in the eye to occupy the space where the lens is removed, the client may have the head elevated slightly and is not permitted to lie flat because this would push the iris toward the anterior chamber and obstruct the flow of aqueous fluid. Intense pain in the eye or near the brow is an indication of intraocular hemorrhage or rising IOP, and is reported immediately.

RETINAL DETACHMENT

In **retinal detachment,** the sensory layer becomes separated from the pigmented layer of the retina.

Pathophysiology and Etiology

Retinal separation is associated with a hole or tear in the retina caused by stretching or degenerative changes (Fig. 49-18). Retinal detachment may follow a sudden blow, penetrating injury, or eye surgery. Tumors, hemorrhage in front of or behind the retina, and loss of vitreous fluid are particularly likely to lead to retinal detachment. This condition may also be a complication of other disorders, such as advanced diabetic changes in the retina. In many instances, the cause of retinal detachment is unknown. Retinal separation is more common after 40 years of age.

The separation of the two layers of the retina deprives the sensory layer of its blood supply. Vision is lost in the affected area because the sensory layer no longer can receive visual stimuli. Vitreous fluid moves between the separated layers of the retina, holding the layers apart and causing further separation.

Assessment Findings

Many clients notice definite gaps in their vision or blind spots. They describe the sensation that a curtain is being drawn over their field of vision and they often see flashes of light. Seeing spots or moving particles, called *floaters,* is common. Complete loss of vision may occur in the affected eye. The condition is not painful, but clients usually are extremely apprehensive. When the retina is inspected with an ophthalmoscope, the tissue appears gray in the detached area.

Medical Management

In a few select cases, an office procedure called *pneumatic retinopexy* is performed. Before the procedure, the client must recline for about 16 hours to allow the separated retina to fall back toward the choroid. Then, 0.5 to 1 mL of

Nursing Care Plan 49-1

POSTOPERATIVE MANAGEMENT OF THE CLIENT UNDERGOING EYE SURGERY

Assessment

Clients having eye surgery require the usual preoperative care. Frequently, they have surgery in ambulatory care settings, so preoperative assessments may be done before the day of surgery. Obtain preoperative vital signs to have a baseline for postoperative monitoring.

Depending on the type of surgery, it is important to ask the client about medications. Check to ensure that instructions about withholding any medications before surgery were followed. Examples include the following:

■ Anticoagulation therapy withheld as ordered. For example, if the client takes warfarin (Coumadin), a prothrombin time of 1.5 is the desired level before surgery.

■ Aspirin withheld for 5 to 7 days

■ Nonsteroidal anti-inflammatory drugs (NSAIDs) withheld for 3 to 5 days

In addition, check the preoperative orders and administer eye drops as ordered.

PC: Ophthalmic Hemorrhage or **Increased Intraocular Pressure** (IOP)

Expected Outcome: Bleeding and IOP will be managed and minimized.

Interventions	Rationales
Report sudden or intense pain immediately.	Pain may indicate hemorrhage or increased IOP, which may require emergency surgery.
Instruct client to avoid coughing, vomiting, straining at stool, bending forward, or lifting anything heavier than 5 lb.	Avoiding these activities prevents the IOP from rising.

Evaluation of Expected Outcome: Client experiences no complications.

Nursing Diagnosis: Pain related to surgery.

Expected Outcome: Client will experience little or no pain or discomfort.

Interventions	Rationales
Acknowledge client's discomfort and administer prescribed analgesic that is appropriate for the level of pain.	Acknowledging and treating the client's pain provide validation and pain relief.
Keep room lights dim. Provide dark glasses if light causes discomfort.	These measures reduce eye sensitivity to light.
If allowed, instruct client to gently use a clean, moist washcloth to remove eye discharge.	This measure promotes increased comfort.

Evaluation of Expected Outcome: Client reports little or no pain.

Nursing Diagnosis: Risk for Infection related to impaired tissue integrity.

Expected Outcome: The incised tissue will heal without evidence of infection.

Interventions	Rationales
Perform conscientious handwashing before an eye assessment or treatment procedure.	Consistent and meticulous handwashing remains the the primary method to reduce or prevent the transmission of microorganisms.

(continued)

Nursing Care Plan 49-1 (Continued)

POSTOPERATIVE MANAGEMENT OF THE CLIENT UNDERGOING EYE SURGERY

Interventions	*Rationales*
Follow principles of asepsis when cleaning the eye or applying a new dressing.	Asepsis prevents infection of operative site.
Keep the tips of all medication applicators clean.	Doing so prevents contamination of equipment and prevents infection of the operative site.

Evaluation of Expected Outcome: The incision heals without evidence of redness, swelling, or unusual drainage.

Nursing Diagnosis: **Risk for Injury** related to compromised vision

Expected Outcome: Client's safety will be maintained.

Interventions	*Rationales*
While client is hospitalized, raise side rails and identify the location of the signal device.	These measures provide client with security and orient the client as to how to get needed assistance.
Encourage client to use a dim light or night light in the room after sundown.	Total darkness presents safety challenges to the visually compromised client. Minimal light provides a light source and prevents injury.
Reorient the confused client. Ask a family member to sit at the bedside if confusion persists.	These measures provide the client with a sense of where he or she is and where things are. Visual compromise can cause confusion. Having someone stay promotes safety.
Apply a shield over the patched eye.	The shield provides additional protection and prevents client from rubbing or accidentally poking the eye.
Assist client to ambulate; ensure the pathway is clear.	Doing so maintains client's safety.

Evaluation of Expected Outcome: Client remains free of injury.

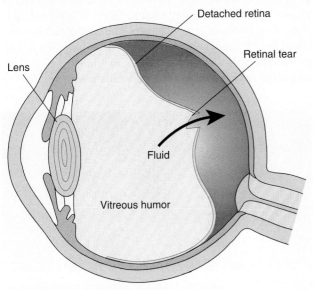

FIGURE 49-18 Retinal detachment. (From Smeltzer, S. C. & Bare, B. G. [2000]. *Brunner & Suddarth's textbook of medical–surgical nursing* [9th ed.]. Philadelphia: Lippincott Williams & Wilkins.)

gas is injected intraocularly into the posterior area of the eye. The gas compresses the retina and holds it in place. To ensure success from the procedure, the client must again assume a restricted position, sometimes up to 8 hours each day for 3 weeks. If pneumatic retinopexy is not appropriate, the physician usually recommends prompt admission to the hospital for surgery.

Surgical Management

Surgical interventions for retinal reattachment include cryosurgery, electrodiathermy, laser reattachment, and scleral buckling. The amount of sight regained depends on the extent of the detachment and the success of the surgery.

Cryosurgery involves the application of a supercooled probe to the sclera. The sclera, choroid, and retina then adhere to one another as a result of scar tissue formation.

With *electrodiathermy*, an electrode needle is inserted into the sclera so that the fluid that has collected underneath the retina can escape. The retina ultimately adheres to the choroid. This method seldom is used.

Laser reattachment involves focusing a laser beam on the damaged area of the retina and causing a small burn. The exudate that forms between the retina and choroid results in adhesion of the retina to the choroid. Laser therapy can be used only when the retinal separation involves a small area.

Scleral buckling is a surgical procedure that shortens the sclera, thus allowing contact between the choroid and retina (Fig. 49-19). A section of the sclera is exposed, opened, and retracted from the choroid. A laser beam or cryosurgery probe is then used to produce adhesion of the retina and choroid. A small silicone patch is placed between the sclera and choroid, and the sclera is pulled over the patch and sutured. The inward displacement of the choroid allows for reattachment of the retina to the choroid.

Before surgery, the client is kept on complete bed rest with the affected eye dependent until surgery is performed. Sedation may be ordered. The eyes are patched and covered with an eye shield. Mydriatic eyedrops are instilled to dilate the pupil and facilitate further examination of the retina.

Nursing Management

Anyone with sudden loss of vision is referred immediately for examination by a physician. If surgery is performed, the client usually is kept on complete bed rest for several days with the head immobilized. The client is not turned or moved without orders. If an air bubble is instilled to promote contact between the retina and choroid, the client is positioned with the face parallel to the floor so that the bubble floats to the posterior of the eye. If floaters are still seen after the eye heals, the nurse can tell the client that they eventually become absorbed or settle to the inferior floor of the eye, out of the line of vision. For additional postoperative nursing management, see Nursing Care Plan 49-1.

ENUCLEATION

Enucleation is the surgical removal of an eye. It is necessary when the eye is destroyed by injury or disease, when a malignant tumor develops (rare), or to relieve pain if the eye is severely damaged and sightless. Sometimes only the contents of the eyeball are removed and the sclera is left in place. Other times, the entire eyeball is removed as well as tissues in the bony orbit.

Medical and Surgical Management

When enucleation is performed, a metal or plastic ball is buried in the capsule of connective tissue from which the eyeball is removed (Fig. 49-20). A pressure dressing is applied to control hemorrhage, a complication of enucleation. After the tissues have healed, a shell-shaped prosthesis is placed over the buried ball. The shell is painted to match the client's remaining eye. The shell is the only portion that is removed for cleaning.

Nursing Management

The nurse observes the client after surgery for signs and symptoms of bleeding or infection. The client usually is allowed out of bed the day after surgery. When healing is complete, in about 2 to 4 weeks, the nurse teaches the client how to insert and remove the prosthetic shell. The prosthesis typically is removed before going to bed and inserted the next morning. The nurse instructs the client to

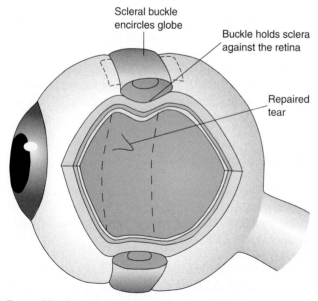

FIGURE 49-19 Scleral buckle. (From Smeltzer, S. C. & Bare, B. G. [2000]. *Brunner & Suddarth's textbook of medical–surgical nursing* [9th ed.]. Philadelphia: Lippincott Williams & Wilkins.)

FIGURE 49-20 Eye prostheses. (**Left**) Anophthalmic ocular prosthesis. (**Right**) Scleral shell. (From Smeltzer, S. C. & Bare, B. G. [2000]. *Brunner & Suddarth's textbook of medical–surgical nursing* [9th ed.]. Philadelphia: Lippincott Williams & Wilkins.)

hold the head over a soft surface, such as a bed or padded table, when removing or inserting the prosthesis to avoid damage if he or she drops the prosthetic eye. The client should clean the shell after removal and keep it in a safe place where it will not become scratched or broken.

GENERAL NUTRITIONAL CONSIDERATIONS

Several studies suggest that carotenoids other than beta-carotene, particularly those found in green leafy vegetables, may protect against macular degeneration. Theorists believe that lutein and zeaxanthin, carotenoids that form the yellow pigment in the macula, may protect the eye against damage by filtering out visible blue light. One study showed that people who ate spinach or collard greens two to four times per week had half the risk of macular degeneration as people who ate them less than once per month.

Studies have shown that vitamins A and C are essential for preventing cataracts. Clinical trials are underway to determine if zinc can reduce the risk of cataracts and macular degeneration.

Advise clients who have cataract surgery to eat soft, easily chewed foods until healing is complete to avoid tearing from excessive facial movements.

GENERAL PHARMACOLOGIC CONSIDERATIONS

Although many nonprescription ophthalmic preparations are available for dry eyes and irritation, an ophthalmologist should assess and treat all eye complaints to detect any underlying pathology.

GENERAL GERONTOLOGIC CONSIDERATIONS

Older adults need to use their glasses or contact lenses when explanations are provided about test procedures.

Teaching aids with large-sized letters are helpful for older clients who are experiencing lens changes associated with aging.

Visual changes can result in accidents and injuries. Assisting older adults with visual deficits with ADLs is essential.

To ensure the safety of older adults with visual impairments, the room should be kept dimly lit at night. Objects, chairs, and footstools are placed away from areas where the client walks, and assistance is given whenever the client is out of bed.

Visual impairment curtails favorite activities such as reading, watching television, and engaging in hobbies or other forms of recreation, resulting in depression and withdrawal.

Critical Thinking Exercises

1. *If a client reports having difficulty seeing, what additional data are important to obtain?*
2. *Discuss preventive measures for transmitting an infectious eye disorder.*
3. *Explain the preoperative and postoperative management of a client undergoing a cataract extraction.*

References and Suggested Readings

Barnie, D. C. (2002). Restoring vision in older patients. *RN*, 65(1), 30–35.

Bullock, B. A. & Henze, R. L. (2000). *Focus on pathophysiology*. Philadelphia: Lippincott Williams & Wilkins.

Polsdorfer, J. R. (1999). Visual impairment. *Gale encyclopedia of medicine*. [On-line.] Available: http://www.findarticles.com/cf_dk/g2601/0014/260100455/print.jhtml

Porth, C. M. (2002). *Pathophysiology: Concepts of altered health states* (6th ed.). Philadelphia: Lippincott Williams & Wilkins.

Scerra, C. (2000). Retinal imaging system works with pupil dilation. *Ophthalmology Times* [On-line.] Available: http://www.findarticles.com/cf_0/m0VEY/18_25/65197577/pl/article.jhtml

Smeltzer, S. C. & Bare, B. G. (2000). *Brunner & Suddarth's textbook of medical–surgical nursing* (9th ed.). Philadelphia: Lippincott Williams & Wilkins.

Smith, S. E. (2000). Time to manage seasonal ocular allergies. *Journal of Ophthalmic Nursing and Technology*, 19(2), 68–73.

Caring for Clients With Ear Disorders

Learning Objectives

On completion of this chapter, the reader will:

- Describe the anatomy and physiology of the ear.
- List types of hearing impairment and the acuity levels for each.
- Name techniques that clients with impaired hearing use to communicate with others.
- Give examples of support services available for the hearing impaired.
- Discuss the role of the nurse in caring for clients with a hearing loss.
- Name conditions that involve the external ear.
- Explain the technique for straightening the ear canal of adults to facilitate inspection and the administration of medication.
- Discuss methods for preventing or treating disorders of the external ear.
- Name conditions that affect the middle ear.
- Describe nursing interventions appropriate for managing the care of a client with ear surgery.
- Explain the pathophysiology of Ménière's disease, and name some consequences of this inner ear disorder.
- Discuss the nursing management of clients with Ménière's disease.

Ear disorders occur throughout the life cycle. Many ear disorders result in hearing loss, a common sensory deficit among older adults. Hearing aids can compensate for some but not all forms of hearing loss. Nurses play a pivotal role in preventing hearing loss by reducing the severity and frequency of ear infections among children and advocating for measures that reduce exposure to loud noise.

ANATOMY AND PHYSIOLOGY

The ear (Fig. 50-1) is divided into three areas: the outer, middle, and inner sections. Sound is perceived because of a chain reaction involving all three areas of the ear. The inner ear also helps maintain balance.

Outer Ear

The outer ear, or *auricle,* consists of the *pinna,* the fleshy external projection of the ear, and the *external acoustic meatus,* a 1-inch canal that extends to the *tympanic mem-*brane, or eardrum. The outer ear collects sound waves and directs them inward. The external acoustic meatus contains the glands that produce *cerumen,* a waxy substance that lubricates the ear canal, protects the eardrum, and helps prevent external ear infections. Chewing and talking help to move cerumen to the outer area of the external acoustic meatus, where it is easily washed away.

Middle Ear

The middle ear is a small, air-filled cavity in the temporal bone. The *eustachian tube* extends from the floor of the middle ear to the pharynx and is lined with mucous membrane. It equalizes air pressure in the middle ear. A chain of three small bones, the *malleus,* the *incus,* and the *stapes,* stretches across the middle ear cavity from the tympanic membrane to the *oval window.* They move when struck by sound waves transmitted from the outer ear. When these bones are set in motion, the footplate of the stapes, which is very flexible, strikes the oval window, agitating the fluid in the inner ear.

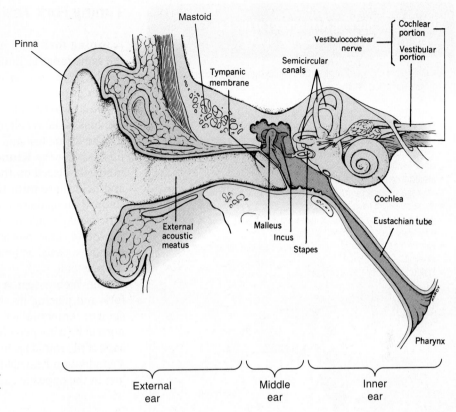

FIGURE 50-1 Diagram of the ear, showing the external, middle, and internal subdivisions.

Inner Ear

The inner ear, or *labyrinth,* consists of a series of cavities and canals that contain fluid. It contains the *cochlea,* which provides for hearing, and the *semicircular canals,* which promote balance, and the *vestibulocochlear nerve (cranial nerve VIII).*

The fluid motion created by the vibrating stapes excites the nerve endings in the sensitive sound receptors of the *organ of Corti* located in the cochlea. The impulses are then converted to nerve impulses and transmitted along the cochlear nerve to the brain, where sound is perceived.

Nerve receptors for balance are found both in the vestibule and semicircular canals. They transmit information about motion through the vestibular nerve, which joins with the cochlear nerve to form the eighth cranial nerve, the vestibulocochlear nerve (formally called the *auditory* or *acoustic nerve*).

ASSESSMENT

Although family practice physicians assess and treat many ear disorders, they refer some clients to *otolaryngologists,* physicians who specialize in the diagnosis and treatment of ear, nose, and throat disorders. An *audiologist* is a paraprofessional with special training in performing hearing tests, measuring hearing loss, and recommending methods

for improving the perception of sound. Box 50-1 outlines the nursing assessment.

Basic Auditory Acuity Tests

One general method is used to assess a client's gross auditory acuity. The method is referred to as the *whisper test.* For this test, the examiner covers the untested ear with his or her palm and stands 1 to 2 feet from the client's uncovered ear. He or she whispers a number or a phrase and asks the client to repeat it. The examiner provides several numbers to ensure valid test results. Another technique is to sit beside the client and bring a ticking watch toward the ear. The client should perceive the sound at the same time as the nurse, who is assumed to have normal hearing.

Otoscopic Examination

An otoscopic examination involves inspecting the external acoustic canal and tympanic membrane using an **otoscope,** a handheld instrument with a light, lens, and optional speculum for inserting into the client's ear (Fig. 50-2). If normal, the canal appears smooth and empty. The normal tympanic membrane is intact, looks pearly gray, and transmits light. Excessive cerumen interferes with inspection.

BOX 50-1 ● Nursing Assessment of the Ear and Basic Hearing Acuity

- Obtain client's appraisal of his or her hearing, including whether the client experiences tinnitus.
- Observe for actions that suggest a hearing problem such as leaning forward, turning the head, or cupping a hand to the ear to hear better.
- Document the use of a hearing aid.
- Ask client about allergies, a history of upper respiratory and middle ear infections, high fevers, or exposure to loud sounds, because all these can cause hearing loss.
- Inspect external ear for signs of infection, such as swelling, redness, drainage, or evidence of trauma.
- Shine a penlight into the ear to grossly inspect the ear canal; straighten the ear canal by gently pulling the ear up and back for an adult and downward and backward for small children.
- Palpate the areas in front of and behind the ear lobe for tenderness and swelling.
- Perform a basic hearing acuity test.

Tuning Fork Tests

A **tuning fork** is an instrument that produces sound in the same range as human speech. It is used to screen for conductive or sensorineural hearing loss. A **conductive hearing loss** involves interference in the transmission of sound waves to the inner ear. **Sensorineural hearing loss** is the result of nerve impairment.

The Rinne test and Weber test identify types of hearing loss. For the **Rinne test** (Fig. 50-3), the tuning fork is struck, placed on the mastoid process behind the ear, and held there until the client indicates the sound has stopped. Immediately after that, the still vibrating tuning fork is held beside the ear and the client again says when the sound stops. Normally, air conduction beside the ear measures twice as long as by bone conduction through the mastoid.

The **Weber test** is performed by striking the tuning fork and placing its stem in the midline of the client's skull or center of the forehead (Fig. 50-4). A person with normal hearing perceives the sound equally well in both ears. If the sound seems lateralized to one ear, it suggests a conduction hearing loss in that ear or a sensorineural loss in the opposite ear.

FIGURE 50-2 Technique for using the otoscope.

FIGURE 50-3 The Rinne test for both air and bone conduction of sound.

FIGURE 50-4 The Weber test for bone conduction of sound.

Romberg Test

The **Romberg test** is used to evaluate a person's ability to sustain balance. The client stands with feet together and both arms extended. The client closes his or her eyes. Swaying, losing balance, or arm drifting are abnormal responses. Because central nervous system lesions cause similar abnormal results, additional testing is needed to confirm an inner ear dysfunction.

Diagnostic Studies

Audiometry

Audiometry is done by an audiologist. Audiometric testing measures hearing acuity precisely. During the test, controlled intensities of sound, measured in **decibels**

(dB), are projected to one ear at a time through a headset. The client indicates when the sound is heard. The lowest level of sound that normal individuals can first perceive is 20 dB; painful sounds occur at 120 dB. Hearing acuity is determined by measuring the intensity at which a person first perceives sound.

Caloric Stimulation Test

A **caloric stimulation test** assesses vestibular reflexes of the inner ear that control balance. Warm (40°C) or cool (25°C) water or air is instilled into the external meatus of each ear separately. The fluid alters the temperature of the temporal bone and creates convection currents in the fluid of the inner ear that simulate movement of the head. **Nystagmus,** a quivering movement of the eyes, is the expected response. Slight dizziness also may be experienced. A diminished response in one eye is significant for an inner ear disorder such as Ménière's disease (discussed later).

Electronystagmography

Electronystagmography is a more precise method for evaluating vestibular function, the mechanisms that facilitate maintaining balance. It is performed in conjunction with caloric stimulation. When the fluid is instilled within the ear, a machine records the duration and velocity of the eye movements with electrodes attached superiorly, inferiorly, and laterally about the eyes.

HEARING IMPAIRMENT

Hearing impairment is described as mild, moderate, severe, or profound, depending on the intensity of sound required for a person to hear it (Table 50-1). Diminished hearing results from a conductive loss, sensorineural loss, or both. Conductive hearing loss occurs from conditions such as an accumulation of cerumen in the external acoustic meatus or failure of the tiny ear bones to vibrate. Sensorineural hearing loss includes such etiolo-

TABLE 50-1	HEARING ACUITY		
HEARING RANGE	**DECIBELS (DB)**	**WITHOUT A HEARING AID**	**WITH A HEARING AID**
Normal	20–120	Can hear faint to painful sounds	Unnecessary
Mild impairment	40–120	Cannot hear unvoiced consonants such as "s" and "f"	Helpful, but not necessarily worth the expense
Moderate impairment	60–120	Cannot hear conversational volume unless others talk loudly	Beneficial for restoring ability to hear normal conversations
Severe impairment	70–120	Misses most conversational content	Amplifies 40-dB sounds to 75 dB, but also amplifies nonspeech and background noise
Profound impairment	90–120	Depends heavily on speech reading	Helps hearing vowels, but amplified speech and background noise are painful
Total deafness	120	Hears only painfully loud sounds or vibrations created by loud sounds	Not useful for understanding speech

gies as atherosclerosis, a tumor of the vestibulocochlear nerve, infections, and drug toxicity. Clients with a hearing impairment often have **tinnitus,** in which the client hears buzzing, whistling, or ringing noises in one or both ears. Box 50-2 elaborates on causes of conductive and sensorineural hearing loss. Hearing loss also can result from repeated exposure to excessive noise, such as live concerts, high volumes from stereos or headphones, or loud work environment (machinery or jackhammers).

Hearing loss seriously impairs the ability to protect oneself and communicate with others. The age at which hearing loss occurs plus the severity of the impairment have extensive consequences. For example, hearing loss during the first 3 years of life, the most critical period for learning to make sounds, affects language acquisition at the word, phrase, and sentence levels. If uncorrected, hearing deficits can lead to depression and social isolation.

Medical Management

Besides treating the cause of the hearing loss, medical management includes a recommendation for a hearing aid, a battery-operated device that fits in the external ear and amplifies sound. Clients with a conductive hearing loss benefit more from the use of a hearing aid because the

---

BOX 50-2 ● Common Causes of Conductive and Sensorineural Hearing Loss

CONDUCTIVE HEARING LOSS
- External ear conditions
  - Impacted ear wax or foreign body
  - Otitis externa
- Middle ear conditions
  - Trauma
  - Otitis media
  - Otosclerosis
  - Tumors

SENSORINEURAL HEARING LOSS
- Trauma
  - Head injury
  - Noise
- Central nervous system infections (e.g., meningitis)
- Degenerative conditions
  - **Presbycusis** (impairment of hearing in old age)
- Vascular
  - Atherosclerosis
- Ototoxic drugs
- Tumors
- Ménière's disease

MIXED CONDUCTIVE AND SENSORINEURAL HEARING LOSS
- Middle ear conditions
- Temporal bone fractures

(Adapted from Porth, C. M. [2002]. *Pathophysiology: Concepts of altered health states* [6th ed., p. 1298]. Philadelphia: Lippincott Williams & Wilkins.)

---

structures that convert sound into energy and facilitate perception of sound in the brain continue to function.

Some clients with hearing deficits learn **sign language** (Fig. 50-5), a method for communication that uses a hand-spelled alphabet and word symbols, and **speech reading,** also called *lip reading.*

Many technologic devices have been developed to promote communication. Some television programs are transmitted using closed-caption inserts in which the dialogue is printed on the bottom of the screen or a person who simultaneously signs is displayed in a corner of the screen. Some theaters provide headsets that amplify actors' voices to individual patrons. Telephones can be adapted with a hearing amplifier that increases sound from incoming callers. Another device for people with severe hearing impairment is a telecommunication device for the deaf (TDD). This device is a combination special typewriter and telephone used to call someone else with a TDD. A TDD business directory is available, or the TDD user can call a relay center and the center will communicate for the TDD user. Computer modems also facilitate communication.

Many other products allow the hearing impaired to perceive (rather than hear) sound. For example, light-activated alarms in smoke detectors, alarm clocks, door-bells, and telephones flash a light when sound is produced. Hearing dogs, like guide dogs for the blind, are specially trained to warn their owners when certain sounds occur.

Surgical Management

Sensorineural hearing loss usually is irreversible. It is somewhat improved with a **cochlear implant,** a device that is surgically placed in the inner ear and connected to a receiver in the bone behind the ear (Fig. 50-6). Even with a cochlear implant, clients frequently have difficulty understanding and learning speech.

Nursing Management

The nurse observes for signs of hearing impairment such as leaning forward, turning and cupping the ear to hear better, and asking that words be repeated. He or she assesses gross hearing using the techniques described earlier. The nurse also determines the clarity of the client's speech. He or she refers a client for the diagnosis and subsequent treatment of a hearing impairment, and speech therapy. Many people reject the idea that their hearing is impaired. Some consider it a sign of aging and deterioration. If the client fears that wearing a hearing aid is a stigma, the nurse describes the various types of hearing aids that are available, some of which fit almost unnoticeably in the ear (Fig. 50-7). The nurse also stresses

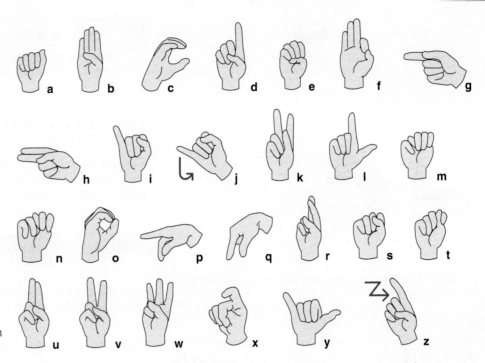

FIGURE 50-5 The alphabet in sign language.

the importance of avoiding the purchase of a hearing aid from a mail order catalogue or a company salesman.

If a hearing impairment exists, the nurse obtains information about its severity and the methods used to understand the speech of others. When a client hears poorly, the nurse determines the communication method the client prefers: speech reading, signing, writing, or typing. Suggestions for oral communication are listed in Nursing Guidelines 50-1. If the client uses a hearing aid, the nurse safeguards the instrument, assists the client with its insertion, and helps maintain its function.

To protect their self-esteem, some clients with a hearing impairment nod their heads as if they are following the conversation or laugh along with others to conceal the fact that they do not understand what has been said. The nurse encourages clients with a hearing loss to be forthright and inform others about the hearing deficit. In addition, he or she identifies assistive hearing devices and aids for communication discussed earlier. The nurse advises clients to maintain previously established relationships because a physical impairment in unlikely to affect genuine friendships.

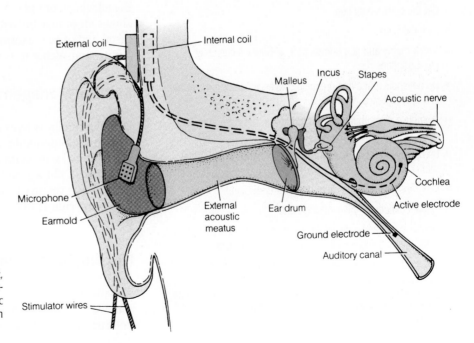

FIGURE 50-6 With a cochlear implant, sound is passed from the external transmitter to the inner coil by magnetic conduction and is then carried over an electrode to the cochlea.

FIGURE 50-7 Examples of hearing aids: (**A**) in-the-ear, (**B**) behind-the-ear, and (**C**) body aid.

The nurse uses illustrations, pamphlets and written directions to aid teaching and includes a family member. He or she asks the client to repeat information and demonstrate technical skills. The nurse initiates a referral to a community agency to evaluate if and how well the client is performing self-care after discharge.

NURSING GUIDELINES 50-1

Communicating With People Who Have a Hearing Loss

- Eliminate background noise as much as possible.
- Stand or sit on the side of the client's better ear.
- Ensure that there is adequate natural or artificial light.
- Get the client's attention.
- Face the client.
- Speak clearly and at a normal pace without exaggerating pronunciations.
- Do not shout, but avoid dropping conversational volume at the end of a sentence.
- Promote a clear image of your mouth; do not chew gum or cover your mouth.
- Use gestures and facial expressions to enhance what is being said orally.
- Rephrase whatever the client does not understand.
- Remain patient, positive, and relaxed.
- Provide paper and pencil if the client communicates by sign language or has speech that is difficult to understand.
- Use a support person who can communicate by signing.

(Adapted from Trychin, S. [1993]. *Communication issues related to hearing loss.* Bethesda, MD: Self Help for the Hard of Hearing People, Inc.)

Stop, Think, and Respond ● BOX 50-1
What recommendations can you make for someone to prevent injury to the ears or hearing loss?

DISORDERS OF THE EXTERNAL EAR

Various disorders such as impacted cerumen, injury from foreign objects, or otitis externa affect the external acoustic meatus. If these disorders are not treated carefully and adequately, they may spread to the middle ear.

● IMPACTED CERUMEN

Impacted cerumen is accumulated ear wax that obstructs the external acoustic meatus.

Pathophysiology and Etiology

Impacted cerumen is more common among people who have excessive thick or dry cerumen. Both qualities interfere with drainage toward the proximal end of the meatus, where cerumen normally leaves the ear during regular shampooing and showering. The trapped cerumen interferes with the transmission of sounds carried on air waves.

Assessment Findings

The client reports having a sense of fullness in the ears and diminished hearing. The client asks that words be repeated, misinterprets questions, or raises the volume on the television or radio. Visual inspection with an otoscope shows an orange-brown accumulation of cerumen in the distal end of the external acoustic meatus. Audiometric, Rinne, and Weber tests reveal conductive hearing loss.

Medical Management

Dried cerumen is hydrated by instilling 1 or 2 drops of half-strength peroxide, warm glycerin, or mineral oil, or it is softened with commercial agents, such as carbamide peroxide (Debrox) and triethanolamine (Cerumenex). Cerumen is removed mechanically by irrigating the ear if the eardrum is intact or using an instrument called a *cerumen spoon.*

Nursing Management

The nurse inspects the ears and implements measures to remove excessive cerumen. Ear drops can be warmed by holding the container in the hand for a few moments or placing it in warm water. If irrigation or instillation of liquids is ordered, the nurse warms the liquid to body temperature. Cold or hot liquids cause dizziness, and the potential for injury exists if the liquid is hot. The nurse avoids inserting the irrigating syringe too deeply so as to close off the auditory canal. He or she directs the flow toward the roof of the canal rather than the eardrum.

● FOREIGN OBJECTS

Pathophysiology and Etiology

Foreign objects find their way into the ear either by accident or by deliberate insertion. Sharp objects can scratch the skin or cause blunt penetration of the eardrum. Insect stings cause local inflammation of the tissue.

Assessment Findings

The client describes discomfort, diminished hearing, feeling movement, or hearing a buzzing sound. On gross inspection, there is evidence of abrasion from trauma or an insect, or an object is seen. Inspection with a penlight or otoscope reveals swelling and redness in the auditory canal.

Medical Management

Mineral oil is instilled into the ear to smother an insect. Solid objects are removed with a small forceps.

Nursing Management

The nurse instructs clients to clean the ears with a face cloth rather than inserting objects into the ears. A hat with earflaps or a scarf is recommended when venturing into the woods or other areas with a high insect population.

● OTITIS EXTERNA

Otitis externa is an inflammation of the tissue in the outer ear.

Pathophysiology and Etiology

Inflammation usually is caused by an overgrowth of pathogens. The microorganisms tend to follow trauma to the lining of the ear, or their growth is supported by retained moisture from swimming. Another possibility is that a hair follicle becomes infected, causing a furuncle or an abscess to develop.

Assessment Findings

The tissue in the external ear looks red. Sometimes it is difficult to see the tympanic membrane because of swelling. Clients describe discomfort that increases with manipulation during the examination. Hearing is reduced because of swelling. In severe infections, a fever develops and the lymph nodes behind the ear enlarge.

Otoscopic examination reveals diffuse or confined inflammation, swelling, and pus. A culture of drainage identifies the specific pathogen.

Medical Management

Treatment includes warm soaks, analgesics, and antibiotic ear medication.

Nursing Management

The nurse instructs the client to carry out the medical treatment and provides health teaching to prevent recurrence. For example, he or she advises swimmers to wear soft plastic ear plugs to prevent trapping water in the ear. If chewing produces or potentiates discomfort, the nurse encourages the client to temporarily eat soft foods or consume nourishing liquids. Above all, the nurse advises the client to avoid the use of nonprescription remedies unless they have been approved by the physician and to contact the physician if symptoms are not relieved in a few days.

DISORDERS OF THE MIDDLE EAR ●

● OTITIS MEDIA

Otitis media is an inflammation or infection in the middle ear. Clients may have acute or chronic forms of either serous otitis media, also known as secretory or non-suppurative otitis media, or the purulent or suppurative type. Although otitis media is more common among young children, adults can and do develop middle ear infections.

Pathophysiology and Etiology

Serous otitis media, a collection of pathogen-free fluid behind the tympanic membrane, results from irritation associated with respiratory allergies and enlarged adenoids. Purulent otitis media usually results from the spread of microorganisms from the eustachian tube to the middle ear during upper respiratory infections.

When fluid or pus collects in the middle ear, pressure increases, which causes the eardrum to bulge and spontaneously rupture in some cases. Rupture results in a jagged tear of tissue that heals slowly and sometimes incompletely. Scarring interferes with the vibration of the eardrum, causing diminished hearing. Clients with perforated eardrums are prone to repeated infections.

Other potentially serious complications can occur. Because the middle ear connects with the mastoid process, a part of the temporal bone, pathogens that are unresponsive to antibiotic therapy can spread, causing **mastoiditis,** or they can travel deeper in the inner ear, causing **labyrinthitis.** Infection also may extend to the meninges, causing meningitis, or brain abscess may result from its extension to the brain. If septicemia occurs, the infection can spread to the large veins at the base of the brain and cause lateral sinus thrombosis. Facial nerve damage and facial paralysis may result from the infection. With prompt and adequate treatment, complications are rare.

Assessment Findings

The client often describes a history of having had a recent upper respiratory infection or seasonal allergies. Signs and symptoms vary widely depending on the type and severity of the inflammation, but may include a fever, tinnitus, malaise, severe earache, and diminished hearing. Tenderness behind the ear indicates mastoiditis. The eardrum looks red and bulging. Pressure in the middle ear or dysfunction of inner ear structures can cause nausea, vomiting, and dizziness. If the tympanic membrane perforates, fluid drains into the external acoustic canal and pain is relieved.

The white blood cell count shows an elevated number of neutrophils and eosinophils. If the eardrum has ruptured and drainage is present, the cultured drainage reveals a specific infectious microorganism.

Medical and Surgical Management

Prompt treatment usually prevents rupture of the eardrum. In some cases, the fluid is aspirated by needle. Antibiotics are given to control the infection. The overuse of antibiotics, however, has created another problem: microorganisms are becoming resistant and, for some infections, the available antibiotics are of limited benefit.

To reduce the consequences of spontaneous rupture of the eardrum, subsequent scarring, and hearing loss, the physician performs a **myringotomy,** an incisional opening of the eardrum. The incised opening facilitates drainage of the purulent material, eases the pressure, and relieves the throbbing pain. The incision heals readily with little scarring.

Plastic surgery (**myringoplasty**) usually is successful in repairing the perforated eardrum. In one technique, the edges of the perforation are cauterized and a patch of blood-soaked absorbable gelatin sponge (Gelfoam) is used as a scaffolding over which new tissue grows until it has filled in the defect. Chronic infections are prevented if the eardrum is repaired. In the case of mastoiditis, a **mas-**

toidectomy is performed to remove the diseased tissue. With early and effective antibiotic therapy, mastoiditis is rare.

Nursing Management

After myringotomy, the discharge from the ear is bloody and then purulent. To remove the drainage, the nurse wipes the external ear repeatedly with a dry sterile cotton applicator. An alternative is to insert a loose (not tightly packed) cotton pledget in the external ear to collect drainage. The nurse changes the cotton when it becomes moist.

● OTOSCLEROSIS

Otosclerosis is the result of a bony overgrowth of the stapes and a common cause of hearing impairment among adults. Fixation of the stapes occurs gradually over many years.

Conductive

Pathophysiology and Etiology

The underlying cause of otosclerosis is unknown. The condition, which is more common in women than in men, usually becomes apparent in the second and third decades of life. It seems to be accelerated during pregnancy. Most clients have a family history of the disease, which indicates a possible hereditary relationship.

Otosclerosis interferes with the vibration of the stapes and the transmission of sound to the inner ear. Although hearing loss in otosclerosis is of the conductive type, when and if progression of the disease involving the cochlea of the inner ear occurs, a mixed type of hearing loss develops.

Assessment Findings

Signs and Symptoms

A progressive, bilateral loss of hearing is the most characteristic symptom. The client notices the hearing loss when it begins to interfere with the ability to follow conversation. There is particular difficulty hearing others when they speak in soft, low tones, but hearing is adequate when the sound is loud enough. Tinnitus appears as the loss of hearing progresses. It is especially noticeable at night, when surroundings are quiet, and can be quite distressing to the client.

The eardrum appears pinkish-orange from structural changes in the middle ear. When the Rinne test is performed, the sound is heard best when the tuning fork is applied behind the ear. The sound lateralizes to the more affected ear when the Weber test is performed.

Diagnostic Findings

Audiometric tests reveal the type and severity of hearing loss. A computed tomography (CT) scan demonstrates the location and extent of excessive bone growth.

Medical and Surgical Management

Although otosclerosis has no cure, a hearing aid helps. The level of restored hearing depends greatly on the severity of the sensorineural involvement. The outcome is best when the hearing loss is purely conductive. If the surgical treatment is selected, a **stapedectomy** is performed on the ear most affected. In this procedure, all or part of the stapes is removed and a prosthesis is inserted that can vibrate the oval window (Fig. 50-8). Once the stapes is freed or replaced, the client experiences an immediate, dramatic improvement in hearing. Hearing temporarily diminishes after surgery because of swelling, but eventually returns. Complications include dislodgment of the prosthesis and continued hearing loss, infection, dizziness, and facial nerve damage. Depending on the outcome of surgery, the procedure may be repeated for the opposite ear.

Nursing Management

The nurse uses selected alternatives for communicating with the client as identified earlier in Nursing Guidelines 50-1, and provides the preoperative client with an explanation of what to expect in the immediate postoperative period. The nurse tells the client that activity is restricted for 24 hours or more after surgery and that hearing may be temporarily the same as or worse than before surgery.

After surgery, the nurse positions the client on the nonoperative side. He or she takes care to prevent dislodgment of the prosthesis as a result of coughing, sneezing, or vomiting. Nausea and dizziness are common problems. The nurse assesses facial nerve function by checking symmetry when the client smiles or frowns.

N U R S I N G   P R O C E S S

● **The Client Recovering From Stapedectomy**

Assessment

After the client returns from surgery, nursing assessments include taking vital signs and monitoring for complications, drainage from the affected ear, and level of discomfort. It is important that the nurse report any elevation in temperature.

Diagnosis, Planning, and Interventions

Impaired Comfort (pain, nausea, vertigo) related to tissue disruption

Expected Outcome: Client will experience relief of discomfort to at least a tolerable level.

- Administer prescribed analgesic and assess again in 30 minutes. *Ongoing assessment determines effectiveness of pain medication. Response to pain and pain medication is unique for each client.*
- Give an antiemetic for nausea or vomiting. *Antiemetics promote relief of nausea.*
- Validate client's feelings of discomfort. *This measure promotes the nurse–client relationship and reassures the client that his or her needs are important.*
- Provide small, frequent sips of fluid or light food. *Doing so prevents nausea.*
- Limit head movement and avoid jarring the bed. *Movement aggravates vertigo. Limiting movement minimizes pain, dizziness, and nausea.*

Risk for Infection related to impaired tissue integrity secondary to the surgical incision

Expected Outcome: Client will remain free of a secondary infection.

- Adhere strictly to aseptic principles when changing a dressing or cleaning the ear. *Using aseptic technique reduces the introduction and transmission of microorganisms and protects the client from exposure to pathogens.*
- Administer prescribed antibiotics. *Appropriate and timely administration of antibiotics promotes a consistent blood level needed to treat or prevent infection.*
- Instruct client to keep his or her hands away from the dressing or packing. *Doing so maintains integrity of the dressings and prevents contamination from opportunistic infections.*
- Keep external ear and surrounding skin meticulously clean and free of purulent drainage. *This measure pro-*

Fat

FIGURE 50-8 A wire prosthetic stapes is positioned in the middle ear.

motes healing and prevents infection through reduction of microorganisms.

Risk for Injury related to vertigo

Expected Outcome: Client will be free of injury.

- Encourage client to use the side rails and handrails for support when preparing to ambulate. *Side and hand rails prevent client from falling or causing injury to the affected ear. Basic safety measures prevent injury.*
- Walk with the client who is dizzy. *Assistance promotes the client's safety and reduces the chance for injury.*

Evaluation of Expected Outcomes

The client remains comfortable, as evidenced by minimal complaints of pain, and no complaints of nausea or vertigo. He or she has no signs or symptoms of infection. The client experiences mild vertigo but maintains safety. The nurse discusses the prescribed medical regimen and restrictions with the client or a family member. He or she includes one or more of the following in a teaching plan:

- Avoid blowing the nose because this action can dislodge the prosthesis.
- Avoid high altitudes or flying.
- Do not lift heavy objects, strain when defecating, or bend over at the waist; these activities increase pressure in the middle ear.
- Do not get water in the ear. Avoid swimming, showering, and washing the hair until approved by the physician.
- Follow the physician's instructions for keeping the ear clean.
- Stay away from people with respiratory infections. If a head cold occurs, contact the physician immediately.
- Notify the physician immediately if severe pain, excessive drainage, a sudden loss of hearing, or fever occurs.
- Adhere to the restriction of activities recommended by the physician until told otherwise.

DISORDERS OF THE INNER EAR

● MÉNIÈRE'S DISEASE

Ménière's disease is a term given to the episodic symptoms created by fluctuations in the production or reabsorption of fluid in the inner ear. This ear disease is analogous to glaucoma of the eye—there is too much circulating fluid (Smeltzer & Bare, 2000).

Pathophysiology and Etiology

The cause of the excessive fluid production is unknown. There appears to be a malabsorption of fluid in the endolymphatic sac, although some clients may have a blockage in the endolymphatic duct. "Regardless of the cause,

endolymphatic hydrops, a dilation in the endolymphatic space, develops" (Smeltzer & Bare, 2000, p. 1595).

Several theories attempt to explain Ménière's disease. These include abnormal hormonal and neurochemical influences that affect blood flow to the labyrinth, electrolyte disturbances, allergic reactions, and autoimmune responses. A last theory suggests that abnormally high levels of metabolites (e.g., glucose, insulin, triglycerides, cholesterol) destroy the microvasculature of the inner ear (Porth, 2002).

Ménière's disease typically is unilateral, appears during middle age, and occurs equally in men and women. It causes a triad of hearing loss, vertigo, and tinnitus (Porth, 2002). When the fluid accumulates, it dilates the cochlear duct, which diminishes hearing. It also affects equilibrium as the vestibular system becomes damaged, and tinnitus occurs. At times, the client is symptom free except for permanent, residual hearing loss as the number of attacks increase. Occasionally, clients recover spontaneously.

Assessment Findings

The client periodically experiences severe vertigo, tinnitus, and progressive hearing loss. Nausea and vomiting accompany the vertigo. Nystagmus of the eyes may occur, caused by an imbalance in vestibular control of eye movements (Porth, 2002). Some clients experience preattack symptoms of headache and a full feeling in the ear.

An attack lasts from a few minutes to weeks and can occur with alarming suddenness. Some clients are reluctant to leave their homes for fear they will have an attack in public. Continued employment becomes impossible for some clients.

A caloric stimulation test and electronystagmography demonstrate a difference in eye movement response. A CT scan or magnetic resonance imaging (MRI) rules out other possible causes of the symptoms, such as a tumor that involves the vestibulocochlear nerve. Audiometry identifies the type and magnitude of the hearing deficit.

Medical and Surgical Management

Treatment aims at reducing fluid production in the inner ear, facilitating its drainage, and treating the symptoms that accompany the attack. A low-sodium diet lessens edema. Smoking is contraindicated to prevent vasoconstriction, which interferes with fluid drainage. Treatment of the allergy or avoidance of the allergen is recommended. Bed rest may be necessary during acute attacks. Specific drug therapy may include the following:

- Meclizine (Antivert)—an antihistamine often prescribed because it suppresses the vestibular system
- Diazepam (Valium) or other tranquilizers—may be ordered for acute episodes to help control vertigo;

these are used only for short-term therapy because of the addictive potential

- Promethazine (Phenergan)—an antiemetic to help control the nausea and vomiting; has an antihistamine effect
- Hydrochlorothiazide or other diuretics—may decrease the fluid in the endolymphatic system and relieve symptoms (Smeltzer & Bare, 2000)

If clients become extremely incapacitated, surgery becomes an option. Surgeries range from decompression of the endolymphatic sac to insertion of intraotologic catheters to vestibular nerve section. Box 50-3 presents a brief description of specific surgical procedures.

Nursing Management

The nurse obtains a history of symptoms, their duration, and complete medical, drug, and allergy histories. He or she assesses gross hearing and performs the Weber and Rinne tests. It also is important to determine the extent and effect of the client's disability.

The client with Ménière's disease requires a great deal of emotional support because of the unpredictability of the attacks and the resulting impairments. During an attack, the nurse administers prescribed drugs, limits movement, and promotes the client's safety. He or she assists the client with activities of daily living because the least amount of motion can produce severe vertigo.

BOX 50-3 ● **Surgical Procedures for Ménière's Disease**

Endolymphatic Sac Decompression—A shunting procedure that involves the insertion of a shunt or drain in the endolymphatic sac to equalize pressure in the endolymphatic space. This procedure is safe and usually is the first choice. It is done as an outpatient procedure.

Middle and Inner Ear Perfusion—Antibiotics, such as gentamycin or streptomycin (considered to be ototoxic), are infused into the middle and inner ear. This procedure decreases vestibular function and vertigo, but holds a high risk for significant hearing loss. Clients usually stay overnight. Clients may experience a period of imbalance for several weeks.

Intraotologic Catheters—A catheter is inserted in the external ear canal through or around the tympanic membrane to the round window, for the purpose of instilling medications. Potential treatments are for sudden hearing loss, vertigo, tinnitus, and slowly progressive sensorineural hearing loss.

Labyrinthectomy—Excision of the labyrinth through the transcanal or transmastoid route assists in eliminating vertigo. Auditory function of the inner ear is destroyed, and potential complications include facial nerve injury and total hearing loss.

Vestibular Nerve Section—This procedure has the highest success rate in eliminating vertigo and is used for clients who are incapacitated by Ménière's disease and already have significant hearing loss. Cutting the nerve prevents the brain from receiving input from the semicircular canals. The procedure requires a brief hospital stay.

(Adapted from Smeltzer, S. C. & Bare, B. G. (2000). *Brunner & Suddarth's textbook of medical–surgical nursing*, [9th ed.]. Philadelphia: Lippincott Williams & Wilkins.)

The nurse is available, empathic, and responsive to the client. Trust and confidence develop when the client does not feel abandoned or required to convince caregivers of the necessity for attention. Clients are comforted when the nurse acknowledges that dealing with temporary or permanent hearing loss is a challenge.

If a low-sodium diet is recommended, the dietitian provides a list of foods to avoid or a specific diet to follow. If an allergy is suspected as the cause of the disorder, the nurse advises the client to take the prescribed antihistamines as directed and to avoid known allergens. If a hearing aid is recommended, the nurse refers the client to an audiologist for instructions on its use and care.

Stop, Think, and Respond ● BOX 50-2

*A nurse admits a client with Ménière's disease who is having an acute episode. After assessing the client, the nurse selects **Risk for Deficient Fluid Volume** as the best nursing diagnosis. Complete the diagnostic statement with expected outcomes.*

● OTOTOXICITY

Ototoxicity describes the detrimental effect of certain medications on the eighth cranial nerve or hearing structures. Signs and symptoms of ototoxicity include tinnitus and sensorineural hearing loss. Vestibular toxicity includes sign and symptoms of light-headedness, vertigo, nausea, and vomiting. Drugs associated with ototoxicity include salicylates, loop diuretics, quinidine, quinine, and aminoglycosides. Box 50-4 lists selected ototoxic medications. It is important that nurses are knowledgeable about the ototoxic effects of certain medications, and that they carefully monitor the dosage and frequency of administration, as well as assessing the client for changes in hearing.

● ACOUSTIC NEUROMA

An **acoustic neuroma** is a benign Schwann cell tumor that progressively enlarges and adversely affects cranial nerve VIII (the vestibular and cochlear nerves). Most acoustic tumors arise in the auditory canal and extend into the cerebellar region, pressing on the brain stem.

Pathophysiology and Etiology

The cause of acoustic neuroma is unknown. Men and women are equally affected. Acoustic neuromas account for 5% to 10% of intracranial tumors (Smeltzer & Bare, 2000). The tumor usually is unilateral. Hearing

BOX 50-4 ● Selected Ototoxic Substances

DIURETICS
ethacrynic acid
furosemide
acetazolamide

CHEMOTHERAPEUTIC AGENTS
cisplatin
nitrogen mustard

ANTIMALARIALS
quinine
chloroquine

ANTI-INFLAMMATORY AGENTS
salicylates (aspirin)
indomethacin

CHEMICALS
alcohol
arsenic

AMINOGLYCOSIDE ANTIBIOTICS
amikacin
gentamicin
kanamycin
netilmicin
neomycin
streptomycin
tobramycin

OTHER ANTIBIOTICS
erythromycin
minocycline
polymyxin B
vancomycin

METALS
gold
mercury
lead

MRI with contrast agents is done to determine the location and extent of the tumor. Cerebrospinal fluid (CSF) studies demonstrate increased pressure and the presence of proteins.

Medical and Surgical Management

Surgical removal of the tumor is the usual treatment. Acoustic neuromas do not respond well to chemotherapy or radiation therapy. The challenge of this surgical procedure is to remove the tumor and retain facial nerve function. Usually hearing loss already has occurred, so destruction of the hearing mechanism that occurs with the surgical approach is not a consideration. If the client has little or no hearing loss, however, the suboccipital or middle cranial fossa approach is used, with close monitoring of cranial nerve VIII function. Complications of acoustic neuroma excision include the following:

- Facial nerve paralysis
- CSF leak
- Meningitis
- Cerebral edema
- Increased intracranial pressure

Nursing Management

The assessment of a client with acoustic neuroma includes evaluating hearing function, observing the client's facial movements, and testing for facial sensation. If the client has hearing deficits, refer to Nursing Guidelines 50-1 for measures to communicate with people with a hearing loss. For clients with vertigo, the nurse takes measures to protect the client from injury.

After surgery, the nurse implements the aforementioned measures as well as monitoring the client for signs of increased intracranial pressure, including restlessness, confusion, or unresponsiveness, pupillary changes, bradycardia, hypertension, and respiratory changes. It also is important that the nurse maintain strict asepsis to prevent transmission of microorganisms. Clients are at risk for wound infection and meningitis.

loss occurs secondary to compression of the cochlear nerve or interference with the blood supply to the nerve and cochlea.

Assessment Findings

Signs and symptoms vary according to the size and location of the tumor. The client may exhibit or experience any or all of the following signs and symptoms—usually unilateral:

- Hearing loss (usually gradual)
- Impaired facial movement
- Altered facial sensation
- Tinnitus
- Vertigo with or without balance disturbance

Initial audiometric studies reveal significant differences in hearing and presence of tinnitus and vertigo.

 GENERAL PHARMACOLOGIC CONSIDERATIONS

Nonprescription preparations are available for softening hardened cerumen. Refer the client to a physician if hearing remains diminished.

Many commonly administered medications are potentially ototoxic, such as furosemide (Lasix), cisplatin, salicylates (aspirin), and many antibiotics. Nurses need to be aware of these potential effects, monitoring the prescribed dosages and the client for signs of impaired hearing.

GENERAL GERONTOLOGIC CONSIDERATIONS

Older clients form drier cerumen and experience an increased incidence of impaction in the external acoustic meatus.

Hearing loss is common as adults age. Options in the style of prescribed hearing aid are limited by the client's ability to care for and maintain it.

The older adult with a hearing impairment may become disoriented and confused in strange surroundings. Frequent contact and reorientation prevent confusion.

Critical Thinking Exercises

1. *Describe techniques that promote communication when interacting with clients who have a hearing deficit.*
2. *What cues can a nurse observe in an older client who has possible hearing loss?*

References and Suggested Readings

Aschenbrenner, D. S., Cleveland, L. H., & Venable, S. J. (2002). *Drug therapy in nursing.* Philadelphia: Lippincott Williams & Wilkins.

Bullock, B. A. & Henze, R. L. (2000). *Focus on pathophysiology.* Philadelphia: Lippincott Williams & Wilkins.

Cavenish, R. (1998). Clinical snapshot: Adult hearing loss. *American Journal of Nursing, 98*(8), 50–51.

Grossan, M. (2000). Safe, effective techniques for cerumen removal. *Geriatrics, 55,* 83–86.

McConnell, E. A. (1998). Communicating with a hearing-impaired patient. *Nursing, 28*(1), 32.

Porth, C. M. (2002). *Pathophysiology: Concepts of altered health states* (6th ed.). Philadelphia: Lippincott Williams & Wilkins.

Smeltzer, S. C. & Bare, B. G. (2000). *Brunner & Suddarth's textbook of medical–surgical nursing* (9th ed.). Philadelphia: Lippincott Williams & Wilkins.

Tupper, S. (1999). When the inner ear is out of balance. *RN, 62*(11), 36–40.

chapter **51**

Introduction to the Gastrointestinal System and Accessory Structures

<table>
<tr><td colspan="2">

Words to Know

</td></tr>
<tr>
<td>

barium enema
barium swallow
cholangiography
cholecystography
colonoscopy
endoscopic retrograde
   cholangio-
   pancreatography
enteroclysis
esophagogastro-
   duodenoscopy
flexible sigmoidoscopy
gallbladder series

</td>
<td>

lower gastrointestinal
   series
panendoscopy
percutaneous liver
   biopsy
peristalsis
proctosigmoidoscopy
PY test
radionuclide imaging
ultrasonography
upper gastrointestinal
   series

</td>
</tr>
</table>

Learning Objectives

On completion of this chapter, the reader will:

- Identify major organs and structures of the gastrointestinal system.
- Discuss important information to ascertain about gastrointestinal health.
- List facts in the client's history that provide pertinent data about the present illness.
- Discuss physical assessments that provide information about the functioning of the gastrointestinal tract and accessory organs.
- Describe common diagnostic tests performed on clients with gastrointestinal disorders.
- Explain nursing management of clients undergoing diagnostic testing for a gastrointestinal disorder.

The gastrointestinal (GI) system (Fig. 51-1) may be arbitrarily divided into two sections: the upper GI tract and the lower GI tract. The upper GI tract begins at the mouth and ends at the jejunum. The lower GI tract begins at the ileum and ends at the anus. Accessory structures include the peritoneum, liver, gallbladder, and pancreas. The primary functions of the GI tract are digestion (Table 51-1) and distribution of food.

ANATOMY AND PHYSIOLOGY

Mouth

Food normally enters the GI system at the mouth, where it is chewed (masticated) before being swallowed. Food that contains starch undergoes partial digestion when it mixes with the enzyme *salivary amylase*, which the *salivary glands* secrete (Table 51-2).

Esophagus

The *esophagus* begins at the base of the pharynx and ends at the opening between the esophagus and stomach. Layers of muscle tissue surround the esophagus. They consist of striated muscle tissue in the proximal esophagus, striated and smooth muscle in the mid-esophagus, and smooth muscle in the lower esophagus. Coordinated movement of these muscle layers propels food into the stomach. These wavelike contractions are known as **peristalsis.** An *upper esophageal sphincter* or *hypopharyngeal sphincter* prevents food or fluids from re-entering the pharynx.

Stomach

The stomach temporarily holds ingested food and prepares it by mechanical and chemical action to pass in semi-liquid form into the small intestine. The opening between

729

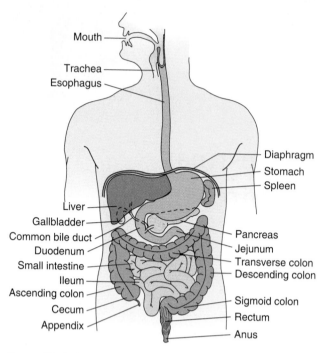

FIGURE 51-1 Organs of the gastrointestinal tract.

the esophagus and stomach is called the *lower esophageal sphincter* or *cardiac sphincter*. The opening between the stomach and duodenum is called the *pyloric sphincter*. Both sphincters are circular bands of muscle fibers. When contracted, these sphincters keep stomach contents enclosed (or confined). When the pyloric sphincter relaxes, stomach contents flow to the duodenum.

Gastric secretions that contain digestive enzymes are released continuously but increase when food is eaten. Gastric secretions are acidic because they contain hydrochloric acid (HCl). The contractions of the stomach mix the food with the gastric secretions and move the mixture of semiliquid food called *chyme* to the small intestine

by peristalsis. The time required for the stomach to empty depends on the amount and composition of food. Fats, for example, delay stomach emptying.

Small Intestine

The small intestine is divided into three portions: duodenum, jejunum, and ileum. The *duodenum*, which is approximately 10 inches long, is the first region of the small intestine and the site where bile and pancreatic enzymes enter. These secretions continue to promote the chemical breakdown of food and transform chyme to an alkaline state. Peristalsis mechanically propels the mixture, which is semiliquid at this point, into the jejunum and ileum, which have a combined length of approximately 23 feet.

The primary function of the small intestine is to absorb nutrients from the chyme. Absorption of different nutrients occurs at different sites in the small intestine (Table 51-3). When a part of the small intestine is diseased or removed surgically, absorption in that area is diminished or lost altogether.

The *ileocecal valve* lies at the distal end of the small intestine and regulates the flow of intestinal contents, which are liquid at this point, into the large intestine. It also prevents the reflux of bacteria from the large intestine, preserving the relative sterility of the small intestine.

Large Intestine

The large intestine, which is approximately 4 to 5 feet long and 2 inches in diameter, receives waste from the small intestine and propels waste toward the *anus,* the opening from the body for elimination. The large intestine absorbs water, some electrolytes, and bile acids. The cecum, colon, rectum, and anal canal make up the struc-

TABLE 51-1	SELECTED DIGESTIVE ENZYMES/SECRETIONS		
LOCATION	**ENZYME**	**SUBSTANCE THE ENZYME ACTS ON**	**PRODUCTS OF ENZYMATIC ACTION**
Salivary glands	Salivary amylase	Starch	Smaller carbohydrates
Stomach	Pepsin	Proteins	Polypeptides (process activated by HCl)
	Gastric lipase	Triglycerides (lipids)	Glycerides and fatty acids
	HCl	Proteins	Smaller polypeptides
Pancreas	Trypsin	Proteins and polypeptides	Smaller polypeptides, amino acids
	Nuclease	Nucleic acids	Nucleotides (base + sugar + phosphate)
	Pancreatic amylase	Starch	Smaller carbohydrates
	Pancreatic lipase	Lipids, especially triglycerides	Glycerides, free fatty acids, glycerol
Small intestine	Peptidases	Peptides	Amino acids
	Lactase, maltase, sucrase	Disaccharides	Monosaccharides
	Intestinal lipase	Fats	Glycerides, fatty acids, glycerol
Liver	Bile	Fats	Glycerides, fatty acids, glycerol

HCl, hydrochloric acid.

TABLE 51-2	HOW ORAL STRUCTURES PARTICIPATE IN DIGESTION
STRUCTURE	**CONTRIBUTION TO THE DIGESTIVE PROCESS**
Teeth	Reduce food to sizes appropriate for swallowing; break down dense particles
Tongue	Places food in proper position for swallowing; mixes secretions to moisten food
Salivary glands	Moisten and lubricate foods in the mouth; add ptyalin enzyme for digestion of starches
Muscles of mastication	Provide movement for the grinding of food to smaller particles; provide more surface area for the digestive enzymes to act

(From Bullock, B. A. & Henze, R. L. [2000]. *Focus on pathophysiology*, [p. 722]. Philadelphia: Lippincott Williams & Wilkins.)

tures of the large intestine through which fecal material passes.

The *cecum* is a pouchlike structure at the beginning of the large intestine. The *appendix*, a narrow blind tube at the tip of the cecum, has no known function in humans.

The colon is divided into the *ascending, transverse, descending,* and *sigmoid* colons and *rectum.* In the colon, the unabsorbed material becomes fecal matter, which is composed of water, food residue, microorganisms, digestive secretions, and mucus. Water is reabsorbed by means of diffusion across the intestinal membrane as the mixture moves through the colon. By the time the mixture reaches the descending and sigmoid colon, the portion of the bowel adjacent to the rectum, it is a formed mass. The rectum holds and retains fecal matter through the contraction of the internal and external anal sphincters. As fecal mass accumulates, it distends the rectal wall, creating the urge to defecate. When the external anal sphincter relaxes, the fecal matter is expelled through the anus.

If any portion of the large intestine becomes diseased or is surgically removed, its absorptive function is diminished or lost. This may result in the passage of loose stools and potential fluid and electrolyte imbalance. Passage of liquid stool, which contains many bile salts, makes the client especially vulnerable to skin breakdown in the perianal area. If stool remains in the large intestine too long, constipation results. The client may then strain to evacuate hard, solid stool, which can disrupt skin integrity.

Accessory Structures

The three accessory digestive organs are the liver, gallbladder, and pancreas. Although not an accessory structure itself, the peritoneum encloses the abdominal organs.

Peritoneum

The *peritoneum,* a membrane that lines the inner abdomen, encloses the viscera and the serous fluid that it secretes. It allows the abdominal organs to move about without creating friction. The walls of the digestive organs normally prevent the gastric and intestinal contents from escaping into the peritoneal cavity. Any perforation that allows material to seep out of the digestive tract is serious because the microorganisms and enzymes can cause a severe inflammation and infection of the surrounding tissue. This condition is known as *peritonitis.*

Liver

The *liver,* the largest glandular organ in the body, weighs between 1 and 1.5 kg (2 to 3 lbs.). It is located in the right upper abdomen just under the diaphragm, which separates the liver from the right lung. The liver is involved in many vital, complex metabolic activities. It forms and releases bile; processes vitamins, proteins, fats, and carbohydrates; stores glycogen; contributes to blood coagulation; metabolizes and biotransforms many chemicals (including drugs), bacteria, and foreign matter; and forms antibodies and immunizing substances (gamma globulin). See Chapter 55 for more information.

Gallbladder

The *gallbladder* is attached to the mid-portion of the undersurface of the liver. It normally has a thin wall and holds approximately 60 mL of bile. The liver forms approximately 1 L of bile each day. When the bile reaches the gallbladder from the common hepatic duct, water and minerals are absorbed from the bile to form a more concentrated product. Gallbladder contraction, triggered by ingested food (especially fats), causes bile to be released first through the cystic duct and then the common bile duct into the duodenum, where it aids in the absorption of fats, fat-soluble vitamins, iron, and calcium. Bile also activates the pancreas to release its digestive enzymes and an alkaline fluid that neutralizes stomach acids that reach the duodenum.

Pancreas

The *pancreas* is both an *exocrine gland,* one that releases secretions into a duct or channel, and an *endocrine gland,* one that releases substances directly into the bloodstream. As an endocrine organ, it produces the hormones insulin and glucagon (see Chap. 58). As an exocrine organ, it produces various protein-, fat-, and carbohydrate-digesting enzymes. At the appropriate time for digestion, the pancreatic enzymes are released in inactive forms and transported to the duodenum, where they are activated.

TABLE 51-3	SITES OF AND REQUIREMENTS FOR ABSORPTION OF DIETARY CONSTITUENTS AND MANIFESTATIONS OF MALABSORPTION		
DIETARY CONSTITUENT	**SITE OF ABSORPTION**	**REQUIREMENTS**	**MANIFESTATIONS**
Water and electrolytes	Mainly small bowel	Osmotic gradient	Diarrhea Dehydration Cramps
Fat	Upper jejunum	Pancreatic lipase Bile salts Functioning lymphatic channels	Weight loss Steatorrhea Fat-soluble vitamin deficiency
Carbohydrates Starch	Small intestine	Amylase Maltase Isomaltase α-dextrins	Diarrhea Flatulence Abdominal discomfort
Sucrose	Small intestine	Sucrase	
Lactose	Small intestine	Lactase	
Maltose	Small intestine	Maltase	
Fructose	Small intestine		
Protein	Small intestine	Pancreatic enzymes (e.g., trypsin, chymotrypsin, elastin)	Loss of muscle mass Weakness Edema
Vitamins A	Upper jejunum	Bile salts	Night blindness Dry eyes Corneal irritation
Folic acid	Duodenum and jejunum	Absorptive; may be impaired by some drugs (i.e., anticonvulsants)	Cheilosis Glossitis Megaloblastic anemia
B_{12}	Ileum	Intrinsic factor	Glossitis Neuropathy Megaloblastic anemia
D	Upper jejunum	Bile salts	Bone pain Fractures Tetany
E	Upper jejunum	Bile salts	Uncertain
K	Upper jejunum	Bile salts	Easy bruising and bleeding
Calcium	Duodenum	Vitamin D and parathyroid hormone	Bone pain Fractures Tetany
Iron	Duodenum and jejunum	Normal pH (hydrochloric acid secretion)	Iron-deficiency anemia Glossitis

(From Porth, C. M. [2002]. *Pathophysiology: Concepts of altered health states* [6th ed., p. 853]. Philadelphia: Lippincott Williams & Wilkins.)

ASSESSMENT

Many conditions can disrupt the normal function of the GI system. In addition to disorders of the GI tract and accessory organs, many disorders involving other organ systems can affect GI function. As a result, the client with a GI disorder may experience a wide variety of health problems that involve disturbances of ingestion, digestion, absorption, and elimination. Accurate recording of the client's health history and physical assessment findings help the healthcare team to diagnose and treat GI disorders.

History

The objective of the history is to identify the client's specific problem and its possible cause. The history includes the chief complaint, a focus assessment of current nutritional, metabolic, and elimination patterns, and past history.

The nurse gathers as much data as possible about why the client has sought treatment and current symptoms. This includes how long the symptoms have been present and what appears to cause or be related to them. Pertinent information to elicit includes which types of food produce distress, and when symptoms are most likely to occur. The nurse also determines what measures, if any, the client uses to relieve the symptoms, and the effects of these measures.

During GI assessment, the focus is on nutritional, metabolic, and elimination patterns, including quality of the client's appetite; problems associated with chewing or swallowing; what and how much the client eats each day; discomfort before, during, or after food consumption; nutritional supplements, if any, that the client uses (e.g., vitamins, herbs, home remedies); weight gain or loss; and bowel elimination patterns (usual consistency and color of stools, visible blood, stool frequency, effort or pain with passage of stool). After obtaining a current health history, the nurse obtains a history of all past medical and surgical disorders and their treatment. He or she compiles a family history of illnesses and causes of death. Family history of digestive disorders is especially important because several, such as colorectal cancer, have a hereditary link. The nurse also explores the client's work history to evaluate the possibility of exposure to environmental toxic wastes or radioactive materials.

The nurse obtains a complete allergy history, including adverse reactions to foods, because food allergies can cause various GI symptoms. The medication history includes prescription and nonprescription drugs, especially those affecting GI function. For each drug, the nurse lists the name, dose, frequency, and reason for taking.

Stop, Think, and Respond ● BOX 51-1

A client says that she has been experiencing nausea and occasional vomiting for several days. What questions should you ask to gain more information?

Physical Examination

General Appearance

The nurse assesses the client's overall physical condition and measures weight, height, and vital signs. He or she evaluates general appearance with regard to age and body size and assesses hygiene, energy, breathing pattern, emotional attitude, and mental status to the degree that they may affect the client's general appearance.

Skin

Using natural sunlight or bright artificial light, the nurse inspects the skin for any abnormal color, such as a yellowish tint indicating jaundice. In very dark-skinned clients, he or she inspects the hard palate, gums, conjunctiva, and surrounding tissues for discoloration. If the skin appears jaundiced, the nurse inspects the sclera to see if it

is yellow (see Chap. 11). Inspection of the skin of the face and abdomen is necessary to look for other abnormalities, such as *spider angiomas* (superficial red discolorations consisting of blood vessels that assume a spider-shaped pattern), distended abdominal veins ("caput medusae"), and scars. The nurse also assesses for dryness of the oral mucosa and skin turgor. Mucous membranes may be dry and skin turgor may be poor in clients who are dehydrated as a result of fluid losses from the GI tract.

Mouth

The nurse examines the lips for sores, cracks, lesions, or other abnormalities. Using a tongue blade and a flashlight, he or she inspects the mouth for inflammation, sores, swellings, or discolorations. Assessment of the quality of oral care is essential and includes evaluating for missing teeth and partial plates, bridges, or dentures. If the client has dentures, the nurse asks if they fit well and whether the client can eat regular food. If the client can eat only soft foods, the nurse communicates this information to the physician and dietary department.

Abdomen

The nurse continues the physical assessment by having the client lie supine for an abdominal examination. Abdominal areas typically are described in quadrants (right upper, right lower, left upper, and left lower), with the umbilicus as the center point for both horizontal and vertical divisions. The nurse then observes the abdomen's contour, noting whether it is flat, round, concave, or distended, as well as the effort associated with breathing. Distention may cause dyspnea as a result of upward pressure on the diaphragm (see Chap. 3).

Abdominal auscultation is done before palpation because palpation disrupts normal bowel sounds. Using a stethoscope, the nurse listens over each quadrant for bowel sounds, which sound like gurgles. He or she describes the location, pitch quality, and frequency, which usually is every 5 to 30 seconds. Listening for a full 5 minutes over each quadrant is important to confirm absence of bowel sounds. Measurement of abdominal girth is done at the widest point (usually at the umbilicus). Using a pen, the nurse marks the measurement location on the abdomen to ensure that additional examiners use the same reference point.

Next is abdominal palpation to determine if it is soft or firm and to detect masses and areas of pain or tenderness. If the client reports tenderness, the nurse probes the lower liver margin. An enlarged liver may be felt below the right lower rib cage. Pain or discomfort in this area may suggest a liver disorder, gallbladder or intestinal disease, or a pancreatic disorder. The nurse percusses the abdomen to elicit changes in sounds from dullness over an area with a solid mass, such as the liver, to resonance over less dense structures or those filled with air.

Anus

The nurse examines the anal area for external hemorrhoids, skin tags, or fissures (small tears in the anal opening). He or she inspects the skin surrounding the anus for breaks, lesions, rash, inflammation, and drainage. If and when stool passes, the nurse examines its characteristics. The shape, color, and consistency of stool usually are helpful in the differential diagnosis of GI disorders. Foods and medications alter the color of stool (Table 51-4).

Diagnostic Tests

Radiographic Studies

Radiographic studies are used to identify the location and structural appearance of organs or other space-occupying masses (air, fluid, tumors, foreign objects) in the abdomen, chest, or GI system. Radiographic studies involve the use of radiopaque contrast media. One radiographic study, *fluoroscopy,* may be used to observe the shape and contour of empty organs and how these hollow structures fill with and evacuate radiopaque dye (contrast medium).

BARIUM SWALLOW OR UPPER GASTROINTESTINAL SERIES

Sometimes the terms *barium swallow* and *upper GI series* are used interchangeably. Strictly speaking, a **barium swallow** is fluoroscopic observation of the client actually swallowing a flavored barium solution and its progress down the esophagus. Barium swallow facilitates the identification of structural abnormalities of the esophagus as well as swallowing discoordination and oral aspiration. An **upper gastrointestinal series** also includes radiographic observation of the barium moving into the stomach and the first part of the small intestine.

Structural abnormalities in the esophagus include tumors, strictures, varices, and hiatal hernia. Structural abnormalities below the esophagus include gastric tumors, peptic ulcers, and numerous gastric disorders (see

Chap. 54). The examination may take as little as 20 minutes if only a barium swallow is performed. If stomach filling and emptying need to be observed, the test may take approximately 1 hour.

For several days before the procedure, the client is on a low-residue diet. Usually, he or she takes nothing by mouth (NPO) for 8 to 12 hours before the test. A laxative may be given to clean out the GI tract. Smoking stimulates gastric motility, so the client is asked not to smoke the day of the procedure. With rare exceptions (e.g., anticonvulsants, insulin), all medications are withheld.

Barium is very constipating. Once any test using barium is over, the nurse encourages the client to drink fluids liberally to dilute the barium and promote its elimination from the GI tract. He or she advises the client that stools will appear white, streaky, or clay colored from the barium. The nurse must wait to obtain stool specimens until the client has fully excreted the barium. In some cases, a laxative may help with evacuation. In all cases, failure to have a bowel movement within a reasonable time must be reported to the physician because the retained barium may cause a blockage.

SMALL BOWEL SERIES

A small bowel series is fluoroscopy of the small intestine after the ingestion of a contrast medium. It is used to identify tumors, inflammation, or obstruction in the jejunum or ileum. It is performed like an upper GI series, but the client must swallow more barium for the small intestine to be well visualized. If the healthcare provider suspects an obstruction or *fistula* (a leaking channel between two structures), he or she substitutes a water-soluble contrast medium such as methylglucamine diatrizoate (Gastrografin) for the barium. The test takes 5 to 6 hours, which is when the contrast medium reaches the lower portion of the small intestine. When a small bowel series fails to detect subtle small bowel disease, enteroclysis may be indicated.

ENTEROCLYSIS

Also known as a *small bowel enema,* **enteroclysis** requires nasal or oral placement of a flexible feeding tube, the tip of which is positioned in the proximal jejunum. This study uses two contrast media. First, 500 to 1000 mL of a thin barium suspension is infused through the tube, followed by methylcellulose. The two contrast media fill in and pass through the intestinal loops. The examiner observes the intestine continuously by fluoroscopy and takes periodic x-rays of the various sections of the small intestine. Even with normal motility, this process can take up to 6 hours (Smeltzer & Bare, 2000). If sedation is administered to ensure the client's comfort, he or she requires monitoring accordingly. Risk for aspiration of the contrast media is increased if the client vomits while under sedation. Therefore, positioning of the client on

TABLE 51-4	FOODS AND MEDICATIONS THAT ALTER STOOL COLOR

ALTERING SUBSTANCE	COLOR
Meat protein	Dark brown
Spinach	Green
Carrots and beets	Red
Cocoa	Dark red or brown
Senna	Yellow
Bismuth, iron, licorice, and charcoal	Black
Barium	Milky white

(From Smeltzer, S. C. & Bare, B. G. [2000]. *Brunner & Suddarth's textbook of medical–surgical nursing* [9th ed., p. 797]. Philadelphia: Lippincott Williams & Wilkins.)

his or her side and availability of a suction apparatus are critical.

BARIUM ENEMA OR LOWER GASTROINTESTINAL SERIES

A **barium enema** or **lower gastrointestinal series** is used to identify polyps, tumors, inflammation, strictures, and other abnormalities of the colon. It is performed in the radiology department. The radiographic technologist rectally instills 1 to 1.5 L of barium solution. He or she observes the rectum, sigmoid colon, and descending colon fluoroscopically during filling. To facilitate this process, the examiner directs the client to make multiple position changes. The client must retain the barium during this test, which may take up to 30 minutes.

During the test, the client may experience abdominal cramping and a strong urge to defecate. The nurse reassures the client that most people can retain the instilled barium throughout the test. Radiographs are taken again after the client expels the barium. In some cases, air is instilled to compress the barium residue against the wall of the lower intestine to aid in detecting mucosal defects. Stool specimens are not collected until the barium has been expelled completely.

Twenty-four to 72 hours before the barium enema, the client follows certain restrictions and procedures to reduce the formation of stool and remove any residual stool:

- Low-residue diet 1 to 2 days before the test
- Clear liquid diet the evening before the test
- A laxative the evening before the test
- NPO after midnight
- Cleansing enemas the morning of the test (if not contraindicated by inflammation or active bleeding)

The amount of fluids is not restricted, and the client usually does not have to withhold oral medications. The client may have up to three cleansing enemas (or until the evacuated solution appears clear) before the procedure. After the examination is complete, the client may resume eating. The nurse encourages the client to rest and to drink fluids liberally. He or she also monitors the passage of stool and informs the client that feces will appear white until the barium is completely eliminated.

ORAL CHOLECYSTOGRAPHY OR GALLBLADDER SERIES

Oral **cholecystography** or **gallbladder series** identifies stones in the gallbladder or common bile duct and tumors or other obstructions. The test also determines the ability of the gallbladder to concentrate and store a dyelike, iodine-based, radiopaque contrast medium. After the dye is absorbed, it goes to the liver, is excreted into the bile, and passes into the gallbladder, making it radiographically visible. Radiography of the gallbladder should be performed before other GI examinations in which barium is used because residual barium tends to obscure the image of the gallbladder and its ducts.

To prepare for this test the client swallows six dye tablets—one every 5 minutes after the evening meal with a total of 250 mL of water or more. The nurse instructs the client that he or she may not eat or drink until the test is complete. If the tablets cause nausea and vomiting, the nurse should notify the physician so that more tablets can be administered or the test rescheduled. Once the initial radiographs are obtained, a fatty test meal is given and additional radiographs taken to determine the gallbladder's ability to empty.

CHOLANGIOGRAPHY

Performed in the radiology department or during surgery, **cholangiography** determines the patency of the ducts from the liver and gallbladder. It is used when the gallbladder is not distinctly visualized with an oral cholecystogram, vomiting interferes with the retention of the oral dye, or the status of the ductal system needs to be determined during or after surgery.

The dye for cholangiography usually is instilled intravenously (IV). Other routes include infusion through a T-tube surgically placed in the common bile duct, a cannula advanced through the skin at a site below the rib margin, or an endoscope inserted through the upper GI tract into the sphincter of Oddi (where the common bile duct empties into the duodenum).

The client must sign a consent form. The nurse must ask if the client is allergic to iodine or shellfish. The nurse checks physician orders to determine if the client needs a cleansing enema. The client may need to restrict food and fluids for several hours before the examination. The nurse informs the client that he or she may experience a warm sensation and nausea when the dye is instilled. After the procedure, the client may eat and drink. The nurse encourages the client to drink liberally to promote dye excretion.

RADIONUCLIDE IMAGING

Radionuclide imaging detects lesions of the liver or pancreas and assists in evaluating gastric emptying. A radionuclide is a radioactive natural or synthetic element, such as technetium. Once the radionuclide is injected IV or ingested orally, the radiologist may examine a body organ by passing the radionuclide imaging scanner over the structure. This test is helpful in demonstrating the size of the organ, as well as defects or lesions such as tumors. Specialized radionuclide studies are done to identify sites of bleeding or inflammation in the GI tract. Radionuclides have rather short half-lives, lasting a few hours to days, during which they emit radiation, which usually is less than with diagnostic radiography.

Pretest measures include weighing the client to calculate the radionuclide dose and determining pregnancy and lactation. Breast milk may be pumped and discarded so that the nursing child remains safe from radioactivity. The test is contraindicated in pregnant women.

COMPUTED TOMOGRAPHY

Computed tomography (CT) scanning may be performed to detect structural abnormalities of the GI tract. These tests help detect metastatic lesions that might not be apparent on regular GI radiographs. Oral barium sulfate or IV calcium phosphate may be given to provide contrast for the hollow GI organs examined by CT scan. The client is NPO for 6 to 8 hours before the CT test. Before the test, the bowel may be cleaned to reduce stool and gas. Drugs may be administered to decrease peristalsis or improve gastric motility.

Nonradiographic Studies

MAGNETIC RESONANCE IMAGING

Magnetic resonance imaging (MRI) uses magnetic energy rather than radiation to visualize soft tissue structures. It is used to examine GI structures when CT scanning is inadequate. Oral contrast agents are used to enhance the evaluation of GI disorders, such as abscesses or bleeding.

The client is NPO for 6 to 8 hours before the MRI. He or she must remove any metal objects, credit cards, wristwatch, jewelry, and the like. IV fluids, if required, must be infused by gravity during MRI because the changes in electrical charges during the test can affect mechanical infusers or pumps. The nurse informs clients that the scanner, a narrow, tunnel-like machine that will enclose them during the test, makes loud repetitive noises while the test is in progress. Clients who tend to be claustrophobic (fear enclosed spaces) may need sedation because it is imperative that they lie still and not panic during the test.

ULTRASONOGRAPHY

In **ultrasonography** (also called *ultrasound*), high-frequency sound waves are directed through the body, where they bounce off nearby structures, such as the liver and pancreas. The returning sound waves are then interpreted and recorded electronically. Ultrasonography, which shows the size and location of organs and outlines structures and abnormalities, helps detect cholecystitis, cholelithiasis, pyloric stenosis, and some disorders of the biliary system. It may be useful in detecting changes caused by appendicitis. Although the client can drink water before ultrasonography, the nurse discourages drinking through a straw, smoking, or chewing gum. In these activities, the client may swallow air and thereby distort sound wave transmission.

PERCUTANEOUS LIVER BIOPSY

In a procedure called **percutaneous liver biopsy,** the physician obtains a small core of liver tissue by placing a needle through the client's lateral abdominal wall directly into the liver. The tissue is then examined microscopically to detect abnormalities, which may include malignant changes, infectious or inflammatory processes, liver damage ("cirrhosis"), and signs of rejection in clients who have received a liver transplant.

The client must have coagulation studies before the procedure. A major complication after a liver biopsy is bleeding. The procedure is performed at the bedside or in the radiology department. Ultrasound or CT scanning is performed before or during the biopsy to identify an appropriate site for placement of the biopsy needle. The client usually receives a sedative and anesthetic to promote comfort and cooperation.

When assisting with a percutaneous liver biopsy, the nurse ensures that the biopsy equipment is assembled and in order. He or she assists the client to a supine position with a rolled towel beneath the right lower ribs. Before the physician inserts the needle, the nurse instructs the client to take a deep breath and hold it to keep the liver as near to the abdominal wall as possible. After specimen cells are obtained, they are placed in a preservative. The nurse makes sure that the specimen container is labeled and delivered to the laboratory (Nursing Guidelines 51-1).

GASTROINTESTINAL ENDOSCOPY

Gastrointestinal endoscopy is the direct visual examination of the lumen of the GI tract. It facilitates evaluation of the appearance and integrity of the GI mucosa and detects lesions. It provides access for therapeutic procedures. GI endoscopy is performed using a flexible fiberoptic endoscope. Diagnostic uses include obtaining biopsies of the mucosa, obtaining samples of fluids found in the GI tract, and injecting dyes for radiographic purposes. Therapeutic uses include inserting tubes and drains, electrocautery, and injecting medications. Among the variations of GI endoscopy (Box 51-1) are **proctosigmoidoscopy, esophagogastroduodenoscopy** (EGD) (Fig. 51-2), small bowel enteroscopy, peritoneoscopy, **colonoscopy, flexible sigmoidoscopy, panendoscopy,** and **endoscopic retrograde cholangiopancreatography** (ERCP).

Before an endoscopic procedure, the client follows dietary and fluid restrictions and bowel preparation pro-

---

NURSING GUIDELINES 51-1

Client Care After Liver Biopsy

- Assist the client to roll on right side after procedure, placing a small pillow under the costal margin.

- Instruct client to remain in this position for several hours to prevent the release of blood, bile, or both.

- Ask the client to avoid coughing or straining while immobilized.

- Take vital signs every 15 minutes for the first hour, then every 30 minutes for the next 2 hours, or until client is stable. Changes in vital signs may indicate bleeding.

- Teach the client to avoid heavy lifting or strenuous activity postprocedure.

During an endoscopic procedure, the nurse monitors respirations and vital signs. Assessing the client's level of pain and discomfort during the procedure is important, as is medicating the client as indicated. After the test, the nurse monitors the client for complications, especially signs of perforation. These include fever, abdominal distention, abdominal or chest pain, vomiting blood, or bright red rectal bleeding. The nurse offers the client food and fluids, unless the procedure was an EGD. After an EGD, the client may not have food or fluids until the gag reflex returns. Once the gag reflex is present, the nurse may introduce clear fluids and advance the diet to regular foods and fluids according to the client's tolerance. Occasionally, the client may complain of a sore throat after EGD. If the client's gag reflex has returned, the nurse may offer saline gargles, ice chips, or cool drinks.

LABORATORY TESTS

Depending on the suspected or confirmed diagnosis, various blood and urine tests may be ordered. Laboratory tests may include a complete blood count, urinalysis, serum bilirubin, cholesterol, serum ammonia level, prothrombin time, protein electrophoresis, and enzymes, such as amylase, lipase, aspartate aminotransferase, and lactic acid dehydrogenase. Common tumor marker blood studies include carcinoembryonic antigen and alphafetoprotein. Tests specific to the GI system are described in the following sections.

Gastric Analysis. Analysis of gastric fluids assists in determining problems with the secretory activity of the gastric mucosa. It also helps to evaluate gastric retention in clients who may have partial or complete pyloric or duodenal obstruction. For 8 to 12 hours before the test, the client is NPO. A small nasogastric tube is inserted into the stomach. Gastric contents are aspirated every 15 minutes for at least 1 hour and analyzed for acidity (pH), volume, and cytology if indicated.

cedures if the examination involves the lower GI structures. For the client undergoing an EGD, it is necessary for the client to spray or gargle with a local anesthetic. For an EGD and a colonoscopy, the client receives an anxiolytic agent [e.g., midazolam (Versed)] before the procedure to provide sedation and relieve anxiety.

FIGURE 51-2 Esophagogastroduodenoscopy. (From Smeltzer, S. C. & Bare, B. G. [2000]. *Brunner & Suddarth's textbook of medical–surgical nursing* [9th ed.]. Philadelphia: Lippincott Williams & Wilkins.)

PY Test. The **PY test** uses ¹⁴C-urea capsules to detect *Helicobacter pylori*, the bacteria associated with peptic ulcer disease. This test is simple and straightforward (Fig. 51-3). The client takes a ¹⁴C-urea capsule, waits approximately 10 minutes, and blows up a balloon. The air in the balloon is then transferred to a special vial for analysis. If gastric urease, an enzyme not normally present in human cells, is identified in the balloon air, the client most likely has *H. pylori* infection. This breath analysis is 90% accurate.

Clients having this test must avoid antibiotics or bismuth for 1 month, proton pump inhibitors and sucralfate for 2 weeks, and food and fluids for 6 hours before the test. To ensure accurate test results, the nurse advises the client not to handle or chew the test capsule but instead to swallow it intact.

Hydrogen Breath Testing. This test involves collecting a breath sample before and at intervals after ingestion of a carbohydrate solution. The two major gases in expired air are hydrogen and carbon dioxide. Elevated hydrogen levels in the expired breath sample indicate carbohydrate malabsorption. The type of solution used for the test depends on the suspected type of malabsorption. Lactose malabsorption (lactose intolerance) is a common disorder investigated using this technique.

Stool Analysis. Stool specimens are collected to identify white blood cells (indicating inflammation), red blood cells (indicating GI blood loss), and fat (indicating malabsorption). They also are collected to identify infection. Routine cultures may reveal bacterial infections (e.g., *Salmonella, Shigella, Campylobacter*). Placement of the specimen in a specific preservative to detect parasites and their ova allows diagnosis of parasitic infections (e.g., *Giardia, Cryptosporidium*).

Stool specimens that require examination for microorganisms should be fresh and warm for analysis. Only a small amount of stool needs to be collected; it always should be placed in a covered container. Eating red meat or other foods containing peroxidase within the previous 3 days may produce a false-positive result in some tests used for detecting occult blood.

NURSING PROCESS

● Diagnostic Testing for a Gastrointestinal Disorder

Assessment

The nurse interviews the client to determine past familiarity with the test or similar procedure. He or she asks the client to discuss previous experiences or current expectations. If the client is responsible for self-preparation before the test, the nurse explores those preparations. He or she reviews the client's history and explores any data on prior hypersensitivity or allergy to test preparations. In particular, the nurse asks about reactions to radionuclide or iodine-based contrast medium (dye) signaled by allergy to seafood. In some situations, the nurse labels an allergic client's chart and applies a special band or tag to the client's identification bracelet.

The nurse takes vital signs and weighs the client if required before the procedure. He or she encourages the client to empty the bladder before some tests. Recording other essential baseline data is important for later comparison and identification of serious reportable changes or complications (e.g., rectal bleeding). In addition, the nurse must record the client's informed consent. The client and family members need teaching and reassurance about the test's purpose and procedure. They also need to know care measures to be implemented after the test.

Diagnosis, Planning, and Interventions

Anxiety related to lack of knowledge of test procedure or possible test findings
Expected Outcomes: (1) Client will demonstrate knowledge of the test procedure. (2) Client will express feelings of relief from anxiety.

- Review test preparations. *Such review ensures that the client understands and carries out preparations as required.*
- Provide printed directions. *Printed directions reinforce verbal instructions.*
- Encourage client to express fears. *Expressing feelings assists in alleviating fear and clarifying misconceptions.*

FIGURE 51-3 The breath test that indicates *Helicobacter pylori* is performed in three easy steps: (1) the client takes a ¹⁴C-urea capsule and waits about 10 minutes. (2) The client blows up a balloon. (3) The client waits while the air in the balloon is analyzed for gastric urease.

- Discuss the client's perceptions of the test and explain what to expect during and after. *Having knowledge of the client's understanding provides an opportunity to reinforce the knowledge and to clarify expectations for the test.*
- Respect the client's individuality and remain non-judgmental and supportive. *Respect makes the client more likely to ask questions without fear of ridicule.*

Pain related to test procedure

Expected Outcome: Client will state no or minimal discomfort.

- Use pillows or blankets for positioning to relieve discomfort if the client has physical problems that cause pain (e.g., arthritis). *Supportive positioning alleviates and relieves pain.*
- Medicate the client with opioid analgesic or sedative if ordered before the procedure. *Analgesia or conscious sedation reduces pain and discomfort during the procedure.*
- Tell the client to inform test personnel if he or she experiences pressure or cramping during the instillation of test fluids. *Test personnel can slow the instillation or take other measures to relieve discomfort.*
- Teach the client to expel gas and test fluids from the bowel when he or she experiences the urge. *Ignoring the urge to expel bowel contents increases pain and discomfort.*

Risk for Deficient Fluid Volume related to fluid restriction or loss associated with diarrhea or vomiting

Expected Outcome: Client will maintain fluid volume balance as evidenced by normal findings on intake and output records.

- Weigh client and monitor the color and amount of urine. *These data provide a baseline for the client's response to tests, fluid loss related to diarrhea or vomiting, or both.*
- Monitor pulse rate and blood pressure. *Changes may indicate dehydration.*
- Report dizziness and confusion. *Such findings may indicate dehydration.*
- Administer oral fluids as soon as possible. *These fluids replace fluid loss.*
- When testing is complete, monitor intake and output and encourage liberal intake. *These measures ensure that client is taking in adequate fluids.*

Risk for Constipation related to barium retention

Expected Outcome: Client achieves regular bowel elimination pattern within 2 to 3 days.

- Encourage client to drink at least 2000 mL of fluid per 24 hours after tests, using barium. *This amount provides sufficient fluid to facilitate evacuation of stool.*
- Administer post-test laxative or enema if ordered. *A laxative or an enema promotes faster evacuation of barium.*
- Monitor stool passage, observing the stool for barium. *Stools with barium appear light-colored or white-streaked.*
- Report diminished or hyperactive bowel sounds. *Such sounds may indicate barium retention.*

Evaluation of Expected Outcomes

The client reports minimal anxiety and pain, maintains adequate fluid balance, and evacuates all barium. Normal bowel elimination resumes, as evidenced by one bowel movement of soft-formed brown stool per day

GENERAL NUTRITIONAL CONSIDERATIONS

Observe for weight loss or failure to gain weight in clients with GI problems. Many GI tests require at least an 8-hour fast beforehand. Repeated or multiple tests performed over days can compound potential or existing nutritional problems.

Encourage adequate fluid intake to promote dilution and elimination of dyes and other test substances.

If the client receives a local anesthetic that suppresses the gag reflex, withhold food and fluids until the reflex returns.

Observe for subsequent signs and symptoms of intolerance in clients whose test required ingesting a special solution, such as a carbohydrate solution. For instance, clients tested for lactose intolerance may experience cramping, abdominal distention, and diarrhea after ingestion of the substrate used for testing.

GENERAL PHARMACOLOGIC CONSIDERATIONS

Depending on the test procedure, the client's medication regimen, and physician's orders, some, all, or none of the client's medications may be withheld before and during testing.

For certain diagnostic tests of the GI tract, the bowel may be cleaned or the client may receive various cleansing medications orally to promote clear visualization of internal structures. In such cases, the client may take cleansing preparations orally or by enema.

Polyethylene glycol/electrolyte (GoLYTELY, NuLytely, Colyte) may be used for bowel cleansing in preparation for GI diagnostic examination. The solution is reconstituted with water and the client instructed to drink 240 mL every 10 minutes until 4 L is consumed or fecal returns are clear. Allow the client to drink only clear liquids after administration of the solution begins.

The ingestion of a large amount of polyethylene glycol/electrolyte solution is required to produce watery stools. This type of solution, however, usually is not associated with increased risk for fluid and electrolyte imbalance.

Alternative medications used for bowel preparation include those that contain a large amount of phosphorus (e.g., Phosphosoda, Visicol). These medications work by creating an osmotic diarrhea. As a result, risk for fluid and electrolyte imbalance is increased. Take measures to ensure adequate fluid intake during the bowel cleansing process.

Before biopsy procedures, clients at risk for serious bleeding may receive precautionary vitamin K, which promotes blood clotting. If sedative, IV medications or dyes, or general anesthetics are administered, monitor the client appropriately.

Emergency medications must be kept stocked and oxygen must be readily available in case the client experiences an adverse reaction to the dye or drugs administered during the test.

GENERAL GERONTOLOGIC CONSIDERATIONS

Fluid balance for clients, especially older adults, may be precarious, given the fluid restrictions and multiple enemas or laxatives required for GI tests.

Older adults are at higher risk for dehydration when undergoing a lower GI series or endoscopic examinations of the bowel than are younger people because they tend to have fewer physiologic reserves to compensate for fluid loss. A history of vomiting or diarrhea or diuretic therapy may compound the potential for fluid deficit.

The older adult usually has less control of the rectal sphincter than a younger adult because of age-related changes in innervation, a diminished awareness of the filling reflex, and decreased muscle tone.

To detect fluid volume deficit, weigh the client and observe the color and amount of urine.

Explain the diagnostic examination to the older adult in simple language, allowing ample time to answer questions. Repeated explanations and assurances may be necessary to ease the older adult's anxiety.

After the diagnostic test, the older adult may experience dizziness or confusion from the stress of the examination or enduring 6 to 8 hours without food or fluids. Provide nourishment as soon as possible after the examination, and give assistance with ambulation when necessary.

Critical Thinking Exercise

1. *A client is preparing for an EGD. This includes withholding food and fluids for 6 to 12 hours and receiving a sedative before the test. In addition, the nurse will spray the client's throat with a local anesthetic or the client will gargle with the local anesthetic. What precautions does the nurse take before the client goes for the EGD?*

References and Suggested Readings

Bickley, L. S. & Hoekelman, R. A. (1999). *Bates' guide to physical examination and history taking* (7th ed.). Philadelphia: Lippincott Williams & Wilkins.

Bullock, B. A. & Henze, R. L. (2000). *Focus on pathophysiology.* Philadelphia: Lippincott Williams & Wilkins.

Smeltzer, S. C. & Bare, B. G. (2000). *Brunner & Suddarth's textbook of medical–surgical nursing* (9th ed.). Philadelphia: Lippincott Williams & Wilkins.

Caring for Clients With Disorders of the Upper Gastrointestinal Tract

Learning Objectives

On completion of this chapter, the reader will:

- Discuss assessment findings and treatment of disorders that affect eating, disorders of the esophagus, and gastric disorders.
- Describe nursing management of a client with a nasogastric or gastrointestinal tube or gastrostomy.
- List suggestions for relieving upper gastrointestinal discomfort.
- Discuss the nursing management of clients undergoing gastric surgery.

Digestion begins in the mouth and continues in the stomach and small intestine, with food traveling through the esophagus in between. The nurse is responsible for managing the care of clients with disorders affecting the upper gastrointestinal (GI) tract (see Fig. 51-1).

DISORDERS THAT AFFECT EATING

● ANOREXIA

Simple **anorexia,** or lack of appetite, is a common symptom of many diseases. Prolonged anorexia may lead to serious consequences, such as malnutrition.

Pathophysiology and Etiology

The appetite center, which stimulates or suppresses the appetite, is located in the hypothalamus. Pleasant or noxious food odors, effects of drugs, emotional stress,

fear, psychological problems, or illnesses may affect appetite.

Brief periods of anorexia are not life-threatening but can cause temporary malnutrition. During periods of reduced food consumption, most people have a sufficient reserve of stored glycogen, which provides energy through the process of *glycogenolysis,* the conversion of glycogen to glucose. Hormones such as glucagon, glucocorticoid hormones from the adrenal cortex, and thyroid hormones stimulate the liver to carry out *gluconeogenesis,* which depends on the use of stores of fat-soluble vitamins. Selective reabsorption by the kidneys can temporarily maintain electrolyte balance.

Assessment Findings

Signs and Symptoms

Hunger usually is absent, and clients describe having no desire for food. Some clients state that they feel nauseous when they smell food or even think about eating.

741

Some eat a small amount only because they feel they should or others coerce them to do so. Amounts of weight loss vary, depending on how long the anorexia and reduced food intake have lasted. Eventually the client may show signs of *hypovitaminosis* (vitamin deficiency). The body does not store any water-soluble vitamins (B vitamins, including folic acid and vitamin C) except for B_{12}. Therefore, deficiencies in these vitamins may be seen in more acute phases of illness. The body does store fat-soluble vitamins (A, D, E, and K) but requires fat absorption to do so. Chronic illnesses and those that directly affect fat absorption (e.g., cystic fibrosis, pancreatitis, liver disease) result in deficiency of the fat-soluble vitamins.

Diagnostic Findings

Depending on the chronicity of the anorexia, hemoglobin level and blood cell counts may be reduced. Red blood cells (RBCs) may become abnormally enlarged. Serum albumin, electrolyte, and protein levels may be low, with accompanying cardiac dysrhythmias. For example, an elevated U wave on the electrocardiogram may indicate potassium deficiency.

Medical and Surgical Management

Management depends on the cause. Short-term anorexia (less than 1 week) usually requires no medical intervention. Persistent anorexia may require various approaches, such as a high-calorie diet, high-calorie supplemental feedings, tube feedings, and total parenteral nutrition (TPN). Psychological support, psychiatric treatment, or both may be essential for the client whose anorexia is linked with *anorexia nervosa,* a psychiatric disorder, instead of a defined organic disease (see Chap. 16).

Nursing Management

To maintain sufficient nutrition and sustain normal body weight, the client must eat an adequate quantity of food. In assisting the client to meet this goal, the nurse monitors weight daily. He or she also obtains a complete medical and allergy (drugs and food) history from the client or a family member and compiles a dietary history, including a description of the client's eating patterns and food preferences. For more information, see Nursing Guidelines 52-1.

Additional nursing measures depend on any consequences of anorexia. In the case of altered bowel patterns (diarrhea or constipation) from reduced bulk secondary to liquid supplements, potential interventions include the following:

NURSING GUIDELINES 52-1

Managing Care of the Client With Anorexia

- Provide foods that the client likes during meals.
- Offer nourishing beverages (egg nog, milk shakes, and commercial concentrates such as Ensure or Instant Breakfast) as between-meal snacks.
- If the client is hospitalized or in another healthcare facility, encourage family members to bring favorite foods that can be refrigerated or reheated.
- Conduct a daily caloric count if necessary to determine total caloric intake and the amount of vitamins, minerals, fats, proteins, and carbohydrates in the client's diet.
- Keep serving sizes and containers small to avoid overwhelming the client.
- Serve and keep hot foods hot and cold foods cold.
- Encourage eating in the company of others.
- Formulate a nutritional plan with the client and dietitian that promotes weight gain (approximately 600 calories per meal).
- If necessary, arrange for supplementation based on documented deficiencies in the client's intake.
- Consult the physician and dietitian in cases of prolonged anorexia.

- Keep a record of the client's bowel movements.
- If the client experiences diarrhea, consult with the physician and dietitian about changing the type of supplement.
- If the client is constipated, change formula to one that contains fiber to add bulk to stools.
- Dilute the formula temporarily until the client adjusts to the concentrated contents.
- Assist the client and dietitian to increase dietary fiber.
- Administer a prescribed stool softener to promote ease and frequency of bowel elimination.

● NAUSEA AND VOMITING

Nausea and vomiting are common and often coexisting problems. If these symptoms are prolonged, weakness, weight loss, nutritional deficiency, dehydration, and electrolyte and acid-base imbalances may result.

Pathophysiology and Etiology

Some of the more common causes of nausea and vomiting include drugs, infections and inflammatory conditions of the GI tract, intestinal obstruction, systemic infections, lesions of the central nervous system, food poisoning, emotional stress, early pregnancy, and uremia. Nausea usually precedes vomiting and usually results from distention of the duodenum. Increased salivation and peripheral vasoconstriction, which causes cold, clammy skin and tachycardia, accompany nausea. The vomiting center, located in the medulla, is particularly sensitive to parasympathetic neurotransmitters released in response to gastric irritation. The Valsalva maneuver, which accompanies the forceful expulsion of stomach contents, causes dizziness, hypotension, and bradycardia.

Assessment Findings

Signs and Symptoms

The client describes an unpleasant feeling, identified as nausea, which usually is associated with loss of appetite and refusal to eat. When a client vomits, others may observe him or her retching while he or she evacuates the stomach contents. The process occurs once or several times in succession.

The client who experiences excessive fluid loss (dehydration) with vomiting may complain of excessive thirst and report decreased or no urine production. Eyes and oral mucosa appear dry or dull, and poor skin turgor reflects fluid loss (see Chap. 22).

The client's history may include ingestion of noxious substances, such as excessive amounts of alcohol, presumably contaminated food, or drugs that commonly cause GI side effects. Exposure to other people with similar symptoms suggests a bacterial or viral cause.

When vomiting is secondary to intestinal obstruction, the abdomen is distended, tender, and firm to touch. Bowel sounds may be absent or hypoactive.

Diagnostic Findings

Prolonged vomiting may lead to low levels of serum sodium and chloride. Bicarbonate levels may rise to compensate for the loss of chloride and accumulation of metabolic acids. The hematocrit value, if high, is secondary to the hemoconcentration that accompanies dehydration.

Medical and Surgical Management

Sometimes nausea and vomiting are short-lived and do not require medical intervention. In some instances, intravenous (IV) fluids, electrolyte replacement, and drug therapy are necessary. Elimination of the cause necessitates various interventions, ranging from stopping a drug to surgical intervention for intestinal obstruction. Symptomatic relief may be achieved by administering an antiemetic agent (Drug Therapy Table 52-1), providing IV fluid and electrolyte replacement, and temporarily restricting food intake until the cause of vomiting is eliminated.

N U R S I N G   P R O C E S S

● **The Client With Nausea and Vomiting**

Assessment

The nurse obtains a complete medical, dietary, drug, and allergy history. In addition, he or she compiles a list of symptoms that occurred before and along with the nausea and vomiting, how long the problem has existed, and the frequency, color, and amount of vomited material. Because the cause may be unknown, the nurse lists the foods and where the client ate in the past 24 hours. In addition, he or she assesses general appearance, weight, and vital signs. Documenting intake and output and monitoring for signs of fluid volume deficit are additional essential assessment requirements (see Chap. 22).

Diagnosis, Planning, and Interventions

Deficient Fluid Volume related to prolonged vomiting and decreased intake of oral fluids

Expected Outcome: Fluid balance will be restored as evidenced by intake of 1500 to 3000 mL/day with similar fluid loss.

● Offer clear fluids in small amounts. *Slow introduction of fluids allows client to develop tolerance and determine if he or she can advance the diet.*
● Recommend commercial over-the-counter beverages such as GatorAde. *GatorAde replaces fluids and electrolytes.*
● Inform physician if urine output is below 500 mL/day or serum electrolyte levels are abnormal. *Such findings indicate severe dehydration and the need for IV replacement fluids.*
● Monitor weight daily. *Daily monitoring helps to determine trends in weight loss or gain.*
● Assess skin turgor and mucous membranes. *Decreased skin turgor and dry mucous membranes indicate dehydration.*

Imbalanced Nutrition: Less than Body Requirements related to nausea and vomiting

Expected Outcome: Client's nutritional status will be adequate as evidenced by maintenance of weight and normal electrolyte and blood values.

● When client tolerates clear fluids, advance diet to full liquids, then to soft, bland foods, such as creamed soups, crackers, or toast. *Advancing diet slowly helps client develop tolerance for fluids and food.*
● Collaborate with the dietitian to provide nutritional foods. *The dietitian can help create a plan that assists client to increase caloric intake with foods that he or she can tolerate.*

DRUG THERAPY TABLE 52-1 | ANTIEMETIC MEDICATIONS

DRUG CATEGORY AND EXAMPLES/ MECHANISM OF ACTION	SIDE EFFECTS	NURSING CONSIDERATIONS
Serotonin Receptor Antagonist		
Ondanestron (Zofran) Blocks receptors for 5HT₃, which affects the neural pathways involved in nausea and vomiting	Headache, dizziness (low blood pressure), myalgia (muscle aches and pains), malaise, fatigue, drowsiness	Review client's allergy history before administering medication. Provide oral drug form q8h around the clock for 1 to 2 days after chemotherapy or radiation to prevent nausea and vomiting. Caution client about side effects that may make activities such as driving a car or operating other machinery hazardous.
Phenothiazine		
Prochlorperazine (Compazine) Inhibits the CTZ and vomiting center in the brain	Drowsiness, hypotension, changes in heart rhythms, photophobia, blurred vision, dry mouth, discolored urine	Tell client that this drug is for short-term control of nausea and vomiting and should be used exactly as directed. Explain side effects and advise client not to save any medicine for a later date or give any to anyone else. Monitor older clients because effects of drug may lead more rapidly to dehydration than in younger clients.
Antihistamines		
Hydroxyzine (Atarax, Vistaril) Blocks H₁ receptors, decreasing stimulation of the CTZ and vomiting center	Drowsiness, tremor, dry mouth, hypersensitivity reaction (includes difficulty breathing), tremors, loss of coordination, sore muscles, or muscle spasms	Take full health history to help determine underlying cause of nausea and vomiting. Give by deep intramuscular injection in volume prescribed to control vomiting. Report breathing problems, tremors, muscle problems and incoordination.
Promethazine (Anergan, Phenergan) Blocks H₁ receptors, decreasing stimulation of the CTZ and vomiting center	Dizziness, drowsiness, poor coordination, confusion, restlessness, excitation, epigastric distress, thickened bronchial secretions, urinary frequency, dysuria	Take drug and health history. Because this drug interacts with several others, review potential for drug interactions; for example, do not administer medication if client is taking monoamine oxidase inhibitor. Do not give to a client with a lower respiratory tract disorder. Advise client to avoid drinking alcohol when taking this medication.
Dimenhydrinate (Dramamine) Inhibits vestibular stimulation in the ear, thereby relieving motion sickness	Drowsiness, confusion, nervousness, restlessness, headache, dizziness, vertigo, tingling, heaviness and weakness of hands, epigastric discomfort, low blood pressure, nasal stuffiness, chest tightness, rash, photosensitivity	Advise client not to take if pregnant or lactating. Review client history for glaucoma, peptic ulcer, bronchial asthma, heart problems because drug may pose a danger. Urge client to avoid alcohol because serious sedation could result. Advise client to report breathing problems, tremors, loss of coordination, visual disturbances or hallucinations, and irregular heartbeat.

CTZ, chemoreceptor trigger zone.

● Discourage caffeinated or carbonated beverages. *Such drinks may decrease appetite and lead to early satiety.*

Evaluation of Expected Outcomes

The client has an oral intake of 2500 mL and an output of 2600 mL. Weight is maintained or restored to preillness level. Serum electrolyte levels and other laboratory test results are within normal limits.

● CANCER OF THE ORAL CAVITY

Cancer cells undergo changes in structure and appearance. They multiply, eventually forming a colony of abnormal and dysfunctional cells (see Chap. 20). When cancer affects the oral cavity, cells in the lips, mouth, or pharynx undergo malignant changes. When cancers of the oral cavity are detected early, the rate of cure is fairly good.

Pathophysiology and Etiology

Development of oral cancers is linked with smoking, chewing tobacco, and drinking alcohol in excess. Lip cancer is associated with pipe smoking and prolonged exposure to wind and sun. As cancer cells in the oral cavity increase, the mass may distort a client's appearance; exert pressure on surrounding tissue, making it difficult to masticate (chew); cause local pain; or produce *dysphagia* (difficulty swallowing). The most common oral cancer is squamous cell carcinoma. Malignant growths can be found anywhere in the oral cavity, but cancers usually occur on the lips, sides of the tongue, or floor of the mouth. Untreated, cancerous growths may extend into nearby tissue, such as the middle ear or nasal sinuses; infiltrate regional lymph nodes; or invade large blood vessels, such as the carotid arteries, that are near the oral cavity. Serious hemorrhage ("carotid blowout") and death may result when cancer cells invade an artery that becomes ulcerated or when necrosis follows radiation therapy.

Assessment Findings

The early stage of oral cancer is characteristically asymptomatic. At first, the client may notice a lesion, lump, or other abnormality of the lips or mouth. Other changes, such as pain, soreness, and bleeding follow. If a lesion is on the tongue, the client commonly experiences difficulty eating or tasting food. Pain and numbness also follow. Dentists and oral hygienists may be the first to notice changes in mouth tissues, such as *leukoplakia,* a white patch on the tongue or inner cheek that may become cancerous. A biopsy of the lesion discloses malignant cells, which confirms the diagnosis of oral cancer.

Medical and Surgical Management

Treatment depends on the location and type of tumor, extent (or stage) of involvement, and the client's physical condition. In cases of hemorrhage, transfusions are given to replace lost blood. Ligation of the bleeding vessel usually is necessary. Drugs such as antianxiety agents are prescribed to relieve the client's apprehension.

Surgical treatment of most oral cancers includes tumor excision alone or with follow-up radiation therapy. Chemotherapy usually is not beneficial for primary tumors. Surgical excision may result in complete cure, provided that it is performed early. A neck dissection is performed if the cancer has spread to the lymph nodes near the jaw or below the ears. Cancer of the tongue usually involves radical surgery to remove part or all of the tongue. Excision of the tumor from parts of the jaw or palate is disfiguring.

For clients with advanced disease, treatment is palliative only. Chemotherapy or radiation therapy is used to relieve pain and temporarily decrease tumor size. A tracheostomy and tube feedings are instituted to maintain an adequate airway and provide nourishment.

Nursing Management

General nursing management of the client with oral cancer is much the same as for any client with cancer (see Chap. 20). The focus of attention, however, is on maintaining a patent airway, promoting adequate fluid and food intake, and supporting communication that the tumor or treatment may have impaired. To review care of the client needing airway management, refer to Chapter 28 and the discussion of endotracheal intubation and tracheostomy care.

Nurses collaborate with speech pathologists to address communication problems. They must be patient when the client chooses to communicate by speaking and clarify or repeat what he or she says if speech is not understandable. Nurses may substitute written forms for communicating if speech is impaired. They also offer the client pencil and paper, a Magic Slate, or an alphabet board, or suggest that the client use hand signals.

When the client returns from the operating room after oral surgery, he or she should be positioned flat, either on the abdomen or side, with the head turned to the side to facilitate drainage from the mouth. After recovery from the anesthetic, the client is positioned with the head of the bed elevated, which makes it easier for the client to breathe deeply and cough up secretions. It also controls edema in the operative area.

After oral surgery, there should be equipment for suctioning, administration of oxygen, and tracheostomy at the client's bedside. If the client does not have a tracheostomy, a tracheostomy tray must be nearby for emergency use because respiratory distress or airway obstruction requires immediate attention. If the client has a tracheostomy, the nurse suctions secretions from the cannula and cleans it on a regular basis.

The nurse should not irrigate the client's mouth until the client is awake and alert. When and if mouth irrigation is carried out, the nurse should turn the client's head to the side to allow the solution to run in gently and flow out into an emesis basin. The nurse instills only a small amount of solution and then waits for the fluid to drain before administering more. In addition, he or she suctions the mouth as necessary to remove secretions, blood, or irrigating solution.

The client must not receive oral liquids or foods until a written order exists. The nurse observes the client's ability to swallow small amounts of liquid. In cases of coughing or other difficulty, the nurse must suction the liquid from the mouth immediately.

The client may receive prescribed antiemetics if he or she experiences nausea or vomiting. If the client has a gastric tube, the nurse checks it for patency. Clients should not use a straw because it causes the client to swallow air, which can distend the stomach.

The client's emotional response to radical oral surgery is a real and difficult problem. Extensive surgery of the mouth and adjacent structures is not only disfiguring but incapacitating. It interferes with communication, eating, and control of saliva. Although healthcare providers explain the extent of surgery before the operation, many clients and families cannot grasp all the ensuing effects. The first time family members or clients see the effects of surgery, the experience usually is traumatic. The nurse needs to promote effective coping and therapeutic grieving at this time. Responses may range from crying or extreme sadness and avoiding contact with others to refusing to talk about the surgery or changes in appearance. Allowing the client time to mourn, accept, and adjust to losses is essential. To facilitate adaptation, the client needs opportunities to express feelings. Nurses must observe severely depressed clients closely. Clients who are suicidal need psychological evaluation and counseling. In addition, the nurse provides time for family members to express fears, ask questions, and grieve. It may help to refer clients and family members to support groups and counselors.

Nutritional management is a particular challenge when caring for clients with oral cancer. If the client can take oral nourishment, a nutritional consultation may be necessary to modify the diet according to the client's ability to chew and swallow. Because oral tissues are sensitive, the client should avoid hot and cold liquids and spicy foods. The nurse can consult with the physician about prescribing a topical anesthetic mouthwash containing lidocaine (Xylocaine), which numbs the tissues, or a systemic analgesic to relieve pain. Providing nourishment by a route other than the mouth may be necessary.

> ### Stop, Think, and Respond ● BOX 52-1
>
> *A client comes to the clinic with complaints of difficulty chewing and swallowing. What questions should you ask?*

Gastrointestinal Intubation for Feedings or Medications

At some time during the care of the client with oral cancer, as well as when caring for others with GI disorders, the nurse may have to perform GI intubation, which is the insertion and management of GI tubes. GI intubation is done to provide nutrition, medications, or both; perform **gastric decompression,** which is removal of gas and fluids from the stomach; lavage the stomach to remove ingested toxins; diagnose GI disorders, a process that may include aspiration of gastric contents for analysis; treat GI obstruction; or apply pressure to a GI bleed. Examples of different types of GI intubation include **nasogastric intubation** (tube passes through nose into stomach via esophagus), **orogastric intubation** (tube passes through mouth into the stomach), **nasoenteric intubation** (tube passes through the nose, esophagus, and stomach to the small intestine), **gastrostomy** (tube enters the stomach through a surgically created opening into the abdominal wall), and **jejunostomy** (tube enters jejunum or small intestine through a surgically created opening into the abdominal wall). See Table 52-1.

GI tubes are advanced to the upper GI tract by way of the mouth or nose or introduced directly into the stomach or small intestine through the abdominal wall. A gastric tube lies in the stomach; an intestinal tube extends past the pylorus. When placed directly into the upper GI

TABLE 52-1	NASOGASTRIC, NASOENTERIC, AND FEEDING TUBES			
TUBE TYPE	**LENGTH**	**SIZE (FRENCH)**	**LUMEN**	**OTHER CHARACTERISTICS**
Nasogastric Tubes				
Levin (plastic or rubber)	125 cm	14–18	Single	Circular markings serve as guidelines for insertion.
Gastric sump Salem (plastic)	120 cm	12–18	Double	Smaller lumen acts as a vent.
Moss	90 cm	12–16	Triple	Tube contains both a gastric decompression lumen and a duodenal lumen for postoperative feedings.
Sengstaken-Blakemore (rubber)			Triple	Two lumens are used to inflate the gastric and esophageal balloons.
Nasoenteric Decompression Tubes				
Miller-Abbott (rubber)	300 cm	12–18	Double	One lumen uses tungsten or air for balloon inflation.
Harris	180 cm	14, 16	Single	Tip is tungsten weighted.
Cantor (rubber)	300 cm	16	Single	Bag is tungsten weighted.
Baker (plastic)	270 cm	16	Double	One lumen is used for balloon inflation.
Nasoenteric Feeding Tubes				
Dobhoff or Keofeed II (polyurethane or silicone rubber)	160–175 cm	8–12	Single	Tip is tungsten weighted, radiopaque.

tract through an incision in the abdominal wall, the tube is referred to as a *gastrostomy tube.*

The nasal route is the preferred route for passing a tube when the client's nose is intact and free from injury. The type of tube selected depends on the reason for placing the tube (Box 52-1). In general, smaller tubes are used for feeding because they tend to be more easily tolerated by clients; larger tubes are used for decompression because they allow for evacuation of large pieces of debris or blood clots from the upper GI tract.

NURSING PROCESS

● The Client Receiving Tube Feedings

Assessment

Before beginning a tube feeding, the nurse determines why the client requires it: such as to improve nutritional and hydration status for chronic illness. Evaluating renal

---

BOX 52-1 ● Uses of Gastrointestinal (GI) Tubes

Gastrointestinal tubes come in several types, depending on their uses. Among common GI tubes used for decompression are the Levin tube and the Salem sump. Narrower, more flexible tubes, such as Keofeed, Dubbhoff gastrostomy, jejunostomy, and others, are made of polyurethane or silicone and are used for administering liquid nourishment.

Feeding tubes are longer than Levin tubes and terminate in the upper, small intestine. Their advantages include ease of insertion, more comfort for the client, reduced potential for vomiting and aspiration because the formula is instilled below the pylorus, and extended use because they may remain in the same nostril for up to 4 weeks. Their disadvantage is that distal location is difficult to assess without a chest or abdominal radiograph.

FEEDING METHODS
Liquid nourishment is administered by bolus, intermittent, cyclic, or continuous methods. Depending on institutional policy and individual feeding orders, the feeding tube is flushed with water at various intervals to ensure patency. Many tube feeding formulas are available to suit a client's different nutritional needs. Nursing observation of tolerance of the feeding is essential to determine which tube and formula are best for the client.

Bolus tube feedings
- Allow introduction of 250 to 400 mL formula through the tube in a short period (usually 15–30 minutes)
- Administered by syringe or gravity flow system attached to the distal end of the feeding tube

Intermittent tube feedings
- Allow delivery of between 250 and 400 mL formula over 30 to 60 minutes
- Delivered by gravity flow system or an electronic feeding pump

Continuous tube feedings
- Allow formula to be administered at lower rates—usually 1.5 mL/minute over a longer time (usually 12–24 hours)
- Delivered by gravity flow system or an electronic feeding pump

Cyclic tube feedings
- Allow formula to be administered continuously for 8 to 12 hours during sleep followed by a 16- to 12-hour pause
- Ensure adequate nutrition during weaning from tube to oral feeding
- Alternated with oral food intake until client can take most nutrition orally

---

function and checking for any digestive issues are essential, as is assessing previous stool patterns, present weight, and any vomiting.

Diagnosis, Planning, and Interventions

When a client is receiving tube feedings, medications, or both (Table 52-2), the nurse's role is to ensure that the lungs remain free of liquid substances, the client does not acquire an infection, and intake and output are appropriate for the client's age and size. Additional objectives include providing adequate nutrition, promoting appropriate stool patterns (amount, consistency, and frequency), and preserving intact skin and nasal mucosa. Efforts to keep the mucous membranes, which tend to dry from mouth breathing and restricted oral fluids, moist also are important. Frequent mouth care may relieve discomfort from dryness and unpleasant tastes and odors. Ice chips and analgesic throat lozenges, gargles, or sprays may help if the client's mouth and throat become sore. Providing mouth care after removal of the tube is an important nursing intervention, as is informing the client that a sore throat (an aftereffect of intubation) may persist for several days.

The client is at risk not only for dry mouth but also fluid volume deficit resulting from insufficient fluid intake. The nurse must be aware of the client's normal fluid needs and whether the formula alone can meet them. Observation for signs and symptoms of dehydration is very important. For example, if urine output is less than 500 mL/day, the nurse needs to administer formula and additional water as ordered.

While ensuring adequate hydration, the nurse also needs to protect the client from infections that stem from microbes in the tube-feeding formula. Signs and symptoms of infection include diarrhea, fever, or abnormal white blood cell count. Interventions to prevent infection include washing hands before handling equipment; keeping feeding formula refrigerated or unopened until it is

TABLE 52-2	MEDICATION ADMINISTRATION BY WAY OF FEEDING TUBE
TYPE	**PREPARATION**
Liquid	None
Simple compressed tablets	Crushed and dissolved in water
Buccal or sublingual tablets	Give as intended
Enteric-coated tablets	Cannot be crushed; change in form required
Time-release tablets	Some can be opened; cannot be crushed because doing so may release too much drug too quickly (overdose); check with pharmacist

ready for use; warming bolus, intermittent, or cyclic feeding formula to room temperature just before administering; hanging continuous formula-feeding containers with only the volume for 4 to 6 hours; flushing the tubing with water before adding more formula and after giving a bolus or intermittent feeding or medications; discarding any premixed formula after 24 hours; thoroughly cleaning and drying all equipment used for bolus feedings (i.e., syringe, feeding adapters, tubing, containers) after each use; and replacing the infusion container and tubing used for a continuous tube feeding every 24 hours or as directed by agency policy.

The plan of care contains the following diagnoses, outcomes and interventions.

Imbalanced Nutrition: Less than Body Requirements related to inadequate dietary intake
Expected Outcome: Nutrition will be adequate as evidenced by stable body weight.

● Maintain feeding schedule, drip rate, and amount administered by gravity drip, bolus feeding, or continuous controlled pump. *Feeding at set rate and amount ensures the client will receive the appropriate amount, calories, and nutrients, and assists client to digest the feeding without discomfort.*
● Aspirate and measure residual content before each intermittent feeding or every 4 to 8 hours for continuous feedings. Delay feeding if residual content measures more than 100 mL or 10% to 20% of the hourly amount of a continuous feeding. Readminister the residual amount. *Measuring the residual content ensures that the client digests feedings and will not be overfed. Readministering residual amounts ensures that the client does not lose nutrients and digestive enzymes.*
● Maintain tube function by:
  ● Administering 15 to 30 mL of water before and after medications and feedings (every 4 to 6 hours with continuous feedings). *This measure ensures tube patency and decreases the risk for bacterial infection and crusting or blockage of the tube.*
  ● Changing tube feeding container and tubing per agency policy. *Regular changes prevent blockage and infection.*
  ● Monitor weight daily. *Daily monitoring checks for trends in weight loss or gain.*
  ● Consult with physician and dietitian if client experiences any problems with tube feeding, such as nausea, bloating, diarrhea, or cramping. *Such problems may indicate poor tolerance of feeding, wrong formula for client, or other issues.*

PC: Aspiration
Expected Outcome: The nurse will manage tube feedings to reduce risk for aspiration during feedings or vomiting episodes.

● Check tube placement and gastric residual prior to feedings. *Checking prevents improper infusion and assists to prevent vomiting.*

● Place client in semi-Fowler's position during and 30 to 60 minutes after an intermittent feeding, and at all times for a continuous feeding. *Proper positioning prevents regurgitation.*
● Stop feeding if client vomits or aspiration is suspected. *In these cases, cessation prevents further problems and allows for treatment of the immediate problem.*

Risk for Diarrhea related to hypertonic feeding solutions, lack of dietary fiber, high carbohydrate and electrolyte content, or other factors (e.g., gastroenteritis, deficient fluid volume)
Expected Outcome: Client will have normal bowel patterns with formed stool.

● Consult with physician about decreasing the infusion rate. *A decreased infusion rate provides time for carbohydrates and electrolytes to be diluted, preventing increased fluid from the vascular system going to the jejunum.*
● Administer feedings at room temperature. *Cold or warm feedings stimulate peristalsis.*
● If possible, administer feedings continuously. *Bolus or intermittent feedings cause sudden distention of the small intestine.*
● Instruct client to remain in semi-Fowler's position during and after feedings (as discussed previously). *This position slows movement of feeding into the intestine.*
● Consult with physician and dietitian if diarrhea persists. *Client may require a different formula if all other possible causes for diarrhea are ruled out.*

Evaluation of Expected Outcomes

The client maintains his or her weight. Lungs are clear to auscultation, and the client has not vomited. Bowel patterns are normal with formed stool.

Gastrointestinal Intubation for Decompression

The larger GI tube is used to relieve abdominal distention caused by problems after surgery, episodes of acute upper GI bleeding, or symptoms associated with intestinal obstruction, or for diagnostic purposes. It is inserted by following the same procedure as is used for insertion of a feeding tube (Fig. 52-1).

Some tubes, such as a gastric sump tube, have a double lumen, one of which serves as a vent, allowing a small amount of air to be drawn in when the tube is connected to suction. Sump tubes decrease the possibility of the stomach wall adhering to and obstructing the tube openings during gastric decompression. A common problem associated with vented tubes is leakage from the vent lumen. The nurse may prevent this by keeping the vent above the level of the client's stomach. Newer gastric sump tubes have a one-way antireflux valve that allows air to enter but prevents gastric contents from escaping. In many cases, decompression tubes are connected to a source of suction, which is discussed in Nursing Guidelines 52-2.

1. Mark the nasogastric tube at a point 50 cm from the distal tip; call this point "A."

2. Have the client sit in a neutral position with head facing forward. Place the distal tip of the tubing at the tip of the client's nose (N); extend tube to the tragus (tip) of the ear (E) and then extend the tube straight down to the tip of the xiphoid (X). Mark this point "B."

3. To locate the point between A and X, identify the midpoint (M). The nasogastric tube is passed to point M to ensure optimum placement in the stomach.

FIGURE 52-1 Measuring length of nasogastric tube for placement into stomach.

Gastrostomy Tubes for Long-Term Feeding

A client with a gastrostomy has a transabdominal opening into the stomach that provides long-term access for administering fluids and liquid nourishment. Creating a gastrostomy is a relatively minor procedure that can be performed surgically or endoscopically.

GENERAL CONSIDERATIONS

Surgical placement of a gastrostomy involves laparotomy and surgical creation of an external stoma through which a gastrostomy tube is placed. When a **percutaneous endoscopic gastrostomy** (PEG) is performed, an endoscope is introduced orally and advanced into the stomach so that the physician can see the correct location for the

---

NURSING GUIDELINES 52-2

Managing the Care of a Client Needing GI Suction and Decompression

- Locate the suction source, usually a wall outlet or portable machine.

- Adjust the suction level on the wall outlet or portable machine to provide the amount and frequency of suction specified by the physician.

- Select intermittent high, low, or continuous suction when using a Salem sump tube; select low intermittent suction when using a Levin tube because the single lumen may adhere to the lining of the stomach during continuous suction. (If the tube is used only to obtain specimens for diagnostic purposes, manual suction may be achieved by attaching a syringe to the end of the tube and drawing back on the plunger.)

- Insert the gastric decompression tube in accord with accepted standards and connect it to the suction.

Maintain Safe Suction

- Observe the amount and quality of the gastric contents being suctioned and the client's response.

- Monitor the procedure frequently because abdominal or gastric distention caused by suction failure may have serious consequences, such as strain on surgical sutures or vomiting around the tube.

- Check equipment frequently to make sure it is operating properly. If the suction is not operating satisfactorily, obtain another suction machine.

Maintain Tube Patency

- If the decompression tube is occluded, irrigate or replace it.

- First review the client's chart. The physician may order irrigation on an as-needed basis.

- When irrigating the tube, use normal saline solution to prevent disturbance of electrolyte balance. Also use a large syringe to instill the irrigant into the distal end of the tube.

- After the fluid is instilled, remove it by gently pulling back on the plunger.

- Document the amount of solution used and the amount of fluid returned on the client's intake and output record.

Ensure Client Comfort

- Provide ice chips sparingly because water pulls electrolytes into the gastric secretions, which are then removed by suction, increasing the risk for an electrolyte disturbance.

tube. This location also is identified on the external abdominal surface before an incision is made. Two physicians or one physician and a specially trained nurse usually perform the PEG, which can be done either in the endoscopy suite or at the bedside with the client needing minimal sedation (Fig. 52-2). Because of the reduced risks, endoscopic placement is preferred to surgical laparotomy unless the client has ascites, is morbidly obese, or has had previous gastric surgery. If the client's condition eventually improves, the gastrostomy tube is removed and the opening closes over time. Rarely, the gastrostomy opening may require surgical closure.

Gastric feedings are administered by bolus, intermittent, cyclic, or continuous methods, using the same techniques described previously. Bolus feedings are not given through tubes inserted below the pylorus because such placement causes abdominal cramping and diarrhea. Intermittent, cyclic, or continuous feedings simulate the normal passage of food into the small intestine and usually are well tolerated.

Gastrostomy feeding devices may be skin-level devices (known as *buttons*) or tubes. Some tubes have a double lumen to allow infusion of two different fluids at once, such as administration of medications and delivery of feeding formula without interruption. For stabilization, most gastrostomy tubes have an external bumper and a firm internal bumper or an inflatable balloon. The advantage of the firm internal bumper is that it is difficult to dislodge accidentally. The disadvantage is that it may be difficult or painful to remove when replacement is desired. The advantage of the balloon-style internal bumper is that it is relatively painless and easy to replace. Disadvantages include relative ease of accidental dislodgment and gradual loss of fluid from the inflated balloon, resulting in leakage. The volume of fluid placed in the balloon is measured regularly and replaced as necessary.

NURSING MANAGEMENT

Before insertion of a PEG tube, the nurse weighs the client, assesses vital signs, auscultates bowel sounds, and offers an opportunity to empty the bladder. Other activities include determining the client's perception of the procedure, clarifying information, and checking that proper consent forms are signed and in order. The nurse prepares the client's skin and conducts other ordered preprocedural activities, such as inserting an IV line and administering sedatives.

The nurse monitors vital signs (i.e., respiratory rate, oxygen saturation, heart rate and rhythm) throughout the procedure according to institutional protocol. He or she monitors and documents the client's tolerance of the procedure. Monitoring of vital signs and response to the procedure continues in the postprocedural period. The nurse observes the stoma and surrounding skin for signs of infection and checks dressings frequently for evidence of bleeding and drainage.

The nurse must examine the appearance and volume of the drainage from the gastrostomy tube during the first 24 hours when the tube may be temporarily attached to gravity drainage. He or she auscultates bowel sounds and palpates the abdomen lightly for signs of distention and tenderness. He or she inspects the oral mucosa for excessive dryness. In addition, the nurse notes the client's tolerance of the instilled formula when tube feeding is initiated, promptly reporting abdominal distention, vomiting, fever, and severe pain to the physician. Another important nursing intervention is to monitor the characteristics and pattern of bowel elimination and trends in daily weight.

FIGURE 52-2 (A) Percutaneous endoscopic gastrostomy (PEG). **(B)** Detail of abdomen and PEG tube, showing catheter fixation. (From Smeltzer, S. C. & Bare, B. G. [2000]. *Brunner & Suddarth's textbook of medical–surgical nursing* [9th ed.]. Philadelphia: Lippincott Williams & Wilkins.)

Accidental removal of the gastrostomy device necessitates immediate replacement. Clients who have recently placed gastrostomy devices (less than 2 weeks) do not have a well-established tract and are at high risk for inadvertent replacement into the peritoneum instead of the stomach. If fluids are administered into this device, the resulting peritonitis may be life-threatening. For this reason, the nurse notifies the physician immediately and takes steps to ensure proper placement of the replacement device. For clients with well-established tracts, the nurse can maintain patency of the tract by inserting a clean catheter (i.e., Foley) and inflating the balloon to hold the catheter in place. The diameter of the replacement device should be the same as that of the device that was removed. The nurse notifies the physician so a new feeding device can be inserted. It is safe to administer gastric feedings through a catheter until it is replaced.

DISORDERS OF THE ESOPHAGUS

Various disorders can affect the esophagus. Examples include gastroesophageal reflux disease (GERD), esophageal diverticulum, hiatal hernia, and cancer. Esophageal varices, which result from hypertension in the portal venous system, are discussed in Chapter 55.

● GASTROESOPHAGEAL REFLUX DISEASE

Gastroesophageal reflux disease is a common disorder that develops when gastric contents flow upward into the esophagus. All adults and children normally have some degree of reflux, especially after eating. Gastroesophageal reflux is considered a disease process only when it is excessive or causes undesirable symptoms, such as pain or respiratory distress.

Pathophysiology and Etiology

GERD results from an inability of the lower esophageal sphincter (LES; also called *cardiac sphincter*) to close fully, allowing the stomach contents to flow freely into the esophagus. Obesity and pregnancy increase susceptibility to GERD because of the upward pressure that increased abdominal girth associated with these conditions places on the diaphragm.

Assessment Findings

Signs and Symptoms

The most common symptoms associated with GERD are epigastric pain or discomfort (**dyspepsia**), burning sensation in the esophagus (**pyrosis**), and regurgitation. Other symptoms include difficulty swallowing (dysphagia), painful swallowing (**odynophagia**), inflammation of the lining of the esophagus (**esophagitis**), aspiration pneumonia, and respiratory distress. Clients with esophagitis related to GERD may experience bleeding from the lining of the esophagus, manifested by vomited blood (*hematemesis*) or tarry stools (*melena*). Sometimes *occult* (hidden) *bleeding* for long periods produces iron-deficiency anemia. Because the esophagus is anatomically close to the heart, clients with epigastric pain may think they are having a heart attack. Until a myocardial infarction is ruled out as a cause for the discomfort, it is considered a potential diagnosis. Prolonged or severe esophagitis can lead to scarring and stricture formation. In these events, the client may report a sensation of feeling food "stick" in the esophagus for varying periods.

Diagnostic Findings

Barium swallow findings show inflammation or stricture formation from chronic esophagitis. Upper endoscopy with biopsy confirms esophagitis. Tests of stool may show positive findings of blood. Twenty-four–hour esophageal monitoring allows for observation of the frequency of reflux episodes and their associated symptoms. Bronchoscopy with analysis of fluids found in the lungs and nuclear medicine scans may be used to test for aspiration.

Medical and Surgical Management

Medications used to control esophageal reflux are discussed in Drug Therapy Table 52-2. The most common surgical procedure performed for GERD is **fundoplication,** a procedure that tightens the LES by wrapping the gastric fundus around the lower esophagus and suturing it into place. Fundoplication may be performed using laparoscopic technique, endoscopic technique, or open laparotomy. Esophageal strictures may be managed by endoscopic dilatation. Recurrent strictures may require repeat dilatation. In some cases, clients are taught self-dilatation using a tapered flexible dilator in the home setting.

Nursing Management

The nurse educates the client with GERD about diet and lifestyle changes needed to reduce the reflux symptoms. Dietary management, which consists of avoiding foods and beverages that lower pressure in the LES (e.g., alcohol, peppermint, licorice, caffeine, high-fat foods), may control mild symptoms. Additional measures include losing weight, avoiding tight-fitting garments, elevating the head of the bed, stopping smoking, and avoiding food and drink for several hours before bedtime. Nurses must advise pregnant clients that symptoms of GERD usually re-

DRUG THERAPY TABLE 52-2	MEDICATIONS USED TO TREAT PROBLEMS IN THE UPPER GI TRACT

DRUG CATEGORY AND EXAMPLES	MECHANISM OF ACTION	SIDE EFFECTS	NURSING CONSIDERATIONS
Antacids			
calcium carbonate (Tums)	Neutralize gastric acid to relieve heartburn and sour stomach	Constipation, hypercalcemia, hypophosphatemia	Avoid using in large amounts for a prolonged time. These drugs may be used as calcium supplements.
aluminum hydroxide (AlternaGEL, Gaviscon)		Constipation, indigestion	Do not administer to clients on a sodium-restricted diet. Do not administer with tetracycline.
aluminum hydroxide with magnesium hydroxide (Maalox, Mylanta)		Hypermagnesemia, hypophosphatemia	Observe for central nervous system depression and other symptoms of hypermagnesemia, especially in clients with renal failure.
Histamine-2 Antagonists			
cimetidine (Tagamet)	Suppress gastric acid by blocking H_2 receptors	Blood abnormalities (agranulocytosis, neutropenia, thrombocytopenia), diarrhea, dizziness, sleepiness, headache, confusion, increased plasma creatinine level, cardiac rhythm disturbances, erectile dysfunction (reversible), rash	Give drug with meals and at bedtime. Urge client to report sore throat, fever, unusual bruising/bleeding, or dizziness.
ranitidine (Zantac)		Headache, GI disturbance, insomnia, nausea/vomiting, rash, blood abnormalities, erectile dysfunction	Give drug with meals and at bedtime. Encourage regular checkups. Urge client to report sore throat, fever, unusual bruising/bleeding, dizziness, severe headache, or muscle/joint pain.
famotidine (Pepcid)		Headache, dizziness, diarrhea, constipation, muscle cramps, erectile dysfunction	Give drug with meals and at bedtime. Encourage regular checkups. Advise client to report sore throat, fever, unusual bruising/bleeding, dizziness, severe headache, or muscle/joint pain.
Antiulcer Agents			
sucralfate (Carafate)	Protect ulcers from acid and pepsin	Dizziness, insomnia, vertigo, constipation, GI discomfort, dry mouth, rash, back pain	Give drug to client with an empty stomach 1 hour before or 2 hours after meals and at bedtime. Do not administer concurrently with an antacid or H_2 antagonist. Advise client to report severe gastric pain.
Proton Pump Inhibitors			
omeprazole (Prilosec)	Suppress gastric acid by blocking enzymes associated with the final step of acid production	Headache, fatigue, dizziness, depression, abdominal pain, cramps, gas, nausea, diarrhea, flulike symptoms, rash, arthralgia	Give before meals to prevent upset stomach. Instruct client to swallow capsule whole without breaking, opening, or crushing contents. Caution client not to drive car or operate machinery if side effects are severe.

(continued)

| | DRUG THERAPY TABLE 52-2 | MEDICATIONS USED TO TREAT PROBLEMS IN THE UPPER GI TRACT (Continued) |

DRUG CATEGORY AND EXAMPLES	MECHANISM OF ACTION	SIDE EFFECTS	NURSING CONSIDERATIONS
lanisoprazole (Prevacid)		Diarrhea, abdominal pain, nausea/vomiting, constipation, dry mouth, headache, dizziness, vertigo, insomnia, upper respiratory symptoms (reversible), rash	Give drug before meals. Arrange for client to be medically monitored while taking drug. Advise client to report worsening symptoms, severe headache, fever, or chills.
GI Motility Agents *metoclopramide (Reglan)*	Stimulate upper GI tract and gastric emptying without stimulating release of gastric acid	Restlessness, drowsiness, fatigue, extrapyrimidal symptoms, parkinson-like reactions, nausea, diarrhea	Instruct client not to use alcohol or sleeping pills because resulting sedation may be dangerous. Advise client to report severe depression, diarrhea, and involuntary tremors or tics of the face, eyes, arms, and legs.
cisapride (Propulsid)		Headache, abdominal pain, diarrhea, constipation, nausea/vomiting, serious cardiac dysrhythmias from potential drug interactions, runny nose	Assess medication history and for gallbladder disease, GI bleeding or obstruction, pregnancy, or lactation. Give 15 minutes before each meal and at bedtime. Instruct client not to use alcohol or sleeping pills because resulting sedation may be dangerous.
bethenechol (Urecholine)		Abdominal discomfort, salivation, nausea/vomiting, sweating, flushing	Administer on an empty stomach. Monitor bowel function, especially in older adults.
Anticholinergics *atropine sulfate (Atropine)*	Relax smooth muscles of GI tract and inhibit gastric secretions	Blurred vision, dilated pupils, cycloplegia, dizziness, nervousness, insomnia, dry mouth, increased intraocular pressure, palpitations, heart rhythm changes, life-threatening paralytic ileus, urinary retention, intolerance to heat	Assess for health conditions that may contraindicate therapy. Give 30 minutes before meals. Be sure client has adequate fluid intake. Keep room temperature cool but comfortable. Tell client to report eye pain, abnormal heartbeats, difficulty swallowing, or breathing problems.
dicyclomine HCl (Bentyl)		Constipation, dry mouth, blurred vision, sensitivity to light, difficulty urinating, irregular heartbeat, intolerance to heat	Ensure adequate fluids. Keep room temperature stable to prevent problems resulting from heat intolerance. Tell client to report eye pain, abnormal heartbeats, difficulty swallowing, breathing problems, and so forth. Assess for health conditions that contraindicate therapy (glaucoma, bronchial asthma).
propantheline bromide (Pro-Banthine [Can])		Constipation, dry mouth, blurred vision, sensitivity to light, difficulty urinating, irregular heartbeat, intolerance to heat	

solve after delivery. The nurse teaches the client how to self-administer medications to control reflux. He or she emphasizes strict compliance with drug therapy to reduce symptoms. The nurse also teaches about the importance of controlling severe GERD to prevent possible complications, such as esophageal stricture formation and esophageal cancer. He or she closely observes for postoperative abdominal distention and nausea because many clients cannot belch or vomit after fundoplication.

Stop, Think, and Respond ● BOX 52-2

You are assigned to care for a client with GERD. After lunch, the client tells you that he needs to take a nap. What should you advise?

● ESOPHAGEAL DIVERTICULUM

A **diverticulum** is a sac or pouch in one or more layers of the wall of an organ or structure. Esophageal diverticula (plural) are found at the junction of the pharynx and the esophagus or in the middle or lower portion of the esophagus.

Pathophysiology and Etiology

The most common esophageal diverticulum, known as *Zenker's diverticulum,* occurs at the pharyngeal–esophageal juncture. Men are more likely than women to have this condition. Diverticula result from a congenital or an acquired weakness of the esophageal wall. They trap food and secretions, which then narrows the lumen, interferes with the passage of food into the stomach, and exerts pressure on the trachea. The trapped food decomposes in the esophagus, causing esophagitis or mucosal ulceration.

Assessment Findings

The client has foul breath and experiences difficulty or pain when swallowing, belching, regurgitating, or coughing. Auscultation of the middle to upper chest may reveal gurgling sounds. A barium swallow determines the structural abnormalities in the esophagus. Esophagoscopy usually is contraindicated secondary to the risk of esophageal perforation.

Medical and Surgical Management

For mild symptoms, treatment usually includes a bland, soft, semisoft, or liquid diet to facilitate passage of food. Eating four to six small meals a day is recommended. Clients with more severe symptoms may require surgical excision of the diverticulum. If the diverticulum is at the lower esophagus, it is repaired through a thoracic (chest) approach. The surgical approach for an esophageal diverticulum at the junction of the pharynx and esophagus usually is above the clavicle (collarbone).

Nursing Management

The nurse explains that oral hygiene will not alleviate the foul breath. He or she provides instructions for dietary modifications or arranges a consultation with a dietitian. See the section on Nursing Management of hiatal hernia and Nursing Care Plan 52-1 as well.

● HIATAL HERNIA

A **hiatal** or **diaphragmatic hernia** is a protrusion of part of the stomach into the lower portion of the thorax. There are two types of hiatal hernias (Fig. 52-3):

- *Axial or sliding*—The junction of the stomach and esophagus and part of the stomach slide in and out through the weakened portion of the diaphragm.
- *Paraesophageal*—The fundus is displaced upward, with greater curvature of the stomach going through the diaphragm next to the gastroesophageal junction.

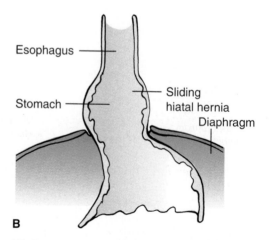

FIGURE 52-3 (A) Paraesophageal hiatal hernia. **(B)** Sliding hiatal hernia.

Pathophysiology and Etiology

A hiatal hernia results from a defect in the diaphragm at the point where the esophagus passes through it. It is particularly common in women. There is congenital muscle weakness or weakness resulting from trauma. Factors that increase intra-abdominal pressure also contribute to the potential for hiatal hernia and include multiple pregnancies, obesity, and loss of muscle strength and tone that occurs with aging. When the upper portion of the stomach slips from its usual position and becomes trapped, gastroesophageal reflux occurs.

Assessment Findings

The client describes having heartburn, belching, and a feeling of substernal or epigastric pressure or pain after eating and when lying down. He or she may report increased symptoms when bending at the waist. If scars form, swallowing becomes difficult. As food distends the esophagus, the client may vomit. Reflux does not usually accompany gastroesophageal hernias, because the gastroesophageal sphincter remains intact. Sliding hernias, however, are often associated with reflux. A barium swallow confirms the diagnosis by outlining the abnormal positioning of the stomach. An esophagoscopy shows the extent of irritation and scarring in the esophagus.

Medical and Surgical Management

Medical management of hiatal hernia is the same as that of GERD. The narrowed esophagus is stretched endoscopically, but the procedure may need to be repeated often. Clients who do not respond to a rigid medical regimen are treated surgically, which involves restoring the stomach to its proper position and repairing the diaphragmatic defect.

N U R S I N G   P R O C E S S

● The Client With an Esophageal Disorder

Assessment

The nurse asks the client about his or her appetite, particularly changes, difficulty swallowing, and problems after meals, such as discomfort, bloating, regurgitation, and belching. If the client indicates that he or she has pain after meals, the nurse asks if the pain follows every meal or certain foods, if other things (e.g., a particular position) seem to aggravate it, and if the pain is a burning sensation or associated with stomach fullness or pressure. In addition, the nurse determines if the client has experienced any weight loss. Finding out if the client has tried antacids or other over-the-counter medications to relieve symptoms also is important. The nurse weighs the client and checks for signs of malnutrition and dehydration. When completing the history, he or she asks about past infections, exposure to irritants, and alcohol and tobacco use.

Diagnosis, Planning, and Interventions

For clients who undergo thoracic surgery to repair a hiatal hernia, nursing care is the same as for a client who had chest surgery (see Chap. 28). Regardless of the surgical approach, postoperative care will likely involve intubation for gastric decompression to prevent stomach distention and avoid pressure on the surgical repair (see Nursing Guidelines 52-2). When managing nonsurgical care of clients with hiatal hernia or other esophageal disorders, the care plan includes, but is not limited to, the following.

Imbalanced Nutrition: Less than Body Requirements related to difficulty swallowing
Expected Outcome: Client will consume adequate nutrients to gain or maintain weight.
- Encourage client to eat frequent, small, well-balanced meals. *This meal plan provides adequate nutrition without overloading the upper GI system.*
- Instruct client to eat slowly and to chew food thoroughly. *Slow eating and thorough chewing promote easy passage of food to the stomach through the esophagus.*
- Suggest that the client avoid foods that cause discomfort. *Clients with GERD should avoid foods that decrease LES pressure (e.g., caffeine, chocolate).*
- Record daily weights. *A daily record reveals trends in weight gain or loss.*
- Instruct client to avoid alcohol or tobacco products. *They may suppress the appetite and can irritate the digestive tract.*

Pain related to pressure, reflux of gastric secretions, or difficulty swallowing
Expected Outcome: Client will experience relief from epigastric discomfort.
- Tell client to avoid very hot or cold fluids or spicy foods. *These foods stimulate esophageal spasm and secretion of hydrochloric acid in the stomach.*
- Inform client to remain upright for at least 2 hours after meals. *An upright position helps prevent reflux.*
- Discourage client from eating before bedtime. Raise the head of the bed on blocks 4 to 8 inches. *These measures help to prevent reflux.*
- Tell client to avoid activities that may involve the Valsalva maneuver (e.g., lifting heavy objects, straining for bowel movements). *The Valsalva maneuver increases intra-abdominal pressure and may cause the stomach to wedge above the diaphragm.*
- Instruct client to take medications as prescribed. *Excessive antacids may cause rebound stomach acidity. Prescribed medications reduce acidity effectively, prevent esophageal irritation, and relieve pain.*

Evaluation of Expected Outcomes

The client consumes adequate nutrients as evidenced by maintenance of weight and adherence to small, frequent meals. He or she states relief from epigastric pain.

● CANCER OF THE ESOPHAGUS

Esophageal cancer is a serious condition. Clients usually do not experience symptoms until the disease has progressed to interfere with swallowing and passage of food, leading to weight loss.

Pathophysiology and Etiology

Esophageal cancer affects men more often than women. Clients usually are diagnosed in the fourth or fifth decade of life. The tumor usually is a squamous cell carcinoma, although some tumors are classified as adenocarcinomas. A strong correlation exists among esophageal cancer, alcohol abuse, and cigarette smoking. As the cancer advances, the mass occupies space and interferes with swallowing. If the tumor grows unchecked, it may obstruct passage of food into the stomach, promoting the possibility of aspiration, or the tumor may ulcerate, leading to occult or frank blood loss.

Assessment Findings

Symptoms usually develop slowly. Beginning symptoms are mild, with vague discomfort and difficulty swallowing some foods. Weight loss accompanies progressive dysphagia. As the disease continues, solid foods become almost impossible to swallow, and the client resorts to consuming liquids only. He or she may experience regurgitation of food and liquids. The tumor also may hemorrhage, resulting in hemoptysis. By the time swallowing difficulty is pronounced, the cancer may have invaded surrounding tissues and lymphatics. Expansion of the tumor causes back pain and respiratory distress. Pain is a late symptom. The client also exhibits weight loss and weakness.

A barium swallow demonstrates a filling defect caused by a space-occupying mass. A biopsy of tissue removed during esophagoscopy reveals malignant cells. A bronchoscopy may be done to determine if the cancer cells have affected the trachea.

Medical and Surgical Management

Clients who are not candidates for surgery are treated with palliative measures and, possibly, endoscopic laser surgery to destroy some of the tumor. Esophageal dilatation may be used to enlarge the obstructed area. A prosthesis (stent placement) may be inserted at the tumor site to widen the narrowed area or when a fistula forms at the tumor site.

When surgery is a curative option, the type depends on the tumor location, extent of the lesion, and evidence of metastasis. If the tumor is in the lower third of the esophagus, the surgeon removes the affected area and attaches the remaining two thirds to the stomach. If the tumor is in the upper two thirds of the esophagus, the surgeon removes the affected area and replaces that portion of esophagus with a section of jejunum or colon.

Nursing Management

The nurse must consult with the dietitian before instituting measures for weight reduction or gain as ordered. A major nursing goal is adequate or improved nutrition and eventually stable weight. The nurse encourages small, frequent meals. If the client has difficulty swallowing, the nurse ensures that the client receives soft foods or high-calorie, high-protein semiliquid foods. The client needs to refrain from consuming foods that contain significant air or gas, such as soufflés and carbonated drinks. To reduce bloating, the client should avoid drinking from straws or narrow-necked bottles to reduce the volume of air trapped in the esophagus or stomach. The client should receive liquid supplements between meals.

The nutritional needs of the client with inoperable cancer of the esophagus are met with nasogastric or gastrostomy tube feedings or TPN. In such cases, essential nursing management involves caring for the skin at the tube insertion site, preventing infection, administering nourishment, maintaining tube patency, and preparing the client or family for self-care or home care after discharge. (See the earlier sections on GI intubation and gastrostomy.)

Clients who return from esophageal or gastric surgery need to be turned and to perform deep breathing and coughing every 2 hours. They also must know how to support the surgical incision for coughing and deep breathing. The nurse may use an incentive spirometer to motivate the client and provide immediate feedback on respiratory efficiency. The client must ambulate to mobilize secretions, increase depth of respiration, and promote expulsion of intestinal gas.

To avoid gastric distention, the client should not have oral nourishment until bowel sounds resume and are active. The nurse provides oral liquids, when allowed, to thin secretions. To minimize dyspnea, the nurse gives frequent, small meals and does not allow the client to lie down immediately after eating.

The nurse explains the rationale underlying the prescribed treatment and instructs the client and family to adhere to the therapeutic regimen, follow the necessary dietary modifications, and attend medical follow-up appointments regularly. He or she emphasizes that the client should inform the physician immediately of worsening symptoms, steady weight loss, difficulty swallowing soft foods, abnormal bleeding, or other new problems.

GASTRIC DISORDERS

● GASTRITIS

Gastritis is inflammation of the stomach lining (gastric mucosa). It may be acute or chronic.

Pathophysiology and Etiology

The causes of gastritis include dietary indiscretions; reflux of duodenal contents; use of aspirin, steroids, nonsteroidal anti-inflammatory drugs (NSAIDs), alcohol, or caffeine; cigarette smoking; ingestion of poisons or corrosive substances; food allergies; infection; and gastric ischemia secondary to vasoconstriction caused by a stress response. Gastric secretions are highly acidic. *Parietal cells* in the stomach increase acid production (hydrochloric acid) in response to seeing, smelling, and eating food. The parasympathetic vagus nerve releases histamine and acetylcholine, chemicals that also stimulate the parietal cells. An increasing level of acid triggers the conversion of pepsinogen to pepsin, creating a chemical mixture strong enough to digest the stomach wall. Because mucus protectively coats the stomach lining, however, pepsin normally has little effect.

Prostaglandin E, a lipid compound secreted in the stomach, apparently promotes the production of mucus, which contains buffering substances and mechanically bars penetration by stomach acids. The submucosal layers of the stomach can become inflamed, however, when irritating substances reduce or penetrate the mucous layer. Consequently, the client experiences epigastric discomfort, often described as *heartburn*. The mucus-producing cells usually heal and regenerate in 3 to 5 days. Chronic irritation leads to ulceration.

Assessment Findings

Usually the client complains of epigastric fullness, pressure, pain, anorexia, nausea, and vomiting. When a bacterial or viral infection causes the gastritis, the client may experience vomiting, diarrhea, fever, and abdominal pain. Drugs, poisons, toxic substances, and corrosives can cause gastric bleeding. Clients may describe seeing blood in emesis or note a darkening of their stool color. Chronic gastritis may give rise to no symptoms or symptoms similar to mild indigestion.

A complete blood count may reveal anemia from chronic blood loss. Stool testing for occult blood often detects RBCs. In difficult cases, gastroscopy may be performed to visualize the mucosa and obtain specimens, which are examined for pathogens or cellular abnormalities.

Medical and Surgical Management

Treatment depends on the cause and symptoms. Ingestion of poisons requires emergency treatment. In acute cases, eating is restricted and IV fluids are given to correct dehydration and electrolyte imbalances, particularly if vomiting is severe. Antiemetics are prescribed to control nausea and vomiting, and antibiotics may be prescribed to inhibit or destroy infection.

The usual treatment of chronic gastritis is the avoidance of irritating substances, such as alcohol and NSAIDs. Some clients may wish to avoid spicy foods, high-fat foods, and caffeine, depending on the degree to which these items aggravate their symptoms. Various drugs, such as antacids, histamine-2 antagonists, and proton pump inhibitors may be prescribed.

Nursing Management

The nurse monitors the client's symptoms. Evaluating the client's response to dietary modifications and prescribed medications is important. The nurse observes the color and characteristics of any vomitus or stool that the client passes. In addition, he or she teaches about diet, drug therapy, and the need for continued medical follow-up. For complications such as ulcer formation, refer to the section on Nursing Management of peptic ulcer disease.

● PEPTIC ULCER DISEASE

A **peptic ulcer** is a circumscribed loss of tissue in an area of the GI tract that is in contact with hydrochloric acid and pepsin. Most peptic ulcers occur in the duodenum; however, they may develop at the lower end of the esophagus, in the stomach, or in the jejunum after the client has had surgery at the spot where the stomach and the jejunum were sutured. Gastric ulcers are more likely to recur and have the highest incidence for undergoing malignant changes. Men are affected more frequently by peptic ulcer disease (PUD) than women are. The highest incidence occurs during middle life, but the condition can occur at any age.

Pathophysiology and Etiology

PUD occurs when the normal balance between factors that promote mucosal injury (gastric acid, pepsin, bile acid, ingested substances) and factors that protect the mucosa (intact epithelium, mucus, and bicarbonate secretion) is disrupted. The single greatest risk factor for the development of PUD is infection with the organism *Helicobacter pylori.* Transmission of these bacteria is thought to be by fecal–oral or oral–oral pathways. *H. pylori,* a gram-negative microorganism, is present in the gastric or duodenal mucosa of 80% to 90% of clients with PUD. The bacteria, which shelter themselves in the bicarbonate-rich mucus, are a factor in chronic gastritis and PUD. The mechanism by which this microorganism makes the mucosa more susceptible to erosion is not yet completely understood. It appears that *H. pylori* secrete an enzyme that theoretically depletes gastric mucus, making it more vulnerable to injury.

Family history is thought to be an additional risk factor for the development of PUD. A genetic component may exist, as demonstrated by the high incidence among first-degree relatives. Another explanation is the clustering of infection with *H. pylori* in families. Other risk factors include chronic use of NSAIDs, cigarette smoking, and physiologic stress. PUD resulting from physiologic stress is seen most often in the intensive care unit and may accompany increased intracranial pressure (Curling's ulcer), burns (Cushing's ulcer), and sepsis.

Ulcers develop when there is prolonged hyperacidity or chronic reduction in mucus. Once gastric acid has penetrated the mucosal layer, the acid begins to digest the stomach wall (Fig. 52-4). Histamine, released from the injured cells, aggravates the condition by triggering hypersecretion of more hydrochloric acid and pepsin.

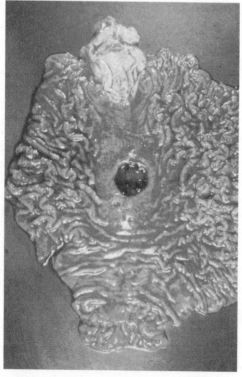

FIGURE 52-4 Gastric ulcer. (From Rubin, E. & Farber, J. L. [1999]. *Pathology* [3rd ed.]. Philadelphia: Lippincott Williams & Wilkins.)

The body responds with the inflammatory process. Capillary permeability is increased; the mucosa swells and bleeds easily.

Because food dilutes stomach acid, clients with PUD experience more discomfort when the stomach is empty than after eating food. Unless the process is controlled, the erosion can lead to an obstruction from scar formation or penetrate the entire thickness of the stomach wall, spilling gastric contents into the peritoneal cavity, a process that may be accompanied by hemorrhage.

Aging and chronic stomach inflammation, as in recurrent gastric ulcers, cancer of the stomach, or a long history of alcoholism lead to atrophy of the glandular epithelium of the stomach. The chronic gastric inflammation causes the parietal cells to secrete less hydrochloric acid, resulting in hypochlorhydria (reduced gastric acidity) or achlorhydria (absence of hydrochloric acid). In addition, the gastric mucosa produces intrinsic factor, which the body requires for the absorption of vitamin B_{12}. Chronic gastric inflammation inhibits the production of intrinsic factor, leading to poor absorption of this essential nutrient. As a result, the client is at high risk for pernicious anemia (see Table 52-1).

Assessment Findings

Signs and Symptoms

Most clients with PUD have abdominal pain, which usually is confined to the epigastrium and does not radiate. Clients most often describe it as having a "burning" quality. They often complain of pain that disturbs sleep and also occurs 1 to several hours after meals. Eating food may relieve the pain. Back pain suggests that the ulcer is irritating the pancreas. Approximately 20% of clients may have bleeding as the first sign of the ulcer. Hemorrhage, hematemesis, or melena may occur. Protracted vomiting secondary to scarring and resultant obstruction also are seen among those who have ignored earlier symptoms.

Diagnostic Findings

The diagnosis is suggested by the history and confirmed by results of an upper GI series or esophagogastroduodenoscopy. To differentiate between benign and malignant ulcers, a gastric washing or biopsy for cytologic analysis may be performed. Typically, the hemoglobin level and RBC count are low from chronic blood loss. Vomiting alters electrolyte levels.

Medical and Surgical Management

The effectiveness of dietary therapy in treating PUD is unknown. Foods known to increase acid production include milk and milk products, alcohol, caffeinated beverages, and decaffeinated coffee. Clients are provided with small, frequent meals and instructed to avoid eating foods that they find particularly irritating.

In the presence of *H. pylori,* eradication therapy is initiated, which includes the use of a combination of antibiotics (e.g., tetracycline), metronidazole (Flagyl), and bismuth salts. Treatment may also include histamine (H₂) antagonists, proton pump inhibitors, cytoprotective agents, and antacids. The following list provides examples of drugs used to treat PUD:

- *Antibiotics:* Tetracycline, amoxicillin, and clarithromycin exert bactericidal effects to eradicate *H. pylori.*
- *Amebicides:* Metronidazole (Flagyl) assists in the eradication of *H. pylori.*
- *Bismuth salts:* Bismuth salicylate (Pepto-Bismol) suppresses *H. pylori* and assists in healing mucosal lesions.
- *Antacids:* These drugs initially are used to buffer stomach acid. They are not absorbed from the GI tract and therefore do not produce alkalosis, even when given in large doses.
- *Histamine (H₂) antagonists:* Cimetidine (Tagamet), famotidine (Pepcid), nizatidine (Axid), and ranitidine (Zantac) block H₂ receptors and decrease acid secretion in the stomach.
- *Cytoprotective agents:* Sucralfate (Carafate) forms a seal over the ulcer, protecting it from irritation. Misoprostol (Cytotec), a synthetic prostaglandin, is used to sustain the mucosal layer especially among clients who require large doses or long-term treatment with aspirin or NSAIDs.
- *Proton pump inhibitors:* Omeprazole (Prilosec), lansoprazole (Prevacid), esomeprazole (Nexium), rabeprazole (Acifex), and pantoprazole (Protonix) block the final step in acid production at the surface of parietal cells.

Obstruction resulting from edema and inflammation often subsides when gastric intubation is used concurrently with treatment for the ulcer. Treatment of hemorrhage includes complete rest, blood transfusions, and gastric lavage with saline solution. Iced saline solution no longer is used because of its potential to cause hypothermia. Nothing is given by mouth, and IV fluids are administered until the bleeding has stopped. Endoscopic laser therapy or endoscopic injections of epinephrine or anhydrous alcohol into the ulcer bed may be used to control bleeding if more conservative measures are unsuccessful. Ulcers that persist despite medical interventions, repeatedly recur, cause severe hemorrhage, create unrelieved obstruction, cause perforation, or are predisposed to malignant changes justify surgical interventions as described in Table 52-3.

If a total **gastrectomy** (removal of the stomach) is performed, the client receives vitamin B₁₂ injections or intranasal vitamin B₁₂ for life because, without the stomach, the intrinsic factor necessary for absorption of vitamin B₁₂

no longer is produced. B₁₂ therapy usually is not necessary for 1 or 2 years after surgery because the body uses very small amounts of this vitamin and body reserves usually are sufficient for several years. Older adults, however, might be at risk.

Clients with a gastrojejunostomy are at risk for developing the dumping syndrome when they begin to take solid food. The **dumping syndrome,** which produces weakness, dizziness, sweating, palpitations, abdominal cramps, and diarrhea, results from the rapid emptying (dumping) of large amounts of hypertonic chyme (a liquid mass of partly digested food) into the jejunum. This concentrated solution in the gut draws fluid from the circulating blood into the intestine, causing hypovolemia. The drop in blood pressure can produce syncope. As the syndrome progresses, the sudden appearance of carbohydrates in the jejunum stimulates the pancreas to secrete excessive amounts of insulin, which in turn causes hypoglycemia.

Nursing Management

The nurse must explore each symptom of PUD in depth. For example, if pain occurs, the nurse determines its type, onset in relation to eating food, location, and duration. A dietary history must include relevant questions pertaining to foods that cause distress, the amount of food eaten at each meal, and whether eating food relieves pain.

For a client to continue eating, it may be necessary to modify ingredients, temperature, or consistency of foods, as well as to use smaller portions on smaller plates. Clients need nutritional supplements. If the client is receiving tube feedings, reinstilling the gastric residual is necessary because it contains partially digested nutrients and essential electrolytes.

In addition, the nurse notes the client's bowel patterns and stool characteristics. He or she also evaluates the client's emotional status and response to activity. The nurse monitors the nonsurgical client closely for medical complications, which includes assessing vital signs and fluid status. Refer to Nursing Guidelines 52-3 for assessment of gastric pH. For a discussion of appropriate nursing management of a surgical client, refer to the Nursing Management section that accompanies the discussion of cancer of the stomach.

N U R S I N G   P R O C E S S

● The Client With a Gastric Disorder

Assessment

The nurse asks about current symptoms, looking for specific information about such symptoms as indigestion, fullness, heartburn, nausea, vomiting. How long has the

TABLE 52-3	SURGICAL PROCEDURES TO TREAT PEPTIC ULCER DISEASE

PROCEDURE   **DEPICTION**

Vagotomy–a branch of the vagus nerve is cut to reduce gastric acid
secretion.

Pyloroplasty–the pylorus is repaired or reconstructed to expand the stomach
outlet narrowed by scarring or improve gastric motility and emptying.

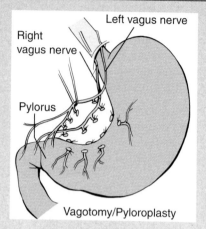

Antrectomy–The antrum (lower portion of the stomach, including the
pylorus) is removed to eliminate a benign ulcer in the lesser curvature of
the stomach if the ulcer has not healed after 12 weeks of medical treatment or is recurring.

Gastroduodenostomy (Billroth I)–Part of the stomach is removed, while the
remaining portion is connected to the duodenum. Usually, a vagotomy also is
performed. This procedure is done to remove an ulcerated area in the
stomach that is prone to hemorrhage, perforation, and obstruction.

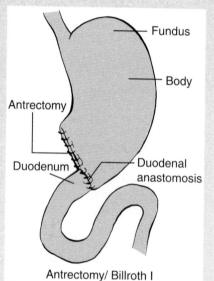

Gastroduodenostomy (Billroth II)–Same as Billroth I, except the remaining
portion is connected to the jejunum in cases of extensive duodenal
inflammation or perforation.

Total gastrectomy–The entire stomach is removed and the esophagus is
joined to the jejunum to remove an ulcer high in the stomach near the gastroesophageal junction. It is performed to treat a gastric
malignancy.

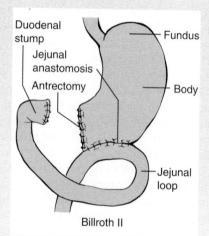

Assessing the pH of Aspirated Fluid

Purpose: To evaluate the effectiveness of antacid or histamine-2 antagonist therapy in peptic ulcer disease by aspirating stomach fluid and testing gastric pH. Desired pH range is 3 to 5.

- Obtain a pH test kit.
- Put on gloves.
- Verify that the distal tip of the client's nasogastric tube is in the stomach and has not migrated to the intestine.
- Use a separate syringe for withdrawing the test specimen because antacid residue or irrigating solution in the nasogastric tube will falsely raise the gastric pH.
- Connect the syringe to the tube.
- Instill a small amount of air to clear fluid from the gastric tube just before aspirating.
- Aspirate a small amount of fluid.
- Drop a sample of the gastric fluid onto a pH color indicator strip.
- Compare the color on the test strip with the color guide supplied in the test kit.
- Record the findings.

client had these symptoms? When do they occur? For example, does the client experience problems before or after eating or with certain foods? Do situations such as stress make the problems worse? Does anything relieve the problem? Having the client provide a record of dietary intake for the last 72 hours may be useful. Also, the nurse asks about previous gastric problems and treatments/surgery. In addition, he or she assesses for signs of abdominal discomfort/pain, malnutrition, and dehydration.

Diagnosis, Planning, and Interventions

Risk for Deficient Fluid Volume related to vomiting, diarrhea, bleeding, or all these factors
Expected Outcome: Client will maintain adequate fluid balance.

- Assist client to set a goal for minimum oral liquid intake during waking hours. *Involving the client in planning helps to meet his or her needs.*
- Provide fluids with calories and electrolytes hourly. Offer different choices. *Frequent fluid intake maintains fluid balance. Various choices prevent monotony.*
- Monitor fluid intake and output. *This record helps indicate trends in fluid balance and early signs of dehydration.*

Deficient Knowledge about dietary management and gastric disorder
Expected Outcome: Client will demonstrate knowledge of dietary management as evidenced by appropriate choices of foods and fluids.

- Review client's fluid and nutritional needs. *Understanding of fluid and nutritional needs promotes better compliance and intake.*
- Provide a list of foods and substances to avoid. *Doing so may help prevent gastric irritation.*
- Review medications with client, including reasons for medications, schedule, and side effects and their management. *Such review promotes better compliance and outcomes.*

Evaluation of Expected Outcomes

Fluid intake is 2000 mL/24 hours, with a urine output of 1850 mL/24 hours. Nutritional intake is adequate as evidenced by maintenance of preillness weight. The client adheres to medical regimen as evidenced by appropriate choice of foods and fluids and compliance with medication schedule.

● CANCER OF THE STOMACH

Pathophysiology and Etiology

Cancer of the stomach is a malignancy characterized by either an enlarged mass or ulcerating lesion that expands or penetrates several tissue layers. Stomach malignancies are most common among natives of Japan, African Americans, and Latinos. Heredity and chronic inflammation of the stomach appear to be contributing factors. Although a single etiology has not been identified, *achlorhydria* (absence of free hydrochloric acid in the stomach), which may promote bacterial growth, and chronic ingestion of toxins such as food preserved with nitrates or cooked over charcoal, are being linked to stomach cancer. When gram-negative microorganisms proliferate in the stomach, they produce a high level of nitrate reductase. This enzyme converts gastric nitrates to nitrites, which eventually become nitrosamines—known carcinogens. Stomach cancer often spreads to the lymph nodes and metastasizes to the spleen, liver, pancreas, or colon.

Assessment Findings

Early symptoms are vague. As the tumor enlarges, symptoms include a prolonged feeling of fullness after eating, anorexia, weight loss, and anemia. Stool usually contains occult blood. Pain is a late symptom. A barium swallow or computed tomography (CT) scan and a tissue biopsy obtained by gastroscopy or open laparotomy assist to confirm the diagnosis. Gastric analysis may disclose no free hydrochloric acid. CT scanning or ultrasonography helps determine the depth of the cancer.

Medical and Surgical Management

A subtotal (partial) or total gastrectomy is the only curative approach. The type and extent of surgery usually depend on tumor location, symptoms, and any metastasis. A subtotal gastrectomy preserves more normal digestion. Even though surgery may not achieve a complete cure, it still may be performed to control bleeding or relieve obstruction at the cardiac or pyloric junction. Chemotherapy with drugs such as 5-fluorouracil (5-FU) or doxorubicin (Adriamycin) and palliative radiation also may be used.

Nursing Management

The nurse's role in management of gastric cancer includes teaching the public, especially susceptible ethnic groups or clients with a family history of stomach cancer, how to change their dietary habits to reduce the predisposition for this disease. The nurse also may instruct high-risk groups, such as those who have undergone vagotomy or must take medications to reduce hydrochloric acid formation, on the early warning signs of cancer and the value of frequent health assessments. Nursing roles in managing clients undergoing surgery for gastric cancer are extensive. See Nursing Care Plan 52-1 and Client and Family Teaching Box 52-1.

GENERAL NUTRITIONAL CONSIDERATIONS

Because fat delays gastric emptying, limit high-fat foods such as nonlean meats, high-fat dairy products, and rich desserts in clients with nausea.

Limit liquids with meals to minimize the feeling of fullness. Encourage a liberal intake of fluid between meals.

Hot foods may contribute to nausea.

Intermittent cyclic and bolus tube feedings are physiologically preferable to continuous feedings for long-term use because they resemble a more normal pattern of intake, allowing hormone and enzyme levels to rise and fall rather than being constantly stimulated. Continuous feedings, however, may be preferred to decrease the risk of aspiration.

Fat malabsorption, gastric stasis, and diarrhea are common after a vagotomy. Replacing some dietary fat with medium-chain triglycerides (MCT) minimizes diarrhea and provides readily absorbed fat calories. Many commercial products, such as Osmolite and Isocal, contain MCT as the fat source. MCT oil can be used in place of vegetable oil in cooking, but it is unpalatable and expensive.

GENERAL PHARMACOLOGIC CONSIDERATIONS

H_2 antagonists, such as ranitidine, cimetidine, or famotidine, are used for the short-term treatment of duodenal and gastric ulcers for managing GERD. They decrease healing time and reduce the incidence of surgical intervention for the management of PUD.

Antacids may be given two to four times per day or as frequently as every 1 to 2 hours. They are not administered within 1 hour of the H_2 antagonists or many other oral medications because they may decrease absorption of the other drug. Antacids may cause diarrhea or constipation. Most antacids contain a combination of magnesium hydroxide and aluminum hydroxide. The magnesium component may tend to cause diarrhea in some clients. In such cases, switching to an aluminum-only antacid (e.g., AlternaGEL) or a calcium-containing antacid (e.g., Tums) may be helpful.

Sucralfate is administered 2 hours after an H_2 antagonist to ensure the absorption of the H_2 antagonist. It is given for 4 to 6 weeks to ensure ulcer healing.

For hospitalized clients who self-administer a prescribed antacid, the nurse:
- Demonstrates how to measure the drug in a medicine cup
- Explains the importance of antacids in the treatment of dyspepsia
- Explains the time of day the drug is to be taken (i.e., every hour, every 2 hours on the even hour)
- Makes sure that the client has a clock or watch
- Periodically checks the supply of the drug and measuring cups
- Checks that the client is taking the medication.

Although sodium bicarbonate (baking soda) is an antacid, it is readily absorbed from the GI tract and in large doses may produce alkalosis. Avoid sodium bicarbonate in clients for whom antacids have been prescribed to treat gastric disorders.

Consult the physician for changes in drug orders if a client cannot retain oral medications.

Never crush and administer an enteric-coated drug through any type of enteral feeding tube (nasogastric, nasoenteric, or gastrostomy).

GENERAL GERONTOLOGIC CONSIDERATIONS

Severe and prolonged episodes of vomiting can be especially serious for older adults whose nutritional and fluid intake may be marginal; more profound electrolyte imbalances and severe dehydration can result.

Anorexia and weight loss are common in the older adult and can result from ill-fitting dentures or dysphagia (caused by oropharyngeal dysphagia), or may be a manifestation of depression.

Oropharyngeal dysphagia occurs in approximately 50% of institutionalized older adults and is manifested by difficulty swallowing, drooling or leakage of fluids from the mouth, and coughing or choking while eating or drinking.

With age, the salivary glands become less active and the numbers of taste buds are reduced, contributing to anorexia in the older adult.

Consider food preferences, economic status, and the inability of the older adult to chew because of tooth loss or ill-fitting dentures when modifying a diet.

The older adult has a diminished gag reflex. This places the elderly client at greater risk for aspiration.

As individuals age, the gastric mucosa becomes thinner, predisposing older adults to superficial gastritis and gastric ulcers.

Older adults are more prone to developing gastritis, gastric bleeding, and gastric ulcers because many regularly take drugs to treat osteoarthritis (e.g., aspirin or NSAIDs) or vascular or cardiac conditions (e.g., anticoagulant medications).

The incidence of hiatal hernia increases with age. Approximately 60% of individuals older than 70 years of age develop hiatal hernia. Hiatal hernia is more likely to develop in older women than in older men.

The older adult is at increased risk for pernicious anemia because a degeneration of the gastric mucosa results in a loss of parietal cells. The

Nursing Care Plan 52-1

THE CLIENT UNDERGOING GASTRIC SURGERY

Preoperative Assessment

In addition to performing assessments for the client with a GI disorder:

- Obtain a complete health, drug, tobacco, and allergy history.
- Ask approximately how long symptoms have lasted, whether eating is normal, and how much weight, if any, the client has lost.
- Assess bowel sounds for presence and quality.
- Ask about food intolerance and current dietary management.
- Determine bowel elimination patterns and stool characteristics.
- Assess understanding of diagnostic tests, scheduled surgery, and preparations for surgery.

Nursing Diagnosis: Anxiety related to test results, diagnosis, and surgical procedure

Expected Outcome: Anxiety will be mild as evidenced by a calm demeanor, appropriate questions, and expressions of fear.

Intervention	Rationale
Provide time for client to verbalize fears and express needs related to diagnosis and surgery.	Being present and supportive encourages communication.
Allow client to express his or her personal reaction to the threat to well-being.	Expressing feelings without being judged can help reduce fears.
Explain tests, procedures, and surgery, using nonmedical speech and allowing time for questions.	Education helps to increase coping skills.
Keep client informed of progress and explain delays or changes in plans.	Adequate explanations make clients feel more secure and less anxious.
If surgery is emergent (such as in GI hemorrhage), provide explanations to family members and anticipate questions and concerns that client will have after surgery.	Family members will have decreased anxiety and be less anxious and better able to provide support when seeing client after surgery.

Evaluation of Expected Outcome: Client is less anxious, expressing fears and questions about diagnosis and surgery.

Nursing Diagnosis: Deficient Knowledge related to preoperative preparations

Expected Outcome: Client will demonstrate exercises satisfactorily and acknowledge the purpose of equipment and procedures that may be used after surgery.

Intervention	Rationale
Using nonmedical language, instruct client about common postoperative equipment: intravenous (IV) line, infusion pump, nasogastric suction, oxygen, urinary catheter, wound drain, cardiac monitor, and pulse oximeter.	Providing understandable explanations helps client learn information effectively.
Prepare client by explaining reasons for postoperative treatments and procedures, such as frequent assessment of vital signs and performance of breathing exercises.	Such explanation promotes postoperative compliance with needed treatments and procedures.
Explain postoperative administration of analgesics to reduce and manage pain.	Clients fear pain—understanding that pain will be managed will reduce fear.
Evaluate client's learning through return demonstrations of deep breathing, coughing, moving legs, and turning, as well as verbalization of instructions.	Having client provide explanations and demonstrations reinforces instructions and helps nurse determine if client needs further teaching.

(continued)

Nursing Care Plan 52-1 (Continued)

THE CLIENT UNDERGOING GASTRIC SURGERY

Evaluation of Expected Outcome: Client can discuss the surgical procedure and demonstrate how to turn, deep breathe, cough, and splint incision.

Postoperative Assessment Refer to Standards for Postoperative Care in Chapter 25. When the client returns from surgery:

■ Assess vital signs.

■ Review the chart about the type of surgery performed and the client's progress during surgery and in the postanesthesia recovery unit.

■ Inspect the surgical dressing for drainage and tubes or catheters for placement, patency, and type of drainage.

■ Carefully observe nasogastric tube drainage for evidence of bleeding. Although the nasogastric tube may contain a small amount of dark blood when the client first returns from the operating room, the drainage should promptly return to the yellow-green of normal gastric secretions.

■ Inspect the IV site and note the current rate and progress of fluid infusion.

■ Document fluid intake and output as well as level of consciousness and comfort.

■ Closely monitor the client for change in vital signs, especially fluctuations in blood pressure (BP may increase initially in response to shock), increased pulse rate, and elevated temperature; extreme restlessness; difficulty breathing (increased respiratory rate, cyanosis); severe pain, especially after an analgesic has been given or in an area other than the operative site; abdominal distention or rigidity; excessive or absent nasogastric output; urinary output less than 35 mL/hour if catheterized or failure to void within 8 hours of surgery; failure to pass flatus or stool more than 48 hours after surgery; profuse diaphoresis; excessive bloody drainage from the nasogastric tube, surgical drains, or surgical dressing; separation of the surgical wound edges; and unusual color or odor of drainage.

Nursing Diagnosis: **Imbalanced Nutrition, Less than Body Requirements** related to poor nutritional intake before surgery and changed GI system after surgery

Expected Outcome: Client will achieve optimal caloric intake to maintain weight.

Interventions	Rationales
Assess client for changes in physiologic status that will interfere with nutrition.	Malnutrition contributes to poor recovery from surgery.
Administer total parenteral nutrition (TPN) as ordered (see Chap. 24).	TPN provides adequate calories, nutrition, and fluid replacement and supports metabolic needs.
Administer nasogastric feedings as ordered (see section in this chapter).	Nasogastric feedings provide adequate calories, nutrition, and fluid replacement and support metabolic needs.
When bowel sounds return, advance oral diet as ordered and tolerated. Encourage small, frequent meals.	An advanced diet provides opportunity for client to eat and adjust. Small, frequent meals prevent fullness and nausea.
Monitor food intake.	Such monitoring helps identify trends in client's nutritional status.
Weigh client twice a week.	Weighing determines weight loss, gain, or maintenance.
Report laboratory values such as low blood cell and hemoglobin counts and decreased iron, serum protein, transferrin, or ferritin level.	Such findings may indicate malnutrition.

(continued)

Nursing Care Plan 52-1 (Continued)

THE CLIENT UNDERGOING GASTRIC SURGERY

Evaluation of Expected Outcome: Client attains optimal nutrition as evidenced by reasonable weight and tolerance of six small meals of soft foods and liquids.

PC: **Dumping syndrome**

Expected Outcome: The nurse will minimize and manage problems associated with dumping syndrome.

Interventions	Rationales
Offer small, frequent feedings low in simple sugars.	Small frequent feedings delay entry of foods into the jejunum, allowing time for dilution and absorption.
Withhold oral fluids at meals. Provide fluids 1 hour after meals.	These measures avoid rapid emptying of food from the stomach.
Encourage client to lie down for about 30 minutes after a meal.	Lying down for 30 minutes helps food to remain longer in the stomach.
Maintain bed rest if dizziness and weakness occur.	Bed rest decreases other symptoms, such as nausea, vomiting, and palpitations.

Evaluation of Expected Outcome: Client does not have any signs or symptoms of dumping syndrome and follows dietary restrictions.

52-1 *Client and Family Teaching*
The Client With Stomach Cancer

The type and extent of teaching depends on the surgery that is performed. If tube or gastrostomy feedings, tracheostomy care, and suction techniques will continue after discharge, the nurse involves the client and a family member in practicing these procedures while the client is still hospitalized. He or she identifies where medical supplies can be purchased and offers a referral for home care from a local community agency. Other points to instruct the client and family about in the discharge teaching plan include the following:

- Adhere to the diet (e.g., foods to eat or avoid) recommended by the physician. Also adhere to the dietary, fluid, and positional modifications to avoid the dumping syndrome.
- Take medications exactly as prescribed. Follow the directions on the label, paying particular attention to when you should take the drug (e.g., before, after, or with food or meals).
- Monitor weight weekly. Report any significant weight loss to the physician.
- Keep appointments for periodic medical follow-up.

loss of parietal cells decreases the production of the intrinsic factor and absorption of vitamin B_{12}, leading to pernicious anemia.

Critical Thinking Exercises

1. *An older adult is admitted to a healthcare facility because of unexplained weight loss. What assessments are appropriate?*
2. *A man is diagnosed with a peptic ulcer. He tells you that he had an ulcer many years ago, and that he watched his diet carefully and used antacids, and eventually the symptoms subsided. He asks if he should start doing this again. What should you advise him?*

References and Suggested Readings

Bowers, S. (1999). Nutrition support for malnourished, acutely ill adults. *MedSurg Nursing, 8*(3), 145–166.

Bullock, B. A. & Henze, R. L. (2000). *Focus on pathophysiology.* Philadelphia: Lippincott Williams & Wilkins.

National Institutes of Health. (1994). NIH consensus statement: *Helicobacter pylori* in peptic ulcer disease. Washington, DC: Department of Health and Human Services.

Resto, M. A. (2000). Gastroesophageal reflux disease. *American Journal of Nursing, 100*(9), 24D, F, H.

Smeltzer, S. C. & Bare, B. G. (2000). *Brunner & Suddarth's textbook of medical–surgical nursing* (9th ed.). Philadelphia: Lippincott Williams & Wilkins.

Caring for Clients With Disorders of the Lower Gastrointestinal Tract

Words to Know

abdominoperineal
  resection
appendectomy
appendicitis
colectomy
Crohn's disease
diverticula
diverticulitis
diverticulosis
encopresis
fissure
fistula
fistulectomy
fistulotomy
hemorrhoidectomy
hemorrhoids
hernia
hernioplasty

herniorrhaphy
inflammatory bowel
  disease
irritable bowel
  syndrome
intussusception
paralytic ileus
peritonitis
pilonidal sinus
segmental resection
short bowel syndrome
skip lesions
spastic colon
tenesmus
toxic megacolon
ulcerative colitis
ulcerative proctitis
volvulus

Learning Objectives

On completion of this chapter, the reader will:

- List factors that contribute to constipation and diarrhea.
- Explain the symptoms of irritable bowel syndrome.
- Contrast Crohn's disease and ulcerative colitis.
- Describe the features of appendicitis and peritonitis.
- Describe the nurse's role as related to tubes for intestinal decompression.
- Differentiate diverticulosis and diverticulitis.
- Identify factors that contribute to the formation of an abdominal hernia.
- Discuss nursing management for a client with constipation, diarrhea, inflammatory bowel disease, acute abdominal inflammatory disorders, intestinal obstruction, or surgical repair of a hernia.
- Describe warning signs of colorectal cancer.
- List common problems that accompany anorectal disorders.

The lower gastrointestinal (GI) tract includes the small and large intestines from the duodenum to anus (see Fig. 51-1). The material that moves down the lower GI tract consists of food residues, microorganisms, digestive secretions, and mucus. The mixture of these substances composes feces. Disorders of the lower GI tract usually affect movement of feces toward the anus, absorption of water and electrolytes, and elimination of dietary wastes.

ALTERED BOWEL ELIMINATION

People differ greatly in their bowel habits. Normal bowel patterns range from three bowel movements per day to three bowel movements per week. In differentiating normal from abnormal, the consistency of stools and the comfort with which a person passes them are more reliable indicators than is the frequency of bowel elimination. The type and amount of food a person consumes greatly affect stool consistency. High-fiber diets, such as those containing whole grains, fresh fruits, and uncooked vegetables, form an increased residual of cellulose, an insoluble, indigestible product, in the bowel. Cellulose absorbs water. The combination of cellulose and water increases and softens fecal volume, which speeds the passage of feces through the lower GI tract.

Diseases or disorders of the lower GI system usually manifest themselves as changes in bowel elimination. The most common problems are constipation and diarrhea. Irritable bowel syndrome is a motility problem in which constipation and diarrhea are alternately present. The following sections address these conditions.

• CONSTIPATION

Pathophysiology and Etiology

Constipation is a condition in which stool becomes dry, compact, and difficult and painful to pass. Normally, fecal matter collects in the rectum and presses on the internal anal sphincter, creating an urge to defecate (eliminate stool). Peristalsis and distention of the colon facilitate the signal to release stool. The gastrocolic reflex facilitates stool passage by accelerating peristalsis. This reflex is most active after eating, particularly after the first meal of the day.

A diet low in fiber predisposes clients to constipation because the stools produced are small in volume and dry. The lower GI tract propels low-volume stools more slowly. Whenever stool remains stationary in the large intestine, moisture continues to be absorbed from the residue. Consequently, retention of stool, for any number of reasons, causes stool to become dry and hard.

Constipation may result from insufficient dietary fiber and water, ignoring or resisting the urge to defecate, emotional stress, use of drugs that tend to slow intestinal motility, or inactivity. It may stem from several disorders, either in the GI tract or systemically. Anatomic disorders of the colon, rectum, and anus, which predispose the client to constipation, include strictures (e.g., secondary to disease or intestinal resection), anal stenosis, and anterior displacement of the anus.

Impaired GI motility also may lead to chronic constipation. Motility may be impaired in the absence of other disorders (intestinal pseudo-obstruction) or as a result of visceral myopathies, musculoskeletal disorders, neuropathy, or spinal cord lesions. Systemic disorders that predispose clients to constipation include hypothyroidism, diabetes, pheochromocytoma, porphyria, and hypercalcemia (resulting from hyperparathyroidism and excessive production of vitamin D). Constipation may also result from chronic use of laxatives ("cathartic colon") because such use can cause a loss of normal colonic motility and intestinal tone. Laxatives also dull the gastrocolic reflex. Chronic lead poisoning or concurrent medications may also result in constipation.

Assessment Findings

Signs and Symptoms

Bowel elimination is infrequent or irregular. Clients describe feeling bloated. The abdomen may be tympanic or distended, and bowel sounds may be hypoactive. The client experiences rectal fullness, pressure, and pain when he or she attempts to eliminate stool. What he or she passes usually is hard and dry. Rectal bleeding may result as the tissue stretches and tears while the person tries to pass the hard, dry stool. When a practitioner inserts a gloved and lubricated finger in the rectum, the stool may feel like small rocks, a condition referred to as *scybala*.

Sometimes, when he or she has been constipated for a long time, the client may begin passing liquid stool around an obstructive stool mass (**encopresis**), a phenomenon sometimes misinterpreted as diarrhea. The liquid stool results from dry stool stimulating nerve endings in the lower colon and rectum, which increases peristalsis. The increased peristalsis sends watery feces from higher in the bowel than the retained stool. This symptom is most common in residents of nursing homes and school-aged children who have a long-standing history of constipation, stool-withholding behavior, or both.

Diagnostic Findings

A thorough history and physical examination are necessary to determine the underlying cause and need for further diagnostic testing. Frequently, treatment is based on findings of the history and physical examination, precluding the need for a more aggressive approach. Abdominal radiography helps to determine the extent of the constipation. A barium enema is performed if a structural abnormality is suspected. Anorectal motility studies may be performed to confirm a motility disorder.

Medical and Surgical Management

Treating the cause provides the best relief. For quick symptomatic relief, the physician prescribes an enema or a laxative in oral or suppository form, followed by prophylactic administration of a stool softener. Dietary management also is promoted.

N U R S I N G P R O C E S S

• The Client With Constipation

Assessment

In addition to completing the assessments performed on the client with a GI disorder (see Chap. 51), the nurse obtains a complete history as well as a drug history, including the frequency with which the client uses laxatives or enemas. In discussing bowel elimination, the nurse must determine the client's definition of constipation. Some clients are unaware that a daily bowel movement is not necessarily a rigid standard for proper bowel function.

The nurse obtains a description of the bowel elimination pattern, asking about frequency, overall appearance and consistency of stool, blood in the stool, pain, and effort necessary to pass stool. He or she asks the client to keep a record of bowel elimination. In addition, the nurse assesses dietary habits, fluid intake, and activity level. Physical examination includes the anal area, looking for fissures, redness, and hemorrhoids. The nurse auscultates the abdomen for bowel sounds and palpates for distention and masses. Finally, he or she inspects the stool or gently inserts a lubricated, gloved finger in the anal canal to assess the characteristics of the unpassed stool.

Diagnosis, Planning, and Interventions

Major goals of nursing management are restoring normal bowel function, relieving rectal discomfort and anxiety, and helping the client understand how to maintain normal bowel function. To make these goals measurable, the nurse must add specific criteria.

When constipation is related to dietary habits, decreased fluid intake, stress, lack of exercise, or other factors, the nurse suggests a high-fiber diet that includes plenty of raw fruits and vegetables, whole-grain breads, and coarse brans and cereals (Box 53-1). Teaching clients to drink eight or more full glasses of water and fruit juice daily promotes regularity because fructose is a natural laxative. In addition, the nurse urges the client to schedule time to exercise each day because such activity promotes intestinal motility.

The client must respond quickly to the urge to defecate and allow sufficient time to evacuate the bowel. The nurse encourages the client to use the toilet at regular intervals even without the urge to defecate, particularly after meals, when the gastrocolic reflex is most active. He or she helps the client and family understand the need for privacy during bathroom times. Instructing the client to avoid excessive straining to have a bowel movement also is necessary.

The nurse discourages self-treatment with daily or frequent enemas or laxatives. Chronic use of such products causes natural bowel function to be sluggish. In addition, laxatives containing stimulants can be habit forming, requiring continued use in increasing doses. The nurse teaches about the use of fiber supplements, such as those containing psyllium. Agents considered "natural" sometimes contain ingredients that lead to chronic laxative dependence. The client must discuss any medication he or she uses for control of chronic constipation with the physician or nurse practitioner. If long-term treatment with stool softeners is indicated, the nurse provides a list of safe medications, such as those containing mineral oil, magnesium, or nonabsorbable sugar (i.e., sorbitol, lactulose).

Diagnoses, outcomes, and interventions are as follows.

Constipation related to immobility or inadequate fluid intake as evidenced by infrequent passage of stool and abdominal distention

Expected Outcomes: Client attains a normal pattern of elimination, and stools are soft and easily passed.

- Review usual pattern of elimination. *Constipation has many possible reasons; assessing usual pattern is the first step in identifying the cause.*
- Review current medications. *Many medications affect bowel elimination.*
- Encourage client slowly to increase dietary fiber intake to 25 g/day. Bran cereals, fresh fruits and vegetables, and beans are excellent sources. Remind client to add these foods gradually. *Fiber absorbs water in the colon and forms a gel, adding bulk and easing defecation. Adding fiber gradually helps to avoid bloating, gas, and diarrhea.*
- Instruct client to increase fluids to six to eight glasses per day. *This intake prevents hard, dry stools.*
- Encourage client to be out of bed, increase activity, or develop a regular exercise program. *Activity increases peristalsis and promotes bowel elimination.*
- Administer laxatives, suppositories, and enemas as ordered. *Treatments should be used only as ordered to avoid cathartic bowel.*

Pain related to rectal distention, difficulty passing stool, or anal tears

Expected Outcome: Client will state reduced or no rectal discomfort.

- Apply lubricant in rectum and around anus with glove. *Lubricant provides emollient action for passage of stool and healing of anal tears.*
- Assist client to soak rectal area in tub of warm water. *Soaking in a warm tub relieves pain, helps to heal anal tears, and soothes rectal distention.*

BOX 53-1 ● Dietary Modifications for Common Intestinal Problems

HIGH-FIBER DIET TO MANAGE CONSTIPATION

Adding fiber to the diet relieves constipation by adding bulk and moisture to the stool. The following foods increase dietary fiber:

- Bran and whole grains (100% bran, rolled oats, granola, wheat germ, brown rice, cornmeal)
- Legumes (dried peas, beans, lentils; split peas; black-eyed peas; pinto, kidney, navy beans; red or yellow lentils)
- Seeds and nuts (sesame, sunflower, poppy, crunchy peanut butter, popcorn)
- Fruits: raw (apples with skin, pears, oranges, melons, berries) and dried (prunes, dates, raisins)
- Vegetables: raw (sprouts, spinach, carrots, peppers, broccoli, cabbage) and steamed (peas, potatoes with skin)

LOW-RESIDUE DIET TO MANAGE DIARRHEA

Reintroducing food after a bout of diarrhea usually calls for a low-residue diet to reduce the volume of stool. The following foods may be used to manage diarrhea:

- Dairy products (all forms of milk, yogurt, pudding, cottage cheese) unless client is lactose intolerant
- Meat and meat substitutes (baked, steamed, roasted or pressure-cooked poultry without skin; tuna or salmon; poached or boiled eggs)
- Fruits and vegetables (strained, cooked, steamed without skins or seeds, applesauce, bananas)
- Grains (products made with refined flour such as white bread or soda crackers)

Evaluation of Expected Outcomes

The client has soft, formed stool every 2 days. He or she reports feeling more comfortable after warm soaks and application of lubricant.

● DIARRHEA

Pathophysiology and Etiology

Diarrhea is the frequent passage of liquid or semiliquid stool. It results from increased peristalsis, which moves fecal matter through the GI tract much more rapidly than normal. The swift velocity causes intestinal cramping and decreases the time available for water to be absorbed from stool in the large intestine. Consequently, the stool is either very soft or liquid.

Three major problems associated with severe or prolonged diarrhea include dehydration, electrolyte imbalances, and vitamin deficiencies. When diarrhea results from a disease that causes malabsorption, the client is at risk for a nutritional deficiency. The sudden onset of acute abdominal pain or a rise in temperature may indicate perforation of the bowel.

Diarrhea may be related to bacterial or viral infections affecting the intestine; lactose intolerance; food allergies or intolerance; uremia; intestinal disease such as diverticulitis, ulcerative colitis, malabsorption, or intestinal obstruction; rapid addition of fiber to the diet; consumption of highly spiced or seasoned food; overuse of laxatives; and adverse effects of drugs, especially antibiotics or concentrated tube-feeding formulas. The most common cause is infection by bacterial, parasitic, or viral agents. The client may give a history of contacts with ill people in his or her household, foreign travel, or use of water from an impure source (e.g., lakes, streams). The client also may mention long-standing abdominal pain or diarrhea or a family history of metabolic or inflammatory disorders.

Diarrhea also may result from several metabolic disorders and diseases such as cystic fibrosis, pancreatic insufficiency, or inflammatory bowel disease. It may be caused by surgical resection of large portions of the small bowel (short bowel syndrome). Other causes include immunoglobulin A deficiency, overeating, concurrent medication (especially antibiotics), and irritable bowel syndrome.

Assessment Findings

Signs and Symptoms

Stools are watery and frequent. In severe cases, blood and mucus pass with the stool. The client usually experiences urgency (**tenesmus**) and abdominal discomfort. Bowel sounds are hyperactive. Skin around the anus may become excoriated from contact with fecal matter and products of the digestive process (e.g., gastric acid, bile salts). Fever may be present. Infectious diarrhea typically has a sudden onset, with accompanying generalized malaise.

Diagnostic Findings

Routine stool cultures are obtained to identify bacterial infections as the cause for infectious diarrhea. They do not identify parasites, however, which necessitates the use of other measures. Stool specimens obtained to identify parasites and their ova are placed in special preservatives and analyzed separately by the microbiology department. Several samples may be needed because parasites are not typically shed with each stool. Routine ova and parasite analysis may identify amebic infections; however, such infections may require serologic (blood) tests.

Blood in the stool may be common with certain infections and disease processes. Nurses typically test stool specimens, collecting a specimen from the client (e.g., Hemoccult testing). A proctosigmoidoscopy or colonoscopy may be performed to identify chronic inflammation or alteration in the mucosal layer of the large intestine. These studies often are carried out to identify the cause of chronic inflammation. An upper GI series with small bowel follow-through allows for radiologic examination of the small bowel and identification of inflammation. Upper GI endoscopy allows for identification of malabsorptive disorders such as celiac disease.

Medical and Surgical Management

Treatment of diarrhea that is mild or of short duration, such as that caused by dietary changes or acute illness, involves resting the bowel by limiting intake to clear liquids for one or two meals and gradually advancing to a regular diet. When diarrhea persists and stools are frequent and large, or if the person is very young, elderly, or debilitated, medical treatment may include one or more of the following measures:

- Administration of an antidiarrheal agent, such as diphenoxylate hydrochloride with atropine sulfate (Lomotil), loperamide hydrochloride (Imodium), or a combination product such as kaolin and pectin (Kaopectate)
- Fluid and electrolyte replacement by either the oral or intravenous (IV) route
- Dietary adjustments, which may involve eliminating foods that cause diarrhea
- Total parenteral nutrition (TPN) if diarrhea is severe and prolonged and if the introduction of oral fluid and food results in another episode of diarrhea

Chronic diarrhea depletes the bowel of helpful organisms and allows yeasts and fungi to thrive unchecked. To recolonize the bowel, capsules or granules containing *Lactobacillus acidophilus* (Bacid or Lactinex) are prescribed. These agents are referred to as *probiotics.*

NURSING PROCESS

● The Client With Diarrhea

Assessment

In addition to conducting the assessments performed on the client with a GI disorder (see Chap. 51), the nurse obtains a complete health, dietary, allergy, and drug history. Including a history of newly prescribed drugs, such as antibiotics, is important, as is the pattern of laxative and enema use. The nurse asks about any recent incidence of constipation because diarrhea can result from an impacted fecal mass. He or she observes emotional status because anxiety affects bowel motility. To help determine a cause-and-effect relationship, the nurse asks about the onset of diarrhea in relation to the possibility of eating tainted foods. Learning that others who ate the same food have similar symptoms may support the possibility of food-related diarrhea. Asking the client about recent foreign travel is important. Drinking unsanitary water or consuming uncooked food washed with contaminated water may transmit some intestinal pathogens.

Depending on the severity and duration of the diarrhea, the nurse may need to examine the anal area for redness or other tissue changes. Abdominal auscultation helps identify characteristics of bowel sounds. The nurse palpates for distention and masses, monitors the frequency and characteristics of stools, and measures the volume of liquid stools to assess fluid loss. He or she also assesses for signs of dehydration, electrolyte imbalance, and metabolic acidosis (see Chap. 22). Baseline data collection includes recording daily weights and taking vital signs. Reporting the sudden onset of acute abdominal pain to the physician immediately is essential.

Diagnosis, Planning, and Interventions

The nurse provides a list of foods and beverages to avoid. If medication is prescribed, he or she explains its purpose and routine for use and identifies common side effects. Cautioning the client to avoid self-treatment of diarrhea and to consult the physician if the diarrhea does not respond to dietary restrictions and antidiarrheal medications is essential. The nurse advises the client with an underlying GI disorder (e.g., Crohn's disease, ulcerative colitis) to consult the physician or nurse practitioner before using drugs that affect motility (e.g., loperamide, diphenoxylate hydrochloride). Use of these drugs in diseases that affect bowel mucosa may cause dangerous complications. The nurse also advises the client to contact the physician if diarrhea is prolonged or accompanied by severe abdominal pain, blood or mucus passes with stool, fever develops, or urine output decreases. The care plan may include the following.

Diarrhea related to an enteric infection, as manifested by frequent liquid stools and abdominal cramping
Expected Outcome: Client will develop a normal bowel elimination pattern of one soft, formed stool every 1 to 3 days and will not experience pain or cramping.

● Encourage client to withhold foods until the acute attack subsides. *Withholding food rests the bowel and slows peristalsis.*
● Give clear liquids as tolerated. *Drinking clear liquids prevents dehydration.*
● Advance oral intake as tolerated, offering bland foods initially. *Bland foods are more easily digested. Slow introduction of low-residue foods prevents excessive peristalsis.*
● Teach client to avoid caffeinated and carbonated beverages. *Such beverages stimulate GI motility.*
● Administer antidiarrheal medications as ordered for prolonged diarrhea. *These medications slow intestinal motility and inhibit peristalsis.*
● Encourage client to rest in a comfortable position with legs bent toward the abdomen. *This position relaxes abdominal muscles and reduces discomfort.*
● Advise client to avoid carbonated beverages or drinking with a straw. *These increase volume of swallowed air, which in turn increases gas and cramping.*

Risk for Deficient Fluid Volume related to frequent passage of watery stools and inadequate fluid intake
Expected Outcome: Client's output will not exceed fluid intake.

● Assess hydration status by monitoring intake and output, skin turgor, and moisture of mucous membranes. *Assessment provides a baseline.*
● If diarrhea is severe, offer water, clear liquids, and electrolyte solutions (e.g., Gatorade) as allowed. *These substances replace fluids and electrolytes and prevent dehydration.*
● Report urine output of less than 240 mL in 4 hours. *Such a finding indicates dehydration.*
● Monitor the number and consistency of stools. *A record documents stool output and provides a baseline to guide fluid replacement.*
● Observe for symptoms of sodium and potassium loss, such as weakness, abdominal or leg cramping, or dysrhythmias. Note results of blood chemistry testing. *Excessive diarrhea causes severe loss of electrolytes.*

Risk for Imbalanced Nutrition: Less than Body Requirements related to anorexia and malabsorption secondary to rapid passage of stool through the GI tract
Expected Outcome: Client maintains adequate nutritional intake and maintains body weight.

● Notify physician if client cannot tolerate resuming a progressive diet. *This client may require other medical interventions.*

- Instruct client to avoid spicy, fatty foods and milk or milk products if he or she is lactose intolerant. *These foods stimulate GI motility.*
- Weigh client as indicated. *A record provides a baseline for monitoring weight loss, particularly for clients with prolonged diarrhea.*

Risk for Impaired Skin Integrity related to mechanical and chemical trauma to the rectum

Expected Outcome: Client's perianal tissue will remain intact.

- Assist with or administer perianal care after each bowel movement. Provide or use premoistened, nonirritating, non–alcohol-based wipes rather than paper for the anal area. *These measures prevent perianal excoriation.*
- Apply a medicated ointment, such as one containing vitamins A and D or zinc oxide, if perianal area is reddened. *The ointment minimizes excoriation of the perianal skin.*
- If perianal skin becomes excoriated or desquamated, apply a wound hydrogel. *Moisture-barrier ointments protect against further excoriation and promote healing.*

Evaluation of Expected Outcomes

The client's bowel elimination pattern is normal, as evidenced by one to two soft, formed stools every 2 days. The client states that he or she has no pain or cramping. Urine output does not exceed fluid intake. Weight remains stable. Skin remains intact with no signs of redness or excoriation.

● IRRITABLE BOWEL SYNDROME

Irritable bowel syndrome (IBS), sometimes referred to as **spastic colon,** is a paroxysmal motility disorder primarily affecting the colon. It is not a disease but a cluster of symptoms that occur despite the absence of a disease process. Persons with IBS experience alternating periods of constipation and diarrhea. One or the other elimination pattern predominates. Women are affected more often than men.

Pathophysiology and Etiology

Fluctuating intestinal motility tends to be the underlying factor that produces symptoms (Fig. 53-1). Because the autonomic nervous system affects motor function in the GI tract, neuron stimulation and inhibition influence bowel motility. When a parasympathetic neurotransmitter (e.g., acetylcholine) is released, intestinal motility increases and diarrhea results. An opposite effect occurs when the smooth muscle of the gut responds to sympathetic neurotransmission. In many clients, IBS appears to intensify with stress.

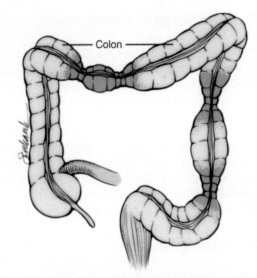

FIGURE 53-1 In irritable bowel syndrome, the spastic contractions of the bowel are visible in x-ray contrast studies. (From Smeltzer, S. C. & Bare, B. G. [2000]. *Brunner & Suddarth's textbook of medical–surgical nursing* [9th ed.]. Philadelphia: Lippincott Williams & Wilkins.)

The cause of IBS is unknown, although some factors appear to be associated with it. These include heredity; psychological stress or illness; a diet high in rich, stimulating, or irritating foods; alcohol consumption; smoking (Smeltzer & Bare, 2000); and intolerance of lactose and other sugars (Porth, 2002). These factors are not definitive for all individuals with IBS. Many cases appear to have no precipitating factors.

Assessment Findings

Signs and Symptoms

Most clients with IBS describe having chronic constipation with sporadic bouts of diarrhea. Some report the opposite pattern, although less commonly. Most clients experience various degrees of abdominal pain that defecation may relieve. Many clients suffer with belching and flatulence (intestinal gas). In general, symptoms do not awaken individuals from sleep. Some clients with IBS report anxiety, insecurity, depression, or anger.

Weight usually remains stable, indicating that when diarrhea occurs, malabsorption of nutrients does not accompany it. When loose stools are inspected, although passed frequently, they usually are of low volume and may contain mucus. Blood usually is not found in the stool because the bowel is not locally inflamed.

Diagnostic Findings

Radiographic and endoscopic tests rule out other disorders with similar symptoms, such as peptic ulcer disease, colorectal cancer, diverticulosis, or inflammatory bowel disease.

Medical and Surgical Management

Dietary changes reduce flatulence and abdominal discomfort. By trial and error, the client eliminates common food sources that cause discomfort or intestinal gas, such as beans or cabbage. At the same time, a high-fiber diet or a bulk-forming agent, such as products containing psyllium (e.g., Metamucil), is prescribed to regulate bowel elimination. The fiber draws water into constipated stool and adds bulk to watery stool. An anticholinergic, such as dicyclomine (Bentyl), has an antispasmodic effect if taken before meals. Either a prescription or nonprescription antidiarrheal is used for temporary relief from diarrhea.

Nursing Management

Most clients with IBS are not hospitalized. Nurses become involved in their care during diagnostic testing, follow-up visits, or hospitalization for a concurrent problem. During these encounters, the nurse gathers a comprehensive database of symptoms, helps manage the problems associated with constipation and diarrhea, explains therapeutic treatments, evaluates the client's understanding of the regimen for self-care, and monitors the response to therapy. For more specific nursing interventions, refer to the preceding discussions of clients with constipation and diarrhea.

Stop, Think, and Respond ● BOX 53-1

A neighbor confides that she has IBS. She wonders if you can provide her with any tips about managing her condition. What is your best response?

INFLAMMATORY BOWEL DISEASE   ●

Inflammatory bowel disease (IBD) is a chronic illness characterized by exacerbations and remissions. **Ulcerative colitis** and **Crohn's disease** collectively comprise IBD. These two distinct disorders are grouped together because of their similar symptoms and treatments. Their characteristics are summarized in Table 53-1. Because of the similarity in presenting symptoms and results of diagnostic procedures, differential diagnosis may be difficult. Unlike IBS, IBD does not resolve without medical intervention.

● CROHN'S DISEASE

Crohn's disease is also called *granulomatous colitis, ileitis,* and *regional enteritis.* This chronic inflammatory condition can occur in any portion of the GI tract but predominantly affects the bowel in the terminal portion of the ileum. Its general onset is in young adulthood.

Pathophysiology and Etiology

The inflammation in Crohn's disease extends transmurally through all the layers of the bowel, but the submucosal layer is most involved. Hyperemia (increased blood supply), edema, and ulcerations characterize affected areas. Endoscopic examination shows inflamed areas alternating with healthy tissue. The inflamed areas occur randomly, a phenomenon described as **skip lesions.** The

---

TABLE 53-1	CHARACTERISTICS OF INFLAMMATORY BOWEL DISEASE	
CHARACTERISTICS	**CROHN'S DISEASE**	**ULCERATIVE COLITIS**
Onset of symptoms	Gradual	Abrupt
Location	Diffuse	Localized
Distribution	Can occur at any location in the GI tract, most commonly found in the ileum	Rectum to cecum
Type of lesion	Patchy, positioned between areas of normal tissue, and referred to as *skip lesions*	Continuous from rectum to cecum, without areas of healthy tissue
Extent of inflammation	May extend through all bowel layers; may be visible in the large intestine or invisible if located in the higher GI tract	Limited to mucosal lining
Blood in stool	Occult	Visible
Weight loss	Common	Less common
Perianal disease	Typical (fistula formation, abscesses)	Atypical
Extraintestinal symptoms (joint pain, skin lesions, inflammatory conditions of the eyes)	Common	Less common but can occur
Biopsy findings	Signs of chronic inflammation; granulomas	Signs of chronic inflammation; granulomas rare
Carcinogenesis	Rare	Common
Surgery	Does not relieve chronicity	Curative

bowel is described as having a "cobblestone" appearance because of the deep ulcerations that form among the edematous tissue (Fig. 53-2).

Because Crohn's disease is a transmural inflammatory process, inflammation can extend beyond the lining of the bowel. As a result, inflammatory channels containing blood, mucus, pus, or stool may develop. Such an inflammatory channel is called a **fistula;** two or more are referred to as *fistulae*. Fistulae may form a channel between the bowel and the skin surface (enterocutaneous fistulae). Common sites for enterocutaneous fistulae are perianal and perilabial sites. Inflammation also may extend between the bowel and other pelvic organs (e.g., vagina), between the bowel and bladder, or between loops of bowel (enterovaginal, enterovesical, and enteroenteric fistulae, respectively). Fistulae also may form between the rectum and vagina in women, as evidenced by passage of stool from the vagina. Chronic inflammation in Crohn's disease also may lead to scarring and stricture formation and eventual obstruction of the lumen.

The cause of Crohn's disease is unknown. Because incidence is increased among family members, a genetic predisposition is presumed. Other possible contributing factors include allergic and autoimmune responses triggered by diet or infectious microbial antigens. Recurrent attacks on the tissue are believed to result from an exaggerated immune response, which explains the chronic nature of the disease. The role of stress in the development of symptoms and subsequent exacerbations has not been defined. As with any chronic illness, stress may influence the client's ability to cope with symptoms. This issue is certainly confused by the fact that many clients with IBD also may have IBS. Diarrhea as a response to anxiety may be confused with exacerbation of the disease.

Assessment Findings

Signs and Symptoms

Usually, onset is insidious, and the course of the disease varies. Usually, most clients have abdominal pain, disten-

FIGURE 53-2 Crohn's disease. (From Rubin, E. & Farber, J. L. [1999]. *Pathology* [3rd ed.]. Philadelphia: Lippincott Williams & Wilkins.)

tion, and tenderness in the lower abdominal quadrants, especially on the right side. Pain may be associated with eating. The client may have a history of chronic diarrhea and fatigue. Growth failure is a common early symptom in children and adolescents. Fever may be present. As Crohn's disease progresses, anorexia, weight loss, dehydration, and signs of nutritional deficiencies occur. Symptoms gradually increase in some clients, whereas acute exacerbations alternate with remissions in other clients. The symptoms may go into remission spontaneously.

The systemic nature of this disease is evidenced by symptoms outside the GI tract, referred to as *extraintestinal manifestations of IBD*. They include arthritis, arthralgias, skin lesions (erythema nodosum and pyoderma gangrenosum), inflammation in the eyes (uveitis, conjunctivitis, and iritis), and disorders of the liver and gallbladder. Usually, extraintestinal manifestations become quiescent when the bowel disease is under control.

During the physical examination, palpation may reveal an abdominal mass. Inspection of the perineum and perianal areas may reveal scars from previous fissures, skin tags, or evidence of fistulae or perianal abscesses.

Diagnostic Findings

Stool cultures fail to reveal an etiologic microorganism or parasite, but occult blood and white blood cells (WBCs) often are found in the stool. Results of blood studies indicate anemia from chronic blood loss and nutritional deficiencies. The WBC count and erythrocyte sedimentation rate may be elevated, confirming an inflammatory disorder. Serum protein and albumin levels may be low because of malnutrition. Low serum levels of the fat-soluble vitamins also reflect the client's malnourished state.

All these laboratory findings do not confirm IBD because they can be associated with several other disorders, especially acute infections. Abnormal serum electrolyte levels and a disturbed acid-base balance may accompany severe diarrhea. The recent development of serologic tests (Prometheus Laboratories, Inc., San Diego, California) for IBD may be helpful in some cases. These tests allow for the identification of certain antibodies common to those with Crohn's disease (anti-*Saccharomyces* antibodies, or ASCAs) and those with ulcerative colitis (antineutrophil cytoplasmic antibodies, or ANCAs). These tests do not confirm IBD because clients with IBD may not test positive for the antibodies, and some individuals who do not have IBD may test positive. These tests may, however, serve as an important adjunct to other diagnostic tests.

Barium enema findings may show inflammation in the large intestine, but confirmation of the diagnosis requires endoscopic examination (colonoscopy or sigmoidoscopy). Endoscopic evaluation allows for identification of mucosal abnormalities (e.g., skip lesions, ulcerations, cobblestone appearance). Biopsies taken during colonoscopy or sigmoidoscopy are examined under the microscope for evidence of chronic inflammation and possible granuloma.

A granuloma is an aggregate of inflammatory cells and, when identified on biopsy, confirms the diagnosis of Crohn's disease. The absence of a granuloma does not rule out the diagnosis of Crohn's disease.

Clients with Crohn's disease are vulnerable to intestinal perforation during barium enema and endoscopy because of poor integrity of the bowel wall. They are monitored accordingly. Esophagogastroduodenoscopy with biopsy is indicated when inflammation is suspected in the upper GI tract. An upper GI series with small bowel follow-through allows for radiographic examination of the small intestine and identification of inflammation that endoscopy cannot evaluate.

Medical Management

Treatment is supportive. The dietary approach varies. A high-fiber diet may be indicated when it is desirable to add bulk to loose stools. A low-fiber diet may be indicated in cases of severe inflammation or stricture. A high-calorie and high-protein diet helps replace nutritional losses from chronic diarrhea. The client may need nutritional supplements, depending on the area of the bowel affected. When the small intestine is inflamed, some clients experience lactose intolerance, requiring avoidance of lactose-rich foods.

Some clients need an elemental diet formula, such as Tolerex, Vivonex, or Peptamen, that reduces proteins, fats, and carbohydrates to an easily absorbed form. Elemental diets effectively induce remission in Crohn's disease without medications. Unfortunately, clients are not allowed to eat or drink normally while on the elemental diet, making this treatment modality unacceptable for many. In addition, elemental formulas are not very palatable. Some may need to be administered through a naso-gastric tube. Success with elemental diet therapy requires extensive education and client motivation. Newly introduced polymeric diets (Modulen, Nestle, U.S.A.) may provide the benefit of inducing remission and are more palatable. TPN may become necessary to provide intestinal rest. IV fluids, electrolytes, and whole blood are given to correct anemia and restore fluid and electrolyte balance.

Drug therapy involves supplementary vitamins, iron, antidiarrheal drugs, anti-inflammatory corticosteroids and 5-acetylsalicylic acid (5-ASA) medications, immune modulating agents, and antibiotics (Drug Therapy Table 53-1). Vitamin and iron supplements are used for known deficiencies and malabsorption. Antidiarrheal agents, such as diphenoxylate (Lomotil) and loperamide (Imodium), usually are used sparingly and only when clients do not have an infection. Decreasing motility in cases of infection predisposes clients with IBD to **toxic megacolon,** a complication that is discussed in the section on ulcerative colitis.

Considered first-line treatment for IBD, 5-ASA drugs contain salicylate, which is bonded to a carrying agent that allows the drug to be absorbed in the intestine. These drugs work by decreasing the inflammatory response. The 5-ASA medications include sulfasalazine (Azulfidine), olsalazine (Dipentum), and mesalamine (Asacol, Pentasa). Mesalamine also is available in enema or suppository form (Rowasa) and may be used to treat distal disease. Folic acid usually is recommended for clients taking sulfasalazine, which interferes with absorption of this nutrient. Corticosteroids (prednisone) are used during acute exacerbations of symptoms and when 5-ASA drugs cannot control the symptoms. Hydrocortisone is available in enema form (Cortenema) and is effective in controlling distal disease without posing a high risk for systemic side effects. Long-term corticosteroid use is undesirable because of the potentially severe side effects; the dose usually is tapered and discontinued when the symptoms are in remission.

Failure to maintain remission necessitates the use of an immune-modulating agent such as mercaptopurine (6-MP) or azathioprine (Imuran). These agents often allow clients to discontinue corticosteroids without exacerbating symptoms. Other immune modulators are cyclosporine (Sandimmune), tacrolimus (Prograf), and methotrexate (MTX). Antibiotics such as metronidazole (Flagyl) and ciprofloxacin (Cipro) are effective adjuncts to treating Crohn's disease, especially related fistulae.

Approved in 1998 for the treatment of moderate to severely active and fistulizing Crohn's disease, infliximab (Remicade) has proven safe and effective in achieving and maintaining remission in many clients with Crohn's disease. This drug fits into a new classification of medications known as biologic agents. Infliximab is an antibody that interferes with the inflammatory process early in the immune response. It is given IV over 2 hours in an outpatient or inpatient setting. Repeat infusions may help to sustain remission.

Surgical Management

Surgical treatment is reserved for complications such as intestinal obstruction, perforation, or fistula formation. The need for surgical intervention is common in Crohn's disease. In fact, more than 75% of clients with Crohn's disease require surgery within 20 years of the onset of symptoms, and 90% require surgery within 30 years. Unlike surgical treatment for ulcerative colitis, removing the inflamed portion of the intestine does not alter disease progression or recurrence. Many clients who undergo surgery for Crohn's disease require additional surgery within a few years.

Surgical removal of a large amount of intestine results in the loss of absorptive surface, called **short bowel syndrome.** Massive bowel resection results in dependence on TPN, possibly for life. Removal of the colon requires a permanent ileostomy because the disease tends to recur in any rectal pouch. Ileostomy is discussed in Chapter 54.

DRUG THERAPY TABLE 53-1	AGENTS FOR DISORDERS OF THE LOWER GI TRACT

DRUG CATEGORY AND EXAMPLES	SIDE EFFECTS	NURSING CONSIDERATIONS
Antidiarrheals		
bismuth subsalicylate (Pepto-Bismol)	Constipation, dark discoloration of oral mucous membranes and stools	Do not administer to clients who are allergic to aspirin or salicylates.
kaolin and pectin (Kaopectate)	Constipation, abdominal pain	This drug may interfere with absorption of nutrients and other drugs.
diphenoxylate with atropine sulfate (Lomotil)	Sedation, dizziness, dry mouth, paralytic ileus, constipation	Monitor closely for proper bowel function. Advise client not to drive or operate dangerous machinery while taking this drug.
loperamide (Imodium)	CNS depression, abdominal pain and distention, nausea, vomiting, constipation	If necessary and prescribed, administer naloxone to counteract CNS depression from overdosage. Avoid prolonged use.
Laxatives, Cathartics, and Bulk-Forming Agents		
bisacodyl (Dulcolax)	Abdominal cramps, nausea, vomiting, rectal irritation (from suppository form)	Advise client that prolonged use creates dependence. Do not administer within 1 hour of milk or antacids.
magnesium preparations (milk of magnesia, magnesium citrate, magnesium oxide)	Abdominal cramps, diarrhea, nausea, vomiting	Monitor serum magnesium levels and avoid prolonged use. Explain that these drugs may interfere with absorption of histamine-2 antagonists, phenytoin, steroids, and some antibiotics.
mineral oil polyethylene glycol (GoLYTELY, Colyte)	Leakage of oil from rectum, diarrhea, abdominal cramps	Mineral oil may cause lipid pneumonitis if aspirated. Do not administer to clients who are vomiting and therefore at risk for aspiration. Prolonged use in high doses may result in poor absorption of fat-soluble vitamins. Monitor serum levels of these vitamins.
psyllium (Metamucil, Citrucel)	Nausea, vomiting, abdominal distention and cramps Nausea, vomiting, diarrhea, intestinal gas, abdominal cramps	Administer for bowel evacuation prior to GI testing. Explain that large amounts may be administered. Compliance may be difficult. Do not give if client has intestinal obstruction or fecal impaction. Some forms require reconstitution with water.
Anti-inflammatory 5-Acetylsalicylic Acid Medications		
sulfasalazine (Azulfidine), olsalazine (Dipentum), mesalamine (Pentasa, Asacol, Rowasa)	Headache, diarrhea, abdominal pain and cramps, malaise, hair loss, rash, harmless orange discoloration of urine, bone marrow suppression, photosensitivity, decreased sperm motility (sulfasalazine)	These drugs are contraindicated in clients allergic to salicylates. Continued GI symptoms may indicate an exacerbation of the disease and should be reported to the physician. Routine blood tests to monitor for bone marrow suppression are indicated. Encourage application of sunscreen to prevent skin damage (sulfasalazine). Decreased sperm motility is reversible with discontinuing sulfasalazine. Clients taking Asacol may report passing the tablets whole in the stool, which is not harmful. They should notify the physician if this occurs repeatedly.
Anti-inflammatory Corticosteroids		
prednisone, methylprednisolone (Medrol)	Cushingoid appearance, hypertension, acne, water retention,	Monitor closely for side effects, especially with long-term use.

(continued)

DRUG THERAPY TABLE 53-1	AGENTS FOR DISORDERS OF THE LOWER GI TRACT (Continued)

DRUG CATEGORY AND EXAMPLES	SIDE EFFECTS	NURSING CONSIDERATIONS
	weight gain, hair loss, increased appetite, hypokalemia, gastric irritation, ulcer formation, adrenal suppression, decreased resistance to infection, complications associated with prolonged use (osteoporosis, development of cataracts, growth retardation, peptic ulceration, hyperglycemia)	Administer with food to decrease gastric irritation. Encourage low-sodium diet to minimize water retention. Clients with diabetes may have increased insulin needs; monitor blood glucose levels. Abrupt withdrawal may precipitate addisonian crisis, which may be fatal. Caution clients that drug should be weaned. Monitor blood pressure. Monitor linear growth in children. Instruct clients taking prednisone to wear a bracelet or necklace that states they are taking prednisone and may need additional corticosteroids during a medical crisis. Clients taking corticosteroids may not have a normal immune response to infection. Monitor closely for signs of infection, prevent exposure through universal precautions, and encourage consultation with physician regarding routine immunizations. Encourage regular physical examinations to monitor for long-term side effects. Clients should consider a calcium supplement to help prevent osteoporosis.
Immune-Modulating Agents		
mercaptopurine, 6-MP (Purinethol), azathioprine (Imuran)	Bone marrow suppression, increased vulnerability to infection, rash, arthralgias, hepatic dysfunction, nausea, vomiting, diarrhea, pancreatitis, hair loss, development of neoplasms	Encourage client to undergo routine blood tests used to screen for bone marrow suppression and hepatic dysfunction. Clients taking these agents may not have a normal immune response to infection. Monitor closely for signs of infection, prevent exposure through universal precautions, and encourage client to consult the physician before routine immunizations. Drugs may be teratogenic: women of childbearing age should consult their physician before considering pregnancy. Sexually active females should use appropriate birth control. Drugs may be toxic to infants when transmitted through breast milk.
Biologic Agents		
infliximab (Remicade)	Infusion-related reactions: pruritus, rash, chest pain, hypotension, hypertension, dyspnea; other potential side effects: headache, nausea, vomiting, fatigue, fever, autoantibody, lupus-like syndrome, lymphoproliferative disorders, increased susceptibility to infection	Drug is currently approved for a single dose in moderate to severely active Crohn's disease and is being investigated for multidose use to maintain remission in both Crohn's disease and ulcerative colitis. Clients often are given acetaminophen (Tylenol) and diphenhydramine (Benadryl) before the infusion to minimize side effects. Clients with a history of previous infusion reaction may be pretreated with prednisone. Drug is administered intravenously over 2 hours: monitor client for infusion reaction every 1/2 hour during the infusion. Should a reaction develop, discontinue the infusion and notify the ordering physician. Instruct client to continue routine medications unless otherwise directed by physician. Encourage client to undergo routine medical follow-up care. Clients taking this medication may not have a normal immune response to infection. Monitor closely for signs of infection, prevent exposure through universal precautions, and encourage client to consult physician before routine immunizations. Safety during pregnancy and breast-feeding has not been established.

CNS, central nervous system.

Nursing Management

A health history assists in determining the onset, duration, and nature of the client's GI problems. Medical, drug, allergy, and diet histories also are important. Nursing care focuses on monitoring the client for complications, managing fluid and nutrition replacement, supporting the client emotionally, and teaching about diet and medications.

The nurse determines the average number of stools the client passes each day and their appearance. Providing regular skin care to avoid breakdown is essential (see Nursing Process: The Client With Diarrhea). In addition, the nurse asks the client about weight loss and whether any foods increase the frequency of bowel movements or cause discomfort. The client will require assistance to maintain adequate nutritional intake. The nurse monitors the client's intake and collaborates with the dietitian to replace uneaten food with something more acceptable.

Physical examination includes auscultating and lightly palpating the abdomen and inspecting the rectal area. The nurse takes vital signs, weighs the client, and measures and documents intake and output. Advising the client to report whenever a bowel movement occurs is important so it can be inspected and a sample sent to the laboratory for occult blood and other analysis.

● ULCERATIVE COLITIS

In **ulcerative colitis,** the chronic inflammation usually is limited to the mucosal and submucosal layers of the colon. The disease is most common in young and middle-aged adults but can occur at any age. Some clients experience prolonged remission, whereas others experience mild to severe (and potentially life-threatening) exacerbations of symptoms.

Pathophysiology and Etiology

Although the exact cause is unknown, some believe that multiple factors trigger ulcerative colitis, including genetic predisposition, infection, allergy, and abnormal immune response. The connection between the disease and a malfunction of the immune system is supported by the fact that clients with ulcerative colitis often have other coexisting immune-related disorders such as ankylosing spondylitis and other extraintestinal manifestations.

Inflammation usually begins in the rectum and extends proximally and continuously. As a rule, no healthy tissue appears between inflamed areas, as in Crohn's disease. When inflammation remains confined to the most distal area of the large intestine, the client has **ulcerative proctitis.** When inflammation extends beyond the sigmoid colon, the client has ulcerative colitis.

The lining of the colon tends to bleed easily. Ulceration may extend to the muscular layer of the bowel wall. Superficial abscesses form in depressions in the mucosa. Poor integrity of the bowel wall may lead to *toxic megacolon,* a complication in which the colon dilates and becomes atonic (lacks motility). The thin bowel wall is vulnerable to perforation under these conditions, leading to peritonitis, septicemia, and the need for emergency surgical repair.

Assessment Findings

Signs and Symptoms

The onset of the disease usually is abrupt. The client experiences severe diarrhea and expels blood and mucus along with fecal matter. Cramps accompany diarrhea. Eating precipitates cramping and diarrhea, resulting in anorexia and fatigue. The urge to defecate may come so suddenly and with such urgency that the client is incontinent. Some clients experience such incontinence during sleep. Despite intense tenesmus, the client may expel very little stool.

Diagnostic Findings

Laboratory findings are similar to those described in the section on Crohn's disease. Barium enema reveals evidence of inflammation. Definitive diagnosis requires proctosigmoidoscopy or colonoscopy with biopsy. Endoscopic examination and biopsy of the lining of the colon reveals characteristic inflammatory lesions. Biopsies of the intestinal mucosa reveal evidence of chronic inflammation. These diagnostic studies usually are withheld in cases of toxic megacolon because of the high risk for perforation.

Medical and Surgical Management

Medical treatment aims toward achieving and maintaining remission. The diet is kept as normal as possible but modified to increase caloric and nutritional content. The client is instructed temporarily to refrain from eating foods associated with discomfort. If all foods cause discomfort, the symptoms are likely from the disease itself and not food. The client may be given TPN and intermittent lipid infusions to rest the bowel completely. The use of an elemental diet, as described with Crohn's disease, has not proved effective for ulcerative colitis.

Blood transfusions and iron are given to correct anemia. The client also may need parenteral fluids and electrolytes. Because frequent bowel movements interfere with absorption of nutrients, supplementary vitamins are prescribed.

Medications used to treat Crohn's disease also are used to treat ulcerative colitis (see section on Crohn's Disease and Drug Therapy Table 53-1). Corticosteroids, given orally, IV, or rectally, are used if the disease does not respond to other measures. Because of unacceptable side effects associated with long-term use of corticosteroids, the dose is tapered and discontinued according to the client's response. When tapering corticosteroids without exacerbating the disease becomes impossible, immunomodulating agents (azathioprine, 6-mercaptopurine) are used to decrease the immune response and allow tapering. The goals of therapy are to induce and retain remission, allow the client to be as healthy as possible when contemplating elective surgery, or both.

Surgery is necessary when the disease does not respond to medical treatment or with complications such as dysplastic tissue (a precancerous condition), perforated colon, or hemorrhage. Removal of the colon under elective, nonemergent circumstances offers the client the best possible outcome and is the definitive cure. The current standard treatment is ileoanal pull-through and anastomosis (see Chap. 54). This procedure typically is done in two stages, several weeks apart. In the first stage, the colon is removed, and a rectal "pouch" is created from a section of the ileum. The rectal mucosa is removed to create a temporary ileostomy. In the second stage, the surgeon closes the ileostomy and connects the intestine to the rectum, allowing the client to defecate normally. When an emergency colectomy is performed (i.e., for toxic megacolon or perforation), an anastomosis (rejoining of the bowel) may be impossible, necessitating creation of a permanent ileostomy.

Nursing Management

The nurse obtains a health history to identify the nature of the abdominal pain, number and frequency of stools, anorexia, and weight loss. He or she asks the client about dietary patterns, including daily amounts of alcohol and caffeine. The nurse auscultates the abdomen for bowel sounds and their characteristics and palpates the abdomen to determine any pain or tenderness.

The nurse compiles a comprehensive database and conducts frequent focused assessments to identify early changes in the symptoms, which may herald rapidly progressing complications. Until the disease is confirmed, preparing clients for diagnostic tests is necessary. The nurse needs to question radiographic and endoscopic protocols for harsh laxatives and cleansing enemas when the client is experiencing severe diarrhea because bowel irritation and stimulation tend to aggravate the client's symptoms.

Once the diagnosis is confirmed, the physician orders drug and fluid therapy. If antispasmodics and opiates are prescribed, the nurse must exercise great caution when administering them because they may trigger the development of toxic megacolon. The nurse reports any sudden

onset of abdominal distention, severe pain, or fever in a client with acute ulcerative colitis. In addition, he or she observes the client receiving steroids for subtle changes because these drugs mask inflammatory symptoms accompanying complications. The dosage and frequency of steroids gradually are tapered when clients no longer need them. The nurse teaches the client about the disease and measures for self-care as soon as he or she is well enough to learn (Client and Family Teaching Box 53-1).

ACUTE ABDOMINAL INFLAMMATORY DISORDERS

Appendicitis and peritonitis are among disorders known as *acute abdominal inflammatory disorders.*

53-1 *Client and Family Teaching*
Inflammatory Bowel Disease

The nurse should include the following topics in the plan for teaching the client and family about IBD:

- Special dietary modifications and the importance of complying with them
- Name, purpose, dosage, and adverse effects of prescribed drugs
- Use of medications to control symptoms rather than cure the disease
- Importance of keeping all follow-up physician and laboratory appointments so potentially dangerous complications of disease and side effects of medications can be monitored
- Techniques for rectal hygiene and skin care
- Signs to report immediately to the physician such as more frequent bowel movements, extreme fatigue, severe abdominal pain, visible blood in the stool, adverse drug effects, or weight loss
- Recommendations for regular medical checkups, even when symptoms subside, because clients with ulcerative colitis have an increased risk for the development of colon cancer

Clients who are discharged and need high levels of care, such as enteral feeding or TPN, require extensive teaching specific to their home care needs. Central venous catheter care and maintenance of TPN are a few examples of these special learning needs. The nurse thoroughly covers all technical procedures for the client or significant other to perform and allows time for the client or caregiver to perform them with nursing supervision before discharge. The nurse makes a referral to a home care agency to provide continuity of care and to ease the transition from acute care to home care.

● APPENDICITIS

Appendicitis is inflammation of a narrow, blind protrusion called the *vermiform appendix* located at the tip of the cecum in the right lower quadrant (RLQ) of the abdomen (Fig. 53-3). Appendicitis can occur at any age but is most common in adolescents and young adults. It is difficult to diagnose at its onset because the initial symptoms resemble a host of other disorders such as gastroenteritis, Crohn's disease, ovarian cyst, tubal pregnancy, and inflammation of the kidney or ureter.

Pathophysiology and Etiology

The inflammation begins when the opening of the appendix narrows or becomes obstructed. The obstruction

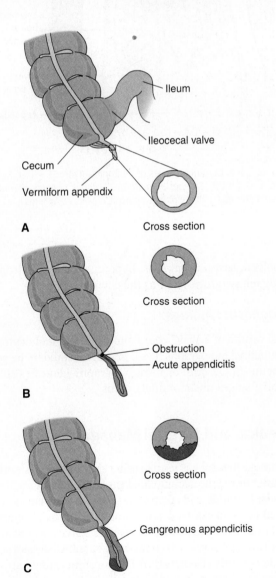

A

Ileum
Ileocecal valve
Cecum
Vermiform appendix
Cross section

B

Cross section
Obstruction
Acute appendicitis

C

Cross section
Gangrenous appendicitis

FIGURE 53-3 (**A**) Normal appendix. (**B**) Acute appendicitis resulting from obstruction (note the narrowing in the cross section). (**C**) Appendicitis and gangrene.

may result from a hard mass of feces, called a *fecalith*, a foreign body, local edema, or a tumor. The blockage interferes with the drainage of secretions from the appendix, and they accumulate in the confined space. The appendix enlarges and distends, and the swelling compresses surrounding blood vessels. The locally damaged cells are then easily infected with bacteria from within the intestinal lumen. Unless the inflammation resolves, the appendix can become gangrenous or rupture, spilling bacteria throughout the peritoneal cavity.

Assessment Findings

An attack of abdominal pain is the most frequent symptom. At first, the pain is generalized throughout the abdomen or around the umbilicus. Later, the pain localizes in the RLQ at McBurney's point, an area midway between the umbilicus and the right iliac crest. Often the pain is worse when manual pressure near the region is suddenly released, a condition called *rebound tenderness*. Fever, nausea, and vomiting may be present. The abdomen is tense, and the client usually flexes the right hip to relieve the discomfort.

A WBC count reveals moderate leukocytosis. When a differential count of leukocytes is performed, it shows an ever-increasing number of immature neutrophils, indicating a progressive worsening of the inflammatory condition. A computed tomography (CT) scan or abdominal ultrasound shows enlargement at the cecum.

Medical and Surgical Management

Antibiotics are given, and the client is restricted from eating or drinking while a decision is made about surgery. IV fluids are prescribed to meet the client's fluid needs. Analgesics may be withheld initially to avoid masking symptoms that may affect the diagnosis. If symptoms worsen, the surgeon performs an **appendectomy** to remove the appendix before it spontaneously ruptures. The appendix has no known function in the body. Its removal results in cure with no physiologic changes.

Nursing Management

The nurse assesses vital signs and the client's pain to detect early changes in the symptoms. If ordered, the nurse administers IV fluid therapy and observes the client's response to antibiotics. When analgesics are withheld, the nurse is empathetic and facilitates comfort with positioning, imagery, and distraction.

When surgery is indicated, preparing the client quickly is important to avoid delay that may cause surgical complications. Soon after surgery, if no complications occur, the client ambulates and tries light nourishment. Convalescence may be rapid, although postoperative progress depends on the client's age, general physical condition, and extent of complications. A healthy young adult usually can return to normal activities soon. Clients need to avoid heavy lifting or unusual exertion, however, for several months. For more specific nursing interventions when caring for a client undergoing surgery, see Chapter 25.

Stop, Think, and Respond ● BOX 53-2

An older adult client presents with vague symptoms of lower abdominal pain, nausea, and one episode of vomiting. In the initial assessment, what is an important question to ask?

● PERITONITIS

Pathophysiology and Etiology

In **peritonitis,** the peritoneum, a serous sac lining the abdominal cavity, becomes inflamed. Peritonitis may be caused by perforation of a peptic ulcer, the bowel, or the appendix; abdominal trauma, such as gunshot or knife wounds; IBD; ruptured ectopic pregnancy; or infection introduced during peritoneal dialysis, a procedure used to treat kidney failure. Refer to Figure 53-4 for common causes of peritonitis.

Spillage of chemical contents and bacteria inflames the peritoneum, which leads to localized abscess formation or generalized inflammation. When generalized peritonitis occurs, vascular fluid shifts to the abdomen, lowering blood pressure and producing hypovolemic shock or septic shock. If the condition is not treated promptly or adequately, death may follow.

Assessment Findings

Signs and Symptoms

Symptoms include severe abdominal pain, distention, tenderness, nausea, and vomiting. Fever may be absent initially, but the temperature rises as infection becomes established. The client avoids moving the abdomen when breathing because movement increases pain. He or she may draw the knees up toward the abdomen to lessen the pain. Lack of bowel motility typically accompanies peritonitis. The abdomen feels rigid and boardlike as it distends with gas and intestinal contents. Bowel sounds typically are absent. The pulse rate is elevated, and respirations are rapid and shallow. If the peritonitis is un-

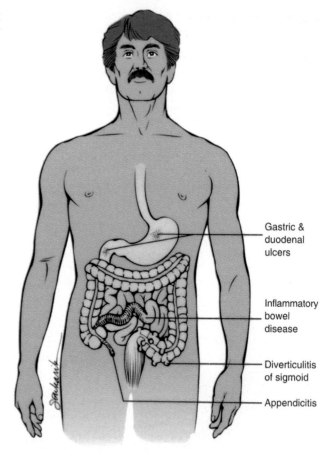

FIGURE 53-4 Common causes of peritonitis. (From Smeltzer, S. C. & Bare, B. G. [2000]. *Brunner & Suddarth's textbook of medical–surgical nursing* [9th ed.]. Philadelphia: Lippincott Williams & Wilkins.)

Gastric & duodenal ulcers

Inflammatory bowel disease

Diverticulitis of sigmoid

Appendicitis

resolved, severe weakness, hypotension, and a drop in body temperature occur as the client nears death.

Diagnostic Findings

The results of a WBC count show marked leukocytosis. Abdominal radiographs reveal free air and fluid in the peritoneum. A CT scan or ultrasonography identifies structural changes in abdominal organs.

Medical and Surgical Management

A nasogastric tube is used to relieve abdominal distention by suctioning the accumulated gas and stagnant upper GI fluids. IV fluids and electrolytes replace substances relocated in the peritoneal cavity and lost through vomiting and drainage from gastric intubation. Large doses of antibiotics are prescribed to combat infection. Analgesics such as meperidine (Demerol) or IV morphine sulfate are ordered to relieve pain and promote rest. The perforation is surgically closed so that intestinal contents can no longer escape.

Nursing Management

The nurse monitors the acutely ill client while completing preparations for diagnostic tests or surgery. He or she administers analgesics and infuses IV fluids with secondary administrations of antibiotics. If ordered, a nurse passes a nasogastric tube and connects it to suction (see Chap. 52). The client may need a urinary retention catheter. The nurse assesses the circulatory status by taking vital signs frequently and monitoring central venous and pulmonary artery pressures.

For the client who has had surgery, the nurse assesses the client's vital signs, fluid balance, the incision, dressing, and drains. Assessing the client's pain level is important, as is medicating according to the medical orders. For clients who have prolonged recovery time, TPN may be initiated.

Clients are fearful of the emergent nature of the peritonitis and subsequent surgery. The nurse provides frequent explanations and emotional support. Clients also need monitoring for continued abdominal infection. If the client experiences abdominal distention, fever, changes in level of consciousness, or deviations in vital signs, the nurse must notify the physician quickly. Refer to Chapter 25 for further management of the postoperative client.

INTESTINAL OBSTRUCTION ●

Intestinal obstruction occurs when a blockage interferes with the normal progression of intestinal contents through the intestinal tract. The causes are classified as mechanical or nonmechanical (adynamic) and as partial or complete. The severity depends on the region of the bowel affected, degree to which the lumen is obstructed, and degree to which blood circulation to the intestine is impeded (Smeltzer & Bare, 2000). An intestinal obstruction is extremely dangerous and may be fatal if not treated promptly.

Pathophysiology and Etiology

Mechanical obstructions result from a narrowing of the bowel lumen with or without a space-occupying mass. A mass may include a tumor, *adhesions* (fibrous bands that constrict tissue), incarcerated or strangulated hernias, **volvulus** (a kinking of a portion of intestine), **intussusception** (a telescoping of one part of the intestine into an adjacent part), or impacted feces or barium (Table 53-2).

The intestine can become adynamic (lacking peristalsis, a condition referred to as **paralytic ileus**) from an absence of normal nerve stimulation to intestinal muscle fibers. Paralytic ileus is common 12 to 36 hours after abdominal surgery. It also can result from inflammatory conditions (e.g., peritonitis), electrolyte disturbances

TABLE 53-2	MECHANICAL CAUSES OF OBSTRUCTION
CAUSE AND COURSE OF EVENTS	**APPEARANCE**
Adhesions—Loops of intestine adhere to areas that heal slowly or scar after abdominal surgery. The adhesions cause the intestinal loop to kink 3 to 4 days later.	
Intussusception—One part of the intestine slips into another lower part (like a telescope shortening). The intestinal lumen narrows.	
Volvulus—The bowel twists and turns on itself, obstructing the intestinal lumen. Gas and fluid accumulate in the trapped bowel.	
Hernia—The intestine protrudes through a weakened area in the abdominal muscle or wall. Intestinal flow and blood flow to the area may be completely obstructed.	
Tumor—A tumor in the intestinal wall extends into the intestinal lumen; or a tumor outside the intestine causes pressure on the intestinal wall. The lumen becomes partially obstructed; if the tumor is not removed, complete obstruction results.	

(e.g., hypokalemia), or adverse drug effects (e.g., narcotics, cholinergic blockers). Even a vascular embolus or low blood flow during shock can interfere with the neuromuscular function of the bowel.

When the intestinal contents cannot move freely, the portion above the obstruction distends, whereas the portion below the obstruction is empty. If the obstruction is complete, no gases or feces are expelled rectally. Both forward and reverse peristalsis becomes forceful in an attempt to clear the obstruction. Stasis of the accumulating volume and the violent muscular peristaltic contractions potentiate the risk for intestinal rupture.

Locally, the increased pressure pushes electrolyte-rich fluid from the intestine and capillaries into the peritoneal cavity. Failure of the mucosa to reabsorb the secretions contributes to water and electrolyte imbalances and shock. Increasing pressure on the bowel from severe distention and edema impairs circulation and leads to necrosis and eventually gangrene of a portion of the bowel. Perforation of the gangrenous bowel, which results from pressure against weakened tissue, causes the intestinal contents to seep into the peritoneal cavity, resulting in peritonitis.

Small bowel obstruction and large bowel obstruction are similar in terms of development and resulting pathophysiology. Dehydration occurs more slowly with large intestine obstruction, however, because the colon can absorb the fluid contents and distend to a considerably greater size.

Assessment Findings

Signs and Symptoms

Nausea and abdominal distention are common. When an obstruction occurs high in the GI tract, the client usually vomits whatever contents are in the stomach and small intestine. The emesis appears to contain bile or fecal material. If the obstruction is lower in the GI tract, vomiting may not occur. The client may have one or two bowel movements soon after the intestine has been obstructed because he or she is expelling the material already past the obstruction. The client may experience severe intermittent cramps. Sudden, sustained pain, abdominal distention, and fever are symptoms of perforation.

In a nonmechanical obstruction, peristalsis is absent; therefore, bowel sounds are not heard. In a mechanical obstruction, the bowel sounds usually are high-pitched above the obstructed area. Pulse and respiratory rates are elevated. Blood pressure falls, and urine output decreases if shock develops.

Clinical symptoms associated with large bowel obstruction occur more slowly. Constipation may be the only symptom for many days. Eventually the client experiences abdominal distention. It is possible to see loops of bowel outlined through the abdominal wall, and the client complains of lower abdominal cramps and pain. Fecal vomiting also may occur. The client can have symptoms of shock.

Diagnostic Findings

A radiographic study of the abdomen shows air and fluid collecting in a segment of the intestine. A barium enema (used when the risk of perforation is low) pinpoints the location of the obstruction. Tests of serum electrolytes may indicate low levels of sodium, potassium, and chloride. Metabolic alkalosis is evidenced by arterial blood gas results. A complete blood count (CBC) shows an increased WBC count in instances of infection. The hematocrit level is elevated if dehydration develops.

Medical and Surgical Management

While diagnostic tests are done to determine the cause and appropriate treatment for the client's obstruction, the client receives medical support. The client receives nothing by mouth (NPO). IV fluids with electrolytes are administered to correct fluid and electrolyte imbalances, and antibiotics are ordered to treat infection.

To relieve intestinal distention, cramping, and vomiting and to reduce the potential for intestinal rupture with peritonitis, intestinal decompression is begun. Intestinal decompression is accomplished by suctioning large amounts of accumulated secretions and gas through a nasogastric tube or longer intestinal tube, which may or may not be weighted. Nasogastric tubes are used when the obstruction is partial or located high in the small intestine.

Before surgery, decompression alone may be sufficient to relieve a nonmechanical obstruction or symptoms in clients who are undergoing surgery for mechanical obstruction. In some cases, mechanical obstructions are treated during colonoscopy by removing obstructing polyps or destroying benign tumors with laser therapy or electrocautery. Most mechanical obstructions, however, require surgery. Usually, a section of the obstructed bowel is removed and then the proximal and distal sections are reconnected (bowel resection and anastomosis). A temporary or permanent ostomy (see Chap. 54) may be performed in some cases.

Nursing Management

In addition to the assessments performed on the client with a GI disorder, the nurse obtains complete medical, drug, and allergy histories, assesses fluid intake and output, and takes vital signs. Documenting all symptoms and obtaining detailed information about each is important. For example, if vomiting has occurred, the nurse gathers information regarding its onset, amount, and color. If an intestinal tube has been inserted, the nurse monitors its progress (Nursing Guidelines 53-1).

The care of a client with an intestinal obstruction involves managing pain, maintaining fluid balance to prevent deficits related to fluid shifts and losses from vomiting, and helping the client deal with fear related to severe, possibly life-threatening symptoms and an unstable condition. The nurse also manages pain by maintaining the patency of the decompression tube and administering a prescribed narcotic analgesic as long as blood pressure and respiratory rate indicate that doing so is safe. The nurse maintains uninterrupted infusion of IV fluids and shortens the siege of vomiting by maintaining intestinal decompression, even though intestinal fluid is lost in the suctioning. It is crucial to monitor urinary output hourly and to report output below 50 mL/hour, a finding that may indicate that the client is going into shock.

NURSING GUIDELINES 53-1

Managing Care of a Client With an Intestinal Tube

Preparations

- Auscultate and examine the abdomen for bowel sounds, distention, and tenderness.

- To provide a baseline for reference, measure abdominal girth, placing a measuring tape about the largest diameter of the abdomen.

- Mark the measuring location on the skin (with an indelible marker) to facilitate consistency when obtaining future comparison measurements.

- Assemble all the equipment the physician will need. If a weighted double-lumen tube is selected, label the tip of the adapter leading to the lumen through which tungsten gel is instilled to avoid confusing which lumen to use for suction.

Tube Advancement

- After the physician inserts the tube, ambulate the client, if possible, to facilitate tube passage through the pylorus. When a radiographic image indicates that the tube has advanced beyond the stomach, position the client as follows:

  –On the right side for 2 hours, then

  –On the back in a Fowler's position for 2 hours, then

  –On the left side for 2 hours.

- Observe the lines or numbers on the tube periodically to evaluate the tube's progressive movement and approximate anatomic location.

- Advance the tube several inches at specified intervals as directed to avoid tension as it descends into the intestine.

- Stabilize or tape the tube to the nose after a radiographic image verifies that the tube has reached the obstruction. Coil the excess length, securing it to the bedding or the client's hospital gown.

- Attach the proximal end to suction.

- Prepare for radiography to be performed daily to evaluate progress toward relieving the obstruction.

Removal

- Remove the tube once the obstruction is relieved or another treatment replaces intubation.

- Disconnect the tube from suction.

- If removing a weighted tube, withdraw the tungsten gel by aspirating it with a 10-mL syringe. Remove the tungsten gel in the other types of tubes after the tube is withdrawn.

- Withdraw 6 to 10 inches of the tube between 10-minute pauses. When the tube is in the esophagus, as determined by 18 inches of length remaining in the client, flush the tube with a small amount of air to remove debris.

- Clamp the tube to prevent secretions from being deposited in the client's upper airway and instruct the client to hold the breath while the tube exits the esophagus.

- If removing a Cantor-like or Harris-like tube, grasp the bag of tungsten gel with a forceps and withdraw it from the client's mouth when it reaches the oropharynx.

- Once the tungsten gel is removed from the bag, remove the tube from the client's nose. Provide nasal and oral hygiene immediately afterward.

DIVERTICULAR DISORDERS

Diverticula are sacs or pouches caused by herniation of the mucosa through a weakened portion of the muscular coat of the intestine or other structure (Fig. 53-5). They can appear anywhere in the GI tract (see Chap. 52).

● DIVERTICULOSIS AND DIVERTICULITIS

Asymptomatic diverticula are called **diverticulosis.** When the diverticula become inflamed, the term **diverticulitis** is used. Diverticula are common in the colon, especially in the sigmoid area in people older than 50 years of age.

Pathophysiology and Etiology

The incidence of diverticula is higher in individuals who have a low intake of dietary fiber. There also may be a congenital predisposition. It is thought that most diver-

Diverticula

FIGURE 53-5 Intestinal diverticula, particularly common in the sigmoid colon of older adults, usually do not cause symptoms except for occasional rectal bleeding. They may become inflamed and infected from fecal matter that becomes lodged in the pouchlike herniations.

ticula result from weakness in the muscular coat associated with aging.

Diverticula become inflamed when fecal material becomes trapped in one or more blind pouches. The inflammation causes swelling of the tissue in the area. If the localized swelling involves several diverticula in one area, the edema may be severe enough to cause an intestinal obstruction. Abscesses form when the inflamed tissue becomes infected with intestinal bacteria present in the bowel. The swollen tissue has the potential to rupture into the peritoneal cavity or form a fistular connection with an adjacent organ such as the bladder.

Assessment Findings

Constipation alternating with diarrhea, flatulence, pain and tenderness in the left lower quadrant, fever, and rectal bleeding may occur. A palpable mass may be felt in the lower abdomen. When the diverticula bleed, the stools appear maroon and are sometimes described as resembling "currant jelly."

A barium enema shows an irregular mucosal wall. A colonoscopy helps visualize the areas of inflammation. A CT scan may be used as an alternative to a barium enema or colonoscopy because both require an aggressive bowel preparation that may be contraindicated when the large intestine is acutely inflamed. Risk for perforation is increased. A CBC shows leukocytosis. A stool specimen may reveal occult blood.

Medical and Surgical Management

Diverticula noted during routine examination require no treatment if they do not cause symptoms. Avoiding foods that contain seeds of any kind is recommended. A high-fiber diet supplemented with bran or prescription of a bulk-forming agent (e.g., Metamucil) helps to avoid constipation.

When symptoms occur, the diet is temporarily adjusted to low-residue foods. If the inflammation is severe and accompanied by pain and local tenderness, the client is maintained on IV fluids for several days with no oral intake. As the inflammation subsides under antibiotic therapy, oral fluids and food are reintroduced.

If the diverticulitis does not respond to medical treatment, or if complications such as perforation, intestinal obstruction, or severe bleeding occur, surgery becomes necessary. The portion of colon that contains the diverticula is removed, and the continuity of the bowel is reestablished by joining the remaining portions of the colon. Depending on the location and extent of the disease and whether there is intestinal obstruction, a temporary colostomy may be necessary (see Chap. 54). The continuity of the bowel is restored, and the colostomy is closed 3 to 6 weeks later.

Nursing Management

In addition to the assessments performed on the client with a GI disorder, the nurse obtains a history of symptoms, diet, drug use, and allergies and asks questions regarding pain, bowel elimination, and diet habits. He or she takes vital signs to establish a baseline and to determine if the client is febrile. The nurse examines the abdomen for pain, tenderness, and masses.

Explaining the underlying pathology and rationale for treatment is important. Because dietary compliance reduces the potential for recurrences, consulting the dietitian for teaching is useful. If surgery becomes necessary, the nurse prepares the client before surgery and manages the postoperative care. A dietary consult or a list of foods to eat or avoid is necessary. The nurse includes the following points in the teaching plan:

- Follow the diet recommended by the physician, which will probably reduce pain and discomfort.
- Bran adds bulk to the diet. Unprocessed bran can be sprinkled over cereal or added to fruit juice.
- Avoid the use of laxatives or enemas except when recommended by the physician.
- Avoid constipation. Do not suppress the urge to defecate.
- Drink at least 8 to 10 large glasses of fluid each day.
- Take prescribed medications as directed, even if symptoms improve.
- Exercise regularly if the current lifestyle is somewhat inactive.
- If severe pain or blood in the stool occurs, see a physician immediately.

ABDOMINAL HERNIA

Although **hernia** refers to the protrusion of any organ from the cavity that normally confines it, the term most commonly is used to describe the protrusion of the intestine through a defect in the abdominal wall. Certain areas in the abdominal wall are weaker than other areas and more vulnerable to the development of a hernia. These areas include the inguinal ring, the point on the abdominal wall where the inguinal canal begins; the femoral ring at the abdominal opening of the femoral canal; and the umbilicus.

If the protruding structures can be replaced in the abdominal cavity, it is a *reducible hernia*. Placing the client in a supine position and applying manual pressure over the area may reduce the hernia. An *irreducible* or *incarcerated hernia* is one in which the intestine cannot be replaced in the abdominal cavity because of edema of the protruding segment and constriction of the muscle opening through which it has emerged. If the process continues without treatment, the blood supply to the trapped segment of bowel can be cut off, leading to gangrene. This development is referred to as a *strangulated hernia.*

Pathophysiology and Etiology

The most common abdominal hernias are *inguinal, umbilical, femoral,* and *incisional* (Box 53-2), with inguinal hernias the most common type. Inguinal hernias are more prevalent in men than women. Umbilical and femoral hernias are more frequent among women than men.

A hernia develops when intra-abdominal pressure increases, such as while straining to lift something heavy, having a bowel movement, or coughing or sneezing forcefully. When the pressure increases, a segment of intestine moves into a weak area of abdominal muscle. In the areas that are naturally predisposed to weakness, the abdominal wall may be thin or stretched from an inadequate amount of collagen. Such a condition may be present at birth or develop as a result of aging, abdominal surgery, or obesity.

At first, the defect in the abdominal wall is small. As the hernia persists and the organs continue to protrude, the defect grows larger. Eventually the bowel becomes

trapped in the weakened pouch. If the blood supply to the bowel is compromised, it becomes gangrenous.

Assessment Findings

A hernia initially causes swelling on the abdomen with no other symptoms. When the client coughs or bears down, the protrusion is more obvious. Sometimes the swelling is painful, but the pain subsides when the hernia is reduced. Incarcerated hernias cause severe pain, and if not treated, may become strangulated. In this case, the client suffers extreme abdominal pain. The severe pressure on the loop of intestine protruding outside the abdominal cavity causes intestinal obstruction.

Medical and Surgical Management

When a hernia forms, it tends to enlarge, leading to serious complications. Surgery is the only method of eliminating a hernia. Some clients, either because they are unwilling to have or are not candidates for surgery, may wear a truss, an apparatus that presses over the hernia and prevents protrusion of the bowel. The client also may lie supine while manual pressure is applied over the protruding area to reduce the hernia periodically. Some clients learn to do this themselves.

A **herniorrhaphy,** the surgical repair of a hernia, is the recommended treatment. When a herniorrhaphy is performed, the protruding intestine is repositioned in the abdominal cavity and the defect in the abdominal wall is repaired. Herniorrhaphy is performed under local, spinal, or general anesthesia. Some types of hernias can be treated using a laparoscopic approach. When a hernia is neglected for many years, the tissues in the area weaken, and postoperative healing may be impaired. Obese people who have put off surgical repair for a prolonged period are especially prone to recurrence of the hernia, despite surgical repair. For these cases, the surgeon also may perform a **hernioplasty.** The weakened area is reinforced with wire, fascia, or mesh. The obese client usually is advised to lose weight before the surgery to lessen the possibility of recurrence.

Strangulation is an acute emergency. Unless surgery is performed promptly, blood flow to the intestine is impaired. If necrosis occurs, the gangrenous part of the intestine must be excised and portions of the intestine reconnected.

Nursing Management

If the client is managing herniation with a truss and not undergoing surgery, nursing care centers primarily on teaching. The nurse educates the client about ways to avoid constipation, control a cough, and perform proper body mechanics. The client needs to know the signs of

---

BOX 53-2 ● **Types of Hernias**

Inguinal—Protrusion of the hernial sac contains the intestine at the inguinal opening.
  Direct—Hernia extends through inguinal ring; it follows spermatic cord in males and round ligament in females.
  Indirect—Protrusion follows the posterior inguinal wall; it often descends into the scrotum in males.
Umbilical—Hernia occurs in the umbilical region, through which the hernial sac protrudes. This type occurs in children when the umbilical orifice fails to close shortly after birth. It may occur in obese adults who have prolonged abdominal distention.
Femoral—Intestines descend through the femoral ring where the femoral artery passes into the femoral canal, below the inguinal ligament. Incidence of strangulation is high.
Incisional—This type occurs through the scar of a surgical incision when healing is impaired. Careful surgical technique, particularly prevention of wound infection, can prevent incisional hernias. Obese, older, or malnourished clients are prone to the development of incisional hernias.

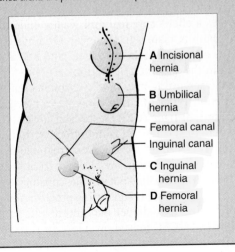

A Incisional hernia
B Umbilical hernia
Femoral canal
Inguinal canal
C Inguinal hernia
D Femoral hernia

incarceration and strangulation of the hernia. The nurse teaches the client how to wear a truss and observe for and treat skin irritation from friction caused by continuous rubbing. Advising the client to keep the skin clean and dry or to use cornstarch to absorb moisture is an important intervention. The nurse also explains that compression from a truss may produce localized edema from interference with lymphatic and venous blood flow.

When surgery is scheduled, the nurse prepares the client and manages postoperative care (see Chap. 25). The assessment of clients undergoing surgery includes obtaining a complete medical and drug history because malnutrition, diabetes, or concurrent use of corticosteroids or antimetabolite cancer drugs can affect wound healing. The nurse also obtains the client's allergy history, especially to seasonal inhalants (i.e., ragweed pollen), and smoking history because sneezing and coughing can increase intra-abdominal pressure after surgery and place the client at risk for weakening the surgical repair. Before surgery, the nurse takes vital signs, auscultates the lungs to identify infectious or respiratory risk factors, and documents the client's weight and duration of the hernia. These factors influence the potential for postoperative healing complications. The client's previous surgical experience may affect how the client feels about this surgery. The nurse also assesses the client's urinary and bowel patterns to determine if the client has any preexisting problems affecting elimination. After surgery, the nurse inspects the scrotum of male clients because it is common for edema to follow surgical repair.

Hernia repairs are performed mainly on an outpatient basis. Therefore, the nurse teaches measures to the client and significant others who will provide care after discharge. The nurse needs to reinforce verbal instructions with written instructions about signs and symptoms of possible complications (i.e., bleeding, infection) and the need to report these symptoms to the physician. The instructions include techniques for avoiding constipation and straining to have a bowel movement. The nurse also includes instructions to avoid strenuous exertion and heavy lifting until the physician determines that the client can safely undertake such activities. For clients who perform heavy physical labor, it is essential to explore how they may modify the manner in which they perform their jobs, take an extended sick leave, or apply for a temporary leave of absence. The nurse explains to those whose work is sedentary or light that they usually can return to full employment with few activity restrictions within a few weeks.

CANCER OF THE COLON AND RECTUM

Intestinal malignancies may develop anywhere in the lower GI tract. Approximately 75% of cases develop in the lower sigmoid colon and rectum. Colorectal cancer ranks second among causes of cancer deaths in the United States. The incidence of the disease increases with age. The American Cancer Society recommends annual fecal occult blood testing every 5 years and colonoscopy every 10 years for colorectal cancer screening in individuals older than 50 years of age. This screening may be done for younger clients who have risk factors, such as a family history of colorectal cancer or ulcerative colitis.

Pathophysiology and Etiology

Many malignant colorectal tumors develop from benign adenomas in the mucosal and submucosal intestinal layers. It is believed that genetic, environmental, and lifestyle factors spark the transformation from a benign to a cancerous state. Catalysts seem to include chronic bowel inflammation, as in ulcerative colitis, and a lifetime pattern of eating low-fiber, high-fat foods.

Having a blood relative with this disease is a high-risk factor. Genetic testing may be carried out to identify some types of familial colon cancer. At some point, the normal cells undergo mutation, which affects their proliferation and growth pattern. Some believe that an *oncogene,* a genetic messenger that stimulates tumor growth, is not adequately suppressed. Without growth inhibition, the neoplastic cells reproduce rapidly and later proceed to invade the muscle wall. Other research suggests that a gene mutation interferes with the ability of colon cells to copy their DNA molecule correctly.

Although the malignant growth remains in situ (confined to its site of origin), it may change the shape of the stool, compressing it or making it appear pencil-like as it passes by the protruding mass. Untreated, the cancer extends to other organs by way of the mesentery lymph nodes or portal vein leading to the liver.

Assessment Findings

The chief characteristic of cancer of the colon is a change in bowel habits, such as alternating constipation and diarrhea. Occult or frank blood may be present in the stool. Sometimes a client may feel dull, vague abdominal discomfort. Pain is a late sign of cancer. On physical assessment, the abdomen feels distended, and a mass may be palpated in the abdomen or rectum.

Genetic screening may detect chromosomal markers for particular types of colon cancer. An elevated carcinoembryonic antigen (CEA) test result suggests a tumor. Unfortunately, a CEA test is not effective in identifying colorectal cancer in its earliest, most treatable stages. Unless the malignant growths are elevated from the mucosal wall, a barium enema may not provide conclusive evidence either. A tissue sample taken during proctosigmoidoscopy or colonoscopy may detect malignant cells in the area of the biopsy. A CBC may show a low erythrocyte count from chronic blood loss.

Medical and Surgical Management

When polyps are discovered during endoscopic examination, they are removed and examined. Even if the polyps are benign, the client continues to undergo periodic radiographic and endoscopic examinations to identify recurrent polyps for early malignant changes. An exception to this rule is the finding of juvenile polyps in young children. These benign growths do not tend to recur. The primary treatment of colorectal cancer is surgical, but sometimes treatment involves a combination of surgery, radiation therapy, and chemotherapy.

An encapsulated colorectal tumor may be removed without taking away surrounding healthy tissue. This type of tumor, however, may call for partial or complete surgical removal of the colon (**colectomy**). Occasionally, the tumor causes a partial or complete bowel obstruction. If the tumor is in the colon and upper third of the rectum, a **segmental resection** is performed. In this procedure, the surgeon removes the cancerous portion of colon and rejoins the remaining portions of the GI tract to restore normal intestinal continuity.

Cancers in the lower third of the rectum are treated with an **abdominoperineal resection**—wide excision of the rectum and creation of a sigmoid colostomy. The surgical procedures used to treat cancers in the middle third of the rectum vary. A low resection with a temporary colostomy usually is attempted to preserve the anal sphincter. Radiation therapy is indicated in many cases of colon cancer, whereas chemotherapy usually is reserved for those with evidence of lymphatic infiltration or metastasis. If the cancer metastasizes, a colostomy may be performed to relieve an intestinal obstruction. In some cases the obstruction is relieved or bleeding is controlled with laser surgery.

Nursing Management

The nurse advises and prepares clients for routine colorectal screening. He or she follows standard guidelines for collecting stool specimens and sending them to the laboratory for analysis (Box 53-3). The nurse advises anyone who is asymptomatic but whose stool test results are positive for blood to undergo a colonoscopy, the next step in cancer detection. Nursing management of the client with a colostomy is discussed in Chapter 54.

ANORECTAL DISORDERS

Clients with anorectal disorders usually experience localized pain and bleeding, and thus seek medical attention. They also may have problems with perianal itching, tenderness, and swelling. They may delay defecation secondary to pain and other discomfort.

BOX 53-3 ● Testing Stool for Occult Blood

Seven to 10 days before and throughout the test, the nurse:
- Tells the client not to drink alcohol or take aspirin, NSAIDs, vitamin C, or iron preparations
- Checks with physician if anticoagulants, steroids, colchicines (used to treat gout), or cimetidine (for peptic ulcer treatment) have been prescribed

Two days before and throughout the test, the nurse:
- Advises client to consume a high-fiber diet and to avoid red meat, substituting with poultry and fish
- Informs client to avoid turnips, cauliflower, broccoli, cantaloupe, horseradish, and parsnips

During the test, the nurse or client:
- Collects stool within a toilet liner or bedpan
- Uses an applicator stick and removes a sample from the center of the stool
- Applies a thin smear of stool onto the test area supplied with the screening kit
- Takes care to cover the entire space
- Places two drops of developer solution onto the test area
- Waits precisely 60 seconds
- Observes for a blue color, indicating a positive reaction (for more valid results, test samples from several stools over 3 to 6 days)

● HEMORRHOIDS

Hemorrhoids are dilated veins outside or inside the anal sphincter (Fig. 53-6). Thrombosed hemorrhoids are veins that contain clots.

Pathophysiology and Etiology

Chronic straining to have a bowel movement or frequent defecation with chronic diarrhea likely weakens the tissue supporting the veins. Clients whose work requires prolonged sitting are at increased risk for the development of hemorrhoids. Pregnancy, prolonged labor, portal hypertension, or other intra-abdominal conditions that inter-

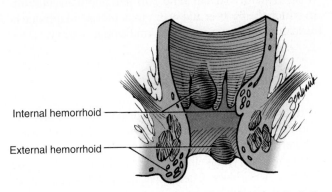

FIGURE 53-6 Internal and external hemorrhoids. (From Smeltzer, S. C. & Bare, B. G. [2000]. *Brunner & Suddarth's textbook of medical–surgical nursing* [9th ed.]. Philadelphia: Lippincott Williams & Wilkins.)

fere with venous blood return can cause or aggravate the condition. The veins near the anal sphincter probably are displaced downward from their natural location as the result of a loss of supporting tissue. Without adequate connective tissue and smooth muscle support, the veins dilate and fill with blood. Dry stool passes by the engorged hemorrhoids, which stretches and irritates the mucosa, giving rise to the local symptoms of burning, itching, and pain. Passing dry, hard stool causes the hemorrhoids to bleed.

Assessment Findings

External hemorrhoids may cause few symptoms, or they can produce pain, itching, and soreness of the anal area. They appear as small, reddish-blue lumps at the edge of the anus. Thrombosed external hemorrhoids are painful but seldom cause bleeding.

Internal hemorrhoids cause bleeding but are less likely to cause pain, unless they protrude through the anus. The amount of bleeding varies from an occasional drop or two of blood on toilet tissue or underwear to chronic loss of blood, leading to anemia. Internal hemorrhoids usually protrude each time the client defecates but retract after defecation. As the masses enlarge, they remain outside the sphincter.

An anoscope, an instrument for examining the anal canal, or a proctosigmoidoscope allows visualization of internal hemorrhoids. A colonoscopy rules out colorectal cancer, which has similar symptoms.

Medical Management

Small external hemorrhoids may disappear without treatment, or the client may obtain relief through symptomatic treatment. The physician may recommend warm soaks, an ointment that contains a local anesthetic for the relief of pain and itching, topical astringent pads to relieve swelling, a diet that corrects or prevents constipation, and a stool softener. In some cases the hemorrhoid is ligated (tied off) with a rubber band. Infrared photocoagulation, in which the protein and water in hemorrhoidal tissue is destroyed, is an alternative to traditional surgery.

Surgical Management

A **hemorrhoidectomy,** the surgical removal of hemorrhoids, may be necessary in chronic and severe cases. The procedure is performed using conventional surgery or laser surgery; the client receives a local anesthetic or regional nerve block. Internal packing of lubricated gauze, external gauze dressing, or a perineal pad is applied to absorb blood. A T-binder holds the absorbent material in place.

Nursing Management

The nurse gathers a complete history, including drug and allergy histories. Because bleeding accompanies many colorectal disorders, it is important to ask the client to describe the bleeding as well as other related symptoms. The nurse determines if there is a history of constipation or alternating diarrhea and constipation, and if the client uses any prescription or nonprescription drugs. In addition, the nurse obtains a diet history, paying particular attention to the type of foods (especially fiber) included in the diet. The physical examination involves putting on gloves, draping the client, and inspecting the anus.

Health teaching is focused on self-management. The nurse reviews the physician's home care instructions, demonstrates wound care to the client or responsible caregiver and provides an opportunity for returning the demonstration, provides dietary recommendations and offers a list of high-fiber foods, instructs about stool softeners as indicated, emphasizes the importance of an active lifestyle and increased fluid intake, and cautions against the prolonged use of laxatives.

● ANORECTAL ABSCESS

An anorectal abscess is an infection with a collection of pus in an area between the internal and external sphincters.

Pathophysiology and Etiology

The original source of the infection may be microorganisms harbored in the intestine itself. An anorectal abscess is common among clients with Crohn's disease. Anorectal infections, however, also are transmitted from others through anal intercourse or foreign bodies inserted into the rectum.

Usually, infectious microorganisms invade anal crypts, small tubular cavities in the anal skin and rectal mucosa. A purulent exudate collects, and the pressure causes pain and swelling. The abscess eventually may develop into a fistulous tract.

Assessment Findings

Clients with an anorectal abscess experience pain that is aggravated by walking and sitting or other activities that increase intra-abdominal pressure such as coughing, sneezing, and straining to have a bowel movement. A swollen mass is evident in the anus. Fever and abdominal pain develop if the abscess has extended into deeper tissues. Foul-smelling drainage may leak from the anus if the abscess spontaneously ruptures. A culture of anal drainage reveals the infectious microorganism.

Medical and Surgical Management

Analgesics and sitz baths are prescribed to relieve symptoms. Antibiotic therapy is used to treat gonorrheal, staphylococcal, streptococcal, or other drug-sensitive bacteria. An incision and drainage to remove the infected material may be necessary. If a fistula has formed, deeper excision and removal of the fistulous tract are necessary. Because fistula formation frequently is associated with Crohn's disease, additional diagnostic testing may be necessary to determine the presence of this condition.

Nursing Management

To limit the spread of infectious microorganisms, the nurse instructs the client to practice scrupulous handwashing after each bowel movement, to use separate hygiene articles, to cleanse the bathtub after each use, and to use a condom if having anal intercourse. Refer to the nursing management of a client with an anorectal disorder for specific nursing interventions.

● ANAL FISSURE

An anal **fissure** (fissure in ano) is a linear tear in the anal canal tissue.

Pathophysiology and Etiology

Constipation is the leading cause of anal fissures. Other factors that may lead to formation of a slitlike tear include eversion of the anus during vaginal delivery and trauma to the anus, such as during anal intercourse or through the insertion of foreign bodies or medical instruments. When the anal canal is excessively stretched, the skin rips apart, exposing the underlying tissue.

Assessment Findings

Severe pain and bleeding on defecation are common. If constipation was not an original problem, it becomes one. Most clients with an anal fissure are reluctant to defecate because of the associated pain. The torn area may be visible when the anus is visually inspected, and the irregular surface of the fissure may be felt during a digital examination. Anoscopy provides evidence of the altered integrity of the anal mucosa.

Medical and Surgical Management

Treatment includes applying anesthetic creams, ointments, or suppositories; taking sitz baths and analgesics; and preventing constipation. Surgical excision of the area may be necessary.

Nursing Management

The nurse includes the following in the plan of care:

- Teach the client how to insert a suppository.
- Instruct the client in how to take a sitz bath.
- Discuss strategies to relieve constipation.

Refer to Nursing Care Plan 53-1 for more information.

● ANAL FISTULA

An anal fistula (fistula in ano) is a tract that forms in the anal canal.

Pathophysiology and Etiology

When healing of an anorectal abscess is inadequate, an inflamed tunnel develops, connecting the area of the original abscess with perianal skin (Fig. 53-7). Purulent material drains from the opening.

Assessment Findings

The client reports pain on defecation. The opening of the fistula appears red, and pus leaks from the external opening of the fistula or can be expressed if the area is compressed. If the fistula is superficial, it feels cordlike on palpation. A proctosigmoidoscopy or colonoscopy may identify Crohn's disease, which predisposes the client to an anorectal abscess or anal fistula.

Medical and Surgical Management

Antibiotics are prescribed to treat infection. Treatment of underlying Crohn's disease often allows for resolution of the fistula without surgical intervention. Most simple low-lying fistulae can be managed by **fistulotomy.** This procedure involves incising the fistula along with partial sphincter division and is reserved for those fistulae that arise from relatively normal surrounding tissue. Another surgical procedure, referred to as **fistulectomy,** involves an excision of the fistulous tract. This type usually is the recommended surgery.

Nursing Care Plan 53-1

THE CLIENT WITH AN ANORECTAL CONDITION

Assessment

Include the following questions in the health history:

- Do you have any burning, itching, or pain in the anorectal area? If so, when do these symptoms occur—with defecation? How long do they last? Do you have any other discomfort, such as abdominal cramps?
- Is any blood in the stool or on the toilet tissue when you wipe the rectum? How much? Is the blood bright or dark red?
- Is there mucus or pus from the rectal area?
- What is your stool pattern?
- Do you use laxatives? If so, how often?
- What is your typical diet?
- Do you exercise regularly? If so what is the exercise?
- Do you sit or stand for long periods?

Nursing Diagnosis: **Risk for Constipation** related to fear of painful elimination

Expected Outcome: Client identifies measures that prevent or treat constipation.

Interventions	Rationales
Instruct client, unless contraindicated, to increase intake of water to 2 L/day.	Such fluid intake prevents hard, dry stools and eases defecation.
Provide a list of high-fiber foods.	A high-fiber diet promotes bulk of stool and prevents constipation.
Instruct client in use of laxatives or stool softeners as ordered.	Prolonged use of these measures is not encouraged; they should be used only as indicated.
Teach the client to heed the urge to have a bowel movement.	This measure prevents constipation.

Evaluation of Expected Outcome: Client practices measures that prevent constipation, as evidenced by increased fluid and fiber intake and the passage of soft, formed stools.

Nursing Diagnosis: **Acute Pain** related to surgical procedure

Expected Outcome: Client will report that pain management regimen relieves his or her pain.

Interventions	Rationales
Administer pain medications as ordered.	Medications promote ongoing pain relief.
Encourage client to rest in a comfortable position that removes pressure from surgical site, or to use a flotation device.	These measures relieve pressure and decrease pain at the surgical site.
Apply ice and analgesic ointments as indicated.	These measures promote pain relief.
Use warm compresses or sitz baths three to four times daily as indicated.	Warmth through compresses or baths relaxes the rectal sphincter spasm and soothes irritated tissues.

Evaluation of Expected Outcome: Client states that positioning and use of sitz baths relieve pain.

(continued)

Nursing Care Plan 53-1 (Continued)

THE CLIENT WITH AN ANORECTAL CONDITION

Nursing Diagnosis: **Risk for Ineffective Therapeutic Regimen Management** related to knowledge deficit

Expected Outcome: Client will demonstrate ability to manage therapeutic regimens.

Interventions	*Rationales*
Instruct client to cleanse perianal area with warm water and to dry with cotton wipes.	These measures prevent infection and irritation.
Teach client how to do sitz baths at home, using warm water, three to four times each day.	Sitz baths promote healing, decrease skin irritation, and relieve rectal spasms.
Instruct client to take a sitz bath after each bowel movement.	Sitz baths also help keeps the perianal area clean.
Encourage client to follow diet and medication instructions.	Encouragement promotes compliance with therapeutic regimen and prevents complications.
Encourage moderate exercise.	Activity promotes healing and normal stool patterns.

Evaluation of Expected Outcomes: (1) Incision heals without complications. (2) Client has no signs of infection and eats a diet high in fiber. (3) Vital signs are normal. (4) Stools are soft-formed and regular.

If a sphincter division compromises fecal continence, a noncutting seton may be placed into the fistula to allow for drainage of the fistula and to minimize the risk for future abscesses. A *seton* is a nonabsorbable suture or drain that is passed from the cutaneous opening of the fistula into the lumen of the anal canal and then back out onto the skin, where it is tied to itself. The seton can be gradually tightened to cut through the sphincter or left in place as a drain.

Nursing Management

The nurse teaches the client to self-administer medications, keep the anal region clean, and avoid transferring microorganisms to other hygiene articles that they share with family members (e.g., bar soap). For surgical nursing care, refer to Nursing Care Plan 53-1.

● PILONIDAL SINUS

Pilonidal means "a nest of hair." A **pilonidal sinus** is an infection in the hair follicles in the sacrococcygeal area above the anus (Fig. 53-8). Other local infections, such as osteomyelitis and furuncles of the skin, also have common presenting signs and symptoms and must be ruled out. The terms *pilonidal sinus* and *pilonidal cyst* are both used to describe the condition.

Pathophysiology and Etiology

The condition typically occurs after puberty. People who have a deep intergluteal cleft and those who have abundant hair in the perianal and lower back regions are predisposed to the condition. Inadequate personal hygiene, obesity, and trauma to the area also contribute to its development.

A sinus or cyst begins to form when the skin deep in the cleft softens as a result of being chronically moist. Stiff hairs then irritate and pierce the soft, macerated skin, becoming embedded in it. The irritation inflames the tissues. Infection readily follows because the break in the skin allows microorganisms to enter. Several channels may lead from the sinus to the skin.

Hypertrophied papilla

Fistula

FIGURE 53-7 Anal fistula.

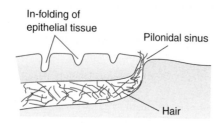

FIGURE 53-8 (**A**) Pilonidal sinus on lower sacrum about 5 cm (2 in) above the anus in the intergluteal cleft. (**B**) Note: hair particles emerge from the sinus tract, and localized indentations (pits) can appear on the skin near the sinus openings. (From Smeltzer, S. C. & Bare, B. G. [2000]. *Brunner & Suddarth's textbook of medical–surgical nursing* [9th ed.]. Philadelphia: Lippincott Williams & Wilkins.)

Assessment Findings

Pain and swelling at the base of the spine and purulent drainage occur. On inspection, the sinus opening may be located in the gluteal fold. Dilated pits of the hair follicles in the sinus are a unique characteristic.

Medical and Surgical Management

The abscess is drained, and the tissue is incised. The sinus and all its connecting channels are laid open, and purulent material and hair are removed. Packing is inserted into the cavity, and the wound heals by secondary intention. In some cases, the wound edges are approximated. Healing by primary intention, however, sometimes allows the purulent material to reform and collect, causing another abscess. Because the infection is localized, systemic antibiotics usually are not prescribed.

Nursing Management

The nurse teaches the client how to minimize discomfort and facilitates postoperative bowel elimination. As appropriate, the nurse instructs a family member in the procedures of removing the packing, cleaning the incised tissue, and redressing the area. See Nursing Care Plan 53-1 for additional nursing management.

GENERAL NUTRITIONAL CONSIDERATIONS

A *high-fiber diet* is a vague term that does not quantify or qualify fiber content. Daily guidelines call for consuming between 6 and 11 servings of breads, cereals, and grains. This number includes several servings of high-fiber bread (at least 2 to 5 g of fiber per serving) and a serving of high-fiber cereal (at least 5 g of fiber per serving).

Encourage clients to consume approximately one-half cup of dried peas or beans (legumes) daily. These food items are low-fat, high-fiber alternatives to meat protein.

Teach clients to consume two to four servings of fruit daily. The skin and seeds contain most of the fiber; fresh whole fruit is higher in fiber than is canned fruit or fruit juice.

Encourage clients to eat between three and five servings of vegetables daily. The less peeling and scraping of the vegetables that is done, the higher the fiber content will be. Because vegetables vary greatly in their fiber content, clients should choose a variety.

Clients should consider slowly adding coarse, unprocessed wheat bran, a natural laxative, to the diet. They should start with 1 teaspoon daily and work up to 2 to 3 tablespoons daily to decrease the likelihood of flatus, distention, cramping, and diarrhea. They can mix wheat bran with juice or milk; add it to muffins, quick bread, or casseroles; or sprinkle it over cereal, applesauce, or other foods.

Calcium-fortified orange juice is an excellent source of readily absorbed calcium for clients who are lactose intolerant. An 8-oz glass provides approximately the same amount of calcium as an 8-oz glass of milk, plus a significant amount of folic acid, potassium, and vitamin C.

Encourage the client with diarrhea to consume potassium-rich foods as tolerated. Examples of such foods include bananas, canned apricots and peaches, apricot nectar, orange juice, grapefruit juice, tomato juice, fish, potatoes, and meat.

For clients with diverticulosis, a high-fiber diet excludes foods with husks and seeds (nuts, popcorn, cucumbers, strawberries, raspberries, tomatoes, corn, and breads containing sesame or poppy seeds). These foods become trapped in the diverticula. In addition to lactose intolerance, some clients with Crohn's disease develop wheat or gluten intolerance during exacerbations of the disease, further complicating nutritional management.

GENERAL PHARMACOLOGIC CONSIDERATIONS

Narcotics and sedatives decrease peristalsis and can result in constipation. Assess bowel function daily. The client may require a stool softener to minimize the constipating effects of these drugs.

Habitual use of laxatives can decrease muscle tone in the large intestine, resulting in constipation.

The misconception that a daily bowel movement is necessary may contribute to the overuse of laxatives. Teach the client about normal bowel patterns, which vary from one to three stools daily to one bowel movement every 3 days.

GENERAL GERONTOLOGIC CONSIDERATIONS

Constipation is a common problem in older adults and often results from inadequate intake of dietary fiber, lack of exercise, and decreased fluid intake.

Encourage older adults to schedule regular health examinations, including screenings for colorectal cancer, because its incidence increases with age.

The gastric mucosa (mucous lining of the stomach) atrophies with age, resulting in decreased production of gastric acids.

With age, peristaltic action of the GI tract decreases; therefore, the risk for constipation in the older adult increases.

Constipation can occur in an older adult who feels rushed when defecating or cannot get to the toilet in time.

An older adult with prolonged constipation or constipation that shifts to diarrhea must be checked for a fecal impaction. Liquid feces may ooze around the impacted feces, giving the appearance of diarrhea.

Older adults with appendicitis may not display the type of acute pain that younger adults with the condition experience. Severe pain may be absent, minimal, or referred in the older adult, causing a delay in diagnosis and a greater incidence of complications.

Critical Thinking Exercises

1. *The admitting department notifies the nursing unit to expect a client with ulcerative colitis. Based on the characteristics of the disease process, what assessments are essential to obtain at the time of admission?*

2. *As you assist an older adult with using a bedpan, you notice blood on the toilet tissue. What other data are appropriate to gather at this time?*

References and Suggested Readings

Heitkemper, M. & Jarrett, M. (2001). Irritable bowel syndrome. *American Journal of Nursing, 101*(1), 26–32.

Heppel, J. & Kelly, K. (1999). Surgical treatment of inflammatory bowel disease. In T. Yamada & D. H. Alpers (Eds.), *Inflammatory bowel disease.* [On-line.] Available: http://www.gastro.org/public/ibd.html.

Levine, C. D. (1999). Toxic megacolon: Diagnosis and treatment challenges. *AACN Clinical Issues: Advanced Practice in Acute and Critical Care, 10,* 492–499.

Porth, C. M. (2002). *Pathophysiology: Concepts of altered health states* (6th ed.). Philadelphia: Lippincott Williams & Wilkins.

Rayhorn, N. (1999). Understanding inflammatory bowel disease. *Nursing '99, 29*(12), 57–61.

Smeltzer, S. C. & Bare, B. G. (2000). *Brunner & Suddarth's textbook of medical–surgical nursing* (9th ed.). Philadelphia: Lippincott Williams & Wilkins.

Yamada, T., Alpers, D. H., Laine, L., Owyang, C., & Powell, D. W. (1999). *Textbook of gastroenterology* (3rd ed.). Philadelphia: Lippincott Williams & Wilkins.

Caring for Clients With an Ileostomy or Colostomy

Words to Know

abdominoperineal
   resection
appliance
colostomy
continent ileostomy
   (Kock pouch)
double-barrel colostomy
effluent
enterostomal therapist

ileoanal reservoir
   (anastomosis)
ileostomy
loop colostomy
ostomate
ostomy
segmental resection
single-barrel colostomy
stoma

Learning Objectives

On completion of this chapter, the reader will:

- Differentiate between ileostomy and colostomy.
- Discuss preoperative nursing care of a client undergoing ostomy surgery.
- List complications associated with ostomy surgery.
- Discuss postoperative nursing management of a client with an ileostomy.
- Describe the components used to apply and collect stool from an intestinal ostomy.
- Cite reasons for changing an ostomy appliance.
- Summarize how to change an ostomy appliance.
- Explain how stool is released from a continent ileostomy.
- Describe the two-part procedure needed to create an ileoanal reservoir.
- Discuss various types of colostomies.
- Explain ways that clients with descending or sigmoid colostomies may regulate bowel elimination.

The term **ostomy** refers to an opening between an internal body structure and the skin. The most common intestinal ostomies are the **ileostomy,** an opening from the distal small intestine, and the **colostomy,** an opening from the colon (Table 54-1). Fecal material exits through a **stoma,** an opening on the exterior abdominal surface. Most ostomies are created in response to an inflammatory bowel disorder that fails to respond to medical treatment or complications such as rupture of a portion of intestine, irreversible obstruction, compromised blood supply to the intestine, or cancerous tumor. Whether an ostomy is temporary or permanent, each client requires an individually adapted plan of care that incorporates preparation for surgery, recovery from surgery, and knowledge required for ongoing self-care.

ILEOSTOMY

In the usual surgical procedure for a conventional ileostomy, the entire colon and rectum (total colectomy) are removed. The terminal end of the ileum is brought out through a separate area on the right lower quadrant of the abdomen slightly below the umbilicus, near the outer border of the rectus muscle (Fig. 54-1). The cut end is everted and sutured to the skin, a process referred to as creating a *matured* stoma. When an ileostomy is performed, the stoma continually releases stool and gas. The fecal material discharged from an ileostomy is liquid or mushy and contains digestive enzymes.

TABLE 54-1	TYPES OF INTESTINAL OSTOMIES		
TYPE	STOMA LOCATION	FECAL CONSISTENCY	FECAL CONTROL
Conventional ileostomy	Lower abdomen	Liquid	Never
Continent ileostomy	Lower abdomen	Liquid	By siphoning
Ascending colostomy	Middle right abdomen	Semiliquid	Never
Transverse colostomy	Center of the abdomen below the belt line	Semiliquid	Never
Descending colostomy	Middle left abdomen	Soft	Sometimes
Sigmoid colostomy	Lower left abdomen	Formed	Usually

● THE OSTOMY APPLIANCE

The matured stoma promotes healing and provides a smooth peristomal area that permits the immediate postoperative application of an **appliance,** the collection device worn over a stoma. Clients with an ileostomy always wear an appliance, which requires frequent emptying. Ostomy suppliers provide various appliances to meet the individual needs of the **ostomate** (client with an ostomy). All appliances consist of one-piece or two-piece devices with a pouch for collecting feces and a faceplate, or disk, that is attached to the abdomen with an opening through which the stoma protrudes (Fig. 54-2). The faceplate adheres to the skin either with self-adhesive backing or another bonding substance such as an adhesive powder, paste, or wafer. Karaya gum is a common component in ostomy supplies. It becomes gelatinous when in contact with moisture and is used in place of an adhesive. Karaya gum protects the skin as well as promotes adhesion of the ostomy appliance. Karaya gum rings are used around the stoma. They are pulled or pushed into any shape and are ideal for correcting problems created by an ill-fitting appliance. Unlike rings made of rigid material, a karaya gum ring fits snugly around the stoma without injuring it.

A disposable, or temporary, appliance is preferred in the immediate postoperative phase because the size of the stoma changes over time as a result of swelling from the procedure itself. The size of the stoma may change rapidly and differ from one appliance change to the next. After the stoma heals and reaches its final size and shape, a permanent (reusable) appliance is fitted.

Reusable equipment consists of a sturdier pouch with a custom-sized faceplate and "O" ring. The pouch is designed to fasten into position when pressed over the ring, much like snapping a lid on a plastic margarine tub. The pouch has a clamp at the bottom, which can be released when the pouch needs to be emptied. The pouch may be fastened to a belt for more security. The belt supports the weight of the liquid fecal material and prevents the faceplate from being pulled away from the abdominal skin. Foam rubber, gauze, or flannel padding is placed under a belt if the belt cuts into the flesh. The client requires two sets of permanent appliances so that one can be cleaned periodically. Disposable equipment may be appropriate for some clients. Disposable bags, faceplates, and attachment rings are replaced with new ones with each change of the ostomy appliance (usually daily with bathing).

FIGURE 54-1 An ileostomy.

FIGURE 54-2 The ostomy appliance. (From Smeltzer, S. C. & Bare, B. G. [2000]. *Brunner & Suddarth's textbook of medical–surgical nursing* [9th ed.]. Philadelphia: Lippincott Williams & Wilkins.)

● PREOPERATIVE PERIOD

Surgical Management

Before surgery, the physician explains the purpose for the surgical procedure along with its benefits and risks. He or she describes the appearance and function of the stoma, where it will be placed, and its required care. The physician carefully marks the site to ensure that it is away from bony prominences, skin creases, and scars; is within the rectus abdominis muscle; is unobstructed; and is visible to the client. Clients benefit from preoperative interactions with an enterostomal therapy nurse (also known as an **enterostomal therapist**). This nurse assists with marking placement of the stoma and collaborates with the surgeon regarding placement and the client's educational needs.

The physician identifies potential risks from the total colectomy, such as possible bladder and sexual dysfunction secondary to parasympathetic nerve injury. Sexual dysfunction in men after a total colectomy is unusual but does occur in some clients undergoing this procedure. If such dysfunction persists after a colectomy, operative and nonoperative options are available to facilitate erection. Young male clients may wish to collect and store sperm for later use if they plan to have children. A colectomy may slightly diminish fertility in women; however, this procedure does not preclude the ability to achieve a full-term pregnancy with a normal vaginal delivery.

Cleansing of the bowel before surgery is carried out using dietary restrictions in combination with laxative or lavage agents (e.g., GoLYTELY, NuLytely, Colyte), depending on the client's condition (i.e., presence or absence of obstruction) and according to the surgeon's preference. Opinions vary regarding the need for antibiotic prophylaxis. Most surgeons order a combination of intravenous (IV) antibiotics (i.e., a third-generation cephalosporin and metronidazole) before surgery and continue administration after surgery.

Whenever possible, prednisone should be tapered and discontinued before surgery to avoid negative effects of the drug on tissue healing. A preoperative "stress dose" of IV steroid (i.e., hydrocortisone) is given to clients who have been on prednisone within the previous 6 months to prevent adrenal crisis. Adrenal crisis is potentially life-threatening and can result from the abrupt withdrawal of corticosteroids or significant stress after the client has been treated with corticosteroids. See Chapter 57 for additional information on adrenal crisis.

Immunosuppressive agents such as azathioprine, 6-mercaptopurine, and cyclosporine should be discontinued 3 to 4 weeks before surgery to prevent negative effects on tissue healing. Aspirin-containing compounds are discontinued at least 1 week before surgery to minimize the risk of bleeding. Blood samples are taken before surgery, and the client's blood is typed and cross-matched for replacement of losses that occur during surgery.

NURSING PROCESS

● Preoperative Ileostomy Care

Assessment

The nurse obtains complete medical, allergy, diet, and drug histories. Asking the client if he or she has been taking corticosteroids is important—if so, the nurse needs to monitor the client closely for signs and symptoms of adrenal insufficiency such as weakness, lethargy, hypotension, nausea, and vomiting as dosages are tapered. The nurse performs a physical assessment, paying particular attention to inspecting the skin over the abdomen, auscultating bowel sounds, and getting the client's vital signs and weight. In addition, the nurse checks the preoperative laboratory test results to determine if blood cell counts and serum electrolyte levels are within normal ranges. Obtaining a description of preoperative preparations the client may have been asked to perform, such as dietary modifications and antibiotic therapy, is important. The nurse implements the medical orders for cleansing the bowel, inserting a nasogastric tube, and preparing the client for surgery.

Referral to community and professional resources before surgery may positively affect the client's postoperative quality of life. Resources for education and support include the medical and surgical teams and the lay public (e.g., the Crohn's and Colitis Foundation of America, the United Ostomy Association).

Healthcare teams hold several views about beginning ostomy instructions before surgery. Some believe that such teaching helps clients to accept the ostomy. Others believe that this type of teaching creates premature stress and anxiety. Often, an enterostomal therapist provides ostomy instruction, whether before or after surgery. He or she is certified to care for ostomates and manage their unique problems. The enterostomal therapist also is an excellent resource for nurses providing direct care to ostomates. If the client expresses a readiness to learn or asks questions about ostomy care, the nurse provides information about ostomy equipment and general principles of ostomy management. The nurse also can arrange a preoperative visit with the enterostomal therapy nurse.

Diagnosis, Planning, and Interventions

Anxiety related to change in health status and fear of the unknown

Expected Outcome: Client will experience reduced anxiety.

● Provide an overview of preoperative procedures, using explanations the client understands. *Explanations enable the client to know what to expect.*

● Allow time for the client to ask questions and express fears. *Adequate time and support promote communication and assist the client to verbalize anxiety.*

- Assess previous positive coping skills and assist client to access them again. *Past successful coping methods are likely to be effective now.*

Disturbed Body Image related to the stoma and altered bowel elimination

Expected Outcome: Client verbalizes what the changes will be and their benefit to future health.

- Encourage the client to discuss feelings about the stoma. *Such discussion enables the client to express concerns and fears about the fecal diversion.*
- Inform the client that an assigned staff nurse will be there when the client first views and touches the stoma. *Such information gives reassurance that a familiar nurse will be available to answer questions and give support.*
- If the client expresses interest, provide a list of appropriate community resources. *Knowing that others have experienced the same surgery and can share their experience and offer advice and support may help the client.*

Evaluation of Expected Outcomes

The client verbalizes fears and demonstrates positive coping skills. He or she discusses what physical changes to expect.

● POSTOPERATIVE PERIOD

Surgical Management

The rectum is packed with gauze during surgery to absorb drainage and promote gradual healing. The rectal pack usually is removed in 5 to 7 days. Afterward, irrigations may be ordered to promote healing. A nasogastric tube is used for gastrointestinal (GI) decompression until normal bowel motility resumes. Fluid, electrolyte, and nutritional balances are maintained with IV fluids until oral nourishment is possible. Within several days, the nasogastric tube is removed and oral feedings begin. Antibiotic therapy continues. Analgesics are prescribed for pain relief. Wound healing is monitored, and complications that develop are managed.

Possible postoperative complications include intestinal obstruction; bleeding; and impaired blood supply to, stenosis of, or prolapse or excessive protrusion of the stoma. Intestinal obstruction, a serious complication, may result from a twisted, strangulated, or incarcerated segment of the remaining intestine or a bolus of poorly chewed or inadequately digested food. When a collection of food causes obstruction, the physician may attempt to correct the problem by irrigating the stoma. If the bowel is twisted or strangulated, surgical intervention is necessary.

Prolapse or protrusion of the ileostomy is fairly common. If it is moderate (1 or 2 inches), no treatment is required. A severe prolapse of the stoma is a serious complication, however. If edema occurs, it may cause an obstruction and restrict stomal blood supply. Stomal necrosis results if the prolapse is not promptly and skillfully managed. Once the stoma prolapses, recurrence is likely.

N U R S I N G   P R O C E S S

● The Client Recovering From Ileostomy Surgery

Assessment

Reviewing the medical record for information regarding the type of surgery and any problems during or immediately after surgery is very important. Postoperative assessments include obtaining vital signs; inspecting the dressing and stoma for bleeding and signs of infection (Table 54-2); monitoring the rate and progress of fluid and blood infusions; checking the function of the gastric suction; measuring intake and output; and inspecting the collection appliance, special drains, packing, or tubes. The nurse records all immediate postoperative findings to provide a database. For a step-by-step discussion of how to replace an ostomy appliance, see Nursing Guidelines 54-1.

TABLE 54-2	**CHARACTERISTICS OF HEALTHY AND UNHEALTHY STOMAS**	
CHARACTERISTICS	**HEALTHY STOMA**	**UNHEALTHY STOMA**
Color	Bright pink or red	Dusky blue or black
Size	Comparable in diameter to the intestine from which it has been formed; may be somewhat large after surgery because of edema	Larger or smaller in comparison to size after resolution of postoperative edema
Opening	Patent, unobstructed	Tight or narrow
Surface	Moist, shiny with an overlying layer of mucus; may bleed slightly when being cleansed	Dull, dry; excessive bleeding
Length	Protrudes from or is just flush with the skin	Protrudes beyond 2 inches from the skin or retracts beneath it
Sensation	Painless	Peristomal burning
Function	Regular passage of feces	Sparse or absent elimination of feces

NURSING GUIDELINES 54-1

Changing an Ostomy Appliance

Assemble clean gloves, scissors, ostomy belt, stoma gauge, faceplate, pouch, adhesive or protectant (e.g., karaya paste), and cleaning materials such as gauze pads, water, or adhesive solvent.

- Wash hands and put on gloves.

- Empty pouch when it is one-third full.

- Change the faceplate only when needed, that is, if it becomes loose or tight or client experiences discomfort. If the faceplate is changed too frequently, skin around stoma may become raw and excoriated secondary to removal of protective layers of epithelium with the faceplate.

- If the ostomy appliance is being replaced routinely, schedule the change when the gastrocolic reflex is less active. For many clients, this time is early in the morning, before eating, or 2 or 3 hours after mealtime.

- Gently ease the faceplate from the skin. If the faceplate was applied with adhesive, roll the adhesive from the skin and appliance. If it does not roll off, use a small amount of solvent, which chemically loosens the adhesive bond. Because some solvents irritate the skin, apply solvent sparingly between the body and faceplate using a sprayer, medicine dropper, or gauze pad. Avoid rubbing, which may further irritate skin. Clean the area with soap and water and pat dry after a solvent has been used.

- Inform the client that the most common causes of discomfort are reactions to the adhesive or solvent used to remove it or irritation from leaking fecal drainage. In such cases, the client may experience stinging, tingling, or itching immediately after an appliance change. These sensations should quickly subside. If a sensation is prolonged or intensified, remove the appliance regardless of whether it has been on for 1 hour or several days. When using a new adhesive product, remember to patch test it first on nonirritated skin at the inner aspect of the client's forearm.

- After removing the faceplate and pouch, protect the peristomal area from drainage by placing a tissue cuff around the stoma or using a receptacle such as a small paper cup to collect the drainage. Use a soapy washcloth to clean the skin around the stoma and wipe the soap from the skin. Pat the area or allow it to air dry.

- Inspect the stoma and skin carefully. If excoriation is observed, use a temporary appliance or hydrocolloid dressing, such as DuoDERM or Tegabsorb, to cover the excoriated skin to promote moist healing.

- Create an even surface for reapplying the pouch by filling irregular hollows in the peristomal skin with karaya paste before replacing the faceplate.

- Measure the circumference of the stoma and cut a comparable hole in the faceplate, allowing ⅛-inch margin to account for potential swelling in a new stoma.

- Secure the pouch to the faceplate. Be sure to smooth out ridges or openings in the closure. Also be sure to seal the pouch.

- Peel the backing from the faceplate.

- Affix the faceplate to the skin.

In logical steps and at a pace that promotes comprehension, the nurse teaches the client and another family member about managing the ostomy, adopting dietary modifications, recognizing how drug therapy affects bowel elimination, and adjusting to various surgery-related changes, such as possible sexual dysfunction (Box 54-1). Additional aspects to include in the teaching plan are discussed in Client and Family Teaching Box 54-1.

Diagnosis, Planning, and Interventions

In addition to the measures discussed in the following, postoperative care includes standard pain management (see Chap. 21) and postoperative interventions (see Chap. 25).

Risk for Impaired Skin Integrity related to effects of fecal material and adhesives on the skin

Expected Outcome: Client will maintain intact peristomal skin.

- Demonstrate safe, gentle removal of the pouch. *This type of removal prevents skin irritation.*
- Gently cleanse the peristomal area with warm water and mild soap. *Gentle cleansing minimizes skin irritation and abrasions.*
- Teach the client to apply a skin barrier, such as a wafer, gel, paste, or powder. *The skin barrier protects the peristomal skin from digestive enzymes and bacteria.*

Risk for Infection related to fecal contamination of the surgical wound

Expected Outcome: Client's wound is free from infection.

- Apply dressing securely, covering the surgical wound completely. *The dressing protects the incision from contact with fecal material.*
- Change the ostomy pouch when it is loose and leaking. *Changing at the correct time minimizes the risk of fecal drainage entering the incision.*
- When drainage leaks near the incision, wipe it away from the incision and change the dressing if soiled at all. *These measures keep fecal drainage away from incision, ensuring that the dressing always is clean.*

BOX 54-1 ● Sexual Modifications for Ostomates

- Always practice good hygiene. Bathe and apply a fresh pouch before having sex.
- Disguise the pouch by enclosing it within a purse-string cloth cover.
- When anticipating sexual activity, avoid eating or drinking substances that activate the bowel or create a lot of gas.
- Fashion a cummerbund with a pocket or fold into which the pouch can be held.
- Remove the belt and temporarily secure the pouch to the skin with tape.
- If accidents happen, cultivate a sense of humor that may similarly relieve the anxiety of the sexual partner as well.
- Consult with members of a local ostomy group who also may provide support and counseling regarding sexual matters.

54-1 *Client and Family Teaching*
Postoperative Ileostomy Care

The nurse discusses the following issues with the client and his or her family:

- Restrict oral intake only with medical supervision.
- Eat slowly and chew food well with the mouth closed to help lessen the development of gas.
- Avoid foods that cause discomfort, excessive gas, or loose stools.
- Drink extra fluids, especially in warm weather.
- Dilate the stoma if the volume of stool decreases for some unexplained reason. To do this, cut the nail on the index or little finger, cover the finger with a finger cot, lubricate it thoroughly, and then insert the finger gently into the stoma for a few minutes.
- Clean the pouch thoroughly to prevent odors.
- Use an internal odor-absorbing substance or one that can be added to the pouch to control lingering or stubborn odors.
- Use an old or disposable pouch when medications or offending foods that cause disagreeable odors are excreted.
- Slip a plastic cover over the pouch to act as a second barrier against escaping odors.
- Check with a physician before self-administering any drug, especially a laxative or antidiarrheal agent.

- Allow a small amount of air to be trapped in the pouch. *Liquid feces will then drain to the bottom of the pouch, placing less tension on it.*
- Make several pinhole-sized punctures at the upper edge of the pouch. *Punctures allow excess gas to escape and decrease tension on the pouch.*

Risk for Deficient Fluid Volume related to decreased appetite, vomiting, or increased loss of fluids and electrolytes from ileostomy

Expected Outcome: Client maintains adequate fluid and electrolyte balance.

- Assess fluid balance. *This evaluation determines any deficits.*
- Examine serum and urine test results for sodium and potassium levels. *Review may indicate imbalances and other potential problems (e.g., acidosis, cardiac dysrhythmias).*
- Observe skin turgor and appearance of the tongue. *Poor skin turgor and dry tongue indicate fluid deficits.*

Risk for Sexual Dysfunction related to altered body image

Expected Outcome: Client will plan modifications for maintaining sexual fulfillment.

- Encourage client and partner to verbalize fears and concerns about intimacy. *Discussion allows client and partner to express feelings and explore needs.*
- Reassure the client who is not experiencing sexual dysfunction that intercourse will not harm the healed ostomy. *Fear can interfere with sexual relations; reassurance assists clients to reestablish sexual relationships.*
- Recommend alternative sexual positions. *Different positions may enable the client to avoid embarrassment about the stomal appearance until he or she is more comfortable.*
- Refer clients who experience sexual dysfunction to a sexual therapist, enterostomal therapist, or advanced practice nurse. *Clients and partners may need assistance to determine problems and solutions, including alternative methods to achieve sexual satisfaction.*

Ineffective Coping related to disturbed body image and altered bowel function

Expected Outcome: Client will cope effectively with body changes.

- Ensure privacy when teaching and providing ileostomy care. *Privacy allows client to get used to changes without fear of embarrassment in front of others.*
- Help client to set realistic goals and identify personal skills and knowledge. *Participation in the care plan allows the client to make decisions and move toward independence.*
- Use empathetic communication, allowing time for client to express fears and concerns. *A supportive environment promotes coping.*
- Refer client to support networks, such as ostomy groups or other ostomates. *Resources help client to problem solve and increase coping skills.*

- Observe for signs of wound infection: wound drainage, abdominal pain, and elevated temperature. *These signs indicate possible wound infection.*

Bowel Incontinence related to loss of sphincter control and change in intestinal motility

Expected Outcome: Client will not experience leaking from the appliance or soiling with fecal material.

- Instruct the client how to prepare the drainage pouch for a secure fit around the stoma, leaving an extra $\frac{1}{8}$ inch in the appliance opening. (Use a gauge for measuring, provided by the manufacturer.) *Accurate preparation provides room for stoma clearance and potential swelling.*
- Press the adhesive faceplate around the stoma for about 30 seconds. *This measure ensures secure attachment of the pouch to the peristomal skin.*
- Demonstrate frequent emptying of the pouch. *Frequent emptying prevents tension on the pouch and skin from the weight of the drainage.*
- Use the following measures to avoid leaking:
  - Press the adhesive faceplate from the stomal edge outward. *This technique prevents the formation of wrinkles.*
  - Ask client to remain inactive for 5 minutes. *This period allows time for body heat to strengthen the adhesive bond.*

Evaluation of Expected Outcomes

Peristomal skin is not reddened, there is no evidence of edema or drainage, and the client does not complain of burning sensations. The incision heals without infection. Stool is contained in the ostomy pouch. The client maintains adequate fluid balance as evidenced by balanced intake and output, good skin turgor, moist tongue and mucous membranes, and normal serum and urine sodium and potassium levels. The client reports that he or she has attained satisfactory sexual performance. He or she also demonstrates coping skills as evidenced by interest in self-care, ability to seek assistance, and ability to maintain relationships.

CONTINENT ILEOSTOMY (KOCK POUCH)

A **continent ileostomy** or **Kock pouch** is the creation of an internal reservoir for the storage of GI **effluent** (discharged fecal material or liquid feces). The reservoir stores this effluent for several hours until the client removes it with a catheter. Doing so eliminates the need for an external appliance.

Surgical Management

After removing the diseased portion of the ileum, the surgeon forms a reservoir with a portion of the terminal ileum and creates a nipple valve by telescoping (intussusception) the distal ileal segment into the reservoir. The surgeon then forms a permanent external stoma and anchors it to the abdominal wall (Fig. 54-3).

During the operation, the surgeon inserts a temporary catheter through the nipple valve and sutures the catheter in place so that its end protrudes from the external stoma.

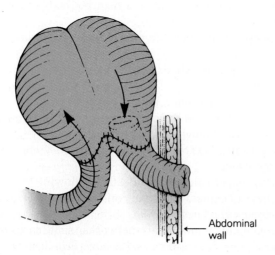

FIGURE 54-3 Continent ileostomy.

Then the surgeon packs the perineal area from which the lower intestine was removed with gauze. The packing remains in place for about 1 week.

Nursing Management

The nurse reinforces the perineal packing, as needed, during the postoperative period. In addition, the nurse checks the abdominal dressing for drainage and connects the stomal catheter, if ordered, to low, intermittent suction that empties the reservoir continuously, thereby preventing tension on healing suture lines. He or she checks the ileal catheter frequently for signs of obstruction: lack of fecal drainage, the client's complaint of feeling full in the area of the ileal pouch, or leakage of liquid stool around the catheter. The nurse notes the color and amount of drainage, observes the size and color of the stoma, and administers either routine or as-needed irrigations of the ileal catheter with small amounts of normal saline solution if the catheter appears to be obstructed, according to physician's orders. He or she keeps the skin clean around the stoma, changes the gauze dressing over the stoma when it becomes wet with mucus or serosanguineous drainage, and changes the dressing every 6 to 8 hours as drainage decreases.

The nurse also monitors ileal output carefully during the entire postoperative period. As GI function resumes, the initial amount of ileal drainage usually is high. If excessive fluids and electrolytes are lost, parenteral fluid and electrolyte replacement is necessary. When ileal drainage stabilizes, about 10 to 14 days after surgery, the physician removes the ileal catheter. The reservoir then holds the accumulating effluent until the nurse or client siphons it. Initially the reservoir is emptied every 2 to 4 hours. As the capacity of the reservoir increases (usually in about 6 months), the client or caregiver performs the procedure three or four times daily.

The nurse includes the following information in the teaching plan:

- To care for the stoma and catheter, assemble a clean catheter, lubricant, basin, tissues, irrigating syringe and solution, and gauze dressing.
- Sit on or beside the toilet or on the side of the bed.
- Warm the catheter to body temperature and lubricate the tip. Insert it about 2 inches into the stomal opening.
- Expect resistance when the catheter reaches the nipple valve (about 2 inches), which controls the retention of waste matter. Gently push the catheter a little further into the ileal pouch. At the same time, exhale, cough, or bear down as if to pass stool until fecal material begins to drain.
- Direct the external end of the catheter into a basin or the toilet about 12 inches below the stoma.

- Allow 5 to 10 minutes for drainage to cease; then remove the catheter, clean it with soapy water, and store it in a sealable plastic bag until needed again.
- Wash the area around the stoma and pat the skin dry.
- Place an absorbent pad or dressing over the stoma.

For additional nursing management, refer to the discussion that addresses similar problems experienced by a client with ileoanal reservoir. For tips on how to manage an obstructed catheter, see Box 54-2.

ILEOANAL RESERVOIR

The **ileoanal reservoir** (also called an ileoanal **anastomosis;** Fig. 54-4) is a procedure that maintains bowel continence. It is performed on selected clients who have chronic ulcerative colitis or whose disease does not affect the anorectal sphincter. Besides allowing the client to control bowel elimination, this procedure, as opposed to a conventional ileostomy with total colectomy, preserves innervation to the male genitalia. Subsequently, the client is unlikely to experience bladder dysfunction, erectile dysfunction, or infertility.

Surgical Management

An ileoanal anastomosis is performed in two stages. In the first stage, the surgeon creates a temporary ileostomy, removes a large length of diseased colon down to the terminal section of the rectum above the anal sphincter, joins several distal loops of healthy ileum to form a pouch for holding stool, and connects the ileal reservoir to the anal cuff. After the first stage of surgery, clients experience an almost continuous discharge of mucus from the anus and a frequent discharge of fecal material from the ileostomy. Initially, the client cannot control the frequent watery discharge.

The second stage is done 2 or 3 months later. At this time, the surgeon closes the temporary ileostomy and reunites the two sections of ileum. The area where the two sections of bowel are joined is called an *anastomosis.* The anastomosis establishes a normal flow of fecal material

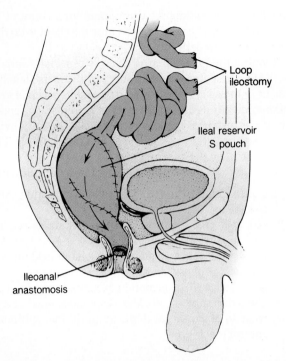

FIGURE 54-4 An ileoanal anastomosis joins a section of ileum to create an ileal reservoir. The distal end of the ileum is sutured above the anus. Intestinal effluent is temporarily discharged through the proximal stoma of a loop ileostomy until the second stage of surgery is performed.

through the ileum to the reservoir. The fecal material, which is stored in the ileal reservoir, is then expelled from the anus. Control is achieved as edema subsides and the anal sphincter becomes stronger.

Nursing Management

The preoperative assessment of a client having an ileoanal reservoir (both stages) is essentially the same as for the client with an ileostomy. The postoperative assessment after the first stage of ileoanal reservoir surgery includes making the same observations and assessments as those for an ileostomy. In addition, the nurse inspects the anal area for drainage and checks the drain or drainage tube in the presacral area if there is one. After the second stage, when the ileostomy is closed and the ileum is connected to the anal reservoir, the nurse inspects the anal area and the operative sites for drainage.

The postoperative plan of nursing care involves measures pertaining to general surgery and related client problems, such as risk for fluid volume deficit, risk for bowel incontinence, and impaired perianal skin integrity (refer to Nursing Process: The Client Recovering From Ileostomy Surgery). To reduce the risk for bowel incontinence, the nurse instructs the client to perform perineal exercises four to six times a day to re-establish anal sphincter control and enlarge the ileoanal reservoir. These exercises involve tightening the anus as if trying to prevent a bowel

---

BOX 54-2 ● **Unblocking the Catheter in a Continent Ileostomy**

If the catheter used to drain fecal matter or mucus from the internal reservoir becomes obstructed, suggest the following measures:

- Bear down as if to have a bowel movement.
- Rotate the catheter tip inside the stoma.
- Milk the catheter.
- If these are not successful, remove the catheter, rinse it, and try again.
- Notify the physician if these efforts do not result in any drainage.
- Never wait longer than 6 hours without obtaining drainage.

movement and holding the contraction for a count of 10 before relaxing. The nurse should urge the client to do this exercise for 10 repetitions.

Keeping the perianal area clean is especially important. After first-stage ileoanal surgery, the nurse teaches the client to use a squirt bottle to clean the perianal area and avoid skin irritation. After the second-stage repair, the nurse instructs the client to cleanse the anus with warm, soapy water to remove mucus, stool, or both. The client also must dry the area well.

The nurse teaches the client and family the following:

- Continue performing perineal strengthening exercises daily.
- Apply protective ointments or creams as recommended by the physician.
- Inspect the anal area daily using a hand-held mirror. Contact the physician if the anal area becomes sore or skin changes (e.g. ulceration, bleeding) are apparent.
- Use a thin sanitary shield or disposable, lined underwear to absorb fecal drainage until anal sphincter control is achieved.

COLOSTOMY

A colostomy is an opening in the large bowel created by bringing a section of the large intestine out to the abdomen and fashioning a stoma. A cancerous lesion, an ulcerative inflammatory process, multiple polyposis (condition of numerous polyps), and traumatic injury to the bowel are indications for a colostomy.

Types

A temporary or permanent colostomy may be created in the ascending, transverse, descending, or sigmoid areas of the colon (Fig. 54-5). The consistency of the fecal material ranges from semiliquid to formed depending on the intestinal area from which the colostomy is formed (see Table 54-1). Regular irrigations may control a sigmoid colostomy, and sometimes a descending colostomy, thus eliminating the need for the client to constantly wear an appliance.

The stoma may be found anywhere from the lower right, center, to middle or lower left positions on the abdomen. The terms *single-barrel, double-barrel,* and *loop* are used to describe the appearance of the colostomy.

Surgical Management

Single-Barrel Colostomy

The term **single-barrel colostomy** indicates that the ostomy has a single stoma through which fecal matter passes. The colon is cut above the diseased area, and the healthy end is brought through the abdominal wall to form the ma-

FIGURE 54-5 Various colostomies.

tured stoma. The diseased portion of the bowel is removed, with the remaining distal end closed for later reconnection (**segmental resection**). For tumors in the lower third of the sigmoid, that portion, the rectum, and anus may be surgically removed through a perineal incision in a procedure referred to as an **abdominoperineal resection.** After performing an abdominoperineal resection, the surgeon leaves a drain or pack in the perineal area for about 1 week, after which it is removed and irrigations of the perineal wound may be ordered.

Double-Barrel Colostomy

A **double-barrel colostomy,** which is performed most often in the transverse section of the large intestine, contains both a proximal and distal stoma. Each stoma is everted and sutured in place. The proximal stoma expels the fecal material. The distal stoma leads from the lower portion of the cut bowel to the anus. Because fecal drainage has been diverted, the distal portion of the bowel does not pass feces. The distal stoma and the anus may expel mucus. When a double-barrel colostomy has been performed, the physician is asked to identify the distal and proximal stomas. A diagram is provided in the medical record, and the nurse may duplicate it on the nursing care plan. This information is essential when assessing bowel function and whether irrigations are required. Irrigation (Nursing Guidelines 54-2) may be ordered for both the proxi-

NURSING GUIDELINES 54-2

Standard Colostomy Irrigation

Colostomy irrigation begins on the fourth or fifth postoperative day. Standard irrigation is a scheduled irrigation, using 500 to 1500 mL tepid water. Check physician orders. Try to use colostomy irrigation equipment that the client will use at home.

■ Ask client to sit on a toilet seat or chair near the toilet.

■ Prepare the irrigation, purging air from the tubing.

■ Place the irrigation sheath over the stoma, directing the sheath into the toilet.

■ Lubricate the distal end of the catheter.

■ Hang the container of irrigant so that the bottom of the solution bag is about 12 inches above the stoma.

■ Gently insert the catheter tip into the stoma and advance it 2 to 3 inches.

■ If there is resistance, remove the catheter, release the tubing clamp, and gently reinsert the catheter while the solution is flowing.

■ Allow the irrigant to flow slowly and gradually into the stoma.

■ If the client complains of cramping, clamp the tubing and ask the client to take a few deep breaths.

■ Once the cramping subsides, continue the irrigation.

■ If water escapes from the stoma during the irrigation, clamp the tubing until it stops. If a catheter tip is used instead of a cone, introduce the catheter further into the stoma, but no more than 6 inches.

■ When the prescribed amount of solution is instilled, remove the catheter. The client may remain sitting or walk around (clamp the distal end of the irrigation sheath). Complete drainage usually takes 30 minutes.

■ If the irrigant fails to return properly, gently massage the lower abdomen or have the client take several deep breaths and relax or reposition his or her body. Notify the physician if these measures do not work.

■ Document the procedure, including the amount of irrigant used, appearance of returns, and client's response.

Irrigating bag with fluid

Cone attached to irrigating catheter

mal and distal portions of the bowel, or for the proximal portion only.

A double-barrel colostomy often is temporary and usually performed to rest a portion of the bowel to treat a disorder such as acute diverticulitis, chronic constipation, or inflammatory bowel disease. The interval before reestablishing the continuity of the bowel may be 16 months or longer. When the diseased portion of the bowel is removed or healed, the bowel is reconnected and functions normally. In the meantime, the stoma may need irrigation (Box 54-3) or alternative methods for regulating bowel elimination (Box 54-4).

Stop, Think, and Respond ● BOX 54-1

A client calls the doctor's office 4 months after a double-barrel colostomy. He tells the triage nurse that the stool is more liquid than usual and that he is emptying the pouch every 4 hours. What questions does the triage nurse need to ask?

Loop Colostomy

A **loop colostomy** indicates that a loop of bowel has been lifted through the abdomen and is supported in place with a glass rod or plastic butterfly device. About 24 to 72 hours

BOX 54-3 ● Alternatives to Standard Irrigation

If the client has a double-barrel colostomy, irrigate the proximal stoma in the same manner as a single-barrel colostomy. To irrigate the distal stoma, try the following:

● Have the client sit on a toilet or a bedpan because the irrigation fluid and a small amount of mucus will leave by way of the anus. During the immediate postoperative period, necrotic tissue also may be expelled.

● Use a bulb syringe, short catheter, container of solution, plastic sheath or apron, and an emesis basin as another technique for irrigation. This method calls for several instillations of 250 to 500 mL solution at a time, sometimes twice a day. Some clients have found this method effective for controlling spillage for 24 hours or more. It may be used as an alternate choice when the standard method cannot be used.

BOX 54-4 ● Regulating Bowel Elimination Without Irrigating

Some ostomates learn to regulate bowel elimination without irrigating frequently. The following tips may be encouraging to new ostomates, who may be able to establish regular elimination patterns.

- Insert a suppository, such as glycerin or bisacodyl (Dulcolax), into the stoma. The suppository should be recommended by the physician. Up to 7 days or more of daily use may be needed before a regular elimination pattern is established. Initially movements may occur three or four times daily, but each day movements should decrease until only one or two movements occur daily.

Other methods to stimulate bowel elimination and a regular schedule include:

- Drinking prune or fruit juice
- Eating fiber-rich foods and dried fruits and performing mild exercise
- Using a stool softener, mineral oil, or milk of magnesia if recommended by the physician

---

after surgery, the anterior wall of the loop is opened at the client's bedside or in a treatment room, either by incising the bowel or using a cautery machine to form the stoma. The posterior wall of the bowel is left intact, which results in a proximal and distal opening to the bowel.

By delaying the opening of the intestinal loop, the initial healing of the incision occurs without danger of contamination. Opening the bowel does not cause any discomfort because the bowel lacks pain receptors. When a loop colostomy is opened, the bed and client's clothing are well protected. Preparing the client for the pungent odor of cauterized tissue, which subsides shortly, and the initial gush of fecal material is important. A temporary ostomy pouch initially is used to receive the flow of liquid feces.

Nursing Management

Preoperative nursing management is similar to that for clients having an ileostomy. Because a colostomy may be performed for cancer of the colon or rectum, however, the client may be more anxious about the procedure. Postoperative cancer treatment options also may serve to increase the client's anxiety.

NURSING PROCESS

● **Care After Colostomy Surgery**

Assessment

After the client returns from surgery, assessments include taking vital signs, checking dressings, and monitoring nasogastric tubes and IV infusions. The nurse reviews the client's chart for the type of colostomy and the location of the stoma(s). If an abdominoperineal resection was per-

formed, he or she checks the drain or packing in the perineal area and notes the characteristics of the drainage.

The nurse monitors vital signs every 4 hours or as ordered. He or she takes the client's temperature by a route other than rectal. The nurse reports a sudden elevation in temperature over 38.3°C (101°F) or an increase in pain and abdominal tenderness or distention to the physician immediately. The nurse also checks the surgical dressing frequently in the early postoperative period and observes the characteristics of the stoma. Monitoring urine output and the volume of suctioned gastric secretions is important. If urine output is markedly decreased or less than 500 mL/day, the nurse informs the physician immediately.

Diagnosis, Planning, and Interventions

The nurse performs standard postsurgical measures to maintain the airway and relieve pain and anxiety. He or she performs nasogastric decompression (see Chap. 52) and monitors fluid and electrolyte status. The nurse may need to measure fluids lost through decompression and replace them by administering additional IV fluids. An indwelling catheter may be used to relieve abdominal pressure and prevent urine retention during the first few days after surgery.

The nurse teaches how to care for the colostomy by demonstrating the irrigating procedure and, if possible, outlining nonirrigation methods for keeping the ostomy patent and establishing a regular pattern of bowel elimination. The time between the use of these methods and eventual regularity is unique to each client. Natural methods are the least predictable for regulating the bowel, but many clients learn to recognize subtle clues that the bowel will be moving. They then have sufficient time to reach a bathroom and eliminate in private.

The nurse also demonstrates skin and stoma care and appliance application and removal. To provide ample learning time, he or she divides material that the client must learn into small units. After demonstrating one aspect of care, the client returns the demonstration. The nurse then adds additional material when the client feels self-confident. Reinforcing verbal information and demonstrated skills with printed material that may be available from ostomy associations or the enterostomal therapy nurse is an important intervention. In addition, the nurse arranges a dietary consultation to discuss nutrition and food modifications. The nurse includes the following points in the teaching plan:

- Changes in the size and color of the stoma vary with activity and emotional status. Anger or extreme annoyance may cause the stoma to turn red or purple. Small beads of blood may ooze from the surface. Fright may cause the stoma to blanch. These reactions are normal and insignificant as long as the tissues revert to their normal state when the cause is alleviated.
- Eat a regular diet, but avoid gas-forming foods to control intestinal gas.

- In most cases, increasing fiber in the diet and drinking extra water correct constipation.
- Diarrhea may be related to diet. Characteristics of diarrhea include both increased stool output and liquid nature of the stool. One or two loose stools per day does not necessarily indicate a problem. Eliminating food items that result in diarrhea may help to control the problem. If diarrhea persists for more than 2 days, the client should contact the physician.
- Eat slowly with the mouth closed and chew food well to decrease gas that results chiefly from swallowing air rather than from digestion.
- With the exception of tight clothing, no adjustments are necessary in clothing worn. Clients who require firm support (e.g., those who wear girdles, have back problems, wear braces) may find a stoma shield helpful in preventing irritation or undue pressure on the stoma.
- Check body weight weekly. Contact the physician if there is a sudden weight loss or gain.
- Perform irrigations at approximately the same time each day. The best time to irrigate is after a meal because food in the digestive tract stimulates peristalsis and defecation.
- The physician may recommend that the schedule for irrigations gradually progress to every other day, every third day, or even twice a week. If constipation occurs, contact the physician regarding a change in the irrigation schedule.
- Do not restrict travel or activities outside the home. Changes in stool pattern may be normal when daily routine is altered. Preassembled kits that contain all materials needed for irrigation and changes of the colostomy appliance are available. If traveling by air, take ostomy supplies in carry-on luggage to prevent their loss if luggage is misdirected or lost. Necessary items also may be assembled individually and placed in waterproof containers.

Risk for Bowel Incontinence related to unpredictable bowel elimination pattern

Expected Outcome: Client will not experience accidental soiling.

- Instruct the client how to keep the ostomy appliance intact. *Proper application prevents accidental soiling.*
- Schedule colostomy irrigation or suppository insertion for a descending or sigmoid colostomy. *These measures assist with maintaining predictable bowel elimination.*

Risk for Diarrhea or **Constipation** related to changes in bowel motility

Expected Outcome: Client will maintain expected consistency of feces according to location of the colostomy.

Diarrhea

- Instruct client to keep a record of food intake, noting time of problems with loose stools or diarrhea. *A food record helps identify specific foods that irritate the GI tract.*

- Inform client about the need to reduce or eliminate offending foods. *Such information helps prevent diarrhea.*
- Teach client to report prolonged problems with increased stool volume, watery stool consistency, nausea, vomiting, or abdominal pain to the physician. *Ostomates can experience gastroenteritis.*

Constipation

- Gently dilate the stoma with a lubricated-gloved finger. *Dilation assists with expelling stool.*
- Advise client to increase fluid intake. *Increased intake will add fluid to stool, making it easier to pass.*
- Encourage client to eat regular meals. *Dieting or fasting can decrease stool volume and slow elimination.*
- Provide high-fiber, nonirritating foods. *Such foods increase stool bulk and moisture.*
- Offer foods such as coffee or stewed prunes. *These foods promote elimination.*
- Consult with physician if preceding measures fail. *Client may benefit from irrigation, suppository, or laxative.*

Evaluation of Expected Outcomes

The client reports a predictable stool pattern and no problems with soiling. Stool consistency is as expected and the client has not had constipation or diarrhea.

 GENERAL NUTRITIONAL CONSIDERATIONS

A low-fiber diet may be prescribed for 6 to 8 weeks after ostomy surgery to prevent irritation and slow transit time. Thereafter, small amounts of foods containing fiber are added individually to the diet so that the client's tolerance can be evaluated. Foods not tolerated initially may be reintroduced weeks or months later.

One to 2 quarts of fluid are needed to replace liquid lost from decreased water reabsorption from the bowel. Reassure the client that extra fluids do not contribute to watery stools but are excreted as urine. Fluid restriction should not be used to control liquid feces. Likewise, the client may need extra sodium.

Foods that may produce odorous gas include beans, corn, chocolate, coconut, green pepper, legumes, onions, vegetables of the cabbage family, beets, simple sugars, pork, oat bran, dark rye and pumpernickel breads, carbonated beverages, beer and other alcoholic beverages, and fried foods.

Because they may be linked to stomal obstruction in clients with ileostomy, clients should avoid fibrous vegetables (celery, cabbage), bamboo shoots, nuts, and foods with kernels, especially popcorn.

Parenteral injections or intranasal administrations (Nascobal) of vitamin B_{12} are used to prevent deficiencies in clients who have had most or all of the ileum removed because this area is responsible for B_{12} absorption. Clients may not need such replacement for several months after surgery because the body stores vitamin B_{12}.

Decreased absorption of bile salts allows their passage in the stool. When in contact with the skin surface, these bile salts can lead to excoriation. The physician may prescribe cholestyramine to bind and inactivate these bile salts. Occasionally, lack of bile salt absorption leads to poor fat absorption. A low-fat diet or a diet supplemented with medium-chain triglycerides may be used to minimize these symptoms and to maintain proper nutrition.

GENERAL PHARMACOLOGIC CONSIDERATIONS

Some medications, especially vitamins, antibiotics, and antituberculosis drugs, cause particularly strong odors that cling to the appliance. The client can obtain a list of drugs that may leave an odor on an ostomy appliance from an ostomy association or ostomy appliance manufacturers.

Clients with an ileostomy should avoid enteric-coated products and some modified-release drugs, such as slow-release beads and layered tablets. These products may pass through without being absorbed. When changing the ileostomy appliance, check for undissolved—and therefore unabsorbed—capsules. Such findings mean that the client has not received the desired effect of the medication; contact the physician.

Some preparations such as Slow-K (potassium chloride) leave a "ghost" of the wax matrix coating, but that does not indicate the drug has been unabsorbed. Clients with an ileostomy may need monthly vitamin B_{12} injections or intranasal B_{12} because the terminal ileum may be compromised to such an extent as to interfere with dietary absorption of the vitamin.

GENERAL GERONTOLOGIC CONSIDERATIONS

Teach ostomy care as appropriate for the client's age and prior understanding. Presenting the material in brief sessions is best. Supplement the instructions with illustrations and written directions.

Teach a family member or another responsible person how to perform ostomy care in case the client cannot temporarily assume responsibility for this task. Always provide the telephone number of an individual to contact (i.e., the enterostomal therapist) if problems occur after discharge.

Older adult ostomates with chronic disorders such as poor vision and arthritis may encounter difficulty in changing the appliance, performing skin care, irrigating the colostomy stoma, and caring for the permanent appliance. Consult with an enterostomal therapist about which equipment may best meet the client's needs. If the older adult will be

permanently unable to assume care for an ostomy, healthcare professionals need to arrange for daily care. Depending on the situation, a family member, visiting nurse, or home healthcare nurse needs to assume this responsibility. In some instances, transfer to a skilled nursing facility or nursing home may be necessary.

Ostomates are particularly vulnerable to emotional distress, including loss of self-esteem, poor body image, and increased anxiety. Actively listen to expressed concerns and fears over adjusting to and caring for the ostomy and rejection from family and friends. Some clients benefit from professional psychological support in coping with a new body image. Sexuality issues surface during puberty and continue throughout the client's adulthood. Never assume that an older adult is not concerned about the effects of the ostomy on sexuality. Provide an opportunity to discuss sexual concerns. Support groups are available.

Critical Thinking Exercises

1. *In what ways does the care of a 20-year-old client with an ileostomy differ from that of a 60-year-old client with a colostomy?*

2. *A client with an ileostomy is disturbed by the need to empty liquid stool from his appliance so frequently. He intends to reduce his intake of fluids. What information is important to give this client?*

3. *What recommendations are appropriate for the client with a colostomy who has been experiencing an unusual amount of intestinal gas?*

References and Suggested Readings

Ball, E. M. (2000). Part two: A teaching guide for continent ostomy. *RN, 63*(12), 35–38.

Bryant, D. & Fleischer, I. (2000). Changing an OSTOMY appliance. *Nursing 2000, 30*(11), 51–55.

Moskovitz, D. N., Maunder, R. G., Cohen, Z., McLeod, R. S., & MacRae, H. (2000). Use of community resources before surgery for inflammatory bowel disease is associated with postsurgical quality of life. *Canadian Journal of Gastroenterology, 14,* 95–98.

Thompson, J. (2000). Part one: A practical ostomy guide. *RN, 63*(11), 61–66.

Vaccari, J. (1999). Consult stat: Certain drugs may not work in ileostomy patients. *RN, 62*(2), 69–70, 75.

Young, M. (2000). Caring for patients with coloanal reservoirs for rectal cancer. *MEDSURG Nursing, 9,* 193–197.

Caring for Clients With Disorders of the Liver, Gallbladder, or Pancreas

Words to Know

alpha fetoprotein
ascites
balloon tamponade
biliary colic
caput medusae
cholecystitis
choledocholithiasis
cholelithiasis
cholestasis
cirrhosis
Cullen's sign
esophageal varices
fetor hepaticus
hepatic encephalopathy
hepatic lobectomy
hepatitis

hepatorenal syndrome
injection sclerotherapy
laparoscopic
    cholecystectomy
lithotripsy
open cholecystectomy
pancreatectomy
    (partial, total)
pancreatitis
portal hypertension
radical pancreatoduo-
    denectomy (Whipple
    procedure)
steatorrhea
T-tube
Turner's sign

Learning Objectives

On completion of this chapter, the reader will:

- List common findings manifested by clients with cirrhosis.
- Discuss common complications of cirrhosis.
- Identify the modes of transmission of viral hepatitis.
- Describe nursing measures after liver biopsy.
- Discuss nursing management for clients with a medically or surgically treated liver disorder.
- Identify factors that contribute to, signs and symptoms of, and medical treatments for cholecystitis.
- Name techniques of gallbladder removal.
- Discuss nursing management for clients with a T-tube.
- Summarize the nursing management of clients undergoing medical or surgical treatment of a gallbladder disorder.
- Describe the treatment and nursing management of pancreatitis.
- Describe the treatment of pancreatic carcinoma.
- Explain the nursing management of clients undergoing pancreatic surgery.

The liver, gallbladder, and pancreas play important roles in digestion. They also are responsible for many other physiologic activities (see Chap. 51). Their poor function impairs the digestive process and the client's overall nutritional status.

DISORDERS OF THE LIVER

The *liver* has two major lobes (right and left) and two small lobes (caudate and quadrate), which are found on its undersurface (Fig. 55-1). The liver is supported by intra-abdominal pressure and various attachments called *mesenteries,* which connect the liver to the adjacent intestines,

abdominal wall, and diaphragm. Unless it is abnormally enlarged, the liver usually is not palpable.

The liver has various functions (Box 55-1) and a rich blood supply. It receives arterial blood from the hepatic artery, an indirect branch of the aorta. The portal vein transports blood from the intestinal tract to the liver. After blood has traversed vascular pathways inside the liver, the hepatic veins collect the blood and transport it to the inferior vena cava and then back to the heart (Fig. 55-2).

Microscopically, the liver's internal structure includes smaller branches of the hepatic artery, the hepatic and portal veins, the lymphatics, and the bile ducts. The cellular constituents of the liver are the hepatic parenchymal cells, which perform most of the liver's metabolic func-

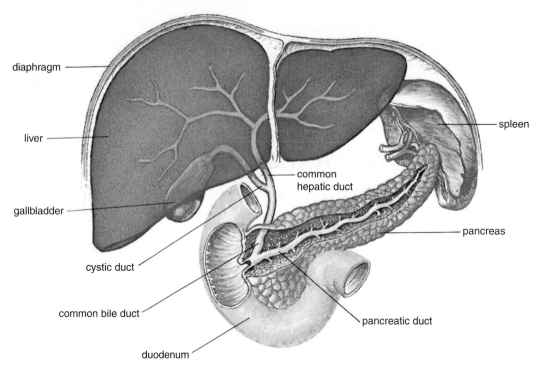

FIGURE 55-1 The liver and biliary system. (From Smeltzer, S. C. & Bare, B. G. [2000]. *Brunner & Suddarth's textbook of medical–surgical nursing* [9th ed.]. Philadelphia: Lippincott Williams & Wilkins.)

tions, and the Kupffer cells, which engage in the liver's immunologic, detoxifying, and blood-filtering actions.

● JAUNDICE (ICTERUS)

Jaundice, also called *icterus,* is a greenish-yellow discoloration of tissue. It is a sign of disease, but it is not itself a unique disease. Jaundice accompanies many diseases that directly or indirectly affect the liver and is probably the most common sign of a liver disorder.

BOX 55-1 ● **Functions of the Liver**

- Metabolizes glucose
- Regulates blood glucose concentration
- Converts glucose to glycogen to glucose to maintain normal glucose levels
- Synthesizes amino acids from the breakdown of protein or from lactate that muscles produce during exercise to form glucose (*gluconeogenesis*)
- Converts ammonia (byproduct of gluconeogenesis) into urea
- Metabolizes proteins and fats
- Stores vitamins A, B$_{12}$, D, and some B-complex vitamins, as well as iron and copper
- Metabolizes drugs, chemicals, bacteria, and other foreign elements
- Forms and excretes bile
- Excretes bilirubin
- Synthesizes factors needed for blood coagulation (e.g., prothrombin, fibrinogen)

Jaundice results from an abnormally high concentration of the pigment *bilirubin* in the blood. Normally, total bilirubin concentration ranges from 0.2 to 1.3 mg/dL. If the serum bilirubin level exceeds 2.5 mg/dL, jaundice is visible, notably on the skin, oral mucous membranes, and (especially) sclera.

To understand the scope and significance of jaundice, it is important to know how bile is formed and excreted. Bilirubin is produced in the liver, spleen, and bone marrow. It also results from hemoglobin metabolism and is a byproduct of hemolysis (red blood cell [RBC] destruction). The reticuloendothelial system also produces bilirubin. The liver removes bilirubin from the body, excreting it in *bile,* of which bilirubin is the major pigment. Thus, serum contains a normal amount of bilirubin. Serum bilirubin levels increase when (1) there is excessive destruction of RBCs or (2) the liver cannot excrete bilirubin normally.

There are two forms of bilirubin. *Indirect* or *unconjugated bilirubin* binds with protein as it circulates in the blood. This form normally circulates in the blood; when its level is elevated, the usual cause is increased hemolysis. The other form of bilirubin is *direct* or *conjugated bilirubin,* which circulates freely in the blood until reaching the liver. The liver conjugates direct bilirubin with glucuronide. The conjugated bilirubin is excreted in the bile. As the bile enters the bile ducts and moves into the intestine, bacterial enzymes transform the direct bilirubin into *urobilinogen.* Some urobilinogen is changed into *urobilin,* the brown pigment of stool; some is excreted in

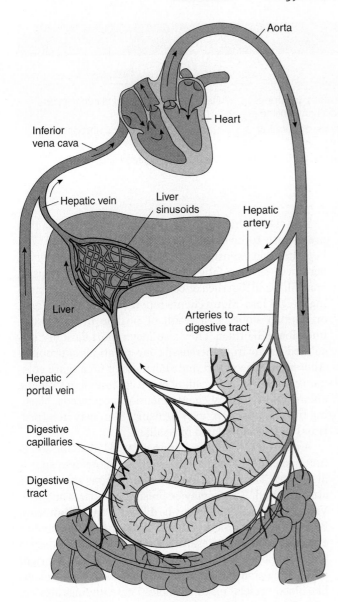

FIGURE 55-2 Hepatic blood supply and circulation.

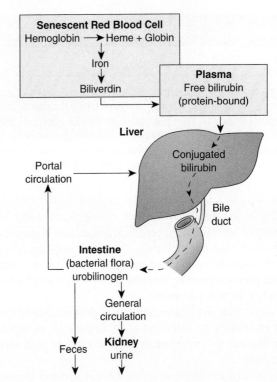

FIGURE 55-3 Formation, circulation, and elimination of bilirubin.

● CIRRHOSIS

Cirrhosis is a degenerative liver disorder caused by generalized cellular damage.

Pathophysiology and Etiology

Once liver cells are irreversibly damaged, nonfunctional fibrous connective scar tissue replaces them, which leads to considerable anatomic distortion and partial or complete occlusion of blood channels in the liver. The liver becomes increasingly unable to carry out its many functions. This leads to disturbances in digestion and metabolism, defects in blood coagulation, fluid and electrolyte imbalances, and impaired ability to metabolize hormones and detoxify chemicals. Because bile begins to drain into the intestine, the client experiences fat malabsorption and an inability to absorb fat-soluble vitamins (A, D, E, and K). Portal hypertension, esophageal varices, ascites, and hepatic encephalopathy are complications of advanced cirrhosis (see later discussion).

There are several types of cirrhosis: Laënnec's, postnecrotic, and cardiac. *Alcoholic* or *Laënnec's cirrhosis,* the most common type, results from chronic alcohol intake and is frequently associated with poor nutrition. It also can follow chronic poisoning with certain chemicals (e.g., carbon tetrachloride, a cleaning agent) or ingestion of hepatotoxic drugs (e.g., acetaminophen). Alcoholic cirrhosis is characterized by necrotic liver cells, which

the urine; and some is carried back to the liver by the bloodstream for re-excretion in the bile (Fig. 55-3).

There is no direct test for indirect bilirubin levels. They are calculated by subtracting direct bilirubin levels from total bilirubin levels. For example, if the total bilirubin level is 1.0 mg/dL and the conjugated bilirubin level is 0.1 mg/dL, then the indirect bilirubin level is 0.9 mg/dL.

There are three forms of jaundice: (1) *hemolytic jaundice,* caused by excess destroyed RBCs (see Chap. 39); (2) *hepatocellular jaundice,* caused by liver disease; and (3) *obstructive jaundice,* caused by a block in the passage of bile between the liver and intestinal tract (Table 55-1). Because unconjugated and conjugated bilirubin are distinct and can be differentiated, they are important in the differential diagnosis of diseases that produce jaundice.

TABLE 55-1	TYPES OF JAUNDICE	
TYPE	**DESCRIPTION**	**CHANGES IN BILIRUBIN LEVELS**
Hemolytic	Hemolytic processes (e.g., multiple blood transfusions, pernicious anemia, sickle cell anemia) cause an overproduction of bilirubin.	Elevated unconjugated bilirubin levels
Hepatocellular	Liver cells damaged by viral infections, medications, or chemical toxicity cannot clear bilirubin from the blood.	Elevated conjugated and unconjugated bilirubin levels
Obstructive	Gallstones, inflammation, or tumors obstruct the bile duct, causing reabsorption of bile into the blood.	Elevated conjugated bilirubin levels

gradually are replaced by scar tissue. Eventually the amount of scar tissue exceeds functional liver tissue. The liver takes on a characteristic "hobnail" appearance, in which there are islands of normal tissue, regenerating tissue, and scar tissue. The disease develops over a long period of 30 years or more.

Postnecrotic cirrhosis results from destruction of liver cells secondary to infection (e.g., hepatitis), metabolic liver disease, or exposure to hepatotoxins or industrial chemicals.

In *biliary cirrhosis,* scarring occurs around the bile ducts in the liver. The cause usually is related to chronic biliary obstruction and infection.

The prognosis for clients with cirrhosis is based on bilirubin and albumin levels, presence of ascites (accumulation of serous fluid in the peritoneal cavity), neurologic involvement, and nutritional status. See Table 55-2 for further information.

Assessment Findings

Signs and Symptoms

Signs and symptoms of cirrhosis increase in severity as the disease progresses (Box 55-2). The clinical manifestations are categorized as compensated and decompensated. *Compensated cirrhosis* is less severe, and signs and symptoms are more vague. As the disease progresses, it is referred to as *decompensated cirrhosis.* Signs and symptoms are very pronounced and indicate liver failure.

The client's history often correlates with factors that predispose to cirrhosis, such as chronic alcohol use, hepatitis, and exposure to toxins. The client typically experiences chronic fatigue, anorexia, dyspepsia, nausea, vomiting, and diarrhea or constipation, with accompanying weight loss. Many clients report passing clay-colored or whitish stools as a result of no bile in the gastrointestinal (GI) tract. They also may report dark or "tea-colored" urine from increased concentrations of urobilin. Abdominal discomfort and shortness of breath are common complaints as a result of organ compression from the enlarged liver. Many clients mention nosebleeds, bleeding from the gums, or easy bruising. Skin may itch (pruritus) from accumulated bile salts.

A client with cirrhosis has an enlarged liver and sometimes an enlarged spleen, causing the abdomen to appear distended. The skin, sclera, or oral mucous membranes are jaundiced. Edema may be present in the legs and feet. Veins over the abdomen may be dilated (**caput medusae**). Because the dysfunctional liver cannot fully metabolize estrogen, men may present with *gynecomastia* (enlarged breasts) and testicular atrophy. *Palmar erythema* (bright pink palms) and *cutaneous spider angiomata* (tiny, spider-like blood vessels) may be visible. These findings also are related to an inability to inactivate estrogen.

Diagnostic Findings

A liver biopsy, which reveals hepatic fibrosis, is the most conclusive diagnostic procedure. The biopsy is obtained percutaneously with mild sedation on the nursing unit

TABLE 55-2	CHILD'S CLASSIFICATION OF HEPATOCELLULAR FUNCTION IN CIRRHOSIS		
GROUP DESIGNATION	**A (LEAST SEVERE)**	**B**	**C (MOST SEVERE)**
Serum bilirubin (mg/dL)	Below 2.0	2.0–3.0	Over 3.0
Serum albumin (g/dL)	Over 3.5	3.0–3.5	Under 3.0
Ascites	None	Easily controlled	Poorly controlled
Neurologic disorder (degree of encephalopathy)	None	Minimal	Advanced coma
Nutrition	Excellent	Good	Poor with "wasting"

(From Sherlock, S. & Dooley, J. [1997]. *Diseases of the liver and biliary system* [10th ed, p. 162]. Oxford: Blackwell.)

BOX 55-2 ● Clinical Manifestations of Cirrhosis

COMPENSATED
Intermittent mild fever
Vascular spiders
Palmar erythema (reddened palms)
Unexplained epistaxis
Ankle edema
Vague morning indigestion
Flatulent dyspepsia
Abdominal pain
Firm, enlarged liver
Splenomegaly

DECOMPENSATED
Ascites
Jaundice
Weakness
Muscle wasting
Weight loss
Continuous mild fever
Clubbing of fingers
Purpura (due to decreased platelet count)
Spontaneous bruising
Epistaxis
Hypotension
Sparse body hair
White nails
Gonadal atrophy

(Nursing Guidelines 55-1) or through a surgical incision. It also can be performed in the radiology department with ultrasound or computed tomography (CT) to identify appropriate placement of the trochar or biopsy needle.

Certain blood tests provide information about liver function (Box 55-3). Prolonged prothrombin time (PT) and low platelet count place the client at high risk for hemorrhage. The client may receive intravenous (IV) administration of vitamin K or infusions of platelets before liver biopsy to reduce the risk of bleeding. Other tests used to examine the liver include CT, magnetic resonance imaging (MRI), and radioisotope liver scan, all of which may demonstrate the liver's enlarged size, nodular configuration, and distorted blood flow.

Medical and Surgical Management

No specific cure for cirrhosis exists. The principal aim of therapy is to prevent further deterioration by abolishing underlying causes and to preserve whatever liver function remains. Various approaches are used to relieve associated symptoms. Vitamins and nutritional supplements promote healing of liver cells. Improved nutritional status helps the client feel better. Malnutrition is treated with enteral or parenteral feedings. Because absorption of the fat-soluble vitamins is impaired, special attention is given to their supplementation (see Table 52-1). Vitamin K

also is used to correct coagulopathy, which results from prolonged PT and partial thromboplastin time (PTT). Vitamin B complex, vitamin C, and iron also may be prescribed. IV albumin may be given if hypoproteinemia is severe. The client *must not* consume alcohol.

Protein intake is restricted in clients with advanced liver disease because it increases the ammonia in the intestine, precipitating hepatic encephalopathy (see Complications of Cirrhosis, later). Lactulose is administered to detoxify ammonium and to act as an osmotic agent, drawing water into the bowel, which causes diarrhea in some clients. Antacids may be used to reduce gastric disturbances and decrease the potential for GI bleeding. Potassium-sparing antidiuretics such as spironolactone are used to treat ascites (see Complications of Cirrhosis, later).

Transfusions of platelets may be necessary to correct thrombocytopenia (low platelet count). Packed RBCs may be administered in cases of anemia or blood loss. Cholestyramine may be prescribed to bind bile salts and relieve pruritus. Additional measures to relieve pruritus include skin care and routing cleansing with a nondrying agent. Skin is patted dry, and moisturizing lotion is applied immediately after bathing. Ursodeoxycholic acid (Actigall) may be used to promote bile flow from the liver. Sodium intake is carefully regulated and often restricted because of the potential for water retention, which can lead to edema, circulatory congestion, and heart failure. Fluid intake also may be restricted. Liver transplantation is an option for treating liver failure as well as chronic liver disease (Box 55-4).

Nursing Management

If the client has active alcoholism, the nurse monitors vital signs closely. A rise in blood pressure (BP), pulse, and temperature correlates with alcohol withdrawal; the nurse must recognize and treat these appropriately along with the other presenting symptoms (see Chap. 17).

The nurse weighs the client daily and keeps an accurate record of intake and output. If the abdomen appears enlarged, the nurse measures it according to a set routine (Fig. 55-4). Because of the anorexia that accompanies severe cirrhosis, the client may better tolerate frequent, small, semisolid or liquid meals rather than three full meals a day.

Careful evaluation of the client's response to drug therapy is important because the liver cannot metabolize many substances. The nurse reports any change in mental status or signs of GI bleeding immediately because they indicate secondary complications.

The nurse provides educational information specific to the liver disorder. He or she can refer the client to the American Liver Foundation (or a similar organization) for information about available support groups. The nurse

NURSING GUIDELINES 55-1

Assisting With a Percutaneous Liver Biopsy

1. Explain that the purpose of the procedure is to obtain a small sample of liver tissue for a differential diagnosis of liver disease or to evaluate the extent of liver disease.

2. Check results of coagulation studies (PTT, PT, and platelet count).

3. Check that the informed consent form has been signed.

4. Instruct client to lie supine with the right arm behind the head.

5. Tell client that the site will be cleansed and then draped with a sterile barrier.

6. The physician will instruct the client to take a deep breath and hold it while the needle is introduced, sample obtained, and needle withdrawn—this takes only a few seconds.

7. Monitor vital signs throughout the procedure.

8. Place a pressure dressing over the biopsy site. Instruct client to lie on the right side for several hours.

9. Continue to monitor vital signs according to agency policy.

10. Monitor the biopsy site frequently for bleeding, swelling, or hematoma.

11. Assess breath sounds regularly. Report diminished breath sounds immediately.

12. Assess the abdomen for distention or rigidity. Report if the client is experiencing abdominal pain.

13. Instruct client to avoid coughing or straining.

14. Instruct client to avoid heavy lifting and strenuous activity for 1 week.

emphasizes the need for abstinence from alcohol and all nonprescription drugs unless approved by the physician. In addition, he or she contacts social services about referrals to alcohol or drug cessation programs. Additional teaching depends on the type and cause of the disorder and the physician's prescribed or recommended home care. For additional nursing management, see Nursing Care Plan 55-1 and Client and Family Teaching Box 55-1.

Complications of Cirrhosis

Portal Hypertension

The portal system consists of gastric veins from the stomach, the mesenteric vein from the intestines, the splenic vein from the spleen and pancreas, and the portal vein. All these veins drain into and through the liver and out the hepatic veins into the inferior vena cava.

In the scarred cirrhotic liver, intrahepatic veins may be compressed. Consequently, blood backs up into the portal system, which is the venous pathway through the liver. This congestion and increased fluid pressure are called **portal hypertension.** As the normal pathway for blood is obstructed, the collateral veins become distended and engorged with blood (Fig. 55-5). These distended collateral vessels develop primarily in the esophagus (esophageal varices) and rectum (hemorrhoids) and on the abdominal surface (caput medusae).

BOX 55-3 ● Common Blood Test Findings in Cirrhosis

Blood studies of clients with cirrhosis are likely to show:
- Increased unconjugated and conjugated bilirubin levels
- Increased enzyme levels of AST (SGOT), ALT (SGPT), and GGT
- Low RBC count—cells appear large
- Decreased leukocytes and thrombocytes
- Low fibrinogen level
- Prolonged PT
- Decreased platelet count
- Low serum albumin level
- Increased globulin level
- Hypokalemia

ALT, alanine transaminase; AST, aspartate phosphatase; GGT, gamma glutamyltransferase; PT, prothrombin time; RBC, red blood cell; SGOT, serum glutamic-oxaloacetic transaminase; SGPT, serum glutamic-pyruvic transaminase.

BOX 55-4 ● Liver Transplants and Organ Donation

The United Network for Organ Sharing (UNOS) is a nonprofit organization that advances organ availability and transplantation by uniting and supporting communities for the client's benefit. The UNOS administers the Organ Procurement and Transplantation Network, adding clients who need transplants to a national waiting list and generating a list of potential recipients when a donor organ becomes available. The UNOS bases its list of potential recipients on such factors as genetic similarity, organ size, medical urgency, and time on the waiting list.

Many transplanted livers are from cadaver donors. Some centers, however, now have "living related donor" programs, in which portions of livers for transplantation come from living donors. In either type of transplant, recipients need life-long immunosuppressant therapy to suppress the immune system and prevent rejection of the transplanted organ.

The organs available are nowhere close to the number needed. Many potential recipients succumb to liver failure while waiting for donor organs. Transplantation costs are high, and the condition of potential recipients is fragile, jeopardizing the chances for successful transplantation. The decision to do a liver transplantation is based on careful scrutiny and assessment of the client, with consideration of the potential for success and improved quality of life.

Methods of treating portal hypertension aim to reduce fluid accumulation and venous pressure. Sodium is restricted. A diuretic, usually an aldosterone antagonist such as spironolactone (Aldactone), is prescribed (Drug Therapy Table 55-1). Diuretics such as furosemide (Lasix) also may be given to promote urinary excretion of excess fluids. These diuretics must be administered with caution, however, because long-term use can cause sodium depletion. Administration of a beta-adrenergic blocker, such as propranolol (Inderal), reduces BP and lowers pressure in the portal system.

A *surgical shunt* may be created. This procedure uses a graft to decompress the portal system by diverting blood flow into the systemic circulation. It is not frequently performed, however, because of the high incidence of complications and shunt failure. An alternative, nonsurgical method of shunt placement is a *transjugular intrahepatic*

portosystemic shunt (TIPS). This invasive radiologic procedure involves the creation of a tract from the hepatic to the portal vein. In TIPS, a cannula with an expandable stent is inserted into the portovenous system through the jugular vein. The stent serves as the intrahepatic shunt between the hepatic vein and portal circulation to relieve portal hypertension. TIPS may be carried out using conscious sedation or anesthesia (see Chap. 25).

Esophageal Varices

Dilated, bulging esophageal veins are referred to as **esophageal varices.** A single dilated, bulging esophageal vein is called a *varix.* Esophageal varices overfill as a result of portal hypertension. They are especially vulnerable to bleeding because they lie superficially in the mucosa, contain little protective elastic tissue, and are easily traumatized by rough food or chemical irritation. Figure 55-6 depicts the pathogenesis of esophageal varices.

Esophageal bleeding is a cardinal sign of esophageal varices. It may be slight but chronic, or massive and rapid. Massive bleeding from esophageal varices is a life-threatening medical emergency requiring immediate intervention. Once bleeding begins, clotting disorders common to liver damage occur. Barium swallow or esophagoscopy confirm the diagnosis of esophageal varices.

Measures to treat portal hypertension reduce the potential for bleeding varices. In addition, a soft diet and elimination of alcohol, aspirin, and other locally irritating substances may prevent varices. Antitussives and stool softeners are prescribed when the client is symptomatic, to reduce coughing or straining, which increases vascular pressure.

Esophageal varices also are treated with injection sclerotherapy or variceal banding. In **injection sclerotherapy,** the physician passes an endoscope orally to locate the varix. He or she then passes a thin needle through the endoscope into the varix and then directly injects a sclerosing agent (sodium tetradecyl, sodium morrhuate). The sclerosing agent solidifies and stops circulation to the varix.

In *variceal banding* (*variceal band ligation*), another endoscopic procedure, the physician uses a device with small rubber bands at the end of the endoscope. After locating the varix, the physician places a rubber band over it. The band restricts blood flow to the varix, which sloughs off after a few days. Persistent portal hypertension allows varices to form again, making it necessary to repeat sclerotherapy or banding procedures regularly.

Acute hemorrhage from esophageal varices is life-threatening. Resuscitative measures include administration of IV fluids and blood products. IV octreotide (Sandostatin) is started as soon as possible. Octreotide reduces pressure in the portal venous system and is preferred to the previously used agents, vasopressin or terlipressin. Urgent endoscopy is indicated to allow for treatment with sclerotherapy or banding. If a skilled

FIGURE 55-4 To measure abdominal girth, place a tape measure around the largest diameter of the abdomen. Make guide marks on the skin so that future measurements are obtained from the same site.

(*text continued on page 818*)

Nursing Care Plan 55-1

THE CLIENT WITH A LIVER DISORDER

Assessment

- Obtain complete diet, drug, and allergy histories and a history of symptoms from client or family. Depending on the circumstances, in-depth questioning may be necessary. Contributing factors may include exposure to toxic chemicals, history of hepatitis, or long-term alcohol abuse.
- Pay special attention to ventilation, abdominal size, weight, and any jaundice or other symptoms of liver disease.
- Analyze food intake and fluid records.
- Review laboratory and diagnostic studies and the physician's progress notes daily to assess client's response to therapy.

Nursing Diagnosis: **Fatigue** related to malnutrition and liver disease

Expected Outcome: Client will report improved energy and adhere to plan to conserve energy.

Interventions	Rationales
Assess client's ability to perform activities of daily living and pattern of fatigue.	Data provide a baseline for comparison and help nurse and client to target ways to conserve energy.
Assist client to set small, short-term goals that will be easy to achieve.	Such goals help the client accomplish tasks without being overwhelmed or exhausted.
Encourage client to separate essential and nonessential tasks and to delegate.	Doing so creates a realistic picture of what must be done and who should do it.
Encourage the client to limit demands on his or her time.	Doing so helps the client set priorities and balance demands with available energy.
Teach strategies for energy conservation such as sitting instead of standing in the shower, storing items within easy reach, and breaking large tasks into smaller ones.	These strategies enhance energy and give a client more control over activities.
Offer a high-protein (if client does not have severe liver disease) and high-calorie diet.	Inadequate nutrition contributes to fatigue.
Encourage client to rest frequently.	Inadequate sleep contributes to fatigue.

Evaluation of Expected Outcome: Client participates in appropriate activities, gradually increases activities, and reports feeling stronger and more energetic.

Nursing Diagnosis: **Imbalanced Nutrition: Less than Body Requirements** related to loss of appetite, nausea, and vomiting

Expected Outcome: Client will identify nutritional requirements and consume adequate nutrition.

Interventions	Rationales
Encourage client to eat six small meals a day.	Small, frequent meals reduce the sensation of fullness and the stimulus for vomiting.
Consult the dietitian for ways to provide nutritional meals that complement the prescribed diet.	Such meals will provide foods that the client is likely to eat within dietary restrictions.
Provide high-carbohydrate snacks or supplements to meals.	Doing so provides additional calories.

(continued)

Nursing Care Plan 55-1 (Continued)

THE CLIENT WITH A LIVER DISORDER

Interventions	Rationales
Offer highest-calorie meal when the client's appetite is greatest.	Clients with liver disease usually are hungriest at breakfast, so providing the highest-calorie meal at the beginning of the day would be most logical.
If vomiting is a problem, administer antiemetics before meals.	Antiemetics prevent nausea and vomiting.
Monitor food intake and ask dietitian to calculate caloric intake.	Tracking nutritional intake provides a record of foods the client best tolerates at different times of day.
Ask family members to assist with meal planning and preparation, adapting to the client's cultural preferences.	These measures enhance the client's ability to eat preferred foods and meet nutritional requirements within dietary restrictions.

Evaluation of Expected Outcome: Client reports improved appetite, identifies appropriate foods that meet dietary requirements, and demonstrates appropriate weight gain.

Nursing Diagnosis: **Ineffective Breathing Pattern** related to ascites and liver enlargement

Expected Outcome: Client will breathe without effort.

Interventions	Rationales
Assess respiratory pattern, noting what causes and relieves dyspnea.	Assessing the cause of dyspnea helps the nurse provide relief measures and improve client's ventilatory efforts.
Place client in an upright or semi-Fowler's position.	These positions facilitate lung expansion by reducing pressure on the diaphragm.
Schedule rest periods before and after activity.	Rest reduces metabolic and oxygen requirements.
Provide supplemental oxygen if client becomes short of breath.	Oxygen therapy decreases dyspnea by reducing the central drive mediated by chemoreceptors in the carotid bodies.

Evaluation of Expected Outcome: Client reports decreased shortness of breath and improved comfort with breathing.

Nursing Diagnosis: **Excess Fluid Volume** related to peripheral edema, ascites, and sodium retention

Expected Outcome: Client will maintain fluid balance.

Interventions	Rationales
Assess location and extent of edema. Measure and record abdominal girth daily.	These measures help locate changes in peripheral edema and ascites.
Monitor weight daily.	Weight reflects changes in body fluid volume.
Restrict sodium and fluid intake as ordered.	Such restrictions reduce peripheral edema and ascites.
Administer prescribed diuretics and potassium.	These measures promote fluid excretion through the kidneys to maintain fluid and electrolyte balance.
Monitor serum albumin levels. Administer protein supplements as ordered.	Low albumin levels can cause severe peripheral edema because they lead to impaired movement of fluid from interstitial spaces to intravascular spaces.

(continued)

Nursing Care Plan 55-1 (Continued)

THE CLIENT WITH A LIVER DISORDER

Interventions	*Rationales*
Maintain IV infusion rates carefully.	Doing so prevents inadvertent infusion of excess fluid volumes.
Encourage client to turn at least every 2 hours when in bed.	Edematous tissue is vulnerable to ischemia and pressure ulcers.

Evaluation of Expected Outcome: Client maintains fluid balance, as evidenced by stable BP, adequate urine output, and decreased peripheral edema and ascites.

Nursing Diagnosis: **Ineffective Protection** related to risk for impaired blood coagulation, bleeding from portal hypertension, and infection

Expected Outcome: Client will not demonstrate evidence of new bleeding or infection.

Interventions	*Rationales*
Carefully monitor vital signs.	Changes may indicate the onset of bleeding or infection.
Notify physician promptly when client has signs of infection: fever, chills, or drainage.	Prompt treatment reduces the risk of morbidity and mortality.
Monitor bleeding times, clotting studies, and platelet counts.	Abnormal results indicate increased risk for bleeding.
Teach client to avoid aspirin or nonsteroidal anti-inflammatory drugs and to use electric razors and soft toothbrushes.	These drugs can cause GI bleeding, and aspirin interferes with platelet function. Electric razors and soft toothbrushes can minimize unnecessary trauma.
Practice aseptic measures and teach family members to do so.	Asepsis reduces the risk of infection.
Observe stools for color and consistency. Test stool for occult blood.	Tests detect blood in stool.
Note any complaints of anxiety, epigastric fullness, weakness, and restlessness.	These findings may indicate bleeding and early shock.
Monitor for ecchymosis, epistaxis, petechiae, and bleeding from gums.	These findings indicate altered clotting mechanisms.
Monitor client carefully during blood transfusions.	Doing so can help detect a transfusion reaction.
Administer vitamin K as ordered.	Vitamin K promotes clotting.

Evaluation of Expected Outcome: Client does not exhibit any new signs of bleeding or infection. Vital signs are stable, and laboratory values are normal.

Nursing Diagnosis: **Impaired Skin Integrity** related to pruritus, jaundice, bleeding tendencies, and edema

Expected Outcome: Skin will remain intact

Interventions	*Rationales*
Provide frequent skin care, avoiding drying soaps and alcohol-based lotions.	Skin care removes waste products deposited in skin and prevents drying.
Encourage client to keep fingernails short and smooth.	Doing so prevents excoriation and infection from scratches.
Turn client at least every 2 hours, massaging bony prominences with emollients.	Turning and massage mobilize edema and improve circulation.

(continued)

Nursing Care Plan 55-1 (Continued)

THE CLIENT WITH A LIVER DISORDER

Interventions	Rationales
Use nonallergenic bed linens; instruct family to avoid harsh detergents.	These measures decrease skin irritation.

Evaluation of Expected Outcome: Skin remains intact with no evidence of pressure ulcers.

Nursing Diagnosis: **Chronic Pain** related to liver enlargement and ascites

Expected Outcome: Client will report increased level of comfort.

Interventions	Rationales
Encourage client to remain on bed rest when experiencing abdominal discomfort, changing position frequently.	These measures relieve pressure and promote comfort.
Administer prescribed analgesics.	These drugs relieve chronic pain.
Explain the pain management regimen.	Adequate explanations help the client understand implementation of the pain-control plan.
For client receiving opioids, monitor sedation and respiratory status when dose is increased.	Usually, clients receiving long-term opioids develop a tolerance to the respiratory depressant effects. They still require monitoring for sedation and respiratory problems.
Instruct client in nonpharmacologic techniques to relieve pain.	Other interventions supplement pain medications and improve comfort level.

Evaluation of Expected Outcome: Client reports that pain medication is effective and that comfort is improved.

PC: **Hepatic Encephalopathy**

Expected Outcome: The nurse will minimize and manage problems associated with hepatic encephalopathy.

Interventions	Rationales
Assess cognitive and neurologic status at least every 8 hours.	Baseline data provide a means by which to determine changes.
Restrict dietary protein as ordered.	Protein is a source of ammonia, which contributes to encephalopathy.
Give small and frequent feedings high in carbohydrates.	Carbohydrates provide energy and spare protein breakdown.
Restrict medications that increase encephalopathy.	Sedatives, hypnotics, and opioids may precipitate hepatic encephalopathy and increase confusion.
Monitor laboratory results, especially ammonia levels.	Increased ammonia levels indicate hepatic encephalopathy, which can lead to coma.
Administer medications that reduce serum ammonia levels, such as lactulose.	Reduced serum ammonia levels are a key goal.
Identify potentially dangerous items and modify the environment.	Doing so promotes the client's safety.
Report any new or sudden increase in mental confusion.	Confusion indicates increased hepatic encephalopathy and possible coma. It requires immediate medical intervention.

(continued)

Nursing Care Plan 55-1 (Continued)

THE CLIENT WITH A LIVER DISORDER

Interventions	*Rationales*
Orient client to name, place, time, and date as needed.	Doing so reinforces reality and provides the client with cues about the world.
If hepatic coma develops, monitor respiratory status and initiate measures to prevent complications.	Clients in hepatic coma are at increased risk for pneumonia and infection.
Implement measures to prevent skin breakdown and pressure.	These clients are at increased risk for skin breakdown and pressure ulcers.

Evaluation of Expected Outcome: Client remains free from injury.

---

endoscopist is not available or bleeding is too rapid to permit endoscopy, **balloon tamponade** with a Sengstaken-Blakemore tube may be useful in compressing the varices and stemming the flow of blood (Fig. 55-7). Unfortunately, this method usually allows only temporary relief

55-1 *Client and Family Teaching* The Client With Cirrhosis

The following topics are appropriate for a teaching plan:

- Follow the diet recommended by the physician.
- Consult a dietitian if you require a special diet (i.e., a low-sodium diet to prevent edema and ascites). Many metabolic liver disorders require highly specialized diets and necessitate extensive teaching from nursing and nutritional staff. Some diets require routine monitoring and home care.
- Avoid situations that could further damage the liver, such as drinking alcohol, taking tranquilizers, or inhaling chemicals such as benzene or vinyl chloride, which are toxic.
- Rest frequently, especially if activity causes fatigue.
- Avoid exposure to people with known infections.
- Continue skin care.
- Avoid nonprescription drugs (especially aspirin and products that contain it because they contribute to bleeding problems) unless approved by the physician.
- Be prepared for rejection as a blood donor because of liver disease.
- Contact the physician immediately about vomiting of blood, tarry stools, extreme fatigue, yellow skin, light-colored stools, or dark urine.

from hemorrhage, necessitating endoscopy with sclerotherapy or banding after the client's condition is stabilized.

Ascites

Ascites is collection of fluid in the peritoneal cavity. Undoubtedly, portal hypertension is a major underlying factor in the development of ascites. It leads to a cascade of events, referred to as the **hepatorenal syndrome,** that ultimately alter fluid distribution and interfere with fluid excretion.

Increased pressure in the portal system forces serum proteins into the peritoneal cavity. The proteins draw plasma from the circulating blood by osmosis. The kidneys respond to decreases in blood volume and renal BP by initiating the renin–angiotensin–aldosterone system (see Chap. 35). In response, the body conserves sodium ions, which further contributes to fluid retention. Low renal blood volume also may suppress antidiuretic hormone, causing water to be reabsorbed rather than eliminated as urine. These combined factors promote fluid accumulation in the abdomen. Ascites is visible as extensive and massive abdominal swelling.

Abdominal paracentesis may be performed to remove ascitic fluid. Abdominal fluid is rapidly removed by careful introduction of a needle through the abdominal wall, allowing the fluid to drain. This usually eases severe discomfort caused by distention and relieves breathing difficulty secondary to a high volume of abdominal fluid pressing on the diaphragm and lungs. Up to 6 to 8 L of fluid may be removed over 60 to 90 minutes. IV albumin is simultaneously infused to pull fluid back into the vascular space. Monitoring of BP and urine output is crucial to evaluate the effects of the fluid shifts. Diuretic therapy is prescribed if the circulatory volume becomes excessive.

Additional treatment includes maintenance diuretic therapy and a sodium-restricted diet. The potassium-sparing diuretic spironolactone (Aldactone) may be

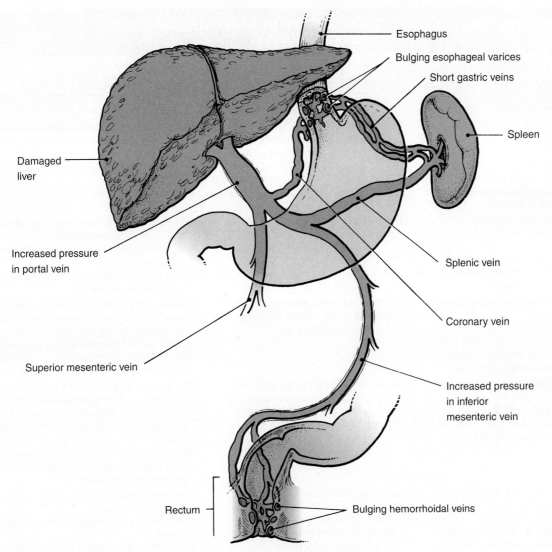

FIGURE 55-5 In portal hypertension, collateral vessels become dilated.

chosen because it specifically antagonizes the hormone aldosterone. Reversing the effects of aldosterone causes the excretion of sodium and water, retention of potassium, and reduction of ascitic fluid.

If ascites repeatedly develops despite conservative treatment, the physician may surgically insert an internal catheter to redirect the ascitic fluid back into the vascular space. See the section on portal hypertension for more information.

Hepatic Encephalopathy

Hepatic encephalopathy is a central nervous system (CNS) manifestation of liver failure that often leads to coma and death. This neurologic complication is related to an increased serum ammonia level, but not singularly. Ammonia forms in the intestine by bacterial action on ingested proteins. The liver normally detoxifies ammonia by converting it to urea, which the kidneys then excrete in urine. A failing liver, as in advanced cirrhosis, can no longer break down ammonia, causing it to accumulate in the blood. Ammonia can cross the blood-brain barrier and enter brain cells, where it interferes with brain metabolism, cell membrane pump mechanisms, and neurotransmission.

Indications of CNS effects include disorientation, confusion, personality changes, memory loss, a flapping tremor called *asterixis,* a positive Babinski reflex, sulfurous breath odor (referred to as **fetor hepaticus**), and lethargy to deep coma. Symptoms usually worsen after the client eats a high-protein meal or has active GI bleeding because both dietary protein and digested blood cells increase ammonia volume in the intestine. In addition to an elevated serum ammonia level, electroencephalography may show abnormal waveforms.

Treatment includes eliminating dietary protein, removing residual protein (such as blood if the client had a

DRUG THERAPY TABLE 55-1	SELECTED MEDICATIONS USED FOR LIVER, GALLBLADDER, AND PANCREATIC DISORDERS	
DRUG CATEGORY AND EXAMPLES/ MECHANISM OF ACTION	**SIDE EFFECTS**	**NURSING CONSIDERATIONS**
For Liver Disorders		
Procoagulant vitamin K (AquaMEPHYTON, Mephyton, Konakion) Promotes blood coagulation in bleeding conditions resulting from liver disease	Dizziness, transient hypotension, rapid and weak pulse, diaphoresis, flushing, skin rash, anaphylaxis	Instruct client not to take additional vitamin supplements unless specifically directed to do so by the physician. Assess adequacy of therapy by measuring prothrombin time.
Aminoglycoside antibiotic kanamycin (Kantrex) Decreases intestinal bacteria, thereby decreasing serum ammonia level	Diarrhea, cramping, ototoxicity, nephrotoxicity	Administer orally to decrease intestinal bacteria and serum ammonia levels. Note that discoloration does not indicate the loss of potency. Assess adequacy of therapy by measuring serum ammonia levels.
Laxative and ammonia reduction agent lactulose (Cephulac, Chronulac, Constilac, Duphalac, Heptalac, Portalac) Degrades intestinal bacteria	Diarrhea, cramping, abdominal distention, flatulence, nausea, vomiting, belching, hypernatremia	Because acidic stools excoriate the perianal area, perform careful cleansing after bowel movements to maintain skin integrity. Monitor serum sodium level for hypernatremia. Assess adequacy of therapy by measuring serum ammonia levels.
Bile acid sequestrant cholestyramine (Questran) Reduces pruritus by binding bile salts for excretion in feces	Headache, anxiety, vertigo, dizziness, insomnia, fatigue, tinnitus, constipation, hematuria, dysuria, skin rash, muscle and joint pain	Give all other drugs at least 1 hour before or 4 hours after cholestyramine because drug interferes with absorption of fat-soluble vitamins (A, D, E, and K), as well as many other drugs. Mix powder with liquid. Taking the medication in its dry form causes esophageal irritation and severe constipation.
Potassium-sparing diuretic cironolactone (Aldactone, Spirotone) Promotes excretion of sodium and water, particularly in cases of ascites	Headache, drowsiness, lethargy, confusion, ataxia, diarrhea, gastric bleeding, cramping, vomiting, urticaria, skin eruptions, hyperkalemia, dehydration, hirsutism, agranulocytosis	To enhance absorption, give with meals. Protect drug from light. Monitor serum electrolytes, intake and output, weight. Administer in the morning to prevent nocturia. Avoid potassium supplements and salt substitutes.
Immune agents interferon alfa-2b, recombinant (Intron A) Promotes virus-fighting capacities	Dizziness, confusion, paresthesia, lethargy, depression, insomnia, anxiety, fatigue, amnesia, malaise, hypotension, chest pain, anorexia, nausea, diarrhea, abdominal pain, dyspepsia, constipation, stomatitis, gingivitis, transient impotence, gynecomastia, leukopenia, anemia, thrombocytopenia, dyspnea, cough, rash, pruritus, alopecia, dermatitis, flulike symptoms (fever, fatigue, chills, headache, muscle aches), back pain, diaphoresis	Administer intramuscularly or subcutaneously for chronic hepatitis. Administer at bedtime to minimize daytime drowsiness. Monitor for flulike symptoms. Monitor blood studies for hematologic side effects. Explain to the client the increased risk for infection when taking this drug. Advise avoiding contact with those who have an acute illness and those who have recently received oral polio vaccine. The client should not receive vaccines prepared with live virus, unless specifically instructed to do so by the physician.
Immunosuppressives cyclosporine (Sandimmune) Prevent rejection of transplanted organ	Tremor, headache, seizures, confusion, paresthesia, hypertension, gum hyperplasia, nausea, vomiting, diarrhea, nephrotoxicity, hepatotoxicity, anemia, leukopenia, thrombocytopenia, hemolytic anemia, acne, flushing, infection, hirsutism, anaphylaxis, gynecomastia	Administer from a glass container or dropper to minimize adherence of the drug to container walls. Monitor cyclosporine blood levels to ensure that the client's level is within therapeutic range. Monitor renal function, blood urea nitrogen (BUN) and creatinine levels. Monitor liver enzyme levels for hepatotoxicity.

(continued)

DRUG THERAPY TABLE 55-1	SELECTED MEDICATIONS USED FOR LIVER, GALLBLADDER, AND PANCREATIC DISORDERS (Continued)

DRUG CATEGORY AND EXAMPLES/ MECHANISM OF ACTION	SIDE EFFECTS	NURSING CONSIDERATIONS
		Because the client is at increased risk for infection when taking this drug, advise against contact with those who have an acute illness and those who have recently received oral polio vaccine. The client should not receive vaccines prepared with live virus, unless specifically instructed to do so by the physician.
tacrolimus (Prograf, FK-506) Prevent rejection of transplanted organ	Headache, tremor, insomnia, paresthesia, hypertension, peripheral edema, diarrhea, nausea, constipation, abnormal liver function test, anorexia, abdominal pain, abnormal renal function, elevated creatinine or BUN levels, oliguria, hyperkalemia, hypokalemia, hyperglycemia, hypomagnesemia, anemia, leukocytosis, thrombocytopenia, pleural effusion, dyspnea, atelectasis, pruritus, rash, back pain, ascites, anaphylaxis	Monitor for neurotoxicity and nephrotoxicity, especially in clients who receive high doses, or who have renal dysfunction. Monitor serum magnesium and electrolyte levels and blood glucose levels. Monitor liver enzymes. Inform client of an increased risk for infection when taking this drug. The client should avoid contact with those who have an acute illness and those who have recently received oral polio vaccine. The client should not receive vaccines prepared with live virus, unless specifically instructed to do so by the physician.
For Gallbladder Disease *Gallstone-dissolving agents* chenodiol—also called chenodeoxycholic acid (Cheodiol, Chenix) Suppresses hepatic synthesis of cholesterol and cholic acid	Diarrhea, cramping, heartburn, constipation, nausea, anorexia, epigastric distress, elevated liver enzymes, possible hepatotoxicity	Administer orally to dissolve gallstones; may require long-term therapy for effectiveness. Monitor the client's liver enzyme levels. Avoid administering during pregnancy.
ursodiol (Actigall) Suppresses hepatic synthesis of cholesterol and inhibits intestinal absorption of cholesterol	Headache, fatigue, anxiety, depression, sleep disorders, rhinitis, nausea, vomiting, dyspepsia, metallic taste, abdominal pain, biliary pain, diarrhea, constipation, flatulence, cough, pruritus, rash, dry skin, urticaria, alopecia, myalgia, back pain	Administer orally to dissolve cholesterol-related gallstones; may require long-term therapy for effectiveness and may be helpful in promoting bile flow in liver disease. Monitor the client's liver enzyme levels.
For Pancreatic Disorders *Pancreatic enzymes* pancreatin (Creon, Boglan, Panazyme, Donnazyme, Entozyme) pancrelipase (Pancrease, Cotazym, Creon 10 and Creon 20, Protilase, Ultrase, Viokase, Zymase) Promote digestion and fat, protein, and carbohydrate absorption	Anorexia, nausea, diarrhea, allergic reactions, perianal irritation	Administer with meals and with snacks. Monitor stool consistency. Open capsules and sprinkle onto a small quantity of soft food. Do not crush or chew enteric-coated preparations. Expect dosage to vary with degree of malabsorption, amount of fat in diet, size of the meal and enzyme activity of individual preparations (300 mg pancrelipase/17 g dietary fat). Cautious use in history of allergy to pork products or enzymes.

recent GI hemorrhage), and depleting intestinal microorganisms with drugs, laxatives, and enema therapy. Antibiotics, such as neomycin or kanamycin (Kantrex), which are poorly absorbed from the GI tract, are prescribed to destroy intestinal microorganisms and thereby decrease ammonia production. The administration of lactulose (Cephulac) reduces the serum ammonia concentration. In the colon, lactulose splits into lactic acid and acetic acid, attracts ammonia from the blood, and forms a compound that can be eliminated in the feces. Levodopa (L-dopa) is a precursor of dopamine that restores normal neurotransmission in the brain. Supportive measures include

Portal hypertension results from
increased resistance
to portal flow and increased
portal venous inflow.

↓

Pressure gradient increases
between portal vein and
inferior vena cava.

↓

Venous collateral circulation develops
from high portal system pressure to
systemic veins, forming esophageal,
gastric, and hemorrhoidal varices.

↓

Varices may rupture,
causing life-threatening hemorrhage.

FIGURE 55-6 Pathogenesis of esophageal varices.

administering IV fluids containing electrolytes and multivitamins or total parenteral nutrition (TPN).

The prognosis for clients with hepatic encephalopathy is grim. Only a few survive without a liver transplant.

● HEPATITIS

Hepatitis is inflammation of the liver. The disease may be acute or chronic.

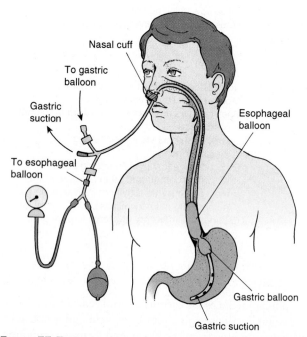

FIGURE 55-7 The Sengstaken-Blakemore tube has three separate openings: one lumen inflates the gastric balloon, another inflates the esophageal balloon, and the third one is used to aspirate blood from the stomach.

Labels: Nasal cuff; To gastric balloon; Gastric suction; To esophageal balloon; Esophageal balloon; Gastric balloon; Gastric suction

Pathophysiology and Etiology

The liver may become inflamed shortly after exposure to hepatotoxic chemicals or drugs, after lengthy alcohol abuse, or by invasion with an infectious microorganism. The most common cause of hepatitis is a viral infection, which is the focus of this discussion. The letters A, B, C, D, and E identify the viruses that infect the liver (Table 55-3). The modes of transmission and incubation periods differentiate each virus.

Once the virus invades the *hepatocytes* (liver cells), it alters their structure. An immune reaction ensues, in which the infected cells become inflamed and dysfunctional. The active disease process affects the uptake, conjugation, and excretion of bilirubin.

Most people recover from acute infection, but a few suffer from chronic active hepatitis and subsequent liver damage. In chronic persistent hepatitis (most common with hepatitis B, C, and D), liver damage does not worsen, but it does not improve, and the liver remains enlarged. Some clients may develop cirrhosis. Others deteriorate rapidly with liver failure and die unless liver transplantation is performed. Invasion of the transplanted liver by the virus is common, but it usually takes years before the newly transplanted liver develops cirrhosis.

Hepatitis B and C commonly are associated with hepatocellular carcinoma. Therefore, routine monitoring (e.g., blood test for alpha-fetoprotein and ultrasound) should be carried out for clients with chronic forms of these diseases.

A sixth viral type is hepatitis G, which is considered to be non-A, non-B, and non-C. It occurs 14 to 145 days after a blood transfusion. It cannot be identified as can the other types, and thus is designated type G. It is similar to hepatitis C.

Other types of hepatitis include:

- *Autoimmune hepatitis*—results from an abnormal immune system response. Treatment of this uncommon form consists of the administration of corticosteroids and immune-modulating agents (azathioprine or 6-mercaptopurine) (see Drug Therapy Table 53-1). Without treatment, many of these clients will die or require a liver transplant.
- *Toxic hepatitis*—develops when certain chemicals toxic to the liver (e.g., chloroform, phosphorus, carbon tetrachloride) cause liver necrosis. Treatment includes removing the toxin and treating symptoms. If liver damage is severe and prolonged, the prognosis is not good without a liver transplant.
- *Drug-induced hepatitis*—occurs when a drug reaction damages the liver. This form of hepatitis can be severe and fatal. Examples of drugs that may cause a severe reaction are anesthetic agents, antidepressants, or anticonvulsants. High-dose corticosteroids are administered to treat the reaction. Liver transplantation may be necessary.

TABLE 55-3	FORMS OF VIRAL HEPATITIS				
TYPE	**CAUSE**	**MODE OF TRANSMISSION**	**INCUBATION**	**SIGNS AND SYMPTOMS**	**OUTCOME**
Hepatitis A (previously called *infectious hepatitis*)	Hepatitis A virus (HAV)	Oral route from feces and saliva of infected persons; water, food, and equipment contaminated with HAV	3–5 weeks	May occur with or without symptoms; flu-like illness Preicteric phase: headache, malaise, fatigue, anorexia, fever Icteric phase: dark urine, jaundice, tender liver	Usually mild with full recovery; fatality rate <1%; no carrier state or increased risk of chronic hepatitis, cirrhosis, or hepatic cancer
Hepatitis B (previously called *serum hepatitis*)	Hepatitis B virus (HBV)	Infected blood or plasma; needles, syringes, surgical or dental equipment contaminated with infected blood; also sexually transmitted through vaginal secretions and semen of carriers or those actively infected	2–5 months	Arthralgias, rash; may occur without symptoms	May be severe; fatality rate 1% to 10%; carrier state possible; increased risk of chronic hepatitis, cirrhosis, and hepatic cancer; some infected people become carriers
Hepatitis C (previously called *non-A, non-B hepatitis–NANB*)	Hepatitis C virus (HCV)	Infected blood or blood products; sexual contact	2–20 weeks	Similar to HBV, although less severe and without jaundice	Frequent occurrence of chronic carrier state and chronic liver disease; increased risk of hepatic cancer
Hepatitis D (also called *delta hepatitis*)	Hepatitis D virus (HDV)	Same as HBV; cannot infect alone; occurs as dual infection with HBV	2–5 months	Similar to HBV	Similar to HBV with greater likelihood of carrier state, chronic active hepatitis, and cirrhosis
Hepatitis E	Hepatitis E virus (HEV)	Fecal–oral routes; low risk of person-person contact; found more in countries with poor sanitation and water quality	2–9 weeks	Similar to HAV—very severe in pregnant women	Similar to HAV—very severe in pregnant women

Assessment Findings

Signs and Symptoms

The signs and symptoms of the various forms of hepatitis sometimes are indistinguishable. The three phases of all forms of hepatitis are as follows:

1. *Preicteric phase:* nausea; vomiting; anorexia; fever; malaise; arthralgia; headache; right upper quadrant (RUQ) discomfort; enlargement of the spleen, liver, and lymph nodes; weight loss; rash; and urticaria
2. *Icteric phase:* jaundice, pruritus, clay-colored or light stools, dark urine, fatigue, anorexia, and RUQ discomfort; symptoms of the preicteric phase may continue
3. *Posticteric phase:* liver enlargement, malaise, and fatigue; other symptoms subside

Not all clients with hepatitis experience all the listed symptoms, and the severity of any one symptom may vary. Even though the symptoms are categorized, not all clients with hepatitis necessarily develop jaundice.

Diagnostic Findings

Serologic analysis can detect specific viral antibodies. Ribonucleic acid (RNA) testing may be performed to identify the virus itself. Test results may take up to 1 week. The white blood cell count may be elevated. Evidence of **cholestasis** (ineffective bile drainage) is seen with elevated bilirubin levels. Hepatic aminotransferase (alanine aminotransferase [ALT] and aspartate aminotransferase [AST]) levels rise during the incubation period and begin to fall once symptoms appear. Chronic disease may result in persistent elevation of the transaminases. A prolonged PT or PTT reflects poor synthetic liver function. Additional indicators of poor synthetic function include low blood glucose and serum albumin levels. Liver biopsy and histologic examination of the specimen allow for evaluation of the severity of the disease by identifying inflammation, fibrosis, and cirrhosis.

Medical and Surgical Management

Treatment is symptomatic and includes bed rest, a balanced diet of small feedings at intervals, and IV fluid administration if the client is extremely ill or has a low oral fluid intake. Supplementation of vitamins, especially the fat-soluble vitamins, is necessary regardless of oral intake because these vitamins are poorly absorbed. In some cases, antiemetics are given to relieve vomiting, but usually drug therapy is avoided until the liver recovers.

Recombinant interferon alfa-2b (Intron A, Roferon) may be given to clients with chronic hepatitis B, C, and D to force the virus into remission. It frequently is administered in combination with ribavirin (Rebetol), a synthetic antiviral also used to treat respiratory syncytial virus infection. The combination therapy increases the likelihood of a sustained virus-free response (more than 6 months). Ribavirin may cause birth defects, so clients of childbearing age need to be counseled about using strict birth control methods while taking this drug (Chene & Decker, 2001).

For clients with chronic disease who do not respond to medical treatment, a liver transplantation may be performed. This involves total removal of the diseased liver and transplantation of a healthy liver in the same location. Immunosuppression must be done for transplantation to succeed. Immunosuppressant agents include cyclosporine, tacrolimus, serolimus, corticosteroids, and azathioprine. The goal is to find immunosuppressive agents that effectively reduce rejection of transplanted organs and cause the fewest side effects. See Box 55-4 for more information.

Nursing Management

The nurse practices preventive techniques to control the spread of hepatitis viruses and teaches the family and general public how to reduce the risk of infection (Nursing Guidelines 55-2). Nursing care in the early stages focuses on maintaining physical rest, supporting nutritional intake, and preventing complications. Before discharge, the nurse teaches self-care measures to promote health and avoid transmitting the infection to others. The client must avoid alcohol and drugs that can further damage the liver. For clients who develop chronic active or persistent hepatitis and require liver transplants, see Nursing Process: The Client Having Surgery for a Liver Disorder (later).

Stop, Think, and Respond ● **BOX 55-1**

You are assigned to a client who is recovering from abdominal surgery. She tells you that the client in the next room has chronic hepatitis, and she is afraid she will catch it. Which answer would best help this client?

- *"Don't worry, dear. That kind of hepatitis can only be transmitted sexually."*
- *"There are many kinds of hepatitis—do you know which kind she has?"*
- *"Hospital staff always use precautions to prevent any possibility of transmission of infectious diseases to other clients."*
- *"There is no problem—that client is not a carrier of the disease."*

● TUMORS OF THE LIVER

A tumor of the liver is an abnormal mass of cells in the liver. Liver tumors may be benign or malignant (see Chap. 20). If malignant, the tumor may be a primary lesion (classified as a *hepatoma*) or a metastasis.

Pathophysiology and Etiology

Primary malignancies (hepatomas) are rare but appear to have an increased incidence in people with previous hepatitis B or D virus infections or cirrhosis, especially those with the postnecrotic form. The most common liver malignancy is a metastatic lesion from the breast, lung, or GI tract. Causes of benign liver tumors are tuberculosis and fungal and parasitic infections. Oral contraceptives and anabolic steroids also have been implicated in the development of benign hepatic lesions.

Tumor cells grow at an accelerated rate. They function in a disorganized manner and eventually impair the liver's physiologic activities. They may obstruct bile flow,

NURSING GUIDELINES 55-2

Techniques for Preventing Viral Hepatitis

Preventing Hepatitis A*

- Receive hepatitis A virus (HAV) vaccine, especially when considered at high risk (healthcare workers, day-care workers, foreign travel).

- Obtain immune globulin (IG) injection if exposed (in household or sexual contacts with infected individuals) to hepatitis without previous immunization.

- Observe Standard Precautions. Wear gloves if hands come into contact with body fluids; wear gown and face shield if body fluids may be splashed.

- Require child care staff to wear gloves during diaper changes and to perform adequate handwashing.

- Perform conscientious handwashing, even after removing gloves.

- Screen food handlers.

- Avoid eating from public salad bars and buffets that do not have sneeze guards or other hygienic devices and practices to prevent food contamination.

- Use liquid soap dispensers and hand dryers in public restrooms rather than bar soap and cloth towels.

- Avoid placing fingers and hand-held objects in mouth.

- Do not share cigarettes, eating utensils, or beverage containers.

- Avoid eating raw seafood or seafood harvested from possibly polluted water.

- Use a pocket mask when giving pulmonary resuscitation.

- Drink bottled water in underdeveloped countries. Avoid ice unless it was made from bottled water.

Preventing Hepatitis B†

- Receive hepatitis B virus (HBV) vaccine, especially if in a high-risk category (dialysis, blood dyscrasias, IV drug abuser, homosexual, healthcare worker, school teacher).

- Adhere to American Academy of Pediatrics guidelines for immunization.

- Obtain hepatitis B immune globulin (HBIG) if exposed to HBV and not previously vaccinated within 24 hours but no later than 7 days after blood contact.

- Observe Standard Precautions (wear gloves if hands may come into contact with body fluids; wear gown and face shield if body fluids may be splashed).

- Do not recap needles.

- Dispose of needles and other sharp objects in a puncture-resistant container.

- Use a condom when engaging in sexual intercourse.

- Do not share razors, fingernail tools, toothbrushes, or any personal care item that may come into contact blood or body fluids.

- If contemplating surgery, investigate the possibility of donating and storing your own blood for later use.

- Wear a mouth shield when giving mouth-to-mouth resuscitation.

---

*Prevention of hepatitis A also prevents hepatitis E; no vaccine or postexposure treatment is available for hepatitis E.
†Prevention of hepatitis B also prevents hepatitis C and D; no vaccine or postexposure treatment is available for hepatitis C or D.

---

leading to jaundice, liver failure, portal hypertension, and ascites.

Assessment Findings

Symptoms can be vague and confused with those of cirrhosis. Jaundice is common. Once the tumor is sufficiently large, the client may report pain in the RUQ. Weight loss and debilitation are common. The client usually experiences bleeding tendencies. Eventually, the abdomen becomes distended from liver enlargement and related ascites.

Alpha fetoprotein, a serum protein normally produced during fetal development, is a marker indicating a primary malignant liver tumor. Total bilirubin and serum enzyme (ALT, AST, alkaline phosphatase) levels are elevated. A liver scan, ultrasonography, MRI, or CT scan identifies the tumor and its location. A biopsy, performed

to identify the specific type of tumor cells, also can define and disclose damage to adjacent liver tissue.

Medical and Surgical Management

If the tumor is confined to a single lobe of the liver, a **hepatic lobectomy** may be attempted to remove primary malignant or benign tumors. Metastatic tumors usually are considered inoperable because they often are scattered throughout the liver. The frequency of metastasis and poor survival rate usually eliminate liver transplantation as a therapeutic option. Sometimes biliary ducts obstructed by disease are bypassed with percutaneous biliary or transhepatic drainage. A catheter is inserted under fluoroscopy through the abdominal wall, past the obstruction, into the duodenum. This procedure relieves the pressure and pain caused by bile buildup and decreases jaundice and pruritus. In some cases *cryosurgery* or *cryoablation* is used. This technique uses liquid nitrogen at −196°C to destroy tumors. Two or three freeze-and-thaw cycles are administered through probes inserted with open laparotomy. The effectiveness of this procedure is still being evaluated (Smeltzer & Bare, 2000).

For malignant tumors, short-term improvement may be achieved using IV chemotherapy or infusions directly into the hepatic artery or in the peritoneum. Doxorubicin hydrochloride (Adriamycin) and 5-fluorouracil (5-FU) are common choices for drug therapy. Unfortunately, results from chemotherapy tend to be transient. Radiation therapy may be administered to reduce pain and discomfort.

Nursing Management

In the terminal stages of the disease, the nurse keeps the client as comfortable as possible by administering analgesics, supporting ventilation compromised by ascites, and reducing discomfort from pruritus. When the liver fails and coma develops, the nurse institutes safety measures and continues performing total care. While the client is alert, the nurse provides support for the client and the family as both begin grieving their potential losses. As appropriate, he or she makes referrals for hospice care. Additional nursing management depends on symptoms and treatment.

Teaching includes the following points:

- Follow the diet recommended by the physician.
- Plan rest periods during the day.
- Avoid heavy lifting.
- Take medications exactly as prescribed. Follow directions on the label, particularly with regard to taking the drug before, after, or with food or meals.
- Record weight weekly or as recommended by the physician. Report any significant weight gain or loss to the physician.
- Contact the physician about significant increase in abdominal size, fever, nausea, vomiting, vomiting of blood (bright red, coffee ground), tarry stools, difficulty concentrating or changes in level of consciousness, jaundice, or swelling of the ankles.
- Make and keep appointments for periodic follow-up office visits.

NURSING PROCESS

● The Client Having Surgery for a Liver Disorder

Assessment

The nurse determines if the client will be undergoing a lobectomy or a liver transplantation (see Chap. 25 for perioperative nursing management). Postoperative assessments include checking vital signs and the function of drains and tubes. Observation for potential complications (hemorrhage, shock, infection, rejection in cases of transplant, electrolyte imbalances, and hepatic coma) is constant. In addition, the nurse observes the client with cirrhosis for signs of alcohol withdrawal. Standard postsurgical assessments include evaluating breathing pattern, airway patency, and pain.

Diagnosis, Planning, and Interventions

Risk for Deficient Fluid Volume related to hemorrhage from surgical site and fluid loss from drainage, tubes, or both
Expected Outcome: Client will maintain fluid balance as evidenced by adequate urine output and normal BP and pulse.

- Monitor intake and output at least every 8 hours. *Urine output less than 30 mL is inadequate for renal function and indicates hypovolemia.*
- Monitor vital signs at least every 4 hours; do so more frequently if client is hypovolemic. *Hypovolemia causes hypotension and decreased oxygenation.*
- Monitor IV infusion replacement solutions and rates. *Fluids replace intravascular volume and promote kidney function.*
- Monitor serum and urine osmolality, serum sodium, blood urea nitrogen (BUN), creatinine, and hematocrit levels. *Decreased intravascular volume will elevate these fluid volume levels.*

Hyperthermia related to infection, rejection, or both
Expected Outcome: Body temperature will be below 101°F.

- Monitor temperature frequently. Report elevation above 101°F immediately. *This finding may indicate wound infection and require cultures. It also can indicate a need to change immunosuppressant drugs if rejection is suspected after liver transplantation.*
- If client is diaphoretic, assist with bathing and changing into dry clothes. *These measures increase comfort and minimize shivering caused by water evaporation from the skin.*
- If client is shivering, cover with light blanket. If client is not shivering, cover with a sheet only. *Shivering increases body temperature. A light blanket will prevent shivering. A sheet should be sufficient to keep a client who is not shivering covered but not too warm.*
- Administer antipyretics as ordered. *They help reduce fever, which enhances the immune response.*
- Notify physician if client's mental status changes. *This finding can indicate septic shock.*
- Place client on hypothermia blanket as ordered. *Cooling blankets are used if temperature rises to 105°F to control fever.*

Imbalanced Nutrition: Less than Body Requirements related to anorexia, impaired use of proteins and carbohydrates, and nausea, vomiting, and sluggish peristalsis

Expected Outcome: Weight will remain stable, and the client will tolerate oral feedings.

- Initially administer nutrition by IV access. *Client will not tolerate oral liquids until bowel sounds resume and he or she passes flatus or stool.*
- After removal of the nasogastric tube, give small sips of clear liquids. *Small sips prevent nausea and vomiting.*
- Progress diet to full liquids and then soft foods. *Advancing the diet as tolerated prevents nausea, vomiting, or gastric discomfort.*

Evaluation of Expected Outcomes

Fluid balance is adequate as evidenced by moist mucous membranes, good skin turgor, intake of 2400 mL and output of 2300 mL, BP of 136/88 mm Hg, and pulse rate of 84 beats/minute. Body temperature remains below 101°F. The client tolerates food, nourishment meets metabolic needs, and the client's weight stabilizes.

DISORDERS OF THE GALLBLADDER ●

Several disorders affect the *biliary system* (Box 55-5), which refers to the *gallbladder* and *bile ducts,* which carry bile (Fig. 55-8). These disorders impair the drainage of bile into the duodenum.

● CHOLELITHIASIS AND CHOLECYSTITIS

Cholelithiasis denotes stones that form in the gallbladder. Gallstone formation represents the most common abnormality of the biliary system. If the stones are located in the common bile duct, the condition is re-

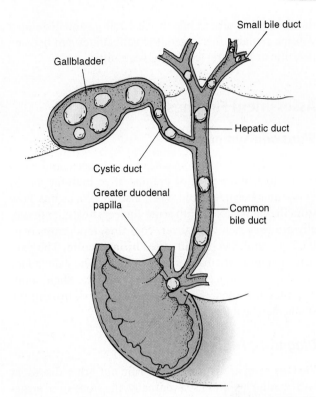

FIGURE 55-8 Gallstones may form in many locations within the biliary tree.

ferred to as **choledocholithiasis.** The formation of stones often leads to **cholecystitis,** an inflammation or infection of the gallbladder. Cholecystitis may be chronic or acute.

Pathophysiology and Etiology

Cholelithiasis and cholecystitis are intimately related and almost always coexist. Their incidence increases progressively with age. Gallstones are more frequent in women than in men, particularly women who are middle-aged or have a history of multiple pregnancies, diabetes, and obesity. The cause of cholelithiasis remains unestablished, but bile stasis, dietary factors, and infection are suspected. The formation of pigmented stones is associated with hemolytic anemia, which increases free bilirubin (see Chap. 39). Cholesterol-type stones are linked to a high-fat diet or predisposition to hypercholesterolemia.

Symptoms tend to develop when one or more gallstones partially or totally impair the passage of bile, causing the gallbladder to become inflamed, swollen, and distended with bile. Each time the person eats fatty foods, *cholecystokinin,* a hormone secreted by the small intestine, stimulates the gallbladder to send bile for its digestion. The gallbladder responds by contracting forcefully. Discomfort results from a combination of the inflammation and contractile spasms. Digestion problems result from

---

BOX 55-5 ● **Terms Related to the Biliary System**

Cholecystitis: inflammation of the gallbladder
Cholelithiasis: the presence of calculi in the gallbladder
Cholecystectomy: removal of the gallbladder
Cholecystostomy: opening and drainage of the gallbladder
Choledochotomy: opening into the common duct
Choledocholithiasis: stones in the common duct
Choledocholithotomy: incision of common bile duct for removal of stones
Choledochoduodenostomy: anastomosis of common duct to duodenum
Choledochojejunostomy: anastomosis of common duct to jejunum
Lithotripsy: disintegration of gallstones by shock waves
Laparoscopic cholecystectomy: removal of gallbladder through endoscopic procedure
Laser cholecystectomy: removal of gallbladder using laser rather than scalpel and traditional surgical instruments

the reduced or absent bile. If the swelling and distended volume remain unrelieved, the gallbladder can become necrotic or rupture, leading to peritonitis.

Assessment Findings

Signs and Symptoms

Initially, clients experience belching, nausea, and RUQ discomfort, with pain or cramps after high-fat meals. Symptoms become acute when a stone blocks bile flow from the gallbladder. With acute cholecystitis, clients usually are very sick with fever, vomiting, tenderness over the liver, and severe pain called **biliary colic.** The pain may radiate to the back and shoulders. The gallbladder may be so swollen that it becomes palpable. Slight jaundice may be noted. The urine appears dark brown; the stools may be light-colored.

Diagnostic Findings

Various tests are performed to rule out other disorders with similar symptoms. Eventually, the stones and structural changes in the gallbladder are imaged by means of *cholecystography* (gallbladder imaging), ultrasonography, CT scan, or radionuclide imaging. Percutaneous transhepatic cholangiography distinguishes jaundice caused by liver disease from jaundice caused by gallbladder disease. Endoscopic retrograde cholangiopancreatography (ERCP) locates stones that have collected in the common bile duct. Magnetic resonance cholangiopancreatography is a noninvasive technique that uses MRI to detect gallstones and gallbladder disorders.

Clients with jaundice have elevated bilirubin levels. Leukocytosis findings correlate with inflammation. In addition, serum liver enzymes may be elevated. The PT may be prolonged as a result of interference with absorption of vitamin K.

Medical and Surgical Management

When the gallbladder is acutely inflamed, the client takes nothing by mouth. Instead, a nasogastric tube is inserted, and antibiotics and parenteral fluids are prescribed until the inflammation subsides. Treatment of mild or chronic cholecystitis involves a low-fat diet. To relieve pain and discomfort, analgesics, anticholinergics, and even nitroglycerin are prescribed. Fat-soluble vitamins may be ordered to compensate for their reduced absorption. A bile-binding resin, such as cholestyramine (Questran), is prescribed to relieve pruritus.

Clients who are a surgical risk and whose gallstones appear radiolucent on diagnostic studies receive oral bile acids, either chenodeoxycholic acid (chenodiol, Chenix, or CDCA) or ursodeoxycholic acid (ursodiol, Actigall, or UDCA), in an attempt to dissolve the gallstones. These drugs, which may take between 6 and 12 months to be effective, are only moderately successful. The success rate is greatest when the stones are small, but the rate of recurrence within 5 years is high.

Dissolving the stones by direct contact may be attempted by instilling a solvent, methyl-tert-butyl ether, into the gallbladder or common bile duct through a percutaneously placed catheter. If successful, the stones clear in hours or a few days. The rate for recurrence is unknown at this time.

Lithotripsy, a nonsurgical procedure using shock waves generated by a machine called a *lithotriptor,* may be tried to break up some types of gallstones. The shock waves are directed at the gallbladder while the anesthetized client lies in a specially designed water tank. After the shock waves fragment the gallstones, endoscopy or direct contact dissolution removes the fragments.

Stones in the common bile duct can be removed by performing a *sphincterotomy* (opening of the sphincter of Oddi where the common bile duct joins the duodenum) using an endoscope. The stone is snared or retrieved using a basket-like attachment on the endoscope. Other nonsurgical techniques for removing gallstones are pictured in Figure 55-9.

Laparoscopic cholecystectomy is the preferred surgical procedure for gallbladder removal. It is the treatment of choice for about 80% of clients with gallbladder disease. The procedure requires general anesthesia, but the surgery is performed with an endoscope inserted in one of three or four small puncture sites in the abdomen (Fig. 55-10). After inflating the abdomen with carbon dioxide to displace abdominal structures and provide a better view, the surgeon drains the gallbladder, dissects the vessels and ducts, and then grasps and removes the gallbladder. Next, the surgeon staples the puncture sites closed and covers the incisions with a light dressing.

Most clients return home in the evening or the morning after the procedure. Although a nasogastric tube may have been inserted during surgery, it is removed before the client is awake and alert. Mild analgesics are administered to relieve minor discomfort. The client may eat food once the effects of the anesthetic subside. A prolonged recovery period usually is unnecessary. Most clients resume normal activities within 1 week.

For some clients, laparoscopic removal is inappropriate. When the gallbladder is extremely distended and fragile from inflammation and infection or contains unusually large or multiple stones, its removal through a small abdominal opening may be impossible or dangerous. In these cases, the surgeon performs an **open cholecystectomy.** This procedure involves a laparotomy (abdominal incision). A *Penrose drain,* a wide, flat rubber tube, or a *vacuum drain,* a plastic tube connected to a bulb or other collecting device, is inserted in the wound to re-

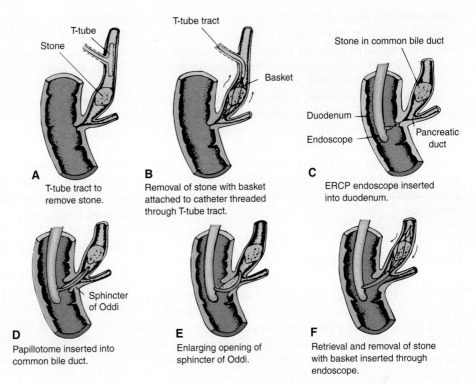

FIGURE 55-9 Nonsurgical techniques for removing gallstones. (From Smeltzer, S. C. & Bare, B. G. [2000]. *Brunner & Suddarth's textbook of medical–surgical nursing* [9th ed.]. Philadelphia: Lippincott Williams & Wilkins.)

A T-tube tract to remove stone.

B Removal of stone with basket attached to catheter threaded through T-tube tract.

C ERCP endoscope inserted into duodenum.

D Papillotome inserted into common bile duct.

E Enlarging opening of sphincter of Oddi.

F Retrieval and removal of stone with basket inserted through endoscope.

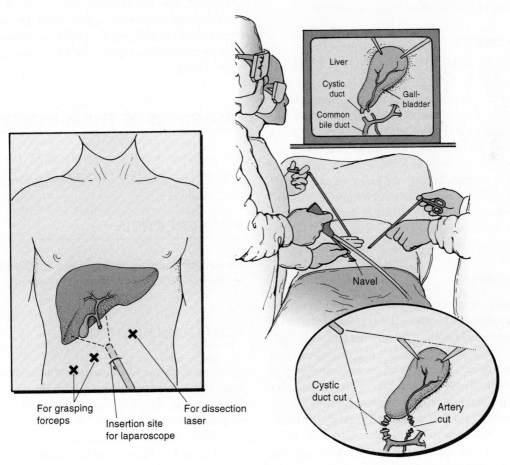

FIGURE 55-10 In laparoscopic cholecystectomy, the abdominal organs are viewed on a television monitor while the gallbladder is removed.

move serosanguineous fluid. After surgery, clients experience a lengthy period of gastric decompression and acute postoperative pain and about 1 week of hospitalization. A 6-week recovery period follows after discharge. See Nursing Care Plan 55-2.

During cholecystectomy, a *choledochotomy,* surgical opening and exploration of the common bile duct, may be performed. A **T-tube** (a tube used to drain bile) usually is inserted while the surgical wound heals (Fig. 55-11). The T-tube is brought through the abdomen near the incision and connected to gravity drainage. Bile salts such as dehydrocholic acid (Decholin) may be prescribed to promote drainage.

Nursing Management

During an attack of biliary colic, the nurse ensures that the client rests, monitors the client's ability to digest a bland liquid diet, and administers prescribed antispasmodics or analgesics. If gastric decompression is required, the nurse inserts a nasogastric tube and connects it to suction (see Chap. 52). If lithotripsy or another procedure is initiated to remove the stones, close observation of the client after the procedure for increased pain, shock, or signs of internal bleeding is important.

Same-Day Surgery

When outpatient or laparoscopic surgery is scheduled, the nurse instructs the client about presurgical procedures, laboratory testing, and the consent form. On the day of surgery, the nurse completes preoperative skin preparation, inserts an IV line, and administers sedation. After the client recovers from anesthesia and before discharge, the nurse provides intensive instruction to the client and the accompanying caregiver regarding self-care. Giving written instructions for reference is useful. In accord with agency policy, the nurse performs follow-up measures, such as telephoning the client the day after surgery to inquire about recovery progress.

Cholecystectomy

The nurse asks the client to describe symptoms experienced before admission such as the type and location of pain or discomfort. He or she asks whether and which specific foods cause pain or discomfort and discusses other problems, such as nausea, vomiting, or abdominal cramping. The nurse inspects the skin and sclera for jaundice and palpates the abdomen for tenderness. Routine presurgical and postsurgical assessments are necessary when the client returns from surgery (see Nursing Care Plan 55-2). If a T-tube is in place after an open cholecystectomy, the nurse monitors and records the drainage and maintains tube patency by keeping the collector below the level of the incision. This prevents bile from flowing back into the duct. A physician's order is necessary to clamp a T-tube. As healing occurs, the physician may direct that the T-tube be clamped temporarily before a meal and reopened later after eating.

The nurse measures bile drainage every 8 hours or according to agency policy. If more than 500 mL of bile drains within 24 hours or if drainage is significantly reduced, the nurse notifies the physician. Preventing tension on the tubing is important because it may become dislodged internally. A return of normal color to stool and urine indicates that bile is being deposited normally in the GI tract.

Client and Family Teaching

Diet and drug regimens are among the many aspects of care for clients with gallbladder disease. The client should meet with a dietitian and needs a complete list of foods to avoid. He or she also needs to know how to read the labels of all food products to determine their fat content.

When applicable, the nurse explains the purpose of drug therapy, the schedule to follow for its administration, and the potential side effects. He or she must inform the client to continue the medication even if symptoms disappear, and that frequent monitoring of the effect of drug therapy is necessary. The nurse also reinforces the importance of notifying the physician immediately of severe pain, jaundice, or fever or if the color of the stools or urine changes.

DISORDERS OF THE PANCREAS

The pancreas is in the upper abdomen. Disorders of the pancreas can affect both exocrine and endocrine functions.

● PANCREATITIS

Pancreatitis, inflammation of the pancreas, may be acute or chronic with a long history of relapse and recurrences.

ACUTE PANCREATITIS

Acute pancreatitis ranges from mild to severe and can be fatal. Characteristics of the mild form are inflammation and edema of the pancreas. Although the client is very ill, pancreatic function usually returns to normal within 6 months. In the severe form, more generalized and complete enzymatic digestion of the pancreas occurs. The tissue becomes necrotic, and the client develops many local and systemic complications.

Nursing Care Plan 55-2

THE CLIENT HAVING GALLBLADDER SURGERY

Postoperative Assessment

See Chapter 25 for perioperative management. When the client returns from surgery:

- Assess vital signs.
- Review chart for type of surgery and client's progress during surgery and in the post-anesthesia recovery unit.
- Inspect surgical dressing for drainage and tubes or catheters for placement, patency, and type of drainage.
- Carefully observe nasogastric tube for type and amount of drainage. If there is a T-tube, monitor drainage for amount. If there is a Penrose drain, observe and change dressing as needed.
- Inspect IV site; note current rate and progress of fluid infusion.
- Document fluid intake and output, as well as level of consciousness and comfort.
- Closely monitor for the following complications:
  - Change in vital signs, especially BP fluctuations, increased pulse rate, and elevated temperature
  - Change in respiratory status, including difficulty breathing and increased respiratory rate
  - Abdominal discomfort
  - Urine output less than 35 mL/hour if catheterized, or failure to void within 8 hours of surgery
  - Jaundice

Nursing Diagnosis: Pain related to surgical incision

Expected Outcome: Client will report that analgesics relieve pain.

Interventions	Rationales
Administer analgesics as ordered.	Timely administration provides maximum and effective pain control.
Teach client to splint incision when moving or coughing.	Splinting reduces pain and discomfort.
Maintain patency of nasogastric and T-tubes if present.	Doing so maintains drainage flow, preventing pressure of accumulated fluids and reducing pain.

Evaluation of Expected Outcome: Client reports decreased abdominal pain and demonstrates good splinting technique when moving or coughing.

Nursing Diagnosis: Risk for Ineffective Breathing Pattern related to proximity of incision (if an open cholecystectomy) to lungs, inhibiting deep breathing

Expected Outcome: Client will report comfort with breathing and exhibit unlabored breathing and effective respirations.

Interventions	Rationales
Place client in upright or semi-Fowler's position.	These positions facilitate lung expansion.
Encourage client to deep breathe, cough, and splint incision at least every 2 hours.	These measures provide for lung expansion and mobilize secretions.

(continued)

Nursing Care Plan 55-2 (Continued)

THE CLIENT HAVING GALLBLADDER SURGERY

Interventions	Rationales
If client has shallow breaths, instruct him or her to use incentive spirometer.	It promotes deeper breathing and more lung expansion.
Ambulate client as soon as possible four times a day, increasing distance each time. Encourage client to sit at least twice a day.	Ambulation and sitting prevent pulmonary complications and promote lung expansion.
Auscultate lung sounds at least every 8 hours.	Auscultation detects retained secretions and atelectasis early, helping prevent respiratory complications.

Evaluation of Expected Outcome: Client demonstrates adequate lung function, as evidenced by ability to take deep breaths and cough and no signs of respiratory complications.

Nursing Diagnosis: **Impaired Skin Integrity** related to altered biliary drainage after surgery and insertion of T-tube, Penrose drain, or both

Expected Outcome: Incision and skin around T-tube and drain will remain intact and not be irritated.

Interventions	Rationales
Inspect all drainage tubes to ensure they are connected to drainage bags, appropriately covered with sterile dressings, and fastened to client's clothing to prevent dislodgement or kinking.	Doing so prevents bile from leaking onto skin.
Keep drainage collector for T-tube below incision and maintain connection to gravity drainage.	These measures promote drainage of bile through T-tube.
Change dressings frequently as needed. Apply protectants such as zinc oxide or petrolatum to skin around drainage tubes.	These measures prevent skin irritation.
Observe sclerae for jaundice. Report abdominal pain, nausea, vomiting, bile drainage around T-tube, or clay-colored stools.	These findings may indicate obstruction of bile drainage.

Evaluation of Expected Outcome: Skin around drainage tubes remains intact and free of irritation.

Nursing Diagnosis: **Imbalanced Nutrition: Less than Body Requirements** related to high metabolic needs and decreased ability to digest fatty foods

Expected Outcome: Client will maintain weight and optimal nutritional status.

Interventions	Rationales
Offer a diet low in fats and high in carbohydrates and proteins. Instruct client that fats are restricted for 4 to 6 weeks after surgery.	Initially bile is drained and unavailable for fat digestion. As the biliary ducts dilate to accommodate the bile volume once held by the gallbladder, sufficient bile will be released into the GI tract to emulsify fats and allow for digestion.
Administer vitamins A, D, E, and K as indicated.	These fat-soluble vitamins are needed for adequate nutritional intake.
Consult with dietitian if client is having difficulty meeting nutritional needs.	Doing so provides client with a resource for nutritional information and alternatives to dietary restrictions.

(continued)

Nursing Care Plan 55-2 *(Continued)*

THE CLIENT HAVING GALLBLADDER SURGERY

Interventions	Rationales
Instruct client to weigh himself or herself weekly.	This provides a record of weight maintenance, loss, or gain.
Encourage client to increase activity.	Increased activity promotes appetite.
Instruct client to maintain a record of nutritional intake and any problems with GI symptoms during or after meals.	This method helps client to track and avoid foods that cause GI symptoms.

Evaluation of Expected Outcome: Client reports that weight remains stable and that he or she is tolerating the diet very well.

Nursing Diagnosis: **Risk for Ineffective Therapeutic Regimen Management** related to insufficient knowledge for self-care

Expected Outcome: Client will demonstrate knowledge of discharge instructions as evidenced by adequate wound care and repetition of dietary and medication instructions.

Interventions	Rationales
Reinforce diet instructions as above, with rationales as to why client must restrict fat.	Knowledge improves understanding of and compliance with dietary restrictions.
Provide verbal and written information that the client can understand about any prescriptions.	Clients learn in various ways. Presenting understandable information promotes learning.
Demonstrate and have client or family member return demonstration of wound care, dressing changes, and care of T-tube and drainage collector.	Return demonstrations allow the nurse to determine the client or family member's ability and knowledge, reinforce instructions, and correct misconceptions.
Instruct client or family member to notify the physician if wounds appear red or swollen or have purulent drainage, or if T-tube output increases.	Such findings indicate infection or obstruction below the T-tube, which needs early intervention.
Explain that initially stools may be loose and frequent.	Bile will initially trickle continuously into the digestive system because the gallbladder no longer stores bile.
Instruct client to notify physician of clay-colored stools, dark brown urine, or jaundice.	These findings indicate obstruction and require early intervention.
Recommend that the client avoid lifting anything over 5 lb for at least 1 month.	This will prevent incisional hernia formation.

Evaluation of Expected Outcome: Client manages self-care at home as evidenced by proper wound healing, compliance with dietary and medication regimen, and no complications.

Pathophysiology and Etiology

Primarily, the pancreas becomes inflamed when the organ's own enzymes—especially trypsin—cause the pancreas to digest itself (*autodigestion*). Autodigestion develops when there is reflux of bile and duodenal contents into the pancreatic duct, which activates the exocrine enzymes that the pancreas produces. Swelling of the opening to the pancreatic duct impairs or even obstructs the release of bicarbonate, which neutralizes chyme as it enters the small intestine. It also obstructs the release of the enzymes trypsin, which digests proteins; amylase, which digests carbohydrates; and lipase, which digests fats. As the enzymes accumulate in the gland, they begin to digest the pancreatic tissue itself. Eventually, destruction of the pancreas leads to impairment of endocrine functions.

The causes of acute pancreatitis vary widely. Known causes include structural abnormalities, abdominal trauma, infections, metabolic disorders (e.g., hyperlipidemia, hypercalcemia), vascular abnormalities, inflammatory bowel disease, hereditary factors, ingestion of alcohol or certain other drugs, or refeeding after prolonged fasting or anorexia. Sometimes, however, acute

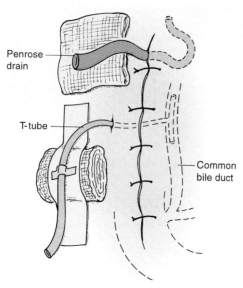

FIGURE 55-11 After an open cholecystectomy, a wound drain removes exudates from the area formerly occupied by the gallbladder and a T-tube diverts bile, which the liver is still forming.

pancreatitis develops without any of these predisposing factors or other identifiable causes.

Complications from severe acute pancreatitis are serious and sometimes fatal. Hyperglycemia results from an imbalance of glucagon, insulin, and somatostatin. Necrosis and hemorrhage of the gland, peritonitis, severe fluid and electrolyte imbalance, shock, pleural effusion, acute respiratory distress syndrome, and blood coagulation problems ensue. When lipase digests the fatty tissue around the pancreas, calcium binds with the released fatty acids. In rare cases, this reduces the level of circulating calcium to a dangerous degree, resulting in tetany and convulsions. Pancreatic cysts and abscesses also can develop.

Assessment Findings

Signs and Symptoms

The most common complaint of clients with pancreatitis is severe mid- to upper-abdominal pain, radiating to both sides and straight to the back. Nausea, vomiting, and flatulence usually are present. The client may describe the stools as being frothy and foul-smelling, a sign of **steatorrhea,** increased fat in the stool, from poor fat digestion. The symptoms, which worsen after the client eats fatty foods or drinks alcohol, are relieved when the client sits up and leans forward or curls into a fetal position.

Physical examination may reveal jaundice. Bowel sounds are diminished or absent with accompanying distention, and the abdomen is tender to palpation. The client may be hypotensive, indicating hypovolemia and shock caused by the release of large amounts of protein-

rich fluid into the tissues and peritoneal cavity. A bluish-gray discoloration to the skin about the umbilicus (**Cullen's sign**) or on the flanks (**Turner's sign**) indicates that the injured pancreas is releasing blood. The client may be feverish and tachycardic. Breathing is shallow from severe pain. Chvostek's sign (facial twitching when the skin over the facial nerve is tapped) and Trousseau's sign (spasms of the fingers when a blood pressure cuff is inflated) indicate low calcium levels.

Diagnostic Findings

Elevated serum and urine amylase, lipase, and liver enzyme levels accompany significant pancreatitis. If the common bile duct is obstructed, the bilirubin level is above normal. Blood glucose levels and white blood cell counts can be elevated. Serum electrolyte levels (calcium, potassium, and magnesium) are low. Pancreatic edema and necrosis appear on CT scan with vascular enhancement. Various endoscopic examinations and ultrasound may be performed to assist the differential diagnosis and to determine the presence of pancreatic cysts, abscesses, and pseudocysts (fibrous capsules filled with fluid, blood, enzymes, pus, and tissue debris).

Medical and Surgical Management

Medical treatment concentrates on relieving pain, reducing pancreatic secretions, restoring fluid and electrolyte losses, and preventing or treating systemic complications such as respiratory distress syndrome, acute (renal) tubular necrosis, and bleeding abnormalities. The client usually receives nothing by mouth, and a nasogastric tube is inserted and connected to suction. This relieves nausea, distention, and vomiting and reduces stimulation of the pancreas by gastric contents that otherwise may enter the duodenum. Along with general fluid therapy for hydration purposes, IV albumin may be given to pull fluid trapped in the peritoneum back into the circulation. Administration of diuretics is necessary if circulating fluid is excessive.

Atropine or other anticholinergics are given to reduce the activity of the vagus nerve, which stimulates the pancreas. IV antibiotic therapy is prescribed to prevent localized abscesses or to treat systemic sepsis. If pseudocysts develop, they may be located by CT scan and drained by percutaneous needle aspiration. Improvement, if it is forthcoming, usually occurs in about 1 week. A clear liquid diet is prescribed initially, with a slow progression to a low-fat diet. Alcohol, caffeine, and pepper, which are digestive stimulants, are withheld. If pancreatic exocrine function is impaired, pancreatic enzyme replacement therapy is administered with meals to promote digestion.

In severe cases, surgical management involves opening the abdomen to debride necrotic tissue. Every 2 to 3 days, the process is repeated to prevent the spread of infection. Multiple sump drains, inserted into the cavity to remove debris, are attached to continuous irrigation (Fig. 55-12). If acute cholecystitis or obstruction of the common duct is thought to be a coincidental or inciting factor, drainage and simple stone removal may be necessary.

Nursing Management

Nursing management involves monitoring the client for life-threatening changes and alcohol withdrawal if substance abuse is part of the client history. It also entails performing the prescribed treatment measures. The nurse is responsible for inserting a nasogastric tube, maintaining its patency, and infusing IV fluids. If gastric decompression is prolonged, the client can receive jejunal feedings of a low-fat formula or TPN. The nurse must monitor blood glucose levels closely. Clients with acute pancreatitis require frequent administrations of analgesics. Most clients with acute pancreatitis are severely ill. The nurse must continuously monitor intake and output, especially urine volume. If the physician inserts a pulmonary artery or central venous catheter, the nurse monitors pressure mea-

surements. Cardiac monitoring is continuous because electrolyte imbalances can produce dysrhythmias. The nurse continues to perform other assessments, including vital signs, lung sounds, serum electrolyte values, and observes for bleeding tendencies. If the client develops severe respiratory problems, he or she may require intubation and mechanical ventilation. The nurse must report any sudden change in the client's general condition or symptoms (i.e., pain or abdominal distention) to the physician immediately.

When surgery is performed, the nurse infuses irrigation solution and ensures that suction is functioning effectively. He or she also provides skin care if pancreatic drainage leaks from the sump drain sites.

CHRONIC PANCREATITIS

Pathophysiology and Etiology

Chronic pancreatitis is prolonged and progressive inflammation of the pancreas. In most cases, alcohol is the cause. Alcohol can lead to edema of the duodenum and decrease the tone of the sphincter of Oddi. Consequently, duodenal contents can move into the pancreatic duct. Other causes include hereditary predisposition, hyperparathyroidism, hypertriglyceridemia, autoimmune pancreatitis, trauma, and anatomic abnormalities. In about 20% of cases, no particular cause is identifiable. With chronicity, the gland undergoes fibrotic scarring from the recurring inflammation. The pancreas hardens, and exocrine and endocrine functions are partly or completely lost as pancreatic tissue is destroyed.

Assessment Findings

Signs and Symptoms

In chronic pancreatitis, the client has severe to persistent pain, weight loss, and digestive disturbances, such as flatulence, vomiting, and diarrhea. If pseudocysts form, they contribute to the severity of the symptoms by putting pressure on adjacent organs or by rupturing. If secondary diabetes develops, the client may experience increased appetite, thirst, and urination. A firm mass may be palpated in the upper left quadrant. The urine may be dark; the stools may be light-colored and foul-smelling. Fatty streaks appear in the stool. With the loss of plasma proteins from the blood, peripheral edema and ascites develop.

Diagnostic Findings

Abnormal laboratory findings are the same for chronic pancreatitis as for acute disease. CT scans, MRI, ultrasound, and endoscopic retrograde studies of the pancreas

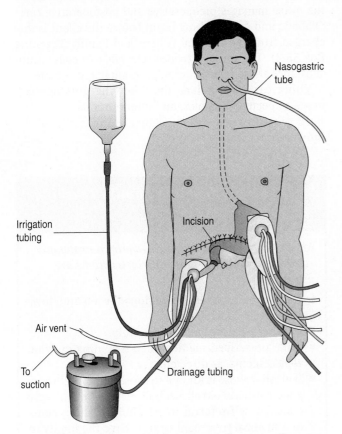

FIGURE 55-12 Multiple sump tubes are used after pancreatic surgery. Triple-lumen tubes consist of ports that provide tubing for irrigation, air venting, and drainage. (From Smeltzer, S. C. & Bare, B. G. [2000]. *Brunner & Suddarth's textbook of medical–surgical nursing* [9th ed.]. Philadelphia: Lippincott Williams & Wilkins.)

Nasogastric tube

Irrigation tubing

Incision

Air vent

To suction

Drainage tubing

show diagnostic results similar to those in clients with acute pancreatitis. Results of a glucose tolerance test show an impaired ability to metabolize carbohydrates because of malfunctioning endocrine cells in the islets of Langerhans.

Medical and Surgical Management

Treatment depends on the cause and whether the pancreatic duct is obstructed. If the duct is not obstructed, treatment consists of abstinence from alcohol, a clear liquid to bland, fat-free diet, and correction of associated biliary tract disease or hyperparathyroidism. The client who adheres to treatment may have good results.

Drug therapy with meperidine (Demerol) is ordered in deference to morphine sulfate (morphine causes spasm of the sphincter of Oddi). Narcotics are prescribed cautiously. The focus is on management of pain using non-opioid methods. Treatment for insulin and digestive enzyme deficiencies includes diet, insulin, and pancreatic enzyme replacement therapy. Such therapy uses pancreatic enzymes, such as pancreatin (Creon, Bioglan, Panazyme, Donnazyme, Entozyme) or pancrelipase (Pancrease, Cotazyme, Creon 10 and Creon 20, Protilase, Ultrase, Viokase, Zymase, Pancreacarb), which help digest and absorb fats, proteins, and carbohydrates.

When surgery is part of treatment, some or all of the pancreas (**partial** or **total pancreatectomy**) may be removed. If there is scarring, with stricture and stenosis of portions of the pancreatic duct, various surgical measures can be performed to attempt reconstitution of the duct. A pancreaticojejunostomy (joining of the pancreatic duct to the jejunum) can relieve ductal obstruction. Pancreatic autotransplantation is a recent surgical development. It involves excision and relocation of the pancreas. During this procedure, innervation is severed, effectively treating pain symptoms. Although exocrine function is lost, necessitating enzyme replacement, endocrine function and normal insulin production are preserved.

NURSING PROCESS

● The Client With Pancreatitis

Assessment

Initial assessment includes a history of symptoms the client experienced before admission as well as a complete medical history. The nurse asks about the frequency and amount of alcohol ingestion and determines when the client had his or her last drink as a method of evaluating if or how soon withdrawal symptoms may occur. For reliability, it is essential to involve family members in compiling assessment data (if possible), especially if the client's condition is serious. During the interview, the nurse obtains a description of pain with respect to location, type, severity, and circumstances that aggravate or relieve it. The physical examination includes gentle palpation of the abdomen, especially the epigastric area, for pain, tenderness, distention, or rigidity.

The nurse includes an immediate evaluation of vital signs because shock often is an outstanding symptom of acute pancreatitis. A description of the client's general appearance is important, as well as inspection of the skin for Cullen's and Turner's signs. Periodic weights provide a comparison for when more serious symptoms occur. The nurse instructs the client to save stool for inspection or laboratory testing. The nurse may initiate blood glucose testing.

Diagnosis, Planning, and Interventions

The nurse administers prescribed analgesics. The client may exhibit or develop tolerance as a result of cross-addiction to alcohol or chronic use of analgesics. The nurse must monitor for signs of alcohol withdrawal, which may develop within the first 24 hours of admission. He or she also implements measures to manage nutrition and blood glucose levels and administers insulin as indicated. The client requires therapeutic skin care to prevent breakdown from frequent, loose stools. If surgery is planned, the nurse manages preoperative and postoperative care. Diabetic and diet teaching begin before the client is discharged from the hospital (Client and Family Teaching Box 55-2). The nurse provides referrals to a community substance abuse rehabilitation program if appropriate.

Other care can include the following nursing diagnoses, expected outcomes, and interventions.

Pain related to distention, edema, and irritation of the inflamed pancreas

55-2 *Client and Family Teaching* **Pancreatitis**

Most clients with pancreatitis require a prolonged recovery period. The following instructions are usual:

- Follow the written instructions for a bland, low-fat, calorie-controlled diet.
- Eat four or more small meals daily.
- Take prescribed medications, including enzyme replacements, as directed.
- If alcohol abuse is known to cause acute or chronic pancreatitis, avoid all alcoholic beverages. Strongly consider self-referral to Alcoholics Anonymous or a medical treatment center. Urge the family to attend Al-Anon meetings. (If insulin administration is necessary because of diabetes mellitus, see Chap. 58.)

Expected Outcome: Client will report reduced pain.

- Administer analgesics as ordered. *Prompt administration of analgesics provides a therapeutic level of analgesia and promotes pain relief.*
- Withhold oral feedings. *Doing so limits the reflux of bile and duodenal contents into the pancreatic duct, preventing activation of the exocrine enzymes produced by the pancreas.*
- Instruct client to remain on bed rest. *Bed rest reduces metabolic rate and thus decreases secretion of pancreatic and gastric enzymes.*
- Report unrelieved pain or sudden increased intensity of pain. *Increased pain stimulates secretion of pancreatic enzymes. Sudden increased pain may indicate pancreatic rupture.*
- Administer anticholinergic medications as ordered. *They reduce gastric and pancreatic secretions.*
- Maintain continuous nasogastric drainage. *Drainage removes gastric contents and prevents gastric secretions from entering the duodenum.*

Ineffective Breathing Pattern related to severe pain and pancreatic distention, edema, and inflammation

Expected Outcome: Client will maintain adequate lung function as evidenced by improved breathing patterns and clear lungs.

- Position client with head of bed elevated or in semi-Fowler's position. *These measures reduce pressure on the diaphragm from abdominal distention and promote lung expansion.*
- Reposition client at least every 2 hours. *Repositioning prevents atelectasis and pooling of respiratory secretions.*
- Monitor pulse oximetry. Report episodes of desaturation to physician. *Pulse oximetry helps show changes in respiratory status and promotes early interventions.*
- Encourage client to deep breathe and cough every 2 hours. *Deep breathing and coughing clear the airway and reduce atelectasis.*

Deficient Fluid Volume related to vomiting, decreased fluid intake, fever, diaphoresis, and fluid shifts

Expected Outcome: Client will be adequately hydrated as evidenced by sufficient urine output and normal BP and skin turgor.

- Monitor intake and output at least every 8 hours. *This record can show if fluid loss is excessive.*
- Monitor serum electrolytes and BUN levels. *Findings might indicate a need for fluid and electrolyte replacements.*
- Administer IV fluids and electrolytes as ordered. *Replacing fluids and electrolytes restores fluid balance.*
- Administer plasma, albumin, and blood products as ordered. *Clients with severe pancreatitis lose large amounts of blood and plasma, which decreases effective circulating blood volume.*

Diarrhea related to impaired fat and protein digestion

Expected Outcome: Client experiences decreased diarrhea.

- Monitor number and characteristics of stools. *Such monitoring provides a baseline for determining fluid and electrolyte loss from stools.*
- Maintain low-fat diet if client is allowed food. *Decreased fat intake reduces the amount that the client cannot properly digest.*
- Administer antidiarrheal medications if ordered. *They assist in decreasing diarrhea and, in turn, reduce fluid and electrolyte losses.*

Risk for Injury related to alcohol withdrawal

Expected Outcome: Client remains uninjured with stable vital signs and no seizures.

- Monitor client for signs of CNS stimulation, such as agitation or belligerence. Observe for signs of hand tremors and emotional lability. *Such findings may indicate that the depressant effects of alcohol are wearing off.*
- Report if client's heart rate is over 100 beats/minute, diastolic BP is greater than 100 mm Hg, or temperature is above 100°F (36.6°C). *Such findings may indicate signs of alcohol withdrawal and the need for medical intervention.*
- Minimize environmental stimuli. *Extraneous lights and noise can increase agitation and possibly cause confusion.*
- Administer prescribed sedatives. *They provide appropriate sedation as the client withdraws from the effects of alcohol.*
- Provide a safe environment for the client if he or she is extremely agitated or at risk for seizures. Place client near nurses' station if he or she requires close observation. *Anticipating safety needs prevents harm to the client. If the client is near the nurses' station, the nurses can more closely monitor his or her activities.*
- Pad side rails and keep oral suction available. *If the client has a seizure or becomes extremely agitated, padded side rails, other safety measures, and immediate availability of suction can prevent further injury.*
- If a seizure occurs, initiate seizure precautions by protecting, but not restraining, the client. Observe the client throughout the seizure. After the seizure, ensure that the airway is clear and administer oxygen briefly according to agency policy. *Restraining a client during a seizure can cause more injury. Staying with the client during and after the seizure provides protection for the client and ensures that his or her airway is patent.*

Evaluation of Expected Outcomes

The client reports relief of pain, with an increased ability to sleep and rest more comfortably. He or she breathes deeply at a rate of 12 to 20 breaths/minute and maintains adequate pulmonary ventilation, as evidenced by clear lungs and 95% saturation by pulse oximetry. Fluid intake and output are balanced as evidenced by urine output of at least 50 mL/hour and normal BP and skin turgor. The client reports fewer stools and that stools have more form. Alcohol withdrawal occurs without hypertension or seizures.

● CARCINOMA OF THE PANCREAS

Carcinoma of the pancreas may occur in the gland's head, body, or tail. Some tumors are primary lesions, whereas others are metastases from other locations. Because tumors of the head of the pancreas tend to cause obstructive jaundice, they usually are diagnosed earlier. Nevertheless, most are discovered late in the disease and invariably have a lethal prognosis.

Pathophysiology and Etiology

When sufficient malignant cells accumulate, they block the pancreatic duct, producing symptoms similar to chronic pancreatitis. There is some question as to whether the pancreatitis is a precursor or consequence of tumor development. Tumors in the body or tail of the pancreas can press on the portal vein and lead to the formation of varices and bleeding. Once a tumor develops, it tends to grow rapidly. By the time symptoms are serious enough for the client to seek medical assistance, the tumor may have spread to adjacent structures, such as the liver or spleen.

Besides pancreatitis, factors that correlate with pancreatic cancer include diabetes mellitus, a high-fat diet, and chronic exposure to carcinogenic substances (i.e., petrochemicals). Although data are inconclusive, a relationship may exist between cigarette smoking and high coffee consumption (especially decaffeinated coffee) and the development of pancreatic carcinoma.

Assessment Findings

Signs and Symptoms

Symptoms may not appear until the disease is far advanced. The most common symptoms are left upper abdominal pain that may be referred to the back, jaundice, anorexia, and weight loss. The client may describe light-colored stools but dark urine, typical symptoms of obstructive jaundice. Pruritus may accompany jaundice.

A mass may be palpated in the left upper quadrant. The mass may be a tumor or an enlarged gallbladder, which tends to expand as a result of obstructed passage of bile. Ascites may be present in late stages of the disease. Some clients develop thrombophlebitis from pancreatic tumor products, which increase the blood's coagulability.

Diagnostic Findings

Abdominal ultrasonography or CT scan demonstrates pancreatic enlargement but does not indicate the underlying cause. A biopsy obtained by ERCP or percutaneous needle aspiration provides evidence of malignant cells.

Elevated serum amylase, alkaline phosphatase, and bilirubin levels support the evidence that the pancreas is diseased, but they do not confirm carcinoma. The level of carcinoembryonic antigen is elevated, but this elevation is a less specific tumor marker than is CA 19–9.

Medical and Surgical Management

The prognosis is poor. In some cases, resection of a tumor at the head of the pancreas is possible by **radical pancreatoduodenectomy (Whipple procedure)** (Fig. 55-13). This surgical procedure involves removing the head of the pancreas, resecting the duodenum and stomach, and redirecting the flow of secretions from the stomach, gallbladder, and pancreas into the jejunum. The tumor may be irradiated during surgery, or radioactive seeds may be implanted. Because metastasis to the spleen is so common, some surgeons also may perform a splenectomy. Rather than do an extensive resection, others are inclined to do a total pancreatectomy. This radical surgery then creates a malabsorption syndrome and historically brittle diabetes, which must be treated after surgery. Some complications associated with this surgery include bleeding tendencies caused by a vitamin K deficiency and liver and kidney failure.

A cholecystojejunostomy, a rerouting of pancreatic and biliary drainage, may be done to relieve obstructive jaundice. This measure is considered palliative only. For inoperable tumors, radiation therapy or chemotherapy with 5-fluorouracil (5-FU) or mitomycin (Mutamycin) may be tried. These treatments do not cure the disease. Despite surgery, chemotherapy, or radiation therapy, most clients die within 3 to 12 months after the onset of symptoms.

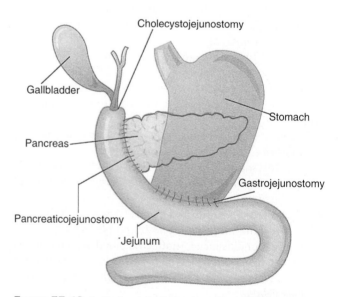

FIGURE 55-13 Radical pancreatoduodenectomy (Whipple's procedure). (From Smeltzer, S. C. & Bare, B. G. [2000]. *Brunner & Suddarth's textbook of medical–surgical nursing* [9th ed.]. Philadelphia: Lippincott Williams & Wilkins.)

Nursing Management

Nursing management for those treated medically is the same as for any client with a terminal malignant disorder (see Chap. 20). Clients undergoing palliative surgery require care similar to that of clients having general abdominal surgery. If clients have severe anorexia and weight loss they are poor risks for immediate surgery. These clients may receive preoperative IV fluids, TPN, or a special diet to improve nutritional status and correct any fluid or electrolyte imbalances. Most surgical clients have a nasogastric tube inserted. Once the biliary obstruction is relieved, the color of the skin, stools, and urine returns to near normal. Clients undergoing the Whipple procedure or one of its variations require more intensive nursing management because of the profoundly invasive nature of the procedure.

Initially, the nurse evaluates the client's general physical condition and obtains a history of all symptoms present before admission. He or she asks about the onset of symptoms, weight loss, bleeding tendencies, and the type of pain or abdominal discomfort. Physical examination includes inspection for jaundice, a visual examination of stools and urine, and palpation of the abdomen for tenderness and distention. Laboratory tests include blood or urine samples for analysis and detection of glucose. The nurse records vital signs and weight and assesses nutritional status.

The nurse observes the client after surgery for complications such as shock, pancreatic abscess formation, and hemorrhage. See Chapter 25 for postoperative nursing management measures for pain control, anxiety, and impaired skin integrity. Immediate postoperative assessments include vital signs and a review of the chart for the type and extent of surgery. The nurse also checks the surgical dressing and all drains and tubes for patency, as well as noting the amount and color of drainage throughout the entire postoperative course.

Close observation for signs of bleeding, such as easy bruising, blood in the urine or stool, or bleeding from the incision, drains, or tubes, is important. The nurse also monitors for signs of infection (elevated temperature, increased pain, abdominal distention, abdominal tenderness, and purulent drainage from the incisional site).

The surgery for carcinoma of the pancreas is very serious, with potentially major complications and poor outcomes. Nursing diagnoses can include the following:

- **Acute Pain** related to surgical procedure
- **Deficient Fluid Volume** related to hemorrhage and loss of fluids
- **Ineffective Breathing Pattern** related to abdominal discomfort and drainage tubes
- **Risk for Infection** related to invasive procedure and poor physical condition

- **Risk for Imbalanced Nutrition: Less than Body Requirements** related to high metabolic requirements and decreased ability to digest food
- **Risk for Injury** related to failure to consume adequate calories or get enough insulin
- **Anticipatory Grieving** related to shortened life span and poor prognosis

Clients who have surgery for pancreatic carcinoma and their significant others require diligent and caring attention. The nurse providing care focuses on:

- Assessing pain with a rating scale from 0 to 10
- Administering medications as prescribed
- Emptying drainage collection devices before they become full, taking care to avoid contaminating the drainage port
- Replacing fluids as ordered
- Monitoring serum electrolyte levels
- Auscultating lung sounds
- Instructing client to splint abdomen when turning or moving
- Encouraging client to deep breathe and cough at least every 2 hours
- Using aseptic technique to change or reinforce dressings when they become moist
- Following agency policy for changing IV sites, tubing, and infusing solutions
- Reassigning staff with potentially infectious symptoms to assignments that do not require direct client care or advising them to take sick leave
- Discouraging family or friends who may be ill from visiting until they are well
- Monitoring blood glucose levels several times each day
- Administering IV solutions, TPN, or both per orders
- Monitoring oral and IV caloric intake
- Teaching client about pancreatic enzyme replacement and a low-fat diet
- Providing support to client and family members as they begin to cope with the prognosis
- Helping client and family gain access to support services, hospice, and other organizations for palliative care and support

Care for clients with pancreatic tumors also must consider the psychological and emotional outcomes. If the client is discharged home, he or she and the family members require extensive teaching and home health services. The teaching plan should address schedules and techniques for administering prescribed medications, how to check the blood glucose level, recommended diet, importance of drinking fluids and eating, skin care (particularly around the incision), and the future schedule for follow-up visits, radiation therapy, or chemotherapy. The nurse also must review with the client and family symptoms to report to the physician: jaundice, dark urine, bleeding tendencies, vomiting, tarry stools, increased pain, swelling of the extremities, abdominal enlargement, decreased urine output, weight loss, and calf pain.

GENERAL NUTRITIONAL CONSIDERATIONS

A high-protein diet of 1.5 to 2.0 g/kg is used to promote liver cell regeneration in clients with hepatitis. To spare protein, 3000 to 4000 calories is recommended. Fat is allowed as tolerated. Small, frequent meals help maximize intake.

For clients with cirrhosis, there often is a small margin of error regarding protein intake. Too much protein may precipitate hepatic encephalopathy; too little protein intake results in body protein catabolism, with the same effect as eating too much protein. As little as 0.74 g/kg of protein (normal Recommended Dietary Allowance for protein is 0.8 g/kg) may achieve positive nitrogen balance without promoting CNS symptoms. Tolerance and intake are monitored closely; protein allowance is determined on a meal-to-meal basis for critical clients.

Some studies suggest that specially formulated mixtures of amino acids may help prevent encephalopathy by correcting the abnormal amino acid profiles seen in clients with cirrhosis. Although clients with chronic encephalopathy may benefit from these supplements that are high in branched-chain amino acids, controlled studies have failed to confirm that they are beneficial to clients with acute encephalopathy.

Coffee, both regular and decaffeinated, causes a significant increase in plasma cholecystokinin, the hormone that stimulates gallbladder contraction. Clients with symptomatic gallstones should avoid coffee. All other diet modifications are based on individual tolerance, including fat intake. Although eating fat bothers some clients with gallbladder disease, some studies show that fat intolerance is no more common among clients with gallbladder disease than among the general population.

If motility and absorption are not impaired, malnourished clients may be given nasojejunal feedings of an elemental formula during an acute attack of pancreatitis; their extremely low fat content causes only minimal pancreatic stimulation. TPN is used cautiously; some clients with pancreatitis cannot tolerate a high-glucose concentration even with insulin coverage. IV lipids are used sparingly when pancreatitis is related to hyperlipidemia.

GENERAL PHARMACOLOGIC CONSIDERATIONS

Many drugs are potentially hepatotoxic. Liver impairment may occur in some persons with normal, short-term doses, prolonged use, or high doses. Examples of drugs capable of causing hepatotoxicity are the penicillins, acetaminophen (Tylenol), methotrexate, and allopurinol (Zyloprim).

Oral bile acids given to dissolve gallstones can be hepatotoxic; frequent monitoring of liver function is necessary.

When chenodiol (Chenix) is prescribed to dissolve gallstones, about 2 years of therapy with the drug is necessary.

Barbiturates, narcotics, and any drug metabolized or detoxified by the liver are contraindicated or used with caution in clients with liver disease.

The effectiveness of a conventional pancreatic enzyme such as pancrelipase (Ilozyme) is increased when the gastric pH is 4 or above; but enteric-coated preparations such as pancreatin (Panteric) require a pH of under 4 to 5 to avoid being broken down in the stomach.

Clients with carcinoma of the head of the pancreas usually require vitamin K before surgery to correct a prothrombin deficiency.

GENERAL GERONTOLOGIC CONSIDERATIONS

Although hepatitis A commonly is found in younger people, older adults may contract hepatitis through contact with younger people who have the disease, such as grandchildren, waiters, or supermarket or nursing home employees.

Older adults may recover more slowly from surgery on the gallbladder. They also are more prone to develop postoperative complications, such as pneumonia and thrombophlebitis, because of an inability to move about in bed, adequately perform deep breathing exercises, and ambulate shortly after surgery.

Disease of the gallbladder is common in older adults. The incidence of gallstones is greater in older women than in men. Approximately 33% of the abdominal surgeries performed in adults older than 70 years of age are for disorders of the gallbladder and biliary tree.

With age, the liver loses weight, becomes more fibrous, and takes on a brownish color. However, function is not significantly affected unless disease is present.

Although recurrent severe pain is the predominant symptom of chronic hepatitis in young to middle-aged adults, older adults report the pain with chronic hepatitis as mild or absent.

Hepatitis B vaccination is not routinely given to older adults. In general, older adults should receive the vaccine only if they are traveling to areas where they may be exposed to the disease. Immunogenecity is somewhat reduced in the older adult.

Critical Thinking Exercises

1. *A client has jaundice. What questions can you use to help determine the cause?*
2. *How would you reassure someone who is interested in becoming a nurse, yet has reservations because of potentially acquiring a blood-borne disease, such as hepatitis B?*
3. *What are the differences between a laparoscopic cholecystectomy and an open cholecystectomy?*

References and Suggested Readings

Ambrose, M. S. & Dreher, H. M. (1996). Pancreatitis: Managing a flare-up. *Nursing, 26*(4), 33–40.

Aronson, B. S. (1999). Update on acute pancreatitis. *MEDSURG Nursing, 8,* 9–16.

Chappell, S. M. (1997). Anxiety in liver transplant patients. *MEDSURG Nursing, 6,* 98–103.

Chene, B. L. & Decker, A. P. (2001). Battling hepatitis C. *RN, 64*(4), 54–58.

Coyne, P. J. (1998). Assessing and treating the pain of pancreatitis. *American Journal of Nursing, 98*(11), 14, 16.

Elta, G. H. (1999). Approach to the patient with gross gastrointestinal bleeding: Acute upper gastrointestinal bleeding. In T. Yamada, D. H. Alpers, C. Owyang, L. Laine, & D. W.

Powell (Eds.), *Textbook of gastroenterology.* Philadelphia: Lippincott Williams & Wilkins.

Farrar, J. A. & Kearney, K. (2001). Acute cholecystitis. *American Journal of Nursing, 101*(1), 35–36.

Finlay, T. (1996). Making sense of the care of patients with pancreatitis. *Nursing Times, 92*(32), 38–39.

Fischbach, F. (2000). *A manual of laboratory and diagnostic tests* (6th ed.). Philadelphia: Lippincott Williams & Wilkins.

Holcomb, S. S. (2000). Reviewing acute pancreatitis. *Nursing 2000, 30*(4), 32–35.

Kirton, C. A. (1996). Physical assessment. Assessing for ascites. *Nursing96, 26*(4), 53.

Klainberg, M. (1999). Clinical snapshot: Primary biliary cirrhosis. *American Journal of Nursing, 99*(12), 38–39.

Meissner, J. E. (1996). Caring for patients with liver cancer. *Nursing96, 26*(1), 52–53.

Porth, C. M. (2002). *Pathophysiology: Concepts of altered states* (6th ed.). Philadelphia: Lippincott Williams & Wilkins.

Roberts, A. (1996). Systems of life: The pancreas. *Nursing Times, 92*(28), 42–44.

Smeltzer, S. C. & Bare, B. G. (2000). *Brunner & Suddarth's textbook of medical–surgical nursing* (9th ed.). Philadelphia: Lippincott Williams & Wilkins.

Tasota, F. J. (2000). Eye on diagnostics: Reading liver function values. *Nursing2000, 30*(6), 73–75.

Warren, M. L. (1999). Taking a hard look at cirrhosis. *Nursing 99, 29*(12), 32–34.

chapter 56

Introduction to the Endocrine System

Learning Objectives

On completion of this chapter, the reader will:

- Identify the chief function of the endocrine glands.
- Describe the general function of hormones.
- Explain the relationship between the hypothalamus and the pituitary gland.
- Discuss the regulation of levels of hormones.
- List endocrine glands and the hormones they secrete.
- Outline information to include when taking the health history of a client with an endocrine disorder.
- Describe physical assessment findings that suggest an endocrine disorder.
- List examples of laboratory and diagnostic tests that identify endocrine disorders.
- Discuss the nursing management of clients undergoing diagnostic tests to detect endocrine dysfunction.

The endocrine glands (Fig. 56-1) secrete **hormones,** chemicals that accelerate or slow physiologic processes, directly into the bloodstream. This characteristic distinguishes endocrine glands from exocrine glands, which release secretions into a duct. Hormones circulate in the blood until they reach receptors in target cells or other endocrine glands (Fig. 56-2). They play a vital role in regulating homeostatic processes such as:

- Metabolism
- Growth
- Fluid and electrolyte balance
- Reproductive processes
- Sleep and awake cycles

Table 56-1 presents an overview of the hormones involved in the endocrine system.

Stop, Think, and Respond ● BOX 56-1

Give an example of hormones that affect metabolism, growth, fluid and electrolyte balance, reproductive processes, and sleep and awake cycles.

ANATOMY AND PHYSIOLOGY

Pituitary Gland

Many endocrine glands respond to stimulation from the **pituitary gland** (or **hypophysis**), which is connected by a stalk to the **hypothalamus** in the brain (Fig. 56-3). The pituitary is divided into three lobes: the anterior lobe

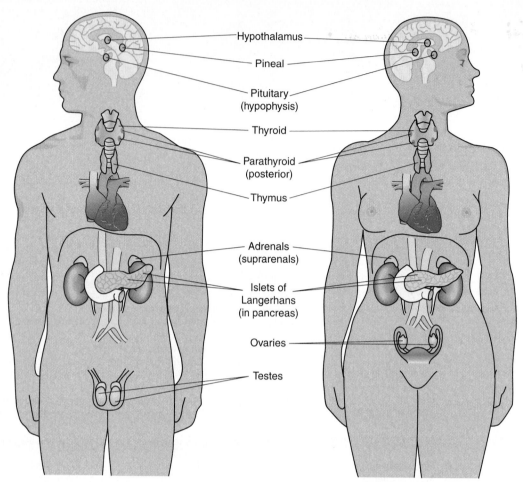

FIGURE 56-1 The glands of the endocrine system. (From Smeltzer, S. C. & Bare, B. G. [2000]. *Brunner & Suddarth's textbook of medical–surgical nursing* [9th ed.]. Philadelphia: Lippincott Williams & Wilkins.)

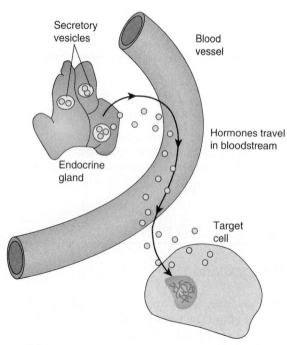

FIGURE 56-2 Transmission of hormones.

(**adenohypophysis**), intermediate lobe (pars intermedia), and posterior lobe (**neurohypophysis**). The pituitary gland is called the *master gland* because it regulates the function of other endocrine glands. The term is somewhat misleading, however, because the hypothalamus influences the pituitary gland.

Hypothalamus

The hypothalamus, a portion of the brain between the cerebrum and the brain stem, stimulates and inhibits the pituitary gland. It sends nerve impulses to the posterior lobe of the pituitary gland and releasing factors to the anterior lobe. When stimulated, each lobe secretes various hormones (Fig. 56-4).

Hormone Regulation

A feedback loop controls hormone levels. A **feedback loop** is a mechanism that turns hormone production off and on (Fig. 56-5). Feedback can be either negative or positive. Most hormones are secreted in response to negative

TABLE 56-1	ENDOCRINE HORMONES		
GLAND	**HORMONE RELEASED**	**HORMONE FUNCTION**	**HORMONE REGULATOR**
Posterior pituitary	**Antidiuretic hormone** (ADH)	Increases water absorption from kidney; raises blood pressure	Hypothalamic secretions, blood osmolarity
	Oxytocin	Stimulates contraction of pregnant uterus and release of breast milk after childbirth	Hypothalamic secretions, uterine stretch, suckling
Anterior pituitary	**Somatotropin** (growth hormone)	Stimulates bone and muscle growth; promotes protein synthesis and fat mobilization	Hypothalamic secretions
	Prolactin	Promotes production and secretion of milk after childbirth	Hypothalamic hormones
	Thyroid-stimulating hormone (TSH)	Stimulates production and secretion of thyroid hormones	Blood thyroxine levels; hypothalamic secretions
	Adrenocorticotropic hormone (ACTH)	Stimulates adrenal cortex to secrete cortisol and other steroids	Corticotropin-releasing hormone (CRH) from the hypothalamus; blood cortisol levels
	Luteinizing hormone (LH) in females and interstitial cell–stimulating hormone (ICSH) in males	Initiates ovulation and the secretion of sex hormones in both genders	Hypothalamic secretions, estrogen and testosterone levels
	Follicle-stimulating hormone (FSH)	Stimulates development of ovum in ovaries and sperm in testes	Hypothalamic secretions, progesterone
Thyroid	Tetraiodothyronine (thyroxine or T_4 and triiodothyronine or T_3)	Increases oxygen consumption and heat production; stimulates, increases, and maintains metabolic processes	TSH regulated by thyrotropin-releasing hormone (TRH) from the hypothalamus
	Calcitonin	Inhibits calcium release from bone, thus lowering blood calcium levels	Blood calcium concentrations
Parathyroids	Parathyroid hormone (PTH)	Increases blood calcium by stimulating calcium release from bone; decreases blood phosphate level	Calcium concentrations in blood
Thymus	Several thymosin and thymopoietin hormones; thymic humoral factor; thymostimulin; factor thymic serum	Stimulates T-cell development in thymus and maintenance in other lymph tissue; involved in some B cells developing into antibody-producing plasma cells	Not known
Pineal gland	Melatonin	Involved in circadian rhythms; antigonadotropic effect; exposure to light decreases release	Exposure to light–dark cycles
Adrenal medulla	Epinephrine (adrenaline)	Constricts blood vessels in skin, kidneys, and gut, which increases blood supply to heart, brain, and skeletal muscles, leads to increased heart rate and blood pressure; stimulates smooth muscle contraction; raises blood glucose levels	Sympathetic nervous system
	Norepinephrine	Constricts blood vessels; increases heart rate and contraction of cardiac muscles; increases metabolic rate	Sympathetic nervous system

(continued)

TABLE 56-1	ENDOCRINE HORMONES (Continued)		
GLAND	HORMONE RELEASED	HORMONE FUNCTION	HORMONE REGULATOR
Adrenal cortex	Corticosteroids Glucocorticoids	Regulates blood glucose by affecting carbohydrate metabolism; affects growth; decreases effects of stress and anti-inflammatory agents	ACTH; stress and serum electrolyte concentrations
	Mineralocorticoids (mainly aldosterone)	Regulates sodium, water, and potassium excretion by the kidney	Renin and angiotensin
	Gonadocorticoids (mainly androgens–male sex hormones)	Contribute to secondary sex characteristics (particularly after menopause)	ACTH
Pancreas (islets of Langerhans)	Insulin	Lowers blood sugar; increases glycogen storage in liver; stimulates protein synthesis	Blood glucose concentrations
	Glucagon	Stimulates glycogen breakdown in liver; increases blood sugar (glucose) concentration	Blood glucose and amino acid concentration
Ovary follicle	Estrogens	Develop and maintain female sex organs and characteristics; initiates building of uterine lining	FSH and LH
Ovary (corpus luteum)	Progesterone and estrogens	Influences breast development and menstrual cycles; promotes growth and differentiation of uterine lining; maintains pregnancy	FSH
Testes	Androgens (mainly testosterone)	Develop and maintain male sex organs and characteristics; aid sperm production.)	FSH and ICSH

Note: Words in bold type are key terms.
(Adapted from Campbell, N. A. [1996]. *Biology* [4th ed.]. Redwood City, CA: Benjamin/Cummings.)

feedback; a decrease in levels stimulates the releasing gland. In positive feedback the opposite occurs, keeping concentrations of hormones within a stable range at all times. Most endocrine disorders result from overproduction or underproduction of specific hormones.

Thyroid Gland

The **thyroid gland** is located in the lower neck anterior to the trachea (Fig. 56-6). It is divided into two lateral lobes joined by a band of tissue called the *isthmus*. The thyroid concentrates iodine from food and uses it to synthesize **tetraiodothyronine** (thyroxine or T_4) and **triiodothyronine** (T_3). These two hormones regulate the body's metabolic rate. Another hormone, **calcitonin,** inhibits the release of calcium from bone into the extracellular fluid. A rise in the serum calcium level stimulates the release of calcitonin from the thyroid gland.

Parathyroid Glands

The **parathyroid glands** are four small, bean-shaped bodies embedded in the lateral lobes of the thyroid (Fig. 56-7). The upper parathyroids are found posteriorly at the junction of the upper and middle thirds of the thyroid. The lower parathyroids typically lie among the

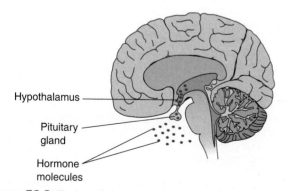

Hypothalamus

Pituitary gland

Hormone molecules

Figure 56-3 The hypothalamus regulates pituitary activity.

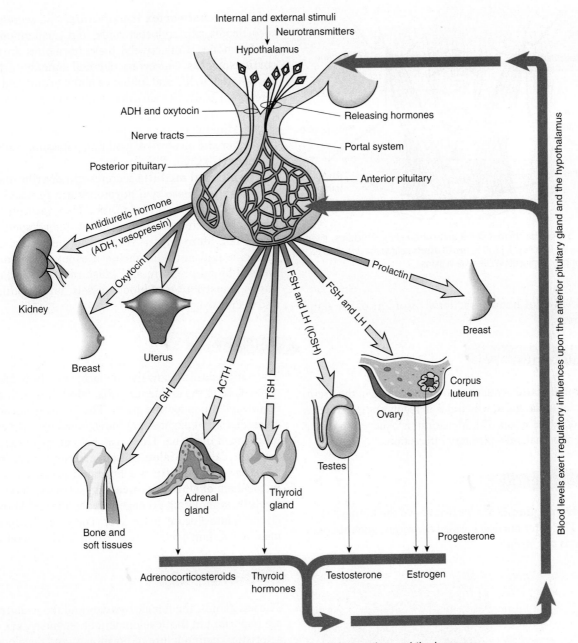

FIGURE 56-4 The pituitary gland, the relationship of the brain to pituitary action, and the hormones secreted by the anterior and posterior pituitary. (From Smeltzer, S. C. & Bare, B. G. [2000]. *Brunner & Suddarth's textbook of medical–surgical nursing* [9th ed.]. Philadelphia: Lippincott Williams & Wilkins.)

FIGURE 56-5 A feedback loop regulates hormone levels.

branches of the inferior thyroid artery. They secrete **parathormone,** which regulates the metabolism of calcium and phosphorus.

Thymus Gland

The **thymus gland** is located in the upper part of the chest above or near the heart. It secretes **thymosin,** which aids in developing T lymphocytes, a type of white blood cell involved in immunity (see Chap. 41). The thymus gland is large during childhood but usually

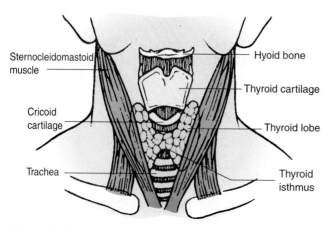

Figure 56-6 The thyroid gland and surrounding structures. (From Weber, J. W. & Kelley, J. [2003]. *Health assessment in nursing* [2nd ed.]. Philadelphia: Lippincott Williams & Wilkins.)

shrinks by adulthood. Functional disorders of the gland are rare.

Pineal Gland

The **pineal gland** is attached to the thalamus in the brain. It secretes **melatonin,** which aids in regulating sleep cycles and mood (see Chap. 15). Melatonin is believed to play a role in hypothalamic–pituitary interaction.

Adrenal Glands

The **adrenal glands** are located above the kidneys (Fig. 56-8). The outer portion is called the *cortex,* and the inner portion is the *medulla.*

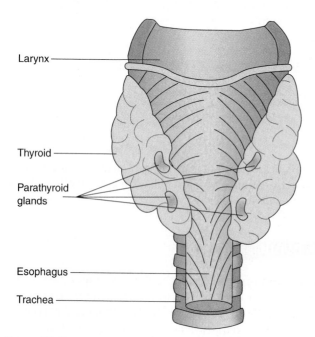

Figure 56-7 The parathyroid glands.

The **adrenal cortex** manufactures and secretes glucocorticoids, mineralocorticoids, and small amounts of sex hormones. Collectively, these hormones are called **corticosteroids.** Glucocorticoids and mineralocorticoids are essential to life and influence many organs and structures of the body. Glucocorticoids affect body metabolism, suppress inflammation, and help the body to withstand stress. Mineralocorticoids, primarily aldosterone, maintain water and electrolyte (sodium, potassium, chloride) balances (see Chap. 22).

The **adrenal medulla** secretes epinephrine and norepinephrine. These two hormones are released in response to stress or threat to life. They facilitate what has been referred to as the *fight-or-flight response* (see Chap. 12). Many organs respond to the release of epinephrine and norepinephrine. Responses include increased blood pressure and pulse rate, dilation of the pupils, constriction of blood vessels, bronchodilation, and decreased peristalsis.

Pancreas

The **pancreas** lies below the stomach, with the head of the gland close to the duodenum (Fig. 56-9). It is both an exocrine and an endocrine gland. The exocrine portion secretes digestive enzymes that the common bile duct carries to the small intestine. The hormone-secreting cells of the pancreas, called the **islets of Langerhans,** release insulin and glucagon. **Insulin** is a hormone necessary for the metabolism of glucose. **Glucagon** increases blood sugar levels by stimulating **glycogenolysis,** the breakdown of glycogen into glucose, in the liver. Together, glucagon and insulin maintain a relatively constant level of blood sugar.

Ovaries and Testes

The sex glands, the female **ovaries** and the male **testes,** are important in the development of secondary sex characteristics, manufacture of hormones, and development of the ovum (female) and sperm (male).

The testes produce the hormone **testosterone,** which is involved with the development and maintenance of male secondary sex characteristics, such as facial hair and a deep voice. The ovaries produce **estrogen** and **progesterone.** The functions and roles of these hormones are discussed in Chapters 59 and 61.

ASSESSMENT

History

The health history becomes important in the diagnosis of many endocrine disorders. Some endocrine disorders are inherited or have a tendency to occur in families; there-

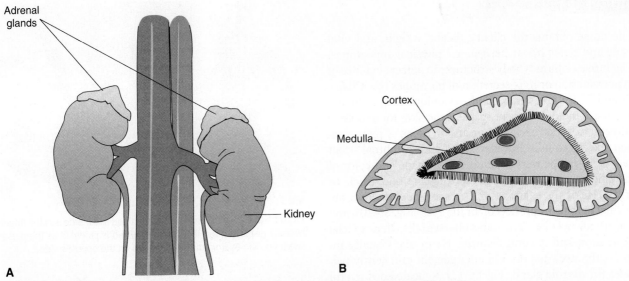

FIGURE 56-8 (**A**) The adrenal glands sit on top of each kidney. (**B**) Each gland is composed of the outer cortex and the inner medulla, both of which secrete specific hormones. (From Porth, C. M. [2002]. *Pathophysiology: Concepts of altered health states* [6th ed.]. Philadelphia: Lippincott Williams & Wilkins.)

fore, a complete family history is essential. The nurse also obtains diet and drug histories.

The nurse documents an allergy to iodine, a component of contrast dyes, or seafood, and informs the physician. He or she also reports whether the client has had a test that used iodine (e.g., intravenous pyelography, gallbladder series) within the past 3 months. This informa-

tion is essential before initiating a thyroid test. The nurse identifies the current symptoms. Sometimes the symptoms of endocrine disorders are vague or resemble other physical or mental disorders. Examples are fatigue, personality changes, inability to sleep, and frequent urination. At other times, symptoms are dramatic, such as a change in mental acuity or sudden weight loss.

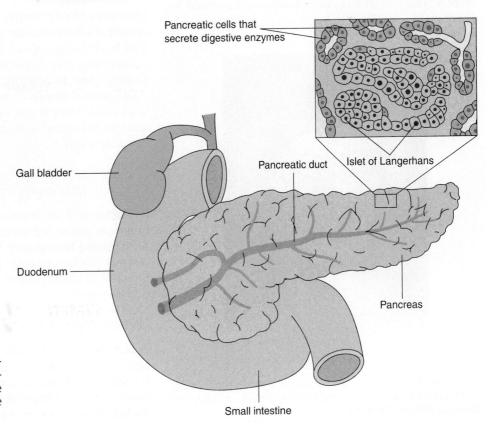

FIGURE 56-9 The pancreas secretes hormones from the isles (singular, islet) of Langerhans. Digestive enzymes are released from the common bile duct.

Physical Examination

The nurse obtains the client's height, weight, and vital signs and notes his or her general physical appearance. The nurse examines body structures to detect evidence of hypersecretion or hyposecretion of hormones (see Chaps. 57 and 58 for assessment findings unique to specific endocrine glands). He or she inspects the skin for excessive oiliness, dryness, excessive or absent areas of pigmentation, excessive hair growth or loss, and skin breaks that heal poorly. The nurse examines the shape and color of the nails and determines whether they are thin, thick, or brittle. He or she examines the eyes for *exophthalmos,* abnormal bulging or protrusion of the eyes (Fig. 56-10), and periorbital swelling. The nurse observes the client's facial expression and general features. He or she visually inspects the neck for thyroid enlargement and gently palpates the thyroid gland (Fig. 56-11). Repeated or forceful palpation of the thyroid can result in a sudden release of a large amount of thyroid hormones, which can have serious implications. The nurse notes the pulse rate and rhythm. He or she examines the extremities for edema and changes in pigmentation, auscultates the lungs for abnormal sounds, and examines outstretched hands for tremors. The nurse also determines if the client has experienced any loss of motor function or decreased sensitivity to pain or touch in the extremities.

The nurse assesses the client's mental and emotional status and evaluates his or her demeanor (e.g., dull, apathetic, extremely nervous). He or she determines the client's ability to process information and respond to questions.

FIGURE 56-10 Exophthalmos in a person with hyperthyroidism. (From Rubin, E. & Farber, J. L. [1999]. *Pathology* [3rd ed.]. Philadelphia: Lippincott Williams & Wilkins.)

FIGURE 56-11 With the head slightly tilted to the side and the fingers laterally displacing the thyroid, the thyroid is palpated as the person swallows. The examination is repeated on the opposite side.

Diagnostic Tests

The type and extent of laboratory and diagnostic testing depends on the tentative medical diagnosis. Because the physical symptoms may be vague, multiple and varied laboratory tests may be necessary to ultimately determine the etiology of the client's symptoms. A complete blood count and chemistry profile are performed to determine the client's general status and to rule out disorders.

Hormone Levels

Measuring blood hormone levels helps evaluate the functioning of some endocrine glands. These tests include cortisol levels (morning and evening) to determine adrenal hyperfunction or hypofunction, antidiuretic hormone (ADH) levels to determine the presence or absence of ADH, testosterone levels to detect increased or decreased total testosterone levels, and total thyroxine to identify diseases associated with increased or decreased thyroid hormone levels.

Radiography, Computed Tomography Scan, Magnetic Resonance Imaging

Radiographs of the chest or abdomen are taken to detect tumors as well as to determine organ size and placement. A computed tomography (CT) or magnetic resonance imaging scan is performed to detect a suspected pituitary tumor or to identify calcifications or tumors of the parathyroid glands.

Radionuclide Studies

A **radionuclide** is an atom with an unstable nucleus that emits electromagnetic radiation as alpha, beta, or gamma particles. A radioactive iodine uptake test (RAI, ^{131}I uptake) or thyroid-stimulating hormone test are radionuclide studies performed to determine thyroid function.

A **radioimmunoassay** determines the concentration of a substance in plasma. Venous blood samples are required for radioimmunoassay tests. A radioactively labeled substance (e.g., hormone, protein, antibodies, antigens) is combined in the laboratory with a blood sample to determine the quantity of the substance to be identified. For example, a T$_3$ determination by radioimmunoassay evaluates thyroid function.

A **nuclear scan** uses a radioactive substance that is taken orally or injected intravenously. The dose of the radioactive substance is larger than the dose used for radionuclide studies. Certain endocrine organs are visualized or their activity determined by means of special equipment. Examples of scans include thyroid scan, adrenergic tumor scan, and parathyroid scan.

NURSING MANAGEMENT

The nurse prepares the client for laboratory and diagnostic testing. He or she explains the general purpose of the test, type of test, and how it will be performed. The nurse encourages the client and family to ask questions and discuss the results with the physician.

Nurses must consult the institution's procedure manual and the physician's orders for the required preparation for each diagnostic procedure. Some tests, such as a CT scan, require no special preparation other than a general explanation. Some tests require fasting; others require temporary elimination of certain foods from the diet.

The nurse explains to the client how to participate in the test. For example, some tests require the client to save all voided urine for some time or to return for additional testing.

If a client is anxious about the use of radioactive materials for tests, the nurse offers assurance that these substances are safe and ordinarily pose no danger to the client or others.

GENERAL NUTRITIONAL CONSIDERATIONS

Some health foods, especially sea salt and kelp, are high in iodine. A diet history includes the use of any type of health food or health food supplements.

GENERAL PHARMACOLOGIC CONSIDERATIONS

If a client has recently taken a drug that contains iodine or has had radiographic contrast studies that used iodine, thyroid test results may be inaccurate. Other drugs (e.g., salicylates, corticosteroids) also affect the results of thyroid tests. Be sure to enter all drugs the client is taking or has taken within the past 3 months on the laboratory request slip.

GENERAL GERONTOLOGIC CONSIDERATIONS

Older adults may forget the instructions for a diagnostic test. Nurses may give printed directions to outpatients and, when possible, review them with a family member. This is especially important if test preparation or participation in the test is complicated.

When obtaining a drug history before a diagnostic examination in an older adult, it may be necessary to consult a family member or the caregiver to confirm drugs the client is taking or those he or she has taken within the last several months.

Critical Thinking Exercises

1. *Explain why the pituitary gland is considered the master gland. Give some examples that support the terminology.*
2. *Discuss the meaning and purpose of a feedback loop.*

References and Suggested Readings

Alesci, S., Koch, C. A., Bornstein, S. R., et al. (2001). Adrenal androgens regulation and adrenopause. *Endocrine Regulations, 35,* 95–100.

A quick check of the endocrine system. (2000). *Nursing, 30*(8), Critical Care, 32cc10–32cc11.

Bullock, B. L. & Henze, R. L. (2000). *Focus on pathophysiology.* Philadelphia: Lippincott Williams & Wilkins.

Cohen, B. J. & Wood, D. L. (2000). *Memmler's structure and function of the human body* (7th ed.). Philadelphia: Lippincott Williams & Wilkins.

Fischbach, F. T. (1999). *A manual of laboratory diagnostic tests* (6th ed.). Philadelphia: Lippincott Williams & Wilkins.

Fuller, J. & Schaller-Ayers, J. (1999). *Health assessment: A nursing approach* (3rd ed.). Philadelphia: Lippincott Williams & Wilkins.

Habib, K. E., Gold, P. W., & Chrousos, G. P. (2001). Neuroendocrinology of stress. *Endocrinology and Metabolism Clinics of North America, 30,* 695–728.

Hormone-disrupting chemicals. (1998). *HealthFacts, 23*(11), 1–4.

Jabbour, S. A. (2001). Steroids and the surgical patient. *Medical Clinics of North America, 85,* 1311–1317.

Kirsten, D. (2000). The thyroid gland: Physiology and pathophysiology. *Neonatal Network: Journal of Neonatal Nursing, 19*(8), 11–26, 37–40.

Porth, C. M. (2002). *Pathophysiology: Concepts of altered health states* (6th ed.). Philadelphia: Lippincott Williams & Wilkins.

Settle, M. (2000). The hypothalamus. *Neonatal Network: Journal of Neonatal Nursing, 19*(6), 9–14.

Walsh, J. (1998). How your hormones are affected by what you eat—the debate rages. *Environmental Nutrition, 21*(2), 1, 4.

Watson, R. (2000). Assessing endocrine system function in older people. *Nursing Older People, 12*(9), 27–28.

Wills, R., Norton M., & Winward, D. S. (1999). The endocrine system and steroids. *Surgical Technologist, 31*(9), 10–22.

Zouboulis, C. C. (2000). Human skin: An independent peripheral endocrine organ. *Hormone Research, 54,* 230–242.

Caring for Clients With Disorders of the Endocrine System

Words to Know

acromegaly
addisonian crisis
adrenalectomy
adrenal insufficiency
carpopedal spasm
Chvostek's sign
cushingoid syndrome
Cushing's syndrome
diabetes insipidus
goiter
hyperparathyroidism
hyperplasia
hyperthyroidism
hypoparathyroidism
hypophysectomy
hypothyroidism
myxedema
pheochromocytoma
Simmonds' disease
syndrome of
  inappropriate
  antidiuretic hormone
  secretion
tetany
thyroiditis
thyrotoxic crisis
Trousseau's sign

Learning Objectives

On completion of this chapter the reader will:

- Describe the physiologic effects of hyposecretion and hypersecretion of the pituitary, thyroid, parathyroid, and adrenal glands.
- Identify assessment findings for clients experiencing endocrine disorders.
- Discuss the basic nursing management of clients experiencing endocrine disorders.
- Identify symptoms of emergency conditions resulting from endocrine disorders.
- Discuss use of the nursing process in the management of a client with hypothyroidism, hyperthyroidism, Addison's disease, and diabetes insipidus.

A disorder of any endocrine gland can profoundly affect the other endocrine glands, as well as many major body systems. When caring for clients with endocrine disorders, the nurse must consider not only the management of the endocrine disorder itself, but the effects of the disorder on other organs and systems.

DISORDERS OF THE PITUITARY GLAND

Pituitary disorders usually result from excessive or deficient production and secretion of a specific hormone. When oversecretion of growth hormone (GH) occurs before puberty (when the ends [epiphyses] of the long bones are fully united), *gigantism* results. *Dwarfism* occurs when secretion of GH is insufficient during childhood.

Refer to a pediatric text for further discussion of gigantism and dwarfism.

Oversecretion of GH during adulthood results in *acromegaly.* Conversely, an absence of pituitary hormonal activity causes panhypopituitarism, or *Simmonds' disease.*

● ACROMEGALY (HYPERPITUITARISM)

Pathophysiology and Etiology

Acromegaly is a condition in which GH is oversecreted after the epiphyses of the long bones have sealed. It results from **hyperplasia** (increased number of cells) or a tumor of the anterior pituitary. The most common pituitary tumor is an *adenoma,* which is benign. As with other cranial tumors, a benign pituitary tumor becomes a space-occupying lesion and can affect other cerebral structures (see Chap. 45).

Assessment Findings

Signs and Symptoms

A client with acromegaly has coarse features, a huge lower jaw, thick lips, a thickened tongue, a bulging forehead, a bulbous nose, and large hands and feet (Fig. 57-1). When the overgrowth is from a tumor, headaches caused by pressure on the sella turcica are common. Partial blindness may result from pressure on the optic nerve. The heart, liver, and spleen may be enlarged. Despite enlarged tissues, muscle weakness is common, and hypertrophied joints become painful and stiff. Osteoporosis of the spine and joint pain develop. Many men experience erectile dysfunction, and women may have amenorrhea (absence of menstruation), increased facial hair, and deepened voices (Fig. 57-2).

Diagnostic Findings

Skull radiography, magnetic resonance imaging (MRI), and computed tomography (CT) scan reveal pituitary enlargement. Bone radiographs show thickened long bones and skull bones. Radioimmunoassay shows increased plasma levels of GH. Results of a glucose tolerance test show the same or increased levels of GH in a client with acromegaly and decreased GH levels in a person who does not have the disorder.

Medical and Surgical Management

Acromegaly is treated by surgical removal of the pituitary gland (**hypophysectomy**) or by radiation therapy with consequent destruction of the pituitary. Even if the

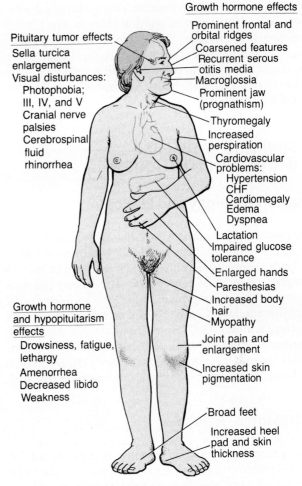

FIGURE 57-2 Clinical manifestations of acromegaly.

Growth hormone effects
- Prominent frontal and orbital ridges
- Coarsened features
- Recurrent serous otitis media
- Macroglossia
- Prominent jaw (prognathism)
- Thyromegaly
- Increased perspiration
- Cardiovascular problems:
  - Hypertension
  - CHF
  - Cardiomegaly
  - Edema
  - Dyspnea
- Lactation
- Impaired glucose tolerance
- Enlarged hands
- Paresthesias
- Increased body hair
- Myopathy
- Joint pain and enlargement
- Increased skin pigmentation
- Broad feet
- Increased heel pad and skin thickness

Pituitary tumor effects
- Sella turcica enlargement
- Visual disturbances:
  - Photophobia;
  - III, IV, and V Cranial nerve palsies
- Cerebrospinal fluid rhinorrhea

Growth hormone and hypopituitarism effects
- Drowsiness, fatigue, lethargy
- Amenorrhea
- Decreased libido
- Weakness

FIGURE 57-1 A 64-year-old man with acromegaly. Note the prominent, "lantern-like" jaw, the large zygomatic arches and supraorbital ridges, and the sloping "beetle brow." The bony overgrowth often results in a comparative hollowing of the temporal region. The nose and ears are enlarged, and the latter may be calcified. The skin folds are exaggerated, the skin is tough and oily, and there is enlargement of the sebaceous glands and pores.

disease is arrested successfully, physical changes are irreversible. If radiation therapy removes or destroys the tumor, replacement therapy with thyroid hormone, corticosteroids, and sex hormones is necessary.

Medical treatment includes bromocriptine mesylate (Parlodel), an antiparkinsonism drug that inhibits release of GH in clients with acromegaly. Parlodel is used alone or in conjunction with pituitary irradiation or surgery to reduce the serum GH level.

Nursing Management

Nursing priorities include correcting the fluid volume excess or deficit, relieving pain, and improving nutrition. The nurse carefully measures fluid intake and output, weighs the client daily, and observes for signs of fluid volume excess or deficit. He or she notifies the physician of a sudden or steady weight loss or gain. Skeletal changes can cause mild to severe musculoskeletal pain. The nurse evaluates such pain, noting type and location. He or she gives analgesics as ordered and notes whether the client reports relief from pain.

The client may experience severe psychological stress because of the prominent physical changes, erectile dysfunction, and decreased libido. The nurse discusses such issues to help the client cope with changes. If the client expresses concern over sexual dysfunction, the nurse brings it to the physician's attention. Referral to a sex therapist could be indicated.

● SIMMONDS' DISEASE (PANHYPOPITUITARISM)

Pathophysiology and Etiology

Simmonds' disease is a rare disorder caused by destruction of the pituitary gland followed by no pituitary hormonal activity. Events such as postpartum emboli, surgery, tumor, and tuberculosis can destroy pituitary function. This disease usually affects the hormones of the anterior pituitary: GH (bones and muscles), adrenocorticotropic hormone (ACTH; adrenals), thyroid-stimulating hormone (TSH; thyroid), follicle-stimulating hormone (FSH; ovaries), luteinizing hormone (LH), interstitial cell-stimulating hormone (testes), and prolactin (breasts).

Assessment Findings

The gonads and genitalia atrophy. Because of the impaired pituitary stimulus, the thyroid and adrenals fail to secrete adequate hormones. Signs and symptoms of hypothyroidism, hypoglycemia, and adrenal insufficiency (Addison's disease—see later discussion) are apparent. The client ages prematurely and becomes extremely cachectic. Results of laboratory tests show decreased hormone levels (e.g., thyroid, corticosteroid, reproductive hormones).

Medical Management

Treatment includes administration of substitute hormones for the glands that depend on the pituitary for stimulation. If untreated, the disease is fatal. GH replacement is necessary only for children. Deficiency of TSH requires replacement with levothyroxine (Synthroid) or liothyronine (Cytomel) for the client's lifetime. Male clients receive testosterone and female clients receive estrogen; both sexes receive FSH and LH.

Nursing Management

The nurse administers all hormone replacements as prescribed. Teaching the client to adhere to the medication schedule and never to omit a dose is important. The nurse monitors blood hormone levels and assesses mental status, emotional state, energy level, and appetite. He

or she is alert to any alterations in nutrition. Most clients with Simmonds' disease better tolerate four to six small meals per day as opposed to three regular meals.

● DIABETES INSIPIDUS

Diabetes insipidus is an endocrine disorder that develops when antidiuretic hormone (ADH) from the posterior pituitary gland is insufficient.

Pathophysiology and Etiology

Diabetes insipidus can result from head trauma that damages the pituitary or from primary or metastatic brain tumors. In some congenital incidences, symptoms occur shortly after birth. Diabetes insipidus also can occur after *hypophysectomy,* surgical removal of the pituitary. ADH, secreted by the posterior pituitary, regulates the reabsorption of water in the kidney tubules. Lack of ADH secretion causes the client to produce large volumes of dilute urine.

Assessment Findings

Urine output may be as high as 20 L/24 hours. Urine is dilute, with a specific gravity of 1.002 or less. Limiting fluid intake does not control urine excretion. Thirst is excessive and constant. The need frequently to drink and void limits activities. Weakness, dehydration, and weight loss develop.

In a fluid deprivation test, fluids are withheld for 8 to 12 hours, and urine specific gravity and osmolarity are determined at the beginning and end of the test. Failure to concentrate urine during the period of fluid deprivation is characteristic of this disorder. Urinalysis reveals virtually colorless urine of low specific gravity. The 24-hour urine output is abnormally large.

Medical Management

Desmopressin (DDAVP) nasal solution and lypressin (Diapid) nasal spray are synthetic drugs with ADH activity that reduce urine output to 2 to 3 L/24 hours (Nursing Guidelines 57-1). If the client cannot take oral fluids to meet the excessive fluid volume loss, intravenous (IV) fluids are necessary.

Nursing Management

Nursing measures to correct fluid volume deficit include closely monitoring the rate of IV infusions to ensure that the prescribed amount is given over the required period and measuring fluid intake and output. If the client is acutely ill or extremely dehydrated, fails to take oral fluids, or is beginning to receive medical treatment, the nurse measures urine output every 30 minutes. He or she weighs the client daily to identify weight gain or loss and observes for signs of fluid excess or deficit. The nurse notifies the physician of sudden or steady weight gain or loss. He or she reassures the client that symptoms are controllable with treatment.

● SYNDROME OF INAPPROPRIATE ANTIDIURETIC HORMONE SECRETION

The **syndrome of inappropriate antidiuretic hormone secretion** (SIADH) is characterized by renal reabsorption of water rather than its normal excretion.

Pathophysiology and Etiology

Causes of SIADH include lung tumors, central nervous system (CNS) disorders, brain tumors, cerebrovascular accident, head trauma, and drugs such as vasopressin, general anesthetic agents, oral hypoglycemics, and tricyclic antidepressants. The continued release of ADH increases fluid volume and causes *hyponatremia* (decreased serum sodium level).

Assessment Findings

Water retention, headache, muscle cramps, and anorexia develop. As the condition worsens, the client experiences nausea, vomiting, muscle twitching, and changes in level of consciousness (LOC). Diagnosis is based on symptoms and a history of a disorder associated with SIADH. Serum sodium levels and serum osmolarity are decreased. Urine sodium levels and osmolarity are high.

Medical Management

When possible, treatment aims at eliminating the underlying cause. Osmotic diuretics, such as mannitol (Osmitrol), and loop diuretics, including furosemide (Lasix), help to correct water retention. Severe hyponatremia is treated with IV administration of a 3% hypertonic sodium chloride solution.

Nursing Management

The nurse closely monitors fluid intake and output and vital signs. He or she carefully assesses LOC and immediately reports any changes to the physician. The nurse checks closely for signs of fluid overload (confusion, dyspnea, pulmonary congestion, hypertension) and hyponatremia (weakness, muscle cramps, anorexia, nausea, diarrhea, irritability, headache, weight gain without edema).

The nurse gives the client and family extensive information about the medication schedule and adverse effects of drug therapy, especially if several medications are prescribed. He or she stresses the importance of adhering to the medication schedule and not omitting a dose.

DISORDERS OF THE THYROID GLAND

Thyroid disorders are difficult to detect because symptoms are vague until the disease advances to a severe level. Treatment often is long term, and the client requires periodic follow-up to monitor response. Thyroid disorders include hyperthyroidism, thyrotoxic crisis, hypothyroidism, thyroid tumors, and endemic and multinodular goiters.

● HYPERTHYROIDISM

Hyperthyroidism also is called *Graves' disease, Basedow's disease, thyrotoxicosis,* or *exophthalmic goiter.*

Pathophysiology and Etiology

There is no one etiologic factor for hyperthyroidism. Researchers have suggested that it may be autoimmune or inherited. Hypersecretion of thyroid hormones accompanies thyroid tumors, pituitary tumors, and hypothalamic malignancies. It also may result from stress or infection. The metabolic rate increases because of the oversecretion of the thyroid hormones thyroxine (T_4) and triiodothyronine (T_3). Both T_4 and T_3 increase the metabolic rate. Hyperthyroidism is more common in women than in men.

Assessment Findings

Signs and Symptoms

Symptoms vary from mild to severe. Clients with well-developed hyperthyroidism characteristically are restless despite feeling fatigued and weak, highly excitable, and constantly agitated. Fine tremors of the hands occur, causing unusual clumsiness (Fig. 57-3). The client cannot tolerate heat and has an increased appetite, but loses weight. Diarrhea also occurs. Visual changes, such as blurred or double vision, can develop. *Exophthalmos,* seen in clients with severe hyperthyroidism, results from enlarged muscle and fatty tissue surrounding the rear and sides of the eyeball (see Fig. 56-10). Neck swelling caused by the enlarged thyroid gland often is visible. Table 57-1 compares the signs and symptoms of hyperthyroidism and hypothyroidism.

Diagnostic Findings

The protein-bound iodine, free T_3, thyroglobulin, and serum T_3 and T_4 levels are elevated. The TSH level is decreased. Thyroid ultrasonography shows an enlarged thyroid gland. A thyroid scan indicates an increased uptake of radioactive iodine (RAI; ^{131}I and ^{123}I). Results of an RAI uptake study show an increased uptake of iodine.

Medical and Surgical Management

Antithyroid drugs, such as propylthiouracil (PTU, Propyl-Thyracil) and methimazole (Tapazole), are given to block the production of thyroid hormone. Potassium iodide (Lugol's solution) is prescribed in combination with an antithyroid drug. Antithyroid medications are avoided during pregnancy because they can induce hypothyroidism, or cretinism, in the fetus. Drug Therapy Table 57-1 discusses these and other drugs used to treat thyroid disorders.

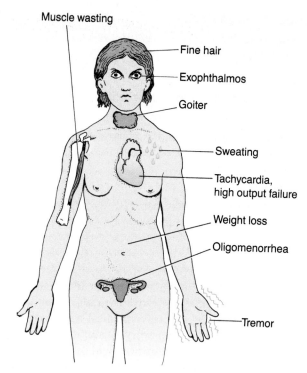

FIGURE 57-3 Clinical manifestations of hyperthyroidism.

^{131}I is used to destroy hyperplastic thyroid tissue by radiation. The thyroid is quick to remove iodine, including RAI, from the bloodstream. Antithyroid drugs are given for 6 months or more before administration of ^{131}I. If symptoms do not improve, a second and perhaps a third dose of ^{131}I is given. About 6 to 8 weeks after the initial dose of ^{131}I, most clients notice some remission of symptoms. The extended time lag before relief of symptoms is a disadvantage of this treatment method. A more common and unfortunate result of treatment is hypothyroidism because accurately determining the precise amount of thyroid tissue that radiation will destroy is very difficult. This complication may not develop until long after the administration of ^{131}I, and clients must remain under medical supervision for many years.

TABLE 57-1	**SYMPTOMS OF THYROID DYSFUNCTION**	
BODY SYSTEM OR FUNCTION	**HYPERTHYROIDISM**	**HYPOTHYROIDISM**
Metabolism	Increased, with symptoms of increased appetite, intolerance to heat, elevated body temperature, weight loss despite increased appetite	Decreased, with symptoms of anorexia, intolerance to cold, low body temperature, weight gain despite anorexia
Cardiovascular system	Tachycardia, moderate hypertension	Bradycardia, moderate hypotension
Central nervous system	Nervousness, anxiety, insomnia, tremors	Lethargy, sleepiness
Skin and skin structures	Flushed, warm, moist	Pale, cool, dry; face appears puffy, hair coarse; nails thick and hard
Ovarian function	Irregular or scant menses	Heavy menses, may be unable to conceive, loss of fetus also possible
Testicular function		Low sperm count

DRUG THERAPY TABLE 57-1	AGENTS FOR THYROID DISORDERS		
DRUG CATEGORY AND EXAMPLES	**MECHANISM OF ACTION**	**SIDE EFFECTS**	**NURSING CONSIDERATIONS**
Antithyroid Agents *methimazole (Tapazole)* *propylthiouracil (PTU)*	Inhibits synthesis of thyroid hormones	Paresthesias, nausea, agranulocytosis, bleeding, rash, diarrhea, vomiting	Caution clients to avoid use during pregnancy. Monitor results of blood tests for bone marrow depression. Administer in three equal doses every 8 hours. Alert client to notify the physician of fever, sore throat, unusual bleeding or bruising, or malaise.
Iodides *strong iodine solution* *(Lugol's solution)*	Inhibits synthesis and release of T_3 and T_4	Iodism: metallic taste, burning mouth, sore teeth and gums, nausea, abdominal pain, diarrhea, rash	Monitor for symptoms of acute iodine toxicity: vomiting, abdominal pain, diarrhea, circulatory collapse. Dilute with fruit juice or water. Advise client to drink solution with a straw to avoid staining teeth.
Radioactive Iodine *sodium iodine ^{131}I and [123]I*	Used in diagnostic scans; destroys thyroid tissue in hyperthyroidism and thyroid malignancies	Allergy to iodine, nausea, vomiting	Follow precautions for body fluids for 24 hours after diagnostic testing. Monitor for signs of hypothyroidism.
Beta-Adrenergic Blockers *propranolol (Inderal)*	Reduces symptoms of hyperthyroidism—tachycardia, tremors, nervousness	Nausea, vomiting, diarrhea, constipation, bradycardia, congestive heart failure, dysrhythmias, hypoglycemia	Monitor cardiac function. Administer with meals. Instruct client not to discontinue abruptly. Assess blood glucose level regularly for clients with diabetes.
Thyroid Hormone Replacement Drugs *thyroid dessicated (Armour thyroid, S-P-T, Thyrar, Thyroid Strong)* *thyroid hormones T_3 and T_4 in their natural state* *liothyronine (T_3, Cytomel, Triostat)* *liotrix (Thyrolar)*	Increases metabolic rate of body tissues	Hyperthyroidism: tachycardia, tremors, headache, nervousness, insomnia, diarrhea, weight loss, heat intolerance	Monitor response closely. Monitor thyroid function tests. Advise client that drug usually is required for lifetime. Administer drug as a single daily dose before breakfast. Thyroid preparations interact with digitalis, estrogen, beta blockers, glucagon, and anticoagulants.

Subtotal thyroidectomy (partial removal of the thyroid gland) is an effective treatment for hyperthyroidism. *Total thyroidectomy* (removal of the thyroid gland) may be performed if a neoplastic tumor is present. Clients commonly receive antithyroid drug therapy for several weeks before surgery to prevent a dramatic release of thyroid hormones into the bloodstream during surgery. Single thyroid nodules less than 3 cm in diameter can be removed by minimally invasive endoscopic techniques in which the surgeon makes three to four small incisions in the neck rather than the typical single incision, which is several inches long.

Complications of thyroidectomy include the following:

- Accidental removal of or alteration in the blood supply to the parathyroid glands, which are embedded in thyroid tissue, resulting in hypocalcemia
- Hemorrhage caused by the vascularity of the thyroid and surrounding tissue
- Thyrotoxicosis (or thyroid storm) as a result of excessive secretion of thyroid hormones during surgical excision
- Damage to the recurrent laryngeal nerve, which affects the function of the vocal cords. If the recurrent

laryngeal nerve is damaged either temporarily or partially, breathing may be impaired because the vocal cords cannot open properly during inspiration; the voice may sound weak, hoarse, or breathy; and aspiration and pneumonia may occur if the vocal cords do not close completely during swallowing.

Nursing Management

The nurse monitors heart rate and blood pressure (BP) regularly. He or she records the client's sleep pattern and daily weights. The nurse promotes rest and helps the client avoid excess physical stimulation. Increased caloric intake can compensate for increased metabolism. The nurse informs the client that effects of antithyroid therapy usually are not apparent until the thyroid gland has secreted the excess thyroid hormone into the bloodstream. This process may take several weeks or more. If RAI is used to destroy thyroid tissue, the nurse tells the client that it does not seriously affect other tissues. Possible transient effects after use of ^{131}I and ^{123}I are nausea, vomiting, malaise, fever, and gland tenderness. Nursing Care Plan 57-1 discusses care of the client undergoing thyroid surgery.

● THYROTOXIC CRISIS

Pathophysiology and Etiology

Thyrotoxic crisis, an abrupt and life-threatening form of hyperthyroidism, is thought to be triggered by extreme stress, infection, diabetic ketoacidosis, trauma, toxemia of pregnancy, or manipulation of a hyperactive thyroid gland during surgery or physical examination. Although rare, this condition may occur in clients with undiagnosed or inadequately treated hyperthyroidism.

The oversecretion of T_3 and T_4 is followed by a release of epinephrine. Metabolism is markedly increased. The adrenal glands produce excess corticosteroids in response to the stress created by this hypermetabolic state.

Assessment Findings

The temperature may be as high as 41°C (106°F). The pulse rate is rapid, and cardiac dysrhythmias are common. The client may experience persistent vomiting, extreme restlessness with delirium, chest pain, and dyspnea.

The diagnosis is based on the symptoms and a recent medical history that indicates symptoms of severe hyperthyroidism. Laboratory tests, such as serum T_3 and T_4 determinations, may be used to confirm the diagnosis. In thyrotoxic crisis, serum thyroid determinations are markedly elevated.

Medical Management

Immediate treatment is necessary. Antithyroid drugs (e.g., propylthiouracil, methimazole) are used to block the synthesis of thyroid hormones. An IV corticosteroid may be given to replace depletion that results from overstimulation of the adrenals during the hypermetabolic state. IV sodium iodide prevents the thyroid gland from releasing thyroid hormones. Propranolol (Inderal), a beta blocker, reduces the effect of thyroid hormones on the cardiovascular system. Supportive therapy includes IV fluids, antipyretic measures, and oxygen therapy.

Nursing Management

The client with thyrotoxic crisis is acutely ill. The nurse monitors vital signs, especially the temperature, frequently. Failure to respond to an antipyretic drug requires other measures, such as a cooling blanket or ice application. A cool room also may help reduce body temperature. The nurse gives all therapeutic treatment measures as ordered because the situation must be corrected as soon as possible.

● HYPOTHYROIDISM

Hypothyroidism occurs when the thyroid gland fails to secrete adequate thyroid hormones.

Pathophysiology and Etiology

This condition may originate in the thyroid (primary hypothyroidism) or in the pituitary, in which case insufficient TSH is secreted. Regardless of the cause, the result of inadequate thyroid hormone secretion is a slowing of all metabolic processes (see Table 57-1). Severe hypothyroidism is called **myxedema.** Advanced, untreated myxedema can progress to myxedema coma. Signs of this life-threatening event are hypothermia, hypotension, and hypoventilation. A client with hypothyroidism experiencing infection, trauma, or excessive chills, or taking narcotics, sedatives, or tranquilizers, can lapse into a myxedema coma.

Assessment Findings

Signs and Symptoms

Signs and symptoms are opposite in many respects to those of hyperthyroidism. Metabolic rate and physical and mental activity slow down. The client is lethargic, lacks energy, dozes frequently during the day, is forgetful,

(text continued on page 862)

Nursing Care Plan 57-1

THE CLIENT UNDERGOING THYROID SURGERY

Assessment

■ Obtain complete medical, drug, and allergy histories.

■ Check and compare present weight with preillness weight.

■ Measure vital signs each shift and more often if findings are abnormal.

■ Perform a physical examination, but avoid palpating the thyroid gland (manipulation releases excess thyroid hormones).

■ Determine client's preoperative compliance with antithyroid drug therapy.

■ Explore client's knowledge of the operative procedure and perioperative care.

Nursing Diagnosis: Anxiety related to perception of pending surgery

Expected Outcome: Anxiety will be reduced to a tolerable level as evidenced by a rating below 5 on a scale from 0 to 10, uninterrupted sleep, no restlessness or purposeless activity, and moderate emotional responses.

Interventions	Rationales
Be calm and confident during interactions with client.	A nurse who conveys expertise helps reduce anxiety and builds a sense of security.
Interact with client frequently and respond promptly to requests for assistance.	Trust develops when a client obtains attention and support in a reasonable amount of time.
Give client opportunities to talk and ask questions about the surgery and subsequent health management issues.	If a nurse is receptive to questions, the client is more likely to verbalize concerns about the impending procedure.
Encourage the presence of those who give the client emotional support.	Significant others with whom the client has emotional bonds potentiate security.

Evaluation of Expected Outcomes: Client reports decreased anxiety.

Nursing Diagnosis: Deficient Knowledge related to unfamiliarity with perioperative measures that reduce potential postoperative complications

Expected Outcome: Client will demonstrate breathing and leg exercises and the technique for postoperative head support.

Interventions	Rationales
Provide routine instructions for deep breathing and leg exercises (see Chap. 25).	These measures decrease the potential for pneumonia, thrombi, and other complications.
Show client how to support the neck with the hands when rising to sit (Fig. 57-4).	Supporting the head avoids straining neck muscles or the surgical incision.

Evaluation of Expected Outcomes: Client performs exercises and supports the head as taught before surgery.

Nursing Diagnosis: Risk for Ineffective Breathing Pattern related to compression of the trachea from edema of the glottis, accumulated blood in the operative area, recurrent laryngeal nerve damage, or retained secretions

Expected Outcome: Breathing will be regular, noiseless, and effortless with an SpO_2 of at least 90%.

(continued)

Nursing Care Plan 57-1 (Continued)

THE CLIENT UNDERGOING THYROID SURGERY

Interventions	*Rationales*
Elevate the head of the bed 30° or more.	Head elevation reduces edema.
Apply an ice bag to the neck if prescribed.	It promotes vasoconstriction, thereby reducing edema and bleeding.
Place a tracheostomy set in client's room.	Having a means for establishing a patent airway is an emergency life-saving measure.
Assemble oral/pharyngeal suction equipment at client's bedside and suction client if he or she cannot raise respiratory secretions.	Suctioning clears the airway of substances that compromise movement of gases into and out of the lungs.
Observe for dyspnea and restlessness.	Increased breathing effort is evidence of a compromised airway.
Report signs of respiratory distress to the nurse in charge and the physician.	Sharing information aids in collaborative efforts to prevent complications.

Evaluation of Expected Outcomes: Client maintains normal ventilation, with no airway obstruction.

PC: **Hemorrhage**

Expected Outcome: The nurse monitors to detect, manage, and minimize signs of hemorrhage.

Interventions	*Rationales*
Monitor vital signs every 1 to 4 hours.	Tachycardia and hypotension suggest cellular hypoxia and fluid volume deficit secondary to bleeding.
Inspect the surgical dressing frequently for bleeding.	Gauze dressing material wicks blood from the surgical incision.
Check the back of the neck for bloody drainage.	Gravity causes blood to drain posteriorly, which interferes with its visibility on the surface of the surgical dressing.
Attend to client's complaints of fullness in or around the surgical incision.	Blood may accumulate beneath the sutured incision rather than drain externally.
Place suture or staple removal equipment in client's room or stock equipment in a clean utility room.	The incision may need to be opened to remove clotted blood or ligate blood vessels that continue to bleed.

Evaluation of Expected Outcomes: There is no evidence of excessive bleeding in or around the operative site.

Nursing Diagnosis: **Impaired Verbal Communication** related to hoarseness secondary to recurrent laryngeal nerve damage

Expected Outcome: Client will regain normal volume and quality of speech.

Interventions	*Rationales*
Minimize unnecessary vocalizations for client.	Resting the voice reduces strain on the vocal cords.
Deliver bedside humidification.	Inhalation of moist air helps relieve hoarseness.
Provide an alternate means (pad of paper, magic slate, alphabet board) for the client to ask questions or make needs known.	Written communication provides a substitute for verbal interactions.

(continued)

Nursing Care Plan 57-1 *(Continued)*

THE CLIENT UNDERGOING THYROID SURGERY

Interventions	Rationales
Ensure that client has access to a signal cord or bell with which to summon a caregiver.	A light or bell signals a need for assistance and is essential when a client cannot call for help.
Assess the quality of client's voice periodically every 2 to 4 waking hours for the first 2 postoperative days.	The nurse must report a weakening of the voice or loss of the ability to project sounds.

Evaluation of Expected Outcomes: Speech is at the presurgical volume.

Nursing Diagnosis: **Risk for Aspiration** related to recurrent laryngeal nerve damage

Expected Outcome: Lungs will be free of food or liquids.

Interventions	Rationales
Prepare oral/pharyngeal suction equipment.	Suctioning provides a way to clear the airway.
Have client sit upright.	An upright position promotes the mechanics of swallowing and a more forceful cough if substances enter the airway.
Provide thickened substances initially.	Watery food and beverages are more difficult to swallow.
Encourage client to place a very small amount in his or her mouth at any one time.	Controlling ingested substances increases the potential success for swallowing the mass.

Evaluation of Expected Outcomes: Client does not experience respiratory distress, and lungs are clear on auscultation.

Nursing Diagnosis: **Pain** related to tissue trauma secondary to operative procedure

Expected Outcome: Client will report an increased comfort level within 30 minutes of a pain-relieving intervention.

Interventions	Rationales
Administer analgesics as prescribed.	They interfere with pain transmission and perception.
Place pillows under the head, neck, and shoulders.	Pillows support the operative area, preventing excessive muscular pulling and possible separation of the incision.
Maintain head support when client's position is changed.	Head support reduces muscle contraction and tension on the surgical incision.

Evaluation of Expected Outcomes: Client is comfortable or pain free.

PC: **Tetany**

Expected Outcome: The nurse will monitor to detect, manage, and minimize tetany.

Interventions	Rationales
Observe for spontaneous spasm of the fingers or toes, mouth twitching or jaw tightening when you tap the cheek anteriorly to the earlobe (Chvostek's sign), and spasm of the fingers toward the wrist when you inflate a BP cuff midway between systolic and diastolic pressures for 3 minutes (Trousseau's sign).	Tetany develops when the parathyroid glands, which regulate blood calcium levels, are accidentally removed during a thyroidectomy. Hypocalcemia results in neuromuscular hyperexcitability.

(continued)

Nursing Care Plan 57-1 (Continued)

THE CLIENT UNDERGOING THYROID SURGERY

Interventions	Rationales
Note crowing respirations and dyspnea.	Manifestations of hypocalcemia include symptoms caused by laryngeal spasm.
Be prepared to implement seizure precautions.	Seizures may occur when the blood calcium level falls below normal.
Have calcium gluconate for IV administration available if prescribed by the physician.	Calcium replacement controls symptoms of tetany.

Evaluation of Expected Outcomes: No complications develop.

PC: Thyrotoxic Crisis

Expected Outcome: The nurse will monitor to detect, manage, and minimize thyrotoxic crisis.

Interventions	Rationales
Assess for hyperthermia, tachycardia, chest pain, cardiac dysrhythmias, and altered level of consciousness.	Excess levels of thyroid hormones raise body temperature and accelerate cardiac activity by increasing the rate of metabolism.
Notify the physician if symptoms of thyrotoxic crisis develop.	Collaborative measures are necessary to control symptoms and their consequences.
Implement measures to reduce body temperature such as administering antipyretics or placing client on an aquathermia pad.	Measures to reduce body temperature help prevent complications such as seizures and brain damage.
Follow medical orders for measures to reduce heart rate and dysrhythmias.	Tachycardia increases myocardial demands for oxygen; unless managed, it can lead to myocardial infarction, acute heart failure, or cardiac arrest.

Evaluation of Expected Outcomes: No complications develop.

and has chronic headaches. The face takes on a masklike, unemotional expression, yet the client often is irritable. The tongue may be enlarged and the lips swollen, and there may be edema of the eyelids. Temperature and pulse rate are decreased; the client is intolerant to cold. Weight increases despite a low caloric intake. The skin is dry, and hair characteristically is coarse and sparse and tends to fall out. Menstrual disorders are common. Constipation may be severe. The voice is low pitched and hoarse, and speech is slow. Hearing may be impaired. The client may experience numbness or tingling in the arms or legs that is unrelieved by position change.

Hypothyroidism may lead to an enlarged heart caused by pericardial effusion and an increased tendency toward atherosclerosis and heart strain. Anemia also may be present. Early recognition of hypothyroidism is difficult because many of the symptoms are nonspecific and may not be sufficiently dramatic to bring the client to the physician. This condition can go untreated for years.

Diagnostic Findings

In primary hypothyroidism, levels of TSH are increased because of the negative feedback to the pituitary gland (see Chap. 56). The RAI uptake may be decreased. The T_3 and T_4 levels show no response in primary untreated hypothyroidism but may show a response if hypothyroidism results from failure of the pituitary to secrete TSH.

Medical Management

Hypothyroidism is treated with thyroid replacement therapy (see Drug Therapy Table 57-1). Thyroid hormone in the form of desiccated thyroid extract, or with one of the synthetic products, such as levothyroxine sodium (Synthroid) or liothyronine sodium (Cytomel), are oral thyroid preparations. A low dose of thyroid hormone is given initially and then increased or decreased as needed.

FIGURE 57-4 After a thyroidectomy, the client uses the hands to support the head while rising to a sitting position. This type of support helps avoid strain to the neck muscles and surgical incision.

NURSING PROCESS

● The Client With Hypothyroidism

Assessment

The nurse obtains medical, drug, and allergy histories and a thorough description of symptoms. He or she checks vital signs and weight. During physical examination, the nurse observes for symptoms of hypothyroidism: lethargy, fatigue, anorexia, weight gain, hair loss, brittle nails, and cold intolerance.

Once a definitive diagnosis is made, the nurse observes for adverse effects of thyroid replacement therapy. Dyspnea, rapid pulse rate, palpitations, precordial pain, hyperactivity, insomnia, dizziness, and gastrointestinal (GI) disorders—in other words, signs of hyperthyroidism—may be seen if the dose of thyroid hormone is too high. Once replacement therapy has begun, a dramatic change may be seen in a few weeks.

Diagnosis, Planning, and Interventions

Activity Intolerance related to fatigue and depressed cognitive processes
Expected Outcome: Client will demonstrate increased activity tolerance.

- Assess activity tolerance. *Altered metabolism from reduced secretion of thyroid hormone compromises client's ability to perform physical activities.*
- Allow adequate rest between activities. *Conserving energy increases endurance.*
- Assist with hygiene and other self-care activities as needed. *Such assistance extends the client's tolerance until he or she can progress to independent self-care.*

Constipation related to decreased bowel function
Expected Outcome: Stools will be moist and easily and regularly passed.

- Assess bowel elimination patterns and stool characteristics. *A record of bowel elimination and stool characteristics helps determine the need for measures to promote defecation.*
- Provide high-fiber foods. *Fiber increases stool bulk and promotes additional water in the intestinal mass. Bulky stool creates pressure in the rectum, which causes the stimulus to defecate.*
- Encourage adequate fluid intake. *Moist stool is expelled more easily than dry stool.*
- Encourage increased physical activity (e.g., short walks) within client's tolerance. *Physical activity promotes the movement of intestinal contents toward the rectum and anus.*

Risk for Imbalanced Body Temperature related to hyposecretion of thyroid hormones
Expected Outcome: Body temperature will be maintained.

- Assess body temperature; report deviations from usual values. *Decreased metabolism lowers body temperature; reduced muscle contraction from inactivity interferes with the generation of body heat.*
- Provide extra warmth with blankets or clothing. *Layers of fabric that trap and hold warm air next to the body surface conserve or increase body heat.*
- Protect client from exposure to cold or drafts. *Body heat is lost through convection as air currents pass over the warmer areas of exposed skin.*

Deficient Knowledge related to need for lifelong thyroid replacement therapy
Expected Outcome: Client will verbalize the need for daily hormone replacement and describe the consequences of overdosage or underdosage.

- Teach reasons for hormone replacement therapy. *Pharmacologic replacement is necessary when the thyroid gland does not produce adequate endogenous thyroid hormone.*
- Explain therapeutic effects. *When the level of thyroid hormone is adequate, fatigue, lethargy, weight gain, impaired cognition, tendency to feel cold, altered physical features, bradycardia, and hypotension gradually resolve.*
- Teach signs of overdosage and underdosage. *Lack of compliance can prolong recovery and delay health restoration if self-administration of thyroid replacement is erratic or discontinued. An overdosage can increase metabolic processes, causing nervousness, tremor, tachycardia, hypertension, and insomnia.*
- Assist client to develop a schedule for taking medication each day. *Such a schedule helps the client avoid missing one or more doses.*
- Explain the need for continued follow-up to monitor hormone status. *Response to thyroid replacement therapy is evaluated through laboratory tests that measure*

TSH, T_3, and T_4 levels and regular medical examinations by the prescribing physician.

● Recommend that the client obtain and wear a Medic Alert tag at all times. *It helps healthcare personnel to assess an unconscious client more readily if they are aware of a pre-existing health problem.*

PC: Myxedema and **Myxedema Coma**

Expected Outcome: The nurse will monitor to detect myxedema or myxedema coma and will manage and minimize these conditions should they develop.

● Assess for decreased pulse, respirations, BP, and temperature. *Changes in vital signs accompany decreased metabolism.*

● Cover client with warm blankets if temperature is below normal. *The heat from warmed cotton blankets is conducted to the skin and superficial blood vessels.*

● Assess for changes in LOC, difficulty waking, or increasing confusion. *Profound hypothyroidism slows all body functions, including the ability to remain awake and alert.*

● Monitor oxygenation status using a pulse oximeter. *A stuporous or comatose client may be unable to protect his or her airway, causing the blood oxygen saturation (SpO_2) to fall below 90%.*

● Administer oxygen as prescribed to maintain SpO_2 at or above 90%. *Maintaining SpO_2 at 90% ensures that the arterial oxygen pressure (PaO_2) is between 80 and 100 mm Hg.*

● Maintain a patent airway using an oral or pharyngeal airway. *An artificial airway keeps the tongue from obstructing the upper airway.*

● Consult with the physician or respiratory therapist if client requires endotracheal intubation and mechanical ventilation. *An endotracheal tube maintains an airway and provides a means to oxygenate a client who does not breathe adequately.*

● Implement medical directives for IV fluids and administration of vasopressors and thyroid replacement hormone. *Clients with myxedema or myxedema coma are treated with IV administration of levothyroxine and vasopressors.*

● Carefully administer analgesics; avoid administering sedatives or hypnotics. *CNS depressants interfere with the client's neurologic status and subsequent assessment of it.*

Evaluation of Expected Outcomes/Teaching Plan

Client reports feeling rested and meets self-care needs. He or she has regular stools without discomfort. The client reports feeling comfortable, not cold, in a normal temperature setting. He or she describes the medication regimen, possible side effects, and precautions. The client does not develop myxedema or myxedema coma, or, if it develops, the nurse collaborates with the physician to restore a normal physiologic state.

Symptoms associated with hyperthyroidism and hypothyroidism often affect learning and retention ability.

The nurse carefully explains the treatment regimen, including the dose of the medications and possible adverse effects. If a special diet has been recommended, the nurse obtains a dietary consultation and reviews sample diets with the client. A teaching plan includes the following:

● Weigh self weekly; keep a record of symptoms and weight in case the medication dose needs adjustment.
● Avoid stressful situations.
● Maintain good nutrition.
● Notify the physician if symptoms worsen or adverse drug effects occur.

● THYROID TUMORS

Tumors of the thyroid can cause hyperthyroidism. They are more commonly benign, but all nodules must be evaluated.

Pathophysiology and Etiology

A *follicular adenoma* is the most common benign thyroid lesion. A lump is most likely to be benign for adult women with symptoms of hyperthyroidism or hypothyroidism. *Papillary carcinoma* is the most common malignant lesion; it usually occurs in clients who received radiation treatments to the head or neck region in the past. It tends to spread only to nearby lymph nodes and rarely to other parts of the body. The cure rate of thyroid cancer depends on the type of tumor present.

Assessment Findings

Symptoms are vague, and the client may be unaware of the lesion. Often a routine physical examination reveals a nodular thyroid. As the tumor enlarges, the client often notices a swelling in the neck. Benign tumors cause symptoms of hyperthyroidism in some clients. Malignant tumors can cause voice changes, hoarseness, and difficulty swallowing.

Biopsy of the lesion confirms the diagnosis. Thyroid cancer is suspected when the gland is firm and palpable and when results of RAI studies show poor concentration in the suspect area.

Medical and Surgical Management

If there are no symptoms of hyperthyroidism with a benign nodule, treatment usually is not needed. The nodule is examined yearly. If the enlargement causes such symptoms as difficulty swallowing and noticeable neck swelling, surgical removal of the lesion is considered. Although treatment of malignant lesions varies, a thyroidectomy (total or subtotal) typically is performed. A modified or radical neck dissection is indicated if there is metastasis. After a thyroidectomy, replacement therapy (consisting of thyroid hormones) is given to supply thyroid hormones and to suppress pituitary TSH so that it no longer stimulates growth of residual thyroid tissue. [131]I is administered to destroy remaining thyroid tissue as well as to treat lymph node metastasis, if present.

Nursing Management

If the thyroid tumor is malignant, the physician explains the planned treatment and expected outcome. The nurse provides emotional support, especially if the tumor has metastasized and radical surgery is necessary. When RAI is used after surgery, the client is isolated and placed on radiation precautions (see Chap. 20). The nurse handles body fluids carefully to prevent spread of contamination.

● ENDEMIC AND MULTINODULAR GOITERS

The word **goiter** refers to an enlarged thyroid gland.

Pathophysiology and Etiology

An *endemic goiter* is caused by a deficiency of iodine in the diet, by the inability of the thyroid to use iodine, or by relative iodine deficiency caused by increasing body demands for thyroid hormones. *Nontoxic goiter* (also called *simple* or *colloid goiter*) is an enlarged thyroid, usually with no symptoms of thyroid dysfunction. *Nodular goiters* contain one or more areas of hyperplasia. This type

of goiter appears to develop for essentially the same reasons as an endemic goiter.

Assessment Findings

The thyroid gland enlarges. The client has a sense of fullness in the neck area. Continued gland enlargement eventually results in difficulty swallowing and breathing as the thyroid presses on the trachea and esophagus. When the gland has enlarged, it is visible as a swelling in the neck. Nodular goiters also produce enlargement, but the gland has an irregular surface on palpation (Fig. 57-5).

A thyroid scan shows an enlarged gland and a decreased uptake of [131]I. Tests of thyroid function are performed, but results may or may not be abnormal and, thus, are inconclusive.

Medical Management

Treatment depends on the cause. If the diet is deficient in iodine, foods high in iodine, such as seafood or iodized salt, are recommended. Potassium iodide to supplement iodine intake may be given. In some instances, a thyroidectomy is recommended, especially when the gland is grossly enlarged.

Nursing Management

If the client has respiratory distress because of the enlarged thyroid, the nurse closely observes respiratory status and elevates the head of the bed to relieve respiratory symptoms. He or she provides a diet high in iodine and iodized salt. Natural iodine content is highest in seafoods; it is also found in varying amounts in bread, milk, eggs,

A   **B**   **C**

FIGURE 57-5 Thyroid abnormalities. (**A**) Diffuse toxic goiter (Graves' disease) with exophthalmos. (**B**) Diffuse nontoxic goiter. (**C**) Nodular goiter. (From Judge, R. D., Zuidema, G. D., & Fitzgerald, F. T. [Eds.]. [1982]. *Clinical diagnosis* [4th ed.]. Boston: Little, Brown.)

meat, and spinach. A soft diet may be necessary if the client has difficulty swallowing.

● THYROIDITIS

Thyroiditis, inflammation of the thyroid gland, can be acute, subacute, or chronic.

Pathophysiology and Etiology

Acute thyroiditis, most common in children, appears to result from bacterial infection of the gland. *Subacute thyroiditis* can follow an upper respiratory viral infection and is relatively rare. More common is *Hashimoto's thyroiditis,* a chronic form of thyroiditis, believed to be an autoimmune disorder.

Assessment Findings

Signs and symptoms of acute thyroiditis include high fever, malaise, and tenderness and swelling of the thyroid gland. Subacute thyroiditis produces symptoms of a swollen and painful gland, chills, fever, and malaise approximately 2 weeks after a viral infection. Hashimoto's thyroiditis is manifested by an enlarged thyroid and, in some cases, symptoms of hypothyroidism.

In acute thyroiditis, laboratory test results show an elevated white blood cell (WBC) count and normal thyroid function. In subacute thyroiditis, the results of some thyroid tests, such as T_3 and T_4, are elevated. The RAI study shows a decreased iodine uptake. In Hashimoto's thyroiditis, there are high titers of antithyroid antibodies, and RAI studies show increased iodine uptake.

Medical and Surgical Management

Acute thyroiditis requires administration of appropriate antibiotics. The treatment of subacute thyroiditis is symptomatic and includes analgesics for pain and discomfort. Corticosteroids also may be prescribed to reduce inflammation. The treatment of Hashimoto's thyroiditis includes thyroid hormone replacement therapy. Surgery is required if the gland becomes excessively large.

Nursing Management

Management depends on the type of thyroiditis and severity of symptoms. The nurse gives antipyretics for fever. He or she elevates the head of the bed if the client has difficulty breathing. The nurse offers a soft diet if the gland is markedly enlarged and the client has difficulty swallowing.

If a client has undergone surgery (see Nursing Care Plan 57-1), before discharge the nurse instructs the client in the care of the surgical wound and to avoid excessive strain on the wound until it is healed. Because the incision is made in a neck crease, the healed scar is barely visible. If a client appears concerned about scarring, the nurse may suggest that the client wear clothing that covers the neck until the scar is almost invisible.

The nurse discusses the symptoms of hypothyroidism, hyperthyroidism, and hypoparathyroidism with instructions to notify the physician immediately if they occur. If medication is prescribed, the nurse reviews the dosage and adverse effects of each drug. A teaching plan includes techniques for wound care, the need to take thyroid replacement medication in the morning at the same time each day to avoid insomnia and CNS stimulation, and side effects that require notification of the physician (chest pain, tachycardia, and dyspnea).

> **Stop, Think, and Respond ● BOX 57-1**
> *When reviewing a client's medical record, you read that the physician has detected an enlarged thyroid gland. What are some possible causes?*

DISORDERS OF THE PARATHYROID GLANDS

When the parathyroid gland dysfunctions, hyperparathyroidism or hypoparathyroidism develops. Calcium and phosphorus levels are affected.

● HYPERPARATHYROIDISM

Hyperparathyroidism can be a primary or secondary condition.

Pathophysiology and Etiology

The most common cause of *primary hyperparathyroidism* is an adenoma of one of the parathyroid glands. In primary hyperparathyroidism, excessive secretion of parathyroid hormone (parathormone) results in increased urinary excretion of phosphorus and loss of calcium from the bones. The bones become demineralized as the calcium leaves and enters the bloodstream. Renal stones may develop as calcium becomes concentrated in the urine.

In *secondary hyperparathyroidism,* the parathyroid glands secrete excessive parathormone in response to hypocalcemia (low serum calcium level), which may result from vitamin D deficiency, chronic renal failure, large doses of thiazide diuretics, and excessive use of laxatives and calcium supplements.

Assessment Findings

Signs and Symptoms

Excessive calcium in the blood depresses the responsiveness of the peripheral nerves, accounting for fatigue and muscle weakness. The muscles become hypotonic (loss of or decrease in muscle tone). Cardiac dysrhythmias may develop. Because the bones have lost calcium, there is skeletal tenderness and pain on bearing weight; the bones may become so demineralized that they break with little or no trauma (pathologic fractures). Other possible effects include nausea, vomiting, and constipation. Large amounts of calcium and phosphorus passing through the kidneys predispose the client to the formation of stones in the genitourinary tract, pyelonephritis, and uremia.

Diagnostic Findings

The diagnosis is based on elevated serum calcium and decreased serum phosphorus levels without other causes of hypercalcemia. The results of a 24-hour urine test show increased urine calcium levels. Skeletal radiographs show calcium loss from bones. An MRI or a CT scan identifies a parathyroid adenoma if present. Parathormone levels are elevated in hyperparathyroidism.

Medical and Surgical Management

Secondary hyperparathyroidism is managed by correcting the cause (e.g., vitamin D therapy for a vitamin D deficiency, correction of renal failure, calcium-restricted diet). Sodium and phosphorus replacements often are ordered. Hormone replacement with synthetic calcitonin (Calcimar) is avoided because it is associated with allergic reactions and drug resistance. The latter is caused by antibodies that neutralize the hormone.

The only treatment for primary hyperparathyroidism is surgical removal of hypertrophied gland tissue or of an individual tumor of one of the parathyroid glands. Before surgery, the physician determines the number of glands to be removed, based on the cause of hyperparathyroidism and laboratory and diagnostic test results. One or more of the parathyroids is left in place because they are necessary for calcium and phosphorus metabolism.

Nursing Management

The nurse closely measures the client's intake and output. He or she observes for signs of urinary calculi from hypercalcemia, flank pain, and decreasing urine output. The nurse encourages a large volume of fluid to keep the urine dilute. He or she assesses the client's ability to perform self-care, provides a safe environment to prevent falls and other injury, encourages frequent rest periods, and monitors fatigue level.

The primary nursing responsibility is teaching the client about the effects of the disease, the planned medical management, and the importance of following the prescribed treatment. If the client undergoes surgery, the nursing management is similar to that for thyroid surgery. In addition, the nurse observes the client for symptoms of hypoparathyroidism.

● HYPOPARATHYROIDISM

Hypoparathyroidism is a deficiency of parathormone that results in hypocalcemia.

Pathophysiology and Etiology

Parathormone regulates calcium balance by increasing calcium absorption from the GI tract and bone resorption of calcium. Hypocalcemia affects neuromuscular functions. It causes hyperexcitability, resulting in spastic muscle contractions and *paresthesias* (abnormal sensations).

The most common causes of hypoparathyroidism are trauma to the glands and inadvertent removal of all or nearly all these structures during thyroidectomy or parathyroidectomy. The idiopathic form of this disorder is rare but may be autoimmune in origin or caused by the congenital absence of the parathyroids.

Assessment Findings

Signs and Symptoms

The main symptom of acute and sudden hypoparathyroidism is **tetany.** The client may report numbness and tingling in the fingers or toes or around the lips. A voluntary movement may be followed by an involuntary, jerking spasm. Muscle cramping may be present. Tonic (continuous contraction) flexion of an arm or a finger may occur. If a nurse taps the client's facial nerve (which lies under the tissue in front of the ear), the client's mouth twitches and the jaw tightens. The response is identified as a positive **Chvostek's sign** (see Chap. 22). The nurse may elicit a positive **Trousseau's sign** by placing a BP cuff on the upper arm, inflating it between the systolic and diastolic BP, and waiting 3 minutes. The nurse observes the client for spasm of the hand (**carpopedal spasm**), which is evidenced by the hand flexing inward (see Chap. 22).

Laryngeal spasm can occur in the larynx, causing dyspnea, with long, crowing respirations as air tries to get past the constriction. Cyanosis may be present, and the client is in danger of asphyxia and cardiac dysrhythmias. Nausea, vomiting, abdominal pain, and seizures can develop.

In chronic hypoparathyroidism, the client experiences neuromuscular irritability, constipation or diarrhea, numbness and tingling of the arms and legs, loss of tooth enamel, and muscle pain. Positive Chvostek's and Trousseau's signs may or may not be elicited, depending on the degree of hypocalcemia.

Diagnostic Findings

The serum calcium level is decreased, the serum phosphorus level is increased, and the urine levels of both are decreased. In chronic hypoparathyroidism, radiographs show increased bone density.

Medical Management

Tetany and severe hypoparathyroidism are treated immediately by the administration of an IV calcium salt, such as calcium gluconate. Endotracheal intubation and mechanical ventilation may be necessary if acute respiratory distress occurs. Bronchodilators also are used. Parathyroid replacement therapy is not the usual treatment because of its associated incidence of allergic reactions. If it is used, drug resistance develops in approximately 2 weeks.

Long-term treatment after trauma to or inadvertent removal of the parathyroids includes administration of oral calcium, vitamin D, or vitamin D_2 (calciferol), which increases the serum calcium level. The dose is related to the degree of hypocalcemia, which is determined by frequent monitoring of serum and urine calcium levels. A diet high in calcium and low in phosphorus usually is recommended.

Nursing Management

The nurse is alert for signs of tetany and assesses for Chvostek's and Trousseau's signs. He or she monitors the client with chronic hypoparathyroidism for increasing severity of symptoms. The nurse is prepared to administer IV calcium salt and observes the client during such administration for adverse effects, such as flushing, cardiac dysrhythmia (usually a bradycardia), tingling in the arms and legs, and a metallic taste. Local tissue necrosis may occur if the IV fluid escapes into surrounding tissues. The nurse monitors serum calcium levels to determine the effectiveness of therapy.

If the client has chronic hypoparathyroidism, the nurse obtains complete medical, drug, and allergy histories. He or she examines the client for symptoms of the disorder, primarily for the effect of hypocalcemia on the CNS. The nurse assesses the arms and legs for evidence of muscle

spasm. He or she auscultates the lungs because the client may have dyspnea or other respiratory difficulty. During assessment of vital signs, attention to heart rate and rhythm is particularly important.

The nurse keeps an emergency tracheostomy tray, mechanical ventilation equipment, artificial airway, and endotracheal intubation equipment at the client's bedside if hypocalcemia is severe. He or she inserts an IV line for the emergency administration of calcium. The nurse observes frequently for respiratory distress and notifies the physician immediately if this problem occurs.

Until hypocalcemia is corrected, the nurse must assist the client with activities of daily living (ADLs). Movement, noise, and other environmental disturbances can trigger muscle contractions or convulsions. Thus, minimizing all forms of stress is essential until serum calcium levels approach normal and symptoms are relieved.

Clients who require lifetime treatment of the disorder need careful review of the prescribed treatment. Because normal calcium levels depend on drug and diet therapy, the nurse must stress the importance of these two aspects of treatment. Consultation with a dietitian may be necessary to provide a list of foods to include or avoid in the prescribed diet. The nurse gives the client a list of the symptoms of hypercalcemia and hypocalcemia, either of which can occur if the dose of the prescribed drug is too high or too low or if the drug is omitted. He or she emphasizes the need to contact the physician immediately about any symptoms. The nurse reminds the client that the physician may need periodically to adjust the dose of the drug; therefore, recognizing the symptoms associated with hypercalcemia and hypocalcemia is essential. For more teaching points, see Client and Family Teaching Box 57-1.

 57-1 *Client and Family Teaching*
Hypoparathyroidism

The nurse develops a teaching plan that includes the following points:

- Take drugs at the doses and intervals prescribed.
- Never increase, decrease, or omit drug doses unless advised by the physician. Increasing the dose can cause symptoms of hypercalcemia; decreasing or omitting the dose can cause the original symptoms to return.
- If nausea, vomiting, or severe diarrhea develops, contact the physician.
- Adherence to the recommended diet is necessary. Read food labels carefully so that you include foods that are part of the diet and avoid those that are not.

DISORDERS OF THE ADRENAL GLANDS

Adrenal dysfunction includes pathology of the outer portion of the adrenal gland, the *cortex,* which synthesizes and secretes the hormones known as *steroids:* mineralocorticoids, glucocorticoids, and androgens or estrogens. Disorders of the adrenal glands also involve the *medulla,* the inner portion, which secretes the catecholamines norepinephrine (noradrenaline) and epinephrine (adrenaline). Proper secretion of these hormones is essential to life.

● ADRENAL INSUFFICIENCY (ADDISON'S DISEASE)

Adrenal insufficiency is classified as either primary or secondary.

Pathophysiology and Etiology

Primary adrenal insufficiency (Addison's disease) results from destruction of the adrenal cortex by diseases such as tuberculosis. It also may be an autoimmune disorder, in which antibodies formed by the client's immune system destroy adrenal tissue. In many instances, the cause is unknown.

The consequences of decreased adrenal cortical function include decreased available glucose and hypoglycemia. The glomerular filtration rate of the kidneys slows dramatically, causing decreased urea nitrogen excretion.

Secondary adrenal insufficiency is the result of surgical removal of both adrenal glands (*bilateral adrenalectomy*), hemorrhagic infarction of the glands, hypopituitarism (caused by pituitary failure or surgical removal of the pituitary), or suppression of adrenal function by the administration of corticosteroids. Clients with secondary adrenal insufficiency after bilateral adrenalectomy or surgical removal of the pituitary gland do not experience true adrenal insufficiency because corticosteroids are administered to replace the hormones no longer secreted by the adrenals.

Assessment Findings

Signs and Symptoms

Decreased or absent adrenocortical hormones lead to symptoms of adrenal insufficiency, which are the same in primary and secondary adrenal insufficiency (Box 57-1). Clients with primary adrenal insufficiency usually experience symptoms gradually. Clients with secondary adrenal insufficiency develop symptoms suddenly or over several days to weeks.

BOX 57-1 ● Signs and Symptoms of Adrenal Insufficiency

- Increased urinary excretion of sodium and retention of potassium followed by dehydration and reduced blood plasma volume
- Weakness, fatigue, dizziness, hypotension, postural hypotension, hypothermia
- Vascular collapse because of poor myocardial tone, decreased cardiac output, weak and irregular pulse
- Weight loss, anemia, anorexia, gastrointestinal symptoms
- Nervousness, periods of depression
- Hypoglycemia from a deficiency of the hormones that facilitate the conversion of protein into glucose; episodes of hypoglycemia may occur 5 to 6 hours after eating—the period before breakfast is especially dangerous
- Abnormally dark pigmentation, especially of exposed areas of the skin and mucous membranes, and decreased hair growth (primary adrenal insufficiency)

Diagnostic Findings

A dose of synthetic ACTH, cosyntropin (Cortrosyn), is administered intramuscularly as a screening test for adrenal function. In primary adrenal insufficiency, an absent or a low cortisol response indicates adrenal insufficiency. In secondary insufficiency, the decrease in serum cortisol levels is less significant.

The serum cortisol level is decreased. Serum sodium and fasting blood glucose levels are low, and serum potassium, calcium, and blood urea nitrogen levels are increased. The WBC count often is elevated. A glucose tolerance test shows evidence of hypoglycemia. In Addison's disease, the glucose level in the bloodstream does not rise as high as normal and returns to its fasting level more quickly than it would under normal conditions. The fasting blood glucose level may be low. Radiographs of the adrenals show calcification. An abdominal CT scan reveals atrophy of the adrenal glands.

Medical Management

Clients with primary adrenal insufficiency require daily corticosteroid replacement therapy for the rest of their lives. Fludrocortisone (Florinef), a synthetic corticosteroid preparation that possesses glucocorticoid and mineralocorticoid properties, frequently is selected for replacement therapy. An additional glucocorticoid can be necessary, depending on the client's response to therapy.

Treatment for secondary adrenal insufficiency caused by bilateral adrenalectomy or pituitary failure is the same as treatment for primary adrenal insufficiency. Treatment of secondary adrenal insufficiency resulting from discontinuation of corticosteroid therapy or hemorrhagic infarction of the gland varies and depends on the ability of the adrenals to return to normal function.

If the client is not given or does not take the medication, acute adrenal crisis can develop (see next section). This also applies to clients on long-term corticosteroid therapy for the treatment of disorders such as allergies, rheumatoid arthritis, and collagen diseases who abruptly discontinue taking their prescribed steroid. If the drug is to be discontinued, the dose must be tapered over time. Client and Family Teaching Box 57-2 discusses important information to teach clients receiving corticosteroid therapy.

NURSING PROCESS

● The Client With Addison's Disease

Assessment

The nurse obtains a complete health history that includes presence or absence of weight loss, salt craving, nausea and vomiting, abdominal cramps, diarrhea, muscle weakness, and decreased stress tolerance. The nurse takes vital signs frequently. Hypoglycemia may be seen in clients with primary adrenal insufficiency. These clients must never receive insulin by error because insulin would lower the blood glucose to a critically low level that could result in brain damage, coma, or death.

Diagnosis, Planning, and Interventions

Nursing management of the client with primary adrenal insufficiency is essentially the same as that of the client with secondary adrenal insufficiency because the major problem in both types is a lack of adrenal cortical hormones. The client with secondary adrenal insufficiency because of surgery (bilateral adrenalectomy, surgical removal of the pituitary) has a controlled deficiency that hormone replacement therapy corrects.

Risk for Deficient Fluid Volume related to inadequate fluid intake, fluid loss secondary to inadequate adrenal hormone secretion

Expected Outcome: Fluid intake will be 1500 to 3000 mL/day.

● Keep careful records of fluid intake and urine output. *Data collection is necessary to determine if a problem is developing.*

● Weigh client daily on the same scale, at a similar time, with similar clothing. *Consistency in data collection helps the nurse accurately compare assessment findings.*

● Notify the physician if dehydration, signs of hyponatremia, or progressive weight loss occurs. *The physician and nurse collaborate to manage a client's problem.*

● Encourage client to drink fluids and eat the prescribed diet to maintain fluid and electrolyte balance. *Fluid and nutritional needs are easier to meet orally than parenterally.*

● If serum sodium levels are decreased, instruct client to add salt to food. If excessive perspiration occurs, increase fluid and salt intake. *Salt is sodium chloride. Sodium is an electrolyte that attracts water and reduces its excretion. Increasing oral fluid intake compensates for unusual loss of body fluid.*

PC: Hypoglycemia

Expected Outcome: The nurse will monitor to detect, manage, and minimize episodes of low blood glucose.

● Minimize any reason for fasting, such as before a diagnostic test. *Eating carbohydrates regularly maintains the blood glucose level.*

● Observe for symptoms of hypoglycemia: hunger, headache, sweating, weakness, trembling, emotional instability, visual disturbances, and, finally, disorientation, and loss of consciousness. *Physiologic and emotional changes accompany a low blood glucose level.*

● Check client's blood glucose level with a glucometer 30 minutes before each meal, at bedtime, and whenever the client is symptomatic. *Checking capillary blood glucose provides a numeric assessment of the blood glucose level.*

● Follow agency protocol for raising blood glucose level, which may include offering the client a glass of grape juice if the level is below 80 mg/dl and rechecking the level in 15 minutes. If the blood glucose level continues to be low, repeat administration of grape juice. *Glucose found in carbohydrate sources like grape juice raises the blood glucose level fairly quickly.*

● Give client milk and graham crackers when the blood glucose level is above 80 mg/dl. *Milk and graham crackers contain forms of carbohydrate that take longer to absorb and tend to maintain the blood glucose level for an extended period.*

● Contact the physician if the client continues to be symptomatic and the blood glucose level is below 80 mg/dl. *Regulation of blood glucose level may require parenteral administration of glucose, which the nurse cannot implement independently.*

● Instruct client to remain in bed. *Dizziness and fainting may accompany the low blood glucose level; maintaining bed rest protects the client from injuries from a fall.*

● Offer five or six small meals per day rather than three regular meals to control hypoglycemic episodes; if client is eating three meals per day, give between-meal snacks of milk and crackers. *Eating carbohydrates frequently and regularly helps stabilize blood glucose levels within a normal range.*

Fatigue related to fluid, electrolyte, and glucose imbalances

Expected Outcome: Client will demonstrate endurance to meet self-care needs independently.

● Assist with bathing and grooming as needed. *The nurse helps the client until the client can resume total self-care.*

● Provide rest between activities. *Rest replenishes energy.*

● Control environmental stimuli to promote rest. *Stimulation interferes with client's ability to relax physically and become refreshed.*

Risk for Injury related to hypotension, muscle weakness
Expected Outcome: Client will experience no injuries or falls.

- Tell client to lie down if he or she becomes dizzy when rising or changing position. *Blood tends to pool temporarily in dependent areas, causing a deficit in the brain when assuming an upright positioning.*
- Take client's BP if symptoms such as weakness and faintness occur. *Measuring BP provides objective data for assessing hemodynamic changes.*
- Keep side rails raised. *They remind the client that he or she should not ambulate independently.*
- Instruct client to ask for assistance getting out of bed. *Assistance can support and reposition the client if syncope develops.*
- Emphasize the importance of getting out of bed slowly. *Moving quickly aggravates symptoms of hypotension and potentiates the risk for fainting and falling.*

Evaluation of Expected Outcomes

Fluid intake approximates output; electrolytes remain within normal limits. The client has sufficient energy for ADLs. No injuries occur.

● ACUTE ADRENAL CRISIS (ADDISONIAN CRISIS)

Clients with either primary or secondary adrenal insufficiency are at risk for **addisonian crisis,** a life-threatening endocrine emergency.

Pathophysiology and Etiology

Acute adrenal crisis occurs when the adrenal glands suddenly fail. Because the hormones of the adrenal cortex are prominent in effecting the body's adaptive reactions to stress, clients with Addison's disease may develop acute adrenal crisis when faced with extreme stress. Even uncomplicated surgery requires more physiologic adaptive ability than a client with Addison's disease usually possesses. Salt deprivation, infection, trauma, exposure to cold, overexertion, or any abnormal stress can cause adrenal crisis. Acute adrenal crisis can occur when corticosteroid therapy is suddenly stopped. If the condition is untreated, coma and death result.

Assessment Findings

Adrenal crisis may be sudden or gradual. It may begin with anorexia, nausea, vomiting, diarrhea, abdominal pain, profound weakness, headache, intensification of hypotension,

57-2 *Client and Family Teaching* Corticosteroid Therapy for Adrenal Insufficiency

The nurse explains adrenal insufficiency and the importance of lifetime corticosteroid replacement. A teaching plan includes the following points:

- Lifetime corticosteroid replacement therapy is necessary. Never omit, increase, or decrease a dose. If the prescribed drug is not taken, adrenal insufficiency, which is life-threatening, will occur.
- The body has limited ability to handle stress of any kind. Seek medical attention for dosage readjustment whenever there is stress. Examples of stress include an infection, a motor vehicle accident (even if not noticeably hurt), a family crisis, and a heavy work load.
- Avoid exposure to infections and excessive fatigue.
- If an infection (e.g., sore throat, upper respiratory tract infection) or other type of illness occurs, contact the physician immediately. An increased medication dose may be necessary.
- Vomiting, diarrhea, or any other condition that prevents the medication from being taken orally or interferes with proper drug absorption requires immediate medical attention. Parenteral administration will be necessary. (The physician instructs the client on the procedures to follow if the medication cannot be taken orally.)
- Wear identification, such as a Medic Alert tag or bracelet, stating that the wearer has adrenal insufficiency. If an accident or other problem occurs, medical personnel must be made aware of the need for corticosteroids.
- Follow the diet recommended by the physician.

restlessness, or fever. Unless the corticosteroid dose is increased to meet the demand, the client progresses to acute adrenal crisis. The BP markedly decreases, and shock develops.

Diagnosis is based on symptoms and history. Case finding can show an omission of daily corticosteroid therapy. (See section on Diagnostic Findings for adrenal insufficiency.)

Medical Management

Adrenal crisis is an emergency; death may occur from hypotension and vasomotor collapse. Corticosteroids are given IV in solutions of normal saline and glucose. Antibiotics are administered because of an extremely low resistance to infection.

Nursing Management

Two important nursing tasks are the recognition of signs and symptoms of adrenal crisis and the accurate administration of corticosteroid drugs. A client with a diagnosis of adrenal insufficiency is a candidate for acute adrenal crisis; therefore, the nurse constantly observes such clients for this problem. He or she administers the correct dose of corticosteroid therapy at the correct time. Doses must never be omitted or abruptly discontinued because this can result in adrenal crisis. Once the condition is recognized, the nurse takes vital signs frequently, paying special attention to heart rate and rhythm. He or she observes for signs of hyponatremia and hyperkalemia. The nurse keeps the client warm and as quiet as possible until treatment is instituted and the condition is stabilized.

● PHEOCHROMOCYTOMA

Pheochromocytoma is a tumor of the adrenal medulla that causes hyperfunction.

Pathophysiology and Etiology

A pheochromocytoma usually is a benign tumor. Hyperfunction causes the adrenal gland excessively to secrete the catecholamines epinephrine and norepinephrine. Exercise, emotional distress, trauma such as surgery, manipulation of the tumor, and postural changes can trigger episodes. Excessive secretion of epinephrine leads to hypertension and increases the potential for cerebrovascular accident, palpitations, and tachycardia.

Assessment Findings

Symptoms include elevated BP (intermittent or, more frequently, persistent), tremors, nervousness, sweating, headache, nausea, vomiting, hyperglycemia, polyuria, and vertigo. The level of vanillylmandelic acid in a 24-hour urine specimen is markedly increased. Urinary catecholamine determination on the same or a different specimen may be elevated. CT, MRI, ultrasonography, aortography, and retrograde pyelography reveal the tumor. A drop in BP after phentolamine (Regitine) injection supports the presence of a pheochromocytoma.

Medical and Surgical Management

Treatment involves surgical removal of the tumor by means of *unilateral adrenalectomy* (removal of one adrenal gland). Phentolamine is given before and during surgery to control hypertension. Alpha-adrenergic blockers, such as phenoxybenzamine (Dibenzyline), are used to control hypertension before surgery or when surgery is contraindicated, or to treat a malignant pheochromocytoma. Medical treatment includes metyrosine (Demser), an enzyme inhibitor that reduces synthesis of catecholamines to decrease hypertensive attacks.

Nursing Management

The nurse monitors the BP closely when initiating drug therapy or during dose changes. He or she notifies the physician of a sudden decrease in BP. If the client undergoes adrenalectomy, the nurse assesses for signs and symptoms of acute adrenal insufficiency (see earlier discussion).

● CUSHING'S SYNDROME (ADRENOCORTICAL HYPERFUNCTION)

Cushing's syndrome is an endocrine disorder that results from excessive secretion of hormones by the adrenal cortex.

Pathophysiology and Etiology

An overproduction of adrenocortical hormones results from (1) overproduction of ACTH by the pituitary gland, with resultant hyperplasia of the adrenal cortex and excessive production and secretion of glucocorticoids, mineralocorticoids, and androgens; (2) benign or malignant tumors of the pituitary gland or adrenal cortex; or (3) prolonged administration of high doses of corticosteroids. Those clients who take corticosteroids are advised to remain compliant and avoid discontinuing their self-administration abruptly to avoid addisonian or adrenal crisis. When these types of medications are no longer necessary, they are discontinued gradually (see section on Adrenalectomy later in this chapter).

Hyperadrenalism affects most body systems and causes many changes in appearance and physiology. The term **cushingoid syndrome** refers to the physical changes that accompany this disorder (Fig. 57-6). Examples of physiologic alterations include suppression of the inflammatory response, hyperglycemia, hypokalemia, hypernatremia with subsequent weight gain and elevated BP, peptic ulcer, demineralization of bones, and muscle weakness. Increased levels of androgenic hormone cause women to acquire male secondary sex characteristics. Both sexes experience decreased sexual drive. Many suffer from depression, and the endocrine imbalance may cause psychosis.

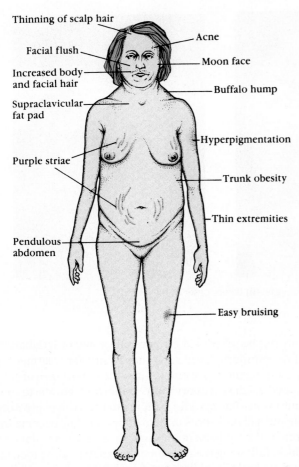

Thinning of scalp hair

Facial flush

Increased body and facial hair

Supraclavicular fat pad

Purple striae

Pendulous abdomen

Acne

Moon face

Buffalo hump

Hyperpigmentation

Trunk obesity

Thin extremities

Easy bruising

FIGURE 57-6 The symptoms of Cushing's disease. (From Beyers, M. & Dudas, S. [Eds.]. [1984]. *The clinical practice of medical surgical nursing* [p. 71]. Boston: Little, Brown.)

Assessment Findings

Signs and Symptoms

Physical examination reveals muscle wasting and weakness resulting from extensive protein depletion. Carbohydrate tolerance is lowered, and signs and symptoms of diabetes mellitus develop (see Chap. 58). Fat is redistributed, leading to facial fullness and the characteristic moon face and buffalo hump. The skin is thin, and the face is ruddy. The client has increased susceptibility to wounds, and healing is prolonged; however, the immunosuppressive effects of the disorder usually mask symptoms of infection.

Because the blood vessels are fragile, the client bruises easily, and striae often form over extensive skin areas. The bones become so demineralized that the client may have backache, kyphosis, and collapse of the vertebrae. He or she retains sodium and water, and peripheral edema and hypertension develop. The client reports mood changes and difficulty coping with stressors that were manageable in the past. The family may report serious

mental changes. In women, Cushing's syndrome produces masculinization with hirsutism and amenorrhea. These sexual changes and alterations in appearance are reversible when adrenocortical hormone levels return to normal (Fig. 56-7).

Diagnostic Findings

Diagnosis is tentatively based on the physical changes. Urine levels of 17-hydroxycorticosteroids (17-OHCS) and 17-ketosteroids (17-KS) almost always are increased. Plasma and urine cortisol levels are elevated. An overnight dexamethasone suppression test is used as an initial screening. The client takes 1 mg oral dexamethasone; the next morning plasma cortisol levels are obtained. If these results are above normal (5 mg/dl), 0.5 mg dexamethasone is given every 6 hours, and 24-hour urine collections are tested for 2 consecutive days. Clients without the disorder will have decreased 17-OHCS and 17-KS levels; these levels remain elevated in those with Cushing's syndrome.

To determine whether the symptoms of Cushing's syndrome are the result of pituitary stimulation, plasma ACTH is measured in conjunction with the administration of dexamethasone. If ACTH levels subsequently are found to be low or normal and the cortisol level is elevated, it suggests that the adrenal gland alone is hyperfunctioning. If both the ACTH and cortisol levels are elevated, a pituitary or hypothalamic etiology is more likely.

Laboratory blood test results also reveal increased serum sodium, decreased serum potassium, and increased blood glucose levels. Abdominal radiographs, CT scan, or MRI may show adrenal enlargement, and an IV pyelogram may show changes in the renal shadow caused by an abnormally large adrenal gland.

Medical and Surgical Management

Treatment depends on whether a tumor or adrenal hyperplasia causes the disorder. It is directed toward removing the cause and lowering plasma cortisol levels. Radiation therapy to or removal of the pituitary may be used for adrenal hyperplasia. Bilateral adrenalectomy may be preferred if both adrenals are involved.

Drug therapy includes diuretics for edema as well as an antihypertensive agent. A diet low in sodium and carbohydrates controls edema and blood glucose level. Antibiotics are used to treat infection.

If cushingoid syndrome results from exogenous administration of a corticosteroid preparation, the drug is slowly withdrawn by tapering the dose over days or weeks. In some instances, as in the treatment of a disorder such as leukemia, or to prevent rejection of transplanted organs, the syndrome is allowed to persist.

FIGURE 57-7 Progressive facial changes in a woman with Cushing's disease: (**A**) before onset of the illness, (**B**) preoperative, and (**C**) 1 year after surgery.

NURSING   PROCESS

● **The Client With Cushing's Syndrome**

Assessment

The nurse obtains thorough medical, drug, and allergy histories and observes for symptoms of an adrenal disorder: altered skin pigmentation and integrity, decreased energy level, mental changes, sexual dysfunction, and changes in mood, appetite, weight, and bowel patterns. He or she monitors vital signs every 4 hours and tests the blood or urine (or both) for glucose three or four times per day. If the urine tests positive for glucose or the blood glucose level is elevated, the nurse reports the information to the physician.

Because the client is at risk for the development of peptic ulcers, the nurse observes the color of each stool and tests the stool for occult blood. If the client reports epigastric pain or discomfort or the stool has a black appearance or tests positive for blood, the nurse makes the physician aware of the assessment findings.

Diagnosis, Planning, and Interventions

If corticosteroid therapy has caused a cushingoid appearance and the dose is to be tapered over time, the nurse gives the client and family a detailed explanation of the tapering schedule. He or she reviews the directions printed on the prescription container and emphasizes the importance of strictly following the tapering schedule. The client may find it helpful to use a calendar to enter the dosage for each day of the tapering schedule. The nurse can write the entire tapering schedule on a card and instruct the client to cross off each day.

Depending on many factors, such as age and severity of the disorder, clients with Cushing's syndrome may or may not be scheduled for adrenalectomy or irradiation of the pituitary. Until such time as further treatment is scheduled, the nurse emphasizes the importance of continued medical supervision. Important points to emphasize include avoiding trauma to the skin; contacting the physician if sores or cuts do not heal or become infected, if easy bruising occurs, or if stools are dark or black; following the recommended diet; reading food labels carefully; avoiding exposure to infection; avoiding nonprescription drugs (unless approved by the physician); weighing self weekly; and reporting marked weight gain or edema to the physician.

Diagnoses, expected outcomes, and interventions include, but are not limited to, the following.

Excess Fluid Volume related to sodium and water retention

Expected Outcome: Fluid volume will be normal as evidenced by equivalent fluid intake and output volumes, reduced or no dependent edema, consistent daily weights, and BP measurements within normal limits.

- Examine extremities for increased or decreased edema. *Fluid retention is manifested by swelling in dependent areas, pitting when pressure is applied to the skin over a bone, tight-fitting shoes or rings, the appearance of lines in the skin from stockings, and seams in the shoes or areas where they lace.*

- Measure intake and output daily, weekly, or as ordered. *Acutely ill clients require more frequent assessment. A gain of 2 lb in 24 hours suggests 1 L of water retention.*

- Assess vital signs each shift; report systolic BP that exceeds 139 mm Hg or diastolic BP that exceeds 89 mm Hg. *Hypertension is defined as a consistently elevated BP above 139/89 mm Hg (see Chap. 35). One factor that contributes to hypertension is excess circulatory volume.*

- Administer prescribed diuretics. *They promote the excretion of sodium and water.*

● Provide a sodium-restricted diet at the level prescribed by the physician. *Limiting sodium reduces the potential for fluid retention.*

Risk for Impaired Skin Integrity related to thinning of skin and edema

Expected Outcome: Skin will remain intact.

● Inspect the skin daily, especially over bony prominences, for open lesions or ulcers. *The skin is thin and fragile and prone to breaking down with minimal trauma.*

● Encourage client to change positions frequently. *Relieving pressure on capillaries helps maintain a supply of oxygenated blood to cells and tissues. Cells deprived of oxygenated blood are prone to cellular death.*

● Handle client gently; use interventions that relieve pressure on the skin. *Gentleness reduces the potential for skin abrasions, and interventions that cushion the weight and force of gravity against body surfaces help prevent the development of pressure ulcers.*

● Exercise care when performing tasks that may damage the skin, such as removing tape when discontinuing an IV infusion. *The skin's fragility increases its potential for injury.*

Fatigue related to muscle wasting and protein depletion

Expected Outcome: Client will demonstrate energy to complete ADLs.

● Provide frequent rest periods between activities. *Rest restores energy and improves endurance.*

● Assist client with activities when muscle wasting or pain secondary to osteoporosis is severe. *The nurse relieves client of responsibilities until the client can safely and comfortably manage self-care.*

Risk for Infection related to suppressed inflammatory response and immune function

Expected Outcome: Client will be free from infection.

● Observe for signs and symptoms that indicate infection: a skin injury that does not heal, increased temperature, sore throat, or cough. *Signs of infection or inflammation are less dramatic in these clients than in others. What may appear to be a minor problem could be masking a more serious problem.*

● Make every effort to prevent exposing the client to infectious microorganisms. *Microorganisms are spread by direct and indirect contact. A client with suppressed defenses is more likely to succumb to an infection.*

● Immediately notify the physician if an infection is suspected. *The nurse collaborates with the physician on medical interventions.*

Risk for Injury related to demineralization of bones

Expected Outcome: Client will be safe from injury such as bone fracture.

● Protect client from falls by applying supportive slippers and keeping the environment free of clutter and water spills. *The force of a fall is more likely to cause a fracture when the bones are porous. Environmental safety reduces the potential for injury.*

● Use side rails and instruct client to seek assistance when getting out of bed. *Assistance reduces the incidence and consequences of a fall.*

Risk for Self-directed Violence related to mood changes and depression

Expected Outcome: Client's mood will stabilize with no depressive symptoms.

● Assess mental status, including suicidal ideation, regularly. *A depressed client is likely to appear sad, be tearful, have difficulty sleeping or sleep more than expected, neglect hygiene, have a poor appetite and reduced energy, and lack interest in the future. Clients who entertain thoughts of suicide usually admit to their despair when openly questioned.*

● Explain that a depressed mood is a common symptom of the disorder or side effect of corticosteroid therapy. *Depressed clients may blame themselves for their inability to cope with stressors. Providing information as to the cause of the depressed mood may help the client to persevere with the treatment regimen.*

● Maintain safety by removing items that could be used for suicide, checking on client frequently, transferring client to a room close to the nursing station, and offering to stay with the client when he or she is feeling self-destructive. *Eliminating the opportunity or methods by which the client can harm himself or herself may prevent a suicide attempt.*

● Collaborate with the physician about a referral to a mental health practitioner or agency. *Counseling, drug therapy, and psychotherapy after discharge provide long-term measures for keeping a client safe from self-harm.*

Disturbed Body Image related to changes in appearance

Expected Outcome: Client will express a positive self-image.

● Provide client opportunities to express feelings over physical changes. *Verbalizing feelings with a supportive person increases the client's ability to cope with stress.*

● Explain that when the cause of the disorder is eliminated, some physical changes gradually improve, but others, such as striae and kyphosis, are permanent. *Being honest and sharing accurate information promotes the client's trust and confidence.*

● Offer suggestions such as wearing loose clothing, a hat, or cap, to help disguise physical changes that the client finds difficult to tolerate. *Although the client's perception of physical changes probably is more exaggerated than others', he or she may feel more confident in social situations with techniques that minimize changes in appearance.*

Evaluation of Expected Outcomes

Fluid volume is normal, with no evidence of edema, hypertension, or weight gain. The client meets self-care needs without fatigue. Temperature and WBC count are within normal limits. Skin is intact. The client is free from injury, such as pathologic fractures. He or she demonstrates normal range of moods and denies suicidal ideation. The client copes effectively with physical changes.

● HYPERALDOSTERONISM

The secretion of aldosterone, a mineralocorticoid, is regulated by serum levels of potassium and sodium, the renin–angiotensin mechanism, and ACTH. The hypersecretion of aldosterone creates extreme electrolyte imbalances.

Pathophysiology and Etiology

The cause of primary hyperaldosteronism may be a benign aldosterone-secreting adenoma of one of the adrenals, an adrenal malignant tumor, or unknown. Pregnancy, congestive heart failure, narrowing of the renal artery, and cirrhosis can cause secondary hyperaldosteronism.

Excessive secretion of aldosterone results in increased reabsorption of sodium and water and excretion of potassium by the kidneys. Figure 57-8 presents an overview of the renin–angiotensin–aldosterone cycle.

Assessment Findings

Headache, muscle weakness, increased urine output, fatigue, hypertension, and cardiac dysrhythmias are seen. Serum potassium levels are decreased and serum sodium levels are increased in the absence of other causes, such as diuretic therapy or diarrhea. The serum bicarbonate, serum aldosterone, and plasma renin levels are increased. CT or MRI may rule out or locate an adrenal tumor. Adrenal venography may identify small tumors that CT scanning fails to reveal.

Medical and Surgical Management

If the cause is an adrenal tumor, unilateral adrenalectomy may be performed. Medical management may include administration of spironolactone, a potassium-sparing diuretic, and an antihypertensive agent to control BP. A sodium-restricted diet may be necessary.

Nursing Management

The nurse monitors vital signs every 4 hours or as ordered. He or she reports marked elevations to the physician. The nurse measures fluid intake and output and weighs the client every 2 to 7 days. Daily examination of the extremities for edema is essential. The nurse observes for signs of hypokalemia and hypernatremia (see Chap. 22).

● ADRENALECTOMY

Adrenalectomy is surgical removal of the adrenal gland(s), usually to remove a cancerous tumor. In some instances, removal of the ovaries, testes, and both adrenal glands (which secrete male and female hormones), is considered to control cancers of the breast and prostate, which depend on hormones for growth.

The adrenals are surgically approached by means of an abdominal incision or a flank incision under and following the position of the 12th rib. The abdominal incision usually is long because adequate exposure is needed to access the adrenals, which lie posteriorly. The flank incision is the same surgical approach used for kidney surgery.

Nursing Management

Preoperative Period

Major goals include reduced anxiety and an understanding of preparations for surgery and possible postoperative events. The nurse keeps the client on bed rest and minimizes anxiety. The client who requires surgery to halt progression of a metastatic disease may be anxious as well as depressed and needs time to discuss the surgery and anticipated results. If the client has a pheochromocytoma, the nurse monitors BP frequently before surgery. When bilateral adrenalectomy is scheduled, the nurse may start IV administration of a solution containing a corticosteroid

FIGURE 57-8 The renin–angiotensin–aldosterone cycle.

preparation the morning of surgery. Some surgeons prefer to initiate corticosteroid administration during removal of the adrenals. Additional preparations are the same as for the client having general surgery (see Chap. 25).

Postoperative Period

When the client returns from surgery, the nurse reviews the surgical record because postoperative observations and management depend on whether one or both adrenal glands were removed. In addition to the complications associated with general anesthesia, the nurse observes for such problems as hemorrhage, atelectasis, and pneumothorax because the adrenals are located close to the diaphragm and inferior vena cava. He or she monitors vital signs frequently and closely observes for signs of adrenal insufficiency (addisonian crisis, adrenal crisis), which may occur when:

- The prescribed dose of a corticosteroid preparation is inadequate to meet the client's needs (bilateral adrenalectomy).
- The remaining adrenal gland does not produce sufficient hormone to meet the client's needs (unilateral adrenalectomy).
- The prescribed dose of a corticosteroid preparation is not given.

If symptoms of adrenal insufficiency occur, the nurse notifies the physician immediately. He or she should never omit administering a prescribed corticosteroid because corticosteroid replacement is essential to life. Acute adrenal insufficiency is managed with infusions of IV solutions, glucose, and cortisol. Client and Family Teaching Box 57-3 provides detailed instructions for postdischarge management of the client who has undergone bilateral adrenalectomy.

N U R S I N G   P R O C E S S

● The Client Undergoing an Adrenalectomy

Assessment

The nurse checks vital signs as soon as the client returns to the unit to establish a database. He or she conducts other routine postoperative assessments, such as examining the dressing over the incision and the patency and characteristics of fluid from incisional drains, noting LOC, checking infusion of IV fluids, auscultating the lungs and abdomen, checking breathing, identifying level of pain, measuring intake and output, and checking whether the client is performing leg exercises. The nurse closely observes for acute adrenal crisis evidenced by hypotension and shock, nausea, vomiting, dehydration, muscle weakness, and hypoglycemia. He or she monitors blood studies

for electrolyte imbalances and assesses closely for any signs of infection. Throughout the postoperative period, the nurse continues to monitor pulse, BP, temperature, breath sounds, blood glucose levels, and urinary output.

Diagnosis, Planning, and Interventions

Pain related to tissue trauma
Expected Outcome: Pain will be eliminated or reduced to a tolerable level within 30 minutes of a nursing intervention.

- Assess pain whenever assessing vital signs. *Pain assessment is the fifth vital sign; assess pain whenever you take vital signs and more often if indicated.*
- Give an analgesic promptly before pain increases. *Giving an analgesic before pain becomes intolerable more easily relieves and controls pain.*
- Assess and note client's response to the analgesic. *The nurse is obligated to manage the client's pain; the client may require additional measures if the analgesic is ineffective.*
- Offer comfort measures such as massage, skin care, and emotional support. *Nonpharmacologic approaches complement and supplement pain-relieving medications.*

Ineffective Airway Clearance related to inadequate coughing secondary to incisional pain
Expected Outcome: The airway will be clear as evidenced by normal breath sounds and respiratory rate and effort.

- Support the incision firmly when turning or changing client's position. *Movement of the skin and tissue underlying the incision stimulates nociceptors that transmit pain impulses to the CNS. Limiting pain facilitates movement, circulation, and breathing.*
- Apply firm support over the incision when the client deep breathes and coughs. *Pressing on the incision with a pillow or folded bath blanket promotes fuller lung expansion and more effort when coughing, both of which help to maintain a patent airway.*
- Change client's position every 2 hours. *Movement helps prevent stasis of respiratory secretions.*
- Encourage deep breathing and coughing every 2 hours. *Deep breathing and coughing open and clear respiratory passages.*
- Encourage adequate (2000 mL) intake of oral fluids. *When oral fluids are absorbed, they contribute to the volume in all fluid compartments. Adequate oral intake thins mucus.*
- Consult with physician about the need for suctioning or aerosolized respiratory treatments if the lungs sound congested or sputum is thick and difficult to raise. *Suctioning is a mechanical means to remove retained secretions; it is useful if the client's natural cough is ineffective. Respiratory treatments provide medications that dilate the bronchi and thin mucoid secretions so they are more easily expelled.*

Risk for Infection related to decreased cortisol secretion or immunosuppression secondary to steroid therapy replacement

Expected Outcome: The wound is clean and dry, with no signs of infection.

- Observe strict aseptic technique for all procedures, such as changing the dressing on the surgical wound. *Medical asepsis reduces microorganisms; surgical asepsis uses techniques in which microorganisms are absent or destroyed before contact with a susceptible host.*
- Notify the physician if vital signs change, purulent drainage is on the dressing, or analgesics do not control pain. *The nurse reports findings that may require medical interventions.*
- Inspect the wound during each dressing change. Notify the physician about excessive redness, swelling of the suture line, or purulent drainage. *Impaired skin from an incision increases the potential for infection. Nurses must report abnormal wound characteristics immediately.*

Risk for Injury related to postural hypotension and weakness secondary to adrenal insufficiency

Expected Outcome: Client will be free from injury.

- Assist with ambulatory activities and observe for weakness and dizziness. *Until client's condition is stable and BP is normal, he or she requires assistance.*
- Notify the physician of continued hypotension or weakness. *Persistent symptoms may represent an impending adrenal crisis, which requires more definitive medical treatment.*

Evaluation of Expected Outcomes

Client reports pain relief and improved comfort. Lungs are clear to auscultation; client coughs and breathes effectively. There is no evidence of infection. Safety is maintained; the client is injury free.

57-3 *Client and Family Teaching*
Discharge Instructions After Adrenalectomy

The nurse teaches the client about the:

- Function of the adrenal glands and importance of adhering to the prescribed treatment regimen
- Care of the surgical wound until healed
- Medication schedule
- Need for obtaining adequate rest, eating a well-balanced diet, complying with ongoing medical supervision, avoiding infections and stressful situations, carrying identification indicating surgical removal of the adrenal glands, and seeking immediate medical help if unable to take the prescribed corticosteroid drug or if symptoms of adrenal insufficiency and adrenal crisis develop

---

DISORDERS OF THE OVARIES AND TESTES

Disorders associated with the female and male reproductive systems are covered in Chapters 59 and 61, respectively.

GENERAL NUTRITIONAL CONSIDERATIONS

Clients with hyperthyroidism may need 4500 to 5000 calories/day or more to maintain normal weight. A liberal protein intake of 100 g or more, combined with a liberal carbohydrate intake, is recommended. Clients experiencing steady weight loss despite eating large amounts of food often are frustrated and discouraged. Encourage frequent meals and the intake of nutritionally dense foods (fortified milkshakes, foods fortified with skim milk powder, eggs, cheese, butter, or milk).

Until normal metabolism is restored, clients with myxedema experience weight gain even if calorie intake is low. After hormone replacement therapy begins, the client may still need to follow a low-calorie diet to attain or maintain normal weight. A high-fiber intake helps alleviate constipation and promotes satiety. Additional diet modifications, such as low fat, low cholesterol, and low sodium, are necessary if the client has cardiovascular complications.

Clients with hyperparathyroidism should drink at least 3 to 4 L of fluid daily to dilute the urine and prevent renal stones from forming. It is especially important that the client drink fluids before going to bed and periodically throughout the night to avoid concentrated urine.

In addition to calcium and vitamin D supplements, clients with hypoparathyroidism may be prescribed a high-calcium, low-phosphorus diet, even though the diet is difficult to achieve because milk and milk products (the richest sources of calcium) also are high in phosphorus. Clients with Addison's disease who are treated with cortisone may require a high sodium intake (at least 4 to 6 g/day). A high sodium intake is contraindicated in clients receiving fludrocortisone (Florinef) because it is a sodium-retaining hormone. Potassium requirements are determined on an individual basis. Frequent meals, including a large bedtime snack, that are high in protein and moderate in carbohydrates are recommended to avoid hypoglycemia. Concentrated sugars are restricted.

GENERAL PHARMACOLOGIC CONSIDERATIONS

Substances that contain iodine, such as some cough medicines and dyes administered for radiographs of the gallbladder, IV pyelograms, and bronchograms, can interfere with the results of some thyroid tests.

The most serious adverse effect of antithyroid drugs is agranulocytosis, which occurs most often in the first 2 months of therapy and necessitates discontinuing the drug. Instruct the client to report sore throat, fever, chills, headache, malaise, weakness, or unusual bleeding or bruising.

Antithyroid drugs are administered every 8 hours around the clock, unless directed otherwise by the physician.

During initial therapy with a thyroid replacement, the most common adverse reaction is signs of hyperthyroidism (which would indicate drug overdosage). Other adverse reactions are rare.

The dosage of thyroid replacement medication may need to be decreased or increased over time until the optimal dose is attained. A full therapeutic response to thyroid hormone replacement therapy may not be evident until the client has concluded several weeks of therapy. Early effects may be observed within 48 hours of the initial dose.

Florinef is a mineralocorticoid with some glucocorticoid activity. It commonly is prescribed after a bilateral adrenalectomy and for the management of adrenocortical insufficiency. The more common adverse reactions to Florinef include frontal and occipital headache, arthralgia, edema, and hypertension. Dosage increases may be necessary during stressful periods to prevent drug-induced adrenal insufficiency.

GENERAL GERONTOLOGIC CONSIDERATIONS

Changes in hormone levels may accompany aging. Although levels of T_4 tend to remain constant, levels of T_3 may decrease with age. Parathyroid hormone levels tend to increase with age. Older adults have an increased incidence of nodules and small goiters on the thyroid gland.

The symptoms of thyroid disease in older adults often are atypical or minor and easily attributed to other problems. For example, the older adult may not experience restlessness or hyperactivity and may not appear nervous. Symptoms seen most often in older adults include anorexia, weight loss, palpitations, angina, and atrial fibrillation. The most reliable thyroid function test to diagnose hyperthyroidism in an older adult is a serum T_4 level.

Hypothyroidism is difficult to identify in older adults because symptoms closely resemble normal aging—for example, anorexia, constipation, weight loss, muscular weakness and pain, joint stiffness, apathy, and depression.

Dosages of thyroid replacement drugs are lower in older adults, and drug therapy is initiated slowly and increased cautiously. The older adult receiving thyroid replacement therapy is at increased risk for adverse reactions associated with cardiac function.

Critical Thinking Exercises

1. *When caring for a client receiving fludrocortisone (Florinef) orally after bilateral adrenalectomy, nurses have a team conference to review the client's potential for acute adrenal insufficiency. What information is appropriate to discuss?*
2. *A client had a thyroidectomy this morning. It is now 8:00 PM, and she complains of difficulty swallowing clear liquids and a fullness in her throat. Her BP is normal, but her pulse rate is elevated. You see no drainage on the surface of her dressing. What actions would you take at this time?*

References and Suggested Readings

A quick check of the endocrine system. (2000). *Nursing, 30*(8), Critical Care, 32cc10–32cc11.

Carr, S. (2001). Acromegaly management in the community. *Nursing Times, 97*(2), 32–33.

Clayton, L. H. & Dilley, K. B. (1998). Cushing's syndrome. *American Journal of Nursing, 98*(7), 40–41.

Clement, B. (1998). Parathyroid physiology. *Seminars in Perioperative Nursing, 7,* 186–192.

Coskeran, P. (1999). Management and treatment of patients with acromegaly. *Nursing Times, 95*(13), 50–52.

Eisenberg, A. A. & Redick, E. L. (1999). Caring for a patient after resection of pituitary adenoma. *Nursing, 29*(12), Critical Care, 32cc1–32cc2, 32cc4–32cc6.

Ezzone, S. A. (1999). Clinical focus: SIADH. *Clinical Journal of Oncology Nursing, 3*(4), 187–188.

Heater, D. W. (1999). If ADH goes out of balance: Diabetes insipidus. *RN, 62*(7), 44–46, 50.

Incredibly easy! Understanding goiter. (2001). *Nursing, 31* (8), 78.

Johnson, D. (1998). Review of endocrine physiology. *Seminars in Perioperative Nursing, 7,* 142–151.

Jordan, S. & White, J. (1998). The immune system: Hyperthyroidism. *Nursing Times, 94*(24), 48–51.

Kaye, J., Morton, J., Bowcutt, M., et al. (2000). Stress, depression, and psychoneuroimmunology. *Journal of Neuroscience Nursing, 32*(2), 93–100.

Levin, N. A. & Greer, K. E. (2001). Cutaneous manifestations of endocrine disorders. *Dermatology Nursing, 13,* 185–186, 189–196, 201–202.

Nayback, A. M. (2000). Hyponatremia as a consequence of acute adrenal insufficiency and hypothyroidism. *Journal of Emergency Nursing, 26,* 130–133.

Nickolaus, M. J. (1999). Diabetes insipidus: A current perspective. *Critical Care Nurse, 19*(6), 18–30.

Sabol, V. K. (2001). Addisonian crisis: This life-threatening condition may be triggered by a variety of stressors. *American Journal of Nursing, 101*(7), Advanced Practice Extra, 24AAA, 24CCC–24DDD.

Terpstra, T. L. & Terpstra, T. L. (2000). Syndrome of inappropriate antidiuretic hormone secretion: Recognition and management. *MEDSURG Nursing, 9*(2), 61–70.

Williams, M. (1998). Disorders of the adrenal gland. *Seminars in Perioperative Nursing, 7,* 179–185.

Caring for Clients With Diabetes Mellitus

Words to Know

diabetes mellitus	ketones
diabetic ketoacidosis	Kussmaul respirations
diabetic nephropathy	lipoatrophy
diabetic retinopathy	lipohypertrophy
fasting blood glucose	lipolysis
glycosuria	metabolic syndrome
glycosylated hemoglobin	oral glucose tolerance
hyperglycemia	test
hyperosmolar hyper-	polydipsia
glycemic nonketotic	polyphagia
syndrome	polyuria
hypoglycemia	postprandial glucose
insulin independence	random blood glucose
ketoacidosis	renal threshold
ketonemia	

Learning Objectives

On completion of this chapter, the reader will:

- Define and distinguish the two types of diabetes mellitus.
- Identify the three classic symptoms of diabetes mellitus.
- Explain the source of ketones.
- Name three laboratory methods used to diagnose diabetes mellitus.
- Describe the methods used to treat diabetes mellitus.
- Explain the cause of diabetic ketoacidosis.
- List three main goals in the treatment of diabetic ketoacidosis.
- Identify two physiologic signs of hyperosmolar hyperglycemic nonketotic syndrome.
- Describe the treatment of hyperosmolar hyperglycemia nonketotic syndrome.
- Explain the cause and treatment of hypoglycemia.
- List common complications of diabetes mellitus.
- Differentiate between the symptoms of hypoglycemia and hyperglycemia.
- Discuss the nursing management of the client with diabetes mellitus.

Diabetes mellitus, a metabolic disorder of the pancreas, affects carbohydrate, fat, and protein metabolism. This disease is reaching epidemic proportions in the United States. Some believe that diabetes in adults is one consequence of **metabolic syndrome,** which includes obesity, especially in the abdominal area; high blood pressure (BP); elevated triglyceride, low-density lipoprotein, and blood glucose levels; and a low high-density lipoprotein level (see Chap. 33).

Although no age group is exempt from diabetes, the American Diabetes Association (2002) indicates that 90% to 95% of affected persons acquire the disease as adults. Current estimates are that 16,000,000 people in the United States have diabetes, with one third being undiagnosed (Insulin-Free World Foundation, 2000). Incidence is increased among African Americans, Latinos, Native Americans, and Asian Americans (including Pacific Islanders). The World Health Organization predicts that, as a result of longer life expectancies, diabetes will affect 300,000,000 people worldwide by 2025. At present, diabetes is the seventh leading cause of death in the United

States. Because of the chronic nature of diabetes, affected persons experience many debilitating and life-threatening complications before death. Research is providing exciting discoveries, however, that may eventually cure at least one form of this disease.

DIABETES MELLITUS

The Expert Committee on the Diagnosis and Classification of Diabetes Mellitus (1997) has identified and described the two major forms of diabetes mellitus:

- Type 1—insulin-dependent diabetes mellitus (IDDM), also referred to as *juvenile diabetes* because it affects children and adolescents, is characterized by no insulin production by the beta cells in the islets of Langerhans of the pancreas (Fig. 58-1).
- Type 2—non–insulin-dependent diabetes mellitus (NIDDM) is characterized by insulin resistance or insufficient insulin production. Although NIDDM

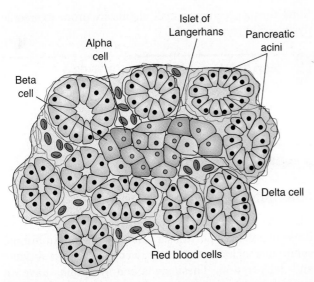

Alpha cell

Islet of Langerhans

Pancreatic acini

Beta cell

Delta cell

Red blood cells

FIGURE 58-1 Islet of Langerhans in the pancreas. (Guyton, A. C. & Hall, J. E. [1996]. *Textbook of medical physiology* [9th ed.]. Philadelphia: W.B. Saunders.)

is more common in aging adults (half of affected clients are older than 55 years), type 2 diabetes also is being detected in obese children.

Hyperglycemia, an elevated blood glucose level, is associated with other disorders or their management. For example, pancreatitis (see Chap. 55) causes both exocrine and endocrine disturbances. When production of adrenocortical hormones is excessive, as in Cushing's syndrome (see Chap. 57), or with the administration of glucocorticoid drugs for immunosuppressive purposes, secondary diabetes develops. Impaired glucose metabolism and hyperglycemia also are associated with drugs like loop and thiazide diuretics, levodopa, and oral contraceptives, and with the administration of total parenteral nutrition. A normal blood glucose level is restored once these diabetogenic regimens are discontinued.

Pathophysiology and Etiology

Type 1 Diabetes Mellitus

Insulin has three functions: (1) it carries glucose into body cells as their preferred source of energy, (2) it promotes the storage of glucose as glycogen, and (3) it inhibits the breakdown of glycogen back into glucose. In type 1 diabetes, the islet cells, or endocrine portion of the pancreas, cease to produce insulin. Without insulin, the blood glucose level rises beyond its normal range, and the body breaks down fat and protein as alternative sources of cellular energy (Porth, 2002). The breakdown of fat, known as **lipolysis,** results in the accumulation of fatty acids and **ketones,** metabolic byproducts of fat metabolism. When ketones accumulate in the blood, clients with diabetes are prone to developing a form of metabolic

acidosis known as **ketoacidosis.** In type 1 diabetes, keto-acidosis develops quite suddenly because of the total cessation of insulin production.

Type 1 diabetes is considered an autoimmune disorder. As reported by several sources, such as the *New York Times* on January 15, 2002 (Kolata, 2002), Dr. Denise Faustman and her colleagues at Massachusetts General Hospital have shown that a genetic mutation causes killer (CD8) T-cell lymphocytes to attack and destroy the insulin-producing islet cells. The hypothesis is that the B-cell lymphocytes and macrophages of people with type 1 diabetes lack a protein marker, known as major histocompatibility complex, or MHC, that helps the T cells identify natural cells as "self." Consequently, the T cells misidentify islet cells as unnatural and subsequently destroy them. This same research has now found a way to destroy the islet-attacking T cells using tumor necrosis factor-alpha (TNF-alpha) and stimulate the growth of new islet cells. This discovery may eventually mean that type 1 diabetes can be cured rather than controlled with daily injections of insulin. Faustman's research also may help in curing other autoimmune diseases.

Type 2 Diabetes Mellitus

Diabetes mellitus, especially type 2, runs in families, although a specific diabetic gene has not been isolated. When this form of the disease is manifested, the beta cells of the islets of Langerhans secrete insulin into the bloodstream, but the blood glucose level remains elevated because of peripheral insulin resistance and increased conversion of glycogen to glucose by the liver. Insulin resistance is linked to obesity, especially intra-abdominal obesity, a cofactor in metabolic syndrome. The correlation of obesity and insulin resistance helps explain how dieting and weight loss control type 2 diabetes and delay, reduce, or eliminate the need for medication to treat the disease.

The lack of response to the usual amount of insulin causes the beta cells to secrete even more insulin. Despite hyperinsulinemia, however, the blood glucose level remains elevated. Eventually, the overstimulation exhausts the beta cells, resulting in a decline in insulin production, and the client with type 2 diabetes also becomes insulin deficient.

An excessive level of glucose in the blood leads to **glycosuria,** glucose in the urine, and urinary excretion. Glycosuria appears when the blood glucose level rises above 180 mg/dl. At this level, the kidneys' **renal threshold,** the ability to reabsorb glucose and return it to the bloodstream, is impaired. The hypertonicity from concentrated amounts of glucose in the blood pulls fluid into the vascular system, resulting in **polyuria,** excessive urine production. The client experiences urinary frequency accompanied by increased excreted urine. Because so much water is lost, **polydipsia,** excessive thirst, develops.

While the needed glucose is being wasted, the body's requirement for fuel continues. The person with diabetes feels hungry and eats more (**polyphagia**). Despite eating more, he or she loses weight as the body uses fat and protein to substitute for glucose. Ketones, chemical intermediate products in fat metabolism, such as beta-hydroxybutyric acid, acetoacetic acid, and acetone, cause ketoacidosis when they accumulate.

The bicarbonate buffer system buffers ketones. Thus, **ketonemia** (increased ketones in the blood) causes a decreased alkali (base) reserve, leading to acidosis. **Kussmaul respirations** (fast, deep, labored breathing) are common in ketoacidosis (Fig. 58-2). Acetone, which is volatile, can be detected on the breath by its characteristic odor. If treatment is not initiated, the outcome of ketoacidosis is circulatory collapse, renal shutdown, and death. Ketoacidosis is more common in clients with diabetes who no longer produce insulin, such as those with type 1 diabetes. Clients with type 2 diabetes are more likely to develop hyperosmolar hyperglycemic nonketotic syndrome (HHNKS; see later discussion) because with limited insulin, they can use enough glucose to prevent ketosis, but not enough to maintain a normal blood glucose level.

Infection, failure to eat, vomiting, and stress invite ketosis because they increase the demand for insulin that the pancreas cannot accommodate in diabetes. In addition, clients with diabetes mellitus are at increased risk for vascular disorders such as atherosclerosis, cerebrovascular accidents, myocardial infarction, peripheral vascular disease with decreased ability to heal, renal failure, blindness, and neuropathy. Female clients are prone to complications during pregnancy; male clients are prone to erectile dysfunction (see Chap. 61).

Stop, Think, and Respond ● BOX 58-1

Identify some differences between type 1 and type 2 diabetes mellitus.

Assessment Findings

Signs and Symptoms

The three classic symptoms of both types of diabetes mellitus are polyuria, polydipsia, and polyphagia. Additional symptoms include weight loss, weakness, thirst, fatigue, and dehydration. These signs and symptoms have an abrupt onset in clients with type 1 diabetes. Clients with type 2 diabetes have a gradual onset of symptoms. Some develop skin, urinary tract, and vaginal infections, possibly because the elevated blood glucose level supports bacterial growth. There may be changes in visual acuity manifested by blurred vision because the hypertonicity of body fluid affects the cells in the lens and retina (Porth, 2002).

Diagnostic Findings

Although diabetes mellitus is a highly complex disease, screening for its detection is relatively simple. Normally,

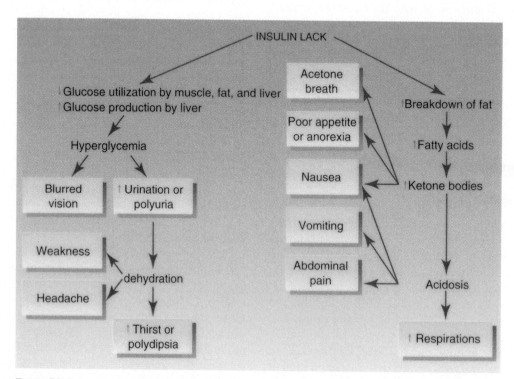

FIGURE 58-2 Abnormal metabolism that causes signs and symptoms of diabetic ketoacidosis: ↑, increased; ↓, decreased. (Pearce, M. A., Rosenberg, C. S., & Davidson, M. D. [1991]. Patient education. In M. B. Davidson [Ed.], *Diabetes mellitus: Diagnosis and treatment* [3rd ed.]. New York: Churchill Livingstone.)

urine contains no detectable glucose or ketones; in diabetes, one or both may be present. Because the body fails to use glucose adequately, it excretes glucose in the urine. If the body metabolizes fats faster than it can use the ketone bodies, ketone bodies also appear in the urine. The relative ease of these urinary tests facilitates early detection of diabetes (Nursing Guidelines 58-1).

Because glycosuria and ketonuria may not become evident until glucose exceeds the renal threshold, blood tests are helpful in establishing the diagnosis. Blood tests such as a random blood sugar, fasting blood glucose, postprandial glucose, and the oral glucose tolerance test are based on measuring glucose intolerance (Table 58-1). Another method of testing for blood glucose is with a glucometer (Fig. 58-3). A glucometer measures capillary blood glucose from a finger stick blood sample. Close monitoring of blood glucose levels can delay the onset of complications associated with diabetes. Many physicians now recommend self-monitoring of blood glucose levels with a glucometer for clients taking insulin, clients with unstable diabetes, or clients with frequent hypoglycemic episodes. Self-monitoring with a glucometer is helpful for those taking an oral hypoglycemic agent to determine the effects of diet, exercise, and medications.

Once a client with diabetes receives a treatment regimen to follow, the physician can assess the effectiveness of treatment and the client's compliance by obtaining a glycosylated hemoglobin, or hemoglobin A1c, test. The results of this test reflect the amount of glucose that is stored in the hemoglobin molecule during its life span of 120 days. Normally, the level of glycosylated hemoglobin is less than 7%. According to the American Diabetes Association, a hemoglobin A1c of 7% is the equivalent of

---

NURSING GUIDELINES 58-1

Performing Urine Glucose Testing

Method: Test-tape and Diastix

- Client empties the bladder to eliminate glucose and ketones that have been stored in the bladder for hours; save this specimen in case the client cannot void later.

- Encourage the client to drink water; ask the client to void in 30 minutes.

- For the client with an indwelling catheter, clamp the catheter for 30 minutes and take the specimen directly from the catheter, not the drainage bag.

- Test the second voided specimen to detect current concentration of glucose and ketones.

- Dip the testing strip into the urine and wait for the recommended time.

- Observe the color change and document the results.

TABLE 58-1	DIAGNOSTIC TESTS FOR DETECTING GLUCOSE INTOLERANCE	
TEST	**IMPLEMENTATION**	**DIAGNOSTIC RESULT**
Random blood glucose	Blood specimen is drawn without preplanning.	≥200 mg/dl in the presence of symptoms is suggestive of diabetes mellitus.
Fasting blood glucose	Blood specimen is obtained after 8 hours of fasting.	In the nondiabetic client the glucose level will be between 70 and 110 mg/dl. In the diabetic client glucose is ≥ 110 mg/dl but <126 mg/dl.
Postprandial glucose	Blood sample is taken 2 hours after a high-carbohydrate meal.	In the nondiabetic client, the glucose level will be between 70 and 110 mg/dl. In the client with diabetes mellitus, the result is ≥140 mg/dl but <200 mg/dl.
Oral glucose tolerance test	Diet high in carbohydrates is eaten for 3 days. Client then fasts for 8 hours. A baseline blood sample is drawn and a urine specimen is collected. An oral glucose solution is given and time of ingestion recorded. Blood is drawn at 30 minutes and 1, 2, and 3 hours after the ingestion of glucose solution. Urine is collected simultaneously. Drinking water is encouraged to promote urine excretion.	In the nondiabetic client, the glucose returns to normal in 2 to 3 hours and urine is negative for glucose. In the diabetic client, blood glucose level returns to normal slowly; urine is positive for glucose.
Glycosylated hemoglobin or Hemoglobin A1c	Single sample of venous blood is withdrawn.	The amount of glucose stored by the hemoglobin is elevated above 7.0% in the newly diagnosed client with diabetes mellitus, in one who is noncompliant, or in one who is inadequately treated.

FIGURE 58-3 Examples of blood glucose monitors. (Smeltzer, S. C. & Bare, B. G. [2000]. *Brunner & Suddarth's textbook of medical–surgical nursing* [9th ed.]. Philadelphia: Lippincott Williams & Wilkins.)

an average blood glucose level of 150 mg/dL. Amounts of 8% or greater indicate that control of the client's blood glucose level has been inadequate during the previous 2 to 3 months.

Medical Management

Treatment depends on many factors, such as the type of diabetes and the ability of the pancreas to manufacture insulin, and involves combinations of the following:

- Diet and weight loss
- Exercise
- Insulin
- Oral antidiabetic agents
- Pancreas transplantation
- Islet cell transplantation

Diet and Weight Loss

Diet is a major component of treatment for every person with diabetes. Formulation of a diabetic diet depends on the client's sex, age, height and weight, activity level, occupation, state of health, former dietary habits, and cultural background. When dietary allowances (calories, percentages of carbohydrates, fats, and proteins) are prescribed, the client is given a diet prescription and a list of substitutions and exchanges to vary the diet. For example, the physician determines that the client with dia-

betes may have 1500 calories per day. The calories are then distributed according to the percentage of carbohydrates, fats, and proteins that equal the total prescribed caloric amount. A dietitian provides the client with a list of foods in six different categories—starch/bread, meat, vegetable, fruit, milk, and fat—and indicates how many items from each category the client can consume for breakfast, lunch, dinner, and snacks (Fig. 58-4). The dietitian gives the client a list of foods in each category and their equivalent amounts. The client can then exchange or substitute one food for another in the specified amount for variety (Fig. 58-5).

Dietary modifications alone can control type 2 diabetes for some clients. These clients have a mild form of diabetes, with the pancreas producing some insulin. The client with diabetes who is overweight is placed on a weight reduction diet because diabetes is less easily controlled in the presence of obesity. Even a moderate weight loss improves the body's use of insulin.

Exercise

Exercise helps metabolize carbohydrates, thus decreasing insulin requirements. It improves circulation, which is compromised in the client with diabetes. Exercise also lowers cholesterol and triglyceride levels and improves muscle tone. An exercise program for the client with diabetes specifies the type of exercise and the length of time to perform it. The program is tailored according to the client's needs and lifestyle. Most important, the client needs to exercise consistently each day. Sporadic periods of exercise are discouraged because wide fluctuations in blood glucose levels can occur. It is necessary to regulate food and insulin requirements during times of increased activities.

Insulin

All clients with type 1 diabetes must rely on insulin therapy. The goal of pancreas and islet cell transplantation (see later discussion), which is performed only for clients with type 1 diabetes, is that the client will acquire **insulin independence**—that is, the client's own naturally produced insulin will regulate blood glucose levels within consistently normal ranges. Better yet, clients with type 1 diabetes eventually may be cured using Dr. Faustman's recent findings on a technique for reversing autoimmu-

	1 Starch/Bread	2 Meat	3 Vegetable	4 Fruit	5 Milk	6 Fat
Breakfast	2			1	1	1
Snack time						
Lunch	2	1	1	1		1
Snack time				1		
Dinner	2	2	1	1		2
Snack time	1			1	1	

FIGURE 58-4 A diabetic meal plan for 1500 calories.

Bran cereals, concentrated	1/3 cup
Bran cereals, flaked (Bran Buds, All Bran)	1/2 cup
Bread	1 oz
Bulgur, cooked	1/2 cup
Cooked cereals	1/2 cup
Cornmeal, dry	1 1/2 tsp
Grapenuts	3 tbsp
Grits, cooked	1/2 cup
Pasta, cooked	1/2 cup
Rice (white or brown), cooked	1/2 cup
Shredded Wheat	1/2 cup
Unsweetened cereals	3/4 cup
Wheat germ	3 tsp
Lentils, cooked	1/3 cup
Baked beans	1/4 cup
Beans and peas, cooked (kidney, split)	1/3 cup
Corn	1/2 cup
Corn on cob	6" 1
Lima beans	1/2 cup
Peas, green (canned or frozen)	1/2 cup
Plantain	1/2 cup
Potato, baked (3 oz)	1 small
Potato, mashed	1/2 cup
Squash, winter (acorn, butternut)	3/4 cup
Yam, sweet potato, plain	1/3 cup

FIGURE 58-5 Sample of starch/bread categories.

nity and stimulating islet cells once again to proliferate and produce insulin. Additional possibilities for eliminating the need for exogenous insulin include gene therapy or transplantation of stem cells. Until then, clients with type 1 diabetes continue to require daily, multiple, or continuous injections of insulin. Clients with type 2 diabetes eventually may become dependent on insulin therapy when other antidiabetic agents are no longer effective.

TYPES OF INSULIN

Human forms of insulin are gradually replacing purified insulin extracts from beef and pork pancreas. There are two methods for deriving human insulin: genetic engineering using strains of *Escherichia coli*, a microorganism found in the gastrointestinal tract, and chemical modification of pork insulin, which differs from human insulin by just one amino acid (Porth, 2002). Human insulin appears to cause fewer allergic reactions than insulin obtained from animal sources; however, clients who switch from animal to synthesized human insulin must be monitored for low blood glucose levels initially because the human form of insulin is used more effectively.

Gastrointestinal juices inactivate insulin; therefore, insulin must be injected. Pharmaceutical companies are working on an inhaled form of insulin and one that can be absorbed through a topical skin patch; however, these are not yet available. Table 58-2 includes commonly used insulin preparations, which are divided into four categories: rapid acting, short acting, intermediate acting, and long acting. Some clients with type 2 diabetes maintain glycemic control with a once-daily injection of an intermediate-acting insulin or combination of intermediate-acting and short-acting insulin in a 70:30 or 50:50 proportion. Clients with type 1 diabetes may self-administer three to four injections or more throughout the day unless they use an insulin pump (discussed later).

TABLE 58-2	INSULIN PREPARATIONS		
INSULIN	**ONSET (HR)**	**PEAK (HR)**	**DURATION (HR)**
Rapid acting			
insulin lispro (Humalog) aspart (Novalog)	5–15 min	1–2	3–4
Short acting			
regular insulin (Humulin R, *Clear* Novolin R, Iletin II Regular)	30 min–1 hr	1–3	6–8
Intermediate acting			
isophane insulin suspension *Cloudy* (NPH, Humulin N, Novolin N)	1–1.5	4–12	24
insulin zinc suspension (Lente)	1–2.5	7–15	24
Long acting			
extended insulin zinc suspension (Ultralente, Humulin U)	4–8	8–10	18–30
glargine (Lantus) *Clear Cannot be mixed*	2–4	No peak	≥24
Insulin Mixtures			
Humulin 50/50	15 min	2–4	20–22
Humulin 70/30	30 min	7–12	16–24
Novolin 70/30	30 min		
Humalog 75/25	15 min	2	20–22

Stop, Think, and Respond ● BOX 58-2

Identify which of the following insulins is rapid acting, short acting, intermediate acting, and long acting: glargine (Lantus), Lente, lispro (Humalog), Novolin R.

ADMINISTRATION OF INSULIN

Insulin is prescribed in units. U100 means that 1 mL contains 100 units of insulin. The physician specifies both the dosage and the type of insulin to be used. When combining two types of insulin in the same syringe, the short-acting regular insulin is withdrawn into the syringe *first* and the mixture is administered within 15 minutes to ensure that the onset, peak, and duration of each separate insulin remains intact. Glargine (Lantus) insulin cannot be mixed with other types of insulin in the same syringe. Combination mixtures of insulin, such as Humulin 70/30, Novolin 70/30, and Humulin 50/50, eliminate the need for mixing insulins from two separate vials.

Regular insulin can be administered intravenously (IV) and subcutaneously. The IV route is used to (1) treat severe hyperglycemia or (2) prevent or control elevated blood sugar by adding it to a total parenteral nutrition solution that contains a high concentration of glucose. The subcutaneous route is used most commonly for administering insulin (Fig. 58-6). Insulin is absorbed more rapidly when injected in the abdomen than in the arms or legs. Clients with diabetes are taught to use the abdomen as the preferred site for self-administration (Fig. 58-7). Sub-

FIGURE 58-7 Inserting the needle into the skin.

cutaneous injection sites require rotation to avoid **lipoatrophy,** breakdown of subcutaneous fat at the site of repeated injections, and **lipohypertrophy,** buildup of subcutaneous fat at the site of repeated injections, either of which eventually interferes with insulin absorption in the tissue. Because insulin is an anabolic hormone, it also causes weight gain.

Other techniques for injecting insulin subcutaneously include an insulin pen, jet injector, or insulin pump.

Insulin Pen. An insulin pen is a device in which a cartridge containing 150 to 300 units of insulin is loaded into an injecting pen with a needle attached. Once the device is loaded, the client (1) selects the number of units for injection by dialing in the dose in 1- to 2-unit increments, (2) cleans and pierces the skin, and (3) injects the programmed amount.

Jet Injector. A jet injector uses high pressure and rapid speed, rather than a needle, to instill insulin through the skin. The pressure transforms the liquid into a fine mist that is distributed over a wide area of tissue, resulting in faster absorption (Fig. 58-8). Although a jet injector offers several advantages, such as reducing pain at the site and

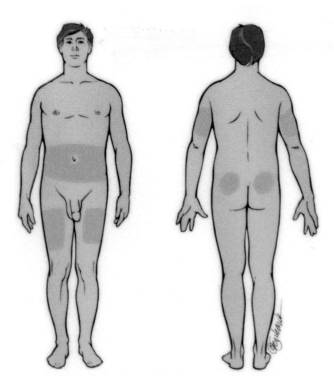

FIGURE 58-6 Suggested areas for insulin injection.

FIGURE 58-8 (**A**) Needle produces a pool of insulin beneath the skin, which is slowly absorbed. (**B**) Jet injector produces an insulin mist beneath the skin, which is absorbed more quickly.

eliminating the use of needles and their appropriate disposal, the cost tends to make this form of administration less attractive.

Insulin Pump. An insulin pump provides a means for delivering insulin by continuous infusion. The device has three components: pump, tubing, and needle (Fig. 58-9). The pump itself contains a reservoir for rapid-acting or short-acting insulin, a battery-operated infuser, and a computer chip that enables a person to regulate basal (continuous) and premeal bolus doses in 0.05- to 0.1-unit increments. The pump, which is worn in a pouch or belt holder, is attached to tubing with a needle. The needle is inserted in the subcutaneous tissue of the abdomen and can remain in the same site for up to 3 days. Clients who are interested in controlling their diabetes with an insulin pump need to consider both its advantages and disadvantages (Table 58-3).

Oral Antidiabetic Agents

Oral antidiabetic drugs are prescribed for clients with type 2 diabetes who meet the following criteria:

- Fasting blood glucose level less than 200 mg/dl
- Insulin requirement of less than 40 units/day
- No ketoacidosis
- No renal or hepatic disease

Before 1995, only one category of drugs, the sulfonylureas, was used to lower the blood glucose level. Since then, many new drugs have been developed that help control type 2 diabetes by various mechanisms. Recently developed drug categories include biguanides, alpha-glucosidase inhibitors, thiazolidinediones, and meglitinides. Drug Therapy Table 58-1 lists examples of oral hypoglycemic drugs.

SULFONYLUREAS AND MEGLITINIDES
Sulfonylureas such as glyburide (DiaBeta, Glynase, Micronase) and glipizide (Glucotrol) were modified from

FIGURE 58-9 (A) Diagram of an insulin pump showing syringe in place inside pump and connection of pump through tubing to needle site. **(B)** Actual insertion site. (Smeltzer, S. C. & Bare, B. G. [2000]. *Brunner & Suddarth's textbook of medical–surgical nursing* [9th ed.]. Philadelphia: Lippincott Williams & Wilkins.)

sulfa-containing antibiotics when it was found that some such drugs reduced the blood glucose level. The sulfonylureas, which have evolved through several generations, and the meglitinides, nonsulfonylureas such as repaglinide (Prandin), are described as being "insulin releasers" because they stimulate the pancreas to secrete more insulin. Although they are effective drugs, they tend to cause weight gain, hypoglycemic reactions, and *secondary failure,* a phenomenon in which the pancreas cannot continue making sufficient insulin, perhaps as a result of the gland's overstimulation. Repaglinide has a short duration

TABLE 58-3	INSULIN PUMP CONSIDERATIONS
ADVANTAGES	**DISADVANTAGES**
Resembles the normal pancreatic release of insulin Decreases the necessity for multiple daily injections in different sites Helps maintain consistent blood sugar levels; reduces the potential for episodes of hyperglycemia and ketoacidosis Provides more flexibility for eating food at varying times during the day Facilitates the instillation of smaller doses than those of insulin syringes	Requires high motivation to control diabetes by frequently checking blood glucose levels and adjusting the infusion Creates a potential for hyperglycemia if the pump fails, the tubing becomes kinked or obstructed, or the needle is displaced Interferes or creates a nuisance factor when participating in active sports, sexual intercourse, or bathing; the pump can be temporarily disconnected without removing the needle, but doing so stops the delivery of insulin until it is reconnected

DRUG THERAPY TABLE 58-1	ORAL HYPOGLYCEMIC AGENTS

DRUG CATEGORY AND EXAMPLES	MECHANISM OF ACTION	SIDE EFFECTS	NURSING CONSIDERATIONS
First-Generation Sulfonylureas			
acetohexamide (Dymelor), chlorpropamide (Diabinese), tolazamide (Tolinase), tolbutamide (Orinase)	Stimulates insulin release in type 2 diabetes	Anorexia, nausea, vomiting, hypoglycemia	Give before breakfast and evening meal. Monitor serum and urine glucose levels. Avoid administering to pregnant women.
Second-Generation Sulfonylureas			
gilmepride (Amaryl), glipzide (Glucotrol), glyburide (DiaBeta, Glynase Pres Tab, Micronase)	Stimulates insulin release; are more potent than first-generation sulfonylureas	Increased risk of cardiovascular mortality, anorexia, nausea, vomiting, heartburn, diarrhea, hypoglycemia, allergic skin reactions, insulin "burn out"	Give before breakfast. Monitor urine and serum glucose levels. Avoid administering to pregnant women. Caution client to avoid alcohol. Teach client appropriate diet, exercise, signs and symptoms of hypoglycemia and hyperglycemia, avoidance of infection. Do not abruptly discontinue medication.
Alpha-Glucosidase Inhibitors			
acarbose (Precose), miglitol (Glyset)	Delays digestion of carbohydrates Effects are additive to sulfonylureas in type 2 diabetes	Abdominal pain, flatulence, diarrhea, hypoglycemia	Give three times a day 15 min before each meal. Monitor urine and serum glucose levels. Inform client of gastrointestinal side effects.
Biguanide Compound			
Metformin (glucophage)	Improves use of insulin in type 2 diabetes	Anorexia, nausea, heartburn, diarrhea, lactic acidosis, hypoglycemia, allergic skin reactions, flatulence	Monitor urine and serum glucose levels. Avoid administering to pregnant women. Caution client to avoid use of alcohol. Instruct client not to discontinue medication.
Insulin-Enhancing Agents			
rosiglitazone (Avandia), piaglitazone (Actos)	Increases effects of circulating insulin	Headache, pain, liver injury, hypoglycemia, hyperglycemia, infections, fatigue	Give once daily in morning.
Meglitinides			
repaglinide (Prandin)	Stimulates insulin release	Upper respiratory infections, hypoglycemia, hyperglycemia, headache	Monitor urine and serum glucose levels. Teach client appropriate diet, exercise, signs and symptoms of hypoglycemia and hyperglycemia, avoidance of infection.

of action, making hypoglycemia less common than with sulfonylureas, but must be taken with each meal.

BIGUANIDES AND THIAZOLIDINEDIONES

Metformin (Glucophage) is the only biguanide approved for use. The thiazolidinediones (TZDs), which include rosiglitazone (Avandia) and pioglitazone (Actos), are the newest drugs used for type 2 diabetes. The biguanides and TZDs are categorized as "insulin sensitizers"—they help tissues use available insulin more efficiently. Metformin does not promote weight gain like the sulfonylureas, nor does it trigger a low blood glucose level. It may, however, cause upset stomach, flatulence, and diarrhea, and it is associated with a small risk for lactic acidosis. TZDs, on the other hand, are known to cause weight gain, edema, and liver damage; in fact, troglitazone (Rezulin), a third TZD, was withdrawn from the market after its initial approval because several deaths were related to its use. Anyone taking a TZD should have liver function tests performed every 2 months during the first year of treatment.

ALPHA-GLUCOSIDASE INHIBITORS

Alpha-glucosidase inhibitors include drugs such as miglitol (Glyset) and acarbose (Precose). Alpha-glucosidase is an intestinal enzyme that breaks down complex carbohydrates into glucose, a simple sugar. When this enzyme is inhibited, the process of forming glucose is slowed and glucose is absorbed more slowly from the small intestine. Consequently, blood glucose is balanced with the body's available insulin. Drugs in this category must be taken 15 minutes before each meal. They are most effective in reducing postprandial (after a meal) hyperglycemia. Occasionally, clients with type 1 diabetes take both insulin and an alpha-glucosidase inhibitor because this category of drug tends to equalize blood glucose levels and prevents swings between hyperglycemia and hypoglycemia.

Unfortunately, a person who develops hypoglycemia while taking an alpha-glucosidase inhibitor cannot respond to the first line of treatment, which is drinking fruit juice, because the drug interferes with the conversion of the carbohydrate in the juice to glucose. The better treatment, in this case, is to give glucose either in tablets or by injection because glucose requires no further breakdown for absorption.

Stop, Think, and Respond ● BOX 58-3

Name at least one oral antidiabetic agent in each of the following categories: (1) promotes release of insulin, (2) enhances response to insulin (insulin sensitizer), and (3) slows the breakdown of complex carbohydrates.

Pancreas Transplantation

Replacing the pancreas involves a whole or partial organ transplant. The usual candidate is a client with type 1 diabetes who has renal failure and will benefit from a combined kidney and pancreas transplant. Clients with type 2 diabetes are not offered the option of a pancreas transplant because usually their problem is insulin resistance, which does not improve with a transplant.

Because the pancreas is both an exocrine and endocrine gland, transplanting it requires providing a means for exocrine enzymatic drainage and venous absorption of insulin. Exocrine drainage is accomplished by establishing a duodenal or urinary bladder connection with the transplanted pancreas. Insulin is released into the portal vein, which carries blood to the liver. Although bladder connections have a lower incidence of organ rejection, they also tend to cause urologic complications and are used less often than originally.

As with any transplant, lifelong immunosuppressive drug therapy also is required because without it, the new organ is destroyed. Because type 1 diabetes can be managed with insulin, many believe that the risks involved

with immunosuppression outweigh the benefit that can be achieved with a pancreas transplant, unless a kidney transplant also is necessary.

Islet Cell Transplantation

Some clients with type 1 diabetes are recipients of islet cell transplants, rather than a transplant of the entire organ or part of the organ. Islet cells, which are the insulin-producing components of the pancreas, have been harvested from human organ donors and from pigs. Two human pancreases are necessary to obtain sufficient numbers of islet cells for transplantation. Furthermore, the cells from the donor pancreases must be used within 12 hours of harvesting to remain viable (Gottlieb, 2000).

After the pancreas is harvested, the islet cells are separated from the tissue and injected through the abdominal wall into the client's peritoneal cavity, where they begin to release insulin. The current practice is to avoid including a steroid with other immunosuppressive drugs. Steroids raise the blood glucose to levels the new islet cells have difficulty overcoming. Currently, islet cell transplantation surgeons use a combination of tacrolimus (Prograf), sirolimus (Rapamune), and dacliximab (Zenapax) to prevent rejection. Although only a few islet cell transplantations have been performed, most recipients require no or very little insulin and can eat whatever they want.

Nursing Management

The nurse obtains a complete medical, drug, and allergy history, including a list of all symptoms and their duration. He or she determines when the client was diagnosed with diabetes and if others in the family also are diabetic. If the client is a diagnosed diabetic, the nurse asks the client to identify his or her prescribed treatment regimen and when he or she last consumed food and self-administered drugs. The nurse weighs the client and performs a complete head-to-toe physical examination because diabetes affects many systems. The nurse looks for physical changes associated with diabetes:

- Changes in the skin over insulin injection sites, impaired skin areas that appear to be healing poorly; ulcerations or evidence of skin or soft tissue infection
- Vital signs, peripheral pulses, temperature of the extremities, inspection of the extremities for edema or changes in color
- Decreased visual acuity and visual changes such as blurred vision
- Muscle atrophy, weakness, or loss of sensation

See Nursing Care Plan 58-1 for managing the care of a client with diabetes mellitus.

(text continued on page 893)

Nursing Care Plan 58-1

THE CLIENT WITH DIABETES MELLITUS

Assessment

Determine the following:

- Evidence of polyuria, polydipsia, polyphagia
- Current weight
- Vital signs, especially blood pressure in lying, sitting, and standing positions
- Blood glucose level before each meal and bedtime
- Any ketones or albumin in the urine
- Serum electrolyte, cholesterol, lipid, triglyceride, blood urea nitrogen, and creatinine levels
- Condition of the skin and feet
- Any abnormal sensations such as pain, tingling, burning, numbness
- Visual acuity and last date of ophthalmic examination
- Knowledge of therapeutic management

Nursing Diagnosis: **Imbalanced Nutrition: More than Body Requirements** related to altered satiety, decreased activity, and habituation of preillness eating habits

Expected Outcome: Client will adhere to his or her prescribed calorie-controlled diet.

Interventions	*Rationales*
Provide three meals and snacks within prescribed caloric limits.	Restriction of calories promotes weight loss and balances glucose with naturally produced or parenterally administered insulin.
Suggest free foods such as up to 1 cup of raw vegetables like cucumbers, radishes, celery, or zucchini; unlimited sugar-free drinks; or low-sodium bouillon, if the client becomes hungry between meals or snacks.	Free foods contain *fewer* than 20 calories per serving; their consumption provides negligible calories.
Encourage client to drink 8 ounces of water before eating a meal.	Water is calorie free, distends the stomach, and provides a feeling of fullness.
Advise client to eat slowly and wait 15 seconds between chewing thoroughly, swallowing, and taking the next bite.	Slowed eating prolongs the pleasure of eating and allows time for the brain to sense satiation.

Evaluation of Expected Outcome: Client eats the prescribed diet and verbalizes understanding of restrictions and allowances.

PC: **Hypoglycemia**

Expected Outcome: The nurse will monitor for, manage, and minimize hypoglycemia.

Interventions	*Rationales*
Test capillary blood glucose level with a glucometer 30 minutes before each meal and at bedtime.	Hypoglycemia is more likely before the client consumes food.
Monitor for signs of hypoglycemia such as shakiness, diaphoresis, hunger, and disturbed cognition.	Low blood glucose level causes physiologic stimulation and diminishes the ability to think clearly.
Follow agency policy for administering a quick-acting source of simple carbohydrate according to lower limit of blood glucose level.	Simple carbohydrates are absorbed quickly and tend to raise the blood glucose level high enough to eliminate the symptoms of hypoglycemia.

(continued)

Nursing Care Plan 58-1 *(Continued)*

THE CLIENT WITH DIABETES MELLITUS

Interventions	*Rationales*
Recheck the capillary blood glucose level within 15 to 30 minutes after treating a hypoglycemic episode.	Rechecking the level helps determine the client's response to the nursing intervention.
Repeat the administration of simple carbohydrate if the client continues to be symptomatic; reassess capillary blood glucose level.	The client may need additional simple carbohydrate to successfully raise blood glucose.
Notify the physician if the client's symptoms continue after two attempts to raise the blood sugar with oral substances.	Parenteral interventions to raise the blood glucose level are medically prescribed.
Offer client complex carbohydrates when hypoglycemia is controlled.	Complex carbohydrates are digested and absorbed more slowly than simple carbohydrates, which reduces the potential for another hypoglycemic episode.
Withhold insulin when the client must fast before laboratory or diagnostic procedures.	Eating and administration of insulin are timed according to insulin's onset, peak, and duration of action.
Ask a second nurse to double-check the vial of insulin and the number of units in the syringe before administering the injection.	Double-checking helps avoid errors in insulin administration. Giving more than the prescribed amount or mistaking rapid-acting or short-acting insulin for intermediate- or long-acting insulin can cause hypoglycemia.

Evaluation of Expected Outcome: Client eats the prescribed diet and verbalizes understanding of restrictions and allowances.

PC: Hyperglycemia
Expected Outcome: The nurse will monitor for, manage, and minimize hyperglycemia.

Interventions	*Rationales*
Monitor capillary blood glucose levels before each meal and at bedtime; check urine for ketones if glucose levels are elevated.	Elevated blood glucose level before a client eats suggests that he or she is not compliant with the diet and may require a higher dose of an oral antidiabetic agent or coverage with rapid-acting or short-acting insulin. Ketonuria increases the potential for DKA.
Assess for clinical signs and symptoms of hyperglycemia such as thirst, increased urination, and sleepiness.	Hyperglycemia has a gradual onset with symptoms similar to the undiagnosed state; hyperglycemia can progress to DKA or HHNKS.
Administer insulin or oral antidiabetic agents as prescribed.	Insufficient insulin results in elevated blood glucose level.
Implement medical orders for insulin administration according to a sliding scale established by the physician.	Insulin lowers blood glucose level.
Notify the physician if the client with hyperglycemia is noninsulin dependent.	Modifications in the diet or changes in antidiabetic medications are medically prescribed.
Reinforce the importance of compliance with the prescribed diet, exercise, and medication regimen.	These measures manage hyperglycemia.

Evaluation of Expected Outcome: Blood glucose levels are within 80 to 120 mg/dl in a nonfasting state.

Nursing Diagnosis: **Risk for Imbalanced Fluid Volume** related to hyperglycemia and polyuria
Expected Outcome: Client will maintain proper fluid balance.

(continued)

Nursing Care Plan 58-1 (Continued)

THE CLIENT WITH DIABETES MELLITUS

Interventions	Rationales
Monitor intake and output.	A deficit in fluid intake or excess urine output suggests a deficit in fluid volume.
Provide at least 1500 to 3000 mL of fluid per day.	The average fluid requirement per 24 hours is 1500 to 3000 mL.

Evaluation of Expected Outcome: Client is well-hydrated as evidenced by a fluid intake of between 1500 to 3000 mL with a similar urine output.

Nursing Diagnosis: **Risk for Injury** related to orthostatic hypotension and impaired vision secondary to neuropathy and retinopathy
Expected Outcome: Client will be free from injury.

Interventions	Rationales
Assist client when rising from a sitting or laying position.	Autonomic neuropathy causes orthostatic hypotension and the potential for fainting and falling.
Have client dangle on the side of the bed before ambulating.	Dangling allows a period during which blood flow increases in the brain.
Keep the floor dry and the environment free of clutter.	Retinopathy may interfere with the client's ability to see potential safety hazards.

Evaluation of Expected Outcome: There is no evidence of trauma.

Nursing Diagnosis: **Risk for Impaired Skin Integrity** related to loss of sensation in feet and impaired blood circulation
Expected Outcome: Skin will remain intact.

Interventions	Rationales
Examine skin and feet daily.	Client may be insensitive to injuries and slow to heal because of peripheral neuropathy and vascular disturbances.
Assess skin for signs of breakdown, poor healing, change in color or temperature, or infection.	Impaired blood supply compromises the integrity of the integument.
Dry client's skin well after bathing, especially in areas of the body that are dark and moist.	Fungal infections are common in creases and folds of skin.
Rotate insulin injection sites; give each injection 1/2 to 1 inch away from the previous injection.	Rotating injection sites prevents lipoatrophy and lipohypertrophy.
Inspect inside the client's shoes for foreign objects or disrepair.	Friction or pressure can impair the integrity of the feet.
Provide foot care with daily hygiene.	Care of the feet prevents injury and skin breakdown.

Evaluation of Expected Outcome: Skin is warm, dry, and intact, with no evidence of tissue breakdown in the feet.

Nursing Diagnosis: **Risk for Ineffective Management of Therapeutic Regimen** related to insufficient knowledge regarding diabetes self-management
Expected Outcome: Client will verbalize and demonstrate knowledge of diabetes and self-management techniques.

(continued)

Nursing Care Plan 58-1 (Continued)

THE CLIENT WITH DIABETES MELLITUS

Interventions	*Rationales*
Assess client's ability and willingness to learn about diabetes and self-management.	Teaching is more effective when the learner is capable and motivated to acquire information.
Teach client about insulin and how to self-administer using proper technique.	Clients learn in various ways: verbal explanations, reading information, seeing a demonstration, or using a hands-on application.
Allow client opportunities to practice administering insulin.	Practice promotes self-confidence and develops expertise.
Show client how to monitor blood glucose using a glucometer.	Using the same method as the client will use after discharge increases knowledgeable self-management.
Arrange for the dietitian to teach client about his or her exchange diet.	Dietitians are experts in diet therapy.
Review the importance of exercise and methods for daily activity.	Exercise reduces blood glucose level, helps with weight loss, and improves circulation.

Evaluation of Expected Outcome: Client demonstrates knowledge and skills to independently manage his or her disease.

The nurse monitors the client's blood glucose level before meals and at bedtime. He or she tests the urine for ketones if the blood glucose level is high. The nurse administers prescribed medications and evaluates the client's response to their effects. If hypoglycemia develops, the nurse uses quick-acting sources of glucose to raise the client's blood glucose level. The nurse initiates or reinforces information the client must know to manage his or her condition independently. He or she refers the client to a diabetic educator if one is available; consultation with a dietitian may be appropriate. The extent of the teaching program depends on whether the client has been diabetic for some time or is newly diagnosed; even those who have had the disorder for years may have inaccurate ideas about their disorder and treatment regimen.

Before teaching begins, the nurse confers with the physician regarding:

- Type of diet for the client to follow
- Medication regimen (insulin or oral antidiabetic agent)
- Materials for insulin administration, such as needle and syringe, insulin pen, insulin jet, or insulin pump
- Technique for monitoring blood glucose levels, self-testing devices (glucometer), and the suggested brand to use
- Materials for and frequency of urine testing
- Additional information, such as skin care, signs of diabetic ketoacidosis (DKA), hyperosmolar hyperglycemic nonketotic syndrome (HHNKS), and hypoglycemia (discussed later)

Whenever possible, the nurse includes the family in a diabetic teaching program because one or more family members may assume some or all responsibility for the treatment regimen. To allow the client and family member time to understand information, the nurse presents material in small increments. He or she may choose to begin teaching by explaining diabetes, why treatments are necessary, and the various methods of treatment. The nurse uses audiovisual materials to enhance learning. Because the treatment of diabetes is highly individualized, he or she emphasizes that the treatment of one person cannot be compared with that of another.

If the client requires insulin, the nurse identifies that the preferred site for injections is the abdomen and uses a chart to explain how to rotate injection sites. The American Diabetes Association, in its 1998 Clinical Practice Recommendations, advocates rotating insulin injections in only one anatomic region to ensure consistent rates of absorption. Abdominal injections are absorbed most quickly and have the least rate variability. If the physician has recommended the use of a glucometer to monitor blood glucose levels, the nurse allows time for the client to use the glucometer and monitor his or her own blood glucose levels. Additional teaching topics include the following:

- Signs and symptoms of hyperglycemia and hypoglycemia
- The importance of weight reduction, if necessary
- Methods of terminating hypoglycemia, such as grape or orange juice, Prolycen (a commercial prod-

uct containing glucose), 2 or 3 teaspoons of honey, hard candy, and glucose tablets
- Problems that require contacting the physician, such as skin infection, pain in the extremities, visual problems, change in color or temperature of the skin of the extremities, frequent episodes of hypoglycemia, prolonged nausea and vomiting, and illness
- The importance of following an exercise regimen suggested by the physician. The nurse stresses that during exercise, the client needs to have some food or other physician-approved form of glucose if symptoms of hypoglycemia occur. This is especially important for clients taking insulin or those subject to episodes of hypoglycemia while taking an oral antidiabetic agent.
- How to integrate the dietary exchange list throughout the day
- The information that is printed on food labels to promote compliance with the prescribed diet
- The definitions of products labeled as "low calorie" and "dietetic" and that these terms are not synonymous with "no sugar." They may contain sugar.
- The importance of drinking adequate water, especially in warm weather, when exercising, and when perspiring
- Foot care
- The necessity for regular appointments with an ophthalmologist for comprehensive eye examinations
- The need to consult the physician regarding dosage adjustments for insulin or oral antidiabetic agent if the client becomes ill or cannot eat

ACUTE COMPLICATIONS OF DIABETES MELLITUS

Some clients, despite careful control of their disease, develop one or more serious complications over time. Some complications can be controlled when detected in the early stages.

● DIABETIC KETOACIDOSIS

Diabetic ketoacidosis (DKA), a type of metabolic acidosis, occurs when there is an acute insulin deficiency or an inability to use whatever insulin the pancreas secretes.

Pathophysiology and Etiology

DKA can develop despite the client's compliance with the prescribed treatment regimen. Clients who develop DKA often have a severe, hard-to-control form of the disease

(brittle diabetes). Occasionally, a client admitted to the hospital in DKA has undiagnosed diabetes. Other causes of this serious event are infection and noncompliance with the treatment regimen. (See the discussion of ketoacidosis under Pathophysiology of Diabetes Mellitus.)

When the amount of glucose transported across cell membranes decreases, the liver increases its production of glucose. The blood glucose level becomes extremely elevated. The kidneys attempt to excrete the glucose, which is well beyond the renal threshold. In the process, excessive amounts of water, sodium, and potassium are excreted as well. The client becomes dehydrated; the skin is warm, dry, and flushed. Stored fat is broken down, causing ketones to accumulate in the blood and urine. As ketones mount, the pH of the blood becomes acidotic. The client begins breathing rapidly and deeply in an attempt to eliminate carbon dioxide and prevent it from forming carbonic acid, which would contribute even more to the acidotic state. If the condition is severe and prolonged, the client becomes comatose. Death results with untreated or ineffective treatment of DKA.

Assessment Findings

Early symptoms are vague and become more definite and serious as increasing ketones accumulate in the bloodstream. Weakness, thirst, anorexia, vomiting, drowsiness, and abdominal pain develop. The cheeks are flushed, and the skin and mouth are dry. The breath has an odor of acetone. Kussmaul respirations often are evident. The pulse is rapid and weak. The blood pressure is low. The client may become unresponsive, but restless. Blood glucose levels are elevated to 300 to 1000 mg/dl or more. Urine contains glucose and ketones. The blood pH ranges from 6.8 to 7.3. The serum bicarbonate level is decreased to levels from 0 to 15 mEq/L. The compensatory breathing pattern can lower the partial pressure of carbon dioxide in arterial blood ($PaCO_2$) to levels of 10 to 30 mm Hg. Serum sodium and potassium levels reflect the degree of dehydration (i.e., they may be elevated because they are concentrated in a low volume of body fluid); however, intracellular levels are low, but they are unmeasurable.

Medical Management

Treatment depends on the severity of DKA. The main goals of treatment are to (1) reduce the elevated blood glucose, (2) correct fluid and electrolyte imbalances, and (3) clear the urine and blood of ketones. To accomplish these goals, insulin is given IV. Insulin reduces the production of ketones by making glucose available for oxidation by the tissues and by restoring the liver's supply of glycogen. Regular insulin is added to an IV solution and infused continuously. The amount of insulin and the rate of infusion depend on the blood glucose levels, but the rate may be in the range of 5 U/hour. Isotonic fluid is instilled at a high volume, for example, 250 to 500 mL per hour for several hours. The rate is adjusted once the client becomes rehydrated and diuresis is less acute. As insulin begins to lower the blood glucose level, the IV solution is changed to include one with glucose. This helps to avoid the potential for hypoglycemia. Potassium replacements are given despite elevated serum levels to raise intracellular stores. Periodic monitoring of serum electrolytes and blood glucose levels is necessary. The urine is tested for glucose and ketones.

Nursing Management

The nurse monitors IV infusions closely and takes vital signs frequently. Older adults and those with cardiopulmonary or renal disorders are prone to fluid overload. The nurse inserts an indwelling urinary catheter and monitors urine output to ensure that replaced potassium has a means for excretion. Besides checking serum electrolyte findings, the nurse attaches cardiac leads and observes the client's heart conduction pattern to detect evidence of hyperkalemia such as peaked T waves. Blood glucose level is measured frequently; the urine is similarly checked for the presence of ketones. He or she keeps the physician informed of the client's response, or lack of response, to therapy. See Nursing Care Plan 58-1 for additional nursing care.

● HYPEROSMOLAR HYPERGLYCEMIC NONKETOTIC SYNDROME

Hyperosmolar hyperglycemic nonketotic syndrome (HHNKS), an acute complication of diabetes, is characterized by hyperglycemia without ketosis. It is not unusual to find the blood glucose level well over 500 mg/dl, but the pH of the blood remains within the normal range of 7.35 to 7.45. Fluid and electrolyte imbalances accompany HHNKS.

Pathophysiology and Etiology

HHNKS often results from a serious illness during which metabolic needs exceed the limits of available insulin. Because of persistent hyperglycemia, fluid moves from the intracellular compartment to the extracellular compartment. Diuresis occurs with a subsequent loss of sodium and potassium. Because the client still is secreting some insulin, which can transport glucose in the cells, fat metabolism is minimal or unaffected; hence, ketosis does

not develop. HHNK syndrome is more common in undiagnosed or older clients with type 2 diabetes. It also occurs among clients who do not have diabetes who receive drugs that elevate blood glucose, or who require kidney dialysis or total parenteral nutrition.

Assessment Findings

Hypotension, mental changes, extreme thirst, dehydration, tachycardia, and fever develop. Neurologic signs include paralysis, lethargy, coma, and seizures. Symptoms of hypokalemia and hyponatremia usually are present. Physical examination reveals dry mucous membranes and poor skin turgor. Blood glucose levels are exceedingly high and serum potassium and sodium levels are low. The serum osmolarity is increased.

Medical Management

Treatment includes the administration of insulin and correction of fluid and electrolyte imbalances. A central venous pressure manometer is used to monitor the client's response to fluid replacement.

Nursing Management

The nurse measures the client's blood glucose level and assesses for electrolyte imbalances and dehydration. He or she implements medical orders for insulin, fluids, and electrolyte replacement and closely monitors the client's response to treatment. The nurse's priority areas for evaluation include hydration status, intake and output, skin turgor, vital signs, and electrolyte studies. The nurse observes the client's neurologic and cognitive symptoms; cognition may be significantly impaired in the early stages of care. The nurse protects the client's safety if cognition is impaired and judgment is poor. Additional management depends on symptoms (see Nursing Care Plan 58-1).

● HYPOGLYCEMIA

Hypoglycemia, a low blood glucose level, is always a potential adverse reaction when administering medications for diabetes.

Pathophysiology and Etiology

When too much insulin (hyperinsulinism) is in the bloodstream relative to the amount of available glucose, hypoglycemia occurs. The blood glucose level falls below

60 mg/dl. Because glucose is the primary source of cellular energy, especially for the brain, hypoglycemia tends to manifest as neurologic changes such as confusion, difficulty processing information, anxious feelings, emotional irritability, and headache. The client feels hungry, a homeostatic mechanism to stimulate eating. If the condition is untreated, seizures, permanent brain damage, or death can occur.

Hypoglycemia occurs when a client with diabetes is (1) not eating at all and continues to take insulin or oral antidiabetic medications, (2) not eating sufficient calories to compensate for glucose-lowering medications, or (3) is exercising more than usual, which lowers available blood glucose. Alcohol consumption also interferes with the liver's ability to synthesize glucose from noncarbohydrates, placing clients with diabetes who drink at higher risk for hypoglycemia.

Assessment Findings

Signs and Symptoms

The pattern of symptoms varies somewhat depending on the degree of hypoglycemia, the individual reaction, and the type of insulin taken. Initial symptoms include weakness, headache, nausea, drowsiness, nervousness, hunger, tremors, malaise, and excessive perspiration. Some clients have characteristic personality or behavior changes. Confusion and dizziness can occur. If hypoglycemia is not corrected, symptoms can progress to difficulty with coordination. The client may complain of double vision. If left untreated, unconsciousness and seizures can develop.

Although symptoms vary, each client tends to have a uniquely repetitious pattern when hypoglycemia devel-

ops. The manifestation of hypoglycemic symptoms usually is quite rapid, with unconsciousness or seizures occurring shortly after onset.

When a client with diabetes is found unconscious, DKA or hypoglycemia needs to be ruled out. These conditions are direct opposites: in ketoacidosis, the blood glucose level is high; in hypoglycemia, it is low. The nurse and client must be familiar with the symptoms of hypoglycemia and hyperglycemia to recognize and differentiate the complication as it is developing and treat it appropriately (Table 58-4).

Diagnostic Findings

Diagnosis is based on symptoms, client history, and blood glucose levels. The history is important in differentiating between DKA and hypoglycemia. If the client had insulin and has not eaten, it is most likely that hypoglycemia is present. If the client has eaten and has not taken or received insulin, DKA is more likely. Recognition of hypoglycemia must be immediate; therefore, a bedside glucometer test, as well as sharp assessment skills, are important.

Medical Management

The medical treatment for a hypoglycemic reaction is administration of 15 to 20 g of simple carbohydrate as soon as possible. Some sources for quickly available concentrated carbohydrate include sweetened fruit juice, honey, candy, cake frosting, sugar, or glucose tablets. If the client is unconscious, glucose gel can be applied in the buccal cavity of the mouth. If the client does not respond

TABLE 58-4	CHARACTERISTICS OF HYPERGLYCEMIA AND HYPOGLYCEMIA	
CHARACTERISTIC	HYPERGLYCEMIA	HYPOGLYCEMIA
Predisposing factors	Insufficient or omitted insulin Concurrent infection Dietary indiscretion	Excessive insulin Unusual exercise Too little food
Onset	Slow; hours to days	Sudden; minutes
Mental status	Drowsy	Disoriented; eventually becomes comatose
Skin	Flushed, dry, hot	Pale, moist, cool
Blood pressure	Low	Normal
Pulse	Rapid, weak	Normal or slow, bounding
Respiration	Air hunger	Normal to rapid, shallow
Hunger	Absent	Often present
Thirst	Present	Absent
Vomiting	Present	May be absent
Urine glucose	Present in large amounts	Absent in second voided specimen
Response to treatment	Slow	Rapid

(Adapted from Lilly Research Laboratories, *Diabetes mellitus*.)

fairly quickly and the blood glucose level continues to be low, glucagon, a hormone that stimulates the liver to release glycogen, or 20 to 50 mL of 50% glucose is prescribed for IV administration. Once the hypoglycemic symptoms are relieved, the client with diabetes is given complex carbohydrates such as graham crackers and milk to sustain and prolong an adequate level of blood glucose.

Nursing Management

If the client is conscious and can swallow, the nurse gives grape juice or sweetened orange juice, candy, warm tea or coffee with sugar, a cola beverage, honey, or an oral source of glucose. He or she implements medical orders for parenteral medications such as IV glucose or parenteral glucagon. Whenever a client with diabetes mellitus is on a hospital unit, quick-acting carbohydrates are stocked and available. In a severe reaction, the nurse may provide more than an initial offering of carbohydrate and monitors the client's blood glucose level to evaluate the effect. If the symptoms do not abate and the blood glucose level remains low, the nurse collaborates with the physician concerning additional medical measures.

Above all, the nurse stays with the hypoglycemic client until the pronounced symptoms are corrected. When an episode of hypoglycemia occurs, the regulation of glucose metabolism may be tenuous for about 24 hours. The nurse observes the client at frequent intervals for further episodes of hypoglycemia.

The nurse can prevent hypoglycemia by:

- Ensuring that the meal is served within 15 minutes of administering rapid-acting insulin, and within 30 minutes of giving short-acting insulin
- Ensuring that the client eats the prescribed diet and between-meal snacks
- Informing the physician immediately if nausea, vomiting, or diarrhea occur, or if the client refuses to eat
- Administering the correct type and dose of insulin at the prescribed times
- Asking a colleague to check the label on the insulin vial and the number of units in the insulin syringe against that which is ordered before administering insulin, to avoid a medication error

Additional nursing management of hypoglycemia depends on the symptoms presented (see Nursing Care Plan 58-1).

CHRONIC COMPLICATIONS OF DIABETES MELLITUS

Although clients with diabetes can develop many complications, extremely common ones include peripheral neuropathy, nephropathy, retinopathy, and vascular changes.

● PERIPHERAL NEUROPATHY

Neuropathy is a general term that refers to pathologic changes in nerves. Neuropathies in clients with diabetes can affect motor, sensory, and autonomic nerves. Neuropathies develop 10 or more years after the onset of diabetes, but the incidence increases with the duration. Because their onset is gradual, the client usually is oblivious to the development in early stages.

Pathophysiology and Etiology

Neuropathy results from poor glucose control and decreased blood circulation to nerve tissue. Manifestations of peripheral neuropathies are more common among clients with diabetes who smoke and whose blood glucose level is poorly controlled. Because nitric acid dilates blood vessels, some believe that consistently elevated blood glucose levels lower nitric acid levels, impair circulation, and subsequently damage peripheral nerves.

Motor Neuropathy

When motor nerves are affected, the muscles weaken and atrophy. Joint support is diminished. The feet widen. Eventually bone structure is affected, resulting in skeletal deformities, usually in the feet and ankles, with subsequent changes in gait. Areas of skin and soft tissue that are subjected to friction and pressure are prone to ulcerate (Fig. 58-10). If there is infection or impaired healing, portions of the affected extremity may require amputation (see Chap. 67).

FIGURE 58-10 Neuropathic ulcers occur on pressure points in areas with diminished sensation in diabetic polyneuropathy. Pain is absent (and therefore the ulcer may go unnoticed). (Smeltzer, S. C. & Bare, B. G. [2000]. *Brunner & Suddarth's textbook of medical–surgical nursing* [9th ed.]. Philadelphia: Lippincott Williams & Wilkins.)

Sensory Neuropathy

Neuropathy involving sensory nerves leads to *paresthesias,* abnormal sensations like prickling, tingling, burning, or needle-like pain in the feet, legs, and sometimes hands. In severe cases, feeling is totally lost. This lack of sensitivity increases the potential for soft tissue injury without the client's awareness.

Autonomic Neuropathy

Neuropathy of autonomic nerves that affect organ functioning has several consequences. *Gastroparesis,* atony of the stomach, retards the movement of food from the stomach. If nerves that innervate the bladder are affected, the client does not sense the urge to void, and retained urine supports bacterial growth, causing frequent urinary tract infections. Incontinence also may occur when the bladder is overfilled. According to the American Diabetes Association, up to 50% of men with diabetes develop erectile dysfunction when nerves that promote erection become impaired. When autonomic nerves that affect cardiovascular function fail to function effectively, episodes of orthostatic hypotension occur. Clients with diabetes often do not sense the chest pain of angina as acutely as those without diabetes, which delays or interferes with prompt assessment and treatment of coronary artery disease and myocardial infarction.

Assessment Findings

Signs and Symptoms

Pain is one of the leading symptoms that accompany motor and sensory nerve changes. Skeletal muscles in the extremities become smaller. The feet swell and become insensitive to temperature or other tactile stimuli. Disturbing sensations develop that often are intensified by maintaining a position for an extended period, such as occupational tasks that require standing in place, holding the steering wheel while driving, or performing a repetitive motion like knitting. The client may report digestive, urinary, and sexual dysfunction and dizziness when rising.

Diagnostic Findings

A neurologic examination validates that when a tuning fork is in contact with the skin of the extremities, the client has diminished vibratory sense. Loss of protective sensation, the ability to sense and differentiate hot and cold, sharp and dull, and soft and rough stimuli, occurs. This is demonstrated with a screening test in which areas of the feet are touched with a nylon filament that delivers 10 g of force without the client's perception. Electromyo-graphy studies demonstrate a slowed conduction of electrical stimulation along nerves (see Chap. 44).

Medical Management

Diet, exercise, and medication control blood glucose levels. Several medications can reduce pain, such as non-narcotic analgesics or a tricyclic antidepressant such as imipramine (Tofranil). Anticonvulsants like gabapentin (Neurontin), carbamazepine (Tegretol), or phenytoin (Dilantin) also provide pain relief. Nonpharmacologic pain relief can be facilitated with transcutaneous electrical nerve stimulation. Elastic compression stockings, increasing dietary sodium, administration of fludrocortisone (Florinef), which increases fluid volume, or a trial with an antihypotensive agent such as midodrine (ProAmatine), help reduce orthostatic hypotension. Small, frequent meals or administration of metoclopramide (Reglan) are recommended for the relief of symptoms associated with gastroparesis. Antibiotic therapy, increased oral fluid intake, and urinating every 3 hours helps eliminate urinary tract infections. Various options are available for men who are concerned about erectile dysfunction (see Chap. 61).

Several pharmaceutical companies are developing drugs that might reverse diabetic neuropathies. Clinical trials include aldose reductase inhibitors (ARI), which reduce the conversion of high blood glucose to sorbitol, which is known to damage nerve and renal cells, and insulin-like growth factor-1, a protein that promotes neural conduction and regrowth of nerve axons. Neither drug category has been approved for general use, however; in fact, one study on a promising ARI has been suspended because the drug caused renal toxicity in high doses.

Nursing Management

The nurse implements a teaching plan for the management of diabetes and its potential complications. If possible, the primary care nurse refers the client for classes with a diabetes educator. The nurse stresses foot care (Client and Family Teaching Box 58-1) and advises the client with peripheral autonomic neuropathy to rise slowly from a lying or sitting position, to drink generous fluids, and to wear knee-high or thigh-high elastic stockings during waking hours. The nurse emphasizes compliance with prescribed medications and warns the client to avoid taking more than the recommended doses of analgesics. For digestive problems, he or she explains that consuming a large volume of food at any one sitting and eating fatty foods delays stomach emptying. The nurse refers clients with erectile dysfunction to a urologist.

58-1 *Client and Family Teaching*
Foot Care in Diabetes

The nurse instructs the client and family as follows:

- Inspect the feet daily for blisters, corns, calluses, long or ingrown nails, or any reddened areas; use a mirror if necessary to visualize all aspects of the foot.
- Wash the feet daily in warm (not hot) water.
- Dry the feet thoroughly, being careful to dry between the toes.
- Keep toenails short and cut straight across.
- Apply a moisturizer to feet daily.
- Do not use razor, abrasive, or commercial products to remove corns or calluses.
- Use lamb's wool between toes that overlap.
- Wear well-fitting shoes that fit comfortably when first worn; do not wear rubber, plastic, or vinyl shoes that cause the feet to perspire. Consult physician about wearing sneakers.
- Never go barefoot.
- Visit a podiatrist regularly for foot care.
- Wash, dry, and cover any injuries with sterile gauze and call healthcare provider immediately for evaluation.
- Notify the physician about a blister, abrasion, or foot injury.

● DIABETIC NEPHROPATHY

Diabetic nephropathy refers to the progressive decrease in renal function that occurs with diabetes mellitus. Clients with type 1 diabetes are most likely to develop diabetic nephropathy, but clients with type 2 diabetes also are affected.

Pathophysiology and Etiology

Nephropathy is a consequence of glomerular deterioration resulting in impaired filtration of blood during urine formation (see Chap 63). There are five stages of nephropathy, each characterized by a successive progression of renal dysfunction (Table 58-5). Essentially, the glomeruli excrete blood proteins, especially albumin, and lose their ability to excrete nitrogen waste products.

Poor glucose control contributes to the onset of nephropathy. Although hypertension is an eventual consequence of diabetic nephropathy, when it occurs in the prediabetic or prenephropathic state, it accelerates the onset and progression of renal damage. Nephropathy is associated with retinopathy and systemic vascular changes (discussed later).

Assessment Findings

In the early stages, the client does not manifest any obvious signs and symptoms. Eventually, he or she notices swelling of the feet and hands, most likely from the loss of albumin, a colloid that pulls water into the vascular system. The blood pressure increases gradually. The client feels tired and weak.

A routine urinalysis or dip with a chemical strip detects albumin in the urine. The blood urea nitrogen and serum creatinine become elevated. The renal creatinine clearance is decreased.

TABLE 58-5	STAGES OF DIABETIC NEPHROPATHY		
STAGE	CHARACTERISTICS	EFFECTS	AVERAGE ONSET AFTER DIAGNOSIS OF DIABETES
Stage I	Hyperfiltration Glomerular hypertrophy	Blood flow through kidneys is increased. Kidneys are enlarged.	10 yr
Stage II	Microalbuminuria	Albumin, a blood protein, is excreted in small amounts.	
Stage III	Gross albuminuria	Large amount of albumin is excreted; urine consistently tests positive for its presence. Blood pressure becomes elevated. Excretion of nitrogen wastes is impaired.	15 yr
Stage IV	Advanced dysfunction	Severe impairment of glomerular filtration is evidenced by excessive proteinuria, hypertension, and rise in blood urea nitrogen and creatinine levels.	
Stage V	End-stage renal failure	Kidney functions are severely impaired; dialysis or renal transplantation is necessary.	20–25 yr

Medical Management

Controlling both blood glucose levels and hypertension can prevent or delay the development of diabetic nephropathy. The National Heart, Lung, and Blood Institute recommends that clients with diabetes maintain their BP at or below 130/85 mm Hg. The target BP of clients with diabetes who already have developed proteinuria is at or lower than 125/75 mm Hg. Angiotensin-converting enzyme (ACE) inhibitors like captopril (Capoten) and angiotensin II receptor antagonists such as losartan (Cozaar) slow the progressive nature of nephropathy. A moderate reduction in dietary protein is beneficial. Smoking cessation is strongly recommended.

A new drug, aminoguanidine (Pimagedine), an advanced glycosylation end-product inhibitor, is under study. Results indicate that the yet-unapproved drug prevents or reduces damage to the glomeruli from excess glucose and decreases the urinary excretion of albumin. Research also has shown that aminoguanidine lowers blood lipid levels and slows retinal changes, raising the hope that, if the drug is approved, it can prevent or treat multiple complications of diabetes.

Nursing Management

The nurse monitors the client's blood glucose and hemoglobin A1c results. He or she checks the urine with a test strip to detect evidence of albuminuria. The nurse provides additional teaching if the client's blood glucose level is not controlled. He or she refers the client to programs that assist with smoking cessation or discusses the possibility of nicotine patches or gum to control further habituation. The nurse explains the therapeutic regimen associated with prescribed antihypertensive drugs and dietary measures for lowering BP and complications from vascular disease (see Chap. 35). Because nephropathy is progressive, the nurse encourages the client to keep appointments for regular medical follow-up.

● DIABETIC RETINOPATHY

Diabetic retinopathy refers to pathologic changes in the retina that are experienced by persons with diabetes. On average, it develops 10 or more years after the onset of diabetes. The earlier retinopathy develops, the more likely it is that vision will rapidly deteriorate.

Pathophysiology and Etiology

Diabetic retinopathy is a consequence of inadequately controlled blood glucose levels, which cause vascular changes in the retina (Fig. 58-11).

A

B

FIGURE 58-11 (**A**) In the normal eye, the light circular area over which several blood vessels converge is the optic disc, where the optic nerve meets the back of the eye. (**B**) In diabetic retinopathy, the fundus photograph shows characteristic waxy-looking lesions, microaneurysms, and hemorrhages.

There are two types: (1) nonproliferative retinopathy is the milder manifestation, and (2) proliferative retinopathy, the more severe form, can lead to blindness. In nonproliferative retinopathy, *microaneurysms,* outpouchings in retinal capillaries, develop from high vascular pressure and compromised circulation. The stasis of blood flow interferes with transferring substances between the retina and blood vessels. The deprived retinal cells swell.

In the more advanced, proliferative form, damaged blood vessels are replaced with new ones that grow along the surface of the retina. The newer blood vessels, however, are more fragile. They tend to rupture and leak blood into the vitreous, the gel-like fluid that fills the posterior portion of the eye. Inelastic scar tissue forms, which alters the shape of the retina, causes distorted vision, and pulls at the retina, increasing the potential for retinal detachment.

Assessment Findings

Clients with nonproliferative and proliferative retinopathy may not experience any visual changes for some time.

When symptoms do occur, the client reports blurred vision, no vision in spotty areas, or seeing debris floating about the visual field.

Visual acuity is diminished. Ophthalmic examination reveals swelling near the macula of the eye, an area lateral to the optic nerve that provides acute central vision. Fluorescein angiography documents changes in retinal blood vessels photographically (see Chap. 49).

Medical Management

The client with diabetes is referred for an ophthalmic evaluation within 3 to 5 years after diagnosis. Some physicians may suggest yearly ophthalmic examinations. If there is evidence of retinal vessel changes, an ACE inhibitor like lisinopril (Prinivil) is prescribed to dilate the retinal blood vessels and improve blood flow. If vitreous hemorrhage already has occurred, some physicians prefer to let the condition resolve on its own, which may take up to 18 months. A more expeditious technique is to seal leaking or newly forming blood vessels with laser photocoagulation. A vitrectomy, removal of bloodied vitreous, also improves the clarity of vision. Physicians hope that within 1 to 2 years, when clinical trials are complete, a drug called Vitrase will be available for use. Vitrase has been shown to clear the bloodied vitreous after intraocular injection in approximately 1 month. Researchers also hope to provide physicians in the near future with a genetically engineered form of angiopoietin, a vascular growth factor that stimulates the repair of leaky retinal blood vessels.

Nursing Management

The nurse encourages clients with diabetes to follow their therapeutic regimen to facilitate tight glucose control. He or she teaches clients about complications associated with diabetes and encourages regular ophthalmic examinations. When medications are prescribed, the nurse explains their purpose, techniques for self-administration, side effects, and symptoms that are important to report to the prescribing physician.

● VASCULAR DISTURBANCES

Vascular disturbances affect many tissues and organs, as described in previous discussions of peripheral neuropathy, diabetic nephropathy, and retinopathy. In clients with diabetes, however, all the arteries and arterioles are more susceptible to accelerated atherosclerotic and arteriosclerotic changes than in clients without diabetes.

Pathophysiology and Etiology

A consistent finding in clients with diabetes is thickening of the arterial walls. The incidence of coronary artery disease also is increased. One possible explanation for obesity among clients with diabetes is that the brain may be insensitive to leptin, a chemical that signals satiation. A lack of response to leptin promotes overeating, which contributes to hyperlipidemia.

Assessment Findings

Peripheral vascular changes are one of the most common complications associated with diabetes (see Chap. 33). Because of a decreased blood supply, the extremities are pale and cool. Leg cramps can occur. Gangrene develops if blood supply to the extremities is markedly diminished. Uncontrolled infection leads to skin ulcers. Clients with diabetes are likely to develop chest discomfort when the coronary arteries are affected. Myocardial infarctions occur at a much earlier age than among the nondiabetic population.

Hyperlipidemia and elevated triglyceride levels correlate with the predisposition to atherosclerosis. Angiography and Doppler ultrasonic flow studies indicate peripheral vascular disease.

Medical and Surgical Management

Atherosclerosis is managed with lipid-lowering measures such as a low-fat diet, exercise, and medications. Vasodilators are prescribed to combat the effects of arteriosclerosis. Drugs that reduce platelet aggregation (e.g., aspirin) are prescribed prophylactically. Smoking cessation is advised. Impaired skin is managed with aggressive measures to promote healing (see Chap. 33). Uncontrolled gangrene of the extremities can result in amputation. The lower extremities are involved most often. Any type of surgery or hospitalization is an enormous stressor. The diabetic client's glucose levels increase, with a concomitant increased demand for insulin. The healthcare team closely monitors the client's blood glucose levels. Either higher doses of insulin or antidiabetic drugs are prescribed, or elevated blood glucose levels are covered by administering rapid-acting or short-acting insulin before meals and at bedtime.

Nursing Management

Nursing management is geared toward the type of vascular disturbance and the signs and symptoms the client experiences.

GENERAL NUTRITIONAL CONSIDERATIONS

Nutrition therapy is the cornerstone of treatment for all clients with diabetes, regardless of weight, blood glucose levels, or use of medication. There no longer is one diabetic diet that is appropriate for all individuals; meal plans are individualized according to the assessment data and treatment goals. Traditional assumptions that sugar causes blood glucose levels to rise too high and too quickly no longer hold true. Today, consistency in the total amount of carbohydrate consumed is considered a more important factor influencing blood glucose level than is the type of carbohydrate eaten.

Because most clients with type 1 diabetes are of normal weight, calorie allowances are calculated for weight maintenance. Weight loss is the focus of nutrition intervention for clients with type 2 diabetes. A low-calorie diet may immediately improve clinical symptoms; even a mild to moderate weight loss (e.g., 10 to 20 lb) can lower blood glucose levels and improve insulin action. Because gradual weight loss is easier to maintain than rapid loss, and because weight fluctuations can be detrimental to long-range goals, a 1/2- to 1-lb loss per week is recommended.

Diet recommendations issued by the American Diabetes Association in 1994 state that saturated fat intake should provide less than 10% of total calories to reduce the risk of cardiovascular disease, and that polyunsaturated fat provide up to 10% of total calories. The percentage of total fat in the diet is determined by assessment data; 30% of calories from total fat may be appropriate for normal-weight clients with normal lipid levels, whereas lower-fat diets may promote weight loss in obese clients. Unless the client has nephropathy, protein recommendations for diabetic clients are the same as for the general public, approximately 10% to 20% of total calories. The remainder of calories in the diet is provided by carbohydrates; consistency in the total amount of carbohydrates consumed daily is emphasized.

The nutrition recommendations for diabetes are merely guidelines; the actual content of the diet depends on the client's assessment data and ability and willingness to change eating habits. The diet should be designed so that a minimal amount of adjustment is needed. Goals can best be met by providing information in stages, beginning with basic information and progressing to in-depth details, if the client is so motivated. Some clients never progress beyond basic information, which is acceptable as long as goals are met.

The use of exchange lists simplifies meal planning, eliminates the need for daily calculations, and offers variety. Clients are given a meal pattern that specifies how many servings from each food exchange are allowed at each meal and snack. Factors that influence which and how many exchanges are allowed at what times include the total calorie allowance, the type of medication used, and the client's preferences and lifestyle.

Elderly diabetic clients who are not treated with medication may simply be told to avoid "sugar."

GENERAL PHARMACOLOGIC CONSIDERATIONS

The three important properties of insulin are onset, when the insulin first begins to act in the body; peak, the time when insulin is exerting maximum action; and, duration, the time the insulin remains in effect.

Oral antidiabetic agents usually are used to treat clients whose diabetes can be controlled by 40 or fewer units of insulin per day.

The measurement of insulin must be accurate because clients may be sensitive to minute dose changes. Observe the client for signs of hypoglycemia at the expected onset and again at the peak of action.

Hospital policy may dictate the actions to take when a client taking insulin or an oral antidiabetic agent experiences hypoglycemia. Most hospitals approve of the administration of oral glucose, fruit juice, Karo syrup and water, ginger ale, and others substances if the client can safely swallow. The unconscious or semiconscious client requires IV administration of 50% dextrose or glucagon.

Observe the client receiving an oral antidiabetic agent for signs of hypoglycemia. The time when the reaction might occur is not predictable and could be from 30 to 60 minutes to several hours after the drug is ingested.

Make certain that the client understands that insulin and the oral antidiabetic drugs are used to control hyperglycemia, but do not cure diabetes.

The sulfonylureas may interact with other drugs such as diuretics, antihypertensives, and thyroid preparations and, depending on the specific drug, may increase or decrease the effects of the sulfonylurea.

The oral antidiabetic drugs may be used in conjunction with insulin therapy in some clients with insulin-dependent diabetes; this reduces the insulin requirement and decreases the incidence of hypoglycemic reactions.

Use of alcohol with the oral hypoglycemic drugs may result in abdominal cramps, nausea, flushing, headache, and hypoglycemia.

GENERAL GERONTOLOGIC CONSIDERATIONS

Diabetes mellitus is especially prevalent among older adults. Many older clients with diabetes can learn to care for themselves if they receive sufficient time, instruction, and help in overcoming disabilities.

Although it is useful for a family member to learn how to care for the older adult with diabetes, be certain actively to include the client unless it is evident that the client cannot safely assume responsibility for his or her own treatment.

Some older clients experience difficulty in administering their insulin because of problems such as decreased visual acuity or arthritis. Evaluate the client's ability to self-administer insulin before developing a teaching program.

A variety of aids, such as a magnifier that fits over the syringe, are available for clients who experience difficulty in preparing insulin for injection.

The eating and sleeping habits of older adults often differ from those of young or middle-aged persons. Take this into consideration when planning meals and selecting the proper type and dosage of insulin or oral hypoglycemic agent.

Good foot care is especially important in the older adult because other diseases common in this population, such as peripheral vascular disease and osteoarthritis, increase the risk of complications related to the feet. The client should consult a podiatrist at regular intervals.

Cognitive problems such as depression, dementia, or Alzheimer's disease can interfere with the management of diabetes.

Because older adults usually take several drugs, review all drugs (both prescription and nonprescription) for any that may interact with the oral antidiabetic drugs.

Critical Thinking Exercises

1. *A client with diabetes mellitus has not followed the diet prescribed by his physician. What information would you include*

in a teaching plan for this client? What approach would you take to reinforce the importance of diet in the management of diabetes?

2. *Explain the differences between the signs and symptoms of hyperglycemia and hypoglycemia.*

References and Suggested Readings

American Diabetes Association. (2002). One step closer to a cure. [On-line.] Available: http://ada.yellowbrix.com/pages/ada/Story.nsp?story_id=26991107&ID=ada.

Beebe, C. & O'Donnell, M. (2001). Educating patients with type 2 diabetes. *Nursing Clinics of North America, 36,* 375–386.

Braun, L. T. (2001). Lipid disorders in type 2 diabetes. *Nursing Clinics of North America, 36,* 291–302.

Brosnan, C. A., Upchurch, S., & Schreiner, B. (2001). Type 2 diabetes in children and adolescents: An emerging disease. *Journal of Pediatric Health Care, 15,* 187–193.

Camporeale, J. (2001). Client challenge: Teaching an insulin-dependent blind patient about self-care. *Home Healthcare Nurse, 19,* 247–250.

Chu, J. (2001). A breath of fresh insulin: Inhaled insulin may be a welcome answer for millions. *American Journal of Nursing, 101*(10), 30.

Chyun, D. A. (2001). Diabetes and coronary heart disease: A time for action. *Critical Care Nursing, 21*(1), 10, 12, 14–16.

Clarke, P. (2001). Developments in insulin therapy and diabetes management. *Journal of Diabetes Nursing, 5*(2), 56–58.

Colwell, L., Quinn, L. (2001). Glycemic control and heart disease. *Nursing Clinics of North America, 36,* 321–331.

Conlon, P. C. (2001). A practical approach to type 2 diabetes. *Nursing Clinics of North America, 36,* 193–202.

Creviston, T. & Quinn, L. (2001). Exercise and physical activity in the treatment of type 2 diabetes. *Nursing Clinics of North America, 36,* 243–272.

Cromie, W. J. (2001). Adult stem cells effect a cure. *Harvard Gazette Archives.* [On-line.] Available: http://www.news.harvard.edu/gazette/2001/08.16/01-stemcells.html.

Cunningham, M. A. (2001). Glucose monitoring in type 2 diabetes. *Nursing Clinics of North America, 36,* 361–374.

Cypress, M. (2001). Acute complications. *RN, 64*(4), 26–32.

Expert Committee on the Diagnosis and Classification of Diabetes Mellitus. (1997). The report of the Expert Committee on the Diagnosis and Classification of Diabetes Mellitus. *Diabetes Care, 20,* 1183–1197.

Fain, J. A. (2001). Lowering the boom on hyperglycemia. *Nursing, 21*(8), 48–50.

Fritschi, C. (2001). Preventive care of the diabetic foot. *Nursing Clinics of North America, 36,* 303–320.

Gottlieb, S. (2000). Islet cell transplantation more successful than previously thought. *British Medical Journal.* [On-line.] Available: http://www.findarticles.com/cf_dis/m0999/7257_321/64980320/print.jhtml.

Hardman, L. & Young, F. T. (2001). Combating hyperosmolar hyperglycemic nonketotic syndrome. *Nursing, 31*(3), Hospital Nursing: 32hn1–32hn2, 32hn4.

Insulin-Free World Foundation. (2002). [On-line.] Available: http://www.insulin-free.org

Kolata, G. (2002, January 15). Doctors advance in helping body repair itself. *New York Times.* [On-line.] Available: http://www.nytimes.com.

MGH researchers first to identify genetic malfunction in type I diabetes. (1999). *Science Daily.* [On-line.] Available: http://www.sciencedaily.com/releases/1999/11/991125091030.htm.

Ogden. V. (1999). Promoting good foot care in type 2 diabetes. *Journal of Community Nursing, 13*(8), 10, 12, 14+.

Porth, C. M. (2002). *Pathophysiology: Concepts of altered health states* (6th ed.). Philadelphia: Lippincott Williams & Wilkins.

Plummer, E. S. (2001). Diabetes update: Chronic complications. *RN, 64*(5), 34–36, 38–40.

Quinn, L. (2001). Diabetes emergencies in the patient with type 2 diabetes. *Nursing Clinics of North America, 36,* 341–360.

Quinn, L. (2001). Pharmacologic management of the patient with type 2 diabetes. *Nursing Clinics of North America, 36,* 217–242.

Quinn, L. (2001). Type 2 diabetes: Epidemiology, pathophysiology, and diagnosis. *Nursing Clinics of North America, 36,* 175–192.

Rezabek, K. M. (2001). Medical nutrition therapy in type 2 diabetes. *Nursing Clinics of North America, 36,* 203–216.

Ruiz, E. K. (2001). Diabetes update: Type 2 disease in children. *RN, 64*(10), 44–48, 50, 82–83.

Sammer, C. E. (2001). How should you respond to hypoglycemia? *Nursing, 31*(7), 48–50.

Simple therapy cures mice of type I diabetes. (2001). *Focus, News from Harvard Medical, Dental & Public Health Schools.* [On-line.] Available: http://www.med.harvard.edu/publications/Focus/2001/Jul13_2001/immunology.html

Springett, K. (2001). Foot ulceration in diabetic patients. *Primary Health Care, 11*(8), 27–31.

Study offers new theory on treating type I diabetes. (2002). *Society for Women's Health Research.* [On-line.] Available: http://www.womens-health.org/faustmanpr.html.

Tamborlane, W. & Nattrass, M. (2001). Insulin analogues. *Journal of Diabetes Nursing, 5*(3), 93.

Treatment could end daily jabs . . . type 1 diabetes could be conquered in 10 years. (2001). *Nursing Times, 97*(5), 8.

Uzun, S. & Inanc, N. (2001). Determining optimal needle length for subcutaneous insulin injection. *Journal of Diabetes Nursing, 5*(3), 83–87.

Williams, J. A. (2001). Diabetes update: We make foot exams a priority. *RN, 64*(5), 40.

chapter **59**

Caring for Female Clients With Disorders of Pelvic Reproductive Structures

Words to Know

amenorrhea
carcinoma in situ
cervicitis
conization
cystocele
dilatation and curettage
dysmenorrhea
dyspareunia
endometrial ablation
endometriosis
fertilization
fibroid tumors
fistula
gynecologic examination
hormone replacement
  therapy
hysterectomy
implantation
Kegel exercises
libido
menarche

menopause
menorrhagia
menstrual diary
menstruation
metrorrhagia
oligomenorrhea
oophorectomy
ova
ovulation
Papanicolaou test
pelvic inflammatory
  disease
premenstrual
  syndrome
rectocele
salpingo-
  oophorectomy
sterility
toxic shock syndrome
vaginitis

Learning Objectives

On completion of this chapter, the reader will:

- Name three reproductive processes associated with sexual maturation.
- Explain the processes of ovulation, fertilization, implantation, and menstruation.
- Name at least four conditions that deviate from normal menstrual patterns.
- Describe the purpose of and how to keep a menstrual diary.
- Discuss therapeutic techniques for managing menstrual disorders.
- Discuss the nurse's role in caring for clients with menstrual disorders.
- List several physiologic consequences of menopause and the benefits of hormone replacement therapy.
- Name four infectious and inflammatory conditions common in women and one cause for each.
- Describe the signs and symptoms that differentiate three types of vaginal infections.
- Discuss methods that may help prevent vaginal infections or their recurrence.
- Describe the technique for inserting vaginal medications.
- Name at least four aspects of nursing care for clients with pelvic inflammatory disease.
- Give at least two suggestions that can help women avoid toxic shock syndrome.
- List four structural abnormalities of the female reproductive system and their effects on fertility or sexuality.
- Discuss methods the nurse can use to help a client decide on an appropriate treatment for endometriosis.
- List three problems experienced by women who develop vaginal fistulas, and related nursing management.
- Give examples of appropriate information when teaching a client to use a pessary.
- Explain the term *carcinoma in situ* and how it applies to the prognosis of women with gynecologic malignancies.
- Identify the most common reproductive cancers and methods for early diagnosis.
- Discuss nursing diagnoses and potential complications among clients who undergo a hysterectomy, and nursing interventions important to include in their care.
- Give two reasons that explain the high lethality associated with ovarian cancer.
- Name three possible causes of vaginal cancer.
- Discuss the nursing management of and appropriate discharge instructions for a client who has a radical vulvectomy for vulvar cancer.

Diseases or disorders of pelvic reproductive structures can profoundly affect a woman's health and sexuality. Some common problems for which adult women seek healthcare include disturbances in menstruation, infectious and inflammatory disorders, structural abnormalities, and benign and malignant tumors of the reproductive system.

ANATOMY AND PHYSIOLOGY

External and Internal Structures

The female reproductive system consists of external and internal structures. The external structures include the breasts (see Chap. 60) and female genitalia (Fig. 59-1). The genitalia comprise the vaginal orifice (opening), labia majora, labia minora, and clitoris.

The internal structures of the female reproductive system (Fig. 59-2) consist of two ovaries, two fallopian tubes, the uterus, and the vagina. The two ovaries (female gonads) lie behind and slightly below the ends of the fallopian tubes. Each ovary contains thousands of **ova** (sing., *ovum*), all of which are present at birth. The ovaries secrete two hormones: estrogen, which is responsible for secondary sexual characteristics such as breast development and the preparation of the uterus for conception, and progesterone (discussed later).

After **puberty,** which is the onset of sexual maturation, and up to **menopause,** the termination of female fertility, three processes occur: ovulation, pregnancy, and menstruation.

Ovulation

The role of the internal reproductive structures is to release and transport ova and to support the implantation and nourishment of a fertilized ovum. The cyclical release of an ovum is known as **ovulation** and occurs under the influence of pituitary hormones.

Ovulation is initiated monthly by the anterior pituitary hormone known as follicle-stimulating hormone (FSH). It triggers the maturation of a follicle in one of the ovaries and an increased production of ovarian estrogen. A second pituitary hormone, luteinizing hormone (LH), causes the mature follicle to rupture, thereby releasing an ovum from the ovary (Fig. 59-3). After the ovum is released, movement of the cilia at the end of the fallopian tube combined with muscular contractions of the tube itself draw the ovum toward the uterus.

Meanwhile, the endometrium, the inner lining of the uterus, becomes thick and vascular in response to the secretion of estrogen. The ruptured follicle is transformed into the corpus luteum, a small body filled with yellow fluid. The corpus luteum secretes progesterone, a hormone that sustains the lining of the uterus should fertilization occur.

Pregnancy

Pregnancy occurs as a result of fertilization and implantation. **Fertilization,** the union of an ovum and a spermatozoon (pl., *spermatozoa*), normally occurs in the fallopian tube. At the moment a sperm penetrates the ovum, the number of chromosomes is complete, making it possible for an embryo to develop. The fertilized ovum, or zygote, then proceeds down the uterus and attaches itself in the endometrium, a process referred to as **implantation.** Once fertilization and implantation occur, the pituitary production of FSH is inhibited so that ovulation is temporarily halted.

Menstruation

If the ovum is not fertilized, the production of progesterone by the corpus luteum begins to decrease until it changes from a yellow to a white spot on the ovary (corpus albicans). Without the high level of progesterone, the endometrium degenerates and is shed, a process referred to as **menstruation.** Menstruation begins about 2 weeks after ovulation. Menstrual flow usually lasts 4 to 5 days, with a normal loss of 30 to 60 mL of blood. Women who have a heavy menses, or menstrual flow, lose more blood.

External female genitalia.

- Mons pubis
- Prepuce
- Clitoris
- Labia majora
- Urinary meatus
- Labia minora
- Vaginal introitus
- Hymen
- Perineum
- Anus

FIGURE 59-1 Female external genitalia.

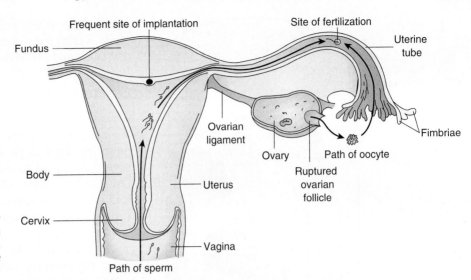

FIGURE 59-2 Schematic drawing of female reproductive organs, showing path of ovum from ovary into fallopian tube, path of spermatozoa, and the usual site of fertilization and implantation.

After menstruation, the endometrium becomes thicker and more vascular again in preparation for a possible pregnancy. Because of these hormone-dependent changes, the microscopic characteristics of the uterus are in a cyclical state of transition. Thus, it is important that each gynecologic specimen sent to the laboratory is marked with the date of the beginning of the client's last menstrual period (LMP).

ASSESSMENT

Health History

To ensure a thorough baseline history, the nurse obtains the following information:

- General health and family history
- Age of **menarche,** the first menstruation
- Date of client's LMP, description of the menstrual pattern and flow, other symptoms associated with menstruation
- Risks for sexually transmitted diseases (see Chap. 62)
- Pregnancy history: number of pregnancies, live births, stillborn births; type of fetal abnormalities
- Abortion history
- Contraceptive practices
- Age of menopause, associated symptoms, and use of hormone replacement therapy (HRT)
- Date of last gynecologic and breast examination, including mammograms and Papanicolaou tests
- Prior treatments or surgery for a gynecologic disorder
- Drug, allergy, substance abuse, and smoking history
- Symptoms of present disorder, such as painful intercourse or characteristics of vaginal discharge, and duration

Gynecologic Examination (Pelvic Examination)

A physician, clinical nurse specialist, physician's assistant, or nurse practitioner performs the **gynecologic examination,** an inspection and palpation of pelvic reproductive structures. Inspection of the external genitalia and adjacent structures occurs first, followed by the inspection of the vaginal wall and cervix using a bivalve speculum (Fig. 59-4). Next, one or two fingers of a lubricated, gloved hand are placed into the vagina. By vaginal–abdominal palpation, the structures beyond the vaginal orifice are examined and the position, size, and contour of the uterus, ovaries, and other pelvic structures are assessed (Fig. 59-5). At the end of the examination, a gloved finger is inserted into the rectum to palpate the posterior surface of the uterus.

In preparation for the test, the nurse obtains examination gloves, lubricant, several sizes of bivalve speculums, a light source, and materials for obtaining a Papanicolaou test (discussed next). The nurse is sensitive to the fact that many women dislike having gynecologic examinations because they anticipate discomfort, are embarrassed, and have anxiety over possible diagnoses.

Diagnostic Tests

Cytologic Test for Cancer (Papanicolaou Test)

A **Papanicolaou test** (Pap test) is an important cancer screening tool. It involves obtaining a sample of exfoliated cells (dead cells that are shed). The specimens, which are best obtained 2 weeks after the first day of the LMP, are removed by scraping and brushing tissue during the pelvic examination. The test is used mainly to detect early cancer of the cervix and secondarily to determine estrogen activity as it relates to menopause or endocrine abnormalities. See Box 59-1 for the classification system.

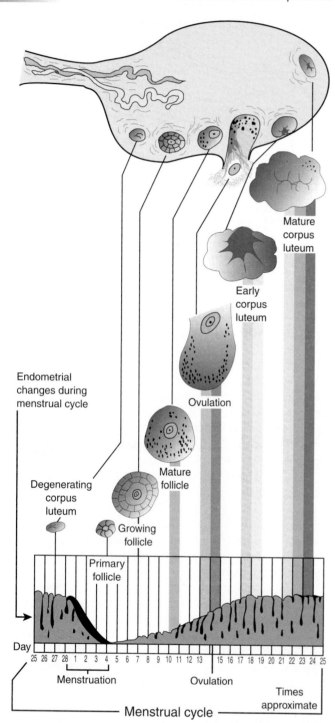

Endometrial changes during menstrual cycle

Mature corpus luteum

Early corpus luteum

Ovulation

Degenerating corpus luteum

Mature follicle

Growing follicle

Primary follicle

Day
25 26 27 28 1 2 3 4 5 6 7 8 9 10 11 12 13 15 16 17 18 19 20 21 22 23 24 25

Menstruation   Ovulation

Times approximate

Menstrual cycle

FIGURE 59-3 One menstrual cycle and the corresponding endometrial changes. (Smeltzer, S. C. & Bare, B. G. [2000]. *Brunner & Suddarth's textbook of medical–surgical nursing* [9th ed.]. Philadelphia: Lippincott Williams & Wilkins.)

The American Cancer Society recommends that all women have an initial Pap test at 18 years of age (or earlier if sexually active). Women should then have them yearly for 3 years, then every 3 years if the results for the three prior tests are normal. The nurse advises the client to avoid intercourse for 2 days and douching for 1 day before the test. When assisting with the examination, the nurse obtains the required materials, prepares the client, and labels and preserves the specimens (Fig. 59-6).

Cervical Biopsy

A cervical biopsy is performed when results from a Pap test are positive or questionable. Tissue is obtained by punching out multiple small samples or by **conization,** removing a larger cone-shaped section of cervical tissue. Conization is an invasive surgical procedure that is performed on an outpatient basis; it also is used to treat early-stage cervical cancer.

If the client is premenopausal, the nurse schedules the biopsy for 1 week after the end of a menstrual period, when the cervix is least vascular. He or she tells the client that cramps and slight spotting may occur afterward. The nurse recommends a mild analgesic for discomfort and advises the client to report severe pain or heavy bleeding.

Endometrial Smears and Biopsy

Diagnosing cancer of the endometrium, the inner lining of the uterus, is accomplished by aspirating endometrial tissue specimens or performing an endometrial biopsy. Of the two, the endometrial biopsy is more accurate. A smear is obtained by inserting a flexible cannula through the cervix and into the uterine cavity. The cannula is attached to a syringe that is used to aspirate secretions. This procedure usually is performed without anesthesia.

To obtain a biopsy specimen, a dilating instrument called a *uterine sound* is inserted through the cervical opening. A tissue sample is then obtained with a scraping instrument called a *curette,* or by aspiration. This procedure can be performed in the physician's office without anesthesia.

Dilatation and Curettage

Dilatation and curettage (D and C) is a surgical procedure in which the cervix is stretched open and the endometrium scraped (curettage). Dilatation and curettage is done to diagnose or treat various gynecologic problems (e.g., abnormal uterine bleeding) and to remove fetal and placental tissue. Samples of endometrial scrapings are obtained when the client is under general or light intravenous (IV) anesthesia. A vaginal and cervical pack usually is left in place and a sterile perineal pad applied before the client leaves the operating room. See Nursing Guidelines 59-1 for examples of discharge instructions.

Endoscopic Examinations

Endoscopic examinations are diagnostic procedures that use a lighted instrument inserted into the body for the pur-

A   **B**   **C**

FIGURE 59-4 Technique for speculum examination of the vagina and cervix. (**A**) Examiner uses a gloved left hand to spread apart labia while grasping the speculum with the right hand and turning it counterclockwise before insertion. (**B**) Insertion of the speculum, with the blades spread apart. (**C**) The cervical os. (Smeltzer, S. C. & Bare, B. G. [2000]. *Brunner & Suddarth's textbook of medical–surgical nursing* [9th ed.]. Philadelphia: Lippincott Williams & Wilkins.)

pose of visualizing structures not otherwise accessible. They are less invasive and more economical than using surgical techniques.

CULDOSCOPY

Culdoscopy, performed under local or general anesthesia, allows visualization of the uterus, broad ligaments, and fallopian tubes by inserting an endoscope through an incision made in the posterior vaginal wall. Ectopic pregnancy and pelvic masses can be visualized. Afterward, the

nurse observes the client for signs of internal bleeding and symptoms of shock.

LAPAROSCOPY

Laparoscopy is an examination of the interior of the abdomen using a special endoscope called a *laparoscope* (Fig. 59-7). It is inserted through a small incision located one-half inch below the umbilicus. Two or three liters of carbon dioxide or nitrous oxide gas are introduced into the peritoneal cavity to separate the intestines from the pelvic organs and facilitate visualization. Laparoscopy is used to detect an ectopic pregnancy, perform a tubal ligation, obtain ovarian tissue for biopsy, and detect pelvic abnormalities. The nurse can tell the client undergoing laparoscopy that she will experience discomfort in the shoulder as a result of the instillation of gas. The nurse checks the incisional sites for bleeding afterward and relieves discomfort by administering a prescribed analgesic.

COLPOSCOPY

A colposcopy is a procedure used to visualize the cervix and vagina. A speculum is inserted into the vagina, and the

FIGURE 59-5 Bimanual examination of the pelvis. (Smeltzer, S. C. & Bare, B. G. [2000]. *Brunner & Suddarth's textbook of medical–surgical nursing* [9th ed.]. Philadelphia: Lippincott Williams & Wilkins.)

BOX 59-1 ● Papanicolaou Classification System

Papanicolaou findings are described using the following numerical system:
Class 1—No atypical or abnormal cells
Class 2—Atypical cells but no evidence of malignancy
Class 3—Suggestive of but not conclusive for malignancy
Class 4—Strongly suggestive of malignancy
Class 5—Conclusive for malignancy

FIGURE 59-6 (**A**) With the speculum in place, the examiner uses the Ayre spatula to obtain cervical secretions. (**B**) He or she places the spatula tip in the cervical os and rotates the spatula 360°. (**C**) Examiner smears material that clings to the spatula smoothly on a glass slide and promptly places in a solution. (**D**) He or she rotates the cytobrush in the cervical os and rolls it onto a glass slide. (Smeltzer, S. C. & Bare, B. G. [2000]. *Brunner & Suddarth's textbook of medical–surgical nursing* [9th ed.]. Philadelphia: Lippincott Williams & Wilkins.)

surface areas are examined with a light and magnifying lens (colposcope). A cervical biopsy and Pap test can be taken at this time.

Hysterosalpingogram

A *hysterosalpingogram* is a radiographic examination that visualizes the uterus and fallopian tubes. It is used to detect deviations such as adhesions and to determine fallopian tube patency, other tubal abnormalities, or congenital malformations of these structures. A cannula is inserted into the cervix and contrast media injected. Fluoroscopic or radiographic films are then taken. Bowel preparation usually is necessary to clear the intestine of gas and fecal material that interferes with proper visualization of the uterus and fallopian tubes.

Abdominal Ultrasonography (Sonogram)

Ultrasonography aids in visualizing soft tissue by recording the reflection of sound waves. An abdominal ultrasound detects pelvic abnormalities such as tumors and the size and location of fetal and placental tissue. The nurse instructs the client to drink at least 1 quart of water 45 minutes to 1 hour before the test and not to void until after the test is completed. A full bladder facilitates the transmission of the ultrasound waves and elevates the bowel away from the other pelvic organs. Solid food may be restricted for 6 to 8 hours to avoid obscuring the image with gas and intestinal contents.

Laboratory Tests

Various laboratory tests, such as a complete blood cell count, hemoglobin, and serum electrolytes, are ordered to obtain a baseline of the client's health status. Culture and sensitivity tests are ordered if an infection is suspected. Ovarian hormone activity is evaluated by tests such as total urine estrogen and urine pregnanediol.

DISORDERS OF MENSTRUATION

● PREMENSTRUAL SYNDROME

Premenstrual syndrome (PMS), also known as *late luteal dysphoric disorder,* is a group of physical and emotional symptoms that occur in some women 7 to 10 days

before menstruation. Its cause is unknown; however, it has been proposed that PMS results from excess estrogen, deficient progesterone, or both; hypothalamic–pituitary dysregulation; or the effect of reproductive hormones on brain chemicals such as endorphins, melatonin, and serotonin. Women experience several symptoms, including weight gain; headache; nervousness; irritability; personality changes; depression; abdominal bloating; pain or tenderness of the breasts; breast enlargement; craving for sweets; swelling of the ankles, feet, and hands; anxiety; or increased physical activity. Diagnosis is based on data from a **menstrual diary** (Fig. 59-8) in which the client keeps daily recordings of her symptoms for at least 2 months. The classic finding is that the client is symptom free during the period between the onset of menstruation and ovulation.

Treatment of PMS depends on the severity and type of symptoms experienced. Hormonal drug therapy aims at manipulating the cyclic fluctuation in estrogen and progesterone. This is accomplished with oral contraceptives, progesterone therapy, synthetic androgens, or gonadotropin-releasing hormone (GnRH) analogs such as histrelin (Supprelin) and nafarelin (Synarel) for 6 months. In some instances, short-term therapy with tranquilizers or antidepressants is indicated. Non-narcotic analgesics, such as mefenamic acid (Ponstel), ibuprofen (Motrin), and naproxen (Anaprox), are given for discomfort.

The nurse encourages clients to make healthy lifestyle changes such as exercising, eating nutritiously, and managing stress more effectively to augment the medical treatment. He or she explains how to maintain an accurate menstrual diary and helps the client identify dietary sources of sodium so that she can restrict salt consumption during the second half of her menstrual cycle. The nurse explains drug therapy using oral contraceptives and stresses the importance of taking nonsteroidal anti-inflammatory drugs (NSAIDs) with food or after meals to avoid gastric distress. He or she tells the client who takes a GnRH analog that, because estrogen levels are pharmacologically suppressed, she may experience vaginal dryness that can make intercourse uncomfortable and a loss of bone density similar to osteoporosis (see nursing management of menopause for additional interventions).

● DYSMENORRHEA

Dysmenorrhea is painful menstruation and may be primary or secondary. Primary dysmenorrhea usually is idiopathic, and no abnormality is found. Secondary dysmenorrhea is a result of other disorders such as endometriosis, displacement of the uterus, or fibroid uterine tumors. Symptoms are lower abdominal pain and cramping, which may become more severe with fatigue, cold, and tension. Dysmenorrhea is treated with mild non-

FIGURE 59-7 Laparoscopy. (Smeltzer, S. C. & Bare, B. G. [2000]. *Brunner & Suddarth's textbook of medical–surgical nursing* [9th ed.]. Philadelphia: Lippincott Williams & Wilkins.)

Diagnostic Diary A: Evaluation of PMS Symptoms

NAME _____

YEAR _____

Grading of Symptoms:
0—*No Symptoms*   2—*Moderate Symptoms*
1—*Mild Symptoms*   3—*Severe Symptoms (i.e., Disabling)*

DAY OF CYCLE	1	2	3	4	5	6	7	8	9	10	11	12	13	14	15	16	17	18	19	20	21	22	23	24	25	26	27	28	29	30	31
DATE																															
MENSES																															

PSYCHOLOGICAL SYMPTOMS

Depression																															
Anxiety																															
Irritability																															
Lethargy																															
Insomnia																															
Forgetfulness																															
Confusion																															

PHYSICAL SYMPTOMS

Swelling																															
Breast tenderness																															
Abdominal bloating																															
Palpitations																															
Weight gain																															
Constipation																															
Headache																															
Rhinitis																															

PAIN SYMPTOMS (Usually NOT associated with PMS)

Menstrual cramps																															
Painful intercourse																															
Pelvic pain																															
Backache																															

Morning weight (lb)																															

FIGURE 59-8 Example of a diary kept by the client to track premenstrual symptoms. (Chihal, H. J. [1990]. *Premenstrual syndrome: A clinic manual* [2nd ed., pp. 80–81]. Dallas, TX: Essential Medical Information Systems.)

narcotic analgesics and by treating the underlying cause if one is identified.

For symptomatic relief of pain and discomfort, suggest local applications of heat, such as a warm shower, heating pad, or water bottle. Demonstrate how to assume a knee–chest position (Fig. 59-9) to relieve discomfort caused by retroversion (backward tilt) of the uterus. Encourage the client to obtain adequate rest, nutrition, and relief from stress to facilitate coping with periodic discomfort.

● AMENORRHEA AND OLIGOMENORRHEA

Amenorrhea is the absence of menstrual flow. *Primary amenorrhea* is the term used when a woman of reproductive age has never menstruated. If menstruation stops after menstrual cycles have occurred, it is called *secondary amenorrhea*. Secondary amenorrhea occurs normally during pregnancy, after menopause, sometimes throughout lactation, and when the ovaries or uterus are surgically removed. **Oligomenorrhea** is infrequent menses. It is perfectly normal for adolescent girls to experience oligomenorrhea for 1 year or more before they establish regular menses.

Oligomenorrhea and amenorrhea usually are caused by endocrine imbalances resulting from pituitary disorders or hypothyroidism, the stress response, or severely lean body mass. Female athletes, women with anorexia nervosa, or women with debilitating diseases can have such low levels of estrogen that menstruation ceases. Treatment focuses on correction of the underlying cause. Clients with eating disorders (see Chap. 16) require referral to appropriate psychiatric specialists.

● MENORRHAGIA

Menorrhagia is excessive bleeding at the time of normal menstruation. It may be quantified as menstrual flow that lasts more than 7 days, that requires the use of an additional two pads per day, or that extends 3 or more days longer than usual. It can be caused by endocrine, coagulation, or systemic disorders.

Symptomatic relief is accomplished with NSAIDs, progestins, and oral contraceptives with combinations of estrogen and progestin. NSAIDs reduce prostaglandins, biologic chemicals that exist in endometrial tissue, where they exert a stimulating effect on the uterus. Progestins, natural and synthetic forms of progesterone, transform the proliferative endometrium into a secretory endometrium that simulates a pregnant state. When combination oral contraceptives are administered, they produce a "pill period," which is characterized by light menstrual bleeding.

A D and C is performed for symptomatic relief; however, effectiveness sometimes lasts only 1 to 2 months. **Endometrial ablation** (detachment of the lining of the uterus) by photodynamic therapy or uterine balloon therapy is a potential nonsurgical alternative. When photodynamic therapy is used, a photosensitive substance is applied to endometrial tissue, after which a laser probe is inserted through the cervix. The absorption of laser light by the tissue causes the endometrium to slough, in contrast to being removed with a surgical curette. Uterine balloon therapy produces the same effect by introducing a heated balloon into the uterus for 8 minutes (Fig. 59-10). Both of these procedures are gaining popularity because they are cost-effective. The post-treatment course is similar to that after a D and C. See Client and Family Teaching Box 59-1 for education guidelines.

● METRORRHAGIA

Metrorrhagia is vaginal bleeding at a time other than a menstrual period. The amount of blood is not important; the fact that it occurs unexpectedly is significant. Irregular bleeding often is due to an erratic stimulation of or response to pituitary or ovarian hormones, especially in adolescent girls and perimenopausal women. Some women spot for a day or two midway between menstrual periods. This functional bleeding is attributed

FIGURE 59-9 Knee–chest position.

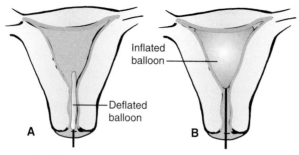

FIGURE 59-10 Uterine balloon therapy. (**A**) Insertion of the catheter. (**B**) Infusion and heating of fluid within the balloon.

to ovulation and is not considered abnormal. However, other causes for atypical bleeding include uterine malignancies, cervical irritation, or breakthrough bleeding that occurs with HRT or low-dose oral contraceptives. Intermenstrual or postcoital (after intercourse) bleeding needs to be evaluated promptly. Treatment depends on the underlying cause.

The nurse advises the client with unexplained bleeding to see a physician. For metrorrhagia or any menstrual disorder, the role of the nurse is the same: gather appropriate information; assist with gynecologic examinations; offer suggestions for relieving discomfort; instruct clients about their drug therapy; prepare clients for surgical interventions; care for them during recovery; and provide specific health-teaching instructions.

59-1 *Client and Family Teaching* Education After Dilatation and Curettage

Following a D and C, the nurse instructs the client as follows:

- Expect slight cramping and a dark, bloody discharge for a few days to several weeks.
- Report bright red bleeding, foul vaginal drainage, a fever, or pain that is intolerable despite mild analgesia.
- Change soiled perineal pads frequently and avoid tampons.
- Shower rather than take tub baths for 3 or 4 days.
- Refrain from strenuous exercises and heavy household cleaning for 4 to 5 days, after which full activity may be resumed.
- Wipe from front to back after bowel elimination to avoid introducing microorganisms into the vaginal canal or urethra.
- Delay intercourse and douching for 1 to 2 weeks or until the physician indicates that they may be resumed.

Stop, Think, and Respond ● BOX 59-1

What are the differences between primary and secondary amenorrhea and menorrhagia and metrorrhagia?

MENOPAUSE

Menopause ("change of life") is the cessation of the menstrual cycle. The climacteric or perimenopausal period refers to the time during which ovarian activity gradually ceases; the postmenopausal period begins 1 year after menstruation ceases. Menopause normally occurs between the ages of 45 and 55 years. Surgical menopause, which results when the ovaries are removed, occurs at any age.

Menopause is a natural physiologic process. The changes in hormone levels that accompany menopause cause a variety of reproductive and systemic effects. Some women have symptoms so mild and transitory that they go unnoticed; other women experience severe symptoms. Some women seek health care to reduce the risk for osteoporosis and cardiovascular disease that occur when estrogen production decreases.

Physiology

Menopause occurs when ovarian function diminishes. Levels of estrogen and progesterone are reduced, ovulation gradually ceases, menstruation becomes irregular until it stops, and natural reproductive capacity ends. As the levels of estrogen and progesterone drop, the hypothalamus attempts to raise them by releasing GnRH, which stimulates the anterior pituitary gland to release FSH and LH. The surge of hypothalamic–pituitary stimulation is thought to be responsible for altered temperature, sleep, and mood-regulating mechanisms. Estrogen deficiency causes thinning of the vaginal walls, breast and uterine atrophy, and loss of bone density. The risks for heart disease and stroke increase with estrogen reduction. Depression, should it occur, is thought to be related more to an individual's perception of the social or psychological implications of menopause rather than biologic factors.

Assessment Findings

Changing menstrual patterns, including irregular periods and scanty or sometimes unusually copious menstrual flow, signal the onset of menopause. Vasomotor disturbances such as hot flashes and sweats, sleep disturbance, irritability or depression, vaginal dryness, diminished **libido** (interest or desire for sex), or **dyspareunia** (discomfort during intercourse) are not uncommon and often are the symptoms for which women seek treatment. A cytologic examination of vaginal and cervical smears (Pap test) shows a decrease in estrogen production.

Medical Management

The decision to administer **hormone replacement therapy** (HRT), or estrogen combined with progestin, is made for each client on an individual basis. If HRT is indicated, it is prescribed in the lowest appropriate dose. It is believed that estrogen in small doses can help prevent osteoporosis and reduce the atherosclerotic process. The slight risk of endometrial or breast cancer is outweighed by the seriousness of future myocardial infarction, stroke, hip fracture, and kyphosis.

It may be necessary to treat some of the symptoms associated with menopause. Vaginal itching and drying is prevented or reduced by drugs such as an estrogen or cortisone cream or ointment. Low-dose androgens are added to the hormone replacement regimen to restore an interest in sexual activity. Antidepressants or minor tranquilizers are prescribed for women experiencing emotional problems.

Nursing Management

The nurse collects a database that includes a menstrual, reproductive, and sexual history and prepares and supports the client during physical and diagnostic examinations. Health teaching addresses topics such as normal developmental changes during middle adulthood (see Chap. 8), coping strategies, health promotion techniques, methods to achieve symptomatic relief, and treatment-related information.

Because normal and abnormal structural changes are easily confused, the nurse recommends regular gynecologic and breast examinations during and after menopause. The nurse also gives the following suggestions:

- Use bland skin creams or lotions to reduce skin dryness.
- Plan an exercise program to prevent weight gain and loss of calcium from the bones.
- Increase calcium intake by eating calcium-rich foods, or take a supplement.
- Take HRT by the oral, transdermal, or vaginal route, as prescribed.
- Discuss breakthrough bleeding or menses that may occur with HRT with the physician. Changing the dose or using a different combination of hormones may eliminate this effect.
- Cultivate new interests and hobbies or resume those that have been abandoned because of other responsibilities.

INFECTIOUS AND INFLAMMATORY DISORDERS OF THE FEMALE REPRODUCTIVE SYSTEM

● VAGINITIS

Vaginitis is a condition in which the vagina is inflamed.

Pathophysiology and Etiology

Vaginal inflammation is caused by chemical or mechanical irritants such as feminine hygiene products, allergic reactions, age-related tissue changes (atrophic vaginitis with menopause), and the most common etiology, infections. The pathogenic microorganisms frequently associated with vaginitis are the bacteria *Gardnerella vaginalis,* the protozoan *Trichomonas vaginalis,* and the yeast (fungus) *Candida albicans* (also see Chap. 62).

Although the vagina is self-protected by mucus-secreting cells and an acidic environment (pH of 3.5 to 4.5), the tissue still may become disrupted. Some situations predispose to vaginitis because they alter one or the other protective mechanism. For example, antibiotics or frequent douching eliminate the bacilli that promote an acidic vaginal environment. Decreased estrogen at menopause reduces the thick, moist consistency of vaginal tissue. Pregnant women, those with unregulated diabetes, and those who take oral contraceptives containing estrogen have an excess of glycogen in vaginal mucus, which supports the growth of microorganisms.

Assessment Findings

An abnormal vaginal discharge is the primary symptom of vaginal infection, and the characteristics of the discharge often are indicative of the infecting organism (Table 59-1). The discharge often is accompanied by itching, burning, redness, and swelling of surrounding tissues. Diagnosis is confirmed by visual and microscopic examination of secretions.

Medical Management

Infectious vaginitis is remedied by using drugs to which the microorganism is particularly sensitive. They include antifungal, antiprotozoal, and antibiotic agents (Drug Therapy Table 59-1). In some cases, the sexual partner also is infected and the vaginitis recurs if both are not treated simultaneously.

Atrophic vaginitis is relieved with estrogen replacement administered as a topical cream. If the client has diabetes mellitus, regulating blood glucose is an important aspect of treatment.

TABLE 59-1	CHARACTERISTICS OF VAGINAL INFECTIONS			
MICROORGANISM	COLOR OF DISCHARGE	CONSISTENCY	ODOR	OTHER SYMPTOMS
Candida albicans	Curdy white	Thick	Strong	Burning with urination
Trichomonas vaginalis	Yellow-white	Foamy	Foul	Severe itching
Gardnerella vaginalis	Gray-white	Watery	Fishy	More discharge after intercourse

Nursing Management

The nurse informs the client not to douche before the physical examination because washing away the secretions removes the characteristics of the vaginal discharge and interferes with obtaining an adequate diagnostic smear. After diagnosis, the nurse may insert the first dose of vaginal medication while teaching the client how to repeat the technique. Nonprescription drugs for the treatment of yeast infections are available. The nurse informs clients that although these drugs usually are effective, the initial diagnosis of vaginitis is best made by a physician.

DRUG THERAPY TABLE 59-1	AGENTS TO TREAT VAGINITIS		
DRUG CATEGORY AND EXAMPLES	MECHANISM OF ACTION	SIDE EFFECTS	NURSING CONSIDERATIONS
Antiprotozoal			
metronidazole (Flagyl)	Antiprotozoal–trichomonicidal Mechanism of action unknown Used to treat trichomoniasis and *Gardnerella vaginalis*	Headache, dizziness, ataxia, unpleasant metallic taste, anorexia, nausea, vomiting, diarrhea, darkening of urine	This drug is contraindicated in first trimester of pregnancy. Sexual partner may need to be treated. Instruct client to complete therapy. Administer with food if gastrointestinal upset occurs. Advise client to avoid alcoholic beverages and alcohol-containing products—a severe reaction may occur. Alert client that darkening of the urine may occur.
Antifungal			
clotrimazole (Gyne-Lotrimin), meconazole (Monistat), terconazole (Terazol), tioconazole (Vagistat)	Disrupts fungal cell membrane, causing cell death Used in the treatment of candidiasis	Cramping, nausea, vomiting, slight urinary frequency, erythema, stinging	Obtain culture before initiating therapy. Administer cream or vaginal tablets high into vaginal canal; instruct client to remain recumbent for 10–15 min or administer at bedtime. Treatment continues through menses if necessary. Instruct partner to use a condom to prevent reinfection. Partner may need treatment. Client should use a sanitary pad to prevent staining underwear.
Antibiotic			
sulfisoxazole (Gantrisin)	Prevents cell replication by competing with the enzyme involved in the synthesis of intracellular proteins Used to treat vaginitis, *Chlamydia trachomatis*	Headache, nausea, vomiting, abdominal pain, agranulocytosis, photosensitivity, hematuria	Discontinue immediately if hypersensitivity reaction occurs. Administer medication on an empty stomach with a full glass of water. Complete drug therapy as ordered. Inform client of potential side effects. Tell client to report blood in urine, rash, fever, difficulty breathing, drowsiness, nausea, vomiting, or diarrhea.

The nurse emphasizes the importance of completing the course of therapy.

The nurse also informs the client to avoid routine douching when asymptomatic, but to combat vaginitis, the client may douche once or twice a day for 1 week with a solution of 1 tablespoon of white vinegar to 1 pint of water (Reeder et al., 1992). Taking *Lactobacillus acidophilus* in capsule form or eating yogurt containing active cultures of lactobacilli can replenish normal vaginal microorganisms. Sitz baths are recommended to relieve itching, burning, and swelling of the vulva and perineum. Skin protectants containing zinc oxide promote healing. The nurse offers additional suggestions for preventing a recurrence of vaginal infections, as presented in Client and Family Teaching Box 59-2.

● CERVICITIS

Cervicitis is an inflammation of the cervix.

Pathophysiology and Etiology

Cervical inflammation is caused by infectious microorganisms, decreased estrogen levels during menopause, or trauma during gynecologic procedures, or occurs as a consequence of inserting tampons or vaginal medication applicators. Streptococcal, staphylococcal, gonorrheal, and chlamydial (see Chap. 61) infections are the most common etiologies. The potential is greater during pregnancy and after childbirth, when the microorganisms can enter cervical tissue through small lacerations. The infection can travel upward through uterine and tubal structures, leading to pelvic inflammatory disease (see later discussion). Inflammation and subsequent formation of scar tissue increase the potential for ectopic pregnancy or difficulty conceiving. Chronic cervicitis decreases the amount and quality of cervical mucus and alters the pH, both of which are underlying causes of infertility.

Assessment Findings

Early cervicitis may fail to produce any symptoms. The client eventually spots or bleeds intermenstrually or develops a vaginal discharge. Dyspareunia (painful intercourse) or slight bleeding after sexual intercourse may occur. Severe cervicitis sometimes causes a sensation of weight in the pelvis.

Diagnosis is made by visual examination of the cervix. Microscopic examination of cervical smears identifies the causative microorganism.

Medical Management

Douches and local or systemic antibiotics are the treatment of choice for acute cervicitis. Chronic cervicitis is treated with electrocautery. Frank bleeding requires cervical or vaginal packing or electric coagulation of the bleeding vessel. Healing often takes 6 to 8 weeks. Severe chronic cervicitis is treated by conization (removal of the diseased portion of the cervical mucosa). This outpatient procedure uses an instrument that simultaneously cuts tissue and coagulates the bleeding area. Dilatation is done if there is cervical stenosis. Successful treatment eliminates the inflammation, relieves the symptoms, and aids fertility.

Nursing Management

The nurse schedules treatment procedures 5 to 8 days after the end of the menstrual period to reduce the potential for bleeding. The nurse positions the client as for a gynecologic examination and explains that a momentary cramping sensation may be felt during the electrocautery procedure. After electrocautery, the nurse instructs the client to:

● Rest more than usual for 1 to 2 days.
● Avoid straining or heavy lifting.
● Rest in bed and report if slight bleeding does occur; frank bleeding requires a return visit to the physician.

59-2 *Client and Family Teaching*
Preventing Vaginal Infections

The nurse teaches the client to do the following:

■ Bathe daily with particular attention to perineal hygiene.
■ Wipe from front to back after voiding and bowel movements.
■ Avoid feminine hygiene products and douching more than once per week.
■ Wear cotton undergarments and change them daily.
■ Refrain from wearing layers of clothing, such as underwear plus pantyhose plus slacks, that increase warmth and interfere with air circulation about the genital area.
■ Change from a wet swimsuit as soon as possible.
■ Wash hands and devices that are inserted into the vagina, such as medication applicators, douche tips, and diaphragms, and store them in clean containers.
■ Change sanitary pads before they become saturated; substitute a sanitary pad for a tampon at night.
■ Use a condom or avoid intercourse if either client or her sex partner has genitourinary symptoms.

- Expect a grayish-green, malodorous discharge about 3 weeks after cautery.
- Anticipate slight bleeding about the 11th day.
- Return for a follow-up visit to the physician in 2 to 4 weeks.
- Abstain from sexual relations until tissues are healed.
- Plan for healing that may take 6 to 8 weeks.

● PELVIC INFLAMMATORY DISEASE

Pelvic inflammatory disease (PID) is an infection of the pelvic organs except the uterus. These include the ovaries (oophoritis), fallopian tubes (salpingitis), pelvic vascular system, and pelvic supporting structures.

Pathophysiology and Etiology

Microorganisms enter pelvic structures through the cervix from the vagina (Fig. 59-11). The cause usually is bacterial, with gonococci and *C. trachomatis* being the most common pathogens. The infection travels up the uterus to the fallopian tubes (salpingitis) and ovaries (oophoritis) and can result in pelvic abscess or peritonitis as pus from the infected tubes leaks into the abdomen.

Assessment Findings

Signs and symptoms include an infectious malodorous discharge, backache, severe or aching abdominal and pelvic pain, a bearing-down feeling, fever, dyspareunia, nausea and vomiting, menorrhagia, and dysmenorrhea. Some women experience milder symptoms such as pain during a pelvic examination. Severe infection may cause urinary symptoms.

Diagnosis is based on symptoms as well as a gynecologic examination. A culture and sensitivity test of the vaginal discharge is obtained to identify the causative microorganism. Ultrasonography, magnetic resonance imaging (MRI), or computed tomography (CT) may disclose a pelvic abscess.

Medical Management

Hospitalization with complete bed rest often is necessary. Parenteral or oral antibiotics are administered as soon as culture and sensitivity tests are obtained. IV fluids are ordered if the client is dehydrated, and antipyretics are used if the temperature is elevated. A ruptured pelvic abscess requires emergency surgery.

NURSING PROCESS

● The Client With Pelvic Inflammatory Disease

Assessment

The nurse obtains a complete medical, drug, and allergy history and asks the client to describe all symptoms. A vaginal smear may be necessary. If the client is an outpatient, the nurse instructs the client to refrain from douching for 48 hours before being examined. If the client is admitted to the hospital and a vaginal smear is ordered, the nurse inquires if the client has douched within the last 48 hours.

Diagnosis, Planning, and Interventions

The nurse's role in caring for a client hospitalized with PID includes, but is not limited to the following:

PC: Sepsis related to systemic spread of pathogenic microorganisms

A Spread of bacterial infection

B Spread of gonorrhea

C Spread through blood via circulatory system

FIGURE 59-11 (**A**) Bacteria spread from the vagina and uterus through the lymphatics. (**B**) Gonorrhea spreads from the vagina and uterus through the tubes and ovaries. (**C**) Bacteria can also reach the reproductive organs through the bloodstream. (Smeltzer, S. C. & Bare, B. G. [2000]. *Brunner & Suddarth's textbook of medical–surgical nursing* [9th ed.]. Philadelphia: Lippincott Williams & Wilkins.)

Expected Outcome: The nurse will monitor to detect, manage, and minimize sepsis if it occurs.

- Monitor vital signs and results of white blood cell counts. *Increased temperature, pulse rate, and leukocytosis indicate an infectious process.*
- Maintain IV site and administer parenteral fluids and antibiotic therapy as scheduled. *The nurse implements prescribed medical therapy for treating an infectious process.*
- Keep client in a semisitting position. *Keeping the upper body elevated facilitates pelvic drainage and minimizes upward extension of infection.*

Risk for Infection Transmission related to direct or indirect contact with infectious microorganisms

Expected Outcome: No nosocomial infections will occur among other clients or staff that can be traced to the client with the primary infection.

- Provide client with a private room with a toilet and sink. *Separating the client from others confines the source of transmission to one location.*
- Follow contact isolation precautions. *Contact isolation is a category of transmission-based precautions for controlling the spread of infectious microorganisms found in wound drainage and other body fluids.*
- Wrap and dispose soiled perineal pads in a lined biohazard container. *Confining objects that are heavily contaminated with infectious microorganisms reduces the potential for transmitting them to other susceptible people.*
- Bag soiled linen according to infection control policies of the institution. *Linen that has been in contact with a person with infectious body fluids is contained in specially marked bags to avoid transmitting pathogens to personnel who handle laundry.*
- Leave a disposable stethoscope and paper thermometers in the room for assessments. *Instruments used for frequent assessments are restricted to the infectious client and then destroyed.*
- Wash hands after removing gloves. *Handwashing reduces the number of pathogens on the skin, which tend to grow and multiply in the warmth of latex or vinyl gloves.*
- Clean the cover on the blood pressure cuff with a disinfectant when the client is discharged. *A disinfectant destroys microorganisms on the surface of objects in the environment.*
- Instruct housekeeping personnel to damp mop the client's room after cleaning other clients' rooms and change the mop head when finished. *A principle of medical asepsis is to always clean the most heavily soiled area last. Changing the mop head prevents spreading microorganisms to other areas.*

Acute Pain related to inflamed tissue and pelvic congestion

Expected Outcome: Client's comfort will be maintained within a level of tolerance.

- Administer prescribed analgesic. *Analgesics relieve pain by various biochemical mechanisms.*

- Provide diversional activities to distract client from pain. *Distraction reduces pain perception by providing alternative stimuli to the brain.*
- Position for comfort and limit unnecessary activity. *An uncomfortable position and movement tend to increase pain intensity.*

Risk for Impaired Skin Integrity related to excoriating potential of vaginal drainage

Expected Outcome: Vulvar and perineal tissue will be intact.

- Wash the perineum well with soap and water every 4 hours. *Removing drainage from contact with the skin promotes skin integrity.*
- Pat or blot the skin dry. *Touching the skin gently rather than vigorously reduces trauma to the skin. Keeping the skin dry reduces the potential for maceration.*
- Change perineal pads frequently. *Changing perineal pads frequently increases the potential for absorbing and wicking drainage from the skin surface.*

Evaluation of Expected Outcomes

Expected outcomes are that vital signs and white blood cell count are normal. Infection control measures are effective. The client's pain or discomfort is relieved or eliminated. The genital tissue is free of redness and excoriation.

After discharge from the hospital, the nurse tells the client to temporarily abstain from sexual intercourse to prevent extending the infection and infecting the partner. In addition, the nurse explains that preventing subsequent episodes of PID can be accomplished by seeking medical attention when symptoms of infection, such as a feeling of pressure in the pelvic area, burning on urination, or vaginal drainage, first appear. Early treatment prevents the infection from moving up the reproductive tract and resulting in complications such as peritonitis, abscess formation, and obstruction of the fallopian tubes. When early treatment of acute PID is delayed or inadequate, the infection may become chronic.

● TOXIC SHOCK SYNDROME

Toxic shock syndrome (TSS), a type of septic shock (see Chap. 23), is a life-threatening systemic reaction to the toxin produced by several kinds of bacteria. Some causative microorganisms include *Staphylococcus aureus*, *Streptococcus pyogenes*, and *Clostridium sordellii*. TSS also occurs in men and in nonmenstruating women with soft tissue and postoperative infections.

Pathophysiology and Etiology

TSS is associated with the use of superabsorbent tampons that are not changed frequently and internal contraceptive devices that remain in place longer than necessary. The syndrome occurs when virulent bacteria reproduce suddenly and abundantly in the body and remain unchecked by normal physiologic defense mechanisms. The bacteria produce chemicals that cause blood vessels to dilate, which keeps the major portion of the blood volume in the periphery, reduces cardiac output, and causes severe hypotension (shock). The toxin also seems to inhibit the ability of affected cells to use oxygen (Porth, 2002).

Assessment Findings

Signs and Symptoms

A sudden onset of high fever, chills, tenderness or pain in the muscles, nausea, vomiting, diarrhea, hypotension, hyperemia (increased redness and congestion) of vaginal mucous membranes, disorientation, and headache occurs. The skin is warm despite the fact that the client is in shock. A rash that first appears on the palms of the hands or the body a few hours after the infection later results in a shedding of the superficial layer of the skin (desquamation). The pulse is rapid and thready.

Diagnostic Findings

The infecting microorganism is found in cultures of specimens from the vagina, blood, urine, or other sites. The blood urea nitrogen, serum creatinine, and serum bilirubin levels are increased. The serum enzymes aspartate aminotransferase (AST) and alanine aminotransferase (ALT) are elevated. The platelet count may be decreased.

Medical Management

Circulation is supported with IV fluids while combating the infection with IV antibiotic therapy. Some drugs that are used include oxacillin (Prostaphlin), nafcillin (Nafcil), and methicillin (Staphcillin). Potent adrenergic drugs such as dopamine (Intropin) or dobutamine (Dobutrex) are given to counteract peripheral vasodilation and maintain renal perfusion. Oxygen is given to promote aerobic metabolism at the cellular level.

Nursing Management

The nurse frequently assesses vital signs. He or she administers the first dose of antibiotics immediately and as ordered thereafter. The nurse applies pressure to venipuncture or injection sites to control bleeding and oozing if the platelet count is low. He or she carefully measures intake and output and reports any sudden decrease in the urinary output or a urinary output of less than 500 mL/ day to the physician.

Before discharge, the nurse teaches preventive measures such as using perineal pads rather than tampons or changing tampons frequently. He or she tells clients who use a diaphragm, vaginal sponge, or cervical cap for birth control to remove the device within 24 hours after use. The nurse emphasizes handwashing and keeping vaginal devices clean.

STRUCTURAL ABNORMALITIES

● ENDOMETRIOSIS

Endometriosis is a condition in which tissue that histologically and functionally resembles that of the endometrium is found outside the uterus. The atypical locations for endometrial tissue include the ovaries, the pelvic cavity, and occasionally the abdominal cavity.

Pathophysiology and Etiology

The cause of endometriosis is not clearly understood. It may result from remnants of embryonic tissue that remain in the abdominal cavity. Another possible cause is retrograde menstruation, in which the fallopian tubes expel fragments of endometrial tissue that eventually become implanted outside the uterus.

The ectopic tissue responds to stimulation by estrogen and, perhaps, to progesterone. The tissue bleeds when the endometrium of the uterus is shed, but unfortunately there is no outlet for the extrauterine bleeding. The trapped blood causes pain and ultimately adhesions in the peritoneal cavity. If the fallopian tubes are affected, they may become occluded and result in **sterility,** an inability to conceive. If endometrial tissue is enclosed in an ovary, a chocolate cyst (named because of its collection of dark blood) develops. Occasionally this cyst ruptures, spilling old blood and endometrial cells into the pelvic or abdominal cavity. The condition is naturally relieved when endometrial tissue atrophies after menopause or regresses during pregnancy.

Assessment Findings

Severe dysmenorrhea and copious menstrual bleeding are typical symptoms. The client may experience dyspareunia and pain on defecation. Rupture of a chocolate cyst results in severe abdominal pain that can mimic other abdominal pathologies such as appendicitis or bowel obstruction.

A pelvic examination reveals fixed, tender areas in the lower pelvis. Restricted mobility of the uterus from adhesions may be noted. A laparoscopy confirms the diagnosis.

Medical and Surgical Management

Endometriosis is cured by natural or surgical menopause. Many women are managed medically as long as possible, however, to maintain the potential for having children later. Estrogen–progestin contraceptives are administered to keep the client in a nonbleeding phase of her menstrual cycle for about 9 months. The goal is to control the ectopic tissue so that the client is symptom free for several years. The progestin norethindrone (Norlutin) and the synthetic androgen danazol (Danocrine) are effective in causing atrophy of endometrial tissue.

Without destroying the possibility for childbearing, surgery is performed to remove the cysts, as much of the ectopic tissue as possible, and lyse adhesions caused by bleeding. Laparoscopy is used to remove small areas of endometrial tissue as well as relieve adhesions. Endometriosis that is widespread throughout the pelvic organs, however, may necessitate a panhysterectomy, removal of the uterus, both fallopian tubes, and ovaries.

Nursing Management

The nurse obtains a complete reproductive history, asking the client to describe all symptoms, including their duration; type and location of pain; number of days of menses; amount of menstrual flow; and regularity or irregularity of the menstrual cycle. He or she offers information on methods for relieving menstrual pain (see discussion of dysmenorrhea) and assists the client through the decision-making process as it applies to family planning and medical or surgical treatment of endometriosis before natural menopause. Some techniques for resolving decisional conflict include the following:

- Reinforce or clarify explanations of treatment options and the consequences of each option.
- Emphasize that the condition does not require an immediate decision and avoid giving advice or influencing the client's opinions.
- Suggest that the client include her significant other in discussion of options.
- Offer the option of seeking a second medical opinion.
- Suggest listing the pros and cons of each option to help determine which choice is most compatible with her values and goals.

The nurse emphasizes the importance of adhering to the prescribed medication schedule, if that is the client's choice, and the importance of regular gynecologic evaluations. He or she instructs the client to seek care if pain increases, the menstrual flow is extremely heavy, or pregnancy occurs. Refer to the information on nursing management of clients undergoing a hysterectomy (later in this chapter) for those who choose that treatment option.

● VAGINAL FISTULAS

A **fistula** is an unnatural opening between two structures. The opening may be between a ureter and the vagina (ureterovaginal fistula), between the bladder and the vagina (vesicovaginal fistula), or between the rectum and the vagina (rectovaginal fistula; Fig. 59-12).

Pathophysiology and Etiology

Vaginal fistulas are caused by cancer, radiation treatment, surgical or obstetric injury, congenital anomaly, or a complication of ulcerative colitis. They result in the continuous drainage of urine or feces from the vagina. The vaginal wall and the external genitalia become excoriated and often infected. The client may not void through the urethra because urine does not accumulate in the bladder.

Assessment Findings

The client reports that urine or stool leaks from the vagina. Diagnosis is made by physical examination of the vaginal wall. A sterile probe is inserted if the fistula is easily seen or a dye (usually ethylene blue) is used to detect the exact location of the fistula. When a vesicovaginal fistula is suspected, the colored dye is injected into the bladder through a urethral catheter. A ureterovaginal fistula requires IV administration of the dye. An IV pyelogram (IVP) detects the flow of radiopaque dye through the lower genito-

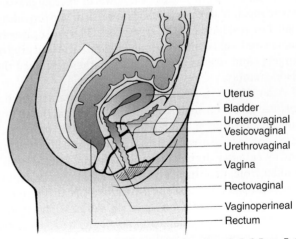

FIGURE 59-12 Types of vaginal fistulae. (Smeltzer, S. C. & Bare, B. G. [2000]. *Brunner & Suddarth's textbook of medical–surgical nursing* [9th ed.]. Philadelphia: Lippincott Williams & Wilkins.)

urinary tract. A rectovaginal fistula is located by looking for fecal drainage on the posterior vaginal wall.

Medical and Surgical Management

Surgery is performed after inflammation and edema have disappeared. This may require months of treatment. Sometimes the tissues are in such poor condition that surgical repair is not possible. In the meantime, or if the fistula cannot be repaired, symptomatic treatment to reduce the risk for infection and manage skin excoriation is provided.

NURSING PROCESS

● **The Client With a Vaginal Fistula**

Assessment

The nurse obtains the client's history and performs a physical assessment. He or she asks the client to describe the characteristics of the vaginal drainage. While wearing gloves, the nurse inspects the vaginal meatus and vault as well as the condition of the perianal skin. He or she helps the client discuss the lifestyle changes that have accompanied the vaginal fistula.

Diagnosis, Planning, and Interventions

The nurse's focus when managing the care of a client with a vaginal fistula includes implementing and teaching measures for maintaining skin integrity, helping the client maintain self-esteem, and offering suggestions for promoting sexuality if the client experiences sexual repercussions as a consequence of the condition. The nurse administers neomycin (Mycifradin), kanamycin (Kantrex), or another prescribed antibiotic to clean the bowel of microorganisms before repair of a rectovaginal fistula. He or she provides a light, low-residue diet to keep stool soft. The nurse gives an enema and a cleansing vaginal irrigation the morning of surgery, and inserts an indwelling catheter to keep the bladder empty.

After surgery, serosanguineous vaginal drainage on the perineal pad is normal. No urine or feces from the vagina indicates healing of the repaired fistula. The nurse prevents pelvic pressure and stress on the suture line by monitoring catheter drainage closely. The pressure of a full bladder from an obstructed catheter may break down the surgical repair and cause the fistula to reappear. The nurse prevents and relieves pressure on perineal structures. Warm perineal irrigations and heat-lamp treatments are effective in promoting healing and lessening discomfort. Douches used during the postoperative time frame remove drainage, keep the suture area clean, and lessen chances of infection. About the third or fourth postoperative day,

a rectal suppository or a stool softener may be ordered to prevent straining during a bowel movement.

Specific diagnoses, expected outcomes, and interventions include, but are not limited to the following:

Risk for Situational Low Self-Esteem related to leaking of urine and stool and body and environmental odors
Expected Outcome: Client's self-esteem will be maintained or restored as evidenced by a positive self-image and self-confidence.

- Recommend wearing disposable, absorbent incontinence briefs or perineal pads with protective panties, and changing and laundering clothing or bed linens as soon as possible. *Measures that absorb the drainage and keep clothing and the environment clean help to control odors that may be socially unacceptable.*
- Let the client know that commercial deodorizers are available for use in the home. *Pleasant fragrances disguise odors that may linger in the home.*
- Recognize positive attributes when they are demonstrated. *Acknowledging the client's strengths elevates self-esteem.*
- Affirm that the client is capable of managing odor and elimination problems. *Instilling a sense of control increases self-esteem.*
- Provide genuine feedback on self-care and hygiene measures. *Compliments, when they are deserved, improve self-esteem.*

Risk for Impaired Skin Integrity related to continuous skin contact with urine or stool
Expected Outcome: Skin will remain intact or skin integrity will be restored.

- Advise daily bathing and frequent perineal hygiene with premoistened disposable wipes. *Removing drainage from contact with the skin promotes skin integrity.*
- Apply a skin protectant, such as collodion, over intact skin, or a skin barrier, such as zinc oxide or karaya paste, to excoriated skin. *Commercial skin products reduce contact with irritating drainage.*
- Teach client how to take sitz baths and administer cleansing douches. *Water that is in motion helps to loosen debris and reduce contact with the skin.*
- Explain that mixing a perfumed scent with a fecal or urine odor may intensify the odor as well as irritate the area. *Colognes and perfumes contain alcohol, which promotes evaporation of drainage that contains unpleasant odors. Alcohol irritates excoriated skin.*
- Inform client that powders may cake and cause irritation or a superficial skin infection. She may use a thin dusting of plain cornstarch but must wash it off thoroughly when the area becomes soiled with feces or urine. *Talc tends to attract moisture and take on the consistency of paste. Applying a light layer of cornstarch reduces friction when two skin surfaces move over one another.*

Sexual Dysfunction related to embarrassment over vaginal drainage

Expected Outcome: Client will engage in satisfying sexual activity.

- Recommend scheduling sexual intercourse to allow for hygienic preparation (e.g., bathing, perineal care). *Being clean promotes mutual sexual response between client and partner.*
- Point out that attractive lingerie, soft music, and scented candles may overcome emotional barriers to sex. *Modifications in clothing and the environment promote eroticism.*
- Suggest reclining on an absorbent, disposable pad. *Planning measures that prevent soiling of bed linen decreases self-consciousness.*
- Propose substituting the shower, private swimming pool, or a hot tub as a place for intercourse. *Having intercourse while water is flowing helps reduce attention on the drainage.*
- Encourage using alternate means of reaching orgasm other than vaginal intercourse (e.g., manual or mechanical stimulation). *Orgasm is possible using alternative methods.*

Evaluation of Expected Outcomes

Expected outcomes are that the client demonstrates a positive self-image and self-confidence. Skin remains intact. The client pursues satisfying sexual activities.

● PELVIC ORGAN PROLAPSE

The term *prolapse* indicates a structural protrusion. Women experience any number of problems of this nature in the vagina. They include cystocele, rectocele, enterocele, and uterine prolapse (Fig. 59-13).

A **cystocele** is the bulging of the bladder into the vagina. Herniation of the rectum into the vagina is called a **rectocele.** An enterocele is a protrusion of the intestinal wall into the vagina. A uterovaginal prolapse is the downward displacement of the cervix anywhere from low in the vagina to outside the vagina.

Pathophysiology and Etiology

Pelvic organ prolapse is a consequence of congenital or acquired weaknesses in the muscles and fascia that are needed to support pelvic structures. Common causes include unrepaired postpartum tears; stretching during pregnancy and childbirth or with tumorous masses, ascites, and obesity; and postmenopausal atrophy. As the pelvic floor relaxes, the uterus, rectum, intestine, and bladder, alone or in combination, herniate downward. Structural displacement of the bladder and bowel leads to alterations in urinary and bowel elimination. Uterine tissue that protrudes below the vaginal orifice is subject to irritation from clothing or rubbing against the thighs while walking; ulceration and infection frequently follow. Clients with severe uterovaginal prolapse are at greater risk for cervical cancer.

The functional consequences of pelvic organ prolapse can be disruptive. The client often experiences difficulty standing for long periods, walking with ease, lifting, and other activities that are hard to avoid.

Assessment Findings

Signs and Symptoms

Clients with a cystocele may experience stress incontinence—a little urine seeps every time the woman coughs, sneezes, laughs, bears down, or strains. Cystitis (inflammation of the bladder), discussed in Chapter 65, results from the stagnation of urine in the bladder. Constipation often is a problem for those with a rectocele. In some instances, the client has to put her finger into the vagina and apply pressure to the posterior vaginal wall to reduce the herniation before being able to evacuate stool. Symp-

FIGURE 59-13 (A) Cystocele. **(B)** Rectocele. **(C)** Enterocele. (Smeltzer, S. C. & Bare, B. G. [2000]. *Brunner & Suddarth's textbook of medical–surgical nursing* [9th ed.]. Philadelphia: Lippincott Williams & Wilkins.)

toms of a uterovaginal prolapse include backache, pelvic pain, fatigue, and a feeling that "something is dropping out," especially when lifting a heavy object, coughing, or standing for prolonged periods.

Diagnostic Findings

Diagnosis is confirmed during a pelvic examination and visual inspection of the vagina. Urinary tests are performed to reproduce stress incontinence or to determine the volume at which a client senses an urgent need to void. A Pap test determines the client's estrogen status.

Medical and Surgical Management

A pessary, which is a firm, doughnut-shaped or ring device, may be inserted in the upper vagina to reposition and give support to the uterus when surgery cannot be done or the client declines surgery. **Kegel exercises,** also known as *pelvic floor strengthening exercises* (see Chap. 65), are recommended when there is stress incontinence.

Surgical repairs are done transvaginally. The surgical repair of a cystocele is called *anterior colporrhaphy.* Repair of a rectocele is called *posterior colporrhaphy.* Repair of the tears (usually old obstetric tears) of the perineal floor is called *perineorrhaphy.* A vaginal hysterectomy (see later discussion) is done to remove a completely prolapsed uterus.

Nursing Management

The nurse obtains a comprehensive medical history, including the chief complaint and symptoms; inserts a catheter for diagnostic testing; assists with the pelvic examination and collection of specimens; and provides appropriate health teaching based on the physician's plan for treatment. He or she shows the client how to remove, clean, and reinsert a pessary, including the following information:

- Remove the pessary and then thoroughly wash it with warm, soapy water, followed by rinsing and drying.
- Inspect the pessary to be sure that all secretions have been removed.
- Apply a sterile lubricant to the pessary before it is reinserted. Discomfort may indicate that it has been inserted incorrectly, the pessary has moved, or that it is causing irritation. Contact the physician if these problems occur.
- See the physician immediately if a white or yellow discharge from the vagina develops. It may indicate an infection.
- Assume the knee–chest position for a few minutes once or twice a day to keep the pelvic organs and the pessary in good position.

- Avoid heavy lifting and straining when having a bowel movement.

The nurse tells clients not wishing to manage their own pessary to see their physician at least every 2 months or sooner if vaginal discharge or changes in voiding develop.

After an anterior colporrhaphy, some women have temporary difficulty voiding or emptying the bladder completely. For this reason, clients are discharged with a retention catheter in place or are taught to perform clean intermittent catheterization (see Chap. 65) for 7 to 10 days until they can void sufficiently to empty the bladder. The client learns Kegel exercises after surgical repairs.

● UTERINE DISPLACEMENT

In some women, the uterus, which normally is flexed about 45° anteriorly with the cervix positioned posteriorly, is displaced. Anteflexion describes a uterus that is bent forward on itself. In retroflexion, the uterus tilts backward (the opposite of anteflexion). Retroversion, the most common displacement, refers to the posterior tilt of the uterus while the cervix tilts anteriorly (Fig. 59-14).

Pathophysiology and Etiology

Displacement usually is congenital; sometimes backward displacement is from childbearing or scar tissue that forms in clients who have endometriosis or PID. Positional displacement may not cause any noticeable problems, or it may be the underlying reason for discomfort during men-

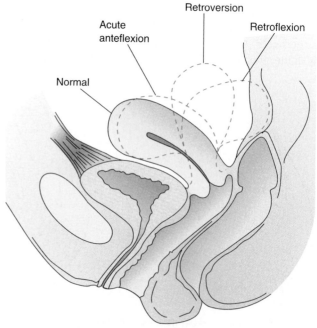

FIGURE 59-14 Variations in uterine position.

struation and intercourse. Some cases of infertility are caused by retrodisplacement of the uterus.

Assessment Findings

Clients with a malpositioned uterus describe having backache, dysmenorrhea, or dyspareunia. Sometimes the client seeks a medical examination to investigate the reason pregnancy has not occurred. A bimanual pelvic examination locates the abnormal position of the uterus.

Medical and Surgical Management

If the displacement causes severe discomfort, or if the sterility can be corrected, abdominal surgery is performed to relocate and suture the uterus to a more natural position. Age or complicating diseases sometimes make surgery too great a risk. Under such circumstances, the displacement is reduced by inserting a pessary, which repositions the uterus, and having the client assume the knee–chest position several times a day.

Nursing Management

The nurse performs an initial interview, collects pertinent data, and assists with the gynecologic examination. If surgery is performed, the nurse assesses the client for complications, manages wound drains, maintains patency of the indwelling catheter, inspects vaginal packing, and notes the condition of dressings. He or she includes deep breathing, pain management, and early ambulation in the postoperative management.

If a pessary is used to correct the prolapse, the nurse shows the client how to remove, clean, and reinsert it. He or she explains how to assume a knee–chest position and describes activity level and hygiene measures. The nurse schedules medical follow-up or instructs the client to do so.

TUMORS OF THE FEMALE REPRODUCTIVE SYSTEM

● UTERINE LEIOMYOMA

A *leiomyoma*, sometimes shortened to *myoma*, is a benign uterine growth principally consisting of smooth muscle and fibrous connective tissue. Myomas, which are the most common tumor in the female pelvis, often are referred to as **fibroid tumors.**

Pathophysiology and Etiology

Estrogen is believed to stimulate the development of fibroids. Tumors may be small or large, single or multiple. Growth usually is slow except during pregnancy. They shrink during and after menopause. Fibroids can occur in various locations in the uterus: subserous (below the serous membrane), intramural (within the wall), and submucosal (below the mucous membrane; Fig. 59-15). The latter are associated most frequently with excessive menstrual bleeding.

Assessment Findings

When symptoms exist, menorrhagia is most common. There can be a feeling of pressure in the pelvic region, dysmenorrhea, anemia (from loss of blood), and malaise.

Benign uterine tumors may be detected during a pelvic examination. A Pap test is done to rule out a malignancy. A sonogram reveals uterine and fibroid size. Microscopic examination of the excised tumor confirms the diagnosis.

Medical and Surgical Management

Several factors govern the treatment of benign uterine tumors. A symptomatic tumor in a woman who wishes to have children is watched closely. The client receives a gynecologic examination every 3 to 6 months. A Pap test is repeated every 6 to 12 months.

When the client has abnormal bleeding, a D and C is performed to determine the cause of or to control the

FIGURE 59-15 Submucosal, intramural, and subserosal leiomyomas.

bleeding. Although a D and C does not remove the tumor, it may make more extensive surgery unnecessary. A myomectomy (surgical removal of the tumor only) through an abdominal incision or with a laparoscope inserted through the cervical canal, preserves the uterus if the tumor is benign or a woman of childbearing years wishes to become pregnant in the future. A hysterectomy is performed when symptoms are severe and incapacitating, if the client is past childbearing years, or a future pregnancy is not wanted.

Nursing Management

The nurse assists with the gynecologic examination, reinforces medical explanations, and provides preoperative instructions. During the postoperative time frame, the nurse assists in the safe recovery of the client who undergoes surgery similar to that discussed for cervical and endometrial cancer.

● CERVICAL AND ENDOMETRIAL CANCER

Cervical cancer, which affects the lowest portion of the uterus, is the second most frequent malignancy of the female reproductive system (breast cancer is first). Cancer of the endometrium affects the lining of the uterus, usually in the area of the fundus or corpus, and is more common in postmenopausal women.

Pathophysiology and Etiology

Cancer of the cervix has its peak incidence among women between the ages of 35 and 50 years and is associated with the following risk factors:

- Being born to mothers treated with diethylstilbestrol (DES) while pregnant
- Becoming sexually active at an early age
- Having multiple sexual partners or having intercourse with a high-risk man (one who has had multiple partners or penile condyloma [warts])
- Acquiring genital infections caused by the human papilloma virus (HPV)
- Having chronic cervicitis secondary to uterine prolapse
- Having a history of cigarette smoking
- Having had pelvic radiation

The risk of endometrial cancer increases after the age of 50 years, especially among those women taking estrogens without the addition of progesterone for 5 or more years during and after menopause. Other risk factors in-

clude early menarche, late menopause, never having been pregnant (nulliparity), and obesity.

Cervical and endometrial cancers probably begin as premalignant lesions that later undergo malignant changes. The localized malignancy is referred to as **carcinoma in situ.** Untreated, it subsequently invades other areas of the uterus and adjacent tissue.

Assessment Findings

Signs and Symptoms

Bleeding is the earliest and most common symptom of both endometrial and cervical cancer. In early cervical cancer, spotting occurs first, especially after slight trauma such as douching or intercourse. The bleeding from endometrial cancer can be mistaken for menorrhagia in premenopausal women. Late symptoms for both include pain, symptoms of pressure on the bladder or bowel, and the generalized wasting associated with advanced cancer.

Diagnostic Findings

All vaginal bleeding is investigated, first by a gynecologic examination, then by diagnostic tests. Cervical cancer is detected with Pap tests and biopsies of suspect tissue. Cells obtained by endocervical aspiration or endometrial biopsy during a hysteroscopy identify abnormal cells higher in the uterus. Radiography, MRI, or CT scanning is used to determine if there is metastasis; a barium study or IVP is ordered to determine bowel or bladder metastasis. Both types of cancer are classified according to stages (Table 59-2).

TABLE 59-2		STAGES OF UTERINE CANCERS
TYPE	**STAGE**	**DESCRIPTION**
Cervical	0	Carcinoma in situ
	I	Limited to the cervix
	II	Extends beyond the cervix to the upper two thirds of the vagina
	III	Involves the lower third of the vagina and is fixed to the pelvic wall
	IV	Involves the rectum, bladder, or extends beyond the true pelvis
Endometrial	0	Cancer in situ
	I	Confined to the corpus
	II	Involves the corpus and cervix
	III	Extends outside the uterus, but not the true pelvis
	IV	Involves the rectum, bladder, or extends outside the true pelvis

[Adapted from the Federation Internationale de Gynecologie et Obstetrique (FIGO).]

Medical and Surgical Management

Treatment of cervical and endometrial cancer depends on the stage of the tumor. Prognosis depends on how early the cancer is diagnosed. Methods for treating cervical and endometrial cancer include one of various **hysterectomy** (removal of uterus) procedures (Box 59-2), external or internal radiation therapy (Fig. 59-16), and chemotherapy (see Chap. 20).

The uterus is removed using an abdominal or vaginal approach—the choice usually depends on the pathology and the client's condition. An abdominal approach always is used for a radical hysterectomy. The vaginal approach has fewer complications, reduced recovery time, and a lower cost. Laparoscopically assisted vaginal hysterectomy, a combination of surgical and endoscopic techniques, is being used to perform vaginal hysterectomies that otherwise would have been performed abdominally.

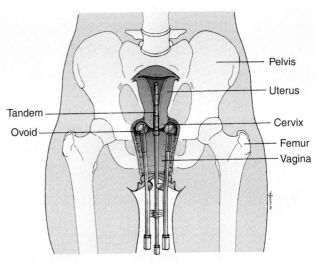

FIGURE 59-16 Placement of tandem and ovoids for internal radiation therapy. (© J. Wolfe.)

Nursing Management

A major role of the nurse is educating all women to have regular gynecologic examinations and Pap tests. Theoretically, all uterine cancers begin in situ. Therefore, regular cytologic (cell) examinations increase the potential for an early diagnosis before invasion occurs. Specific nursing management depends on the selected treatment. In the interim between diagnosis and treatment, the nurse offers emotional support and information about the various options for treatment. See Chapter 20 for discussion of radiation therapy or chemotherapy and nursing management techniques.

Preoperative and Postoperative Care

Preoperative preparations vary depending on the surgeon's preference and the planned surgical approach (abdominal or vaginal). A douche is given before a vaginal hysterectomy, and an enema is given before either surgery. The nurse inserts an indwelling catheter before surgery and administers an antibiotic, usually one of the cephalo-

sporins, during or after surgery to prevent infection. For general postoperative care, refer to perioperative standards of care discussed in Chapter 25; for postoperative care specific to an abdominal hysterectomy, refer to Nursing Care Plan 59-1.

Client and Family Teaching

Depending on the client's treatment, the teaching plan includes some or all of the following:

- Take any prescribed medications as ordered. Seek care if adverse drug effects occur.
- Avoid heavy lifting, sexual intercourse, vigorous physical exercise, and douching until permitted by the physician.
- Ambulate at intervals and avoid sitting in one position for a prolonged period.
- Clean the incision as directed.
- Seek medical care if any of the following signs and symptoms occur: fever; redness, swelling, pain, or drainage of the incision; vaginal discharge that has a foul odor; vaginal bleeding; pain in the chest, abdomen, or legs.
- Avoid constipation and straining to have a bowel movement. Drink plenty of fluids. If constipation occurs, contact the physician.

● OVARIAN CYSTS AND BENIGN OVARIAN TUMORS

A cyst is a membranous sac filled with fluid, cells, or both. Ovarian cysts, which are benign, are filled with fluid. Benign ovarian tumors are noncancerous growths of solid tissue.

(text continued on page 930)

BOX 59-2 ● Types of Hysterectomies

Total hysterectomy—Removal of the entire uterus and cervix

Subtotal hysterectomy—Removal of the uterus only, with a stump of the cervix left intact

Panhysterectomy—Removal of the uterus, fallopian tubes, and ovaries

Radical hysterectomy—Removal of the uterus, cervix, ovaries, and fallopian tubes; part of the upper vagina and some pelvic lymph nodes also may be removed at this time

Pelvic exenteration—Removal of all reproductive organs, rectum, colon, bladder, distal ureters, iliac blood vessels, and pelvic lymph nodes and peritoneum

Nursing Care Plan 59-1

THE CLIENT WITH A TOTAL ABDOMINAL HYSTERECTOMY

Assessment

- Assess vital signs and level of consciousness.
- Evaluate pain intensity.
- Monitor condition of the dressing, location of drains (nasogastric, wound), and patency of urinary catheter.
- Regularly check the type, volume, and rate of IV fluid, and the location and appearance of the IV site.
- Note the presence of antiembolic stockings.

Nursing Diagnosis: Acute Pain related to tissue trauma

Expected Outcome: Pain will be reduced to a tolerable level within 30 minutes of a nursing intervention.

Interventions	Rationales
Assess type of pain, intensity, and location each time you assess vital signs and as needed.	Pain assessment is the fifth vital sign.
Administer analgesics as ordered.	They reduce pain perception.
Implement nonpharmacologic interventions, such as distraction, imagery, and repositioning, to augment analgesia.	Substituting alternative stimuli to the brain decreases pain perception.

Evaluation of Expected Outcome: Client reports decreased discomfort; pain is adequately controlled.

PC: Thrombophlebitis

Expected Outcome: The nurse will monitor to detect, manage, and minimize thrombophlebitis.

Interventions	Rationales
Remove and reapply antiembolic stockings every 8 hours.	Antiembolic stockings support valves in veins and reduce venous stasis.
Encourage active leg exercises every 2 to 4 hours.	Skeletal muscle contraction propels venous blood toward the heart.
Assess for Homans' sign bilaterally every shift.	Homans' sign indicates the possibility of a thrombus in the lower extremities.
Do not place pillows beneath the knees or raise the knees with the electric bed.	Bending the knees interferes with venous circulation and promotes venous stasis and clot formation.
Ambulate as much as possible.	Walking requires skeletal muscle contraction, which promotes venous circulation.

Evaluation of Expected Outcome: Homans' sign is negative bilaterally.

PC: Urinary Retention

Expected Outcome: The nurse will monitor to detect, manage, and minimize urinary retention.

(continued)

Nursing Care Plan 59-1 (Continued)

THE CLIENT WITH A TOTAL ABDOMINAL HYSTERECTOMY

Interventions	Rationales
Measure intake and output every shift.	Intake and output facilitates assessment of fluid status.
Palpate the lower abdomen for distention.	The bladder is palpable when distended with urine.
Measure the volume of each voiding.	Voiding small amounts can indicate urinary retention with overflow.
Encourage a liberal fluid intake.	Urinary elimination is related to fluid intake.
Report to the physician bladder distention in the absence of voiding.	Medically prescribed interventions such as inserting a straight or indwelling catheter require an order from the physician.

Evaluation of Expected Outcome: Client voids in sufficient quantity.

PC: Abdominal Distention, Paralytic Ileus

Expected Outcome: The nurse will monitor to detect, manage, and minimize abdominal distention.

Interventions	Rationales
Palpate the abdomen every 4 hours for signs of rigidity.	The abdomen loses its soft quality as it distends with gas.
Encourage ambulation.	Movement promotes intestinal peristalsis, which moves gas toward the rectum.
Report abdominal discomfort, nausea, abdominal distention, or diminished or faint bowel sounds to the physician.	Elimination of intestinal gas may be facilitated by using a rectal tube, which must be medically ordered.

Evaluation of Expected Outcome: Abdomen is soft; bowel sounds are normal; client passes flatus rectally.

PC: Vaginal Hemorrhage

Expected Outcome: The nurse will monitor to detect, manage, and minimize hemorrhage.

Interventions	Rationales
Record the number of perineal pads used.	Counting perineal pads facilitates the assessment of blood loss.
Assess blood pressure and pulse every 15 minutes if bleeding seems severe.	Blood pressure falls and pulse rate increases in relation to loss of circulating blood volume.
Record the color of bloody drainage.	Bright red bleeding correlates with arterial bleeding; dark red blood is more likely venous.
Report excessive bleeding or passage of blood clots to the physician.	A blood transfusion or an increased rate of IV fluid may be necessary to maintain blood volume to prevent shock.

Evaluation of Expected Outcome: Client has normal postoperative vaginal drainage; vital signs are within normal range.

Nursing Diagnosis: Risk for Disturbed Body Image related to misconceptions about physical and sexual consequences of hysterectomy

Expected Outcome: Client will maintain an accurate body image after surgery.

(continued)

Nursing Care Plan 59-1 (Continued)

THE CLIENT WITH A TOTAL ABDOMINAL HYSTERECTOMY

Interventions	Rationales
Give client an opportunity to verbalize perceptions and fears.	Clients are less apt to discuss personal problems or fears if they sense that the nurse does not have time to engage in a discussion.
Clarify that a hysterectomy does not physically compromise libido or ability to achieve orgasm or cause premature aging, depression, or masculinization.	Many women accept common myths and misperceptions as fact.

Evaluation of Expected Outcome: Client has a realistic understanding of the physical outcomes of surgery.

Nursing Diagnosis: Deficient Knowledge related to onset of menopause secondary to removal of ovaries in premenopausal women

Expected Outcome: Client will understand the consequences that accompany removal of the ovaries and methods for stabilizing reproductive hormone levels.

Interventions	Rationales
Discuss the physiologic effects of surgical menopause.	Besides the cessation of menstruation, hot flashes, emotional irritability, predisposition to osteoporosis, and increased cardiac risks also accompany hysterectomy.
Explain the action, frequency of administration side effects, and benefits of HRT.	Providing exogenous hormones reduces the deficit of endogenous hormone production.

Evaluation of Expected Outcome: Client accurately paraphrases health teaching related to surgical menopause.

Pathophysiology and Etiology

The exact etiologic mechanism for the variety of ovarian cysts and tumors is essentially unknown, but endocrine dysfunction has been implicated in some types. Follicular cysts are thought to develop when a ripening ovum fails to be released. Another type forms when the corpus luteum fails to regress after ovulation and continues to produce progesterone. Chocolate cysts are secondary to endometriosis. Ovarian cysts and benign tumors tend to affect menstruation and fertility, depending on the specific type. Some benign tumors have a potential to become malignant (Porth, 2002).

Assessment Findings

The client may experience pressure in the lower abdomen, backache, menstrual irregularities, and pain, which can be mistaken for appendicitis, ureteral stone, or other abdominal disorders. Clients with tumors associated with or influenced by hypothalamic, pituitary, or adrenal hormones can develop hirsutism (growth of facial hair), atrophy of the breasts, and sterility.

Tumors and cysts may be detected during a pelvic examination. Ultrasonography and laparoscopy are used to determine tumor size. Surgery is the only means for confirming a diagnosis of a benign tumor or cyst.

Medical and Surgical Management

Some ovarian cysts and benign tumors require no treatment or are treated with oral contraceptives to provide symptomatic relief. If the cyst ruptures, surgery, which can entail complete **oophorectomy** (removal of the ovary), removal of the tissue (oophorocystectomy) only, or a **salpingo-oophorectomy** (removal of the ovary and fallopian tube), is required.

Nursing Management

The nurse explains measures for relieving menstrual discomfort and provides referrals to support groups that are devoted to infertile women. The preoperative preparation and postoperative management are the same as for any client having abdominal surgery and a general anesthetic (see Chap. 25). After surgery, some women develop abdominal distention, which is relieved by ambulating, inserting a rectal tube, or applying an abdominal binder. The nurse informs the client who has had surgery but not a hysterectomy to continue having regular gynecologic examinations and Pap tests because she is still at risk for uterine cancer.

● CANCER OF THE OVARY

Although other types of female reproductive system cancers occur with greater incidence, ovarian tumors are the leading cause of death from gynecologic malignancies (National Institutes of Health, 1994). Tumors of the ovary are so lethal largely because they present with nonspecific symptoms and therefore frequently are far advanced and inoperable by the time they are diagnosed.

Pathophysiology and Etiology

It is believed that some ovarian tumors have a hereditary link, whereas others arise from ovarian cysts. Recent research has shown that the more times a woman ovulates during her lifetime, the greater the risk for ovarian cancer. Certain individuals in the population tend to develop ovarian cancer more often than others. They include nulliparous women, those with a family history of ovarian cancer, and those who have been diagnosed with other types of cancer such as endometrial, colon, or breast cancer.

Malignant tumors of the ovary are classified according to the type of cell from which they originate. Most are epithelial, followed by germ cell (an ovum) tumors. Other types are very rare.

Assessment Findings

In the beginning, clients experience vague lower abdominal discomfort. As the tumor grows larger, urinary frequency and urgency may develop because of pressure on the bladder. Later, ascites, weight loss, severe pain, and gastrointestinal symptoms occur.

A mass may be felt during a pelvic examination. Many physicians believe that ovarian enlargement found on pelvic examination requires surgical exploration. Laboratory studies measuring tumor marker antigens, such as alpha-fetoprotein, carcinoembryonic antigen, and CA 125, are ordered. Transvaginal and transabdominal ultrasound and Doppler imaging of ovarian vessels are used in an effort to detect early-stage ovarian cancer. An abdominal CT scan, proctoscopy, barium study, chest radiograph, and IVP are done to detect metastasis to other areas. A positive diagnosis is made by microscopic examination.

Medical and Surgical Management

Preventive measures are recommended to at-risk populations. They include having at least two full-term pregnancies followed by breast-feeding and using oral contraceptives for more than 5 years. In addition, prophylactic bilateral oophorectomy is recommended for women at risk for hereditary ovarian cancer syndrome after they reach the age of 35 years or after childbearing is completed. After diagnosis of a malignant tumor, the diseased ovary is removed. A total hysterectomy may or may not be performed. If both ovaries are removed, HRT may be prescribed.

Surgical treatment, which reduces the tumor load, is followed by chemotherapy. The current antineoplastic drug regimen of choice is a combination of cisplatin (Platinol) and paclitaxel (Taxol), although combinations of other drugs such as cyclophosphamide (Cytoxan) and carboplatin (Paraplatin) may be used as alternatives (National Institutes of Health, 1994). The use of radiation therapy rather than chemotherapy is controversial at this time.

Nursing Management

Only a small percentage of clients with malignant tumors of the ovary survive 5 or more years despite intensive treatment. The emotional effects of the diagnosis require support and understanding on the part of the nurse and other members of the health team. Many of these clients are young, the treatment is difficult, and the prognosis is poor. Preoperative and postoperative nursing care is similar to that of others who undergo abdominal surgery (see preoperative and postoperative care in the nursing management discussion of the client with cervical and endometrial cancer). See Nursing Care Plan 59-1 for nursing diagnoses and interventions for the client undergoing a total abdominal hysterectomy.

● CANCER OF THE VAGINA

Cancer of the vagina is rare and usually seen in women older than 40 years of age.

Pathophysiology and Etiology

The incidence of vaginal cancer is higher among women infected with the human papilloma virus (HPV), a sexually transmitted microorganism (see Chap. 62), and among those who use a pessary but neglect to remove and clean it. Studies have shown a relationship between taking diethylstilbestrol (DES) during early pregnancy and the development of vaginal carcinoma in the (young) female offspring. DES no longer is used to treat problems associated with pregnancy.

The upper posterior third of the vagina is the most common site of vaginal cancer. Metastatic lesions may occur in the cervix or adjacent areas such as the vulva, uterus, or rectum.

Assessment Findings

Abnormal vaginal bleeding usually is the predominant symptom. Dyspareunia also may occur. Visual examination of the vaginal canal discloses the lesion. A biopsy then confirms the diagnosis.

Medical and Surgical Management

Cancer of the vagina is treated according to the extent of the tumor. Most clients undergo laser photovaporization treatments, although a partial or total vaginectomy is a possibility. Radiation therapy also is used. Complications, such as fistulas and bleeding, arise from the tumor itself and from radiation therapy. These complications are difficult to correct and control.

Nursing Management

The poor prognosis and complications associated with vaginal cancer and its treatment present a nursing challenge. The nurse keeps the client as comfortable as possible and changes bedding and clothing frequently. Urine or fecal drainage from the fistulas make odors difficult to control, but a room deodorizer and frequent gown and linen changes help.

The nurse encourages all women who took DES during a pregnancy to tell their daughters and advise them to have complete gynecologic examinations regularly. After treatment, clients may profit from techniques to reduce the discomfort during sexual intercourse that is caused by narrowing of the vagina. Some suggestions include using K-Y gel or prolonged foreplay to lubricate the vagina, having one's sex partner dilate the vagina with fingers before penetration with the penis, and taking a slower pace during sexual activities.

● CANCER OF THE VULVA

Cancer of the vulva, the external female genitalia, is relatively rare. It usually occurs in women older than 60 years of age, but cases among younger women have arisen recently. Vulvar cancer is highly curable when diagnosed in an early stage.

Pathophysiology and Etiology

Infections with carcinogenic agents like HPV and herpes simplex virus type 2 increase the risk for vulvar cancer (see Chap. 62). These infections are treatable, but not curable, which explains the lifelong threat of genital cancer.

Atypical cells, which appear as white or pigmented raised patches, most commonly involve the labia majora. The cancer also occurs in the labia minora, clitoris, and Bartholin glands. Because of the widespread presence of the viruses in the vulvar epithelium and their potential for carcinogenesis, multiple cancerous sites may coexist or occur again after treatment. Although the cancer is slow growing, it can and does spread to the vagina, urethra, and anus through regional lymph nodes.

Assessment Findings

Pruritus and genital burning are the most frequent early symptoms. Later, a bloody discharge, enlarged lymph nodes, ulceration and swelling of the vulva, and a visible mass develop. Eventually, the client experiences severe pain. As the cancer ulcerates, a bloody and sometimes purulent discharge from the vulva occurs.

The lesions are first noted during inspection of the genitalia. Application of acetic acid tends to accentuate the abnormal tissue. Biopsy confirms the diagnosis.

Medical and Surgical Management

Vulvectomy (removal of the vulva) with or without the removal of lymph nodes (radical vulvectomy) is the standard for treatment. Laser photovaporization is being used as an alternative, however, to preserve the cosmetic appearance of the genitalia, especially if the lesions do not exceed a depth of 3 mm. The efficacy of preoperative chemotherapy plus radiation before surgery for advanced disease is being investigated.

When cancer of the vulva is inoperable, wet dressings and perineal irrigations with a deodorizing solution help to control the odor and the infection that usually occur in the ulcerating neoplasm. Narcotic analgesics usually are necessary in the terminal stage of the disease.

N U R S I N G   P R O C E S S

● The Client With Cancer of the Vulva Undergoing Surgery

Assessment

The nurse determines the location and level of discomfort or pain. He or she checks for signs of infection and Homans' sign, as well as the status of peripheral circulation and integrity of the skin. The nurse discusses the client's perception of body image and explores concerns she may have about sexual function.

Diagnosis, Planning, and Interventions

The nurse offers emotional support while the client awaits the results of the biopsy. If surgery is the selected method of treatment, the nurse provides appropriate preoperative and postoperative care.

Before surgery, the nurse instructs the client to begin initial skin preparation by washing the lower abdomen, genitalia, perineum, and upper thighs with antibacterial soap for several days before surgery. On the day of surgery, the nurse inserts a Foley catheter and provides standard teaching for deep breathing and leg exercises. Antibiotic therapy may begin before the operative procedure.

The nurse plans measures to prevent postoperative complications, manage pain, relieve edema in the lower extremities, prevent wound infection, and preserve and restore skin integrity. The nurse also intervenes therapeutically to assist the client in maintaining an acceptable body image, preparing for the resumption of sexual function, and performing self-care activities after discharge. Refer to perioperative standards of care in Chapter 25.

Other nursing measures include, but are not limited to the following diagnoses, expected outcomes, and interventions:

Acute Pain related to tissue trauma and swelling
Expected Outcome: Pain will be relieved to a tolerable level within 30 minutes of a nursing intervention.

- Administer prescribed analgesics liberally. *Pain is best relieved by administering analgesia before pain becomes severe.*
- Apply an air or eggcrate mattress to the bed. *These mattresses promote comfort by distributing pressure more evenly.*
- Place client in a semirecumbent position. *It relieves pressure on the sutures.*
- Modify client's position at least every 2 hours. *Any position becomes uncomfortable if maintained for a prolonged period.*
- Use as many pillows as necessary to promote comfort. *Pillows support, elevate, and relieve pressure.*
- When in a lateral position, bend and support the upper leg on pillows. *Bending and supporting the upper leg in a lateral position prevents tension on the operative area.*

PC: Thrombophlebitis
Expected Outcome: The nurse will monitor to detect, manage, and minimize risk for the development of thrombophlebitis.

- Assess for and report calf pain on dorsiflexion or calf tenderness. *Calf pain or tenderness indicates the possible development of a blood clot.*
- Remove and reapply antithrombotic stockings or pneumatic leg compression device at regular intervals

each day. *Compression of valves in the veins prevents venous stasis.*

- Ensure that client performs leg exercises while in bed and ambulates as tolerated. *Skeletal muscle contraction promotes venous circulation.*
- Administer prescribed anticoagulants; monitor laboratory tests for therapeutic levels. *Anticoagulants interfere with blood clotting; dosages of anticoagulants are based on assessments of the partial thromboplastin time, prothrombin time, or international normalized ratio.*

Ineffective Tissue Perfusion related to compromised lymphatic and venous circulation secondary to excision of lymph nodes and ligation of blood vessels
Expected Outcome: Dependent edema will be absent by discharge.

- Elevate the lower extremities whenever possible. *Gravity promotes venous and lymphatic circulation.*
- Dangle the client's legs the evening of surgery and assist to ambulate daily. *Skeletal muscle movement that is required for ambulation promotes venous circulation.*

Risk for infection related to compromised skin integrity in close proximity to the rectum
Expected Outcome: Client will remain free of infection.

- Perform conscientious handwashing before caring for the wound. *Handwashing is the best method for preventing the transmission of microorganisms.*
- Inspect and change perineal dressing following principles of asepsis. *Using aseptic principles reduces the potential for transmitting pathogens.*
- Cleanse the anus with moistened antiseptic wipes after bowel elimination. *Stool contains pathogens that can be introduced into the wound.*
- Empty surgical drains and catheter drainage bag aseptically. *A tube or catheter provides a portal through which microorganisms can enter the body.*
- Observe and record the appearance and amount of drainage. *Evidence of purulent drainage suggests infection.*

Impaired Skin Integrity related to unresolved tissue healing
Expected Outcome: The wound will become approximated.

- Irrigate the wound with sterile saline, hydrogen peroxide, or a medically prescribed antiseptic solution at least three times daily. *Removing wound debris facilitates healing.*
- Dry the wound with a heat lamp or hair dryer. *Pressure or friction increases pain and can disrupt healing.*
- Give warm sitz baths after sutures have been removed. *Sitz baths increase circulation to the area and promote healing.*
- Cover intact skin with a transparent or air and water occlusive dressing. *Intact skin is protected from contact with moist drainage.*
- Support surgical drain during periods of ambulation. *An unsupported drain may be displaced from internal areas of the wound.*

- Explore the need to refer the client for home health nursing. *Home health nursing services are necessary if family or a significant member is unavailable for post-discharge wound care.*

Risk for Disturbed Body Image related to emotional distress secondary to amputated genitalia

Expected Outcome: Client will maintain a positive self-image.

- Ensure privacy when assessing the wound or carrying out treatment measures. *Privacy demonstrates respect for the client's dignity.*
- Keep client clean, odor free, and well groomed. *Attention to personal appearance promotes feeling attractive.*
- Listen when client expresses emotions regarding her changed appearance. *Verbalizing feelings relieves stress.*
- Encourage significant others to be genuinely attentive and to express acceptance through hand holding, sitting close, or other actions. *Touching is a nonverbal method for expressing continued regard for one another.*

Risk for Sexual Dysfunction related to anatomic changes in external genitalia

Expected Outcome: Client will find satisfactory techniques for experiencing sexual intimacy.

- Act as a liaison for information between the client and her surgeon as to the physical consequences of surgery. *Clients sometimes are reluctant to discuss sexual issues.*
- Role play or encourage discussions regarding sexual issues between the client and significant other. *Role playing can help client communicate sensitive issues.*
- Explore the idea of using a vaginal dilator, liberal lubrication, and a side-lying position for intercourse once healing is complete. *Alternative sexual practices promote comfort and pleasure during sexual activities.*
- Suggest that the client seek a referral from her physician to a sexual counselor if sexual issues are unresolved. *Sexual counselors have expertise in helping clients resolve problems with sexuality.*

Evaluation of Expected Outcomes

Expected outcomes are that pain is reduced or eliminated. The calves are of normal size and nontender. There is no dependent edema. Temperature is normal, with no wound tenderness or purulent drainage; white blood cell count is normal. The wound heals and the skin becomes intact. The client interacts with others and resumes previous lifestyle activities. The client can experience sexual intimacy.

Before discharge, the nurse instructs the client on the following measures for self-care:

- Wound healing will take as long as 6 months.
- Elevate the legs and wear antiembolic stockings to reduce dependent edema in the lower extremities.
- Eat a high-protein diet with sources of vitamin C to promote healing.
- Try to stand and straddle the toilet when attempting to void after the catheter is removed in 7 to 10 days so that urine is directed into the toilet rather than down the leg or perineum.
- After urination, cleanse the periurethral area with water or normal saline in a plastic drink container with a spout.
- Continue to take the prescribed stool softener after discharge.
- Take a sitz bath using a portable basin after each bowel movement.
- Report any unusual odor, fever, fresh bleeding, separation of the wound margin, inability to void or constipation, and perineal pain.

GENERAL NUTRITIONAL CONSIDERATIONS

Although some studies suggest that megadoses of vitamin B$_6$ relieve PMS symptoms, large doses (i.e., 500 mg) can cause sensory neuropathy, which disappears after supplement use stops. Until the relationship between nutrients and PMS is more clearly defined, discourage self-medicating with megadoses of vitamins and minerals.

Soy is rich in naturally occurring compounds called *phytoestrogens* (plant estrogens), which are similar to the body's own estrogen. Some studies suggest that increasing the intake of soy products may help alleviate menopausal symptoms such as hot flashes and vaginal dryness. Interestingly, women from Asian countries, where soy intake is high, report a low incidence of menopausal symptoms.

GENERAL PHARMACOLOGIC CONSIDERATIONS

Estrogen therapy can cause nausea and vomiting, pigmentation of the nipple and areola, and uterine bleeding. Stress incontinence may occur. Sodium may be retained, leading to excessive storage of interstitial fluid and edema. Diuretics and a low-sodium diet help relieve this situation. Large doses of estrogen sometimes cause the mobilization of calcium into the bloodstream, damaging the kidney when it excretes the excess calcium.

Because synthetic estrogen hormones cause thromboembolic phenomena, instruct the client to contact the physician if tenderness, pain, swelling, or redness occurs in the legs. If vaginal bleeding occurs during hormonal therapy, the client should contact the physician because the dose may need to be adjusted.

When androgen therapy is prescribed, clients may have increased bone pain after the first few injections. As therapy continues, pain frequently lessens, some recalcification of bone occurs, and the client has an increased appetite and gains weight. Androgen therapy may cause fluid retention, increased libido, and distressing symptoms of virilization, such as deeper voice and increased facial and body hair.

To prevent loss of bone mass in postmenopausal women who cannot tolerate HRT, the drug alendronate (Fosamax) may be prescribed. Alendronate acts to prevent bone resorption. Do not give the drug with milk or milk products because calcium inhibits absorption of the drug. The drug is best absorbed when given in 8 ounces of water on arising in the morning. Instruct the client to avoid lying down and to remain upright for at least 30 minutes after taking the drug to prevent dyspepsia and esophageal irritation.

When antibiotics are taken for a long time or if repeated courses of antibiotic therapy are necessary, an overgrowth of yeastlike fungi that usually exists in small numbers in the vagina can occur, resulting in vaginitis.

GENERAL GERONTOLOGIC CONSIDERATIONS

Older women may develop perineal pruritus. Effort is required to discover the cause of the pruritus; it may require asking questions about diet, type of clothing worn, vaginal discharge, and so on. The client also may be tested for glucose in the blood and urine, and a pelvic examination may be performed to rule out other abnormalities, such as cervicitis, cystocele, rectocele, or cancer of the vulva, cervix, or uterus.

When an older client has a uterine prolapse, surgery may not be considered because of complicating chronic disorders. A pessary may be used to return the uterus to its normal position in the pelvis.

The female genitalia changes during aging. The vulva atrophies, causing a loss of vascularity and elasticity. This can result in irritation or excoriation of the tissue. Pubic hair thins and the labia majora and minora became smaller.

Vaginal flora changes with age, causing the environment to become more alkaline and predisposing the older woman to vaginitis.

Hot flashes, which occur in approximately 75% of all perimenopausal women, are accompanied by increased perspiration, vasodilation, and a 10% to 20% increase in pulse rate. Estrogen, progesterone, combinations of the two, or clonidine may be used to alleviate symptoms.

Critical Thinking Exercises

1. *When a client says she has "female problems," what information is important to ask?*
2. *What nursing activities are appropriate when a woman has a pelvic examination during which a Papanicolaou test will be performed?*

References and Suggested Readings

Ahlgrimm, M., Battistini, M., Ravnikar, V., et al. (1998). Beyond hormones: Other treatments for menopausal symptoms. *Patient Care, 32*(8), 28–30, 32, 37+.

Andrist, L. C. (2001). Vaginal health and infections. *Journal of Obstetric, Gynecologic, and Neonatal Nursing, 30,* 306–315.

Barrow, C. (1999). Balloon endometrial ablation as a safe alternative to hysterectomy. *American Operating Room Nurses Journal, 70*(1), 79–80.

Christman, N. J., Oakley, M. G., & Cronin, S. N. (2001). Developing and using preparatory information for women undergoing radiation therapy for cervical or uterine cancer. *Oncology Nursing Forum, 28*(1), 93–98.

Clark, A. (1999). Menorrhagia: The treatment options. *Nursing Times, 95*(42), 44–45.

Duffy, M. S. (2001). Recent surgical approaches to gynecologic oncology. *Nursing Clinics of North America, 36,* 603–615.

Egan, M. E. & Lipsky, M. S. (2000). Diagnosis of vaginitis. *American Family Physician, 62,* 1095–1104.

FDA clears uterine balloon to treat excessive bleeding. (1998). *OR Manager, 14*(2), 10.

Gamel, C., Hengeveld, M., & Davis, B. (2000). Informational needs about the effects of gynaecological cancer on sexuality: A review of the literature. *Journal of Clinical Nursing, 9,* 678–688.

Holmquist, N. D. (2000). Revisiting the effect of the Pap test on cervical cancer. *American Journal of Public Health, 90,* 620–623.

Kim, K. H. & Lee, K. A. (2001). Symptom experience in women after hysterectomy. *Journal of Obstetric, Gynecologic, and Neonatal Nursing, 30,* 472–480.

Lee, C. O. (2000). Gynecologic cancers: Part I. Risk factors. *Clinical Journal of Oncology Nursing, 4*(2), 67–71, 89–90.

Lee, C. O. (2000). Gynecologic cancers: Part II. Risk assessment and screening. *Clinical Journal of Oncology Nursing, 4*(2), 73–77.

Lucas, B. D. (1999). Five reasons to consider a hysterectomy. *Patient Care, 33*(14), 34–36.

Napoli, M. (2001). A call for more research: What we don't know about hysterectomy is as significant as what we do know. *American Journal of Nursing, 101*(9), 35.

National Institutes of Health. (1994, April 5–7). *Ovarian cancer: Screening, treatment, and followup* (NIH Consensus Statement 12, 3). Bethesda, MD: Author.

Porth, C. M. (2002). *Pathophysiology: Concepts of altered health states* (6th ed.). Philadelphia: Lippincott Williams & Wilkins.

Reeder, S. J., Martin, L. L., & Koniak, D. (1992). *Maternity nursing: Family, newborn, and women's health care* (17th ed.). Philadelphia: J. B. Lippincott.

Reich, H. (2001). Issues surrounding surgical menopause: Indications and procedures. *Journal of Reproductive Medicine, 46*(3, Suppl.), 297–306, 333–336.

Robb-Nicholson, C. (2000). By the way, doctor. . . . Differences between vaginal and abdominal hysterectomy. *Harvard Women's Health Watch, 8*(3), 7.

Robotham, M. (1999). Pelvic pain: Hidden troubles. *Nursing Times, 95*(32), 32–33.

Rovner, E. S. (2000). Pelvic organ prolapse: A review. *Ostomy/Wound Management, 46*(12), 24–37.

Sato, F., Miyake, H., Nishi, M., et al. (2000). Early normal menstrual cycle pattern and the development of uterine leiomyomas. *Journal of Women's Health and Gender-Based Medicine, 9,* 299–302.

Scott, L. D. & Hasik, K. J. (2001). The similarities and differences of endometritis and pelvic inflammatory disease. *Journal of Obstetric, Gynecologic, and Neonatal Nursing, 30,* 332–341.

Seiser, B. V. (2001). Ovarian cancer strategies for nurse practitioners. *Journal of the American Academy of Nurse Practitioners, 13,* 359–363.

Sharts-Hopko, N. C. (2001). Hysterectomy for nonmalignant conditions. *American Journal of Nursing, 101*(9), 32–41.

Smith, C. B. (1999). Abnormal uterine bleeding: How to sort out benign from more troubling causes. *Consultant, 39,* 1266–1268.

Trotto, N. E. (2001). Ovarian cancer screening: An ongoing challenge. *Patient Care, 35*(14), 14–16.

Wellbery, C. (1999). Diagnosis and treatment of endometriosis. *American Family Physician, 60,* 1753–1762, 1767–1768.

Wolff, L. L. (1999). Dysmenorrhea. *Journal of the American Academy of Nurse Practitioners, 11,* 125–133.

Caring for Clients With Breast Disorders

Words to Know

breast abscess
breast cancer
breast reconstruction
breast self-examination
clinical breast examination
fibroadenoma
fibrocystic breast disease
lumpectomy
lymphedema
mammography
mammoplasty
mastalgia
mastitis
mastopexy
modified radical
   mastectomy
partial (or segmental)
   mastectomy
reduction
   mammoplasty
sentinel lymph node
   mapping
simple (or total)
   mastectomy
subcutaneous
   mastectomy

Learning Objectives

On completion of this chapter, the reader will:

- List four common signs and symptoms in all breast disorders.
- Describe three techniques for obtaining a breast biopsy.
- Name two infectious and inflammatory breast disorders and explain how they are acquired.
- Discuss health teaching that may help prevent or eliminate infectious and inflammatory breast disorders.
- Compare and contrast two benign breast disorders.
- Explain how and when to perform breast self-examination.
- Give the current recommendations for mammography.
- Name groups at high risk for developing breast cancer.
- List common signs and symptoms of and three methods for treating breast cancer.
- Describe six surgical techniques used to remove a malignant breast tumor.
- Give two criteria that are used when selecting a mastectomy procedure.
- Name a serious complication of breast cancer treatment.
- Discuss the nursing management of clients who undergo surgical treatment for breast cancer.
- List four sites to which breast cancer commonly metastasizes.
- Describe three elective cosmetic breast procedures for clients with a mastectomy.
- Describe three cosmetic breast procedures that women with nondiseased breasts may elect.

The breasts are part of the female reproductive system, and they respond to the hormonal cycle associated with ovulation, menstruation, and pregnancy. Their primary function is to produce milk, a process referred to as *lactation.*

ANATOMY AND PHYSIOLOGY

The breasts contain the mammary glands, a network of ducts that carry milk to the nipple (Fig. 60-1). Each mammary gland consists of 15 to 20 lobes divided by *adipose tissue.* The adipose tissue determines the size of the breast

but not the amount of milk produced. The breasts manufacture milk from elements in the blood. Prolactin, a hormone produced by the anterior pituitary gland, stimulates milk production. The breasts have an abundant supply of blood vessels and lymphatics. The axillary lymph nodes and the internal mammary lymph nodes drain the breasts.

Estrogen secreted by the ovaries causes the growth and development of the mammary system. Further growth and development that occurs during pregnancy is hormone dependent. Prolactin promotes the production of milk. Progesterone, secreted by the placenta, stimulates the development of alveoli, which secrete the milk. Estrogen, also secreted by the placenta, stimulates increased pro-

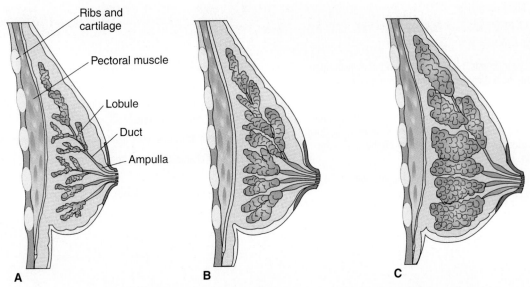

FIGURE 60-1 Breast structures. (**A**) Nonpregnant woman, (**B**) pregnant woman, and (**C**) lactating woman.

duction of tubules and ducts to transport the milk to the lactiferous duct, which drains at the nipple.

ASSESSMENT

Breast Examination

Clinical breast examination is performed when the client has a gynecologic examination, before a mammogram, or during the annual physical examination. The examiner notes breast size and symmetry and any unusual changes in the skin of the breasts and nipples. The examiner looks for masses, dimpling, flattening, rashes, ulcerations, or discharge from the nipple. Using the flat part of the fingertips, the examiner palpates the breasts and axillae for masses, lymph nodes, tenderness, and other abnormalities, with the client lying down, arm raised over the head.

Disorders of the breast are manifested by one or more signs or symptoms in Box 60-1 among adult women of all age groups. Therefore, regular **breast self-examination** (BSE), described and illustrated in Nursing Guidelines 60-1, is an important way for women to discover early

breast changes, initiate early treatment, and improve outcomes of breast disorders. Because breast cancer can occur in men also, examination of the male breasts and axillae should be included in the annual physical examination.

Mammography

Mammography (mammogram) is a radiographic technique used to detect cysts or tumors of the breast, some of which may be too small to palpate. Mammography is used as a screening test for breast cancer (Fig. 60-2). The National Cancer Institute recommends that women begin receiving annual mammograms at 40 years of age (Box 60-2). The need for mammograms before age 40 years depends on factors such as a family history of breast cancer, a past history of benign breast disease, incisional or excisional breast biopsies, or other conditions that interfere with accurate BSEs.

Ultrasonography

Ultrasonography (ultrasound) often is used with a mammogram to differentiate fluid-filled cysts from other types of breast lesions. It involves the use of high-frequency sound waves to produce a visual picture. It has been especially useful for women with very dense breasts, such as younger women and those on hormone replacement therapy.

When a mammogram is scheduled, the nurse explains the radiographic procedure and instructs the client to omit using a deodorant with aluminum hydroxide or body talc the day of the test to avoid artifacts on the x-ray film. If the client forgets or was not provided with this information,

---

BOX 60-1 ● Signs and Symptoms Common to Breast Disorders

- Pain, tenderness, fullness of the breast
- Breast mass(es)
- Nipple discharge
- Change in breast appearance

NURSING GUIDELINES 60-1

Teaching Breast Self-Examination

- Examine your breasts 3 days after the end of menstruation or monthly on a date of your choice if you no longer menstruate.

- Begin the examination in the shower when the breasts are wet and soapy and again after the shower when lying down with a folded towel under the shoulder on the side being examined.

- Use light, medium, and firm pressure applied with the pads of three fingers when checking each breast.

- Move your fingers in circles, spokes of a wheel, or rows, but follow the same technique with each BSE.

- Feel every part of each breast, including the nipple area and the armpit to the collar bone.

- Raise your arms over your head and look at the breasts in a mirror.

- Look for changes in breast shape, size, and contour; puckering (dimpling) of the skin; or areas that appear red.

- Squeeze each nipple and look for liquid drainage.

the nurse provides a premoistened wipe to cleanse the axillae just before the test. The nurse determine how often the client performs BSEs and has her demonstrate or describe the technique. For women who are unfamiliar with BSE, the nurse instructs and demonstrates how to perform BSE. He or she ensures privacy throughout the examination and advises clients to have their mammograms at the same health agency or arrange for records to be transferred so that previous mammogram results can be compared.

Stop, Think, and Respond ● BOX 60-1

A 52-year-old woman tells you she has never had a mammogram and has heard they are painful. How would you respond to her?

BOX 60-2 ● Guidelines for Mammography

The National Cancer Institute recommends that all women have a mammogram:

- Initially at age 40
- Every 1 to 2 years thereafter
- Women at higher than average risk of breast cancer should seek expert medical advice about screening before age 40 and the frequency of screening.

(Source: National Cancer Institute. [2001]. NCI Statement on Mammography Screening. [On-line.] Available: http://newscenter.cancer.gov/pressreleases/mammstatements31jan02.html.)

FIGURE 60-2 A client undergoing mammography.

Breast Biopsy

A breast biopsy is performed to determine if a breast lesion is malignant. A specimen of tissue from the breast may be obtained in one of three ways: incisional biopsy, excisional biopsy, or aspiration biopsy.

Incisional Biopsy

Incisional biopsy is performed in the operating room, where one or more sections of tissue are removed. The specimen is frozen quickly and examined microscopically by a pathologist while the client remains anesthetized. If the tissue is negative (i.e., benign), the remainder of the benign tissue is removed (if it had not been completely removed for biopsy), the incision closed, and the client sent to the recovery room. If the removed specimen is found to be malignant, the surgeon may then perform the surgical procedure that offers the best chance of cure. The decision to operate immediately when there is a malignancy is thoroughly discussed with the client before surgery.

Excisional Biopsy

Some surgeons prefer an excisional biopsy, which is removal of the entire lesion. A pathologist examines the excised specimen later and more comprehensively. Clients may be discharged from the hospital before the results of the biopsy are obtained, or they may remain hospitalized. If the lesion is malignant, the biopsy results and the proposed treatment are discussed with the client.

Aspirational Biopsy

Aspirational biopsy, a procedure usually performed on an outpatient basis, uses a needle and syringe to obtain a sample of the suspect tissue. A local anesthetic is first injected around the area, and a sample of tissue is removed. A pathologist examines the tissue sample. Sometimes this procedure is done in the hospital under mammographic guidance to ensure an accurate sample of suspect tissue.

Nursing Management

The nurse allows the client time to ask questions and listens to concerns before the breast biopsy is performed. The client may have concerns about not only the procedure but the results of the biopsy and a possible diagnosis of cancer.

An aspiration biopsy usually causes minimal discomfort after the procedure, but there may be redness and soreness in the area. The nurse instructs the client to notify the physician if drainage or bleeding from the biopsy site is more than slight or if increased redness, pain, or fever occurs. Incisional and excisional biopsies require sutures, but pain usually is minimal and can be relieved with a mild analgesic.

The nurse provides instructions regarding wound care, use of a mild analgesic, wearing a supportive brassiere, and timing of a follow-up appointment. He or she reviews the signs and symptoms that suggest wound infection.

INFECTIOUS AND INFLAMMATORY BREAST DISORDERS

● MASTITIS

Mastitis, an inflammation of breast tissue, is most common in women who are breast-feeding. It may occur in one or both breasts. Although it can occur at any time, it is most common during the second or third postpartum week.

Pathophysiology and Etiology

Breast inflammation is caused or contributed to by one or more plugged lactiferous ducts or an infectious agent that enters through cracked or fissured nipples. Ducts become plugged as a consequence of infrequent nursing, failure to alternate breasts at each feeding, or a poorly nursing infant.

Lactating breasts have an elaborate blood supply and ductal system that easily supports microbial growth. If an infection develops, the most common causative microorganism is *Staphylococcus aureus,* which often is resistant to antibiotic therapy. The infectious process results from inadequate maternal handwashing or an infant infected by microorganisms on the hands of nursery personnel or by organisms on the mother's skin.

Assessment Findings

Fever and malaise accompany breast tenderness, pain, and redness. The breast later becomes swollen, firm, and hard. A crack in the nipple or areola develops, and the axillary lymph nodes enlarge. Rarely, a breast abscess develops. A culture and sensitivity test on expressed breast milk identifies the infectious agent.

Medical Management

Appropriate antibiotic therapy based on culture and sensitivity tests is given for 10 days. For organisms that are penicillin resistant, oxacillin (Prostaphlin), cephalosporins such as cefazolin (Kefzol), or vancomycin (Vancocin) are given. Analgesics are prescribed for pain. Heat also can be applied locally. To prevent engorgement and maintain lactation, the breasts are emptied using a breast pump. Recent research indicates treatment of nipples infected with *S. aureus* with systemic antibiotics decreases mastitis (Livingstone & Stringer, 1999).

Nursing Management

The nurse assists with taking the health history (which includes identifying allergies to antibiotics), prepares the client for a physical examination, and collects the specimen of breast milk using standard precautions and aseptic principles. Client teaching includes information for self-administering antibiotic medications, principles of medical asepsis, and techniques to promote comfort and temporary alternatives to breast-feeding. Specific instructions include the following:

- Take antibiotics for the full time prescribed.
- Report side effects from the medication such as rash, gastrointestinal upset, and opportunistic infections in the mouth or vagina.
- Perform scrupulous handwashing before touching the breast.
- Bathe or shower regularly and apply lotion to dry or cracked nipples.
- Wear a supportive brassiere.
- Avoid wearing breast shields, which trap breast milk and moisture around the nipple.
- Apply warm soaks to the breast or let warm water from a shower flow over the breast.
- Express milk with a breast pump until the infection is resolved sufficiently to resume breast-feeding.

● BREAST ABSCESS

A **breast abscess** is a localized collection of pus in breast tissue.

Pathophysiology and Etiology

When an abscess occurs in the breast, it most frequently is a complication of postpartum mastitis. Purulent exudate accumulates in a confined, local area of breast tissue. *S. aureus* again is the most common cause.

Assessment Findings

The client experiences the signs and symptoms of mastitis; in the case of an abscess, however, pus may drain from the nipple. The diagnosis is based on physical examination of the breast. A culture and sensitivity of nipple drainage identifies the infecting microorganism and indicates to which antibiotics it is sensitive.

Medical and Surgical Management

The client usually is hospitalized and placed on contact isolation precautions because the soiled dressings are highly infectious. The client is started on intravenous (IV) antibiotic therapy. The abscess may be incised, drained, and packed.

Nursing Management

The nurse removes and reapplies dressings following aseptic principles. To avoid irritating the skin from frequent removal of tape, the nurse uses a binder to hold the dressing in place. He or she applies zinc oxide to the surrounding skin to avoid maceration from irritating drainage or wound compresses. To reduce swelling, the nurse supports the arm and shoulder with pillows. He or she instructs the client not to shave axillary hair on the side with the abscess until healing is complete.

The mother who is temporarily separated from her newborn needs emotional support. The nurse helps the client pump her breasts to remove milk and prevent engorgement. If the mother decides to terminate breast-feeding, the nurse applies a tight-fitting brassiere.

BENIGN BREAST LESIONS

● FIBROCYSTIC BREAST DISEASE

Fibrocystic breast disease, also called *mammary dysplasia* (abnormal development of breast tissue) or *chronic cystic mastitis,* is a benign breast condition that affects women primarily between the ages of 30 and 50 years.

Pathophysiology and Etiology

Fibrocystic disease results from hormonal changes during the menstrual cycle. Caffeine and nicotine also may aggravate the condition.

When the disorder develops, single or multiple breast cysts appear in one or both breasts (Fig. 60-3). The cysts increase in size and become increasingly tender in proportion to the secretion of estrogen. Cyst formation tends to continue throughout the reproductive years. Some disappear, although others may remain permanently. The condition resolves with menopause.

FIGURE 60-3 Depiction of single and multiple breast cysts.

Although a correlation between fibrocystic disease and breast cancer was reported years ago, current studies have indicated no cause-and-effect relationship between the two conditions. Women with fibrocystic disease, however, may mistake a cancerous mass for a fibrocystic mass and delay medical diagnosis, perform BSE less vigorously because of breast tenderness, or fail to palpate a malignant mass disguised by scar tissue from a previous incisional biopsy.

Assessment Findings

Signs and Symptoms

Fibrocystic disease of the breast may cause no symptoms, but many women report having tender or painful breasts and feeling one, but more often multiple lumps within breast tissue. The symptoms are most noticeable just before menstruation and usually abate during menstruation. The size of the cyst often changes with the menstrual cycle, becoming larger before menstruation. Activities, such as weight training, can increase **mastalgia** (breast pain).

Diagnostic Findings

A preliminary diagnosis is made by examination of the breasts. The characteristic breast mass of fibrocystic disease is soft to firm, movable, and unlikely to cause nipple retraction. Fluid from the cysts is aspirated for cytologic examination, or an incisional biopsy is performed. If the results are questionable, mammography and ultrasonography are performed to distinguish a cystic lesion from a solid malignant tumor.

Medical and Surgical Management

Mild discomfort is relieved with an analgesic such as aspirin or ibuprofen (Advil). For severe symptoms, oral contraceptives or danazol (Danocrine), a synthetic androgen, and bromocriptine (Parlodel), a semisynthetic ergot derivative that mimics prolactin inhibitory factor, are prescribed (Drug Therapy Table 60-1). Occasionally, one or more cysts are removed surgically. Widespread disease that causes severe discomfort is treated with partial mastectomy. Care is taken to preserve the areola to provide a cosmetic appearance to the breast after surgery.

Nursing Management

The nurse obtains a health history and asks focused questions about the characteristics and timing of symptoms in relation to the menstrual cycle. During diagnostic examinations, the nurse prepares and supports the client, labels tissue or fluid specimens, and arranges for laboratory analysis.

The nurse teaches the client with fibrocystic disease to:

- Perform BSE monthly using the same technique each time, and become familiar with the feel and location of cystic masses.
- Schedule a breast examination with a physician every 6 months or whenever a new or unusual lump develops.
- Follow the American Cancer Society's Breast Advisory Committee's Guidelines for mammography (see Box 60-2).
- Wear a well-fitting, supportive brassiere day and night.
- Take mild analgesics or prescription medications according to label directions.
- Apply cold compresses to the breasts when symptomatic.
- Avoid smoking, coffee, chocolate, and caffeinated soft drinks.
- Restrict activities that may cause trauma to the breasts such as playing soccer or other sports in which the breasts are unprotected.
- Consult with the physician about taking vitamin E supplement or oil of evening primrose (a herbal preparation), which some clients have found helpful.

● FIBROADENOMA

A **fibroadenoma** is a solid, benign breast mass composed of connective and glandular tissue (Fig. 60-4). This type of breast lesion usually occurs in women during late adolescence and early adulthood, but occasionally is found in older women.

Pathophysiology and Etiology

The cause of fibroadenomas is unknown. There may be a hormonal influence, however, because the mass grows during pregnancy and shrinks after menopause.

Classically, the benign tumor is a single nodule that grows slowly in nonpregnant women until it reaches a fixed, stable size. It usually does not enlarge and regress with each menstrual cycle, like those in fibrocystic disease, and it, too, is not considered precancerous.

Assessment Findings

A fibroadenoma presents as a painless, nontender lump in the breast. The lesion usually is encapsulated, mobile, and firm when palpated. If the size of the mass is large, the breasts may appear asymmetric.

DRUG THERAPY TABLE 60-1	AGENTS FOR SEVERE FIBROCYSTIC DISEASE		
DRUG CATEGORY AND EXAMPLES	**MECHANISM OF ACTION**	**SIDE EFFECTS**	**NURSING CONSIDERATIONS**
Synthetic Androgen danazol (Danocrine)	Decreases estrogen and progesterone levels by suppressing follicle-stimulating hormone and luteinizing hormone	Acne, deepened voice, weight gain, flushing, vaginitis, enlarged clitoris, nervousness, emotional lability, fluid retention, headache, fatigue, liver dysfunction	Arrange for periodic history and physical exam; long-term use increases chances of side effects and medical supervision is required. Cancer should be ruled out before treatment is initiated. Client should begin taking the hormone during her menstrual period to ensure she is not pregnant. Instruct client to use a nonhormonal form of birth control. Inform client of possible side effects, that masculinizing can occur, and to report any unusual developments.
Progestins medroxyprogesterone (Provera, Amen)	Hinders estrogen's effect on breast tissue	Breakthrough bleeding, spotting, amenorrhea, rash, acne, weight gain, edema, depression, thrombophlebitis, migraine, loss of vision, photosensitivity	Arrange for periodic history and physical exam as noted above. Have client mark drug administration days on the calendar. Inform client of possible side effects, including signs and symptoms of thrombophlebitis and embolism. Instruct client to use a reliable method of birth control and sunscreen and to report any visual disturbances.
Estrogen and Progesterone Combinations estradiol and norethindrone (Ortho-Novum 10/11)	Oral contraceptives suppress ovarian secretion of estrogen and oppose estrogen's effect on breast tissue	Headache, dizziness, thromboembolism, nausea, breakthrough bleeding, depression, anxiety	Continued medical supervision is required; arrange for physical examination, Papanicolaou tests, and breast examinations at least yearly. Discuss side effects with client; instruct on signs and symptoms of thrombophlebitis and embolism. Instruct client not to smoke and to report any side effects.
Ergot Derivative bromocriptine (Parlodel)	Binds with prolactin-secreting cells of the anterior pituitary; inhibits the release of prolactin	Nausea, vomiting, diarrhea, constipation, headache, drowsiness, nasal congestion, hypotension	Administer initial dose at bedtime and with meals thereafter. Advise client to change positions slowly and to use a reliable contraceptive. Report any side effects.

FIGURE 60-4 Fibroadenoma.

Ultrasound can reveal physical characteristics unique to a fibroadenoma versus malignant mass with a higher degree of accuracy than mammography (Greenfield et al., 2001). In the case of very young women—an atypical age for breast cancer—an excisional biopsy is performed only if the mass changes or becomes larger. If the mass is detected in a woman with a higher risk for developing breast cancer, such as one with a family history or in an older age group, a biopsy is performed to validate that the tissue is indeed benign.

Medical and Surgical Management

Based on the diagnostic findings, the client and her physician decide either to continue to observe the mass or excise it. Surgery involves removal of the benign tumor but not a mastectomy. The client is discharged a few hours after recovery from anesthesia.

Nursing Management

The nurse provides emotional support while the diagnosis is tentative because finding a mass in the breast conjures up fears that it may be malignant. The nurse teaches the client as follows:

- Continue monthly BSE and follow recommendations for mammography.
- Consult a physician if the characteristics of the mass change or if a pregnancy occurs.

If surgery is performed, the nurse should include the following instructions:

- Keep the wound clean and covered until the incision heals.
- Wear a firm, supportive brassiere to reduce incisional discomfort.
- Follow label directions for taking a mild non-narcotic analgesic to relieve minor pain that may last 1 to 3 days.
- Contact the surgeon to schedule a postoperative evaluation or call immediately if there is exceptional incisional pain or if swelling, wound drainage, or a fever develops.

MALIGNANT BREAST DISORDERS

● CANCER OF THE BREAST

One woman in eight develops **breast cancer,** a mass of abnormal cells. The risk for breast cancer in women increases with age. Although breast cancer does occur in men, the ratio is approximately 1:150 cases in women. In terms of cancer-related deaths in women, breast cancer is second only to lung cancer. When the disease is discovered and treated early, the 5-year survival rate for small lesions is at least 80%.

Pathology and Pathophysiology

Certain factors appear to increase the risk for development of breast cancer. Being female, being older than 50 years of age, and having a family history of breast cancer are the most common risk factors. Relatives of women with breast cancer who carry a defective gene (BRCA1 and BRCA2) are very likely to develop breast cancer. Additional factors include exposure to ionizing radiation in childhood or adolescence, previous breast cancer, a history of colon or endometrial cancer, chronic alcohol consumption, early menarche, late menopause, obesity, and having no children or having children after 30 years of age. White women are at higher risk for breast cancer than are African Americans, but African-American women are more likely to die of it. More than 50% of women diagnosed with breast cancer demonstrate none of the identified risk factors other than age (Machia, 2001).

Each normal breast contains 15 to 20 lobes connected by ducts to smaller lobules (see Fig. 60-1). The most common malignancy is ductal carcinoma (75%), followed by infiltrating lobular carcinoma (5% to 10%), medullary carcinoma (6%), mucinous carcinoma (3%), tubular ductal carcinoma (2%), and inflammatory breast cancer (1% to 2%). Some malignant breast tumors are hormone dependent, meaning that estrogen or progesterone enhances tumor growth. Regardless of the type or its etiology, untreated cancer spreads elsewhere through the axillary lymph nodes.

Assessment Findings

Signs and Symptoms

The primary sign of breast cancer is a painless mass in the breast, most often in the upper outer quadrant (Fig. 60-5). The tumor may have been developing in situ for as long as 2 years before becoming palpable. Other signs of breast cancer include a bloody discharge from the nipple, a dimpling of the skin over the lesion, retraction of the nipple, peau d'orange (orange peel) appearance of the skin, and a difference in size between the breasts (Fig. 60-6). The lesion may be fixed or movable, and axillary lymph nodes may be enlarged. Many of these signs depend on several factors, such as the type, location, and duration of the tumor.

Diagnostic Findings

Mammography detects breast lesions earlier than they can be palpated. The radiologist often can differentiate between a benign and malignant tumor on the radiograph. Biopsy and microscopic cell examination confirm the diagnosis. Even in women who are 65 years of age or older, regular mammograms ensure an early diagnosis and a decreased mortality rate from breast cancer (McCarthy et al., 2000).

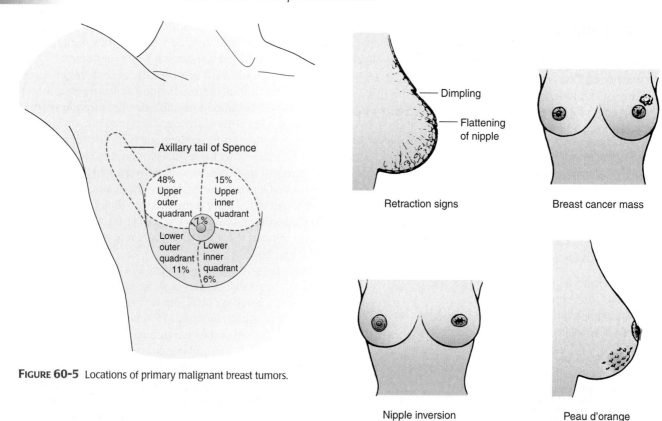

FIGURE 60-5 Locations of primary malignant breast tumors.

FIGURE 60-6 Signs and symptoms of breast cancer.

Medical and Surgical Management

Treatment depends on the stage of the breast tumor (Fig. 60-7). It includes surgery, which may be combined with chemotherapy (including hormone therapy) and radiation therapy. Clinical trials using immunotherapy are in progress.

Surgery

Surgery is performed immediately after obtaining the results of the biopsy or shortly thereafter. The type of surgery recommended depends on the stage of the tumor and the client's informed decision about treatment options (Table 60-1). The current trend is to perform the least mutilating procedure necessary to obtain a favorable prognosis. Compared with more extensive types of mastectomy procedures, breast-conserving surgeries such as lumpectomy, partial mastectomy, and segmental mastectomy have demonstrated equivalent outcomes in terms of survival rate for treatment of early-stage breast cancer (National Institutes of Health, 1990).

Removal of the ovaries enhances the prognosis for women whose tumors are hormone stimulated. The additional surgery inhibits the growth of the primary tumor or metastatic tissue derived from the primary tumor elsewhere in the body.

A new technique, sentinel lymph node mapping, is being done to determine whether complete removal of axillary lymph nodes is necessary. **Sentinel lymph node mapping** involves identifying the first (sentinel) lymph nodes through which the breast cancer cells would spread to regional lymph nodes in the axilla. The sentinel lymph nodes are located by injecting a nuclear isotope around the breast tumor followed by the instillation of blue dye. After excising the breast tumor, the surgeon passes a Geiger counter over the perimammary tissue to find the area of most intense radioactivity. A small incision is made and the surgeon follows the blue dye to the sentinel lymph nodes. The sentinel lymph nodes are removed with a minimum of surrounding tissue and investigated for cancer cells. No cancer cells in the sentinel lymph nodes suggests that all lymph nodes are free of cancer cells. Validating the lack of lymph node metastasis allows the surgeon to preserve more breast, axillary tissue, and chest muscle. Leaving many normal lymph nodes intact reduces the potential for complications, such as lymphedema (discussed later), delayed wound healing, and altered skin sensation, from the extensive disruption of lymphatic circulation.

In extensive surgical procedures such as modified radical mastectomy (radical mastectomy no longer is the standard of practice for the surgical treatment of breast cancer), drains are inserted to remove serous fluid that collects under the skin. Removing fluid promotes healing and reduces the potential for infection. Also, a skin graft

Stage I: Tumors are less than 2 cm in diameter and confined to breast.

Stage II: Tumors are less than 5 cm, or tumors are smaller with mobile axillary lymph node involvement.

Stage IIIa: Tumors are greater than 5 cm, or tumors are accompanied by enlarged axillary lymph nodes fixed to one another or to adjacent tissue.

Stage IIIb: More advanced lesions with satellite nodules, fixation to the skin or chest wall, ulceration, edema, or with supra-clavicular or intraclavicular nodal involvement.

Stage IV: All tumors with distant metastases.

FIGURE 60-7 Breast cancer stages.

may be required to close the wound if a radical mastectomy is performed. Pressure dressings are applied to both the donor and recipient graft sites.

Lymphedema, soft tissue swelling from accumulated lymphatic fluid, occurs in some women after breast cancer surgery. The condition is a consequence of removing or irradiating the axillary lymph nodes. It is evidenced by temporary or permanent enlargement of the arm and hand on the side of the amputated breast. Impaired lymphatic circulation predisposes to disfigurement, reduced range of motion, heaviness of the limb, skin changes, infection, and, in severe cases, tissue necrosis that may require amputation of the limb.

Depending on circumstances, chemotherapy and chemotherapy plus radiation therapy are common surgical adjuncts. The choice depends on factors such as the the type of cancer and stage of the tumor, any metastasis, and the client's age. Bone marrow transplantation may be used if the breast cancer resists other forms of treatment.

Chemotherapy

The goal of chemotherapy is to destroy any cancer cells that may have metastasized before or during surgery. One or more of the following drugs are given:

- An antiestrogen drug, such as tamoxifen (Nolvadex), for postmenopausal women whose tumors are hormone dependent
- An antiprogestin drug, mifepristone (RU486), which blocks progesterone-dependent breast cancers as determined by progesterone receptor assay on excised tissue
- Androgen therapy for advanced breast cancer in postmenopausal women using testolactone (Teslac)
- Single or combined antineoplastic agents, such as cyclophosphamide (Cytoxan), doxorubicin (Adriamycin), 5-fluorouracil (5-FU), methotrexate (Folex), and prednisone (Deltasone). Antineoplastic drugs also are combined with drugs mentioned earlier that influence hormonal physiology.

Radiation Therapy

Radiation therapy can be given before or after surgery. If the surgeon finds that the axillary nodes contain cancer cells, there is chest wall involvement, or the tumor is larger than 5 cm, a series of radiation treatments usually is ordered prophylactically even after a modified radical mastectomy. Side effects of radiation therapy include fatigue, skin redness similar to a bad sunburn,

Stop, Think, and Respond ● BOX 60-2

A client has had a modified radical mastectomy. While trying to teach her how to care for the incision, she avoids looking at the wound. How can you help her cope with the change in body image?

TABLE 60-1	SURGICAL PROCEDURES FOR BREAST CANCER

PROCEDURE	DESCRIPTION	ILLUSTRATION
Lumpectomy	Only the tumor is removed; some axillary lymph nodes may be excised at the same time for microscopic examination.	Axillary dissection
Partial or segmental mastectomy	The tumor and some breast tissue and some lymph nodes are removed.	
Simple or total mastectomy	All breast tissue is removed. No lymph node dissection is performed.	
Subcutaneous mastectomy	All breast tissue is removed, but the skin and nipple are left intact.	

(continued)

TABLE 60-1	SURGICAL PROCEDURES FOR BREAST CANCER (Continued)

PROCEDURE	DESCRIPTION	ILLUSTRATION
Modified radical mastectomy	The breast, some lymph nodes, the lining over the chest muscles, and the pectoralis minor muscle are removed.	
Radical mastectomy	The breast, axillary lymph nodes, and pectoralis major and minor muscles are removed. In some instances, sternal lymph nodes also are removed.	

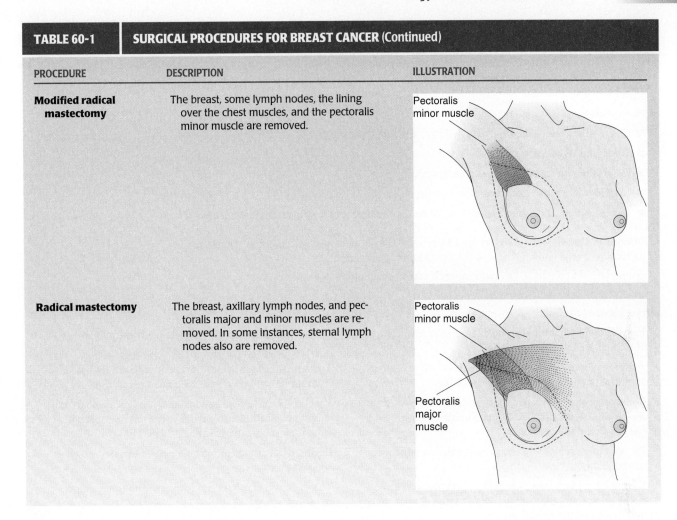

rash, minor discomfort, or pain (see Chap. 20). Some develop pneumonitis, rib fractures, and breast fibrosis.

Stop, Think, and Respond ● BOX 60-3

What measures would you recommend to your client receiving radiation therapy to decrease skin irritation to the radiated area?

Nursing Management

The nurse encourages anyone who detects breast changes to see a physician immediately. The nurse prepares the client for surgery and assists with her or his safe recovery. Men who undergo a mastectomy do not face the extreme physical changes, but they still require emotional support because of the diagnosis. For breast-conserving procedures, nursing care focuses on wound management and discharge instructions. Refer to Nursing Care Plan 60-1 for more specific information in managing the care of the client undergoing a modified radical mastectomy.

The nurse prepares the client for common side effects of chemotherapy like nausea, vomiting, changes in taste, alopecia (hair loss), mucositis, dermatitis, fatigue, weight gain, and bone marrow suppression. Some clients also experience mild short-term memory loss and difficulty with thought processes, known as "chemo-brain." It is not known whether this results from the chemotherapy or the depression that frequently accompanies a cancer diagnosis. Administering antiemetics and anxiolytic medications before a chemotherapy treatment helps to lessen the potential for vomiting. The nurse provides instructions about when and how to take medications at home to alleviate nausea and mouth sores and to boost the white blood cell or red blood cell production. If alopecia is likely, the nurse offers the client a list of wig suppliers (usually provided through the American Cancer Society). Catalogs are available, through the American Cancer Society, to purchase scarves, turbans, or hats to camouflage the hair loss.

Most clients are not hospitalized long after mastectomy. Therefore, providing early discharge instructions and making arrangements for home care are important inter-

(text continued on page 952)

Nursing Care Plan 60-1

THE CLIENT UNDERGOING A MODIFIED RADICAL MASTECTOMY

Assessment

- Discuss the client's medical, drug, allergy, and family history.
- Take vital signs and weight.
- Determine the location of the breast lesion.
- Establish what diagnostic tests were performed before admission (if any).
- Discuss information the physician has given the client about the type and extent of surgery.

Nursing Diagnoses: Anxiety and **Fear** related to undergoing an unfamiliar experience and the potential consequences of the disease and its treatment

Expected Outcome: Client will indicate increased emotional comfort.

Interventions	Rationales
Provide an opportunity for the client to express feelings and discuss concerns.	Verbalizing helps the client deal openly with feelings.
Answer all questions; consult with other team members about matters that involve their expertise.	Presenting facts provides the client with reality-based information and reduces exaggerated perceptions.
Collaborate with physician on arranging for a visit from a Reach to Recovery or I Can Cope volunteer sponsored by the American Cancer Society.	People who have recovered from a similar diagnosis and surgery can serve as role models and answer questions from their own personal experiences.
Do not stifle crying; stay with client when emotions are overwhelming.	Crying relieves tension when a person can find no other coping strategy.
Encourage client's significant other or whomever the client turns to for support to remain with client as much and as long as possible.	The presence of others who provide emotional support reduces anxiety.
Keep client informed of the routine that will be followed in preparation for surgery and postoperative care.	Dealing with unexpected events heightens anxiety; knowledge facilitates a sense of control.

Evaluation of Expected Outcome: Anxiety is reduced.

Nursing Diagnosis: Deficient Knowledge related to surgical routines

Expected Outcome: Client will be able to paraphrase the preoperative and postoperative routine.

Interventions	Rationales
Explain that the arm on the surgical side may be elevated and movement away from the body (abduction) may be temporarily restricted.	Elevation reduces edema. Abduction is temporarily restricted until healing progresses.

Evaluation of Expected Outcome:

- Client demonstrates an understanding of the type of surgery and potential postsurgical treatment modalities; preoperative preparations; and postoperative management, including coughing, deep breathing, and leg exercises.
- Client openly discusses and asks questions about surgery.

PC: Hemorrhage and **Shock**

Expected Outcome: The nurse will monitor to detect, manage, and minimize hemorrhage and shock.

(continued)

Nursing Care Plan 60-1 *(Continued)*

THE CLIENT UNDERGOING A MODIFIED RADICAL MASTECTOMY

Interventions	Rationales
Obtain vital signs according to agency routines. Do not take blood pressure on the arm on the side of the mastectomy.	The circulation of blood and lymph can be further compromised if the arm on the side of the mastectomy is used to measure blood pressure, to take blood specimens, or for intravenous (IV) infusions or injections.
Check color and amount of blood loss from the wound and drain, if one is present.	An increase in the volume or change to bright red color suggests excessive or arterial blood loss.
Feel underneath client's side or back for obscured bleeding.	Gravity can cause blood to drain posteriorly.
Administer IV fluids or blood transfusions at the rate prescribed.	Fluid replacement offsets fluid losses.

Evaluation of Expected Outcome: Bleeding is controlled; shock does not occur.

Nursing Diagnosis: **Risk for Ineffective Breathing Pattern** and **Ineffective Airway Clearance** related to pain, weak cough, and bulky dressing

Expected Outcome: Client will breathe effortlessly and be well oxygenated.

Interventions	Rationales
Instruct client to deep breathe and cough every 2 hours during waking hours or use an incentive spirometer.	Deep breathing distends alveoli and promotes increased gas diffusion.
Splint incision to reduce discomfort.	Pain or fear of pain interferes with deep breathing.
Administer oxygen as prescribed.	Supplemental oxygen provides a higher concentration than found in room air.
Instruct client to self-administer analgesia before deep breathing and coughing if a patient-controlled analgesia (PCA) pump is available.	Pain is more adequately controlled when an analgesic is given before severe pain develops.

Evaluation of Expected Outcome: Gas exchange is adequate as evidenced by an SpO_2 of 90% or greater and clear lung sounds.

Nursing Diagnosis: **Acute Pain** related to tissue trauma
Expected Outcome: Discomfort will be controlled within a tolerable level.

Interventions	Rationales
Administer pain medication liberally according to prescribed dose and frequency.	Clients have the right to pain relief.
Avoid giving injections in the arm on the same side as the surgery.	Circulation of blood and lymph is impaired, which can affect the absorption of parenteral medication and increases the potential for infection.
Monitor response to analgesia 30 minutes after administration or more frequently if PCA is in use.	The nurse is obligated to use additional measures to reduce the client's pain until it is at her or his tolerable level.
Pin the tubing of the drain or the drain collection chamber to the client's gown.	Stabilizing the drain helps prevent it from pulling at the insertion site and increasing discomfort.
Implement nursing techniques such as changing positions, relaxation, distraction, and guided imagery (see Chap. 21).	Nonpharmacologic measures supplement or complement analgesia.
Collaborate with the physician if pain control is inadequate.	The nurse consults with the physician to determine possible changes in the type of analgesic, its dose, or frequency.

Evaluation of Expected Outcome: Pain is reduced.

(continued)

Nursing Care Plan 60-1 *(Continued)*

THE CLIENT UNDERGOING A MODIFIED RADICAL MASTECTOMY

Nursing Diagnoses: **Impaired Skin Integrity** and **Risk for Infection** secondary to surgical wound

Expected Outcome: The incision will heal; no infection will develop.

Interventions	Rationales
Limit movement, especially abduction, of the arm on the side of surgery until the wound edges are intact.	Activity can disrupt the approximation of the incision.
Inspect the wound for swelling, unusual drainage, odor, redness, or separation of the suture line.	Wound infections are accompanied by signs of inflammation and a delay in healing.
Empty and re-establish negative pressure in closed wound drains at least once per shift.	Negative pressure (suction) pulls fluid from the incisional area, which facilitates healing.
Administer antibiotic therapy as prescribed.	Antibiotics destroy or inhibit the growth of microorganisms.
Monitor the trend in temperature and white blood cell counts.	A fever and leukocytosis suggest that an infection is developing.
Allow the client to shower after the sutures and drains are removed.	Hygiene reduces the number of microorganisms on the skin.

Evaluation of Expected Outcome: Incision heals without complications.

Nursing Diagnosis: **Risk for Ineffective Tissue Perfusion (lymphedema)** related to compromised flow of lymphatic fluid

Expected Outcome: Soft tissue in the arm on the side of surgery will be comparable with the opposite arm in color, size, and temperature.

Interventions	Rationales
Do not take blood pressures, give injections, administer IV infusions, or have blood drawn from the arm on the side of the mastectomy.	Procedures that affect the circulation in the affected arm can contribute to ineffective tissue perfusion.
Support and elevate the arm on the side of the mastectomy with pillows so it is kept higher than the heart.	Elevation promotes gravity drainage of fluid trapped in the soft tissue.
Place the arm in a sling when the client ambulates initially; eventually the arm can be positioned at the client's side.	A sling prevents stasis of fluid in distal areas of the arm.
Show the client how to squeeze and release a soft rubber ball or a rolled pair of cotton socks several times a day.	Venous blood and lymph circulate with contraction of skeletal muscles.
Remove and reapply an elastic roller bandage from the fingers to the axilla twice a day, or insert the affected arm into a pneumatic sleeve, an air-filled device that mechanically pumps the arm, for a half-hour or the prescribed amount of time twice a day.	An elastic roller bandage or pneumatic sleeve compresses the valves in veins to promote circulation.
Assess the hand for swelling, dusky color, delayed nail blanching, coldness, and tingling and report abnormal findings.	The nurse is responsible for reporting abnormal findings to reduce the potential for complications.

Evaluation of Expected Outcome: The circulation is maintained in the operative arm; both arms are of comparable size.

(continued)

Nursing Care Plan 60-1 *(Continued)*

THE CLIENT UNDERGOING A MODIFIED RADICAL MASTECTOMY

Nursing Diagnosis: **Impaired Physical Mobility** related to alteration in pectoral chest muscles

Expected Outcome: Client will achieve full range of arm motion.

Interventions	Rationales
Start active exercises of the affected arm on the first or second postoperative day, or later if the physician indicates a need to postpone them (skin grafts may need additional time to heal).	Active exercise reduces the potential for contractures.
Begin with flexing and extending the fingers, wrist, and elbow. Later, encourage the client to use the affected arm to perform oral hygiene, hair combing, and face washing.	Exercise gradually restores the ability to flex, extend, and abduct the arm.
Show the client how to face and "finger-walk" up a wall in the room. Mark the client's progress with masking tape so that the height can be exceeded with subsequent efforts.	Finger-walking increases the ability to raise the arm. Marking progress provides an incentive to meet or exceed heights during previous exercises.
Loop a rope or cord around a shower rod and raise and lower each arm in pulley fashion.	Modification in the technique for performing arm exercises facilitates rehabilitation.
Tie a string or rope to a doorknob and have the client turn the rope in a circular fashion.	Turning a rope promotes circumduction.

Evaluation of Expected Outcome: Client improves the use of the arm and hand of operative side. The client performs postmastectomy exercises.

Nursing Diagnosis: **Risk for Injury** related to change in center of gravity secondary to extensive removal of chest tissue

Expected Outcome: The client will not fall.

Interventions	Rationales
Assist the client during periods of ambulation.	The nurse supports the client when or if client loses balance.
Walk on the client's unaffected side.	The client is more likely to drift toward the side of the body that is heavier.
Instruct the client to keep the shoulders level and the muscles relaxed when walking.	Clients tend to accommodate for the change in the center of gravity by leaning to the side.

Evaluation of Expected Outcome: The client remains injury free.

Nursing Diagnosis: **Risk for Dysfunctional Grieving** related to loss of breast

Expected Outcome: Client will express grief and deal with losses in an appropriate amount of time.

Interventions	Rationales
Avoid trying to diminish the significance of the loss.	Grief work involves dealing with the reality of a significant loss.
Acknowledge client's grief and reinforce that feeling angry or sad is normal and expected.	Validating client's feelings gives permission for him or her to experience true emotions.

(continued)

Nursing Care Plan 60-1 (Continued)

THE CLIENT UNDERGOING A MODIFIED RADICAL MASTECTOMY

Interventions	Rationales
Stay with client and ensure privacy during emotional periods.	The nurse's presence provides support. Ensuring privacy demonstrates respect for the client's dignity.
Avoid administering prescribed sedatives or tranquilizers as a substitute for spending time with the client.	Numbing the mind interferes with grieving.
Encourage sharing with those who can be empathic, such as another breast cancer survivor.	Sharing the significance of a loss with a person who has survived a similar experience provides a bond for healing.

Nursing Diagnoses: Risk for Disturbed Body Image, Ineffective Coping, and **Sexual Dysfunction** related to perceived loss of physical attractiveness and sexual desirability

Expected Outcome: Client will accept body changes, use positive coping strategies, and experience satisfactory sexual activity.

Interventions	Rationales
Suggest that client pad a bra with one or two cotton socks until a prosthesis is fitted in 6 to 8 weeks.	Padding a bra gives the outward appearance that the client has both breasts. Purchasing a prosthetic bra is delayed until the tissue heals.
Inform client that cosmetic breast reconstruction is an option to discuss with the surgeon.	Cosmetic breast reconstruction provides an alternative for simulating natural breast tissue.
Advocate that client and sexual partner openly express to each other how the surgery has affected them emotionally.	Open communication facilitates mutual understanding and acceptance of body change.
Discuss methods for dealing with the removed breast during sexual activities such as using no or low lighting during intercourse or wearing the upper portion of lingerie.	Modifying sexual activities reduces self-consciousness.

Evaluation of Expected Outcomes: Client adjusts to the loss of the breast.

ventions. Information that nurses commonly must address is as follows:

- Explain wound and drain care or arrange for home health nursing.
- Assess availability of family assistance at home.
- Look for and report any signs of infection or impaired wound healing such as drainage or significant pale or dusky appearance to the skin around the incision.
- Stress continuation of arm exercises (Fig. 60-8).
- Arrange for follow-up examinations by the surgeon.
- Instruct client on the self-administration of prescribed drug therapy.
- Tell client to expect some residual numbness or tingling on the chest wall and the inner side of the arm from the axilla to the elbow, which may take as long as 1 year to resolve.
- Suggest applying cream or lotion to the arm if the skin tends to be dry.

- Explain that when selecting a prosthesis, those that are filled with fluid assume natural contours like the other breast, feel like normal breast tissue, and even radiate body warmth.
- Advise against lifting or carrying objects that weigh more than 15 lb and making vigorous repetitive movements with the affected arm.
- Discourage sleeping on the affected arm or wearing constrictive clothing that impairs circulation.
- Reinforce that blood pressure measurements, injections, blood donations, and IV infusions are contraindicated in the arm on the side of the mastectomy.
- Recommend wearing gloves while doing yard or housework to prevent injuries that may heal slowly or become infected.
- Advise using an electric razor for shaving axillary hair.
- Instruct to continue to perform monthly BSE on the intact breast and have the intact breast clinically ex-

1. *Wall handclimbing.* Stand facing the wall with feet apart and toes as close to the wall as possible. With elbows slightly bent, place the palms of the hand on the wall at shoulder level. By flexing the fingers, work the hands up the wall until arms are fully extended. Then reverse the process, working the hands down to the starting point.

2. *Rope turning.* Tie a light rope to a doorknob. Stand facing the door. Take the free end of the rope in the hand on the side of surgery. Place the other hand on the hip. With the rope-holding arm extended and held away from the body (nearly parallel with the floor), turn the rope, making as wide swings as possible. Begin slowly at first; speed up later.

3. *Rod or broomstick lifting.* Grasp a rod with both hands, held about 2 feet apart. Keeping the arms straight, raise the rod over the head. Bend elbows to lower the rod behind the head. Reverse maneuver, raising the rod above the head, then return to the starting position.

4. *Pulley tugging.* Toss a light rope over a shower curtain rod or doorway curtain rod. Stand as nearly under the rope as possible. Grasp an end in each hand. Extend the arms straight and away from the body. Pull the left arm up by tugging down with the right arm, then the right arm up and the left down in a see-sawing motion.

FIGURE 60-8 Arm exercises following surgery for breast cancer.

amined each year by a physician, along with obtaining a mammogram.

● METASTATIC BREAST CANCER

Despite treatment even in the early stages of breast cancer, some women develop metastatic disease. *Metastasis* means the migration of cancer cells from one part of the body to another. Malignant cells are spread by direct extension, through the lymphatic system, bloodstream, and cerebrospinal fluid.

Pathophysiology

Lymph nodes most commonly are involved in metastasis, with skeletal and pulmonary involvement following in order of frequency. The brain and liver also may become involved. Once metastasis occurs, the prognosis is less favorable, but some metastases progress slowly, whereas others are more rapid.

Assessment Findings

Signs and Symptoms

Metastases often cause pain in the new site. When bone becomes involved, pathologic fractures (a fracture after slight or no trauma) are possible.

Diagnostic Findings

Radiographs of the lungs, spine, or other areas of the body are used to detect metastases. Magnetic resonance imaging or computed tomography scanning also may be performed. These studies are done before or after treating the primary tumor. Lymph node dissection is performed either at the time of breast surgery or later to evaluate metastasis to the lymph nodes draining the breasts.

Medical Management

Treatment aims at providing the greatest period of palliation (relieving symptoms without curing the disease) for the client. It varies with the physician and specific type of metastasis. Large doses of estrogen or testosterone sometimes alleviate the pain, weight loss, and malaise of metastatic cancer. Intramuscular androgen (testosterone) therapy is used especially when metastases are to bone. All forms of treatment carry the possibility of unpleasant effects and complications. For palliative purposes, radiation therapy may be used to treat regional or distant metastases (especially to bone) or local tumor recurrence of the chest wall. Sometimes surgery, chemotherapy, or

radiation is used to slow the growth of the new malignant site.

Nursing Management

For nursing care of the client undergoing chemotherapy or radiation and caring for the terminally ill client with cancer, see Chapters 20 and 26.

● BREAST CANCER PREVENTION

Three options are available to women with increased risk for developing breast cancer: (1) long-term follow-up, (2) bilateral prophylactic mastectomy, and (3) chemoprevention with tamoxifen (Nolvadex). Those who choose long-term follow-up receive an annual mammogram with a clinical breast examination and monthly BSE. Prophylactic bilateral mastectomy is the more invasive of the three options. Clients considering this option are informed that removing the breasts reduces the risk for breast cancer, but does not eliminate the risk completely.

A breast cancer preventive study, funded by the National Cancer Institute—the lead agency in the United States for cancer research—has determined that taking the drug tamoxifen can reduce the risk of breast cancer in women who are at high risk by 49% (1998). Besides reducing the risk of breast cancer, tamoxifen preserves bone mineral density, thus preventing osteoporosis. It also lowers the low-density lipoprotein cholesterol levels, although it is still unknown if it decreases the incidence of myocardial infarction in women. On the other hand, tamoxifen can have detrimental effects. It increases the incidences of endometrial cancer, deep vein thrombosis, pulmonary embolism, and cataracts. Other side effects are increased hot flashes, cold sweats, vaginal discharge, genital itching, and pain with intercourse.

Raloxifene (Evista), a drug used to prevent osteoporosis, is being studied to determine its effect in reducing the risk of breast cancer. Because the results are not yet in, it is not recommended as a preventive measure for breast cancer.

COSMETIC BREAST PROCEDURES

Some women undergo various cosmetic breast procedures, collectively referred to as **mammoplasty,** for several reasons, but primarily to improve their appearance.

● BREAST RECONSTRUCTION

Breast reconstruction is a surgical procedure in which the area of a mastectomy is refashioned to simulate the contour of a breast and optionally to create a nipple and an areola. The procedure is accomplished by using either an artificial implant filled with saline or autogenous (self) tissue. Reconstruction can begin at the time of mastectomy if sufficient skin is spared, or it can be performed later.

Artificial Implants

Before an implant can produce an optimum cosmetic appearance, the skin and tissue on the chest wall are expanded to provide a large enough space to fill and approximate the size of the remaining breast. Tissue expansion is achieved by stretching the chest wall over several months with an inflatable or saline-filled pocket (Fig. 60-9).

Although there has been no definitive proof of a correlation between silicone implants and connective tissue and autoimmune diseases, silicone implants no longer are used except in clinical studies. Saline implants now are used for breast enhancement procedures.

Autogenous Tissue

Reconstructing the breast with autogenous tissue provides a more natural look and feel to the breast. The tissue is harvested similarly to a "tummy tuck" (abdominoplasty) from the rectus abdominis muscle along with its adjoining skin and fat (Fig. 60-10). Other donor sites, such as a portion of the latissimus dorsi or gluteal muscles, may be used. Removing donor tissue tends to leave a physical deformity, parts of which may be more obvious than others.

Muscle flap from rectus abdominus

FIGURE 60-10 Autogenous breast reconstruction.

If a woman desires a nipple, it is reconstructed from tissue from the opposite nipple, the ear, or toe. Tissue for the areola is selected from a site with a similar color, like the inner thigh or vaginal labia. It also may be created by pigmented tattoo.

● REDUCTION MAMMOPLASTY

A **reduction mammoplasty** is an overnight surgical procedure in which glandular breast tissue, fat, and skin are removed bilaterally to decrease the size of large, pendulous breasts. Most candidates for a reduction mammoplasty wear a size D cup or larger brassiere and experience discomfort in the shoulders or back, skin irritation beneath the breasts, difficulty in finding suitable clothing, self-consciousness, or low self-esteem.

To reduce the size of the breasts, an incision is made around the nipple through which tissue is removed. The loose skin is tightened to reposition the areola and nipple. The client is discharged with a bulky chest dressing and sometimes a small wound drain.

Syringe connected to inflation port

FIGURE 60-9 Tissue expander and breast implant.

● OPPOSITE BREAST REDUCTION

The size of a reconstructed breast is limited by the amount of tissue that remains; thus, there may be potential asymmetry. Opposite breast reduction is a surgical procedure that is performed to reduce the volume of a healthy breast so it more closely resembles the size of a reconstructed breast. The procedure, although done for different reasons, is the same as a reduction mammoplasty.

● BREAST LIFT

Ptosis, or drooping, of the breast(s) is corrected with a breast lift or, more technically, **mastopexy.** The sagging skin and low nipple placement that accompany weight loss or aging are corrected in a procedure similar to reduction mammoplasty, although the incision and scar line are smaller and the recovery time is shorter. In some cases, the size or contour of the breast is enhanced with breast augmentation techniques.

● BREAST AUGMENTATION

Women who wish to enlarge their breasts may choose breast augmentation, which is similar to reconstructing the breast using an artificial saline implant. When caring for women who undergo this procedure, the nurse maintains the client in a semi-Fowler's position after cosmetic breast surgery to promote drainage from the operative site. He or she gives analgesics for pain and inspects the operative site for changes in color and temperature. To minimize stretching of the tissues and suture line, the nurse maintains dressings and assists the client to use a support brassiere. He or she provides clients undergoing cosmetic breast surgery with information that applies to the type of surgery being performed. General guidelines are as follows:

- Have a mammogram to verify that there are no malignancies before having any cosmetic surgery.
- Continue to perform BSE and have clinical breast examinations (inspection and palpation) by the physician.
- Expect reduced sensation in the nipple, a certain amount of scarring, and temporary discomfort when moving the arms and shoulders after cosmetic breast surgery.
- Wear a soft brassiere for 3 to 6 weeks after surgery except when bathing or taking a shower.
- Avoid activities, such as vigorous sports, that may result in injury to the the breasts until healing is complete.

GENERAL NUTRITIONAL CONSIDERATIONS

Although once suspected as a risk factor, studies have failed to prove that a high-fat diet increases the risk of breast cancer. Studies on the protective role of fruits and vegetables, soy, and fiber also are inconclusive. The strongest link between diet and breast cancer is with alcohol: drinking more than one alcoholic drink per day may increase the risk of breast cancer by 40%. It is possible that the greatest effect of nutrition on breast cancer occurs during puberty or adolescence, when breasts are still forming.

GENERAL PHARMACOLOGIC CONSIDERATIONS

Metastases of breast cancer to soft tissue and bone may respond to antineoplastic drugs. These drugs may cause bone marrow depression, granulocytopenia, anemia, nausea and vomiting, hypotension, dermatitis, malaise, diarrhea, and stomatitis.

Pain management is an important issue in managing clients with breast cancer metastases. The opioid analgesics morphine and fentanyl are the drugs most often used for relief of cancer pain. Morphine can be given orally, rectally, subcutaneously, intravenously, intramuscularly, and by epidural catheter. Fentanyl (Duragesic) is given transdermally for pain. Clients taking these drugs must be monitored for adverse reactions that include excessive sedation, confusion, weakness, hypotension, constipation, dry mouth, nausea, vomiting, and anorexia.

When a client is taking danzol (Danocrine) for fibrocystic breast disease, amenorrhea may occur, especially with higher doses. Treatment with danazol for fibrocystic disease usually continues for 4 to 6 months and may continue up to 9 months, if necessary, to eliminate cystic lesions. Inform the client to notify the healthcare provider if regular menses do not resume within 90 days after discontinuing the drug.

GENERAL GERONTOLOGIC CONSIDERATIONS

Many breast disorders that are hormonally influenced regress after menopause.

The risk for breast cancer increases with age. Older adult women need to continue performing monthly BSE and have yearly clinical breast examinations and mammograms.

With age, the breast tissue atrophies, causing sagging and hanging of the breast. Fibrotic changes may cause some retraction of the nipple in older women.

In the older client, surgery for breast cancer may be limited to a lumpectomy or simple mastectomy.

Occasionally, breast tumors that have been present for years become more evident with age, making detection easier.

Critical Thinking Exercises

1. *How might the signs and symptoms differ among women with fibrocystic breast disease, fibroadenomas, and malignant breast tumors?*
2. *What advice is appropriate for preventing breast cancer?*

References and Suggested Readings

Baron, R. H. (1999). Sentinel lymph node biopsy in breast cancer and the role of the oncology nurse. *Clinical Journal of Oncology Nursing, 3*(1), 17–22.

Breast imaging: mammograms still rule. (2000). *Harvard Women's Health Watch, 7*(10), 5–6.

Davis, B. S. (2001). Lymphedema after breast cancer treatment. *American Journal of Nursing, 101*(4), Continuing Care Extra: 24AAAA–24DDDD.

Erikson, V. S., Pearson, M. L., Ganz, P. A., et al. (2001). Arm edema in breast cancer patients. *Journal of the National Cancer Institute, 93*, 96–111.

Fontenot, B. (1999). Nutrition and fibrocystic breast disease: Is there a connection? *Nutrition Forum, 16*(1), 3–4.

Greenfield, L. J., Mulholland, M. W., Oldhan, K. T., et al. (2001). *Surgery: Scientific principles and practice* (3rd ed.). Philadelphia: Lippincott Williams & Wilkins.

Hall, A. M. & Hooper, C. (1999). The frequency of breast screening in older women. *Professional Nurse, 15*, 155–159.

Harcourt, D. & Rumsey, N. (2001). Psychological aspects of breast reconstruction: A review of the literature. *Journal of Advanced Nursing, 35*, 477–487.

Harmer, V. (2000). The surgical management of breast cancer. *Nursing Times, 96*(48), 34–35.

Judkins, A. F. & Akins, J. (2001). Breast cancer: Initial diagnosis and current treatment options. *Nursing Clinics of North America, 36*, 527–542.

Livingstone, V. & Stringer, S. J. (1999). The treatment of *Staphylococcus aureus* infected sore nipples: A randomized comparative study. *Journal of Human Lactation, 15*, 241–246.

Machia, J. (2001). Breast cancer: Risk, prevention, and tamoxifen. *American Journal of Nursing, 101*(4), 26–36.

Mautner, B. D., Schmidt, K. V., & Brennan, M. B. (2000). New diagnostic techniques and treatments for early breast cancer. *Seminars in Oncology Nursing, 16*, 185–196.

McCarthy, E. P., Burns, R. B., Freund, K. M., et al. (2000). Mammography use, breast cancer stage at diagnosis, and survival among older women. *Journal of the American Geriatrics Society, 48*, 1226–1233.

McMasters, K. M., Tuttle, T. M., Carlson, D. J., et al. (2000). Sentinel lymph node biopsy for breast cancer: A suitable alternative to routine axillary dissection in multi-institutional practice when optimal technique is used. *Journal of Clinical Oncology, 18*, 2560–2566.

Miers, M. (2001). Understanding benign breast disorders and disease. *Nursing Standard, 15*(50), 45–52.

National Cancer Institute. (1998). Breast Cancer Prevention Trial shows major benefit, some risk. [On-line.] Available: http://newscenter.cancer.gov/pressreleases/prevtrial.htm.

National Institutes of Health. (1990, June 18–21). Early stage breast cancer: Consensus statement. (Vol. 8, No. 6). Bethesda, MD: Author.

Pacewicz, K. (1999). Breast reconstruction. *Journal of Gynecologic Oncology Nursing, 9*(1), 23–24.

Pruthi, S. (2001). Detection and evaluation of palpable breast mass. *Mayo Clinic Proceedings, 76*, 641–648.

Ruot-Worley, J. (2001). Augmentation mammoplasty: Implications for the primary care provider. *Journal of the American Academy of Nurse Practitioners, 13*, 304–309.

Sarwer, D. B., Nordmann, J. E., & Erbert, J. D. (2000). Cosmetic breast augmentation surgery: A critical overview. *Journal of Women's Health and Gender-Based Medicine, 9*, 843–856.

Thomas, S. & Greifzu, S. P. (2000). Oncology today: Breast reconstruction. *RN, 63*(4), 45–48.

Wilmoth, M. C. (2001). The aftermath of breast cancer: An altered sexual self. *Cancer Nursing, 24*, 278–286.

Wolfe, S. (1997). The great mammogram debate. *RN, 60*(8), 40–44.

Zack, E. (2001a). Mammography and reduced breast cancer mortality rates. *MEDSURG Nursing, 10*(1), 17–21.

Zack, E. (2001b). Sentinel lymph node biopsy in breast cancer: Scientific rationale and patient care. *Oncology Nursing Forum, 28*, 997–1007.

Caring for Clients With Disorders of the Male Reproductive System

Words to Know

benign prostatic
  hyperplasia
cryptorchidism
digital rectal
  examination
ejaculation
epididymitis
impotence
orchiectomy
orchiopexy
orchitis

prostatectomy
prostate-specific
  antigen
retrograde ejaculation
semen
spermatogenesis
testicular self-
  examination
transillumination
tumor markers
vasectomy

Learning Objectives

On completion of this chapter, the reader will:

- List the external and internal structures of the male reproductive system.
- Identify at least three possible consequences of disorders that affect the male reproductive system.
- Give four examples of structural disorders that affect the male reproductive system.
- Explain the technique and purpose for performing testicular self-examination.
- List three infectious or inflammatory conditions and how they are acquired.
- Discuss two erectile disorders and explain their effects on fertility and sexuality.
- Identify two methods for treating impotence.
- Describe the nursing plan of care for a client who receives a penile implant.
- Explain how prostatic hyperplasia compromises urinary elimination, and the symptoms it produces.
- Discuss the nursing management of a client undergoing a prostatectomy.
- Compare and contrast three male reproductive cancers in terms of age of onset, incidence, and treatment outcomes.
- List home care instructions after a vasectomy.

The physiologic functions of the male reproductive structures include generation of gender-specific sexual characteristics and the manufacture and transportation of sperm and seminal fluid. The lower urinary tract and reproductive system structures are so closely associated that disorders frequently affect both systems. Congenital or acquired structural abnormalities, infectious and inflammatory conditions, erection disorders, benign prostatic enlargement, and cancer are all threats to male reproductive health.

ANATOMY AND PHYSIOLOGY

External and Internal Structures

The external male genitalia consists of the penis and scrotum. The testes (sing., *testis*) lie within the scrotum and are responsible for **spermatogenesis,** sperm production, and secretion of testosterone. Testosterone is the male sex hormone that affects the development and maintenance of secondary male sex characteristics. The structures that extend from the testes, the epididymides (sing., *epididymis*), vas deferens (or ductus deferens), seminal vesicles, prostate gland, and bulbourethral (Cowper's) glands (Fig. 61-1), form a complex secretory and ductal system. Their functions are to nurture and enhance the motility of sperm and ensure their survival once they are released from the body. The prostate gland is an accessory sex organ that surrounds the urethra at the neck of the bladder. It secretes fluid that neutralizes acidic vaginal secretions.

Spermatogenesis and Ejaculation

Under the influence of follicle-stimulating hormone and testosterone, sperm are manufactured and sustained in the seminiferous tubules of the testes until they are motile—a process that takes approximately 64 days. They then pass into the epididymides and vas deferens, where they complete their maturation. The seminal vesicles that empty into the vas deferens produce seminal fluid, which adds volume to the sperm and nourishes them after ejaculation.

Ejaculation is the discharge of **semen,** the fluid that contains the sperm, from the body. The process of ejaculation results from rhythmic contraction of the muscles of the vas deferens and the penis during orgasm and sexual climax. The normal volume of ejaculate is 2.5 to 6 mL, which contains an average of 400 million spermatozoa (Bullock & Henze, 2000). A count of less than 20 to 50 million spermatozoa per milliliter results in infertility.

ASSESSMENT

History

The nurse obtains a general health and family history (see Chap. 4) and a detailed sexual history. A sexual history includes questions that elicit information about:

- Risks for sexually transmitted diseases (STDs)
- Contraceptive practices
- Ability to achieve or sustain an erection
- Pain during sexual intercourse
- Premature ejaculation or other concerns of a sexual nature
- Inability of a sex partner to conceive
- Prior treatment (including drug therapy, diagnostic tests, or surgery) that relate to the genitourinary system.

Physical Examination

The nurse inspects the external genitalia, looking for abnormalities such as skin lesions and urethral discharge. He or she palpates the testes for tumors and examines the scrotum. **Transillumination,** shining a light through the scrotum, provides clues about the density of scrotal tissue. A **digital rectal examination** (DRE) is performed to assess the prostate for size as well as evidence of tumor (Fig. 61-2). Yearly DREs are recommended for men older than 40 to 50 years of age.

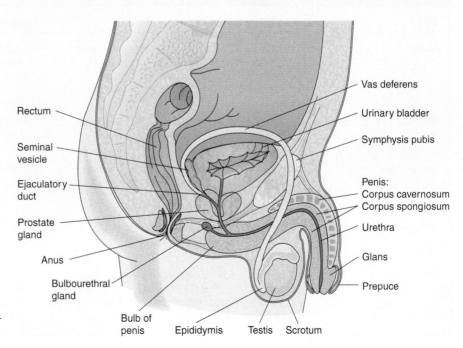

FIGURE 61-1 Anatomy of the male reproductive system.

Labels: Rectum, Seminal vesicle, Ejaculatory duct, Prostate gland, Anus, Bulbourethral gland, Bulb of penis, Epididymis, Testis, Scrotum, Vas deferens, Urinary bladder, Symphysis pubis, Penis: Corpus cavernosum, Corpus spongiosum, Urethra, Glans, Prepuce

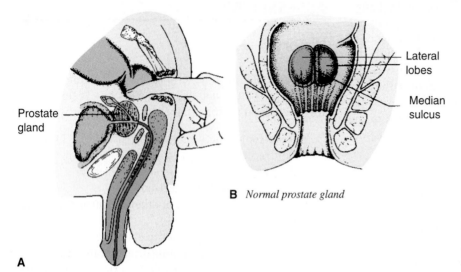

B *Normal prostate gland*

Lateral
lobes

Median
sulcus

A

FIGURE 61-2 (**A**) Palpation of the prostate gland during digital rectal examination (DRE). (**B**) The prostate is round with a palpable median sulcus or groove that separates the two lobes.

Diagnostic Tests

Several diagnostic tests commonly are performed to evaluate the male genitourinary tract. See Box 61-1 for appropriate nursing care.

Transrectal Ultrasonography

Transrectal ultrasonography (sonogram) is a test in which a lubricated probe is inserted into the rectum to obtain a view of the prostate gland from various angles. The test is indicated in cases in which the prostate gland is enlarged or the blood level of prostate-specific antigen (see later discussion) is elevated.

Cystoscopy

In a cystoscopy, an illuminated optical instrument called a *cystoscope* is inserted into the meatus to inspect the bladder, prostate, and urethra. This aids in evaluating the degree of encroachment by the prostate on the urethra.

BOX 61-1 ● **Nursing Management of the Client Undergoing Genitourinary Diagnostic Testing**

Test	Preprocedure Care	Postprocedure Care
All tests	Explain procedure, answer questions in a calm and reassuring manner. Use techniques of therapeutic communication to provide an opportunity for client to express concerns. Talk with client and inform him of each step as test proceeds.	Assist client to resume a comfortable position and clean up gels or lubricants. Answer questions about when test results will be available and when normal activity can resume. Provide written post-test instructions, if applicable.
Ultrasound of the prostate	Assure client that test is not painful; administer or have client self-administer an enema; encourage client to focus on breathing slowly to reduce anxiety.	Assist client in removing excess lubricant. Explain that client may resume normal activities.
Prostatic biopsy	Inform client that a local anesthetic may be used to minimize discomfort; administer or have client self-administer an enema if a rectal approach is used.	Provide information about site care. Instruct client that sitz baths and a mild analgesic will reduce discomfort. Tell client that a prophylactic antibiotic will be given and stress that medication be taken as ordered.
Testicular biopsy	Inform client that a local anesthetic will be administered.	In the case of an incisional rather than a needle biopsy, instruct the client to refrain from tub baths until the sutures are removed.
Cystoscopy	Inform client that he will experience bladder fullness and a strong desire to void. Inform client that an anesthetic lubricant will be instilled into the urethra to minimize discomfort and facilitate passage of cystoscope.	Instruct client to monitor voiding pattern and to report any bleeding or difficulty urinating. Inform client that prophylactic antibiotics will be given and stress that medication be taken as ordered.

Tissue Biopsy

A needle biopsy of prostatic tissue is obtained for analysis by the perineal or rectal approach. A testicular biopsy is obtained for evaluation of spermatozoa production or to diagnose a testicular malignancy.

Cultures

Cultures are obtained from urethral secretions, skin lesions, or urine. Prostatic fluid can be expressed during a DRE and also sent for culture.

Fertility Tests

Fertility studies include a semen analysis to determine the sperm count, sperm motility, and any abnormal sperm. Other laboratory tests may include measuring the level of plasma luteinizing hormone (LH), which is necessary for the release of testosterone from the testes. A decrease in the blood level of LH may be responsible for decreased testosterone production and infertility.

Tumor Markers

Tumor markers are substances synthesized by tumors that are released into the circulation in excessive amounts. The **prostate-specific antigen** (PSA) assay is a blood test that detects prostate cancer. Although an elevated PSA does not always indicate a malignancy, it now is possible to differentiate free PSA in total PSA. High percentages of free PSA are associated more often with benign disease, whereas low percentages of free PSA indicate malignancy. Regular PSA tests assist in the early diagnosis and staging of prostatic cancer, and in evaluating the effectiveness of the cancer treatment. Other blood test findings that suggest cancer are elevated levels of alpha-fetoprotein, beta-human chorionic gonadotropin (bHCG), and total urine estrogens. Alkaline and acid phosphatase blood tests determine if prostatic cancer has spread to the bone.

Stop, Think, and Respond ● BOX 61-1

What health teaching is important to provide men to ensure early diagnosis and treatment of disorders that affect the male reproductive system?

STRUCTURAL ABNORMALITIES

Structural abnormalities of the male genitalia may be congenital or acquired. These various abnormalities, including cryptorchidism, torsion of the spermatic cord, disorders of the foreskin, and benign scrotal swelling, often require surgical repair. Nursing management after these surgeries is similar.

● CRYPTORCHIDISM

Cryptorchidism is a condition in which one or both testes fail to descend into the scrotum. The undescended testis or testes may lie in the inguinal canal, in the abdominal cavity, or, rarely, in the perineum or femoral canal. The scrotum essentially is empty, but otherwise the client is asymptomatic. During childhood or at puberty, undescended testes occasionally find their way into the scrotum without treatment. At least one testis must be in the scrotum to ensure production of sperm.

The cause of undescended testes is unknown. The longer the testis remains undescended during childhood, however, the greater is the potential that fertility will be compromised. If the condition is not corrected by 2 years of age, the seminiferous tubules atrophy and fibrose. Some clients are treated with a short trial of androgen hormone therapy when the condition is diagnosed. If a response is not noted within a brief period (3 to 6 weeks), surgery to secure the testis in the scrotum, called **orchiopexy**, is performed (Kelley, 1997). A second consequence of undescended testes is a 20% to 40% greater risk for testicular cancer (see later discussion).

Nurses teach all men, especially those who have had cryptorchidism, to perform **testicular self-examination** (Fig. 61-3) to detect any abnormal mass in the scrotum. The nurse instructs clients to examine the testicles monthly, preferably when warm, such as in the shower.

After surgery, the nurse inspects the dressing and checks for a rubber band secured to the upper thigh. The rubber band provides traction on the relocated testes. The nurse ensures that the traction remains taut.

● TORSION OF THE SPERMATIC CORD

Torsion means "to twist." In this case, it is the spermatic cord that twists, kinking the artery and compromising blood flow to the testicle (Fig. 61-4). The condition occurs in prepubescent boys and in men whose spermatic cords are congenitally unsupported in the tunica vaginalis, the membrane surrounding the testes. Clients report a sudden, sharp testicular pain, with visible local swelling. The pain may be so severe that nausea, vomiting, chills, and fever occur. Torsion may follow severe exercise, but it also may occur during sleep or after a simple maneuver such as crossing the legs. Physical examination reveals an extremely tender testis. Elevation of the scrotum intensifies the pain by increasing the degree of twist.

Immediate surgery is necessary to prevent atrophy of the spermatic cord and preserve fertility. The torsion is reduced, excess tunica vaginalis is excised, and the testis is anchored with sutures in the scrotum. A prophylactic procedure may be performed on the opposite side.

Preoperatively, the nurse administers prescribed analgesia to relieve pain. After surgery, he or she applies a scro-

Lump

A

B

C

Spermatic
cord

1. Use both hands to palpate the testis. The normal
   testicle is smooth and uniform in consistency.

2. With the index and middle fingers under the
   testis and the thumb on top, roll the testis gently
   in a horizontal plane between the thumb and
   fingers (**A**).

3. Feel for any evidence of a small lump or
   abnormality.

4. Follow the same procedure and palpate upward
   along the testis (**B**).

5. Locate and palpate the epididymis (**C**), a cord-like
   structure on the top and back of the testicle that
   stores and transports sperm. Also locate and
   palpate the spermatic cord.

6. Repeat the examination for the other testis,
   epididymis, and spermatic cord. It is normal to
   find that one testis is larger than the other.

7. If you find any evidence of a small, pea-like lump
   or if the testis is swollen (possibly from an
   infection or tumor), consult your physician.

FIGURE 61-3 Testicular self-examination should be performed monthly.

tal support, especially when the client is out of bed. The nurse inspects the dressing for signs of drainage and gives antibiotics if medically ordered. He or she reports any sudden onset of pain to the physician.

● PHIMOSIS AND PARAPHIMOSIS

Phimosis and paraphimosis are conditions that occur among uncircumcised male clients when the opening of the foreskin is constricted. Phimosis refers to an inability

to retract the foreskin (prepuce); paraphimosis is a strangulation of the glans penis from an inability to replace the retracted foreskin. These phimotic conditions often are caused by a congenitally small foreskin; however, chronic inflammation at the glans penis and prepuce secondary to poor hygiene or infection also are etiologic factors. Clients with phimosis report pain with erection and intercourse and difficulty cleaning under the foreskin. Clients with paraphimosis experience painful swelling of the glans. If the condition continues, severe edema and urinary retention may occur. Circumcision is recommended to relieve these conditions permanently; if

FIGURE 61-4 Torsion of the spermatic cord.

surgery is not indicated, the client is instructed to wash under the foreskin daily and seek care if he cannot retract the tissue.

HYDROCELE, SPERMATOCELE, AND VARICOCELE

The suffix, *cele,* indicates a swelling. Hydrocele, spermatocele, and varicocele all present as a swelling of the scrotum (Fig. 61-5), but in each case, the conditions are somewhat different. Often, hydrocele and spermatocele are not clinically significant and do not require treatment; however, varicoceles are thought to be an underlying cause of male infertility and may be surgically repaired (Table 61-1).

INFECTIOUS AND INFLAMMATORY CONDITIONS

PROSTATITIS

Prostatitis is an inflammation of the prostate gland and is most often caused by microorganisms that reach the prostate by way of the urethra. *Escherichia coli* and microbes that cause STDs (see Chap. 62) often are responsible, but in some instances no evidence of bacterial infection is found. Occasionally, a psychosexual problem may be the suspected cause of the client's symptoms. In any case, inflammation causes glandular swelling and tenderness. Because the prostate surrounds the urethra, a combination of genitourinary problems develops. Clients experience perineal pain or discomfort, an unusual sensation preceding or following ejaculation, low back pain, fever, chills, dysuria, and urethral discharge. Treatment consists of up to 30 days of antibiotic therapy, mild analgesics, and sitz baths.

The nurse stresses that sexual partners also need to be treated. He or she tells the client to avoid caffeine, prolonged sitting, and constipation, and regularly to drain the prostate gland through masturbation or intercourse. The nurse instructs the client to comply with antibiotic therapy and use a mild analgesic for pain.

EPIDIDYMITIS AND ORCHITIS

An inflammation of the epididymis (**epididymitis;** Fig. 61-6) and testis (**orchitis;** Fig. 61-7) occurs alone or simultaneously (epididymo-orchitis). Common causes are an extension of the infectious agent causing prostatitis or an infection elsewhere in the body. Noninfectious epididymitis may result from long-term indwelling

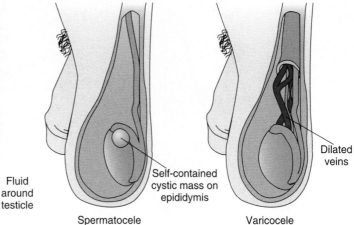

FIGURE 61-5 Causes of scrotal swelling.

Hydrocele — Fluid around testicle

Spermatocele — Self-contained cystic mass on epididymis

Varicocele — Dilated veins

TABLE 61-1	COMPARISON OF HYDROCELE, SPERMATOCELE, AND VARICOCELE

CONDITION AND ETIOLOGY	DESCRIPTION	SIGNS AND SYMPTOMS	DIAGNOSTIC AIDS	MEDICAL AND SURGICAL MANAGEMENT
Hydrocele				
Congenital defect, injury, infection, lymph obstruction, tumor, side effect of radiation, or unknown cause	Accumulation of as much as 100 mL of lymphatic fluid between the testis and tunica vaginalis	Swollen testicle, heaviness in scrotum or lower back; may be asymptomatic, pain if testicular blood flow is impaired	Palpation, transillumination	No treatment if asymptomatic; aspiration of fluid as a temporary measure; surgical excision of fluid-filled sac; treatment of primary condition (i.e., infection)
Spermatocele				
Unknown cause	Epididymal, sperm-containing cyst	Small, freely movable mass; usually asymptomatic, may be painful if large	Palpation, transillumination	No treatment unless cyst is large and causes pain
Varicocele				
Incompetent valves in the spermatic veins	Venous dilation with damage to elastic fibers and hypertrophy of vein walls	Feeling of heaviness in scrotum; may be asymptomatic or have pain and swelling	Palpation, auscultation of venous rush, ultrasound, blood flow studies	No treatment, surgical ligation, or sclerosing

catheter use or genitourinary procedures such as cystoscopy or prostatectomy. Orchitis without epididymal involvement is associated with a viral mumps infection that occurs after puberty and may result in testicular atrophy and sterility. Bilateral epididymitis frequently leads to permanent azoospermia (absence of sperm), especially when the infection recurs frequently or becomes chronic.

The chief complaint is pain and swelling in the inguinal area and scrotum. Fever and chills occur with bacterial infections, and the urine contains pus and bacteria. Inspection reveals a markedly swollen testis and epididymis and scrotal skin that is red and tense. It is important to differentiate epididymitis from testicular torsion because torsion is a surgical emergency. Treatment consists of bed rest, scrotal elevation, analgesics, anti-inflammatory agents, and comfort measures such as local cold applications. Antibiotic therapy is initiated to eliminate the infectious agent. An epididymectomy (excision of the epididymis) is performed on clients who have recurrent, chronic, or intractable infections, but this results in sterility if it is performed bilaterally.

The nurse elevates the scrotum with a folded towel, a four-tail bandage, or adhesive taped across the upper

FIGURE 61-6 Acute epididymitis.

FIGURE 61-7 Acute orchitis.

thighs (Fig. 61-8) to relieve pain by lessening the weight of the testes. He or she places an ice bag under the tender scrotum, not on top of it or leaning against it. The nurse avoids keeping the cold bag constantly next to the skin because it may damage tissue. He or she may use a routine such as on 60 minutes, off 30 minutes. As with any infection, the nurse encourages copious fluid intake.

Home care includes instructions to continue taking prescribed antibiotics, take sitz baths, apply local heat after scrotal swelling subsides, and avoid lifting and sexual intercourse until symptoms are relieved. Nurses also advocate for infant and childhood immunizations against infectious diseases, such as mumps, to reduce potential adult complications such as orchitis.

ERECTION DISORDERS

● IMPOTENCE

Impotence is the inability to achieve or maintain an erection that is sufficiently rigid for sexual activity. There must be multiple or persistent incidences of failed erection for the disorder to be considered pathologic. It often is a consequence of inadequate blood flow to the penis or rapid emptying of blood once it accumulates. Aging, testosterone insufficiency, side effects of drug therapy, atherosclerosis, hypertension, and complications of diabetes mellitus are common causes. Impotence also may be related to anxiety or depression. A nocturnal penile tumescence test is used to determine if the client is experiencing spontaneous erections during sleep. The test involves applying paper bands about the shaft of the penis at bedtime and observing if the bands are broken in the morning. Absence of nocturnal erec-

FIGURE 61-8 Technique for scrotal elevation.

Double-faced tape, except at end

tions supports a physical rather than emotional cause for impotence.

Several approaches exist to help restore sexual function. Substituting other drugs for those that cause impotence or treating the contributing cause may restore potency (erectile ability). Some elect to facilitate penile engorgement by attaching a vacuum device to the penis or self-injecting drugs such as papaverine (Pavatine), phentolamine (Regitine), or alprostadil (Caverject) into the corpus cavernosa to achieve an erection. The drug sildenafil (Viagra) facilitates penile erection by producing smooth muscle relaxation in the corpus cavernosa, facilitating an inflow of blood. Sildenafil is taken orally about 1 hour before sexual activity. It has no erectile effect without sexual stimulation. Apomorphine (Uprima), a dopamine agonist, is an older drug used in the treatment of Parkinson's disease (see Chap. 45) that is now an alternative to sildenafil for the treatment of erectile dysfunction. This drug, which is administered as a nasal spray, has some advantages over sildenafil: (1) it acts within 15 to 25 minutes of administration, and (2) it is safer for men with coronary artery disease.

Vascular surgery is an option for some clients, but many clients choose a surgically implanted penile prosthesis (Fig. 61-9). One type contains a saline reservoir that is pumped to fill the implant when sexual activity is desired and the other type maintains the penis in a semierect state at all times. The nurse informs the client before surgery that when a pump-type of implant is inserted, the erect penis tends to be shorter than experienced in pre-illness erections because the cylinders do not fill the glans portion of the penis.

If the client prefers to self-inject a vasodilator, the nurse provides instruction on technique, suggested frequency of injections, and side effects. If the client undergoes a penile implant, the nurse assesses for pain, swelling, bleeding, and surgical complications like infection. The nurse reinforces the information the physician identifies as possible complications after discharge, such as:

- Erosion of penile or urethral tissue from a mis-sized implant, pressure, and friction of the implanted cylinders that is evidenced by seeing the implant through the skin
- Erosion of scrotal, bowel, or bladder tissue if an implant with a fluid reservoir is used detected by changes in scrotal skin texture and elimination
- Migration of the cylinders, pump, or reservoir from their intended location that is accompanied by pain, tenderness, and dysfunction of components that are part of the device
- Malfunction of the device characterized by underinflation, bulging of the cylinders during inflation, and loss of fluid from the implant that can occur with migration, accidental trauma such as a fall, or aggressive or improper use of the device

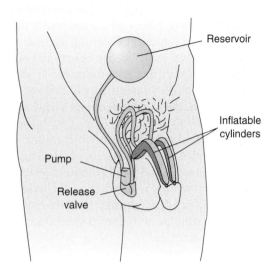

FIGURE 61-9 Examples of penile implants.

The nurse implements measures to ensure a safe recovery and provides instructions to promote self-care (Nursing Care Plan 61-1).

● PRIAPISM

Priapism is a condition in which the penis becomes engorged and remains persistently erect without any sexual stimulation. The underlying etiology usually is a vascular problem, a medical condition that causes blood to thicken, or a side effect of medications, including those prescribed to treat impotence. The engorged penis produces significant discomfort and interferes with arterial blood flow and, in some cases, urinary elimination. If the erection lasts longer than 6 hours, the tissue may be sufficiently damaged to result in impotence.

Treatment options include administering vasoconstrictive medications such as terbutaline (Brethine) or phenylephrine (Neo-Synephrine) or draining the trapped blood with a needle placed in the side of the penis. If these interventions fail, emergency surgery is performed to shunt blood temporarily out of the corpus cavernosum. Healthcare providers must extend respect for the client's feelings and understandable embarrassment throughout interactions.

BENIGN PROSTATIC HYPERPLASIA ●

When the number of cells in a structure increases, the condition is referred to as *hyperplasia*. If the cells are nonmalignant, it is called *benign hyperplasia*. Thus, **benign prostatic hyperplasia** (BPH) indicates that the prostate gland contains more than the usual number of normal cells. When the gland enlarges, the condition is known as *benign prostatic hypertrophy*.

Pathophysiology and Etiology

BPH occurs as men age. The outward expansion of the gland is of no clinical importance. Inward encroachment, however, diminishes the diameter of the prostatic section of the urethra and interferes with emptying the bladder (Fig. 61-10).

Assessment Findings

Signs and Symptoms

The symptoms of BPH appear gradually. At first, the client notices that it takes more effort to void. Eventually, the urinary stream narrows and has decreased force. The bladder empties incompletely. As residual urine accumulates, the client has an urge to void more often and nocturia occurs. Because residual urine is a good culture medium for bacteria, symptoms of cystitis (inflammation of the bladder) may develop (see Chap. 65).

Diagnostic Findings

A DRE reveals an enlarged and elastic gland. Cystoscopy exposes the extent of the infringement on the urethra and the effects on the bladder. Intravenous and retrograde pyelograms and blood chemistry tests give information about possible damage to the upper urinary tract from urinary retention. Measurement of a significant quantity of residual urine adds to the data that confirm the diag-

Nursing Care Plan 61-1

POSTOPERATIVE MANAGEMENT OF THE CLIENT WITH A PENILE IMPLANT

Assessment

- Determine level of consciousness and vital signs.
- Check the condition of dressing and incision.
- Assess the client's level of pain.
- Evaluate the amount of penile and scrotal swelling.
- Check the status of the IV infusion (type of solution, drip rate, location of IV site).
- Note the urinary catheter and volume of urine elimination.
- Assess the client's knowledge of postoperative care and discharge instructions.

Nursing Diagnosis: **Acute Pain** related to tissue injury and swelling

Expected Outcome: Pain will be eliminated or reduced to the client's level of tolerance.

Interventions	Rationales
Assess level of discomfort as needed and whenever you assess vital signs.	An assessment of pain level is the fifth vital sign.
Administer analgesia as prescribed.	Clients have the right to pain relief.
Elevate genitalia with a rolled towel.	Elevation reduces swelling.
Apply an ice pack to the incision and replace as needed.	Facilitating vasoconstriction with an ice pack reduces swelling and pain.
Suspend linen over lower pelvis with a bed cradle.	A cradle prevents pressure on painful tissue from the weight of bed linen.

Evaluation of Expected Outcome: Pain is relieved and comfort is maintained.

PC: **Risk for Bleeding** related to inadequate hemostasis

Expected Outcome: The nurse will monitor for, manage, and minimize incisional bleeding.

Interventions	Rationales
Assess for frank bleeding or an enlarging hematoma around the incision, usually at the base of the penis where it joins the scrotum.	A large amount of obvious blood or its collection in the skin and underlying tissue indicates significant blood loss.
Ensure that the implant is semirigid.	Implant rigidity provides localized pressure that reduces bleeding.

Evaluation of Expected Outcome: Blood loss is minimal and swelling of the genitalia remains within acceptable limits.

Nursing Diagnosis: **Risk for Urinary Retention** related to urethral compression

Expected Outcome: Client will void without difficulty and empty his bladder with each voiding.

Interventions	Rationales
Monitor frequency and amount of each voiding.	Urinary retention is evidenced by the absence of voiding or voiding small, frequent amounts.

(continued)

Nursing Care Plan 61-1 *(Continued)*

POSTOPERATIVE MANAGEMENT OF THE CLIENT WITH A PENILE IMPLANT

Interventions	*Rationales*
Palpate the lower abdomen.	The bladder is palpable when it is distended with urine.
Report an inability to void or lack of sufficient quantity per voiding.	Catheterization may be required to empty the bladder, or the physician may choose to order a medication to induce voiding.

Evaluation of Expected Outcome: Client voids in sufficient quantities; the bladder remains nonpalpable.

Nursing Diagnosis: **Risk for Impaired Skin Integrity** related to dermal deterioration secondary to a tight prosthesis

Expected Outcome: Skin in the operative area will remain supple and intact.

Interventions	*Rationales*
Look for pale, thin skin near the glans penis.	The prosthesis occupies space, stretches the skin, and reduces the diameter of blood vessels.
Report signs of inadequate capillary perfusion and skin erosion.	Prolonged interruption of blood flow causes tissue necrosis.

Evaluation of Expected Outcome: Skin in the operative area will remain supple and intact.

Nursing Diagnosis: **Risk for Situational Low Self-Esteem** related to possible spectator curiosity concerning the outcome of the surgical procedure.

Expected Outcome: Client retains positive self-esteem.

Interventions	*Rationales*
Explain the purpose for genital inspection.	Genital inspection is performed for the purpose of assessing local tissue response rather than satisfying curiosity.
Provide privacy and draping during genital assessments.	The client has the right to privacy and to be treated with dignity.
Avoid unprofessional comments about the client's reasons for or outcome of surgery.	The client's decision for elective surgery is private and personal.
Provide opportunities for the client to privately share his feelings about his changed appearance.	Clients are more likely to openly discuss their feelings when they feel secure that others will not overhear the conversation.
Describe techniques for concealing the semierect appearance of the penis, such as wearing untucked shirts and pleated trousers or pants with an elastic waist.	Disguising the state of semierection decreases self-consciousness in social situations.

Evaluation of Expected Outcome: Client's self-esteem is undisturbed.

Nursing Diagnosis: **Risk for Ineffective Therapeutic Regimen Management** related to lack of knowledge concerning postoperative course after discharge

Expected Outcome: Client will acquire knowledge to ensure recovery without complications.

(continued)

Nursing Care Plan 61-1 (Continued)

POSTOPERATIVE MANAGEMENT OF THE CLIENT WITH A PENILE IMPLANT

Interventions	*Rationales*
Explain that the penis should be taped against the skin in a straight position for 1 week or longer, but can be untaped for voiding.	Taping acts as a splint to keep the penis from moving about while healing takes place.
Identify the period for sexual abstinence (usually 3 to 6 weeks).	Sexual intercourse is safe once healing is complete.
Instruct on how to inflate and deflate an inflatable prosthesis.	An erect penis facilitates vaginal penetration; the client empties the penile implant after intercourse.
Inform client to avoid tight-fitting underwear.	Pressure and friction can cause tissue erosion and curvature of the penis.
Advise client to avoid contact sports.	The force of physical contact may alter the position or integrity of the penile implant.
Explain that the client must avoid heavy lifting for at least 3 weeks.	Straining can disrupt internal sutures and reconstructed tissue.
Emphasize the need to report persistent pain and swelling.	Pain and swelling are common signs of infection, erosion, and migration.

Evaluation of Expected Outcome: Client can verbalize discharge instructions and receives written information to which he can refer for self-care at home.

---

nosis. The PSA test results may be slightly elevated. Transrectal ultrasonography indicates prostatic size and helps rule out the possibility that a malignancy is causing the enlargement.

Medical and Surgical Management

In the early stages of BPH, the progression of prostatic enlargement is monitored with periodic DREs. Drug therapy is the second line of treatment (Drug Therapy Table 61-1). Terazosin (Hytrin), an alpha-adrenergic blocker, helps relax the muscles in the prostate and relieve urinary symptoms. Finasteride (Proscar), an androgen hormone inhibitor, can be used to decrease symptoms and also appears to arrest the progression of prostate enlargement in some clients.

Some men have found that taking saw palmetto, a herbal substance from the fruit of the palm tree, relieves the symptoms of benign prostatic hyperplasia. Saw palmetto interferes with the enzyme that converts testosterone to dihydrotestosterone. When dihydrotestosterone is inhibited, the stimulus for growth of the prostate gland is reduced. This herb also may inhibit cyclooxygenase, an enzyme that plays a role in inflammation, which may explain the manner in which the symptoms of prostatitis are relieved (Hulisz & Plant, 2000). Before self-administering any substance that is considered alternative therapy, clients should discuss the matter with their physicians.

Other forms of treatment are used when glandular enlargement results in pronounced symptoms. The aim of all surgical procedures for BPH is to enlarge the bladder outlet (Table 61-2). Surgeries preformed through the urethra include transcystoscopic urethroplasty, transurethral prostatectomy (TURP), transurethral incision of the prostate (TUIP), and transurethral laser incision of the prostate (TULIP). Operations such as suprapubic,

FIGURE 61-10 Comparison of normal prostate and enlarged prostate.

DRUG THERAPY TABLE 61-1	**AGENTS FOR BENIGN PROSTATIC HYPERPLASIA**

DRUG CATEGORY AND EXAMPLES	MECHANISM OF ACTION	SIDE EFFECTS	NURSING CONSIDERATIONS
Hormonal Agents			
finasteride (Proscar)	Inhibits the conversion of testosterone into a potent androgen (dihydrotestosterone) on which the prostate depends; causes the gland to shrink	Loss of libido, impotence, decreased ejaculate, adverse effects on fetal development	Monitor urinary output. Avoid handling the drug if pregnant. Instruct to use a condom to prevent fetal exposure. Explain that sexual changes are reversible after drug is discontinued. Inform client that it may take 6 months or longer to achieve full benefit.
Alpha-Adrenergic Blockers			
terazosin (Hytrin)	Reduces the tone of smooth muscle in the bladder neck and prostatic urethra	Hypotension, dizziness, nausea, urinary frequency, incontinence, edema, fatigue, headaches	Monitor urinary elimination patterns and postural blood pressure changes. Administer drug at bedtime to reduce orthostatic hypotension. Warn to change position slowly. Weigh regularly for evidence of fluid imbalance.

retroperitoneal, or perineal prostatectomy are preformed through an external incision (Fig. 61-11). In almost all cases, a continuous bladder irrigation is ordered after TURP to remove blood clots and residual tissue.

After a TURP, clients experience **retrograde ejaculation,** a condition in which the semen is deposited in the bladder rather than discharging through the urethra at the time of orgasm, rendering the client sterile. After a TURP and open prostatectomies, men may have temporary or permanent urinary incontinence, depending on the procedure used and the surgeon's technical skill. Perineal surgical approaches often result in permanent impotence, although some nerve-sparing techniques are being developed.

TABLE 61-2	**INVASIVE PROCEDURES FOR PROSTATIC ENLARGEMENT**

PROCEDURE	DESCRIPTION
Transurethral Approaches	
Transcystoscopic urethroplasty	The balloon tip of a catheter is inflated for 10 to 20 minutes to stretch the prostatic urethra.
Urethral stent or coils	A flexible tube is permanently placed in the urethra to dilate the lumen.
Thermotherapy	A heated instrument inserted in a urethral catheter destroys prostatic tissue but preserves the urethra.
Transurethral resection of the prostate (TURP)	Part of the prostate is removed with a cutting instrument inserted through an endoscope.
Transurethral incision of the prostate (TUIP)	No tissue is removed; the bladder outlet is enlarged by making an incision in the prostate, which relieves pressure on the urethra.
Transurethral laser incision of the prostate (TULIP)	A laser is used to incise and destroy prostate tissue.
Open Surgical Approaches	
Suprapubic prostatectomy	The prostate gland is removed by making a midline abdominal incision into the bladder. A suprapubic catheter, also known as a cystostomy tube, and a Foley catheter are inserted.
Retropubic prostatectomy	The prostate gland is removed through an abdominal incision, but the bladder is not entered.
Perineal prostatectomy	The prostate gland is removed through an incision made between the scrotum and anus.
Radical prostatectomy	The prostate gland and its capsule, seminal vesicles, and lymph nodes are removed through a retropubic or perineal incision; this procedure is reserved for clients with prostatic cancer.

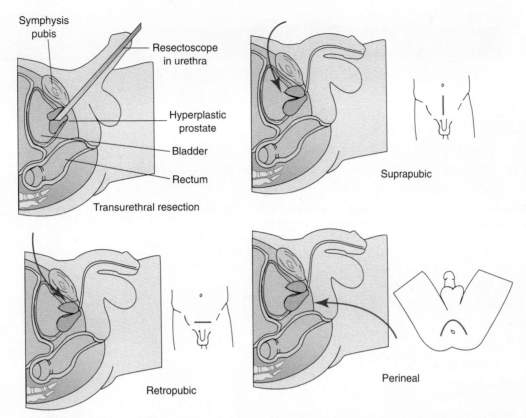

FIGURE 61-11 Examples of prostatectomy techniques.

Nursing Management

For the client who is not yet a candidate for surgery, the nurse teaches how to maintain optimal bladder emptying (Client and Family Teaching Box 61-1).

61-1 *Client and Family Teaching* Optimal Bladder Function

The nurse instructs the client as follows:

- Void often and assist bladder emptying by leaning forward on toilet and "bearing down" (Valsalva maneuver), or pressing down on the bladder while seated on the toilet (Credé's maneuver).
- Drink frequent small volumes of oral fluids so that the bladder does not become extremely full at any one time.
- Note any signs and symptoms of acute urinary obstruction and urinary infection such as distended bladder, lower abdominal discomfort, inability to urinate, small and frequent urination, fever and chills, and flank pain that indicate a need for medical attention.

The surgical client requires support and information to allay anxiety and promote a postoperative period that is free of complications. The nurse teaches deep breathing and leg exercises and explains that the client will have continuous bladder irrigation for at least 24 hours after surgery.

Urethral catheterization before surgery is necessary for clients with sudden or acute retention. If difficulty is encountered while inserting a urethral catheter, a coudé catheter, which has a curved tip, and instillable anesthetic lubricant are used to facilitate the procedure. If the catheter cannot be passed urethrally, a temporary suprapubic catheter is required to relieve bladder distention. For care after a prostatectomy, see Nursing Care Plan 61-2.

MALIGNANCIES OF THE MALE REPRODUCTIVE SYSTEM

● CANCER OF THE PROSTATE

Prostatic cancer is most common in men older than 50 years of age. In fact, it is the third most common cause of death from cancer in men of all ages and is the most common cause of death from cancer in men older than 75 years of age. Prostatic cancer grows slowly and has a high survival rate if detected early.

(text continued on page 976)

Nursing Care Plan 61-2

THE CLIENT UNDERGOING A PROSTATECTOMY

Assessment

Determine the following before surgery:

■ Medical, drug, and allergy history

■ Symptoms such as urgency, frequency, hesitancy, nocturia, decreased urinary stream

■ Previous episodes of urinary tract infections

■ Discomfort that is associated with an acute, sudden episode of urinary retention because this problem may require immediate preoperative attention

■ Vital signs

■ Weight

Determine the following after surgery:

■ Level of consciousness

■ Vital signs

■ Level of discomfort

■ Location of urinary catheter(s)

■ Volume and color of urine

PC: **Risk for Hemorrhage** related to inadequate hemostasis

Expected Outcome: The nurse will monitor to detect, manage, and minimize excessive bleeding.

Interventions	Rationales
Monitor vital signs every 15 minutes until stable and then every 4 hours.	Hypotension and tachycardia suggest a loss of blood volume.
Assess color of urine and status of dressing, if there is one, at least every 4 hours.	A change from burgundy to bright red, like catsup, suggests fresh bleeding.
Maintain traction on the urinary catheter for at least 6 hours after surgery.	Traction provides pressure on blood vessels, which facilitates hemostasis.
Discourage straining to have a bowel movement, attempts to void with the catheter in place, and lifting heavy objects.	Bearing down increases blood pressure, which can trigger fresh bleeding.
Report signs of hypovolemic shock to the physician.	The physician determines the medical measures such as administering blood transfusions and medications for stabilizing the client's condition.

Evaluation of Expected Outcome: Client's urine is light pink, clear, or amber.

PC: **Anemia** related to postoperative bleeding

Expected Outcome: The nurse will monitor to detect, manage, and minimize anemia.

Interventions	Rationales
Monitor laboratory test results when a complete blood count (CBC) is performed.	Low erythrocyte, hemoglobin, and hematocrit results indicate that the client may require the replacement of blood.

(continued)

Nursing Care Plan 61-2 (Continued)

THE CLIENT UNDERGOING A PROSTATECTOMY

Interventions	Rationales
Assist with administering whole blood or packed cells as prescribed by the physician.	Transfusions of whole blood or packed cells replace depleted cells and intravascular fluid volume faster than the bone marrow can reproduce erythrocytes.

Evaluation of Expected Outcome: Client's hemoglobin is at least 10 g/dl.

Nursing Diagnosis: **Risk for Urinary Retention** related to obstruction of urinary catheter with tissue debris and blood clots or urethral stricture

Expected Outcome: Catheter will remain patent.

Interventions	Rationales
Instill bladder irrigation solution at a rate to maintain light pink or clear urine (Fig. 61-12).	Irrigating solution dilutes blood cells and tissue debris and facilitates removal from the bladder by gravity drainage.
Encourage client to drink about one glass of water every hour while awake.	A generous fluid intake keeps the urine dilute and the catheter patent.
Palpate bladder and assess true urine volume every 4 hours, whenever client complains of pain, or if urine leaks around catheter.	The bladder is not palpable unless distended. True urine volume is assessed by subtracting the volume of irrigating solution from the total urinary output. Pain and leaking fluid suggest accumulated urine with no appropriate outlet.
Avoid dependent loops and kinks in urinary catheter, never clamp urinary catheter, and do not allow client to lie on the drainage tubing.	Interference with gravity drainage results in urine accumulation in the bladder.
Keep drainage bag below the level of the bladder.	Fluid (urine in this case) flows by gravity from higher to lower locations. If the urinary drainage bag is above the bladder, urine flows backward into the bladder.

Evaluation of Expected Outcome: Urine drains freely from the catheter or with spontaneous voiding.

PC: **Hyponatremia** related to absorption of bladder irrigation solution

Expected Outcome: The nurse will monitor to detect, manage, and minimize hyponatremia.

Interventions	Rationales
Analyze if there is a realistic relationship between the amount of instilled irrigation solution and the drainage volume.	A deficit in irrigation volume suggests systemic absorption of a portion of the full amount.
Monitor and report if client develops weakness, muscle cramps, nausea, vomiting, confusion, seizures, or elevated blood pressure.	Hyponatremia is manifested in physical signs and symptoms.
Slow or interrupt the bladder irrigation if you suspect hyponatremia or fluid excess; report assessment data to the physician.	The nurse collaborates with the physician when management of the client's problems involves medical interventions.

Evaluation of Expected Outcome: Client's serum sodium level is 135–145 mEq/L.

Nursing Diagnosis: **Acute Pain** related to tissue injury or bladder spasms

Expected Outcome: Pain will be controlled within the client's level of tolerance.

(continued)

Nursing Care Plan 61-2 (Continued)

THE CLIENT UNDERGOING A PROSTATECTOMY

Interventions	*Rationales*
Check that catheter is patent and draining before administering medication.	Obstruction in the flow of urine contributes to pain.
Administer a prescribed antispasmodic, such as a belladonna and opium suppository, or prescribed medications like oxybutynin (Ditropan) or propantheline (Pro-Banthine), or an analgesic for incisional pain.	Anticholinergics relieve bladder spasms. Analgesics interfere with the perception of pain.
Explain that the large balloon holding the catheter in place, traction on the catheter, and the volume of instilling irrigant tend to produce the urge to void, but an effort to do so contributes to discomfort.	Offering the client an explanation helps to alleviate the anxiety concerning the cause of discomfort.
Use nursing measures such as placing a rolled towel beneath the scrotum, assisting with the application of an athletic support, suggesting the use of a recliner rather than sitting on a hard surface, changing position, and diversional activities.	Alternative measures enhance the response to drug therapy.

Evaluation of Expected Outcome: Pain and discomfort are tolerable.

Nursing Diagnosis: **Risk for Infection** related to impaired tissue and potential contamination of catheters and incisional drains

Expected Outcome: Client will be free of infection as evidenced by progressive wound healing, no fever, no purulent drainage, expected white blood cell count, and urine free of bacteria.

Interventions	*Rationales*
Practice conscientious handwashing before providing nursing care.	Handwashing is the single most important method to reduce the potential for spreading microorganisms.
Keep ports used for emptying drainage clean.	A contaminated port provides a portal for microorganisms that can ascend to other structures in the urinary tract.
Reinforce or change moist dressings using surgical asepsis.	Moisture on a dressing wicks microorganisms into the wound.
Keep perineum clean after a bowel movement for clients with a perineal prostatectomy.	Stool contains many bacteria that can easily enter a perineal wound because of its close proximity to the anus.
Report tenderness, unusual drainage, foul odor, and fever.	An infection produces a cluster of common signs and symptoms.

Evaluation of Expected Outcome: There is no evidence of infection; vital signs are normal.

Nursing Diagnosis: **Risk for Impaired Skin Integrity** related to leaking urine from suprapubic catheter

Expected Outcome: Skin will remain free of redness and excoriation around the catheter site.

Interventions	*Rationales*
Clean skin around suprapubic catheter with mild soap and water; dry skin thoroughly (Nursing Guidelines 61-1).	Wet skin causes maceration of tissue. Strong soaps can irritate the skin.
Apply and change drain gauze around suprapubic catheter as it becomes moist.	A drain gauze absorbs moisture.

(continued)

Nursing Care Plan 61-2 (Continued)

THE CLIENT UNDERGOING A PROSTATECTOMY

Interventions	Rationales
Enclose the suprapubic catheter in an ostomy appliance.	Ostomy equipment can be used as a means to collect urine and prevent contact between the skin and urine.
Consult an enterostomal therapist on substances such as karaya that can be applied to the skin.	Karaya provides a moisture-resistant barrier and protects the skin.

Evaluation of Expected Outcome: Skin remains intact or the wound heals normally.

Nursing Diagnosis: **Urge or Total Urinary Incontinence** related to altered urinary sphincter or nerve damage secondary to surgical procedure if nerves have been spared

Expected Outcome: Client will disguise incontinence or regain continence.

Interventions	Rationales
Provide absorbent pads or underwear.	Absorbing urine reduces embarrassment associated with incontinence.
Teach pelvic floor–strengthening exercises (Nursing Guidelines 61-2).	Pelvic floor exercises strengthen the muscles that promote urinary continence.
Suggest using a penile clamp (Fig. 61-13).	A penile clamp compresses the urethra externally, preventing incontinence.

Evaluation of Expected Outcome: Continence problems are controlled.

Nursing Diagnosis: **Sexual Dysfunction** related to structural changes secondary to surgical procedure

Expected Outcome: Sexual activity will be satisfactory.

Interventions	Rationales
Provide information on support groups.	Others who have experienced sexual dysfunction after prostatectomy may be both supportive and influential in solving sexual problems.
Clarify information concerning potential sexual consequences of the specific surgical procedure.	Sexual problems may be temporary or permanent depending on the type of prostatectomy that is performed.

Evaluation of Expected Outcome: Client resumes sexual activity, when appropriate, or adapts to sexual changes.

Nursing Diagnosis: **Risk for Ineffective Therapeutic Regimen Management** related to lack of knowledge about care after discharge

Expected Outcome: Client will refer to written instructions that correlate with drug teaching, wound and catheter care, and medical follow-up.

Interventions	Rationales
Emphasize ongoing medical care.	Medical follow-up ensures progressive recovery and monitoring for developing complications.
Advise client to avoid self-administering aspirin.	Aspirin interferes with platelet aggregation, which promotes bleeding.

(continued)

Nursing Care Plan 61-2 (Continued)

THE CLIENT UNDERGOING A PROSTATECTOMY

Interventions	*Rationales*
Explain drug action, frequency of drug administration, and side effects of medications that will be taken after discharge.	Knowledge about discharge medications promotes compliance and safe use of prescribed drugs.
Demonstrate and have client return demonstration for catheter and wound care.	Appropriate catheter and wound care reduces the potential for infection.
Identify when client can resume activity, including sexual intercourse.	Physical exertion increases the potential for bleeding.
Suggest consuming 10–12 glasses of oral fluid each day, increasing dietary fiber, or using a mild laxative or stool softener.	Preventing constipation decreases the potential for bleeding if effort is required to eliminate stool.
Instruct client to immediately report pain in the pelvis or perineum, cloudy or bloody urine that persists despite drinking fluids, or fever or chills.	Unusual signs and symptoms indicate the possibility of a developing complication.

Evaluation of Expected Outcome: Client demonstrates an understanding of perineal exercises, medication schedule, activities to avoid, when to contact physician, and wound care.

Pathophysiology and Etiology

The cause of prostatic cancer is unknown, but there seems to be a relationship with increased testosterone levels and a diet that is high in fat. Having two or more blood relatives with prostatic cancer increases the risk for developing the disease. Most prostatic carcinomas occur in the periphery of the gland. As it enlarges, it causes genitourinary symptoms similar to a variety of other conditions (e.g., BPH and cystitis). If untreated, tumor cells spread by way of the bloodstream and lymphatics to the pelvic lymph nodes and bone, particularly the lumbar vertebrae, pelvis, and hips.

FIGURE 61-12 A three-way system for bladder irrigation.

Assessment Findings

Signs and Symptoms

At first, no symptoms occur, and none may develop for years. When the tumor grows large enough, it compromises urinary flow and causes frequency, nocturia, and dysuria (difficult or painful urination). The first symptoms of metastases may be back pain or pain down the leg from nerve sheath involvement. When pain develops, the disease often is in an advanced stage.

Diagnostic Findings

Rectal examination detects a prostatic nodule. A PSA greater than 4 ng/mL is the basis for performing more definitive diagnostic procedures, and a PSA above 10 ng/mL indicates a prostatic malignancy. A PSA greater than 80 ng/mL indicates advanced metastatic disease. Researchers are now finding that measuring insulin-like growth factor-1 and insulin-like growth factor binding protein-3 is a more sensitive test for prostate cancer that may identify cases that PSA alone fails to detect (Holly, 1998; Kurek et al., 2000; Wolk et al., 2000).

NURSING GUIDELINES 61-1

*Managing the Care of a Client With a Suprapubic Catheter**

Purpose: To drain urine from the bladder through a catheter that is inserted through the anterior abdominal wall and anchored with external skin sutures. The client may or may not have a urethral (Foley) catheter as well.

- Stabilize the catheter by taping it to the skin of the abdomen.
- Keep the catheter connected to a sterile drainage system.
- Keep the drainage system below the level of the insertion site.
- Empty the urine from the bag periodically to reduce tension on the catheter and skin.
- Record the urine output from the suprapubic catheter separate from voided urine output or output from another catheter.
- Keep the skin clean and dry at the insertion site to avoid skin irritation and compromised skin integrity.
- For "trial voiding":
  - Clamp the catheter for 4 hours.
  - Have the client void naturally.
  - Unclamp the suprapubic catheter.
  - Measure the residual urine.
- Collaborate with the physician on removing the suprapubic catheter when the residual urine is repeatedly <100 mL.
- To remove the catheter:
  - Offer an analgesic 30 minutes before proceeding.
  - Wash hands and don gloves.
  - Empty the urinary drainage and record amount.
  - Remove gloves, rewash hands.
  - Position the client on his back.
  - Free the tape from the skin.
  - Open a package of sterile gloves and suture removal kit.
  - Remove the skin sutures.
  - Pull gently on the catheter until it is free.
  - Place a sterile dressing over the insertion site.
  - Remove gloves and wash hands.
  - Change the dressing when it becomes moist until the site heals in approximately 2 days.

---

*A suprapubic catheter also may be called a *cystostomy tube.*

NURSING GUIDELINES 61-2

Teaching Pelvic Floor–Strengthening Exercises

- Squeeze the pelvic floor muscles (those used to stop urination and hold back a bowel movement) for up to 10 seconds—longer is not better.
- Relax completely for 10 seconds—less is not better.
- Repeat sequence as many times as possible in 5 minutes or a cycle of 15 contractions followed by relaxation.
- Interrupt exercises when muscles can no longer be contracted tightly.
- Perform exercises in the morning and evening.
- Perform shorter pelvic floor exercises four or five times during the day:
  - Squeeze pelvic floor muscles and hold for one second.
  - Relax for 1 second.
  - Repeat five times in succession within 2 minutes.
- Continue long and short exercises for 3 to 4 months or until continent.

(Adapted from the Pelvic Floor Retraining Team, Incontinence Clinic, Beth Israel Hospital, Boston, MA, and The Prostate Cancer Infolink [1995].)

intravenous pyelogram (IVP) and other renal function studies detect kidney damage caused by long-standing urethral obstruction and urinary retention (if present).

Medical and Surgical Management

The tumor size, microscopic characteristics, and any metastases are used to establish the stage, which in turn determines treatment (Table 61-3). The client's age and gen-

Transrectal ultrasound confirms the presence of a mass. The definitive diagnosis is made by biopsy and microscopic examination of tissue. Sometimes the malignancy is detected after microscopic examination of tissue removed during a TURP or open prostatectomy for BPH.

Pelvic or spinal radiographs, bone scan, and magnetic resonance imaging (MRI) or computed tomography (CT) scanning detect metastases to bones. An elevated serum acid phosphatase is associated with bone metastasis. An

FIGURE 61-13 Penile clamp. Clamp is molded to comfortably fit penis and gently compress urethra.

TABLE 61-3	STAGING AND TREATMENT OF PROSTATE CANCER	
STAGE	TREATMENT	5-YEAR SURVIVAL RATE
Stage A1: Cancer is found incidentally with <5% malignant cells	Observation	98%
Stage A2: Tumor is not palpable, biopsy is positive	Observation, surgery, or radiation therapy	90%
Stage B: Tumor is palpable, confined to prostate	Surgery or radiation therapy	77%
Stage C: Local extension of tumor but no distant metastasis	Radiation therapy or combination of surgery, radiation and hormone therapy	60%
Stage D: Distant metastasis	Medical therapy	26%

eral health status also are considered when planning treatment. Treatment regimens include observation, surgery, radiation, hormone therapy, or a combination of these.

Surgery

If the nodule is localized, an open suprapubic prostatectomy is the treatment of choice. A radical prostatectomy, performed through a perineal or retropubic approach, is the surgical preference if the tumor is large enough to be palpated or if it has spread to adjacent tissue.

When a radical prostatectomy is performed, the entire prostate, its capsule, and the seminal vesicles are removed. The bladder neck is sutured to the membranous urethra over an indwelling urethral catheter, which is left in place for 10 to 14 days. Potential complications of this surgery include a 25% to 50% chance of impotence, difficulty with urinary control, and genital and lower extremity edema. A TURP may be done if the client has urethral obstruction and his physical status is not amenable to treatment. Occasionally, permanent suprapubic drainage may need to be established.

A bilateral orchidectomy (surgical removal of the testes) may be performed to eliminate the production of testosterone in men with advanced prostatic carcinoma (stage D). Permanent side effects are impotence, loss of libido, hot flashes, and possible psychological disturbances. Many men do not accept surgical castration and low levels of testosterone are achieved with hormone therapy.

Radiation Therapy

Radiation therapy (see Chap. 20) may be used alone or in conjunction with other treatment modalities, especially when there is local metastasis. Possible side effects include impotence, diarrhea, and urinary frequency and urgency.

Hormone Therapy

Men with stage D carcinoma of the prostate are candidates for hormone therapy (Drug Therapy Table 61-2). With the use of antiandrogenic (male) hormones or estrogenic hormones, the progression of the malignancy may be retarded and there may be a prolonged period of palliation (comfort). Estramustine (Emcyt) is a combination of estrogen and an antineoplastic drug that also is used for palliative treatment.

DRUG THERAPY TABLE 61-2	HORMONAL AGENTS FOR PROSTATIC CANCER		
DRUG	MECHANISM OF ACTION	SIDE EFFECTS	NURSING CONSIDERATIONS
diethylstilbestrol (DES)	Synthetic estrogen that reduces testosterone levels	Breast enlargement, nausea, vomiting, photosensitivity, elevated blood sugar	Offer small, frequent meals to offset nausea. Monitor blood sugar, especially in clients with diabetes mellitus. Recommend using a sunscreen or wearing protective clothing.
flutamide (Eulexin)	Blocks androgens	Breast enlargement, impotence, diarrhea, anemia, leukopenia, thrombocytopenia, jaundice	Instruct clients that periodic blood tests are required. Observe if urine is dark yellow.
goserelin acetate (Zoladex)	Inhibits pituitary gonadotropin secretion, which reduces testosterone to castration levels	Hot flashes, impotence, loss of libido	Administer as a monthly injection or subcutaneous implant. Use a local anesthetic before administering injection. Repeat injection every 28 days. Drug resistance occurs after 2 to 3 years of therapy.

Feminizing side effects occur with hormone therapy. The client's voice may become higher, hair and fat distribution may change, and breasts may become tender and enlarged. Libido and potency also are diminished. When estrogens are used in lower doses, the client may not experience these problems.

NURSING PROCESS

● The Client With Prostatic Cancer

Assessment

The nurse obtains a health history from the client and focuses on identifying information such as changes in patterns of urinary elimination (frequency, urgency, and nocturia), hematuria, low back pain, and a family history of prostatic cancer. After extensive surgical treatment for prostatic cancer, the nurse assesses the client for signs of infection, urinary incontinence, and sexual dysfunction and reinforces health teaching that aids in the detection of metastasis.

Diagnosis, Planning, and Interventions

Refer to Chapter 25 for general preoperative and postoperative standards of care. Radical prostatectomy is similar to other prostatectomy procedures and the same immediate postoperative nursing diagnoses and interventions apply. Diagnoses, expected outcomes, and interventions for clients with prostatic cancer include, but are not limited to, the following.

Risk for Infection related to home care of Foley catheter
Expected Outcome: Client will be free of a urinary tract infection as evidenced by clear urine without bacteria or white blood cells.

- Tell client to use soap and water to clean around the urethral meatus and several inches of the catheter at least twice a day. *Medical asepsis decreases the growth of microorganisms that can ascend upward into the urinary tract.*
- Demonstrate and have the client return the demonstration for keeping the connection between the catheter and leg bag clean when changing and replacing leg bags for routine cleaning. *Keeping connections and equipment clean reduces the portals for microbial entry into the urinary tract.*
- Tell the client or caregiver to clean the leg bag by using soap and water and then rinsing it with a 1:7 solution of vinegar and water. *Vinegar is a weak acid (acetic acid) that chemically interferes with the growth of microorganisms.*

Total Urinary Incontinence related to surgical compromises to internal and external urinary sphincter muscles
Expected Outcome: Urinary control will be reestablished within 3 months after surgery or client will use equipment to collect urine.

- Teach pelvic floor retraining exercises (see Nursing Guidelines 61-2) if incontinence is not permanent. *Pelvic floor retraining exercises improve sphincter tone and bladder control.*
- For permanent incontinence, show the client how to apply a penile clamp or an external catheter connected to a leg bag. *Devising a method for mechanically controlling urinary incontinence or collecting urine unobtrusively decreases social embarrassment.*

Sexual Dysfunction related to temporary impotence when pudendal nerve (responsible for erection and orgasm) is spared
Expected Outcome: Client will use alternatives other than intercourse for sexual pleasure until potency resumes.

- Explain to the client and sexual partner that it may take from 3 to 12 months for sexual potency to return. *Providing a timeline helps the client and his sexual partner cope with temporary sexual dysfunction.*
- See interventions for impotence for additional suggestions. *Various alternatives to sexual intercourse may be useful for managing sexual dysfunction.*

PC: Impotence related to pudendal nerve damage secondary to non–nerve-sparing radical perineal prostatectomy
Expected Outcome: The nurse will assist the client and sexual partner to manage and minimize erectile dysfunction.

- Recommend demonstrating sexual feelings in ways other than intercourse. *Intimacy is communicated in many different ways. Becoming asexual is counterproductive.*
- Discuss the use of manual stimulation or a mechanical vibrator if it does not compromise the sex partner's moral values. *Stimulating the clitoris of the female manually or with a vibrator is an alternative method to sexual penetration for promoting female orgasm.*

PC: Metastasis
Expected Outcome: The nurse will assist the client to manage and minimize the possibility of a recurrence of the primary cancer or metastasis.

- Explain that the PSA level will decrease after prostatectomy; a subsequent rise indicates the cancer has reoccurred. *Having regular PSA levels after treatment aids in the early detection of cancer recurrence or metastasis.*
- Clarify that repeat lymph node biopsies may be part of the surgical follow-up. *One method by which cancer cells are spread is the lymphatic system.*
- Inform the client that blood tests for measuring serum acid phosphatase are used to monitor evidence of bone metastasis. *A rise in acid phosphatase is a tumor marker for a client who has been treated for cancer of the prostate.*

Evaluation of Expected Outcomes

Expected outcomes for the client who is treated for cancer of the prostate are no evidence of infection and urinary continence. The client finds acceptable techniques for sexual expression when impotence is permanent. He identifies techniques that assist in monitoring for a recurrence of the primary cancer or its metastatic spread.

As the client recovers, the nurse promotes increased self-care, and provides instructions for home management. The discharge plan of care includes, but is not limited to, the following:

- Maintain medical follow-up.
- Take medications as prescribed.
- Decrease dietary fat and increase fiber.
- Exercise regularly to increase lean body mass and decrease insulin levels, which is a catabolic hormone that promotes weight gain.
- Join a support group to learn more about the disease process and clinical trials of research.
- Consult with the family physician or oncologist before self-treating with herbal supplements such as saw palmetto, which some believe is beneficial in relieving disorders of the prostate gland.

● CANCER OF THE TESTES

Cancer of the testes is a rapidly metastasizing malignancy seen in men between the ages of 18 and 40 years. Although this cancer is relatively rare, it is the most common type in men between 15 and 34 years of age and is the leading cause of death from cancer in men between 25 and 34 years of age. Significant advancement in treatment in recent years, however, has resulted in a high cure rate even in clients with metastatic disease.

Pathophysiology and Etiology

The incidence is higher among men with a history of cryptorchidism regardless of whether an orchiopexy was performed. Although the exact etiology is unknown, one possible explanation is that the cells in the undescended testis or testes degenerate earlier than occurs with natural aging. The degenerative process then leads to abnormal cellular changes. In most cases, only one testicle is affected, but the other may become cancerous if the tumor is not diagnosed early.

Nearly all testicular tumors involve the sperm-forming germ cells. Those that consist of immature germ cells are called *seminomas; nonseminomas* develop among more mature, specialized germ cells. Nonseminomas grow more rapidly and tend to metastasize at a faster rate; therefore, treatment is more aggressive.

Assessment Findings

Gradual or sudden swelling of the scrotum or a lump felt on palpation always deserves prompt medical attention. The tumor usually presents as a hard, nontender nodule of the testis with additional coexisting symptoms (Box 61-2). Unless discovered early through testicular self-examination, the first symptoms may be those of tumor metastasis. They may include abdominal pain, general weakness, and aching in the testes.

Tumor markers include elevated levels of alpha-fetoprotein and bHCG. An IVP may show lymph node enlargement that displaces the ureters. Lymphangiography also is used to detect lymph node involvement. A CT scan or MRI can detect metastases. Because biopsy risks spreading the highly malignant tumor cells, surgery is recommended immediately.

Medical and Surgical Management

Treatment of testicular tumors depends on the stage of the disease (Table 61-4) and includes surgery, chemotherapy, and radiation. An autologous (self-donated) bone marrow transplantation may be recommended for recurrent disease or for clients who are resistant to drug therapy. Before medical or surgical treatment, however, the topic of sperm banking should be discussed. Locating a sperm bank and then collecting and banking sperm, which may take as long as 12 to 24 days, is omitted if the delay would jeopardize the outcome of treatment.

Surgery

A radical inguinal **orchiectomy** (removal of the testis) and ligation of the spermatic cord is performed. Clients with nonseminomas usually undergo a radical retroperitoneal lymph node dissection as well. If only one testis is removed, sexual activity, the libido, and fertility usually are unaffected. After a radical lymph node dissection, libido and erections are preserved, but surgical disruption of nerve pathways results in impaired ejaculation. New nerve-sparing techniques are being developed that preserve ejaculatory function, and therefore fertility, in most clients.

Chemotherapy

A multiple antineoplastic drug regimen usually is instituted after surgery. The types of drugs, the frequency of their administration, and the duration of therapy depend on the type of tumor and if metastasis has occurred. Chemotherapy, which usually is aggressive initially, is

---

BOX 61-2 ● Signs and Symptoms of Testicular Cancer

- Testicular lump that is hard or granular
- Increase in the size of one testicle
- Heavy or dragging feeling in the scrotum
- Dull ache in the groin or above the pubis
- Diminished sensitivity to testicular pressure

TABLE 61-4	STAGING AND TREATMENT OF GERM CELL TUMORS OF THE TESTIS	
STAGE	TREATMENT	SURVIVAL RATE
Stage I: Tumor confined to the testis	Orchiectomy, retroperitoneal lymph node dissection	95%
Stage II: Involvement of testis plus retroperitoneal nodes	Orchiectomy, retroperitoneal lymph node dissection, possible chemotherapy	93%
Stage III: Distant metastasis	Orchiectomy, retroperitoneal lymph node dissection, four cycles of chemotherapy, surgery to resect residual masses	70%

modified as the tumor markers show a response. Sperm tend to be destroyed or mutated when exposed to toxic cancer drugs, but spermatogenesis eventually resumes.

Radiation

Seminomas are sensitive to radiation, and most clients receive radiation to the retroperitoneal lymph nodes. For clients with nonseminomas, radiation is considered an adjunct to lymphadenectomy and chemotherapy.

Nursing Management

Preoperative Period

One of nursing's chief concerns is responding to the client's emotional distress over having a life-threatening diagnosis, being unfamiliar with the surgical experience, and confronting alterations in body image and sexuality. All clients are understandably concerned over the potential change in their sexual image and fertility; however, it may be of even greater concern to men in this age group. The nurse provides private opportunities for the client to ask questions and uses therapeutic communication techniques to encourage the client to verbalize his feelings.

Postoperative Period

Refer to Chapter 25 for postoperative standards of care. After an orchiectomy the nurse applies a scrotal support. If drains have been inserted, they are connected to closed (Jackson-Pratt) or open (machine) suction. The nurse gives prophylactic antibiotics to prevent infection. He or she manages pain, which may be severe after a radical lymph node dissection, with narcotic analgesics. If pain is not relieved and nursing measures to augment the effect of analgesics are inadequate, the nurse collaborates with the physician to modify drug therapy.

As the client's comfort improves, the nurse may discuss the effects of the diagnosis and treatment and again provide opportunities for the safe expression of anxiety, fear, and grief. The nurse advises the client that a testicular prosthesis can be inserted at a later date if he desires and that fertility may be regained in 2 to 3 years after drug therapy is discontinued, and sooner when surgery or radiation is used. The nurse provides the client with names of local support groups and encourages him to contact them for emotional support after discharge.

Client and Family Teaching

A teaching plan includes the following instructions:

- Drink plenty of fluids and eat a well-balanced diet to avoid constipation.
- Obtain adequate rest; avoid fatigue and heavy lifting.
- Wash the incision with warm soap and water. Report any redness, drainage, pain, or swelling of the incision or scrotum.
- Take any prescribed medication exactly as directed.
- Perform self-examination of the remaining testicle every month and immediately report any changes.
- Seek care if any of the following occur: fever, chills, adverse drug effects, weight loss, or anorexia.

For clients who are concerned about future reproduction, the nurse discusses issues as appropriate for the client's particular situation. If a client has banked sperm, the nurse informs him that normal pregnancies have occurred with sperm stored up to 10 years. For clients for whom treatment has proceeded without collecting and storing sperm, the nurse identifies other pregnancy options, such as donor insemination or adoption. He or she may suggest contacting the department of social services to become a foster parent, volunteering as a Big Brother, or leading a scout troop or youth group to compensate for the inability to raise biologic children.

● CANCER OF THE PENIS

Penile cancer is rare and occurs more often in men who are uncircumcised. The cause is unknown but it is thought that chronic irritation leads to a precancerous skin lesion that eventually undergoes malignant changes. Medical attention is sought when the lesion, which typically has been present for years, becomes infected. Biopsy confirms the existence of malignant cells and lymphangiography identifies if the lymph nodes are involved. The tumor is staged using MRI and CT scanning.

Treatment includes tumor excision, chemotherapy, external or interstitial radiation therapy, or all three. In some cases, the penis is partially or completely amputated and the scrotum and testes excised. Full amputation of the penis requires the insertion of a permanent drainage tube in the perineal tissue to empty the bladder. The 5-year survival rate for cancer of the penis is less than 50%.

ELECTIVE STERILIZATION

A **vasectomy** is a minor surgical procedure done in a physician's office or clinic. It involves the ligation of the vas deferens and results in permanent sterilization by interrupting the pathway that transports sperm (Fig. 61-14). On occasion, the client may complain of impotence, although the procedure has no effect on erection or ejaculation. It may take several weeks or more after surgery before the ejaculatory fluid is free of sperm, and the client is informed to use a reliable method of contraception until sperm no longer are present. The client may wish to consider banking sperm before undergoing the procedure. Some men feel ambivalent about having this procedure and the nurse provides the client with an opportunity to express these feelings.

The nurse reinforces the following important information for home care after a vasectomy:

- Expect some bruising and incisional soreness after the local anesthetic wears off.
- Apply ice packs to the scrotum to reduce swelling; remove the cold application after 20 minutes and replace again after the tissue rewarms.
- Take a mild analgesic, such as aspirin or acetaminophen, for discomfort.
- Wear an athletic support for several days for comfort.
- Resume usual activities in 2 to 3 days, but avoid strenuous exercise for up to 5 days.
- Resume sexual activity when comfort allows, usually in 1 week.
- Use a reliable method of contraception until the physician indicates that sperm no longer are present, which may be determined after 10 or more ejaculations.
- Report severe pain, fever, or swelling at the top of the testes.

A vasovasostomy is a surgical attempt to reverse a vasectomy by restoring patency and continuity to the vas deferens; a vasoepididymostomy connects the stump of the vas deferens directly to the epididymis. It may take from 3 to 6 months after reversal procedures before sperm counts and motility are normal. Lack of success usually is the result of either scar formation or sperm leakage from the surgical connection.

GENERAL NUTRITIONAL CONSIDERATIONS

Studies show a high-fat diet may increase the risk of prostate cancer by 30% to 50%. Other risk factors include living an inactive lifestyle and being overweight.

GENERAL PHARMACOLOGIC CONSIDERATIONS

Platinum-based drugs such as cisplatin (Platinol) are very effective in treating certain forms of testicular cancer. They almost always are combined with other antineoplastic drugs.

Other drugs used in combination with cisplatin in treating testicular cancer include etoposide (VePesid) and bleomycin (Blenoxane). Bleomycin can cause pulmonary toxicity in those taking high doses of the drug or in those older than 70 years of age. Some clients taking bleomycin for testicular cancer have developed Raynaud's phenomenon (see Chap. 33).

Cisplatin is extremely nephrotoxic and the client must be kept well hydrated. Administration of at least 3,000 mL of fluid per 24 hours is necessary if the client's condition permits. Report any evidence of fluid retention such as edema, weight gain, difficulty breathing, or bubbly lung sounds. Irreversible ototoxicity can occur. Audiometric testing is recommended before the first dose and before each subsequent dose. Ototoxicity can occur after a single dose.

Chemotherapy for cancer increases the risk for infection, anorexia, vomiting, and hair loss.

Drugs such as epoetin (Epogen) and filgrastim (Neupogen) can stimulate the development of red and white blood cells whose production has been suppressed with antineoplastic drugs.

Administration of antiemetic drugs before chemotherapy can reduce or eliminate the incidence of nausea and vomiting. Some chemotherapeutic agents, such as cisplatin, however, can cause severe nausea and vomiting that does not respond well to antiemetics and that can persist for up to 7 days after treatment.

Certain medications such as antihypertensive drugs (e.g., methyldopa, spironolactone), antidepressants, narcotics, and cimetidine can cause sexual dysfunction in men. If impotence or sexual dysfunction occurs, obtain a thorough drug history to determine if the sexual dysfunction is an adverse reaction to a drug and could be corrected by the use of a different medication.

All chemotherapeutic agents are capable of causing an anaphylactoid reaction. Report any of the following symptoms to the primary healthcare provider: any skin rash, hives, difficulty breathing, wheezing, tachycardia, or hypotension.

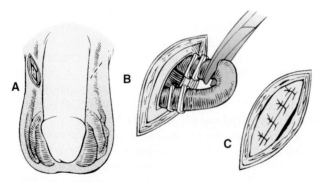

FIGURE 61-14 Vasectomy procedure. (**A**) An incision is made to expose the vas deferens. (**B**) The vas deferens is isolated and severed. (**C**) The severed ends are occluded with sutures or sealed with electrocautery.

GENERAL GERONTOLOGIC CONSIDERATIONS

When an older man develops a varicocele when none existed before, the congestion of blood may be caused by pressure from a urologic tumor.

Impotence increases as men age; 15% to 25% of all men experience impotence by age 65 years. More than half of all men 75 years of age or older are chronically impotent.

Sperm and testosterone production gradually decreases as men age. This phenomenon possibly is the result of degenerative changes in the vascular system in the testes.

There are greater numbers of older than middle-aged men who are uncircumcised because many were born at home and the procedure was not performed. Therefore, the incidence of phimosis, paraphimosis, balanoposthitis, and penile cancer is more common in older men.

Along with a decrease in sperm production, the volume and viscosity of seminal fluid decreases with age. A loss of muscular tone causes the scrotum to become more pendulous. As the scrotum drops, there is an increased risk of trauma and injury to this area.

Impotence is not a normal part of aging. If impotence occurs, other causes should be explored such as adverse reactions to medication, atherosclerosis, or psychological problems.

Critical Thinking Exercises

1. *Assume you are attending a team conference to plan the care of a client who is having a suprapubic prostatectomy. What nursing interventions are appropriate?*

2. *Describe the typical client who acquires prostatic hypertrophy versus one who develops testicular cancer.*

References and Suggested Readings

Allison, L. (2000). Clinical effectiveness: Testicular self-examination. *Professional Nurse, 15,* 710–713.

Anchors, N. (1998). Growth hormone IGF-1 and prostate cancer. *Life Extension Magazine, 4*(5), 42–44.

Bullock, B. L. & Henze, R. L. (2000). *Focus on pathophysiology.* Philadelphia: Lippincott Williams & Wilkins.

Cerrato, P. L. (2000). Complementary therapies: Diet and herbs for BPH? *RN, 63*(2), 63–64.

Chow, R. D. (2001). Benign prostatic hyperplasia: Patient evaluation and relief of obstructive symptoms. *Geriatrics, 56*(3), 33–38.

Clenney, T. L. & Higgins, J. C. (1999). Vasectomy techniques. *American Family Physician, 60,* 137–146, 151–152.

Cohen, B. J. & Wood, D. L. (2000). *Memmler's structure and function of the human body* (7th ed.). Philadelphia: Lippincott Williams & Wilkins.

DuFour, J. L. (2001). Short communications: Assessing and treating epididymitis. *Nurse Practitioner: American Journal of Primary Health Care, 26*(3), 23–24.

Epperly, T. D. & Moore, K. E. (2000). Health issues in men: Part I. Common genitourinary disorders. *American Family Physician, 61,* 3657–3664.

Gleich, P. (2001). Scrotal masses: Benign or serious? *Consultant, 41,* 369–372.

Held-Warmkessel, J. (2001). Treatment of advanced prostate cancer. *Seminars in Oncology Nursing, 17,* 118–128.

Holly, J. (1998). Insulin-like growth factor-1 and new opportunities for cancer prevention. *Lancet, 351,* 1373–1374.

Holman, J. R. & Stuessi, K. A. (1999). Adult circumcision. *American Family Physician, 59,* 1514–1518.

Hulisz, D. & Plant, R. (2000). Popular herbal remedies: Examining their effectiveness and potential for drug interactions and adverse reactions. American Council on Pharmaceutical Education. [On-line.] Available: http://www.continuing-education.com/pharmacy/herbs/index.html.

Iwamoto, R. R. & Maher, K. E. (2001). Radiation therapy for prostate cancer. *Seminars in Oncology Nursing, 17,* 90–100.

Junnila, J. & Lassen, P. (1998). Testicular masses. *American Family Physician, 57,* 685–692.

Kelley, W. N. (1997). *Textbook of internal medicine* (3rd ed.). Philadelphia: Lippincott-Raven.

Kinkade, S. (1999). Testicular cancer. *American Family Physician, 59,* 2539–2544.

Klingman, L. (1999). Assessing the male genitalia. *American Journal of Nursing, 99*(7), 47–50.

Kloner, R. A. (2001). Erectile dysfunction and cardiovascular risk factors. *Hospital Practice, 36*(8), 41–44, 49–51.

Kurek, R., Tunn, W., Eckart, O., et al. (2000). The significance of serum levels of insulin-like growth factor-1 in patients with prostate cancer. *British Journal of Urology, 85,* 125–129.

Maliski, S. L., Heilemann, M. V., & McCorkle, R. (2001). Mastery of postprostatectomy incontinence and impotence: His work, her work, our work. *Oncology Nursing Forum, 28,* 985–992.

Marsche, P. S. (2001). The role of surgery in the treatment of prostate cancer. *Seminars in Oncology Nursing, 17,* 85–89.

Nelson, S. A. & Schumann, L. (1998). Continuing education forum: Differentiating prostate disorders. *Journal of the American Academy of Nurse Practitioners, 10,* 415–425.

Neuhouser, M. L., Kristal, A. R., Patterson, R. E., et al. (2001). Dietary supplement use in the Prostate Cancer Prevention Trial: Implications for prevention trials. *Nutrition and Cancer, 39*(1), 12–18.

Patten, E. (2000). Apomorphine effectively treats erectile dysfunction. [On-line.] Available: http://www.plsgroup.com/dg/1CFCD6.htm.

Poole, G., Poon, C., Achille, M., et al. (2001). Social support for patients with prostate cancer: The effect of support groups. *Journal of Psychosocial Oncology, 19*(2), 1–16.

Sneddon, D. (2000). Assessing and treating erectile dysfunction. *Journal of Community Nursing, 14*(11), 4–6, 8.

Stevermer, J. J. & Easley, S. K. (2000). Treatment of prostatitis. *American Family Physician, 61,* 2961–2964, 3015–3022, 3025–3026.

Weaver, J. (2001). Combating complications of transurethral surgery. *Nursing, 31*(7), Hospital Nursing: 32hn1–32hn2, 32hn4.

Weinrich, S. (2001). The debate about prostate cancer screening: What nurses need to know. *Seminars in Oncology Nursing, 17,* 78–84.

Wolk, A., Andersson, S., Mantzoros, C., et al. (2000). Can measurement of IGF-1 and IGFBP-3 improve the sensitivity of prostate screening? *Lancet, 356,* 1902.

Caring for Clients With Sexually Transmitted Diseases

Learning Objectives

On completion of this chapter, the reader will:

- Name five common sexually transmitted diseases (STDs) and identify those that are curable.
- List seven STDs that by law must be reported.
- Give two reasons why statistics on reportable STDs are not totally accurate.
- Discuss several contributing factors to the transmission of STDs.
- Give two reasons why women acquire STDs more often than men.
- Name the most common and fastest-spreading STD.
- Explain two ways STDs are spread.
- Discuss methods that are helpful in preventing STDs.
- Discuss information that is important to teach clients about using condoms.
- Give the classification of the infectious microorganism that causes each of the common STDs.
- Identify complications that are common among clients who acquire each of the most common STDs.
- Name drugs used to treat the common STDs.

Sexually transmitted diseases (STDs), also known as **venereal diseases,** are a diverse group of infections spread through sexual activity with an infected person, and represent a significant public health problem. Some, such as acquired immunodeficiency syndrome (AIDS; see Chap. 43), hepatitis (see Chap. 55), and skin infestations with lice and mites (see Chap. 69), are spread by additional routes as well. The pathogens that cause STDs include bacteria, fungi, parasites, protozoans, and viruses. Besides AIDS, the five most common STDs are chlamydia, gonorrhea, syphilis, genital herpes, and genital warts. Of these, chlamydia, gonorrhea, and syphilis are easily cured with early and adequate treatment. Social, sexual, and biologic factors contribute to the high incidence of venereal disease, and include the following:

- Ignorance of how STDs are transmitted or prevented
- Asymptomatic sex partner(s)
- Casual sex with partner(s) about whom little is known
- Sex with high-risk partner(s), like those who use intravenous (IV) drugs, are bisexual, or have sex with prostitutes
- Multiple concurrent or sequential sex partner(s)
- Failure to use contraceptive techniques that also reduce the risk for acquiring STDs
- Sexual contact during the period between infection and the manifestation of symptoms
- Failure to seek early treatment
- Noncompliance with treatment or instructions to refrain from sexual contact until treatment is complete

● Mutation and resistance of microorganisms to anti-microbial drug therapy

EPIDEMIOLOGY

Epidemiology is the study of the occurrence, distribution, and causes of human diseases. The Centers for Disease Control and Prevention (CDC) has the awesome task of gathering disease statistics such as the incidence of STDs. Determining the exact incidence of these diseases is difficult because only a few are reportable by law (Box 62-1), and some go untreated, treated and unreported, or misdiagnosed or undiagnosed. Women acquire STDs more often than men, probably because the moist, warm vaginal environment is conducive to microbial growth and because the vagina, as a receptive orifice, is more readily traumatized during sexual activity. Table 62-1 lists common STDs and their estimated incidence in the United States.

Obtaining a sexual history (Nursing Guidelines 62-1) is a crucial component of assessment of clients presenting with signs or symptoms of an STD, and asking questions nonjudgmentally is essential. In addition to curing the infection when possible (some STDs are not curable), treatment consists of education and counseling to reduce the client's risk for contracting an STD in the future (Nursing Guidelines 62-2), and screening, counseling, and, if indicated, treating their sexual partner(s).

COMMON SEXUALLY TRANSMITTED DISEASES

● CHLAMYDIA

Chlamydia is the most common and fastest-spreading bacterial STD in the United States. The number of new cases and reinfections amounts to as many as 3 million annually (Sexually Transmitted Disease Information Center, 2000).

TABLE 62-1	COMMON STDs AND ESTIMATED INCIDENCE IN THE UNITED STATES
STD	NUMBER OF CASES/YEAR
Chlamydia	3,000,000
Condyloma acuminata	5,500,000
Gonorrhea	650,000
Genital herpes	1,000,000
Syphilis	70,000
AIDS	40,000
Hepatitis B	120,000

(From Centers for Disease Control and Prevention. [2001]. Tracking the hidden epidemics: Trends in STDs in the United States 2000. [On-line.] Available: http://www.cdc.gov/std.)

Pathophysiology and Etiology

The causative microorganism is a bacterium, *Chlamydia trachomatis,* that lives inside the cells it infects. The disease is spread by sexual intercourse or genital contact without penetration.

The microorganism invades the reproductive structures (see discussion of pelvic inflammatory disease [PID] in Chap. 59), the urethra in women, and the urethra and epididymis in men (see discussion of nongonococcal urethritis in Chap. 65). The tissue irritation, which may be permanent despite successful eradication of the bacteria, puts those with chlamydial infections at greater risk for acquiring other STDs, such as AIDS. Untreated chlamydia can cause sterility in infected women; infected pregnant women can transmit the microorganism to their infants during birth.

BOX 62-1 ● **Reportable STDs**

By federal law, the following STDs must be reported to the Department of Public Health:
● Gonorrhea
● Syphilis
● Chlamydia
● Chancroid
● Granuloma inguinale
● Lymphogranuloma venereum
● Acquired immunodeficiency syndrome

NURSING GUIDELINES 62-1

Obtaining a Sexual History From the Client With an STD

■ Has the client had new or multiple sexual partners in recent weeks?

■ Was a condom used during sexual activity?

■ Is there a past history of STD?

■ Has the client engaged in vaginal, anal, or oral sex?

■ Was the client the receptive partner in anal or oral sex?

■ Is there a history of infection with human immunodeficiency virus?

■ Is there a history of employment as a sex worker?

■ Are drugs and alcohol used?

■ Is there a possibility of pregnancy?

NURSING GUIDELINES 62-2

Methods for Reducing the Risk for STDs

- Abstain from sexual activities.

- Have monogamous sex with an uninfected partner.

- Use latex condoms with nonoxynol-9 (a spermicide) when having oral, vaginal, or anal intercourse.

- Combine the use of male condoms with a spermicide when having vaginal intercourse, or use a female condom.

- Urinate and wash the genital and perineal areas before and immediately after having sexual intercourse.

- Wash your hands and any areas where there has been direct contact with semen or vaginal mucus.

- Refuse or terminate sexual activity that causes trauma to the genitals, internal reproductive structures, anus, and elsewhere.

- If infected, report the information to all sexual partners and encourage them to seek medical diagnosis and treatment.

- Avoid unprotected sex until you and sex partners have completed treatment.

Chlamydial infections also can be spread to the eyes by **autoinoculation** (self-transmission to another area of the body), usually by unwashed hands. Ophthalmic infections, which are more common in underdeveloped countries where flies are the vector for transmitting the microorganism, can cause granulation of the cornea and blindness.

Assessment Findings

As many as 75% of all infected women and 25% of all infected men are asymptomatic. Symptoms, if they occur, may appear 1 to 3 weeks after infection. They include a sparse, clear urethral discharge, redness and irritation of the infected tissue, burning on urination, lower abdominal pain in women, or testicular pain in men.

Diagnosis is made by microscopic examination and culture of secretions. A test kit is available that identifies the microorganism in approximately 15 minutes. It is common practice to test clients for chlamydia, gonorrhea, and syphilis because it is not unusual for clients to have concurrent infections with more than one STD.

Medical Management

Antimicrobial drugs, such as doxycycline (Vibramycin), the tetracyclines, erythromycin, clarithromycin (Biaxin), and azithromycin (Zithromax) are used for treatment.

Nursing Management

The nurse sensitively obtains a sexual history, follows precautions for preventing infection transmission, assists in collecting a specimen for microscopic analysis, explains the course of treatment, and discusses methods for preventing transmission and reinfection (Nursing Care Plan 62-1 and Nursing Guidelines 62-3).

● GONORRHEA

Gonorrhea is a common STD with the highest incidence in the 15- to 24-year-old age group. Many women are asymptomatic, a factor that contributes to the spread of the disease.

Pathophysiology and Etiology

The infection is caused by a bacteria, *Neisseria gonorrhoeae,* which can be transmitted heterosexually or homosexually. The microorganism invades the urethra, vagina, rectum, or pharynx, depending on the nature of sexual contact; it can spread throughout the body.

In untreated men, the localized infection may spread to the prostate, seminal vesicles, and epididymis. Urethral strictures may develop, requiring periodic dilatation of the urethra or, possibly, reconstructive urethral surgery. In women, the infection may progress upward to the cervix, endometrium, and fallopian tubes, and symptoms of PID (see Chap. 58) may develop. Gonorrhea also can be transmitted to an infant's eyes at the time of birth.

Assessment Findings

Signs and Symptoms

In men, symptoms usually appear 2 to 6 days after infection. Urethritis with a purulent discharge and pain on urination are the most common signs and symptoms. A small proportion of men are asymptomatic. More than half of infected women experience no symptoms. When symptoms do occur, women have a white or yellow vaginal discharge, intermenstrual bleeding due to cervicitis, and painful urination. An anal infection is accompanied by painful bowel elimination and a purulent rectal discharge; the throat is sore when the pharynx is infected. If the microorganism disseminates (scatters) throughout the body, the client may manifest a skin rash, fever, and painful joints.

Diagnostic Findings

Specimens of drainage from infected tissue are examined microscopically immediately after they are collected or are

Nursing Care Plan 62-1

THE CLIENT WITH AN STD

Assessment

Determine the following:

- Vital signs
- Health history with a focus on the onset and course of current symptoms
- Similar symptoms in sexual partner(s)
- Presence of oral, vaginal, rectal, or genitourinary lesions
- Characteristics of discharge (vaginal, urethral, rectal), if any is evident
- Evidence of skin rash or abnormal appearance of integument
- Accompanying symptoms such as joint or abdominal pain or pain during intercourse
- Failure to become pregnant if pregnancy is desired
- Drug and allergy history

Nursing Diagnosis: Situational Low Self-Esteem related to shame or guilt about acquiring an STD

Expected Outcome: Client's self-esteem will be positive.

Interventions	Rationales
Avoid being judgmental.	Negative responses from others lower self-esteem.
Affirm client's good judgment in seeking treatment.	Acknowledging a positive action helps increase client's self-esteem.
Assure client that medical information is confidential and, although some STDs are reported, access to such information is carefully guarded.	Keeping personal information confidential helps the client avoid any public ridicule.
Refer client to a support group for people who have acquired a similar STD.	Members of support groups have similar problems and help others cope with medical, emotional, and social issues.

Evaluation of Expected Outcome: Client's self-esteem remains at the same level as before he or she required medical treatment for STD.

Nursing Diagnosis: Acute Pain related to inflammation and changes in the skin and mucous membranes

Expected Outcome: Pain will be relieved to client's level of tolerance.

Interventions	Rationales
Provide a prescribed analgesic.	Analgesics relieve pain by various physiologic mechanisms.
Administer prescribed antimicrobials specific to the infectious microorganism.	Discomfort usually is relieved when the infection resolves.
Advise regular bathing.	Bathing removes irritating drainage.
Recommend wearing loosely woven cotton underwear and full-cut, nonconstricting outer clothing.	Cotton is a natural fiber that wicks drainage away from the body. Nonconstricting clothing allows air to circulate between the skin and outerwear and avoids friction.

(continued)

Nursing Care Plan 62-1 *(Continued)*

THE CLIENT WITH AN STD

Evaluation of Expected Outcome: Client is comfortable; symptoms are reduced or relieved.

Nursing Diagnoses: Impaired Skin Integrity and **Impaired Mucous Membranes** related to inflammation of local tissues and scratching secondary to infectious process

Expected Outcomes: (1) Skin lesions will heal. (2) Integrity of mucous membranes will be restored.

Interventions	Rationales
Provide information on appropriate topical skin applications.	Various over-the-counter and prescription medications can be applied to the skin to relieve inflammation, reduce itching, lubricate the skin, and dry lesions.
Advise client to pat rather than rub skin dry.	Patting reduces friction and the itch–scratch–itch cycle.
Reinforce compliance with medical treatment.	Taking prescribed medications according to directions ensures eradication or control of the infecting microorganism.

Evaluation of Expected Outcomes: Skin and mucous membranes are intact; no lesions are evident.

Nursing Diagnosis: Risk for Infection Transmission related to infectious drainage and viral shedding

Expected Outcome: The infection will remain confined and not be transmitted to any other susceptible host.

Interventions	Rationales
Follow Standard Precautions before diagnosis and Contact Precautions after diagnosis is confirmed.	Standard Precautions reduce the risk of transmission of a blood-borne infection before a diagnosis is made. Transmission-based precautions interfere with the routes by which specific pathogens are spread.
Advise client to have all sexual partners tested and treated.	STDs often are transmitted between both sexual partners; to eradicate the infection, sexual partners must be treated as well.
Identify methods for preventing STDs such as abstinence, barrier and chemical types of contraceptives, and voiding and washing after sexual intercourse.	STDs are spread by direct contact; methods that prevent direct contact reduce the potential for disease transmission.
Recommend early prenatal care to pregnant women.	Some STDs can be transmitted during childbirth.
Explain how to manage articles used for personal hygiene and items to avoid sharing with noninfected people.	Keeping personal hygiene items separate from others and preventing indirect contact with contaminated items can reduce the potential for disease transmission.
Direct client to take medications as prescribed and return for medical follow-up.	Compliance and medical follow-up help ensure that the infection responds to treatment.

Evaluation of Expected Outcome: No other person acquires the STD from the infected person.

Nursing Diagnosis: Anxiety related to possible consequences of STD

Expected Outcome: Client will feel comfortable when he or she acquires realistic information.

(continued)

Nursing Care Plan 62-1 (Continued)

THE CLIENT WITH AN STD

Interventions	Rationales
Explain the cause of the STD and how to avoid potential consequences or complications.	Accurate knowledge dispels inaccurate beliefs and misconceptions.
Instruct client infected with carcinogenic (cancer-causing) viruses to have regular cancer screening examinations.	These examinations in risk-prone clients facilitate early diagnosis and optimistic prognosis.

Evaluation of Expected Outcome: Client feels self-assured and confident about managing the STD.

Nursing Diagnosis: **Ineffective Sexuality Patterns** related to shame about revealing the risk for an STD to sexual partner(s)

Expected Outcome: Client will resume sexual relationships with modifications that help to avoid STD transmission.

Interventions	Rationales
Role-play situations in which client communicates his or her STD status to a significant other.	Role-playing with an uninvolved person helps a person rehearse and prepare for a situation that evokes anxiety.
Suggest that the client and sexual partner(s) discuss and select methods that will facilitate sexual activity without transmitting the STD.	Open communication facilitates a mutual plan for reducing the potential for disease transmission.

Evaluation of Expected Outcome: Client discusses and implements modifications for sexual expression.

Nursing Diagnoses: **Risk for Ineffective Therapeutic Regimen Management** and **Risk for Noncompliance** related to lack of knowledge or abandoning recommendations

Expected Outcomes: (1) Client will understand the regimen for curing or controlling the STD. (2) Client will comply with the plan of care.

Interventions	Rationales
Provide specific client teaching that is appropriate for the particular STD.	STDs result from various pathogens; treatment varies.
Stress completing the full course of drug therapy.	Drug therapy may cure or slow the progression of the STD and relieve symptoms.
Provide client with a telephone number for obtaining objective and authoritative information.	Clients may be more inclined to ask questions about an STD and its treatment if their identity can remain anonymous.
Schedule an appointment for follow-up care.	Medical follow-up promotes compliance with therapeutic regimen.

Evaluation of Expected Outcomes: Client paraphrases the plan for treatment and carries out prescribed interventions.

NURSING GUIDELINES 62-3

Educating the Client With an STD

- Take prescribed medication according to label directions for the full length of time that it is prescribed.

- Stop having sex until retesting indicates that the infection is gone.

- Urge any and all sex partners to be examined and follow-through with concurrent treatment.

- Use a condom, a contraceptive barrier device, consistently and correctly (Nursing Guidelines 62-4) before any and all sexual contact after completing medical treatment.

- Do not assume that successful treatment means there is any permanent immunity; reinfection can and does occur if preventive sexual practices are not implemented.

- Seek treatment as soon as possible if the symptoms continue or if they recur after successful treatment.

inoculated on a culture medium and incubated to reveal the causative organism.

Medical Management

Because of the increasing resistance of *N. gonorrhoeae* to penicillin, gonorrhea is now treated with a single intra-muscular dose of ceftriaxone (Rocephin) or a single oral dose of ciprofloxacin (Cipro). Coinfection with chlamydia is common and clients also are given oral doxycycline (Vibramycin) for 7 to 10 days. Clients with complicated gonococcal infections, as in PID or disseminated infection, are hospitalized and treated with IV multiple-drug therapy. Repeat therapy with different antibiotics may be required.

Nursing Management

The nursing management and client teaching are similar to those provided clients with chlamydia. However, when a culture is collected from a woman, the vaginal speculum is moistened with water rather than lubricated, which may destroy the gonococci and cause inaccurate test results (see Nursing Care Plan 62-1).

● SYPHILIS

Syphilis is a curable STD that also can be transmitted from the blood of an infected person, directly from the lesion, or across the placenta to an unborn infant. The incidence of syphilis in the United States has risen in certain groups, particularly young African-American men and women. The disease has been declining in the

NURSING GUIDELINES 62-4

Teaching Clients How to Use a Condom

- Purchase condoms that are made in the United States because they are of high quality and have been tested for reliability.

- Select condoms that are lubricated with a spermicide or silicone.

- Natural-membrane condoms are porous and although they act as a barrier to sperm, viruses may pass through.

- Keep condoms in a cool, dry place.

- Discard condoms beyond their expiration date or if they are more than 5 years old.

- Never unroll or examine a condom before its use or use one that appears to have deteriorated.

- Unroll the condom over the erect penis while pinching the space at the condom tip.

- Use additional water-based lubricant to reduce friction and prevent tearing the condom; avoid oil-based lubricants, which can weaken latex.

- Remove the condom from the vagina before the penis becomes limp.

- Dispose of the condom in a lined container.

- Apply a new condom for each sex act.

- Breakage and slipping rates may be higher during anal sex.

- Condom breakage rate can be reduced by using a silicone-based lubricant; silicone does not deteriorate latex.

(Adapted from American Social Health Association. [2001]. Condoms—do's and don'ts. [On-line.] Available: http://www.ashastd.org/stdfaqs/condom_dd.html.)

United States since 1995, however, with a record low number in 1998 (Centers for Disease Control and Prevention, 1999).

Pathophysiology and Etiology

The spirochete *Treponema pallidum* is the causative microorganism of syphilis. The time between infection and the first occurrence of symptoms is about 21 days. If untreated, syphilis progresses through three distinct stages: primary, secondary, and tertiary. Syphilis is infectious only during the primary and secondary stages. In the third stage, the client becomes demented and dies from complications involving other organ systems.

Assessment Findings

Signs and Symptoms

In the primary (early) stage, a **chancre** (painless ulcer) appears on the genitals, anus, cervix, or other parts of the body (Fig. 62-1). At first, the lesion resembles a small papule, which later ulcerates. The chancre heals in several weeks and, if treatment has not been initiated, the client progresses to the secondary stage of syphilis.

Symptoms of secondary syphilis include fever, malaise, rash, headache, sore throat, and lymph node enlargement. Late, or tertiary, syphilis is noninfectious because the microorganism has invaded the central nervous system (CNS) as well as other organs of the body. Symptoms of tertiary syphilis include **tabes dorsalis** (a degenerative condition of the CNS that results in loss of peripheral reflexes and of vibratory and position senses), ataxia, and **neuropathic joint disease,** also called **Charcot's joints.** Cardiovascular complications include aortic aneurysm and aortic valve insufficiency.

Diagnostic Findings

Diagnosis is made by detecting the spirochete in microscopic examination of scrapings from the chancre, by a positive Venereal Disease Research Laboratory (VDRL) test or rapid plasma reagin (RPR) on blood serum, and a positive fluorescent treponemal antibody absorption test (FTA-ABS). Occasionally, the FTA-ABS test is falsely positive in clients with systemic lupus erythematosus, a connective tissue disease, and rheumatoid arthritis. When a person develops CNS symptoms, the cerebrospinal fluid is examined.

Medical Management

Penicillin is used to treat primary and secondary syphilis. Clients who are allergic to the penicillins are given tetracycline or doxycycline. Follow-up examinations and laboratory tests are recommended 3, 6, and 12 months after initial treatment. Those with tertiary syphilis require larger doses of penicillin. The response is poor in those with cardiovascular syphilis.

Nursing Management

The nurse gathers health information and a sexual history, asks about the client's allergy history in anticipation of antibiotic treatment, prepares the client for diagnostic laboratory tests, supports the client emotionally at the time the diagnosis is confirmed, and informs the client that case-finding is reported to the department of public health. (See Nursing Care Plan 62-1 for more on nursing management.)

● HERPES INFECTION

Herpes infection is a highly contagious STD that is controllable but not curable. It increases the risk for cervical cancer and infection with human immunodeficiency virus (HIV).

Pathophysiology and Etiology

Although **herpes simplex virus** type 2 (HSV-2), also known as **genital herpes,** is primarily responsible for genital and perineal lesions, herpes simplex virus type 1 (HSV-1), associated with cold sores around the nose and lips, also can cause anogenital lesions. One in five people older than 12 years of age are infected with the virus that causes genital herpes (Sexually Transmitted Disease Information Center, 2000). Transmission of these viruses is either by direct contact with oral or genital secretions from a person during an active stage of the disease, sexual contact during periods of asymptomatic viral shedding, or autoinoculation. Either virus may be

FIGURE 62-1 Syphilitic chancres. (**A**) Penile chancre. (**B**) Vulvar chancre.

introduced into the eye, the mouth, the genital area, or a skin site.

Genital herpes increases the risk for cervical cancer and HIV infection. Transmission also can occur from mother to infant during a vaginal birth and carries a neonatal mortality rate of 50%.

Herpes recurs because after the initial infection, the virus remains dormant in the ganglia of the nerves that supply the area. Symptoms usually are more severe with the initial outbreak. Subsequent episodes usually are shorter and less intense. When the virus is active, shedding viral particles are infectious.

Most victims have at least 1 outbreak per year, and many clients report 5 to 10 outbreaks per year. Some clients note that stress, emotional situations, exposure to sunlight, menstruation, and fever reactivate the disease.

Assessment Findings

After a short incubation period, HSV-2 causes single or multiple vesicles on the penis, prepuce, buttocks, thighs, introitus, or cervix (Fig. 62-2). The HSV-2 lesions burn and itch before becoming fluid-filled blisters. The vesicles rupture in 1 to 3 days and are followed by painful, reddened ulcers that scab over and eventually disappear. The outbreak may be accompanied by swelling of the inguinal lymph nodes, flulike symptoms, and headache. The initial attack lasts 3 to 4 weeks; subsequent attacks usually last 10 days.

Diagnosis of HSV-1 and HSV-2 infection is tentatively made by inspecting the lesions. Smears and scrapings from the lesions are examined microscopically using special stains to confirm the clinical impression.

Medical Management

Because an outbreak of HSV-1 infection often is self-limiting, treatment may be unnecessary. If treated, either type of herpes responds to the antiviral drugs acyclovir

(Zovirax) and valacyclovir (Valtrex) (Drug Therapy Table 62-1). IV acyclovir is used if there is a severe episode of HSV-2 or if the client is immunocompromised. Acyclovir and valacyclovir shorten subsequent active episodes and tend to reduce the frequency of outbreaks. Cesarean delivery is performed on pregnant women with active lesions.

Nursing Management

The nurse collects appropriate health and sexual data, uses Standard Precautions when inspecting lesions, obtains specimens, and provides related health teaching. More on nursing management appears in Nursing Care Plan 62-1.

The nurse instructs clients with HSV-2 infections to:

- Inform all potential sexual partners of the HSV infection, even if it is in an inactive state.
- Use a condom during sexual activity even if the disease is dormant.
- Avoid sexual contact if there is any question that the infection is active; condoms do not protect skin and mucous membrane that is left exposed.
- Keep lesions dry using alcohol, peroxide, witch hazel, and warm air from a hair dryer.
- Check with the physician about taking warm baths with Epsom salts or baking soda to relieve discomfort.
- Wear loose clothing that promotes air circulation about the genitals.
- Perform thorough handwashing after direct contact with lesions, and keep any personal hygiene articles, like a towel, separate to avoid inadvertent use by others.
- Use a separate towel to pat lesions dry and another when drying other body parts to avoid autoinoculation.
- Have annual Papanicolaou smears to detect cervical cancer.
- Investigate stress management strategies because reducing stress tends to decrease the frequency of outbreaks.

● VENEREAL WARTS

Venereal (genital) **warts,** also called **condylomas,** are an STD that tends to recur even after treatment. Anyone can become infected with venereal warts, but people with AIDS as well as others with an immunodeficiency are particularly susceptible. One-fourth of the people in the United States carry the virus and are infectious, but do not manifest symptoms.

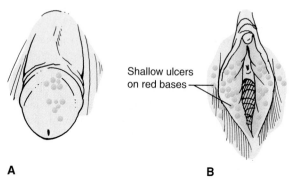

Shallow ulcers on red bases

A   **B**

FIGURE 62-2 Herpes genitalis lesions. (**A**) Penile lesions. (**B**) Vulvar lesions.

DRUG THERAPY TABLE 62-1	AGENTS TO TREAT STDs

DRUG CATEGORY AND EXAMPLES/USE	SIDE EFFECTS	NURSING CONSIDERATIONS
Antibiotics		
	Allergy, anaphylaxis (applies to all antibiotics listed below)	Inquire about allergies and past reactions to medications. Be aware that clients allergic to cephalosporins also may be allergic to penicillin antibiotics. Inform client to seek treatment if rash, hives, fever, or difficulty breathing occur.
penicillin G: syphilis, gonorrhea	Allergy, stomatitis, nausea, vomiting, diarrhea, rash, fever, wheezing, pain at injection site	Give intramuscularly into gluteus maximus only. Massage site. Have client wait for 30 min after injection in case allergic reaction occurs.
erythromycin: syphilis, gonorrhea, chlamydia, chancroid, lymphogranuloma venereum, prophylactically to prevent eye infection in newborns	Allergy, abdominal cramps, diarrhea, vomiting, rash, emotional lability, altered thinking, ototoxicity, hepatitis	Reassure client that emotional and cognitive side effects, should they occur, are temporary. Report tinnitus and jaundice.
doxycycline: syphilis, gonorrhea, granuloma inguinale, lymphogranuloma venereum	Allergy, anorexia, nausea, vomiting, diarrhea, sensitivity to light, liver failure, discoloration of developing teeth, liver damage	Suggest taking with meals if gastrointestinal upset occurs. Inform client to report dark-colored urine or light-colored stools. Use a sunscreen. Strongly encourage client to return for all follow-up visits to ensure that organism has been eradicated.
ceftriaxone: gonorrhea	Allergy, anorexia, nausea, vomiting, diarrhea, rash, fever, decreased hematocrit, disulfiram-like reaction with alcohol	Avoid alcohol during and for 3 days after drug therapy. Inform client of possible side effects and to report unusual fatigue.
tetracycline: syphilis, gonorrhea, chlamydia	Allergy, nausea, vomiting, diarrhea, discoloration of developing teeth, phototoxicity, superinfections	Take on an empty stomach. Avoid antacids, dairy products, and iron supplements. Do not use outdated drugs because they are nephrotoxic. Use a sunscreen. Report appearance of oral or vaginal yeast infections.
ciprofloxacin: gonorrhea	Headache, dizziness, nausea, diarrhea, vomiting	Take on an empty stomach and avoid antacids within 2 hr of antibiotic dose. Drink plenty of water. Report any side effects.
Antivirals		
acyclovir: decreases severity and frequency of herpes outbreaks	Transient burning at application site	Apply with a rubber glove or finger cot. Inform client that drug does not cure the disease. Clients should avoid sexual activity during outbreaks and wear a condom at other times.
Caustics		
podophyllum resin: venereal warts	Peripheral neuropathy, thrombocytopenia and leukopenia when absorbed systemically, irritation of normal tissue	Highly toxic and should be applied only by the physician. Surrounding skin may be protected with petroleum jelly. Use minimal amount possible. Warn client that local irritation may occur in 12–48 hr.

Strongly encourage all clients to return for all follow-up visits to ensure that organism has been eradicated.

Pathophysiology and Etiology

The **human papillomavirus** (HPV) causes venereal warts. HPV is transmitted by genital–genital, genital–anal, or genital–oral contact with an infected person and is contagious as long as the warts are present. Sexual penetration is not necessary to transmit HPV, and the warts also can be spread to other body areas by autoinoculation. The virus is contagious as long as the warts are present. Warts can grow in the mouth and throat of infants infected at birth. There is an increased risk of cancer of the vulva, vagina, and cervix in women with genital warts. Cervical infection with HPV is associated with more than 80% of cases of invasive cervical cancer (National Institute of Allergy and Infectious Diseases, 1998).

Assessment Findings

Genital warts usually are painless and appear as a single lesion or cluster of soft, fleshy growths on the genitalia (Fig. 62-3) or cervix, in the vagina, or on the perineum, anus, throat, or mouth. Sometimes the warts are so small that they are inconspicuous; however, they can become large and raised—resembling a cauliflower. Large venereal warts may narrow or obstruct the urethra, vagina, anus, or throat.

Venereal warts turn white when vinegar is applied to the lesion. The highlighted tissue is then examined with a magnifying glass.

Medical and Surgical Management

Warts are removed in various ways: laser therapy, electrocautery (heat), cryosurgery (freezing), or treating them with chemicals. Three major drugs are used to eradicate the warts: trichloroacetic acid, podophyllum solution in tincture of benzoin, and 5-fluorouracil (5-FU). Eradication does not mean the condition is cured; the person is temporarily noncontagious once the warts are destroyed.

Nursing Management

Nurses provide information about STD transmission to sexually active people and prepare affected individuals for medical examination, diagnosis, and treatment. Nursing management is discussed further in Nursing Care Plan 62-1.

The nurse tells clients with venereal warts to:

- Avoid intimate contact until the warts are removed.
- Advise all sexual contacts to be examined and treated.
- Seek treatment at an STD clinic or with a private physician when, and if, the warts return.
- Use a condom even when the lesions are absent, and suggest that the sex partner wash his or her genitals or other skin areas immediately after intimate contact.
- Provide information about the diagnosis and treatment in future health histories, especially if a pregnancy occurs.
- Avoid stress and genital trauma, which appear to be factors in reactivating the virus (Porth, 2002).
- Obtain yearly examinations for the possibility of reproductive cancers.

Stop, Think, and Respond ● BOX 62-1

Which STD is associated with the following signs?

1. *Painless ulceration on the genitals or other areas of sexual contact*
2. *Discharge from the vagina, urethra, or both; burning on urination; and abdominal pain in women*
3. *Cluster of soft, fleshy growths about the genitals or other places of sexual contact*
4. *Burning and itching about the genitals before an outbreak of multiple vesicles that become painful after rupture*

OTHER SEXUALLY TRANSMITTED DISEASES ●

● GRANULOMA INGUINALE

Granuloma inguinale, or donovanosis, is caused by *Calymmatobacterium granulomatis* and is relatively uncommon in the United States. The infection is characterized by lesions in the genital, inguinal, and anal areas;

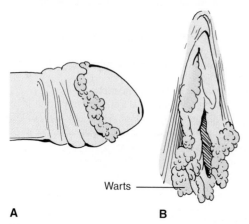

FIGURE 62-3 Venereal warts. (**A**) Penile warts. (**B**) Vulvar warts.

A   B

Warts

it is treated with antimicrobials, usually tetracycline or sulfisoxazole (Gantrisin).

● CHANCROID

Chancroid is caused by the *Haemophilus ducreyi* bacillus. The infection is characterized by the appearance of a macule, followed by vesicle–pustule formation, and, finally, a painful ulcer. It is treated and cured with erythromycin or tetracycline.

● LYMPHOGRANULOMA VENEREUM

Lymphogranuloma venereum, caused by a strain of *C. trachomatis,* is characterized by a small erosion or papule and enlargement of adjacent lymph nodes. The affected lymph nodes can become necrotic. The usual site of infection is the genital area. The infection is treated with tetracycline.

GENERAL PHARMACOLOGIC CONSIDERATIONS

Obtain an allergy history before administration of any antimicrobial agent. Inform the physician of an allergy to any antimicrobial agent, so that he or she can order a different drug.

Explain the prescribed drug regimen to the client. Information includes the number of capsules or tablets per dose, the time of day to take the drug, food restrictions (if any), and possible adverse effects. Emphasize the importance of completing a course of therapy.

Both doxycycline and azithromycin are contraindicated during pregnancy.

Monitor clients receiving penicillin for at least 30 minutes after a parenteral injection to watch for a possible allergic reaction. Symptoms of an allergic reaction include pruritus, difficulty breathing, hypotension, sweating, and tachycardia.

Observe the client closely for an allergic reaction, which can occur at any time during antibiotic administration. If an allergic reaction occurs, contact the primary healthcare provider immediately.

GENERAL GERONTOLOGIC CONSIDERATIONS

Nurses must abandon biases that older adults are sexually inactive. Therefore, when taking a health history, nurses must include questions about sexuality and behaviors that put them at risk for STDs.

Older clients who are sexually active have the same risks of acquiring an STD as other age groups.

Some older clients have limited knowledge about STDs and therefore may not recognize the symptoms or seek treatment.

Older adults who are not in monogamous relationships may not understand that barrier and chemical contraceptives are appropriate for preventing STDs.

Syphilis causes approximately 10% of cases of heart disease in those older than 50 years of age. The most frequently seen valvular disorder as the result of syphilis is aortic insufficiency. Damaged valves may need to be replaced with a ball-valve prosthesis.

Some older adults with an STD are embarrassed and may not seek medical attention. Careful assessment is necessary to help the older adult obtain medical treatment as quickly as possible.

Critical Thinking Exercises

1. *Discuss STD information that is appropriate to provide for a person who confides that he or she is having unprotected sexual intercourse with more than one person.*
2. *Explain information a person who has never used a condom should know.*

References and Suggested Readings

American Social Health Association. (2001). Facts & answers about STDs. [On-line.] Available: http://www.ashastd.org/stdfaqs/syphilis.html.

Bielan, B. (2001). Clinical snapshot: Herpes simplex. *Dermatology Nursing, 13,* 372.

Centers for Disease Control and Prevention. (1999). Syphilis continues to retreat: Nation sets sights on elimination. [On-line.] Available: www.cdc.gov/nchstp/od/nchstp/html.

Centers for Disease Control and Prevention. (2001). Tracking the hidden epidemics: Trends in STDs in the United States 2000. [On-line.] Available: http://www.cdc.gov/std.

Chapin, K. (1999). Probing the STDS. *American Journal of Nursing, 99*(7), Advanced Practice Nursing Extra: 24AAA–24BBB, 24DDD.

Chard, S. (1998). Diagnosing and treating genital herpes. *Nursing Times, 94*(46), 58–62.

Coombes, R. (2000). Return of the dirty dozen . . . sexually transmitted infections. *Nursing Times, 96*(36), 12–13.

Davis, A. (1998). Chlamydia: The most common sexually transmitted infection. *Nursing Times, 94*(5), 56–58.

Edwards, M. (1999) Your role in the management of chlamydia. *Practice Nurse, 18,* 293–294, 297.

Gleave, T. (2000). Keeping an eye on chlamydia. *Nursing Times, 96*(27), 51.

Hinds, P. (2000). Improving screening practices in the fight against chlamydia. *Community Nurse, 6*(8), 31–32.

Kobayashi, A., Miaskowski, C., Wallhagen, M., et al. (2000). Recent developments in understanding the immune response to human papilloma virus infection and cervical neoplasia. *Oncology Nursing Forum, 27,* 643–653.

National Institute of Allergy and Infectious Diseases. (1998). Fact sheet: STD statistics. [On-line.] Available: http://www.naid.nih.gov/factsheets/stdstats.htm.

Norton, N. J. (1998). Combatting infection: Coping with HPV . . . human papilloma virus. *Nursing, 28*(9), 73–74.

Parini, S. M. (1998). Combatting infection: Understanding sexually transmitted diseases, Part II. *Nursing, 28*(4), 26, 28.

Porth. C. M. (2002). *Pathophysiology: Concepts of altered health states* (6th ed.). Philadelphia: Lippincott Williams & Wilkins.

Resnick, S. D. (2001). Skin signs of sexually transmitted diseases in adolescents. *Adolescent Medicine: State of the Art Reviews, 12,* 285–303.

Scipio-Bannerman, J. (1998). Chlamydia infections on the rise. *Nursing Spectrum (Washington, DC, Baltimore Metro Edition), 8*(23), 20.

Sexually Transmitted Disease Information Center. (2000). Sexually transmitted disease statistics. Journal of the American Medical Association (JAMA) Women's Health STD Information Center. [On-line.] Available: http://www.ama-assn.org/special/std/support/stdstat.htm.

Sheff, B. (2001). Microbe of the month: *Chlamydia trachomatis. Nursing, 31*(1), 71.

Sheff, B. (2000). Microbe of the month: *Neisseria gonorrhoeae. Nursing, 30*(7), 76.

Swanson, J. M. (1999). The biopsychosocial burden of genital herpes: Evidence-based and other approaches to care. *Dermatology Nursing, 11,* 257–260.

Thomas, D. J. (2001). Sexually transmitted viral infections: Epidemiology and treatment. *Journal of Obstetric, Gynecologic, and Neonatal Nursing, 30,* 316–323.

Weston, A. (1998). Striking back at syphilis. *Nursing Times, 94*(3), 30–32.

Weston, A. (1998). Warts and all. *Nursing Times, 94*(3), 26–28.

Wright, S. (1999). Sexually transmitted diseases. *Nursing Standard, 13*(46), 37–43.

chapter

63

Introduction to the Urinary Tract

Words to Know

blood urea nitrogen
costovertebral angle
creatinine
creatinine clearance test
cystogram
cystometrogram
cystoscope
cystoscopy
excretory urogram
intravenous pyelogram
postvoid residual

renal arteriogram
retrograde pyelogram
ultrasonography
urinalysis
urine protein test
urine specific gravity
urodynamic studies
uroflowmetry
urography
voiding
    cystourethrogram

Learning Objectives

On completion of this chapter, the reader will:

● Name the parts of the urinary system.
● Define the primary functions of the kidney and other structures in the urinary system.
● List tests performed for the diagnosis of urologic and renal system diseases.
● Identify laboratory tests performed to diagnose urologic and renal system diseases.
● Discuss nursing management for a client undergoing diagnostic evaluation of the urinary tract.

The urinary system consists of the kidneys, renal pelves (sing. *pelvis*), ureters, urinary bladder, and urethra. The kidneys have many functions (Box 63-1), including excreting excess water and nitrogenous waste products of protein metabolism; assisting in maintenance of acid-base and electrolyte balance; producing the enzyme *renin,* which helps regulate blood pressure; and producing the hormone *erythropoietin,* which stimulates red blood cell production. The remainder of the urinary system is involved in the transport (ureters and pelves), storage (bladder), and excretion (urethra) of urine.

Urologic nursing assessment focuses on changes in urine production, transport, storage, and elimination. Other responsibilities of urologic nurses involve caring for clients with conditions that affect the reproductive systems, discussed in Chapters 59 and 61.

ANATOMY AND PHYSIOLOGY

The upper urinary tract is composed of the kidneys, renal pelves, and ureters. The lower urinary tract consists of the bladder, urethra, and pelvic floor muscles (Fig. 63-1). The two kidneys are paired, bean-shaped organs located

in the upper abdomen on either side of the vertebral column. They span from the level of the 12th thoracic vertebra to the 3rd lumbar vertebra. A thin, fibrous capsule encloses each kidney; the peritoneum separates the kidney from the abdominal cavity anteriorly. The blood supply to each kidney consists of a renal artery and renal vein. The renal artery arises from the aorta and the renal vein empties into the vena cava. The kidneys receive 25% of the total cardiac output.

A cross-section of the kidney (Fig. 63-2) helps to illustrate the inner structures. The two main areas are the renal pelves and the parenchyma. The *parenchyma* is made up of a cortex (outer layer) and a medulla (inner core). Within each cortex are microscopic nephrons that carry out the functions of the kidneys. Each kidney contains about 1 million *nephrons,* which are the smallest functioning units of the kidney. Each nephron consists of the *glomerulus, afferent arteriole, efferent arteriole, Bowman's capsule, distal* and *proximal convoluted tubules,* the *loop of Henle,* and the *collecting tubule* (Fig. 63-3). The medulla contains calyces (pyramids), cone-shaped structures that open to the pelvis, a large funnel-like structure in the center of the kidney. The renal pelvis then empties into the ureter, which carries urine to the bladder for storage.

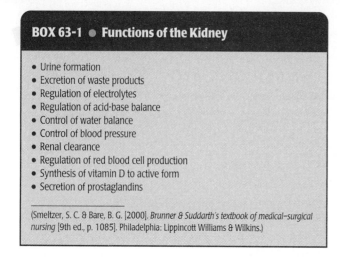

BOX 63-1 ● Functions of the Kidney

- Urine formation
- Excretion of waste products
- Regulation of electrolytes
- Regulation of acid-base balance
- Control of water balance
- Control of blood pressure
- Renal clearance
- Regulation of red blood cell production
- Synthesis of vitamin D to active form
- Secretion of prostaglandins

(Smeltzer, S. C. & Bare, B. G. [2000]. *Brunner & Suddarth's textbook of medical–surgical nursing* [9th ed., p. 1085]. Philadelphia: Lippincott Williams & Wilkins.)

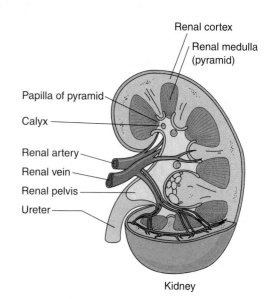

Kidney

FIGURE 63-2 Internal structure of the kidney. (Adapted from Willis, M. C. [1996]. *Medical terminology: The language of healthcare.* Baltimore: Williams & Wilkins.)

The bladder, urethra, and pelvic floor muscles form the urethrovesical unit. The urinary bladder, located just behind the pubis, is a hollow, muscular organ. Its shape and size vary with the amount of urine it contains as well as the person's age. In general, adult bladders hold 300 to 500 mL of urine. The urethra is a hollow tube that begins at the bladder neck and ends at the external meatus. It serves as a conduit during urination and has a sphincter mechanism to prevent urine leakage. The male urethra extends approximately 24 cm (10 inches) from the bladder neck through the prostate and the penile shaft to the glans penis. The female urethra extends about 4 cm (1.5 to 2 inches) from the bladder neck to the external meatus, anterior to the vagina. The pelvic floor muscles constitute the final part of the urethrovesical unit. These muscles form a sling that supports the bladder and urethra, rectum, and some reproductive organs.

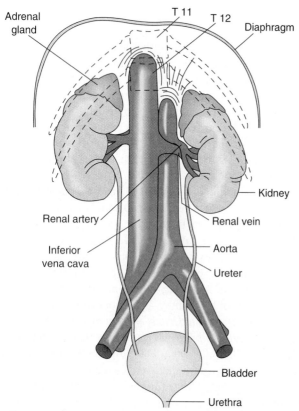

FIGURE 63-1 Kidneys, ureters, and bladder. The right kidney is usually lower than the left.

FIGURE 63-3 Representation of a nephron.

There are three steps in the complex process of urine formation:

- *Glomerular filtration*—involves the filtration of plasma by the glomerulus (see Fig. 63-3). Filtered substances include water, sodium, chloride, bicarbonate, potassium, glucose, urea, creatinine, and uric acid.
- *Tubular reabsorption*—the filtrate enters Bowman's capsule and then moves through the tubular system of the nephron and is either reabsorbed (placed back into the systemic circulation) or excreted as urine.
- *Tubular secretion*—the formed urine drains from the collecting tubules, into the renal pelves, and down each ureter to the bladder.

The filtrate that is secreted as urine usually contains water, sodium, chloride, bicarbonate, potassium, urea, creatinine, and uric acid. Amino acids and glucose typically are reabsorbed and not excreted in the urine. Protein molecules, except for periodic small amounts of globulins and albumin, also are reabsorbed. Transient proteinuria in small amounts (<150 mg/dL) is not considered a problem. Persistent and elevated proteinuria may indicate glomerular damage. Glycosuria (glucose in the urine) occurs when the glucose concentration in the blood and glomerular filtrate exceeds the ability of the tubules to reabsorb the glucose (Porth, 2002; Smeltzer & Bare, 2000).

Urine flows from the renal pelvis through the ureter into the bladder. Peristaltic waves help to move the urine to the bladder. Normally, urine flows in one direction because of this peristaltic action and because the ureters enter the bladder at an oblique angle (Bullock & Henze, 2000). Reflux of urine (urine that flows backward) can occur secondary to an overdistended bladder or other problems, and may cause infections (see Chapter 65).

The desire to urinate comes from the feeling of bladder fullness. A nerve reflex is triggered when approximately 150 mL of urine accumulates. During urination, the bladder muscle contracts and the sphincter muscles relax, forcing urine out of the bladder and urethra through the urethral meatus. If there is any interference or abnormality of these muscles, the bladder may not empty completely or empty uncontrollably (incontinence).

Stop, Think, and Respond • BOX 63-1

What factors influence the amount of urine produced?

ASSESSMENT

History

The nurse obtains information about general health, childhood and family illnesses, past medical history, allergies, sexual and reproductive health, exposure to toxic

chemicals or gas, and history of present complaint (Box 63-2). Box 63-3 describes risk factors for renal or urologic disorders. In addition to the client's chief complaint and medical history, a medication history is important. Older clients in particular may be taking multiple medications, which may affect renal function. The nurse also obtains information about voiding patterns, which may indicate renal or urologic problems (Table 63-1).

Physical Examination

Before beginning the physical examination, the nurse asks the client to void. Inspection includes observing the abdomen for scars, symmetry, abdominal movements, and pulsations. Examining the back and noting any bulging, bruising, or scars are important steps. The experienced examiner auscultates the abdomen for bruits (abnormal vascular sounds heard over a blood vessel). In addition, he or she percusses the area over the bladder beginning 2 inches above the symphysis pubis and moving toward the base of the bladder (Fig. 63-4). Percussion usually produces a tympanic sound; it produces a dull sound if the bladder is filled. The nurse can palpate the suprapubic area but can palpate the bladder only if it is moderately distended. Assessing the kidneys for tenderness or pain is done by lightly striking the fist at the **costovertebral angle** (CVA), which is the area where the lower ribs meet the vertebrae (Fig. 63-5). Normally, the client experiences a dull thud. Pain or tenderness may indicate a renal disorder. The nurse also assesses for signs of electrolyte and water imbalance (see Chap. 22).

In addition to evaluating the client's general health, the nurse evaluates the client for signs or symptoms of:

- Periorbital edema (swelling around the eyes)
- Edema of the extremities
- Cardiac failure
- Mental changes

BOX 63-2 • Assessing the Chief Complaint

- Voiding changes or disturbances
- Urine volume changes
- Irritative voiding symptoms (frequency, urgency, nocturia, dysuria)
- Obstructive voiding symptoms (hesitancy, straining, residual urine, retention, urinary stream force and size)
- Urinary incontinence (total overflow, stress, urge, functional)
- Urine characteristics changes (color, hematuria, clarity, odor, pH)
- Systemic manifestations (fever, weight loss)
- Gastrointestinal signs and symptoms (nausea, vomiting, diarrhea, abdominal cramping, distention)
- Pain (type, location, severity, local, referred, colic, spasms)
- Masses of the flank, abdomen, or genital areas (polycystic kidneys, hydronephrosis, renal cell carcinoma)
- Abnormal abdominal or genital appearance
- Sexual or reproductive dysfunction

BOX 63-3 ● Risk Factors for Various Renal or Urologic Disorders

Risk Factor	Possible Renal or Urologic Disorder
Childhood diseases: "strep throat," impetigo, nephrotic syndrome	Chronic renal failure
Advanced age	Incomplete emptying of bladder, leading to urinary tract infection
Instrumentation of urinary tract, cystoscopy, catheterization	Urinary tract infection, incontinence
Immobilization	Kidney stone formation
Occupational, recreational, or environmental exposure to chemicals (plastics, pitch, tar, rubber)	Acute renal failure
Diabetes mellitus	Chronic renal failure, neurogenic bladder
Hypertension	Renal insufficiency, chronic renal failure
Systemic lupus erythematosus	Nephritis, chronic renal failure
Gout, hyperparathyroidism, Crohn's disease	Kidney stone formation
Sickle cell anemia, multiple myeloma	Chronic renal failure
Benign prostatic hypertrophy	Obstruction to urine flow, leading to frequency, oliguria, anuria
Radiation therapy to pelvis	Cystitis, fibrosis of ureter, or fistula in urinary tract
Recent pelvic surgery	Inadvertent trauma to ureters or bladder
Obstetric injury, tumors	Incontinence
Spinal cord injury	Neurogenic bladder, urinary tract infection, incontinence

All of these signs or symptoms may indicate urinary tract disorders. The nurse also obtains vital signs and weight.

Diagnostic Tests

In the male client, diseases and disorders of the reproductive system also affect the urinary system. In addition to the diagnostic tests discussed in the following sections, tests that may be performed on the male client are discussed in Chapters 61 and 62.

Radiography

An x-ray study of the abdomen includes x-rays of the kidneys, ureters, and bladder (KUB). It is performed to show the size and position of the kidneys, ureters, and bony pelvis as well as any radiopaque urinary calculi (stones), abnormal gas patterns (indicative of renal mass), and anatomic defects of the bony spinal column (indicative of neuropathic bladder dysfunction). An x-ray of the pelvis, chest, or other area may reveal metastatic bone lesions that could be a result of renal or bladder tumors.

Ultrasonography

Renal **ultrasonography** identifies the kidney's shape, size, location, collecting systems, and adjacent tissues. Other uses include identification of renal cysts or obstruction sites, assistance in needle placement for renal biopsy or nephrostomy tube placement, and drainage of a renal abscess. There are no contraindications to this procedure. It is not invasive, does not require the injection of a radiopaque dye, and does not require fasting or bowel preparation for a renal or bladder sonogram.

Computed Tomography Scan and Magnetic Resonance Imaging

A computed tomography (CT) scan or magnetic resonance imaging (MRI) of the abdomen and pelvis may be obtained to diagnose renal pathology, determine kidney size, and evaluate tissue densities with or without contrast material. An iodine-based contrast medium may be injected intravenously (IV) after the initial scan to enhance the images, especially when vascular tumors are suspected. The CT scan also is useful in identifying calculi, congenital abnormalities, obstruction, infections, and polycystic disease. An MRI produces sharp images of the kidneys and can delineate the renal cortex from the medulla. It also is useful in identifying bladder tumors, staging renal cell carcinoma, and imaging the vascular system.

Angiography

A renal angiogram (**renal arteriogram**) provides details of the arterial supply to the kidneys, specifically the location and number of renal arteries (multiple vessels to the kidney are not unusual) and the patency of each renal artery. A catheter is passed up the femoral artery into the aorta to the level of the renal vessels. Contrast medium is then injected into the catheter and serial x-rays are taken. The radiopaque dye first outlines the aorta in the area of the renal artery, then enters the renal artery and the kidney. A series of x-rays is taken. The catheter tip also may be passed into each renal artery for additional images. The procedure lasts 30 to 90 minutes. This procedure is contraindicated if a client is allergic to iodine contrast material.

The nurse must ask the client about allergy to iodine or seafood and any previous dye reactions. He or she reviews pertinent laboratory tests (blood urea nitrogen [BUN], creatinine) to assess renal function, records vital signs, and assesses peripheral pulses. The nurse instructs the client to void before the procedure. If ordered, he or she administers a sedative to promote relaxation before the procedure. After the procedure, the physician applies a pressure dressing to the femoral area, which remains in place for several hours. The nurse palpates the pulses in the legs and feet at least every 1 to 2 hours for signs of arterial occlusion. Monitoring the pressure dressing is im-

TABLE 63-1	PROBLEMS ASSOCIATED WITH CHANGES IN VOIDING	
PROBLEM	**DEFINITION**	**POSSIBLE ETIOLOGY**
Frequency	Frequent voiding—more than every 3 hours	Infection, obstruction of lower urinary tract leading to residual urine and overflow, anxiety, diuretics, benign prostatic hyperplasia, urethral stricture, diabetic neuropathy
Urgency	Strong desire to void	Infection, chronic prostatitis, urethritis, obstruction of lower urinary tract leading to residual urine and overflow, anxiety, diuretics, benign prostatic hyperplasia, urethral stricture, diabetic neuropathy
Dysuria	Painful or difficult voiding	Lower urinary tract infection, inflammation of bladder or urethra, acute prostatitis, stones, foreign bodies, tumors in bladder
Hesitancy	Delay, difficulty in initiating voiding	Benign prostatic hyperplasia, compression of urethra, outlet obstruction, neurogenic bladder
Nocturia	Excessive urination at night	Decreased renal concentrating ability, heart failure, diabetes mellitus, incomplete bladder emptying, excessive fluid intake at bedtime, nephrotic syndrome, cirrhosis with ascites
Incontinence	Involuntary loss of urine	External urinary sphincter injury, obstetric injury, lesions of bladder neck, detrusor dysfunction, infection, neurogenic bladder, medications, neurologic abnormalities
Enuresis	Involuntary voiding during sleep	Delay in functional maturation of central nervous system (bladder control usually achieved by 5 years of age), obstructive disease of lower urinary tract, genetic factors, failure to concentrate urine, urinary tract infection, psychological stress
Polyuria	Increased volume of urine voided	Diabetes mellitus, diabetes insipidus, diuretics, excess fluid intake, lithium toxicity, certain types of kidney disease (hypercalcemic and hypokalemic nephropathy)
Oliguria	Urine output less than 400 mL/day	Acute or chronic renal failure (see Chap. 64), inadequate fluid intake
Anuria	Urine output less than 50 mL/day	Acute or chronic renal failure (see Chap. 64), complete obstruction
Hematuria	Red blood cells in the urine	Cancer of genitourinary tract, acute glomerulonephritis, renal stones, renal tuberculosis, blood dyscrasia, trauma, extreme exercise, rheumatic fever, hemophilia, leukemia, sickle cell trait or disease
Proteinuria	Abnormal amounts of protein in the urine	Acute and chronic renal disease, nephrotic syndrome, vigorous exercise, heat stroke, severe heart failure, diabetic nephropathy, multiple myeloma

FIGURE 63-4 Bladder percussion.

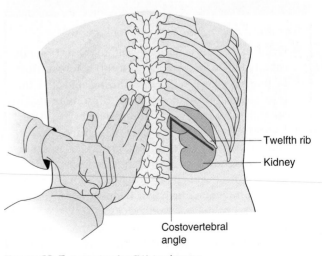

Twelfth rib

Kidney

Costovertebral angle

FIGURE 63-5 Assessing for CVA tenderness.

portant to note frank bleeding or hematoma formation. If either condition occurs, the nurse immediately notifies the physician. Another important assessment is for hypersensitivity responses to contrast material. Clients remain on bed rest for 4 to 8 hours. The nurse also monitors and documents intake and output. See Client and Family Teaching Box 63-1 for education points.

Cystoscopy

Cystoscopy is the visual examination of the inside of the bladder using an instrument called a *cystoscope*. When the urethra is examined, the procedure is called *cystourethroscopy*. The **cystoscope** consists of a lighted tube with a telescopic lens (Fig. 63-6). Cystoscopy is used to identify the cause of painless hematuria, urinary incontinence, or urinary retention. It is useful in the evaluation of structural and functional changes of the bladder. The cystoscope is inserted through the urethra into the bladder. Local anesthesia is usual; however, spinal or general anesthesia also may be used. The procedure lasts 30 to 45 minutes. The size of the cystoscope is graded in the French (F) scale; usually, one that is 20 to 24 F is used in adults. Biopsy samples (tissue examination), cell washings (cytologic analysis), and urine samples may be obtained.

Preoperative sedatives or antispasmodics may be ordered. Cystoscopy can aggravate any abnormality of the urinary tract. A urine culture should be obtained before testing. If a urinary infection was present before the cystoscopy, chills, fever, and possibly septicemia may occur. The nurse observes the client for these and other symptoms and reports findings to the physician. Clients receive antibiotics after a cystoscopy. The nurse records vital signs before and after the procedure. If general anesthesia is used, he or she should monitor vital signs every

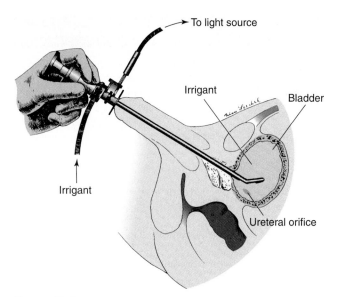

FIGURE 63-6 Cystoscopic examination.

15 to 30 minutes until the client is stable. Significant prostatic obstruction may result in pain and complete urinary retention after a cystoscopy. The nurse administers medications for pain or bladder spasms postprocedure as ordered.

Stop, Think, and Respond ● BOX 63-2

A client having a cystoscopy has the potential for complications. What are these?

Intravenous Pyelogram and Retrograde Pyelogram

An **intravenous pyelogram** (IVP) is a radiologic study used to evaluate the structure and function of the kidneys, ureters, and bladder. It locates the site of any urinary tract obstructions and is helpful in the investigation of the causes of flank pain, hematuria, or renal colic. It is based on the ability of the kidneys to excrete a radiopaque dye (also called a *contrast medium*) in the urine. The IV radiopaque dye outlines the kidney pelves, ureters, and bladder as the blood containing the dye passes through the urinary tract. Synonymous terms for this procedure are **excretory urogram** and IV **urography.** After the IV injection of contrast material, radiographs of the urinary tract are taken after 1 minute (kidney visualization), at 3 to 5 minutes (renal collecting system visualization), at 10 minutes (ureters visualization), and at 20 to 30 minutes (bladder filling visualization). A postvoiding film shows the emptying of the bladder.

Because radiopaque dye usually contains iodine, the physician may inject a minute amount of the radiopaque dye IV and observe the client for 5 to 10 minutes to determine any allergy to iodine. Radiopaque dyes that do not contain iodine, called *nonionic contrast agents,* are available and produce fewer allergic reactions.

63-1 *Client and Family Teaching*
The Client Undergoing Renal Angiography

The nurse reviews the following points:

- Drink extra fluids on the day before the test; do not eat any food or fluids (per protocol) before testing; IV fluids will be given before, during, and after the test; medication will be given to promote relaxation; local anesthesia is administered.

- Expect a burning sensation or feeling of heat, pain, or nausea while contrast material is injected. These reactions are normal and transient.

- Remain on strict bed rest for 4 to 8 hours or more as per protocol. A urinal or bedpan must be used in the meantime.

- Drink extra fluids (2000 to 3000 mL over the 24-hour postprocedure period).

A **retrograde pyelogram** may be performed if better visualization of the complete ureter and renal pelvis is needed. A flexible radiopaque ureteral catheter is inserted in each ureteral orifice (opening at the terminal end of the ureter), which lie on the lower posterior wall of the bladder. This is done during a cystoscopy. Visualization of the ureters and renal pelves is possible after sterile contrast medium is instilled into the renal collecting system. This procedure also is used to evaluate ureteral stent or catheter placement. Retrograde pyelography carries a risk of sepsis and severe urinary tract infection.

An IVP is scheduled before any barium test or gallbladder series that uses contrast material (iodine). If the client already is scheduled for barium studies of the upper or lower gastrointestinal tract, these diagnostic tests probably will be delayed until urologic studies are completed. It may take several days for barium to be removed from the gastrointestinal tract, and its presence can distort IVP findings. Nursing Guidelines 63-1 provide information on the care of the client undergoing a pyelogram.

After the IVP or retrograde pyelogram, the nurse instructs the client to consume an adequate fluid intake. In addition, the client continues to receive IV fluid replacement. The nurse monitors and documents the intake and output, making sure that urine output is at least 30 mL/hour. Clients who are dehydrated are at high risk for renal failure from the toxic effect of the contrast medium on the kidney tissues. The nurse also monitors vital signs. If additional radiographic films are to be taken in the next 24 hours (if the excretory function of the kidney is abnormal), the physician or radiology department provides instructions regarding the food and fluid intake.

The client undergoing a retrograde pyelogram may experience a dull ache caused by distention of the renal pelves with the radiopaque dye. The nurse observes the client for signs and symptoms of pyelonephritis (see Chap. 64) 24 to 48 hours postprocedure because of the instrumentation and injection of material. If there are any symptoms, the nurse reports them to the physician and obtains a urine specimen for culture and analysis. Antibiotic agents are administered as directed.

Biopsy

Biopsies of urinary tract tissue are taken to diagnose cancer, assess prostatic enlargement, diagnose and monitor progression of renal disease, and assess and evaluate treatment of renal transplant rejection. Bladder biopsies are obtained during cystoscopy. Information about prostate biopsy can be found in Chapter 61. Table 63-2 describes renal biopsy techniques. Renal biopsy carries the risk of postprocedure bleeding because the kidneys receive up to 25% of the cardiac output each minute.

The nurse reassures the client undergoing a renal biopsy and explains the procedure and its purpose. In addition, he or she records vital signs and reviews pretest coagulation studies, urinalysis, IVP, and renal scan. After

---

NURSING GUIDELINES 63-1

Care of Client Undergoing Intravenous or Retrograde Pyelogram

- Check the client's allergy history, especially to intravenous contrast dye (iodine) or seafood. Inquire about previous reactions to x-ray studies that used contrast media. Report allergies to the physician or radiology department personnel.

- Instruct the client to fast from food for 8 to 12 hours before the pyelogram. Fluid is permitted.

- Cleanse the bowel so that there is no interference with visualization of the kidneys on the radiographic film. It is important that the bowel preparation is effective because poor cleansing of the intestinal tract may require that the test be repeated. Clients with a peptic ulcer or ulcerative colitis usually require modification of the bowel-cleansing preparation.

- Document baseline vital signs.

- Explain the procedure and its purpose. Tell clients that a series of x-rays will be taken after injection or instillation of IV contrast material and that the entire test requires 1 to 1½ hours to complete.

- Caution clients that they may experience burning, hot flushing sensations, unpleasant (metallic) taste in the mouth, or nausea or vomiting as the contrast is given. Half the clients experience nausea or vomiting. Reassure clients that these reactions are transient.

- Encourage adequate fluid intake postprocedure and voiding within 8 hours postprocedure. A burning sensation on voiding and small amounts of blood-tinged urine are normal and should disappear after the third voiding.

- Advise the use of warm tub baths to decrease urethral discomfort or spasms after a retrograde pyelogram. These reactions should disappear within 24 hours.

- Instruct the client to abstain from alcohol 48 hours postprocedure to avoid irritating the bladder.

- Discuss taking antibiotics for 1 to 3 days postprocedure. Teach the client to report flank pain, chills, fever, dysuria, or bleeding. Advise client to notify physician should symptoms present.

---

the procedure, the client remains on bed rest. The nurse observes the urine for signs of hematuria. It is important to assess the dressing frequently for signs of bleeding, monitor vital signs, and evaluate the type and severity of pain. Severe pain in the back, shoulder, or abdomen can indicate bleeding. The nurse notifies the physician of these signs and symptoms immediately. He or she also assesses the client for difficulty voiding. The nurse needs to encourage the client to have adequate fluid intake after the biopsy. If the client is to be discharged the following day, the nurse instructs him or her to:

- Maintain limited activity for several days to avoid bleeding.
- Complete prophylactic antibiotic therapy as indicated.

TABLE 63-2	TECHNIQUES FOR RENAL BIOPSY
TYPE OF BIOPSY	**DESCRIPTION**
Needle biopsy	• Minimally invasive • Renal tissue is removed through a needle • Useful when CT or MRI findings are inconclusive
Fine-needle aspiration biopsy	• Minimally invasive • Performed under local anesthesia in the operating room • Needle placement guided by fluoroscopy
Open biopsy	• Small incision made into flank • Usually performed if needle biopsy tissue samples are not satisfactory

• Report signs of systemic infection (fever, malaise), urinary tract infection (dysuria, frequency, discolored urine, malodorous urine), or bleeding (hematuria, lightheadedness, flank pain, or rapid pulse). Advise the client to notify the physician immediately should symptoms occur.

Cystogram and Voiding Cystourethrogram

A **cystogram** evaluates abnormalities in bladder structure and filling through the instillation of contrast dye and radiography. A **voiding cystourethrogram** (VCUG) is similar to a cystogram except the client is instructed to void (the urine contains the radiopaque dye), and a rapid series of x-rays are taken. Urinary tract infection is a contraindication to a cystogram or VCUG.

Urodynamic Studies

Urodynamic studies evaluate bladder and urethral function and are performed to assess causes of reduced urine flow, urinary retention, and urinary incontinence. Two of the main tests are uroflowmetry and cystometrogram.

    Uroflowmetry (determination of the urinary flow rate) is performed to evaluate bladder and sphincter function. This noninvasive procedure measures the time and rate of voiding, the volume of urine voided, and the pattern of urination. The results are compared with normal flow rates and urinary patterns. Results vary by age

and sex. See Table 63-3 for normal uroflowmetry values. The client usually is catheterized afterward for the postvoid residual. A **postvoid residual** is the amount of urine left in the bladder after voiding and provides information about bladder function. Normal postvoid residual is 0 to 30 mL; however, retention of up to 100 mL may be acceptable in the older adult.

    A **cystometrogram** (CMG) evaluates the bladder tone and capacity. A retention catheter is inserted into the bladder after the client voids. The bladder is slowly filled with sterile saline and the client indicates at what point the first urge to void is felt and when the bladder feels full. These measurements indicate whether the client's bladder capacity is normal. Most clients feel a mild urge to void at approximately 120 mL and a strong urge to void at about 250 mL. By comparison, clients with a neurogenic bladder (see Chap. 65) may not feel an urge to void till 500 mL or more has been instilled. In many instances the client with a neurogenic bladder never feels an urge to void and instillation is terminated at this point. The client is assessed for bladder contractions that he or she cannot control, leakage around the catheter, or leakage of urine when asked to cough. Pressures within the bladder are also assessed. The client may be given antibiotics for a day or two after a CMG.

Laboratory Tests

URINALYSIS

Much information about systemic diseases and the condition of the kidneys and lower urinary tract can be learned by **urinalysis,** a study of the components and characteristics of the urine. Urinalysis also is useful in monitoring the effects of treatment of known urinary or renal conditions. The characteristics of normal urine and possible causes contributing to abnormal results are listed in Table 63-4. A clean-catch midstream specimen from the first voiding of the morning is preferred. See Nursing Guidelines 63-2 for instructing the client how to collect a clean-catch specimen.

URINE CULTURE AND SENSITIVITY

When infection is suspected, a urine specimen may be taken for culture by collecting a clean-catch midstream specimen or by urinary catheterization. It is important that the urine specimen not be contaminated by skin bacteria. The container is labeled with the client's name and the time and date of the voiding. To prevent the growth

TABLE 63-3	NORMAL URINE FLOW RATES		
GENDER	**YOUNG ADULT**	**MIDDLE-AGED ADULT**	**OLDER ADULT**
Male	21 mL/second	12 mL/second	9 mL/second
Female	18 mL/second	15 mL/second	10 mL/second

TABLE 63-4	URINALYSIS CHARACTERISTICS	
CHARACTERISTIC AND NORMAL VALUE	**ABNORMAL FINDINGS**	**POSSIBLE CAUSES**
Color: yellow	Colorless	Overhydration, diabetes insipidus, chronic renal disease, diuretic therapy, diabetes mellitus
	Red, pink	Hematuria, foods (beets, rhubarb, blackberries), drugs (phenothiazines, rifampin)
	Dark yellow or orange	Bilirubin, dehydration, drugs (multiple vitamins, pyridium, azogantrisin)
	Green	*pseudomonas* infection, bilirubin, drugs (methylene blue, amitriptyline, vitamin B complex)
	Brown	Dehydration, urobilinogen, drugs (Cascara, Flagyl)
	Dark brown to black	Melanin, drugs (Macrodantin, Quinine, Methyldopa)
Clarity: clear	Cloudy	Phosphaturia
	Turbid	Pyuria, bacteriuria, parasitic disease
	Hazy	Mucus
	Smoky, milky	Prostatic fluid, sperm, lipids
	Pinkish precipitates	Hyperuricemia
Specific gravity: 1.003–1.029	Dilute (1.00–1.010) or concentrated (1.029–1.030)	Low: diabetes insipidus, kidney disorders High: false reading due to pus, albumin, protein, glucose, or dextran in urine
pH: 4.5–7.5	>7.5	Urinary tract infection, metabolic acidosis, Cushing's syndrome, low-protein diet with large vegetable intake, diet high in dairy and citrus fruit, drugs (sodium bicarbonate, thiazides)
Ketones: none	Ketonuria	Starvation, fasting, abnormal carbohydrate metabolism, diabetes mellitus, pregnancy, pernicious anemia, vomiting, high-protein diet
Protein: none	Proteinuria	Cancer, severe heart failure, renal disease, glomerulonephritis, nephrotic syndrome, trauma, fever, heavy exercise
Glucose: none	Glycosuria	Diabetes mellitus, gestational diabetes
Red blood cells: 0–3 RBCs/high-power field	>3 RBCs/high-power field	Renal disorders (glomerulonephritis, calculus, cancer, trauma, cysts), systemic disease (lupus, sickle cell, hypertension)
White blood cells: 0–4/high-power field	>4/high-power field	Urinary tract infection (acute pyelonephritis, cystitis, urethritis), renal disease, urinary stones
Bilirubin: none	Bilirubinuria	Hepatitis, biliary obstruction
Urobilinogen: <1 mg/dL	>1 mg/dL	Hepatitis, cirrhosis, congestive heart failure, hemolytic anemia
Casts: 0–2 hyaline casts/low-power field	>2/low-power field	Granular casts (glomerulonephritis, renal disease); fatty casts (nephrotic syndrome); cellular casts (glomeruli or tubule infection); hyaline casts (fever, strenuous exercise, congestive heart failure)
Crystals: none to few	Many	Urolithiasis, chronic renal failure, gout, urinary tract infection
Bacteria: negative per high-power field	Positive	Urinary tract infection, pyelonephritis, cystitis

of bacteria in the urine and decomposition, the nurse ensures delivery of the urine specimen immediately to the laboratory or refrigerates it promptly until it can be taken to the laboratory.

24-HOUR URINE COLLECTION

Sometimes the entire 24-hour volume of urine is collected, such as a 24-hour urine for 17-ketosteroids. The client is initially instructed to void and discard the urine. The collection bottle is marked with the time the client voided. Thereafter, all the urine is collected for the entire 24 hours. The last urine is voided at the same time the test originally began. The entire specimen is refrigerated to prevent bacterial growth. To prevent any part of the spec-

imen from being lost or contaminated, the nurse tells the client to use separate receptacles for voiding and defecation. If any urine is discarded by mistake or lost while defecating, the nurse stops the test. The loss of even a small amount of urine can invalidate the test.

URINE SPECIFIC GRAVITY

Urine specific gravity is a measurement of the kidney's ability to concentrate and excrete urine. The specific gravity measures urine concentration by measuring the density of urine and comparing it with the density of distilled water. The density of distilled water is 1 (1 mL of distilled water weighs 1 g). The number, weight, and size of urine solutes (particles) determine its specific gravity (density).

NURSING GUIDELINES 63-2

Instructing Client on Obtaining a Clean-Catch Midstream Specimen

Tell the client to:

- Wash hands and remove the lid from the specimen container without touching the inside of the lid.

- Open antiseptic towelette package and cleanse the urethral area. Tell the female client to hold labia apart with one hand and wipe down one side of the urethra with the first towelette and discard, wipe down the other side with the second towelette and discard, and wipe down the center with the third towelette and discard. Emphasize wiping one time only, from front to back. Tell the male client to retract foreskin if uncircumcised and to clean the urethral meatus in a circular motion using each towelette one time.

- Instruct the client to begin voiding into the toilet, urinal, or bedpan; tell the female client to continue to hold labia apart while voiding.

- Tell the client to void 30 to 50 mL of the midstream urine into the collection container and then finish urinating into the toilet, bedpan, or urinal. Emphasize not to contaminate the container.

- Tell the client to carefully replace the lid, dry the container if necessary, and wash his or her hands.

Normally, the specific gravity is inversely proportional to urine volume. On a hot day, a person who is perspiring profusely and taking little fluid has low urine output with a high specific gravity. Conversely, a person who has a high fluid intake and who is not losing excessive water from perspiration, diarrhea, or vomiting has copious urine output with a low specific gravity. When the kidneys are diseased, the ability to concentrate urine may be impaired and the specific gravity remains relatively constant, no matter what the water needs of the body are or how much the client drinks.

URINE PROTEIN

The **urine protein test** is used to identify renal disease. Normally, protein is minimally present in the urine. An increase in urine protein levels also may be seen with salt depletion, strenuous exercise, fever, or dehydration. Proteinuria in an individual urine specimen may be detected by dipping a test reagent stick (dipstick method) in the urine and comparing color changes with the provided color chart.

CREATININE CLEARANCE TEST

A **creatinine clearance test** is used to determine kidney function and creatinine excretion. **Creatinine** is a substance that results from the breakdown of phosphocreatine (an amino acid waste product), which is present in

muscle tissue. It is filtered by the glomeruli and is excreted at a fairly constant rate by the kidney. The total amount of excreted creatinine is called *creatinine clearance.* The renal tubules increase creatinine secretion with any decrease in glomerular filtration (renal failure). Muscle necrosis and atrophy greatly increase urinary creatinine owing to accompanying protein catabolism. For this test a 4-, 12-, or 24-hour urine specimen and a sample of blood (serum creatinine) are collected. The blood sample is obtained either at the midpoint or at the beginning and end of urine collection (varies per protocol). Both urine and blood samples are sent to the laboratory.

BLOOD CHEMISTRIES

When the nephrons fail to remove waste products efficiently from the body, the blood chemistry is altered. Deterioration in renal function is manifested by rises in the **blood urea nitrogen** (BUN) and creatinine values, both of which are protein breakdown products. Table 63-5 shows normal values of common blood studies performed on clients with signs and symptoms of a urinary system disorder, as well as renal implications regarding abnormal results. A moderate decrease in renal function occurs, however, before these values rise.

NURSING PROCESS

● The Client Undergoing Diagnostic Testing for a Renal or Urologic Disorder

Assessment

The nurse interviews the client to determine past experience with the test or other urologic procedures. He or she asks the client to discuss the nature of past experiences and expectations for the current tests. If the client had preparations before the test, the nurse checks to see that preparations are complete. He or she also reviews the client's history and determines if there is any allergy history to contrast agents, if applicable.

The nurse takes the client's vital signs and weighs the client if required. Depending on the test, the nurse asks the client to void. If informed consent is required (necessary for invasive procedures), the nurse checks for the signed consent form. Client and family members need teaching and reassurance about the purpose of the test and what the procedure involves. They also need to know the care required after the procedure.

Diagnosis, Planning, and Interventions

Clients undergoing diagnostic testing often are anxious and worried. Clients having urologic testing may feel embarrassed and afraid that the testing will be painful. It is important to provide privacy, reassurance, and information and to maintain a professional and empathic attitude.

TABLE 63-5	NORMAL SERUM VALUES AND RENAL DISEASE	
PARAMETER	**NORMAL VALUE**	**CHANGE SEEN IN RENAL DISEASE**
Calcium	8.8–10 mg/dL	Decreased in renal failure
Carbon dioxide combining power	23–30 mmol/L	Decreased in acute renal failure
Magnesium	1.3–2.1 mEq/L	Decreased in chronic renal disease
Phosphate, inorganic phosphorus	2.7–4.5 mg/dL	Increased in renal failure
Potassium	3.5–5.0 mEq/L	Increased in renal failure
Total protein	6.0–8.0 g/dL	Increased in poor renal function; decreased in nephrotic syndrome
Sodium	135–148 mmol/L	Decreased in severe nephritis; increased in renal disease
Blood urea nitrogen	7–18 mg/dL	Increased in renal disease and urinary obstruction
Creatinine	Male: 0.7–1.3 mg/dL Female: 0.6–1.1 mg/dL	Increased in renal disease or insufficiency
Albumin	>60 yr: 3.4–4.8 g/dL <60 yr: 3.5–5 g/dL	Decreased in renal failure
Chloride	98–107 mEq/L	Decreased in renal failure (onset)
Uric acid	Male: 4.5–8 ng/dL Female: 2.5–6.2 ng/dL	Increased in renal failure

Anxiety and **Fear** related to uncertainty of outcomes of diagnostic testing and the undertaking of an unfamiliar experience

Expected Outcome: Client will verbalize reduced apprehension about diagnostic testing.

- Assess client's level of anxiety. *A high level of fear interferes with learning and cooperation.*
- Explain or re-explain the test, diagnostic procedure, equipment, tubes, or drains to be used. *Thorough understanding of what is expected promotes compliance and cooperation and decreases fear.*
- Use simple language with client or significant others, especially with outpatient procedures or tests. *Using words and language that the client can understand promotes understanding and cooperation.*
- Answer questions about testing or consult with other health team members in matters that involve their expertise. *Additional information provides clarification, promotes understanding, and reduces anxiety.*
- Acknowledge appropriateness of client's feelings; correct any misinterpretations. Avoid false reassurances. Encourage client to verbalize thoughts and feelings. *Acknowledgment of a client's fears conveys acceptance of the client and allows him or her to focus on instructions and what is expected.*
- Provide a calm, nonthreatening environment. Respond to client's needs as quickly as possible. Encourage significant other(s) to stay with the client. *These measures convey calm and promote client's ability to cope.*

- Administer sedative medications as ordered. *Medication reduces anxiety and assists the client to proceed with the test.*

Deficient Knowledge related to diagnostic procedures, tests, and preprocedure and postprocedure care

Expected Outcome: Client will be able to demonstrate or verbalize an understanding of diagnostic procedure, test, and precare and postcare.

- Provide for physical comfort and quiet atmosphere for the client (or significant other) without disruptions. *Doing so allows for concentration on topic and limits distractions.*
- Assess client's knowledge base; explain the purpose of and discuss the procedure or test. *These steps incorporate prior knowledge and promote learning.*
- Move from general to specific details (i.e., radiologic site, required medications, equipment, IV lines, anesthesia, precare and postcare, catheters or drains used). *Doing so provides a foundation of knowledge and proceeds to more specific information.*
- Discuss home care (i.e., fluid intake, medication use, signs and symptoms of genitourinary infection) and postprocedure conditions requiring physician follow-up (i.e., frank bleeding, inability to urinate, increased pain, or fever). *The nurse provides essential information for home care and builds on the foundation of information about the procedure.*
- Discuss concerns about radiographic exposure or refer concerns to the physician or radiologist. *Expressing*

concerns reduces their effects and provides a means to access other resources.

- Encourage questions, repetition of information, return demonstration (as appropriate) from the client or significant other. *Repetition of information and return demonstrations internalize information and behaviors.*

Evaluation of Expected Outcomes

The client reports a decrease in his or her fear and demonstrates a better understanding of the tests, procedures, or both. The client complies with instructions.

GENERAL NUTRITIONAL CONSIDERATIONS

Dietary intake can affect urine characteristics as well as urinary tract disorders and their management. An acid ash or basic ash diet may be ordered in conjunction with drug therapy to help alter urine pH. Drug therapy is a more effective and consistent means of altering urinary pH.

A high-protein, low-carbohydrate diet can cause ketonuria. Megadoses of vitamin C can interfere with certain laboratory tests, such as for glycosuria and fecal occult blood. Asparagus has a weak diuretic action and produces a pungent urine odor.

GENERAL PHARMACOLOGIC CONSIDERATIONS

Nephrotoxicity may occur with the administration of certain drugs and is potentially serious because it decreases urinary excretion of the drug and increases the risk of drug toxicity.

Some drugs may have an effect on the outcome of urinary tract tests as well as the appearance of the urine. For example, nitrofurantoin may color the urine brown and methylene blue may color the urine a pale blue-green. Contamination of urine with povidone–iodine can cause a false-positive hematuria result (dipstick method). Other drugs can affect urine pH, such as ammonium chloride and mandelic acid, both of which can cause acidic urine, whereas sodium bicarbonate, thiazide diuretics, acetazolamide, and potassium citrate promote alkaline urine.

Aminoglycosides such as gentamicin can result in increased levels of BUN and serum creatinine, indicating nephrotoxicity. Signs of nephrotoxicity may not occur until the client has received 5 or more days of therapy. Nephrotoxicity from the use of the aminoglycosides is reversible if the drug is discontinued as soon as the symptoms appear.

Diuretic therapy can result in increased sodium, chloride, and magnesium levels with 24-hour urine electrolyte testing.

GENERAL GERONTOLOGIC CONSIDERATIONS

The older client may have difficulty following directions when collecting a 24-hour urine specimen. The directions may need to be repeated and the client supervised at frequent intervals.

Age-related changes in kidney function, such as decreased glomerular filtration rate and thickening of the renal tubules, can alter the excretion of drugs in older adults, increasing the risk of drug toxicity.

Nephrotoxicity is more likely to occur in older adults than in younger adults receiving prolonged or high doses of nephrotoxic drugs. It is important for the nurse to identify and report signs of nephrotoxicity (increased BUN or serum creatinine levels, oliguria, or proteinuria).

Critical Thinking Exercises

1. *A client is scheduled for a cystoscopy and retrograde pyelogram. He is very nervous and asks many questions about the procedure. What could you do to try to decrease his anxiety?*
2. *A client has possible renal disease and is scheduled for many tests on her upper and lower urinary tract and gastrointestinal tract. What would you do to be sure one test does not interfere with another test?*

References and Suggested Readings

Albaugh, J. (1999). Unlocking the mystery of urodynamics. *Urologic Nursing, 19,* 202, 206–208.

Bullock, B. A. & Henze, R. L. (2000). *Focus on pathophysiology.* Philadelphia: Lippincott Williams & Wilkins.

Fischbach, F. (2002). *Nurses' quick reference to common laboratory and diagnostic tests* (3rd ed.). Philadelphia: Lippincott Williams & Wilkins.

Porth, C. M. (2002). *Pathophysiology: Concepts of altered health states* (6th ed.). Philadelphia: Lippincott Williams & Wilkins.

Smeltzer, S. C. & Bare, B. G. (2000). *Brunner & Suddarth's textbook of medical–surgical nursing* (9th ed.). Philadelphia: Lippincott Williams & Wilkins.

Stark, J. (1998). Interpretation of BUN and serum creatinine. *Critical Care Clinics of North America, 10,* 491–496.

Weber, J. R. (2001). *Nurses' handbook of health assessment* (4th ed.). Philadelphia: Lippincott Williams & Wilkins.

Caring for Clients With Disorders of the Kidneys and Ureters

Words to Know

acute renal failure
acute tubular necrosis
anasarca
anuria
arteriovenous fistula
arteriovenous graft
azotemia
bruit
calciuria
calculus
casts
chronic renal failure
colic
dialysate
dialysis
dialyzer
disequilibrium syndrome
end-stage renal disease
extracorporeal shock
   wave lithotripsy
glomerulonephritis

hematuria
hemodialysis
hydronephrosis
nephrectomy
nephrolithiasis
nephrostomy tube
nocturia
oliguria
osteodystrophy
periorbital edema
peritoneal dialysis
pyelonephritis
pyeloplasty
pyuria
thrill
uremia
uremic frost
ureteral stent
ureterolithiasis
ureteroplasty
urolithiasis

Learning Objectives

On completion of this chapter, the reader will:

- Differentiate between pyelonephritis and glomerulonephritis.
- Name three problems the nurse manages when caring for clients with glomerulonephritis.
- Explain the pathophysiology and associated renal complications of polycystic disease.
- Give examples of conditions that predispose to renal calculi.
- Identify methods for eliminating small renal calculi and larger stones.
- Discuss the nursing management of a client with a nephrostomy tube.
- Describe conditions that cause a ureteral stricture.
- Explain the classic triad of symptoms associated with renal cancer.
- Discuss problems the nurse manages when caring for a client with a nephrectomy.
- Differentiate acute and chronic renal failure.
- Explain at least five pathophysiologic problems associated with chronic renal failure.
- Describe sources of organs for kidney transplantation.
- Identify at least three nursing methods for managing pruritus.
- Explain the purposes and methods of dialysis.
- Discuss nursing assessments performed when caring for clients undergoing dialysis.

The most common urologic disorders are infectious and inflammatory conditions. Those that affect the kidneys are extremely dangerous because damage to the nephrons can result in permanent renal dysfunction. The same is true of other upper urinary tract disorders such as kidney and ureteral stones and tumors. The consequences can lead to acute or chronic renal failure.

INFECTIOUS AND INFLAMMATORY DISORDERS OF THE KIDNEY

Infectious and inflammatory disorders of the kidney affect structures such as the renal pelvis, the nephrons, or both.

● PYELONEPHRITIS

Pyelonephritis is an acute or chronic bacterial infection of the kidney and the lining of the collecting system (kidney pelvis). *Acute pyelonephritis* presents with moderate to severe symptoms that usually last 1 to 2 weeks. If the treatment of acute pyelonephritis is unsuccessful and the infection recurs, it is termed *chronic pyelonephritis*.

Pathophysiology and Etiology

Bacteria ascend to the kidney and kidney pelves by way of the bladder and urethra. Normal fecal flora such as *Escherichia coli, Klebsiella pneumoniae, Proteus mirabilis,*

Streptococcus fecalis, Pseudomonas aeruginosa, and *Staphylococcus aureus* are the most common bacteria that cause acute pyelonephritis. *E. coli* accounts for about 85% of infections. Additional risk factors for chronic pyelonephritis, such as urinary obstruction and reflux (Fig. 64-1), are listed in Box 64-1.

In acute pyelonephritis, the inflammation causes the kidneys to grossly enlarge. The cortex and medulla develop multiple abscesses. The renal calyces and pelves also can become involved. Resolution of the inflammation results in fibrosis and scarring. Chronic pyelonephritis develops after recurrent episodes of acute pyelonephritis. The kidneys manifest irreversible degenerative changes and become small and atrophic. If destruction of nephrons is extensive, renal failure develops. Renal dysfunction may not occur for 20 or more years after the onset of

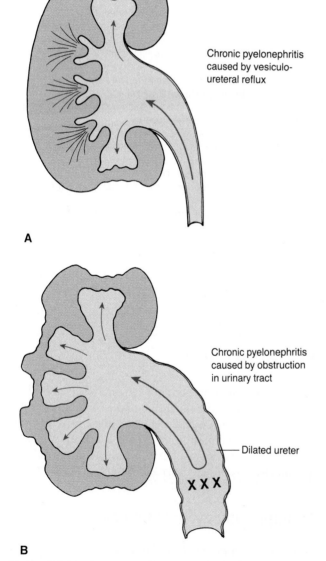

A

B

FIGURE 64-1 Causes of chronic pyelonephritis include vesiculo-ureteral reflux (**A**) and Urinary tract obstruction (**B**).

Polar scar

Chronic pyelonephritis caused by vesiculo-ureteral reflux

Chronic pyelonephritis caused by obstruction in urinary tract

Dilated ureter

BOX 64-1 ● **Risk Factors for Pyelonephritis**

ACUTE PYELONEPHRITIS
- Instrumentation of the urethra and bladder (catheterization, cystoscopy, urologic surgery)
- Inability to empty the bladder
- Pregnancy
- Urinary stasis
- Urinary obstruction (tumors, strictures, calculi, prostatic hypertrophy)
- Diabetes mellitus
- Other renal disease (polycystic kidney disease)
- Neurogenic bladder (stroke, multiple sclerosis, spinal cord injury)
- Women with increased sexual activity, diaphragm, spermicide use, failure to void after intercourse, history of recent urinary infection
- Men who perform anal intercourse, infection with HIV

CHRONIC PYELONEPHRITIS
- Recurrent episodes of acute pyelonephritis
- Chronic obstruction (e.g., strictures and stones)
- Reflux disorders that allow urine to flow backward up the ureters

---

the disease. About 10% to 15% of clients with chronic pyelonephritis require dialysis.

Stop, Think, and Respond ● **BOX 64-1**

Explain why a client with an indwelling catheter is at risk for acute pyelonephritis.

Assessment Findings

Signs and Symptoms

Flank pain or tenderness, chills, fever, and malaise occur in clients with acute pyelonephritis. Frequency and burning on urination are present if there is accompanying cystitis (bladder infection). Some clients with chronic pyelonephritis are asymptomatic; others have a low-grade fever and vague gastrointestinal complaints. Polyuria and nocturia develop when the tubules of the nephrons fail to reabsorb water efficiently.

Diagnostic Findings

A urinalysis demonstrates multiple abnormalities. The chief abnormality is **pyuria,** or pus (a combination of bacteria and leukocytes) in the urine (Box 64-2). A urine culture identifies the causative microorganism. A cystoscopy, or intravenous pyelogram (IVP) or retrograde pyelogram, demonstrates obstruction or damage to structures of the urinary tract. An x-ray of the kidneys, ureters, and bladder may reveal calculi, cysts, or tumors in the kidney or other urinary structures. The diagnosis of chronic pyelonephritis is based on a history of repeated acute pyelonephritis. Serum creatinine and blood urea nitrogen (BUN) levels, if elevated, indicate impaired renal function.

Medical and Surgical Management

Treatment of acute pyelonephritis includes relieving fever and pain and prescribing antimicrobial drugs such as trimethoprim-sulfamethoxazole (Septra) or ciprofloxacin (Cipro) for 14 days. Antispasmodics and anticholinergics such as oxybutynin (Ditropan) and propantheline (Pro-Banthine) are additional pharmacologic interventions that relax the smooth muscles of the ureters and bladder, promote comfort, and increase bladder capacity. Symptoms usually disappear within a few days of antibiotic therapy. Four weeks of drug therapy is prescribed for clients with a history of frequent relapsing infections with the same microorganism.

The goal of treatment for chronic pyelonephritis is to prevent progressive kidney damage. When possible, any urinary tract obstruction is relieved. An effort is made to improve the client's overall health. A **nephrectomy,** the surgical removal of a kidney, is performed if severe hypertension develops and if the other kidney has adequate function.

Nursing Management

The nurse obtains complete medical, drug, and allergy histories and assesses vital signs, reporting abnormal findings such as elevated temperature or blood pressure. Continued and regular monitoring of vital signs is important to detect any evidence of changes. A physical examination helps the nurse determine the location of discomfort and any signs of fluid retention such as peripheral edema or shortness of breath. The nurse observes and documents the characteristics of the client's urine. A clean-catch urine specimen is collected for urinalysis and urine culture. The nurse measures intake and output. Encouraging a liberal daily fluid intake of approximately 2000 to 3000 mL helps to flush the infectious microorganisms from the urinary tract. The nurse administers prescribed medications. He or she evaluates laboratory test results such as BUN, creatinine, serum electrolytes, and urine culture to determine the client's response to therapy. If chronic pyelonephritis develops, the treatment often is lengthy. Poor health and prolonged medical therapy are discouraging. The nurse urges the client to follow the recommendations of the physician and adhere to the prescribed medication regimen.

Client and family teaching includes the following information from the nurse:

- Explanation of the disease, its cause, related risk factors, treatment, and preventive measures
- Discussion of the purpose, dosage, side effects, and toxic effects of all prescribed medications
- Instructions to complete the entire regimen of antimicrobial therapy as indicated, even if symptoms abate
- Reinforcement of the importance of consuming a large volume of oral fluids daily
- Suggestions to consume acid-forming foods such as meat, fish, poultry, eggs, grains, corn, lentils, cranberries, prunes, plums, and their juices to prevent calcium and magnesium phosphate stone formation
- Recommendation to avoid alcohol and caffeine products if bladder spasms are present or until a clinical response to therapy is verified
- Explanation of the purpose and protocols for diagnostic procedures
- Teaching how to collect a clean-catch urine specimen for subsequent medical follow-up at 2 weeks and 3 months after treatment
- Referring client to resources where blood pressure can be monitored intermittently
- Identification of the signs of recurring or worsening pyelonephritis or lower urinary tract infection (frequency, urgency, burning, cloudy urine, and fever) and emphasis on the need to consult the primary care provider
- Discussion of methods to prevent reinfection—women should wipe from front to back after defecation and wear cotton undergarments. The nurse tells all clients to void every 2 to 3 hours when awake and before and after intercourse.

• ACUTE GLOMERULONEPHRITIS

The term *nephritis* describes a group of inflammatory but noninfectious diseases characterized by widespread kidney damage. **Glomerulonephritis** is a type of nephritis that occurs most frequently in children and young adults; however, it can affect people of any age. The exact incidence of the disease is unknown, but it occurs twice as often in men as in women. Most clients recover spontaneously or with minimal therapy without sequelae. Some develop chronic glomerulonephritis.

Pathophysiology and Etiology

Symptoms of acute glomerulonephritis appear about 2 to 3 weeks after an upper respiratory infection with group A beta-hemolytic streptococci. Impetigo (skin infection) and viral infections such as mumps, hepatitis B, or human immunodeficiency virus also may precede acute glomerulonephritis (Smeltzer & Bare, 2000). The relationship between the infection and acute glomerulonephritis is not clear. Microorganisms are not present in the kidney when symptoms appear, but the glomeruli are acutely inflamed. Most believe that the inflammatory response is from antigen–antibody stimulation in the glomerular capillary membrane. The disruption of membrane permeability causes red blood cells (RBCs) and protein molecules to filter from the glomeruli into Bowman's capsule and eventually become lost in the urine. Refer to Figure 64-2 for more information.

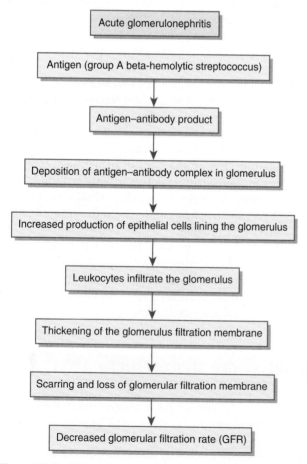

FIGURE 64-2 Sequence of events in acute glomerulonephritis.

Assessment Findings

Signs and Symptoms

About 50% of clients with glomerulonephritis have no symptoms. Early symptoms may be so slight that the client does not seek medical attention. Occasionally the onset is sudden with pronounced symptoms such as fever, nausea, malaise, headache, generalized edema, or **periorbital edema,** puffiness around the eyes. Some clients experience pain or tenderness over the kidney area and mild to moderate hypertension. In some instances, a routine physical examination reveals the disorder. More often, the client or family notices that the person's face is pale and puffy and that slight ankle edema occurs in the evening. The appetite is poor, and **nocturia** (urination during the night) may be present. Irritability and shortness of breath also develop. As the condition progresses, the client develops **hematuria** (blood in the urine), anemia (from the hematuria), convulsions associated with hypertension, congestive heart failure, **oliguria** (low urine output of 100 to 500 mL/day), and perhaps **anuria** (<100 mL of urine over 24 hours). Fluid retention and hypertension contribute to visual disturbances, often as a result of papilledema or hemorrhage in the eye, and epistaxis (nosebleeds).

Diagnostic Findings

Gross or microscopic hematuria gives the urine a dark, smoky, or frankly bloody appearance. Laboratory findings include proteinuria (primarily as albumin in the urine) and an elevated anti-streptolysin O titer from the recent streptococcal infection. There is decreased hemoglobin, slightly elevated BUN and serum creatinine levels, and an elevated erythrocyte sedimentation rate. If renal insufficiency develops, serum electrolyte levels indicate hyperkalemia, hypermagnesemia, hypocalcemia, and dilutional hyponatremia. Percutaneous renal biopsy reveals cellular changes characteristic of an antigen–antibody response and the extent of damage that already has occurred.

Medical Management

No specific treatment exists for acute glomerulonephritis. Treatment is guided by the symptoms and the underlying abnormality. Treatment may consist of bed rest, a sodium-restricted diet (if edema or hypertension is present), and antimicrobial drugs to prevent a superimposed infection in the already inflamed kidney. Penicillin may be used to abolish any remaining streptococci from the recent infection. Diuretics to reduce edema and antihypertensive agents for severe hypertension may be necessary. Vitamins are added to the diet to improve general resistance, and oral iron supplements may be needed to counteract anemia. Corticosteroids and immunosuppressive agents may be given to treat a rapidly progressive inflammatory process. Any increase in hematuria, proteinuria, or blood pressure indicates a need for aggressive treatment The client is not considered cured until the urine is free of protein and RBCs for 6 months. Return to full activity usually is not permitted until the urine is free of protein for 1 month.

Nursing Management

The client must maintain bed rest when the blood pressure is elevated and edema is present. The nurse collects daily urine specimens to assist with evaluating the client's response to treatment. He or she assesses blood pressure every 4 hours or as ordered. Encouraging adequate fluid intake and measuring intake and output are important nursing interventions. Although the diet may be restricted in sodium and protein, it is necessary for the client to have adequate carbohydrate intake to prevent the catabolism of body protein stores.

The nurse provides teaching based on the following guidelines:

- Identify the specific amount of sodium that is allowed and sources of sodium to avoid.
- Explain the purpose of diuretic therapy or other prescribed medications, the dosing regimen, and side effects.
- Recommend regular blood pressure monitoring.
- Caution client to avoid contact with persons who have infections.
- Emphasize compliance with medical appointments and the necessity for repeated urinalyses.
- Advise client to contact the physician if urinary volumes diminish, there is unexplained weight gain, or headaches or nosebleeds occur.

● CHRONIC GLOMERULONEPHRITIS

Chronic glomerulonephritis is a slowly progressive disease characterized by inflammation of the glomeruli, causing irreversible damage to the nephrons. The course of the disease is highly variable. Some clients live for years with no or occasional symptomatic episodes. In other clients, the disease is rapidly fatal unless they receive dialysis to take care of the renal failure.

Pathophysiology and Etiology

A small number of those with chronic glomerulonephritis are known to have had repeated acute glomerulonephritis, but many do not have that history. Complications of autoimmune connective tissue disorders, such as lupus erythematosus (see Chap. 67) and Goodpasture's syndrome (a rare disease that includes progressive glomeru-

lonephritis, hemoptysis, and marked RBC destruction), also may cause chronic glomerulonephritis.

The chronic inflammation leads to ever-increasing bands of scar tissue that replace nephrons, the vital functioning units of the kidney. Decreased glomerular filtration eventually can lead to renal failure. Chronic glomerulonephritis accounts for approximately 40% of people on dialysis.

Assessment Findings

Signs and Symptoms

Some clients do not experience symptoms until renal damage is severe. Generalized edema known as **anasarca** is a common finding. Anasarca is caused by the shift of fluid from the intravascular space to interstitial and intracellular locations. The fluid shift results from depletion of serum proteins, particularly albumin, which is lost in the urine. Clients remain markedly edematous for months or years. They may feel relatively well, but the kidney continues to excrete albumin. The fluid burden and subsequent renal failure contribute to fatigue, headache, hypertension, dyspnea, and visual disturbances.

Diagnostic Findings

Low RBC volume is detected through complete blood counts. Its underlying cause is the excretion of erythrocytes in the urine and reduced production of erythropoietin. **Azotemia,** accumulation of nitrogen waste products in the blood, is evidenced by elevated BUN, serum creatinine, and uric acid levels. The urine contains protein (albumin), sediment, **casts** (deposits of minerals that break loose from the walls of the tubules), and red and white blood cells. The urinary creatinine clearance is reduced. Serum electrolyte changes indicate nephron dysfunction.

Chest radiography and echocardiography evaluate cardiac size because cardiac enlargement is common. A percutaneous kidney biopsy may be performed in the early stage to confirm the diagnosis and to determine the severity of the disorder. In late stages, the kidneys are too small to safely perform a biopsy.

Medical Management

Treatment is nonspecific and symptomatic. Management goals include the following:

- Controlling hypertension with medications and sodium restriction
- Correcting fluid and electrolyte imbalance
- Reducing edema with diuretic therapy
- Preventing congestive heart failure
- Eliminating urinary tract infections with antimicrobials

Renal failure eventually may necessitate dialysis or kidney transplantation, discussed later in this chapter.

NURSING PROCESS

● The Client With Chronic Glomerulonephritis

Assessment

Assessment includes monitoring fluid and electrolyte balance by checking blood values, intake and output, and skin turgor, and looking for any edema. It also is important to assess the client's neurologic, cardiac, and mental status.

Diagnosis, Planning, and Interventions

Caring for the client with chronic glomerulonephritis involves close observation for changes in fluid and electrolyte status and kidney function. Clients may experience anxiety or depression and require emotional support. Diagnoses, expected outcomes, and interventions include, but are not limited to, the following:

Excess Fluid Volume related to decreased glomerular filtration

Expected Outcome: Client will maintain a fluid volume within normal limits as evidenced by urine output greater than 500 mL/day, systolic blood pressure less than 140 mm Hg, reduced proteinuria, and no crackles, gurgles, or S_3 heart sound.

- Weigh client daily at the same time on the same scale with client wearing similar clothing each time. *Changes in body weight reflect changes in body fluid volume. Consistent conditions provide a baseline and database for observing changes and determining treatment.*
- Measure intake and output. *Accurate measurements provide a database for evaluating fluid balance.*
- Plan with client to proportionately distribute restricted fluid volumes over 24 hours. *The nurse must carefully plan fluid restriction to maintain intravascular volume and cardiac workload. Involving the client in planning promotes his or her compliance with restrictions.*
- Monitor blood pressure, heart rate, and lung and heart sounds each shift. Notify the physician of significant changes. *Changes in these parameters indicate changes in fluid volume.*
- Assess for edema, tight rings or shoes, or clothes that do not fit comfortably. *Renal failure causes dependent edema, as evidenced by pitting edema and tight rings or shoes.*
- Request that the dietitian instruct the client on sodium restriction and adequate caloric intake. *Restricted sodium promotes excretion of excess fluid. Clients require adequate caloric intake to maintain energy levels and proper nutrition.*
- Suggest herbs or spices that increase the palatability of food. *Decreased sodium reduces the flavor of food. Adding herbs and spices helps enhance food flavor.*

- Administer prescribed diuretics. *They promote diuresis, decrease edema, and increase renal blood flow.*

Activity Intolerance related to fatigue, anemia, retention of waste products, and generalized edema

Expected Outcome: Client will demonstrate the need to balance rest and activity.

- Avoid clustering nursing tasks and physical activities. *Spacing activities conserves energy.*
- Provide periods of rest and promote uninterrupted sleep at night. *Adequate rest conserves energy levels and decreases fatigue.*
- Facilitate an adequate nutritional intake that includes some complete protein and iron-rich foods. *Complete proteins provide a positive nitrogen balance needed for growth and healing. Although some protein is necessary for complete nutrition, clients with decreased kidney function have difficulty excreting waste products from protein metabolism, so there is need to restrict protein intake. Iron-rich foods enhance hemoglobin formation, increasing the blood's oxygen-carrying capacity and enhancing energy levels and activity tolerance.*
- Eliminate any unnecessary activities of daily living (ADLs). Assist client with ADLs when he or she shows evidence of tachycardia or dyspnea. *Reducing activities and providing assistance decrease oxygen consumption and conserve energy.*

Evaluation of Expected Outcomes

Urine output is 650 mL/day. Systolic blood pressure is 132 mm Hg. Bilateral breath sounds are clear and heart sounds are normal. The client plans rest periods in the day and reduces commitments. He or she also demonstrates understanding of appropriate diet, as evidenced by food choices.

The nurse evaluates the client's ability to manage home care and the availability of a support system before developing discharge plans. If the client lacks a support system from the family or extended family members, the nurse consults with the physician for a referral to a social agency or home health care agency. He or she develops a teaching plan with the following instructions:

- Follow the diet and fluid regimen recommended by the physician and as outlined by the dietitian.
- Take medications exactly as directed on the container label. Do not omit or discontinue any medication unless ordered to do so by the physician. Do not take nonprescription drugs unless a physician approves their use.
- Monitor and record temperature and weight daily. (In some instances, clients may be asked to monitor their blood pressure.)
- Follow the physician's recommendations as to physical activity and exercise. Take frequent rest periods if fatigue occurs.
- Contact the physician with any question about the medication, if symptoms become worse, or if fever, chills, blood in the urine, weight gain, swelling of the

arms or legs or periorbital edema, difficulty in breathing, difficulty in thinking, severe fatigue, excessive sleepiness, constipation, loss of appetite, or an upper respiratory infection occurs.

- Emphasize that frequent follow-up visits and laboratory tests are necessary to monitor response to treatment.

CONGENITAL KIDNEY DISORDERS: POLYCYSTIC DISEASE

Individuals may be born with various malformations of renal structures. Most of these are unpredictable because they are the result of errors in fetal development. Polycystic disease, however, is the result of a hereditary trait.

The two manifestations of polycystic disease are the infantile and adult forms. The infantile form is rare. It may cause fetal death (before delivery), early neonatal death, or renal failure during childhood. The adult form has its onset between 30 to 50 years of age and insidiously progresses to renal insufficiency. Once renal failure develops, polycystic disease usually is fatal within 4 years, unless the client receives dialysis treatment or an organ transplant. Women and men are affected equally. Death usually results from renal failure or the complications of hypertensive cardiovascular disease.

Pathophysiology and Etiology

Adult polycystic kidney disease is inherited as an autosomal dominant trait, which means that an affected parent passes the gene for the disease to his or her children. Each child has a 50:50 chance of acquiring the defective gene (Fig. 64-3). This is opposed to autosomal recessive inheritance, in which a child has a 25% chance of being affected.

As the name implies, this disorder is characterized by the formation of multiple bilateral kidney cysts (Fig. 64-4). The cysts interfere with kidney function and eventually lead to renal failure. The fluid-filled cysts cause great enlargement of the kidneys, from their normal size of a fist to that of a football. As the cysts enlarge, they compress the renal blood vessels and cause chronic hypertension. Bleeding into cysts causes flank pain. People with polycystic disease are much more susceptible to kidney infections and kidney stones. Besides renal failure, other complications include cysts on the pancreas and liver, an enlarged heart, mitral valve prolapse, and brain aneurysm.

Assessment Findings

Hypertension is present in approximately 75% of affected clients at the time of diagnosis. Other symptoms, such as pain from retroperitoneal bleeding, lumbar discomfort,

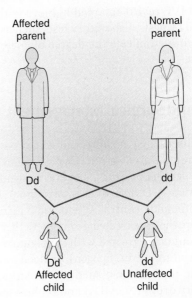

FIGURE 64-3 Inheritance of an autosomal dominant disorder.

and abdominal tenderness, are caused by the size and effects of the cysts. The client may experience **colic** (acute spasmodic pain) when there is ureteral passage of clots or calculi.

A family history of affected members is a presumptive diagnostic indicator. Urinalysis shows mild proteinuria, hematuria, and pyuria. A complete blood count may show decreased or increased RBCs and hematocrit; an increase is seen because erythropoietin production sometimes is accelerated. Abdominal ultrasound, com-

FIGURE 64-4 Normal kidneys in comparison with polycystic kidneys.

puted tomography (CT) scan, magnetic resonance imaging (MRI), and IVP reveal enlarged kidneys with indentations caused by cysts. Laboratory tests such as BUN and serum creatinine indicate the degree of current kidney dysfunction.

Medical and Surgical Management

Polycystic disease has no cure, but some interventions reduce the rate of progression. Hypertension is treated with antihypertensive drugs, diuretic medications, and sodium restriction. Despite these interventions, the hypertension is difficult to control. When and if urinary infections develop, they are treated promptly with antibiotics. Low RBC counts are treated with iron supplements, injections of erythropoietin (Epogen), or blood transfusions. Nephrotoxic medications, such as nonsteroidal anti-inflammatory drugs (NSAIDs) and cephalosporin antibiotics, are avoided at all costs.

Dialysis substitutes for kidney function when renal failure occurs and while the client awaits an organ transplant. Surgical removal of one or both kidneys may be required. Animal research is being conducted using the antineoplastic drug, paclitaxel (Taxol), steroids such as methylprednisolone (Depo-Medrol), and an antihyperlipidemic agent, lovastatin (Mevacor) to evaluate if these drugs slow the rate of disease progression.

Nursing Management

Many clients with polycystic disease are treated as outpatients by primary care physicians or nephrologists, physicians who specialize in the diagnosis and treatment of renal diseases. When hospitalization is necessary, the nurse assesses vital signs, especially blood pressure, and reports any significant elevations. He or she monitors laboratory test results for indicators of renal function. The nurse inspects the urine for signs of bleeding or infection. He or she measures and documents intake and output at least every 8 hours. The nurse reports any decrease in or absence of urine output. For further information about complications or advanced stages, refer to Nursing Process: The Client With Renal Calculi, and the Nursing Management sections in the discussions of the client with renal failure and dialysis.

OBSTRUCTIVE DISORDERS

Urinary obstruction at any point in the urinary tract can occur in clients of all ages for various reasons. Obstructing conditions include urinary tract stones, structures, and tumors. Table 64-1 lists causes of urinary tract obstruction.

● KIDNEY AND URETERAL STONES

Urolithiasis refers to a condition of stones (**calculus;** pl. *calculi*) in the urinary tract. A calculus is a precipitate of mineral salts that ordinarily remain dissolved in urine. About 70% to 80% of renal calculi in the United States are composed of calcium oxalate, calcium phosphate, or both (Porth, 2002). Others are composed of calcium phosphate, uric acid, cystine, and magnesium ammonium phosphate, or struvite (Table 64-2). Stones may be smooth, jagged, or staghorn shaped (Fig. 64-5).

Calculi can occur anywhere in the urinary tract from the kidney pelvis and beyond. When a stone forms, the condition is called *urolithiasis*. **Nephrolithiasis** refers to a kidney stone, the size of which may range from microscopic to several centimeters. **Ureterolithiasis** is a stone in the ureter. Ureteral stones usually are small; some may be no larger than a grain of sand.

Pathophysiology and Etiology

The reason urinary calculi form is not fully understood. Predisposing factors include the following:

- **Calciuria,** excessive calcium in the urine, as may accompany hyperparathyroid disease, administra-

TABLE 64-1	CAUSES OF URINARY TRACT OBSTRUCTION
LEVEL OF OBSTRUCTION	**CAUSE**
Renal pelvis	Renal calculi
	Papillary necrosis
Ureter	Renal calculi
	Pregnancy
	Tumors that compress the ureter
	Ureteral stricture
	Congenital disorders of the ureterovesical junction, and ureteropelvic junction strictures
Bladder and urethra	Bladder cancer
	Neurogenic bladder
	Bladder stones
	Prostatic hyperplasia or cancer
	Urethral strictures
	Congenital urethral defects

(From Porth, C. M. [2002]. *Pathophysiology: Concepts of altered health states* [6th ed]. Philadelphia: Lippincott Williams & Wilkins.)

TABLE 64-2	COMPOSITION, CONTRIBUTING FACTORS, AND TREATMENT OF KIDNEY STONES	
TYPE OF STONE	**CONTRIBUTING FACTORS**	**TREATMENT**
Calcium (oxalate and phosphate)	Hypercalcemia and hypercalciuria Immobilization	Treatment of underlying conditions Increased fluid intake Thiazide diuretics
	Hyperparathyroidism Vitamin D intoxication Diffuse bone disease Milk-alkali syndrome Renal tubular acidosis Hyperoxaluria Intestinal bypass surgery	Dietary restriction of foods high in oxalate
Magnesium ammonium phosphate (struvite)	Urea-splitting urinary tract infections	Treatment of urinary tract infection Acidification of the urine Increased fluid intake
Uric acid (urate)	Formed in acid urine with pH of approximately 5.5 Gout High-purine diet	Increased fluid intake Allopurinol for hyperuricuria Alkalinization of urine
Cystine	Cystinuria (inherited disorder of amino acid metabolism)	Increased fluid intake Alkalinization of urine

tion of calcium-based antacids, and excessive intake of vitamin D
- Dehydration
- Urinary tract infection with urea-splitting organisms such as *P. mirabilis,* which makes urine alkaline, a condition that promotes precipitation of calcium
- Obstructive disorders, such as an enlarged prostate gland, which foster urinary stasis
- Metabolic disorders, such as gout, in which uric acid crystallizes
- Osteoporosis, in which bone is demineralized
- Prolonged immobility from paralysis secondary to spinal injuries or other incapacitating conditions that result in sluggish emptying of urine from the urinary tract

Calculi traumatize the walls of the urinary tract and irritate the cellular lining, causing pain as violent contractions of the ureter develop to pass the stone along. But the ureteral spasms may just as easily hold a stone in place. If a stone totally or partially obstructs the passage of urine beyond its location, pressure increases in the area above the stone. The pressure contributes to pain, and urinary stasis promotes secondary infection. The retained urine distends the renal pelvis, a condition called **hydronephrosis.** Eventually, there may be compression of the glomeruli and tiny arterioles that supply blood to the kidney, which can result in permanent kidney damage.

Assessment Findings

Signs and Symptoms

Symptoms of a kidney or ureteral stone vary with size, location, and cause. Small stones may pass unnoticed; however, sudden, sharp, severe flank pain that travels to the suprapubic region and external genitalia is the clas-

FIGURE 64-5 Staghorn calculi. The kidney shows hydronephrosis and stones that are casts of the dilated calyces. (Rubin, E. & Farber, J. L. [1999]. *Pathology* [3rd ed.]. Philadelphia: Lippincott Williams & Wilkins.)

sic symptom of urinary calculi. The pain is accompanied by renal or ureteral colic, painful spasms that attempt to move the stone. The pain comes in waves that radiate to the inguinal ring, the inner aspect of the thigh, and to the testicle or tip of the penis in men, or the urinary meatus or labia in women. The severity of the pain usually is inversely proportional to the size of the stone. Smaller stones travel more rapidly down the ureter, causing more forceful ureteral spasm and, therefore, greater pain. The severity of the pain can cause nausea, vomiting, and shock.

If an infection develops, the client may experience chills, fever, and serious hypotension. Urinary retention or dysuria may accompany obstruction. The kidney pelvis and ureter may become markedly enlarged as a consequence of urinary obstruction, and a mass may be palpated. The client also may experience renal tenderness.

Diagnostic Findings

Urinalysis shows evidence of gross or microscopic hematuria from trauma as the calculus tears at tissue as it moves downward. In addition, the urinalysis may show a pH conducive to stone formation, increased specific gravity, mineral crystals, and casts. Leukocytes in the urine and an elevated white blood cell count indicate an infectious process. A urine culture identifies specific infectious microorganisms.

Radiography identifies most translucent kidney stones. If visualization is inconclusive, an IVP shows dye-filling defects caused by a stone. The dye stops at a certain point in the ureter and demonstrates enlargement above the obstruction. Kidney ultrasonography also detects obstructive changes. Depending on how long the stone has been pre-

sent, some blood chemistry values, such as serum creatinine, BUN, and serum uric acid, may be elevated. Analysis of the stone content is useful in preventing recurrence.

Medical Management

pyelo- kidney pelvis

Small calculi are passed naturally with no specific interventions. If the stone is 5 mm or less in diameter and moving, the pain is tolerable, and there is no obstruction, the client is managed medically with vigorous hydration, analgesics (including opioids and NSAIDs), antimicrobial therapy, and drugs that dissolve calculi or eventually alter conditions that promote their formation (Drug Therapy Table 64-1).

For larger stones, **extracorporeal shock wave lithotripsy** (ESWL), a procedure that uses 800 to 2400 shock waves aimed from outside the body toward soft tissue to dense stones (Fig. 64-6), may be used. The stones are shattered into smaller particles that are passed from the urinary tract. ESWL is administered with the client in a water bath or surrounded by a soft cushion while under light anesthesia or sedation. Stones also can be pulverized with laser lithotripsy. To do so, a fine wire, through which the laser beam passes, is inserted into the ureter by means of a cystoscope. Repeated bursts of the laser reduce the stone to a fine powder, which is then passed in the urine.

Other stone removal procedures are performed with ureteroscopic approaches in which the endoscope is inserted from the urethra into the upper urinary tract under anesthesia to grasp, crush, and remove stones from the

DRUG THERAPY TABLE 64-1	**AGENTS TO TREAT PYELONEPHRITIS**		
DRUG CATEGORY AND EXAMPLES	**MECHANISM OF ACTION**	**SIDE EFFECTS**	**NURSING CONSIDERATIONS**
Antispasmodics *oxybutinin chloride (Ditropan) flavoxate (Urispas), belladonna and opium suppositories*	Inhibits the action of acetylcholine and relaxes smooth muscle of the ureters and bladder	Dizziness, drowsiness, blurred vision, dry mouth, constipation, increased heart rate, delirium	Do not administer to clients with closed-angle glaucoma or hypotension.
Anticholinergics *propantheline (Pro-Banthine), hyoscyamine (Levsinex), tincture of belladonna*	Reduces spasms and smooth muscle contractions by inhibiting the effects of acetylcholine, thereby increasing bladder capacity	Same as above	Same as above
Oral Antibiotics *trimethoprim-sulfamethoxazole (Bactrim, Septra), ciprofloxacin (Cipro)*	Inhibits bacterial growth and destroys microorganisms	Same as above	Drugs can be used for up to 14 days. Clients do not require hospitalization unless nausea, vomiting, or signs of septicemia develop.

FIGURE 64-6 Methods of treating renal stones. (**A**) Cystoscopy. (**B**) Extracorporeal shock wave lithotripsy (ESWL). (**C**) Percutaneous nephrolithotomy.

kidney pelvis or ureter. Afterward, a catheter or **ureteral stent,** a slender supportive device, is left in place for 3 days to splint the ureter or divert the urine past any possible tear in the ureteral wall (Fig. 64-7). If the stone cannot be removed, a ureteral catheter is left in place for 24 hours to dilate the ureter in the hope that the stone will pass through it or that it will be pulled into the bladder when the catheter is removed.

Stop, Think, and Respond ● BOX 64-2

For healthcare personnel to perform ESWL, the client must be in a clean water bath or surrounded by soft cushions. What concerns might the client have? What are your best responses?

Surgical Management

Calculi that are large or complicated by obstruction, ongoing urinary tract infection, kidney damage, or constant bleeding require surgical removal. Surgical options include a percutaneous nephrolithotomy (see Fig. 64-6), ureterolithotomy, pyelolithotomy, and nephrolithotomy. Drainage of urine from the affected kidney is accomplished with a nephrostomy tube during the postsurgical healing process.

A **nephrostomy tube,** also called a *pyelostomy tube,* is a catheter inserted through the skin into the renal pelvis. A nephrostomy tube is used to manage any obstruction to urine flow above the bladder. The tube is kept in place with a suture through the skin. Unlike the bladder, the kidney pelvis can hold only 5 to 8 mL of urine. If a blood clot or kinking or compression of the tubing impairs urinary drainage for even a short time, hydronephrosis and damage to surgically repaired tissue can result. The client complains of pain if the renal pelvis becomes distended with urine.

Percutaneous Nephrolithotomy

A percutaneous nephrolithotomy is an endoscopic procedure. A nephroscope is tunneled into the kidney through a tiny skin incision while the client is under general anesthesia (Fig 64-8). Ultrasound is used to crush the stone. The fragments are removed through the endoscope.

Ureterolithotomy, Pyelolithotomy, Nephrolithotomy

With the client anesthetized, a suprapubic abdominal or flank incision is made and the stone is removed under direct visualization. A **pyeloplasty,** surgical repair of

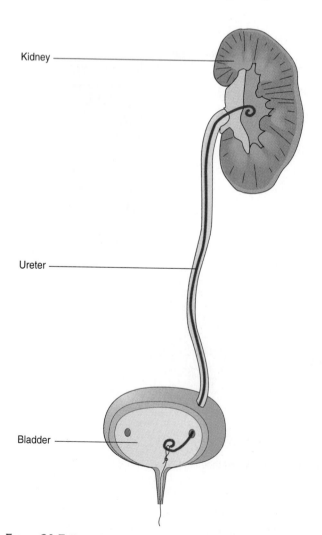

FIGURE 64-7 Example of a ureteral stent; in this case, a double J stent.

FIGURE 64-8 A nephroscope is inserted through a surgically created tunnel when a percutaneous nephrolithotomy is performed.

the ureteropelvic junction or other anatomic anomalies, may be performed at the same time. The additional surgery is done to correct conditions that contribute to the development of stones and prevent their recurrence. A nephrectomy is indicated if a stone has permanently and severely damaged a kidney beyond adequate function. The other kidney must be fully functional.

NURSING PROCESS

● The Client With Renal Calculi

Assessment

The nurse obtains a complete history, including a drug and allergy history, family history, history of immobility, episodes of dehydration, urinary tract infections, and diet. Assessment of pain intensity and location and associated symptoms such as nausea and vomiting is essential. In addition, the nurse monitors vital signs and assesses all urine for stones by straining it through a gauze or wire mesh and closely inspecting it. The nurse must save solid material for laboratory analysis. Urine may show evidence of hematuria. In some instances, the client may experience anuria related to bilateral obstruction and have abdominal distention.

Diagnosis, Planning, and Interventions

Three goals when caring for a client with urinary calculi include improving urinary output, relieving pain, and preventing or treating infection. Clients often are frightened because of the excruciating pain, and thus require emotional support as well as pain management. Typical diagnoses, expected outcomes, and interventions include, but are not limited to, the following.

Pain related to increased pressure in the renal pelvis or renal colic

Expected Outcome: Pain will decrease within 30 minutes of a nursing measure.

● Administer prescribed narcotic analgesic. *It assists in decreasing pain related to ureteral colic during an acute episode and promotes muscle relaxation.*

● Provide supplemental nonpharmacologic interventions such as a comfortable position, guided imagery, and distraction. *These measures promote relaxation, redirect attention, and enhance coping ability.*

● Encourage ambulation and liberal fluid intake when the client is comfortable. *The supine position can increase colic; ambulation relieves it. Increased fluid intake promotes the passage of a stone and prevents urinary stasis or the formation of new stones.*

PC: Hydronephrosis related to ureteral obstruction
Expected Outcome: The nurse will manage and minimize hydronephrosis.

● Monitor intake and output. *This record provides information about kidney function and indicates any complications such as hydronephrosis.*

● Administer antibiotics as ordered. *Antimicrobials treat the cause of urinary tract infection associated with urolithiasis and urinary stasis.*

● Manage a nephrostomy tube by following Nursing Guidelines 64-1. *Proper management ensures that the nephrostomy tube remains in place, urine drains properly, and infection is prevented.*

Risk for Infection related to urinary stasis
Expected Outcome: Urinary tract infection will not develop as evidenced by urine free of pus and microorganisms and normal temperature and white blood cell count.

● Administer antimicrobial therapy as prescribed. *Urinary tract infections potentiate stone formation. Antibiotics treat the infection.*

● Encourage fluid intake to 3000 mL/day unless contraindicated. *Increased hydration flushes bacteria, blood, and other debris, and may expedite stone passage.*

● Maintain patency of all catheters or encourage client to void every 2 to 3 hours. *Adequate urinary flow or frequent voiding prevents urinary stasis and eliminates bacteria, blood, and other particles.*

● Follow aseptic principles when changing dressings or urinary drainage equipment. *Strict asepsis prevents introduction of microbes into the urinary tract.*

Risk for Altered (Renal) Tissue Perfusion related to increased fluid pressure in ureter and kidney pelvis

---

NURSING GUIDELINES 64-1

Managing a Nephrostomy Tube

■ Connect the nephrostomy tube to a closed drainage system.

■ Have a second nephrostomy tube available at the bedside for the physician's use in case the present one is displaced.

■ Secure the tube to the client's flank with tape to ensure that it does not become dislodged.

■ Keep the urine collection bag below the level of insertion.

■ Never clamp the nephrostomy tubing.

■ Check that the nephrostomy and drainage tubing are not kinked or that the client is not compressing the tubing.

■ Use no more than 5 to 8 mL of sterile normal saline to maintain patency if an irrigation is medically ordered.

■ Record the urine output from the nephrostomy tube separately from other urinary volumes.

■ Assess the tube insertion site for bleeding and drainage.

■ Change the dressing around the nephrostomy tube if and when it becomes damp. Apply a skin barrier ointment around the incision to prevent excoriation.

■ Notify the physician immediately if the nephrostomy tube becomes dislodged or if there is an absence of urinary drainage.

Expected Outcome: Kidney will remain adequately perfused with blood as evidenced by normal serum creatinine, BUN, and distribution of radiopaque dye after IVP.

● Monitor laboratory and diagnostic test results. *Elevated BUN, creatinine, and electrolyte levels indicate kidney dysfunction and assist in evaluating hydration status and effectiveness of other interventions.*

● Prepare client safely but quickly for treatment measures that promote urinary drainage if it becomes apparent that kidney function is compromised. *Prompt intervention may prevent serious complications.*

Evaluation of Expected Outcomes

Pain is reduced. Urine output is balanced with intake. Urine is clear. The client is afebrile. Findings from urine and blood tests indicate adequate renal function.

For clients undergoing surgical procedures, the nurse explains the procedure and follows standards for perioperative care in Chapter 25. After lithotripsy, endoscopy, or surgery, the nurse assesses vital signs, measures fluid intake and output, and inspects the color of urine, which may be grossly bloody for a time. After ESWL, the nurse should inspect the flank for ecchymosis, which is expected. The nurse documents the location of discoloration. Clients require analgesics for postprocedural discomfort.

If a ureteroscopy is performed and a urethral catheter is in place, the nurse attaches the catheter to a closed drainage system. Pink-tinged urine may be seen, but if frank blood appears in the urine or the client complains of severe abdominal pain, the nurse must notify the physician immediately. If a ureteral stent is present, the nurse checks for the suture, which extends from the urinary meatus and is used for stent removal. It is important that the client maintain a total daily fluid volume of approximately 3000 mL. For more information, see Client and Family Teaching Box 64-1.

● URETERAL STRICTURE

A stricture is a narrowing of a lumen. A ureteral stricture is the narrowing of a ureter.

Pathophysiology and Etiology

A ureteral stricture is relatively rare, but the incidence is higher among those with chronic ureteral stone formation. The recurrent inflammation and infection cause scar tissue to accumulate in the ureter. Other conditions that can interfere with urine passing through the ureter are congenital anomalies or conditions that mechanically compress the ureter, such as pregnancy or tumors in the abdomen or upper urinary tract.

In many instances the ureter is only partially narrowed. Symptoms develop over time as the area of the

---

 64-1 *Client and Family Teaching*
Renal Calculi

The nurse includes the following recommendations when teaching the client and family:

■ Explain the causes of and methods to prevent renal calculi.

■ Recommend drinking plenty of liquids; water is one of the best.

■ Provide a list of foods (Box 64-3) restricted to small amounts if the stones are composed of calcium oxalate.

■ Review the self-administration of antimicrobial and analgesic drugs and, if prescribed, antigout medications. Discuss the purpose for the medications, dosing schedule, and side effects to report.

■ Discuss catheter or nephrostomy tube care.

■ Teach client how to strain urine if the stone or its fragments have not passed.

■ Advise client to report signs of acute obstruction immediately, such as inability or difficulty in voiding, or pain.

■ Identify signs of infection such as fever, chills, dysuria, frequency, urgency, and cloudy urine. Review the relationship between urinary calculi and infection.

■ Provide discharge teaching after a treatment procedure that includes activity level, hygiene measures, dietary modifications, goals for oral fluid intake, and wound care.

■ Emphasize consulting with the physician before self-administering any over-the-counter medications.

---

ureter above the stricture dilates with urine (*hydroureter*) and the kidney pelvis slowly enlarges. Stasis of urine promotes an upper urinary tract infection.

BOX 64-3 ● Sources of Calcium and Oxalate

Apples	Grapes
Asparagus	Ice cream
Beer	Milk
Beets	Oranges
Berries	Parsley
Black pepper	Peanut butter
Broccoli	Pineapples
Cheese	Rhubarb
Chocolate	Spinach
Cocoa	Swiss chard
Coffee	Tea
Cola	Turnips
Collards	Vitamin C
Figs	Yogurt

Assessment Findings

Flank pain or discomfort and tenderness at the costo-vertebral angle from enlargement of the renal pelvis often develops. The client experiences back or abdominal discomfort, which tends to increase during periods of elevated fluid intake. A voiding cystourethrogram and ultrasonography help to identify structural changes consistent with impaired passage of urine.

Medical and Surgical Management

Various measures are used to treat strictures. Management depends on the location, the density, and the length of the stricture. The ureter can be stretched by inserting a dilator called a *filiform* or *urethral sound,* a curved metal rod, followed by others that are sequentially larger.

If the obstruction persists, the physician performs a **ureteroplasty,** removal of the narrowed section of ureter and reconnection of the patent portions. This is the preferred procedure for a mid-ureteral stricture. A ureteral stent is placed in the ureter to provide support to the walls of the ureter, relieve the obstruction, and maintain the flow of urine through the ureter and into the bladder. Lower ureteral strictures are treated by removing the narrowed portion of the ureter and reimplanting the remaining section into the bladder wall.

Besides correcting strictures, ureteral surgery is performed to remove tumors, repair accidental ligation of the ureter during abdominal surgery (the highest incidence is seen in hysterectomies), and to extricate a ureteral stone that cannot be removed by other means.

Nursing Management

The nurse follows the standards of care for the perioperative client if the client undergoes surgery (see Chap. 25). If a ureteral catheter is inserted before surgery, the nurse measures the urine output from the catheter hourly. He or she must immediately report lack of urine output from the ureteral catheter.

On return from surgery, all urinary drainage tubes and catheters are connected to a closed drainage system or to the type of drainage system ordered by the physician. The main complication associated with ureteral surgery is failure of the ureter to transport urine from the kidney to the bladder. The nurse must contact the physician if:

- Signs of shock appear.
- Urinary output from the ureteral catheter is decreased or absent.
- The client complains of significant abdominal pain, which may indicate leakage of urine into the peritoneal cavity.

- Signs of a urinary tract infection develop, such as fever and chills, or the urine is cloudy or has a foul odor.

Depending on the surgical procedure, the client may need instruction in the care of the ureteral or urethral catheter(s), the management of the drainage collection system, incision care, and a review of the prescribed diet and medication schedule.

TUMORS OF THE KIDNEY

A *hypernephroma* (renal adenocarcinoma) is the most common malignant tumor of the kidney in adults. Squamous cell tumors are second. Men are affected more than women.

Pathophysiology and Etiology

The cause of kidney tumors is unknown. The incidence is higher in older adults, which suggests chronic exposure to a carcinogen whose metabolites involve renal excretion. Bladder cancer (see Chap. 65) is associated with the carcinogenic effects of long-term cigarette smoking. It is possible that renal tumors are similarly initiated through this mechanism or exposure to some other environmental toxin (e.g., asbestos) or volatile solvent (e.g., gasoline). Box 64-4 lists risk factors for renal cancer.

Because the kidneys are deeply protected in the body, tumors can become quite large before causing symptoms. As the tumor enlarges, it occupies space, extending into adjacent renal structures and interfering with urine outflow. Tumor cells tend to metastasize by way of the renal vein and vena cava to the lungs, bone, lymph nodes, liver, and brain. Lung metastases predominate. Sometimes, the first symptom occurs when the hypernephroma has metastasized to other organs.

Assessment Findings

The classic triad of renal cancer is painless hematuria, flank pain, and a palpable mass. Additional symptoms

---

BOX 64-4 ● Risk Factors for Renal Cancer

- Gender: Affects men more than women
- Tobacco use
- Occupational exposure to industrial chemicals, such as petroleum products, heavy metals, and asbestos
- Obesity
- Unopposed estrogen therapy
- Polycystic kidney disease

include weight loss, malaise, and unexplained fever. Later, there is colic-like discomfort during the passage of blood clots.

An abdominal mass found on a routine physical examination or on radiographic examination for other purposes suggests a kidney tumor. An IVP, cystoscopy with retrograde pyelograms, ultrasonography, MRI, renal angiography, and CT scan are used to locate the tumor. Sequential urine samples contain RBCs as well as malignant cells.

Medical and Surgical Management

Nephrectomy, including removal of the tumor, adrenal gland, surrounding perinephric fat, and fascia, is the treatment for a malignant renal tumor. When a tumor arises in the collecting system or the ureter, a complete nephroureterectomy (removal of the kidney and ureter) is done. A cuff of bladder tissue is removed as well because the recurrence rate in any stump of ureter left behind is high. Surgery may be followed by radiation therapy, chemotherapy, or both while the client is still in the hospital or on a postdischarge basis. If extensive metastases are found, only palliative treatment is given. When medical management is limited to palliative treatment because of metastases, the physician explains that the treatment measures are not curative.

Nursing Management

In addition to the standard preoperative preparations, the nurse implements other prescribed procedures that facilitate the postoperative assessment and recovery of the client, such as inserting a urethral catheter and nasogastric tube.

NURSING PROCESS

● The Client Recovering From a Nephrectomy

Assessment

On the client's return from surgery, the nurse assesses vital signs frequently. Inspecting and identifying the type and location of drains or catheters are important measures. The indwelling (Foley) catheter drainage system is placed below the level of the bed. Drains in or around the incision may drain by closed negative pressure (i.e., Jackson-Pratt) or low mechanical suction.

Diagnosis, Planning, and Interventions

PC: Internal Hemorrhage related to bleeding from the ligated renal artery or vein

Expected Outcome: The nurse will manage and minimize hemorrhage.

- Monitor blood pressure and pulse rate every 1 to 4 hours for the first 24 to 48 hours after surgery. *Decreased intravascular volume results in hypotension and tachycardia. Frequent monitoring assists in detecting changes in intravascular volume.*
- Report decreased blood pressure, increased pulse, restlessness, or sudden onset of flank pain. *Death can occur quickly unless the client is immediately returned to surgery to control the bleeding.*
- Administer IV fluids and blood transfusions as ordered. *Isotonic fluids and blood replacement help to restore and maintain intravascular volume.*
- Note and record the color of drainage from each tube and catheter. *Assessment findings direct interventions and provide a means for further comparison and evaluation.*
- Follow the physician's orders concerning postoperative positioning. *Keeping the client from lying on the operative side avoids interference with wound drainage.*
- Contact the surgeon about any frank bleeding or a sudden decrease in urine output. *Although pink-tinged drainage is normal for several days after surgery, frank bleeding, sudden decreased urine, or both indicate complications.*

Pain related to tissue trauma and pressure from urinary obstruction

Expected Outcome: Pain will be relieved to a tolerable level within 30 minutes of an intervention.

- Keep drainage catheters unclamped, unkinked, and below the level of insertion. *Unobstructed urine flow promotes urine elimination and prevents pain related to obstruction.*
- Secure all tubings to reduce movement at the site of insertion or displacement. *This measure reduces pain at the insertion site and promotes comfort.*
- Encourage oral fluids as soon as allowed and tolerated without causing nausea or vomiting. *Fluids dilute the urine and prevent catheter obstruction from sediment or small blood clots, thus reducing potential for pain and discomfort.*
- Irrigate tubings as ordered. *Irrigation promotes urinary flow and reduces potential for pain.*
- Administer prescribed analgesia and supplement drug therapy with nursing measures that promote comfort. *Analgesics and nonpharmacologic methods assist in reducing pain and promote the client's sense of control and participation in self-care.*
- Splint the incision when repositioning the client or during efforts to cough and deep breathe. *Splinting reduces tension on the surgical site and prevents or reduces pain-related movement.*

Risk for Ineffective Breathing Pattern related to incisional pain and restricted positioning; **Risk for Ineffective Airway Clearance** related to weak cough secondary to incisional pain

Expected Outcomes: Breathing rate and depth will be sufficient to maintain blood oxygen saturation (SpO_2) at

90% or above. Secretions will be raised. Lung sounds will be clear in all lobes.

- Encourage client to breathe deeply and cough every 2 hours. Use an incentive spirometer to evaluate effectiveness. *These efforts increase alveolar ventilation and assist in clearing secretions.*
- Use two hands to apply firm support of the incision when the client coughs or performs deep breathing exercises. *This technique splints the incision, reducing pain and promoting the client's ability to breathe deeply and cough.*
- Auscultate the lungs daily; notify the physician of any abnormal or absent breath sounds. *Breath sounds should be clear. Fine, scattered crackles at bases indicate that the client should be more vigorous in deep breathing and coughing. Coarser crackles indicate fluid in the airway; wheezes indicate a partial obstruction. Absent breath sounds require prompt intervention.*

Risk for Infection related to impaired skin integrity and stasis of urine

Expected Outcome: Client will be free of infection as evidenced by normal findings in temperature, urine culture, and white blood cell count.

- Monitor temperature every 4 hours. *Fever usually is the first and only sign of infection.*
- Contact the physician if the client's temperature is above 101°F (38.3°C) or he or she experiences chills, or if purulent drainage or redness, swelling, and warmth at the incision are noted. *Elevated temperatures and incisional signs indicate an infection that requires intervention.*
- Use aseptic technique when changing the surgical dressing or managing the catheter and drainage systems. *Asepsis prevents introduction of microorganisms to the urinary tract or to areas where skin integrity has been lost.*
- Administer antibiotic therapy as prescribed. *Antibiotics treat infections, reducing the risk of further infection.*

Evaluation of Expected Outcomes

The client shows no evidence of hemorrhage. Interventions reduce or eliminate pain. Breathing rate and depth maintain the SpO$_2$ at 90% or above. The client raises secretions, and lung sounds are clear in all lobes. No infections develop.

Clients who have had a nephrectomy usually have the drains (if any) removed before discharge. A dressing over the incision may or may not be required. If the physician orders a dressing applied and changed at home, the nurse shows the client and family how to change the dressing and provides a list of the necessary materials for dressing changes (Client and Family Teaching Box 64-2).

RENAL FAILURE ●

Renal failure is the inability of the nephrons in the kidneys to maintain fluid, electrolyte, and acid-base balance,

64-2 *Client and Family Teaching*
Home Care After Nephrectomy

The teaching plan should include the following:

- Change the dressing as ordered by the physician.
- Wash hands thoroughly before and after each dressing change.
- Drink plenty of fluids and follow the diet recommended by the physician.
- Avoid exposure to others who have possible infections.
- Take prescribed medication as directed on the container. Do not omit a dose.
- Contact the physician immediately if pain, fever, or chills occurs or if the urine becomes bloody, cloudy, or foul smelling.

excrete nitrogen waste products, and perform regulatory functions such as maintaining calcification of bones and producing erythropoietin. There are two types of renal failure: acute and chronic. **Acute renal failure** (ARF) is characterized by a sudden and rapid decrease in renal function. ARF potentially is reversible with early, aggressive treatment of its contributing etiology. **Chronic renal failure** (CRF) is characterized by progressive and irreversible damage to the nephrons. It may take months to years for CRF to develop.

Pathophysiology and Etiology

Acute Renal Failure

Renal failure can develop as a consequence of prerenal, intrarenal, and postrenal disorders (Table 64-3). Prerenal disorders are nonurologic conditions that disrupt renal blood flow to the nephrons, affecting their filtering ability. Intrarenal conditions are conditions in the kidney itself that destroy nephrons. Postrenal disorders usually are obstructive problems in structures below the kidney(s) that have damaging repercussions for the nephrons above.

Acute renal failure progresses through four phases:

1. Initiation phase
2. Oliguric phase
3. Diuretic phase
4. Recovery phase

INITIATION PHASE

The initiation phase begins with the onset of the contributing event. It is accompanied by reduced blood flow to the nephrons to the point of acute tubular necrosis.

TABLE 64-3	CAUSES OF RENAL FAILURE		
PRERENAL	**INTRARENAL**		**POSTRENAL**
Hypovolemic shock	Ischemia		Ureteral calculi
Cardiogenic shock secondary to congestive heart failure	Nephrotoxicity secondary to drugs such as amino-glycosides		Prostatic hypertrophy
Septic shock	Acute and chronic glomerulonephritis		Ureteral stricture
Anaphylaxis	Polycystic disease		Ureteral or bladder tumor
Dehydration	Untreated prerenal and postrenal disorders		
Renal artery thrombosis or stenosis	Myoglobinuria secondary to burns		
Cardiac arrest	Hemoglobinuria secondary to transfusion reaction		
Lethal dysrhythmias			

Acute tubular necrosis refers to the death of cells in the collecting tubules of the nephrons where reabsorption of water, electrolytes, and excretion of protein wastes and excess metabolic substances occurs (Fig. 64-9).

OLIGURIC PHASE

The oliguric phase is associated with the excretion of less than adequate urinary volumes. This phase begins within 48 hours after the initial cellular insult and may last for 10 to 14 days or longer (Porth, 2002). Fluid volume excess develops, which leads to edema, hypertension, and cardio-pulmonary complications. Azotemia, the marked accumulation of urea and other nitrogenous wastes such as creatinine and uric acid in the blood, creates a potential for neurologic changes such as seizures, coma, and death.

Currently there is better treatment of many prerenal causes of ARF. For that reason, some clients excrete urinary volumes greater than 500 mL/day. The urine has a very low specific gravity, however, because it lacks normal amounts of excreted substances such as excess potassium and hydrogen ions, to maintain homeostasis. Consequently, hyperkalemia, metabolic acidosis, and **uremia,** a toxic state caused by the accumulation of nitrogen wastes, develop regardless of the excreted water volume.

DIURETIC PHASE

Diuresis begins as the nephrons recover. Despite an increased water content of urine, the excretion of wastes and electrolytes continues to be impaired. The BUN, creatinine, potassium, and phosphate levels remain elevated in the blood.

RECOVERY PHASE

It may take 1 or more years of recovery while normal glomerular filtration and tubular function are restored. Some clients recover completely, whereas others develop varying degrees of permanent renal dysfunction.

Chronic Renal Failure

CRF is associated more often with intrarenal conditions or is a complication of systemic diseases such as diabetes mellitus and disseminated lupus erythematosus. In CRF, the kidneys are so extensively damaged that they do not adequately remove protein byproducts and electrolytes from the blood and do not maintain acid-base balance. There are three stages of CRF:

- Reduced renal reserve—40% to 75% loss of nephron function
- Renal insufficiency—75% to 90% loss of nephron function
- **End-stage renal disease**—less than 10% of nephron function remains. This is the point at which a regular course of dialysis or kidney transplantation is necessary to maintain life (Box 64-5).

Because damage to the nephrons is slow, declining renal function is less apparent until the end stage. The BUN and serum creatinine levels gradually rise. Hypona-

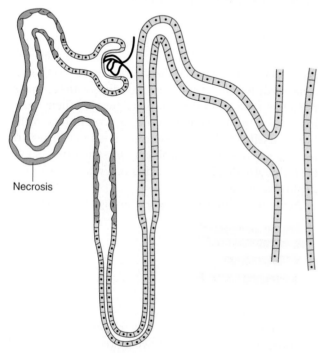

Necrosis

FIGURE 64-9 Acute tubular necrosis.

BOX 64-5 ● Stages of Chronic Renal Disease

STAGE 1
Reduced renal reserve, characterized by a 40% to 75% loss of nephron function. The patient usually does not have symptoms because the remaining nephrons are able to carry out the normal functions of the kidney.

STAGE 2
Renal insufficiency occurs when 75% to 90% of nephron function is lost. At this point, the serum creatinine and BUN rise, the kidney loses its ability to concentrate urine, and anemia develops. The patient may report polyuria and nocturia.

STAGE 3
End-stage renal disease (ESRD), the final stage of chronic renal failure, occurs when there is less than 10% of nephron function remaining. All of the normal regulatory, excretory, and hormonal functions of the kidney are severely impaired. ESRD is evidenced by elevated creatinine and BUN levels as well as electrolyte imbalances. Once the patient reaches this point, dialysis usually is indicated. Many of the symptoms of uremia are reversible with dialysis.

---

tremia is a reflection of diluted sodium ions in an excess volume of water in the blood. Actual electrolyte imbalances include hyperkalemia, hyperphosphatemia, hypermagnesemia, and hypocalcemia. The skin becomes the excretory organ for the substances the kidney usually clears from the body. A precipitate, referred to as **uremic frost,** may form on the skin.

Metabolic acidosis develops because the tubules cannot convert carbonic acid in the blood to water and bicarbonate ions. Erythropoietin production is inadequate, causing anemia. Susceptibility to infection increases as a result of a deficient immune system, particularly cellular immunity (see Chap. 41), as well as a decrease in the white blood cell count. Edema and hypertension are consequences of impaired urinary elimination. **Osteodystrophy,** a condition in which the bones become demineralized, occurs from hypocalcemia and hyperphosphatemia. The parathyroid glands secrete more parathormone to raise blood calcium levels.

Assessment Findings

Signs and Symptoms

In both ARF and CRF, the client has elevated blood pressure and weight gain. Urine output usually is decreased. Those with CRF develop other symptoms as the disease worsens. Facial features appear puffy from fluid retention. The skin is pale. Ulceration and bleeding of the gastrointestinal tract may occur. The oral mucous membranes bleed, and blood may be found in the feces. The client reports vague symptoms such as lethargy, headache, anorexia, and dry mouth. Later, other problems develop such as pruritus and dry, scaly skin. The breath and body may have an odor characteristic of urine. Muscle cramps,

bone pain or tenderness, and spontaneous fractures can develop. Mental processes progressively slow as electrolyte imbalances become marked and nitrogenous wastes accumulate. The client may experience seizures. Table 64-4 lists the systemic manifestations of CRF.

Diagnostic Findings

Laboratory blood tests reveal elevations in BUN, creatinine, potassium, magnesium, and phosphorus. Calcium levels are low. The RBC count, hematocrit, and hemoglobin are decreased. The pH of the blood is on the acidotic side. Urinalysis reveals a decreased specific gravity. An IVP provides evidence of renal dysfunction. In clients with severe renal failure, dye excretion usually is delayed. A percutaneous renal biopsy shows destruction of nephrons. Radiography and ultrasonography demonstrate structural defects in the kidneys, ureters, and bladder. Renal angiography identifies obstructions in blood vessels.

Medical Management

Prevention of ARF is an important function of physicians. Clients at risk for dehydration are adequately hydrated. Risks for dehydration include surgery, diagnostic studies that require fluid restriction and contrast agents, and treatment for cancer or metabolic disorders. Shock and hypotension are treated as quickly as possible with replacement fluids and blood. Treating infections promptly and thoroughly also is important, and greatly assists in preventing sepsis. Continuous monitoring of renal function is very important for clients at risk for ARF. Nurses

TABLE 64-4	**SYSTEMIC COMPLICATIONS OF CHRONIC RENAL FAILURE**
BODY SYSTEM	**COMPLICATION**
Cardiovascular	Congestive heart failure, hypertension, cardiac dysrhythmias, edema
Metabolic	Electrolyte imbalance, metabolic acidosis
Respiratory	Shortness of breath, pulmonary edema
Gastrointestinal	Malnutrition, vitamin deficiencies, anorexia, nausea, bleeding
Integumentary	Dry skin, pruritus
Neurologic	Lethargy, confusion, depression, seizures, coma
Sensory	Peripheral neuropathies
Musculoskeletal	Bone demineralization, muscle cramps, joint pain
Immunologic	Impaired immune function, decreased antibody production, increased incidence of hepatitis B and other infections

are crucial in monitoring renal function, as well as preventing toxic drug effects (Smeltzer & Bare, 2000).

In ARF, measures are taken to quickly remedy the primary cause of renal failure. Renal damage can be limited by aggressively administering parenteral fluids to increase plasma volume, giving vasodilating and diuretic drugs, and infusing dopamine (Intropin) to improve cardiac output and perfuse the renal arteries.

To reduce complications and keep the client alive during the 2 or 3 weeks while the tubules are regenerating, hemodialysis (discussed later), a technique in which the blood is filtered externally with a machine, is performed. When hemodialysis is a temporary measure, the blood is removed and returned through a double-lumen catheter or twin central venous catheters (Fig. 64-10). Another option is peritoneal dialysis, a much slower process (discussed later) in which fluids and electrolytes are removed by osmosis and diffusion across the peritoneum, which acts as a semipermeable membrane.

Fluid and dietary restrictions that include low protein, high calories, low sodium, and low potassium are required as the client is stabilized. Sodium polystyrene sulfonate (Kayexalate), an ion-exchange resin, is prescribed for oral or rectal administration to remove excess potassium when hyperkalemia occurs. An IV infusion of glucose and insulin also facilitates movement of potassium within the cell. Acid-base balance is restored by administering IV sodium bicarbonate if renal function is insufficient to do so.

The medical management of CRF is similar to that for ARF, except the period of treatment is lifelong (unless a kidney transplantation is performed). Rather than administer blood transfusions to correct chronic anemia, epoetin alfa (Epogen) is administered to stimulate bone marrow production of RBCs.

Surgical Management

Some clients in the end stage of CRF are candidates for kidney transplantation. One healthy kidney can perform the work of two. Donors for a transplant are selected from compatible living donors who may or may not be relatives or from organ donors who are brain dead and whose next of kin give permission for harvesting organs. Any potential donor with a history of hypertension, malignant disease, or diabetes is excluded from donation. To facilitate matching a recipient with a donor, a client is placed on a national computerized transplant waiting list. Whenever an organ becomes available, the computer searches for the recipient who is the best match.

When a transplantation is performed, the donor kidney is inserted through an abdominal incision and the nonfunctioning kidneys are left in place unless the client is extremely hypertensive. The blood vessels from the donor kidney are sutured to the iliac artery and vein and the ureter is implanted in the bladder (Fig. 64-11).

Even a perfect match does not guarantee that a transplanted organ will not be rejected. Ironically, even some less than perfectly matched transplanted organs are successful primarily because of immunosuppressive drugs such as:

- azathioprine (Imuran)
- corticosteroids (prednisone)
- cyclosporine—available as a microemulsion (Neoral), which provides a more sustained concentration
- tacrolimus (Prograf; formerly FK-506)—similar to cyclosporine but more potent
- mycophenolate mofetil (CellCept; formerly RS-61433)—specifically for preventing kidney transplant rejection (Smeltzer & Bare, 2000)
- muromonab-CD-3 (Orthoclone OKT3)—a monoclonal antibody

If rejection occurs, the client resumes hemodialysis and waits for another transplant.

Nursing Management

Before conducting an initial interview and physical assessment, the nurse attempts to learn the cause (if known), type (acute versus chronic), and prognosis of the renal disorder. Clients may be unable to give an accurate history because of the effect of renal failure on the thought processes or because they are acutely ill. It may be necessary to obtain information from the family. The nursing care for the client undergoing renal transplantation is complex and specialized. Standard postoperative nursing interventions are applicable (see Chap. 25), with the added consideration of assessing for signs of rejection and prevention of infection. Box 64-6 describes signs and symptoms of transplant rejection.

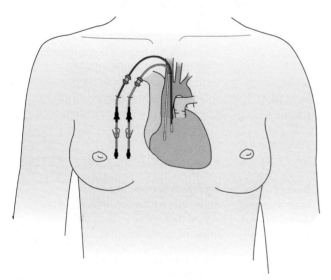

Figure 64-10 Twin catheters used for emergency hemodialysis.

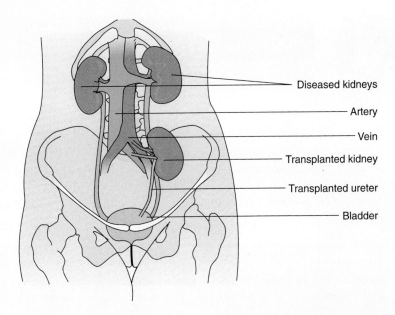

Diseased kidneys

Artery

Vein

Transplanted kidney

Transplanted ureter

Bladder

FIGURE 64-11 Transplanted kidney and ureter.

Nursing care for clients with renal failure is extensive. See Nursing Care Plan 64-1 and Client and Family Teaching Box 64-3 for more information.

> ### Stop, Think, and Respond ● BOX 64-3
>
> *Clients who have a kidney transplant are at risk for infection. What nursing measures help to prevent infection?*

DIALYSIS

Dialysis is a procedure for cleaning and filtering the blood. It substitutes for kidney function when the kidneys cannot remove the nitrogenous waste products and maintain adequate fluid, electrolyte, and acid-base balances.

During dialysis, the client's blood is filtered by diffusion and osmosis (see Chap. 22). Substances such as water, urea, creatinine, and dangerously high levels of potassium move from the blood through the semipermeable membrane to the **dialysate,** the solution used during dialysis that has a composition similar to normal human plasma. Dialysis is performed by hemodialysis and peritoneal dialysis. Either technique can be per-

> ### BOX 64-6 ● Signs and Symptoms of Kidney Transplant Rejection
>
> Oliguria
> Edema
> Fever
> Increasing blood pressure
> Weight gain
> Swelling or tenderness over the transplanted kidney
> Increase in serum creatinine levels

formed at home or in a dialysis center. Each type has advantages and disadvantages (Table 64-5).

● HEMODIALYSIS

Hemodialysis requires transporting blood from the client through a **dialyzer,** a semipermeable membrane filter in a machine (Fig. 64-12). The dialyzer contains many tiny hollow fibers. Blood moves through the hollow fibers. Water and wastes from the blood move into the dialysate fluid that flows around the fibers, but protein and RBCs do not (See Fig. 64-12). The filtered blood is returned to the client. The entire cycle takes 4 to 6 hours and is performed three times a week.

There are several methods for facilitating the removal and return of the client's dialyzed blood. One technique using tunneled central venous catheter access has already been described. Two others more commonly used for clients with CRF are (1) arteriovenous (AV) fistula and (2) AV graft.

Arteriovenous Fistula

An **arteriovenous fistula** is a surgical anastomosis (connection) of an artery and vein lying in close proximity (Fig. 64-13). The vessels usually joined are the cephalic vein and the radial artery or the cephalic vein and brachial artery. Fistulas are preferred over grafts because they have a better record of remaining patent and have fewer complications, such as thrombosis and infection, compared with other access options. They require from 1 to 4 months to mature, however, before being used. Consequently, some fistulas are created prematurely so they are ready when a client eventually requires dialysis.

(text continued on page 1034)

Nursing Care Plan 64-1

THE CLIENT WITH CHRONIC RENAL FAILURE

Assessment

■ Assess fluid status, including problems related to imbalanced intake and output.

■ Monitor nutritional status, making sure the client follows the appropriate restrictions.

■ Assess emotional status to provide relevant support.

Nursing Diagnosis: **Excess Fluid Volume** related to impaired renal function

Expected Outcome: Client will maintain appropriate body weight without excess fluid.

Interventions	Rationales
Weigh client daily under the same conditions: time, clothing, scale.	Information provides a baseline and database for monitoring changes. A gain of 1 kg (2.2 lb) equals 1 L of fluid.
Record output accurately.	Output determines intake. Usually, client is allowed 500 mL intake (equals insensible fluid losses) plus the volume of excreted urine per day.
Assess lung sounds, respiratory rate and effort, and heart sounds. Inspect for jugular vein distention.	Findings provide a baseline and database to determine fluid volume excess, needed interventions, and effects of treatments. Fluid overload may cause pulmonary edema.
Monitor laboratory studies.	Results assist in identifying fluid excess and promote earlier interventions.
Administer prescribed diuretics and antihypertensives.	These drugs reduce fluid excess and decrease cardiac workload.
Prepare client for dialysis.	Dialysis reduces uremic toxins, corrects electrolyte imbalances, and decreases fluid overload.

Evaluation of Expected Outcome: Client demonstrates appropriate urine output/fluid balance as evidenced by stable weight, vital signs within normal range for the client, no edema, and only slightly elevated electrolyte levels.

Nursing Diagnosis: **Imbalanced Nutrition: Risk for Less than Body Requirements** related to anorexia, increased metabolic needs, and dietary restrictions

Expected Outcome: Client will maintain adequate nutritional intake.

Interventions	Rationales
Monitor and record client's dietary intake.	Findings provide a database for nutritional changes and effects of interventions.
Provide frequent small feedings.	They minimize nausea and anorexia and promote the intake of high-calorie, nutritious foods.
Encourage client to be involved with food choices and times for meals.	Involving the client promotes interest and control and considers dietary habits and preferences.
Explain restrictions and provide a list of nutritional needs and acceptable food choices.	Doing so promotes client's understanding of the relationship of food intake to kidney disease and provides a positive approach to dietary restrictions.

(continued)

Nursing Care Plan 64-1 (Continued)

THE CLIENT WITH CHRONIC RENAL FAILURE

Evaluation of Expected Outcome: Client maintains weight, unrelated to fluid volume, following dietary needs and restrictions.

Nursing Diagnosis: **Risk for Impaired Tissue Integrity** related to restricted oral intake and increased nitrogenous wastes in body fluids such as saliva

Expected Outcome: The oral mucosa and lips will remain moist and intact.

Interventions	*Rationales*
Assess mouth for inflammation, ulceration, or bleeding.	Findings provide a database for intervention and evaluation of treatment effectiveness.
Instruct or assist client to provide mouth care after each meal and at bedtime or every 4 hours while awake. Encourage client to swish but not swallow water frequently as desired.	Frequent mouth care removes debris, rinses away nitrogenous wastes in saliva, prevents accumulation of bacteria, and keeps mucous membranes moist.
Provide lanolin-based lip balm for use as needed.	It keeps lips moist and promotes integrity, preventing bleeding and introduction of microorganisms.

Evaluation of Expected Outcome: Client performs frequent mouth care. Mucous membranes and lips remain moist and intact.

Nursing Diagnosis: **Activity Intolerance** related to fatigue, anemia, weakness, retention of nitrogenous waste products, and dialysis procedure

Expected Outcome: Client will participate in activities as tolerated.

Interventions	*Rationales*
Determine cause of activity intolerance.	Knowing the cause assists in planning appropriate interventions.
If able, encourage client to increase activity slowly. Perform range-of-motion exercises as tolerated.	Activity and exercises help maintain or improve muscle tone, strength, and endurance.
Provide periods of rest between activities.	Rest decreases oxygen consumption and improves energy levels.

Evaluation of Expected Outcome: Client participates in activities and can do ADLs with minimal assistance.

PCs: **Hypertension, Azotemia, Electrolyte Imbalances, Anemia**

Expected Outcome: Nurse will minimize and manage potential complications.

Interventions	*Rationales*
Administer prescribed antihypertensive and diuretic medications as ordered.	They lower blood pressure and increase urine output from partially functional kidneys.
Restrict protein intake to foods that are complete proteins (contain all essential amino acids) within prescribed limits.	Complete proteins provide positive nitrogen balance needed for healing and growth.
Provide sufficient calories from carbohydrates and fats.	Doing so prevents catabolism of muscle and body stores of protein.

(continued)

Nursing Care Plan 64-1 *(Continued)*

THE CLIENT WITH CHRONIC RENAL FAILURE

Interventions	*Rationales*
Monitor cardiac rhythm.	Hyperkalemia and other electrolyte imbalances can cause dangerous dysrhythmias.
Restrict sources of potassium usually found in fresh fruits and vegetables.	Hyperkalemia can cause life-threatening changes.
Be prepared to administer glucose and regular insulin.	They promote transfer of potassium from extracellular to intracellular locations.
Restrict sodium intake as ordered.	Doing so prevents excess sodium and fluid accumulation.
Administer calcium supplements, vitamin D supplements, and phosphate binders (Amphogel); at same time, limit phosphorus-containing foods such as dairy products, dried beans, and soft drinks.	CRF causes numerous physiologic changes that affect calcium, phosphorus, and vitamin D metabolism, requiring supplementation and dietary restrictions.
Administer prescribed iron and folic acid supplements or Epogen.	Iron and folic acid supplements are needed for RBC production. Epogen stimulates bone marrow to produce RBCs.

Evaluation of Expected Outcome: Blood pressure is 140/90 mm Hg. BUN and creatinine levels are slightly elevated. Serum electrolyte levels are minimally elevated. RBC and hemoglobin levels are within normal levels.

Nursing Diagnosis: Risk for Impaired Skin Integrity related to scratching secondary to pruritus

Expected Outcome: Skin will remain intact and free of crystals.

Interventions	*Rationales*
Instruct client to limit bathing to less than ½ hour, using lukewarm water and glycerin-based soap. Add emollient to skin two to three times a day.	These measures reduce skin drying while rinsing away nitrogenous waste products. Emollients restore moisture. All measures help to maintain skin integrity.
Keep the environment humidified.	Humidification provides moisture to the skin and prevents drying.
Institute measures that prevent client from scratching, such as keeping fingernails short and encouraging client to use soft clothing and bedding.	These measures prevent trauma to the skin and maintain skin integrity.

Evaluation of Expected Outcome: Client maintains intact skin without evidence of crystals.

Nursing Diagnosis: Risk for Infection related to compromised immune defenses

Expected Outcome: Client will remain free of infection.

Interventions	*Rationales*
Monitor temperature at least every shift. Monitor for signs and symptoms of infection.	Clients with kidney failure are very prone to infection. Chills, malaise, sore throat, redness, drainage, and elevated temperature are all signs of infection.
Restrict contact with family, friends, or staff who may have an infectious disorder.	Doing so prevents spread of microorganisms to immunocompromised client.

(continued)

Nursing Care Plan 64-1 (Continued)

THE CLIENT WITH CHRONIC RENAL FAILURE

Interventions	Rationales
Ensure that all who come in contact with client practice appropriate aseptic technique.	Handwashing, clean environment, and asepsis prevent the spread of microorganisms.

Evaluation of Expected Outcome: Client is afebrile and demonstrates no signs or symptoms of infection.

Nursing Diagnosis: **Situational Low Self-Esteem** related to change in body image, dependency, and role change.

Expected Outcome: Client will seek help as needed and demonstrate improved self-concept.

Interventions	Rationales
Demonstrate acceptance and respect for client.	They promote client's self-acceptance.
Assess client's relationships with significant others.	Doing so identifies client's strengths and support systems.
Encourage client and significant others to discuss changes produced by the disease and its treatments.	Identifying concerns and questions helps arrive at solutions.
Provide information about support groups.	They give an opportunity for clients and families to receive support and understanding. They also assist with coping.

Evaluation of Expected Outcome: Client demonstrates improved self-concept as evidenced by positive coping skills, ability to express concerns, and ability to seek support.

64-3 *Client and Family Teaching*
The Client With Chronic Renal Failure

Develop a teaching plan based on the following:

- Follow the diet and fluid intake recommended by the physician. Do not use salt substitutes (which often contain potassium) unless allowed by the physician.
- Take medications exactly as prescribed by the physician.
- Do not use any nonprescription drug unless use is approved by the physician.
- Measure and record fluid intake and urine output. Limit fluids as recommended.
- Avoid exposure to those with any type of infection (e.g., colds, sore throats, flu).
- Monitor blood pressure as recommended by the physician.
- Keep skin clean and dry. Take brief showers with tepid water, pat skin to dry, use moisturizing lotions or creams like Eucerin, Nivea, Alpha Keri, or Lubriderm. Avoid scratching.
- When doing laundry, use a mild laundry detergent. Use an extra rinse cycle to remove all detergent or add 1 tsp of vinegar per quart of water to the rinse cycle to remove detergent residue.
- Keep a record of daily weight, and report any rapid weight gain to the physician.
- Take frequent rest periods; avoid heavy exercise.
- If any of the following occurs, contact the physician immediately: inability to urinate, slow decrease in daily urine output, weight gain (more than 5 lb or amount recommended by physician), chills, fever, sore throat, cough, blood in the urine or stool, easy bleeding or bruising, lethargy, extreme fatigue, persistent headache, nausea, vomiting, or diarrhea.

TABLE 64-5	COMPARISON OF HEMODIALYSIS AND PERITONEAL DIALYSIS	
TYPE OF DIALYSIS	**ADVANTAGES**	**DISADVANTAGES**

Hemodialysis	Rapid removal of solutes and water
	Takes less time
	
	No risk for peritonitis
	Personnel perform procedure in a
	   dialysis center
		Bulge from fistula or graft is obvious
		Risk for vascular complications, infection, distal ischemia, carpal
		   tunnel syndrome, hypotension, and disequilibrium
		Strict fluid and dietary restrictions
		Lifestyle cycles around dialysis appointments
		Home hemodialysis requires space for the machine and
		   training to use it

Peritoneal	Simple to perform Facilitates independence Easier access No anticoagulation Fewer problems with hypotension or disequilibrium Less rigid dietary and fluid restrictions More flexibility in lifestyle and activities	More time-consuming Weight gain from glucose in the dialysate Peritonitis is a potential complication Requires training and motivation

At the time of dialysis, two venipunctures are performed at either end of the fistula. The distal venipuncture is used to remove blood that is transported to the machine. The proximal needle puncture is used to return the dialyzed blood. When dialysis is completed, the needles are removed and pressure dressings are applied for several hours.

Blood samples are taken before and after dialysis. The client's predialysis and postdialysis weights are compared. Sometimes as much as 10 lbs of fluid is removed. Examples of postdialysis laboratory studies include BUN, creatinine, sodium, potassium, chlorides, and hematocrit. These are used as indicators of the efficiency of dialysis.

Arteriovenous Graft

An **arteriovenous graft** is a type of vascular access method that uses a tube of synthetic material (e.g., Gore-Tex or polytetrafluoroethylene) to connect a vein and artery in the upper or lower arm (see Fig. 64-13). The graft pulsates with blood flow. AV grafts can be used 14 days after their insertion. Although the graft reseals after

Dialyzer
(where filtering
takes place)

Blood flows
back to body

Hemodialysis
machine

Blood flows
to dialyzer

FIGURE 64-12 Hemodialysis machine and dialyzer.

Cephalic vein
Radial artery

Median cubital vein
Graft
Radial artery

FIGURE 64-13 An internal arteriovenous fistula (*top*) is created by a side-to-side anastomosis of the artery and vein. A graft (*bottom*) can also be established between the artery and vein.

each needle puncture, the expected life of the graft is 3 to 5 years with repeated use.

Nursing Management

The nurse assesses and records vital signs before and after hemodialysis as well as weighing the client and obtaining blood for laboratory testing. To prepare for vascular access the nurse:

- Inspects the skin over the fistula or graft for signs of infection
- Palpates for a **thrill** (vibration) over the vascular access or listens for a **bruit,** a loud sound caused by turbulent blood flow (Fig. 64-14). If absent, the nurse postpones further use and reports findings.
- Notes the color of skin and nailbeds and mobility of fingers

FIGURE 64-14 A nurse auscultates the bruit in the client's fistula.

- Washes the skin over the fistula or graft with soap and water or antiseptic
- Avoids puncturing the same site that was used previously
- After dialysis is completed, does not administer injections for 2 to 4 hours. This allows time for the metabolism and excretion of heparin, which is administered during dialysis, to reach safe levels.
- Before discharging the client, observes for disequilibrium syndrome

Disequilibrium syndrome is a neurologic condition believed to be caused by cerebral edema. The shift in cerebral fluid volume occurs when the concentrations of solutes in the blood are lowered rapidly during dialysis. Decreasing solute concentration lowers the plasma osmolality. Water then floods the brain tissue. The syndrome is characterized by headache, disorientation, restlessness, blurred vision, confusion, and seizures. The symptoms are self-limiting and disappear within several hours after dialysis as fluid and solute concentrations equalize. The syndrome can be prevented by slowing the dialysis process to allow time for gradual equilibration of water.

The nurse teaches the client undergoing hemodialysis the following:

- Avoid carrying heavy items in the arm with the fistula or graft.
- Wear clothing with loose sleeves or made of fabrics that will not obstruct blood flow.
- Do not sleep on the vascular access arm.
- Do not permit venipunctures, injections, or blood pressures in the arm with the vascular access.
- Wash the skin over the vascular access daily.
- Assess for a thrill or bruit daily.
- Report signs of an infection or signs of impaired blood flow to dialysis personnel or physician immediately.

● PERITONEAL DIALYSIS

Peritoneal dialysis uses the peritoneum, the semipermeable membrane lining the abdomen, to filter fluid, wastes, and chemicals (Fig. 64-15). The dialysate is instilled and drained from the abdominal cavity by means of a catheter. Substances pass from the tiny blood vessels in the peritoneal membrane into the dialysate. The catheter, which has many perforations, is sutured in place and a dressing is applied. There are three types of peritoneal dialysis: (1) continuous ambulatory peritoneal dialysis (CAPD), (2) continuous cyclic peritoneal dialysis (CCPD), and intermittent peritoneal dialysis (IPD).

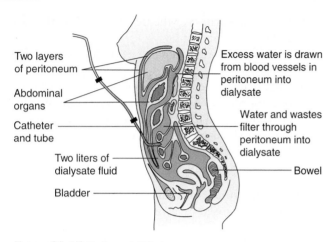

Two layers of peritoneum

Abdominal organs

Catheter and tube

Two liters of dialysate fluid

Bladder

Excess water is drawn from blood vessels in peritoneum into dialysate

Water and wastes filter through peritoneum into dialysate

Bowel

FIGURE 64-15 Peritoneal dialysis.

Continuous Ambulatory Peritoneal Dialysis

When CAPD is performed, approximately 2000 mL of dialysate is instilled by gravity through the catheter in 30 to 40 minutes. The catheter is clamped and the solution dwells for 4 to 6 hours. The instillation bag is lowered below the level of the catheter and unclamped for 30 to 40 minutes to allow time for gravity drainage. The process is repeated about four times a day on a continuous basis.

Continuous Cyclic Peritoneal Dialysis

In CCPD, a machine is connected to the dialysis catheter. It automatically fills and drains dialysate from the abdomen when the person sleeps. CCPD is performed during a 10- to 12-hour period. The peritoneum is filled with solution during the daytime, but it allows the client to go about activities during the day without performing exchanges of dialysate solutions.

Intermittent Peritoneal Dialysis

Treatments for IPD are performed with the same type of machine as that used for CCPD; however, the process occurs periodically, with perhaps several days between dialysis treatments. When IPD is done, sessions may last 24 hours. The total time spent on IPD is between 36 and 42 hours per week.

Nursing Management

The nurse obtains and reviews laboratory test findings before dialysis and records vital signs and weight. If the client is acutely ill, it may be necessary to use a bed scale.

It also may be necessary to weigh the client as often as every 8 hours while the procedure is in progress. Peritonitis is a major complication of peritoneal dialysis. The nurse monitors and reports fever, nausea, vomiting, and severe abdominal pain, rigidity, or tenderness before, during, or after dialysis.

> **Stop, Think, and Respond** ● **BOX 64-4**
> *Consider why a client may not be a good candidate for CAPD.*

Instillation

Dialysate solution is warmed approximately to body temperature. The nurse adds prescribed drugs such as an antibiotic to the dialysate. He or she attaches the bag of dialysate and administration tubing to the abdominal catheter. The nurse instills the solution and clamps the tubing. If the infusion is slow, the nurse asks the client to move from side to side. If this maneuver is unsuccessful, the physician may need to reposition the catheter. Pain in the left shoulder, if it occurs, may be the result of diaphragmatic irritation caused by the high concentration of glucose.

The nurse records the instillation time, the volume and type of dialysate, plus any medications added. He or she monitors blood pressure and pulse frequently. A drop in blood pressure and increased pulse rate are associated with rapid shifts in fluid that may happen because the dialysate has a high concentration of glucose. As long as the client is stable, he or she can change positions, eat, and drink.

Drainage

At the end of the dwell time, the nurse lowers the empty bag used to instill the solution and opens the clamp. He or she observes the appearance of the siphoned fluid—it should be relatively clear. The nurse must report drainage that is cloudy or tinged with blood. The next instillation may relieve abdominal pain at the end of the drainage period. The nurse notifies the physician if marked abdominal distention accompanies pain. In such a case, the nurse must delay the next dialysis cycle until a physician examines the client.

The nurse measures the difference between the volume instilled and the volume removed. If there is a drainage deficit, he or she notifies the physician before instilling more fluid. The nurse weighs the client after the last cycle of drainage.

Client and Family Teaching

When a client performs peritoneal dialysis at home, the nurse provides the following information:

- Keep dialysis supplies in a clean area away from children and pets.
- Avoid using any dialysate solutions that are expired and look cloudy, discolored, or contain sediment.
- Wash hands before handling the catheter.
- Prevent infection by using sterile gloves during cleaning and exchanges of dialysate.
- Wear a mask when performing exchanges if you have an upper respiratory infection.
- Clean the catheter insertion site daily with an antiseptic such as povidone–iodine (Betadine).
- Inspect the catheter insertion site for signs of infection.
- Keep the catheter stabilized to the abdomen above the belt line to avoid constant rubbing.
- Avoid using scissors during dressing changes to prevent puncturing or cutting the catheter.
- Call the physician if:
  - a fever develops.
  - there is redness, pain, or pus draining around the catheter.
  - the external length of the catheter increases.
  - nausea, vomiting, or abdominal pain develop.

GENERAL NUTRITIONAL CONSIDERATIONS

The objectives of dietary intervention for renal disorders are to reduce serum nitrogen levels, reduce hypertension and edema, prevent body catabolism, improve renal function, and prevent or delay the onset of complications. Dietary interventions frequently are adjusted according to the client's laboratory values and clinical symptoms.

Debate continues over whether lowering protein intake prevents or delays the onset of renal failure. Because a low-protein diet is noninvasive, lessens kidney workload, and has the potential to be beneficial, protein restriction remains the cornerstone of dietary treatment for renal insufficiency.

The recommended protein intake for adults with renal insufficiency is 0.6 to 0.8 g/kg, at or slightly below the Recommended Dietary Allowance for protein (0.8 g/kg). Because most Americans consume almost twice as much protein as needed, however, many clients who must follow the diet view it as unrealistically restrictive. Most protein should be from animal sources, which in general have a higher biologic value than plant proteins. Pure sugars and pure fats are used liberally for calories to spare body and dietary protein.

Multiple and complicated restrictions in protein, sodium, potassium, and fluid, compounded by anorexia and taste alterations in CRF, make dietary compliance difficult to achieve and maintain. Factors that appear to improve dietary adherence include strong social support, frequent self-monitoring of protein intake, the use of specially formulated low-protein foods, and adequate guidelines for increasing calorie intake.

Renal diet food lists, called "choices" to distinguish them from diabetic "exchanges," are used to simplify meal planning. Foods are grouped into lists according to their protein, sodium, and potassium content; phosphorus and fluid also may be considered. Portion sizes are specified so that all servings in a list have approximately the same amount of protein, sodium, and potassium. An individualized meal plan specifies the number of choices allowed from each list for each meal and snack; any item may be chosen in a list, but items from one list cannot be substituted for another. The complexity and composition of choice lists vary greatly among institutions.

Once dialysis begins, protein restrictions are liberalized to 1.2 to 1.5 g/kg to account for nutritional losses through the dialysate. Calorie requirements decrease for clients receiving peritoneal dialysis because, on average, 680 cal/day is absorbed from peritoneal dialysate. Potassium, sodium, and fluid allowances are determined on an individual basis.

GENERAL PHARMACOLOGIC CONSIDERATIONS

Nephrotoxic drugs are not administered to a client with renal disease unless the client's life is in danger and no other therapeutic agent is of value.

Give drugs excreted by the kidney with caution to those with renal disease. If the drug is deemed necessary, it may be given in lower than normal doses; observe the client closely for any changes in renal status if normal doses are necessary. Pay special attention to the client's urinary output because this method is a way to determine a change in renal status.

Sodium bicarbonate (baking soda), usually in tablet form, may be used to alkalize the urine of clients with kidney stones to prevent stone recurrence.

GENERAL GERONTOLOGIC CONSIDERATIONS

Acute glomerulonephritis in the older adult usually occurs in those with pre-existing chronic glomerulonephritis. Symptoms in the older adult are subtle and may go undetected.

Urinary obstruction is the most common cause of pyelonephritis in the older adult. When present, the older adult may not experience the fever and difficulty voiding common in younger adults.

The older adult is at high risk for acute renal failure because of a decline in the glomerular filtration rate, loss of nephrons, and reduced glomeruli. Although the aging kidney can recover from acute renal failure, survival rates are only approximately 50%.

Elderly clients often have slightly abnormal renal function test results. Mild abnormalities are caused by the aging process and usually are of no clinical significance.

Elderly clients usually are not considered candidates for kidney transplants, but may be able to use CAPD. Supervision of the procedure by a family member may be necessary. More frequent monitoring of the client's progress is required when this technique is used.

Critical Thinking Exercises

1. *A client with a ureteral stone is experiencing severe pain. Another nurse believes the client has a low pain tolerance. What action is appropriate at this time? Why?*
2. *A client who had a left nephrectomy is having discomfort when coughing, deep breathing, and changing positions. What nursing measures could relieve her discomfort?*
3. *If you had CRF and must decide to have either hemodialysis or peritoneal dialysis when end-stage disease develops, ex-*

plain which choice you would make and the reasons for that choice.

References and Suggested Readings

Astle, S. M. (2001). A new direction for dialysis. *RN, 64*(7), 56–60.

Bullock, B. L. & Henze, R. L. (2000). *Focus on pathophysiology.* Philadelphia: Lippincott Williams & Wilkins.

King, B. (2000). Meds and the dialysis patient. *RN, 63*(7), 54–60.

Marchiondo, K. (1998). A new look at urinary tract infection. *American Journal of Nursing, 98*(1), 16AAA.

McConnell, E. A. (2001). Clinical do's and don'ts: Preventing nosocomial urinary tract infections. *Nursing, 31*(5), 17.

McConnell, E. A. (1998). Myths & facts . . . about end-stage renal disease. *Nursing, 28*(1), 17.

McConnell, E. A. (2001). Myths & facts . . . about kidney stones. *Nursing, 31*(1), 73.

Porth, C. M. (2002). *Pathophysiology: Concepts of altered health states* (6th ed.). Philadelphia: Lippincott Williams & Wilkins.

Rigby, D. (1998). Urinary tract infections: The hidden cause. *Community Nurse, 4*(5), 30–32.

Smeltzer, S. C. & Bare, B. G. (2000). *Brunner & Suddarth's textbook of medical–surgical nursing* (9th ed.). Philadelphia: Lippincott Williams & Wilkins.

Weil, C. M. (2000). Exploring hope in patients with end stage renal disease on chronic hemodialysis. *Nephrology Nursing Journal, 27,* 219–224.

Young, J. (2000). Actionstat: Kidney stone. *Nursing, 30*(7), 33.

Caring for Clients With Disorders of the Bladder and Urethra

Words to Know

cystectomy
cystitis
cystostomy
diverticulum
fulguration
incontinence
interstitial cystitis
litholapaxy

neurogenic bladder
residual urine
retention
stricture
urethritis
urethroplasty
urinary diversion
urosepsis

Learning Objectives

On completion of this chapter, the reader will:

- Differentiate between urinary retention and urinary incontinence.
- Discuss the nursing management of a client with urinary retention and incontinence.
- Describe the pathophysiologic changes seen in cystitis, interstitial cystitis, and urethritis.
- Discuss the cause and treatment of urethral strictures.
- Identify the most common early symptom of a malignant tumor of the bladder.
- Describe various types of urinary diversion procedures.
- Identify components of a teaching plan for a client having a urinary diversion procedure.

Disorders of the bladder and urethra are common and can be the source of severe problems that become chronic, altering a client's lifestyle. Many disorders affecting the bladder and urethra are treated on an outpatient basis; the more serious disorders require hospitalization.

VOIDING DYSFUNCTION

Urinary retention and urinary incontinence are voiding dysfunctions. Urinary **retention** is the inability to urinate or effectively empty the bladder. Urinary **incontinence** is the inability to control the voiding of urine. Clients experiencing either retention or incontinence face temporary or permanent alterations in their ability to urinate normally. These conditions require individualized approaches to solving the problem and sensitivity to the client's needs, both physiologic and psychosocial.

URINARY RETENTION

Pathophysiology and Etiology

Urinary retention may be either acute or chronic. Acute urinary retention is seen in complete urethral obstruction, after general anesthesia, or with the administration of certain drugs such as atropine or a phenothiazine. Chronic urinary retention often is seen in clients with disorders such as prostatic enlargement or neurologic disorders that result in a **neurogenic bladder** (a bladder that does not receive adequate nerve stimulation).

The client with acute urinary retention usually cannot void at all. The client with chronic urinary retention may be able to void but does not completely empty the bladder (retention with overflow) and has a large residual volume. The **residual urine** is urine retained in the bladder after the client voids. The amount may vary from 30 mL to several hundred milliliters.

1039

Assessment Findings

Symptoms of acute urinary retention are sudden inability to void, distended bladder, and severe lower abdominal pain and discomfort. Chronic urinary retention may produce no symptoms because the bladder has stretched over time and accommodates large volumes without producing discomfort. The overstretched bladder does not contract effectively, and the client is unaware that the bladder is not emptying completely. If the amount of residual urine is large, the client may void frequently in small amounts. Signs of a bladder infection (e.g., fever, chills, pain on urination) and dribbling of urine also may be present.

Urinalysis may show an increased number of white blood cells, indicating an acute or chronic bladder infection. Catheterization or ultrasound can determine post-void residual volume.

Medical and Surgical Management

Acute urinary retention requires immediate catheterization. If a catheter cannot be inserted through the urethra, special urologic instruments that dilate the urethra may be used.

Chronic retention is managed by permanent drainage with a urethral catheter, suprapubic **cystostomy** tube (a catheter inserted through the abdominal wall directly into the bladder), or clean intermittent catheterization (CIC). Permanent catheterization of the bladder carries the risk of bladder stones, renal disease, bladder infection, and **urosepsis,** a serious systemic infection from microorganisms in the urinary tract invading the bloodstream. Because the incidence of complications is lower, CIC is the preferred treatment. Other methods, particularly for clients who have lost nervous system control secondary to disease or injury, are to use Credé voiding or abdominal strain (Valsalva voiding). Box 65-1 describes these methods. CIC may not be possible for clients who lack the mobility or cognitive functioning to perform the procedure. Some male clients who cannot perform CIC can avoid the complications of permanent indwelling catheters by undergoing surgery to release the urethral sphincters. Urine then drains freely out the urethra and the client wears a condom catheter. Nursing Guidelines 65-1 provides instructions about the application of a condom catheter. If it is possible to remove the cause, such as excising excess prostatic tissue, surgery is performed. However, surgery does not always result in restoration of normal voiding.

External collection systems for women are available but proper fit is a problem. Women who cannot accomplish CIC usually are treated with a permanent indwelling catheter.

Nursing Management

The conscious client is able to verbalize the pain and discomfort associated with urinary retention. Clients with Alzheimer's disease or psychiatric disorders, or the comatose, anesthetized, or spinal cord-injured client may be unable to communicate or feel the pain and discomfort associated with acute urinary retention. An impor-

---

BOX 65-1 ● Credé or Valsalva Voiding

CREDÉ
Apply gentle downward pressure to the bladder during voiding. This maneuver may be done by the client or family member. The client also may do this by sitting on the toilet and rocking back and forth gently.

VALSALVA
Instruct the client to bear down as with defecation. Do not teach this method to a client with cardiac problems or who may be adversely affected by a vagal response (heart rate slows).

NURSING GUIDELINES 65-1

Application of a Condom Catheter

1. Assess the penis for swelling or skin breakdown.
2. Verify client's willingness to use a condom catheter.
3. Wash and dry the penis well.
4. Wrap the adhesive strip in an upward spiral about the penis, taking care not to wrap it tightly.
5. Roll the wider end of the sheath toward the narrow catheter tip (most condom catheters are packaged this way—rolling the condom is not necessary).
6. Hold approximately 1 to 2 inches (2.5 to 5 cm) of the lower sheath below the tip of the penis and unroll the sheath upward.
7. Secure the upper end of the unrolled sheath to the skin with a second strip of adhesive or a Velcro strap, but not so tightly as to interfere with circulation.
8. Connect the catheter drainage tip to a drainage bag.
9. Keep the penis positioned in a downward position.
10. Assess the penis at least every 2 hours; also check the catheter to make sure it has not become twisted.
11. Empty leg bag (if one is used) when it becomes partially filled, so that the weight of the collected urine does not dislodge the condom.
12. Remove or change the condom catheter daily, or more often as needed, to check skin integrity.
13. Substitute a waterproof garment during periods of nonuse of a condom catheter.
14. Wash the catheter and collection bag with mild soap and water and rinse with a 1 : 7 vinegar and water solution.

tant nursing responsibility is measuring intake and output, palpating the abdomen for a distended bladder, promoting complete urination, and monitoring the voiding pattern of clients.

Stop, Think, and Respond ● BOX 65-1

*If the priority nursing diagnosis for a client with urinary retention is **Urinary Retention** related to high urethral pressure secondary to prostate enlargement, which of the following is a priority nursing intervention?*

1. *Obtain a history from the client about the duration of this problem.*
2. *Ask the client if he has any problems with bowel elimination.*
3. *Initiate a bladder log, which includes information about urine output and fluid intake.*
4. *Catheterize the client to relieve a full bladder and to measure urine output.*

Acute Urinary Retention

Acute retention that is likely to resolve quickly (e.g., after anesthesia) probably will be treated by intermittent catheterization. Clients with acute retention unlikely to resolve without surgical intervention (e.g., retention caused by an enlarged prostate) probably will have an indwelling catheter.

The nurse collaborates with the physician to determine (1) if the catheter is to be left in place or removed after the bladder is emptied, and (2) the size and type of catheter to be used. Catheters are sized according to the French system (e.g., 14 F to 24 F); the higher the number, the larger the diameter of the catheter. Examples of the various types of catheter tips are shown in Figure 65-1.

Clients with an obstruction may be more easily catheterized with a coudé catheter. The curved tip slides over obstructing tissue more readily than the straight-tipped catheter. The nurse selects the appropriate catheter and inserts it under sterile conditions, noting the characteristics and volume of urine returned. If the volume of urine is large (>700 mL), it may be necessary to clamp the catheter before the bladder has emptied completely to prevent bladder spasms or loss of bladder tone. This practice varies, so it is important to check agency policy.

If the client is going to be managed by CIC, the client and the nurse establish the schedule. Clients are catheterized every 4 to 6 hours depending on the amount of urine obtained and the fluid intake. The bladder should not be allowed to get distended beyond 350 mL because bladder overdistention results in loss of bladder tone, decreased blood flow to the bladder, and reduction in the layer of mucin that protects the bladder mucosa. CIC continues until the postvoid residual volume is less than 30 mL. To obtain accurate residual volumes, it is important that clients have the opportunity to void first and that catheter-

FIGURE 65-1 Catheter tips (top to bottom): de Pezzer catheter, Malecot catheter, coudé catheter, Foley catheter, Foley catheter with balloon inflated. The de Pezzer and the Malecot catheters are inserted by the physician with a stylet that temporarily straightens the tip. The Foley and coudé catheters are retained by inflating the balloon.

ization occur immediately after the attempt. The nurse records both the volume voided (even if it is zero) and the volume obtained by catheterization. Postoperative urinary retention usually resolves within 24 to 48 hours.

Chronic Urinary Retention

Chronic urinary retention may go unrecognized. All clients, during an initial health assessment, need to be asked about voiding frequency, the amount (e.g., small, moderate, large) of urine passed each time, the presence of pain or discomfort in the lower abdomen, pain or discomfort on voiding, and difficulty in starting the urinary stream. The examiner gently palpates or percusses the lower abdomen to determine if the bladder is distended. In addition, the nurse obtains a complete medical, drug, and allergy history and reports suspected chronic urinary retention to the physician.

Intermittent Catheterization

Intermittent catheterization performed in the hospital setting is a sterile procedure. When performed by clients or family members in the home, clean rather than aseptic technique is used. A commercially prepared straight catheterization kit is available in hospitals that includes a straight-tipped catheter, sterile gloves, lubricant and a sterile collection container. At home, the client uses a red rubber catheter that can be washed and reused for 2 to 3 months before replacing. Gloves are not required, but clients must wash their hands thoroughly before and after the procedure. The client can drain the urine into a clean container or directly into the toilet bowl. The schedule is usually three to four times per day, although the frequency can be increased depending on residual volume. If more than 400 mL is returned, the client should be catheterized more often. Client education in technique, catheter care, and follow-up care is an important function of the nurse both in the acute and home care settings.

Indwelling Catheters

A urethral indwelling catheter is one route for permanent bladder catheterization. A cystostomy tube, also called a *suprapubic catheter,* is an alternative that is inserted through an abdominal incision into the bladder. Clients require catheter care, including careful cleansing of the urethral meatus or cystostomy site and proximal catheter, maintenance of the integrity of the closed drainage system, proper anchoring of the tube to avoid tension and promote drainage (Fig. 65-2), and scheduled changes of the catheter and drainage system according to facility policy. Nursing Guidelines 65-2 offers additional general management points.

> **Stop, Think, and Respond ● BOX 65-2**
>
> *What methods should a nurse use to prevent the occurrence of a nosocomial infection in the catheterized client?*

● URINARY INCONTINENCE

Urinary incontinence affects many clients and is a major healthcare concern. It is estimated that at least one third of older adults living in the community and one half of older clients in institutions suffer from incontinence. Not only is incontinence a psychosocial problem, it is a physical problem in that skin breakdown and urinary tract infection may result from incontinence. Table 65-1 describes the different types of incontinence.

Pathophysiology and Etiology

Urinary incontinence may result from either bladder or urethral dysfunction (or both). The bladder can contract without warning, fail to accommodate adequate volumes of urine, or fail to empty completely and become overstretched, resulting in overflow incontinence. These conditions result from neurologic disease, bladder outlet obstruction, or trauma in all clients; bladder prolapse or low estrogen levels in women; and prostatic enlargement in men.

Another cause of incontinence is failure of the urethral sphincters to hold urine in the bladder. This may result from trauma, prostate surgery, or relaxed pelvic muscles. Impingement of the spinal nerves, such as in tumors of the spinal cord, herniated disk, or spinal cord injuries, can interfere with the impulse conduction to the brain, resulting in a neurogenic bladder and incontinence. A neurogenic bladder may be spastic, causing incontinence, or it may be flaccid, causing retention.

Assessment Findings

Clients complain of urgency, frequency, leaking small amounts when coughing or sneezing, or complete inability to control urine, depending on the underlying cause. Tests such as a urine culture and sensitivity, cystoscopy, or urodynamics are used to determine the type of incontinence.

FIGURE 65-2 Catheter tubing correctly anchored and attached to closed drainage system. (**A**) Male. (**B**) Female. (**C**) Suprapubic.

NURSING GUIDELINES 65-2

General Principles of Catheterization and Catheter Care

The following general principles apply to the insertion and maintenance of urethral or suprapubic catheters:

- Always use aseptic technique for insertion.

- Thoroughly cleanse the urethral meatus before insertion of a catheter.

- An adult urethra usually takes a size 14-F to 18-F indwelling catheter. A smaller size may be used for intermittent (straight, single) catheterization.

- When inserting an indwelling catheter, test the balloon before insertion.

- Lubricate the catheter with a sterile, water-soluble lubricant and insert.

- Never force a catheter if resistance is felt.

- Never reinsert an indwelling catheter that accidentally becomes dislodged; replace it with a new sterile catheter.

- Catheters are connected to a sterile closed drainage system.

- Keep the drainage bag lower than the catheter.

- Change indwelling urethral catheters according to the physician's orders or agency policy.

- Provide urethral catheter care twice a day and after bowel movements.

- Inspect the cystostomy tube site for leakage of urine around the catheter, bleeding, or signs and symptoms of infection.

- Change the cystostomy dressing once per shift or more often if necessary.

- If a permanent vesicocutaneous (bladder to skin) fistula forms, the size of the cystostomy tube may need to be increased to prevent leakage of urine.

- Unless contraindicated by heart failure or renal disease, encourage clients to drink plenty of fluids (2000 to 3000 mL), especially those that acidify the urine, such as cranberry juice.

- Monitor client for signs and symptoms of urinary tract infection: fever, chills, hypotension, and confusion.

- Monitor fluid balance and laboratory tests that measure kidney function.

Medical and Surgical Management

Treatment is aimed at correcting the disorder causing incontinence (when possible), providing medication to control incontinence, correcting the situational problems that contribute to functional incontinence, or instituting a bladder retraining program. Pharmacologic agents that can improve bladder retention, emptying, and control include drugs such as oxybutynin chloride (Ditropan), which reduces bladder spasticity and involuntary bladder contractions, and phenoxybenzamine hydrochloride (Dibenzaline), which may be useful in treating problems with sphincter control. Bethanechol (Urecholine) helps to increase contraction of the detrusor muscle, which as-

TABLE 65-1	TYPES OF URINARY INCONTINENCE	
TYPE OF INCONTINENCE	**SYMPTOMS**	**CAUSE**
Stress incontinence	Client has involuntary loss of urine from intact urethra, which results from sudden increase in intra-abdominal pressure, such as with sneezing or coughing.	Decreased pelvic muscle tone, primarily seen in women, and associated with multiple pregnancies, obstetric injuries, obesity, menopause, or pelvic disease
Urge incontinence	Client experiences urge to void but cannot control voiding in time to reach a toilet.	Bladder irritation related to urinary tract infections, bladder tumors, radiation therapy, enlarged prostate, or neurologic dysfunction
Total incontinence	Urine is continuously lost from the bladder, which is overdistended and does not empty normally or completely.	Neurologic abnormalities, such as spinal cord lesions or tumors, or obstruction to urine output, such as tumors, enlarged prostate, or urethral strictures
Functional incontinence	Client has intact function of the lower urinary tract but cannot identify the need to void or ambulate to the toilet.	Cognitive impairments, such as brain injury or Alzheimer's disease, or physical limitations, such as rheumatoid arthritis or musculoskeletal injuries
Reflex incontinence	Bladder has uninhibited contractions; involuntary reflexes produce spontaneous voiding, with partial or complete loss of sensation of bladder fullness or urge to void.	Impaired conduction of impulses above reflex arc level secondary to spinal cord injury, tumor, or infection

sists with emptying of the bladder. Sometimes medication to control incontinence results in retention and must be discontinued. Occasionally clients who can easily perform CIC may opt for medication-induced retention and CIC because it allows them to stay dry.

Surgeries to improve urinary control include:

- Bladder augmentation—a procedure that increases the storage capacity of the bladder
- Implantation of an artificial sphincter that can be inflated to prevent urine loss and deflated to allow urination (Fig. 65-3)
- Surgeries to provide better support for urinary structures
- Urethroplasty—surgery to repair structures damaged by trauma

Nursing Management

Goals when caring for a client with urinary incontinence include maintaining continence as much as possible, preventing skin breakdown, reducing anxiety, and initiating a bladder training program. It must be determined if the client is truly incontinent or if situations prevent the client from getting to the bathroom. Such situations include impaired mobility, physical restraints, and use of sedatives. In addition to assessing for functional causes of incontinence, the nurse obtains details regarding the pattern of incontinence and use of medications that may play a role in the problem. It is important to assess for skin breakdown and determine methods the client has used to manage incontinence.

Instruction centers on exercises to increase muscle tone and voluntary control (Kegel exercises), techniques to assist bladder emptying, and bladder training. Refer to Nursing Guidelines 65-3 for teaching Kegel exercises.

FIGURE 65-3 Artificial urinary sphincter. An inflatable cuff is inserted surgically around the urethra or bladder neck. To empty the bladder, the cuff is deflated by squeezing the control pump located in the scrotum.

NURSING GUIDELINES 65-3

Kegel Exercises

Initial Instructions

1. Sit or stand with legs slightly apart.
2. Draw in perivaginal muscles and anal sphincter as when controlling voiding or defecating.
3. Hold this position of contraction for 5 seconds (instruct client to count or time with a watch).
4. Relax contraction for at least 10 seconds.
5. Repeat exercises 5 to 6 times, increasing slowly to 25 times.
6. Repeat the sequence of exercises three to four times a day.
7. Gradually do the exercises for a total of 200 repetitions.

Advanced Instructions

1. Sit on the toilet and begin to urinate.
2. Stop the flow of urine by doing a Kegel exercise.
3. Hold this position for 5 seconds.
4. Relax and begin voiding.
5. Repeat this sequence five times with each voiding.

Success of a bladder retraining program depends not only on the cause of incontinence but on the motivation of the client and the amount of skillful help and encouragement received from the healthcare team.

Bladder Training

One method of bladder training for the client with an indwelling urethral catheter is to alternately clamp and unclamp the catheter. The clamping and unclamping of the catheter begins to re-establish normal bladder function and capacity. In the beginning, the catheter may be unclamped for 5 minutes every 1 or 2 hours. The length of time is gradually increased to every 3 or 4 hours, giving the bladder a chance to fill more completely. When possible, the nurse teaches the client to release the clamp at scheduled times. The catheter eventually is removed.

At this point, or when training clients who have not had an indwelling catheter, the nurse instructs the client to try to void every hour. Usually the client is not able to retain urine longer than an hour, and frequent voiding is necessary to prevent incontinence. Gradually the client lengthens the interval between voidings to 2, 3, or 4 hours. At first, many clients do not empty the bladder and they must be catheterized after voiding to remove residual urine. When the client is catheterized for residual urine, the nurse records the amount removed.

When a client is unable to control the storage and passage of urine or when a bladder training program fails, clients may exhibit varying degrees of anxiety and depression. The nurse needs to offer constant encouragement throughout the bladder training program. Anxiety may be reduced once the client notes the effort, concern, and interest of the healthcare team. If an accident occurs, it is important to change the bed linen promptly and assure the client that accidents are to be expected during the retraining process. Reducing anxiety may, in some instances, contribute to the success of a bladder training program.

Barrier Garments and External Collection Devices

If it is not possible to establish a voiding routine and incontinence persists, the healthcare team works with the client to devise a system of collecting the urine. Male clients can use a condom catheter over the penis and connect the tubing to a closed drainage system or disposable urinary drainage bag. External drainage systems are available for women, but it is difficult to get the devices to fit securely. Male and female clients may choose to wear protective pants with a plastic outside layer and absorbent material inside. These pants can be pinned or snapped in place. Liners also are available and are worn next to the skin. They are nonabsorbent, and thus the urine passes through them to the absorbent layer. For this reason the liners dry quickly and leave the skin dry and free of urine, even though the absorbent material is soaked.

Clients who are incontinent may have problems with odor and maintaining skin integrity. Urea-splitting microorganisms, such as *Micrococcus ureae,* cause the urea in urine to react with water, creating ammonia and causing urine odor, skin breakdown, and ammonia dermatitis. One way to protect the skin is to avoid any contact with urine. When contact is unavoidable, the nurse instructs the client to use soap and water after each episode to clean the skin thoroughly. It also is important to dry the skin completely and apply a skin barrier or moisture sealant to protect the skin. When possible, the nurse encourages the client to expose the affected area to air.

Client and Family Teaching

The nurse encourages clients to actively participate in whatever methods are used to empty the bladder. In addition, the nurse demonstrates procedures as needed for the client and family to understand. A teaching plan is based on the client's individual needs to include one or more of the following:

- Control odors by frequent cleansing of the perineum, changing clothes and incontinence briefs (e.g., Attends, Depends) when they become wet, and using an electric room deodorizer.
- Avoid using perfume or scented powders, lotions, or sprays. Mixing a perfumed scent with a urine

odor may intensify the odor, irritate the skin, or cause a skin infection.
- Wash garments as soon as possible in warm, soapy water.
- Use plastic to cover objects, such as a mattress and chairs, to prevent staining and lingering odors. The plastic must be washed with mild soapy water daily or more often if needed. Instruct the client to place a sheet or blanket between the skin and the plastic.
- Follow the recommendations of the physician about clamping and unclamping the catheter (when this method is prescribed) or changing the catheter or cystostomy tube.
- Keep a record of fluid intake. Drink plenty of fluids during waking hours. Drink most of the required fluids in the morning and early afternoon hours and decrease the intake toward evening.
- Follow the recommended bladder training program. Time is required to achieve success.
- Contact the physician if any of the following occurs: increased discomfort, rash around the perineal area, pain in the lower abdomen, fever, chills, or cloudy urine.

INFECTIOUS AND INFLAMMATORY DISORDERS ●

Infections and inflammations of the bladder and urethra are common. Although usually able to be treated on an outpatient basis, they are a potential source of more complex problems requiring invasive treatment.

● CYSTITIS

Pathophysiology and Etiology

Cystitis is an inflammation of the urinary bladder. The inflammation usually is caused by a bacterial infection. Bacteria can invade the bladder from an infection in the kidneys, lymphatics, and urethra (Fig. 65-4). Because the urethra is short in women, ascending infections or microorganisms from the vagina or rectum are more common. Causes of cystitis include urologic instrumentation (e.g., cystoscopy, catheterization), fecal contamination, prostatitis or benign prostatic hyperplasia, indwelling catheters, pregnancy, and sexual intercourse.

The lining of the bladder provides a natural resistance to most bacterial invasions by preventing an inflammatory reaction from occurring. If bacteria do survive in the bladder, however, they adhere to the mucosal lining of the bladder and multiply. The surface of the bladder becomes edematous and reddened, and ulcerations may develop.

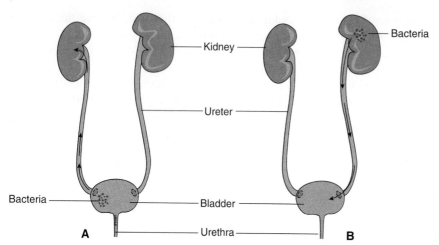

FIGURE 65-4 Urinary tract infection. (**A**) Microorganisms invade the bladder and ascend to the ureter and kidney. (**B**) Microorganisms in the kidney descend the ureter to the bladder.

When urine contacts these irritated areas, the client experiences pain and urgency, which is magnified in the presence of even slight bladder distention.

Assessment Findings

Signs and Symptoms

The symptoms of cystitis include urgency (feeling a pressing need to void although the bladder is not full), frequency, low back pain, dysuria, perineal and suprapubic pain, and hematuria, especially at the termination of the stream (terminal hematuria). If bacteremia is present, the client also may have chills and fever. Chronic cystitis causes similar symptoms, but usually they are less severe.

Diagnostic Findings

Microscopic examination of the urine reveals an increase in the number of red and white blood cells. Culture and sensitivity studies are used to identify the causative microorganism and appropriate antimicrobial therapy. If repeated episodes occur, intravenous pyelogram (IVP) or cystoscopy with or without retrograde pyelograms may be needed to identify the possible cause, such as chronic prostatitis or a bladder **diverticulum** (weakening and outpouching of the bladder wall), which encourages urinary stasis and infection.

Medical Management

Medical management includes antimicrobial therapy and correction of contributing factors. Examples of drugs that may be used include trimethoprim-sulfamethoxazole (Septra, Bactrim) and nitrofurantoin (Macrodantin). Cranberry juice or vitamin C may be recommended to keep the bacteria from adhering to the wall of the bladder and thus promoting their excretion and enhancing the effectiveness of drug therapy. When there is a partial urethral obstruction, no treatment of cystitis is fully effective until adequate drainage of urine is restored by the removal of the obstruction (see discussion of urethral strictures). In some instances, treatment may be prolonged and may need to be repeated.

Nursing Management

The nurse advises the client to drink extra fluids. Cranberry juice provides a less favorable climate for bacterial growth. It is important to emphasize the importance of finishing the prescribed course of therapy. The nurse also instructs the client in the prevention of repeated cystitis (Nursing Guidelines 65-4).

Stop, Think, and Respond ● BOX 65-3

Your 30-year-old client tells you that she has had four urinary tract infections (UTIs) in the past 6 months. What information should you get before providing the client with instructions about preventing future UTIs?

● INTERSTITIAL CYSTITIS

Pathophysiology and Etiology

Interstitial cystitis (IC) is a chronic inflammation of the bladder mucosa. It is more common in women than men. The bladder wall contains multiple pinpoint hemorrhagic areas that join and form larger hemorrhagic areas that may progress to fissuring and scarring of the bladder mu-

Preventing Cystitis

Tell clients with recurrent cystitis to:

- Increase fluid intake to 2 to 3 L a day.
- Avoid coffee, teas, colas, and alcohol.
- Shower rather than bathe in a tub.
- Cleanse perineum after each bowel movement with front-to-back motion.
- Avoid irritating substances such as bubble bath, bath salts, perineal lotions, vaginal sprays, nylon underwear, scented toilet paper.
- Wear cotton underwear.
- Void every 2 to 3 hours while awake.
- Empty bladder completely with each voiding.
- Void after sexual intercourse.
- Notify physician of the following: urgency, frequency, burning with urination, difficulty urinating, or blood in the urine.
- Take medication exactly as prescribed.

cosa. Superficial erosion of the bladder mucosa (Hunner's ulcer) may develop. Eventually, the bladder shrinks from scarring. The cause of IC is unknown, but it has been suggested that there may be a hormonal link because flareups appear to occur before menstruation. Another theory is that IC may be an autoimmune disorder or part of a systemic condition because some persons have a history of migraine headaches, ulcerative colitis, endometriosis, or chronic fatigue syndrome.

Assessment Findings

Symptoms mimic other disorders such as cystitis, bladder cancer, or a sexually transmitted disease (STD). Frequent, painful urination and passing a small volume of urine are the most common symptoms. The pain may be described as searing or burning. The client reports an onset of pain and the need to void as soon as a small amount of urine is present in the bladder.

Cystoscopy reveals a markedly inflamed bladder mucosa with pinpoint hemorrhages and a bladder capacity that is smaller than normal. Filling the bladder during cystoscopy to improve visualization usually results in severe pain.

A voiding cystourethrogram also demonstrates a small bladder capacity. Results of urinalysis usually are normal, but if cystitis is present, an increase in the number of red and white blood cells may be seen; urine cultures are negative. A record of the number of voidings and the amount voided over a 2- or 3-day period, along with the symptoms,

help to confirm the diagnosis. A biopsy of the bladder mucosa reveals an inflammatory process with scarring and hemorrhagic areas and confirms the diagnosis.

Medical and Surgical Management

There is no single effective specific therapy for IC. Antidepressant drugs may relieve pain as well as treat the depression that accompanies the disorder. Other therapies include bladder instillation of DMSO (dimethylsulfoxide) or silver nitrate. Elmiron (pentosan polysulfate) is an orphan drug (a drug that is used for treatment of a disease affecting a small number of persons) that is taken orally. It appears to help in restoration of the bladder mucosa. A more recent treatment uses a laser, inserted into the abdominal cavity with a laparoscope, to sever the sensory (pain) fibers of the bladder. This procedure is used to relieve the severe pain associated with IC. Severe IC can be incapacitating, and a urinary diversion procedure (see later discussion) may offer the only relief of symptoms for a selected group of clients.

Nursing Management

The nurse advises the client to avoid spicy and acidic foods because they may contribute to pain and discomfort. Psychological support is necessary because many times IC has gone undiagnosed and the client has been told that there is nothing wrong. Clients with IC often have their lives severely disrupted by pain and frequent trips to the bathroom, sometimes several times an hour. Some are unable to hold jobs because of the severity of symptoms. Sexual activity is avoided because of fear of pain, straining their relationships and interfering with intimacy. Clients should be referred to a chronic pain center to cope with the pain, and to an IC support group.

● URETHRITIS

Pathophysiology and Etiology

Urethritis (inflammation of the urethra) is seen more commonly in men than in women. Urethritis caused by microorganisms other than gonococci is called *nongonococcal urethritis*. Gonorrhea, an STD, is a specific form of infection that can attack the mucous membrane of a normal urethra (see Chap. 61).

In women, urethritis may accompany cystitis but also may be secondary to vaginal infections. Soaps, bubble baths, sanitary napkins, or scented toilet paper also may cause urethritis.

In men, a common cause of urethritis is infection with *Chlamydia trachomatis* or *Ureaplasma urealyticum,* which causes an STD. The distal portion of the normal male urethra is not totally sterile. Bacteria that normally are present cause no difficulty unless these tissues are traumatized, usually after instrumentation such as catheterization or cystoscopic examination. Under such conditions, bacteria may gain a foothold to cause a nonspecific urethritis. Other causes of nonspecific urethritis in men include irritation during vigorous intercourse, rectal intercourse, or intercourse with a woman who has a vaginal infection.

Assessment Findings

Infection of the urethra results in discomfort on urination varying from a slight tickling sensation to burning or severe discomfort and urinary frequency. Fever is not common, but fever in the male client may be due to further extension of the infection to areas such as the prostate, testes, and epididymis.

The client's history and symptoms often provide a tentative diagnosis. In men, a urethral smear is obtained for culture and sensitivity to identify the causative microorganism. In women, a urinalysis (clean-catch specimen) may identify the causative microorganism.

Medical Management

Treatment includes appropriate antibiotic therapy, liberal fluid intake, analgesics, warm sitz baths, and improvement of the client's resistance to infection by a good diet and plenty of rest. If urethritis is due to an STD, it is treated with appropriate antibiotic therapy (see Chap. 61). Failure to seek treatment for gonococcal urethritis may result in a urethral stricture in men.

Nursing Management

The nurse reinforces the need to complete antibiotic therapy, drink plenty of fluids, and take warm sitz baths and analgesics for pain. Urethritis may be seen in clients with indwelling urethral catheters. To prevent or decrease urethritis, the nurse needs to be vigilant with sterile technique, as well as exercise gentleness when changing catheters. It also is essential to provide frequent perineal care, especially if the client is incontinent of feces. In addition to washing around the anus and buttocks, the nurse also cleans the meatus and labia of the female client. When cleaning the anal area, wiping away from the urethra ensures that there is no contamination. If cotton pledgets are used, the nurse wipes from the urethral meatus to the anus in a single stroke and discards the pledget.

NURSING PROCESS

● **The Client With an Infection of the Bladder or Urethra**

Assessment

The nurse asks the client about present symptoms, specifically seeking information related to the presence of pain and changes in urination, including frequency, urgency, and burning with urination. It also is important to assess the client's sexual practices, including methods of contraception and personal hygiene. The nurse asks the client to void. When the client voids, the nurse measures the volume and checks the urine for color, cloudiness, concentration, odor, and presence of blood.

Diagnosis, Planning, and Interventions

Pain related to infection and inflammation of the bladder and or/urethra

Expected Outcome: The client will express relief of pain and discomfort.

- Assure the client that pain and discomfort will decrease with treatment. *Antibacterial and antispasmodic medications are quickly effective in relieving the pain and discomfort associated with urinary tract infections.*
- Administer analgesics and antispasmodics as indicated. *Prompt administration of prescribed medications ensures that effective blood levels are maintained for treatment of infection. Antispasmodics relieve bladder irritability.*
- Encourage the client to use warm sitz baths two or three times a day to relieve discomfort. *Promotes relief of pain and reduces spasm.*
- Encourage the client to increase daily fluid intake to 2 to 3 L/day, excluding coffee, tea, alcohol, and colas. *Promotes renal blood flow and flushes bacteria from the urinary tract. Coffee, tea, alcohol, and colas are urinary tract irritants.*
- Instruct the client to void at regular intervals, even if uncomfortable. *Frequent voiding promotes emptying the bladder, which contributes to lower bacterial counts, reduction of urinary stasis, and prevention of reinfection.*

Anxiety related to pain, discomfort, and frequent urination

Expected Outcomes: (1) Client will verbalize anxiety related to symptoms. (2) Client will state self-care measures to relieve anxiety.

- Encourage client to talk about his or her symptoms and fears related to the disorder. *Providing an opportunity for the client to discuss concerns and fears assists in relieving anxiety.*
- Provide information that assists in alleviating fears. *Accurate information alleviates fear and corrects misconceptions.*

Deficient Knowledge regarding inflammation and infection of the bladder and urethra related to disease process and treatment

Expected Outcomes: (1) Client will verbalize understanding of condition, prognosis, and treatment. (2) Client will participate in the treatment regimen.

- Review the treatment plan. *Doing so provides a time for the client to ask questions.*
- Instruct client about medications, dosage, frequency, expected effects, and possible side effects. *Providing clients with accurate information promotes adherence to drug regimen.*
- Emphasize the need to complete the entire course of medications, even after symptoms have subsided. *Complete antibiotic therapy eradicates infection and prevents recurrence.*
- Teach client the importance of increased fluid intake. *Increased fluid intake flushes the urinary tract and removes bacteria.*
- Review client's hygiene practices. *Poor hygiene practices, such as back-to-front perineal cleansing, especially after a bowel movement, or soaking in dirty bath water can contribute to the introduction of bacterial contaminants to the urinary tract.*
- Teach client methods to prevent future infections. *Appropriate personal hygiene, increased fluid intake (promotes voiding and dilution of urine), and frequent voiding prevent urinary tract infection.*

Evaluation of Expected Outcomes

The client reports relief of pain and discomfort and states that he or she is adhering to the medication regimen. The client states that he or she is not anxious and feels much better now that there are no symptoms. He or she demonstrates understanding of the treatment plan as evidenced by intake of at least 2 L of water, frequent voiding, and appropriate personal hygiene practices.

Client and Family Teaching

Most cases of cystitis and urethritis are treated in the physician's office. The nurse develops a teaching plan to include the following:

- Take the medication as directed. Do not stop taking the medication even though symptoms have disappeared. It is important to complete the entire course of therapy.
- Take warm tub baths if discomfort is severe.
- Drink at least eight large glasses of fluids per day. Include one or more glasses of cranberry juice in the daily fluid intake. Avoid fluids that are urinary tract irritants, such as coffee, tea, alcohol, and colas. Fluids include water, cranberry juice, clear carbonated beverages, or any food (e.g., flavored gelatin, ice cream) that is liquid at room temperature. If on a special diet (e.g., low-sodium or diabetic diets), check with the physician about drinking juices or beverages or eating foods that are liquid at room temperature. Some of these liquids either must be considered part of the daily dietary allowances or may not be allowed be-

cause they contain substances that must be eliminated from the diet. In some diets, a limited amount of certain liquids may be allowed.

- Notify the physician if symptoms persist after the course of drug therapy is completed, if the symptoms become worse, or if fever or chills occur.
- Follow recommendations preventing future episodes of infection or inflammation.

OBSTRUCTIVE DISORDERS

Obstruction of the lower urinary tract is a blockage in the bladder or in the urethra. Many obstructions are related to congenital anomalies, but in adults, obstructions occur from stones that block the passage of urine, or from a narrowing that occurs as a result of a trauma, inflammation, or infection. Box 65-2 lists general signs of an outflow obstruction.

● BLADDER STONES

Pathophysiology and Etiology

Stones may form in the bladder or originate in the upper urinary tract and travel to and remain in the bladder. Large bladder stones develop in those with chronic urinary retention and urinary stasis. Clients who are immobile (e.g., the unconscious client or those with paraplegia or quadriplegia) also may have a tendency to form bladder stones.

Assessment Findings

Symptoms of bladder stone formation include hematuria, suprapubic pain, difficulty starting the urinary stream, symptoms of a bladder infection, and a feeling that the bladder is not completely empty. Some clients may have few or no symptoms.

Cystoscopy, a kidney–ureter–bladder (KUB) study, IVP, or ultrasound studies detect the presence of bladder stones. Blood chemistries and 24-hour urine collection for serum calcium and uric acid may identify the possible cause of stone formation.

BOX 65-2 ● **Signs of Obstructed Urine Flow**

- Straining to empty bladder
- Feeling that bladder does not empty completely
- Hesitancy
- Weak stream
- Frequency
- Overflow incontinence
- Bladder distention

Medical and Surgical Management

Bladder stones may be removed through the transurethral route, using a stone-crushing instrument (lithotrite). This procedure, called a **litholapaxy,** is suitable for small and soft stones and is performed under general anesthesia. Larger, noncrushable stones must be removed through a surgical (suprapubic) incision into the bladder.

When it is possible to determine the chemical composition of stones that have passed or been removed, dietary treatment may be attempted to adjust the pH of the urine to keep the urinary salts in solution and thus prevent the formation of stones. These diets, however, are not fully effective. Uric acid stones may be prevented by a low-purine diet. Clients with a history of calcium stone formation used to limit their intake of milk and milk products. However, this now is recommended only for clients who have type II absorptive hypercalciuria—approximately half of the clients (Smeltzer & Bare, 2000). Usually, clients are told to increase their fluid intake significantly and to restrict their sodium and protein. Despite dietary changes and urine pH regulation, some clients continue to form stones in the urinary tract.

Nursing Management

The nurse obtains a complete medical, drug, and allergy history, asking the client to describe the symptoms, including the type and location of the pain. Determining if the client is allergic to iodine or seafood is essential because iodine-containing radiopaque substances may be used during diagnostic tests to locate the obstruction. The nurse monitors vital signs every 4 hours or as ordered, and notifies the physician if the client's temperature is higher than 101°F (38.3°C) orally. Intake and output and the color of the urine are documented in the medical record.

If there is any evidence of gross hematuria, the nurse reports it immediately. Encouraging the client to drink fluids (unless contraindicated by heart failure or renal disease) is important because extra fluids help pass stones and reduce the chance of infection or inflammation. The nurse filters the urine for stones by straining all urine through gauze or wire mesh. If solid material is found, it is sent in a labeled container to the laboratory for analysis. If the client has moderate to severe pain, the nurse administers a narcotic analgesic as ordered. If the analgesic fails to relieve at least some of the pain or if the pain becomes worse despite administration of an analgesic, the nurse notifies the physician, and provides details regarding the effects of medical or surgical procedures.

If a litholapaxy successfully removes the stone, a urethral catheter may be left in place to keep the bladder continuously empty for 1 to 2 days after the procedure. The nurse administers antibiotics as ordered. Once oral fluids are tolerated, it is important to encourage the client to drink extra fluids to reduce inflammation of the bladder mucosa. In addition, the nurse monitors the urine output and voiding pattern.

If open removal is required, the bladder is incised and the stone removed. A urethral catheter may be left in place for a week or more to keep the bladder empty and prevent tension on the bladder sutures. In addition to standard postoperative care (see Chap. 25), nursing management involves providing the same care as for the client having a suprapubic prostatectomy (see Chap. 61). The nurse closely monitors the client's voiding once the catheter is removed to prevent urinary retention.

The nurse teaches the client to:

- Strain urine and send any stone found to the laboratory for examination.
- Follow the dietary recommendations.
- Take the prescribed medications as directed.
- Contact the physician if symptoms return.
- Drink plenty of fluids (at least 10 large glasses each day) and exercise regularly.
- Contact the physician if hematuria, burning, chills, fever, or pain occurs.

● URETHRAL STRICTURES

Pathophysiology and Etiology

Strictures of the urethra are caused by infections such as untreated gonorrhea or chronic nongonococcal urethritis. Other causes include trauma to the lower urinary tract or pelvis, such as accidents, childbirth, intercourse, or surgical procedures. Urethral strictures may be congenital.

A **stricture** (narrowing) in the urethra obstructs the flow of urine and can cause complications in the bladder or upper urinary tract. The kidney pelves can become distended with the backflow of urine. The bladder distends when the urethra is obstructed and a diverticulum (outpouching) of the muscular bladder wall may form (Fig. 65-5). In some instances more than one diverticulum may be seen. Urine becomes trapped in the diverticulum, stagnates, and becomes a culture medium for bacteria. For this reason, infection occurs often and is difficult to control until the obstruction is corrected. Men experience urethral stricture more frequently than women, secondary to the anatomic differences and the length of the urethra. A urethral stricture may result in acute or chronic urinary retention.

Assessment Findings

Symptoms include:

- Slow or decreased force of stream of urine
- Hesitancy
- Burning
- Frequency

FIGURE **65-5** Urethral stricture can result in hydroureters, hydronephrosis (dilation of the ureters and kidney), and bladder diverticulum.

FIGURE **65-6** Bougies (**A**) and filiforms (**B**) are used to dilate the urethra.

- Nocturia
- Retention of residual urine in the bladder—may lead to bladder distention and infection

The client may be able to pass more urine after voiding and waiting a few minutes. The final quantity of urine comes from the diverticulum and may be malodorous.

The stricture may be seen on cystoscopy, retrograde pyelogram, and IVP. A voiding cystourethrogram also may show the stricture as well as the presence of a bladder diverticulum.

Medical and Surgical Management

Urethral strictures are treated by dilatation, which is the use of specially designed instruments called *bougies, sounds, filiforms,* and *followers* (Fig. 65-6) that are passed gently into the urethra. Although done gently, the procedure usually is painful. Because forceful stretching of the urethra may cause bleeding and further stricture formation, dilatation begins with a 6-F or 8-F urethral dilator. During subsequent treatments, the physician increases the size of the dilator until 24 F or 26 F can be tolerated. Depending on the cause of the stricture and the response to the therapy, the condition may subside after one or two treatments. However, periodic dilatations usually are required indefinitely or until the condition is corrected surgically.

If dilatation is unsuccessful, a **urethroplasty** (surgical repair of the urethra) may be attempted. The urine is diverted from the urethra by a cystostomy tube until the urethra has been repaired. In one method of reconstructing the urethra, the constricted area is resected, and a mucosal graft (which may be taken from the bladder) is inserted to restore the continuity of the urethra. After

surgery, the client has a splinting catheter in the urethra that remains until healing has occurred. This operation may be performed in two stages: urinary diversion at the first operation and plastic repair at the second.

Nursing Management

The nurse advises the client that the urine may be blood tinged after urethral dilatation and that it may burn when voiding. Sitz baths and non-narcotic analgesics may relieve discomfort. The nurse encourages the client to drink extra fluids for several days after the procedure. It is important for the client to keep appointments for follow-up dilatations and not to wait until there is a marked reduction in the urinary stream or other symptoms of obstruction to return. The nurse instructs the client to take all of the antibiotics and to contact the physician if difficulty voiding or frank bleeding occurs.

If a urethroplasty is performed, it is most important that the urethral catheter remains in place and securely anchored. After surgery, turning and repositioning requires special attention to prevent excessive tension on the urethral catheter.

MALIGNANT TUMORS OF THE BLADDER

Malignant tumors of the bladder are frightening for clients. Bloody urine often is the first sign of a problem and the reason clients seek medical attention.

Pathophysiology and Etiology

Malignant tumors of the bladder are the most common tumors in the urinary system. They occur more frequently in men than in women and usually affect clients 50 years of age or older. Environmental and occupational health hazards thought to be associated with bladder tumors include the following:

- Cigarette smoking and second-hand smoke
- Exposure to industrial dyes, paint, ink, leather, or rubber
- Occupational exposure to sewage
- Coal gas
- Bladder stones
- High urinary pH
- High cholesterol intake
- Pelvic radiation therapy
- Cancers arising from the prostate, colon, and rectum in men (Smeltzer & Bare, 2000)

The most common type of bladder tumor is a transitional cell carcinoma, which develops in the bladder's epithelial lining. The tumors are classified as papillary or nonpapillary. Papillary lesions are superficial and extend outward from the mucosal layer. Nonpapillary tumors are solid growths that grow inward, deep into the bladder wall. This type is more likely to metastasize, usually to the lymph nodes, liver, lungs, and bone. Other types include squamous cell carcinoma and adenocarcinoma.

Assessment Findings

Signs and Symptoms

The most common first symptom of a malignant tumor of the bladder is painless hematuria. Additional early symptoms include UTI with symptoms such as fever, dysuria, urgency, and frequency. Later symptoms are related to metastases and include pelvic pain, urinary retention (if the tumor blocks the bladder outlet), and urinary frequency from the tumor occupying bladder space. If bleeding has been present for some time, the client also may have symptoms of anemia (fatigue, shortness of breath) caused by blood loss.

Stop, Think, and Respond ● BOX 65-4

A 55-year-old man is admitted with blood in the urine. The medical diagnosis is "Rule out bladder cancer." When the nurse admits this client, what is an important question to ask?

Diagnostic Findings

The tumor usually is seen by cystoscopic examination and confirmed by microscopic biopsy. A retrograde pyelogram may be obtained to detect any kidney damage if the tumor is obstructing one of the ureteral orifices. A computed tomography scan and radiographs of the pelvis may show a tumor shadow or bony metastases. Ultrasonography also may show tumor size and location. Routine laboratory tests may be performed to evaluate kidney function and determine the degree of anemia due to persistent hematuria.

Medical Management

Treatment varies according to the grade and stage of the tumor. Metastases usually have not occurred as long as the tumor has not penetrated the muscle wall of the bladder. Small, superficial tumors may be removed by cutting (resection) or coagulation (**fulguration**) with a transurethral resectoscope (the same instrument used in a transurethral resection of the prostate). Bladder tumors removed in this manner have a high incidence of recurrence; consequently, a cystoscopic examination is performed every 2 to 3 months. Clients having no recurrence of the tumor for at least 1 year require cystoscopic examinations every 6 months for the rest of their lives so that recurrence of the tumor or a new malignant growth can be detected early.

Topical application of an antineoplastic drug may be used after resection and fulguration of a tumor. The drug, in liquid form, is instilled into the bladder by means of a catheter (intravesicular injection). Fluid intake usually is limited before and during this procedure so that the drug remains concentrated and in contact with the bladder mucosa for about 2 hours. The client then voids and is given extra oral fluids to flush the drug from the bladder.

Intravesicular injection of BCG (bacillus Calmette-Guérin) Live, a weakened strain of *Mycobacterium bovis,* also may be used. It appears that BCG causes an inflammatory reaction in the bladder wall that in turn destroys malignant cells. Another form of therapy includes the administration of interferon alfa-2a (Roferon-A) injected intravenously (IV) or directly into the bladder. Interferon appears to stimulate the production of lymphocytes and macrophages that may destroy malignant cells.

Photodynamic therapy also may be used in the treatment of bladder cancer. This experimental treatment involves the IV injection of a photosensitizing agent that is absorbed in concentration by malignant cells. A laser, inserted through a cystoscope, is used to destroy those cells that have a high concentration of the photosensitizing agent.

Radiation therapy may be done if surgery is planned for the client. This reduces the size and extent of the tumor and decreases the risk of metastasis.

Surgical Management

A **cystectomy** (surgical removal of the bladder) and a urinary diversion procedure often are necessary when the tumor has penetrated the muscle wall. When a cystectomy is performed, the bladder and lower third of both ureters are removed. If the tumor has extended through the bladder wall, the surgeon may perform a radical cystectomy.

In women, a radical cystectomy usually includes removal of the bladder, lower third of both ureters, uterus, fallopian tubes, ovaries, anterior vaginal wall, and urethra. In men, a radical cystectomy usually includes removal of the bladder, lower third of both ureters, prostate, and seminal vesicles.

Once a cystectomy is performed, urine must be diverted to another collecting system. This is called a **uri-nary diversion.** Although urinary diversion procedures are used for the treatment of bladder tumors, they also are used for extensive pelvic malignancies and severe traumatic injury to the bladder. Some urinary diversions require external ostomy bags to collect the urine—referred to as *cutaneous urinary diversions* (Fig. 65-7). Other types create a reservoir within the body and the reservoir is catheterized to drain the urine—these are called *continent urinary diversions* (Fig. 65-8). In some instances the urine is diverted to the colon and the client voids rectally—this also is referred to as a continent urinary diversion. Each of the procedures has advantages and disadvantages. The

A

Conventional ileal conduit. The surgeon transplants the ureters to an isolated section of the terminal ileum (ileal conduit), bringing one end to the abdominal wall. The ureter may also be transplanted into the transverse sigmoid colon (colon conduit) or proximal jejunum (jejunal conduit).

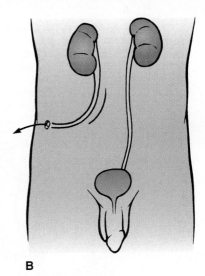

B

Cutaneous ureterostomy. The surgeon brings the detached ureter through the abdominal wall and attaches it to an opening in the skin.

C

Vesicostomy. The surgeon sutures the bladder to the abdominal wall and creates an opening (stoma) through the abdominal and bladder walls for urinary drainage.

D

Nephrostomy. The surgeon inserts a catheter into the renal pelvis via an incision into the flank or, by percutaneous catheter placement, into the kidney.

FIGURE 65-7 Types of cutaneous diversions include (**A**) the conventional ileal conduit, (**B**) cutaneous ureterostomy, (**C**) vesicostomy, and (**D**) nephrostomy.

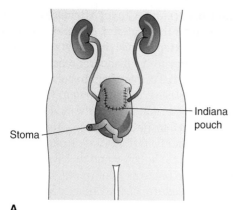

A

Indiana pouch. The surgeon introduces the ureters into a segment of ileum and cecum. Urine is drained periodically by inserting a catheter into the stoma.

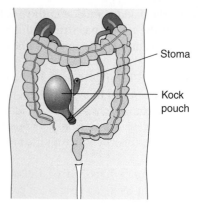

B

Continent ileal urinary diversions (Kock pouch). The surgeon transplants the ureters to an isolated segment of small bowel, ascending colon, or ileocolonic segment and develops an effective continence mechanism or valve. Urine is drained by inserting a catheter into the stoma.

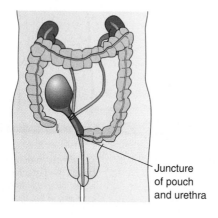

C

In male patients, the *Kock pouch* can be modified by attaching one end of the pouch to the urethra, allowing more normal voiding. The female urethra is too short for this modification.

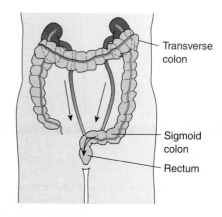

D

Ureterosigmoidostomy. The surgeon introduces the ureters into the sigmoid, thereby allowing urine to flow through the colon and out of the rectum.

FIGURE 65-8 Types of continent urinary diversions include (**A**) the Indiana pouch, (**B** and **C**) the Kock pouch, also called a continent ileal diversion, and (**D**) a ureterosigmoidostomy.

type of procedure used depends on many factors, such as the age and physical condition of the client, the procedure that can produce the best results for the client, and the extent of metastases.

Nursing Management

Preoperative Period

The nurse obtains a complete medical, drug, and allergy history on admission and asks the client or family member to describe all symptoms. The assessment also in-

cludes an evaluation of general physical and emotional status, vital signs, and weight.

Caring for a client during the preoperative period includes reducing anxiety and increasing understanding of the preparations for surgery and postoperative care. The client may display various emotional responses before surgery. Some may appear depressed; others show a mixture of anxiety and depression. The client faces drastic changes in the manner of excreting urine from the body, the diagnosis of cancer, and the changes in body image. The nurse encourages the client to talk about the surgery and the changes that will occur. He or she may suggest a visit from a member of a local ostomy group to provide emotional support as well as information. The enterostomal therapist should meet with the client to discuss placement of the stoma and collection devices. Photographs or drawings are useful in showing the placement of the stoma and urostomy pouch.

The nurse determines the client's ability to manage stoma care or self-catheterization by assessing manual dexterity, level of understanding, and vision. Assessing the client's social support and resources, including whether insurance will cover ostomy supplies, is important. The nurse explains all preoperative preparations to the client and family and gives them time to ask additional questions about the surgery, preparations for surgery, and management after surgery.

Depending on the extent and type of surgery, preoperative preparations may include insertion of a nasogastric tube, placement of IV and central venous pressure lines, administration of cleansing enemas, and adherence to a low-residue diet several days before surgery. Laxatives and enemas and a drug such as kanamycin (Kantrex) or neomycin (Mycifradin) may be given if a ureterosigmoidostomy (see Fig. 65-8) is to be performed. These agents decrease the number of microorganisms in the bowel and lessen the possibility of infection as a complication of connecting the ureters to the bowel. Clients scheduled for an ileal conduit (see Fig. 65-8) or continent urinary diversion procedure also may have the bowel prepared in this manner.

Postoperative Period

Clients undergoing urinary diversion are subject to the same conditions and complications as any surgical client. Refer to Chapter 25 for nursing diagnoses and interventions for managing standard postoperative care. Management issues related specifically to urinary diversion procedures include observing for leakage of urine or stool from the anastomosis, maintaining renal function, assessing for signs and symptoms of peritonitis, maintaining integrity of the urinary diversion and urine collection devices, maintaining skin and stomal integrity, promoting a positive body image, and teaching the client how to manage the diversion.

The nurse checks the client's chart for information regarding the type and extent of surgery and orders for connection of catheters or drains, IV fluids, and analgesics. Clients will have multiple drainage tubes, ureteral stents, and a nasogastric tube. All urinary drainage tubes must be labeled, and the urine output from each catheter or stoma must be measured and recorded hourly.

Maintaining accurate intake and output measurements during the postoperative period is important because it indicates both renal function and the integrity of the urinary diversion structures. Obstruction of urine flow can severely damage the kidneys. If urinary drainage stops or decreases to less than 30 mL/hour, or if the client complains of back pain, the nurse needs to notify the

physician immediately. Inspection of the urine includes checking for color, clarity, and presence of blood. It is essential immediately to report concentrated, cloudy, or bloody urine to the physician. Ureteral stents remain in place for several days after surgery.

The nasogastric tube is connected to low intermittent suction. This prevents distention and pressure on the suture line due to the collection of gas in the bowel. The nasogastric tube is removed once peristalsis has returned and the diet can be advanced. All laboratory reports are reviewed as soon as they are received and abnormalities reported to the physician promptly. The following sections address management issues specific to the most common procedures.

ILEAL CONDUIT

A transparent ostomy bag is applied over the stoma to make stomal assessment easier (Fig. 65-9). The nurse contacts the physician immediately if there is excessive bleeding, changes in the color of the stoma (e.g., from a normal to a cyanotic color), or separation of the stoma edges from the surrounding skin. The nurse uses gauze pads to clean mucus away from the stoma. Because the intestinal anastomosis can leak fecal material or the ileal conduit may leak urine into the peritoneal cavity, he or she observes for and promptly reports symptoms of peritonitis (e.g., abdominal tenderness or distention, fever, severe pain). Management of the urinary stoma is similar to management of a fecal stoma (see Chap. 54). The skin needs protection, the surgical dressings must be changed promptly when they become wet, and the appliances need care and cleansing. Each time he or she changes a temporary drainage bag, the nurse inspects the skin around the stoma for signs of infection and skin breakdown.

CONTINENT URINARY DIVERSION (KOCK POUCH, INDIANA POUCH)

The nurse inspects the stoma for bleeding or cyanosis. He or she may irrigate the pouch, if ordered, to prevent mucus plugs or blood clots. The nurse teaches the client how to perform intermittent self-catheterization (Fig. 65-10). Initially this is done every 1 to 2 hours but eventually will be performed every 4 to 6 hours.

URETEROSIGMOIDOSTOMY

A catheter is inserted in the rectum to drain urine continuously. The nurse checks the amount and color of drainage from the rectal catheter every 1 or 2 hours and inspects the anal and gluteal areas for signs of early skin breakdown. The catheter is removed when peristalsis returns. Because the sigmoid colon reabsorbs urinary constituents, clients are prone to fluid and electrolyte imbalances throughout the postoperative period (as well as for the rest of their lives). Observation for signs of electrolyte losses is essential. The nurse teaches the client exercises to improve sphincter control. Once good control is achieved, the nurse instructs the client to void (rectally) every 2 hours to prevent reabsorption of fluid

FIGURE 65-9 Urostomy pouch and stomadhesive wafer.

and electrolytes. Clients must never have enemas, suppositories, or laxatives.

NURSING PROCESS

● Psychosocial Care of the Client Undergoing Urinary Diversion

Assessment

The nurse assesses the client's knowledge about the effects of surgery on sexual function. Up to 85% of men experience erectile dysfunction after urinary diversion.

FIGURE 65-10 Self-catheterization of a continent urinary diversion through the stoma.

Women may have painful intercourse and lack lubrication. The nurse asks the client about his or her current level of social activity and what changes he or she thinks will occur after surgery. The nurse assesses the client's understanding of long-term postoperative care.

Diagnosis, Planning, and Interventions

Risk for Ineffective Sexuality Patterns related to erectile dysfunction (male) or dyspareunia (female)
Expected Outcome: Client will regain erectile function or ease painful intercourse.

* Tactfully ask the client if he or she has any questions. *Asking provides an opportunity to discuss sexuality issues.*
* Encourage client and partner to share their feelings about alteration in sexual function. *Acknowledging the importance of sexual function and expression may assist the client and partner to seek sexual counseling and to explore alternative methods of expressing sexuality.*
* Discuss alternatives to sexual intercourse such as closeness and giving pleasure to a partner. Provide information about penile prosthesis for men and water-soluble lubricants for women. Inform women that Kegel exercises may ease painful intercourse. Discuss masturbation, either individual or mutual, as an option. *Alternatives to sexual intercourse enable and enhance sexual satisfaction that physical limitations may otherwise impede.*

Disturbed Body Image related to change in appearance and function
Expected Outcome: Client will accept altered appearance and perform self-care.

* Assess client's willingness to look at the stoma. Accept client's response and reinforce that anxiety is normal. Reassure client that nursing staff will provide care until he or she is ready. *Gradual exposure is part of rehabilitation. The nurse supports the client's process.*
* Discuss change in function and let client know what to expect when recovery from surgery is complete. Suggest a visit from an ostomate who can provide valuable personal information, support, and resources. *Providing information and group support assists the client to know that he or she is not alone and will be prepared to care for himself or herself.*
* Help client gain independence by reinforcing that self-care is quite manageable and providing time for practice. *Encouragement and support promote confidence and move the client from a dependent to an independent role.*

Risk for Social Isolation related to fear of accidents or urine odor
Expected Outcome: Client will maintain social relationships.

* Explain that odor-proof pouches or pouches with carbon filters or other odor barriers are available. A few drops of liquid deodorizer or diluted white vinegar also may assist in controlling odors. Suggest avoiding odor-producing foods, such as asparagus, eggs, or cheese. *A client may become socially isolated from the odors pro-*

duced by the urinary diversion. Information about how to control odors will assist the client to implement measures and then to feel that friends, coworkers, and acquaintances will accept him or her.

- Oral ascorbic acid may help to control odors. *Ascorbic acid helps to acidify urine and suppress urine odors.*
- Teach client to care for the pouch and to change it every 3 days if it is a one-piece pouch or every 4 to 7 days if it is a two-piece. *Appropriate care assists in reducing odors and contributes to the client's level of confidence.*
- Tell client to empty the bag before it gets half full to prevent tension on the adhesive wafer and to eliminate source of odors. Inform the client to carry a spare pouch in case adhesive loosens while out. *These measures prevent accidents or embarrassment and provide the client with a sense of control and positive well-being.*
- Suggest drinking cranberry juice or using an appliance deodorant. *These measures reduce odors and assist the client to feel in control.*
- Suggest that the client contact the urostomy association for suggestions and additional support in alleviating anxiety. Instruct client with a ureterosigmoidostomy to avoid gas-forming foods. *Receiving support and accurate information contributes positively to a client's sense of well-being.*

Risk for Ineffective Management of Therapeutic Regimen related to inadequate knowledge about stomal care

Expected Outcome: Client will demonstrate ability to change ostomy pouch.

- Explain procedure for removing the old pouch and fitting and applying a new one. Tell client to change the pouch in the morning before consuming liquids and to insert a tampon or rolled gauze into the stoma to absorb urine during appliance change. Make sure the appliance fits well and the skin is completely dry when applying adhesive wafer. *Knowledge of specific procedures and treatment regimen increases a client's understanding and promotes responsibility for self-care.*
- Picture frame the wafer with paper tape to seal edges. Show the client how to empty the pouch and attach it to an overnight drainage system. *These measures provide more control over the outcome and improve the client's ability to care for himself or herself.*
- Teach client to inspect the periostomal skin each time he or she changes the pouch. Advise using a liquid skin barrier to protect the skin. If abdominal skin must be shaved, use an electric razor. *These strategies prevent skin breakdown and promote early intervention. They also provide the client with the skill and knowledge to adequately care for himself or herself.*

Risk for Ineffective Management of Therapeutic Regimen related to inadequate knowledge about intermittent catheterization of continent urinary diversions (Kock pouch, Indiana pouch)

Expected Outcome: Client will demonstrate ability to catheterize the pouch.

- Identify need for continuous drainage and frequent catheterizations in early postoperative period. Explain need for irrigations (to flush mucus and prevent plugging of catheter). *Understanding the rationales for the procedures promotes learning and ability for self-care.*
- Teach client to self-catheterize by lubricating catheter, inserting it into pouch, and allowing urine to drain into the toilet bowl. *Demonstration of procedures assists the client to develop competence and confidence in the self-care activities.*

Evaluation of Expected Outcomes

The client discusses methods for resuming sexual activity and alternatives to sexual intercourse. He or she states methods to avoid accidents and control urine odor. The client verbalizes a willingness to maintain social activity. He or she correctly changes the ostomy appliance and successfully self-catheterizes continent pouch.

Client and Family Teaching

The material included in a client teaching plan varies according to the type of surgery or the physician's specific discharge orders. In addition to the points discussed previously, the nurse must consider the following when preparing a teaching plan:

- Clients with a ureterosigmoidostomy must know the signs of fluid and electrolyte imbalances. To ensure understanding, give the client a written or printed list of the symptoms.
- Closed collection containers always should be below the level of the stoma. The tubing that connects the catheter or collection appliance to the closed drainage system must be kept straight so that urine does not collect in a curve of the tube. Avoid kinks that prevent the drainage of urine.
- Adequate fluids are necessary. Note the color of the urine. If the urine appears darker than usual, more fluids may be needed. Dark urine, despite an adequate fluid intake, is brought to the attention of the physician.
- Medications are taken as prescribed by the physician. Do not omit or stop taking the drugs. Do not take or use any nonprescription drug without first checking with the physician. Those with a ureterosigmoidostomy must not use laxatives or enemas.
- Odors can be controlled with cranberry juice, yogurt, or buttermilk. Avoid foods that may impart an odor to the urine, such as asparagus, cheese, or eggs.
- The enterostomal therapist recommends skin care techniques. The skin must be kept clean. When the adhesive wafer (to which the urostomy collection bag is attached) is changed, all remaining adhesive is removed before application of a new wafer.
- The continent urostomy should be drained four times a day or as directed by the physician.
- The urinary collection pouch needs to be washed thoroughly after changing. Rinse the pouch with or soak in a solution of vinegar and water if crystals form in the pouch.

- The physician is contacted if any of the following occur:
  - Fever
  - Chills
  - Blood in the urine
  - Failure of a stoma or catheter to drain urine
  - Skin problems around the stoma
  - Weight loss (> 5 lbs)
  - Loss of appetite (more than a few days)
  - Inability to insert the catheter in the continent urostomy
  - Pain in the flank (kidney area or lower abdomen)
  - Signs of fluid or electrolyte imbalance
  - Any unusual symptom or problem

TRAUMA

Trauma to the bladder or urethra is potentially harmful and frequently requires surgical intervention.

Pathophysiology and Etiology

Various types of injury can affect the urinary tract. Gunshot and stab wounds, crushing injuries, and forceful blows can result in tears, hemorrhage, or penetration of one or more parts. Some penetrating bladder injuries are small, whereas others are large with a rapid collection of urine in the peritoneal cavity. Injuries to the kidney area may result in bruising or tearing of the kidney and its capsule. Depending on the severity of the injury, blood and urine may leak into the peritoneal cavity.

Assessment Findings

Signs and Symptoms

Symptoms vary according to the area affected and the type of injury. Anuria, hematuria, pain in the abdomen (which may indicate bleeding or leakage of urine into the abdominal cavity), pain in the bladder or kidney areas, and symptoms of shock may be indicators of urinary tract injury. During treatment of a client with extensive injury, an indwelling catheter may be inserted, and hematuria or lack of urine output may be the first sign of a traumatic injury to the urinary tract. Certain other types of injuries, such as stab or gunshot wounds, may be immediately identified because of outward signs of injury (e.g., entry wounds on skin surface).

Diagnostic Findings

Injury to the urinary tract initially may be overlooked when the client has incurred widespread, massive injuries. Abdominal x-rays, cystoscopy, IVP, and exploratory surgery may be used to identify the type and location of the injury.

Surgical Management

Treatment depends on the type, location, and extent of injury as well as on the condition of the client. For example, a stab wound in the kidney area may require emergency exploratory surgery. Once the kidney is exposed, the physician needs to determine if the trauma to the kidney can be repaired or if the kidney must be removed immediately. Examples of surgeries that may be performed for urinary tract trauma include cystostomy (temporary or permanent), nephrectomy, insertion of a nephrostomy tube, repair (reanastomosis) of the ureter, and cystectomy.

Nursing Management

The most important nursing task is recognition of abnormal findings. Lack of urinary output, diffuse and severe abdominal pain, and hematuria are examples of signs and symptoms that may indicate an injury to the urinary tract. In some instances, the injury may be such that symptoms do not appear for several hours or days after the initial trauma.

Other nursing management depends on the surgical interventions performed and the symptoms the client experiences. In addition, the nurse needs to focus on the client's physical and emotional needs related to the trauma.

GENERAL NUTRITIONAL CONSIDERATIONS

Cranberry juice cocktail sold in grocery stores is only about 25% cranberry juice; the amount needed to acidify the urine is too large to be of practical value. Cranberry juice may be effective against urinary tract infections, however, by preventing bacteria from adhering to the lining of the urinary tract, thus promoting their excretion. Not all bacteria are sensitive to the juice, and protection lasts only as long as the juice is consumed regularly.

Encourage clients with bladder stones to drink 8 ounces of fluid hourly during waking hours, or at least 2 L of fluid daily.

Clients with calcium oxalate stones should limit calcium intake to 1000 mg/day or less (3 cups of milk or less daily). Because fiber interferes with the absorption of oxalate from the gastrointestinal tract, a high-fiber diet is recommended. High intakes of protein and sodium are avoided because they promote urinary calcium excretion.

GENERAL PHARMACOLOGIC CONSIDERATIONS

Antibiotics and sulfonamides are drugs commonly used to treat urinary tract infections. Other drugs used are furan derivatives, nitrofurantoin microcrystals (Macrodantin) and nitrofurantoin (Furadantin), and the acids, methenamine mandelate (Mandelamine) and nalidixic acid (NegGram). An azo dye, phenazopyridine (Pyridium), may be ordered for its soothing effect on bladder mucosa and often is used in conjunction with urinary antimicrobial drugs.

Instruct clients who receive drugs for urinary tract infections to finish the course of therapy even though they may feel improved and be symptom free after several days of therapy. A completed course of therapy is essential to be sure the infection is under control.

Advise clients to follow their physicians' instructions about the medication, such as drinking extra fluids.

 ## GENERAL GERONTOLOGIC CONSIDERATIONS

The older adult may have some form of incontinence. In some, involuntary leakage of urine may occur when the client coughs or sneezes, whereas others may be completely incontinent.

Some older adults may be unable to follow the instructions of a bladder rehabilitation program; others may have involuntary relaxation of the bladder sphincter, making rehabilitation extremely difficult.

Older clients with continence problems must not be treated like infants or scolded for their behavior (e.g., bed-wetting, soiling clothes). Make every effort to help rehabilitate the client. If bladder rehabilitation is not successful, try other methods to keep the client clean, dry, and odor free.

Carefully assess the cause of incontinence in the older adult. Older adults may be incontinent simply because environmental or physical conditions prevent them from maneuvering quickly enough to get to the bathroom before urination occurs. In these situations a change in the environment or an assistive device may alleviate the incontinence.

If the elderly client is incontinent, the perineal area is particularly susceptible to skin breakdown.

Clients must not be made to feel isolated when they have a problem with urinary continence. Planned exercise and social activities should be a part of a bladder rehabilitation program.

Critical Thinking Exercises

1. *A client has recurrent cystitis. Her physician wants to perform a cystoscopy and retrograde pyelograms. She asks you why she needs these tests because the medication she took in the past cured her problem. What explanation would you give?*
2. *Discuss the possible psychosocial effects of interstitial cystitis.*
3. *A client has a ureterosigmoidostomy. What teaching will you do regarding long-term follow-up and care?*

References and Suggested Readings

Bates, P., Getz, B., Gibbs, E., Neu, L., & Pobursky, J. (2000). Clinical conversations: Nurses who work with patients with interstitial cystitis. *Urologic Nursing, 20,* 109–110, 115–118.

Benson, M. & Olson, C. (1999). Continent urinary diversion. *Urologic Clinics of North America 26,* 125–147.

Bullock, B. A. & Henze, R. L. (2000). *Focus on pathophysiology.* Philadelphia: Lippincott Williams & Wilkins.

Gray, M. (2000). Urinary retention: Management in the acute care setting. Part 1. *American Journal of Nursing, 100*(7), 40–47.

Gray, M. (2000). Urinary retention: Management in the acute care setting. Part 2. *American Journal of Nursing, 100*(8), 36–44.

Marchiondo, K. (1998). A new look at urinary tract infection. *American Journal of Nursing, 98*(3), 4–38.

Mayo Clinic. (2001). Overactive bladder: How to keep it from controlling your life. *Women's HealthSource, 5*(11), 1–2.

McConnell, E. A. (2001). Clinical do's and don'ts: Preventing nosocomial urinary tract infections. *Nursing 2001, 31*(5), 17.

McConnell, E. A. (2000). Tech update: New catheters decrease nosocomial infections. *Nursing Management, 31*(6), 52.

Newland, J. A. (1998). Cystitis in women. *American Journal of Nursing, 98*(1), 16AAA.

Peters, K. M. (2000). The diagnosis and treatment of interstitial cystitis. *Urologic Nursing, 20*(2), 101–107, 117–118, 131.

Porth, C. M. (2002). *Pathophysiology: Concepts of altered health states* (6th ed.). Philadelphia: Lippincott Williams & Wilkins.

Rigby, D. (1998). Urinary tract infections: The hidden cause. *Community Nurse, 4*(5), 30–32.

Sienty, M. K. & Dawson, N. (1999). Hospital extra: Preventing urosepsis from indwelling urinary catheters. *American Journal of Nursing, 99*(1), 24C, 24F, 24H.

Smeltzer, S. C. & Bare, B. G. (2000). *Brunner and Suddarth's textbook of medical–surgical nursing* (9th ed.). Philadelphia: Lippincott Williams & Wilkins.

Wooldridge, L. (2000). Ultrasound technology and bladder dysfunction. *American Journal of Nursing, 100*(6), 3–14.

Introduction to the Musculoskeletal System

Words to Know

arthrocentesis
arthrogram
arthroscopy
bone scan
bursa
calcification
cancellous bone
cartilage
cortical bone
diaphyses
epiphyses
joint

ligament
ossification
osteoblasts
osteoclasts
osteocytes
periosteum
red bone marrow
resorption
skeletal muscles
tendon
yellow bone marrow

Learning Objectives

On completion of this chapter, the reader will:

- Describe major structures and functions of the musculoskeletal system.
- Discuss elements of the nursing assessment of the musculoskeletal system.
- Identify common diagnostic and laboratory tests used in the evaluation of musculoskeletal disorders.
- Discuss the nursing management of clients undergoing tests for musculoskeletal disorders.

The musculoskeletal system consists of bones, muscles, joints, tendons, ligaments, cartilage, and bursae. It supports the body and facilitates movement. Other functions include storage of calcium, phosphorus, magnesium, and fluoride; production of blood cells in the bone marrow; and protection and support to body organs, such as the lungs, heart, and brain. Injury to or disease in any part of the musculoskeletal system can cause pain, immobility, or disability and potentially affect quality of life.

ANATOMY AND PHYSIOLOGY

Bones

The human body has 206 bones. The bones of the skeleton are classified as:

- *Short bones,* such as those in the fingers and toes
- *Long bones,* such as the femur and ulna
- *Flat bones,* such as the sternum
- *Irregular bones,* such as the vertebrae

There are two types of bony tissue. The first is **cancellous bone,** or spongy bone, which is light and contains many spaces. The second is **cortical bone,** or compact bone, which is dense and hard. Both types are found in varying amounts in all bones. Cancellous bone is found at the rounded, irregular ends, or **epiphyses,** of long bones. Cortical bony tissue covers bones and is found chiefly in the long shafts, or **diaphyses,** of bones in the arms and legs. The combination of the two types of bony tissue provides strength and support, yet keeps the skeleton light to promote endurance during activity.

Bone is composed of cells, protein matrix, and mineral deposits. The three types of bone cells are osteo*blasts,* osteo*cytes,* and osteo*clasts.* Cells that build bones are called **osteoblasts.** These cells secrete bone matrix (mostly collagen), in which inorganic minerals, such as calcium salts, are deposited. This process of **ossification** and **calcification** transforms the blast cells into mature bone cells, called **osteocytes,** which are involved in maintaining bone tissue. During times of rapid bone growth or bone injury, osteocytes function as osteoblasts to form new bone. **Osteoclasts** are the cells involved in the destruction, resorption, and remodeling of bone.

During growth, bones primarily lengthen. The diameter also increases when osteoclasts break down previously formed bone, however, making the central canal wider. When skeletal growth is complete, the osteoclasts, which are part of the mononuclear phagocyte system (blood cells involved in ingesting particulate matter—or recycling old cells), continue with the remodeling of bones by balancing bone **resorption** with new bone cell replacement. Bone formation and resorption continue throughout life. The greatest activity occurs from birth through puberty. Table 66-1 reviews factors that affect bone formation.

A layer of tissue called **periosteum** covers the bones (but not the joints). The inner layer of periosteum contains the osteoblasts necessary for bone formation. The periosteum is rich in blood and lymph vessels and supplies the bone with nourishment.

Inside bones are two types of bone marrow: red and yellow. **Red bone marrow,** found primarily in the sternum, ileum, vertebrae, and ribs, manufactures blood cells and hemoglobin. Long bones have **yellow bone marrow,** which consists primarily of fat cells and connective tissue. If the blood cell supply becomes compromised, the yellow marrow may take on the characteristics of red marrow and begin producing blood cells.

Muscles

There are three kinds of muscles: skeletal, smooth, and cardiac. **Skeletal muscles** are voluntary muscles; impulses that travel from efferent nerves of the brain and spinal cord control their function. The skeletal muscles promote movement of the bones of the skeleton. Examples of skeletal muscles are the biceps in the arms and the gastrocnemius in the calves.

Skeletal muscle is composed of muscle fibers that contain several myofibers. Sliding filaments called *sarcomeres* make up myofibers. They are the contractile units of skeletal muscle. Impulses from the central nervous system cause the release of acetylcholine at the motor end plate of the motor neuron that innervates the muscle. As a result,

TABLE 66-1	FACTORS THAT AFFECT BONE FORMATION
BONE FORMATION FACILITATORS	**BONE FORMATION RETARDANTS**
Calcium	Estrogen/androgen deficiency
Phosphorus	Vitamin deficiency
Estrogen	Starvation
Testosterone	Diabetes
Calcitonin	Steroids
Vitamins D, A, C	Inactivity/immobility
Growth hormone	Heparin
Exercise	Excess parathyroid hormone
Insulin	

calcium ions are released, and the release stimulates actin and myosin in the sarcomeres to slide closer together, resulting in contraction of the muscle. When calcium is depleted, the actin and myosin fibers move apart, causing relaxation of the sarcomeres, and thus the muscle.

Smooth and cardiac muscles are involuntary muscles; their activity is controlled by mechanisms in their tissue of origin and by neurotransmitters released from the autonomic nervous system. Smooth muscles are found mainly in the walls of certain organs or cavities of the body, such as the stomach, intestine, blood vessels, and ureters. Cardiac muscle is found only in the heart.

Joints

A **joint** is the junction between two or more bones (Table 66-2). Free moving joints, or diarthrodial joints, make up most skeletal joints. They allow certain movements. Terms related to diarthrodial joint movement are presented in Box 66-1. The surfaces of diarthrodial joints are covered with hyaline cartilage, which reduces the friction during joint movement. The space between is the joint cavity, which is enclosed by a fibrous capsule lined

TABLE 66-2	TYPES OF JOINTS	
TYPE	**CHARACTERISTIC**	**EXAMPLE**
Synarthrodial joints	Immovable	At the suture line of skull between the temporal and occipital bones
Amphiarthrodial joints	Slightly movable	Between the vertebrae
Diarthrodial joints (also called *synovial joints*)	Freely movable	Gliding joint: fingers Hinge joint: elbow Pivot joint: ends of radius and ulna Condyloid joint: between the wrist and forearm Saddle joint: between the wrist and metacarpal bone of the thumb Ball and socket joint: hip

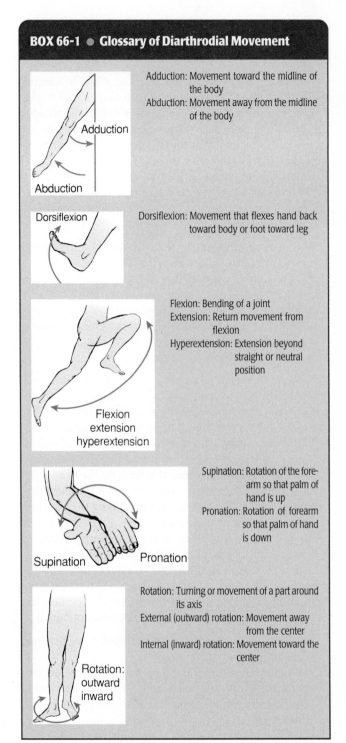

BOX 66-1 ● Glossary of Diarthrodial Movement

Adduction: Movement toward the midline of the body
Abduction: Movement away from the midline of the body

Dorsiflexion: Movement that flexes hand back toward body or foot toward leg

Flexion: Bending of a joint
Extension: Return movement from flexion
Hyperextension: Extension beyond straight or neutral position

Supination: Rotation of the forearm so that palm of hand is up
Pronation: Rotation of forearm so that palm of hand is down

Rotation: Turning or movement of a part around its axis
External (outward) rotation: Movement away from the center
Internal (inward) rotation: Movement toward the center

other is called the *insertion* and is more movable. When a muscle contracts, both attachments are pulled, and the insertion is drawn closer to the origin. An example can be found in the biceps of the arm, which has two origin tendons, attached to the scapula, and one insertion tendon, attached to the radius. When the biceps contracts, the lower arm (with the insertion tendon) moves toward the upper arm (with the origin tendon).

Ligaments

Ligaments consisting of fibrous tissue connect two adjacent, freely movable bones. They help protect the joints by stabilizing their surfaces and keeping them in proper alignment. In some instances, ligaments completely enclose a joint.

Cartilage

Cartilage is a firm, dense type of connective tissue that consists of cells embedded in a substance called the *matrix*. The matrix is firm and compact, thus enabling it to withstand pressure and torsion. The primary functions of cartilage are to reduce friction between articular surfaces, absorb shocks, and reduce stress on joint surfaces.

Hyaline or articular cartilage covers the surface of movable joints, such as the elbow, and protects the surface of these joints. Other types of cartilage include costal cartilage, which connects the ribs and sternum; semilunar cartilage, which is one of the cartilages of the knee joint; fibrous cartilage, found between the vertebrae (intervertebral discs); and elastic cartilage, found in the larynx, epiglottis, and outer ear.

Bursae

A **bursa** is a small sac filled with synovial fluid. Bursae reduce friction between areas, such as tendon and bone and tendon and ligament. Inflammation of these sacs is called *bursitis.*

ASSESSMENT

History

The focus of the initial history depends on whether the client has a chronic disorder or a recent injury. If the disorder is long-standing, the nurse obtains a thorough medical, drug, and allergy history. If the client is injured, the nurse finds out when and how the trauma occurred. He or she compiles a list of symptoms that includes information about the onset, duration, and location of discomfort

with synovial membrane. This membrane produces synovial fluid, which acts as a lubricant.

Tendons

Tendons are cordlike structures that attach muscles to the periosteum of the bone. A muscle has two or more attachments. One is called the *origin* and is more fixed. The or pain. Determining whether activity makes the symptoms better or worse is important. The nurse also identifies associated symptoms, such as muscle cramping or skin lesions, and asks the client if the problem interferes with activities of daily living. If the client has an open wound, the nurse ascertains when the client last received a tetanus immunization.

The nurse must obtain a history of past disorders and medical or surgical treatments as soon as possible. Attention to chronic or concurrent disorders, such as diabetes mellitus, is essential. In addition, the nurse obtains a family history, especially when relatives have had similar symptoms, and an occupational history.

Stop, Think, and Respond ● BOX 66-1

A neighbor calls you and states that he tripped and fell, spraining his ankle. When you arrive to help him, what questions should you ask? What should you observe?

Physical Examination

For a general musculoskeletal assessment, the nurse observes the client's ability to ambulate, sit, stand, and perform activities requiring fine motor skills, such as grasping objects. General inspection includes examining the client for symmetry, size, and contour of extremities and random movements. A spinal inspection includes identifying spinal curvatures (Fig. 66-1):

- *Kyphosis*—exaggerated convex curvature of the thoracic spine (humpback)

- *Lordosis*—excessive concave curvature of the lumbar spine (swayback)
- *Scoliosis*—lateral curvature of the spine

The nurse palpates the muscles and joints to identify swelling, degree of firmness, local warm areas, and any involuntary movements. To test the client's muscle strength, the nurse applies force to the client's extremity as the client pushes against that force. The nurse also must perform a neurovascular assessment (Table 66-3), which includes assessing range of motion for the joints, taking care not to force movement. The nurse notes any abnormal muscle movements such as spasms or tremors. In addition, the nurse:

- Looks for abnormal size or alignment and symmetry, comparing one side with the other
- Inspects and palpates for pain, tenderness, swelling, and redness
- Observes the degree of movement and range of motion, but never persists beyond the point of pain
- Tests for muscle strength
- Inspects for muscle wasting

Depending on the symptoms and findings, additional assessments may include looking for changes in gait and body posture, favoring one side over the other, and ability to bend and twist the trunk, head, and extremities.

If the client has a traumatic injury, physical assessment begins with taking vital signs. Further assessment depends on the type and area of injury. As the nurse conducts the assessment, he or she maintains standard precautions. The nurse needs to cut the clothing from around an injured area if there is no other way to examine the client. Comparing structures and assessment findings on one side of the body with those on the opposite side assists the nurse to determine the degree of injury. Although the nurse must be thorough, it also is important to be gentle, recognizing that assessment techniques may increase the client's pain. The examination includes the following:

- Observing for swelling, external bleeding, or bruising
- Palpating the peripheral pulses
- Evaluating peripheral circulation; assessing peripheral pulse (rate and character), skin coloration (pink, gray, pale, ashen), temperature, and capillary refill time
- Checking the sensation of the injured part
- Looking for broken skin, open wounds, superficial or embedded debris in or around the wound, protrusion of bone or other tissue from the wound
- Examining for injury beyond the original area; for example, auscultating the chest and abdomen if an abdominal or thoracic injury occurred or checking the pupils and mental status if a head injury occurred
- Looking for malalignment of the injured limb
- Assessing for pain, noting the type and location

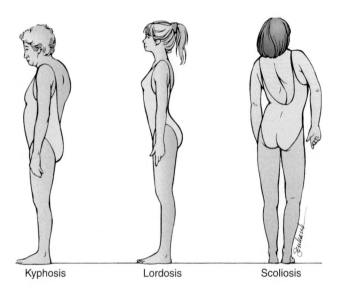

Kyphosis　　Lordosis　　Scoliosis

Figure 66-1 Common spinal curvatures.

TABLE 66-3	NEUROVASCULAR ASSESSMENT FINDINGS IN MUSCULOSKELETAL ASSESSMENT	
ASSESSMENTS	**NORMAL FINDINGS**	**ABNORMAL FINDINGS**
Circulation		
Distal pulses	Present and strong	Absent or weak
Capillary refill	Color returns to compressed nailbed within 3 seconds	Nailbed stays blanched after 3 seconds
Skin color	Similar to color in other body areas	Pale or dusky
Skin temperature	Warm	Cold
Local edema	Absent	+1 to +4 swelling
Sensation		
Arm injury	Can identify pressure applied to the tip of the index finger (median nerve) and the fifth finger (ulnar nerve), web between the thumb (radial nerve)	Numb to touch or feels abnormal sensation, like tingling or burning
Leg injury	Can identify pressure applied to great toe (peroneal nerve) and sole of the foot at the base of the toes (posterior tibial nerve) without observing the stimulus	Same as above
Mobility		
Arm injury	Can spread fingers on affected hand (ulnar nerve) Can press thumb to last digit on affected hand (median nerve) Demonstrates the "hitchhiker's sign" with affected hand, can flex and extend wrist (radial nerve)	Weak or cannot move fingers Cannot approximate thumb to finger Cannot extend thumb
Leg injury	Can flex and extend ankle (peroneal and posterior tibial nerves)	Wrist-drop is apparent. Foot-drop is apparent.
Pain	Proportional to injury but relieved with analgesia or nursing interventions	Constant or increased despite implementation of pain-relieving techniques

The physician needs to examine the client before the nurse touches, cleans, or disturbs open wounds and before moving the injured extremity.

Diagnostic Tests

Radiography, Computed Tomography, and Magnetic Resonance Imaging

Radiographic films, computed tomography, and magnetic resonance imaging help identify traumatic disorders, such as fractures and dislocations, and other bone disorders, such as malignant bone lesions, joint deformities, calcification, degenerative changes, osteoporosis, and joint disease.

Arthroscopy

Arthroscopy is the internal inspection of a joint using an instrument called an *arthroscope.* The most common use of arthroscopy is visualization of the knee joint, a common site of injury. After administering a local or general anesthetic, the physician inserts a large-bore needle into the joint and injects sterile normal saline solution to distend the joint. After inserting the arthroscope, the examiner inspects the joint for signs of injury or deterioration. Joint fluid may be removed and sent to the laboratory for examination. Depending on the findings, the physician sometimes can use the arthroscope to perform therapeutic procedures, such as removing bits of torn or floating cartilage.

Afterward, the client's entire leg is elevated without flexing the knee. A cold pack is placed over the bulky dressing covering the site where the arthroscope was inserted. A prescribed analgesic is administered as necessary. See Nursing Guidelines 66-1 for more discussion.

Arthrocentesis

Arthrocentesis is the aspiration of synovial fluid. The client receives local anesthesia just before this procedure. The physician inserts a large needle into the joint and removes the fluid. Synovial fluid may be aspirated to relieve discomfort caused by an excessive accumulation in the joint space or to inject a drug, such as a corticosteroid preparation. The removed synovial fluid may be sent to the laboratory for microscopic examination or for culture and sensitivity studies. Arthrocentesis also may be performed during an arthrogram or arthroscopy.

Arthrogram

An **arthrogram** is a radiographic examination of a joint, usually the knee or shoulder. The physician injects a local anesthetic and then inserts a needle into the joint space. Fluoroscopy may be used to verify correct placement of the needle. The synovial fluid in the joint is aspirated and sent to the laboratory for analysis. A contrast medium is then injected, and x-ray films are taken. After arthrography, the client is informed that he or she may hear crackling or clicking noises in the joint for up to 2 days. Noises beyond this time are abnormal; the client should report them.

Synovial Fluid Analysis

Synovial fluid is aspirated and examined to diagnose disorders such as traumatic arthritis, septic arthritis (caused by a microorganism), gout, rheumatic fever, and systemic lupus erythematosus. Normally, synovial fluid is clear and nearly colorless. Laboratory examination of synovial fluid may include microscopic examination for blood cells, crystals, and formed debris that may be present in the joint space after an injury. If an infection is suspected, culture and sensitivity studies are ordered. A chemical analysis for substances such as protein and glucose also may be performed.

Bone Densitometry

Bone densitometry estimates bone density. Radiography of the wrist, hip, or spine help to determine bone mineral density. Bone sonometry or ultrasound measures the quantity and quality of heel bone and provides an estimate of bone density.

Bone Scan

A **bone scan** uses the intravenous injection of a radionuclide to detect the uptake of the radioactive substance by the bone. A bone scan may be ordered to detect metastatic bone lesions, fractures, and certain types of inflammatory disorders. The radionuclide is taken up in areas of increased metabolism, which occur in bone cancer, metastatic bone disease, and osteomyelitis (bone infection).

Electromyography

Electromyography tests the electric potential of the muscles and nerves leading to the muscles. It is done to evaluate muscle weakness or deterioration, pain, and disability and to differentiate muscle and nerve problems. The physician inserts needle electrodes into selected muscles and uses electrical current to stimulate the muscles. An oscilloscope records responses to the electrical stimuli. If the client experiences discomfort after the study, warm compresses to the area help relieve the discomfort.

Biopsy

A biopsy is done to identify the composition of bone, muscle, or synovium. The specimen may be removed with a needle or excised surgically while the client is under general anesthesia. Afterward, the nurse observes the site for signs of bleeding or swelling, assesses for pain, applies ice to the site, and administers analgesics as indicated.

Blood Tests

A complete blood count (includes a red blood cell count, hemoglobin level, white blood cell count, and differential) may be ordered to detect infection, inflammation, or anemia. Examples of other diagnostic blood tests and findings of various musculoskeletal disorders include:

- Elevated alkaline phosphatase level, which may indicate bone tumors and healing fractures
- Elevated acid phosphatase level, which may indicate Paget's disease (a disorder characterized by excessive bone destruction and disorganized repair) and metastatic cancer
- Decreased serum calcium level, which may indicate osteomalacia, osteoporosis, and bone tumors
- Increased serum phosphorus level, which may indicate bone tumors and healing fractures
- Elevated serum uric acid level, which may indicate gout (treated or untreated)
- Elevated antinuclear antibody level, which may indicate lupus erythematosus, a connective tissue disorder

Urine Tests

When ordered, the nurse collects 24-hour urine samples for analysis to determine levels of uric acid and calcium excretion. In gout, the 24-hour excretion of uric acid is elevated. Elevated calcium levels are found in metastatic bone lesions and in clients with prolonged immobility.

NURSING MANAGEMENT

Some diagnostic tests are performed while the client is assessed in the emergency department, on an outpatient basis, or after admission for treatment of the disorder. The nurse implements protocols necessary to prepare the client for the diagnostic examination, identifies and sends collected specimens to the laboratory, and manages the client's safe recovery after invasive procedures.

If the client has a chronic disorder, the nurse obtains a general medical history and a description of the current symptoms. He or she compiles drug and allergy histories. An allergy to iodine and seafood may be a contraindication to performing an arthrogram or other test in which a contrast medium is instilled.

No special care is required after most laboratory tests, general radiography, or a bone scan. If the client has had an invasive joint examination, the nurse inspects the area for swelling and bleeding or serous drainage. He or she changes or reinforces dressings as needed. If the client has severe pain in the area, the nurse must notify the physician, who may order the application of ice and an analgesic for pain or discomfort.

In the case of a traumatic injury, the nurse obtains information regarding the injury from the client, the person accompanying the client, or paramedics and ambulance personnel. He or she takes vital signs during the initial examination and at frequent intervals until the client's condition stabilizes. The nurse also checks the neurovascular status of the affected limb, including circulation, motion, and sensation. Keeping the client calm and promoting comfort are essential measures. For example, if the client has an injury of the arm, the nurse prepares a sling to ease pain until treatment can be initiated.

NURSING PROCESS

● The Client With a Musculoskeletal Injury

Assessment

The nurse assesses the client's injury in terms of its location, nature, and effects on mobility. The nurse also determines the circulatory status to the injured area by checking circulation, sensation, and mobility, if it is not contraindicated. Assessing the client's level of pain is es-

sential. The nurse also monitors the client's vital signs and closely observes for signs of shock.

Diagnosis, Planning, and Interventions

The nurse provides a brief, broad overview of diagnostic tests or treatments because the client will find it difficult to comprehend details while anxious. The nurse provides the client and family with information about how long the test or examination will take, where it will be done, and what preparations (if any) are necessary. Allowing the client an opportunity to ask questions or make comments as he or she processes the information is very important. Before carrying out any preliminary activities before a diagnostic test, the nurse describes what is about to be done.

Invasive procedures, such as arthroscopy, and treatment procedures require the client to sign a consent form. The physician is responsible for explaining the purpose of the procedure, its risks and benefits, and available alternatives. The nurse repeats or clarifies the physician's explanations. After an outpatient procedure, the physician often gives the client special instructions for self-care. Because recalling information from memory can lead to confusion or injury, however, the nurse also provides written discharge instructions. Client and Family Teaching Box 66-1 discusses further education points. Additional diagnoses, expected outcomes, and interventions include the following.

Pain related to tissue injury
Expected Outcome: Client will have relief from pain.
- Minimize or avoid moving the painful body part. *Doing so prevents increased pain and helps the client to relax.*
- If the client must be moved from a stretcher, wheelchair, or an examination table, request sufficient help and support the joints above and below the area of discomfort during transfer. *Sufficient support prevents pain and avoids increasing discomfort.*
- Support an acutely or chronically inflamed joint in a comfortable position. *Maintaining a neutral position reduces pain.*
- Elevate a swollen extremity as long as doing so does not potentiate the trauma from an injury. Alternatively, cradle a painful arm in a sling when the client is up and about. *These measures reduce swelling and, subsequently, pain.*
- Observe for signs of respiratory depression if administering a prescribed narcotic analgesic for pain relief. *Opioids may cause respiratory depression and lead to sedation in a client susceptible to shock after a traumatic injury.*
- Notify physician if pain increases or is unrelieved. *Persistent pain may indicate further injury or sequelae to trauma.*

Risk for Impaired Tissue Perfusion related to swelling, inflammation, or inactivity imposed by injury

Expected Outcome: Client will maintain tissue perfusion in the injured area as evidenced by normal neurovascular assessment findings.

- Keep a swollen body part above the level of the heart. *This position promotes venous circulation and relieves edema.*
- Consult with the physician about applying a cold pack if an injury is recent. *Cold reduces circulation to the affected area and may impair neurovascular health.*
- In cases of head injury, elevate the client's head slightly while keeping the neck neutral. *Such positioning reduces the risk of further injury.*
- Report the absence of a peripheral pulse and severe pain immediately. *These findings may indicate ischemia.*

Anxiety related to pain and injury, its treatment, and the potential for altered mobility

Expected Outcome: Client's anxiety will be reduced as evidenced by vital signs within normal range and no signs of being overly alert or easily startled.

- Relieve discomfort as much as possible. *Doing so eliminates at least one aspect of the client's concerns.*
- Call the client by name; be empathic and attentive. *Attention to the client's needs promotes relaxation and comfort.*
- Instill confidence by demonstrating technical skill and competence in explanations or preparations for tests or treatments. *A confident nurse can help reduce a client's anxiety.*

- Speak quietly in simple sentences that the client can understand. *Understanding reduces anxiety.*
- Allow a supportive family member to stay with the client if possible. *This measure can comfort the client.*

Evaluation of Expected Outcomes

The client states that medication and positioning have relieved pain. Neurovascular status remains intact, as evidenced by good perfusion, strong pulses, ability to tense muscles, and appropriate sensation. The client has a calm demeanor and states that he or she feels less anxious.

GENERAL NUTRITIONAL CONSIDERATIONS

Although bone formation and resorption continue throughout life, net bone loss exceeds net bone gain in all people after peak bone mass is attained, sometime between ages 30 and 35 years. An adequate calcium intake before that time helps maximize peak bone mass; the denser the bones, the less susceptible they are to fracture.

Because most North Americans do not eat enough calcium to protect against bone loss, the Institute of Medicine of the National Academy of Sciences has issued new calcium recommendations that are higher than the previous Recommended Dietary Allowances for almost all age groups. The recommendations advise adults younger than 50 years of age to consume 1000 mg of calcium daily; those older than 50 years need 1200 mg daily, which translates to about four servings from the milk group each day. Clients who cannot or are unwilling to consume ample dairy products are not likely to meet their calcium requirement through diet alone.

Nondairy sources of calcium include green leafy vegetables, sardines, canned salmon with bones, broccoli, and calcium-fortified orange juice. With the exception of calcium-fortified orange juice, the body does not absorb calcium from nondairy sources well.

Vitamin D protects against bone loss and decreases the risk of fracture by facilitating the absorption of calcium from food and supplements. Without adequate vitamin D, calcium is excreted, not absorbed, even if calcium intake is adequate. Many people do not consume enough vitamin D because dietary sources are limited to fatty fish and vitamin D-fortified milk and cereals. Skin makes vitamin D when exposed to sunlight, but older skin makes less, and sun exposure does not produce vitamin D during the winter in people living in northern climates. Sunscreen, smog, and clothing block the ultraviolet light that makes vitamin D.

66-1 *Client and Family Teaching* Musculoskeletal Care

The nurse includes the following information:

- Signs or symptoms that clients must report, such as excessive pain or throbbing, prolonged or fresh bleeding, swelling, skin color changes, decrease in sensation, or purulent drainage
- Any special body position that the client must maintain
- When to resume bathing and activity
- How soon the client may return to work
- Purpose of prescribed drugs, how to take them, and possible side effects
- Approximate date for a follow-up appointment with the physician, if one is required
- How to remove and reapply dressings, and how to apply an immobilizer or sling, if one is used
- Demonstrations of the crutch-walking gait and instructions on how to do so safely, if the client must use crutches temporarily

GENERAL PHARMACOLOGIC CONSIDERATIONS

Oral calcium preparations containing vitamin D are better absorbed than those without vitamin D.

Clients should not take oral calcium preparations with other oral drugs because calcium may alter or block the absorption of the other drugs. For example, calcium decreases absorption of tetracycline and phenytoin. Clients should take other drugs 1 to 2 hours after calcium carbonate.

Clients should take oral calcium with meals to enhance absorption as well as to minimize gastric distress.

GENERAL GERONTOLOGIC CONSIDERATIONS

Women older than 45 years of age have a 9% to 10% decrease in cortical bone per decade.

Older adults are more prone to skeletal fractures because bone resorption is more rapid than bone formation.

Maintaining an active lifestyle delays the decline in muscle strength and bone mass among older adults.

With age, the fibrocartilage of intervertebral disks becomes thinner and drier, causing compression of the disks of the spinal column, and the water content of joint cartilage decreases, leading to a height loss of as much as 1.5 to 3 inches (3.75 to 7.5 cm).

Estrogen deficiency, which occurs at menopause, is considered the leading factor in osteoporosis among aging women.

1. *A client for whom you are caring in a nursing home falls. What assessments would you make?*
2. *What signs and symptoms would indicate that the tissue in an injured extremity is not being adequately perfused?*

References and Suggested Readings

Bullock, B. L. & Henze, R. L. (2000). *Focus on pathophysiology.* Philadelphia: Lippincott Williams & Wilkins.

Fischbach, F. T. (2002). *Common laboratory and diagnostic tests* (3rd ed.). Philadelphia: Lippincott Williams & Wilkins.

Kunkler, C. (1999). Neurovascular assessment. *Orthopaedic Nursing 18*(3), 63–71.

O'Hanlon-Nichols, T. (1998). Basic assessment series: Musculo-skeletal system. *American Journal of Nursing, 98*(6), 48–52.

Smeltzer, S. C. & Bare, B. G. (2000). *Brunner and Suddarth's textbook of medical–surgical nursing* (9th ed.) Philadelphia: Lippincott Williams & Wilkins.

Caring for Clients With Orthopedic and Connective Tissue Disorders

Words to Know

ankylosing spondylitis
ankylosis
arthritis
arthrodesis
arthroplasty
avascular necrosis
avulsion fracture
Bouchard's nodes
bursitis
callus
carpal tunnel syndrome
cast
closed reduction
compartment syndrome
contusion
degenerative joint disease
dislocation
ecchymosis
epicondylitis
external fixation
fasciotomy
fracture
gout
hallux valgus
hammer toe
Heberden's nodes

hyperuricemia
internal fixation
involucrum
lupus erythematosus
Lyme disease
open reduction
osseous ankylosis
osteomalacia
osteomyelitis
osteoporosis
osteotomy
Paget's disease
palsy
pannus
rheumatoid arthritis
sequestrum
sprain
strain
subluxation
synovectomy
synovitis
tophi
traction
Volkmann's
    contracture

Learning Objectives

On completion of this chapter, the reader will:

- Differentiate strains, contusions, and sprains.
- Describe the signs and symptoms and common treatments of a fracture.
- Identify the principles for maintaining traction.
- Discuss the complications associated with a fractured hip.
- Describe the difference between rheumatoid arthritis and degenerative joint disease.
- Describe the positioning precautions after a total hip replacement.
- State the pathophysiology of gout, bursitis, and ankylosing spondylitis.
- Explain the inflammatory process associated with Lyme disease.
- Identify the causes of osteomyelitis.
- Discuss the multisystem involvement associated with systemic lupus erythematosus.
- State who is at risk for development of osteoporosis.
- Differentiate between bunions and hammer toe.
- Explain the cause of carpal tunnel syndrome.
- Discuss characteristics of malignant bone tumors.
- Identify reasons for performing orthopedic surgery.
- Describe four principles to follow when wrapping a stump.
- Discuss the nursing management for a client with a sprain, dislocation, or cast; who is in traction or undergoing orthopedic surgery; or with an amputation.

The musculoskeletal system consists of structures the body uses for support and movement. It also protects body organs. Disorders affecting the musculoskeletal system affect the person's ability to perform activities of daily living (ADLs) and to remain active, mobile, and physically fit.

TRAUMATIC INJURIES

STRAINS, CONTUSIONS, AND SPRAINS

A **strain** is an injury to a muscle when it is stretched or pulled beyond its capacity. A **contusion** is a soft tissue injury resulting from a blow or blunt trauma. **Sprains** are injuries to the ligaments surrounding a joint.

Pathophysiology and Etiology

A strain results from excessive stress, overuse, or over-stretching. Small blood vessels in the muscle rupture, and the muscle fibers sustain tiny tears. The client experiences inflammation, local tenderness, and muscle spasms.

In contusions, injury is confined to the soft tissues and does not affect the musculoskeletal structure. Many small blood vessels rupture, causing bruises (**ecchymosis**) or a hematoma (collection of blood). Applying cold packs helps alleviate local pain, swelling, and bruising. A contusion usually resolves within 2 weeks.

Areas most subject to sprains are the wrist, elbow, knee, and ankle. A sprain of the cervical spine is commonly called a *whiplash injury.* Sprains result from sudden, unusual movement or stretching about a joint, common with falls or other accidental injuries. The force twists the joint in a direction it was not designed for or displaces it beyond its normal range of motion (ROM) by partially tearing or rupturing the attachment of ligaments. The damage usually is confined to the ligaments and adjacent soft tissue. In severe traumatic sprains, however, a chip of bone to which the ligament is attached may become detached. At this point, the injury becomes an **avulsion fracture.** A hematoma that may develop subsequently contributes to the pain because the mass exerts additional pressure on nerve endings in the area.

Assessment Findings

The injured area becomes painful immediately, and swelling usually follows. The person typically avoids full weight bearing or using the injured joint or limb. Later, ecchymoses may appear. In cases of extensive ligamental tearing, the joint may be unstable until it heals.

In most cases, diagnosis is made by examination of the affected part and symptoms. Radiographic films may show a larger-than-usual joint space and rule out or confirm an accompanying fracture. Arthrography demonstrates asymmetry in the joint as a result of the damaged ligaments, or arthroscopy may disclose trauma in the joint capsule.

Medical and Surgical Management

Treatment consists of applying ice or a chemical cold pack to the area to reduce swelling and relieve pain for the first 24 to 48 hours. Elevation of the part and compression with an elastic bandage also may be recommended. The acronym RICE refers to *r*est, *i*ce, *c*ompression, and *e*levation—a method for remembering the treatment for strains,

contusions, and sprains. After 2 days, when swelling no longer is likely to increase, applying heat reduces pain and relieves local edema by improving circulation. Full use of the injured joint is discouraged temporarily. Nonsteroidal anti-inflammatory drugs (NSAIDs) ease discomfort.

Continued trauma during healing may result in a permanently unstable joint or the formation of fibrous adhesions that may limit full ROM. Occasionally, a removable splint or light cast is applied for several weeks. A soft cervical collar limits motion if the client has a neck sprain. When sufficient healing has occurred, progressively active exercises are prescribed.

Stop, Think, and Respond ● BOX 67-1

You are at a playground when you notice a man, who has been playing basketball with his son, fall and grab his ankle. He says his ankle hurts very badly, and he does not think that he can walk. What action should you take?

● DISLOCATIONS

Dislocations occur when the articular surfaces of a joint are no longer in contact. The shoulder, hip, and knee commonly are affected. A partial dislocation is referred to as a **subluxation.**

Pathophysiology and Etiology

In adults, trauma usually causes dislocations. Occasionally, diseases of the joint result in dislocations when the ligaments supporting a joint are torn, stretched, or relaxed. Separation of adjacent bones from their articulating joint interferes with normal use and produces a distorted appearance. The injury may disrupt local blood supply to structures such as the joint cartilage, causing degeneration, chronic pain, and restricted movement. **Compartment syndrome** (a condition in which a structure such as a tendon or nerve is constricted in a confined space) also may develop. The syndrome affects nerve innervation, leading to subsequent **palsy** (decreased sensation and movement). If compartment syndrome occurs in an upper extremity, it may lead to **Volkmann's contracture,** a clawlike deformity of the hand resulting from obstructed arterial blood flow to the forearm and hand. The client is unable to extend his or her fingers and complains of unrelenting pain, particularly if attempting to stretch the hand. There also are signs of compromised circulation to the hand.

Another possible complication of dislocations during the healing process involves an insufficient deposit of collagen during the repair stage. The end result is that the ligaments may have reduced tensile strength and future instability, leading to recurrent dislocations of the same joint.

Assessment Findings

The client often reports hearing a "popping" sound when the dislocation occurs. Another common complaint is that the joint suddenly "gave out," implying that it became unstable or nonsupportive. If the dislocation results from trauma, the client usually experiences considerable pain from the injury or the resultant muscle spasm.

On inspection, the structural shape is altered. A depression may be noted about the joint's circumference, indicating that the bones above and below are no longer aligned. If the dislocation affects an extremity, the arm or leg may be shorter than its unaffected counterpart as a result of the displacement of one of the articulating bones. ROM is limited. Evidence of soft tissue injury includes swelling, coolness, numbness, tingling, and pale or dusky color of the distal tissue.

Radiographic films show intact yet malpositioned bones. Arthrography or arthroscopy may reveal damage to other structures in the joint capsule.

Medical and Surgical Management

The physician manipulates the joint or reduces the displaced parts until they return to normal position, then immobilizes the joint with an elastic bandage, cast, or splint for several weeks. Doing so allows the joint capsule and surrounding ligaments to heal. The client may receive a local or general anesthetic before the manipulation is performed. Some dislocations may require surgery, either to correct the dislocation or to repair damage caused by the injury.

Nursing Management

The nurse relieves the client's discomfort by administering prescribed analgesics, elevating and immobilizing the affected limb, and applying cold packs to the injury. He or she performs neurovascular assessments every 30 minutes for several hours and then at least every 2 to 4 hours for the next 1 or 2 days to detect complications such as compartment syndrome. See Chapter 66 (Table 66-3) for more information about neurovascular assessments.

● FRACTURES

A **fracture** is a break in the continuity of a bone. Fractures may affect tissues or organs near the bones as well. Fractures are classified according to type and extent (Box 67-1).

BOX 67-1 ● Types of Fractures

Avulsion—a pulling away of a fragment of bone by a ligament or tendon and its attachment

Comminuted—a fracture in which bone has splintered into several fragments

Compound—a fracture in which damage also involves the skin or mucous membranes

Compression—a fracture in which bone has been compressed (seen in vertebral fractures)

Depressed—a fracture in which fragments are driven inward (seen frequently in fractures of skull and facial bones)

Epiphyseal—a fracture through the epiphysis

Greenstick—a fracture in which one side of a bone is broken and the other side is bent

Impacted—a fracture in which a bone fragment is driven into another bone fragment

Oblique—a fracture occurring at an angle across the bone (less stable than transverse)

Pathologic—a fracture that occurs through an area of diseased bone (bone cyst, Paget's disease, bony metastasis, tumor); can occur without trauma or a fall

Simple—a fracture that remains contained; does not break the skin

Spiral—a fracture twisting around the shaft of the bone

Transverse—a fracture that is straight across the bone

Pathophysiology and Etiology

When force applied to a bone exceeds maximum resistance, the bone breaks. Sudden direct force from a blow or fall causes most fractures; however, some result from indirect force—for example, from a strong muscle contraction, such as during a seizure. A few fractures result from underlying weakness created by bone infections, bone tumors, or more bone resorption than production (as occurs in clients who are inactive or aging).

For 10 to 40 minutes after a bone breaks, the muscles surrounding the bone are flaccid. Then they go into spasm, often increasing deformity and interfering with the vascular and lymphatic circulations. The tissue surrounding the fracture swells from hemorrhage and edema. Healing begins (Fig. 67-1) when blood in the area clots and a fibrin network forms between the broken bone ends. The fibrin network changes into granulation tissue. Osteoblasts, which proliferate in the clot, increase the secretion of an enzyme that restores the alkaline pH. As a result, calcium is deposited and true bone forms. The healing mass is called a **callus.** It holds the ends of the bone together but cannot endure strain. Bone repair is a local process. About 1 year of healing must pass before bone regains its former structural strength, becomes well consolidated and remodeled (reformed), and possesses fat and marrow cells.

Although fractures are common, they are associated with various complications, particularly when they are very complex. Table 67-1 briefly describes the types of possible complications, which include compartment syn-

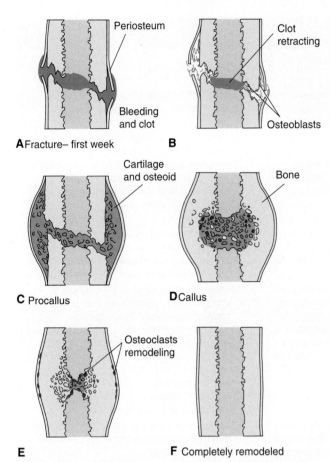

A Fracture– first week

B Periosteum / Bleeding and clot / Clot retracting / Osteoblasts

C Procallus / Cartilage and osteoid

D Callus / Bone

E Osteoclasts remodeling

F Completely remodeled

FIGURE 67-1 Process of bone healing. (**A**) Immediately after a bone fractures, blood seeps into the area, and a hematoma (blood clot) forms. (**B**) After 1 week, osteoblasts form as the clot retracts. (**C**) After about 3 weeks, a procallus forms and stabilizes the fracture. (**D**) A callus with bone cells forms in 6 to 12 weeks. (**E**) In 3 to 4 months, osteoblasts begin to remodel the fracture site. (**F**) If the fractured bone has been accurately aligned during healing, remodeling will be complete in about 12 months.

drome, thromboembolism, fat embolism, delayed healing, nonunion, malunion, infection, and **avascular necrosis** (death of bone from an insufficient blood supply). In addition, any client who is inactive during convalescence is prone to pneumonia, thrombophlebitis, pressure sores, urinary tract infection, renal calculi, constipation, muscle atrophy, weight gain, and depression.

Assessment Findings

Signs and Symptoms

The signs and symptoms of a fracture vary, depending on the type and location. They include the following:

- Pain—One of the most consistent symptoms of a fracture is pain, which may be severe. Attempts to move the part and pressure over the fracture increase pain.

- Loss of function—Skeletal muscular function depends on intact bone.
- Deformity—A break may cause an extremity to bend backward or to assume another unusual position.
- False motion—Unnatural motion occurs at the site of the fracture.
- Crepitus—The grating sound of bone ends moving over one another may be audible (this term also refers to a popping sound caused by air trapped in soft tissue).
- Edema—Swelling usually is greatest directly over the fracture.
- Spasm—Muscles near fractures involuntarily contract. Spasm, which accounts for some of the pain, may cause a limb to shorten when the fracture involves a long bone.

If sharp bone fragments tear through sufficient surrounding soft tissue, there is bleeding and black and blue discoloration of the area. If a nerve is damaged, paralysis may result.

Stop, Think, and Respond ● **BOX 67-2**

You are cross-country skiing with a friend and notice that a person ahead of you has fallen. When you get closer, this person tells you that she has hurt her arm. What signs would indicate that this woman probably has a fractured humerus?

Diagnostic Findings

One or more radiographic views of the area almost always demonstrate altered bone structure. Stress fractures may not be apparent radiographically for a few weeks. A bone scan usually can identify a nondisplaced or stress fracture before radiographic changes are evident. In some instances, a computed tomography (CT) scan or magnetic resonance imaging (MRI) may be necessary.

Medical and Surgical Management

The goal is to re-establish functional continuity of the bone. Treatment includes one or more methods: traction, closed or open reduction, internal or external fixation, or cast application. The treatment method depends on many factors, including the first aid given, the location and severity of the break, and the age and overall physical condition of the client.

Traction

Traction is a method of pulling structures of the musculoskeletal system. For traction to achieve its purpose, it requires *countertraction,* a force opposite to the mechanical pull, that usually is supplied by the client's own weight. Traction is used to relieve muscle spasm, align bones, and

TABLE 67-1	COMPLICATIONS OF FRACTURES

COMPLICATION	DESCRIPTION	NURSING IMPLICATIONS
Shock	Hypovolemic shock related to blood loss and loss of extracellular fluid from damaged tissue. If untreated, the client's condition will deteriorate.	Administer blood and fluid volume replacements as prescribed to prevent further losses.
Fat embolism	Fat globules released after fractures of pelvis or long bones, or after multiple injuries or crushing injuries. Globules combine with platelets to form emboli. Onset is rapid, with client experiencing respiratory distress and cerebral disturbances.	Monitor client for symptoms, which usually occur within 48–72 hours. To prevent fatty emboli, provide early respiratory support, ensure rapid immobilization of fracture, and observe client closely for signs of respiratory and nervous system problems.
Pulmonary embolism	Thromboembolism may occur after fracture or surgery to repair fractures. These lead to pulmonary emboli in some clients and can be fatal.	Promote circulation and prevent venous stasis to avoid pulmonary embolism. Administer low-dose heparin subcutaneously as prescribed to prevent clot formation.
Compartment syndrome	Tissue perfusion in the muscle compartment (muscle covered by inelastic fascia) is compromised secondary to tissue swelling, hemorrhage, or a cast that is too tight. If circulation is not restored, ischemia and tissue anoxia lead to permanent nerve damage, muscle atrophy, and contracture.	Monitor client for signs and symptoms of compartment syndrome such as unrelenting pain, unrelieved by analgesics. Elevate the extremity, apply ice, and perform neurovascular checks to help prevent this complication. As indicated, relieve pressure by loosening cast or preparing the client for a **fasciotomy** (surgical incision of fascia and separation of muscles).
Delayed bone healing	Bone fails to heal at the expected rate. Delayed healing may result from nonunion, characterized by the ends of the fractured bone failing to unite and heal, or it may result from malunion, characterized by the ends of the fractured bone healing in a deformed position.	Delayed union may require surgical intervention to promote bone growth, and correct the incorrect union. If necessary, prepare the client for use of electrical stimulation measures that promote bone growth, or for a bone graft.
Infection	The potential for infection increases with compound fractures, application of skeletal traction, or surgical procedures.	Perform careful assessments and maintain aseptic technique to prevent infections. Monitor for early signs of infection because early detection promotes early correction of the problem.
Avascular necrosis	This condition occurs from interruption of the blood supply to the fracture fragments after which the bone tissue dies; most common in the femoral head.	Be alert for client reports of pain and decreased function of the affected limb. If necessary, prepare the client for surgery, such as bone graft, bone prosthesis, joint replacement, joint fusion, or amputation.

maintain immobilization. The two most common types are skin traction and skeletal traction.

Skin traction is achieved by applying devices to the skin that indirectly affect the muscles or bones. An example is Buck's traction (Fig. 67-2A); another example is Russell traction (see Fig. 67-2B). Skeletal traction is applied directly to a bone by using a wire (Kirschner), pin (Steinmann), or cranial tongs (Crutchfield). General or local anesthesia may be used when inserting these devices. The pull is achieved by connecting the attachment from the client to a system of ropes, pulleys, and weights on an orthopedic bed frame. A Thomas splint with a Pearson attachment often is used to suspend a leg in traction. This is referred to as *balanced suspension traction.*

Figure 67-3 presents an example of skeletal traction with balanced suspension. The principles for maintaining effective traction are discussed in Box 67-2. Nursing care measures for a client in traction are presented in Nursing Guidelines 67-1.

Closed Reduction

In a **closed reduction,** the bone is restored to its normal position by external manipulation. A bandage, cast, or traction then immobilizes the area. X-ray films are taken to ensure correct alignment of the bone. Depending on the site and type of fracture, the client receives a local (nerve block) or general anesthetic for this procedure.

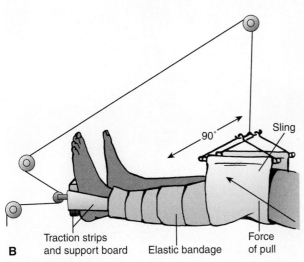

A

B   Traction strips and support board   Elastic bandage   Force of pull   90°   Sling

FIGURE 67-2 Two examples of skin traction: (**A**) Buck's traction and (**B**) Russell traction.

Radiographic studies, taken while the client is still anesthetized, show whether realignments are needed.

Internal Fixation

If **internal fixation** is needed to stabilize the reduced fracture, the surgeon secures the bone with metal screws, plates, rods, nails, or pins. A cast or other method of immobilization is then applied. Open reduction is required when:

- Soft tissue, such as nerves or blood vessels, is caught between the ends of the broken pieces of bone.
- The bone has a wide separation.
- Comminuted fractures are present.
- Patella and other joints are fractured.
- Open fractures are evident.
- Wound debridement is necessary.
- Internal fixation is needed.

External Fixation

In **external fixation,** the surgeon inserts metal pins into the bone or bones from outside the skin surface and then attaches a compression device to the pins. Some complex or comminuted fractures may require an external fixation

Open Reduction

In an **open reduction,** which is performed in the operating room, the bone is surgically exposed and realigned. Usually the client receives a general or spinal anesthetic.

FIGURE 67-3 Skeletal traction with balanced suspension.

NURSING GUIDELINES 67-1

Managing the Care of the Client in Traction

- Assess neurovascular status frequently. Compare assessment findings in the affected limb with those in the unaffected limb.

- Check traction equipment for:
  - Proper alignment (position client so that the body is in an opposite line to the pull of traction)
  - Correct attachment
  - Prescribed amount of weight
  - Freely hanging weights and freely moving ropes over unobstructed pulleys
  - Maintenance of countertraction

- Monitor client for signs of pressure areas.

- Encourage client to be as mobile as possible and to perform exercises as indicated.

- If traction is applied to the lower extremity, observe foot position and prevent footdrop.

- If skeletal traction is applied, follow procedure for pin care.

- Cover tips of any protruding metal pins or rods with corks or other protective material.

FIGURE 67-4 External fixation device.

device to stabilize and position the bone. Because the pin sites are an entry for infection, monitoring for redness, drainage, and tenderness is necessary. Figure 67-4 shows an external fixation device. Nursing Guidelines 67-2 describe pin care.

Casts

A **cast** is a rigid mold that immobilizes an injured structure while it heals. There are basically three types of casts. A *cylinder cast* encircles an arm or leg, leaving the fingers or toes exposed. A *body cast* is a larger form of a cylinder cast that encircles the trunk from about the nipple line to the iliac crests. A *hip spica cast* surrounds one or both legs and the trunk. It may be strengthened by a bar that spans a casted area between the legs (Fig. 67-5). This type of cast is trimmed open in the anal and genital areas to facilitate elimination.

To keep aligned bone fragments from becoming displaced, the cast is applied from the joint above the break to the one below it. The joint is slightly flexed to decrease stiffness. Some fractures (e.g., a stress fracture) do not require surgical reduction or manual manipulation to realign the bone because the fractured bone still remains perfectly aligned. If a closed or open reduction is required, the client receives an analgesic or a general or local anesthetic to relieve pain.

CAST COMPOSITION

Casts usually are made of fiberglass, polyester, or thermoplastic material. Plaster of Paris still is used in some

NURSING GUIDELINES 67-2

Providing Pin Care

Scrupulous pin care assists in preventing localized infection at the pin sites and systemic infection and osteomyelitis:

- Assess pin sites for redness, swelling, increased tenderness, and drainage.

- Examine pins for signs of breakage, bending, or shifting.

- Wearing gloves, use cotton-tipped applicators and saline to cleanse pin sites.

- Use at least one applicator per pin—do not use applicator more than once.

- Clean pin site from pin outward.

- Gently remove crusted areas.

- Avoid applying ointment to pin sites unless specifically ordered.

- Obtain culture if purulent drainage is present.

- Teach client not to touch pin sites.

- Instruct family member in pin care if client is discharged.

Figure 67-5 Spica cast. This client with a spica cast is resting on pillows until the cast dries. His feet are positioned so that they support the desired body alignment. Note the bar ensuring adequate space between the casted legs.

circumstances. Plaster casts require several hours for drying, whereas the other materials dry rapidly. A client with a synthetic cast may bear weight soon after the cast is applied.

When applying the cast, the physician positions the client to ensure proper alignment of the part to be immobilized. The client's buttocks may be supported on a casting frame when a body cast or spica cast is applied so the casting material can be wrapped around the client's trunk. A nurse or an assistant holds the arm or leg in place during application of a cylinder cast (Box 67-3). If the client is awake, healthcare providers explain that the cast material will feel warm during application as a result of being mixed with water.

BOX 67-3 ● Applying a Cast

In general, the physician or nurse practitioner applies a cast as follows:
- Clean and dry the skin surface.
- Cover the skin with stockinette, a tubular knitted material.
- Wrap padding around the limb, especially over bony prominences.
- Apply rolls or strips of cast material over the stockinette and padding.
- Smooth the layers and edges of the cast.
- Fasten the stockinette in cufflike fashion to the outside of the cast.
- Arrange for an x-ray study after casting to check bone alignment.

A wet cast must be kept uncovered so that water can evaporate. Most physicians prefer natural evaporation but may order a cast dryer to speed evaporation. Intense heat never is used. There is a danger not only of burning the client but of cracking the outside of the cast while leaving the inside damp and hospitable to mold. The drying cast should be supported on pillows. If necessary, healthcare personnel can reposition the casted arm or leg with the palms of the hands. Using the fingertips or compressing the cast on a hard surface can lead to a pressure sore later.

CAST WINDOWS

After the cast dries, a cast window, or opening, may be cut. This usually is done when the client reports discomfort under the cast or has a wound that requires a dressing change. The window permits direct inspection of the skin, a means to check the pulse in a casted arm or leg, or a way to change a dressing. Once a window is cut, the solid piece of cast is replaced in its original site and secured with adhesive tape or a roller bandage. Leaving the window open may allow the skin and soft tissue to bulge through the opening.

BIVALVE CASTS

Once a cast has been applied, it may be bivalved, or cut in two (Fig. 67-6). This may be necessary if the arm or leg swells, causing the rigid cast to compress the tissue and interfere with its blood supply. A bivalved cast also

Figure 67-6 (A) A bivalved cast. **(B)** The two halves are rejoined.

may be used for a client who is being weaned from a cast, when a sharp radiograph is needed, or as a splint for immobilizing painful joints when a client has arthritis.

CAST REMOVAL

Casts are removed with a mechanical cast cutter. Cast cutters are noisy and frightening, and the client needs reassurance that the machine will not cut into the skin. Once the cast is off, the skin appears mottled and may be covered with a yellowish crust composed of accumulated body oil and dead skin. The client usually sheds this residue in a few days. Lotions and warm baths or soaks may help to soften the skin and remove debris.

The now uncasted limb feels surprisingly light, and the client may report weakness and stiffness. For some time, the limb will need support. An elastic bandage may be wrapped on a leg, the client may use a cane, and an arm may be kept in a sling until progressive active exercise and physical therapy help the client regain normal strength and motion.

N U R S I N G   P R O C E S S

● **The Client With a Fracture**

Assessment

When caring for the client with a fracture, the nurse assesses for neurovascular and systemic complications.

Diagnosis, Planning, and Interventions

General nursing measures include administering analgesics, providing comfort measures, assisting with ADLs, preventing constipation, promoting physical mobility, preventing infection, maintaining skin integrity, and preparing the client for self-care. Because the client may be discharged shortly after application of an immobilization device or a cast, the nurse reviews care with the client and family. In addition, he or she reinforces instructions regarding exercise and ambulatory activities.

If a client is in traction, he or she requires simple and direct explanations about the traction and its purpose. The nurse points out activities that are allowed or contraindicated and identifies the approximate duration of restrictions. When the traction is discontinued, the nurse prepares the client for further treatment, such as casting (Nursing Guidelines 67-3), and the appearance of the affected area—skin and muscles. He or she reassures the client that, with gradual exercise and use, muscles will regain strength and tone, and joints will be flexible. For more information about managing problems related to casting, refer to Nursing Guidelines 67-3. For information about clients with specific fractures, such as those affecting the clavicle or knee, refer to Table 67-2.

Other responsibilities include, but are not limited to, the following:

Pain related to tissue and bone trauma, swelling, skeletal traction, or cast pressure
Expected Outcome: Client will report relief of pain after analgesics and comfort measures are administered.
- Administer prescribed analgesics. *They provide pain relief. Opioids are used to treat moderate to severe pain, and NSAIDs inhibit the initiation of pain impulses. Often after a traumatic injury, both opioids and NSAIDs are prescribed.*
- Elevate the extremity. *Elevation reduces swelling and pain.*
- Apply ice pack to site of injury as indicated. *Doing so reduces swelling and pain.*
- Change client's position within prescribed limits. *Position changes relieve pressure on bony prominences and promote comfort.*

Risk for Peripheral Neurovascular Dysfunction related to venous stasis, arterial insufficiency, and swelling
Expected Outcome: Client will maintain intact circulation, sensation, and mobility.
- Perform neurovascular assessments frequently, reporting any compromise immediately. *Capillary refill should be brisk (within 3 seconds), skin should be warm and normally colored, and the client should be able to move the extremity. Diminished or absent peripheral pulses, pale or mottled skin, cool to cold skin, or increased pain (especially with movement) can indicate arterial obstruction. Changes in sensation such as numbness, tingling, or prickling may indicate nerve compression and damage, compartment syndrome, or both.*
- Elevate the extremity, if indicated, and maintain proper alignment. *These measures promote circulation and decrease interference with arterial and venous circulation.*
- Encourage client actively to move toes, fingers, and unaffected extremities. *Movement promotes circulation and indicates neurologic and motor function.*
- Apply elastic stockings if indicated. *They promote circulation and decrease risk for deep vein thrombosis.*

Impaired Physical Mobility related to pain, swelling, surgical procedure, or immobilization from traction, cast, or splint
Expected Outcomes: (1) Client will regain or maintain maximum mobility and optimal functional position. (2) Client will have increased strength and function in the affected limb.
- Assess level of mobility. *These data provide a baseline for comparison.*
- Instruct client in active and passive ROM exercises for affected and unaffected extremities, within physical and medical restrictions. *ROM exercises strengthen muscles needed for mobility and function, prevent contractures and deformities, and promote circulation.*
- Teach client how to turn safely, adhering to restrictions. *Doing so encourages client's active participation and prevents further injury.*
- Assist and instruct client in the use of mobility aids (wheelchair, walker, crutches, canes) as needed. *The*

(text continued on page 1083)

NURSING GUIDELINES 67-3

Caring for the Client With a Cast

Before Cast Application

- Inspect the condition of the skin that will be covered with a cast.
- Assess circulation, sensation, and mobility to establish a baseline.
- Evaluate the client's pain level.
- Remove clothing that will be difficult to remove after the cast is applied.
- Explain the procedure to the client. Remember to tell the client that the cast will feel warm—even hot—as it is applied, but that it will not burn the skin.

After Cast Application

- Leave the cast uncovered.
- Assess circulation, sensation, and mobility in exposed fingers and toes every 1 to 2 hours.
- Monitor for signs of complications related to cast application. Report abnormal findings immediately.
- Handle wet cast with the palms of the hands, not the fingers.
- Elevate casted extremity so that it is higher than the heart.
- Reposition the client frequently while cast is drying so that the cast dries as evenly as possible.
- Apply ice packs to the cast where surgery was performed.
- Circle areas where blood seeped through and write the time on the circle.

- Petal cast edges with strips of adhesive tape to prevent chipping and to cover any remaining rough areas.
- Replace windows in the hole from which they were cut to prevent tissue from bulging through the opening.
- Ambulate client as soon as indicated.

Discharge Teaching

- Elevate casted extremity for 24 to 48 hours after cast application, and as indicated.
- If the client has a leg cast, show him or her how to ambulate safely.
- Exercise joints proximal and distal to the cast as indicated to prevent muscle atrophy, weakness, and loss of joint mobility.
- Keep the cast clean and dry. A damp cloth may be used.
- Explain that the skin under the cast may feel itchy, and caution client not to insert objects like straws, combs, eating utensils, knitting needles, and the like.
- Report the following to the physician or nurse: unusual and sudden pain, painful or decreased movement, or persistent pain; fever, foul odors, or increased warmth of extremity; drainage from under the cast; changes in circulation, mobility, or sensation (burning, numbness, tingling, or cold).

Crutch-walking using the three-point, non–weight-bearing gait pattern (three blocks at right). At left, the client positions himself at the bottom of a triangle composed of each crutch and the unaffected leg. In the center, the client advances his unaffected leg forward by supporting himself on the hand grips of the crutches and swinging his hips and the unaffected leg through the crutch opening.

TABLE 67-2	**NURSING CARE FOR SPECIFIC FRACTURES**		
SITE OF FRACTURE	**SIGNS AND SYMPTOMS**	**TREATMENT**	**NURSING MANAGEMENT**
Mandible	Inability to close mouth after trauma to jaw Chin displaced from midline Teeth absent, loose, or broken Lacerations to mouth and tongue Oral pain, swelling, bruising, and bleeding	Fractures are surgically reduced and immobilized with wire loops to stabilize the lower jaw to the upper jaw. Broken teeth are repaired or removed. Oral lacerations are sutured.	Ensure that wire cutters are easily accessible at the client's bedside. Be familiar with how to cut wire loops if client vomits or chokes. Administer antiemetics to treat nausea and prevent vomiting. Administer liquid or semiliquid diet. Assist client to thoroughly clean mouth after each meal and every 2 hours.
Clavicle	After fracture or dislocation, arm on the affected side held close to the chest to reduce pain Affected shoulder appears to slope downward and droop inward Motion restricted Muscle spasm common	Motion can be limited with a sling or clavicular strap. Displaced fractures are immobilized with a figure-8 or Velpeau bandage. Velpeau bandage	Use a layer of stockinette or soft, porous material between skin surfaces. Teach client how to assess circulation, sensation, and mobility frequently. Instruct client to abduct arms or rest elbows on table or chair to relieve axillary pressure.
Rib	Additional injuries—to the lungs, subclavian arteries or veins, liver, or spleen Severe chest pain on inspiration and shallow respirations. The client has other symptoms if other injuries are present.	Clients are treated for the pain that accompanies fractured ribs, especially when breathing. A rib belt or elastic bandage is used to support the injured rib cage, although this restricts chest movement and may cause further lung problems.	Assess for signs and symptoms of pneumonia and atelectasis (collapsed lung) secondary to shallow respirations. Encourage deep breathing. Administer pain medications as indicated.
Upper extremity (fractures ranging from uncomplicated to complex and involving the bone	Pain Compartment syndrome, common complication of forearm fractures, possibly leading to	Extent of injury determines treatment: • Cast with or without closed reduction	Assess neurovascular status frequently. Report abnormal findings immediately.

(continued)

TABLE 67-2	NURSING CARE FOR SPECIFIC FRACTURES (Continued)		
SITE OF FRACTURE	**SIGNS AND SYMPTOMS**	**TREATMENT**	**NURSING MANAGEMENT**
ends, joints, tendons, and ligaments)	Volkmann's contracture, a clawlike deformity of the hand	• Open reduction with internal fixation • Hanging heavy cast that pulls a fractured humerus into alignment	Implement measures to relieve pain and swelling. Pad skin around neck if the client has a hanging cast.
		Hanging arm cast	
Wrist, hand, or finger	Typically results from a fall May involve only the lower radius (e.g., a Colles' fracture in which the distal end of the radius breaks off and becomes displaced) Pain and swelling in the affected area Deformed-looking hand, wrist or finger	Closed reduction with a cast Open reduction with internal fixation Splints applied to fractured fingers	Show client how to use a sling. Teach client how to do active ROM exercises in fingers of affected hand.
Spine	May follow severe injury; if compression fracture, may result from osteoporosis Pain radiating to the leg Tenderness at injury site Muscle spasms Deformity of spinal column Neurologic deficits	Bed rest for an uncomplicated fracture Spinal brace Laminectomy with fusion Cast Head traction: halo brace with rigid vest that allows client to move but immobilizes vertebrae	Teach client to log roll if on bed rest, and as indicated. Assess client's sensation, mobility, and strength in the extremities. Administer pin care if client has a halo brace.
Pelvis (fractures range from minor to severe or crushing injuries)	Tenderness, swelling, and ecchymoses, or more severe symptoms if internal injuries accompany fracture Severed nerves Loss of lower limb function Internal bleeding	Minor fractures: bed rest and comfort measures Severe injuries: multiple-system approach related to the nature of the injuries Pelvic slings, spica casts, or open reduction with internal or external fixation	Assess circulation, sensation, and mobility in the lower extremities. Monitor elimination patterns. Insert an indwelling catheter as necessary. Provide a fracture bedpan. Administer suppositories or small volume enemas as indicated. Assess skin frequently for signs of breakdown. Provide frequent skin care. Administer pain medications as prescribed.

(continued)

TABLE 67-2	NURSING CARE FOR SPECIFIC FRACTURES (Continued)		
SITE OF FRACTURE	**SIGNS AND SYMPTOMS**	**TREATMENT**	**NURSING MANAGEMENT**
Knee (involving kneecap or the ends of the femur or tibia; injuries to the ligaments or tendons)	May follow falls or blows or athletic competition (particularly tears of the cruciate ligaments) Pain, swelling, ecchymoses Inability or limited ability to move or bend the joint	Immobilization with a leg splint Leg immobilizer Arthroscopic surgery to remove bone fragments or to repair ligament tears Open reduction and insertion of wire sutures Removal of patella if fragmented extensively Skeletal traction	Assist client to use ambulatory aids, such as crutches or walker. Teach client to perform active ROM exercises within limitations.
Lower leg (fibula fracture usually occurs with tibial fracture)	Usually results from fall or trauma Pain and swelling Inability to bear weight Ecchymoses and possible deformity Bleeding and protrusion of bone fragments (in compound fractures)	Closed reduction with cast Open reduction with internal fixation	Assess signs and symptoms of compartment syndrome. Urge client to perform active and passive ROM exercises frequently. Assist client to use ambulatory aids.
Ankle	Severe pain Difficulty bearing weight Swelling Protruding bone fragments (severe fractures)	Cast or splint Open or closed reduction and internal fixation followed by casting	Administer pain medications as prescribed. Implement methods to reduce swelling. Assist client to use ambulatory aids. Assess for signs and symptoms of compartment syndrome.
Feet and toes (can occur alone or with other lower extremity fractures)	Pain, swelling, ecchymosis, and difficulty bearing weight Inability to wear shoe Protrusion of small bones (in crushing injuries)	Casting Open reduction with internal fixation Fusion (bones with multiple fractures) Supportive measures: analgesics, cold applications, elevation of foot, and loose-fitting shoes	Assess neurovascular status frequently. Provide cast care as needed. Assist client to use ambulatory aids. Instruct client in safety measures to prevent additional injuries (using nightlights, avoiding narrowed pathways, removing throw rugs, clearing stairways).

client must be aware of the amount of weight bearing allowed. Ambulatory aids assist with non–weight-bearing or partial weight-bearing restrictions. Instruction prevents injury from unsafe use.

Self-Care Deficit: Feeding, Hygiene, Dressing, Toileting related to immobility secondary to traction or casts

Expected Outcome: Client will maintain maximum self-care.

- Assist client to meet self-care needs as indicated. *Limited mobility and ROM prevent client from safely providing self-care; assistance promotes safety.*
- Instruct client to perform self-care activities as much as possible. *Doing so promotes independence.*
- Provide assistive devices as indicated. *They help the client be as independent as possible.*
- Allow client to plan self-care that best meets ongoing needs. *Doing so involves client in care and helps him or her to have control.*

Impaired Tissue Integrity related to puncture wound; compound fracture; pins, wires, screws, or other surgical intervention; or physical immobility

Expected Outcomes: (1) Client will demonstrate adequate wound healing without infection. (2) Skin will remain intact.

- Provide pin care. *It assists in monitoring client for infection and maintains a clean environment.*
- Report any signs of infection in the pin care sites, wounds, or surgical incisions. *Doing so promotes early intervention and prevents further infection.*
- Administer antibiotics as indicated. *Antibiotics treat infection and prevent complications, such as osteomyelitis.*
- Protect bony prominences from pressure by using pressure-relieving techniques under elbows, heels, and coccyx. Massage bony prominences and skin surfaces subjected to pressure unless they remain red when pressure is relieved. *These measures prevent further injury and potential infection and promote circulation to the area.*
- Assess traction frequently to ensure proper alignment and to prevent pressure areas. *Doing so prevents mechanical injury to the skin and tissues.*
- Petal cast edges with waterproof tape. *This measure protects skin from abrasion.*

Risk for Constipation related to immobility and change in toileting methods

Expected Outcome: Client will experience normal bowel elimination.

- Refer to Chapter 53, Nursing Process: The Client With Constipation.

Evaluation of Expected Outcomes

Pain is reduced or relieved. Circulatory status supports tissue perfusion. The client regains mobility and function and achieves the maximum level of self-care. Wounds heal without infection, and the skin is intact. The client reports normal bowel elimination.

● FRACTURED FEMUR

A fracture of the femur commonly occurs in automobile accidents but may occur in falls from ladders or other high places, or in gunshot wounds. Multiple injuries often accompany fractures of the femur, because they usually occur with severe trauma.

Assessment Findings

Severe pain, swelling, and ecchymosis may be seen. The client usually cannot move the hip or knee. If a compound fracture has occurred, an open wound or a protrusion of bone is seen. Radiographic films show the type and location of the fracture.

Medical and Surgical Management

Fractures of the femur usually are treated initially with some form of traction to prevent deformities and soft tissue injury. Skeletal traction or an external fixator is used to align the fracture in preparation for future reduction if the fracture occurred in the lower two-thirds of the femur. Once the femur is aligned, a spica cast may be used to maintain the corrected position.

Nursing Management

Because the client is confined to bed, the nurse implements measures to prevent complications of immobility and inactivity. He or she positions the client in line with the pull exerted by the traction. The nurse cleans pin sites with a prescribed agent to prevent infection (see Nursing Guidelines 67-2).

● FRACTURED HIP

Usually a hip fracture affects the proximal end of the femur (Fig. 67-7). This type of fracture commonly results from a fall and occurs more frequently in older adults with osteoporosis. Usually the falls are not very traumatic, but the client's condition contributes to the resulting fracture. Fractures may occur in the femoral neck (intracapsular or inside the hip joint capsule), between the trochanters (intertrochanteric–extracapsular or out-

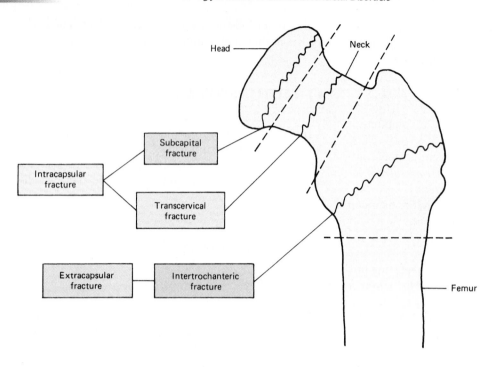

FIGURE 67-7 Types of hip fractures.

side the hip joint capsule), or below the trochanters (subtrochanteric–extracapsular). Older adults are prone to complications after a hip fracture; some die from associated complications.

Assessment Findings

The client reports severe pain that increases with leg movement. The pain frequently radiates to the knee, and the client may have a sensation of pressure in the outer aspect of the hip. Discontinuity of the bone and muscle spasm cause shortening and external rotation of the leg. A large blood loss may accompany subtrochanteric and intertrochanteric fractures, leading to hypovolemic shock. There also may be extensive bruising and swelling in the hip, groin, and thigh. Femoral neck fractures are intracapsular, so bleeding is more likely to be contained within the joint capsule. Radiographic studies reveal the exact location of the fracture, which may be within or outside the joint capsule.

Medical and Surgical Management

Buck's extension or other skin traction may be applied to relieve muscle spasm and pain until surgery is performed. Open reduction–internal fixation, accomplished with a nail or an intramedullary rod (a rod inserted into the center of the bone with wires around the bone for stabilization), is done most commonly for fractures of the hip, particularly extracapsular fractures. Examples of internal fixation devices include the Jewett nail, Richardson hip screw, Moe intratrochanteric plate, Neufeld nail, and

Smith-Petersen nail (Fig. 67-8). Intracapsular hip fractures are prone to nonunion and avascular necrosis from the disrupted blood supply. Therefore, the fractured head and neck may be removed and replaced with a metal device such as an Austin-Moore or Thompson prosthesis. This procedure is referred to as *hemiarthroplasty.* A total hip arthroplasty is discussed later in the chapter.

The bone heals around the metallic device, which in the meantime holds the bone together. Thus, the bone is united immediately, and clients are mobilized much earlier than they are with traction. Plates, bands, screws, and pins may be removed after the bone has healed. More often, they are left in place permanently. The precautions with hemiarthroplasty are greater because the surgeon must dislocate the hip to replace the femoral head.

Nursing Management

Most clients with a fractured hip are older adults and are prone to complications. After surgery, the nurse implements measures to prevent skin breakdown, wound infection, pneumonia, constipation, urinary retention, muscle atrophy, and contractures. The client usually has a wound drain in place for 1 to 2 days after surgery. The nurse monitors the drainage and administers antibiotics as prescribed.

The nurse must show the client how to use the overhead trapeze safely for independent movement and activity. When the client is recumbent, the nurse places a trochanter roll beside the hip to maintain a neutral position so that the repaired hip stays in place. He or she places abductor pillows between the client's legs when turning the client from side to side.

Smith-Petersen nail
with McLaughlin plate

Jewett nail
with overlay plate

Neufeld nail

Massie nail assembly

Moe intertrochanteric plate

FIGURE 67-8 Examples of internal fixation for hip fractures.

If a hip prosthesis has been inserted, the nurse instructs the client to avoid adduction of the affected leg until it has healed. The client must use abductor pillows at all times. Soon after surgery, the nurse or physical therapist assists the client to transfer from the bed to a chair. The chair must have an elevated seat, either with its structure or with pillows, so that the client does not flex the hips beyond 90°. The client usually requires much encouragement and assistance. Eventually the client progresses to ambulating with a walker. Before discharge, the nurse needs to explore ways to ensure safety in the client's home to avoid future injuries and falls.

INFLAMMATORY AND INFECTIOUS DISORDERS

Arthritis is a general condition characterized by inflammation and degeneration of a joint. **Rheumatic disorders** include more than 100 different types of recognized inflammatory disorders, making this collective group the most common orthopedic problem. These disorders involve inflammation and degeneration of connective tissue structures, especially joints. Infectious disorders also may affect the musculoskeletal system, causing temporary or chronic problems with musculoskeletal function. Inflammatory and infectious disorders have the potential to interfere with mobility and ADLs.

Clients with inflammatory and infectious disorders may need assistance with tasks that most people take for granted. These disorders affect a client's physical, psychological, and social functions.

The discussion in this chapter is limited to rheumatoid arthritis, osteoarthritis, gout, bursitis, ankylosing spondylitis, Lyme disease, osteomyelitis, and lupus erythematosus. Many clients with inflammatory and infectious disorders affecting the musculoskeletal system are treated as outpatients. A few may require hospitalization in the acute phase of the disorder, for surgery on a degenerative joint, or for other medical or surgical therapies.

● RHEUMATOID ARTHRITIS

Rheumatoid arthritis (RA) is a systemic inflammatory disorder of connective tissue/joints characterized by chronicity, remissions, and exacerbations. The potential for disability with RA is great and related to the effects on joints, as well as the systemic problems.

Pathophysiology and Etiology

The nature of RA, a crippling disease, is not fully understood. Its cause is unknown, although it is believed to be an autoimmune disease. Genetic predisposition and other factors may be involved. RA strikes in the most productive years of adulthood, usually between 20 and 40 years of age. The disorder also can be found in young children and older adults. Young adult women appear to be affected more than men, but the incidence equalizes as adults age. Typically, RA affects small joints early and involves large joints later (Bullock & Henze, 2000).

The autoimmune reaction from RA occurs primarily in the synovial tissue. Approximately 70% to 80% of people with RA have a substance called *rheumatoid factor* (RF), an antibody that reacts with a fragment of immunoglobulin G (IgG). This self-produced (autologous) antibody forms immune complexes (IgG/RF). It is uncertain why. Theories include viral infections that alter the IgG so that it is seen as foreign, or genetic predisposition. Sixty percent of individuals with RA have other factors known as major histocompatibility complex (MHC) antigen and human leukocyte antigen (HLA) (Porth, 2002).

The autoimmune reaction is described in Figure 67-9. Basically, it seems that lymphocytes in the inflammatory infiltrate of the synovial tissue produce RF. Polymorphonuclear leukocytes, monocytes, and lymphocytes are attracted to the area and cause phagocytosis of the immune complexes. During this process, lysosomal enzymes are released, which cause destructive changes in the joint cartilage (Fig. 67-10). The changes produce more inflammation, which perpetuates the entire process of RA:

1. The inflammatory process (**synovitis**) advances as the congestion and edema develop in the synovial membrane and joint capsule.
2. Synovial tissue experiences reactive hyperplasia.
3. Vasodilation and increased blood flow cause warmth and redness.
4. Increased capillary permeability causes swelling.

5. Rheumatoid synovitis advances, leading to **pannus** formation (destructive vascular granulation tissue, characteristic of RA).
6. Pannus destroys adjacent cartilage, joint capsule, and bone.
7. Pannus eventually forms between joint margins, reducing joint mobility and leading to potential **ankylosis** (joint immobility).
8. Disease progression causes further inflammation and structural changes (Bullock & Henze, 2000; Porth, 2002).

Most clients with RA experience exacerbations and remissions. For some clients, the progression is steady, relentless, and not necessarily responsive to therapy. Box 67-4 lists articular and extra-articular manifestations of RA.

Assessment Findings

Signs and Symptoms

In most clients, onset of symptoms is acute. Joint involvement usually is bilateral and symmetric. Localized symptoms include joint pain, swelling, and warmth; erythema; mobility limitation/stiffness; spongy tissue on joint palpation; and fluid on joints. Over several weeks, more joints become involved. Swelling and pain comes and goes. Fatigue, malaise, anorexia, and weight loss are common. Fever may develop. Tolerance for any kind of stress decreases, as does tolerance for environmental temperature changes. Although dietary iron intake is adequate, clients characteristically have persistent anemia resulting from the effects of RA on the blood-forming organs. Other systemic features include vasculitis, neuro-

FIGURE 67-9 Pathophysiology of rheumatoid arthritis and associated physical signs. (Adapted from Smeltzer, S. C. & Bare, B. G. [2000]. *Brunner & Suddarth's textbook of medical–surgical nursing* [9th ed., p. 1422]. Philadelphia: Lippincott Williams & Wilkins, and Porth, C. M. [2002]. *Pathophysiology: Concepts of altered health states* [6th ed., p. 1369], Philadelphia: Lippincott Williams & Wilkins.)

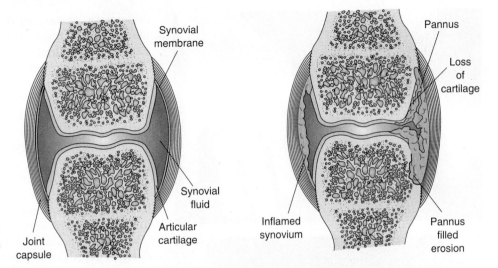

FIGURE 67-10 Joint changes in rheumatoid arthritis.

pathy, scleritis, pericarditis, splenomegaly, and Sjögren's syndrome (dry eyes and mucous membranes).

In some clients, subcutaneous nodules, known as *rheumatoid nodules,* develop. Appearing in more advanced stages of RA, they usually are nontender and movable and

---

BOX 67-4 ● Articular and Extra-articular Manifestations of Rheumatoid Arthritis

- **Subcutaneous nodules:** Firm, freely movable, rubbery or granular nodules caused by deposition of extra-articular granulation tissue. Usually found at joint points such as knuckles and elbows.
- **Synovial cysts:** Called *Baker's cysts* in popliteal fossa; filled with synovial fluid that may be found in periarticular areas in elbow, shoulder, or small joints.
- **Arthritis:** Bilateral involvement of the small joints and later the large joints; hands joints usually are swollen and may be red. Inflammation leads to disability from destruction of cartilage, bone, and tendons. Flexion-contractures are common. Osteoporosis, vertebral compression fractures, and avascular necrosis of the femoral head are common and may relate to treatment with corticosteroids. Usually at least three joint areas are involved.
- **Systemic rheumatoid vasculitis:** Immune complex–mediated inflammation in small and medium-sized arteries. It may be life-threatening if in a critical area. Causes pericardial, cardiac, pulmonary, and other types of lesions. Digital necrosis is common.
- **Compression neuropathy:** Mainly causes peripheral nerve entrapment with carpal tunnel syndrome. Paresthesias, pain, burning, muscle wasting, and weakness are common symptoms.
- **Cardiac disease:** Pericardial lesions and effusions are common and may or may not be symptomatic. Conduction system abnormalities from blockages due to rheumatic nodules around the atrioventricular node may cause heart block.
- **Pleuropulmonary disease:** Pleural effusions or pleuritic chest pain are relatively common. Pulmonary fibrosis or progressive interstitial lung disease may be seen with or without rheumatoid nodules in the lung parenchyma.
- **Episcleritis and scleritis:** Episcleritis is an inflammatory condition of the connective tissue between the sclera and conjunctiva. Scleritis is an inflammatory condition of the sclera and can cause scleral perforation.
- **Sicca syndrome:** A condition of dry eyes and dry mouth that can result from infiltration of the lacrimal and salivary glands with lymphocytes.

---

evident over bony prominences, such as the elbow or the base of the spine.

Muscles weaken and atrophy (shrink), partially from disuse. Connective tissue and neurovascular changes lend a smooth, glossy appearance to the extremities, which may be cold and clammy. Flexion contractures are common.

As the disease progresses, muscle wasting around affected joints accentuates the appearance of swelling. The proximal finger joints swell the most, showing classic deformities (Fig. 67-11), which include the following:

- Swan neck deformity—Hyperextension of the proximal interphalangeal joint with fixed flexion of the distal interphalangeal joint
- Boutonniere deformity—Persistent flexion of the proximal interphalangeal joint with hyperextension of the distal interphalangeal joint
- Ulnar deviation—Fingers deviating laterally toward the ulna

Whether resting or moving, clients in this stage of the disease have considerable chronic pain, which typically is worse in the morning after a night's rest. The symptoms may subside suddenly for no apparent reason. Inflammation leaves joints that were sore and red; the client is not stiff, has no fever, and the pain is gone. Yet the symptoms almost invariably return after the client has had a symptom-free period. Inflammation causes more joint damage, followed by another remission. The pattern of remissions and exacerbations can continue for years.

Without treatment (and sometimes with it), joint destruction may be total. As bony growth replaces the synovial space, the joint loses motion. Once the joint becomes immobile, the pain of the inflammation decreases, but discomfort continues because of contractures and immobility.

Diagnostic Findings

Radiographic films show characteristic joint changes and the extent of damage. Narrowed joint spaces and bony erosions are characteristic of later disease. An

FIGURE 67-11 Rheumatoid arthritis. **(A)** Early. **(B)** Advanced.

arthrocentesis may be done, which is an aspiration of synovial fluid (the client receives a local anesthetic) for microscopic examination. In RA, the synovial fluid usually appears cloudy, milky, or dark yellow, and contains many inflammatory cells, including leukocytes and complement (a group of proteins in blood that affect the inflammatory process and influence antigen–antibody reactions). Arthroscopic examination also may be carried out to visualize the extent of joint damage as well as to obtain a sample of synovial fluid.

A positive C-reactive protein (CRP) test, low red blood cell count and hemoglobin levels in later stages, and positive RF are laboratory findings that support the diagnosis. The erythrocyte sedimentation rate (ESR) may be elevated, particularly as the disease progresses. C4 complement component is decreased. Antinuclear antibody (ANA) test results also may be positive. Serum protein electrophoresis may disclose increased levels of gamma and alpha globulin but decreased albumin.

Medical and Surgical Management

Although RA cannot be cured, much can be done to minimize damage. Treatment goals include decreasing joint inflammation before bony ankylosis occurs, relieving

discomfort, preventing or correcting deformities, and maintaining or restoring function of affected structures. Early treatment leads to the best results.

Optimal health conditions must be maintained because supporting the resistance of the body to the inflammation is one of the few truly therapeutic steps medicine has to offer. Rest, systemic and local, is balanced carefully with exercise. Unless the client has other medical complications, such as diabetes or hypertension, the diet need not be modified.

Local applications of heat and cold are used concurrently with drug therapy to relieve swelling and pain. Drug therapy is not curative but helps relieve pain and, in some instances, suppresses the inflammatory process (Drug Therapy Table 67-1). In early stages, therapeutic doses of NSAIDs or salicylates (aspirin) are given. A new class of NSAIDs, referred to as cyclooxygenase type 2 (COX-2) inhibitors, now are being used as treatment for RA. COX is an enzyme involved in the inflammatory process; COX-2 inhibitors block this enzyme, but do not interfere with the enzyme that protects the stomach lining (Smeltzer & Bare, 2000).

Physicians initiate aggressive pharmacologic treatment after the initial diagnosis. NSAIDs relieve inflammation and pain by inhibiting the production of prostaglandins, which can damage joints. Salicylates also relieve pain and inflammation. Disease-modifying antirheumatic drugs (DMARDs) such as antimalarials (hydroxychloroquine), gold salts (auranofin, aurothioglucose), penicillamine, or sulfasalazine are initiated early. If there are bony erosions, methotrexate (Rheumatrex), an antineoplastic agent, is started. It is faster acting than DMARDs and often is used first in the long-term treatment of RA. Cyclosporine, an immunomodulator, may be added to enhance the effects of methotrexate. Azathioprine (Imuran), an immunosuppressant, may be used in clients with severe classic RA that does not respond to more conventional therapies. Glucocorticoids such as prednisone are used at low doses for short-term relief of pain and inflammation.

For many clients, combination therapy is initiated. Although still considered experimental, early studies show effectiveness (Porth, 2002). A typical drug combination is hydroxychloroquine, azathioprine, and methotrexate or gold plus methotrexate, in addition to an NSAID. As symptoms abate and remission occurs, drug doses are tapered. Biologic response modifiers are now being used to treat RA when other treatments have failed. Etanercept (Enbrel) and infliximab (Remicade) appear to inhibit the progression of structural damage by blocking tumor necrosis factor, which plays a role in the inflammation and destruction of joints in RA. These biologic agents also target specific components of the immune system, while leaving other components intact, which in turn produces fewer side effects (Arthritis Foundation, 2002).

A nondrug therapy approved for clients with RA is Prosorba therapy. This method uses a protein A immunoadsorption column called Prosorba. Blood is taken from

DRUG CATEGORY AND EXAMPLES	MECHANISM OF ACTION	NURSING CONSIDERATIONS
Nonsteroidal Anti-inflammatory Drugs (NSAIDs)		
diclofenac sodium (Voltaron), fenoprofen (Nalfon), ibuprofen (Motrin), indomethacin (Indocin), naproxen (Naprosyn), piroxicam (Feldene), sulinidac (Clinoril)	Blocks undesirable effects of prostaglandins, which contribute to the inflammatory response Reduces pain and inflammation	Give with food or milk. Monitor client for decreased RBC and blood in urine. Assess client for abdominal pain, unusual bleeding or bruising, and tinnitus. Advise client not to take other NSAIDs or salicylates.
Salicylates		
aspirin	Relieves mild to moderate pain Interferes with the inflammatory response	Give with food or milk. Monitor for tinnitus, GI distress, unusual bleeding or bruising, dark-colored stools.
Cyclooxygenase-2 (COX-2) Inhibitors		
celecoxib (Celebrex), rofecoxib (Vioxx)	Blocks the enzyme involved in inflammation, thus relieving pain and inflammation	Do not administer with other NSAIDs. These drugs are less likely to cause gastric symptoms or unusual bleeding or bruising.
Disease-Modifying Antirheumatic Drugs (DMARDs)		
Gold Salts		
auranofin (Ridaura)	Anti-inflammatory, antiarthritic, and immunomodulating	Take with milk or food. May cause abdominal cramps, nausea, vomiting, loose stools, or sun sensitivity.
Immunosuppressant Agents		
azathioprine (Imuran)	Suppresses lymphocyte proliferation, interfering with the inflammatory response	These drugs decrease ability to fight off infection; report fever, chills, or cough.
Antineoplastic Agents		
methotrexate (Rheumatrex)	Interferes with purine metabolism, which then releases adenosine, which is an anti-inflammatory	These drugs may cause nausea and vomiting, loss of appetite, diarrhea, hair loss, unusual bleeding and bruising.
Antirheumatic		
penicillamine (Cuprimine, Depen)	Suppresses immune response by lowering immunoglobulin M associated with rheumatoid factor	Give on empty stomach; withhold food and drugs for 1 hr after administering. Assess for fever after 2–3 wk of therapy. These drugs diminish taste. Use with caution in clients who are allergic to penicillin. Monitor for rash or other skin changes.
Antimalarials		
hydroxychloroquine (Plaquinil)	Reduces inflammation	Give with food or milk. Monitor blood counts. Do not give with other anti-inflammatories or gold compounds. Consult with physician before giving to clients with ophthalmic, neurologic, hepatic, or GI disorders. Inform client that urine will appear brown. Monitor for muscle weakness, visual changes, skin lesions, hypotension, and electrocardiographic changes.
Glucocorticoids		
prednisone (Meticorten), hydrocortisone (Cortef)	Anti-inflammatory and immunosuppressant	Give with food or milk. Decrease dose and frequency gradually. With long-term therapy monitor for GI distress, hyperglycemia, edema, poor wound healing, personality changes, or pathologic fractures.
Biologic-Response Modifiers		
efanercept (Enbrel), infliximab (Remicade)	Reduces inflammatory responses	Do not give live vaccines if client is receiving these medications. Discontinue if client gets a serious infection. Give with caution to clients with multiple sclerosis or other demyelinating disorders.

one arm and run through an apheresis machine to separate plasma from red blood cells and other blood components. The plasma then passes through the Prosorba column, where some of the antibodies associated with RA are removed. The plasma, red blood cells, and other components are rejoined and returned to the client in the other arm. The procedure is done in 12 weekly sessions for 2 to 2½ hours each session. About 30% of the clients who receive these treatments experience limited relief (Arthritis Foundation, 2002; Smeltzer & Bare, 2000).

Another new treatment is the injection of viscosupplements (Hyalgan, Synvisc, and Supartz). These products act as a lubricant, substituting for hyaluronic acid, the substance that provides joint fluid viscosity. Pain relief appears to last 6 to 13 months. Side effects include swelling, redness, or heat at the injection site. Clients allergic to eggs should not receive these injections (Arthritis Foundation, 2002).

Several surgical techniques may be performed to minimize or correct the joint deformities of RA (Box 67-5). Many individuals with various types of arthritis undergo an **arthroplasty,** or reconstruction of the joint, using an artificial joint that restores previously lost function and relieves pain. Reconstructive joint surgery is discussed more fully with the surgical management of degenerative joint disease.

Nursing Management

Nursing management involves teaching clients about the disease and providing information about maintaining general health, relieving pain, reducing stress, decreasing the inflammatory process, and preserving joint mobility. The nurse also instructs clients about the medication regimen, particularly therapeutic and adverse effects. Other nursing activities center on how to apply heat and cold packs locally or how to use a transcutaneous electrical nerve stimulation (TENS) unit to relieve pain in a particular joint. A TENS unit has electrodes that are applied to the skin from a portable stimulation unit that the client learns to operate.

BOX 67-5 ● Surgical Procedures for Rheumatoid Arthritis

Arthrodesis: Fusion of a joint (most often the wrist or knee) for stabilization and pain relief

Arthroplasty: Total reconstruction or replacement of a joint (most often the knee and hip) with an artificial joint to restore function and relieve pain

Osteotomy: Cutting and removal of a wedge of bone (most often the tibia or femur) to change the bone's alignment, thereby improving function and relieving pain

Synovectomy: Removal of enlarged and hypertrophied synovium to prevent the formation of pannus and delay destruction in the joint (most often the fingers, wrist, elbow, and knee)

Nurses collaborate with occupational therapists to provide equipment, utensils, and instruction regarding energy conservation and maintenance of joint alignment. Physical therapists (PTs) plan an appropriate exercise regimen. Home care planning involves providing nursing assistance for ADLs and ensuring that the home environment is safe. Out of consideration for the typical pain and morning stiffness, the nurse teaches the nursing assistant to allow extra time for completing hygiene or other procedures.

When joints are severely inflamed, the use of a splint may reduce but not totally eliminate active motion. Even during an acute episode, the nurse encourages the client to move affected parts gently to help lessen the possibility of ankylosis, muscle wasting, osteoporosis, and the debilitating effects of prolonged rest. Clients must avoid positions of flexion.

The nurse continues to urge the client to eat nutritious, well-balanced meals despite anorexia. As joints become deformed and destroyed, the techniques and equipment used to perform ADLs may require modification. Clients need assistance to deal with chronic pain, changes in function, changes in appearance, and related depression and feelings of helplessness. Education about the disease is essential because many people spend large sums of money on unscientific treatments in hopes of a cure.

Stop, Think, and Respond ● BOX 67-3

A 35-year-old woman recently diagnosed with RA asks you if her disease happened because she experimented with marijuana and drank a lot of alcohol in her adolescence. How would you respond?

● DEGENERATIVE JOINT DISEASE

Degenerative joint disease (DJD), also referred to as osteoarthritis (OA), is the most common form of arthritis. It also is known as the "wear and tear" disease and typically affects the weight-bearing joints. It is characterized by a slow and steady progression of destructive changes in weight-bearing joints and those that are repeatedly used for work. Unlike RA, DJD has no remissions and no systemic symptoms, such as malaise and fever. Table 67-3 compares OA and RA.

Pathophysiology and Etiology

A lifetime of repeated trauma leads to degenerative joint changes. Hips, knees, the spine, and the distal interphalangeal joints in the hands commonly are affected. Risk factors include increasing age, previous joint injury, obesity, congenital and developmental disorders (such as Legg-Calvé-Perthes disease), hereditary factors, and de-

TABLE 67-3	COMPARISON OF RHEUMATOID ARTHRITIS AND OSTEOARTHRITIS	
	RHEUMATOID ARTHRITIS	**OSTEOARTHRITIS**
Age	Usually between ages 20 and 50	Usually after age 40
Sex	More common in women than men	Before age 45, more common in men; after age 45, more common in women, especially in the hands
Onset	May develop suddenly (weeks or months)	Develops slowly over many years
Symptoms		
Pain	General achiness; nocturnal pain; pain at rest	Deep, aching pain with motion early in the disease; later, pain at rest
Stiffness	Morning stiffness that lasts at least 1 hr	Stiffness localized to involved joints, which rarely exceeds 20 min; often related to weather
Joint motion	Decreased	Limited
Other	Depression, fatigue, low-grade fever, anorexia, malaise, weakness, weight loss	Instability of weight-bearing joints; crepitus; crackling
Physical signs	If multiple joints involved, usually symmetric	One or many joints involved; asymmetric
	Joints typically involved are hands (small joints), feet (small joints), wrists, elbows, knees, ankles, shoulders.	Joints typically involved are hands (first carpometa-carpal joint), feet (first metatarsophalangeal joint), hips, knees, cervical and lumbar spine
	Hand deformities include ulnar deviation and subluxation of metacarpophalangeal joints	Joints—bony proliferation or occasional synovitis; local tenderness; crepitus; muscle atrophy; effusions
	Joints may be tender, swollen, and red.	Synovial fluid—high viscosity with mild leukocytosis (<2000 WBC:mm³)
	Synovial fluid is thin and cloudy with elevated protein and polymorphonuclear cell levels.	
Laboratory values	Rheumatoid factor (RF) elevated in 80% of clients with RA	No specific test
	Elevated ESR	ESR and hematologic survey results are normal
	Decreased RBC and C4 complement	No systemic manifestations

creased bone disease. OA may be classified as *primary,* which is disease without a known etiology, or *secondary,* when OA has an underlying cause such as injury or a congenital disorder (Bullock & Henze, 2000).

The degenerative process begins when the cartilage that covers the bone ends becomes thin, rough, and ragged. Malacia or soft spots develop. The cartilage no longer springs back into shape after normal use. As the cartilage wears away, the joint space decreases, so that the bone surfaces are closer and rub together. In an attempt to repair the damaged surface, new bone develops in the form of bone spurs, bone cysts, or osteophytes, which are extended margins of the joints. The joint becomes deformed, and the client experiences pain and limited joint movement. Ankylosis does not occur, but the resulting deformity may partially dislocate the joint. "Degenerative changes are also found in the joint capsule, synovial membrane, ligaments, and muscles and tendons that surround the affected joint" (Bullock & Henze, 2000, p. 832). Figure 67-12 depicts the joint changes seen in osteoarthritis.

Assessment Findings

Early symptoms are brief joint stiffness and pain after a period of inactivity. The pain usually increases with heavy use and is relieved by rest. Later, even rest may not

adequately relieve the pain. Eventually the joint undergoes enlargement and increased limitation of movement. When DJD afflicts the hands, the fingers frequently develop painless bony nodules on the dorsolateral surface of the interphalangeal joints: **Heberden's nodes** (bony enlargement of the distal interphalangeal joints; Fig. 67-13) and **Bouchard's nodes** (bony enlargement of the proximal interphalangeal joints). Crepitus may be heard and

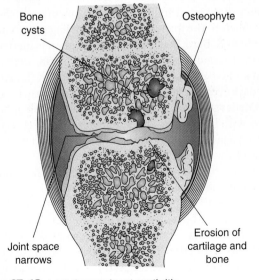

FIGURE 67-12 Joint changes in osteoarthritis.

FIGURE 67-13 Heberden's nodes.

felt when the joint is moved. The ROM of the affected joint becomes progressively limited, and stiffness and pain increase.

Radiographic films demonstrate disruption of the joint cartilage and bony changes. Some clients may have a slightly elevated ESR.

Medical and Surgical Management

Nonpharmacologic treatment includes local rest of the affected joints, which is emphasized more than is total body rest. Heat applied to the painful part may afford some relief. Weight loss is recommended for obese clients. Splints, braces, canes, or crutches may reduce discomfort, relieve pain, and prevent further joint destruction of the affected joints. An exercise program helps to preserve joint ROM and strength. Clients should not engage in activity that places excessive stress on affected joints. A TENS unit may help reduce joint pain.

Large doses of acetaminophen may be used initially, along with nonpharmacologic treatments. Some studies suggest that initial treatment with aspirin and NSAIDs may hasten the progression of cartilage destruction (Smeltzer & Bare, 2000). If acetaminophen is ineffective, however, systemic anti-inflammatory drugs, such as aspirin and NSAIDs, are prescribed. Although these drugs do not prevent or cure DJD, they may decrease its severity. Corticosteroids may be injected into acutely inflamed joints with limited success. When possible, long-term use of these agents is avoided. Use of narcotics is deferred because of the disorder's chronic nature.

Reconstructive joint surgery is performed when mobility and quality of life are compromised. The two joints most frequently replaced are the knee and the hip. Other joints that may be replaced are the shoulder, ankle, wrist, and finger joints. Total joint replacement is not strictly for clients with DJD. This type of procedure also may be done for individuals with RA, trauma, hip fracture, or a congenital deformity.

The materials used in an artificial joint are metal and high-density polyethylene (Fig. 67-14). Special bone cement or a specialized coating on the prosthesis pieces, which promotes bone growth on the implant, holds the prosthesis parts in place. Postoperative complications include hemorrhage, subluxation or dislocation of the artificial hip, infection, thromboembolism, and avascular necrosis. A cemented prosthesis may loosen many years later.

Some clients may want to predonate their own blood for use if a transfusion is needed. Anticoagulant therapy and early ambulation are implemented to prevent clot formation. Clients with a knee or hip replacement may use a continuous passive motion (CPM) machine after surgery. This machine promotes healing and flexibility in the knee or hip joint and increases circulation to the operative area. The physician orders the amount of extension and flexion produced by the machine as well as the frequency of use. The amount of flexion and frequency of movement are increased daily for clients with knee replacements. By discharge, the client's goal is the

FIGURE 67-14 Hip and knee replacement.

ability to bend the knee 90°. The amount of flexion for clients with hip replacements should never exceed 30° in a CPM machine.

Nursing Management

The nurse teaches about the purpose of drug therapy, administration times, and therapeutic and side effects. Because aspirin and NSAIDs can cause gastric bleeding, the nurse advises clients to take the medication with food. It is important that the client maintain moderate activity with instructions about how to regulate the type, vigor, and frequency according to the symptoms experienced. If the client is overweight, he or she needs explanations about dietary changes that promote weight loss. The nurse may need to remind the client to assume good posture to avoid unusual stress on a joint. If the client needs ambulatory aids such as crutches, a cane, or a walker, he or she will need a referral to a PT for fitting and practice.

If a client is scheduled for joint replacement or other surgery, the nurse withholds aspirin before surgery to reduce the risk for excessive bleeding. It is essential to monitor the complete blood count, prothrombin time, and bleeding and clotting times to ensure that the client's ability to control bleeding is not compromised. If the client will use a CPM machine after surgery, it is useful for the client to be fitted for this before surgery.

When the client returns from surgery, the nurse reviews the physician orders concerning movement, turning, or positioning of the extremities. Usually, the head of the bed remains at 45° or less. The client with a total hip replacement needs to have legs abducted and extended because the opposite positions of adduction and flexion beyond 90° can dislocate the prosthetic femoral head from the acetabulum. Clients with a total hip replacement need to sit in an elevated chair or on a seat raised by pillows, so that the flexion remains less than 90°. Ice packs help reduce pain and inflammation to the incisional site (particularly after knee surgery). Box 67-6 provides information about avoiding hip dislocation after total hip replacement.

If CPM devices are prescribed to promote gentle flexion and extension of the knee after knee replacement, the nurse or PT increases the flexion as indicated up to the goal of 90°. If CPM devices are used after hip surgery, the flexion should not exceed 30°.

Preventing postoperative complications after joint replacement is an important role of the nurse. Table 67-4 presents strategies to prevent postoperative complications after joint replacement surgery.

● GOUT

Gout, a painful metabolic disorder involving an inflammatory reaction in the joints, usually affects the feet (especially the great toe), hands, elbows, ankles, and knees.

> **BOX 67-6 ● Avoiding Hip Dislocation After Replacement Surgery**
>
> Until the hip prosthesis stabilizes after hip replacement surgery, the client needs to learn about proper positioning so that the prosthesis remains in place. Dislocation of the hip is a serious complication of surgery that causes pain and necessitates reoperation to correct the dislocation. Desirable positions include abduction, neutral rotation, and flexion of less than 90°. When the client is seated, the knees should be lower than the hip.
> Guidelines for avoiding displacement are as follows:
> - Keep the knees apart at all times.
> - Put a pillow between the legs when sleeping.
> - Never cross the legs when seated.
> - Avoid bending forward when seated in a chair.
> - Avoid bending forward to pick up an object on the floor.
> - Use a raised toilet seat.
> - Do not flex the hip to put on clothing such as pants, stockings, socks, or shoes.

Pathophysiology and Etiology

The disorder tends to be inherited and affects more men than women. Gout may occur secondary to other diseases marked by decreased renal excretion of uric acid. It also has been identified among clients who have received organ transplants and the antirejection drug cyclosporine.

Gout is characterized by **hyperuricemia** (accumulation of uric acid in the blood), caused by alterations in uric acid production, excretion, or both. Hyperuricemia occurs from one or a combination of the following pathologies:

- Primary hyperuricemia
  - Severe dieting or starvation
  - Excessive ingestion of purines (organ meats, shellfish, sardines)
  - Heredity
- Secondary hyperuricemia
  - Abnormal purine metabolism
  - Increased rate of protein synthesis with overproduction or underexcretion of uric acid
  - Increased cellular turnover, as in leukemia, multiple myeloma, and other cancers; some anemias; and psoriasis
  - Altered renal tubular function related to use of diuretics and salicylates and excessive alcohol intake, leading to underexcretion of uric acid (Smeltzer & Bare, 2000)

Urate (a salt of uric acid) crystallizes in body tissues and is deposited in soft and bony tissues, causing local inflammation and irritation. Collections of urate crystals, called **tophi,** are found in the cartilage of the outer ear (pinna), the great toe, hands, and other joints, ligaments, bursae, and tendons. As these deposits accumulate, they destroy the joint, producing a chronically swollen, deformed appearance. The uric acid also may precipitate in urine, causing renal stones.

TABLE 67-4	PREVENTING POSTOPERATIVE COMPLICATIONS AFTER JOINT REPLACEMENT SURGERY	
POTENTIAL COMPLICATION	**POTENTIAL RISK FACTORS**	**PREVENTION STRATEGIES**
Dislocation of prosthesis	Positioning beyond recommended flexion or extension Malfunction of prosthesis	Position client as prescribed. Instruct client to maintain appropriate position. Use pillows, splints, immobilizers, or slings to maintain prescribed position. Report increased pain, swelling, or change in mobility.
Infection	Elderly, debilitated clients Malnourishment Other infections such as urinary tract infections or dental abscesses Incision, wound drains, catheters, or IVs Hematoma	Monitor vital signs. Assess wound appearance and drainage. Practice aseptic technique when changing dressings and emptying drainage devices. Administer prophylactic antibiotics as prescribed. Teach client that for at least 3 months after surgery there is a potential for infection; he or she may require prophylactic antibiotics for dental cleaning or other invasive procedures. Report increased pain, elevated temperature, redness, swelling, or change in drainage from the incision.
Neurovascular compromise	Trauma Edema Immobilization devices	Assess neurovascular status frequently, including color, temperature, capillary refill, pulses, edema, pain, mobility, and sensation. Report client complaints of deep, unrelenting pain; feelings of tightness; numbness; and decreased mobility. Elevate extremity. Release constricting dressings, wraps, casts, or immobilizers.
Deep vein thrombosis	Surgical procedure Immobility	Apply elastic stockings/wraps as prescribed. Assess peripheral pulses. Change position frequently as allowed. Increase activity as indicated. Encourage client to perform passive ROM exercises. Assess for Homans' sign. Prevent pressure on popliteal vessels.

Assessment Findings

Signs and Symptoms

A gout attack is characterized by a sudden onset of acute pain and tenderness in one joint. The skin turns red and the joint swells so that it is warm and hypersensitive to touch. Fever may be present. Tophi may be palpated around the fingers, great toes, or earlobes, particularly if the client has chronic and severe hyperuricemia. The attack may last for 1 or 2 weeks, but moderate swelling and tenderness may persist. A symptom-free period usually is followed by another attack, which may occur any time. Repeated episodes in the same joint may deform the joint.

Diagnostic Findings

Diagnosis usually is based on the obvious clinical signs and hyperuricemia. Synovial fluid aspirated from the joint during arthrocentesis contains urate crystals. The urate deposits also may be identifiable with a radiographic ex-

amination. Elevated uric acid levels in serum and urine (24-hour urine collection) correlate with gout, but these findings are common to other disorders as well.

Medical and Surgical Management

Although gout cannot be cured in the sense of removing the basic metabolic difficulty of constant or recurrent hyperuricemia, the attacks usually can be controlled. The aim of treatment is to decrease sodium urate in the extracellular fluid so that deposits do not form.

Two main treatment approaches involve (1) using uricosuric drugs that promote renal excretion of urates by inhibiting the reabsorption of uric acid in the renal tubules, and (2) decreasing ingestion of purine. The regimen is individualized and may be changed in response to the changes in the course of the disease.

Pain during a severe acute attack may require NSAIDs, such as ibuprofen and indomethacin. Acute attacks of gout also may be treated with colchicine or phenylbutazone. Colchicine is administered every 1 or 2 hours until the pain subsides or nausea, vomiting, intestinal cramping, and diarrhea develop. When one or more of these symptoms occurs, the drug should be stopped temporarily. Drugs used for long-term gout management include colchicine, allopurinol (Zyloprim), probenecid (Benemid), indomethacin (Indocin), and sulfinpyrazone (Anturane). To prevent future attacks, drug therapy continues after the acute attack subsides (Drug Therapy Table 67-2). Salicylates inactivate uricosurics, and clients with a history of gout should not use them.

It is now known that the body can synthesize purines; thus, emphasis on strict diet restriction has decreased, with more focus on the use of uricosuric drugs. The prescribed diet includes adequate protein with limitation of purine-rich foods to avoid contributing to the underlying problem. The diet prescription also is relatively high in carbohydrates and low in fats because carbohydrates increase urate excretion and fats retard it. Overweight clients are encouraged to lose weight. A high fluid intake helps increase excretion of uric acid. Alcohol is restricted because it can trigger an attack.

Surgery may be performed to remove the large tophi of advanced gout. Surgery also may be used to correct crippling deformities that may result from treatment delays or to fuse unstable joints and increase their function.

Nursing Management

The nurse places a bed cradle over the affected joint to protect it from the pressure of the bed linen. If colchicine is prescribed, he or she explains about the hourly administration until side effects occur or acute pain subsides. The nurse instructs the client to report gastrointestinal (GI) symptoms. He or she measures intake and output,

especially when diarrhea accompanies colchicine therapy for acute gout. The nurse provides clear explanations of long-term drug and diet therapy before discharge.

● BURSITIS

Bursitis is an inflammation of the bursa, a fluid-filled sac that cushions bone ends to enhance a gliding movement. The elbow, shoulder, and knee are common sites of bursitis.

Pathophysiology and Etiology

Trauma is the most common cause of acute bursitis. Other causes include infection and secondary effects of gout and RA. Typical of any inflammation, pain and swelling occur with compromised function.

Assessment Findings

Painful movement of a joint, such as the elbow or shoulder, is the most common symptom. A distinct lump may be felt. If the bursa ruptures, tissue in the area may become edematous, warm, and tender.

An x-ray study may reveal a calcified bursa, and aspiration of fluid may demonstrate the following:

- A few leukocytes in transparent fluid if the etiology is trauma
- A large collection of leukocytes if the cause is sepsis
- Colonies of staphylococcal or streptococcal microorganisms

DRUG THERAPY TABLE 67-2	SELECTED ANTIGOUT MEDICATIONS	
DRUG	**MECHANISM OF ACTION**	**NURSING CONSIDERATIONS**
colchicine	Lowers the deposition of uric acid and interferes with leukocytes and kinin formation, thus reducing inflammation Does not alter serum or urine levels of uric acid Used in acute and chronic management	*Acute management:* Administer when attack first begins. Dosage is increased until pain is relieved or diarrhea develops. *Chronic management:* Prolonged use may decrease vitamin B_{12} absorption. Drug causes GI upset in most clients.
probenecid (Benemid)	Uricosuric agent; inhibits renal reabsorption of urates and increases the urinary excretion of uric acid Prevents tophi formation	Be alert for nausea, rash, and constipation.
allopurinol (Zyloprim)	Xanthine oxidase inhibitor; interrupts the breakdown of purines before uric acid forms Inhibits xanthine oxidase because it blocks uric acid formation	Be alert for side effects, including bone marrow depression, vomiting, and abdominal pain.

- Urate crystals in bursitis secondary to gout
- Cholesterol crystals, common in clients with bursitis and RA, which may cause the fluid from the bursa to appear cloudy

Medical and Surgical Management

Joint rest usually is recommended. Salicylates or NSAIDs may be prescribed. If the problem persists, a corticosteroid preparation may be injected into the joint to reduce inflammation. After pain and inflammation are reduced, ongoing therapy involves mild ROM exercises.

Nursing Management

The nurse reviews the prescribed medication and exercise regimens with the client and allows time for questions and answers. He or she advises the client not to traumatize or overuse the recovering joint but to use it normally. Failure to use the joint after pain and inflammation are controlled may result in partial limitation of joint motion.

● ANKYLOSING SPONDYLITIS

Ankylosing spondylitis, or Marie-Strümpell disease, is a chronic connective tissue disorder of the spine and surrounding cartilaginous joints, such as the sacroiliac joints and soft tissues around the vertebrae. Characteristics include spondylosis and fusion of the vertebrae.

Pathophysiology and Etiology

Ankylosing spondylitis usually begins in early adulthood and is more common in men than in women. Its etiology is unknown, although some theorize that an altered immune response occurs when T-cell lymphocytes mistake human cells for similar-appearing bacterial antigens. There also is a strong familial tendency for some affected individuals. Once the inflammation begins, it continues, causing progressive immobility and fixation (ankylosis) of the joints in the hips, and ascends the vertebrae. Respiratory function may be compromised if kyphosis (a hunchback-like spinal curve) develops. In a few cases, there may be extra-articular (nonjoint) manifestations, such as aortitis (inflammation of the aorta), iridocyclitis (inflammation of the iris and ciliary body of the eye), and pulmonary fibrosis.

Assessment Findings

Signs and Symptoms

The most common symptoms are low back pain and stiffness. As the disease progresses, the spine and hips become more immobile, thus restricting movement. The lumbar curve of the spine may flatten. The neck can be permanently flexed. Aortic regurgitation or atrioventricular node conduction disturbances may occur. Lung sounds may be reduced, especially in the apical areas.

Diagnostic Findings

Evidence of inflammation is demonstrated by an elevated ESR. A culture of synovial fluid, however, is negative for causative microorganisms. Elevations of alkaline phosphatase and creatinine phosphokinase levels are common. An HLA test, used for determining inherited tissue markers for immune functions, demonstrates the presence of HLA-B2 in 90% of clients with this disorder. X-ray films or CT scans show erosion, ossification, and fusion of the joints in the spine and hips.

Medical and Surgical Management

Treatment is supportive, the major goal being to maintain functional posture. Aspirin, indomethacin, phenylbutazone, or NSAIDs usually are prescribed for relieving inflammation and pain. Sleeping on a firm mattress (preferably without a pillow) and following a prescribed exercise program may help delay or prevent spinal deformity, especially if begun in the early stages of the disease. A back brace also may be prescribed for some clients. Severe hip involvement may be treated with a total hip replacement.

Nursing Management

The nurse administers prescribed drugs and clarifies information about the disease. He or she encourages the client to perform ADLs as much as possible. The nurse teaches the client to perform mild exercises that reduce stiffness and pain. He or she provides emotional support, recognizing that the client must deal with pain, skeletal changes, and impaired mobility.

● LYME DISEASE

Lyme disease (Lyme borreliosis) gained wide recognition in the 1970s when residents of Lyme, Connecticut experienced an epidemic of progressive symptoms, beginning with a characteristic rash and eventually involving the cardiac, neurologic, and musculoskeletal systems.

Pathophysiology and Etiology

Typically, Lyme disease is prevalent during warmer months, when ticks are abundant, but it may occur at any time. It is most common in the northeast and mid-

Atlantic states, and in other northern areas of the United States, where deer ticks (*Ixodes dammini*) are more prevalent. The ticks feed on white-tailed deer or white-footed mice, and then become carriers of the spirochetal bacterium *Borrelia burgdorferi*. When ticks bite humans, they transmit the bacteria, which results in a chronic inflammatory process and multisystem disease.

Assessment Findings

Signs and Symptoms

If untreated, the disease moves through three stages. Early stage 1 symptoms for about one-third of clients include a red macule or papule at the site of the tick bite, a characteristic bull's-eye rash with round rings surrounding the center, headache, neck stiffness, and pain. Secondary pruritic lesions may accompany fever, chills, and malaise. The initial papule may not develop until 20 to 30 days after the bite. Some clients experience nausea, vomiting, and sore throat.

Midstage symptoms occur as the organism proliferates throughout the body and cardiac and neurologic involvement becomes evident. Cardiac problems include dysrhythmias and heart block. Neurologic symptoms such as facial palsy, meningitis, and encephalitis are possible. Some clients have problems with weakness, pain, and paresthesia (abnormal sensations).

Later symptoms (at least 4 weeks after the bite) include arthritis and other musculoskeletal problems. Joints, particularly knees, become warm, swollen, and painful. Joint erosion may result from the inflammatory process.

Diagnostic Findings

Diagnosis is based on the presenting signs and symptoms. The diagnosis of Lyme disease is assisted by serologic studies for IgG antibodies for *Borrelia*, which can be detected 6 weeks after the tick bite.

Medical and Surgical Management

Treatment includes administering antibiotics and supportive measures. If the disease is treated early, the prognosis is favorable. Permanent multisystem problems may occur if treatment is delayed.

Nursing Management

Nursing management involves teaching the client and family about the disease and its treatment. It is extremely important to educate clients about avoiding Lyme disease (Box 67-7).

BOX 67-7 ● **Tips for Avoiding Lyme Disease**

PERSONAL PROTECTION
- Wear light-colored clothing to increase tick visibility.
- Wear long-sleeved shirts and long pants (tuck pants into socks or boots).
- Treat clothing with tick repellant.
- Wear a hat; pull long hair back so that it does not brush against shrubs or other vegetation.
- Walk in the center of a path surrounded by grass, brush, or woods.
- Do a tick check after being outside—ticks are particularly attracted to hairy areas such as the scalp, groin, and armpits, as well as the back of knees and neck.

ENVIRONMENTAL PROTECTION
- Remove leaf, grass, and brush litter.
- Clear brush and tall grass from around house and other structures, as well as gardens and flower beds.
- Keep grass mowed.
- Place a 3-foot wood chip barrier along lawn edges that border woods.
- Erect fences to keep deer away from houses and gardens.
- Prune low-lying shrubs to let in more sunlight.
- Keep woodpiles neat, dry, and off the ground.
- Keep ground bare under bird feeders, place them away from house, and suspend feeding when ticks are most active.

(Adapted from Wade, C. F. [2000]. Keeping Lyme disease at bay. *American Journal of Nursing, 100*[7], 26–31.)

● OSTEOMYELITIS

Osteomyelitis is an infection of the bone. Limited blood supply, inflammation of and pressure on the tissue, and formation of new bone around devitalized bone tissue make osteomyelitis a difficult and challenging condition to treat. In adults, osteomyelitis may become chronic, greatly affecting quality of life.

Pathophysiology and Etiology

Staphylococcus aureus causes 70% to 80% of bone infections. Other organisms include *Proteus vulgaris* and *Pseudomonas aeruginosa*, as well as *Escherichia coli*. "The incidence of penicillin-resistant, nosocomial, gram-negative, and anaerobic infections is increasing" (Smeltzer & Bare, 2000, p. 1823). Acute osteomyelitis results from bacteria reaching the bone through the bloodstream. Acute localized osteomyelitis occurs when bone is contaminated directly by trauma, such as penetrating wounds or compound fractures. Occasionally, surgical contamination or direct extension of bacteria from an infected area adjacent to the bone, such as the pin sites of skeletal traction, can cause osteomyelitis.

Microorganisms appear to migrate to the area just below the epiphysis of a long bone where the blood supply is more generous, but circulation through the area is limited. As the microorganisms multiply, they spread down to the bone shaft. The pressure from the collecting exudate elevates the periosteum. New bone cells (**involucrum**) are deposited on the periosteum while the underlying bone becomes necrotic. The pocket of necrotic bone (**sequestrum**) may remain sequestered for years or eventually drain by forming a sinus tract through to the skin. The infection tends to linger in a chronic state because it is difficult to penetrate the infected tissue by administering systemic antibiotic drugs.

In its weakened condition, the infected bone is prone to pathologic fracture. The diseased bone may lengthen as bone growth is stimulated, or it may shorten because of the destruction of the epiphyseal plate. Other complications of osteomyelitis include septicemia, thrombophlebitis, muscle contractures, pathologic fractures, and nonunion of fractures.

Assessment Findings

Evidence of an acute infection appears suddenly: high fever, chills, rapid pulse, tenderness or pain over the affected area, redness, and swelling. Chronic infection may be characterized by a persistent draining sinus.

With acute osteomyelitis, laboratory tests usually show an elevated leukocyte count, an elevated ESR, and possibly a blood culture positive for infective organisms. Identification of the causative organism may require an aspiration of subperiosteal pus for culture and sensitivity. Radiographic findings may be inconclusive in the early stages of infection, but later studies demonstrate irregular bone decalcification, bone necrosis, elevation of the periosteum, and new bone formation. Bone scans and MRI are useful in definitive diagnoses.

Radiographic studies for chronic osteomyelitis show large cavities, sequestra or dense bone formations, and raised periosteum. Areas of infection are delineated by bone scan. Blood studies reveal a normal leukocyte count and ESR and possible anemia.

Medical and Surgical Management

Management of osteomyelitis includes the following:

- Immobilization with a cast or immobilizer to decrease pain and prevent fracture. The cast may be windowed to provide access for wound care.
- Application of warm saline soaks to the affected area for 20 minutes several times a day to increase circulation to the affected area
- Identification of the causative organism to initiate appropriate and ongoing antibiotic therapy for infection control. Intravenous (IV) antibiotic therapy is administered for 3 to 6 weeks. Oral antibiotics then follow for as long as 3 months.
- Surgical debridement of the necrotic tissue and sequestrum to remove the infected areas

- Closed irrigation with saline or an antibiotic solution and low suction to the affected area to flush away necrotic tissue
- Antibiotic-impregnated beads may be directly applied in the wound for 2 to 4 weeks
- Bone grafts for the debrided cavity to stimulate bone growth
- Muscle flaps grafted to the affected area to enhance blood supply

Nursing Management

Clients with osteomyelitis experience pain, inflammation, swelling, and impaired mobility because of pain and the inability to bear weight. Caretakers must handle the arm or leg or related area gently to prevent additional pain or fracture. They must protect the infected area from injury. The nurse instructs the client to elevate the area and to bear weight only as indicated. Nursing management includes protecting the skin from breakdown, administering the prescribed antibiotics and pain medications, and informing the client about the expected therapeutic effects and possible side effects. Clients with chronic osteomyelitis require extensive emotional support, related to the long-term nature of this illness.

Stop, Think, and Respond ● BOX 67-4

Which of the following clients is at greatest risk for osteomyelitis?

- *A 65-year-old client recently diagnosed with osteoarthritis*
- *A 70-year-old client who recently sustained an open compound fracture of the tibia after a motor vehicle accident*
- *A 40-year-old client diagnosed with Lyme disease*

● LUPUS ERYTHEMATOSUS

Lupus erythematosus is a diffuse connective tissue disease. The major type is systemic lupus erythematosus (SLE), which, as the name implies, affects multiple body systems such as the skin, joints, kidney, serous membranes of the heart and lungs, lymph nodes, and GI tract.

Pathophysiology and Etiology

Lupus erythematosus is more common in women than in men. Most clients have this disorder in the third or fourth decade of life, but it may be seen in young children and in middle-aged and older adults. It is believed to be autoimmune, but the triggering mechanism is still unknown. There is a strong familial tendency, suggesting that certain inherited cellular antigenic markers confuse the ability of T cells to distinguish self from nonself. By mistake, helper T cells alert B cells to produce antibodies against normal cells, or suppressor T cells may be ineffective in controlling a B-cell response once it has been initiated. The disease may have periods during which it is in a subacute form or even in remission. Exposure to ultraviolet light is a factor in reactivating the disease.

Antibodies destroy connective tissues of the body. Affected structures undergo inflammation, fibrosis, scarring, and dysfunction. Polymorphonuclear leukocytes (neutrophils) engulf the nuclei of attacked cells. Laboratory studies confirm this finding, which is considered diagnostic.

FIGURE 67-15 Characteristic butterfly rash.

Assessment Findings

Signs and Symptoms

According to Porth (2002), SLE is known as the *great imitator* because the clinical signs resemble many other conditions (Box 67-8). Early signs and symptoms of SLE may include fever, weight loss, pain in the joints (arthralgia), malaise, muscle pain, and extreme fatigue. These symptoms are vague and may persist for several months to 2 years before more prominent symptoms develop and the client seeks medical advice.

A prominent sign for about half of the clients with SLE is a red, butterfly-shaped rash on the face over the bridge of the nose and the cheeks (Fig. 67-15). The word *lupus* means "wolf." The term may have been used as a description for the facial rash that, to some, resembled the mask of reddish-brown fur on a wolf. Two other types of skin manifestations may occur with SLE. The first is discoid lupus erythematosus (DLE), which involves a chronic rash with erythematous papules or plaques and scaling. Eventually DLE can lead to scarring and pigmentation changes. The symptoms of DLE are related only to the skin, the most prominent symptom being the appearance of the facial rash. Skin manifestations of the disorder also may be found on the forehead, earlobes, and scalp. Scalp involvement usually results in patchy loss of hair (alopecia). These symptoms also may be seen in people with SLE. The second type is subacute cutaneous lupus erythematosus, which presents with papulosquamous lesions.

Clients also may exhibit behavioral disturbances (confusion, hallucinations, irritability), chest pain (as a result of involvement of the pleura or pericarditis), fluid retention, proteinuria, and hematuria (as a result of renal involvement), progressive weight loss, nausea and vomiting, and, in women, irregular or heavy menses. Other signs of the disease include the following:

- Nonspecific electrocardiographic changes
- A pericardial friction rub
- Pulmonary changes seen on radiographic studies
- Enlargement of the spleen and lymph nodes
- Raynaud's phenomenon (vasospasm of the smaller vessels of the hands and feet resulting in blanching of the skin and, at times, pain and cyanosis of the extremities)
- Musculoskeletal problems, such as arthralgias and arthritis, including joint swelling, tenderness, pain on movement, and morning stiffness

Diagnostic Findings

Diagnosis of SLE is based on presenting symptoms and blood tests. Blood studies show anemia, thrombocytopenia, leukocytosis or leukopenia, and positive ANA. Other laboratory studies may indicate multisystem involvement, such as an elevated creatinine level with kidney involvement. Additional tests, such as a renal biopsy and urinalysis, may be performed to determine the effect of the disorder on other body systems.

Medical Management

There is no specific treatment for this disorder. Medical management aims at producing a remission and preventing or treating acute exacerbations of the disorder. High

---

BOX 67-8 ● Clinical Manifestations of Systemic Lupus Erythematosus

SLE is known as the *great imitator*, with manifestations that resemble many other diseases.

- Constitutional—fevers, fatigue, anorexia, weight loss
- Musculoskeletal—arthritis, muscle weakness and atrophy, avascular necrosis
- Dermatologic—alopecia, photosensitivity, rash
- Cardiovascular—pericarditis, systolic murmurs, valvular complications
- Pulmonary—pleuritis, pneumonitis, pulmonary hypertension
- Renal—nephritis, glomerulonephritis
- Neuropsychiatric—cognitive dysfunction, depression, psychosis

doses of corticosteroids are used initially. Those with severe disease or for whom steroid-related side effects are problematic may be treated with cytotoxic drugs such as azathioprine (Imuran) and cyclophosphamide (Cytoxan). Simple analgesics such as aspirin or an NSAID may be prescribed for fever and joint discomfort. Topical corticosteroids may be used for skin manifestations. Renal impairment may be treated with dialysis or kidney transplantation. Cardiac, GI, and central nervous system complications are treated symptomatically.

NURSING PROCESS

● The Client With Systemic Lupus Erythematosus

Assessment

The nurse reviews the medical record and diagnostic findings to evaluate the stage of disease and appropriate interventions. It is important to assess the client's understanding of the nature of the disorder, its treatment, and the limitations imposed by the disease process. The nurse inspects the skin for rashes, purpuric lesions, and other skin changes and asks about the client's degree of sensitivity to sunlight. Inspection for ulcerations in the mouth and throat (signs of GI involvement) also is necessary. In addition, the nurse listens to the heart for pericardial friction rub and to the lungs for abnormal sounds, which might suggest pleural involvement.

Diagnosis, Planning, and Interventions

Nursing management focuses on measures to minimize exacerbations and to alleviate symptoms. The nurse administers prescribed medications and monitors for side effects. Before discharge, client education efforts involve reminding the client of the need for close medical follow-up and thorough medication instruction (i.e., never abruptly discontinue taking a prescribed corticosteroid without consulting the physician, and follow the dosage regimen exactly, particularly if the drug dose is being decreased gradually).

Because the disease and drugs alter body image, the nurse assists the client to verbalize feelings and implement effective coping mechanisms. If the client desires, the nurse arranges a referral to the Lupus Foundation of America, which is dedicated to providing information about the disease, or to a local support or self-help group.

Because SLE is a chronic disease, treated mainly on an outpatient basis, much nursing management revolves around teaching. Clients and their families need accurate and complete information about the disease, its treatment and prognosis, and self-care measures to increase comfort and promote health. Specific measures are discussed in Client and Family Teaching Box 67-1.

Other nursing care involves, but is not limited to, the following diagnoses, expected outcomes, and interventions.

Chronic Pain related to inflammation and disease progression

Expected Outcomes: (1) Client will experience relief from pain and discomfort. (2) Client will adhere to the prescribed pharmacologic regimen. (3) Client will demonstrate use of alternative methods to reduce pain.

- Administer prescribed analgesic and anti-inflammatory medications. *Pain and discomfort respond to combination drug regimens, which promote comfort and reduce the disease's inflammatory effects.*
- Review the rationale for adhering to the prescribed regimen. *Teaching promotes the client's compliance and may prevent the client from trying unsafe and ineffective therapies.*
- Elevate swollen and painful joints and apply heat or cold as indicated. *Nonpharmacologic methods decrease swelling and promote comfort.*
- Monitor the client if he or she uses braces or splints. *They promote rest to inflamed joints but may cause skin irritation. Frequent monitoring prevents skin breakdown.*
- Balance activity with rest. *Alternating rest and activity conserves energy and promotes productivity and control.*
- Move painful joints gently and slowly while supporting the extremity above and below the joint. *Doing so promotes optimal mobility and reduces pain.*
- Avoid heavy blankets or clothing. *They increase pressure and pain.*

Impaired Physical Mobility related to inflammation, joint problems, pain, or decreased muscle strength

Expected Outcomes: (1) Client will maintain maximal physical function within limitations. (2) Client will increase muscle strength in affected areas or in areas that compensate for physical limitations. (3) Client will retain function with limitation of contractures.

- Assist client to maintain appropriate body alignment and neutral positioning during periods of inactivity. *Doing so prevents contractures and increases mobility.*
- Encourage moderate and progressive exercise as indicated. *Exercise promotes mobility and reduces fatigue.*
- Advise client to use moist heat before performing ROM exercises. *Moist heat relaxes muscles and reduces resistance to ROM exercises.*
- Urge client to wear supportive shoes and to use assistive devices for ambulation as needed. *These measures improve mobility.*
- Recommend sitting in elevated chairs that have arm rests that can help client to stand up. *These chairs improve the client's ability to be more independent.*
- Encourage client to maintain erect posture when sitting, standing, and walking. *Appropriate posture promotes optimal mobility and enhances muscle strengthening.*

Self-Care Deficit (specify bathing/hygiene, dressing/grooming, feeding, toileting) related to exacerbation of disease, inflammation, and decreased mobility

Expected Outcomes: (1) Client will perform self-care activities at highest possible level. (2) Client will identify methods that assist her or him to meet self-care needs.

- Modify clothing so that the client can easily put it on and take it off (e.g., use Velcro fasteners instead of buttons, front fasteners rather than back zippers, elastic shoe laces, cardigan sweaters instead of pullovers). *Ease in changing clothes promotes independence in self-care.*
- Pad handles for easy grasping. *Doing so enhances self-care abilities.*
- Suggest an electric toothbrush, which is easier to handle than a manual toothbrush. *This helps encourage the client to care for self.*
- Provide cooking and eating utensils designed to promote a good grip (particularly useful for clients with hand deformities). *This measure enhances self-care abilities.*
- Identify equipment resources and dealers for wheelchairs, elevated commode seats, and other assistive devices. *Doing so assists the client to plan for changes in lifestyle.*

Disturbed Body Image related to change in appearance and inability to perform tasks and activities

Expected Outcomes: (1) Client will verbalize increased confidence when dealing with changes in appearance and functional abilities. (2) Client will establish realistic future goals.

- Accept client without reservation. *Nonverbal behavior expresses feelings. Facial expressions, tone of voice, or other behaviors promote acceptance or nonacceptance.*
- Avoid nonverbal messages that convey impatience with the client's disabilities. *Clients with disability require more time to finish tasks. Patience promotes independence.*
- Assist client only as needed or requested. *Doing so encourages client to perform self-care as much as possible.*
- Do not overprotect client or increase dependency. *A client involved with his or her own care can make decisions and is better able to identify when he or she needs help.*
- Focus on what the client can do rather than not do. *Emphasizing strengths is essential.*
- Assist client to identify strengths. *Doing so promotes a positive self-image.*
- Encourage client to express fears, misgivings, or other concerns. *Acknowledging feelings assists client to identify resources and use coping mechanisms.*
- Acknowledge feelings of grief and hostility. *Doing so provides an atmosphere of acceptance.*
- Refer client for counseling if he or she withdraws, shows signs of denial, or otherwise exhibits maladaptive behavior. *Doing so provides other resources to increase coping skills.*

Evaluation of Expected Outcomes

The client reports relief of pain and discomfort, adheres to prescribed drug therapy, and uses alternative methods to reduce pain. He or she demonstrates maximal physical function within limitations, showing evidence of increased muscle strength function. The client can perform self-care at the highest possible level and has a plan for meeting future self-care needs as independently as possible. He or she reports self-confidence and acceptance in the face of altered physical appearance and function and states realistic future goals. The client copes realistically and well with the chronicity of the disease.

67-1 *Client and Family Teaching*
Systemic Lupus Erythematosus

The nurse typically addresses the following with the client:

- Lifestyle modifications are necessary as related to musculoskeletal restrictions and systemic involvement. For example, because sunlight tends to exacerbate the disease, avoid sunlight and ultraviolet radiation. When outdoors, apply effective sunscreens with a sun protection factor (SPF) of 15 or higher and wear clothing that covers the arms and legs and a wide-brimmed hat to shade the face. Sunlamps and tanning booths are taboo.
- Pace activities. Because fatigue is a major issue, allow for adequate rest along with regular activity to promote mobility and prevent joint stiffness. Avoid activities that cause severe pain or discomfort.
- Maintain a well-balanced diet and increase fluid intake to raise energy levels and promote tissue healing.
- Avoid crowds when possible and people with known infections, such as colds.
- Periodically review the medication program with your healthcare providers, particularly the effects and adverse effects of medications and related signs and symptoms that require attention and should be reported to the physician (increased severity of symptoms, involvement in other joints or areas of the body, weight loss, prolonged anorexia, nausea, vomiting, fever, cough, shortness of breath, difficult urination, infection, or any other unusual occurrence).
- Take medications exactly as directed and do not stop the medication if symptoms are relieved unless advised to do so by the physician.
- If symptoms become worse, do not increase the dosage unless advised to do so by the physician. Do not use over-the-counter drugs unless a physician approves their use.
- Use nonpharmacologic comfort measures. For instance, a moist form of heat may relieve joint stiffness. Use warm, not hot, soaks, wraps, or towels hot from the clothes dryer and take care not to burn the skin.
- Inform physicians and dentists of current therapy before any treatment, surgery, or drugs are prescribed.

STRUCTURAL DISORDERS

Structural disorders of the musculoskeletal system involve metabolic conditions that alter bone structure. These alterations result in pain, bone deformity, and fracture.

● OSTEOPOROSIS

Osteoporosis, a loss of bone density, occurs principally in older adults and affects more women than men.

Pathophysiology and Etiology

Normally, the processes of bone formation and bone reabsorption occur evenly. In osteoporosis, however, loss of bone substance exceeds bone formation. The total bone mass is reduced, resulting in bones that become progressively porous, brittle, and fragile. Compression fractures of the vertebrae are common. Aging contributes to osteoporosis (the loss of bone mass) in the following ways:

- Levels of calcitonin, which inhibits bone reabsorption and promotes bone formation, decrease with aging.
- Levels of estrogen, which inhibits bone breakdown, decrease in postmenopausal women.
- Levels of parathyroid hormone, which increases bone reabsorption, increase with aging.

Small-framed, thin white women are at greatest risk for osteoporosis. African-American women have a greater bone density and thus are less susceptible to osteoporosis. Men have an increased bone mass and do not have hormonal changes, and thus do not acquire osteoporosis as frequently and get it at a later age (Smeltzer & Bare, 2000).

Other causes of osteoporosis, which may occur in any age group and both sexes, include Cushing's syndrome, prolonged use of high doses of corticosteroids, prolonged periods of immobility, hyperthyroidism, hyperparathyroidism, malabsorption syndromes, renal or liver failure, alcoholism, lactose intolerance, and dietary deficiency of vitamin D and calcium. Some medications interfere with the body's ability to use and metabolize calcium, including thyroid supplements, anticonvulsants, isoniazid, aluminum-containing antacids, tetracycline, and heparin.

Assessment Findings

Clients with osteoporosis frequently complain of lumbosacral pain, thoracic back pain, or both. The bone pain or tenderness results from tiny compression fractures in the vertebrae. Accompanying loss of height is known as *progressive kyphosis* (Fig. 67-16).

FIGURE 67-16 Typical loss of height associated with osteoporosis and aging.

Radiographic examination of the bones shows bone loss once it is 25% or more. Bone deformities (especially in the spine), such as kyphosis and lordosis, and pathologic fractures in long bones also may be seen. Dual-energy x-ray absorptiometry is a test that measures bone mass at the spine and hip. Ultrasonic heel density (bone sonometer) provides baseline information for diagnosing osteoporosis and predicting risk of fracture. Results of laboratory studies usually are normal, but such studies may be performed to rule out other disorders such as multiple myeloma, hyperparathyroidism, or metastatic bone lesions.

Medical Management

A diet rich in calcium and vitamin D throughout life can prevent osteoporosis. Osteoporosis cannot be treated directly, but medical management can slow the rate of bone reabsorption. Bone pain or tenderness may respond to mild analgesics such as aspirin. Oral calcium preparations (calcium gluconate, calcium lactate, calcium carbonate, or dibasic calcium phosphate) may be recommended to supplement dietary calcium. Some of these preparations also contain vitamin D, which is needed for absorption of calcium in the intestine. New medications, such as bisphosphonate–alendronate sodium (Fosamax), inhibit bone resorption. Administration of calcitonin also inhibits bone reabsorption. Hormone replacement therapy for postmenopausal women as well as adequate rest and exercise, especially weight-bearing exercise such as walking, are part of the treatment regimen.

Nursing Management

In providing care for clients with osteoporosis, the nurse emphasizes the need for a nutritious, well-balanced diet that is high in calcium, vitamin D, and protein—all recommended to delay or prevent osteoporosis. He or she especially advises women to drink three glasses of milk daily or eat other dairy products to acquire approximately 1000 to 1500 mg of calcium; those who smoke cigarettes may require more. Orange juice fortified with calcium is a nutritious alternative. If the client takes antacids, the nurse suggests those containing calcium. He or she recommends activity that promotes bone formation, such as regular, aerobic exercise (e.g., walking).

Stop, Think, and Respond ● BOX 67-5

A 45-year-old female client tells you that she has never liked milk and usually avoids dairy products because she thinks they are too fattening. What do you need to assess to ascertain if she is at risk for osteoporosis? What teaching does she need?

● OSTEOMALACIA

Osteomalacia, a metabolic bone disease, is characterized by inadequate mineralization of bone resulting from a calcium or phosphate deficiency.

Pathophysiology and Etiology

The defect in osteomalacia results from insufficient calcium absorption caused by insufficient calcium intake or resistance to the action of vitamin D. Alternatively, it may occur from phosphate deficiency related to increased renal losses or decreased intestinal absorption. Large amounts of new bone fail to calcify. The bone mass is structurally weaker and bone deformities occur. Additional risk factors are identified in Box 67-9.

Assessment Findings

Clients with osteomalacia experience bone pain and weakness. They also complain of tenderness if the bones are palpated. Bone deformities, such as kyphosis and bowing of the legs, occur as the disease advances. Clients exhibit a waddling type of gait, putting them at risk for falls and fractures.

BOX 67-9 ● Risk Factors for Osteomalacia

Dietary deficiencies
Malnutrition, particularly low calcium intake
Malabsorption
Gastrectomy
Chronic renal failure
Anticonvulsant therapy (phenytoin, phenobarbital)
Insufficient vitamin D (no supplements in food and lack of sunlight)
Poverty
Food fads
Lack of nutritional knowledge

(Adapted from Smeltzer, S. C. & Bare, B. G. [2000]. *Brunner and Suddarth's textbook of medical–surgical nursing* [9th ed., p. 1894.]. Philadelphia: Lippincott Williams & Wilkins.)

Radiographic studies demonstrate demineralization of the bone. Serum levels of calcium and phosphorus are low. Alkaline phosphatase levels typically are elevated.

Medical and Surgical Treatment

Treatment aims at correcting the underlying cause. This includes supplements of calcium, phosphorus, and vitamin D; adequate nutrition; exposure to sunlight; and progressive exercise and ambulation. Bone deformities may require braces or surgery for correction.

Nursing Management

The nurse is in a primary role of educating the client about the disease and its treatment and therefore includes teaching in the care plan. He or she teaches the client about methods and medications used to relieve pain and discomfort. The nurse allows the client to verbalize self-concept issues related to deformities and activity restrictions.

● PAGET'S DISEASE

Paget's disease (osteitis deformans) is a chronic bone disorder characterized by abnormal bone remodeling. It affects adults older than 60 years of age. The most common areas of involvement are the long bones, spine, pelvis, and skull.

Pathophysiology and Etiology

In Paget's disease, some skeletal bones are unaffected; other bones are marked by a disturbance in the ratio between bone formation and reabsorption. The excessive osteoclastic activity causes the bones to become soft and bowed initially. Later the bones thicken when compensatory osteoblastic activity resumes. The process of bone turnover continues, resulting in a classic mosaic pattern of bone matrix development. The new bone has high mineral content but is not well formed. This causes the bones to be weak and prone to fracture.

Although the cause of Paget's disease is unknown, the process by which clients with this disorder deposit collagen, a protein in connective tissue, is thought to be defective. This is based on the fact that the affected bones are high in mineral content but poorly constructed. A family history of the disorder is not uncommon. Additional findings indicate a possible link between the disease and a previous viral infection.

Complications include pathologic fractures, paralysis from spinal cord compression, cranial nerve damage, such as deafness from compression of the skull, and kidney stones. Occasionally, the lesions undergo malignant changes.

Assessment Findings

Some clients are asymptomatic with only some mild skeletal deformity. Other clients have marked skeletal deformities, which may include enlargement of the skull, bowing of the long bones, and kyphosis. Bone pain and tenderness on pressure may be elicited. Paget's disease may go undiscovered until an x-ray for another problem reveals the disorder.

Radiographic examination discloses bones in various stages of resorption and remodeling with a mosaic appearance to the bone structure. Pathologic fractures appear and the bones are curved and enlarged. Bone scans usually are done. An elevated serum alkaline phosphatase level and increased urinary hydroxyproline (an amino acid found in collagen) excretion are common. Calcium levels usually are normal.

Medical and Surgical Management

Clients without symptoms usually do not need treatment. Those with symptoms may benefit from drug therapy. Analgesics such as aspirin or NSAIDs usually can control pain. Those with moderate to severe pain may benefit from treatment with calcitonin (Calcimar), a hormone that appears to block the resorption of bone by reducing the number of osteoclasts and decreasing the rate of bone turnover. Treatment with calcitonin usually results in a drop in the serum alkaline phosphatase level and urinary excretion of hydroxyproline, followed by regression of the lesions. Although not an analgesic, calcitonin reduces pain because it seems to promote the regression of lesions. The client still may require analgesics, however, until bone pain is relieved.

A drug used in advanced disease is EHDP or etidronate disodium (Didronel, Didronel IV), given orally or IV. This drug reduces normal and abnormal bone resorption and secondarily reduces bone formation that is coupled to bone resorption. Alendronate sodium (Fosamax) also may be given to reduce bone turnover and relieve pain. When other drugs prove unsuccessful, mithramycin (Mithracin), an antibiotic usually used in cancer treatment for its cytotoxic effect, may be administered.

Surgery may be performed to repair pathologic fractures or relieve neurologic complications.

Nursing Management

The nurse implements prescribed drug therapy and monitors for side effects. If self-care is limited, the nurse assists the client with ADL. Client safety is a priority because strength and balance may be compromised. As appropriate, the nurse also teaches the client how to use ambulatory aids (e.g., a walker or cane), self-administer prescribed drugs, and implement measures to reduce falls within the home. For nursing management of a client who requires surgery, refer to Nursing Care Plan 67-1.

DISORDERS OF THE FEET

Many foot disorders are treated on an outpatient basis or encountered by nurses when caring for clients with other disorders. Foot disorders that commonly affect clients and for which surgery may be performed are bunions and hammer toes.

Hallux valgus, also called *bunions,* is a deformity of the great (large) toe at its metatarsophalangeal joint (Fig. 67-17A). **Hammer toe** is a flexion deformity of the interphalangeal joint and may involve several toes (see Fig. 67-17B).

Pathophysiology and Etiology

Bunions are associated with heredity, arthritis, or improperly fitting shoes. Women tend to be affected more than men. The first metatarsal bone enlarges on the medial side. The metatarsal bone protrudes at an acute angle toward the midline of the body while the great toe points laterally. There is an overgrowth of soft tissue (bursa), which actually is the bunion. The foot widens and the arch flattens. The malalignment results in pain from the stress on the joint, improper support and distribution of body weight, and inflammation of the bursa.

Like bunions, hammer toe also results from wearing poorly fitting shoes. Toes are pulled upward by the shoe, as the ball of the foot is pulled down. Corns (small, round, elevated overgrowths of epidermis) usually develop on

Nursing Care Plan 67-1

THE CLIENT UNDERGOING ORTHOPEDIC SURGERY

Assessment

■ When the client returns from surgery, review orders in the chart regarding immobilization, movement or turning, and positioning of the arm or leg. Inspect the dressing over the incision. If a wound drain is present, assess the patency of the drain and the type and amount of drainage in the collection receptacle. Assess the neurovascular status of the affected extremity. Monitor vital signs frequently until they stabilize, and routinely thereafter. Maintain the infusing IV fluids as ordered. Assess respiratory status. Encourage the client to identify pain levels and the effectiveness of analgesics.

■ Within the first 24 to 72 hours after orthopedic surgery, complications, such as a fat embolus, may occur (see Table 67-1). The symptoms are similar to those of a pulmonary embolus. In addition, petechial hemorrhages may appear on the skin of the chest. Report severe chest pain or unrelieved incisional pain to the physician immediately.

Nursing Diagnosis: Risk for Ineffective Breathing Pattern related to mucus and inability to mobilize secretions from the airway

Expected Outcome: Client will demonstrate effective respiratory rate and depth with clear breath sounds.

Interventions	Rationales
Instruct client to deep breathe and cough every 2 hours until he or she can ambulate.	These measures expand the lungs and mobilize mucus, preventing pooling of secretions.
Encourage client to use an incentive spirometer to increase deep breathing. Evaluate client's efforts.	Increasing respiratory effort improves client's respiratory status.
Turn client at least every 2 hours and encourage activity within the prescribed limits.	Movement facilitates lung expansion and prevents pooling of secretions.
Auscultate lung sounds every 4 hours.	Immobility can cause hypoventilation, predisposing a client to atelectasis, pooling of respiratory secretions, and pneumonia.

Evaluation of Expected Outcome: Client effectively deep breathes and coughs. Lung sounds are clear.

Nursing Diagnosis: Pain related to surgery

Expected Outcome: Client will report relief of pain.

Interventions	Rationales
Gently move client or adjust position.	Gentle handling minimizes discomfort.
Administer analgesics as prescribed. Instruct client in the use of patient-controlled analgesia if ordered.	Regular administration of analgesics controls and prevents escalation of pain.
Elevate affected extremity and use cold applications.	These measures reduce swelling.
Report client's complaints of severe or sudden and unrelenting pain.	These findings may indicate a complication of surgery (see Table 67-1).

Evaluation of Expected Outcome: Client reports pain relief with analgesics and positioning.

(continued)

Nursing Care Plan 67-1 *(Continued)*

THE CLIENT UNDERGOING ORTHOPEDIC SURGERY

Nursing Diagnosis: **Risk for Disuse Syndrome** related to immobility imposed by casting, traction, and non–weight-bearing status

Expected Outcomes: Client will maintain full ROM of unaffected joints, intact skin, good peripheral blood flow, and normal bowel and bladder function.

Interventions	Rationales
Encourage client to do ROM exercises as indicated.	ROM exercises help to maintain muscle strength and tone and prevent contractures.
Position client so that joints are in normal anatomic alignment.	Proper positioning prevents joint deformities and damage to peripheral nerves and blood vessels.
Get client up as soon as indicated, either in chair, ambulating, or on a tilt table.	Early mobilization prevents complications related to prolonged bed rest.
When getting client up after bed rest, do so slowly, monitoring for signs of postural hypotension, tachycardia, nausea, diaphoresis, or syncope.	When sitting or standing after even 3 to 4 days of bed rest, a client can experience postural hypotension.
Turn client every 2 hours; inspect skin for signs of pressure.	Frequent turning relieves pressure and identifies problems, allowing for early intervention.
Apply antiembolism stockings as indicated.	They help prevent deep vein thrombosis (DVT).
Monitor peripheral circulation, particularly noting skin color, pulses, or any swelling.	Prolonged bed rest, orthopedic surgery, and venous stasis can cause DVT and pulmonary embolism.
Monitor bowel function daily. Provide increased fluids and fiber.	Immobilization causes constipation secondary to inactivity and food intake.
Encourage client to increase fluid intake to 2000 mL/day unless contraindicated.	This intake promotes normal bladder function and prevents constipation, kidney stones, and other related complications of prolonged bed rest.

Evaluation of Expected Outcomes:

- Client can maintain full ROM of unaffected joints.
- Skin remains intact without signs of pressure or breakdown.
- Peripheral circulation is adequate to sustain tissue perfusion.
- Client has adequate urine output and regular bowel movements.

Nursing Diagnosis: **Risk for Infection** related to compromised skin integrity

Expected Outcome: Client will remain free of infection.

Interventions	Rationales
Inspect pins or wire sites used in traction or external fixation devices and the surgical incision, or beneath a cast window for signs of infection.	Regular inspection promotes early detection of and prompt intervention for infection.
Practice Standard Precautions and conscientious handwashing.	They prevent infection.
Use aseptic principles when changing dressings and performing pin care.	Asepsis prevents introduction of microrganisms into wounds and incisions.
Keep wound drainage system below the level of the incision.	Doing so prevents backflow of drainage into the incision.
Administer prescribed antibiotics.	They reduce microorganisms and control infection.
Report purulent wound drainage, elevated temperature, chills, and increased white blood count.	These are signs of infection that require intervention.

(continued)

Nursing Care Plan 67-1 (Continued)

THE CLIENT UNDERGOING ORTHOPEDIC SURGERY

Evaluation of Expected Outcome: Client is free of infection, as evidenced by normal temperature, clean incisions and pin sites, and no purulent drainage.

Nursing Diagnosis: **Self-Care Deficit: Bathing and Hygiene, Feeding, Dressing, and Toileting** related to musculoskeletal impairment

Expected Outcome: Client will gradually perform ADLs as independently as possible.

Interventions	Rationales
Collaborate with client to determine tasks that he or she may perform independently.	Doing so promotes independence and provides client with a sense of control.
Plan activities and rest.	Doing so conserves energy and prevents fatigue.
Consult with physical therapist (PT) and occupational therapist (OT) about client's needs related to ADLs.	PT and OT will determine adaptive equipment needed, as well as client's strengths and abilities to master self-care tasks.
Provide pain medication 45 minutes before activity.	Pain relief promotes participation in self-care.

Evaluation of Expected Outcome: Client can partially bathe and feed himself or herself, dress upper body, and use the bedside commode.

---

top of the toes. Calluses (wide, thickened layer of skin) form under the metatarsal area.

Assessment Findings

The malalignment typical of bunions results in pain from the stress on the joint, improper support and distribution of body weight, and inflammation of the bursa. The client complains of pain on walking or flexing the foot, tender-

FIGURE 67-17 Common foot problems: (**A**) Bunion; (**B**) hammertoe.

ness, and redness of the joint. The typical appearance of the foot deformity is obvious. In hammer toe, the foot deformity is evident. Corns and calluses are easily seen. The client complains of discomfort with ambulation.

Radiographic films of the foot reveal the degree of joint deformity.

Medical and Surgical Management

No treatment is necessary for bunions if pain is not severe and the client has little or no difficulty. Low-heeled, properly fitted shoes are recommended. A bunionectomy, the surgical procedure to remove the bunion and correct the deformity, may be performed when the individual has pain and difficulty walking. Treatment of hammer toe includes exercises, wearing properly fitting or open-toed shoes, use of pads to protect the joints, and surgery to correct the malalignment. Both surgeries are performed on an outpatient or short-term admission basis, with the client discharged in the late afternoon or the following morning. Rest, elevation of the foot, and analgesics are prescribed.

Nursing Management

Nursing management of foot disorders includes relieving pain and discomfort, improving mobility, and instructing clients about the necessity for proper foot attire.

NURSING GUIDELINES 67-4

Instructions for a Client After Foot Surgery

Pain Management—Methods to Reduce Pain

- Elevate foot
- Apply ice as instructed
- Take pain medications as prescribed
- Call physician for pain not relieved

Signs of Impaired Circulation to Report to Physician

- Change in sensation
- Inability to move toes
- Toes or foot cool to touch
- Toes or foot are pale or blue

Mobility

- Use assistive devices appropriately
- Adhere to weight-bearing restrictions
- Wear protective shoe over wound dressing

Wound Care

- Keep dressing or cast clean and dry
- Report signs of wound infection—pain, drainage, fever
- Take antibiotics as prescribed
- Change dressing as prescribed

(Adapted from Smeltzer, S. C. & Bare, B. G. [2000]. *Brunner and Suddarth's textbook of medical-surgical nursing* [9th ed.]. Philadelphia: Lippincott Williams & Wilkins.)

Many clients are treated in an outpatient setting. Nurses in these settings usually are charged with teaching the client about the foot condition, treatment, medications, and postoperative care if the client had surgery. Refer to Nursing Guidelines 67-4 for specific nursing actions.

DISORDERS OF THE UPPER EXTREMITY

Frequent sites of injury and pain in the upper extremity include the shoulder, elbow, and wrist. Among disorders frequently encountered are painful shoulder syndrome, epicondylitis, ganglion, and carpal tunnel syndrome.

The shoulder frequently is a site of injury and pain. Common conditions include tendinitis, tears and rupture of the rotator cuff, and bursitis. These result in painful shoulder syndrome.

Epicondylitis (tennis elbow) is a painful inflammation of the elbow. A ganglion is a cystic mass that develops near tendon sheaths and joints of the wrist. **Carpal tunnel syndrome** is a term for a group of symptoms located in the wrist where the carpal bones, carpal tendons, and median nerve pass through a narrow, inelastic canal.

Pathophysiology and Etiology

The primary causes of shoulder injuries are trauma and repeated stress. Injury also is responsible for epicondylitis, which occurs when the tendons of the medial or lateral radial and ulnar epicondyles sustain damage. The injury typically follows excessive pronation and supination of the forearm, such as that which occurs when playing tennis, pitching ball, or rowing. Ganglion cysts form through defects in the tendon sheath or joint capsule and occur most commonly in women younger than 50 years of age.

Carpal tunnel syndrome results from repetitive wrist motion that traumatizes the tendon sheath or ligaments in the carpal canal. The trauma produces swelling that compresses the median nerve against the transverse carpal ligament. Those affected tend to be in occupations that perform repetitive hand movements such as cashiers, typists, musicians, and assemblers.

Signs and Symptoms

Shoulder injuries are marked by pain and inflammation, which can spread to surrounding tissues. In epicondylitis, clients report pain radiating down the dorsal surface of the forearm and a weak grasp. Clients with ganglion cysts experience pain and tenderness in the affected area. Clients with carpal tunnel syndrome describe pain or burning in one or both hands, which may radiate to the forearm and shoulder in severe cases. The pain tends to be more prominent at night and early in the morning. Shaking the hands may reduce the pain by promoting movement of edematous fluid from the carpal canal. Sensation may be lost or reduced in the thumb, index, middle, and a portion of the ring finger. The client may be unable to flex the index and middle fingers to make a fist. Flexion of the wrist usually causes immediate pain and numbness.

Diagnostic Findings

In general, x-ray studies are used to identify abnormalities and rule out fracture and other problems. In carpal tunnel syndrome, results of electromyography, which relies on a mild electrical current to stimulate the nerve, show a delay in motor response in muscles innervated by the median nerve. Other tests are Tinel's sign, which is a test that elicits tingling, numbness, and pain for clients with carpal tunnel syndrome, and Phalen's sign, which involves having the client flex the wrist for 30 seconds to determine if pain or numbness occurs (a positive sign for carpal tunnel syndrome). The examiner percusses the median nerve, located on the inner aspect of the wrist, to elicit this response.

Medical and Surgical Management

Shoulder treatment includes applications of cold (ice) and heat, exercise, anti-inflammatory medications, local injection of corticosteroids, analgesics, NSAIDs, and rest. Surgical intervention may be necessary to repair tears and ruptures. In many cases, clients with injuries of the shoulder or other portions of the upper extremity are referred for physical therapy. Treatment for epicondylitis is similar to that for shoulder injuries, and splinting is added to rest and support the joint structures. Corticosteroids may be injected locally. Treatment of the ganglion cyst includes aspiration of the ganglion, corticosteroid injection, and surgical excision.

Carpal tunnel treatment involves resting the hands when possible and splinting the hand and wrist. NSAIDs and periodic injections of a corticosteroid preparation may relieve the inflammation and discomfort. If conservative treatment fails, surgery to release the pressure of the ligament on the median nerve may be performed.

Nursing Management

The nurse provides information about medications. If the client is taking NSAIDs, the nurse stresses to take these medications with food. If corticosteroid injections are ordered, he or she explains what the client can expect and mentions that the injection itself may cause some discomfort.

The nurse shows clients how to use and care for prescribed splints and braces and perform related ROM exercises. Some clients find that hand exercises are less painful if performed with the hand under warm water. Additional management activities involve exploring ways to perform ADLs or alter job responsibilities to relieve stress and reduce injury to joints.

Key teaching points include the following:

- Rest the joint in a position that reduces stress.
- Support the affected arm joint on pillows while sleeping.
- Apply cold for the first 24 to 48 hours to reduce swelling and pain.
- Gradually increase joint movement.
- Avoid working or lifting above shoulder level. Do not push objects with the arm joint, particularly the shoulder.
- Perform ROM and strengthening exercises as prescribed by the physician or physical therapist

BONE TUMORS

Bone tumors may be malignant or benign. Malignant tumors are primary, originating in the bone, or secondary, originating from elsewhere in the body (i.e., breast, lung, prostate, or kidney) and traveling to the bone (metastasis). Secondary or metastatic bone tumors are more common than primary bone tumors. Benign tumors of the bone also are more common than malignant bone tumors.

● BENIGN BONE TUMORS

Benign bone tumors have the potential to cause fractures of bones. However, they are not life-threatening and usually cause few symptoms.

Pathophysiology and Etiology

Benign tumors usually are the result of misplaced or overgrown clusters of normal bone or cartilage cells that cause the structure to enlarge and impair local function. They grow slowly and do not metastasize. Their growth can weaken the bone structure by compressing or displacing the normal tissue. Types of bone tumors include:

- Osteochondroma—occurs as a large projection of bone at the ends of long bones, developing during growth periods and then becoming a static bone mass
- Enchondroma—a hyaline cartilage tumor that develops in the hand, ribs, femur, tibia, humerus, or pelvis
- Bone cysts:
  - Aneurysmal bone cysts—painful, palpable mass found in long or flat bones and vertebrae
  - Unicameral bone cysts—may cause pathologic fractures in the humerus or femur
- Osteoid osteoma—painful tumor surrounded by reactive bone tissue
- Osteoclastoma—giant cell tumors that may invade local tissue; usually soft and hemorrhagic; may become malignant (Smeltzer & Bare, 2000)

Assessment Findings

Clients with benign bone tumors may experience pain or discomfort that worsens when bearing weight. The bone appears deformed and swelling may appear over the involved area. If the tumor is in a bone of the extremities, movement may be decreased and pathologic fractures may occur easily.

Radiography, bone scans, and biopsy of the tumor determine the diagnosis.

Medical and Surgical Management

Medical management includes treating pain and preventing fractures. Surgery is performed if the tumor does not stop growing, bone deformity is present, or if the pain is interfering with ADLs and mobility.

Curettage (scraping) or local excision is the usual procedure. Bone grafts may need to be done to promote bone growth and healing. Splints or casts are applied until the bone heals. Clients require close monitoring after surgery because benign bone tumors can recur.

Nursing Management

Providing adequate explanations to the client and alleviating anxiety are key nursing responsibilities. The nurse provides adequate explanations to the client, emphasizing the nature of the tumor, prognosis, and treatment. He or she allows time for questions and expressions of fear and anxiety. The nurse administers pain medications as indicated. He or she teaches the client methods to reduce pain and swelling and encourages the client to elevate the affected extremity.

● MALIGNANT BONE TUMORS

Malignant bone tumors are abnormal osteoblasts or myeloblasts (marrow cells) that exhibit rapid and uncontrollable growth.

Pathophysiology and Etiology

Prior exposure to radiation and toxic chemicals has been associated with the genesis of some malignant bone tumors. A hereditary link in which a tumor suppressor gene may be absent or impaired also is suspected because the same type of tumor may appear among siblings in the same family. Primary tumors include osteosarcoma, Ewing's sarcoma, chondrosarcoma, and fibrosarcoma.

Malignant bone tumors usually are located around the knee in the distal femur or proximal fibula; a few are found in the proximal humerus. As the tumor expands, it lifts the periosteum in much the same way as osteomyelitis. Metastasis occurs through the circulatory or lymphatic system. Metastasis to the lungs is common.

Assessment Findings

A pathologic fracture may be the event that leads the client to seek treatment. Clients with malignant tumors of the bone complain of persistent pain, swelling, and difficulty in moving the involved extremity. A limp or abnormal gait may be noted when the client walks. By the time the client experiences symptoms, however, the tumor usually has spread beyond its primary site.

The bone appears abnormal on radiographic examination, MRI, or bone scan. Biopsy identifies abnormal cells. A malignancy of the skeletal system is associated with an elevated serum alkaline phosphatase level.

Medical and Surgical Management

Treatment of primary malignant bone tumors involves surgical removal of the tumor by amputating the extremity or by wide local resection. Radiation therapy and chemotherapy may be used as well. Chemotherapy after surgery aims to destroy tumor cells that escape from the original tumor site.

Nursing Management

Clients with malignant bone tumors require extensive emotional support and information about the disease, treatment, and prognosis. The nurse implements preoperative and postoperative measures for clients who are having surgery. Refer to the section on amputations for specific nursing care for amputees. As in other orthopedic surgeries, general nursing responsibilities include keeping the affected extremity elevated to reduce swelling, assessing neurovascular status frequently (see Chap. 66), and monitoring closely for complications if the affected limb is immobilized after surgery.

ORTHOPEDIC SURGERY

Orthopedic surgery may be performed for various reasons: to correct a deformity, remove a primary bone tumor, align fractured bones (open reduction), repair or replace a joint, insert a bone graft to promote bone healing, or stabilize a bone internally (using rods, pins, screws, nails, or wires).

Preoperative Nursing Management

Before surgery, the nurse obtains a complete medical, drug, and allergy history from the client or a family member. The nurse also assesses the client's physical condition and mental status at the time of the initial interview. Review of the client's chart includes noting the diagnosis, type of surgery to be performed, and any previous treatments, such as traction or drug use. If the client's disorder was treated previously, the nurse needs to determine whether any complications or problems occurred because of or during treatment.

Client goals in the preoperative period focus on helping the client to experience reduced pain; continue to be active, mobile, and injury free; practice measures to reduce the potential for postoperative wound infection; control anxiety at manageable levels; understand instructions;

and comprehend the procedures and rationale of postoperative management (Nursing Guidelines 67-5).

Postoperative Nursing Management

Ideally, postoperative nursing management begins before surgery with demonstrations of deep breathing and coughing exercises and descriptions and demonstrations of the incentive spirometer (if that is likely to be used after surgery). Even if the client will have postoperative physical therapy, the nurse explains and helps the client practice active and isometric leg exercises. He or she also describes other devices that may be used after surgery, such as IV infusions of fluid and blood, oxygen, a wound drain, elastic stockings, or roller bandages. It also is necessary to include a discussion of the possible use of traction or the CPM machine. See Nursing Care Plan 67-1 for additional nursing management of a client having orthopedic surgery.

NURSING GUIDELINES 67-5

Ensuring Complete Care for Clients Before Orthopedic Surgery

- Review the operation and the reason for it.

- Administer prescribed analgesics.

- Relieve the client's discomfort through positioning and joint immobilization.

- Support painful joints and be gentle when moving the client.

- Allow ample time for physical activities because the client with a musculoskeletal disorder needs more time to carry out preoperative routines. Allow the client to use any ambulatory aid that was brought from home.

- Demonstrate use of the overbed trapeze and encourage its use.

- Demonstrate and have the client perform necessary postoperative activities, such as coughing and deep breathing exercises.

- Provide preoperative skin care as indicated by agency policy and procedure. If the client has initiated skin preparation at home, check to be sure the procedures were performed.

- Obtain adequate help when transferring a sedated client who is not in traction from the bed to the surgical stretcher. However, keep a client who is in traction in the hospital bed. Then, without lifting or removing the traction weights, transport the bed to the operating room.

- Administer the IV prophylactic antibiotic if ordered before surgery. (Although laminar airflow in the operating suite has reduced the incidence of postoperative infection, a great risk for infection remains for every client having orthopedic surgery. The number of personnel in the operating room may need to be limited to reduce a potential reservoir of infecting microorganisms.)

Client and Family Teaching

The nurse talks with the client, family, and other significant caregivers about the support system that will be available after discharge. It is important to explore the kinds of assistance the client needs for moving and walking, preparing meals, getting to the physician's office or physical therapy department, and performing other household tasks. The nurse tries to identify modifications that will be necessary in the home environment such as relocating the bed to a ground floor level. In addition, he or she provides information about renting home care equipment, arranging for home delivery of meals through a community agency or church service group, or scheduling transportation with an agency that has a medical van or hydraulic lift available. The nurse may refer the client to a home health care agency or extended care facility. He or she provides printed discharge instructions for future reference and covers the following general points:

- Follow the directions of the physician. Do not resume any activity that has been restricted until told to do so.
- Perform exercises exactly as prescribed by the physician and physical therapist.
- Use the recommended device (walker, cane, crutches) for walking.
- Wear supportive shoes when using crutches, walker, or cane.
- Eliminate safety hazards in the home, such as scatter rugs.
- Eat a nutritious diet and drink plenty of fluids.
- Take prescribed medications as directed; do not use or take any nonprescription drugs unless they have been approved by the physician.
- Notify the physician if the incision has unusual drainage or if fever, chills, sudden onset of pain, redness, or swelling occurs.

AMPUTATION

Amputation is the removal of a limb. It may occur as a result of trauma (traumatic amputation) or in an effort to control disease or disability (therapeutic amputation).

Etiology

The following are conditions for which an amputation may be performed:

- Malignant tumors
- Long-standing infections of bone and tissue that prohibit restoration of function
- Extensive trauma to an extremity

- Death of tissues from peripheral vascular insufficiency or peripheral vasospastic diseases such as Buerger's and Raynaud's diseases
- Thermal injuries
- Deformity of a limb rendering it a useless hindrance
- Life-threatening disorders, such as arterial thrombosis and gas bacillus infections

Medical and Surgical Management

Unless emergency surgery is performed, the client is treated for any disorder that may influence healing (e.g., uncontrolled diabetes mellitus, dehydration, infection, electrolyte imbalances, poor nutrition, chronic respiratory disorders). When it is decided that amputation must be performed as a life-saving measure, the following factors help the surgical team decide at which level to amputate the arm or leg (e.g., above or below the knee, above or below the elbow):

- Amount of tissue that must be removed to eliminate the disorder
- Level at which the blood supply is adequate to preserve circulation to tissue that will remain
- Number of joints that can be preserved
- Length of residual limb that will promote fitting a prosthesis, an artificial limb, for rehabilitation

The levels of some commonly planned amputations include below the knee (BK), above the knee (AK), below the elbow (BE), and above the elbow (AE). The surgical objective is to create a gently tapering stump with muscular padding over the end. Occasionally, knee disarticulations (amputation through a joint), disarticulation at the ankle joint, and partial foot amputations are performed.

Amputation Methods

An amputation may be performed using an open or closed method. In an open amputation (guillotine amputation), the end of the residual limb (or stump) is temporarily open with no skin covering it. Open amputations usually are performed in cases of infection. Skin traction is applied, and the infected area is allowed to drain. The traction must be continuous. The surgeon may arrange the traction so that the client can turn over in bed.

In the more common closed amputation (flap amputation), skin flaps cover the severed bone end. Clients with a closed amputation return from surgery with either a soft compression dressing or rigid plaster shell covering the residual limb. The compression dressing consists of gauze over which elastic roller bandages are wrapped to create pressure to control bleeding. There may be a walking pylon, a type of temporary prosthesis composed of a metal post and molded foot, attached to the rigid plaster shell (Fig. 67-18). It may be weeks before the postoperative client is referred to a prosthetist, a professional who creates and fits artificial limbs.

FIGURE 67-18 Many amputees receive prostheses soon after surgery and begin learning how to use them with the help and support of the rehabilitation team, which includes nurses, physicians, physical therapists, and others.

Arm Amputation

The arms have highly specialized functions. Consequently, the amputation of an arm, particularly the arm with the dominant hand, requires great physical and emotional adjustment during the preoperative as well as postoperative periods. Fortunately, most clients with arm amputations can be measured for a prosthesis shortly after the surgical scar heals.

Three types of prostheses are available for arm amputees: a shoulder harness with cables that attach to a mechanical terminal device, referred to as a *hook;* a semifunctioning cosmetic hand that can be substituted for the hook; and a myoelectric arm.

The hook performs the functions of the hand and fingers when the amputee moves the scapula and expands the chest activating the cables attached from a shoulder harness to the mechanical device. The mechanical terminal device is strong, sturdy, and functional. The cosmetic hand, which can be attached to the same cables as the hook, has the appearance of a natural hand, but it lacks the capacity for performing fine motor skills. The myoelectric arm has a realistic-looking hand that is activated by electrical impulses from muscles in the upper arm. The electrical activity is relayed from electrodes in the shell of the prosthesis to microcircuits in the prosthetic fingers. The myoelectric arm has three advantages: it eliminates the need to wear a harness, the terminal device looks natural, and it has somewhat better function than the cosmetic hand. Despite its advantages, the myoelectric arm is not rugged enough to do the work of the mechanical terminal device.

Leg Amputation

Amputation of a leg is a more common operation than amputation of an arm. The AK amputation is more disabling than a BK amputation; therefore, unless evidence suggests that the knee cannot be saved, every attempt is made to amputate below the knee.

The trend is to have a temporary prosthesis attached to the plaster shell covering the residual lower limb immediately after surgery. It reduces psychological trauma for the client because it promotes a more intact sense of body image after surgery. Also, the walking pylon facilitates early ambulation. Almost immediately, the client is allowed to stand and place a limited amount of weight on the residual limb. As the stump heals and edema disappears, a second cast may be reapplied or a temporary socket made of lightweight polypropylene may be constructed. Ultimately, a conventional prosthesis is custom-made to conform to the stump as well as to the client's needs. Leg prostheses may be held in place by means of a pelvic belt or suction.

Complications

Hematoma, hemorrhage, and infection are potential complications in the immediate postoperative period. Potential complications late in the postoperative course include chronic osteomyelitis (after persistent infection) and, rarely, a burning pain (causalgia), the cause of which is unknown. Pain may result from a stump neuroma, which is formed when the cut ends of nerves become entangled in the healing scar. A neuroma is treated with injections of procaine, a local anesthetic, or reamputation.

Phantom Limb and Phantom Pain

The surgeon informs the client of the potential phenomenon of phantom limb sensation, which is a feeling that the amputated portion of the limb still remains. It is a normal, frequently occurring physiologic response after amputation. Phantom sensations can persist for months or decades, or can come and go. Although clients are aware of phantom sensations, they usually learn to ignore them.

Phantom pain is pain or other discomfort, such as burning, tingling, throbbing, or itching, in the missing limb. Pain felt from the phantom limb can be an extremely serious problem in relation to the client's emotional status and ability to use a prosthesis. Severe, prolonged phantom limb pain may require surgical removal of nerve endings at the end of the stump.

Rehabilitation

The success of the amputee's rehabilitation depends on variables such as age, type of amputation, condition of the stump, physical status, condition of the remaining limb, concurrent debilitating illness, visual motor coordination, motivation, acceptance, and cooperation. Clients vary greatly in their learning capacity and ability to master the use of a prosthesis. The period allotted for training also varies with each client. It is vital that the physician, the nurse, the physical and occupational therapists, the family, and the client maintain realistic expectations throughout the rehabilitation period.

Nursing Management

Nursing management of an amputee can be segmented into two key functions: those before surgery and those after surgery. In general, presurgical nursing management involves considerations for any surgery, specifically taking a complete medical, drug, and allergy history and evaluating the client for mental and emotional acceptance of the surgical procedure.

Assessing motor strength and flexibility of other joints is important to determine potential problems involving rehabilitation. If the client is acutely ill, such as with a gangrenous limb and related fever, disorientation, and electrolyte imbalances, the nurse monitors circulation in the limb for changes, such as severe pain, color changes, and lack of peripheral pulses. It is crucial that the nurse inform the physician of problems as they occur because surgery may become an emergency.

Preoperative Care

Presurgical nursing management includes reducing pain and anxiety and supporting the client as he or she begins to grieve the loss of the limb and adapt to potential changes. The nurse administers narcotic analgesics before surgery to clients with severe pain. Other comfort measures include handling the painful limb gently, elevating a swollen limb, encouraging family presence and support, being available especially at times when the client is alone, helping the client to express concerns, and clarifying misperceptions.

Before surgery, the nurse explains all the routine preoperative preparations and reinforces what the physician has discussed with the client and family regarding the extent of physical disability; the psychological, aesthetic, social, and vocational implications; and the realistic possibilities for prosthetic restoration. The nurse must exercise care in answering questions about prosthetic devices and their use because it always is possible that the amputation may need to involve more of the limb than originally anticipated. In addition, the nurse reviews the postoperative management, such as deep breathing, coughing, positioning, and routine exercises and encourages the client to practice the exercises if time and the client's condition permit.

Clients vary in their reactions to the impending loss of a limb. The amount of grief is thought to be proportional to the symbolic significance of the part and the resultant degree of disability and deformity. Anger and depression are common emotions. The nurse acknowledges the client's feelings and remains objective and nonjudgmental as the client expresses negative emotional responses. Reassuring the client that his or her reaction is normal may provide comfort. The nurse should not shame, criticize, or trivialize the client's behavior.

How well the client can cope usually depends on prior experience and how he or she has dealt with previous losses. The nurse protects the client from additional sources of stress. While the client is preoccupied with the potential loss, the nurse should not make unnecessary demands or expect full participation in the plan of care. The nurse provides assistance with activities that at any other time the client could carry out independently. The nurse also promotes adequate sleep and discusses coping techniques that have been used successfully in the past and encourages their repetition. Fostering communication with family members or friends promotes support.

Client and Family Teaching

Client and family education begins before amputation surgery and extends beyond hospitalization. After surgery, discharge teaching depends on many factors, including the length of hospitalization, the type and location of the amputation, the age and physical condition of the client, and the type of dressing or prosthesis the client wears. The nurse explores factors related to the home environment and determines a plan for continued rehabilitation before discharge. Some clients need to modify their living arrangements, use a wheelchair, or make other accommodations or changes.

If the client has to bandage the stump at home, the nurse teaches both the client and the family how to apply the bandage and how to care for the stump (Nursing Guidelines 67-6), as well as how to wash the bandages, rinse them well, and lay them flat to dry because hanging tends to decrease the elasticity. When the bandages are dry, they must be rolled without stretching. The nurse also should include the following general points in the discharge instructions:

- Follow the physician's recommendations regarding caring for the stump, applying a stump dressing, washing the stump, and elevating the stump when sitting.
- Do not apply nonprescription drugs (ointments, creams, topical pain relievers) to the stump unless the physician has approved the use of a specific product.
- Adhere to the plan of scheduled exercises and complete each group of exercises as outlined by the physical therapist.
- Do not exceed the physician's recommendations regarding weight bearing and joint flexion.
- Eat well-balanced and nutritious meals or follow the diet recommended by the physician. Avoid gaining excess weight during the recovery period

because weight gain may interfere with use of a leg prosthesis.
- Expect that phantom limb sensation, if present, may persist for some time, which is normal.
- Avoid injury to the stump, even though it appears to be healed. Report any skin impairment immediately.
- Continue deep breathing exercises until fully mobile.
- Contact the physician if fever, chills, productive cough, bleeding or oozing from the stump, purulent drainage from the incision, new or different pain in the stump, or any change in the appearance of the stump occurs.

NURSING GUIDELINES 67-6
Stump Care and Bandaging

Stump Care

- Assess the covering over the stump frequently to determine the type and amount of drainage from the incision. Expect some oozing of blood, but if a gauze dressing is used, it may need to be reinforced.

- Keep a tourniquet in plain view at bedside and if hemorrhage occurs, apply it and notify the physician.

- Usually, elevate the stump for the first 24 to 48 hours to prevent edema. In some cases, such as an AK amputation, a slight Trendelenburg position is preferred to elevating the stump on pillows because bending the hip promotes a flexion contracture. A bed board or a firm mattress provides skeletal support.

- If the client has a rigid plaster cast with walking pylon, loosen the harness, which suspends the cast from the waist, when the client is in bed. Slightly tighten the harness when the client is ambulatory.

Bandaging

Before a permanent prosthesis can be made, the stump must shrink and be shaped. This is done with elastic bandages that are wrapped about the stump. Unlike leg stumps, arm stumps do not need as massive a shrinkage over as long a period. Various bandaging techniques are appropriate, but several principles are observed:

- Remove and rewrap the bandage at least twice during the day and before the client retires for the night.

- Bandage joints in a way that promotes a neutral or extended position.

- Avoid circular turns, which act like a tourniquet and interfere with blood flow.

NURSING PROCESS

● Caring for the Client After a Limb Amputation

Assessment

The nurse monitors vital signs to determine any changes, particularly elevations in temperature (indicating possible infection), pulse, and BP. Reviewing the client's medical record provides information about the reason for and type and level of the amputation. The nurse inspects the dressing or plaster shell and, when changing the dressing, assesses the wound for signs of infection, excessive drainage, or separation of wound edges. In addition, the nurse evaluates the client's general condition as well as level of pain and discomfort, and implements measures to relieve it. He or she also implements measures to prevent infection, promote healing, and avoid skin breakdown.

Diagnosis, Planning, and Interventions

Nursing management involves all concerns addressed after any orthopedic surgery (see Nursing Care Plan 67-1). It also includes, but is not limited to, the following:

Risk for Self-Care Deficit (specify bathing/hygiene, dressing/grooming, feeding, toileting) related to impediments imposed by amputation
Expected Outcome: Client will participate in self-care and recuperative measures to the fullest extent possible.

- Encourage clients with leg amputations to assume some of their own care 1 or 2 days after surgery. *Incorporating the client's abilities increases self-care independence.*
- Assist clients with an arm amputation, especially on the dominant side, until they can use the opposite extremity. *It takes time for clients to adjust to having only one upper extremity.*
- Exercise and position the client in proper alignment. *Correct positioning prevents contractures after amputation, maintains skeletal alignment, and promotes active movement of the uninvolved limbs.*
- Work with the PT to implement a program of active and isometric exercises. *These exercises increase the client's abilities and strengths.*

Risk for Disuse Syndrome related to altered mobility after amputation
Expected Outcomes: (1) Client will become progressively mobile and independent. (2) Client will maintain intact skin, adequate tissue perfusion, and normal pulmonary function. (3) Client will develop no complications related to immobility.

- Place client with a leg amputation in the prone position several times a day. *This position promotes stump extension and prevents contractures.*
- Position client so that he or she is in normal anatomic alignment at all times. *Improper positioning may injure peripheral nerves and blood vessels and cause joint deformities.*
- Use a trochanter roll to prevent external rotation of the hip and knee. Avoid placing pillows between the legs. *These measures prevent abduction deformity.*
- Advise the client who is lying on the stomach to adduct the stump so it presses against the other leg. *Adduction stretches flexor muscles and prevents abduction deformity.*

- On the first or second postoperative day, assist client to stand to regain a sense of balance. Stepping on the floor with the temporary prosthesis and weight bearing of about 10% of body weight usually is permitted at this time. *These measures promote strength and balance while preventing injury.*
- Expect the client with a temporary prosthesis to progress to walking with crutches or a walker or in parallel bars 2 to 4 days after the amputation with a high degree of safety (full weight bearing on the unaffected leg). *This measure promotes independence.*
- Provide client with assistive devices. *They help client to be more independent and maintain more mobility.*
- Use antiembolism stockings. *They prevent deep vein thrombosis.*
- Monitor pulmonary status and implement deep breathing and coughing exercises. *Decreased mobility can result in hypoventilation and may lead to atelectasis and pooling of secretions. Pulmonary exercises improve lung expansion and mobilize secretions.*
- Increase fluid intake to 2000 mL (if permitted). *This intake promotes urine output and prevents constipation.*

Risk for Dysfunctional Grieving related to loss of body part
Expected Outcome: Client will state that he or she is beginning to resolve loss and develop strategies for coping without an arm or leg.

- Listen actively and empathetically. *Doing so facilitates communication.*
- Allow clients time to talk about their loss and express feelings of grief, anger, depression, and anxiety. *Grief is hard work and needs time.*
- Discuss each new challenge as it arises. *Providing information and listening to client's feelings assists the client to face new issues.*
- Allow client time to process information. *Providing time allows the client to adjust to new situations.*
- Implement changes gradually. *Doing so gives client time to adjust and adapt.*
- Reinforce progress that has been made. *Doing so provides encouragement and support.*
- Remain available to the client for physical and emotional support. *The nurse can serve as a consistent support system.*
- Foster family involvement because their encouragement often helps motivate a client to face each new problem, accept failure, and develop a determination to overcome obstacles. *Support from significant others can have a positive effect.*
- Ambulate the client with a leg amputation as soon as possible. *Doing so dispels the doubt that permanent disability will prevail.*
- Explore the possibility of a meeting with a rehabilitated amputee. *Someone who has endured a similar experience can serve as a support network.*

Disturbed Body Image related to loss of body part and function

Expected Outcome: Client will progressively adjust to the change in body image.

- Keep in mind that the attitude of staff and family members bears greatly on how clients perceive themselves. *A positive approach promotes a client's positive self-image.*
- Do not treat the client as less than competent. *Focusing on client's strengths and abilities promotes his or her self-image.*
- Avoid nonverbal implications that the client, the stump, or the prosthesis is repulsive. *Being aware of nonverbal behavior indicates how the client feels about himself or herself.*
- Make a point to visit the client frequently, especially when no particular nursing activity must be performed. *Such visits encourage client to feel more positively about himself or herself.*
- Make eye contact during verbal interactions. *The nurse must treat all clients with the same respect.*
- Sit close to the client's bedside and lean forward when talking. *Doing so communicates a personal interest in the client.*
- Offer praise when the client successfully accomplishes a task. *Praise builds self-esteem and self-confidence.*
- If appropriate, explore the client's reasons for refusing to use a prosthesis. *If the problem is amenable to change, the nurse can enlist the help of the surgeon, physical therapist, or prosthetist.*

Evaluation of Expected Outcomes

By discharge, the client reports reduced and manageable pain, no infection, and intact skin; he or she demonstrates optimal participation in self-care. The client experiences increasing mobility along with increasing resolution of grief, greater self-acceptance, and acceptance of current situation. He or she experiences no postoperative complications. The client does not withdraw from social situations, has a positive attitude about the future, and can demonstrate adequate independent self-care.

 ## GENERAL NUTRITIONAL CONSIDERATIONS

Protein requirements increase during prolonged immobility to correct negative nitrogen balance, promote healing, and help prevent skin breakdown and infections. A protein intake of 1.2 g/kg body weight is recommended; the client needs adequate calories to spare protein. A high fiber intake helps prevent constipation.

To reduce the risk of renal calculi, a complication of prolonged immobility and gout, advise clients to drink at least 2 quarts of fluid daily. Drinking fluid before bed and during the night helps keep the urine dilute.

No conclusive evidence has shown that diet therapy can prevent or cure RA. Some studies suggest, however, that a food allergy may cause a small percentage of cases, with dairy products, corn, cereals, citrus fruits, and tomatoes proposed as possible offenders. Other studies suggest that omega-3 fatty acids found in fatty fish (e.g., mackerel, herring, salmon) and, to a lesser extent, in flaxseed, olive, and canola oils may help relieve joint tenderness and fatigue, possibly by inhibiting the inflammatory response of certain prostaglandins. The use of fish oil supplements is not recommended, but eating more dietary sources of omega-3 fatty acids may be beneficial. Malnutrition is common among clients with RA; monitor weight changes. Discourage quack "cures" and self-prescribed supplements.

Gradual weight loss helps reduce serum uric acid levels in clients with gout. Clients should avoid fasting, low-carbohydrate diets, and rapid weight loss because these measures increase the likelihood of ketone formation, which inhibits uric acid excretion.

Excess fiber and protein, caffeine, alcohol, and smoking promote calcium excretion and thereby increase the risk of osteoporosis.

 ## GENERAL PHARMACOLOGIC CONSIDERATIONS

Oral calcium preparations with vitamin D are better absorbed than those without.

Clients should not take oral calcium preparations with other oral drugs because calcium may alter or block absorption of the other drugs. For example, calcium decreases absorption of tetracycline and phenytoin. Clients should take other drugs 1 to 2 hours after calcium carbonate.

Clients may take oral calcium with meals to enhance absorption and minimize gastric distress.

Warn clients with arthritis about drugs, health foods, and certain food substances available in drug form and promoted as cures for arthritis.

Tell clients taking large doses of salicylates the signs of GI bleeding, salicylism, and the possibility of easy bruising and other bleeding tendencies. Signs of salicylism include headache, nausea, vomiting, tinnitus, increased pulse and respiratory rates, fever, mental confusion, and drowsiness.

Large doses of salicylates can interfere with the blood's clotting mechanism. Instruct clients taking these drugs to inform their physicians and dentists of their prolonged and high-dose ingestion of salicylates.

Clients with gout need detailed instructions about their medical regimens in relation to the drugs to take and the importance of increasing their fluid intake to reduce the possibility of urate stone formation in the urinary tract.

Caution clients with diseases of the bones and joints against discontinuing their drugs if and when they begin to feel improved.

Instruct clients taking aspirin for arthritis not to substitute buffered aspirin or enteric-coated aspirin for regular aspirin unless the physician approves the change. Aspirin cannot be used in clients with ulcers, a history of ulcers, or bleeding disorders.

The most common adverse effects of NSAIDs are related to the GI tract: nausea, vomiting, diarrhea, and constipation. GI bleeding, which in some cases is severe, has been reported with the use of these drugs.

Calcitonin may be used in the treatment of Paget's disease and is administered subcutaneously. Some adverse effects associated with calcitonin include nausea (with or without vomiting), inflammation at the injection site, increased urinary frequency, anorexia, diarrhea, and abdominal pain.

 ## GENERAL GERONTOLOGIC CONSIDERATIONS

Women older than 45 years of age have a 9% to 10% decrease in cortical bone per decade.

Older adults are more prone to skeletal fractures because bone resorption takes place more rapidly than bone formation.

Maintaining an active lifestyle delays the decline of muscle strength and bone mass among older adults.

With age, the fibrocartilage of intervertebral disks becomes thinner and drier, causing compression of the disks of the spinal column and leading to a loss of height amounting to as much as 1.5 to 3 inches (3.75 to 7.5 cm).

Estrogen deficiency, which occurs at menopause, is considered the leading factor in osteoporosis among aging women.

Critical Thinking Exercises

1. *A male client had a total hip replacement 3 days ago and wants to use the toilet for a bowel movement. Explain how to assist this client.*

2. *A female client has just returned from the recovery unit after an AK amputation. Fresh blood has saturated the stump dressing. What actions should you take at this time?*

3. *A young man, admitted with a fractured radius, complains of increasing pain in his hand after a cast was applied, despite having received a narcotic analgesic 30 minutes ago. What assessments are important to make at this time?*

References and Suggested Readings

Anderson, L. & Dale, K. (1998). Infections in total joint replacements. *Orthopaedic Nursing, 17*(1), 7–11.

Arthritis Foundation. (2002). Arthritis today: Drug guide. [Online.] Available: www.arthritis.org.

Bryant, G. (2001). Stump care. *American Journal of Nursing, 101*(2), 67–71.

Bullock, B. A. & Henze, R. L. (2000). *Focus on pathophysiology.* Philadelphia: Lippincott Williams & Wilkins.

Hager, C. & Berncick, N. (1998). Fat embolism syndrome: A complication of orthopedic trauma. *Orthopaedic Nursing, 17*(2), 41–46, 58.

Hartzheim, L. A. & Gross, G. L. (1998). Rheumatoid arthritis: A case study. *Nursing Clinics of North America, 33,* 595–602.

Holmes, H. N. (Ed.). *Mastering medical-surgical nursing.* (1998). Springhouse, PA: Springhouse Corporation.

Johnson, B. (1999). Systemic lupus erythematosus. *American Journal of Nursing, 99*(1), 40–41.

Kozuh, J. L. (2000). NSAIDs and antihypertensives: An unhappy union. *American Journal of Nursing, 100*(6), 40–42.

Lappe, J. (1998). Prevention of hip fractures. *Orthopaedic Nursing, 17*(3), 15–26.

Peloso, P. M. (2000). NSAIDs: A Faustian bargain. *American Journal of Nursing, 100*(6), 34–39.

Porth, C. M. (2002). *Pathophysiology: Concepts of altered health states* (6th ed.). Philadelphia: Lippincott Williams & Wilkins.

Ramsburg, K. L. (2000). Rheumatoid arthritis. *American Journal of Nursing, 100*(11), 40–43.

Rodts, M. (1999). Building strong bones. *Orthopaedic Nursing, 18*(5), 9.

Sedlack, C. A., Doheny, M. O., & Jones, J. L. (1998). Osteoporosis prevention in young women. *Orthopaedic Nursing, 17*(3), 53–60.

Sharkey, N. A., Williams, N. I., & Guerin, J. B. (2000). The role of exercise in the prevention and treatment of osteoporosis and osteoarthritis. *Nursing Clinics of North America, 35,* 209–221.

Smeltzer, S. C. & Bare, B. G. (2000). *Brunner and Suddarth's textbook of medical–surgical nursing* (9th ed.). Philadelphia: Lippincott Williams & Wilkins.

Urquhart, B. S. (2001). Emergency: Anterior shoulder dislocation. *American Journal of Nursing, 101*(2), 33–35.

Wade, C. F. (2000). Keeping Lyme disease at bay. *American Journal of Nursing, 100*(7), 26–31.

Williamson, V. (1998). Management of lower extremity fractures. *Orthopaedic Nursing, 17*(5), 84–87.

Yarnold, B. (1999). Hip fracture: Caring for a fragile population. *American Journal of Nursing, 99*(2), 36–41.

chapter **68**

Introduction to the Integumentary System

Words to Know

apocrine glands
debridement
dermis
eccrine glands
epidermis
integument
keratin
melanin
pheromones

pressure sores
sebaceous glands
sebum
shearing
skin tear
stratum corneum
subcutaneous tissue
sweat glands

Learning Objectives

On completion of this chapter, the reader will:

- Name the structures that form the integument.
- List four functions of the integumentary system.
- Identify the purpose of sebum and melanin.
- Differentiate between eccrine and apocrine glands.
- Name at least three facts about the integument that are pertinent to document when obtaining a health history.
- Give the characteristics of normal skin.
- Discuss the criteria for staging pressure sores.
- List characteristics of hair assessed during a physical examination.
- Describe the characteristics of normal nails.
- Name three diagnostic tests performed to determine the etiology of skin disorders.
- Name seven medical and surgical techniques for treating skin disorders.

The **integument** includes structures that cover the body's exterior surface. The primary structure is the skin, which contains sebaceous and sweat glands and sensory nerve endings (Fig. 68-1). The integument also includes accessory structures such as the hair and nails. The structures that make up the integument protect the body from environmental injuries, help to regulate body temperature, serve as sensory organs, and facilitate the synthesis of vitamin D.

ANATOMY AND PHYSIOLOGY

Skin

The skin is composed of two layers: the **epidermis,** the outermost layer, and the **dermis,** which lies below the epidermis. The epidermis contains an outer layer of dead skin cells, the **stratum corneum,** that forms a tough protective protein called **keratin.** The epidermis is constantly shed and replaced with epithelial cells from the dermis. The dermis, or true skin, consists of connective tissue and

contains elastic fibers, blood vessels, sensory and motor nerve fibers, sweat and sebaceous (oil) glands, and hair follicles (roots). The **subcutaneous tissue** is the layer of skin attached to muscle and bone and is composed primarily of connective tissue and fat cells. Skin has a tremendous capacity to stretch with little subsequent damage, as is evident after soft tissue injury and pregnancy.

The color of the skin is determined by a pigment called **melanin,** which is manufactured by melanocytes located in the epidermis. The production of melanin is under the control of the middle lobe (pars intermedia) of the pituitary gland, which secretes melanocyte-stimulating hormone. The more melanin found in the epidermis, the darker the skin color. Exposure to ultraviolet light temporarily stimulates the production of melanin to absorb harmful radiation.

Skin Functions

The skin has four major functions: protection, temperature regulation, sensory processing, and chemical synthesis.

FIGURE 68-1 A cross-section of the skin.

PROTECTION

The skin forms a protective barrier between the outside world and underlying organs and structures of the body. The barrier it provides blocks microorganisms and other foreign substances from contact with the structures below the epidermis. It also prevents a loss of water from structures below the surface of the skin.

TEMPERATURE REGULATION

To maintain an even body temperature, the skin heats or cools the structures below. The body continuously produces internal heat during cellular metabolism. To generate heat and prevent heat loss at the body's surface, erector muscles around shafts of hair contract. Elevation of skin hairs interferes with local air circulation and maintains the warmth of the skin.

Heat dissipates through the skin and through respiration. Heat is lost by four methods (Fig. 68-2):

- *Radiation* is the transfer of surface heat in the environment. An example of radiant heat loss is the escape of heat from the surface of warm skin into cooler air.
- *Conduction* is the transfer of heat through contact. An example of conductive heat loss is placing a cool cloth on warm skin.

A   **B**   **C**   **D**

FIGURE 68-2 Methods of heat loss: (**A**) radiation; (**B**) convection; (**C**) evaporation; and (**D**) conduction.

- *Evaporation* is the loss of moisture or water. Water on the surface of the body is warmed. As the moisture vaporizes, the body is cooled. Evaporation occurs unnoticed (insensible loss) and when there is obvious perspiration.
- *Convection* is the transfer of heat by means of currents of liquids or gasses in which warm air molecules move away from the body. An example of convection is a cool breeze that blows across the body surface.

When the temperature and humidity outside the body rise, radiation, evaporation, and convection are ineffective. The only way heat is transferred under these conditions is by conduction. This is why exposure to warm temperatures and densely saturated moist air can raise the body temperature and result in heat stroke.

SENSORY PROCESSING

The skin serves as a means of monitoring the outside environment, as well as warning of danger. Specialized nerve endings in the skin respond to pressure, pain, heat, and cold.

CHEMICAL SYNTHESIS

The skin forms a chemical substance called 7-dehydrocholesterol, which facilitates the synthesis of vitamin D when the skin is exposed to ultraviolet light (sunlight). Vitamin D is necessary for healthy formation of bones and teeth. Dark-skinned people do not synthesize vitamin D as readily as light-skinned people. Cloudy environments and air pollutants that block sunlight also interfere with vitamin D synthesis. Therefore, vitamin D is added to some food sources, such as milk.

Stop, Think, and Respond ● BOX 68-1

Discuss the importance of keeping the skin intact.

Hair

Hair originates in the hair follicles in the dermis. It is formed from hundreds of strands of keratin linked together with amino acids. Melanin, produced by melanocytes in the hair root, influence hair color. The three types of melanin are brown, black, and yellow. Types of melanin are genetically inherited, as are hair texture, shape, and rate of growth. Scalp hair grows more rapidly than any other. Illness, hormone levels, nutrition, aging, and other factors can affect hair growth and loss.

Hair covers all parts of the body except the palms, soles, dorsum of the fingers, lips, penis, labia, and nipples. In some areas, such as the pubis, axilla, and chest, the hair is more coarse than in other locations. Men of some ethnic groups (e.g., Native Americans) have less facial and body hair than their Euro-American counterparts.

Sebaceous and Sweat Glands

Sebaceous glands are connected to each hair follicle and secrete an oily substance called *sebum*. **Sebum** is a lubricant that prevents drying and cracking of the skin and hair. As sebum fills the glandular duct, it enters the hair follicle, from which it eventually is released. During puberty, sebaceous glands in the forehead, nose, chest, and back become more active.

The two types of **sweat glands** are eccrine and apocrine. **Eccrine glands** release water and electrolytes, such as sodium and chloride, in the form of perspiration. The rate of perspiration is related to body temperature. Adults can produce as much as 3 L under extremely hot conditions. The pH of perspiration is slightly acidic, which helps in providing a hostile environment for microbial colonization. Frequent washing with alkaline soaps removes sebum and reduces the acid mantle of protection.

Apocrine glands are found around the nipples, in the anogenital region, in the eyelids (Moll's glands), in the mammary glands of the breast, and in the external ear canals—where the secretion is referred to as *cerumen*. In lower forms of animals, the apocrine glands release **pheromones,** hormone-like chemicals that communicate reproductive and social information among the species. For example, dogs and other animals release pheromones during urination to mark their territory. The function of apocrine secretions in humans is unknown, although the onset of secretions coincides with puberty. Some speculate that synchronization of menstruation among women in close living conditions such as a dormitory room is the result of apocrine secretions (Arms, 1997; Morofushi et al., 2000).

In general, perspiration, which includes secretions from both eccrine and apocrine glands, is odorless. An odor develops, however, when perspiration mixes with bacteria on the skin.

Nails

Fingernails and toenails are layers of hard keratin that have a protective function. In primates and humans, the nails may be a biologic diversification of claws. Animal species that have claws use them to catch and tear prey, whereas primates and humans developed nails on their fingers and toes because they had a greater biologic need for grasping limbs and manipulating primitive tools or utensils.

The nail root lies buried beneath the nail's exposed surface in a fold of skin (Fig. 68-3). The nails have an abun-

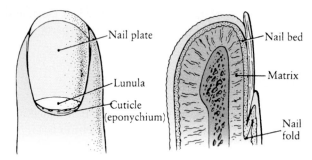

FIGURE 68-3 External and cross-sectional views of a nail.

dant blood supply. Their semitransparent appearance facilitates circulatory assessment.

ASSESSMENT

History

Initial assessment of the client begins with a thorough history. The history is based on symptoms. The nurse includes the following questions:

- When did the disorder first begin and where did it first appear?
- Where are the lesions located?
- Have there been any changes in the disorder since it first appeared (an increase or decrease in symptoms; in appearance or color; in location)?
- Has the problem spread?
- What are the physical sensations pertaining to the disorder (pain, itching, burning, and intensity)?
- Do other physical or emotional problems appear to be associated with the disorder?
- Was a specific event associated with the onset of the disorder?
- What factors appear to make the condition better or worse?
- Do you or anyone in your family have known or suspected allergies?
- What prescription and nonprescription medications have you taken recently?
- Have you made changes in personal products, such as soaps, deodorants, and cosmetics?
- Have there been recent changes in your work or living environment, such as pets, plants, sprays, dust, and pollutants, that might have precipitated this problem?

Physical Examination

During a physical examination, the nurse inspects and palpates the structures of the integument.

Skin Assessment

The nurse examines the skin on all areas of the body. He or she can do so during the head-to-toe assessment or as a focused assessment. Good lighting is essential. The skin should be smooth, unbroken, of uniform color according to the person's ethnic or racial origin, warm, and resilient. It should feel neither wet nor unusually dry.

Color deviations have several possible causes (Table 68-1). While examining the skin, the nurse may detect changes in its structure or integrity such as those listed in Table 68-2. The nurse documents the sites of any abnormalities.

The nurse assesses temperature by placing the dorsum of the hand on the surface of the skin. He or she can detect moisture with the palmar surface. The nurse determines the quality of skin turgor by grasping the skin, such as that over the chest, between the thumb and forefinger. Normally the skin returns to its original position immediately after being released. Tight, shiny skin suggests fluid retention; loose, dry skin may indicate dehydration.

Stop, Think, and Respond ● BOX 68-2

What type of skin lesion does a client have if it is described as follows:

A. *Elevated, round, and filled with serum?*
B. *Flat, round, and red?*
C. *Elevated, solid, with a raised border?*
D. *Elevated, round, raised border, filled with pus?*

Pressure Sore Staging

Pressure sores, also known as *decubitus ulcers,* occur when capillary blood flow to the area is reduced. This may happen when the skin over a bony prominence is

TABLE 68-1	COMMON SKIN COLOR VARIATIONS	
COLOR	**TERM**	**POSSIBLE CAUSES**
Pale, regardless of race	Pallor	Anemia, blood loss
Red	Erythema	Superficial burns, local inflammation, carbon monoxide poisoning
Pink	Flushed	Fever, hypertension
Purple	Ecchymosis	Trauma to soft tissue
Blue	Cyanosis	Low tissue oxygenation
Yellow	Jaundice	Liver or kidney disease, destruction of red blood cells
Brown	Tan	Racial variation, sun exposure, pregnancy, Addison's disease

TABLE 68-2	TERMS FOR VARIOUS SKIN LESIONS		
TYPE OF LESION	**DESCRIPTION**	**EXAMPLES**	**DEPICTION**
Macule	Flat, round, colored	Freckles, rash	Macule
Papule	Elevated, obvious raised border, solid	Wart	Papule
Vesicle	Elevated, round, filled with serum	Blister	Vesicle
Wheal	Elevated, irregular border, no free fluid	Hives	Wheal
Pustule	Elevated, raised border, filled with pus	Boil	Pustule
Nodule	Elevated solid mass, extends into deeper tissue	Enlarged lymph node	Nodule
Cyst	Encapsulated, round, fluid-filled or solid mass beneath the skin	Tissue growth	Cyst

compressed between the weight of the body and a hard surface for a prolonged period. Common locations include the skin over the coccyx and sacrum in the lower spine, the hips, heels, elbows, shoulder blades, ears, and back of head (Fig. 68-4). Prevention of pressure sores first involves identifying persons who are at greatest risk (Box 68-1).

Pressure sores are categorized into one of four stages (Fig. 68-5) depending on the extent of tissue injury.

STAGE I

Stage I pressure sores are characterized by redness of the skin. The reddened skin of a beginning pressure sore fails to resume its normal color, or blanch, when pressure is relieved.

STAGE II

A stage II pressure sore is red and is accompanied by blistering or a shallow break in the skin, sometimes described as a **skin tear.** Impairment of the skin leads to microbial colonization and infection of the wound.

STAGE III

Pressure sores classified as stage III are those in which the superficial skin impairment progresses to a shallow crater that extends to the subcutaneous tissue. Stage III pressure sores may be accompanied by serous drainage from leak-

> **BOX 68-1 ● Risk Factors for Developing Pressure Sores**
>
> - Dehydration
> - Diaphoresis
> - Emaciation
> - Immobility
> - Inactivity
> - Incontinence
> - Localized edema
> - Malnutrition
> - Sedation
> - Vascular disease

ing plasma or purulent drainage (white or yellow-tinged fluid) caused by a wound infection. Although a stage III pressure sore is a significant wound, the area is relatively painless.

STAGE IV

Stage IV pressure sores are the most traumatic and life-threatening. The tissue is deeply ulcerated, exposing muscle and bone (Fig. 68-6). The dead tissue produces a rank odor. Local infection, which is the rule rather than the exception, easily spreads throughout the body, causing a potentially fatal condition referred to as *sepsis.*

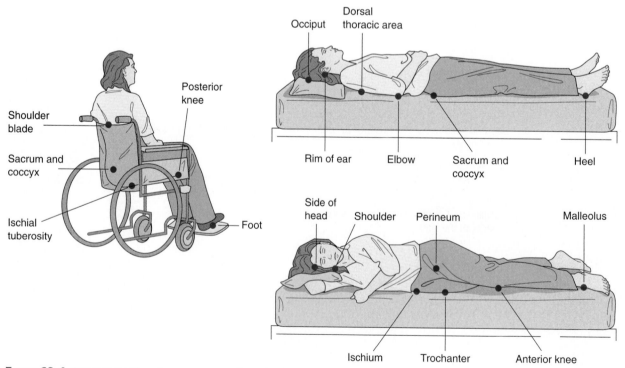

FIGURE 68-4 Common locations for pressure sores in supine, lateral, and sitting positions.

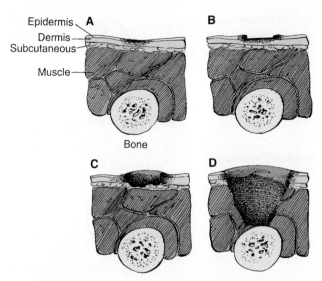

FIGURE 68-5 Pressure sore stages: (**A**) stage I; (**B**) stage II; (**C**) stage III; and (**D**) stage IV.

Once he or she has identified at-risk clients, the nurse implements measures that reduce conditions under which pressure sores are likely to form. Some examples are as follows:

- Turning and repositioning the client frequently
- Keeping client's skin clean and dry
- Massaging bony prominences if the client's skin blanches with pressure relief
- Using a moisturizing skin cleanser rather than soap
- Applying pressure-relieving devices to the bed and chairs
- Padding body areas that are subject to pressure and friction
- Avoiding **shearing,** a physical force that separates layers of tissue in opposite directions, such as when a seated client slides downward

FIGURE 68-6 Example of stage IV pressure sore.

Scalp and Hair Assessment

The nurse assesses the scalp by separating the hair at random areas and inspecting the skin. The scalp normally is smooth, intact, and free of lesions.

Hair assessment not only applies to that which covers the head, but to other locations such as the eyebrows, eyelashes, chest, arms, pubis, and legs. The nurse notes the color, texture, and distribution, keeping sex- and age-related variations in mind. Nits, eggs from a louse infestation, scales, and flaking skin are abnormal findings.

Nail Assessment

Normal nails appear slightly convex with a 160° angle between the nail base and the skin (Fig. 68-7). Concave-shaped nails, referred to as *spooning* because of their characteristic appearance, are a sign of iron deficiency anemia. Clubbing of the nails, evidenced by an angle greater than 160°, suggests long-standing cardiopulmonary disease. Although the thickness of the nail varies from 0.3 to 0.65 mm (Fuller & Schaller-Ayers, 1999), nails thicken when there is a fungal infection and poor circulation. There may be evidence of other nail abnormalities (Fig. 68-8).

The nurse observes the color of the nailbeds. Pink nailbeds suggest adequate oxygenation; however, the nails may be darker in other than Anglo-American clients. To assess tissue perfusion, the nurse compresses the nailbeds, causing them to blanch, and then releases them. Color returns normally in 3 seconds or less. This assessment is called *capillary refill time.*

Diagnostic Tests

The diagnosis of a skin disorder is made chiefly by visual inspection. Some disorders may require additional testing, including the following types:

- Biopsy—performed to identify malignant or premalignant lesions. A biopsy also is of value in helping to identify some skin disorders.

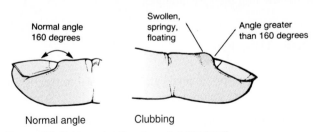

FIGURE 68-7 Normal nail angle and clubbed nail.

Onychorrhexis

- Brittle, fragile, uneven nail edge
- Associated with malnutrition, over-hydration, thyrotoxicosis, chemical damage, radiation, aging

Onychorrhexis

Splinter Hemorrhages

- Blood streaks
- Associated with heart disease, hypertension, rheumatoid arthritis, neoplasms, trauma

Splinter hemorrhage

Onychauxis

- Nail hypertrophy
- Associated with trauma, aging, fungal infections

Onychauxis

Subungual Hematoma

- Blood clot
- Associated with trauma

Subungual hematoma

Beau's Lines

- Tranverse furrows in nail plate
- Associated with malnutrition, severe illness

Beau's lines

FIGURE 68-8 Nail abnormalities.

- Culture and sensitivity tests—performed on lesions that are suspected or known to contain microorganisms.
- Allergy tests—intradermal injection, the scratch test, and the patch test are used to confirm an allergy to one or more substances (see Chap. 41).

MEDICAL AND SURGICAL TREATMENT OF SKIN DISORDERS

Various types of therapies are used in the treatment or management of skin disorders. They include drug therapy, wet dressings, therapeutic baths, surgical excision, radiation therapy, photochemotherapy, hyperbaric oxygenation, and lifestyle changes.

Drug Therapy

Topical and systemic medications are used to treat skin disorders. Some examples are as follows:

- Corticosteroids are applied topically or administered systemically (orally, intramuscularly, intravenously) to relieve inflammatory and allergic symptoms.

When used systemically, corticosteroids can have serious toxic effects; therefore, they are used primarily to relieve acute problems. Continued long-term use brings greater risk and is justified only when the disease itself is serious and other treatments cannot relieve it. Used as directed, topical application of a corticosteroid does not result in the pronounced adverse effects seen with systemic administration, and can be used for longer periods.

- Antihistamines frequently are prescribed when allergy is a factor in causing the skin disorder. They relieve itching and shorten the duration of the allergic reaction.
- Antibiotic, antifungal, and antiviral agents are used to treat infectious disorders. They are applied topically or administered systemically.
- Scabicides and pediculicides are used in the treatment of infestations with the scabies mite and lice.
- Local (topical) anesthetics are applied to relieve minor skin pain and itching.
- Emollients, ointments, powders, and lotions, which may be combined with other agents, soothe, protect, and soften the skin.
- Antiseborrheic agents are applied directly to the scalp or incorporated into shampooing products. They are used to control dandruff.

- Antiseptics are used to reduce bacteria on the skin.
- Keratolytics dissolve thickened, cornified skin such as warts, corns, and calluses. Their action causes the treated area to soften and swell, facilitating removal.

Nurses use Standard Precautions when applying any topical medication to impaired skin or changing dressings that cover an open lesion. Infected, draining, or weeping lesions may require contact precautions as well (see Chap. 19). It is important to apply topical medication as prescribed, such as a thin layer evenly spread over the area, or a thick layer dabbed on the area. The nurse takes care applying medication so that lesions are not broken or skin surfaces abraded.

Wet Dressings

Wet dressings are used to apply a solution to a skin lesion. They have a cooling and soothing effect. The nature of the skin lesion (open or intact) determines whether sterile technique is required. First, a dry dressing consisting of gauze or other porous material is applied to the area. Cotton is not used because of its tendency to stick to wound surfaces. The dressing is then saturated with the prescribed liquid. Dressings can be temporarily anchored with nonallergenic tape or roller gauze.

Some wet dressings are left in place until dry as a method of **debridement,** a technique for removing damaged tissue from a wound. When the dried gauze is removed it usually contains bits of trapped debris in the gauze mesh. Removing dead and dying tissue provides an environment that fosters and promotes regeneration of healthy tissue and closure of the wound.

Therapeutic Baths

A therapeutic bath is one in which various solutions, powders, and oils, but no soap, are added to water into which the client's entire body or only a part is submerged. They are used to relieve inflammation and itching and to aid in the removal of crusts and scales. Examples of products used include corn starch, sodium bicarbonate (baking soda), oatmeal colloid bath preparations, and mineral oil.

The tub or container is filled with lukewarm water. The drug or product is then added and the water stirred so that the preparation mixes thoroughly. A washcloth or a compress is used to apply the solution gently without rubbing the face and any other parts not covered by the solution.

Surgical Excision

When it is necessary to remove a skin lesion, such as a benign or malignant growth, the tissue may be excised conventionally or with a laser, cryosurgery, or electrodesiccation. Surgical excisions are performed under local or general anesthesia.

Laser Therapy

Laser stands for *l*ight *a*mplification by the *s*timulated *e*mission of *r*adiation. Lasers convert a solid, gas, or liquid substance into light. The energy of laser light vaporizes tissue and coagulates bleeding vessels. Lasers also are used to remove tattoos and pigmented skin lesions such as hemangiomas and nevi. When a laser procedure is performed, the eyes must be protected, precautions taken for preventing fires and burns from heated instruments, and vaporized fumes removed.

Cryosurgery

Cryosurgery is the application of extreme cold to destroy tissue. Liquid nitrogen circulates through a probe that is touched to the skin or inserted to the center of the lesion. After application of extreme cold, the area thaws and becomes gelatin-like in appearance. A scab forms at the site. Healing takes approximately 4 to 6 weeks.

Electrodesiccation

Electrodesiccation (or electrosurgery) is the use of electrical energy converted to heat, which destroys the tissue. Plantar warts and skin tumors are examples of disorders treated by this method.

Radiation Therapy

Radiation therapy is used to treat malignant skin lesions. For more information on radiation therapy, see Chapter 20.

Photochemotherapy

Photochemotherapy involves a combination of psoralen methoxsalen and type A ultraviolet light. It is one method used to treat psoriasis, a chronic skin condition (see Chap. 69). The psoralen methoxsalen is taken 1 to 2 hours before exposure to ultraviolet A.

Lifestyle Changes

Some skin disorders grow worse when the person is tired or under emotional stress. Therefore, rest and sleep are an important part of treatment. Diet also is an important part of treatment because certain foods contribute to or aggravate skin disorders in some individuals and therefore must be eliminated from the diet.

GENERAL NUTRITIONAL CONSIDERATIONS

Poor nutrition can lead to changes in skin integrity and turgor.
Nails may soften or develop abnormalities of shape and structure.
Hair may become brittle and thin from poor nutritional status.
Depending on the stage of the pressure sore, protein requirements range from 1 to 1.6 g/kg to promote healing. Calories are increased to spare protein; small, frequent meals help maximize intake. Supplements of vitamins A, C, and zinc may be prescribed. Calorie counts help assess adequacy of intake.

GENERAL PHARMACOLOGIC CONSIDERATIONS

Instruct clients taking antibiotic, antiviral, or antifungal agents to complete the entire prescription, even if the condition clears before he or she finishes all the medication.
As with any medication, drug interactions may occur. If the client is taking medication for another disorder, list all medications the client takes to rule out potential drug interactions.
Suspect a drug allergy whenever the client has a skin rash.

GENERAL GERONTOLOGIC CONSIDERATIONS

Melanin production decreases with aging; older adults develop gray hair.
Facial hair and sometimes chest hair appears in postmenopausal women as a result of decreased production of estrogen.
Loss of skin elasticity and subcutaneous tissue causes wrinkles to form among older adults. Skin in the upper arms becomes fleshy and loose. The eyelids, cheeks, chin, and breasts tend to sag.
The skin becomes dry and flaked as sebum production is reduced.
Small, brown, pigmented, benign lesions, known as *liver spots* or *senile lentigines,* form on the hands and forearms.
Small, yellow or brown, raised lesions called *senile keratoses* appear on the face and trunk. Senile keratoses are precancerous and require close observation by the nurse for any change in size, color, or form. These lesions may be removed by freezing, chemical peel, cauterization, or topical creams.

Critical Thinking Exercise

1. *A client has developed a rash over her arms and thorax. What additional data are important to obtain before contacting the physician?*

References and Suggested Readings

Alora, M. B. T., Dover, J. S., & Arndt, K. A. (1999). Lasers for vascular lesions. *Dermatology Nursing, 11,* 97–102, 105–109.

Andreson, G. P. (1998). As America ages: Assessing the older adult. *RN, 61*(3), 46–56.

Andrychuk, M. A. (1998). Orthopaedic essentials. Pressure ulcers: Causes, risk factors, assessment, and intervention. *Orthopaedic Nursing, 17*(4), 65–83.

Arms, K. (1997). *Biology: A journey into life* (4th ed.). Fort Worth, TX: Harcourt Brace.

Baranoski, S. (2000). Skin tears: Staying on guard against the enemy of frail skin. *Nursing, 30*(9), 41–47.

Fletcher, J. (1998). Wound care: Taking the pressure off. *Nursing Times, 94*(45), 77, 80.

Fuller, J. & Schaller-Ayers, J. (1999). *Health assessment: A nursing approach* (3rd ed.). Philadelphia: Lippincott Williams & Wilkins.

Gordon, K. (1999): Skin care: Itching for a solution . . . atopic eczema. *Nursing Times, 95*(12), 65, 67–68.

Hess, C. T. (1998a). Wound care: Keeping tabs on a pressure ulcer. *Nursing, 28*(1), 18.

Hess, C. T. (1998b). Wound care: Preventing skin breakdown. *Nursing, 28*(7), 28–29.

Hess, C. T. (1998c). Wound care: Treating a stage 3 pressure ulcer. *Nursing, 28*(2), 20.

Kohr, R. (2001). Clinical focus: Wound care. Moist healing versus wet-to-dry. *Canadian Nurse, 97*(1), 17–19.

Kramer, J. D. & Kearney, M. (2000). Patient, wound, and treatment characteristics associated with healing in pressure ulcers. *Advances in Skin and Wound Care, 13*(1), 17–24.

Lawton, S. (2000). Assessing pigmented skin. *Nursing Times, 96*(27), Ntplus: 14.

Lawton, S. (2001). Assessing the patient with a skin condition. *Journal of Tissue Viability, 11,* 113–115.

Lawton, S. (1998). Assessing the skin. *Professional Nurse, 13*(4), Prof Nurse Study: S5–S7, S14.

LeLievre, S. (2000). Skin care for older people with incontinence. *Elderly Care, 11*(10), 36–38.

Makelbust, J. (1999). Preventing pressure ulcers in home care patients. *Home Healthcare Nurse, 17,* 229–238.

Morofushi, M., Shinohara, K., Funabashi, T., et al. (2000). Positive relationship between menstrual synchrony and ability to smell 5alpha-androst-16-en-3alpha-ol (3alpha-androstenol). *Chemical Senses, 25,* 407–411.

Norman, E. M. (1998). Critical questions: Fingernails and microflora. *American Journal of Nursing, 98*(10), Crit Care Extra: 16HH.

Penzer, R. & Finch, M. (2001). Promoting healthy skin in older people. *Nursing Standard, 15*(34), 46–52.

Peters, J. & Watts, J. (1998). Accurate assessment of skin conditions—stop, look and listen. *Practice Nurse, 15,* 525–526, 528–530.

Quick reference guide 7: Dermatological conditions. *Nursing Standard, 13*(46), insert 2p.

Rader, J., Jones, D., & Miller, L. (2000). The importance of individualized wheelchair seating for frail older adults. *Journal of Gerontological Nursing, 26*(11), 24–32.

Twitchen, L. J. & Lowe, A. J. G. (1998). Update. Atopic eczema and wet-wrap dressings. *Professional Nurse, 14,* 113–116.

Whittingham, K. & May, S. (1998). Cleansing regimens for continence care. *Professional Nurse, 14,* 167, 169–172.

Caring for Clients With Skin, Hair, and Nail Disorders

Words to Know

acne vulgaris
alopecia
carbuncle
comedone
dermabrasion
dermatitis
dermatome
dermatophytes
dermatophytoses
erythema
furuncle
furunculosis

herpes zoster
nits
onychocryptosis
onychomycosis
pediculosis
photochemotherapy
podiatrist
pruritus
psoriasis
scabies
shingles

Learning Objectives

On completion of this chapter, the reader will:

- Define and name two types of dermatitis.
- Explain factors that lead to acne vulgaris.
- Differentiate between a furuncle, furunculosis, and carbuncle.
- Describe the appearance and cause of psoriasis.
- List a skin disorder caused by a mite, a fungus, and a virus.
- Discuss factors that promote skin cancer.
- Name two conditions characterized by hair loss, and the etiology for each.
- Describe the appearance of head lice and nits.
- Explain how to remove head lice.
- Discuss factors that promote fungal infections of the nails.
- Name at least three techniques for preventing onychocryptosis (ingrown toenails).

Disorders of the skin, hair, and nails are common. Because self-image is inextricably related to how a person looks, disorders that affect appearance have personal and social consequences. In addition to requiring medical or surgical treatment, clients with disorders of the skin need empathic support while they cope with chronic or acute conditions.

SKIN DISORDERS

● DERMATITIS

Dermatitis is a general term that refers to an inflammation of the skin (Fig. 69-1). It is a common sign of many skin disorders accompanied by a red rash. An associated symptom is **pruritus,** or itching. Dermatitis and pruritus may be localized or generalized. Because both are

nonspecific symptoms, it is essential that the cause be diagnosed and definitively treated. Two common types are allergic and irritant dermatitis.

Pathophysiology and Etiology

Allergic contact dermatitis develops in people who are sensitive to one or more substances, such as drugs, fibers in clothing, cosmetics, plants (e.g., poison ivy), and dyes (Fig. 69-2). Primary irritant dermatitis is a localized reaction that occurs when the skin comes into contact with a strong chemical such as a solvent or detergent.

In clients with allergies, sensitized mast cells in the skin release histamine, causing a red rash, itching, and localized swelling (see Chap. 42). An allergy, however, does not cause irritant dermatitis. Rather, the caustic quality of the substance damages the protein structure of the skin or eliminates secretions that protect it.

FIGURE 69-1 Contact dermatitis of the (**A**) face and (**B**) wrist.

Assessment Findings

The skin response is characterized by dilation of the blood vessels, causing redness and swelling, and sometimes by *vesiculation* (blister formation) and oozing. Itching is a prominent symptom. Primary irritant dermatitis may cause soreness or discomfort from irritation, itching, redness, swelling, and vesiculation.

Diagnosis is made by visual examination of the area. A detailed and thorough history helps to identify the offend-ing substances as well as the type of dermatitis. In difficult cases, a skin patch test may identify an allergic substance.

Medical Management

Treatment of both types of dermatitis is to remove the substances causing the reaction. This is done by flushing the skin with cool water. Topical lotions, such as calamine, or systemic drugs, such as diphenhydramine (Benadryl) or cyproheptadine (Periactin), are prescribed to relieve itching. Moisturizing creams with lanolin restore lubrication. In more severe cases, wet dressings with astringent solutions, such as Burow's solution (aluminum acetate), are prescribed. Corticosteroids taken orally or applied topically also provide relief.

Nursing Management

The nurse advises clients to wear rubber gloves when coming in contact with any substance such as soap or solvents, put all clothes through a second rinse cycle when laundering to remove soap residue, and avoid the use of cosmetics or any topical drug or substance until the etiology of the dermatitis is identified. Measures that reduce itching or preserve the integrity of the skin include the following:

- Keep nails short and clean.
- Use light cotton bedding and clothing that allow normal evaporation of moisture from the skin (avoid wool, synthetics, and other dense fibers).
- Wear white cotton gloves if prone to scratching during sleep.
- Avoid regular soap for bathing; hypoallergenic or glycerin soaps can be used without causing skin irritation or itching.
- Use tepid bath water; pat rather than rub the skin dry.
- Inform the physician if the drug therapy fails to restore skin integrity or relieve itching.

● ACNE VULGARIS

Acne vulgaris, which tends to coincide with puberty, is an inflammatory disorder that affects the sebaceous glands and hair follicles. The severity of the condition varies from minimal to severe.

Pathophysiology and Etiology

Acne is believed to be related to the hormonal changes that occur when secondary sex characteristics are developing. It is aggravated by cosmetics as well as picking and squeezing blemishes that form. Any correlation with specific food items (e.g., chocolate) is more myth than fact.

FIGURE 69-2 Contact dermatitis from shoe material. (Glaxo-Wellcome Co.)

Sebum, keratin, and bacteria accumulate and dilate the follicle. The collective secretions form a **comedone,** or what most refer to as a *blackhead* (Fig. 69-3). The dark appearance is the result of oxidation of the core material. The follicle becomes further distended and irritated, causing a raised papule in the skin. If the follicular wall ruptures, the inflammatory response extends into the marginal areas of dermis. In serious cases, inflamed nodules and cysts develop. Severe acne, if neglected, leads to deep, pitted scars that leave the skin permanently pockmarked. Acne vulgaris improves after adolescence.

Assessment Findings

Comedones and pustules appear on the face, chest, and back, where the skin is excessively oily (Fig. 69-4). Oiliness of the scalp often accompanies acne. Diagnosis is made by visual examination of the affected areas.

Medical Management

Mild cases of acne improve with gentle facial cleansing and nonprescription drying agents containing benzoyl peroxide. Drug therapy includes the topical application of

FIGURE 69-4 Acne of (**A**) the face and (**B**) the chest.

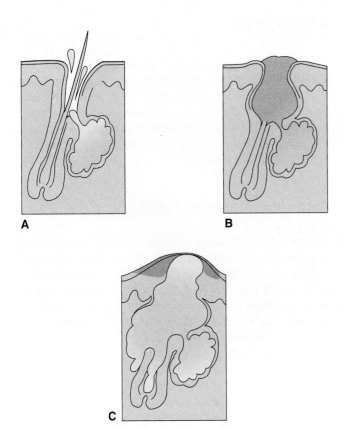

FIGURE 69-3 Acne vulgaris. (**A**) Normal sebaceous gland and hair follicle. (**B**) Comedone formation. (**C**) Pustule formation.

tretinoin (Retin-A) or oral administration of isotretinoin (Accutane). Topical and systemic antibiotics such as tetracycline and erythromycin, in low doses, also are used for severe acne and have produced good results. The comedones can be removed and the pustules drained with special instruments.

Surgical Management

Dermabrasion is a method of removing surface layers of scarred skin. It is useful in lessening scars such as the pitting from severe acne. The outermost layers of the skin are removed by sandpaper, a rotating wire brush, chemicals (chemical face peeling), or a diamond wheel. A local anesthetic, such as an ethyl chloride and Freon mixture, is used during the procedure. Afterward, the skin looks and feels raw and sore, and some crusting from serous exudate occurs. Clients frequently say that the discomfort is much like that from a burn. The client is instructed not to wash the area until it has healed sufficiently. The client also must avoid picking and touching the area because this contact might cause infection or produce marking of the tissues.

Nursing Management

The nurse advises the client to keep the face and hair clean and avoid cosmetics that contribute to oily skin. He or she explains that, above all else, manipulating the lesions worsens the condition. For female clients, the nurse warns about the risk of birth defects associated with oral isotretinoin. He or she explains that women for whom this drug is prescribed must (1) have a negative pregnancy test 2 weeks before beginning therapy, (2) comply with contraceptive measures while taking the drug, and (3) continue reliable contraception for 1 month after discontinuing therapy.

Teaching measures include the following:

- Keep the hair short, clean, and away from the face and forehead.
- Wash the hair frequently; daily shampooing does not damage hair.
- Avoid makeup, lotions, hair sprays, and skin care products unless a physician approves their use.

● FURUNCLES, FURUNCULOSIS, AND CARBUNCLES

A **furuncle** is a boil. **Furunculosis** refers to having multiple furuncles. A **carbuncle** is a furuncle from which pus drains.

Physiology and Etiology

The cause of furuncles and carbuncles is skin infections with organisms that usually exist harmlessly on the skin surface. When an injury such as that caused by squeezing a lesion impairs the integrity of the skin, microorganisms can enter and colonize in the skin. Furunculosis also is associated with diabetes mellitus because an elevated blood glucose level promotes microbial growth. Other factors that predispose to these conditions include poor diet and general health and any disorder that lowers resistance.

Assessment Findings

The lesion, which may appear anywhere on the body, but especially around the neck, axillary, and groin regions, appears as a raised, painful pustule surrounded by erythema. The area feels hard to the touch. After a few days, the lesion exudes pus and later a core. The client also may experience a fever, anorexia, weakness, and malaise. A culture of the exudate identifies the infectious organism.

Medical and Surgical Management

Hot wet soaks are used to localize the infection and provide symptomatic relief. It may be the only treatment necessary. Antibiotics are used in some instances, especially when a fever is present or if the lesion is a carbuncle. Surgical incision and drainage may be necessary.

Nursing Management

The nurse follows strict aseptic technique when applying or changing a dressing to prevent the spread of the infection to other parts of the body or to others. He or she teaches the client also to do so. The nurse informs the client to:

- Never pick or squeeze a furuncle—drainage is infectious, and this practice favors spread of the infection to surrounding tissues or even to the bloodstream.
- Wash hands thoroughly before and after applying topical medications.
- Keep hands away from infected areas.
- Use separate face cloths and towels from those used by others.
- Wash clothing, towels, and face cloths separately from family laundry in hot water and bleach.

● PSORIASIS

Psoriasis is a chronic, noninfectious inflammatory disorder of the skin that affects both men and women. Its onset is in young and middle adulthood. Although there are many types of psoriasis, the most common is plaque psoriasis (Fig. 69-5). Periods of emotional stress, hormonal cycles, infection, and seasonal changes appear to aggravate the condition.

Pathophysiology and Etiology

The cause of psoriasis is unknown, but a genetic predisposition is likely because many report a family history of the disorder. Although the predisposition exists, the disorder seems to require a triggering mechanism such as systemic infection, injury to the skin, vaccination, or injection. This also suggests a link with the immune system. That the disorder has periods of exacerbation and remission strengthens this hypothesis.

In psoriasis, skin cells called *keratinocytes* behave as if there is a need to repair a wound. The cells of the epidermis proliferate faster than normal—so fast, in fact, that the upper layer of cells cannot be shed fast enough to make room for the newly produced cells. The excessive cells accumulate and form elevated, scaly lesions

FIGURE 69-5 Psoriasis on the elbows. (Roche Laboratories)

called *plaque.* The area around the lesion becomes red from the increased blood supply needed to nourish the rapidly developing skin cells.

Assessment Findings

Psoriasis is characterized by patches of **erythema** (redness) covered with silvery scales, usually on the extensor surfaces of the elbows, knees, trunk, and scalp. Itching usually is absent or slight, but occasionally it is severe. The lesions are obvious and unsightly, and the scales tend to shed.

Diagnosis is made by visual examination of the lesions. A skin biopsy reveals increased proliferation of epidermal cells.

Medical Management

Psoriasis has no cure. Symptomatic treatment to control the scaling and itching includes the use of topical agents such as coal tar extract, corticosteroids, or anthralin. Anthralin, a distillate of crude coal tar, is applied to thick plaques; it tends to irritate unaffected skin areas. Topical corticosteroids have proved beneficial. Methotrexate, an antimetabolite used in the treatment of cancer, is prescribed for clients with severe disease that does not respond to other forms of therapy. This drug inhibits the production of cells that divide rapidly (cancer cells, cells composing the skin and mucous membranes) and is capable of reducing plaque formation. Dosage is carefully individualized because the drug causes serious adverse effects.

Etretinate (Tegison) is related to retinoic acid and retinol (vitamin A) and is used to treat psoriasis that does not respond to other therapies. Its use is recommended only for those who can reliably understand and carry out the treatment regimen, are capable of complying with mandatory contraceptive measures, and do not intend to become pregnant. Another method of treatment is the injection of triamcinolone acetonide (Kenacort), a corticosteroid, into isolated psoriatic plaques. This method of treatment is successful in some cases.

Photochemotherapy, a combination of ultraviolet light therapy and a photosensitizing psoralen drug such as methoxsalen (Oxsoralen-Ultra), also has been used for severe, disabling psoriasis that does not respond to other methods of treatment. The extent of exposure is based on the client's skin tolerance. Treatments are given once every other day or less because phototoxic reactions may appear 48 hours or more after light exposure. Once the psoriasis clears, the client is placed on a maintenance treatment program.

Some clients respond well to treatment; others receive only minor relief. The condition tends to recur.

NURSING PROCESS

● **The Client With Psoriasis**

Assessment

The nurse inspects and evaluates the integrity of the skin in a well-lit environment. He or she compares the pathologic appearance of the affected skin with the characteristics of normal skin. The nurse elicits from the client whether there is a family history of psoriasis and determines the onset, duration, and possible triggering factors.

Diagnosis, Planning, and Interventions

The nurse shows acceptance of clients with skin lesions, who need a great deal of understanding and emotional support. He or she explains that treatment usually is for a lifetime, and that the client must follow the plan of therapy. The nurse reassures clients for whom more than one form of treatment has failed that other, untried modalities may offer improved control of symptoms. The nurse instructs the client receiving photochemotherapy to avoid exposure to sunlight for 8 hours after treatment because it takes that long for the body to excrete methoxsalen. Diagnoses, outcomes, and interventions for clients with psoriasis include, but are not limited to, the following.

Impaired Skin Integrity related to decreased protective function of epidermal tissue
Expected Outcome: Client will achieve smoother skin with control of lesions and increased protective skin function.

- Instruct client that repeated trauma to the skin (cuts, abrasions, sunburn) may exacerbate psoriasis. *Giving facts provides a means by which the client can help manage the disorder.*
- Advise client not to pick or scratch lesions. *Disruption of the lesions causes secondary skin trauma.*
- Inspect skin regularly for signs of infection. *Impaired skin integrity provides a portal through which pathogens can enter.*
- Wash affected area with warm water and pat dry. Apply moisturizing or medicated topical ointments as ordered. *Clean, moisturized skin that is not irritated by friction during drying helps maintain skin integrity.*

Disturbed Body Image related to embarrassment of appearance of skin and self-perception of uncleanliness
Expected Outcome: Client will acquire self-acceptance regarding skin changes.

- Inform client that psoriasis has no permanent cure, but the condition usually can be controlled or cleared. *The reality of the prognosis facilitates the development of mechanisms for coping with the skin disorder.*
- Assist client to carry out cosmetic efforts to decrease visibility of lesions. *Camouflaging the skin lesions reduces self-consciousness.*
- Encourage client to join a psoriasis support group. *A support group helps the client understand that many others have the same disorder and similar problems. Group work better facilitates coping than does working alone.*

Evaluation of Expected Outcomes

Expected outcomes are improved integrity and appearance of the skin. Itching is reduced or eliminated. The client understands clearly what the diagnosis of psoriasis means in terms of duration and length of treatment. He or she copes effectively with the altered appearance.

● SCABIES

Scabies is a fairly common infectious skin disease.

Pathophysiology and Etiology

Scabies is caused by infestation with the itch mite (*Sarcoptes scabiei*). Anyone can acquire scabies; it is erroneous to assume that infected people have poor personal hygiene. Outbreaks are common where large groups of people are confined such as nursing homes, military barracks, prisons, boarding schools, and child care centers.

The mites are spread by skin-to-skin contact. In rare cases, scabies is acquired from handling clothing and linen in recent contact with an infected person. Scabies mites do not survive off the body more than 2 days.

Assessment Findings

Signs and Symptoms

Itching is intense, especially at night. Commonly affected areas include the webs and sides of fingers and around the wrists, elbows, armpits, waist, thighs, genitalia, nipples, breasts, and lower buttocks. Excoriation from scratching accompanies the itching. Skin burrows are caused by the female itch mite, which invades the skin to lay her eggs.

Diagnostic Findings

Diagnosis is made by examining the affected areas. Providers, however, often confuse scabies with other skin conditions. Therefore, the American Academy of Dermatology recommends an examination using mineral oil or ink. After dropping sterile mineral oil on the lesion, the skin is scraped onto a slide and examined microscopically to detect the mites, their eggs, or feces. The ink test is performed by applying a blue or black felt-tipped pen to the lesion, which highlights the burrows when the skin surface is wiped.

Medical Management

Scabicides, chemicals that destroy mites, such as lindane (cream or lotion), permethrin cream, and crotamiton cream or lotion, are prescribed. The medication is applied to the skin from the neck down in a thin layer, left on for 8 to 12 hours, and then removed by washing.

Thorough bathing, clean clothing, and the avoidance of contact with others who have scabies are essential in preventing recurrence.

Nursing Management

Before any treatment begins, the nurse advises the client to bathe thoroughly. The nurse then reviews the directions for applying the scabicide medication included with the product. He or she emphasizes the importance of following the directions for complete eradication of the scabies mite. After bathing and applying the medication, the nurse instructs the client to don clean clothing and launder preworn clothing, towels, and bed linen in hot water as soon as possible. He or she tells the client to vacuum furniture and other unwashable items. Last, the nurse explains that itching may continue for 2 to 3 weeks after treatment.

● DERMATOPHYTOSES

Dermatophytoses (tinea) are superficial fungal infections; they have been given many unscientific names. For example, a common term for one dermatophytosis is *ringworm,* which is a misnomer because a worm does not cause the infection. Other examples are *athlete's foot* for a foot infection and *jock itch* for an infection in the groin.

Pathophysiology and Etiology

Dermatophytes (also called *tinea*) are parasitic fungi that invade the skin, scalp, and nails (discussed later). The terms *tinea pedis, tinea capitis, tinea corporis,* and *tinea cruris* identify the skin areas of infection, namely, feet, head, body, and groin, respectively.

Assessment Findings

Tinea corporis appears as rings of papules or vesicles with a clear center in nonhairy areas of the skin (Fig. 69-6). Several clusters of rings may be found in the same general location. The affected skin often itches and becomes red, scaly, cracked, and sore. In tinea pedis, the infection begins in the skin between the toes and spreads to the soles of the feet. Tinea capitis, which is more common in children, invades the hair shaft below the scalp, followed by breaking of the hair, usually close to the scalp.

Diagnosis is made by visual examination of the affected areas. The lesions are scraped and examined microscopically. When a Wood's light is used, the affected areas fluoresce a green-yellow color.

FIGURE 69-6 Tinea corporis of the face, which is commonly referred to as ringworm because of its circular appearance.

Medical Management

Treatment of tinea pedis includes the topical use of antifungal agents, such as benzoic and salicylic acid ointment (Whitfield's ointment), Burow's solution, undecylenic acid, and tolnaftate (Tinactin). Oral griseofulvin (Grisactin), a systemic antifungal agent, also is useful in treatment. The drug may be required for many weeks to eradicate the infection. Tinea capitis may be treated with oral griseofulvin, which is taken with meals. A topical antifungal agent also may be prescribed to destroy fungi present on the hair shafts above the surface of the scalp. Treatment of tinea corporis includes the use of topical antifungal agents for less severe infections. Oral griseofulvin is prescribed for more severe infections. Tinea cruris often responds to topical application of tolnaftate or miconazole (Micatin). Tinea onychomycosis (discussed later) may respond to oral griseofulvin, but long-term therapy usually is necessary.

Nursing Management

If an oral or topical antifungal agent is prescribed, the nurse reviews the directions for use. He or she explains that the infected person must use separate towels, washcloths, grooming articles, and clothing because the disorder is contagious. The nurse stresses that keeping the affected areas dry reduces the spread of the infection. After a bath or shower, the nurse recommends thoroughly drying all areas of the body, including the skin folds. To prevent infection and reinfection of tinea cruris, the nurse suggests avoiding excessive heat and humidity, not wearing tight-fitting clothing or nylon next to the skin (in hot, humid weather), and keeping the skin as dry as possible.

To avoid acquiring or spreading a fungal infection of the feet, the nurse advises against sharing towels and slippers or going barefoot in locker rooms or community bathrooms. He or she recommends keeping the feet (particularly the area between the toes) dry, which increases resistance to the infection. For clients whose feet perspire freely, the nurse advises to apply powder between the toes, keep the area dry, wash and thoroughly dry the feet daily, and put on clean, dry socks and a different pair of shoes after coming home from work or school.

● SHINGLES

Shingles, also known as **herpes zoster,** is a skin disorder that develops years after an infection with varicella (chickenpox). It is more frequent in middle-aged to older adults, as well as in those who are immunocompromised.

Pathophysiology and Etiology

Herpes zoster is an acute reactivation of the varicella-zoster virus, which lies dormant in nerve roots. When aging, cancer, drugs, or acquired immunodeficiency syndrome suppresses a client's immune system, the virus migrates along one or more cranial or spinal nerve routes. Viral reactivation produces inflammatory symp-

toms in the **dermatome,** a skin area supplied by the nerve (Fig. 69-7). Raised, fluid-filled, and painful skin eruptions accompany the inflammation.

If herpes zoster affects the ophthalmic branch of the trigeminal nerve (third cranial nerve), corneal (eye) ulcerations may occur. Involvement of the vestibulocochlear nerve (eighth cranial nerve) can lead to vertigo and permanent hearing loss. Cerebral vasculitis (inflammation of cerebral vessels) is the most serious complication because involvement of the internal carotid arteries can result in a stroke. Rarely, the virus spreads to the brain, resulting in encephalitis.

Susceptible individuals who are exposed to someone in the early stages of herpes zoster infection can acquire varicella. The virus is contagious until the crusts from ruptured lesions have dried and fallen off the skin. Herpes zoster infection also can recur.

Assessment Findings

Initial symptoms include a low-grade fever, headache, and malaise. An area of skin along a dermatome develops a red, blotchy appearance that begins to itch or feel

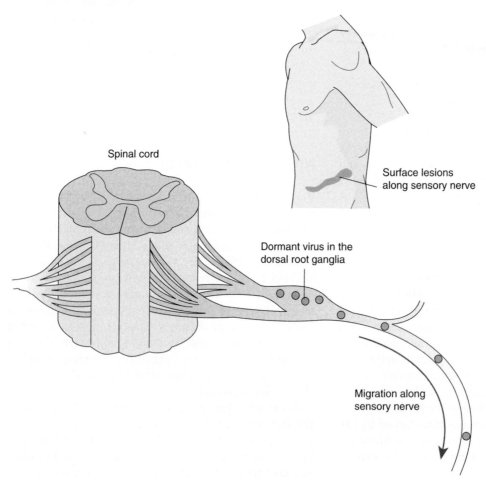

Spinal cord

Surface lesions along sensory nerve

Dormant virus in the dorsal root ganglia

Migration along sensory nerve

FIGURE 69-7 Reactivation of the varicella-zoster virus causing eruptions typical of shingles.

numb. In about 24 to 48 hours, vesicles appear on the skin along the nerve's pathway. Usually the eruptions are unilateral (one side) on the trunk, neck, or head. They become severely painful. Severe itching soon follows. Like chickenpox lesions, the vesicles rupture in a few days and crusts form. Scarring or permanent skin discoloration is possible. Pain (postherpetic neuralgia) and itching may persist for months or as long as 2 years or more. Secondary skin infections may occur from scratching the area.

Diagnosis is made primarily by examination of the lesions and symptoms.

Medical Management

Oral acyclovir (Zovirax), when taken within 48 hours of the appearance of symptoms, reduces their severity and prevents the development of additional lesions. Topical acyclovir also may be applied to the lesions. A brief course of corticosteroid therapy reduces pain. Lesions of the ophthalmic division of the trigeminal nerve require immediate examination and treatment by an ophthalmologist.

Additional treatment is symptomatic. Analgesics and liquid preparations with a drying or antipruritic effect are applied to the affected area once the crusts have fallen off. The skin may be so sensitive that any clothing or application of topical drugs intensifies pain or itching. A narcotic analgesic such as codeine often is necessary during the first few days to weeks.

Nursing Management

The nurse reassigns nursing personnel who have not had chickenpox to avoid contact with a client with herpes zoster. The nurse instructs clients with crusted lesions to avoid contact with immunocompromised people and those who have not had chickenpox. He or she advises the client that application of cool or warm compresses or warm showers may relieve pain and itching; it may be necessary to experiment with both to determine which provides the most relief. The nurse advises the client to wear loose clothing and avoid scratching the area. If oral acyclovir is prescribed, the nurse reviews the dose regimen, as printed on the prescription label.

● SKIN CANCER

Skin cancer is the most common type of cancer in the United States. It can involve any one of three types of cells in the epidermis: squamous cells that are flat and scaly; basal cells that are round; and melanocytes, cells that contain color pigment. One of every seven Americans acquires some form of skin cancer each year.

Pathophysiology and Etiology

Increased exposure to ultraviolet (UV) radiation, especially UVB and UVC, harmful components in the spectrum of sunlight, predisposes to malignant skin changes and other health risks, including cataracts and premature aging of the skin. Fair-skinned people are more susceptible to skin cancer than are dark-skinned people.

Several factors predispose to malignant changes in the skin:

- Thinning layer of ozone, a naturally occurring gas in the earth's atmosphere. Ozone absorbs UVB and UVC radiation (Fig. 69-8). Ozone depletion occurs primarily from the release of chlorofluorocarbons (CFCs) in refrigerants, aerosol propellants, and other industrial pollutants.
- Residence in high-altitude areas where the atmosphere is thinner than at sea level or in areas with a regular cloud cover
- Decreased melanin in skin, especially individuals who sunburn easily and tan minimally; black- or brown-skinned people rarely are affected (Porth, 2002).
- Prolonged, repeated exposure to UV rays such as those who do farming, fishing, road construction,

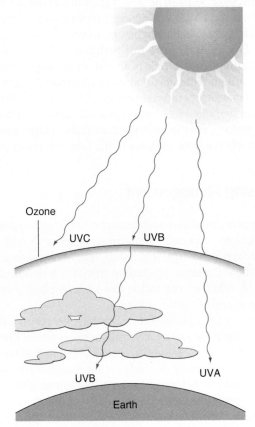

FIGURE 69-8 A layer of ozone shields or reduces the harmful spectrum of ultraviolet wavelengths known as UVC and UVB.

and so on, or those who frequent tanning salons and use sunlamps

- Prior radiation therapy for an unrelated form of cancer
- Ulcerations of long duration and scar tissue (both prone to malignant changes)

Malignant growths of the skin (Table 69-1) usually are primary lesions, that is, they originate in the skin. Prompt removal of the malignant tissue prevents its spread to other parts of the body or tissues.

Assessment Findings

Symptoms vary, but usually the new appearance of a growth or a change in color of the skin is the first symptom the client notices. The lesion can be smooth or rough, flat or elevated, and itchy or tender. It may bleed. Diagnosis is made by visual inspection and confirmed by biopsy.

Medical and Surgical Management

Depending on the size and the location of the lesion, treatment of squamous cell and basal cell carcinomas may involve electrodesiccation, surgical excision, cryosurgery, or radiation therapy. The client is followed regularly for at least 3 to 5 years to be sure regrowth has not occurred.

The treatment of melanoma involves radical excision of the tumor and adjacent tissues, followed by chemotherapy. The administration of melphalan (Alkeran) and prednisone is an example of an initial antineoplastic therapy regimen. Interferon alfa-n3 (Alferon N) has controlled metastases in some persons. Clinical trials of other types of therapies are being conducted. In some instances, skin grafting may be necessary to replace large areas of defect when a wide excision of the tumor is necessary.

Nursing Management

The nurse examines and measures abnormal-appearing skin lesions, especially those in sun-exposed areas such as the face, nose, lips, and hands. The nurse determines facts about the lesion, including when the lesion first was noticed, whether the lesion has undergone any recent changes, and, if so, what kind.

Surgery for a malignant melanoma may involve structures of the head and neck, trunk, or extremities. The specific nursing management of those having radical surgery for this malignancy depends on the original site of the tumor and the extent of surgery. The nurse gives emotional support to those having disfiguring surgery.

The nurse encourages all those with any type of skin change to seek medical attention. He or she advises those in high-risk groups for malignant skin lesions to exam-

ine all areas of their body and scalp for new lesions or changes in moles, other growths, or pigmented lesions. If a client notes any change, he or she should make an appointment for a medical examination as soon as possible.

The nurse educates clients about measures to prevent skin cancer, some of which include the following:

- Always use a sunscreen with a sun protection factor (SPF) of at least 15; higher SPFs are beneficial for clients who sunburn easily.
- Reapply sunscreen at least every 2 hours or more often if swimming or perspiring.
- Use a lip balm with sunscreen.
- Wear a hat with a wide brim and cover the back of the neck.
- Stay in the shade when outdoors.
- Wear tightly woven, but loose-fitting clothing.
- Avoid prolonged sun exposure between 10:00 AM and 4:00 PM.
- Avoid artificial tanning.

The nurse recommends that at-risk clients consult the UV Forecast, a daily report that rates the UV conditions from 0 to 10+ in 30 metropolitan areas. The U.S. Environmental Protection Agency releases the forecast, which radio and television stations broadcast during weather reports as a public service. Depending on the numerical rating, called the UV Index, sun-sensitive people are advised to take protective measures (Fig. 69-9). A sensometer, a credit card–sized device, also is available for a person to determine the UV level in his or her immediate locale.

SCALP AND HAIR DISORDERS

Some conditions are unique to the scalp and hair. They include inflammatory and noninflammatory scalp conditions and disorders that cause hair loss.

● SEBORRHEA, SEBORRHEIC DERMATITIS, AND DANDRUFF

Seborrhea and dandruff are noninflammatory conditions that usually precede or accompany seborrheic dermatitis. Seborrheic dermatitis has an inflammatory component.

Pathophysiology and Etiology

Seborrhea is a dermatologic condition associated with excessive production of secretions from the sebaceous glands. Although seborrhea is not always confined to the scalp, it is one of the primary sites. *Seborrheic dermatitis* presents as red areas covered by yellowish, greasy-appearing scales. *Dandruff,* on the other hand, is loose, scaly material of dead, keratinized epithelium shed from

TABLE 69-1		TYPES OF SKIN CANCER			
TYPE	**INCIDENCE**	**LOCATION**	**APPEARANCE**		**CHARACTERISTICS**
Basal cell carcinoma	Most common, especially in light-skinned individuals Increases with age	Sun-exposed areas	Small, shiny, gray or yellowish plaque that undergoes central ulceration		Slow growing, rarely metastasizes; commonly recurs
Squamous cell carcinoma	Second after basal cell in those with fair skin	Sun-exposed areas such as ears, nose, hands, scalp of bald persons	Scaly, elevated lesion with an irregular border; shallow, large ulcerations form in untreated advanced lesions		Can metastasize through blood and lymph
Malignant melanoma	Increasing in incidence	Arises from pre-existing moles anywhere on the body	Raised brown or black lesion In some cases, satellite lesions occur adjacent to the primary cancer		Poor prognosis because of distant metastases

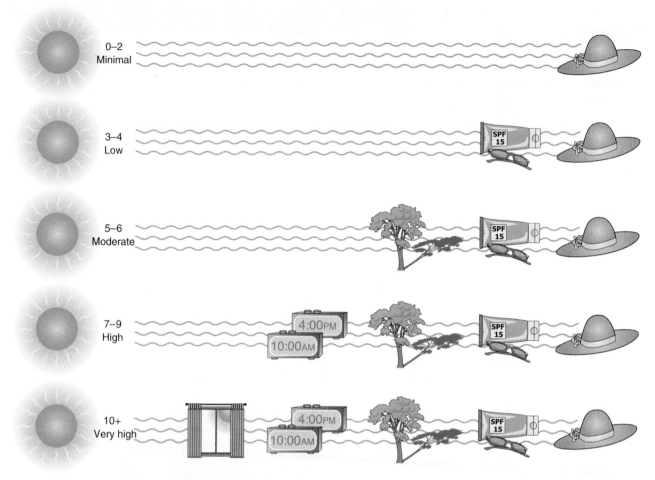

FIGURE 69-9 Sun protection measures based upon the UV index.

the scalp in clients who may or may not have seborrheic dermatitis. Dermatologists believe that a tiny fungus known as *Pityrosporum ovale* causes dandruff. Most people harbor this fungus, yet only some people develop dandruff. Some possible factors for this phenomenon include excessive perspiration, inadequate diet, stress, and hormone activity.

Scalp conditions cause more of a cosmetic rather than a health problem. They usually necessitate retreatment. They do not progress or transform into other serious skin disorders.

Assessment Findings

Clients note that the hair is unusually oily. There may be red or scaly patches on the scalp. White flakes fall from the hair and become more obvious when they collect on the shoulders of dark clothing. The inflamed areas may itch.

No diagnostic testing is necessary unless the condition does not respond to treatment. In that case, a skin biopsy or laboratory blood work is performed to eliminate the possibility that the condition was misdiagnosed.

Medical Management

Frequent shampooing with or without a medicated product helps to reduce oil in the scalp and hair. Effective medicated shampoos contain tar, zinc pyrithione, selenium sulfide, sulfur, or salicylic acid. Some clients require topical applications of corticosteroids.

Nursing Management

The nurse explains the underlying cause. He or she reviews the directions and frequency for using medications. The nurse inform clients that the disorder may recur and that persistent treatment is necessary to control the condition.

● ALOPECIA

Alopecia means "baldness." The condition affects the hair follicles and results in partial or total hair loss. It is normal to shed 50 to 100 hairs a day, which are replaced by new ones from the same hair follicles. In some cases, however, hair loss is excessive, which may be temporary or permanent.

Alopecia is not life-threatening; however, whenever men or women lose their hair, most experience self-consciousness and lose self-confidence. Many spend great sums of money on unscientific methods for restoring hair growth. Although not everyone can be helped, several options are available to clients with hair loss.

Pathophysiology and Etiology

Hair loss can develop for several reasons. In cases of temporary hair loss, possible causes include medications such as antineoplastic drugs, inadequate diet, thyroid disease, tinea infection, improper application of hair care products, and hair styles that pull the hair tightly.

Alopecia areata and androgenetic alopecia are two chronic conditions that are difficult to reverse. Alopecia areata is believed to be an autoimmune disorder characterized by patchy areas of hair loss about the size of a coin. It can progress to total hair loss and even loss of hair from the entire body. Antibodies attack and destroy the hair follicle.

Androgenetic alopecia is a genetically acquired condition; many refer to it as *male pattern baldness.* The term is somewhat inaccurate because it also affects women, although to a milder degree. A person inherits androgenetic alopecia from his or her mother or father. When testosterone, an androgenic hormone, combines with an enzyme, 5-alpha-reductase, in the hair follicle, hair production stops. This condition begins in adolescence or early adulthood and progresses with age.

Assessment Findings

Clients note that their hair is thinning or falling out in patches in several areas of the scalp. Those with a family history of baldness tend to lose hair in the lateral frontal areas or over the vertex of the head (Fig. 69-10). Women report thinning in the frontal, parietal, and crown re-

gions. Primary hair loss is not associated with any other physical health problems.

Diagnostic tests are performed to determine any physical disorder that is contributing to the hair loss. When results are negative, the family history and pattern of hair loss suggest hereditary baldness or an autoimmune disorder.

Medical Management

If a medical disorder causes hair loss, relieving the cause usually restores hair growth. Some drugs can retard hair loss and promote hair growth. One drug is minoxidil (Rogaine); however, the hair growth that is stimulated has a downy texture. If a client discontinues minoxidil, hair growth stops and baldness recurs. Young clients who begin drug therapy when hair loss is minimal obtain the best results. A hair addition is a technique for giving the appearance of more hair by attaching extra hair to the client's natural hair.

Surgical Management

Some balding clients prefer a more permanent solution with hair replacement surgery or other surgical techniques. Hair grafting is a technique for transplanting hair-bearing scalp from the back and sides of the head into bald areas. Each graft contains from one to eight hairs. A bald area that is approximately 3 inches square requires approximately 500 to 600 hair grafts. Unfortunately, because of the progressive nature of androgenetic alopecia, transplanted hairs may not survive permanently.

A procedure that disguises hair loss is a scalp reduction that surgically removes a bald area. A scalp reduction usually is performed along with hair grafts. Another surgical technique is to transfer a skin flap. The flap transfers the greatest amount of hair in a short amount of time. However, the scalp may have to be expanded before surgery to stretch the flap area because the flap remains attached in its original location at one end.

FIGURE 69-10 Patterns of hair loss. (**A** and **B**) Alopecia areata; (**C** and **D**) androgenetic alopecia. **A**   **B**   **C**   **D**

Nursing Management

The nurse supports clients who may not have the financial means for medical or surgical treatment. He or she reassures them that they can cope with hair loss. The nurse suggests consulting a cosmetologist who can provide a haircut and style that minimizes the appearance of hair loss. He or she tells women to opt for loose styling rather than ponytails or braids. The nurse recommends using a conditioner or detangler after shampooing to avoid pulling hair from the head and a wide-toothed comb or brush with smooth tips.

● HEAD LICE

An infestation with lice is called **pediculosis.** Although lice can infest any hairy parts of the body such as the pubic area, they are more likely to be found on and in the hair on the head.

Pathophysiology and Etiology

Lice are crawling brown insects about the size of sesame seeds; they do not fly or jump (Fig. 69-11). Nymphs look like moving dandruff, but they may appear red after feeding. Adult lice and nymphs creep over the skin and feed on human blood. The bites result in itching. Eggs, or **nits,** laid by adult females, are tightly cemented to the side of hair shafts. They appear like small, yellowish-white ovals. Nits hatch in 7 to 10 days. Lice have a life span of approximately 30 days, during which time one female can lay 100 to 400 nits. Researchers believe that lice are developing strains that resist chemical extermination.

Lice are transmitted through direct contact. They cannot survive longer than about 24 hours without blood.

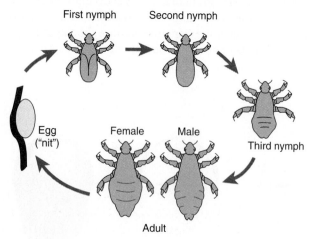

First nymph   Second nymph

Third nymph

Egg ("nit")   Female   Male

Adult

FIGURE 69-11 The life cycle of head lice.

Sharing clothing, combs, and brushes promotes transmission. Anyone can acquire lice, but infestations among school children tend to be difficult to arrest. Many schools have a "zero tolerance" policy for lice infestation; that is, they bar an infected child from attending school until the hair and scalp are free of lice and nits.

Assessment Findings

Itching of the scalp is the most common complaint. Intense scratching can lead to a secondary infection. The adult forms of lice are difficult to see because they quickly move away from light. The nits cling to hairs close to $\frac{1}{20}$ to $\frac{1}{4}$ inch from the scalp.

Diagnosis is made by scalp and hair inspection. Live lice are retrieved with tweezers or the adhesive side of tape.

Medical Management

Nonprescription shampoos, gels, and liquids containing pediculicides are effective. One example is permethrin liquid (Nix), which kills adult forms of lice. Other over-the-counter products such as RID, Pronto, and A-200 contain pyrethrin, a natural insecticide from the chrysanthemum, and piperonyl butoxide. The National Pediculosis Association opposes the use of strong chemicals such as lindane (Kwell), which is neurotoxic, and those that contain benzene, which is carcinogenic, especially in children. Pediculicides are contraindicated in pregnant and nursing women, children younger than 2 years of age, and those who have health conditions such as open wounds, epilepsy, or asthma. Nits and live lice are removed mechanically with a fine-toothed combing tool such as the LiceMeister™.

Nursing Management

The nurse teaches school volunteers and parents how to detect and recognize lice and nits. Those who have not learned this measure may mistake other hair and scalp conditions for lice and unnecessarily stigmatize children who are dismissed from school. Using the information in Nursing Guidelines 69-1, the nurse removes nits and lice and teaches the family to do likewise.

The nurse instructs the client or family not to shampoo or rinse with a conditioner before applying the pediculicide. Conditioner coats the hair and protects the nits. The nurse instructs clients to follow the label directions on the pediculicide; leaving the chemical(s) on for longer than 10 minutes or covering the head with a shower cap does not increase effectiveness and, in fact, may increase the potential for toxicity.

NURSING GUIDELINES 69-1

Removing Nits and Lice

- Cut long hair to make it more manageable.
- Apply the pediculicide to the hair.
- Seat the infested individual where there is good light.
- Comb the hair free of tangles while the hair is damp.
- Divide the hair into sections.
- Lift a 1-inch strand of hair from a hair section.
- Use a special lice comb that has narrow stainless steel teeth (available from the National Pediculosis Association).
- Start at the crown and comb firmly, deeply, and evenly away from the scalp to the end of the hair.
- Pin back or secure the combed strand and hair section before going to another area.
- Redampen the uncombed hair if it begins to dry.
- Dip the comb in water or wipe it with a paper towel periodically to remove dead lice and their eggs, or pull dental floss through the teeth of the comb.
- Deposit debris in a sealable plastic bag.
- Unfasten the sectioned hair and rinse the head thoroughly.
- Assume that some lice will be missed.
- Repeat combings daily until there no longer is any evidence of lice or nits.

Nurses, especially those employed in school systems, can provide clients with important information on detection, elimination, and prevention of reinfestation. Some facts to include are as follows:

- Anyone can become infected; infestation is no reflection on hygiene or living conditions.
- Perform hair inspection whenever there is an outbreak (even if asymptomatic).
- If everyone who is infested with lice follows the prescribed treatment, the outbreak can be controlled and eliminated.
- Pediculicides are contraindicated in pregnant and nursing women, children younger than 2 years of age, and those who have health conditions such as open wounds, epilepsy, or asthma.
- Never use a pediculicide on the eyebrows or eyelashes.
- There is no value in using a pediculicide prophylactically.
- Manual removal is one of the best and safest options for eliminating lice and nits.
- Do not use pediculicides on pets—they do not harbor lice.
- Wash clothing and vacuum furniture, bedding, and carpets.

Stop, Think, and Respond ● BOX 69-1

What information is helpful for parents whose children acquire head lice?

NAIL DISORDERS

The nails, especially toenails, are subject to disorders. Two common conditions include fungal infections, known as *onychomycosis,* and ingrown toenails, technically called *onychocryptosis.*

● ONYCHOMYCOSIS

Onychomycosis is a fungal infection of the fingernails or toenails. A fungus is a tiny, plantlike parasite that thrives in warm, dark, moist environments. Fungi can spread unchecked from one nail to another. They more commonly affect the toenails because conditions inside shoes are perfect for breeding fungi.

Pathophysiology and Etiology

Onychomycosis and tinea pedis (athlete's foot) often occur together. Older adults and immunocompromised clients are at greater risk for fungal infections. The incidence of fungal fingernail infections has increased among women who have artificial nails. Unsanitary cleansing of nail application utensils between customers in salons seems to be the mode of transmission.

The fungi relocate themselves from the surrounding skin to beneath the nail plate. The fleshy portion underneath the nail becomes inflamed. The nail becomes elevated, thickens, loosens, and changes color. Eventually the nail plate is destroyed. The longer the infection is present, the more difficult it is to cure.

Assessment Findings

One or more nails appears grossly different from normal. They are much thicker, causing them to be elevated and distorted. They are yellowed and friable. Because they are difficult to trim, the infected nail(s) may be long and jagged. The pressure and friction from thickened toenails can lead to pain because shoes do not fit comfortably and socks may wear through.

Diagnosis usually is made on the basis of appearance. Microscopic examination of nail scrapings, however, can confirm the diagnosis.

Medical and Surgical Management

Treatment involves prolonged systemic drug therapy with either of two antifungal agents: itraconazole (Sporanox) and terbinafine (Lamisil). Both drugs inhibit fungal enzymes that regulate cell membrane permeability and result in fungal death. Clients take the medications daily for 2 weeks for fingernail infections and 3 weeks for toenail infections. Terbinafine also can be administered in a pulse-dosing regimen consisting of 1 week of medication followed by a 3-week rest period. Repeated pulse dosing is necessary to eradicate the infection. Drug therapy is more than 50% effective. Because nails grow slowly, it may take as long as 12 months before the nail appears normal.

A more radical solution involves removal of the infected nail. This usually is a last resort because it causes permanent cosmetic changes. Surgery is considered when the condition results in chronic pain or causes difficulty in wearing shoes.

Nursing Management

The nurse reinforces that the condition is chronic and to remain compliant with drug therapy for the duration of treatment. He or she explains the dosing regimen, side effects that may develop, and drug interactions. To prevent reinfection, the nurse reminds clients to:

- Alternate pairs of shoes daily.
- Purchase leather shoes that promote evaporation of foot moisture.
- Never go barefoot.
- Wear footwear at communal pools or when showering in gyms or fitness centers.
- Avoid any damage to the skin around the nail, which makes it easier for fungi to colonize.

• ONYCHOCRYPTOSIS

Onychocryptosis is the medical term for an ingrown toenail. This common condition can affect all people, although some are more predisposed than others. It usually affects the inside edge of the great toe. Recurrence tends to be a significant problem.

Pathophysiology and Etiology

Some people have an inherited trait that causes a curvature in the growing nail plate. These clients have a higher incidence of ingrown toenails despite the fit of their shoes or methods for keeping the nails trimmed. The lat-

ter two factors, along with fungal nail infections, explain why most others acquire ingrown toenails. Athletes or those who are physically active seem to have repeated episodes as a result of recurring trauma.

When the nail curves during growth, a corner of the nail becomes trapped under the skin. As the nail grows, it cuts into the flesh at the lateral border of the nail. The trauma causes local inflammation. The impaired skin provides an opportunity for bacteria secondarily to invade the traumatized tissue.

Assessment Findings

The client feels local pressure from the abnormal nail growth. Redness, swelling, and pain occur where the nail pierces the adjacent tissue (Fig. 69-12). The corner of the upper nail is embedded in tissue. Purulent drainage and an odor are evident if the tissue is infected. Some people develop compensatory gait and postural changes in an effort to relieve the pain. Physical examination is sufficient for diagnosis.

Medical and Surgical Management

Treating the infection, if present, is as important as correcting the nail disorder. Local or systemic antibiotic therapy sometimes is prescribed. Applications of hydrogen peroxide are used to loosen and remove exudate. To promote healing, the foot is soaked in warm water and Epsom salts, followed by thorough drying. A wedge of cotton may be inserted to lift the corner of the nail. Clients with diabetes or peripheral vascular disease are referred to a **podiatrist,** a person trained to care for feet. Older clients and those with chronic diseases are especially susceptible to traumatic complications that can impair circulation and necessitate amputation.

FIGURE 69-12 Infected ingrown toenail.

For persistent or recurrent ingrown toenails, surgery is indicated. Various techniques are used to remove the nail border, not the entire nail, and its root. Surgical procedures are done in the physician's office using local anesthesia or a laser to vaporize the abnormal tissue. Chemical cauterization controls bleeding, and no sutures are required. The client temporarily may need to wear a slipper or shoe from which the toe has been cut out until the swelling and discomfort subsides, but he or she can resume most activities immediately.

Nursing Management

The nurse explains how to perform foot-soaking regimens and techniques to relieve the pressure around the ingrown nail. If surgery is performed, the nurse instructs the client how to change the dressing, the frequency of dressing changes, and signs of infection or compromised circulation to report immediately to the surgeon.

The nurse provides the following information to affected clients:

- Wear wide shoes and loose socks with sufficient room for the toes.
- Use nail clippers rather than scissors to trim toenails.
- Trim the toenails so that they are slightly longer than the end of the toes, and do not round off the corners.
- Keep the feet clean and dry.
- Avoid physical activities that involve sudden stops, such as playing basketball, which jams the toes into the front of the shoe.
- Obtain regular foot and nail care from a podiatrist if there is a history of diabetes, diminished vision, or vascular problems.

GENERAL PHARMACOLOGIC CONSIDERATIONS

Ointments, creams, and lotions prescribed for dermatologic disorders must be applied exactly as the physician directs (e.g., sparingly or thick or thin coat covering the lesion). Remind the client that, unless he or she applies the drug exactly as ordered, it may not be of therapeutic value. If the client uses an excessive amount, he or she is wasting the drug.

Drugs prescribed for dermatologic conditions may relieve symptoms but do not necessarily cure the disease. Skin disorders may require long-term therapy, often with a periodic change in prescriptions. This can be discouraging to the client. Encourage persistence in following the physician's instructions.

Warn clients using acne preparations containing benzoyl peroxide that this ingredient is an oxidizing agent and may remove the color from clothing, rugs, and furniture. Thorough handwashing after drug use may not remove all the drug, and permanent fabric discoloration may still occur. Users of products containing benzoyl peroxide should wear disposable plastic gloves when applying the drug.

Clients receiving photochemotherapy for severe psoriasis must follow the physician's directions regarding the timing of taking the drug methoxsalen.

Isotretinoin (Accutane) is used in the treatment of severe acne. Dosage is determined by weight. Warn clients not to increase the dosage of the drug if the acne becomes worse or does not respond to treatment.

GENERAL GERONTOLOGIC CONSIDERATIONS

Advise the elderly client with any type of skin lesion to seek medical attention; caution against self-treatment. Early treatment of skin lesions helps prevent infection and complications.

Explain that excessive drying of the skin may result in pruritus and infection. Encourage older clients to apply creams and lotions to the skin, especially during winter or when living in a hot, dry climate. A daily bath is not necessary.

Carefully assess older debilitated clients or clients with dementia for scabies and head lice. These clients may be unable to inform the nurse of these problems or manifest the typical symptoms. Instead, they may become increasingly confused or agitated.

Critical Thinking Exercises

1. *What health teaching is appropriate for keeping the skin, hair, and nails in healthy condition?*
2. *Name a skin disorder that is more common in younger adults and one that is more common in older adults. Discuss the factors that make these age groups particularly susceptible to the disorder.*

References and Suggested Readings

Aly, R., Forney, R., & Bayles, C. (2001). Treatments for common superficial fungal infections. *Dermatology Nursing, 13,* 91–94, 98–101.

Beltani, V. S. (1999). Managing atopic dermatitis. *Dermatology Nursing, 11,* 171–176, 179–187.

Bielan, B. (2001). Clinical snapshot: Scabies. *Dermatology Nursing, 13,* 300.

Bielan, B. (2000). What's your assessment? . . . Tinea corporis. *Dermatology Nursing, 12,* 350–351.

Cunningham, M. (1999). Acne: A skin condition to take seriously. *Practice Nurse, 18,* 116, 118.

Fishman, T. D. (2000). Wound assessment and evaluation . . . Contact dermatitis. *Dermatology Nursing, 12,* 194–195.

Fogg, D. M. (1999). Clinical issues: Body piercing; perineal preps; insects in the OR; wound classification systems; recommended practices. *American Operating Room Nurses Journal, 70,* 120, 122–124.

Gradewell, C. (2000). Teaching patients to cope with psoriasis. *Practice Nurse, 20,* 543–544, 546, 548.

Herbert, J. (1998). A guide to dry skin problems. *Journal of Community Nursing, 12*(11), 22–24.

Letuzua, M. (2001). Addressing alopecia: Helping patients with cancer deal with hair loss. *American Journal of Nursing, 101*(4), Critical Care Extra: 24LL.

Lowe, J. (2000). Skin care: Over exposed . . . dermatitis. *Nursing Times, 96*(3), 55–56.

Madison, L. K. (2001). Shingles update: Common questions in caring for a patient with shingles. *Dermatology Nursing, 13,* 51, 54–55.

McDonald, N. (1999). Alopecia areata: Identification and current treatment approaches. *Dermatology Nursing, 11,* 356–359, 363–366.

McMichael, A. J. (1999). A review of cutaneous disease in African-American patients. *Dermatology Nursing, 11,* 35–36, 41–47.

Mulinari-Brenner, F. & Bergfeld W. F. (2001). Hair loss: An overview. *Dermatology Nursing, 13,* 269–272, 277–278.

Nelson, L. M. (1998). Hospital nursing. ABCDs of melanoma: Spelling out the dangers. *Nursing, 28*(8), 32hn1–32hn3.

O'Donoghue, M. N. (1999). Update on acne therapy. *Dermatology Nursing, 11,* 205–208.

Porth, C. M. (2002). *Pathophysiology: Concepts of altered health states* (6th ed.). Philadelphia: Lippincott Williams & Wilkins.

Price, J. H., Burkhart, C. N., Burkhart, C. G., et al. (1999). School nurses' perceptions of and experiences with head lice. *Journal of School Health, 69*(4), 153–158.

Schleicher, S. M. (1999). Treating psoriasis: A stepwise approach. *Emergency Medicine, 31*(7), 42–44, 47, 51–52.

Scott, F. (2000). Shingles: Diagnosis and treatment. *Nursing Times, 96*(50), 36–37.

Stewart, K. B. (2000). Combating infection: Stopping the itch of scabies and lice. *Nursing, 30*(7), 30–31.

Venna, S., Fleisher, A. B., Jr., & Feldman, S. R. (2001). *Dermatology Nursing, 13,* 257–262, 265–266.

Watts, J. (1999). Help psoriasis sufferers manage skin care. *Practice Nurse, 18,* 667–668.

Weiss, P. A. & O'Rourke, M. E. (1999). Cutaneous manifestations of cancer and cancer treatment. *American Journal of Nursing, 99*(4, Suppl.), 13–16, 34–36.

Winslow, E. H. & Jacobson, A. F. (2000). Research for practice: Can a fashion statement harm the patient? *American Journal of Nursing, 100*(9), 63, 65.

Caring for Clients With Burns

Words to Know

allograft	eschar
autograft	full-thickness graft
closed method	heterograft
debridement	open method
epithelialization	slit graft
escharotomy	split-thickness graft

Learning Objectives

On completion of this chapter, the reader will:

- Explain how the depth and percentage of burns are determined.
- Name three life-threatening complications of serious burns.
- Differentiate between open and closed methods of wound care for burns.
- Name three sources for skin grafts.
- List at least three priority nursing diagnoses for the care of a client with burns.

According to the American Burn Association (2000), there were more than 1 million burn injuries in the United States in 2000, a decrease from the last reported data in 1993. Currently, approximately 4500 people die from burns each year. The risk for acquiring a burn injury is highest among children and adults older than 60 years. The most common causes of burns in older adults are smoking materials, scaldings, and lighting trash fires or furnaces (National Fire Protection Association, 2001).

BURN INJURIES

A burn is a traumatic injury to the skin and underlying tissues. Heat, chemicals, or electricity cause burn injuries. Burns caused by electricity are characteristically the most severe because they are deep. Furthermore, electricity moving through the body follows an undetermined course from entrance to exit, causing major damage in its path.

Pathophysiology and Etiology

The immediate initial cause of cell damage is heat. The severity of the burn is related to the temperature of the heat source, its duration of contact, and the thickness of the tissue exposed to the heat source. The location of the burn also is significant. Burns in the perineal area are at increased risk for infection from organisms in the stool. Burns of the face, neck, or chest have the potential to impair ventilation. Burns involving the hands or major joints can affect dexterity and mobility.

Thermal injuries cause the protein in cells to coagulate. Chemicals such as strong acids, bases, and organic compounds yield heat during a reaction with substances in cells and tissue. They subsequently liquefy tissue and loosen the attachment to nutritive sublayers in the skin. Electrical burns and lightning also produce heat, which is greatest at the points of entry to and exit from the body. Because deep tissues cool more slowly than those at the surface, it is difficult initially to determine the extent of internal damage. Cardiac dysrhythmias and central nervous system complications are common among victims of electrical burns.

The initial burn injury is further extended by inflammatory processes that affect layers of tissue below the initial surface injury. For example, protease enzymes and chemical oxidants are proteolytic, causing additional injury to healing tissue and deactivation of tissue growth factors. Neutrophils, whose mission is to phagocytize debris, consume available oxygen at the wound site, contributing to tissue hypoxia. Injured capillaries thrombose, causing localized ischemia and tissue necrosis. Bacterial colonization, mechanical trauma, and even topically applied antimicrobial agents further damage viable tissue.

Serious burns cause various neuroendocrine changes within the first 24 hours. Adrenocorticotropic hormone and antidiuretic hormone are released in response to stress and hypovolemia. When the adrenal cortex is stimulated, it releases glucocorticoids, which cause hyperglycemia, and aldosterone, a mineralocorticoid, which causes sodium retention. Sodium retention leads to peripheral edema as a result of fluid shifts and oliguria. The client eventually enters a hypermetabolic state that requires increased oxygen and nutrition to compensate for the accelerated tissue catabolism.

After a burn, fluid from the body moves toward the burned area, accounting for edema at the burn site. Some of the fluid is then trapped in this area and rendered unavailable for use by the body, leading to fluid loss. Fluid also is lost from the burned area, often in extremely large amounts, in the forms of water vapor and seepage. Decreased blood pressure follows. If physiologic changes are not immediately recognized and corrected, irreversible shock is likely. These changes usually happen rapidly and the client's status may change from hour to hour, requiring that clients with burns receive intensive care by skilled personnel.

Fluid shifts, electrolyte deficits, and loss of extracellular proteins like albumin from the burn wound affect fluid and electrolyte status. Anemia develops because the heat literally destroys erythrocytes. The client with a burn experiences hemoconcentration when the plasma component of blood is lost or trapped. The sluggish flow of blood cells through blood vessels results in inadequate nutrition to healthy body cells and organs.

Myoglobin and hemoglobin are transported to the kidneys, where they may cause tubular necrosis and acute renal failure.

The release of histamine as a consequence of the stress response increases gastric acidity. The client with a burn is prone to developing gastric ulcers.

Inhalation of hot air, smoke, or toxic chemicals, accompanying injuries such as fractures, concurrent medical problems, and the client's age increase the mortality rate from burn injuries.

Depth of Burn Injury

One method for determining the extent of injury is to assess the depth of the burn. Burn depth is classified as follows:

1. Superficial (first degree)
2. Partial thickness (superficial and deep second degree)
3. Full thickness (third and fourth degree; Fig. 70-1)

Burn depth is determined by assessing the color, characteristics of the skin, and sensation in the area of the burn injury (Table 70-1).

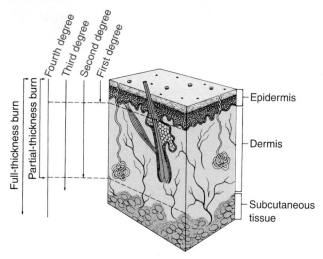

FIGURE 70-1 Depths of burn injury.

A *superficial burn* is similar to a sunburn. The epidermis is injured, but the dermis is unaffected. Although the burn is red and painful, it heals in less than 5 days, usually spontaneously with symptomatic treatment.

A *partial-thickness burn* is classified as either *superficial* or *deep partial thickness,* depending on how much dermis is damaged. A superficial partial-thickness burn heals within 14 days with possibly some pigmentary changes, but no scar; it requires no surgical intervention (Fig. 70-2A). A deep partial-thickness burn takes more than 3 weeks to heal, may need debridement, is subject to hypertrophic scarring, and may require skin grafts (see Fig. 70-2B).

A *full-thickness burn* destroys all layers of the skin and consequently is painless (Fig. 70-3). The tissue appears charred or lifeless. If not debrided, this type of burn injury leads to sepsis, extensive scarring, and contractures. Skin grafts are necessary for a full-thickness burn because the skin cells no longer are alive to regenerate. The most serious burn can involve muscle and bone.

Zones of Burn Injury

Determining the depth of a burn is difficult initially because there are combinations of injury zones in the same location (Fig. 70-4). The *zone of coagulation,* which is at the center of the injury, is the area where the injury is most severe and usually deepest. The area of intermediate burn injury is referred to as the *zone of stasis.* It is here that blood vessels are damaged, but the tissue has the potential to survive. If circulation is secondarily impaired, however, injured tissue in the zone of stasis can convert to a zone of coagulation. The *zone of hyperemia* is the area of least injury, where the epidermis and dermis are only minimally damaged. Because the early appearance of the burn injury can change, the estimate of burn depth may be revised in the first 24 to 72 hours.

TABLE 70-1	DEPTH OF BURN INJURIES	
TYPE	DEPTH	CHARACTERISTICS
Superficial (first degree)	Epidermis and part of dermis	Painful with pink or red edema, but subsides quickly; no scarring
Superficial partial thickness (second degree)	Epidermis and dermis, hair follicles intact	Mottled pink to red, painful, blistered or exuding fluid, blanches with pressure
Deep partial thickness (second degree)		Variable color from patchy red to white, wet or waxy dry, does not blanch with pressure, sensitive to pressure only
Full thickness (third degree)	Epidermis, dermis, subcutaneous tissue	Red, white, tan, brown, or black; leathery covering (eschar); painless
Full thickness (fourth degree)	Epidermis, dermis, subcutaneous tissue; may include fat, fascia, muscle, and bone	Black; depressed; painless; scarring

Extent of Burn Injury

Besides determining the burn depth and zones, the severity of a burn also is determined by assessing the percentage of burn injury. The "Rule of Nines" (Fig. 70-5) is a quick initial method of estimating how much of the client's skin surface is involved. Special charts and graphs, such as the one shown in Figure 70-6, provide more precise estimates for determining the percentage of the total body surface area (TBSA) that is burned. A quick assessment technique is to compare the client's palm with the size of the burn wound. The palm is approximately 1% of a person's TBSA.

Stop, Think, and Respond ● BOX 70-1

Using the Rule of Nines, calculate the TBSA that is burned if the burn includes one arm and the anterior chest.

Assessment Findings

Skin color ranges from light pink to black depending on the depth of the burn. There may be edema or blistering. The client experiences pain in all areas except those of

FIGURE 70-2 (**A**) Superficial second-degree burn. (**B**) Full-thickness second-degree burn.

FIGURE 70-3 Third-degree burn.

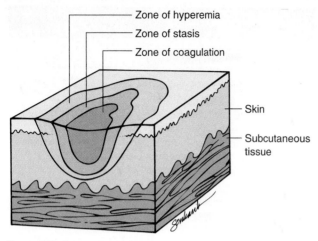

FIGURE 70-4 Zones of burn injury.

full-thickness burns. Clients with extensive burns may exhibit symptoms of hypovolemic shock, such as hypotension, tachycardia, oliguria, or anuria. Breathing may be compromised (Box 70-1). In electrical burns, there usually are entrance and exit wounds.

Diagnosis is made by physical inspection. Radiographs identify secondary injuries such as fractures or compromised lung function in inhalation injuries.

Medical Management

The outcome of a burn injury depends on the initial first aid provided and the subsequent treatment in the hospital or burn center. Any one of three complications—

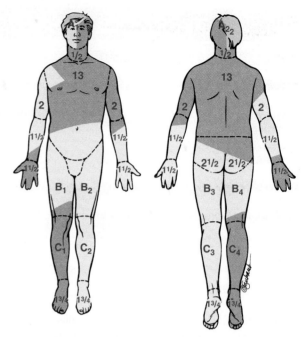

FIGURE 70-6 Sample chart for estimating percentage of body surface area burned (indicated by shading). (Courtesy of Crozer-Chester Medical Center, Upland, PA)

inhalation injury, hypovolemic shock, and infection—can be life-threatening. Clients with major burns are transported to a regional burn center (Box 70-2).

Initial First Aid

At the scene of a fire, the first priority is to prevent further injury to the affected person. If the clothing is on fire, the client is placed in a horizontal position and rolled in a blanket to smother the fire. Laying the client flat prevents the fire, hot air, and smoke from rising toward the head and entering the respiratory passages. The client is taken to a hospital immediately thereafter for examination. During transport, those who have been burned around the face or neck or who may have inhaled smoke, chemicals, steam, or flames are observed closely for respiratory difficulty. Inhalation of such substances can damage or severely irritate the mucous membrane lining

FIGURE 70-5 Rule of nines.

BOX 70-1 ● **Signs of Heat or Smoke Inhalation Injury**

- Sore throat
- Singed nasal hairs, eyebrows, eyelashes
- Hoarseness
- Carbon in sputum
- Soot around mouth or nose
- Shortness of breath
- Stridor

BOX 70-2 ● Criteria for Major Burns

- Full-thickness burn greater than 10%
- Partial-thickness burn greater than 25%
- Burn in a critical location (face, eyes, ears, hands, perineum/genitalia, feet)
- Burn complicated by inhalation or electrical injury, fractures, or other major trauma
- Preexisting medical disorder (e.g., diabetes, heart disease)
- Age younger than 2 years or older than 60 years
- Circumstances of burn suggest abuse (child abuse, spouse abuse)

Stop, Think, and Respond ● BOX 70-2

Using the Parkland-Baxter formula, determine what volume of fluid is required during the first 24 hours of treatment for a client who weighs 168 lbs and has acquired a burn of 40% TBSA.

the respiratory passages, resulting in edema of the respiratory passages. In addition, secretion of mucus may be excessive, which also makes breathing difficult. Oxygen is administered, and intravenous (IV) fluid therapy is begun en route.

Acute Care

When the client with a burn arrives, the medical team works quickly to assess the extent of burn injury and additional trauma such as fractures, head injury, and lacerations. Team members implement several aspects of burn treatment, including maintaining adequate ventilation and initiating fluid resuscitation. If the client has difficulty breathing or if there is edema of the face and neck, an endotracheal tube is inserted.

Blood samples are drawn. Fluid resuscitation begins according to the severity of the burn injury (Table 70-2). IV analgesics are administered for pain, which often is severe. An indwelling urethral catheter is inserted and attached to a closed drainage system to facilitate evaluation of fluid resuscitation. Tetanus immunization and antibiotics are administered.

Wound Management

Staphylococcus aureus, Pseudomonas aeruginosa, and *Candida albicans* are the most common microorganisms causing infection in burned tissue. As soon as possible, all clothing is removed. The body hair around the perimeter of the burns is shaved because hair is a source of bacterial wound contamination. When the head, neck, and upper chest are burned, singed eyebrows and eyelashes are clipped, scalp hair is shaved, the lips and mouth are cleansed, and the lips are lubricated. Eye ointments or irrigations are used to remove dirt and to lubricate the lid margins.

The burned areas are cleansed to remove debris. After cleansing, topical antimicrobial medications are applied. Wound management includes the **open method**, in which the wound is left uncovered, or the **closed method**, in which the wound is covered. The closed method involves the use of one or more types of dressing materials (Table 70-3). The final step is closing the wound with a skin graft or skin substitute or applying cultured skin.

OPEN METHOD

The open method (exposure method), which exposes the burned areas to air, has been virtually abandoned since the advent of effective topical antimicrobials. It still is used on a small scale, however, for burned areas such as

TABLE 70-2	FLUID RESUSCITATION FORMULAS		
FORMULA	FLUIDS	AMOUNT*	EXAMPLE FOR 220-LB VICTIM WITH 50% BURN
Brooke (modified)	Lactated Ringer's	2 mL/kg/% burn	10,000 mL†
	Second 24 hours	0.3–0.5 mL/kg/% burn	1500–2500 mL
	Colloid (plasma, albumin, dextran)		
	5% Glucose/water	Approximate evaporative losses	2000 mL (avg.)
Parkland-Baxter	Lactated Ringer's	4 mL/kg/% burn	20,000 mL†
Evans‡	Saline	1 mL/kg/% burn	5000 mL
	Colloid	1 mL/kg/% burn	5000 mL
	5% Glucose/water	Approximate evaporative losses	2000 mL (avg.)

*Goal: Establish urine output of 50 mL/hour.
†Half of fluid volume given in first 8 hours; remaining half in next 16 hours; time is calculated from time of burn injury, not time fluid resuscitation begins.
‡Maximum of 10,000 mL over 24 hours if calculation exceeds this amount.

TABLE 70-3	OPEN AND CLOSED METHODS OF BURN CARE	
TYPE	**ADVANTAGES**	**DISADVANTAGES**
Open method	Reduces labor-intensive care Causes less pain during wound care Facilitates inspection Decreases expense	Contributes to wound dessication (dryness) Promotes loss of water and body heat Exposes wound to pathogens Contributes to pain during repositioning Compromises modesty
Closed method	Maintains moist wound Promotes maintenance of body temperature Decreases cross-contamination of wound Provides wound debridement during dressing removal Keeps skin folds separated Reduces pain during position changes	Requires more time Adds to expense Enhances growth of pathogens beneath dressings Interferes with wound assessment Causes more blood loss with removal Can interfere with circulation if tightly applied

the face and perineum to which it is difficult to apply dressing materials.

If the open method is used, the client is placed in isolation in a bed with sterile linen. Health team members and visitors wear sterile gowns and masks. The skin of the client with a burn is sensitive to drafts and temperature changes; therefore, a bed cradle or sheets are placed over the client. The room is kept warm and humidified.

A hard crust forms over a partial-thickness burn in 2 or 3 days, and **epithelialization** (regrowth of skin) is completed in about 2 or 3 weeks. At this time, the crust falls off, is debrided, or is loosened by whirlpool baths. **Eschar**, a hard, leathery crust of dehydrated skin, forms in areas of full-thickness burns. If the eschar constricts the area and impairs circulation, an **escharotomy** (an incision into the eschar) is done to relieve pressure on the affected area (see Fig. 70-3). A dressing may be used to cover the exposed areas as the eschar is removed. New skin cannot grow beneath eschar.

CLOSED METHOD

The closed method is the current preferred method of wound management. First, the burn area is covered with nonadherent and absorbent dressings, which consist of gauze impregnated with petroleum jelly or ointment-based antimicrobials and fluffed gauze pads. The final covering is an occlusive or semiocclusive dressing made of polyvinyl, polyethylene, polyurethane, and hydrocolloid materials. Occlusive dressings prevent bacteria from contact with the wound but are minimally permeable to water and oxygen. Various topical antimicrobials are applied to the burn wound to discourage the growth of pathogens or control or eliminate any infection that develops.

Stop, Think, and Respond ● **BOX 70-3**

If a person is seriously burned, which method of wound management would you expect the burn unit to use? Give at least three reasons for your answer.

ANTIMICROBIAL THERAPY

Three major antimicrobials are used to treat burns: silver sulfadiazine (Silvadene) 1% ointment, mafenide (Sulfamylon), and silver nitrate (AgNO$_3$) 0.5% solution. Other commonly used drugs are povidone-iodine (Betadine), gentamicin (Garamycin) 0.1% cream, nitrofurazone (Furacin), mupirocin (Bactroban), clotrimazole (Lotrimin), and ciclopirox (Loprox). Povidone-iodine is contraindicated with some skin substitutes that are discussed later because it can damage new tissue growth in the wound bed.

Topical antimicrobials have various advantages and disadvantages, and no one preparation appears superior to another. All drugs are applied using sterile technique. Because infection is the rule rather than the exception, the client may require systemic antibiotics and antifungals. Some examples include amphotericin B (Fungizone) and penicillin G (Pfizerpen).

Surgical Management

Additional treatment modalities to promote healing include debridement, skin grafting, application of a skin substitute, and application of cultured skin.

Debridement

Wound **debridement** is the removal of necrotic tissue. Debridement is accomplished in one of four ways:

1. Naturally as the nonliving tissue sloughs away from uninjured tissue
2. Mechanically when dead tissue adheres to dressings or is detached during cleansing
3. Enzymatically through the application of topical enzymes to the burn wound
4. Surgically with the use of forceps and scissors during dressing changes or wound cleansing

After dead tissue is removed, it is imperative that the healthy tissue be covered with a skin graft, a temporary skin substitute, or cultured skin.

Skin Grafting

Superficial burns heal when keratinocytes from the periphery and beneath the dermis proliferate to regenerate the epidermis (Schulz et al., 2000). Skin grafting is necessary for deep partial-thickness and full-thickness burns because the skin layers responsible for regeneration have been destroyed. Unassisted healing, that is, healing without the use of skin grafts or skin substitutes, results in the proliferation of granulation tissue. Granulation tissue contains fibroblasts, which create hypertrophic scars that contract and pull the edges of the wound together, causing contractures. Wounds that are greater than 2 cm may not be able to granulate fully, resulting in a chronic open wound (Schulz et al., 2000).

The purposes of a skin graft are to:

- Lessen the potential for infection
- Minimize fluid loss by evaporation
- Hasten recovery
- Reduce scarring
- Prevent loss of function

SOURCES FOR SKIN GRAFTS

Several sources are available for skin grafting. An **autograft** uses the client's own skin, which is transplanted from one part of the body to another. Only autograft or skin transplanted from one identical twin to another can become a permanent part of the client's own skin.

An **allograft** or homograft is human skin obtained from a cadaver. Allografts temporarily cover large areas of tissue. Although allografts slough away after approximately 1 week, they last for the critical period until the client's own skin can be used for skin grafting. Cadaver skin usually is in short supply; although the tissue is screened for human immunodeficiency virus and hepatitis, concerns remain that it could be a source of other pathogens.

A **heterograft** or xenograft is obtained from animals, principally pigs. Like allografts, heterografts are temporary and serve the same purposes. Allografts and heterografts are rejected in days to weeks and must be removed and replaced at that time.

TYPES OF AUTOGRAFTS

Human skin from the client with a burn is harvested under general anesthesia. Either a split-thickness or full-thickness graft is removed. In a **split-thickness graft,** the epidermis and a thin layer of dermis are harvested from the client's skin. Split-thickness autografts vary in thickness (0.008 to 0.024 inch), size, and shape and usually are obtained from the buttocks or thighs. A dermatome, a scalpel, or another special instrument is used to remove the skin from the donor site. Split-thickness autografts have more successful outcomes than other types; however, their cosmetic appearance is less than desirable, they are less elastic, and hair does not grow from their surface.

A **full-thickness graft,** which may be 0.035 inch thick, includes epidermis, dermis, and some subcutaneous tissue. This type of graft is used when the burned area is fairly small or involves the hands, face, or neck. Full-thickness grafts are more comparable in appearance to normal skin and can tolerate more stress once they become permanently attached to the burn wound.

A **slit graft** (also called a *lace* or an *expansile graft*) is used when the area available as a donor site is limited, as in clients with extensive burns. The skin is removed from the donor site and passed through an instrument that slits it; thus, a smaller piece of skin is stretched to cover a larger area (Fig. 70-7).

Harvesting the client's own tissue has several disadvantages: (1) it compounds the client's pain because it creates a new wound, (2) the donor site has the potential for scarring and atypical pigment changes, (3) there is a potential for donor site infection, (4) there is a delay in wound closure while waiting for the donor site to heal and be reharvested, and (5) delays caused by waiting for harvest sites to heal increase costs and challenge the client's ability to cope with a prolonged hospitalization. It may be virtually impossible to harvest sufficient skin to close totally a full-thickness burn wound that is greater than 60% TBSA (Schulz et al., 2000).

Once the skin graft heals, pressure garments made of elasticized cloth or plastic are applied over the grafted area (Fig. 70-8). These garments smooth the grafted skin, reducing scarring and the potential for wound contractures. The client may need to wear a pressure garment for up to 2 years.

Skin Substitutes

Scientists are creating alternative materials referred to as *skin substitutes* that cover the wound and promote healing. These bioengineered coverings promote wound healing by interacting directly with body tissues. Skin substitutes can be applied all over the burn wound as soon as the skin

FIGURE 70-7 A slit graft. The slits allow for stretching to cover a larger area of tissue.

FIGURE 70-8 Elastic pressure garments. (Used with permission of Jobst Institute, Inc., Toledo, Ohio.)

is cleaned and debrided instead of having to wait until enough skin is available for grafting purposes.

One example of a skin substitute is Biobrane, a nylon–silicone membrane coated with a protein derived from pig tissue (Fig. 70-9). Another is Integra, a two-layer membrane: One is a synthetic epidermal layer; the other contains cross-linked collagen fibers that mimic the dermal layer of skin. The pseudodermal layer becomes a perma-

FIGURE 70-9 Biobrane dressing applied to lower extremity partial-thickness burn. (Used with permission of Dow Hickman Pharmaceuticals.)

nent cover; the outer layer, which provides a barrier against pathogens, is removed in 2 to 3 weeks and replaced with a thin autograft. The thin autograft heals in only a few days and provides a better cosmetic appearance.

Cultured Skin

Another alternative to wound closure is to culture the client's skin in a laboratory. Cultured skin is a wound closure product that is developed by growing the client's own skin cells in a laboratory culture medium. From a piece of postage stamp–sized skin, it is possible to grow sufficient skin to cover nearly the entire body in 3 weeks (Strange, 1997). A skin substitute is used to cover the burn wound while the skin culture is growing.

Once sufficient cultured cells are available, they are combined with a fabric material made from collagen that dissolves after it is applied to the wound. The burn wound heals in 2 to 3 weeks without traditional skin grafting. The only current disadvantage to cultured skin is that the pigmentation does not perfectly match the original skin color; however, scientists are working on eliminating that problem.

Nursing Management

Nursing management focuses on assessing the wound and how the burn injury has affected the client's status. The nurse calculates fluid replacement requirements and infuses the prescribed volume according to the agency's protocol. He or she quickly recognizes and efficiently treats signs of shock (see Chap. 23). The nurse administers prescribed analgesics to relieve or reduce pain. He or she cleans the wound, applies an antimicrobial agent, and covers the wound with the prescribed dressing. The nurse monitors the wound to determine any infection. He or she helps the client and family cope with the change in body image and encourages the client to perform exercises that minimize contractures. Before discharge, the nurse teaches the client about the use of a pressure garment and methods for skin care. Refer to Nursing Care Plan 70-1 for additional nursing management.

GENERAL NUTRITIONAL CONSIDERATIONS

Extensive burns are the most severe form of stress that a person can experience. Metabolism may increase as much as 100%; protein catabolism compromises wound healing and immunocompetence.

Weight loss and malnutrition increase morbidity and mortality unless aggressive nutritional support is initiated as soon as possible after fluid resuscitation.

Protein needs increase two to four times above the normal Recommended Dietary Allowance; calorie needs may be 4000 to 5000/day.

Clients with adynamic ileus, impaired swallowing related to facial or neck burns, or bleeding related to a stress ulcer require enteral or parenteral nutritional support.

(text continued on page 1160)

Nursing Care Plan 70-1

THE CLIENT WITH BURNS

Assessment

- Determine the type of burn (thermal, chemical, electrical) and when it occurred.
- Assess vital signs.
- Look for evidence of inhalation injury.
- Determine the oxygen saturation and respiratory effort.
- Evaluate pain intensity.
- Determine the volume and characteristics of urine.
- Note the percentage and depth of burn.
- Auscultate bowel sounds.
- Assess for concurrent medical problems, and review the results of laboratory tests.

Depending on the extent and degree of burns, some or all of the following nursing diagnoses may apply. Diagnoses change as the client progresses through treatment and the stages of healing.

Nursing Diagnoses: **Risk for Ineffective Airway Clearance** related to increased airway secretions; **Risk for Impaired Gas Exchange** related to edema of airway and inhalation of carbon

Expected Outcomes: (1) The airway will be patent. (2) Gas exchange will be adequate as evidenced by clear lung sounds, blood oxygen saturation (SpO_2) greater than 90%, and arterial oxygen pressure (PaO_2) greater than 80 mm Hg.

Interventions	Rationales
Monitor characteristics of respirations and lung sounds frequently.	Frequent focused assessments of respiratory function facilitate early detection of compromised ventilation.
Check respiratory rate before and after administering an opioid analgesic.	Narcotic analgesics depress the respiratory center in the brain.
Measure SpO_2 with a pulse oximeter or analyze arterial blood gas (ABG) results.	The PaO_2 can be determined deductively from the SpO_2; and SpO_2 of 90% or greater suggests that the PaO_2 is at least 80 mm Hg. ABGs provide objective measurements of serum O_2, CO_2, and bicarbonate levels.
Administer oxygen as prescribed.	Supplemental oxygen increases the percentage of inhaled oxygen above that in room air.
Suction the airway cautiously if edema is present.	Suctioning removes accumulated secretions, but the trauma of catheter insertion can worsen edema.
Facilitate ventilation with artificial airways, such as with an endotracheal tube and ventilator.	An artificial airway and ventilator facilitate the maintenance of adequate gas exchange.
Be prepared to assist with an escharotomy if there is a circumferential burn of the chest.	An escharotomy releases constriction and allows greater chest expansion.

Evaluation of Expected Outcomes: Client breathes effortlessly and is well oxygenated.

PC: Hypovolemic Shock

Expected Outcome: Nurse will monitor to detect, manage, and minimize hypovolemia.

Interventions	Rationales
Monitor vital signs every 15 minutes.	Hypotension and tachycardia suggest impending shock.
Measure intake and output hourly.	Hourly measurements facilitate early detection of mismatches between fluid intake and output.

(continued)

Nursing Care Plan 70-1 (Continued)

THE CLIENT WITH BURNS

Interventions	Rationales
Weigh the client daily at the same time with similar dressings.	A loss of 2 lb in 24 hours suggests a 1-L deficit in fluid.
Administer fluids according to the fluid resuscitation formula.	A large volume of fluid is necessary to prevent hypovolemic shock.
Report urine output of < 50 mL/hour.	Urine output <50 mL/hour suggests inadequate renal perfusion due to hypovolemia or other causes.

Evaluation of Expected Outcome: Client does not experience hypovolemic shock.

Nursing Diagnosis: **Acute Pain** related to tissue injury

Expected Outcome: Pain will be within client's level of tolerance.

Interventions	Rationales
Assess pain intensity as needed and whenever you measure vital signs.	Assessing pain is the fifth vital sign.
Administer prescribed IV analgesia.	The IV route facilitates drug distribution when absorption is impaired at other parenteral routes.
Give analgesics prophylactically 30 minutes before dressing changes or debridements.	Preventing severe pain is easier than relieving it.
Implement nonpharmacologic methods of pain relief: imagery, self-hypnosis, and distraction.	Alternative methods for relieving pain supplement pharmacologic methods.
Place client on a CircOlectric bed or other type of turning frame to facilitate turning and repositioning.	Pain is reduced when the bed turns the client mechanically and passively.
Exercise caution and gentleness when removing and reapplying dressings.	Pain is intensified when movement stimulates intact sensory nerves.

Evaluation of Expected Outcome: Client responds to pain-relieving techniques.

Nursing Diagnosis: **Hypothermia** related to impaired ability to regulate body temperature

Expected Outcome: Temperature will be in normal range.

Interventions	Rationales
Reduce evaporation from burn wound by humidifying the environment, preventing drafts, and covering the burn wound with ointment, creams, and dressings.	Impaired skin cannot regulate body temperature; reducing the potential for heat loss helps maintain body temperature.

Evaluation of Expected Outcome: Temperature is normal.

PC: **Infection** related to impaired skin integrity

Expected Outcome: Nurse will monitor to detect, manage, and minimize infection.

Interventions	Rationales
Assess temperature every 4 hours; monitor results of blood counts and cultures.	Fever, leukocytosis, and bacterial growth from a wound culture indicate infection.
Use sterile or clean linen.	Surgical and medical asepsis reduce the potential for infection.

(continued)

Nursing Care Plan 70-1 (Continued)

THE CLIENT WITH BURNS

Interventions	Rationales
Wear sterile or clean caps, gowns, and masks.	Using outer garments reduces the transmission of pathogens from contaminated clothing to the client.
Restrict infectious people from visiting or caring for client.	Limiting contact with sources of infection protects a susceptible host.
Apply and administer prescribed antimicrobial and antibiotic therapy.	Antimicrobials and antibiotics suppress the growth of pathogens.
Inspect burn areas for healing, drainage, formation of eschar, infection, and stability of the skin graft or wound covering. Accurately record all findings.	Direct observation of the wound and comparing normal and abnormal findings help determine the client's response to treatment.

Evaluation of Expected Outcome: Wound infections are eliminated, and the wound heals.

PC: **Skin Graft Disruption**

Expected Outcome: Nurse will monitor to detect, manage, and minimize skin graft disruption.

Interventions	Rationales
Avoid excessive pressure on grafted area; minimize movement.	Relief of pressure and restricting movement promote vascularization.
Assist physician with dressing changes.	Graft disruption is minimized when the nurse assists the physician and client.
Monitor color and odor in the area of grafted tissue.	A pale color suggests ischemia. A dark appearance suggests poor venous outflow. A foul odor suggests colonization with bacteria.

Evaluation of Expected Outcome: The burn wound is covered; skin grafts are viable.

PC: **Gastric and Intestinal Paresis (Hypomotility)** and **Peptic Ulcer**

Expected Outcome: Nurse will monitor to detect, manage, and minimize gastrointestinal hypomotility and peptic ulcer.

Interventions	Rationales
Assess for abdominal distention and status of bowel sounds.	Abdominal distension and diminished or no bowel sounds suggest impaired peristalsis.
Insert a prescribed nasogastric tube; connect it to low intermittent suction.	Negative pressure removes gas and secretions from the upper gastrointestinal tract.
Administer IV histamine antagonists and drugs such as metoclopramide (Reglan).	Histamine antagonists raise the pH of gastric secretions and reduce the potential for gastric mucosal irritation. Metoclopramide promotes stomach emptying.
Instill antacid through nasogastric tube; clamp for 30 minutes before reconnecting to suction.	Antacids neutralize stomach acid.
Assess pH of gastric secretions every shift; report if pH is less than 3.	Drug therapy should raise gastric pH above 3; if not, the physician may choose to include a proton pump inhibitor such as omeprazole (Prilosec) or a cytoprotective agent such as misoprostol (Cytotec).

Evaluation of Expected Outcome: Bowel sounds are active in all abdominal quadrants; client experiences no epigastric distress.

(continued)

Nursing Care Plan 70-1 *(Continued)*

THE CLIENT WITH BURNS

Nursing Diagnosis: **Risk for Constipation** related to fluid loss, decreased oral nutrition, inactivity, and narcotic analgesia

Expected Outcome: Client will pass stool regularly and with ease.

Interventions	Rationales
Monitor bowel elimination.	Infrequent and difficult bowel elimination with passage of dry, hard stool indicates constipation.
Provide a generous volume of oral liquids, fresh fruit and vegetables, and whole grains when the client is allowed oral intake.	Cellulose is undigested fiber and pulls water into the intestine, creating a bulkier, moist stool that is easy to eliminate.
Administer prescribed stool softener or laxatives.	Laxatives promote bowel elimination by increasing intestinal bulk and stimulating motility. Stool softeners draw water into the fecal mass, easing elimination.
Remove any fecal impactions.	Impacted stool is difficult to pass and may require digital removal.

Evaluation of Expected Outcome: Bowel movements are regular; stool is moist and easily passed.

PC: **Anemia** related to destruction of red blood cells (RBCs) and blood loss from stress ulcer

Expected Outcome: Nurse will monitor to detect, manage, and minimize anemia.

Interventions	Rationales
Monitor hemoglobin and hematocrit laboratory results.	Decreased hemoglobin and hematocrit values suggest blood loss.
Check gastric secretions and stool for occult or frank blood.	Identifying the source of blood loss helps the physician prescribe additional medical interventions to alleviate the problem.
Administer whole blood or packed RBCs as prescribed.	Administration of blood helps replace depleted RBCs.
Provide iron-rich food or supplements when it is safe to use the oral route.	The heme component of hemoglobin contains iron.

Evaluation of Expected Outcome: Erythrocyte, hemoglobin, and hematocrit values are within normal ranges.

Nursing Diagnosis: **Risk for Imbalanced Nutrition: Less than Body Requirements** related to increased caloric requirements and inability to ingest food orally

Expected Outcome: Nutritional intake will compensate for a hypercatabolic state.

Interventions	Rationales
Administer total parenteral nutrition (TPN) until tube or oral feedings are initiated.	TPN provides calories and essential nutrients that meet metabolic needs.
Monitor weight loss or gain.	Weighing the client helps determine if dietary management is adequate.
Provide high-protein, iron-rich foods in small, frequent feedings when oral nourishment is allowed.	Protein facilitates cellular growth and repair. Iron prevents nutritional anemia. Small, frequent meals are likely to provide sufficient calories.

(continued)

Nursing Care Plan 70-1 (Continued)

THE CLIENT WITH BURNS

Evaluation of Expected Outcome: Client maintains weight, with no evidence of malnutrition, vitamin deficiencies, electrolyte imbalance, or muscle wasting.

Nursing Diagnosis: **Impaired Physical Mobility** related to pain, bulky dressings, and contracted skin secondary to scar formation

Expected Outcome: Range of motion and muscle strength will be preserved or restored.

Interventions	Rationales
Keep joints in burned areas neutral: extended rather than flexed.	A neutral position facilitates functional use.
Exercise uninvolved joints actively; exercise involved joints during hydrotherapy.	Exercise promotes muscle tone and strength. Exercising in water reduces resistance to work.
Encourage performance of activities of daily living (ADLs), such as brushing teeth and eating.	Performing ADLs is a form of active exercise that maintains the flexibility of joints and muscle tone.

Evaluation of Expected Outcome: Client regains functional use of joints in burn areas.

Nursing Diagnosis: **Risk for Disturbed Thought Processes** related to reduced mental stimulation, sleep deprivation, social isolation, fluid and electrolyte imbalance, narcotic administration, and sepsis

Expected Outcome: Client will remain oriented and have realistic perceptions.

Interventions	Rationales
Assess mental status every shift.	Focused assessments facilitate the early detection of problems.
Reorient the confused client.	Providing facts helps the client reorder thinking.
Have a calendar and clock within client's view.	Environmental cues help prevent disorientation.
Discuss current events; encourage visits from family.	Interacting with others and staying aware of current events help stimulate the mind.
Cluster nursing activities to facilitate continuous sleep.	Sleep deprivation contributes to confusion and disorientation.

Evaluation of Expected Outcome: Client logically processes verbal and environmental cues.

Nursing Diagnoses: **Risk for Ineffective Coping** and **Risk for Ineffective Family Coping** related to inadequate emotional resources for managing multiple stressors

Expected Outcome: Client and family will adapt and use strategies for effective coping.

Interventions	Rationales
Explain methods and reasons for treatment.	Information helps clarify the plan and assists the client to strive to meet goals.
Acknowledge signs of progress.	Objective evidence of progress sustains motivation.
Involve client and family in long-range planning, physical therapy, and vocational rehabilitation.	A client and family who feel they are part of a team willingly participate in achieving goals.
Refer family to counseling for assistance in managing conflicts.	Health professionals with specialized expertise can help clients and family members solve problems.

Evaluation of Expected Outcome: Client and family cope effectively and use resources wisely to manage client's care.

Large supplemental doses of vitamins and minerals, especially vitamin C, the B complex vitamins, iron, and zinc, are prescribed to promote healing and meet increased needs for metabolism.

GENERAL GERONTOLOGIC CONSIDERATIONS

Burns can result in serious complications in the elderly because of diminished renal, cardiac, and respiratory functions associated with the aging process.

Critical Thinking Exercise

1. *Discuss methods used to reduce the potential for infection in a burn wound.*

References and Suggested Readings

American Burn Association. (2000). Burn incidence and treatment in the US: 2000 fact sheet. [On-line.] Available: http://www.ameriburn.org/pub/factsheet.htm.

Badger, J. M. (2001). Understanding secondary traumatic stress. *American Journal of Nursing, 101*(7), 26–33.

Carrougher, G. J. & Cornwell, P. (2000). Nursing forum: Quality outcomes for burn survivors. *Journal of Burn Care and Rehabilitation, 21,* 439.

Clarke, A. & Cooper, C. (2001). Psychosocial rehabilitation after disfiguring injury or disease: Investigating the training needs of specialist nurses. Study 1. *Journal of Advanced Nursing, 34*(1), 18–26.

Clayton, M. C. & Bishop, J. F. (1998). Nursing forum: Perioperative and postoperative dressing techniques for Integra Artificial Skin: Views from two medical centers. *Journal of Burn Care and Rehabilitation, 19,* 358–363.

Cole, M. R. (2000). Burn trauma: More than just skin deep. *Nursing Spectrum (Greater Chicago/NE Illinois, NW Indiana Edition), 13*(17), 32–33.

Docking, P. (1999). Trauma: Electrical burn injuries. *Accident and Emergency Nursing, 7*(2), 70–76.

DuKamp, A. (2000). Managing burn blisters. *Nursing Times, 96*(4), NTPlus: 19–20.

Flynn, M. B. (1999). Identifying and treating inhalation injuries in fire victims. *Dimensions of Critical Care Nursing, 18*(4), 18–23.

Jones, M. L. (2001). Burns. *Practice Nurse, 22*(6), 41–42, 44.

Jordan, K. S. (2000). Fluid resuscitation in acutely injured patients. *Journal of Intravenous Nursing, 23*(2), 81–87.

Kagan, R. J. & Smith, S. C. (2000). Evaluation and treatment of thermal injuries. *Dermatology Nursing, 12,* 334–335, 338–344, 347–350.

McCain, D. & Sutherland, S. (1998). Nursing essentials: Skin grafts for patients with burns. *American Journal of Nursing, 98*(7), 34–39.

McKirdy, L. (2001). Burn wound cleansing. *Journal of Community Nursing, 15*(5), 24, 26–27, 29.

Nagy, S. (1999). Strategies used by burn nurses to cope with the infliction of pain on patients. *Journal of Advanced Nursing, 29,* 1427–1433.

National Fire Protection Association. (2001). Major causes of 1994 through 1998 structure fires. [On-line.] Available: http://www.nfpa.org/.

Nelson, L. A. & Thompson, D. D. (1998). Burn injury. *Plastic Surgical Nursing, 18,* 159–162, 176, 184–187.

Palmer, M. & Collier, S. (1999). Continuing care of burn-injured patients. *Nursing Times, 95*(37), 44–46.

Rose, D. D. & Jordan, E. B. (1999). Perioperative management of burn patients. *Journal of American Operating Room Nurses, 69,* 1211, 1213, 1215–1224+.

Schulz, J. T., III, Tompkins, R. G., & Burke, J. F. (2000). Artificial skin. *Annual Reviews, 51*(1), 231–244. [On-line.] Available: *http://www.AnnualReviews.org.*

Sheridan, R. L. (2000). Evaluating and managing burn wounds. *Dermatology Nursing, 12,* 17–18, 21–28, 30–31.

Strange, C. J. (1997). Second skins. U.S. Food and Drug Administration. [On-line.] Available: http://www.fda.gov/fdac/features/1997/197_skin.html.

Weinberg, K., Birdsall, C., Vail, D., et al. (2000). Pain and anxiety with burn dressing changes: Patient self-report. *Journal of Burn Care and Rehabilitation, 21,* 155–161.

Wiebelhaus, P. & Hansen, S. L. (1999). Burns: Handle with care. *RN, 62*(11), 52–58.

Wiebelhaus, P., Hansen, S., & Hill, H. (2001). Helping patients survive inhalation injuries. *RN, 64*(10), 28–32.

Wiebelhaus, P., & Hansen, S. L. (2001). What you should know about managing burn emergencies. *Nursing, 31*(1), 36–42.

Winfrey, M. E., Cochran, M., & Hegarty, M. T. (1999). A new technology in burn therapy: Integra artificial skin. *Dimensions of Critical Care Nursing, 18*(1), 14–20.

Answers to Stop, Think, and Respond Boxes

1-1: The client has several possible options, depending on his or her needs. Examples include a subacute care unit, a skilled care unit, a rehabilitative care unit, and home care.

2-1: Both Henderson and King focus on the client. Henderson views the nurse as responding to client needs and caring for the client when he or she cannot do so alone. King provides a more holistic view of the client. She sees clients as responding to changes in the environment—her definition would most likely embrace the health–illness continuum (see Chap. 1).

3-1: The nurse would ask questions such as:

- Did the client or family participate in making this decision?
- What prompted this order?
- What other things must the nurse know?

Based on the answers to these questions, the nurse adjusts the care plan accordingly. He or she considers nursing diagnoses such as Death Anxiety, Ineffective Coping, and Spiritual Distress.

4-1: If the client has impaired hearing, speak slowly and deliberately, raising your voice to a level that the client can hear. Determine if the client uses hearing aids, reads lips, or uses sign language. If the client signs, an interpreter can assist with the interview and assessment. If the client is visually impaired, tell the client about his or her surroundings and let the client know what will be done next. Raising your voice is unnecessary unless the client also is hearing impaired.

5-1: The client may regard the nurse's words as a threat—an attempt to scare him into taking his medication, as well as the threat of physical harm. Although the client probably should take the medication, the nurse must use a nonthreatening tone to inform the client about this need. He or she also must find out why the client does not want to take his medication. For example, the medication may make him dizzy or nauseous.

5-2: Several factors are involved. First, the physician should obtain the client's signature after thoroughly explaining the procedure. The nurse may witness the signature, validating that the consent conversation occurred. If the client states that the procedure will accomplish more than may actually be possible, the nurse will need to clarify the physician's explanation or ask the physician to provide more information to the client.

5-3: If you choose the utilitarian approach, you must determine what is the greatest good. If you choose the deontologic approach, you must determine what each person's rights are. Decide which philosophical approach is best, and then use the ethical decision-making model to reach a conclusion.

6-1: New employees benefit from autocratic leadership, in which rules and expectations are clearly defined and communication flows from top to bottom. This style, however, may be intimidating. The new employee may become so worried about breaking the rules that it interferes with his or her ability to learn the important aspects of client care.

6-2: Both the LPN and UAP are responsible and accountable for their actions. The LPN is responsible for assessing that it was appropriate for and that the UAP had the skills to feed this client. The UAP accepted responsibility for this task. If the client had no problems swallowing or other conditions that interfered with eating and if the LPN also knew that the UAP was very experienced in feeding elderly clients, then the delegation was appropriate. In this situation, although the client was harmed, no fault was involved. Something occurred beyond the control of the LPN and UAP. The client had no history of choking or aspirating food, and both the LPN and UAP were appropriate in the delegation and acceptance of responsibility.

7-1: Initiations generally require a potential member to accept a dangerous challenge. If the person accomplishes the challenge, he or she is admitted as a full member of the group.

7-2: Yes. If one sexual partner says "No" and sexual intercourse takes place anyway, it constitutes rape.

8-1: Take the time to educate these clients about the risk factors of overexposure to sun—potential skin cancer, overall loss of skin elasticity, and increased wrinkles. Advise clients to limit their exposure and to always wear sun block to eliminate or reduce harmful sunrays. Eyewear also is important to eliminate harmful rays to the eyes.

8-2: Many women experience depression or anxiety at this time, which is normal. If anxiety or depression persists beyond a reasonable period, however, a client may need professional treatment.

9-1: Older people continue to learn throughout life; however, they may need more time than younger adults. Engaging in mental tasks helps prevent memory decline.

9-2: Signs of hearing loss include the following:
- Cupping the hand behind the ear
- Asking the person to repeat what was said
- Agreeing without waiting for the completion of the sentence
- Speaking in an excessively loud or quiet voice or acting indifferent

10-1: Examples of caregiving skills include bathing, providing oral hygiene, administering medications, giving skin care, changing positions, assisting with ambulation, promoting elimination, providing nourishment and fluids, and administering oxygen.

10-2: Some examples are nurses, nursing assistants, physicians, physical therapists, speech therapists, occupational therapists, pharmacists, rehabilitation counselors, and home health aides or nurses.

10-3: Examples include administering prescribed medications, obtaining specimens for laboratory tests, inserting a catheter, giving an enema, administering intravenous fluid, giving tube feedings, and changing wound dressings.

10-4: "Your family didn't visit you last evening." *(Reflecting)* "You're upset that your family didn't visit." *(Sharing perceptions)* "Did you expect your family to visit you last evening?" *(Direct questioning)* "How did you feel when your family did not visit last evening?" *(Indirect questioning)* "Oh." *(Giving general lead)*

10-5: A laboratory coat implies that the person works in an environment that requires protection of street clothing, such as someone who does research. It also suggests that the person's occupation requires more than secondary education. A ring on the third finger of the left hand informs others that the person is married and not interested in any other romantic relationships. Wearing a badge and gun is nonverbally symbolic that the person has authority for enforcing laws or rules.

11-1: There are several options:
- Ignore the remarks.
- Tell the LPN that she is highly insensitive and does not know what she is talking about.
- Discuss the issues with people who speak English as a second language and who have different cultural values and beliefs.

- Provide information about this client's culture and healthcare practices. Encourage the LPN to learn more from the client about what he understands about his medical problems, their treatment, how he carries out the treatment plan, and what his personal healthcare practices are.

11-2: Nurses must honor the client's beliefs and values. They may provide alternative explanations for the disease process, but they may not disparage the hot/cold theory. Explain the expected effects of the medications ordered by the physician and how the client may use heat and cold to alleviate symptoms. Do not admonish the client for her beliefs that hot foods will help her condition by restoring balance between heat and cold. Unless medically contraindicated, she can have chili peppers and hot coffee.

12-1: The limbic system and the hypothalamus play the greatest role in connecting the mind with physiologic functions.

12-2: Norepinephrine is a stimulating neurotransmitter that promotes activities regulated by the sympathetic division of the autonomic nervous system. Norepinephrine is associated with the following physiologic effects: increased heart rate, increased respirations, elevated blood pressure, hyperalertness, increased blood glucose, dilation of the pupils, dry mouth, slowed peristalsis and digestion, increased muscle tone, and inhibition of urination.

12-3: An infant who is not nurtured could experience mental and physical retardation. The infant may develop a feeling of hopelessness because his or her cries that communicate physical discomfort or a need for attention are unheeded. Eventually, the infant may not even cry or smile because he or she has learned that seeking comfort from another person is fruitless.

12-4: A score of 20 indicates cognitive impairment; a score between 24 and 30 is considered normal.

12-5: Failing one test may create sufficient anxiety to re-examine one's study habits and devote more time and attention to reviewing content for subsequent tests—a positive response. Consistent failure, however, is likely to create distress, evidenced by a lack of self-confidence, a negative self-image, and the stimulus to withdraw from rather than struggle to pass the course. Some believe that students should be grouped according to their innate cognitive abilities so that those who are academically gifted can be challenged and those who have normal or below normal ability can achieve at their own respective levels without feeling inferior. In other words, the stress is balanced according to the person's ability.

12-6: Despite red candy not containing any ingredient that could be considered an aphrodisiac, it is likely that approximately 30 people will report increased sexual desire. This is consistent with the placebo effect. Some might suggest that the red color of the candy may also psychologically suggest "hot," "active," or "stimulating."

12-7: Some other examples might include the smell of gingerbread or chocolate chip cookies, which conjure happy childhood memories. You may correlate the smell of lemons with cleanliness. The smell of ethanol (drinking alcohol) may disgust you because it reminds you of the way an intoxicated person smelled when he or she lost control of his or her temper. (The smell of carnations makes me [the author] sad because it reminds me of going to a funeral home where many floral arrangements surrounded the casket of a loved one.)

13-1: Unconsciously, the manager may feel inadequate, fear personal criticism, or believe that the board will ask him a question that he cannot answer. The emotional stress results in physical symptoms. His illness provides a legitimate excuse from one aspect of his job responsibilities. He lacks insight in recognizing the relationship between his emotional feelings and episodes of diarrhea. When no diagnosis is made, he looks for someone else who can identify his disorder.

14-1: Pain, fever, or palpating a lump in the breast will cause mild anxiety, for which most people will seek a consultation with a physician or health professional. Higher levels of anxiety may develop if a person is robbed or witnesses a violent crime. The person may have difficulty accurately recalling the perpetrator of the crime, the words that were exchanged, or the color, make, and model of the getaway car. The victim may react by becoming paralyzed with fear or hysterical. A witness may struggle with deciding whether to leave the scene to ensure his or her safety, assist the victim, or contact law-enforcement officials.

14-2: Nurses who work in a burn unit continually witness severe physical injuries. They are often unprepared initially for the magnitude of the horror they see. They observe their clients' pain and in some cases even feel responsible for causing it as a consequence of the nursing care they must perform. They respond to their clients' compromised breathing, repeated skin grafts, and altered body image that results from scars and reconstructive surgery. In some cases, they are at the bedside when the burn victim dies. When these nurses go home, they often stifle discussion of their work-related activities and feelings to spare the emotions of their own family. Failing to deal with the psychological effects of their work can eventually lead to a delayed stress response.

14-3: Never combine anxiolytic drugs with alcohol, sleeping medication, narcotic pain medication, or antihistamines. Use caution when driving a vehicle or operating mechanical equipment. Avoid medications, food, and beverages that may contain caffeine or other stimulating chemicals (e.g., appetite suppressants) or drugs that relieve fatigue because they counteract the anxiolytic's desired effect. Never stop taking a benzodiazepine abruptly. Check with the prescribing physician if pregnancy is desired or occurs. Continue taking buspirone for several weeks or longer to evaluate its maximum benefit.

14-4: Clients with congestive heart failure, hypotension, or diabetes who are using beta-adrenergic blockers should be monitored closely for adverse effects as the result of bradycardia, reduced cardiac output, low blood pressure, and hypoglycemia. Nonselective beta-adrenergic blockers are generally contraindicated for clients who have a chronic respiratory disorder such as emphysema or asthma because the drugs may compromise breathing and oxygenation.

15-1: Sociologists have argued whether heredity or environment has the greater influence on human behavior. Those who favor environment would argue that the expression of moods is a learned behavior modeled after others in one's immediate family network.

15-2: Eating hard cheese or fermented meat like pepperoni and drinking beer while taking MAOIs can cause a hypertensive crisis. If the client orders lemonade, pizza without cheese, and ham instead of pepperoni, he or she can avoid a hypertensive crisis.

15-3: Antidepressant drugs have a lengthy lag time before relieving symptoms. It is best to continue taking the prescribed medication for at least 2 to 4 weeks, and sometimes longer, to determine if the drug will be beneficial.

16-1: The client with anorexia nervosa believes that he or she is or may become obese. The person avoids eating and hides or rearranges food on the plate to avoid being confronted about self-starvation. He or she wears bulky clothes to disguise low body weight. The client tends to be cold, and fine hair covers the body to maintain body temperature. Blood pressure and heart rate are low, and the person may faint periodically. Many clients who develop anorexia nervosa are perfectionists driven to achieve. Their family relationships may be dysfunctional, and control over eating is the one facet of life the teenager or young adult can actually control.

16-2: The appetite center is in the hypothalamus, and various neurotransmitters and neurohormones affect it. Norepinephrine and serotonin are two substances that have been known to affect the desire to eat and the amount that is consumed. Recent research, however, also has identified that neurohormones such as leptin and orexin A and B are involved. The conclusion is that eating and eating disorders are very complex. Multiple etiologies and combinations of neurochemicals may activate or suppress appetite.

17-1: The person with alcoholism usually drinks to excess regularly, yet protests that he or she can control drinking. He or she drinks alone and conceals the amount consumed. The person cannot keep resolutions to stop drinking alcohol or reduce the quantity consumed and sometimes cannot recall his or her actions while under the influence of alcohol. He or she has a history of absenteeism from work or school and may spend money for bills or necessities on alcohol instead. There may be legal problems such as arrests for disorderly conduct, physical assault, or DUIL. During periods of abstinence, withdrawal develops.

17-2: Until the person with alcoholism stops denying his or her drinking problem, recovery is impossible. Generally, a spouse, family members, and friends have rescued the client from the consequences of drinking. Once he or she has sought help, the client with alcoholism has acquired some insight that his or her life is out of control.

18-1: Client A's symptoms are more suggestive of delirium; Client B's symptoms resemble the early stages of dementia.

18-2: When a client with schizophrenia becomes delusional, the nurse tells the client that he or she does not share the same belief based on various facts. It is unwise, however, to persist; persistent disagreements may lead the client to perceive a power struggle. The client may become agitated and hostile toward an uncompromising nurse. In addition, when a client is hallucinating, the nurse offers the observation that he or she is not experiencing similar phenomena, but offers to stay with the client until the hallucination subsides or the client can cope with it.

19-1: (1) Susceptible host, (2) infectious agent, (3) reservoir, (4) portal of exit, (5) means of transmission, (6) portal of entry

20-1: Inform the client that you are unsure of the value of vitamin C. Tell him that you will discuss this with his physician and get more information for him. Ask him how much vitamin C he planned to take and how often. Also tell the client that large doses of many vitamins may actually be harmful, so that it is important to have more information before making any decisions about any supplements.

21-1: The nurse should give both clients 75 mg of IM meperidine immediately. Giving less to the client who is calm or delaying the administration of medication for another hour indicates a bias that this client is experiencing less pain than the other, more demonstrative client.

21-2: A more effective dose may be 75 mg or 100 mg.

22-1: The first step is to convert the client's weight in pounds to kilograms by dividing 176 by 2.2 (2.2 lbs equals 1 kg). The converted weight is 80 kg. Using the formula, the client should have 100 mL/kg for the first 10 kg, for a sum of 1000 mL; 50 mL/kg for the next 10 kg, for a sum of 500 mL; and 15 mL/kg for the remaining weight in kg (60), for a sum of 630 mL. Adding 1000 mL, plus 500 mL, plus 630 mL provides a total of 2130 mL/day.

22-2: Client A has signs and symptoms of hypokalemia. Client B has signs and symptoms of hypocalcemia. Client C has signs and symptoms of hypernatremia.

22-3: Using the formula AG (anion gap) = Na + K − (Cl + HCO_3), the anion gap measures 25 mEq/L. This level exceeds the normal range, which indicates metabolic acidosis.

23-1: Client A has cardiogenic shock, Client B has hypovolemic shock, and Client C has distributive, anaphylactic shock.

23-2:
1. Irreversible stage
2. Compensation stage
3. Decompensation stage

24-1: The following supplies are necessary: a 1-liter container of the prescribed solution and primary, unvented, macrodrip tubing; an electronic infusion device may be used as well. A time strip may be attached to the container of fluid to promote hourly assessments.

24-2: A central venous catheter provides an alternative to inserting and replacing a peripheral venous access device every 48 to 72 hours. It allows the infusion of antineoplastic medication into larger veins rather than smaller peripheral veins, which these types of drugs tend to irritate. Filtered tubing is used to prevent the entry of bacteria—many antineoplastic drugs suppress the immune system, causing the client to become a susceptible host for infection.

24-3:
1. Other important assessment data to obtain include the trend in the client's BP and other vital signs since admission, the client's weight compared to admission, whether the client is thirsty, characteristics of oral mucous membranes, 24-hour totals of IV fluid intake volume and output measurements of urine, gastric fluid, and liquid stool. Review the following laboratory test results: complete blood cell, hemoglobin, and hematocrit levels, serum electrolyte levels, and urine specific gravity.
2. If fluid output exceeds fluid intake and assessment findings indicate hypovolemia, the client would most likely benefit from a hypotonic IV fluid solution, such as 5% dextrose in 0.45% saline. The fluid would be transported within blood cells, raising the BP; it would also eventually hydrate other body cells. The physician

also may order the addition of potassium chloride to the solution or a container of Ringer's solution. Potassium is lost in gastric fluid and diarrhea and requires replacement if the client is not consuming food. Ringer's solution contains several electrolytes, not only potassium and chloride, that provide electrolyte replacement. Once the client is rehydrated, the physician may rely on an isotonic solution, such as 0.9% sodium chloride, to maintain fluid balance. Potassium chloride may still be added to the infusing solution to prevent hypokalemia.

25-1: Potential concerns include respiratory problems, including atelectasis and pneumonia; circulatory problems, including thrombophlebitis and embolus; delayed wound healing; wound infection; and delayed metabolism and excretion of anesthetic agents and pain medications.

26-1: This is the bargaining stage. The client may previously have denied that he had a terminal illness and then experienced anger about his diagnosis.

27-1: Assess the client's breath sounds. Observe the respirations, particularly any increased rate or asymmetrical movement. Also monitor vital signs, especially noting a rapid pulse. Monitor the client's cough, noting any blood-tinged, frothy mucus. Following a thoracentesis, clients are at risk for pneumothorax or subcutaneous emphysema. If a large volume was removed with the thoracentesis, the client is at risk for a mediastinal shift, which may cause pulmonary edema or cardiac problems.

28-1: Based on your knowledge and experience, it is appropriate to suggest increasing fluid intake, inhaling steam, or using hot packs. Recommending a decongestant spray would be inappropriate.

28-2: Ask someone to get emergency assistance (call 911 or campus emergency response system). Stay with the woman. Ask her to place her scarf or another piece of clothing at the base of her nose. If possible, get the woman inside a building where it is warmer. If the building has an emergency kit, use it to get bandage supplies to replace the scarf or other clothing. If ice is available, apply an ice pack to the woman's nose. Reassure her that help is coming. Explain that there will be swelling and bleeding, but that the ice pack will help to stop the bleeding and reduce the swelling. Remain with her until help arrives.

29-1: Instruct them in careful handwashing technique. Teach the client to cover his mouth and nose with a tissue when coughing and to wash his hands frequently. In addition, the client must dispose of soiled tissues in a separate container. He should incinerate or dispose of soiled tissues according to the local community's guidelines for disposal of biohazardous waste. The couple must keep the apartment well ventilated.

29-2: Instruct the client to avoid environmental irritants, which include inhaled cigarette smoke. Explain that cigarette smoke contributes to irritation of the bronchial mucosa, leading to increased inflammation and mucus production. Advise the client that continued smoking would also affect his future health. Even though this episode is acute, smoking increases the risk of future episodes of acute bronchitis and eventually chronic bronchitis. If the client expresses interest, refer him or her to a smoking cessation program.

29-3: Possibilities include the following:
- Keep filters clean in air conditioners and furnaces.
- Use washable blankets on the bed.
- Damp mop and dust daily.
- Use lightweight washable cotton or synthetic fiber curtains.
- Keep floors bare except for washable cotton throw rugs.

29-4: Encourage the client to walk regularly and exercise her legs. Suggest that she wear support or antiembolism stockings. Tell her not to cross her legs when sitting and to avoid massaging her legs. If she feels that she has thrombophlebitis again, she needs to see her physician promptly.

29-5: Tell him that he needs to see his physician. A persistent nonsmoker's cough with blood-tinged mucus is a possible sign of lung cancer. Early diagnosis improves a client's chance of survival.

30-1: (A) The mitral valve is between the left atrium and left ventricle. (B) The tricuspid valve is between the right atrium and right ventricle. (C) The pulmonic valve is between the right ventricle and pulmonary artery.

30-2: (A) Pulmonary artery, (B) right atrium, (C) aorta, (D) left atrium

30-3: The sinoatrial (SA) node

30-4: (A) Increased heart rate, (B) increased heart rate, (C) decreased heart rate, (D) increased heart rate, (E) decreased heart rate

30-5: 72 bpm × 65 mL per stroke = 4680 mL or approximately 4.7 L/min; 72 bpm × 70 mL per stroke = 5040 mL or approximately 5 L/min.

31-1: A streptococcal microorganism may cause a severe sore throat, a condition referred to as *strep throat*. This type of infection, if undiagnosed, untreated, or inappropriately treated, can lead to complications such as rheumatic fever and rheumatic carditis. Rheumatic carditis causes changes within the heart that predispose the client to future valvular heart problems. Consulting with a primary health provider such as a physician, physician's assistant, or nurse practitioner is best to determine the cause of the child's sore throat. Treatment with an appropriate antibiotic for the sore throat may prevent complications.

31-2: Certain prior conditions affecting the heart increase the ability of pathogens to colonize endocardial tissue. Most pathogens find their way into the bloodstream through trauma such as during cleaning of the teeth or other procedures involving mucous membranes or other tissues that harbor microorganisms. Administering antibiotics before these procedures helps prevent recurring damage to the inner layer of the heart and heart valves.

31-3: The client is manifesting pulsus paradoxus because the difference between the systolic pressure first heard during expiration is more than 10 mm Hg than that identified during inspiration.

32-1: Terminate the activity immediately and then assess the client's physical status. Ask the client to describe the location and intensity of the chest pain and measure and evaluate vital signs. Use a pulse oximeter to measure the client's oxygen saturation and administer oxygen if the saturation level is less than 90%. Administer a prescribed nitrate or analgesic and modify the care plan with nursing orders to assist the client with hygiene and to provide rest periods intermittently.

32-2: Exercise increases heart rate and the myocardium's demand for oxygen. If either a stenotic or incompetent valve impairs blood circulation through the heart, cardiac output and perfusion of the coronary arteries supplying the myocardium are compromised. The client may experience chest pain. If the heart cannot contract effectively, heart failure may develop. The best way to determine the client's capacity for activity is for the client to undergo an echocardiogram and electrocardiogram while exercising.

33-1: Cardiac risk increases when the total cholesterol level divided by the HDL level is greater than 5. Client C has the lowest cardiac risk (3.8) despite having an elevated total cholesterol level. HDL reduces LDL. Therefore, the higher HDL level offsets the total cholesterol level that exceeds the recommended amount. Client B has a total cholesterol level within the recommended amount, but the HDL level is low. Client B's risk factor is calculated at 5.65. Client A has the highest cardiac risk (5.89) because the total cholesterol level is elevated and the HDL level is less than desired.

33-2: Advise the client to stop or never begin smoking. He or she should ensure that weight is appropriate for height. A physical examination and basic laboratory tests can identify cardiac risks such as hypertension and elevated levels of cholesterol, lipoprotein, and blood glucose, which diet and regular exercise can help minimize. Other diagnostic tests such as a stress electrocardiogram and electron-beam CT also may help determine the client's current cardiac health status. If early disease

is identified, the client must comply with the therapeutic regimen, which may include drug therapy.

34-1: Normal sinus rhythm is characterized by atrial and ventricular rates between 60 to 100 bpm. The conducted impulses occur regularly—they are equally timed rather than long or short pauses occurring between them. The SA node always initiates the heart conduction, as identified by a rounded upright P wave. The time from when the impulse is initiated to when the impulse reaches the AV node, known as the PR interval, is between 0.12 to 0.2 seconds. The ventricles depolarize, as represented by the QRS complex, at 0.12 seconds or less.

34-2: The right ventricle must pump blood to the lungs for oxygenation, and the left ventricle must pump oxygenated blood to all the cells, tissues, and organs of the body. Ineffective ventricular contraction caused by an erratically conducted rhythm impairs cardiopulmonary circulation and cellular oxygenation. Both have potentially fatal consequences unless treated. Most atrial dysrhythmias are not life-threatening unless the ventricular response is too rapid or slow to sustain an adequate cardiac output.

35-1: Ask if she has a history of high BP. Also, ask what she was doing just before you took her BP. Activity increases BP. Retake the BP after the neighbor rests for 10 minutes. If the repeat measurement is similar, write it down, give the written information to the neighbor, and advise her to make an appointment with her primary care physician within 1 month.

36-1: Client A is manifesting signs and symptoms of right-sided heart failure. Client B shows signs and symptoms more suggestive of left-sided heart failure.

36-2: Ask if the client has had his usual dose of digoxin today. When reporting initial assessment findings to the physician, discuss including digoxin or a similar drug in the current medical orders so that there is continuity of drug therapy. When administering the digoxin, assess the apical heart rate and withhold the medication if the heart rate is less than 60 bpm. Report the low heart rate to the physician. Ensure that the client who takes digoxin also has an adequate intake of foods rich in potassium or receives a pharmacologic potassium supplement. The potential for digitalis toxicity increases if the client becomes hypokalemic. Monitor for signs of digitalis toxicity such as anorexia, visual changes, and dysrhythmias; report such findings to the physician. Review the laboratory results of digitalis blood levels and report high or low findings.

37-1: Restlessness and confusion are signs of hypoxia in an older adult. Check Mr. Jones' cardiac and respiratory status, such as lung sounds, heart rhythm, heart sounds, and pulse oximetry. If hypoxia is not causing his symptoms, medications or sensory overload from the ICU may be responsible. As you assess Mr. Jones, re-orient him to his environment and take care of any obvious needs. Document the assessment findings and report the information to the physician.

38-1: The unit of donated blood is compatible. A client with Type A, Rh-positive blood can receive Type A or Type O, Rh-positive or Rh-negative blood. Type A, Rh-positive blood is exactly the same as the client's blood type. Because Rh-negative blood does not contain the Rh protein, however, the client is not at risk for an incompatibility reaction. That does not mean that there are no transfusion-related risks. The client may have other adverse reactions during the blood transfusion and requires close monitoring throughout.

39-1: The Z-track method ensures that the medication does not seep into the subcutaneous tissue. Iron that seeps into subcutaneous tissue can irritate and stain (tattoo) it.

39-2: Sickling causes the abnormally shaped RBCs to occlude small blood vessels. Blockage of small blood vessels in the brain results in cerebral injury from a loss of oxygen to the tissue and ultimately cellular death.

39-3: HbF is present during fetal development and the first 6 months after birth. It does not possess the propensity to sickle; therefore, those who inherit sickle cell disease do not experience symptoms until they are approximately 6 months old. HbA replaces HbF in those who do not inherit sickle cell anemia. Erythrocytes with molecules of HbA remain spherical and move easily throughout the vascular system. In those with sickle cell disease, HbS replaces HbF after approximately 6 months of age. HbS causes RBCs to become sickled when the blood becomes deoxygenated. The altered shape obstructs blood flow within the vascular system.

40-1: Because cancer cells migrate from their site of origin (the breast) to and through the lymphatic system, lymph nodes are removed during some mastectomy procedures. Excising lymph nodes removes cancerous cells and controls the spread of the disease via the lymphatic system. Lymph node removal, however, interrupts the flow of lymph as it returns to the venous system. This condition enables edema in the tissue to surround the location of node removal.

41-1: T-cell lymphocytes perform a cell-mediated response, which involves a cellular attack on an antigen. B-cell lymphocytes are responsible for a humoral response, in which chemicals called antibodies attack an antigen.

41-2: (1) Artificially acquired active immunity, (2) naturally acquired active immunity, and (3) passive immunity

42-1: Possibilities include milk, wheat, eggs, corn, peanuts, fish, strawberries, tomatoes, wool, latex, penicillin, sulfonamides, local anesthetics (e.g., procaine), aspirin, bee venom, cat dander, mold, grasses, poison ivy, and horse serum.

42-2: Diphenhydramine (Benadryl) blocks receptors for histamine, thus limiting and reducing an allergic reaction. Epinephrine (Adrenalin) blocks degranulation of mast cells. Prednisone (Meticorten) blocks the synthesis of leukotrienes and prostaglandins and stabilizes mast cells to prevent further release of histamine. Montelukast (Singulair) is a leukotriene-receptor antagonist that reduces swelling of the airway and promotes breathing by interfering with contraction of bronchial smooth muscles. Cromolyn (Intal, Crolom) is a mast-cell stabilizer taken prophylactically to prevent allergic reactions upon exposure to respiratory allergens.

42-3: Clients who need epinephrine manifest severe hypotension, difficulty breathing, tachycardia, palpitations, widespread swelling of the airway or tissues, and decreased level of consciousness.

42-4: Some measures by which to avoid inhaling allergens are to reduce dust from within the house, select curtains that can be laundered rather than require dry cleaning, use commercial cloths and mops that attract rather than dispense dust in the air, wear a face mask when cleaning, vacuum dust from air and cooling ducts, change furnace filters frequently, and limit outside activities on days when pollen counts are high. To avoid ingested allergens, the client should prepare foods from "scratch," read labels and learn words that mean the same or are related to personal food allergens, and bring a prepared "brown bag" lunch to potlucks or meetings that involve meals.

42-5: The immune system is unstimulated during remissions. The cause may be effective drug therapy, reduced or manageable physical and emotional stressors, or both. Exacerbations may occur when stressors accumulate, if the client is noncompliant with drug therapy, or if age-related changes or pregnancy alters the client's metabolism.

42-6: Unrelenting fatigue and pain can lead to depression, suicidal thoughts, and suicide attempts. They may affect self-esteem, as the person perceives himself or herself as "sick" rather than "well." They may alter role performance, as significant others must assume responsibilities for delegated tasks. Relationships may diminish because social activities exceed the person's comfort and endurance. Spiritual distress is possible, as the person questions the meaning of the burden of coping with a chronic illness.

43-1: Helper T cells recognize antigens and stimulate B cells to produce antibodies.

43-2: Saliva alone cannot transmit HIV/AIDS. Possibility of transmission is remote if there is a mixture of blood and saliva from a person infected with HIV.

43-3: 2C

43-4: The gp 120 protein extends from the capsid and binds to the CD4 receptor of the helper T4 lymphocyte.

43-5: Drug resistance occurs when strains of HIV develop mechanisms that promote their survival. When drug resistance develops, it can also affect the response to similar prescribed drugs. Drug resistance limits the ability to contain HIV and makes a person more susceptible to opportunistic infections. The best advice for people who must take antiretrovirals is to take them exactly as prescribed, never omit or delay any doses or stop taking any of the drugs in the prescribed regimen without consulting the physician, and keep appointments for blood tests.

44-1: The dura mater is the first layer, the arachnoid layer is the middle layer, and the pia mater is the innermost layer.

44-2: (A) Flexion of the arms indicates decorticate posturing. (B) Extension of the arms indicates decerebrate posturing. (C) No motor response is evidence of flaccid posture.

45-1: A client with IICP is usually difficult to arouse. He or she may be restless and confused. The client may have a headache or vomit without experiencing nausea. He or she also may have a seizure. The pupils may respond sluggishly to light and may be unequal. Extremities on one side of the body may be weak. The client may assume decorticate or decerebrate postures. Systolic BP rises, with a difference of more than 40 mm Hg between systolic and diastolic BP. The pulse decreases, and respirations become irregular. Eventually the client may become comatose and unresponsive to even painful stimuli.

46-1: Determine the duration of the client's symptoms. A thrombolytic agent has the best results when it is administered within 3 hours of the onset of stroke. Also measure the client's BP, because severe hypertension is an excluding criterion for use of a thrombolytic. Obtain the client's medical history, focusing on conditions or treatments that could predispose to bleeding. If someone witnessed the client's neurologic changes, inquire as to whether he or she observed a seizure. If there are no medical contraindications for administering a thrombolytic, treatment is ultimately postponed until diagnostic tests determine that the cause of the client's symptoms is an ischemic rather than a hemorrhagic event.

47-1: Although both clients have potentially life-threatening changes, Client A's symptoms suggest an epidural hematoma, which is a consequence of an arterial bleed. Arterial bleeding rapidly increases ICP because the accumulating blood displaces the dura and underlying brain tissue. To prevent herniation of the brainstem, the bleeding must be controlled and the clot must be evacuated. Client B's slower progressive changes suggest a subacute subdural venous bleed. Client B may also require neurosurgery, but the slower venous bleeding allows more time for surgical management before severe neurologic consequences develop.

48-1: Inform the transferring agency about the client's status in the six domains of neurologic impairment: motor, sensory, visual, language, cognitive, and affective. Also, indicate the client's current ability to perform ADLs and any unique interventions that the acute care health team and client have developed.

49-1: The fraction 20/20 is the accepted standard of normal vision. A person with 20/20 vision can see the letters on the line on the Snellen chart designated as 20/20 from a distance of 20 feet. A person with 20/200 visual acuity sees an object 20 feet away that a person with normal vision sees from 200 feet.

49-2: Do not attempt to remove the foreign body. Protect the eye by covering it with something stiff that does not place pressure on the eye (e.g., a metal shield, a paper cup trimmed to approximately 2 inches deep). Provide comfort to the child while arranging for transport to an emergency or urgent care center.

49-3: The most important advice is to encourage the person to have an ophthalmologic examination at least every 2 years, especially after 40 years of age.

50-1: Recommend the following:
- Wear protective devices when exposed to sustained loud noise (as in a work environment).
- Lower the volume on stereos and radios, especially in enclosed areas, and on headphones.
- Have hearing tested if you suspect a hearing deficit.

50-2: The appropriate nursing diagnosis is "**Risk for Deficient Fluid Volume** related to vomiting." An appropriate expected outcome is "The client will demonstrate adequate hydration as evidenced by normal vital signs and adequate urine output."

51-1: Possible questions include the following:
- Does anything trigger the nausea/vomiting, such as odors, food, medications, or activities?
- When do you experience this problem?
- How often have you vomited?
- Do you have a fever, or has fever accompanied the nausea/vomiting?
- What does the vomitus look like?
- Can you keep down any food or fluids?
- Have you changed your diet or medications?
- Have your bowel habits changed?
- Are you in contact with anyone who has had this problem?
- What are you doing to treat this problem?
- What effect do the treatments have?

52-1: Possible questions include the following:
- Has your appetite changed?
- Have you lost weight?
- Do you have any difficulty speaking or forming words?
- Have you noticed any sores or bleeding in your mouth?
- Do you wear dentures?
- When did you last see a dentist?
- Are you having any respiratory difficulties?
- Are you experiencing any pain or discomfort in your mouth or throat?

52-2: Caution the client that lying flat can increase intra-abdominal pressure and promote reflux. Urge the client to delay sleeping for 2 hours or to sleep with the head of the bed elevated at least 12 inches.

53-1: First explain that you are a student nurse and at this point have limited knowledge. Ask her if she receives regular medical care and if she has received adequate information about her condition and its management. You could also suggest that she seek a support group—her primary care provider should be able to give her information to contact appropriate resources.

53-2: Although appendicitis primarily affects adolescents and young adults, it can occur at any age. Ask the client if he or she has had an appendectomy.

54-1: Appropriate questions include the following:
- How long has this been happening?
- What was the previous consistency of the fecal material?
- Have you been around anyone with gastroenteritis?
- Are you experiencing nausea and vomiting?
- Are you eating and drinking normally?
- Are you voiding normally?
- What does the urine look like?
- Are your mucous membranes dry?

55-1: The third response is the best, because it gives correct information without breaking confidentiality. It also provides positive reassurance. The first answer provides only false reassurance. The second response is inappropriate—the client needs general information to allay her fears. The last answer may or may not be correct; it is not information this client needs. It also provides false reassurance.

56-1: Some hormones that affect metabolism include thyroxine, triiodothyronine, epinephrine, and norepinephrine. A hormone that affects growth is somatotropin; hormones such as antidiuretic hormone (ADH) and aldosterone regulate fluid and electrolyte balance. Leuteinizing hormone (LH), follicle-stimulating hormone (FSH), androgens from the adrenal cortex, estrogen, progesterone, and testosterone influence reproductive processes. Melatonin promotes sleep when light in the environment decreases; bright light inhibits its secretion.

57-1: A dietary deficiency of iodine may cause enlargement of the thyroid gland, a disorder referred to as an *endemic goiter.* Enlargement of the thyroid gland also may result from primary hyperfunctioning or hyperfunctioning in response to stimulation from the pituitary gland or hypothalamus. Another possible explanation is that the thyroid gland is swollen from an inflammatory condition like thyroiditis. Diagnostic tests and clinical assessments can help determine the definitive cause.

58-1: Type 1 diabetes occurs before adulthood when the beta cells of the pancreas are destroyed as the result of an autoimmune response and no longer secrete insulin. The person with Type 1 diabetes requires insulin injections to control his or her blood glucose level. Type 2 diabetes is most common in middle-aged or older adults. The beta cells make insulin, but the tissues tend to resist it. Consequently, the client needs oral medications to increase secreted insulin or to improve its use. Some clients with Type 2 diabetes can control their blood glucose level with diet and exercise; others eventually require insulin when the beta cells no longer respond to stimulation.

58-2: Glargine (Lantus) insulin is long acting; Lente insulin is intermediate acting; lispro (Humalog) is rapid acting; and Novulin R is short acting.

58-3: (1) Glyburide (DiaBeta) is a second-generation insulin releaser; it stimulates the beta cells to produce more insulin. (2) Metformin (Glucophage) and rosiglitazone (Avandia) increase the cells' response to insulin. (3) Miglitol (Glyset) and acarbose (Precose) cause a slower breakdown of complex carbohydrates so that the amount of insulin that is available and the level of blood glucose are more evenly balanced.

59-1: Amernorrhea refers to no menstruation. In primary amenorrhea, the female has never menstruated; in secondary amenorrhea, the female has had menstrual cycles but is no longer menstruating. Menorrhagia and metrorrhagia describe vaginal bleeding. The client with metorrhagia has vaginal bleeding at times other than during menstruation. A client with menorrhagia has an excessively heavy flow during menses.

60-1: The procedure may involve some discomfort, but the benefits of early detection of breast cancer far outweigh any temporary discomfort. Annual mammograms for women older than 50 years of age have greatly reduced mortality rates from breast cancer. As women age, the risk for breast cancer increases.

60-2: Provide privacy while dressing the wound. Allow the client to express her feelings about what she perceives. Refer her to Reach for Recovery. Explore options for breast reconstruction with her. Answer questions and address concerns about what lies ahead.

60-3: Use mild soap with minimal rubbing. Avoid perfumed soaps or deodorants. Use lotions, such as Lubriderm, Eucerin, or Aquaphor, for dryness. Use nondrying, antipruritic soap, such as Aveeno, for itching. Avoid tight clothing, underwire bras, excessive heat, and ultraviolet light (including the sun).

61-1: Recommend that males perform monthly testicular self-examinations and report any masses that they palpate. As men reach middle age, they can expect that the physician will perform a digital rectal examination to assess the size and texture of the prostate gland. A prostatic specific antigen test is done during yearly physical examinations to detect prostatic cancer. Other diagnostic tests are performed when the client develops symptoms.

62-1:
1. A painless ulceration, known as a chancre, is a characteristic of syphilis.
2. Discharge from the vagina, urethra, or penis accompanied by burning on urination could be caused by gonorrhea or chlamydia, which have similar symptoms. Because chlamydia is the most common bacterial STD, it is the most likely cause.
3. Genital warts, which erupt from an infection with human papilloma virus, are characterized by the development of soft, fleshy growths around the genitals.
4. An outbreak of multiple fluid-filled vesicles following 1 or 2 days of genital burning and itching suggest an infection with genital herpes.

63-1: Factors that contribute to urine volume include the following:
- Amount of fluid intake
- Kidney function
- Conditions that affect renal and urologic health, such as hypertension, diabetes, infection, neurologic impairment, and cardiovascular problems

63-2: Possible complications include urinary tract infection, secondary to insertion of the cystoscope and introduction of microorganisms, and urinary retention, secondary to edema caused by insertion of the cystoscope, which may obstruct urine flow.

64-1: A client who has an indwelling catheter is at risk for the introduction of pathogens to the urinary tract secondary to improper catheterization technique or improper catheter care. Strict asepsis is essential to prevent urinary tract infections in these clients.

64-2: The following questions are examples. You might find it helpful to research this topic more to understand the client's concerns.
- "If I am going to be in water, will it be cold?" *No, the water will be warm and comfortable.*
- "Will I have to take all of my clothes off if I am going to be in the water?" *Yes, but you will wear a special bathing suit during the procedure. The technicians will make sure that you are not chilled.*

- "Will it hurt?" *Discomfort from multiple shock waves may occur, so the doctor will administer regional or general anesthesia to promote comfort. Pain medication will be available following the procedure.*
- "I have heard there is noise during the procedure." *When the shock waves are aimed at the kidney stone, there is a muffled "firecracker" sound. The physician will let you know when this will happen.*
- "Will I be able to urinate after the procedure?" *Most clients can void after the procedure. Blood will probably appear in the urine for a few days. You may have to strain your urine for several days after the procedure, as small particles will pass within the urine. The physician will want to analyze these particles.*

64-3: Infection may be introduced through the urinary or respiratory tract or surgical incision. Nurses must practice strict aseptic technique and institute protective measures for the client. Examples include protecting the client from exposure by careful handwashing, using masks, and strictly monitoring urine, wound drainage, and attention to drainage tubes. Nurses will need to instruct visitors to wash hands and wear masks while the client is taking immunosuppressant drugs.

64-4: Some reasons may include unwillingness or lack of motivation to perform the procedure, unavailable home support, abdominal contraindications (e.g., multiple surgeries, back problems) that fluid from dialysis would aggravate, immunosuppression (predisposing the client to infection), and other medical conditions that may interfere with the success of CAPD.

65-1: The answer is #4. If the client has acute urinary retention and cannot void, catheterize him as soon as possible to relieve the problem. Find out if the catheter needs to be intermittent or indwelling.

65-2: The nurse should do the following:
- Use scrupulous aseptic technique when inserting the catheter.
- Never disconnect the drainage tubing from the drainage bag for any purpose, including obtaining a urine specimen or transporting or ambulating a client.
- Prevent the drainage bag from touching the floor.
- When raising the drainage bag above the client's bladder, clamp the drainage tube to prevent backflow of urine from the drainage bag to the bladder.
- Ensure a free flow of urine from the bladder to the drainage bag by ensuring that the tube has no kinks or twists and that the loops of the drainage tube are not positioned to allow urine to pool.
- Empty the drainage bag at least every 8 hours (more often if the client is using a leg bag).
- Prevent contamination of the drainage spout. Use a clean drainage receptacle for each client.

- Do not irrigate a catheter without an order. If a catheter must be irrigated, insert a catheter that has a three-way system.
- Wash hands before and after handling the catheter, tubing, or drainage bag.
- Provide perineal care twice a day by washing the perineal area with soap and water. Dry the area well.
- Obtain a urine specimen for culture if there are any signs of infection.

65-3: To determine specific client teaching needs, ask about her sexual history, ability to empty the bladder, hygiene habits, or any known obstructions to urinary flow, such as congenital anomalies, kidney stones, diabetes, or pregnancy.

65-4: The major cause of bladder cancer is cigarette smoke. The nurse needs to ask the client about his smoking, past and present, and any exposure to second-hand smoke.

66-1: Ask about and look for the following:
- When did this happen?
- Is the affected leg/foot in alignment?
- Is the pain sharp, dull, shooting, or throbbing? Is it constant or getting worse?
- Is there swelling, redness, or discoloration?
- Has he tried to bear weight? Has he tried to move the ankle? (Do not ask him to do so.)
- Does he have any numbness or burning or tingling?
- Are pedal pulses present?

67-1: Ask the man to remain recumbent. Elevate the affected ankle as much as possible. Remove any constricting sock. If ice or cold packs are available, apply those to the injury, taking care to protect bare skin. Ask someone to call for assistance, since this man will need further examination to determine the extent of the injury.

67-2: Signs of fracture would be complaints of pain and statements that she cannot move her arm. The arm would appear bent at an awkward angle; the muscles in the upper arm would seem to involuntarily contract.

67-3: Inform this client that the cause of RA remains unknown. Current research points to infectious, genetic, and endocrine factors. Abnormal or altered immunoglobulin G (IGG) antibodies develop when exposed to an antigen. No evidence has suggested that experimentation or abuse of drugs or alcohol leads to the development of RA.

67-4: The client with an open compound fracture of the tibia is most at risk, secondary to the traumatic injury and direct bacterial contamination from the open fracture.

67-5: The assessment must include family history of osteoporosis and skeletal fractures; the client's history of fractures; sources of calcium intake; exercise patterns; menstrual history; and history of smoking, caffeine intake, alcohol, and use of corticosteroids for other medical conditions. Also ask the client about any history of back pain or deformity. Include physical examination of thoracic spine deformities and evidence of loss of height. The client will need information about osteoporosis, risk factors, and measures to prevent or slow the progression of osteoporosis. She also will need diet instructions, taking into account that she does not like milk.

68-1: Intact skin acts as a barrier to microorganisms and prevents the loss of extracellular fluid. An impairment of an extensive area of skin can cause acute pain and alter temperature regulation. Injury to the skin can result in scarring, which may create cosmetic problems for the client.

68-2:
A. Vesicle
B. Macule
C. Papule
D. Pustule

69-1: Begin by reassuring the parents that infestation with head lice occurs in all socioeconomic groups and does not indicate poor hygiene or housekeeping. Explain that lice are insects transferred from an infected person to another through direct skin contact but more likely through contact with lice found on clothing such as hats and collars. Also teach parents that to totally eradicate the infestation, adults, nymphs, and nits must be destroyed. To destroy the lice, they will need to apply a pediculicide and comb the hair daily with a lice comb until all nits are gone. All infected family members require treatment. Objects that may contain lice, such as pillows and clothing, must be washed. Carpets and furniture require meticulous vacuuming.

70-1: One arm is equal to 9 %, and the anterior chest is equal to 18 %, for a total of 27 % TBSA.

70-2: According to the Parkland-Baxter formula, the client should receive 12,218 mL in the first 24 hours. Half (or 6,109 mL) is infused within the first 8 hours of the burn. The time is calculated from the time of the burn, not the time that the client arrived in the ED. The nurse monitors the client's response to fluid resuscitation. He or she adjusts the volume and rate of infusion to promote a urine output of 50 mL per hour.

70-3: Currently, the preferred method of wound management is the closed method. This method has replaced the open method because there are now effective antimicrobials that reduce the potential for infection despite covering the burned surface. The closed method also reduces fluid losses and helps the client maintain normal body temperature, both of which reduce hypercatabolic processes.

Nursing Resources

The Academy for Guided Imagery
P.O. Box 2070
Mill Valley, CA 94942
(800) 726-2070
FAX: (415) 389-9342
http://www.healthy.net/agi

Academy of Medical-Surgical Nurses
East Holly Avenue, Box 56
Pitman, NJ 08071-0056
(856) 256-2323
FAX: (856) 589-7463
http://www.medsurgnurse.org/

Academy of Psychosomatic Medicine
5824 North Magnolia
Chicago, IL 60660
(773) 784-2025
FAX: (773) 784-1304
http://www.apm.org/

Acoustic Neuroma Association
600 Peachtree Pkwy, Suite 108
Cumming, GA 30041
(770) 205-8211
FAX: (770) 205-0239
http://ANAusa.org/

Action on Smoking and Health (ASH)
2013 H Street, NW
Washington, DC 20006
(202) 659-4310
http://www.ash.org

Administration on Aging
U.S. Department of Health and Human Services
330 Independence Avenue, SW
Washington, DC 20201
(202) 619-0724 or (800) 677-1116
FAX: (202) 260-1012
http://www.aoa.dhhs.gov

Adopt a Special Kid
7700 Edgewater Drive, Suite 320
Oakland, CA 94621
(888) 680-7349
FAX: (510) 553-1747
http://www.adoptaspecialkid.org

Adoption Service Information Agency, Inc.
8555 16th St.
Suite 600
Silver Spring, MD
(301) 587-7068

FAX: (301) 587-3869
http://www.asia-adopt.org/

Adoption World, Inc.
820 South 4th St., 2nd Floor
Philadelphia, PA 19147
(215) 336-5135
http://adoptionworld.org

Adult Children of Alcoholics
P.O. Box 3216
Torrance, CA 90510
(310) 534-1815
http://www.adultchildren.org/

Agency for Healthcare Research and Policy
Executive Office Center
2101 East Jefferson Street, Suite 501
Rockville, MD 20852
(301) 594-7195
http://www.ahcpr.gov/

AIDS Action Committee of Massachusetts
131 Clarendon Street
Boston, MA 02116
(617) 437-6200
FAX: (617) 437-6445
http://www.aac.org/

AIDS Drug Assistance Programs (ADAP)
Critical Path AIDS Project
2062 Lombard Street
Philadelphia, PA 19146
(215) 545-2212
FAX: (215) 735-2762
http://www.critpath.org/docs/adap.htm

AIDS Treatment Data Network
611 Broadway, Suite 613
New York, NY 10012
(212) 260-8868
http://www.atdn.org/

AIDS Virus Education and Research Trust (AVERT)
4 Brighton Road
Horsham, West Sussex, RH13 5BA
United Kingdom
44 (0)1403 210202
FAX: 44 (0)1403 211001
http://www.avert.org/

Al-Anon Family Group Headquarters, Inc.
1600 Corporate Landing Parkway
Virginia Beach, VA 23454-5617
(757) 563-1600

FAX: (757) 563-1655
http://www.al-anon.alateen.org/

Alcoholics Anonymous
Box 449, Grand Central Station
New York, NY 10163
(212) 870-3400
FAX: (212) 870-3003
http://www.alcoholics-anonymous.org

**Alexander Graham Bell Association for the Deaf
and Hard of Hearing**
3417 Volta Place, NW
Washington, DC 20007-2778
(202) 337-5220
FAX: (202) 337-8314
http://www.agbell.org

Allergic and Nonallergic Rhinitis
National Jewish Medical and Research Center
1400 Jackson Street
Denver, CO 80206
(800) 222-5864
http://www.njc.org

Alliance for Aging Research
2021 K Street, NW
Suite 305
Washington, DC 20006
(202) 293-2856
FAX: (202) 785-8574
http://www.agingresearch.org/

Alliance of Cardiovascular Professionals
4456 Corporation Lane, #164
Virginia Beach, VA 23462
(757) 497-1225
FAX: (757) 497-0010
http://www.acp-online.org

Alzheimer's Association
919 North Michigan Avenue, Suite 1100
Chicago, IL 60611-1676
(800) 272-3900
FAX: (312) 335-1110
http://www.alz.org

**Alzheimer's Disease Education and Referral
(ADEAR) Center**
P.O. Box 8250
Silver Spring, MD 20907-8250
(800) 438-4380
http://www.alzheimers.org

**American Academy of Allergy, Asthma,
and Immunology**
611 East Wells Street
Milwaukee, WI 53202
(800) 822-2762
http://www.aaaai.org

American Academy of Ambulatory Care Nurses
East Holly Avenue, Box 56
Pitman, NJ 08071-0056
(800) 256-2350
FAX: (856) 589-7463
http://aaacn.inurse.com/default.htm

American Academy of Cardiovascular Perfusion
P.O. Box 3596
Allentown, PA 18106-0596
(610) 395-4853

FAX: same number
http://members.aol.com/Office AACP/home.html

American Academy of Cosmetic Surgery
737 N. Michigan Ave.
Suite 820
Chicago, IL 60611
(312) 981-6760
FAX: (312) 981-6787
http://www.cosmeticsurgery.org/

American Academy of Dermatology
1350 I Street, NW
Suite 880
Washington, D.C. 20005
(202) 842-3555
FAX: (202) 842-4355
http://www.aad.org/

American Academy of Emergency Medicine
611 East Wells Street
Milwaukee, WI 53202
(800) 884-2236
FAX: (414) 276-3349
http://www.aaem.org/

**American Academy of Neurological
and Orthopaedic Surgeons**
2300 South Rancho Dr., Suite 202
Las Vegas, NV 89102
(702) 388-7390
FAX: (702) 388-7395
http://www.aanos.org/

American Academy of Neurology
1080 Montreal Ave.
St. Paul, MN 55116
(651) 695-1940
http://www.aan.com

American Association for the Advancement of Science
1200 New York Ave., NW
Washington, DC 20005
(202) 326-6400
FAX: (202) 371-9526
http://www.aaas.org/

American Association of Clinical Endocrinologists
1000 Riverside Ave., Suite 205
Jacksonville, FL 32204
(904) 353-7878
FAX: (904) 353-8185
http://www.aace.com/

American Association of Critical Care Nurses
101 Columbia
Aliso Viejo, CA 92656-4109
(949) 362-2020
FAX: (949) 362-2020
http://www.aacn.org/

American Association of Diabetes Educators
100 West Monroe
Suite 400
Chicago, IL 60603
(800) 338-3633
FAX: (312) 424-2427
http://www.aadenet.org/

American Association of Echocardiography
1500 Sunday Drive, Suite 102
Raleigh, NC 27607

(919) 787-5181
FAX: (919) 787-4916
http://asecho.org/

American Association of Endocrine Surgeons
c/o Christopher R. McHenry, MD
2500 MetroHealth Drive
Cleveland, OH 44109-1908
(216) 778-4753
FAX: (216) 778-3774
http://www.endocrinesurgeons.org/

American Association of Immunologists
9650 Rockville Pike
Bethesda, MD 20814-3994
http://12.17.12.70/aai/default.asp

American Association of Kidney Patients
3505 E. Frontage Road
Suite 315
Tampa, FL 33607
(800) 749-2257
FAX: (813) 636-9122
www.aakp.org

American Association of Managed Care Nurses, Inc. (AAMCN)
4435 Waterfront Drive
Suite 101
Glen Allen, VA 23060
(804) 747-9698
FAX: (804) 747-5316
www.aamcn.org

American Association of Nephrology Nurses
East Holly Avenue Box 56
Pitman, NJ 08071-0056
(888) 600-2662
FAX: 856-589-7463
http://anna.inurse.com/

American Association of Neuroscience Nurses
4700 West Lake Ave.
Glenview, IL 60025
(888) 557-2266
FAX: 847/375-6333
http://www.aann.org/

American Association of Retired Persons
601 E. St. NW
Washington, DC 20049
(800) 424-3410
http://www.aarp.org/

American Association of Spinal Cord Injury Nurses
75-20 Astoria Blvd.
Jackson Heights, NY 11370
(718) 803-3782
FAX: (718) 803-0414
http://www.aascin.org/

American Association of Tissue Banks
1350 Beverly Rd., Suite 220-A
McLean, VA 22101
(703) 827-9582
FAX: (703) 356-2198
http://www.aatb.org/

American Board of Electroencephalography and Neurophysiology
1701 West Charleston Ave., Suite 105
Las Vegas, NV 89102

(702) 388-4244
FAX: (702) 388-0333
http://www.ecnsociety.com/aben.htm

American Burn Association
625 N. Michigan Ave., Suite 1530
Chicago, IL 60611
(312) 642-9260
FAX: (312) 642-9130
http://www.ameriburn.org/

American Cancer Society
1599 Clifton Road, NE
Atlanta, GA 30329-4251
(404) 320-3333 or (800) ACS-2345
http://www.cancer.org

American Chronic Pain Association
P.O. Box 850
Rocklin, CA 95677
(916) 632-0922
FAX: (916) 632-3208
http://www.theacpa.org

American College of Allergy, Asthma & Immunology
85 West Algonquin Road, Suite 550
Arlington Heights, IL 60005
(800) 842-7777
http://allergy.mcg.edu/

American College of Cardiovascular Nursing
P.O. Box 3345
Riverview, FL 33568-3345
(813) 677-1116
FAX: (813) 671-8912
http://www.accn.net/

American College of Emergency Physicians
1125 Executive Circle
Irving, TX 75038-2522
(800) 798-1822
FAX: (972) 580-2816
http://www.acep.org/

American College of Surgeons
633 N. Clair Street
Chicago, IL 60611-3211
(312) 202-5000
FAX: (312) 202-5001
http://www.facs.org/

American Council for Headache Education
19 Mantua Road
Mount Royal, NJ 08061
(856) 423-0258
FAX: (856) 423-0082
http://www.achenet.org/

American Diabetes Association
1701 N. Beauregard Street
Alexandria, VA 22311
(800) DIABETES
FAX: (703) 549-6995
http://www.diabetes.org

American Dietetic Association
216 West Jackson Blvd.
Chicago, IL 60606
(312) 899-0040
http://www.eatright.org/

American Foundation for AIDS Research (amFAR)
1828 L Street, NW, #802
Washington, DC 20036-5104
(202) 331-8600
FAX: (202) 331-8606
http://www.amFAR.org/

American Foundation of Thyroid Patients
18534 N. Lyford
Katy, TX 77449
(281) 855-6608
http://www.thyroidfoundation.org/

American Gastroenterological Association
7910 Woodmont Avenue
7th Floor
Bethesda, MD 20814
(301) 654-2055
FAX: (301) 652-3890
http://www.gastro.org/

American Hair Loss Council
125 7th St., Suite 625
Pittsburgh, PA 15222
(412) 765-3666
FAX: (412) 765-3669
http://www.ahlc.org/

American Heart Association
National Center
7272 Greenville Avenue
Dallas, TX 75231
(800) 242-8721
http://www.americanheart.org/

American Holistic Nurses' Association
P.O. Box 2130
Flagstaff, AZ 86003-2130
(800) 278-2462
http://ahna.org

American Kidney Stone Management, Ltd
3525 Olentangy River Road
Columbus, Ohio 43214
1-800-637-5188
FAX: (614) 447-9374
http://www.aksm.com

American Liver Foundation
75 Maiden Lane, Suite 603
New York, NY 10038
(800) 465-4837
http://www.liverfoundation.org/

American Lung Association
1740 Broadway
New York, NY 10019
(212) 315-8700 or (800) LUNG USA
http://www.lungusa.org

The American Nurses Association
600 Maryland Avenue, SW
Suite 100 West
Washington, DC 20024
1-800-274-4262
FAX: (202) 651-7001
http://www.nursingworld.org/

American Pain Society
4700 West Lake Avenue
Glenview, IL 60025
(847) 375-4715

FAX: (877) 734-8758
http://www.ampainsoc.org

American Physiological Society
9650 Rockville Pike
Bethesda, MD 20814-3991
(301) 530-7164
http://www.the-aps.org/

American Psychiatric Association
1400 K Street, NW
Washington, DC 20005
(888) 357-7924
FAX: (202) 682-6850
http://www.psych.org/

American Psychological Association
750 First Street, NE
Washington, DC 20002-4242
(202) 336-5510
http://www.apa.com

American Psychosomatic Society
6728 Old McLean Village Drive
McLean, VA 22101-3906
(703) 556-9222
FAX: (703) 556-8729
http://www.psychosomatic.org/

The American Self-Help Clearinghouse
http://mentalhelp.net/selfhelp/

American Social Health Association
P.O. Box 13827
Research Triangle Park, NC 27709
(919) 361-8400
FAX: (919) 361-8425
http://www.ashastd.org/

American Society for Dermatologic Surgery
930 E. Woodfield Road
Schaumburg, IL 60168-4014
(800) 441-2737
http://www.asds-net.org

American Society for Histocompatibility and Immunogenetics
1700 Commerce Parkway
Suite C
Mt. Laurel, NJ 08054
(856) 638-0428
FAX: (856) 439-0525
http://www.ashi-hla.org/index.htm

American Society of Hematology
1900 M Street, NW
Suite 200
Washington, DC 20036
(202) 776-0544
FAX: (202) 776-0545
http://www.hematology.org/

American Society of Interventional Pain Physicians
2831 Lone Oak Road
Paducah, KY 42003
(270) 554-8373
FAX: (270) 554-8987
http://asipp.org

American Society of Pain Management Nurses
7794 Grove Drive
Pensacola, FL 32514
(850) 473-0233

FAX: (850) 484-8762

http://www.aspmn.org

American Society of PeriAnesthesia Nurses

10 Melrose Avenue, Suite 110

Cherry Hill, New Jersey 08003-3696

(877) 737-9696

FAX: (856) 616-9601

http://www.aspan.org

American Society of Plastic Surgeons

444 E. Algonquin Rd.

Arlington Heights, IL

(888) 475-2784

http://www.plasticsurgery.org/

American Speech-Language-Hearing Association

10801 Rockville Pike

Rockville, MD 20852

1-800-498-2071 or 301-897-5700

http://www.asha.org

American Spinal Injury Association

2020 Peachtree Rd., NW

Atlanta, GA 30309-1402

(404) 355-9772

FAX: (404) 355-1826

http://www.asia-spinalinjury.org/

American Stroke Association: A Division of the American Heart Association

7272 Greenville Ave.

Dallas, TX 75231

(888) 478-7653

http://www.strokeassociation.org/

American Thyroid Association

6066 Leesburg Pike, Suite 650

Falls Church, VA 22041

(703) 998-8890

FAX: (703) 998-8893

http://www.thyroid.org/

American Tinnitis Association

P.O. Box 5

Portland, OR. 97207

(800) 634-8978 or (503) 248-9985

FAX: (503) 248-0024

http://www.ata.org

Amputee Resource Foundation of America

6480 Wayzata Boulevard

Golden Valley, Minnesota 55426

http://www.amputeeresource.org/

Amyotrophic Lateral Sclerosis Association of America

27001 Agoura Road, Suite 150

Calabasas Hills, CA 91301-5104

(800) 782-4747 or (818) 880-9007

http://www.alsa.org/

Animated American Sign Language Dictionary

5451 Woodland Lane, SW

Fort Lauderdale, FL 33312

http://www.bconnex.net/~randys/index_nf.html

Anxiety Disorders Association of America

8730 Georgia Avenue, Suite 600

Silver Spring, MD 20910, USA

(240) 487-0120

http://www.adaa.org/

Arthritis Foundation

PO Box 7669

Atlanta, Georgia 30357-0669

1-800-283-7800

http://www.arthritis.org/

Artificial Intelligence Laboratory

Massachusetts Institute of Technology

200 (545) Technology Square

MIT Building NE43

Cambridge, MA 02139

(617) 253-6218

http://www.ai.mit.edu/

Association for the Advancement of Behavior Therapy

305 7th Avenue, 16th Floor

New York, NY 10001-6008

(212) 647-1890

FAX: (212) 647-1865

http://www.aabt.org

Association for the Advancement of Medical Instrumentation

1110 North Glebe Road

Suite 220

Arlington, VA 22201-4795

(703) 525-4890

FAX: (703) 525-1424

http://www.aami.org/

Association for Applied Psychophysiology and Biofeedback

10200 W. 44th Avenue, Suite 304

Wheat Ridge, CO 80033-2840

(303) 422-8436

FAX: (303) 422-8894

http://aapb.org/

The Association for the Cure of Cancer of the Prostate

1250 4th St., Suite 360

Santa Monica, CA 90401

(800) 757-CURE or (310) 458-2873

FAX: (310) 458-8074

http://www.capcure.org/

The Association for Integrative Medicine

Box 1

Mont Clare, PA 19453

(610) 933-8145

http://www.integrativemedicine.org/

Association for Rehabilitation Nurses

4700 West Lake Ave.

Glenview, IL 60025

(800) 229-7530 or (847) 375-4710

FAX: (877) 734-9384

http://www.rehabnurse.org/

Association of Perioperative Registered Nurses

2170 South Parker Road, Suite 300

Denver, CO 80231-5711

(800) 755-2676 or (303) 755-6300

http://www.aorn.org/

Association of Rehabilitation Nurses

4700 W. Lake Ave.

Glenview, IL 60025

(800) 229-7530 or (847) 375-4710

FAX: (877) 734-9384

http://www.rehabnurse.org/

Asthma and Allergy Foundation of America
1233 20th Street, NW
Suite 402
Washington, DC 20036
(202) 466-7643
FAX: (202) 466-8940
http://www.aafa.org

Better Hearing Institute
515 King Street, Suite 420
Alexandria, VA 22314
(703) 684-3391
(703) 684-3394
http://www.betterhearing.org/

Bioethics Network
http://www.bioethics.net

Biorobotics Laboratory
Department of Electrical Engineering
University of Washington
Box 352500
Seattle, WA 98195-2500
(206) 543-2197
FAX: (206) 221-5264
http://brl.ee.washington.edu/BRL/

Blood and Marrow Transplant Information Network
2900 Skokie Valley St., Suite B
Highland Park, IL 60035
(888) 597-7674
FAX: (847) 433-4599
http://www.bmtinfonet.org/

Brain Aneurysm Foundation
295 Cambridge St.
Boston, MA 02114
(617) 723-3870
FAX: (617) 723-8672
http://neurosurgery.mgh.harvard.edu/baf

Breast Implants Information
c/o Food and Drug Administration
HFE-88
Rockville, MD 20857
http://www.fda.gov/cdrh/breastimplants/index.html

Burn Surgery Organization
c/o Brigham & Women's Hospital
Plastic Surgery Department
75 Francis St.
Boston, MA 02115
(617) 732-5465
http://burnsurgery.org

Cancer Information Service (CIS)
National Cancer Institute (NCI)
Building 31, Room 10A31
31 Center Drive, MSC 2580
Bethesda, MD 20892
1-800-422-6237
Cancernet: *http://cancernet.nci.nih.gov*

Cardiac Arrest Survivor Network
http://www.casn-network.com

CDC National Prevention Information Network
P.O. Box 6003
Rockville, MD 20850
(800) 458-5231
FAX: (888) 282-7681
http://www.cdcnpin.org/

Cells Alive
http://www.cellsalive.com/

Center for Food Safety and Applied Nutrition
5100 Paint Branch Parkway
College Park, MD 20740-3835
(888) 723-3366
http://vm.cfsan.fda.gov/list.html

Center for the Study of Anorexia and Bulimia
1 West 91st Street
New York, NY 10024
(212) 595-3449
http://www.4woman.gov/nwhic/references/mdreferrals/csab.htm

Centers for Disease Control and Prevention
1600 Clifton Road, NE
Atlanta, GA 30333
(800) 311-3435
http://www.cdc.gov

The CFIDS (Chronic Fatigue Immune Dysfunction Syndrome) Association of America
P.O. Box 220398
Charlotte, NC 28222-0398
(800) 442-3437
FAX: 704-365-9755
http://www.cfids.org/

Children of Aging Parents (CAPs)
1609 Woodbourne Road, Suite 302A
Levitown, PA 19057
(800) 227-7294
http://www.caps4caregivers.org/

Christopher Reeve Foundation
500 Morris Ave.
Springfield, NJ 07081
(800) 225-0292
FAX: (973) 912-9433
http://www.paralysis.org/

The Compassionate Friends, Inc.
P.O. Box 3696
Oak Brook, IL 60522-3696
(630) 990-0010
FAX: (630) 990-0246
http://www.compassionatefriends.org

Consortium for Spinal Cord Medicine
801 18th St., NW
Washington, DC 20006-3517
(202) 416-7611
FAX: 202-331-1657
http://www.scicpg.org/

Crohn's and Colitis Foundation of America (CCFA)
386 Park Avenue South, 17th Floor
New York, NY 10016-8804
(800) 932-2423
FAX: 212-779-4098
http://www.ccfa.org/

Cultural Diversity in Health Care
http://www.ggalanti.com/index.html

Cystic Fibrosis Research Inc. (CFRI)
Bayside Business Plaza
2672 Bayshore Parkway, Suite 520
Mountain View, CA 94043
(650) 404-9975
FAX: (650) 404-9981
http://www.cfri.org/home.htm

Dermatology Nurses' Association
East Holly Ave., Box 56
Pitman, NJ 08071
(800) 454-4362
FAX: (856) 589-7463
http://www.dna.inurse.com

Diabetes Action Research and Education Foundation
426 C Street, NE
Washington, DC 20002
(202) 333-4520
http://diabetesaction.org/

The Education Center for Prostate Cancer Patients
380 North Broadway, Suite 304
Jericho, NY 11753
(516) 942-5000
FAX: (516) 942-5025
http://www.ecpcp.org/

Eldercare Locator
927 15th Street, NW, 6th floor
Washington, DC 20005
(800) 677-1116
http://www.eldercare.gov/

Emergency Nurses Association
915 Lee Street
Des Plains, IL 60016-6569
(800) 243-8362
http://www.ena.org/

The Endocrine Society
4350 East West Highway, Suite 500
Bethesda, MD 20814
(301) 941-0200
FAX: (301) 941-0259
http://www.endo-society.org/

Endometriosis Association
8585 North 76th Place
Milwaukee, WI 53223
(800) 992-3636
FAX: (414) 355-6065
http://endometriosisassn.org/

Epilepsy Foundation of America
4351 Garden City Drive
Landover, MD, 20785-7223
(800) 332-1000
http://www.efa.org/

Families USA
1334 G Street, NW
Washington, DC 20005
(202) 628-3030
FAX: (202) 347-2417
http://familiesusa.org

Federation of Spine Associations
6300 North River Rd.
Rosemont, IL 60018
(847) 823-7186 or (800) 346-AAOS
FAX: (847) 823-8125
http://www.aaos.org/

The Gerontological Society of America
1030 15th Street NW Suite 250
Washington, DC 20005
(202) 842-1275
FAX: (202) 842-1150
http://www.geron.org

Guillain-Barré Syndrome Foundation International
P.O. Box 262
Wynnwood, PA 9096
(610) 667-0131
FAX: 610-667-7036
http://www.guillain-barre.com/

Health and Human Services Minority HIV/AIDS Initiative
Office of Minority Health Resource Center (OMHRC)
P.O. Box 37337
Washington, DC 20013-7337
301-230-7874 or (800) 444-6472
FAX: 301-230-7198
http://www.omhrc.gov/OMH/AIDS/aidshome_new.htm

Health Resources and Services Administration
Division of Transplantation
5600 Fishers Lane, Room 7C22
Rockville, MD 20857
(301) 443-7577
http://www.hrsa.gov/OSP/dot/dotmain.htm

Healthy People 2010
http://www.health.gov/healthypeople

Hepatitis Foundation International
30 Sunrise Terrace
Cedar Grove, NJ 07009-1423
(973) 239-1035 or (800) 891-0707
FAX: (973) 857-5044
http://www.hepfi.org

Housecall Medical Resources, Inc.
6501 Deane Hill Drive
Knoxville, TN 37919
(865) 292-6261
FAX: (865) 292-6288
http://www.housecall.com/

Hysterectomy Educational Resources & Services (HERS)
422 Bryn Mawr
Bala Cynwyd, PA 19004
(610) 667-7757
FAX: (610) 667-8096
http://www.ccon.com/hers/

Indian Health Service National Diabetes Program
The Reyes Building
5300 Homestead Road, NE
Albuquerque, NM 87110
(505) 248-4182
FAX: (505) 248-4188
http://www.ihs.gov/MedicalPrograms/Diabetes/index.asp

Information Center for Individuals with Disabilities
P.O. Box 750119
Arlington Heights, MA 02475
FAX: (781) 860-0673
http://www.disability.net/

Infusion Nurses Society
220 Norwood Park South
Norwood, MA 02062
(781) 440-9408
FAX: (781) 440-9409
http://www.ins1.org/

The Insulin-Free World Foundation
677 Craig Road, Suite 105
St. Louis, MO 63141-7115
314-991-8004 or (888) 746-4439

FAX: (314) 991-2276
http://www.insulin-free.org/

International Academy of Cardiology
P.O. Box 17659
Beverly Hills, CA 90209
(310) 657-8777
FAX: (310) 275 8922
http://www.cardiologyonline.com/

International Association of Laryngectomees
8900 Thornton Road, Box 99311
Stockton, CA 95209
(866) 425-3678
FAX: (209) 472-0516
http://www.larynxlink.com/

International Association of Sickle Cell Nurses and Physician Assistants
Duke University Medical Center
Box 2916
Durham, NC 27710
(336) 716-4324
http://www.emory.edu/PEDS/SICKLE/parnpage.htm

International Cancer Alliance for Research and Education
4853 Cordell Ave., Suite 11
Bethesda, MD 20814
(301) 654-7933 or (800) 422-7361
FAX: (301) 654-8684
http://www.icare.org

International Food Information Council Foundation
1100 Connecticut Avenue N.W., Suite 430
Washington D.C. 20036
(202) 296-6540
FAX: (202) 296-6547
http://www.ific.org/

International Foundation for Functional Gastrointestinal Disorders
P.O. Box 17864
Milwaukee, WI 53217-8076
(888) 964-2001 or (414) 964-1799
FAX: (414) 964-7176
http://www.iffgd.org

International Hearing Dog, Inc.
5901 East 89th Avenue
Henderson, CO 80640
(303) 287-3277
FAX: (303) 287-3425
http://www.ihdi.org

International Myeloma Foundation
12650 Riverside Dr., Suite 206
North Hollywood, CA 91607-3421
(800) 452-2873
FAX: 818-487-7454
http://www.myeloma.org/

International Ostomy Association
c/o British Colostomy Association
15 Station Road
Reading Berks RG1 1LG
England
44 1189 391537
FAX: 44 1189 569095
http://www.ostomyinternational.org

International Society for Adult Congenital Heart Disease
1500 Sunday Drive, Suite 102
Raleigh, NC 27607
(919) 787-5181

International Society of Endovascular Specialists
1928 East Highland Street, Suite F104-605
Phoenix, AZ 85016
(602) 240-5833
http://isesonline.org/

The International Society of Psychoneuroendocrinology
c/o Dirk Hellhammer, Ph.D.
Center for Psychobiological & Psychosomatic Research
Trier University
Universitaetsring 15
Trier 54286
Germany
49-651-201-2929
FAX: 49-651-201-2934
http://www.ispne.org/

Interstitial Cystitis Association
110 North Washington Street
Suite 340
Rockville, MD 20850
(301) 610-5300 or (800) HELP-ICA
FAX: (301) 610-5308
http://www.ichelp.com

Intracranial Hypertension Research Foundation
6517 Buena Vista Drive
Vancouver, WA 98661
(360) 693-4473
FAX: (360) 694-7062
http://www.IHRFoundation.org/

Joint Center for Sickle Cell and Thalassemic Disorders
Brigham and Women's Hospital
221 Longwood Avenue, Suite 620 LMRC
Boston, MA 02115.
(617) 732-8490
FAX: (617) 975-0876.
http://sickle.bwh.harvard.edu/

The Joint Council on International Children's Services
1320 Nineteenth St., NW
Suite 200
Washington, DC 20036
(202) 429-0400
FAX: (202) 429-0410
http://www.jcics.org

Joslin Diabetes Center
One Joslin Place
Boston, MA 02215
(617) 732-2415
http://www.joslin.harvard.edu

Last Acts
1620 Eye Street NW, Suite 202
Washington, DC 20006
(202) 296-8071;
FAX: (202) 296-8352
http://www.lastacts.org

League of Intravenous Therapy Education
Empire Building, Suite 3
3001 Jacks Run Road

White Oak, PA 15131
(412) 678-5025
FAX: (412) 678-5040
http://www.lite.org/

The Leukemia & Lymphoma Society Inc.
1311 Mamaroneck Ave.
White Plains, NY 10605
(914) 949-5213
FAX: (914) 949-6691
http://www.leukemia.org/

Leukemia Research Foundation
820 Davis St., Suite 420
Evanston, IL 60201
(847) 424-0600
FAX: (847) 424-0606
http://www.leukemia-research.org

Lupus Foundation of America, Inc.
1300 Picard Drive, Suite 200
Rockville, MD 20850-4303
(301) 670-9292 or (800) 558-0121
FAX: (301) 670-9486
http://www.lupus.org/lupus

Lymphoma Research Foundation
215 Lexington Ave.
New York, NY 10016
(800) 235-6848
FAX: (212) 213-1987

**Malignant Hyperthermia Association
of the United States (MHAUS)**
P.O. Box 1069
39 East State Street
Sherburne, New York 13460
(607) 674-7901
http://www.mhaus.org/

Management and Therapy for Sickle Cell Disease
National Institute of Health
National Heart, Lung and Blood Institute
31 Center Dr.
MSC2480, Rm. 4A10
Bethesda, MD 20892-2480
(301) 496-4236
http://www.nhlbi.nih.gov/index.htm

Mental Health Infosearch
http://www.mhsource.com

The Mind/Body Medical Institute
110 Francis Street
Boston, MA 02215
(617) 632-9530
FAX: (617) 632-9545
http://www.mbmi.org/

Mind-Brain Society
http://www.brown.edu/Students/Mind-Brain/

Mothers Against Drunk Driving (MADD)
P.O. Box 541688
Dallas, TX 75354
(800) 438-6233
http://www.madd.org

Multiple Sclerosis Foundation
6350 North Andrews Avenue
Fort Lauderdale, FL 33309-2130
(954) 776-6805 or (800) 225-6495

FAX: (954) 938-8708
http://www.msfacts.org/

Myasthenia Gravis Foundation of America
5841 Cedar Lake Road, Suite 204
Minneapolis, MN 55416
(952) 545-9438 or (800) 541-5454
FAX: (952) 545-6073
http://www.med.unc.edu/mgfa

Narcotics Anonymous
P.O. Box 9999
Van Nuys, CA 91409
(800) 773-9999
FAX: (818) 700-0700
http://www.na.org

National Adrenal Diseases Foundation
505 Northern Boulevard
Great Neck, NY 11021
(516) 487-4992
http://www.medhelp.org/nadf/

National Aging Information Center
330 Independence Ave., SW
Room 4656
Washington, DC 20201
(202) 619-7501
FAX: (202) 401-7620
http://aoa.dhhs.gov/naic/

National Alliance for the Mentally Ill
Colonial Place Three
2107 Wilson Blvd., Suite 300
Arlington, VA 22201
(703) 524-7600
http://www.nami.org

National Anxiety Foundation
3135 Custer Drive
Lexington, KY 40517-4001
(859) 272-7166
http://lexington-on-line.com/naf.html

National Aphasia Association
29 John St., Suite 1103
New York, NY 10038
(800) 922-4622
FAX: (212) 267-2812
http://www.aphasia.org/

**National Association for Anorexia
and Associated Disorders**
P.O. Box 7
Highland Park, IL 60035
(847) 831-3438
FAX: (847) 433-4632
http://www.anad.org/

National Association for Continence (NAFC)
P.O. Box 8310
Spartanburg, SC 29305-8310
(800) BLADDER
FAX: (864) 579-7902
http://www.nafc.org

National Association of Area Agencies on Aging
927 15th Street, NW, 6th Floor
Washington, DC 20005
(202) 296-8130
FAX: (202) 296-8134
http://www.n4a.org/

National Association of Clinical Nurse Specialists
3969 Green Street
Harrisburg, PA 17110
(717) 234-6799
http://www.nacns.org/

National Association of the Deaf
814 Thayer Avenue
Silver Spring, MD 20910
(301) 587-1788 or TTY (301) 587-1789
http://www.nad.org

National Association of Emergency Technicians
408 Monroe Street
Clinton, MS 39056-4210
(800) 34-NAEMT
http://www.naemt.org/

National Association of Hispanic Nurses
1501 16th Street, NW
Washington, DC 20036
(202) 387-2477
FAX: (202) 483-7183
http://www.thehispanicnurses.org/

National Association of Orthopaedic Nurses (NAON)
Box 56
Pitman, NJ 08071-0056
(856) 256-2310
FAX: (856) 589-7463
www.inurse.com/~naon

National Association of the Physically Handicapped
c/o Jerry Snyder, National President N.A.P.H
1375 Dewitt Drive
Akron, OH 44313
(800) 743-5008 (access 01)
http://www.naph.net/

National Association of Rehabilitation Agencies
11250 Roger Bacon Dr., Suite 8
Reston, VA 20190
(703) 437-4377
FAX: (703) 435-4390
http://www.naranet.org/

National Black Nurses Association
8630 Fenton Street, Suite 330
Silver Spring, MD 20910-3803
(301) 589-3200
FAX: (301) 589-3223
http://www.nbna.org/

National Cancer Institute
NCI Public Inquiries Office
31 Center Drive, MSC 2580
Bethesda, MD 20892-2580
(800) 4-CANCER
http://www.cancer.gov/

National Center for Cultural Competence
Georgetown University
Child Development Center
3307 M Street NW, Suite 401
Washington, DC 20007-3935
1-800-788-2066
FAX: (202) 687-8899
http://www.georgetown.edu/research/gucdc/nccc/index.html

National Center for Environmental Health
Mail Stop F-29
4770 Buford Highway, NE
Atlanta, GA 30341-3724
(888) 232-6789
http://www.cdc.gov/nceh/default.htm

National Center for Injury Prevention and Control
Mailstop K65
4770 Buford Hwy. NE
Atlanta, GA 30341
(770) 488-1506
http://www.cdc.gov/ncipc

The National Chronic Fatigue Immune Dysfunction Foundation
103 Aletha Road
Needham, MA 02492
(781) 449-3535
FAX: (781) 449-8606
http://www.ncf-net.org/

National Chronic Pain Outreach Association
7979 Old Georgetown Road, Suite 100
Bethesda, MD 20814-2429
(301) 652-4948
FAX: (301) 907-0745
http://neurosurgery.mgh.harvard.edu/ncpainoa.htm

National Clearing House for Alcohol and Drug Information (NCADI)
P.O. Box 2345
Rockville, MD 20847-2345
(800) 729-6686
http://www.samhsa.gov/centers/clearinghouse/clearinghouses.html

National Coalition Against Domestic Violence
P.O. Box 18749
Denver, CO 80218
(303) 839-1852
FAX: (303) 831-9251
http://www.ncadv.org/

National Commission for Acupuncture and Oriental Medicine
11 Canal Center Plaza, Suite 300
Alexandria, VA 22314
(703) 548-9004
FAX: (703) 548-9079
http://www.nccaom.org

National Council for Adoption
1930 17th St., NW
Washington, DC 2009-6207
(202) 328-1200
FAX: (202) 332-0935
http://www.ncfa-usa.org/

National Council on Alcoholism and Drug Dependence
20 Exchange Place, Suite 2902
New York, NY 10005
(212) 269-7797
FAX: (212) 269-7510
http://www.ncadd.org

National Depressive and Manic Depressive Association
730 North Franklin, Suite 501
Chicago, IL 60610
(800) 826-3632
FAX: (312) 642-7243
http://ndmda.org/

National Diabetes Information Clearinghouse
Office of Communications and Public Liaison
NIDDK, NIH, Building 31, Room 9A04
Center Drive, MSC 2560
Bethesda, MD 20892-2560
(800) 860-8747
http://www.niddk.nih.gov/health/diabetes/ndic.htm

National Digestive Diseases Information Clearing House
2 Information Way
Bethesda, MD 20892-3570
(800) 891-5389 or (301) 654-3810
FAX: (301) 907-8906
http://www.niddk.nih.gov/health/digest/nddic.htm

National Domestic Violence Hotline
PO Box 161810
Austin, TX 78716
(800) 799-7233
http://www.ndvh.org/

National Eating Disorders Association
603 Stewart St., Suite 803, Seattle, WA 98101
(206) 382-3587
http://www.nationaleatingdisorders.org

National Emergency Medical Association
306 W. Joppa Road
Baltimore, MD 21204-4048
410-494-0300
http://www.nemahealth.org/

National Emergency Number Association
422 Beecher Road
Columbus, OH 43236
(614) 741-2080 or (800) 332-3911
FAX: (614) 933-0911
http://www.nena.org/

National Fire Protection Association
1 Batterymarch Park
Quincy, MA 02269
(617) 770-3000
FAX: (617) 770-0700
http://www.nfpa.org/

National Foundation for Depressive Illness
P.O. Box 2257
New York, NY 10116
(800) 239-1265
http://www.depression.org

National Headache Foundation
428 West Saint James Place
2nd floor
Chicago, IL 60614-2750
(888) NHF-5552
FAX: (773) 525-7357
http://www.headaches.org/

National Heart, Lung, and Blood Institute
National Institutes of Health
31 Center Drive, Building 31a
Room 4A03
900 Rockville Pike, Building 31
Bethesda, MD 20892
(301) 496-5166
http://www.nhlbi.nih.gov/index.htm

National Hemophilia Foundation
116 West 32nd Street, 11th Floor
New York, NY 10001

(212) 328-3700 or (800) 42-HANDI
FAX: (212) 328-3777
http://www.hemophilia.org/home.htm

National Institute of Allergy and Infectious Disease
Building 31, Room 7A-50
31 Center Drive MSC 2520
Bethesda, MD 20892-2520
(301) 496-5717
http://www.niaid.nih.gov

National Institute of Arthritis and Musculoskeletal and Skin Diseases
Information Clearinghouse
National Institutes of Health
1 AMS Circle
Bethesda, Maryland 20892-3675
(301) 495-4484 or (877) 22-NIAMS
FAX: (301) 718-6366
http://www.nih.gov/niams

National Institute of Diabetes and Digestive and Kidney Diseases
Office of Communications and Public Liaison
NIDDK, NIH Building 31
Room 9A04 Center Drive, MSC 2560
Bethesda, MD 20892-2560
(301) 496-3583
http://www.niddk.nih.gov/

National Institute of Mental Health (NIMH)
NIMH Public Inquiries
6001 Executive Boulevard, Rm. 8184, MSC 9663
Bethesda, MD 20892-9663
(301) 443-4513
FAX: (301) 443-4279
http://www.nimh.nih.gov/

National Institute of Neurological Disorders and Stroke (NINDS)
National Institute of Health
P.O. Box 5801
Bethesda, MD 20824
(800) 352-9424
http://www.ninds.nih.gov/

National Institute on Aging
Building 31, Room 5C27
31 Center Drive, MSC 2292
Bethesda, MD 20892
(301) 496-1752
http://www.nia.nih.gov/

National Institute on Alcohol Abuse and Alcoholism
6000 Executive Boulevard, Willco Building
Bethesda, MD 20892-7003
http://www.niaaa.nih.gov

National Institute on Deafness and Other Communication Disorders
National Institute of Health
31 Center Drive, MSC 2320
Bethesda, MD 20892
(301) 496-7243
FAX: (301) 402-0018
http://www.nidcd.nih.gov/

National Institute on Drug Abuse
National Institutes of Health
6001 Executive Boulevard, Room 5213
Bethesda, MD 20892-9561

(301) 443-1124
http://www.nida.nih.gov

National Kidney and Urologic Diseases Information Clearinghouse
3 Information Way
Bethesda, MD 20892-3580
(301) 654-4415 or (800) 891-5390
FAX: (301) 907-8906
http://www.niddk.nih.gov/health/kidney/nkudic.htm

National Kidney Foundation
30 East 33rd St., Suite 1100
New York, NY 10016
(212) 889-2210
FAX: (212) 689-9261
http://www.kidney.org

National Lymphedema Network
Latham Square
1611 Telegraph Ave., Suite 1111
Oakland, CA 94612-2138
(510) 208-3200 or (800) 541-3259
FAX: (510) 208-3110
http://lymphnet.org/

National Marrow Donor Program
Suite 500
3001 Broadway Street, Northeast
Minneapolis, MN 55413-1753
(800) 627-7692
http://www.marrow.org/

National Mental Health Association
1021 Prince Street
Alexandria, VA 22314-2971
(703) 684-7722
FAX: (703) 684-5968
http://www.nmha.org/

National Mental Health Consumers' Self-Help Clearinghouse
1211 Chestnut Street, Suite 1207
Philadelphia, PA 19107
(215) 751-1810 or (800) 553-4539
FAX: (215) 636-6312
http://www.mhselfhelp.org/

National Multiple Sclerosis Society
733 Third Avenue
New York, NY 10017
(800) 344-4867
http://www.nmss.org/

The National Parkinson Foundation, Inc.
1501 NW Ninth Avenue
Bob Hope Road
Miami, FL 33136-9990
(800) 327-4545
Fax: (305) 243-4403
http://www.parkinson.org/

National Pediculosis Association, Inc.
50 Kearney Rd.
Needham, MA 02494
(781) 449-NITS
FAX: (781) 449-8129
http://www.headlice.org/

National Psoriasis Foundation
6600 SW 92nd Ave., Suite 300
Portland, OR 97223-7195
(503) 244-7404 or (800) 723-9166

FAX: (503) 245-0626
http://www.psoriasis.org/

National Rehabilitation Association
633 South Washington Street
Alexandria, VA 22314
(703) 836-0850
FAX: (703) 836-0848
http://www.nationalrehab.org/

National Spinal Cord Injury Association
6701 Democracy Blvd., Suite 300-9
Bethesda, MD 20817
(800) 962-9629
FAX: (301) 588-9414
http://www.spinalcord.org/

National Stroke Association
9707 East Easter Lane
Englewood, CO 80112-5112
(303) 649-9299 or (800) STROKES
FAX: 303-649-1328
http://www.stroke.org/

NCCAM Clearinghouse
P.O. Box 7923
Gaithersburg, Maryland 20898
(301) 519-3153 or (888) 644-6226
FAX: (866) 464-3616
http://nccam.nih.gov/

North American Nursing Diagnosis Association
1211 Locust Street
Philadelphia, PA 19107
(215) 545-8105
FAX: (215) 545-8107
http://www.nanda.org

North American Society for Cardiac Imaging
930 Edgecliff Way
Redwood City, CA 94061
(650) 216-6621
FAX: (650) 556-1678
http://www.nasci.org/

Nursing Ethics Network
http://www.nursingethicsnetwork.org/

Office of Minority Health
P.O. Box 37337
Washington, DC 20013-7337
(800) 444-6472
FAX: (301) 230-7198
http://www.omhrc.gov/

Oncology Nursing Society
501 Holiday Drive
Pittsburgh, PA 15220
(412) 921-7373
FAX: (412) 921-6565
http://ons.org/

Organization for Human Brain Mapping
5841 Cedar Lake Road
Suite 204
Minneapolis, MN 55416 USA
(952) 646-2029
FAX: (952) 545-6073
http://www.humanbrainmapping.org/

Organization for Understanding Cluster Headaches (OUCH)
1616 Sixteenth St.
Los Osos, CA 93402
http://www.clusterheadaches.org/

Organization of Parenting Through Surrogacy (OPTS)
P.O. Box 611
Gurnee, IL 60031
(847) 782-0224
http://www.opts.com

Overeaters Anonymous
6075 Zenith Court, NE
Rio Rancho, NM 87124
(505) 891-2664
FAX: (505) 891-4320
http://www.overeatersanonymous.org/

Pan American Health Organization
Regional Office of the World Health Organization
525 23rd Street, NW
Washington, DC 20037
(202) 974-3000
FAX: (202) 974-3663
http://www.paho.org

The Pediatric Endocrinology Nursing Society
P.O. Box 2933
Gaithersburg, MD 20886-2933
http://www.pens.org/

Perivascular Nurse Consultants, Inc.
8013 Bingham Street
Philadelphia, PA 19111
(215) 742-9833
http://www.pncnurse.com

Philippine Nurses Association of America
151 Linda Vista Drive
Daly City, CA 94014
(415) 468-7995
FAX: (415) 468-7995
http://www.pna-america.org/

Pituitary Network Association
P.O. Box 1958
Thousand Oaks, CA 91358
(805) 499-9973
http://www.pituitary.com

Polycystic Kidney Research Foundation
4901 Main Street, Suite 200
Kansas City, MO 64112
(800) PKD-CURE
http://www.pkdcure.org/home.htm

Preventive Cardiovascular Nurses Association
613 Williamson St. Suite 205
Madison, WI 53703
(608) 250-2440
FAX: (608) 250-241
http://www.pcna.net/

P.R.I.D.E. Foundation (Promote Real Independence for the Disabled and Elderly)
391 Long Hill Rd.
Groton, CT 06340
(860) 445-1448
http://members.aol.com/sewtique/pride.htm

Project Inform (Information, Inspiration and Advocacy for People Living with HIV/AIDS)
205 13th Street, #2001
San Francisco, CA 94103
(415) 558-8669 or (800) 822-7422
FAX: (415) 558-0684
http://www.projinf.org/

Recovery, Inc.
802 Dearborn Street
Chicago, IL 60610
(312) 337-5661
FAX: (312) 337-5756
http://www.recovery-inc.com

Research Center for Stroke and Heart Disease
100 High Street
Buffalo, NY 14203
(716) 859-3900
http://www.stroke-heart.org/

RESOLVE (Nationwide Infertility Support Group)
1310 Broadway
Somerville, MA 02144
(888) 623-0744
http://www.resolve.org/

Schizophrenia.com
http://www.schizophrenia.com

Sex Information and Education Council of the United States (SIECUS)
130 West 42nd Street
Suite 350
New York, NY 10036
(212) 819-9770
FAX: (212) 819-9776
http://www.siecus.org

Self-Help for Hard of Hearing People (SHHH)
7910 Woodmont Avenue
Suite 1200
Bethesda, MD 20814
(301) 657-2248
FAX: (301) 913-9413
http://www.shhh.org

Sickle Cell Disease Association of America, Inc.
200 Corporate Pointe
Suite 495
Culver City, CA 90230-7633
(800) 421-8453
http://www.sicklecelldisease.org/

The Simon Foundation for Continence
Box 835-F
Wilmette, IL 60091
1-800-23SIMON
www.simonfoundation.org

Society for Academic Emergency Medicine
901 N. Washington Avenue
Lansing, MI 48906-5137
(517) 485-5484
FAX: (517) 485-0801
http://www.saem.org/

Society for Cardiovascular Pathology
http://scvp.net/

Society for Light Treatment and Biological Rhythms
P.O. Box 591687
174 Cook Street
San Francisco, CA 941159-1687
FAX: (415) 751-2758
http://www.sltbr.org

Society for Neuroscience
11 Dupont Circle, NW, Suite 500
Washington, DC 20036
(202) 462-6688
http://www.sfn.org/

Society for Vascular Nursing
7794 Grow Drive
Pensicola, FL 32514
(800) 536-4786
Fax: (850) 484-8762
http://www.svnnet.org/

Society of Geriatric Cardiology
9111 Old Georgetown Road
Bethesda, MD 20814
(301) 581-3449
FAX: (301) 897-9745
http://www.sgcard.org/

Thyroid Foundation of America, Inc.
Ruth Sleeper Hall, RSL 350
40 Parkman St.
Boston, MA 02114
(617) 726-8500 or (800) 832-8321
FAX: (617) 726-4136
http://www.allthyroid.org

The Thyroid Society
Texas Medical Center
7515 South Main St., Suite 545
Houston, TX 77030
(713) 799-9909 or (800) 849-7643
http://www.the-thyroid-society.org/

Transcultural Nursing Society
c/o Madonna University College of Nursing and Health
36600 Schoolcraft Road
Livonia, MI 48150-1173
(734) 432-5470 or (888) 432-5470
FAX: (734) 432-5463
http://www.tcns.org

Translation Services
AT&T Language Line Services
1-800-752-6096
Provides written and oral translation in 140 languages

United Network for Organ Sharing (UNOS)
1100 Boulders Parkway, Suite 500
PO Box 13770
Richmond, VA 23225-8770
(804) 330-8541
http://www.unos.org/

United Ostomy Association, Inc.
19772 MacArthur Boulevard, Suite 200
Irvine, CA 92612-2405
714-660-8624 or (800) 826-0826
http://www.uoa.org

U.S. Census Bureau
Washington, DC 20233
Street address: 4700 Silver Hill Road
Suitland, MD 20746
301-763-4636
http://www.census.gov/

Us Too (Support group for prostate cancer)
5003 Fairview Ave.
Downer's Grove, IL 60515
(630) 795-1002 or (800) 808-7866
FAX: (630) 795-1602
http://www.ustoo.com/

Volunteers of America
1660 Duke Street
Alexandria, VA 22314-3421
(703) 341-5000 or (800) 899-0089
FAX: (703) 341-7000
http://www.voa.org/

Women in Endocrinology
c/o Ursula B. Kaiser, M.D.
Department of Medicine
Brigham and Women's Hospital
221 Longwood Ave.
Boston, MA 02115
FAX: (617) 732-5764
http://www.women-in-endo.org/

World Health Organization
Avenue Appia 20
1211 Geneva 27
Switzerland
(00 41 22) 791 21 11
FAX: (00 41 22) 791 3111
http://www.who.int/home-page/

World Heart Federation
http://www.worldheart.org/

Wound Ostomy and Continent Nurses Society (WOCN)
4700 W. Lake Ave
Glenview, IL 60025
(866) 615-8560 or (888) 224-WOCN
FAX: (866) 615-8560
http://www.wocn.org

Y-ME National Breast Cancer Organization
212 West Van Buren Street, Suite 500
Chicago, IL 60607
(312) 986-8338 or (800) 221-2141
FAX: 312-294-8597
http://www.y-me.org/

Commonly Used Abbreviations and Acronyms

3DCRT = Three-dimensional conformal radiation therapy

5-DHT = 5-alpha-reductase

5-HT = serotonin

AA = Alcoholics Anonymous

ABG = arterial blood gas

ACC = American College of Cardiology

ACE = angiotensin-converting enzyme

ACF = acute renal failure

ACLS = advanced cardiac life support

ACOA = Adult Children of Alcoholics

ACTH = adrenocorticotropic hormone

ADH = antidiuretic hormone

ADC = AIDS dementia complex

ADLs = activities of daily living

AE = above the elbow

AED = automatic electrical defibrillator

AFP = alpha fetoprotein

AHA = American Heart Association

AI = adequate intake

AICD = automatic implanted cardiac defibrillator

AIDS = acquired immunodeficiency syndrome

AK = above the knee

ALL = acute lymphocytic leukemia

ALP = alkaline phosphatase

ALS = amyotrophic lateral sclerosis

ALT = alanine aminotransferase

AMA = American Medical Association

AML = acute myelogenous leukemia

ANA = American Nurses Association

ANA = antinuclear antibody

ANCAs = antineutrophil cytoplasmic antibodies

ANP = atrial natriuretic peptide

ARDS = acute respiratory distress syndrome

ARI = aldose reductase inhibitor

ASCAs = antisaccharomyces antibodies

ASO = antistreptolysin-O

AST = aspartate aminotransferase

ATN = acute tubular necrosis

ATP = adenosine triphosphate

AV = atrioventricular

BAL = blood alcohol level

BCG = bacilli Calmette-Guérin

BE = below the elbow

BhCG = beta human chorionic gonadatropin

BK = below the knee

BMI = body mass index

BMR = basal metabolic rate

BMT = bone marrow transplant

BP = blood pressure

BPH = benign prostatic hyperplasia

BRAT = bananas, rice, applesauce, toast

BRM = biologic response modifier

BSE = breast self-examination

BUN = blood urea nitrogen

CABG = coronary artery bypass graft

CAD = coronary artery disease

CAP = community-acquired pneumonia

CAPD = continuous ambulatory peritoneal dialysis

CAT = computed axial tomography

CBC = complete blood count

CCPD = continuous cyclic peritoneal dialysis

CDC = Centers for Disease Control and Prevention

CDCA = chenodeoxycholic acid

CEA = carcinoembryonic antigen

CF = cystic fibrosis

CFC = chlorofluorocarbon

CFS = chronic fatigue syndrome

CFTCR = cystic fibrosis transmembrane conductance regulator

CHF = congestive heart failure

CIC = clean intermittent catheterization

CIS = carcinoma in situ

CJD = Creutzfeldt-Jakob disease

CK = creatine kinase

CK-MB = MB isoenzyme of creatine kinase

CLL = chronic lymphocytic leukemia

CMG = cystometrogram

CML = chronic myelogenous leukemia

CNA = certified nurse's aide

CNS = central nervous system

CO = cardiac output

COPD = chronic obstructive pulmonary disease

CPAP = continuous positive airway pressure

CPM = continuous passive motion

CPR = cardiopulmonary resuscitation

CRF = chronic renal failure; corticotropin-releasing factor
CRP = c-reactive protein
CRT = cardiac resynchronization therapy
CSF = cerebrospinal fluid; colony-stimulating factor
CST = cortisol suppression test
CT = computed tomography
CTZ = chemoreceptor trigger zone
CVA = cerebrovascular accident; costovertebral angle
CVP = central venous pressure
D and C = dilatation and curettage
D5W = 5% dextrose in water solution
DASH = Dietary Approaches to Stop Hypertension
DCA = directional coronary atherectomy
DES = diethylstilbestrol
DEXA = dual-energy x-ray absorptiometry
DIC = disseminated intravascular coagulation
DJD = degenerative joint disease
DKA = diabetic ketoacidosis
DLE = discoid lupus erythematosus
DMARD = disease-modifying antirheumatic drugs
DMAST = Dyna Med Anti-Shock Trousers
DMSO = dimethyl sulfoxide
DNA = deoxyribonucleic acid
DNR = do not resuscitate
DPT = diphtheria, pertussis, tetanus
DRE = digital rectal examination
DRG = diagnosis-related group
DSM-IV-TR = Diagnostic and Statistical Manual of Mental Disorders, 4th edition, text revision
DSP = distal sensory polyneuropathy
DST = dexamethasone suppression test
DUIL = driving under the influence of liquor
DVT = deep vein thrombosis
EBCT = electron beam computed tomography
ECF = eosinophil chemotactic factor
ECG = electrocardiogram
ECMO = extracorporeal membrane oxygenator
ECT = electroconvulsive therapy
ED = emergency department
EECP = enhanced external counterpulsation
EEG = electroencephalography
EGD = esophagogastroduodenoscopy
ELISA = enzyme-linked immunosorbent assay
EMG = electromyelogram
EPA = eicosapentaenoic acid
EPS = extrapyramidal symptoms
ERCP = endoscopic retrograde cholangio-pancreatography
ESR = erythrocyte sedimentation rate
ESRD = end-stage renal disease
ESWL = extracorporeal shock wave lithotripsy
EUG = excretory urogram
FAS = fetal alcohol syndrome
FDA = Food and Drug Administration
FSH = follicle-stimulating hormone

FTA-ABS = fluorescent treponemal antibody absorption test
GABA = gamma aminobutyric acid
GAD = generalized anxiety disorder
GCS = Glasgow coma scale
GERD = gastroesophageal reflux disease
GH = growth hormone
GHB = gamma hydroxybutyrate
GI = gastrointestinal
GnRH = gonadatropin-releasing hormone
GTT = glutamyltransferase
GVHD = graft-versus-host disease
HAAT = highly active antiretroviral therapy
HAMD = Hamilton Rating Scale for Depression
HAP = hospital-acquired pneumonia
HAV = hepatitis A virus
HbA = hemoglobin A
HbF = fetal hemoglobin
HbS = hemoglobin S
HBV = hepatitis B virus
HCl = hydrochloric acid
HCV = hepatitis C virus
HDL = high-density lipoprotein
HDV = hepatitis D virus
HEV = hepatitis E virus
HHNKS = hyperosmolar hyperglycemic nonketotic syndrome
HiB = *Haemophilus influenzae* B
HIV = human immunodeficiency virus
HLA = human lymphocyte antigen
HMO = health maintenance organization
HPI = history of present illness
HPV = human papilloma virus
HRT = hormone replacement therapy
HSV-1 = type-1 herpes simplex virus
HSV-2 = type-2 herpes simplex virus
IABP = intra-aortic balloon pump
IBD = inflammatory bowel disease
IBS = irritable bowel syndrome
IC = interstitial cystitis
ICD = integrated delivery system
ICF = intermediate care facility
ICP = intracranial pressure
ICSH = interstitial cell-stimulating hormone
IDDM = insulin-dependent diabetes mellitus
Ig = immunoglobulin
IGF-1 = insulin-like growth factor
IGFBP-3 = insulin-like growth factor binding protein-3
IL = interleukin
IICP = increased intracranial pressure
IL-2 = interleukin-2
IM = intramuscular
INR = international normalized ratio
IOL = intraocular lens
IOP = intraocular pressure
IORT = intraoperative radiation therapy

IPD = intermittent peritoneal dialysis
IPG = impedance plethysmography
IPV = inactivated poliomyelitis
IUG = intravenous urography
IV = intravenous
IVAC = implanted vascular access
IVP = intravenous pyelogram
IVU = intravenous urography
JCAHO = Joint Commission on Accreditation of Healthcare Organizations
KUB = kidney, ureter, bladder
LASIK = Laser-assisted in situ keratomileusis
LES = lower esophageal sphincter
LDH = lactate dehydrogenase
LDL = low-density lipoprotein
LH = luteinizing hormone
LMP = last menstrual period
LOC = level of consciousness
LPN = licensed practical nurse
LVN = licensed vocational nurse
MAB = monoclonal antibodies
MAOI = monoamine oxidase inhibitor
MAST = military antishock trousers
MCH = mean cell hemoglobin
MCHC = mean cell hemoglobin concentration
MCO = managed care organization
MCT = medium-chain triglycerides
MCV = mean cell volume
MDI = metered-dose inhaler
MHC = major histocompatability complex
MI = myocardial infarction
MIDCAB = minimally invasive direct coronary artery bypass
MMR = measles, mumps, rubella
MoAb = monoclonal antibodies
MPHG = metabolite of norepinephrine
MRI = magnetic resonance imaging
MS = multiple sclerosis
MSG = monosodium glutamate
MTBE = methyl-*tert*-butyl ether
NADH = nicotinamide-adenine dinucleotide
NANDA = North American Nursing Diagnosis Association
NCCAM = National Center for Complementary and Alternative Medicine
NCLEX-PN = national licensing examination for practical nurses
NCSBN = National Council of State Boards of Nursing
NIDDM = non–insulin-dependent diabetes mellitus
NIH = National Institutes of Health
NK = natural killer (cell)
NMDA = *N*-methyl-D-aspartate
NMH = neurally mediated hypotension
NNRTI = non-nucleoside reverse transcriptase inhibitor
NPO = nothing by mouth

NRTI = nucleoside reverse transcriptase inhibitor
NS = normal saline
NSAID = nonsteroidal anti-inflammatory drug
OA = osteoarthritis
OAF = osteoclastic-activating factor
OCD = obsessive-compulsive disorder
OIA = optical immunoassay
OPCAB = off-pump coronary artery bypass
OR = operating room
ORIF = open reduction internal fixation
OSHA = Occupational Safety and Health Administration
OT = occupational therapist
PA = pulmonary artery
PAC = premature atrial contraction
PACAB = port access coronary artery bypass
$PaCO_2$ = partial pressure of carbon dioxide
PACU = postanesthesia care unit
PaO_2 = partial pressure of oxygen
PAP = pulmonary artery pressure
PASG = pnenumatic antishock garment
PC = potential complication
PCA = patient-controlled analgesia
PCP = pneumocystis pneumonia
PCR = polymerase chain reaction
PCV = pneumococcal conjugate vaccine
PCWP = pulmonary capillary wedge pressure
PE = pulmonary embolus
PEEP = positive end-expiratory pressure
PEG = percutaneous endoscopic gastrostomy
PENS = percutaneous electrical nerve stimulation
PET = positron emission tomography
PIC = peripheral indwelling catheter
PICC = peripherally inserted central catheter
PID = pelvic inflammatory disease
PMI = point of maximum impulse
PMS = premenstrual syndrome
PNS = peripheral nervous system
PPD = purified protein derivative
PPO = preferred provider organization
PPS = prospective payment systems
PR = peripheral resistance
PRK = photorefractive keratectomy
PRN = prescribed on an as-needed basis
PSA = prostate-specific antigen
PT = physical therapist; prothrombin time
PTCA = percutaneous transluminal coronary angioplasty
PTCRA = percutaneous transluminal catheter rotational ablation
PTSD = post-traumatic stress disorder
PTT = partial thromboplastin time
PTU = propylthiouracil
PUD = peptic ulcer disease
PVC = premature ventricular contraction
RA = rheumatoid arthritis

RAI = radioactive iodine
RAST = radioallergosorbent blood test
RBC = red blood cell
RDA = recommended dietary allowance
RF = rheumatoid factor
RK = radial keratotomy
RLQ = right lower quadrant
RN = registered nurse
RNA = ribonucleic acid
ROM = range of motion
RPR = rapid plasma reagent
RSV = respiratory syncytial virus
RT = reverse transcriptase
RUQ = right upper quadrant
SA = sinoatrial
SAD = seasonal affective disorder
SCLE = subacute cutaneous lupus erythematosus
SIADH = syndrome of inappropriate antidiuretic hormone
SIDS = sudden infant death syndrome
SIV = simian (monkey) immunodeficiency virus
SLE = systemic lupus erythematosus
SNF = skilled nursing facility
SPF = sun protection factor
SpO_2 = saturated oxygen
SRS = stereotactic radiation therapy
SRS-A = slow-reactive substance of anaphylaxis
SSRI = selective serotonin reuptake inhibitor
STD = sexually transmitted disease
SVT = supraventricular tachycardia
TB = tuberculosis
TBSA = total body surface area
TCA = tricyclic antidepressant
TDD = telecommunication device for the deaf
TE = transluminal extraction

TEE = transesophageal echocardiography
TENS = transcutaneous electrical nerve stimulation
TEP = tracheoesophageal puncture
THBO = topical hyperbaric oxygen
THC = tetrahydrocannabinol
TIA = transient ischemic attack
TIPS = transjugular intrahepatic portosystemic shunt
TIQ = tetrahydroisoquinoline
TMD = temporomandibular disorder
TMJ = temporomandibular joint
TMR = transmyocardial revascularization
TNF = tumor necrosis factor
TPA = tissue plasminogen activator
TPN = total parenteral nutrition
TSE = transmissible spongiform encephalopathy
TSH = thyroid-stimulating hormone
TSS = toxic shock syndrome
TUIP = transurethral incision of the prostate
TULIP = transurethral laser incision of the prostate
TUR = transurethral resection
TURP = transurethral resection of the prostate
TZD = thiazolidinedione
UAP = unlicensed assistive personnel
UDCA = ursodeoxycholic acid
UES = upper esophageal sphincter
URI = upper respiratory infection
UTI = urinary tract infection
UNOS = The United Network for Organ Sharing
UV = ultraviolet
VAD = ventricular assist device
VCUG = voiding cystourethrogram
VDRL = Venereal Disease Research Laboratory
WBC = white blood cell
WHO = World Health Organization

Laboratory Values

Laboratory values vary somewhat in different references. Laboratory technique also may alter values. The nurse is responsible for checking reported laboratory values against the normal ranges provided by the laboratory.

ABBREVIATIONS

cu	cubic
dL	decaliter (10 L)
dl	deciliter (100 mL)
g	gram
hpf	high powered field
IU	international unit
L	liter
LPF	low-power field
mcg	microgram
mEq	milliequivalent
mg	milligram
mm	millimeter
mmol	one-thousandth of a mole
mU	milliunit
µg	microgram
µL	microliter; also used for cubic millimeter
µm	micrometer
µU	microunit
ng	nanogram (one billionth of a gram)
pg	picogram (one trillionth of a gram)
torr	measurement equivalent to 1 mm Hg
U	units

SYMBOLS

> greater than
< less than
/ per
µ micro (one-millionth)

COAGULATION TESTS / VALUES

COAGULATION TESTS	VALUES
Bleeding time (Ivy, Duke)	3–10 minutes
Partial thromboplastin time (PTT)	30–45 seconds
Activated partial thromboplastin time (APPT)	16–25 seconds
Prothrombin time (PT)	10–14 seconds or 70%–100% of control
International normalized ratio (INR)	Therapeutic range 2.0–3.0; high therapeutic range 3.0–4.5; over 4.5 critical

HEMATOLOGY / VALUES

HEMATOLOGY	VALUES
Platelet count	150,000–350,000/µL
Reticulocyte count	0.5%–2.5%
Sedimentation rate (ESR)	
Male	0–15 mm/hr
Female	0–20 mm/hr
Complete blood count (CBC)	
Hematocrit	
Male	40%–54%
Female	37%–47%
Hemoglobin	
Male	13.5–17.5 g/dl
Female	12–16 g/dl
Red cell count	
Male	4.6–5.4 million/µL
Female	3.6–5.0 million/µL
White cell count	5,000–10,000/µL
Neutrophils	60%–70% (3000–7000/µL)
Eosinophils	1%–4% (50–400/µL)
Basophils	0.5%–1% (23–100/µL)
Lymphocytes	20%–40% (1000–4000/µL)
Monocytes	2%–6% (100–600/µL)
Erythrocyte indices	
Mean corpuscular volume (MCV)	87–103 µm^3
Mean corpuscular hemoglobin (MCH)	26–34 pg/cell
Mean corpuscular hemoglobin concentration (MCHC)	31%–37%

BLOOD VOLUME

Plasma volume	30–45 mL/kg
Red cell volume	20–35 mL/kg (higher in men than in women)
Total blood volume	55–80 mL/kg

BLOOD CHEMISTRIES / VALUES

BLOOD CHEMISTRIES	VALUES
Alanine aminotransferase (ALT) (formerly SGPT)	7–24 U/L
Ammonia	14–45 µg/dl
Amylase	50–150 µ/L; 25–130 IU/L by enzymatic method
Aspartate aminotransferase (AST) (formerly SGOT)	6–20 µ/L
Bilirubin, total direct (conjugated)	0.2–1.0 mg/dl 0.0–0.2 mg/dl

BLOOD

CHEMISTRIES (Cont.)	VALUES
Bilirubin, indirect (unconjugated)	0.2–08. mg/dl
Anion gap (or R factor)	± 12 mEq/L
Blood gases	
pH	7.35–7.45
$PaCO_2$	35–45 torr
$PvCO_2$	41–45 torr
SO_2	95% or higher arterial blood
	70%–75% mixed venous blood
PaO_2	80 torr or greater
PvO_2	30–40 torr
Blood urea nitrogen (BUN)	7–18 mg/dl
Calcium (total)	8.8–10 mg/dl
Calcium (ionized)	4.4–5.4 mg/dl
Carbon dioxide (CO_2 content)	23–30 mmol/L
Carcinoembryonic antigen (CEA)	up to 2.5 ng/mL
Cephalin flocculation	negative to 1 +
Chloride	98–106 mmol/L
Cholesterol	desirable range 140–200 mg/dl
Coagulant factor assay	
Factor VIII	55%–145% of normal
Factor IX	60%–140% of normal
Creatine kinase (CK)	20–185 U/L
CK isoenzymes	
MM: 100%	
MB: 0%	
BB: 0%	
Creatinine	0.6–1.2 mg/dl
Ferritin	15–300 ng/mL
Folic acid (Folate)	3–17 ng/mL
Formiminoglutamic (FIGLU) Acid excretion test	< 35 mg/day
Glucose (fasting, serum)	70–110 mg/dl
Glucose (postprandial)	< 120 mg/dl
High-density lipoprotein (HDL)	35–85 mg/dl
Insulin	6–24 μU/mL
Ketone bodies	negative
Lactic acid dehydrogenase (LD)	95–200 mU/mL (results vary)
LD isoenzymes	
LD-1	14%–26%
LD-2	29%–39%
LD-3	20%–26%
LD-4	8%–16%
LD-5	6%–16%
Lipase	4–24 U/L
Low-density lipoproteins (LDL)	desirable: < 130 mg/dl
Magnesium	1.3–2.1 mEq/L
Phosphatase, acid	0.15–0.65 BLB (Bersey, Lowry, Block) units
Phosphatase, alkaline	20–70 U/L
Phosphate, inorganic phosphorus	2.7–4.5 mg/dl
Potassium	3.5–5.0 mEq/L
Proteins, total	6.0–8.0 g/dl
Albumin	3.8–5.0 g/dl
Globulin	2.3–3.5 g/dl
Prostate-specific antigen (PSA)	0–4.0 ng/mL
Sodium	135–148 mmol/L
T_3 (free triiodothyronine)	230–660 pg/dL
T_4 (free thyroxine)	0.8–2.4 ng/dL

BLOOD

CHEMISTRIES (Cont.)	VALUES
Triglycerides	desirable: 35–160 mg/mL
Uric acid	3.5–7.2 mg/dL
Vitamin B_{12}	160–1300 pg/mL
Vitamin B_{12} (unsaturated binding capacity)	1000–2000 pg/mL

URINE	VALUES
Acetoacetic acid	negative
Acetone	negative
Albumin (quantitative)	negative
Aldosterone (24-hr specimen)	5–22 μg/24 hr
Bence-Jones protein	negative
Casts	rare/hpf
Color	pale yellow to dark amber
Creatinine clearance	
Male	< 150 mg/24 hr
Female	< 250 mg/24 hr
Glucose	negative to trace
17 hydroxycorticosteroid (as 17-ketogenic steroids or 17 KGS)	male: 3–10 mg/24 hr female: 2–6 mg/24 hr
17-ketosteroids	male: 8–20 mg/24 hr female: 6–15 mg/24 hr
Microscopic examination	RBC—0–1/hpf WBC—0–4/hpf casts—rare/hpf
pH	4.6–8.0
Protein	0–trace
Protein (24 hr)	10–140 mg/L in 24 hr
Specific gravity	1.003–1.035
Turbidity	usually clear (cloudiness not always abnormal)
Volume	600–1,600 mL/24 hr

CEREBROSPINAL FLUID	VALUES
Cell count	0–5 WBC/μL
Chloride	118–132 mEq/L
Color	clear, colorless
Glucose	40–70 mg/dl
Protein	15–45 mg/dl

SEROLOGY	VALUES
Antistreptolysin-O titer (ASLO)	< 160 Todd units
Cold agglutins	< 1:16
C-reactive protein (CRP)	< 0.8 mg/dl
Fluorescent treponemal antibodies (FTA)	negative
Hepatitis-associated antigen (HAA or HBAg)	negative
Heterophile antibodies	< 1:56
VDRL	nonreactive

DRUGS	VALUES
Ethanol	0.3%–0.4% marked intoxication
	0.4%–0.5% alcoholic stupor
	> 0.5% coma
Salicylates	< 100 µg/ml therapeutic range
	> 250 µg/dl toxic range
Digitoxin	14–26 ng/mL therapeutic range
	> 35 ng/mL toxic range
Digoxin	0.5–2.0 ng/mL therapeutic range
	> 2.5 ng/mL toxic range
Lidocaine	1.5–6.0 µg/mL therapeutic range
	> 6 mg/µL toxic range

TESTS FOR AIDS	VALUES
ELISA (Enzyme-linked immunosorbent assay)	positive if antibodies to HIV present
Western blot (WB)	positive if antibodies to HIV present
P24 antigen	negative for HIV
PCR (polymerase chain reaction)	negative for HIV
Murex SUDS (single use diagnostic system) HIV-1 assay	negative (blue result is positive)
T-cell count	644–2201 cells/µL
T4 cells	493–1191 cells/µL
T8 cells	182–785 cells/µL
T4/T8 ratio	> 1.0

Glossary

A

Abdominoperineal resection surgical procedure involving wide excision of the rectum and the creation of a sigmoid colostomy.

Acalculia neurological impairment of a person's ability to perform calculations.

Accelerated hypertension markedly elevated blood pressure accompanied by hemorrhages and exudates in the eyes.

Acceptance fifth stage of Elisabeth Kübler-Ross' five stages of grief in which a dying client accepts his or her fate and makes peace spiritually and with those with whom he or she is close.

Accommodation process in which the lens of the eye changes shape to view objects that are near or distant.

Accountability being answerable for the consequences of one's actions or inactions.

Acetylcholine neurotransmitter released at the nerve endings of parasympathetic nerve fibers, at some nerve endings in the sympathetic nervous system, and at nerve endings of skeletal muscles; also critical for memory and cognition.

Acetylcholinesterase enzyme that inactivates acetylcholine.

Acidosis excessive accumulation of acids or an excessive loss of bicarbonate in body fluids; can occur as a result of either metabolic or respiratory alterations.

Acids substances that release hydrogen into fluid.

Acne vulgaris inflammatory disorder that affects the sebaceous glands and hair follicles.

Acoustic neuroma benign Schwann cell tumor that progressively enlarges and adversely impacts cranial nerve VIII, which consists of the vestibular and cochlear nerves.

Acquired immunodeficiency syndrome infectious and eventually fatal syndrome that profoundly weakens the immune system which is acquired from a pathogen known as the human immunodeficiency virus (HIV).

Acromegaly condition in which growth hormone is over-secreted after the epiphyses of the long bones have sealed.

Active transport movement of dissolved chemicals from an area of low concentration to an area of higher concentration.

Actual diagnosis nursing diagnosis that identifies an existing problem. See also possible diagnosis and risk diagnosis.

Acupuncture technique of healing in which a needle is placed in one or more acupoints to restore the balance and free flow of energy within the body.

Acute bronchitis inflammation of the mucous membranes that line the major bronchi and their branches.

Acute chest syndrome type of pneumonia triggered by decreased hemoglobin and infiltrates within the lungs.

Acute heart failure sudden change in the heart's ability to contract.

Acute pain discomfort that has a short duration (from a few seconds to less than 6 months) and is associated with tissue trauma, including surgery, or some other recent identifiable etiology.

Acute renal failure sudden and rapid decrease in the ability of nephrons within the kidneys to maintain fluid, electrolyte, and acid–base balance, excrete nitrogen waste products, and perform regulatory functions such as maintaining calcification of bones and producing erythropoietin.

Acute retroviral syndrome syndrome that occurs in some cases of primary HIV infection that is often mistaken for "flu" or some other common illness.

Acute tubular necrosis death of cells within the collecting tubules of the nephrons where reabsorption of water, electrolytes, and excretion of protein wastes and excess metabolic substances occurs

Addiction repetitive pattern of drug seeking and drug use to satisfy a craving for a drug's mind-altering or mood-altering effects.

Addisonian crisis life-threatening endocrine emergency when corticosteroid therapy is abruptly discontinued.

Adenohypophysis anterior lobe of the pituitary gland.

Adenoidectomy surgical removal of the adenoids.

Adenoiditis inflammation of the adenoids.

Adenoids lymphoid tissue bodies located in the nasopharynx that protect the body from infection.

Adjuvant drugs medications that are co-administered when treating pain (e.g. improving analgesic effect without increasing dosage, controlling concurrent symptoms, moderating side effects).

Administrative law body of law that creates and enforces rules and regulations concerning the health, welfare, and safety of citizens.

Adolescent moratorium period of time during which persons aged 18 to 27 years continue to live at home and be supported by their parents while working or going to school.

Adrenal cortex outer portion of the adrenal glands; manufactures and secretes glucocorticoids, mineralocorticoids, and small amounts of sex hormones.

Adrenal glands glands located above the kidneys; the outer portion is the cortex, and the inner portion is the medulla.

Adrenal insufficiency decreased adrenal cortical function.

Adrenal medulla inner portion of the adrenal glands; secretes epinephrine and norepinephrine, two hormones released in response to stress or threat to life.

Adrenalectomy surgical removal of the adrenal gland(s), usually to remove a cancerous tumor.

Adrenocorticotropic hormone (ACTH)   substance secreted by the pituitary that stimulates the adrenal glands to secrete corticosteroid hormones.

Advance directives   documents in which a client states in advance his or her wishes regarding life-sustaining treatment and other medical care.

Advocacy   (1) promoting the cause of another person or organization and (2) safeguarding of a client's rights and the supporting of his or her interests.

Affect   verbal and nonverbal behavior that communicates feelings.

Affective learner   person who processes information best when it appeals to his or her feelings, beliefs, and values.

Affective touch   personal contact with a client that is used to communicate concern, caring, and support. See also task-oriented touch.

Afterload   force that the ventricle must overcome to empty its diastolic volume.

Ageism   behaviors and beliefs that depict older adults in negative, inaccurate, or stereotypical ways.

Agnosia   neurologic impairment of a person's ability to recognize objects and sounds.

Agoraphobia   fear of experiencing a panic attack in a public place, which often leads to its victims permanently confining themselves to their homes.

Agranulocytes   leukocytes that do not contain granules.

Agranulocytosis   decreased production of granulocytes, including neutrophils, basophils, and eosinophils.

Agraphia   neurologic impairment of a person's ability to write.

AIDS dementia complex   neurologic condition that causes degeneration of the brain, especially in areas that affect mood, cognition, and motor functions.

AIDS drug assistance programs   state based programs partially funded by Title II of the Ryan White CARE Act that help low- and middle-income clients obtain expensive AIDS medications.

Alcoholism   chronic, progressive multisystem disease characterized by an inability to control the consumption of alcohol.

Aldosterone   hormone that causes retention of sodium and water.

Alexia   neurologic impairment of a person's ability to read.

Alkalosis   excessive accumulation of base or a loss of acid in body fluids; can occur as a result of either metabolic or respiratory alterations.

Allergen   antigen that can cause an allergic response.

Allergic disorder   disorder characterized by a hyperimmune response to weak antigens that are usually harmless.

Allograft   skin graft that uses human skin obtained from a cadaver to temporarily cover large areas of tissue until the client's own skin can be used for skin grafting.

Alloimmunity   immune response waged against transplanted organs and tissues that carry nonself antigens.

Alopecia   condition that affects the hair follicles and results in partial or total hair loss.

Alpha fetoprotein   serum protein normally produced during fetal development that is a marker indicating a primary malignant liver tumor.

Alternative medical systems   healthcare techniques that evolved from non-Western cultures.

Alternative therapy   treatment used instead of conventional medical treatment.

Alveolus (pl. alveoli)   small, clustered sac that begins where the bronchioles end and is the location for the exchange of oxygen and CO_2.

Alzheimer's disease   progressive, deteriorating brain disorder.

Ambulatory surgery   surgery that requires fewer than 24 hours of hospitalization; sometimes referred to as same-day or outpatient surgery.

Amenorrhea   absence of menstrual flow, usually caused by endocrine imbalances resulting from pituitary disorders or hypothyroidism, the stress response, or severely lean body mass.

Anaerobic metabolism   inefficient mechanism for meeting energy requirements used when the amount of oxygen reaching the cells decreases.

Analgesic   controlled substance that interferes with pain perception centrally (at the brain).

Anaphylactic shock   severe allergic reaction that occurs after exposure to a substance to which a person is extremely sensitive.

Anaphylaxis   rapid and profound allergic response characterized by shock, laryngeal edema, wheezing, stridor, tachycardia, and generalized itching.

Anasarca   generalized edema caused by the shift of fluid from the intravascular space to interstitial and intracellular fluid locations.

Androgeny   belief that it is acceptable to perform roles that have been traditionally ascribed to men or women regardless of gender.

Anecdotal record   handwritten, personal account of an incident made at the time of occurrence and updated as needed; used to refresh a nurse's memory.

Anemia   deficiency of either erythrocytes or hemoglobin.

Anergy   inability to mount an immune response.

Anesthesia   partial or complete loss of the sensation of pain with or without the loss of consciousness; may be general, regional, or local.

Anesthesiologist   physician who has completed 2 years of residency in anesthesia and is responsible for administering anesthesia to a client and for monitoring a client during and after the surgical procedure.

Anesthetist   person who administers anesthesia under the supervision of an anesthesiologist.

Aneurysm   stretching and bulging of an arterial wall, usually caused by weakening of the vessel.

Anger   second stage in Elisabeth Kübler-Ross' five stages of grief in which a client responds angrily to impending death and may displace this anger onto others, such as the physician, nurses, family, or God.

Angina pectoris   chest pain of cardiac origin.

Angiocardiography   diagnostic procedure in which a radiopaque dye is injected into a vein and its course through the heart is recorded by a series of radiographic pictures taken in rapid succession.

Angiogenesis   regeneration of myocardial blood vessels.

Angioneurotic edema   acute swelling of the face, neck, lips, larynx, hands, feet, genitals, and internal organs.

Anion gap   difference between sodium and potassium cation (positive ion) concentrations and the sum of chloride and bicarbonate anions (negative ions) in the extracellular fluid.

Anions   negative ions.

Ankylosing spondylitis   chronic, connective tissue disorder of the spine and surrounding cartilaginous joints, such as the sacroiliac joints and soft tissues around the vertebrae.

Ankylosis   joint immobility.

Annuloplasty   surgical repair of the mitral valve leaflets and their fibrous ring.

Anorexia nervosa   eating disorder characterized by an obsession with thinness that is achieved through self-starvation.

Anorexia   lack of appetite.

Antibodies   chemical substances that destroy foreign agents such as microorganisms.

Anticipatory grieving   grieving that occurs before death, often when the dying client and family begin to consider the impact of their potential loss.

Antidiuretic hormone (ADH)   substance secreted by the pituitary in response to low blood volume that promotes reabsorption of water that the kidneys would ordinarily excrete.

Antigens   protein markers on cells.

Antineoplastic   type of drug used to treat cancer that works by interfering with cellular function and reproduction.

Antioxidants   chemicals that block the chemical reactions that cause free radicals.

Anuria   urine output of <100 mL of urine over 24 hours.

Anxiety disorders   group of psychobiologic illnesses that result from the activation of the autonomic nervous system, chiefly the sympathetic division.

Anxiety   vague uneasy feeling, the cause of which is not readily identifiable and which is evoked when a person anticipates nonspecific danger.

Anxiolytics   drugs that relieve the symptoms of anxiety; sometimes referred to as minor tranquilizers.

Aortic regurgitation   backward flow of blood that occurs when the aortic valve does not close tightly.

Aortic stenosis   narrowing of the aortic valve's opening when its cusps become stiff and rigid.

Aortography   diagnostic procedure that detects aortic abnormalities such as aneurysms and arterial occlusions by injecting contrast medium and taking radiographic films of the abdominal aorta and major arteries in the legs.

Aphasia   neurological impairment of a person's ability to speak.

Apheresis   process of separating blood into its components.

Aphonia   complete loss of voice.

Apitherapy   medicinal use of bee venom.

Aplasia   failure to develop.

Apocrine glands   sweat glands found around the nipples, in the anogenital region, in the eyelids (Moll's glands), in the mammary glands of the breast, and in the external ear canals.

Apolipoproteins   proteins on the surface of cholesterol molecules that bind to enzymes which direct cholesterol to sites for metabolism.

Appendectomy   surgical removal of the appendix.

Appendicitis   inflammation of a narrow, blind protrusion called the vermiform appendix located at the tip of the cecum in the right lower quadrant of the abdomen.

Appliance   device worn over a stoma for the collection of feces.

Apraxia   inability to accomplish activities of daily living, such as grooming, toileting, and eating, despite intact motor function.

Arachnoid   middle membrane lying directly below the dura that protects the brain.

Aromatherapy   use of scents to alter emotions and biologic processes.

Arteriography   diagnostic procedure that involves instilling dye, referred to as contrast medium, into an artery.

Arteriosclerosis   loss of elasticity or hardening of the arteries.

Arteriovenous fistula   surgical anastomosis (connection) of an artery and vein lying in close proximity.

Arteriovenous graft   type of vascular access method that uses a tube of synthetic material or polytetrafluoroethylene to connect a vein and artery in the upper or lower arm.

Arthritis   general condition characterized by inflammation and degeneration of a joint.

Arthrocentesis   aspiration of synovial fluid.

Arthrodesis   fusion of a joint, most often the wrist or knee, for stabilization and pain relief.

Arthrogram   radiographic examination of a joint, usually the knee or shoulder.

Arthroplasty   surgical reconstruction of a joint, using an artificial joint that restores previously lost function and relieves pain.

Arthroscopy   internal inspection of a joint by means of an instrument called an arthroscope.

Artificially acquired active immunity   immunity that results from the administration of a killed or weakened microorganism or attenuated toxin.

Asbestosis   fibrous inflammation or chronic induration of the lungs caused by the inhalation of asbestos.

Ascites   collection of fluid in the peritoneal cavity.

Assessment   step in the nursing process that involves the careful observation and evaluation of a client's health status.

Assisted living   type of living arrangement that provides care to residents who require assistance with up to three activities of daily living but also maintains their privacy and dignity.

Asthma   reversible obstructive disease of the lower airway characterized by inflammation of the airway and a hyperresponsiveness of the airway to internal or external stimuli.

Astigmatism   visual distortion caused by an irregularly shaped cornea.

Asystole   cardiac arrest.

Ataxia   neurological impairment of a person's ability to walk.

Atelectasis   disorder in which the alveoli collapse.

Atherectomy   surgical removal of fatty plaque from arteries by inserting a cardiac catheter with a cutting tool at the tip or performing laser angioplasty.

Atheroma   fatty mass within the arterial wall.

Atherosclerosis   condition in which the lumen of the artery fills with fatty deposits, chiefly composed of cholesterol.

Atrial fibrillation   rhythm disorder in which several areas in the right atrium initiate disorganized, rapid impulses causing the atria to quiver rather than contract.

Atrial flutter   rhythm disorder in which a single atrial impulse outside the sinoatrial node causes the atria to contract at an exceedingly rapid rate (200 to 400 times/min).

Atrial natriuretic peptide   hormone-like substance produced in the atrial muscle of the heart released in response to overstretching of the atrial wall to reduce the increased volume of blood filling the heart.

Audiometry   precise measurement of hearing acuity.

Aura sensation, either of weakness, numbness or a hallucinatory odor or sound, that occurs immediately before a tonic-clonic seizure.

Auscultation listening with a stethoscope for normal and abnormal sounds generated by organs and structures such as the heart, lungs, intestines, and major arteries.

Autoantibodies antibodies against self-antigens.

Autocratic leadership style of leadership characterized by strong control by the manager over a work group.

Autograft skin graft that uses a client's own skin, which is transplanted from one part of the body to another.

Autoimmune disorder disorder in which killer T cells and autoantibodies attack or destroy natural cells.

Autoinoculation self-transmission of an infection to another area of the body.

Autologous blood self-donated blood.

Automatic implanted cardiac defibrillator internal electrical device used to restore a life-sustaining cardiac rhythm.

Automaticity ability of heart tissue to initiate electrical stimulus independently.

Automatisms inappropriate, automatic, repetitive movements such as lip smacking and picking at clothing or objects.

Autonomic dysreflexia exaggerated sympathetic nervous system response resulting from a spinal cord injury above T6. Characteristics include severe hypertension, slow heart rate, pounding headache, nausea, blurred vision, flushed skin, sweating, goosebumps, nasal stuffiness, and anxiety.

Autonomy exercising self-direction.

Autophagocytosis process in which portions of a cell are consumed to reduce their size when the cell senses adverse conditions, resulting in a temporary decrease in energy needs and an increase in the potential for survival.

Autoregulation ability of the brain to provide sufficient arterial blood flow despite rising intracranial pressure.

Avascular necrosis death of bone from an insufficient blood supply.

Aversion therapy technique that deters a behavior by causing unpleasant physical reactions when the behavior occurs.

Avulsion fracture severe traumatic sprain in which a chip of bone to which a ligament is attached becomes detached.

Axon nerve fiber that projects and conducts impulses away from the neuron's cell body.

Ayurvedic medicine system of medicine with roots in India whose object is to help individuals become unified with nature to develop a strong body, clear mind, and tranquil spirit.

Azotemia accumulation of nitrogen waste products in the blood, evidenced by elevated BUN, serum creatinine, and uric acid levels.

B

Bacteremia condition resulting from microorganisms escaping the lymph nodes and reaching the bloodstream which may lead to sepsis.

Balloon tamponade tube that is inserted through the esophagus into the stomach, then inflated to compress esophageal varices and control hemorrhage.

Balloon valvuloplasty invasive, nonsurgical procedure to enlarge a narrowed valve opening using a deflated balloon that is threaded through a peripheral blood vessel into the stenotic valve of the heart, then inflated to stretch the opening.

Bargaining third stage in Elisabeth Kübler-Ross' five stages of grief in which a client attempts to negotiate a delay in dying with God or some higher power, usually until after a particularly significant event.

Barium enema radiographic study used to identify polyps, tumors, inflammation, strictures, and other abnormalities of the colon after instilling barium solution rectally.

Barium swallow fluoroscopic observation of a client swallowing a flavored barium solution and its progress down the esophagus to detect structural abnormalities of the esophagus as well as swallowing discoordination and oral aspiration.

Baroreceptors stretch receptors in the aortic arch and carotid sinus that signal the brain to release ADH when blood volume decreases, systolic blood pressure falls, or the right atrium is underfilled, and to suppress ADH when blood volume increases, systolic blood pressure rises, or the right atrium is overfilled.

Basal metabolic rate (BMR) minimum energy a person uses in a resting state.

Bases chemical substances that bind with hydrogen.

Basophils granulocytes that are active in allergic contact dermatitis and some delayed hypersensitivity reactions.

Battle's sign bruising of the mastoid process behind the ear.

Behavioral therapy type of psychotherapy that attempts to extinguish undesirable responses through the learning of other adaptive techniques.

Benign type of tumor that is not invasive or spreading.

Benign prostatic hyperplasia condition in which the prostate gland contains more than the usual number of normal cells.

Beta amyloid starchy component that accumulates in the brains of clients with Alzheimer's disease and injures neurons in the area of the brain responsible for producing acetylcholine, the neurotransmitter that is critical for memory and cognition.

Bicarbonate-carbonic acid buffer system regulates plasma pH by adding hydrogen ions to increase acidity and removing them to promote alkalinity.

Bigeminy pattern in which every other heart beat is a premature ventricular contraction.

Biliary colic upper abdominal pain that may radiate to the back and shoulders.

Binge-eating disorder disorder characterized by an inability to control overeating without engaging in compensating behaviors to prevent weight gain.

Biofeedback technique in which an individual voluntarily controls one or more physiologic functions such as body temperature, heart rate, blood pressure, and brain waves.

Biological-based therapies healing techniques that use natural products such as herbs, aromas, and bee venom.

Bipolar disorder disorder characterized by cycling between depression, euthymia, and euphoria.

Blackouts periods of amnesia involving events and activities while consuming alcohol.

Blended family family in which a married couple are caretakers of children from each spouse's previous marriage(s).

Blood dyscrasias abnormalities in the numbers and types of blood cells.

Blood products components extracted from blood and administered to clients who need specific blood substances but not all the fluid and cellular components in whole blood.

Blood urea nitrogen protein breakdown product; deterioration in renal function is manifested by a rise in its values.

Board of nursing state organization governing the nursing profession responsible for protecting the public, reviewing and approving nursing education programs in the state, forming criteria for granting licensure, overseeing procedures for licensure examinations, issuing or transferring licenses, and implementing disciplinary procedures.

Boarding homes small homes with individual rooms where residents pay for room and board and minimal nursing services.

Body dysmorphic disorder disorder in which a person becomes obsessed with the idea that some feature of his or her body is flawed.

Body mass index mathematical computation based on height and weight used to evaluate a person's size in relation to norms within the adult population.

Body-based therapies healing techniques that use manipulation and movement of the body to improve health and restore biologic functions.

Bone scan study that uses the intravenous injection of a radionuclide to detect the uptake of the radioactive substance by the bone.

Bouchard's nodes bony enlargement of the proximal interphalangeal joints.

Brachytherapy direct internal application of a high dose of radiation on or within a tumor.

Bradydysrhythmia slow abnormal cardiac rhythm.

Bradykinesia slowness in performing spontaneous movements.

Brain mapping technique that compares a client's brain activity patterns (from an EEG or other electronic image) with a computerized database of electrophysiologic abnormalities.

Brain stem part of the central nervous system consisting of the midbrain, pons, and medulla oblongata.

Breast abscess localized collection of pus within breast tissue.

Breast cancer mass of abnormal cells in the breast.

Breast reconstruction surgical procedure in which the area of a mastectomy is refashioned to simulate the contour of a breast and optionally to create a nipple and areola.

Breast self-examination technique for examining one's own breasts for lumps and suspicious changes.

Bronchiectasis chronic obstructive pulmonary disease characterized by chronic infection and irreversible dilatation of the bronchi and bronchioles.

Bronchioles smaller subdivisions of bronchi.

Bronchus (pl. bronchi) one of the two main branches of the trachea.

Brudzinski's sign assessment finding in which flexion of the neck produces flexion of the knees and hips.

Bruit purring or blowing sound caused by blood flowing over the rough surface of one or both carotid arteries.

Bulimarexia eating disorder characterized by a pattern of food restriction and purging to avoid absorbing the food that is consumed.

Bulimia nervosa eating disorder characterized by episodes of secret food binges followed by purging to prevent weight gain.

Bursa small sac filled with synovial fluid that reduces friction between tendon and bone and tendon and ligament.

Bursitis inflammation of the bursa, a fluid-filled sac that cushions bone ends to enhance a gliding movement.

C

Calcification process in which inorganic minerals, such as calcium salts, are deposited in body tissues.

Calcitonin hormone that inhibits the release of calcium from bone into the extracellular fluid.

Calciuria excessive calcium in the urine.

Calculus precipitate of mineral salts that ordinarily remain dissolved in urine.

Callus healing mass that forms after a bone is fractured which holds the ends of the bone together but cannot endure strain.

Caloric stimulation test test that assesses the vestibular reflexes of the inner ear that control balance.

Cancellous bone bony tissue that is light and contains many spaces.

Cancer disease characterized by abnormal, disorganized cell proliferation.

Candidiasis yeast infection caused by the *Candida albicans* microorganism that may develop in the oral, pharyngeal, esophageal, or vaginal cavities or within folds of the skin.

Capitation insurance plan that pays a preset fee per member per month to a healthcare provider, usually a hospital or hospital system, that covers all medical costs incurred and is paid regardless of whether the member requires healthcare services.

Capsid double layer of lipid material that surrounds the genetically incomplete HIV.

Caput medusae dilation of the veins over the abdomen.

Carbuncle deep skin and subcutaneous abscess from which pus drains.

Carcinogens factors or agents that contribute to the development of cancer.

Carcinoma in situ localized malignancy that, if untreated, will subsequently invade other areas.

Cardiac index calculation that reflects the cardiac output in relation to a particular client's body size.

Cardiac output volume of blood ejected from the left ventricle per minute.

Cardiac rehabilitation program following a cardiac event that combines exercise and educational activities to speed recovery and reduce or prevent recurring episodes.

Cardiac resynchronization therapy technique that restores synchrony in the contractions of the right and left ventricles using a biventricular pacemaker.

Cardiac tamponade acute compression of the heart.

Cardiogenic shock shock that occurs when contraction of the heart is ineffective and cardiac output is reduced.

Cardiomyopathy chronic condition characterized by structural changes in the heart muscle.

Cardiomyoplasty surgical procedure in which a client's own chest muscle is grafted to the aorta and wrapped around the heart to augment ineffective myocardial muscle contraction.

Cardioplegia intentional stopping of the heart for a surgical procedure.

Cardiopulmonary bypass technique in which blood is mechanically circulated and oxygenated outside the body.

Caregiver person who performs health-related activities that a sick person cannot perform independently.

Carina lower part of the trachea.

Carpal tunnel syndrome term for a group of symptoms located in the wrist where the carpal bones, carpal tendons, and median nerve pass through a narrow, inelastic canal.

Carpopedal spasm involuntary contraction of hand muscles.

Carrier human or animal that harbors an infectious microorganism but does not show active evidence of the disease.

Cartilage firm, dense connective tissue whose primary functions are to reduce friction between articular surfaces, absorb shocks, and reduce stress on joint surfaces.

Case management system of health care delivery in which a case manager plans and coordinates a client's progress through the various phases of care to avoid delays, unnecessary diagnostic testing, and overuse of expensive resources.

Case method historically early system of nursing care in which one nurse provided all the services that a particular client required, accompanying the client to the hospital, providing care in the home, and performing many household duties as well.

Cast rigid mold that immobilizes an injured structure while it heals.

Casts deposits of minerals that break loose from the walls of renal tubules.

Cataract disorder in which the lens of the eye becomes opaque.

Catecholamines neurotransmitters that stimulate responses by the sympathetic nervous system.

Cation positive charged electrolyte.

Cauda equina small sections of spinal nerves that begin after the end of the spinal cord between the first and second lumbar vertebrae.

Cell-mediated response process that occurs when T cells survey proteins in the body, actively analyze the surface features, and respond to those that differ from the host by directly attacking the invading antigen.

Central nervous system part of the nervous system consisting of the brain and spinal cord.

Central venous infusions infusions that deliver solutions into a large central vein, such as the vena cava.

Central venous pressure pressure produced by venous blood in the right atrium.

Central vision ability to discriminate letters, words, and the details of any image.

Cephalalgia aching in the head.

Cerebellum part of the brain located behind and below the cerebrum that controls and coordinates muscle movement.

Cerebral hematoma bleeding within the skull that forms an expanding lesion.

Cerebral infarction death of brain tissue.

Cerebrovascular accident prolonged interruption in the flow of blood through one of the arteries supplying the brain.

Cerebrum part of the brain consisting of two hemispheres connected by the corpus callosum.

Cervicitis inflammation of the cervix.

Chancre painless ulcer that accompanies first-stage syphilis.

Chancroid sexually transmitted disease caused by the *Haemophilus ducreyi* bacillus and characterized by the appearance of a macule, followed by vesicle–pustule formation and, finally, a painful ulcer.

Charcot's joints neuropathic joint disease, a common finding in tertiary syphillis.

Chemical cardioversion use of drugs to eliminate a dysrhythmia.

Chemical dependence condition of needing to take a drug to avoid withdrawal symptoms.

Chemonucleolysis procedure in which the enzyme chymopapain is injected into the nucleus pulposus to shrink or dissolve a ruptured intervertebral disk and relieve pressure on spinal nerve roots.

Chemoreceptors structures that are sensitive to the pH, CO_2, and oxygen in the blood, and regulate sympathetic nervous system stimulation or inhibition.

Chemotaxis process of attracting migratory cells to a particular area within the body.

Chemotherapy technique that uses antineoplastic (anticancer) agents to treat cancer cells locally and systemically.

Cheyne-Stokes respirations pattern of respiration in which shallow, rapid breathing is followed by a period of apnea.

Chief complaint that which the client perceives to be the health problem that needs treatment.

Chinese medicine medical system developed in China and other Asian countries which views health as the balancing of opposite forces and views illness as a consequence of imbalance.

Chiropractic technique of performing spinal manipulation as a generic method for curing neuromuscular disorders and a host of other diseases.

Chlamydia sexually transmitted disease caused by a bacterium, *Chlamydia trachomatis,* which lives inside the cells it infects; the disease is spread by sexual intercourse or genital contact without penetration and is the most common and fastest spreading bacterial STD in the United States.

Cholangiography test used to determine the patency of the ducts from the liver and gallbladder using a dye that is usually instilled intravenously.

Cholecystitis inflammation or infection of the gallbladder.

Cholecystography test used to identify the presence of stones in the gallbladder or common bile duct and tumors or other obstructions, by observing the ability of the gallbladder to concentrate and store an iodine-based, radiopaque contrast medium.

Choledocholithiasis disorder in which gallstones are located within the common bile duct.

Cholelithiasis disorder in which stones are formed in the gallbladder.

Cholestasis ineffective bile drainage.

Cholesterol fatty (lipid) substance.

Choreiform movements uncontrollable writhing and twisting of the body.

Chronic bronchitis prolonged (or extended) inflammation of the bronchi, accompanied by a chronic cough and excessive production of mucus for at least 3 months each year for two consecutive years.

Chronic fatigue syndrome complex of symptoms primarily characterized by profound lack of energy with no identifiable cause that worsens with physical activity and does not improve with rest.

Chronic heart failure disorder in which another chronic disorder gradually compromises the heart's ability to pump effectively.

Chronic obstructive pulmonary disease broad, nonspecific term that describes a group of pulmonary disorders with symptoms of chronic cough and expectoration, dyspnea, and impaired expiratory airflow.

Chronic pain discomfort that lasts longer than 6 months.

Chronic renal failure progressive and irreversible decrease in the ability of nephrons within the kidneys to maintain fluid, electrolyte, and acid-base balance, excrete nitrogen waste products, and perform regulatory functions such as maintaining calcification of bones and producing erythropoietin.

Chvostek's sign assessment finding in which a client's mouth twitches and jaw tightens following the tapping of the facial nerve.

Cilia hair-like processes whose action moves substances like mucus to prevent irritation to and contamination of the lower airway.

Circulatory overload fluid volume that exceeds what is normal for the intravascular space and has the potential to compromise cardiopulmonary function if it remains unresolved.

Cirrhosis degenerative liver disorder caused by generalized cellular damage.

Civil law body of law that is concerned with disputes between individual citizens and that protects each individual's personal freedoms and property rights.

Client database collection of information from the client's medical and nursing history, physical examination, and diagnostic studies.

Client term used for the recipient of healthcare services that emphasizes the recipient's personal responsibility for health and active partnership in healthcare.

Climacteric abrupt changes in the body at late middle age caused by alterations in the secretion and balance of reproductive hormones.

Clinical breast examination inspection of the breast in which an examiner notes breast size and symmetry and any unusual changes in the skin of the breasts and nipples and palpates the breasts and axillae for masses, lymph nodes, tenderness, and other abnormalities.

Closed head injury injury to the head in which an intact layer of scalp covers the fractured skull.

Closed method burn wound management technique in which the wound is covered. The closed method involves the use of one or more types of dressing materials.

Closed questions questions asked during a client interview that require only "yes" or "no" answers. See also open questions.

Closed reduction procedure in which a fractured bone is restored to its normal position by external manipulation, then immobilized with a bandage, cast, or traction.

Coagulopathies bleeding disorders that involve platelets or clotting factors.

Cochlear implant device that is surgically placed in the inner ear and connected to a receiver in the bone behind the ear to improve hearing.

Codons points on HIV genes where mutations occur.

Cognitive functions abilities of a person involving knowledge, understanding, and perception.

Cognitive learner person who processes information best by listening to or reading facts and descriptions.

Cognitive therapy type of psychotherapy in which a therapist helps a client by altering his or her interpretation of events.

Colectomy partial or complete surgical removal of the colon.

Colic acute spasmotic pain.

Collaboration use of a team effort to achieve client care outcomes.

Collaborative problems complications with a physiologic origin that nurses manage using physician-prescribed and nursing-prescribed interventions.

Collaborator person who works with others to achieve a common goal.

Collateral circulation circulation formed by smaller blood vessels branching off from or near larger occluded vessels.

Colloid solutions solutions containing water and molecules of suspended substances such as blood cells and blood products (e.g. albumin).

Colonoscopy surgical procedure in which an endoscope is used to visually examine the inner surface of the colon.

Colony stimulating factors cytokines that regulate the production, maturation, and function of blood cells.

Colostomy surgically created opening between the colon and the skin.

Comedone skin condition commonly called a blackhead; formed when sebum, keratin, and bacteria accumulate and dilate a hair follicle.

Comfort zone that area of a client's personal space which, when intruded, does not create anxiety.

Commissures area where the cusps of a cardiac valve contact each other.

Commissurotomy surgical procedure in which adhesions are opened in the cardiac valve cusps.

Common law system of laws that uses earlier court decisions, judgments, and decrees as precedents for interpretation of laws; also known as judicial law.

Community-acquired infections diseases that are transmitted from one infected person or reservoir to another, such as TB and meningitis.

Compartment syndrome syndrome in which a structure such as a tendon or nerve is constricted within a confined space.

Compensation stage first stage of shock, during which several physiologic mechanisms attempt to stabilize the spiraling consequences of shock.

Compensation acceleration of regulatory processes in the lungs and kidneys when an imbalance in acids or bases occurs.

Complement system system in which many different proteins are activated in a chain reaction when an antibody binds with an antigen.

Complementary therapy treatment used in addition to conventional medical treatment.

Compulsion anxiety-relieving ritual.

Compulsive overeating eating disorder characterized by eating when not hungry or regardless of feeling full.

Concussion injury resulting from a blow to the head that jars the brain and results in diffuse and microscopic injury to it.

Conductive hearing loss hearing loss that is due to interference in the transmission of sound waves to the inner ear.

Conductivity ability of cardiac tissue to transmit an electrical stimulus from cell to cell within the heart.

Condylomas genital warts, caused by a sexually transmitted disease, which are usually painless and appear as a single lesion or cluster of soft, fleshy growths on the genitalia or cervix, within the vagina, or on the perineum, anus, throat, or mouth.

Congestive heart failure accumulation of blood and fluid within organs and tissues as a result of ineffective heart contraction.

Congregate housing residential center made up of freestanding apartments, private rooms, or both, that provides independent to minimal assistance for seniors or disabled adults.

Conization   surgical removal of a large cone-shaped section of cervical uterine tissue.

Conjunctivitis   inflammation of the conjunctiva.

Conscious sedation   pharmacologically induced state in which clients are free of pain, fear, and anxiety and can tolerate unpleasant procedures while maintaining independent cardiorespiratory function and the ability to respond to verbal commands and tactile stimulation.

Conservatorship   responsibility for managing a client's care and assets appointed by a court when the client is incompetent.

Constitutional law   fundamental freedoms and rights granted by the Constitution to all citizens of the United States.

Continent ileostomy (Kock pouch)   creation of an internal reservoir for the storage of GI effluent.

Contractility   ability of cardiac tissue to stretch as a single unit and recoil.

Contrecoup injury   injury to the head from force that is strong enough to send the brain ricocheting to the opposite side of the skull, resulting in dual bruising.

Contusion   (1) soft tissue injury resulting from a blow or blunt trauma; (2) injury to the head that leads to gross structural injury to the brain and results in bruising and, sometimes, hemorrhage of superficial cerebral tissue.

Conversion disorder   psychobiologic disorder characterized by a sudden loss of motor or sensory function following a stressful event or experience.

Convulsion   seizure characterized by spasmodic contractions of muscles.

Coping mechanisms   unconscious tactics people use to protect themselves from feeling inadequate or threatened.

Cor pulmonale   disorder in which pulmonary disease causes the right ventricle to enlarge or fail.

Corneal transplantation   replacement of abnormal corneal tissue with healthy donated corneal tissue.

Corneal trephine   surgical procedure in which a small hole is produced at the junction of the cornea and sclera to provide an outlet for aqueous fluid.

Coronary artery bypass graft   surgical procedure that improves myocardial oxygenation by bypassing or detouring around the occluded portion of one or more coronary arteries with a relocated blood vessel from a healthy leg vein or chest artery.

Coronary artery disease   arteriosclerotic and atherosclerotic changes in the coronary arteries supplying the myocardium.

Coronary occlusion   closing of a coronary artery that reduces or totally interrupts blood supply to the distal muscle area.

Coronary stent   small, metal coil with mesh-like openings placed within the coronary artery during PTCA that prevents the coronary artery from collapsing.

Coronary thrombosis   blood clot within a coronary artery.

Corpus callosum   band of white fibers that acts as a bridge for transmitting impulses between the left and right hemispheres of the brain.

Cortical bone   bony tissue that is dense and hard.

Corticosteroid hormones   chemicals secreted by the adrenal cortex.

Corticosteroids   collective term for the glucocorticoids, mineralocorticoids, and small amounts of sex hormones manufactured and secreted by the adrenal cortex.

Coryza   rhinitis or the common cold.

Costovertebral angle   area where the lower ribs meet the vertebrae.

Coup injury   injury to the brain caused when the head is struck directly.

Couplets   occurrence of two premature ventricular contractions in a row.

Craniectomy   surgical procedure in which a portion of a cranial bone is removed.

Cranioplasty   surgical procedure in which a defect in a cranial bone is repaired using a metal or plastic plate or wire mesh.

Craniotomy   surgical procedure in which the skull is opened to gain access to structures beneath the cranial bones.

Creatinine   substance that results from the breakdown of phosphocreatine (amino acid waste product), which is present in muscle tissue, is filtered by the glomeruli, and is excreted at a fairly constant rate by the kidney.

Creatinine clearance test   study used to determine kidney function and creatinine excretion.

Credé's maneuver   technique in which the client bends at the waist or presses inward and downward over the bladder to increase abdominal pressure and facilitate emptying the bladder.

Criminal law   body of law concerned with offenses that violate the public's welfare.

Critical pathways   guidelines that standardize important aspects of care such as diagnostic work-ups, nursing care, education, physical therapy, and discharge planning for specific diagnoses or procedures.

Critical thinking   intentional, contemplative, outcome-directed thinking.

Crohn's disease   chronic inflammatory bowel condition that can occur in any portion of the GI tract but predominantly affects the terminal portion of the ileum.

Cross-tolerance   reduced pharmacologic effect when taking sedative-hypnotic drugs developed by alcoholics.

Cryptorchidism   condition in which one or both testes fails to descend into the scrotum.

Crystalloid solutions   solutions that consist of water and uniformly dissolved crystals such as salt (sodium chloride), other electrolytes, and sugar (glucose, dextrose).

Cullen's sign   bluish-gray discoloration to the skin about the umbilicus indicating intraperitoneal bleeding.

Cultural competence   (1) nurse's having an understanding both of his or her own worldview as well as the client's worldview; (2) process in which a nurse consistently tries to work within the cultural context of the client and his or her family and community.

Cultural history   information obtained during a client interview about the client's religious affiliation, cultural background, and health beliefs.

Culture   (1) person's way of perceiving, behaving, and evaluating the world that includes his or her knowledge, beliefs, art, morals, laws, and customs. (2) A test used to identify bacteria within a specimen taken from a person with symptoms of an infection.

Cushing's syndrome   endocrine disorder that results from excessive secretion of hormones by the adrenal cortex.

Cushing's triad   three signs associated with an increase in intracranial pressure: pulse increases initially but then decreases, systolic BP rises, and pulse pressure widens.

Cushingoid syndrome   physical changes that accompany Cushing's syndrome or long-term corticosteroid therapy.

Cutaneous triggering technique in which the client lightly massages or taps the skin above the pubic area to stimulate relaxation of the urinary sphincter.

Cystectomy surgical removal of the bladder.

Cystic fibrosis multisystem disorder affecting infants, children, and young adults that results from a defective autosomal recessive gene; the genetic mutation causes dysfunction of the exocrine glands, involving the mucus-secreting and eccrine sweat glands.

Cystitis inflammation of the urinary bladder.

Cystocele bulging of the bladder into the vagina.

Cystogram study that evaluates abnormalities in bladder structure and filling through the instillation of contrast dye and radiography.

Cystometrogram study that evaluates bladder tone and capacity using a retention catheter that is inserted into the bladder after the client voids and slowly filled with sterile saline until the client indicates at what point the first urge to void is felt and when the bladder feels full.

Cystoscope instrument consisting of a lighted tube with a telescopic lens used to examine the inside of the bladder.

Cystoscopy visual examination of the inside of the bladder using an instrument called a cystoscope.

Cystostomy surgical procedure in which a catheter is inserted through the abdominal wall directly into the bladder.

Cytokines immunologic chemical messengers released by lymphocytes, monocytes, and macrophages.

Cytotoxic T cells lymphocytes that bind to invading cells and destroy them by altering their cellular membrane and intracellular environment and releasing chemicals called lymphokines.

D

Debridement natural, mechanical, enzymatic, or surgical removal of necrotic tissue.

Decerebrate posturing position in which the extremities are stiff and rigid following neurologic trauma.

Decibel unit for measuring the intensity of sound.

Decompensation stage stage in shock that occurs as compensatory mechanisms fail and the client's condition spirals downward into cellular hypoxia, coagulation defects, and cardiovascular changes.

Decorticate posturing position in which the arms are flexed, and the fists clenched, and the legs extended following neurologic trauma.

Decortication surgical removal of the pericardium to allow more adequate filling and contraction of the heart chambers.

Deep vein thrombosis inflammation of a vein deep in the lower extremities accompanied by clot or thrombus formation.

Defibrillation emergency procedure that uses electrical energy to stop a life-threatening ventricular dysrhythmia .

Degenerative joint disease type of arthritis that is characterized by a slow and steady progression of destructive changes in weight-bearing joints and those that are repeatedly used for work.

Dehiscence separation of surgical wound edges without the protrusion of organs.

Dehydration significant reduction of body fluid in both extracellular and intracellular compartments.

Delegation transferring to a competent individual the authority to perform a selected task in a selected situation while retaining accountability for the delegation.

Delegator person who assigns a task to someone.

Delirium sudden, transient state of confusion.

Delusions fixed false beliefs that cannot be changed by logical reasoning and are often persecutory in nature.

Demand (or synchronous) mode pacemaker pacemaker that self-activates when a client's pulse falls below a certain level.

Dementia gradual, irreversible loss of intellectual abilities.

Democratic leadership style of leadership characterized by participation in decision-making by a work group.

Demyelinating disease disorder that causes permanent degeneration and destruction of myelin.

Dendrites threadlike projections or fibers on a neuron that conduct impulses to its cell body.

Denial psychological defense mechanism in which a client refuses to believe certain information; the first stage in Elisabeth Kübler-Ross' five stages of grief.

Deontology theory of ethics that proposes that the rightness of an action is determined entirely by whether or not it follows from an ethical duty.

Dependent edema accumulation of fluid in the body areas most affected by gravity (the feet, ankles, sacrum, or buttocks, in clients who are confined to bed).

Depolarization stage in electrophysiology when positive ions move inside the myocardial cell membranes, and the negative ions move outside.

Depot injections deep intramuscular injections of antipsychotic drugs in an oil suspension that are gradually absorbed over 2 to 4 weeks.

Depression The fourth stage in Elisabeth Kübler-Ross' five stages of grief in which a client realizes the reality of impending death and mourns potential losses such as separation from loved ones, the inability to fulfill future goals, or loss of control.

Dermabrasion method of removing surface layers of scarred skin using sandpaper, a rotating wire brush, chemicals, or a diamond wheel.

Dermatitis general term that refers to an inflammation of the skin.

Dermatome skin area supplied by a nerve.

Dermatophytes parasitic fungi that invade the skin, scalp, and nails.

Dermatophytoses superficial fungal infections.

Dermis layer of skin that lies below the epidermis.

Desensitization (1) form of immunotherapy in which a client receives weekly or twice weekly injections of dilute but increasingly higher concentrations of an allergen; (2) technique for overcoming anxiety by gradually exposing a person to whatever it is that provokes his or her anxiety.

Despair negative developmental outcome in which an older adult views life as disappointing and unfulfilling and anguishes over what might have been.

Detoxification process of stabilizing a client with a sedative drug while alcohol is metabolized from his or her system.

Development ability to perform physical, intellectual, social, and psychological tasks.

Developmental stage period of life during which unique physical and behavioral changes occur.

Developmental tasks   activities that are unique to a particular developmental stage and critical to future development.

Deviated septum   irregularity in the septum that results in nasal obstruction.

Dexamethasone (cortisol) suppression test   blood test that theoretically detects major depression.

Diabetes insipidus   endocrine disorder that develops when antidiuretic hormone from the posterior pituitary gland is insufficient.

Diabetes mellitus   metabolic disorder of the pancreas that affects carbohydrate, fat, and protein metabolism.

Diabetic ketoacidosis   type of metabolic acidosis that occurs when there is an acute insulin deficiency or an inability to use whatever insulin the pancreas secretes.

Diabetic nephropathy   progressive decrease in renal function that occurs with diabetes mellitus.

Diabetic retinopathy   pathologic changes in the retina experienced by persons with diabetes.

Diagnosis-related groups   classifications of diagnoses used for medical reimbursement.

Dialysate   solution used during dialysis that has a composition similar to normal human plasma.

Dialysis   procedure for cleaning and filtering the blood that substitutes for kidney function when the kidneys cannot remove nitrogenous waste products and maintain adequate fluid, electrolyte, and acid-base balances.

Dialyzer   semipermeable membrane filter within a machine that contains many tiny hollow fibers; during dialysis, blood moves through the hollow fibers and water and wastes from the blood move into the dialysate fluid that flows around the fibers, but protein and RBCs do not.

Diaphragm   muscle that separates the thoracic cavity from the abdominal cavity.

Diaphyses   long shafts of bones in the arms and legs.

Diastolic blood pressure   arterial pressure during ventricular relaxation.

Diffusion   process of oxygen and CO_2 exchange through the alveolar-capillary membrane.

Digital rectal examination   technique used to assess the prostate for size as well as evidence of tumor.

Digitalization   method of giving large doses of a digitalis drug at the beginning of treatment to build up therapeutic blood levels of the drug.

Dilatation and curettage   surgical procedure in which the cervix is stretched open and the endometrium is scraped to diagnose or treat various gynecologic problems and to remove fetal and placental tissue.

Diplopia   double vision.

Directed donor blood   blood obtained from specified blood donors among a client's relatives and friends.

Disease   pathologic condition that presents with clinical signs and symptoms.

Disequilibrium syndrome   neurologic condition believed to be caused by cerebral edema; the shift in cerebral fluid volume occurs when the concentrations of solutes within the blood are lowered rapidly during dialysis.

Diskectomy   surgical procedure in which a ruptured intervertebral disk is removed.

Dislocation   injury in which the articular surfaces of a joint are no longer in contact.

Distal sensory polyneuropathy   disorder characterized by abnormal sensations, such as burning and numbness, in the feet and later in the hands.

Distress   excessive, ill-timed, or unrelieved stress.

Distributive shock   shock that occurs when fluid in the circulatory system does not facilitate effective perfusion of the tissue; sometimes called normovolemic shock.

Diverticulitis   inflammation of diverticula.

Diverticulosis   asymptomatic diverticula.

Diverticulum   (pl. diverticula) sac or pouch caused by herniation of the mucosa through a weakened portion of the muscular coat of the intestine or other structure.

Documentation   production of an accurate and thorough written record of client care.

Domestic violence   pattern of physical, sexual, and psychological attacks to control a partner in an intimate relationship.

Dopamine   monoamine neurotransmitter of the sympathetic nervous system and precursor of norepinephrine; excess is associated with distortion of thoughts and sensory perception.

Double-barrel colostomy   creation of an ostomy, often temporary, to the colon that contains both a proximal stoma for expelling fecal material and a distal stoma to the anus.

Doubt   negative developmental outcome of the early childhood stage that may develop due to inability to live up to parental expectations.

Drop factors   ratio of drops to mL delivered by tubing in the administration of IV solution.

Drop size   size of the opening through which fluid passes.

Drug cross resistance   diminished drug response among similar drugs.

Drug resistance   ineffectual response to a prescribed drug because of the survival and duplication of exceptionally virulent mutations.

Dumping syndrome   syndrome in which the rapid emptying of large amounts of hypertonic chyme into the jejunum draws fluid from the circulating blood into the intestine, causing hypovolemia, which can produce syncope. As the syndrome progresses, the sudden appearance of carbohydrates in the jejunum stimulates the pancreas to secrete excessive amounts of insulin, which in turn causes hypoglycemia.

Dura mater   tough outermost membrane that protects the brain.

Durable power of attorney   legal designation of a person to make decisions regarding finances or healthcare when a person becomes incompetent.

Duty   expected action based on moral or legal obligations.

Dysmenorrhea   painful menstruation.

Dyspareunia   discomfort during intercourse.

Dyspepsia   epigastric pain or discomfort.

Dysrhythmia   conduction disorder that results in an abnormally slow or rapid heart rate or one that does not proceed through the conduction system in the usual manner.

E

Eating disorders   disorders in which eating patterns affect healthy weight and result in physiologic imbalances or medical complications.

Ecchymosis bruising.

Eccrine glands sweat glands that release water and electrolytes, such as sodium and chloride, in the form of perspiration.

Echocardiography diagnostic procedure that uses ultrasound waves to determine the functioning of the left ventricle and to detect cardiac tumors, congenital defects, and changes in the tissue layers of the heart.

Ectopic site conductive tissue that initiates an electrical impulse independently of the SA node.

Educator person who provides information.

Effector T cells killer (cytotoxic) T-cell lymphocytes.

Effluent discharged fecal material or liquid feces.

Effusion accumulation of fluid within two layers of tissue.

Ego identity positive developmental outcome of the adolescent stage characterized by exploring alternative value systems, developing a sense of self beyond the family, and eventually adopting values that are compatible with his or her personal beliefs.

Ego integrity positive developmental outcome in which an older adult develops a feeling of personal satisfaction that life has been happy and fulfilling.

Ejaculation discharge of semen from the body.

Elder abuse physical, psychological, social, or financial abuse of an older adult.

Elective electrical cardioversion nonemergency procedure to stop rapid atrial dysrhythmias in which a machine delivers an electrical stimulation that does not disrupt the heart during ventricular repolarization.

Electrocardiography graphic recording of the electrical currents generated by the heart muscle.

Electroconvulsive therapy application of an electric stimulus to one or both temporal regions of the head to produce a brief, generalized seizure; used to treat severe depression.

Electrolytes substances that carry an electrical charge when dissolved in fluid.

Electromagnetic therapy technique of healing using either electricity, magnets, or both.

Electron beam computed tomography radiologic test that produces x-rays of the coronary arteries using an electron beam.

Electronic infusion device machine that regulates and monitors the administration of IV solutions.

Electronystagmography method used to evaluate vestibular function, the mechanisms that facilitate maintaining balance, by measuring the duration and velocity of eye movements during caloric stimulation.

Electrophysiology study procedure that enables a physician to examine the electrical activity of the heart, produce actual dysrhythmias by stimulating structures within the conduction pathway, determine the best method for preventing further dysrhythmic episodes, and, in some cases, eradicate the precise location in the heart that is producing the dysrhythmia.

Embolectomy surgical removal of an embolus.

Embolus moving mass of particles, either solid or gas, within the bloodstream.

Emmetropia normal vision, in which light rays are bent to focus images precisely on the retina.

Empathy intuitive awareness of what a client is experiencing.

Emphysema chronic pulmonary disease characterized by abnormal distention of the alveoli.

Employee or peer assistance programs programs that work with an employing health agency to confidentially treat impaired nurses and help them return to nursing practice as soon as it is safe to do so.

Empyema collection of pus in the pleural cavity.

Emulsion mixture of two liquids, one of which is insoluble in the other; when combined, the two are distributed throughout the mixture as small, undissolved droplets.

Encopresis involuntary passage of liquid stool around an obstructive stool mass.

Endarterectomy surgical removal of the atherosclerotic plaque lining an artery.

Endocannabinoids natural chemicals with marijuana-like properties that activate the appetite center.

Endogenous opiates natural morphine-like substances within the body that modulate pain transmission by blocking receptors for substance P.

Endometrial ablation detachment of the lining of the uterus.

Endometriosis condition in which tissue that histologically and functionally resembles that of the endometrium is found outside the uterus.

Endophthalmitis disorder in which all three layers of the eye and the vitreous are inflamed.

Endoscopic retrograde cholangiopancreatography procedure in which an endoscope is used to visualize the common bile duct and the pancreatic and hepatic ducts through the ampulla of Vater in the duodendum.

Endotoxins harmful chemicals released from within a bacterial cell; probably the major cause of toxic shock.

End-stage renal disease stage in chronic renal failure in which less than 10% nephron function remains and the point at which a regular course of dialysis or kidney transplantation is necessary to maintain life.

Energy therapies techniques that claim to manipulate electromagnetic fields within the body.

Engraftment establishment of bone marrow that has been harvested and reinfused.

Enhanced external counterpulsation noninvasive and nonsurgical therapy that helps relieve angina using a pressure suit that moves blood toward the heart.

Enteroclysis study to determine subtle small bowel disease in which two contrast media fill and pass through the intestinal loops and are observed continuously through fluoroscope and periodic x-rays of the various sections of the small intestine.

Enterostomal therapist nurse who collaborates with the surgeon regarding stomal placement and the ostomate's educational needs.

Enucleation surgical removal of an eye.

Environmental tobacco smoke smoke given off by the burning end of a cigarette, pipe, or cigar and the exhaled smoke from the lungs of a smoker.

Enzyme-linked immunosorbent assay initial HIV screening test that is positive when there are sufficient HIV antibodies.

Eosinophils granulocytes that destroy parasites and play a major role in allergic reactions.

Epicondylitis painful inflammation of the elbow.

Epidemic rapidly spreading infectious disease in a particular region.

Epidermis   outermost layer of skin.

Epididymitis   inflammation of the epididymis.

Epidural hematoma   bleeding within the skull that stems from arterial bleeding, usually from the middle meningeal artery, with blood accumulation above the dura.

Epiglottis   cartilaginous valve flap that covers the opening to the larynx during swallowing.

Epilepsy   chronic recurrent pattern of seizures.

Epinephrine   neurotransmitter of the sympathetic nervous system produced and secreted by the adrenal medulla.

Epiphyses   rounded, irregular ends of long bones.

Epistaxis   nosebleed.

Epithelialization   regrowth of skin.

Epstein-Barr virus   virus that causes infectious mononucleosis.

Equianalgesic dose   oral dose that provides the same level of pain relief as when the drug is given by a parenteral route.

Erythema   redness of the skin.

Erythrocytes   red blood cells.

Erythrocytosis   increase in circulating erythrocytes.

Erythropoietin   hormone released by the kidneys that stimulates erythrocyte production.

Eschar   hard leathery crust of dehydrated skin that forms in areas of full-thickness burns.

Escharotomy   incision into eschar to relieve constricting pressure.

Esophageal varices   dilated, bulging esophageal veins.

Esophagitis   inflammation of the lining of the esophagus.

Esophagogastroduodenoscopy   examination of the esophagus, stomach, and duodenum through an endoscope to inspect, treat, or obtain specimens from any of the upper GI structures.

Essential hypertension   sustained elevated blood pressure with no known cause.

Estrogen   hormone produced by the ovaries.

Ethics   moral principles and values that guide the behavior of honorable people.

Ethmoidal sinuses   honeycomb of small spaces contained in the ethmoid bone, located between the eyes.

Ethnicity   bond or kinship that people feel with their country of birth or place of ancestral origin, regardless of whether they have ever lived outside of the United States.

Ethnocentrism   belief that one's own ethnic heritage is correct and superior to that of others.

Eustress   healthy amount of stress that helps individuals to pursue goals, learn to solve problems, and manage life's predictable and unpredictable crises.

Euthymic   state in which a person is capable of experiencing a variety of feelings, all of which are situationally appropriate.

Evaluation   step in the nursing process that involves the assessment and review of the quality and suitability of care and the client's responses to that care.

Evisceration   protrusion of organs through a separated surgical wound.

Exacerbation   periods of acute flare-ups of the symptoms of a disorder.

Excitability   ability of cardiac tissue to respond to electrical stimulation.

Excretory urogram   radiologic study used to evaluate the structure and function of the kidneys, ureters, and bladder by examining a radiopaque dye as it passes through the urinary tract.

Exertional dyspnea   effort at breathing when active.

Expected outcomes   client goals derived from nursing diagnoses that are measurable, achievable, and developed with the client, family, and other healthcare providers when possible.

Expressive aphasia   neurological impairment of a person's ability to speak.

Extended family   family that includes grandparents, aunts, uncles, and cousins.

External fixation   procedure in which metal pins are inserted into a fractured bone or bones from outside the skin surface and then attached to a compression device.

Extracellular fluid   water in the body located outside cells.

Extracorporeal circulation   technique in which blood is mechanically circulated and oxygenated outside the body.

Extracorporeal shock wave lithotripsy   procedure that uses shock waves to dissolve large kidney stones.

Extramedullary   outside the spinal cord.

Extrapyramidal motor tracts   fibers that originate in the motor cortex and project to the cerebellum and basal ganglia.

Extrapyramidal symptoms   movement disorders associated with certain prescribed drugs.

Extravasation   leaking of an intravenously administered drug into surrounding tissues.

F

Facilitated diffusion   process in which dissolved substances require the assistance of a carrier molecule to pass through a semipermeable membrane.

Factitious disorders   disorders in which people purposefully cause illness-like symptoms.

Fasciculations   involuntary twitching of muscles.

Fasting blood glucose   blood test performed to detect and monitor mellitus.

Fear   feeling of terror in response to someone or something specific that a person perceives as dangerous or threatening.

Feedback loop   mechanism that turns hormone production off and on; negative feedback stimulates a releasing gland in response to a decrease in levels while positive feedback keeps concentrations of hormones within a stable range.

Fertilization   union of an ovum and a spermatozoon.

Fetor hepaticus   sulfurous breath odor.

Fibroadenoma   solid, benign breast mass composed of connective and glandular tissue.

Fibrocystic breast disease   benign breast disorder that affects women primarily between the ages of 30 and 50.

Fibroid tumor   common benign uterine growth.

Fibromyalgia   pain in the fibrous tissues of the body such as muscles, ligaments, and tendons.

Filtration   process that promotes the movement of fluid and some dissolved substances through a semipermeable membrane using pressure differences.

Fissure   tear in tissue.

Fistula   abnormal channel from an organ to the surface of the body or from one organ to another.

Fistulectomy   surgical procedure in which a fistulous tract is excised.

Fistulotomy   surgical procedure involving incision of fistula.

Fixed-rate (or asynchronous) mode pacemaker   pacemaker that produces an electrical stimulus at a preset rate (usually 72 to 80 beats/min), despite the client's natural rhythm.

Flail chest disorder that occurs when two or more adjacent ribs fracture in multiple places and the fragments are free-floating; affects the stability of the chest wall and impairment of chest wall movement.

Flashbacks feelings of reliving a traumatic event.

Flexible sigmoidoscopy procedure in which a flexible fiberoptic sigmoidoscope is used to examine the sigmoid colon.

Focus assessment detailed information about one body system or problem.

Fomites nonliving environment in which an infectious agent can survive and reproduce.

Food binge rapid consumption of many calories.

Foramen magnum opening in the lower part of the skull through which the upper part of the spinal cord connects with the brain and which provides the only extracranial exit for brain tissue.

Formal teaching planned, organized conveying of information. See also informal teaching.

Fracture break in the continuity of a bone.

Free radicals unstable atoms with excessive energy capable of damaging DNA molecules.

Frontal sinuses bony cavities that lie within the frontal bone that extends above the orbital cavities.

Fulguration removal of small, superficial bladder tumors through coagulation with a transurethral resectoscope.

Full-thickness graft skin graft in which the epidermis, dermis, and some subcutaneous tissue are harvested from the client's skin.

Functional assessment determination of how well a client can manage activities of daily living.

Functional nursing task-oriented system of nursing care that evolved in the 1930s in which distinct duties are assigned to specific personnel.

Fundoplication surgical procedure to treat gastroesophageal reflux disorder that tightens the lower esophageal sphincter by wrapping the gastric fundus around the lower esophagus and suturing it into place.

Furuncle skin infection commonly called a boil.

Furunculosis condition of having multiple furuncles, or boils.

G

Gallbladder series test used to identify the presence of stones in the gallbladder or common bile duct and tumors or other obstructions, and to determine the ability of the gallbladder to concentrate and store an iodine-based, radiopaque contrast medium.

Gamma aminobutyric acid inhibitory neurotransmitter.

Gastrectomy surgical removal of the stomach.

Gastric decompression removal of gas and fluids from the stomach.

Gastritis inflammation of the stomach lining.

Gastroesophageal reflux disorder in which there is an upward flow of gastric contents into the esophagus.

Gastrostomy placement of a tube into the stomach via a surgically created opening into the abdominal wall.

Gender role societal determination of behaviors as either feminine or masculine.

Gene therapy technique for fighting cancer that involves replacing altered genes with normal genes, inhibiting defective genes, or introducing substances that destroy defective genes or cancer cells.

General adaptation syndrome nonspecific physiologic cyclical response to stress involving alarm, resistance, and exhaustion.

Generalization acknowledging that common trends exist within a cultural group but understanding that those trends may or may not apply to a particular individual.

Generalized anxiety disorder psychobiologic disorder characterized by chronic worrying on a daily basis for 6 or more months, generally with more than one focus of worry and often with the worrying being out of proportion with reality.

Generalized edema accumulation of fluid in all the interstitial spaces.

Generativity tendency of middle-aged adults to philosophically ponder the purpose for and value of their existence, survey their achievements, and pursue opportunities for self-fulfillment.

Genital herpes sexually transmitted disease caused by herpes simplex virus type 2 that results in genital and perineal lesions.

Genotype testing blood test used to detect drug resistance in which genetic changes in circulating HIV particles are measured.

Gerontology study of aging, including its physiologic, psychological, and social aspects.

Glaucoma eye disorder caused by an imbalance between the production and drainage of aqueous fluid.

Glomerulonephritis inflammatory renal disorder that occurs most frequently in children and young adults that is preceded by an upper respiratory infection with group A beta-hemolytic streptococci, impetigo (skin infection), or viral infections such as mumps, hepatitis B, or HIV.

Glottis opening between the vocal cords in the larynx.

Glucagon hormone that increases blood sugar levels by stimulating the breakdown of glycogen into glucose in the liver.

Glycogenolysis process in which glycogen is broken down into glucose in the liver.

Glycosuria glucose in the urine.

Glycosylated hemoglobin amount of glucose stored within a hemoglobin molecule during its lifespan of 120 days.

Goiter enlarged thyroid gland.

Gonorrhea sexually transmitted disease caused by a bacteria, *Neisseria gonorrhoeae,* which invades the urethra, vagina, rectum, or pharynx, depending on the nature of sexual contact.

Good Samaritan laws laws that provide legal immunity for rescuers who provide first aid in an emergency (outside of a hospital) to accident victims.

Gout painful metabolic disorder involving an inflammatory reaction within the joints that usually affects the feet (especially the great toe), hands, elbows, ankles, and knees.

Granulocytes leukocytes that contain cytoplasmic granules.

Granuloma inguinale sexually transmitted disease caused by a bascillus, *Calymmatobacterium granulomatis,* and characterized by painless nodules in the genital, inguinal, and anal areas.

Growth increase in body size measured by changes in height and weight.

Guardianship court-appointed responsibility for managing a client's care and assets when the client is incompetent.

Guilt negative developmental outcome of the preschool age in response to constant, unwarranted, or harsh discipline without compensating praise.

Gynecologic examination inspection and palpation of pelvic reproductive structures.

H

Hallucinations sensory experiences that others do not perceive; can be auditory, visual, tactile, olfactory, or gustatory (involving taste).

Hallux valgus deformity of the great (large) toe at its metatarsophalangeal joint.

Halo sign blood stain surrounded by a yellowish stain; highly suggestive of a cerebrospinal fluid leak.

Hammer toe flexion deformity of the interphalangeal joint that may involve several toes.

Hardiness effective coping style that includes a sense of having control over sources of stress and the perception of life events as a challenge rather than a threat.

Head-to-toe method technique used for carrying out an examination by beginning at the top of the body and progressing downward. See also systems method.

Health state of complete physical, mental, and social well-being; not merely the absence of disease and infirmity.

Health beliefs client's opinions regarding what causes illnesses, the role of the sick person and the health care professional, what must occur to restore health, and how one stays healthy, often shaped and perpetuated by the client's cultural affiliations.

Health maintenance organization group insurance plans in which each participant pays a preset, fixed fee in exchange for healthcare services.

Health maintenance protecting one's current level of health by preventing illness or deterioration.

Health practices actions that a client takes to restore health or stay healthy, often a product of and perpetuated by the client's cultural affiliations.

Health promotion engaging in strategies to enhance health.

Healthcare delivery system full range of services available to people seeking prevention, identification, treatment, or rehabilitation of health problems.

Healthcare team group of specially trained personnel who work together to help clients meet their healthcare needs.

Hearing perceiving sounds.

Heart block disorders in the conduction pathway that interfere with the transmission of impulses from the sinoatrial node through the atrioventricular node to the ventricles.

Heart failure inability of the heart to pump sufficient blood to meet the body's metabolic needs.

Heberden's nodes bony enlargement of the distal interphalangeal joints.

Helper T cells cells that recognize antigens and form additional T-cell clones that stimulate B-cell lymphocytes to produce antibodies against foreign antigens.

Hematopoiesis manufacture and development of blood cells.

Hematuria blood in the urine.

Heme pigmented, iron-containing portion of hemoglobin.

Hemianopia disorder in which the client is only able to see half of the normal visual field.

Hemiplegia paralysis on one side of the body.

Hemoconcentration high ratio of blood components in relation to watery plasma.

Hemodialysis technique in which blood is transported from a client through a dialyzer, a semipermeable membrane filter within a machine that removes water and wastes from the blood.

Hemodilution reduced ratio of blood components in relation to watery plasma.

Hemodynamic monitoring procedure used to assess the volume and pressure of blood within the heart and vascular system by means of a peripherally inserted catheter.

Hemoglobin iron-containing protein attached to erythrocytes that carries blood.

Hemoptysis expectoration of blood or bloody sputum.

Hemorrhoidectomy surgical removal of hemorrhoids.

Hemorrhoids dilated veins outside or inside the anal sphincter.

Hepatic encephalopathy central nervous system manifestation of liver failure related to an increased serum ammonia level that often leads to coma and death.

Hepatic lobectomy surgical procedure in which a primary malignant or benign tumor confined to a single lobe of the liver is removed.

Hepatitis inflammation of the liver.

Hepatorenal syndrome renal failure associated with liver disease that ultimately alters fluid distribution and interferes with fluid excretion.

Herbal therapy use of plants for treating disease and disorders.

Hernia protrusion of any organ from the cavity that normally confines it; most commonly used to describe the protrusion of the intestine through a defect in the abdominal wall.

Hernioplasty surgical procedure in which the weakened area of a hernia is reinforced with wire, fascia, or mesh to prevent recurrence.

Herniorrhaphy surgical repair of a hernia.

Herpes simplex virus infectious agent responsible for genital and perineal lesions and associated with cold sores around the nose, lips, and anogenital lesions.

Herpes zoster skin disorder (shingles) that develops years after an infection with varicella (chickenpox) due to an acute reactivation of the varicella-zoster virus, which lies dormant in nerve roots.

Heterograft skin graft obtained from animals, principally pigs, to temporarily cover large areas of tissue until the client's own skin can be used for skin grafting.

Hiatal hernia (diaphragmatic hernia) protrusion of part of the stomach through the diaphragm.

High-density lipoprotein lipoprotein that has a higher ratio of protein than cholesterol.

Highly active antiretroviral therapy therapy used to treat HIV with a combination of drugs; sometimes referred to as a "drug cocktail"

Hilus entrance of the bronchi to the lungs.

Histocompatible cells cells whose antigens match an individual's own genetic code.

Histrionic state of being animated, dramatic, and prone to exaggeration.

Hodgkin's disease malignancy that produces enlargement of lymphoid tissue, the spleen, and the liver, with invasion of other tissues such as the bone marrow and lungs.

Holism viewing a person's health as a balance of body, mind, and spirit; considering the client's psychological, sociocultural, developmental, and spiritual needs to restore optimal health.

Homans' sign calf pain that increases on dorsiflexion of the foot.

Home healthcare delivery of healthcare services, for both long-term and short-term health needs, in a client's home.

Homocysteine amino acid created during the metabolism of protein; elevated levels are believed to impair memory and contribute to above-normal cholesterol levels.

Hordeolum (sty) inflammation and infection of the Zeis or Moll gland, a type of oil gland at the edge of the eyelid.

Hormone replacement therapy administration of estrogen combined with progestin to reduce perimenopausal symptoms, prevent osteoporosis, and reduce the atherosclerotic process.

Hormones chemicals secreted by the endocrine glands that accelerate or slow physiologic processes.

Hospice facility for the care of terminally ill clients where they can live out their final days with comfort, dignity, and meaningfulness.

Host person on or in whom a microorganism resides.

Human immunodeficiency virus pathogen that causes acquired immunodeficiency syndrome.

Human papillomavirus infectious agent that causes venereal warts; transmitted by genital–genital, genital–anal, or genital–oral contact with an infected person and contagious as long as the warts are present.

Humor therapeutic use of laughter, which stimulates the immune system and causes the release of neuropeptides.

Humoral response formation of antibodies.

Hydronephrosis condition in which an obstruction of urine from the ureter distends the renal pelvis.

Hyperglycemia elevated blood glucose level.

Hyperlipidemia high levels of fat in blood.

Hypernatremia elevated serum sodium level.

Hyperopia farsightedness; people who are hyperopic see objects that are far away better than objects that are close.

Hyperosmolar hyperglycemic nonketotic syndrome acute complication of diabetes characterized by hyperglycemia without ketosis.

Hyperparathyroidism disorder of the parathyroid gland that affects calcium and phosphorous levels.

Hyperplasia increase in the number of cells.

Hypertension sustained elevation of systolic arterial blood pressure of 140 mm Hg or higher, a sustained diastolic arterial blood pressure of 90 mm Hg or higher, or both.

Hypertensive cardiovascular disease stage of hypertension when elevated blood pressure causes both cardiac abnormality and vascular damage.

Hypertensive crisis potentially fatal condition with symptoms such as extremely elevated blood pressure, headache, nausea, vomiting. sweating, palpitations, visual changes, neck stiffness, sensitivity to light, and tachycardia.

Hypertensive heart disease stage of hypertension when elevated blood pressure causes a cardiac abnormality.

Hypertensive vascular disease stage of hypertension when elevated blood pressure causes vascular damage without heart involvement.

Hyperthyroidism disorder associated with hypersecretion of thyroid hormones in which metabolic rate increases.

Hypertonic solution solution which is more concentrated than body fluid and draws fluid into the intravascular compartment from the more dilute areas within the cells and interstitial spaces.

Hypertrophied turbinates enlargements of the nasal concha that interfere with air passage and sinus drainage, and eventually lead to sinusitis.

Hyperuricemia accumulation of uric acid in the blood.

Hypervolemia high volume of water in the intravascular fluid compartment.

Hypnosis therapeutic intervention that facilitates a physiologic change through the power of suggestion.

Hypochondriasis psychobiologic disorder in which a person is preoccupied with minor symptoms and develops an exaggerated belief that they signify a life-threatening illness.

Hypoglycemia low blood glucose level.

Hypoparathyroidism deficiency of parathormone that results in hypocalcemia.

Hypophysectomy surgical removal of the pituitary gland.

Hypophysis pituitary gland.

Hypothalamus portion of the brain between the cerebrum and the brain stem that stimulates and inhibits the pituitary gland.

Hypothyroidism disorder that occurs when the thyroid gland fails to secrete adequate thyroid hormones.

Hypotonic solution solution that contains fewer dissolved substances in comparison to plasma and is effective in rehydrating clients experiencing fluid deficits.

Hypovolemia low volume of extracellular fluid.

Hypovolemic shock shock that occurs when the volume of extracellular fluid is significantly diminished, primarily because of a loss or reduction in blood or plasma.

Hypoxia decrease in the amount of oxygen reaching the cells.

Hysterectomy surgical removal of the uterus.

I

Ileoanal reservoir (anastomosis) creation of an internal reservoir for the storage of GI effluent.

Ileostomy surgically created opening between the distal small intestine and the skin.

Illness state of being sick; may be viewed as catastrophic (sudden, traumatic), acute, chronic, or terminal.

Imagery psychobiologic technique that uses the mind to visualize a positive physiologic effect.

Immune response target-specific system of defense against infectious, foreign, or cancerous cells carried out primarily by lymphocytes.

Immunoglobulins proteins produced by B lymphocyte plasma cells that bind with antigens and promote the destruction of invading cells; also known as antibodies.

Immunopeptides chemical messengers that relay messages throughout the immune system and the brain.

Immunotherapy use of biologic response modifiers to stimulate the body's natural immune system to restrict and destroy cancer cells.

Impaired nurse   nurse who cares for clients while under the influence of alcohol or other mind-altering or mood-altering drugs.

Impedance plethysmography   test used for diagnosing clots within deep veins by recording blood volume in the arm or leg before and after inflating a BP cuff to stop venous blood flow.

Implantation   process in which a fertilized ovum, or zygote, travels down the uterus and attaches itself within the endometrium.

Implanted pacemaker   permanent electrical device used to manage a chronic bradydysrhythmia.

Implementation   step in the nursing process that involves carrying out the written plan of care, performing the interventions, monitoring the client's status, and assessing and reassessing the client before, during, and after treatments.

Impotence   inability to achieve or maintain an erection that is sufficiently rigid for sexual activity.

Incident report   documentation made by healthcare workers when they make or discover errors, or when an event occurs that results in harm; it identifies the nature of the incident, witnesses, what actions were taken at the time, and the client's condition.

Incompetent   legal term for the inability to understand the risks or benefits of decisions.

Incontinence   inability to control urinary or bowel elimination.

Industry   positive developmental outcome of the school-age stage in which a child enjoys new challenges and is eager to engage in efforts to produce work of high quality.

Infarct   area of tissue that dies from inadequate oxygenation.

Infectious mononucleosis   viral disease that affects lymphoid tissues such as the tonsils and spleen and can involve other organs such as the brain, meninges, and liver as well.

Infectious process cycle   cycle involving the transmission of an infectious disease from a human or animal to a susceptible host. The six components needed for it to occur are an infectious microorganism, reservoir, portal for exit, means of transmission, portal of entry, and susceptible host.

Infective endocarditis   inflammation of the inner layer of heart tissue as a result of an infectious microorganism.

Inferiority   negative developmental outcome of the school-age stage in which a child feels inadequate.

Inflammatory bowel disease   group of chronic illnesses characterized by exacerbations and remissions of inflammation and ulceration of the bowel lining. See also ulcerative colitis and Crohn's disease.

Influenza   acute viral respiratory disease of relatively short duration.

Informal teaching   unplanned, spontaneous conveying of information, usually at the client's bedside or while caring for the client at home. See also formal teaching.

Informed consent   voluntary permission granted by a client, or the client's assigned *medical proxy* for an invasive procedure or surgery.

Infratentorial   below the tentorium (an area between the cerebrum and cerebellum).

Infusion pump   device that exerts positive pressure to infuse IV solutions and adjusts the pressure according to the resistance it meets.

Initiative   positive developmental outcome of the preschool stage in which children feel that others appreciate and encourage their efforts.

Injection sclerotherapy   procedure in which a physician passes an endoscope orally to locate an esophageal varix, then passes a thin needle through the endoscope and injects a sclerosing agent directly into the varix to stop circulation through it.

In-line filter   device that removes air bubbles as well as undissolved drugs, bacteria, and large molecules from an infusing solution.

Insight-oriented therapy   technique that helps clients understand the cause and relationship between their emotional distress and physical symptoms.

Inspection   systematic and thorough observation of a client and specific areas of a client's body.

Insulin   hormone necessary for the metabolism of glucose

Insulin independence   ability of a client's own naturally produced insulin to regulate blood glucose levels within consistently normal ranges.

Integrase   viral enzyme that incorporates a viral code into a host cell's DNA.

Integrated delivery system   network formed by hospitals and other healthcare facilities to reduce the redundancy of healthcare services and increase economic leverage.

Integument   structures that cover the body's exterior surface; the primary structure is the skin, but the integument also includes accessory structures such as the hair and nails.

Intentional tort   deliberate and willful act that infringes on another person's rights or property.

Interferons   chemicals that enable cells to resist viral infection and slow viral replication.

Interleukins   chemicals that coordinate the immune response.

Intermittent claudication   leg pain with exercise.

Internal fixation   procedure in which metal screws, plates, rods, nails, or pins are used to stabilize a reduced bone fracture.

Interstitial cystitis   chronic inflammation of the bladder mucosa.

Interstitial fluid   water located between cells.

Interstitium   structure that lies between the alveoli and contains the pulmonary capillaries and elastic connective tissue.

Interventions   actions for achieving outcomes in a plan of care.

Intimacy   positive developmental outcome of the young adult stage in which a young adult is able to enter into meaningful personal relationships.

Intimate space   physical closeness between two people which is only appropriate for interactions of a very personal nature.

Intra-aortic balloon pump   device that acts as a temporary, secondary pump to supplement ineffectual contraction of the heart's left ventricle.

Intracellular fluid   water located within cells.

Intracerebral hematoma   bleeding within the brain that results from an open or closed head injury or from a cerebrovascular condition such as a ruptured cerebral aneurysm.

Intractable pain   pain that does not respond to analgesic medications, noninvasive measures, or nursing management.

Intramedullary   within the spinal cord.

Intraocular lens implant artificial lens that is inserted in the eye to improve or restore vision.

Intraoperative phase of perioperative care that includes the entire surgical procedure until transfer of the client to the recovery area.

Intravascular fluid water located in the plasma (serum) portion of blood.

Intravenous (IV) therapy parenteral administration of fluids and additives into a vein.

Intravenous pyelogram radiologic study used to evaluate the structure and function of the kidneys, ureters, and bladder by examining a radiopaque dye as it passes through the urinary tract.

Introductory phase stage of the nurse-client relationship during which a nurse and a client get acquainted and the client identifies one or more health problems for which he or she is seeking care.

Intussusception telescoping of one part of the intestine into an adjacent part.

Involucrum new bone cells.

Ions positively and negatively charged substances.

Iridectomy surgical or laser procedure in which holes are made in the iris to increase drainage of aqueous fluid.

Irreversible stage stage in shock that occurs when significant numbers of cells and organ systems become damaged and the client no longer responds to medical interventions.

Irritable bowel syndrome paroxysmal motility syndrome primarily affecting the colon, in which the client experiences alternating periods of constipation and diarrhea.

Ischemia impaired oxygenation of cells and tissues.

Islets of Langerhans hormone-secreting cells of the pancreas that release insulin and glucagon.

Isoenzyme one of several forms of the same enzyme that may exist in cells and is capable of being identified separately from others.

Isolation negative developmental outcome of the young adult stage characterized by an inability to form close relationships with others.

Isotonic solution solution containing the same concentration of dissolved substances normally found in plasma; used to maintain fluid balance when clients temporarily cannot eat or drink.

J

Jejunostomy GI intubation in which the tube enters the jejunum or small intestine via a surgically created opening into the abdominal wall.

Joint junction between two or more bones.

K

Kaposi's sarcoma type of connective tissue cancer common among those with AIDS.

Keratin tough protective protein formed by the outer layer of dead skin cells.

Keratitis inflammation of the cornea.

Keratoplasty corneal transplantation.

Keratotic lesion elevated, darkly pigmented skin plaques that appear as moles on the scalp, face, neck, or trunk.

Kernig's sign inability to extend the leg when the thigh is flexed on the abdomen.

Ketoacidosis form of metabolic acidosis resulting from an accumulation of ketones in the blood.

Ketonemia increased ketones in the blood.

Ketones metabolic by-products of fat metabolism.

Kinesics study of nonverbal techniques of communication such as facial expressions, postures, gestures, and body movements.

Kussmaul respirations fast, deep breathing.

Kyphosis condition in which the thoracic spine takes on an obvious curve.

L

La belle indifference lack of emotion or concern by a person affected with a malady, particularly affiliated with conversion disorder.

Labyrinthitis inflammation of the labyrinth of the inner ear.

Laissez-faire leadership style of leadership characterized by allowing a work group to individually set goals, make decisions, and take responsibility for their own management

Laminectomy surgical procedure in which the posterior arch of a vertebra is removed to expose the spinal cord and allow the removal of a herniated disk, tumor, blood clot, bone spur, or broken bone fragment.

Lanugo fine body hair grown in the absence of subcutaneous fat to help maintain body temperature by reducing heat loss.

Laparoscopic cholecystectomy procedure in which the gallbladder is removed using an endoscope inserted through a small puncture site in the abdomen.

Laryngitis inflammation and swelling of the mucous membrane that lines the larynx.

Laryngoscopy endoscopic examination of the larynx.

Laryngospasm spasm of the laryngeal muscles, resulting in narrowing of the larynx.

Larynx cartilaginous framework between the pharynx and the trachea whose primary function is to produce sound; it also protects the lower airway from foreign objects because of its ability to facilitate coughing.

Laser angioplasty use of short pulses of light to vaporize arterial plaque.

Laws written rules governing conduct and actions.

Leadership ability to guide and influence another person, group, or both to think in a certain way, achieve common goals, or provide inspiration for change.

Learning capacity person's intellectual ability to understand, remember, and apply new information.

Learning needs those skills and concepts that a client and family must acquire to restore, maintain, or promote health.

Learning readiness degree to which a person is in an optimal position to process new information.

Learning style that manner in which a person best comprehends new information.

Left ventricular end-diastolic pressure retrograde pressure from the fluid on the left side of the heart at the end of left ventricular diastole.

Left-sided heart failure heart failure resulting from various conditions that impair the left ventricle's ability to eject blood into the aorta.

Leptin substance manufactured in human fat cells that acts on receptors in the hypothalamus and inhibits food intake.

Leukopenia decreased white blood cell count.

Leukocytes   white blood cells.

Leukocytosis   increased number of leukocytes above normal limits.

Liability   legal responsibility.

Libido   interest in or desire for sex.

Life review   process of looking back at one's life and reviewing decisions, choices, conflicts, and resolutions.

Ligament   fibrous tissue that connects two adjacent freely movable bones and help protect joints by stabilizing their surfaces and keeping them in proper alignment.

Limbic system   ring of structures made up of lobes of the cerebrum, thalamus, hypothalamus, and others that is a physiologic network for emotions, survival and behavioral responses, motivation, and learning.

Lipoatrophy   breakdown of subcutaneous fat at the site of repeated injections.

Lipohypertrophy   buildup of subcutaneous fat at the site of repeated injections.

Lipolysis   breaking down of fat by the body.

Listening   attending to and becoming fully involved in what a client says.

Litholapaxy   surgical procedure in which small bladder stones are removed through the transurethral route, using a stone-crushing instrument (lithotrite).

Lithotripsy   nonsurgical procedure that uses shock waves to break up some types of kidney or gallstones.

Living will   document that states a client's wishes regarding healthcare if he or she is terminally ill.

Lobectomy   surgical removal of a lobe of a lung.

Loop colostomy   procedure in which a loop of bowel is lifted through the abdomen and is supported in place with a glass rod or plastic butterfly device.

Low-density lipoprotein   lipoprotein that has a higher ratio of cholesterol than protein.

Lower gastrointestinal series   study used to identify polyps, tumors, strictures, and other abnormalities of the colon through the fluoroscopic observation of rectally instilled barium solution.

Lumpectomy   surgical procedure in which only a tumor is removed from the breast.

Lung abscess   localized area of pus formation within the lung parenchyma.

Lungs   paired elastic structures enclosed by the thoracic cage that contain the alveoli.

Lupus erythematosus   diffuse inflammatory connective tissue disease.

Lyme disease   chronic inflammatory process and multisystem disease caused by a spirochetal bacterium that is transmitted to humans from deer ticks.

Lymph   watery fluid derived from plasma that exits the walls of capillaries and enters interstitial spaces.

Lymph nodes   clusters of bean-sized structures located primarily in the neck, axilla, chest, abdomen, pelvis, and groin which contain specialized immune defensive cells that trap, destroy, and remove infectious microorganisms, cellular debris, and cancer cells.

Lymphadenitis   inflammation of the lymph nodes.

Lymphangitis   inflammation of the lymphatic vessels.

Lymphatics   vessels that transport lymph.

Lymphedema   disorder in which obstructed lymph circulation causes an accumulation of lymph within soft tissue.

Lymphocytes   white blood cells with immune functions.

Lymphogranuloma venereum   sexually transmitted disease caused by a strain of *C. trachomatis* and characterized by a small erosion or papule and the enlargement of adjacent lymph nodes, which can become necrotic.

Lymphokines   type of cytokines that attracts neutrophils and monocytes to remove debris, promotes the maturation of more T cells when they detect antigens, and directs B cell lymphocytes to multiply and mature.

Lymphoma   group of cancers that affect the lymphatic system.

M

Macrodrip tubing   intravenous therapy tubing that releases large-sized drops of IV solution. See also microdrop tubing.

Macrophages   large phagocytes present in tissues such as the lungs, liver, lymph nodes, spleen, and peritoneum.

Major (unipolar) depression   mood disorder characterized by a feeling of sadness with no obvious relationship to situational events. See also reactive (secondary) depression.

Malignant   type of tumor that is invasive and capable of spreading.

Malignant hypertension   dangerously elevated blood pressure accompanied by papilledema.

Malignant hyperthermia   inherited disorder in which body temperature, muscle metabolism, and heat production increase rapidly, progressively, and uncontrollably in response to stress and some anesthetic agents.

Malingering   deliberately faking an illness to acquire financial compensation, obtain drugs, or be relieved of responsibilities from work or school.

Malpractice   professional negligence resulting from a licensed person's action or lack of action.

Mammography   radiographic technique used to detect cysts or tumors of the breast, some of which may be too small to palpate.

Mammoplasty   collective term for several different cosmetic breast procedures.

Managed care organization   insurer that carefully plans and closely supervises the distribution of healthcare services.

Management   planning, organizing, directing and controlling resources and personnel to meet specific objectives within an organization.

Mania   frenzied state of euphoria.

Massage therapy   technique of applying pressure and movement to stretch and knead soft body tissues to stimulate circulation, relieve physical and psychological tension, and improve mobility or functional use of affected parts of the body.

Mast cells   constituents of connective tissue that contain granules of heparin, serotonin, bradykinin, and histamine; the release of granules causes various allergic and inflammatory manifestations.

Mastalgia   breast pain.

Mastitis   inflammation of breast tissue; most common in women who are breast-feeding.

Mastoidectomy   surgical procedure performed to remove diseased tissue from the mastoid process.

Mastoiditis   inflammation of any part of the mastoid process.

Mastopexy   surgical procedure to correct ptosis, or drooping, of the breast(s).

Maxillary sinuses   cavities on either side of the nose in the maxillary bones; they are the largest sinuses and the most accessible to treatment.

Maze procedure   surgical procedure to treat atrial fibrillation in which a new conduction pathway is created that eliminates the rapid firing of ectopic pacemaker sites in the atria.

Means of transmission   method by which a microorganism is transferred from its reservoir to a susceptible host; the five potential means of transmission are contact, droplet, airborne, vehicle, and vector.

Mediastinum   wall that divides the thoracic cavity into two halves.

Medical durable power of attorney   person with legal authority to make healthcare decisions for a client if he or she is no longer competent or able to make these decisions.

Medication lock   sealed chamber that allows intermittent access to a vein.

Medulla oblongata   part of the brain below the pons that transmits motor impulses from the brain to the spinal cord and sensory impulses from peripheral sensory neurons to the brain; contains vital centers concerned with respiration, heartbeat, and vasomotor activity.

Melanin   pigment that is manufactured by melanocytes located in the epidermis and which determines the color of the skin.

Melanin-concentrating hormone   hormone of which, in animal studies, low levels caused weight loss, while high levels promoted obesity.

Melatonin   hormone that aids in regulating sleep cycles and mood and is believed to play a role in hypothalamic-pituitary interaction.

Memory cells   immunologic cells that convert to plasma cells on re-exposure to a specific antigen.

Menarche   first menstruation.

Ménière's disease   term given to the episodic symptoms created by fluctuations in the production or reabsorption of fluid in the inner ear.

Meninges   membranes that protect the brain and spinal cord.

Menopause   physiologic change in the female reproductive system in which ovulation becomes irregular and eventually ceases.

Menorrhagia   excessive bleeding at the time of normal menstruation.

Menstrual diary   daily written record of a client's premenstrual symptoms.

Menstruation   process that occurs when an ovum is not fertilized, the production of progesterone decreases, and the endometrium degenerates and is shed.

Mental status examination   array of observations and questions that elicit information about a person's cognitive and mental state.

Mentation   mental activity.

Metabolic syndrome   cluster of physiologic alterations that includes obesity, (especially in the abdominal area), high blood pressure, elevated triglyceride and low-density lipoprotein, blood glucose levels, and low high-density lipoprotein level.

Metastasis   spreading of cancer cells to adjacent tissues, from lymph vessels into the tissues adjacent to lymphatic vessels, by transport from blood or lymph systems, or by diffusion within a body cavity.

Methadone maintenance therapy   technique that involves substituting a synthetic addicting drug for another addicting drug to forestall withdrawal, avoid a toxic overdose, or reduce the potential for blood-borne infections.

Metrorrhagia   vaginal bleeding at a time other than a menstrual period.

Microdrip tubing   intravenous therapy tubing that releases small-sized drops of IV solution. See also macrodrop tubing.

Microorganisms   potentially infectious agents that are so small they can only be seen with a microscope; commonly called "germs."

Microphages   small phagocytes present in blood that migrate to tissue as necessary.

Midbrain   forward part of the brain stem that connects the pons and cerebellum with the two cerebral hemispheres.

Midclavicular catheter   peripherally inserted catheter which extends from a superficial vein to the proximal end of the axillary or subclavian vein.

Mid-life crisis   condition experienced by some middle-aged persons in which they view themselves as less likely to accomplish the goals of their youth and, in some cases, relieve feelings of insecurity and unhappiness by having cosmetic surgery, wearing clothing styles more characteristic of younger adults, having extramarital affairs, or abandoning their current lifestyle to seek a more meaningful existence.

Midline catheter   peripherally inserted venous access device inserted from just above or below the antecubital area in the basilic, cephalic, or median cubital vein until the tip rests in the upper arm just short of the axilla; used for clients who have limited peripheral veins or who require an extended period of IV fluid therapy.

Mind-body interventions   techniques that rely on the power of the mind to alter body functions or symptoms.

Minority   group of people who differ from the majority of people within a given society in terms of cultural characteristics (such as religion), physical characteristics (such as skin color), or both.

Mistrust   negative developmental outcome in which a child is unable to rely on and have confidence in others.

Mitral regurgitation   backward flow of blood that occurs when the mitral valve does not close completely; sometimes referred to as mitral insufficiency.

Mitral stenosis   disorder in which the mitral valve does not open properly to facilitate filling of the left ventricle.

Mitral valve prolapse   disorder in which the mitral valve cusps enlarge, become floppy, and bulge backward into the left atrium.

Mitral valve prolapse syndrome   cluster of alterations associated with autonomic nervous system dysfunction in which changes in mitral valve tissue layers cause its cusps to distend, stretching the papillary muscles and leading to valvular incompetence.

Modified radical mastectomy   surgical procedure in which the breast, some lymph nodes, the lining over the chest muscles, and the pectoralis minor muscle are removed.

Modulation   phase of pain impulse transmission during which the brain interacts with the spinal nerves to alter the pain experience by releasing pain-inhibiting neurochemicals.

Monoamine hypothesis   theory that depression results from imbalances in one or more of the monoamine neurotransmitters, serotonin, norepinephrine, and dopamine.

Monocytes   large phagocytes present in tissues such as the lungs, liver, lymph nodes, spleen, and peritoneum.

Mood disorders   conditions in which a person experiences an extreme persistent mood or severe mood swings that interfere with social relationships.

Mood   person's overall feeling state; may be thought of as a continuum with extremes of emotion existing at both ends or poles.

Mortality   death.

Motivation   desire to acquire new information.

Multicratic leadership   style of leadership in which the manager uses a variety of styles and adapts his or her approach to the situation at hand.

Multidrug resistance   ability of some types of bacteria to remain unaffected by several antimicrobial drugs such as antibiotics.

Multifocal PVCs   pattern of premature ventricular contractions originating from more than one ectopic location.

Munchausen's syndrome   syndrome in which a person self-induces an illness to acquire medical treatment.

Munchausen's syndrome by proxy   syndrome in which a person induces an illness in another person—usually his or her own child—to gain attention from medical personnel and sometimes notoriety for being influential in saving the child's life.

Murmur   atypical heart sound.

Myelin   fatty substance that covers and serves as an insulating substance for some axons in the central nervous and peripheral nervous systems.

Myelosuppression   decreased bone marrow function.

Myocardial disarray   alteration in the usual alignment of myofibrils, the contractile component of muscle tissue.

Myocardial oxygen demand   amount of oxygen the heart needs to perform its work.

Myocardial revascularization   surgical procedure that improves the delivery of oxygenated blood to the myocardium for clients who have coronary artery disease using one or more coronary artery bypass grafts.

Myocarditis   inflammation of the myocardium (the muscle layer of the heart).

Myofibrils   contractile component of muscle tissue.

Myopia   nearsightedness; people who are myopic hold things close to their eyes to see them well.

Myringoplasty   surgical repair of a perforated eardrum.

Myringotomy   incisional opening of the eardrum to allow drainage, ease pressure, and relieve pain.

Myxedema   severe hypothyroidism in an adult.

N

Nasal polyps   grapelike growths of tissue that arise from the nasal mucous membranes.

Nasal septum   wall that divides the internal nose into two cavities.

Nasoenteric intubation   GI intubation in which a tube passes through the nose, esophagus, and stomach to the small intestine.

Nasogastric intubation   GI intubation in which a tube passes through the nose and esophagus into the stomach.

Nasopharynx   part of the pharynx that is near the nose and above the soft palate.

Natriuretic factor   hormone produced by the heart, a deficiency of which causes arteries and arterioles to remain in a state of sustained vasoconstriction.

Natural killer cells   lymphocyte-like cells that circulate throughout the body looking for virus-infected cells and cancer cells and release potent chemicals that lethally alter the target cell's membrane, leading to its demise.

Naturally acquired active immunity   immunity that occurs as a direct result of infection by a specific microorganism.

Near death experience   experience in which a person almost dies but is resuscitated.

Near point   closest point at which a person can clearly focus on an object.

Nearing death awareness   phenomenon characterized by a dying client's premonition of the approximate time or date of death.

Negative symptoms   impoverished speech and inability to enjoy relationships or express emotions that are characteristic of schizophrenia.

Negligence   failure to act as a reasonable person would have acted in a similar situation.

Neoangiogenesis   new growth of blood vessels.

Neoplasms   new growths of abnormal tissue; also called tumors.

Nephrectomy   surgical removal of a kidney.

Nephrolithiasis   presence of a kidney stone, the size of which may range from microscopic to several centimeters.

Nephrostomy tube   catheter inserted through the skin into the renal pelvis and used to relieve an obstruction to urine flow above the bladder.

Neuralgia   nerve pain.

Neurally mediated hypotension   disorder in which individuals experience hypotension accompanied by fatigue after standing for more than 10 minutes.

Neurilemma   sheath that covers myelin.

Neuritic plaques   deposits of beta amyloid in the brain.

Neurofibrillary tangles   twisted bundles of nerve fibers in the brain.

Neurogenic bladder   bladder that does not receive adequate nerve stimulation.

Neurogenic shock   shock that results from an insult to the vasomotor center in the medulla of the brain or to the peripheral nerves that extend from the spinal cord to the blood vessels.

Neurohypophysis   posterior lobe of the pituitary gland.

Neurologic deficit   disorder in which one or more functions of the central and peripheral nervous systems are decreased, impaired, or absent.

Neuron   nerve cell.

Neuropathic joint disease   common finding in tertiary syphilis, also called Charcot's joints.

Neuropathic pain   pain that is processed abnormally by the nervous system as a result of damage to either the pain pathways in peripheral nerves or pain processing centers in the brain.

Neuropeptides   neurotransmitters that include chemicals such as substance P, which transmits the sensation of pain, endorphins and enkephalins that interrupt the transmission of substance P and promote a feeling of well-being, and neurohormones released by interactions between the hypothalamus, pituitary, and the endocrine glands they stimulate.

Neurotransmitters chemical messengers that communicate information that affects thinking, behavior, and bodily functions across the synaptic cleft between neurons.

Neutropenia decreased neutrophils.

Neutrophils granulocytes that protect the body through the ingestion and digestion of bacteria and foreign substances.

Nits eggs laid by adult female lice that are tightly cemented to the side of hair shafts.

Nociceptive pain pain that arises from noxious stimuli that are transmitted from the point of cellular injury to the cerebral cortex of the brain.

Nociceptors specialized pain receptors located in the free nerve endings of peripheral sensory nerves.

Nocturia urination during the night.

Nomogram chart that calculates body surface area based on height and weight.

Non-Hodgkin's lymphomas group of 30 subclassifications of malignant diseases that originate in lymph glands and other lymphoid tissue.

Nonpathogens microorganisms that are generally harmless to healthy humans.

Nonverbal communication exchange of information without using words.

Norepinephrine monoamine neurotransmitter produced and secreted by the adrenal medulla whose levels may be low or high among people affected by depression; low levels help to explain why some depressed people develop psychomotor retardation, and high levels help to explain why some depressed people experience psychomotor agitation,

Normal eating consumption of approximately 1500 to 2500 calories per day, usually spread over three meals and two to three snacks, which occurs in response to hunger and ceases when a feeling of comfortable fullness is attained.

Nosocomial infections infections acquired while being cared for in a healthcare agency that were not active, incubatory, or chronic at the time of admission.

Nuchal rigidity pain and stiffness of the neck and an inability to place the chin on the chest.

Nuclear family family that consists of a married man and woman with biologic offspring; also referred to as traditional family.

Nuclear scan study that uses special equipment and a radioactive substance, taken orally or injected intravenously, to visualize certain organs or determine their activities.

Nurse practice acts legal statutes that define nursing practice and set standards for nurses in each state.

Nurse–client relationship relationship which exists during the period when a nurse interacts with clients, sick or well, to promote or restore their health, help them to cope with their illness, or assist them to die with dignity.

Nursing diagnosis step in the nursing process in which the nurse identifies and defines health-related problems.

Nursing orders specific nursing directions given so that all healthcare team members understand exactly what to do for the client.

Nursing process problem-solving approach for planning and implementing client care to achieve desired outcomes; the five steps of the nursing process are assessment, diagnosis, planning, implementation, and evaluation.

Nystagmus uncontrolled oscillating movement of the eyeball.

O

Objective data facts obtained during a client's assessment through observation, physical examination, and diagnostic testing. See also subjective data.

Obsession disturbing, persistent thought.

Obsessive-compulsive disorder psychobiologic disorder manifested by the performance of an anxiety-relieving ritual to terminate a disturbing, persistent thought.

Obstructive shock shock that occurs when the heart or great vessels are compressed.

Odynophagia painful swallowing.

Oligomenorrhea infrequent menses, usually caused by endocrine imbalances resulting from pituitary disorders or hypothyroidism, the stress response, or severely lean body mass.

Oliguria low urine output of 100 to 500 mL/day.

Oncology nursing nursing specialty related to the care of clients with cancer.

Onychocryptosis ingrown toenail.

Onychomycosis fungal infection of the fingernails or toenails.

Oophorectomy surgical removal of the ovary.

Open cholecystectomy surgical procedure in which a gallbladder is removed through an abdominal incision.

Open head injury injury to the head in which the scalp, bony cranium, and dura mater (the outer meningeal layer) are exposed.

Open method burn wound management technique in which the wound is left uncovered.

Open reduction surgical procedure in which a fractured bone is exposed and realigned.

Open-ended questions questions asked during a client interview that require discussion. See also closed questions.

Ophthalmoscopy examination of the fundus or interior of the eye.

Opiate dependence addiction to central nervous system depressant drugs (narcotics) that are either derived from or chemically similar to opium.

Opisthotonos extreme hyperextension of the head and arching of the back.

Opportunistic infections infections in which nonpathogenic or remotely pathogenic microorganisms take advantage of a favorable situation and overwhelm the host; also called superinfections.

Oral glucose tolerance test blood test used to evaluate a client's metabolism of orally ingested glucose.

Orchiectomy surgical removal of the testis.

Orchiopexy surgical procedure in which an undescended testis is secured within the scrotum.

Orchitis inflammation of the testis.

Orexin A neurochemical appetite stimulant that may contribute to binge eating and obesity in humans.

Orexin B neurochemical appetite stimulant that may contribute to binge eating and obesity in humans.

Orogastric intubation GI intubation in which the tube passes through the mouth into the stomach.

Oropharynx part of the pharynx that is near the mouth.

Orthopnea breathing that is eased by sitting upright.

Osmoreceptors specialized neurons that sense the concentration of substances in blood.

Osmosis movement of water through a semipermeable membrane.

Ossification process in which inorganic minerals, such as calcium salts, are deposited in bone matrix.

Osteoblasts cells that build bones.

Osteoclasts cells involved in the destruction, resorption, and remodeling of bone.

Osteocytes mature bone cells involved in maintaining bone tissue.

Osteodystrophy condition in which the bones become demineralized as a result of hypocalcemia and hyperphosphatemia.

Osteomalacia metabolic bone disease characterized by inadequate mineralization of bone, resulting from a calcium or phosphate deficiency.

Osteomyelitis infection of the bone.

Osteoporosis disorder in which bone density decreases, resulting in porous and fragile bones.

Osteotomy procedure involving the cutting and removal of a wedge of bone (most often the tibia or femur) to change the bone's alignment and, as a result, improve function and relieve pain.

Ostomate client with an ostomy.

Ostomy surgically created opening between an internal body structure and the skin.

Otitis externa inflammation of the tissue within the outer ear.

Otitis media inflammation or infection in the middle ear.

Otorrhea leakage of cerebrospinal fluid from the ear.

Otosclerosis disorder characterized by a bony overgrowth on the stapes that is a common cause of hearing impairment among adults.

Otoscope hand-held instrument used to inspect the external acoustic canal and tympanic membrane.

Ototoxicity detrimental effect of certain medications on the eighth cranial nerve or hearing structures.

Ova female sex cells.

Ovaries female endocrine glands important in the development of secondary sex characteristics, the manufacture of hormones, and the development of the ovum.

Ovulation cyclical release of an ovum.

P

P24 antigen test blood test that measures the number of viral particles in the blood and is used to guide drug therapy and follow the progression of a disease.

Pacemaker device that provides an electrical stimulus to the heart muscle to treat a slow abnormal cardiac rhythm.

Packed cells blood solution that has most of the plasma (fluid) removed; used for clients who need cellular replacements but do not need and may be harmed by the administration of additional fluid.

Paget's disease chronic bone disorder characterized by abnormal bone remodeling.

Pain privately experienced, unpleasant sensation usually associated with disease or injury.

Pain disorder disorder in which a person experiences pain in one or more anatomic sites that cannot be linked with any identifiable medical condition; formerly known as somatic pain disorder.

Pain management techniques used to prevent, reduce, or relieve pain.

Pain perception conscious experience of discomfort.

Pain threshold point at which pain-transmitting neurochemicals reach the brain, causing conscious awareness.

Pain tolerance amount of pain a person endures once the pain threshold has been reached.

Palliative treatment treatment that reduces physical discomfort but does not alter a disease's progression.

Palpation assessing the characteristics of an organ or body part by touching and feeling it with the hands or fingertips

Palsy decreased sensation and movement.

Pancreas gland with both exocrine and endocrine functions; the exocrine portion secretes digestive enzymes that the common bile duct carries to the small intestine while the hormone-secreting cells of the pancreas release insulin and glucagon.

Pancreatectomy (partial, total) surgical procedure in which some or all of the pancreas is removed.

Pancreatitis inflammation of the pancreas.

Pancytopenia conditions such as aplastic anemia in which numbers of all marrow-produced blood cells are reduced.

Pandemic rapidly spreading disease infecting large numbers of people throughout the world.

Panendoscopy examination of both the upper and lower GI tracts.

Panic disorder psychobiologic disorder in which a person experiences an abrupt onset of physical symptoms and terror.

Pannus destructive vascular granulation tissue.

Papanicolaou test test in which a sample of exfoliated cells are obtained during a pelvic examination and used to detect early cancer of the cervix, determine estrogen activity as it relates to menopause, or endocrine abnormalities.

Papilledema swelling of the optic nerve.

Paralanguage vocal sounds that communicate a message but which are not words.

Paralytic ileus disorder in which the intestine becomes adynamic from an absence of normal nerve stimulation to intestinal muscle fibers.

Paranasal sinuses extensions of the nasal cavity located in the surrounding facial bones.

Paraplegia paralysis of both legs resulting from spinal injuries at the thoracic level.

Parasympathetic nervous system division of the autonomic nervous system that works to conserve body energy and is partly responsible for slowing heart rate, digesting food, and eliminating body wastes.

Parathormone hormone that regulates the metabolism of calcium and phosphorus.

Parathyroid glands four small bean-shaped bodies embedded in the lateral lobes of the thyroid that secrete parathormone, which regulates the metabolism of calcium and phosphorus.

Paresthesia sensation of numbness and tingling.

Parietal pleura saclike serous membrane that is the outer layer of the lungs.

Parkinsonism cluster of Parkinson-like symptoms that develop from several etiologies.

Paroxysmal nocturnal dyspnea being awakened by breathlessness.

Partial (or segmental) mastectomy surgical procedure in which the breast, axillary lymph nodes, and pectoralis major and minor muscles are removed. In some instances, sternal lymph nodes also are removed.

Passive diffusion process in which dissolved substances such as electrolytes move from an area of high concentration to an area of lower concentration through a semipermeable membrane.

Passive immunity immediate but short-lived immunity that develops when ready-made antibodies are given to a susceptible individual.

Past health history information obtained during a client interview regarding a client's childhood diseases, previous injuries, major illnesses, prior hospitalizations, surgical procedures, and drug history.

Pathogens microorganisms that have a high potential to cause infectious diseases.

Patient-focused care system of nursing care in which an RN partnered with one or more assistive personnel cares for a group of clients.

Pediculosis infestation with lice.

Pelvic inflammatory disease infection of the pelvic organs such as the ovaries, fallopian tubes, pelvic vascular system, and pelvic supporting structures.

Peptic ulcer disease circumscribed erosion of tissue in an area of the GI tract that is in contact with hydrochloric acid and pepsin.

Perception phase of pain impulse transmission during which the brain experiences pain at a conscious level, helps to discriminate the location of the pain, determines its intensity, attaches meaningfulness to the event, and provokes emotional responses.

Percussion tapping a portion of the body to determine if there is tenderness or to elicit sounds that vary according to the density of underlying structures.

Percutaneous endoscopic gastrostomy (PEG) procedure in which an endoscope is introduced orally and advanced into the stomach so that the physician can see the correct location for a gastronomy tube.

Percutaneous liver biopsy procedure in which a small core of liver tissue is obtained by placing a needle directly into the liver through the lateral abdominal wall.

Percutaneous transluminal coronary angioplasty procedure in which a balloon-tipped catheter is inserted into a diseased coronary artery then inflated to compress atherosclerotic plaque.

Perfusion supplying blood to cells, tissues, or organs.

Pericardiectomy surgical removal of the pericardium to allow more adequate filling and contraction of the heart chambers.

Pericardiocentesis needle aspiration of fluid from between the visceral and parietal pericardium.

Pericardiostomy procedure in which a surgical opening is made in the pericardium to drain fluid.

Pericarditis inflammation of the pericardium.

Perioperative entire time span of surgery, including before and after the actual operation.

Periorbital ecchymosis condition in which both eyes are blackened; also called "raccoon eyes."

Periorbital edema puffiness around the eyes.

Periosteum outer layer of bones that is rich in blood and lymph vessels, and supplies the bone with nourishment.

Peripheral nervous system part of the nervous system consisting of all nerves outside the central nervous system.

Peripheral vascular disease disorders that affect blood vessels distant from the large central blood vessels supplying the myocardium or that circulate blood directly in and out of the heart.

Peripheral venous sites superficial veins of the arm and hand; the most common sites for infusing IV fluids.

Peristalsis coordinated wavelike muscular contractions.

Peritoneal dialysis dialysis technique that uses the peritoneum, the semipermeable membrane lining of the abdomen, to filter fluid, wastes, and chemicals.

Peritonitis inflammation of the peritoneum, the serous sac lining the abdominal cavity.

Peritonsillar abscess abscess that develops in the connective tissue between the capsule of the tonsil and the constrictor muscle of the pharynx.

Personal protection order legal document that forbids contact between a batterer and victim.

Personal space distance between two people that is appropriate for one-on-one interactions like interviewing and physical assessment.

Pet therapy use of pets to provide comfort and decrease feelings of loneliness.

Petechiae tiny reddish hemorrhagic spots on the skin and mucous membranes.

Phagocytes white blood cells that engulf and digest bacteria and foreign material.

Phagocytosis process of engulfing and digesting bacteria and foreign material.

Pharyngitis inflammation of the throat.

Pharynx body structure that carries air from the nose to the larynx, and food from the mouth to the esophagus.

Phenotype testing blood test used to detect drug resistance in which a measured amount of antiviral drug is mixed with a virus until there is a quantity that prevents the virus from reproducing.

Pheochromocytoma tumor of the adrenal medulla that causes hyperfunction.

Pheromones hormone-like chemicals that communicate reproductive and social information among a species.

Phlebitis inflammation of the vein.

Phlebothrombosis clot formation with minimal or no venous inflammation.

Pilonidal sinus infection in the hair follicles in the sacro-coccygeal area above the anus.

Phlebothrombosis development of a clot within a vein without inflammation.

Phobic disorder psychobiologic disorder in which a person develops an exaggerated fear.

Phonocardiography graphic representation of normal and abnormal heart sounds.

Photoperiods daytime hours that are short because of fewer hours of sunlight.

Photophobia sensitivity to light.

Phototherapy technique for treating seasonal affective disorder with artificial light that simulates the intensity of sunlight.

Physical assessment examination of a client's body structures.

Physical dependence condition in which a person experiences physical discomfort when a drug that he or she has taken routinely is abruptly discontinued.

Phytoestrogens plant sources of estrogen.

Pia mater delicate inner membrane that adheres to the brain and spinal cord.

Pineal gland gland attached to the thalamus that secretes melatonin, which aids in regulating sleep cycles and mood.

Pitting edema indentations in the skin following compression.

Pituitary gland gland that regulates the function of the other endocrine glands.

Placebo inert or inactive substance that by its very nature cannot alter physiology, but does in a significant number of people.

Placebo effect healing or improvement that takes place simply because an individual believes a treatment method will be effective.

Planning step of the nursing process that involves setting priorities, defining expected outcomes, determining specific nursing interventions, and recording the plan of care.

Plaque fatty deposits chiefly composed of cholesterol.

Plasma liquid, or serum, portion of blood.

Plasma cells B-cell lymphocytes that produce antibodies.

Plasma expanders nonblood solutions that pull fluid into the vascular space and are used as an economical and virus-free substitute for blood and blood products

Platelets disk-like cell fragments in blood that help control bleeding by forming a loose blood clot.

Pleura saclike serous membrane located around the lungs.

Pleural effusion collection of fluid between the visceral and parietal pleurae.

Pleurisy inflammation of the pleura.

Pluripotential stem cells undifferentiated precursors in the bone marrow from which all blood cells develop.

Pneumoconiosis fibrous inflammation or chronic induration of the lungs after prolonged exposure to dust or gases.

Pneumocystic pneumonia type of pneumonia rare among individuals with intact immune systems, but clients infected with HIV are at particular risk for acquiring.

Pneumonectomy surgical removal of an entire lung.

Pneumonia inflammatory process affecting the bronchioles and alveoli.

Pneumothorax air that enters the pleural space causing a lung to collapse.

Podiatrist physician trained to care for feet.

Poikilothermia condition in which the temperature of the body varies with that of the environment.

Point of maximum impulse place on the chest wall where heart pulsations are most strongly felt.

Polarization stage during diastole when positive ions predominate outside myocardial cell membranes and negative ions predominate inside.

Polyarthritis inflammation of more than one joint.

Polydipsia excessive thirst.

Polydrug abuse abuse of more than one substance.

Polymerase chain reaction test test that measures the number of viral particles in the blood and is used to guide drug therapy and follow the progression of HIV infection.

Polyphagia excessive eating.

Polysomnography test that monitors a client's respiratory and cardiac status while he or she is asleep to determine the nature of sleep apnea.

Polyuria excessive urine production.

Pons part of the brain located between the midbrain and medulla.

Portal hypertension congestion and increased fluid pressure in the venous pathway through the liver.

Portal of entry route through which an infectious agent gains entrance into a susceptible host.

Portal of exit route through which an infectious agent exits from a reservoir.

Positive inotropic agents drugs with beta-adrenergic activity that increase the heart rate and improve the force of heart contraction.

Positive symptoms delusions, hallucinations, and fluent but disorganized speech that are characteristic of schizophrenia.

Possible diagnosis nursing diagnosis that identifies problems for which the data are undeveloped or incomplete. See also actual diagnosis and risk diagnosis.

Postvoid residual amount of urine left in the bladder after voiding.

Postoperative phase of perioperative care that begins with admission to the recovery area and continues until the client receives a follow-up evaluation at home or is discharged to a rehabilitation unit.

Postphlebitic syndrome vascular complication which occurs up to 5 years after treatment of thrombophlebitis.

Postprandial glucose blood test used to assess blood sugar following a meal.

Posttraumatic stress disorder disorder that involves a delayed anxiety response 3 or more months after an emotionally traumatic experience.

Power ability to control, influence, or hold authority over an individual or group.

Precordial pain pain in the anterior chest overlying the heart.

Preferred provider organization insurer that creates a community network of providers willing to discount their fees for service in exchange for a steady supply of referred customers.

Preictal phase time immediately before a tonic-clonic seizure consisting of vague emotional changes, such as depression, anxiety, and nervousness.

Preload degree of stretch of the cardiac muscle fibers at the end of diastole.

Premature atrial contraction early electrical impulse initiated by neural tissue in the atrial conduction system.

Premature ventricular contraction ventricular contraction that occurs early and independently in the cardiac cycle before the sinoatrial node initiates an electrical impulse.

Premenstrual syndrome group of physical and emotional symptoms that occur in some women 7 to 10 days before menstruation.

Preoperative phase of perioperative care beginning with the decision to perform surgery and continuing until the client reaches the operating area.

Presbycusis hearing loss associated with aging.

Presbyopia condition in which visual accommodation, the ability to focus an image on the retina, gradually declines with aging, as a result of lens inelasticity.

Pressure infusion sleeve device wrapped around an IV solution bag that exerts a squeezing action to facilitate rapid infusion.

Pressure sores skin impairment that occurs when capillary blood flow to an area is reduced, as when the skin over a bony prominence is compressed between the weight of the body and a hard surface for a prolonged period.

Primary care initial resource, person, or agency that a client contacts about a health need.

Primary nursing   system of nursing care initiated in the 1970s in which an RN assumes 24-hour accountability for a client's care and has total responsibility for the nursing care of assigned clients during his or her shift.

Primary tubing   long tubing used to administer a large volume of IV solution over an extended period or a small volume through a medication lock.

Prion   protein that does not contain nucleic acid that, after undergoing a mutant change, is capable of becoming an infectious agent.

Proctosigmoidoscopy   examination of the rectum and sigmoid colon using a rigid endoscope inserted anally.

Progesterone   hormone produced by the ovaries.

Proptosis   disorder in which an extended or protruded upper eyelid delays closing or remains partially open.

Prospective payment systems   system of healthcare reimbursement that uses financial incentives to decrease total charges by reimbursing on a fixed-rate basis.

Prostatectomy   surgical removal of the prostate.

Prostatic specific antigen   tumor marker whose presence in blood sometimes indicates prostate cancer.

Protease   viral enzyme that cuts long chains of replicated viral particles and releases them into the cytoplasm of a cell.

Protease inhibitor   drug that inhibits the ability of HIV particles to leave the host cell.

Proxemics   use of space when communicating.

Pruritus   itching.

Psoriasis   chronic, noninfectious inflammatory disorder of the skin in which the cells of the epidermis proliferate so quickly that the upper layer of cells cannot be shed fast enough to make room for the newly produced cells.

Psyche   mind.

Psychic numbing   technique for coping with a tragedy in which the affected person avoids dealing with the tragedy and detaches himself or herself from others.

Psychobiologic disorders   those conditions in which evidence supports a link between biologic abnormalities in the brain and altered cognition, perception, emotion, behavior, and socialization.

Psychobiology   study of the biochemical basis of thought, behavior, affect, and mood.

Psychomotor agitation   state characterized by insomnia, pacing, and distractibility.

Psychomotor learner   person who processes information best by doing.

Psychomotor retardation   state characterized by a lack of energy, increased sleep, and little interest in daily events or responsibilities.

Psychoneuroendocrinology   study of how fluctuations in pituitary, adrenal, thyroid, and reproductive hormones alter cognition, perception, behavior, and mood.

Psychoneuroimmunology   study of the connections among the emotions, central nervous system, neuroendocrine system, and immunologic system.

Psychosocial history   information obtained during a client interview about the client's age, occupation, religious affiliation, cultural background, marital status, and home and working environments.

Psychosocial stages   term coined by Erik Erikson for eight periods spanning the life cycle during which a person acquires one of two opposing attributes.

Psychosomatic diseases   medical conditions associated with or aggravated by stress.

Psychotherapy   treatment in which a client talks with a psychiatrist, psychologist, or mental health counselor to cope with emotional problems, gain insight into behaviors, and learn techniques that can improve well-being.

Psychotic depression   extreme form of depressive disorder.

Ptosis   drooping of the eyelids.

Puberty   stage marked by the onset of sexual maturation.

Public space   distance between people that is appropriate for large group interactions such as speeches and meetings with strangers.

Pulmonary capillary wedge pressure   retrograde pressure from the fluid on the left side of the heart at the end of left ventricular diastole.

Pulmonary contusion   crushing bruise of the lung.

Pulmonary edema   fluid accumulation in the interstitium and alveoli of the lungs which interferes with gas exchange in the alveoli.

Pulmonary embolus   thrombus that migrates to the pulmonary circulation.

Pulmonary hypertension   high pressure within pulmonary circulation.

Pulmonary vascular bed   capillary network surrounding the alveoli.

Pulsus paradoxus   disorder characterized by a difference of 10 mm Hg or more between the first Korotkoff sound heralding systolic blood pressure heard during expiration and the first that is heard during inspiration.

Purge   to eliminate nutrients after binging with self-induced vomiting, laxatives, enemas, or diuretics.

PY test   test in which a client's breath is analyzed after consuming ^{14}C-urea capsules to detect *Helicobacter pylori*, the bacteria associated with peptic ulcer disease.

Pyelonephritis   acute or chronic bacterial infection of the kidney and the lining of the collecting system (kidney pelvis).

Pyeloplasty   surgical repair of the ureteropelvic junction.

Pyramidal motor tracts   motor pathways that originate in the motor cortex of the cerebrum, cross over at the level of the medulla, and end in the brain stem and spinal cord.

Pyrosis   burning sensation in the esophagus.

Pyuria   pus (a combination of bacteria and leukocytes) in the urine.

R

R on T phenomenon   premature ventricular contraction whose R wave falls on the T wave of the preceding complex.

Race   biologic differences in physical features such as skin color, bone structure, and eye shape, as opposed to ethnic or cultural differences.

Radiation therapy   technique that uses high-energy ionizing radiation, such as high-energy x-rays, gamma rays, and radioactive particles (alpha and beta particles, neutrons, and protons) to destroy cancer cells.

Radical pancreaticoduodenectomy (Whipple procedure)   surgical procedure to resect a tumor at the head of the pancreas.

Radiofrequency catheter ablation   procedure in which a heated catheter tip destroys dysrhythmia-producing tissue.

Radioimmunoassay   study that determines the concentration of a radioactive substance in blood plasma.

Radionuclide   atom with an unstable nucleus that emits electromagnetic radiation.

Radionuclide imaging   technique used to detect lesions in organs using a radioactive natural or synthetic element that is injected intravenously or ingested orally.

Rape   any forced sexual act in which there is vaginal, oral, or anal penetration, including that performed with an inserted object.

Reactive (secondary) depression   feeling of sadness that can be directly attributed to a situation or cause. See also major (unipolar) depression.

Reality orientation   use of various techniques that reinforce an older adult client's awareness of the date, time, place, names or roles of individuals, and current events.

Receptive aphasia   neurological impairment of a person's ability to understand spoken and written language.

Receptor   structures found on the surface of cells to which chemical messengers attach.

Rectocele   herniation of the rectum into the vagina.

Red bone marrow   substance that manufactures blood cells and hemoglobin.

Reduction mammoplasty   surgical procedure in which glandular breast tissue, fat, and skin are removed to decrease the size of large pendulous breasts.

Reed-Sternberg cells   malignant cells resulting from mutated lymphocytes that are indicative of Hodgkin's disease.

Referred pain   discomfort that is perceived in a general area of the body, but not in the exact site where a diseased organ is anatomically located.

Reflex incontinence   disorder in which a client lacks awareness of the urge to void.

Reflexology   technique of applying manual pressure to reflex centers on the feet and hands to promote natural healing.

Refraction   changing of direction and speed of a ray of light.

Refractory period   time in diastole during which cells are resistant to electrical stimulation.

Regulator T cells   T-cell lymphocytes made up of helper and suppressor cells.

Reiki   Japanese technique of healing by transferring energy through the laying-on of hands.

Relapse   (1) exacerbation of an illness; (2) return of a recovering alcoholic to drinking.

Reminiscence therapy   technique in which older adults are encouraged to talk about past experiences and events.

Remission   asymptomatic periods of a disorder.

Renal arteriogram   study of the arterial supply to the kidneys using radiopaque dye.

Renal threshold   ability of the kidney to reabsorb glucose and return it to the bloodstream.

Renin-angiotensin-aldosterone system   chain of chemicals that increases both blood pressure and blood volume.

Repolarization   stage in cardiac electrophysiology when ions realign themselves in their original position and wait for an electrical impulse.

Reservoir   human, animal, or nonliving environment in which an infectious agent can survive and reproduce.

Residual urine   urine retained in the bladder after the client voids.

Resorption   reduction of bone tissue.

Resource management   using resources (money, supplies, equipment, buildings, and personnel) optimally.

Respiration   exchange of oxygen and CO_2 between atmospheric air and the blood and between the blood and the cells.

Respite care   use of family and friends for brief relief from caretaking responsibilities.

Responsibility   duty to perform a specific task.

Restraint alternatives   protective or adaptive devices for fall protection and postural support that the client can release independently.

Retention   inability to urinate or effectively empty the bladder.

Retinal detachment   disorder in which the sensory layer becomes separated from the pigmented layer of the retina.

Retrograde ejaculation   condition in which semen is deposited in the bladder rather than discharged through the urethra at the time of orgasm.

Retrograde pyelogram   study that provides visualization of the complete ureter and renal pelvis using a radiopaque contrast medium instilled with a uretheral catheter.

Reuptake   reabsorption.

Reverse transcriptase inhibitor   drug that interferes with the human immunodeficiency virus' ability to make a genetic blueprint.

Reverse transcriptase   enzyme that copies RNA into DNA.

Reverse transcription   process in which the enzyme reverse transcriptase copies RNA into DNA.

Rheumatic carditis   inflammatory cardiac manifestations of rheumatic fever in either the acute or later stage.

Rheumatic disorders   term for more than 100 different types of recognized inflammatory disorders that involve inflammation and degeneration of connective tissue structures, especially joints.

Rheumatoid arthritis   systemic inflammatory disorder of connective tissue/joints characterized by chronicity, remissions, and exacerbations.

Rhinitis   inflammation of the nasal mucous membranes; also referred to as coryza or the common cold.

Rhinorrhea   (1) clear nasal discharge. (2) Leakage of cerebrospinal fluid from the nose.

Rhythmicity   ability of cardiac tissue to repeat its cycle with regularity.

Rights   freedoms or actions to which individuals have a just moral or legal claim.

Right-sided heart failure   heart failure that occurs when the right ventricle fails to completely eject its diastolic filling volume.

Rinne test   test used to measure hearing loss by comparing bone conduction and air conduction of sound using a tuning fork.

Risk diagnosis   nursing diagnosis that identifies potential problems. See also actual diagnosis and possible diagnosis.

Risk management   process of reviewing the problems that occur at the workplace, identifying common elements, and then developing methods to reduce the potential for reoccurrence.

Role confusion   negative developmental outcome of the adolescent stage in which a child is reluctant to oppose or question parental or adult views, does not develop true self-identity, and attempts to fulfill the dreams and expectations of others.

Romberg test   test used to evaluate a person's ability to sustain balance.

Rule of one hundreds cluster of signs indicating sedative (alcohol) withdrawal; evidenced by body temperature greater than or equal to 100°F, pulse rate greater than or equal to 100 beats/min, or diastolic blood pressure greater than or equal to 100 mm Hg.

S

Safer sex practices sexual activities in which body fluids are not exchanged.

Salpingo-oophorectomy surgical removal of the ovary and fallopian tube.

Sandwich generation adults who are raising their children while assuming increasing responsibility for their aging parents.

Satiety feeling of comfortable fullness.

Scabies skin disorder caused by infestation with the itch mite.

Schizophrenia thought disorder characterized by deterioration in mental functioning, disturbances in sensory perception, and changes in affect.

Seasonal affective disorder mood disorder characterized by depressive feelings that develop during darker winter months and then disappear in months with more sunlight.

Sebaceous glands glands that are connected to each hair follicle and secrete an oily substance called sebum.

Sebum lubricant released from hair follicles that prevents drying and cracking of the skin and hair.

Secondary care resource, person, or agency that a client is referred to for additional testing, consultation, and diagnosis by their initial contact for a health need.

Secondary gain an indirect benefit from being ill or incapacitated.

Secondary hypertension elevated blood pressure that results from some other disorder.

Secondary tubing short intravenous tubing used to administer smaller volumes of solution through a port in the primary tubing.

Segmental resection (1) surgical procedure in which the cancerous portion of a colon is removed and the remaining portions of the GI tract are rejoined to restore normal intestinal continuity; (2) surgical removal of a lobe segment of the lung.

Seizure brief episode of abnormal electrical activity in the brain.

Semen fluid that contains sperm.

Senescence last stage in the life cycle during which body processes gradually deteriorate.

Sensitivity studies performed to determine which antibiotic inhibits the growth of a nonviral microorganism and will be most effective in treating an infection.

Sensitization development of antibodies to an antigen.

Sensorineural hearing loss hearing loss that is the result of nerve impairment.

Sentinel lymph node mapping/biopsy technique for identifying the first (sentinel) lymph nodes through which breast cancer cells spread to regional lymph nodes in the axilla using a nuclear isotope and blue dye.

Sepsis systemic inflammatory response syndrome resulting from infection.

Septic shock shock associated with overwhelming bacterial infections; also called toxic shock.

Septicemia condition resulting from microorganisms escaping the lymph nodes and reaching the bloodstream, which may lead to sepsis.

Sequela condition that follows a disease.

Sequestrum pocket of necrotic bone.

Serotonin monoamine neurotransmitter that is lower in depressed people.

Serotonin syndrome potentially life-threatening condition that results from elevated levels of serotonin in the blood.

Serum osmolality concentration of substances in blood.

Shame negative developmental outcome of the early childhood stage which may develop in a child due to having disappointed his or her parents.

Shearing physical force that separates layers of tissue in opposite directions, for example, when a seated client slides downward.

Shiatsu application of pressure within various body meridians, or energy channels, to rebalance the body's energy and restore health.

Shingles skin disorder that develops years after an infection with varicella (chickenpox).

Shock life-threatening condition that occurs when arterial blood flow and oxygen delivery to tissues and cells are inadequate.

Short bowel syndrome loss of absorptive surface resulting from the surgical removal of a large amount of intestine.

Sickle cell anemia hereditary disease in which erythrocytes become sickle- or crescent-shaped when oxygen supply in the blood is inadequate.

Sign language method of communication that uses a hand-spelled alphabet and word symbols.

Signs abnormal objective data. See also symptoms.

Silicosis fibrous inflammation or chronic induration of the lungs caused by the inhalation of silica.

Simmonds' disease rare endocrine disorder caused by destruction of the pituitary gland.

Simple (or total) mastectomy surgical procedure in which all breast tissue is removed, but no lymph node dissection is performed.

Single-barrel colostomy opening to the colon that has a single stoma through which fecal matter is released.

Single-parent family family in which one biologic parent provides for the well-being of one or more children.

Sinus bradycardia dysrhythmia that proceeds normally through the conduction pathway but at a slower than usual rate (≤60 beats/min).

Sinus tachycardia dysrhythmia that proceeds normally through the conduction pathway but at a faster than usual rate (100 to 150 beats/min).

Sinusitis inflammation of the sinuses.

Skeletal muscles voluntary muscles that promote movement of the bones of the skeleton.

Skin tear shallow break in the skin.

Skin tenting quality in which skin remains elevated and is slow to return to underlying tissue when pinched.

Skip lesions randomly occurring inflamed areas of the bowel alternating with healthy tissue.

Sleep apnea syndrome phenomenon characterized by frequent, brief episodes of respiratory standstill during sleep.

Slit graft skin graft in which skin is removed from a client's donor site and passed through an instrument that perforates it in multiple places so that a smaller piece of skin can be stretched to cover a larger area.

Social phobia   fear of being in situations in which one must perform in front of or may capture the attention of others.

Social space   distance between people that is appropriate in small group interactions such as lecturing or non-private conversations.

Soma   body.

Somatic pain   pain that arises from mechanical, chemical, thermal, or electrical injuries or disorders affecting bones, joints, muscles, skin, or other structures composed of connective tissue.

Somatic pain disorder   disorder in which a person has combinations of multiple unexplained somatic complaints with no medical explanation.

Somatization   manifestation of unconscious emotional distress through physical symptoms.

Somatoform disorders   conditions in which emotional distress is manifested through physical symptoms.

Spastic colon   paroxysmal intestinal motility disorder characterized by alternating periods of constipation and diarrhea.

Speech reading   perception of conversation by following the movements of a speaker's lips.

Spermatogenesis   sperm production.

Sphenoidal sinuses   bony cavities that lie behind the nasal cavity.

Spinal fusion   surgical procedure in which two or more vertebrae are immobilized.

Spinal shock   loss of sympathetic reflex activity below the level of injury within 30 to 60 minutes of a spinal injury.

Spiritual healing   restoration of health through a higher power such as God or some other metaphysical force.

Splinter hemorrhages   black longitudinal lines in the nails.

Split-thickness graft   skin graft in which the epidermis and a thin layer of dermis are harvested from the client's skin.

Sprain   injuries to the ligaments surrounding a joint.

Stagnation   developmental outcome during middle age characterized by feeling a lack of accomplishment and a lack of commitment to future endeavors.

Stapedectomy   surgical procedure to improve hearing loss in which all or part of the stapes is removed and a prosthesis is inserted.

Starling's law   principle of physiology in which the greater the stretch of the myocardium as the ventricles fill with blood, the stronger is the ventricular contraction.

Status epilepticus   condition marked by a series of tonic-clonic seizures in which the client does not regain consciousness between seizures.

Statute of limitations   designated time in which a person can file a lawsuit.

Statutory law   law that any local, state, or federal legislative body enacts.

Steatorrhea   increased fat in the stool resulting from poor fat digestion.

Stem cells   undifferentiated precursors to various types of cells including lymphocytes, neutrophils, and monocytes.

Stereotyping   mistakenly making the assumption that all people within a particular cultural, racial, or ethnic group share the same values and beliefs, behave similarly, and are basically alike.

Stoma   surgically created opening on the exterior abdominal surface.

Stomatitis   inflammation of the mouth.

Strain   injury to a muscle when it is stretched or pulled beyond its capacity.

Stratum corneum   outer lay of dead skin cells in the epidermis.

Stress   physiologic response to biologic stressors such as surgical trauma or infection, psychological stressors such as worry and fear, or sociologic stressors such as starting a new job or increased family responsibilities.

Stress management   technique for minimizing the harmful effects of stress through relaxation techniques and effective coping strategies.

Stricture   narrowing.

Stridor   high-pitched, harsh sound during respiration, indicative of airway obstruction.

Stroke volume   amount of blood pumped per contraction of the heart.

Subarachnoid space   area between the pia mater and the arachnoid membrane.

Subculture   particular group which shares characteristics that identify it as a distinct entity.

Subcutaneous emphysema   presence of air in subcutaneous tissues.

Subcutaneous mastectomy   surgical procedure in which all breast tissue is removed, but the skin and nipple are left intact.

Subcutaneous tissue   layer of skin attached to muscle and bone that is primarily composed of connective tissue and fat cells.

Subdural hematoma   bleeding below the dura mater that results from venous bleeding.

Subendocardial infarction   infarct that does not extend through the full thickness of the myocardial wall.

Subjective data   information based on statements the client makes about what he or she feels (eg nausea, pain).

Subluxation   partial dislocation.

Substance abuse   use of a drug that is different from its accepted purpose.

Substance P   chemical that transmits the sensation of pain.

Superinfections   infections in which nonpathogenic or remotely pathogenic microorganisms overwhelm the host; also called opportunistic infections.

Supervision   process of guiding, directing, evaluating, and following-up on tasks delegated to others.

Suppressor T cells   cells that limit or turn off the immune response in the absence of continued antigenic stimulation.

Supratentorial   above the tentorium.

Supraventricular tachycardia   atrial dysrhythmia in which the heart rate is dangerously high ($\geq$150 beats/min).

Surgical asepsis   sterile technique.

Susceptibility   potential for infection or disease.

Sweat glands   glands within the dermis that release water and electrolytes or secrete substances such as cerumen.

Sympathectomy   procedure that interrupts or suppresses some portion of the sympathetic nerve pathway.

Sympathetic nervous system   division of the autonomic nervous system that accelerates the expenditure of energy.

Symptoms   feelings of discomfort reported by a client. See also signs.

Synapses junctions between the axon of one neuron and the dendrite of another.

Syncope sudden loss of consciousness.

Syndrome diagnosis nursing diagnosis that is associated with a cluster of other diagnoses.

Syndrome of inappropriate antidiuretic hormone secretion phenomenon that alters fluid and electrolyte balance due to excessive release of ADH.

Synovectomy surgical removal of enlarged and hypertrophied synovium to prevent the formation of pannus and delay destruction within a joint.

Synovitis inflammation of a synovial membrane of a joint.

Syphilis sexually transmitted disease caused by the spirochete *Treponema pallidum* that can be transmitted directly from an infected person or across the placenta to an unborn infant.

Systems method method used for carrying out an examination by assessing each body system separately. See also head-to-toe method.

Systolic blood pressure arterial pressure during ventricular contraction.

T

Tabes dorsalis degenerative condition of the central nervous system that results in the loss of peripheral reflexes and of vibratory and position senses.

Tachydysrhythmias abnormally fast cardiac rhythms.

Tai chi technique developed in China that combines mental and physical exercises for the purpose of integrating body and mind.

Task-oriented touch personal contact with a client that is required when performing nursing procedures. See also affective touch.

Teaching plan organized arrangement of information to be conveyed in a specific time frame.

Team nursing system of nursing care that emerged in the 1950s in which teams made up of an RN team leader, other RNs, LP/LVNs, and nursing assistants provide care to a group of clients.

Telemetry process of sending ECG information over radio waves to a monitor that is distant from the client.

Temporary restraining order legal directive requiring a batterer to avoid all contact with the victim.

Tendon cordlike structures that attach muscles to the periosteum of the bone.

Tenesmus urgent desire to evacuate the bowel.

Tentorium double fold of dura mater in the brain that separates the cerebrum from the cerebellum.

Terminating phase stage of the nurse client-relationship reached when the nurse and client mutually agree that the client's immediate health problems have improved and the nurse's services are no longer necessary.

Tertiary care care provided for clients in facilities where specialists and complex technology are available.

Testes male sex glands, important in the development of secondary sex characteristics, the manufacture of hormones, and the development of sperm.

Testicular self-examination technique for examining one's own testicles to detect any abnormal mass within the scrotum.

Testosterone hormone produced by the testes for the development and maintenance of male secondary sex characteristics, such as facial hair and a deep voice.

Tetany group of signs and symptoms associated with hypocalcemia.

Tetraiodothyronine hormone synthesized by the thyroid gland that regulates the body's metabolic rate.

Tetraplegia paralysis of all extremities due to a high cervical spine injury.

Therapeutic communication using words and gestures to promote a person's physical and emotional well-being.

Third-spacing translocation of fluid from the intravascular or intercellular spaces to tissue compartments, where it becomes trapped and useless.

Thirst mechanism that promotes increased intake of oral fluid.

Thoracentesis aspiration of excess fluid or air from the pleural space.

Thoracotomy surgical opening of the thorax.

Thrill vibration.

Thrombectomy surgical removal of a thrombus (clot).

Thromboangiitis obliterans inflammation of blood vessels associated with clot formation and fibrosis of the blood vessel wall.

Thrombocytopenia decreased platelet count.

Thrombolytic agents drugs that dissolve blood clots.

Thrombophlebitis inflammation of a vein accompanied by clot or thrombus formation.

Thrombosis formation of a blood clot.

Thrombus stationary blood clot.

Thymosin hormone that aids in developing T lymphocytes, a type of white blood cell involved in immunity

Thymus gland gland located in the upper part of the chest above or near the heart that secretes thymosin.

Thyroid gland gland located in the lower neck that concentrates iodine from food and uses it to synthesize tetraiodothyronine (thyroxine or T_4) and triiodothyronine (T_3).

Thyroiditis inflammation of the thyroid gland.

Thyrotoxic crisis abrupt and life-threatening form of hyperthyroidism, thought to be triggered by extreme stress, infection, diabetic ketoacidosis, trauma, toxemia of pregnancy, or manipulation of a hyperactive thyroid gland during surgery or physical examination.

Tilt table test diagnostic test in which a client lays horizontally on a table that is elevated to approximately 70° for 45 minutes while blood pressure and pulse are monitored.

Time management organization and delegation of tasks to make optimal use of one's time.

Tinnitus disorder in which a client hears buzzing, whistling, or ringing noises in one or both ears.

Tolerance condition in which a client needs larger doses of a drug to achieve the same effect as when the drug was first administered.

Tonometry measurement of intraocular pressure.

Tonsillectomy surgical removal of the tonsils.

Tonsillitis inflammation of the tonsils.

Tonsils elliptically shaped lymphoid tissue located on either side of the upper oropharynx that protect the body from infection.

Tophi collections of urate crystals found in the cartilage of the outer ear (pinna), the great toe, hands, and other joints, ligaments, bursae, and tendons in clients with gout.

Topical hyperbaric oxygen   therapy used to treat chronic, non-healing skin lesions by delivering oxygen above atmospheric pressure directly to the wound.

Tort   physical, emotional, or financial injury that occurred because of another person's intentional or unintentional actions, or failure to act.

Tort law   body of law that governs breaches of duty owed by one person to another.

Total parenteral nutrition   hypertonic solution consisting of nutrients designed to meet nearly all the caloric and nutritional needs of clients who are severely malnourished or cannot consume food or liquids for a long time

Toxic megacolon   complication in which the colon dilates and becomes atonic and vulnerable to perforation.

Toxic shock syndrome   life-threatening systemic reaction to the toxin produced by several kinds of bacteria.

Trabeculoplasty   procedure in which a laser beam is directed at the trabecular network in the eye.

Trachea   hollow tube composed of smooth muscle and supported by C-shaped cartilage that transports air from the laryngeal pharynx to the bronchi and lungs.

Tracheitis   inflammation of the trachea.

Tracheobronchitis   inflammation of the mucous membrane that lines the trachea.

Tracheostomy   surgical opening into the trachea into which a tracheostomy or laryngectomy tube is inserted; may be temporary or permanent.

Tracheotomy   surgical procedure that makes an opening into the trachea.

Traction   method of pulling structures of the musculoskeletal system to relieve muscle spasm, align bones, and maintain immobilization.

Traditional family   family that consists of a married man and woman with biologic offspring; also referred to as nuclear family.

Transcultural nursing   specialty in nursing founded by Madeline Leininger in 1977 which emphasizes providing nursing care within the context of another's culture.

Transcutaneous pacemaker   external pacemaker used as a temporary, emergency measure for maintaining adequate heart rate.

Transduction   phase of pain impulse transmission involving the conversion of chemical information in the cellular environment to electrical impulses that move toward the spinal cord.

Transesophogeal echocardiography   ultrasound technique in which a tube with a small transducer is passed internally from the mouth to the esophagus to obtain images of the posterior heart and its internal structures.

Transient ischemic attack   sudden, brief, fleeting attacks of neurologic impairment caused by a temporary interruption in cerebral blood flow.

Transillumination   technique in which a light is shined through tissue.

Transmission   phase of pain impulse transmission during which peripheral nerve fibers form synapses with neurons within the spinal cord and the pain impulses move from the spinal cord to sequentially higher levels in the brain.

Transmission-based precautions   actions taken to interfere with the manner in which a particular pathogen is spread.

Transmural infarction   infarct that extends through the full thickness of the myocardial wall.

Transmyocardial revascularization   laser procedure that improves oxygenation of myocardial tissue by creating channels into which oxygenated blood seeps and is absorbed by the ischemic myocardium.

Transvenous pacemaker   temporary pulse-generating device that is sometimes necessary to manage transient brady-dysrhythmias such as those that occur during acute MIs, after coronary artery bypass graft surgery, or to override tachydysrhythmias.

Triiodothyronine   hormone synthesized by the thyroid gland that regulates the body's metabolic rate.

Trousseau's sign   sign in which the hand spasms after placing a BP cuff on the client's upper arm and inflating it between the systolic and diastolic BP, for 3 minutes.

Trust   positive developmental outcome of the infant stage in which a child has a sense of reliance on and confidence in others.

T-tube   tube used to drain bile while the surgical wound from an opening and exploration of the common bile duct heals.

Tuberculosis   bacterial infectious disease caused by *Mycobacterium tuberculosis.*

Tumor markers   substances synthesized by tumors that are released into the circulation in excessive amounts.

Tumor necrosis factor   type of cytokine used to regulate various autoimmune and inflammatory disorders.

Tuning fork   instrument that produces sound in the same range as human speech; used to screen for conductive or sensorineural hearing loss.

Turbinates (Chonchae)   bones that change the flow of inspired air to moisturize and warm it to a greater degree.

Turner's sign   bluish gray discoloration to the skin on the flanks with acute pancreatitis.

U

Ulcerative colitis   chronic inflammatory condition of the mucosal and submucosal layers of the colon.

Ulcerative proctitis   chronic inflammation of the most distal area of the large intestine.

Ultrasonography   technique that uses high-frequency sound waves to show the size and location of organs and to outline structures and abnormalities.

Uncal herniation   shifting of the brain to the lateral side.

Unintentional torts   injuries caused by another person when the person responsible did not mean to cause any harm; negligence is the principal form of unintentional tort.

Unvented tubing   tubing that does not draw air into a container of solution; used for solutions packaged in plastic bags. See also vented tubing.

Upper gastrointestinal series   fluoroscopic observation of a client swallowing a flavored barium solution and its progress down the esophagus combined with radiographic observation of the barium moving into the stomach and the first part of the small intestine.

Uremia   toxic state caused by the accumulation of nitrogen wastes in the blood.

Uremic frost   precipitate that sometimes forms on the skin during chronic renal failure because it becomes the excretory organ for substances the kidney usually clears from the body.

Ureteral stent   slender supportive device used to splint the ureter or divert urine past a possible tear in the ureteral wall.

Ureterolithiasis   presence of a stone within the ureter.

Ureteroplasty   removal of a narrowed section of ureter and reconnection of the patent portions.

Urethritis   inflammation of the urethra.

Urethroplasty   surgical repair of the urethra.

Urinalysis   laboratory examination of the components and characteristics of urine.

Urinary diversion   diversion of urine either to an external or an internal collecting system.

Urine protein test   laboratory examination used to identify renal disease by detecting an increase in urine protein levels.

Urine specific gravity   measurement of the kidney's ability to concentrate and excrete urine by comparing the density of urine with the density of distilled water.

Urodynamic studies   studies that evaluate bladder and urethral function and are performed to assess causes of reduced urine flow, urinary retention, and urinary incontinence.

Uroflowmetry   study performed to evaluate bladder and sphincter function by measuring the time and rate of voiding, the volume of urine voided, and the pattern of urination.

Urography   radiologic study used to evaluate the structure and function of the kidneys, ureters, and bladder by examining a radiopaque dye as it passes through the urinary tract.

Urolithiasis   condition of stones in the urinary tract.

Urosepsis   serious systemic infection from microorganisms in the urinary tract that invade the bloodstream.

Urticaria   hives.

Utilitarianism   theory of ethics that determines the rightness of an action by its consequences; also referred to as teleologic theory.

Uveitis   inflammation of the uveal tract.

V

Vaginitis   condition in which the vagina is inflamed.

Validation therapy   method of communicating with an elderly client who is confused or disoriented by seeking to reassure the client and gain understanding of the client's behavior or spoken words.

Values   beliefs that individuals find most meaningful.

Valvular incompetence   condition in which the aortic valve does not close tightly.

Valvular regurgitation   leaking of blood backward through a valve that does not close tightly.

Valvuloplasty   surgical procedure in which an incompetent cardiac valve is repaired.

Varicose veins   dilated, tortuous veins.

Vasectomy   surgical procedure involving the ligation of the vas deferens which results in permanent sterilization by interrupting the pathway that transports sperm.

Vasopressors   drugs with alpha-adrenergic activity that increase peripheral vascular resistance and raise blood pressure.

Vegetations   accumulation of inflammatory debris around the valve leaflets of the heart in rheumatic carditis.

Vein ligation   surgical treatment for severe varicose veins in which the affected veins are tied off above and below the area of incompetent valves, but the dysfunctional vein remains.

Vein stripping   surgical treatment for severe varicose veins in which the affected veins are severed and removed.

Vena caval filter   surgically inserted umbrella-like filter used to trap emboli before they reach the heart and lungs.

Vena caval plication procedure   procedure that changes the lumen of the vena cava from a single channel to several small channels through the use of a suture or Teflon clip.

Venereal diseases   diverse group of infections spread through sexual activity with an infected person.

Venipuncture   method for gaining access to the venous system by piercing a vein with one of various devices.

Venography   procedure that uses radiopaque dye instilled into the venous system to identify a filling defect in the area of a clot.

Venous insufficiency   peripheral vascular disorder in which the flow of venous blood is impaired through deep or superficial veins, or both.

Venous reflux   downward flow of venous blood.

Venous stasis ulcer   lesion that forms on the skin when the forward movement of venous blood is impaired.

Vented tubing   intravenous tubing that draws air into a container of solution; used for administering solutions packaged in glass containers to facilitate their flow. See also unvented tubing.

Ventilation   movement of air in and out of the respiratory tract.

Ventricles   (1) hollow structures in the brain that manufacture and absorb cerebrospinal fluid. (2) lower chambers of the heart.

Ventricular assist device   auxiliary heart pump that supplements the heart's ability to eject blood.

Ventricular fibrillation   rhythm of a dying heart; the ventricles do not contract effectively and there is no cardiac output.

Ventricular tachycardia   dysrhythmia in which a single, irritable focus in the ventricle causes the ventricles to beat very fast and cardiac output is decreased.

Ventriculomyomectomy   procedure involving the removal of thickened myocardial muscle from the septum.

Verbal communication   communication that uses words (speaking, reading, and writing).

Vesicants   powerful intravenous antineoplastics that may be particularly damaging in that they cause tissue necrosis if they infiltrate.

Viatical settlement   arrangement in which a terminally ill individual agrees to name a person as beneficiary to his or her life insurance in exchange for immediate cash.

Virchow's triad   slowed circulation, altered blood coagulation, and trauma to the vein.

Virulence   power of a microorganism to produce disease.

Visceral pain   pain that arises from diseased or injured internal organs.

Visceral pleura   saclike serous membrane that covers the lung surface.

Visual acuity   ability to see far images clearly.

Visual field examination   measurement of peripheral vision and detection of gaps in the visual field.

Visually impaired   condition in which visual acuity is between 20/70 and 20/200 in the better eye with the use of glasses.

Vocal cords   folds of tissue within the larynx that vibrate and produce sound as air passes through.

Voice dismissal   technique used to halt a hallucination by saying "stop" or "be gone."

Voiding cystourethrogram   study that evaluates abnormalities in bladder function through the voiding of contrast dye and a rapid series of x-rays.

Volkmann's contracture   claw-like deformity of the hand resulting from obstructed arterial blood flow to the forearm and hand.

Volumetric controller   device that infuses IV solutions using gravity and compressing the tubing at a certain frequency to infuse the solution at a precise preset rate.

Volvulus   kinking of a portion of the intestine.

W

Waiting for permission phenomenon   situation in which some clients who have already accepted death seem to forestall dying when they feel that their loved ones are not yet prepared to deal with their death.

Water loading   technique in which clients with anorexia attempt to demonstrate weight gain by consuming a large volume of water and avoiding urination before being weighed.

Water-hammer pulse   strong radial pulse with quick, sharp beats followed by a sudden collapse of force.

Weber test   test used to measure hearing loss by striking a tuning fork and placing its stem in the midline of the client's skull or center of the forehead; a person with normal hearing perceives the sound equally well in both ears.

Wedge resection   surgical removal of a wedge of diseased tissue from a lung.

Wellness   state that involves good physical self-care, prevention of illness and injury, use of one's full intellectual potential, expression of emotions and appropriate management of stress, comfortable and congenial interpersonal relationships, and concern about one's environment and conditions throughout the world.

Wellness diagnosis   category of nursing diagnoses that begins with the stem "potential for enhanced" and does not include related factors or supporting data.

Western blot   test used to confirm an HIV diagnosis indicated by a positive enzyme-linked immunosorbent assay test.

White-coat hypertension   elevated blood pressure that develops during evaluation by medical personnel as a result of anxiety.

Whole blood   solution containing blood cells and plasma with preservative and anticoagulant added.

Withdrawal   physical symptoms or craving for a drug that occur when a person abruptly stops using a drug that he or she has taken routinely for some time.

Working phase   stage of the nurse-client relationship during which the nurse and client mutually plan the client's care and put the plan into action.

Y

Y-administration tubing   intravenous tubing used to administer whole blood or packed cells that contains two branches: one for blood and one for isotonic (normal) saline.

Yellow bone marrow   bone marrow in long bones that consists primarily of fat cells and connective tissue.

Yoga   technique developed in India that combines mental and physical exercises for the purpose of integrating body and mind.

Index

Page numbers followed by b indicate boxed and display text; those followed by f indicate figures; those followed by t indicate tables.

PROGRAM LICENSE AGREEMENT

Read carefully the following terms and conditions before using the Software. Use of the Software indicates you and, if applicable, your Institution's acceptance of the terms and conditions of this License Agreement. If you do not agree with the terms and conditions, you should promptly return this package to the place you purchased it and your payment will be refunded.

Definitions

As used herein, the following terms shall have the following meanings:

"Software" means the software program contained on the diskette(s) or CD-ROM or preloaded on a workstation and the user documentation, which includes all accompanying printed material.

"Institution" means a nursing or professional school, a single academic organization that does not provide patient care and is located in a single city and has one geographic location/address.

"Geographic location" means a facility at a specific location; geographic locations do not provide for satellite or remote locations that are considered a separate facility.

"Facility" means a health care facility at a specific location that provides patient care and is located in a single city and has one geographic location/address.

"Publisher" means Lippincott Williams & Wilkins, Inc., with its principal office in Philadelphia, Pennsylvania.

"Developer" means the company responsible for developing the software as noted on the product.

License

You are hereby granted a nonexclusive license to use the Software in the United States. This license is not transferable and does not authorize resale or sublicensing without the written approval or an authorized officer of Publisher.

The Publisher retains all rights and title to all copyrights, patents, trademarks, trade secrets, and other proprietary rights in the Software. You may not remove or obscure the copyright notices in or on the Software. You agree to use reasonable efforts to protect the Software from unauthorized use, reproduction, distribution or publication.

Single-User license

If you purchased this Software program at the Single-User License price or a discount of that price, you may use this program on one single-user computer. You may not use the Software in a time-sharing environment or otherwise to provide multiple, simultaneous access. You may not provide or permit access to this program to anyone other than yourself.

Institutional/Facility license

If you purchased the Software at the Institutional or Facility License Price or at a discount of that price, you have purchased the Software for use within your Institution/Facility on a single workstation/computer. You may not provide copies of or remote access to the Software. You may not modify or translate the program or related documentation. You agree to instruct the individuals in your Institution/Facility who will have access to the Software to abide by the terms of this License Agreement. If you or any member of your Institution fail to comply with any of the terms of this License Agreement, this license shall terminate automatically.

Network license

If you purchased the Software at the Network License Price, you may copy the Software for use within your Institution/Facility on an unlimited number of computers within one geographic location/address. You may not provide remote access to the Software over a value-added network or otherwise. You may not provide copies of or remote access to the Software to individuals or entities who are not members of your Institution/Facility. You may not modify or translate the program or related documentation. You agree to instruct the individuals in your Institution/Facility who will have access to the Software to abide by the terms of this License Agreement. If you or any member of your Institution/Facility fail to comply with any of the terms of this License Agreement, this license shall terminate automatically.

Limited warranty

The Publisher warrants that the media on which the Software is furnished shall be free from defects in materials and workmanship under normal use for a period of 90 days from the date of delivery to you, as evidenced by your receipt of purchase.

The Software is sold on a 30-day trial basis. If, for whatever reason, you decide not to keep the software, you may return it for a full refund within 30 days of the invoice date or purchase, as evidenced by your receipt of purchase by returning all parts of the Software and packaging in saleable condition with the original invoice, to the place you purchased it. If the Software is not returned in such condition, you will not be entitled to a re-

HOW TO USE THIS CD

Welcome to the *Introductory Medical-Surgical Nursing* pronunciation glossary CD-ROM!

Included on this CD is a pronunciation glossary of over 1500 terms to aid you in your studying.

The CD should start up automatically when it is put into the computer. If it does not, view the contents of the CD, and double-click on **glossary.exe**.

Access the pronunciation glossary by clicking on the (+) button next to your choice, either by chapter or alphabetically. Then, choose the chapter or letter whose words you want to hear pronounced by clicking on the button or name.

Listen to word pronunciations simply by clicking once on each word you wish to hear.

To go to a different section, click the Menu button to return to view the chapters or letters.

If you want to listen by a different order, click the (-) button to close either Chapters or Alpha, and then click the (+) button for the other choice.

To completely exit the program, click the Exit button.

If you have questions, contact our Tech Support at 1-800-638-3030, Monday–Friday 8:30 to 5:00 EST, or at techsupp@lww.com.

NOTICE TO CONSUMERS
THIS BOOK CANNOT BE RETURNED FOR CREDIT
OR REFUND IF THE SEAL OF THE CD HOLDER
IS BROKEN OR TAMPERED WITH.

fund. When returning the Software, we suggest that you insure all packages for their retail value and mail them by a traceable method.

The Software is a computer assisted instruction (CAI) program that is not intended to provide medical consultation regarding the diagnosis or treatment of any specific patient.

The Software is provided without warranty of any kind, either expressed or implied, including but not limited to any implied warranty of fitness for a particular purpose of merchantability. Neither Publisher nor Developer warrants that the Software will satisfy your requirements or that the Software is free of program or content errors. Neither Publisher nor Developer warrants, guarantees, or makes any representation regarding the use of the Software in terms of accuracy, reliability or completeness, and you rely on the content of the programs solely at your own risk.

The Publisher is not responsible (as a matter of products liability, negligence or otherwise) for any injury resulting from any material contained herein. This Software contains information relating to general principles of patient care that should not be construed as specific instructions for individual patients.

Manufacturers' product information and package inserts should be reviewed for current information, including contraindications, dosages and precautions.

Some states do not allow the exclusion of implied warranties, so the above exclusion may not apply to you. This warranty gives you specific legal rights and you may also have other rights that vary from state to state.

Limitation of remedies

The entire liability of Publisher and Developer and your exclusive remedy shall be: (1) the replacement of any CD which does not meet the limited warranty stated above which is returned to the place you purchased it with your purchase receipt; or (2) if the Publisher or the wholesaler or retailer from whom you purchased the Software is un-

able to deliver a replacement CD free from defects in material and workmanship, you may terminate this License Agreement by returning the CD, and your money will be refunded.

In no event will Publisher or Developer be liable for any damages, including any damages for personal injury, lost profits, lost savings or other incidental or consequential damages arising out of the use or inability to use the Software or any error or defect in the Software, whether in the database or in the programming, even if the Publisher, Developer, or an authorized wholesaler or retailer has been advised of the possibility of such damage.

Some states do not allow the limitation or exclusion of liability for incidental or consequential damages. The above limitations and exclusions may not apply to you.

General

This License Agreement shall be governed by the laws of the State of Pennsylvania without reference to the conflict of laws provisions thereof, and may only be modified in a written statement signed by an authorized officer of the Publisher. By opening and using the Software, you acknowledge that you have read this License Agreement, understand it, and agree to be bound by its terms and conditions. You further agree that it is a complete and exclusive statement of the agreement between the Institution/Facility and the Publisher, which supersedes any proposal or prior agreement, oral or written, and any other communication between you and Publisher or Developer relative to the subject matter of the License Agreement.

Note

Attach a paid invoice to the License Agreement as proof of purchase.